28.10

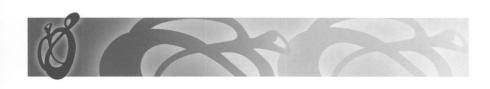

Cardiovascular
Therapeutics
A Companion to *Braunwald's Heart Disease*

Look for these other titles in the Braunwald Heart Disease family

Braunwald's Heart Disease Companions

Pierre Théroux
Acute Coronary Syndromes

Christie M. Ballantyne
Clinical Lipidology

Ziad Issa, John M. Miller, & Douglas Zipes
Clinical Arrhythmology and Electrophysiology

Douglas L. Mann
Heart Failure

Henry R. Black & William J. Elliott
Hypertension

Robert L. Kormos & Leslie W. Miller
Mechanical Circulatory Support

Catherine M. Otto & Robert O. Bonow
Valvular Heart Disease

Marc A. Creager, Joshua A. Beckman & Joseph Loscalzo
Vascular Medicine

Braunwald's Heart Disease Imaging Companions

Allen J. Taylor
Atlas of Cardiac Computed Tomography

Christopher M. Kramer & W. Gregory Hundley
Atlas of Cardiovascular Magnetic Resonance

Ami E. Iskandrian & Ernest V. Garcia
Atlas of Nuclear Cardiology

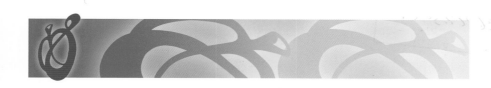

Cardiovascular Therapeutics
A Companion to *Braunwald's Heart Disease*
FOURTH EDITION

Elliott M. Antman, MD
Professor of Medicine
Associate Dean for Clinical/Translational Research
Harvard Medical School
Senior Investigator, TIMI Study Group
Brigham and Women's Hospital
Boston, Massachusetts

Marc S. Sabatine, MD, MPH
Chairman, TIMI Study Group
Brigham and Women's Hospital
Associate Professor of Medicine
Harvard Medical School
Boston, Massachusetts

Section Editors
James de Lemos, MD
John P. DiMarco, MD, PhD
Michael M. Givertz, MD
Suzanne Oparil, MD
Frank M. Sacks, MD
Benjamin M. Scirica, MD, MPH
Piotr Sobieszczyk, MD

ELSEVIER
SAUNDERS

ELSEVIER
SAUNDERS

1600 John F. Kennedy Blvd.
Ste 1800
Philadelphia, PA 19103-2899

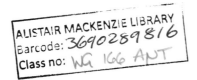
CARDIOVASCULAR THERAPEUTICS:
A COMPANION TO BRAUNWALD'S HEART DISEASE, ED 4

ISBN: 978-1-4557-0101-8

Library of Congress Cataloging-in-Publication Data

Cardiovascular therapeutics: a companion to Braunwald's heart disease / [edited by] Elliott M. Antman, Marc S. Sabatine; section editors, James de Lemos ... [et al.]. – 4th ed.
    p. ; cm.
Includes bibliographical references and index.
ISBN 978-1-4557-0101-8 (hardcover: alk. paper)
I. Antman, Elliott M. II. Sabatine, Marc S. III. Braunwald's heart disease.
[DNLM: 1. Cardiovascular Diseases–therapy. WG 166]
616.1'06–dc23

2012016215

Executive Content Strategist: Dolores Meloni
Content Development Specialist: Julia Bartz
Publishing Services Manager: Patricia Tannian
Project Manager: Carrie Stetz
Design Direction: Steven Stave

Printed in China

Last digit is the print number: 9 8 7 6 5 4 3 2 1

To
Dr. Karen Antman
Drs. Amy and Jeffrey Gelfand
Drs. David and Alicia Antman
Adam, Ethan, and Ryan
Dr. Jennifer Tseng, Matteo, and Natalie

CONTRIBUTORS

William T. Abraham, MD
Associate Director, Cardiac Transplantation, Cardiovascular Institute, University of Pittsburgh, Pittsburgh, Pennsylvania
Implantable Devices for the Management of Heart Failure

Maria Czarina Acelajado, MD
Clinical Associate Professor, Section of Hypertension, Department of Medicine, University of The Philippines, Philippine General Hospital, Manila, The Philippines
Resistant Hypertension

Dominick J. Angiolillo, MD, PhD
Associate Professor of Medicine, Director of Cardiovascular Research, Director, Center for Thrombosis Research, University of Florida College of Medicine, Jacksonville, Florida
Pharmacologic Options for Treatment of Ischemic Disease

Elad Anter, MD
Cardiac Electrophysiology, Division of Cardiovascular Medicine, Beth Israel Deaconess Medical Center; Instructor, Harvard Medical School, Boston, Massachusetts
Nonpharmacologic Treatment of Tachyarrhythmias

Elliott M. Antman, MD
Professor of Medicine, Associate Dean for Clinical/Translational Research, Harvard Medical School; Senior Investigator, TIMI Study Group, Brigham and Women's Hospital, Boston, Massachusetts
Tools for Assessment of Cardiovascular Tests and Therapies

Piero Anversa, MD
Departments of Anesthesia and Medicine, Division of Cardiovascular Medicine, Brigham and Women's Hospital, Harvard Medical School, Boston, Massachusetts
Regenerative Therapy for Heart Failure

Steven R. Bailey, MD
Chief, Division of Cardiology, University of Texas Health Sciences Center, San Antonio, Texas
Percutaneous Treatment for Valvular Heart Disease

Suzanne J. Baron, MD
Interventional Cardiology Fellow, Massachusetts General Hospital, Boston, Massachusetts
Advances in Coronary Revascularization

Eric R. Bates, MD
Professor, Department of Internal Medicine, University of Michigan, Ann Arbor, Michigan
ST-Segment Elevation Myocardial Infarction

Brigitte M. Baumann, MD, MSCE
Head, Division of Clinical Research, Department of Emergency Medicine, Cooper Medical School of Rowan University, Camden, New Jersey
Hypertensive Crisis

Edmund A. Bermudez, MD
Consultant, Florida Cardiac Consultants, Sarasota, Florida
Optimal Timing of Surgical and Mechanical Intervention in Native Valvular Heart Disease

David A. Calhoun, MD
Medical Director, Vascular Biology and Hypertension Program, University of Alabama at Birmingham, Birmingham, Alabama
Resistant Hypertension

Robert M. Califf, MD
Professor of Medicine, Division of Cardiology, Director, Duke University Translational Medicine Institute; Vice Chancellor for Clinical Research, Duke University; Editor-in-Chief, *American Heart Journal*, Raleigh, North Carolina
Tools for Assessment of Cardiovascular Tests and Therapies

David J. Callans, MD
Associate Director of Electrophysiology, University of Pennsylvania Health System, Philadelphia, Pennsylvania
Nonpharmacologic Treatment of Tachyarrhythmias

Niteesh K. Choudhry, MD, PhD
Assistant Professor of Medicine, Division of Pharmacoepidemiology and Pharmacoeconomics, Department of Medicine, Brigham and Women's Hospital, Harvard Medical School, Boston, Massachusetts
Tools for Assessment of Cardiovascular Tests and Therapies

Janice Y. Chyou, MD
Brigham and Women's Hospital, Boston, Massachusetts
Pharmacogenetics

Jay N. Cohn, MD
Professor of Medicine, Cardiovascular Division, University of Minnesota Medical School, Minneapolis, Minnesota
Pharmacologic Management of Heart Failure in the Ambulatory Setting

Wilson S. Colucci, MD
Cardiovascular Section, Boston University Medical Center, Boston, Massachusetts
Strategies for Management of Acute Decompensated Heart Failure

Michael H. Davidson, MD
Clinical Professor of Medicine, Director of Preventive Cardiology, The University of Chicago Pritzker School of Medicine, Chicago, Illinois
Therapy to Manage Low High-Density Lipoprotein Cholesterol and Elevated Triglycerides

James de Lemos, MD
Professor of Medicine, Department of Cardiology, University of Texas, Texas Southwestern Medical Center, Dallas, Texas

G. William Dec Jr., MD
Chief, Cardiology Division, Massachusetts General Hospital; Roman DeSanctis Professor of Medicine, Harvard Medical School, Boston, Massachusetts
Hypertrophic, Restrictive, and Infiltrative Cardiomyopathies

John P. DiMarco, MD, PhD
Professor of Medicine, Director, Heart Rhythm Center, Cardiovascular Division, University of Virginia Health System, Charlottesville, Virginia
Pharmacologic Management of Supraventricular Tachycardias

Kenneth A. Ellenbogen, MD
Kontos Professor of Cardiology, Chairman, Division of Cardiology, Medical College of Virginia, Richmond, Virginia
Role of Implantable Cardioverter-Defibrillators in Primary and Secondary Prevention of Sudden Cardiac Death

Rodney H. Falk, MD
Director, HVMA Cardiac Amyloidosis Program, Brigham and Women's Hospital; Associate Clinical Professor of Medicine, Harvard Medical School, Boston, Massachusetts
Atrial Fibrillation

Bonita E. Falkner, MD
Professor of Medicine and Pediatrics, Thomas Jefferson University, Philadelphia, Pennsylvania
Management of Hypertension in Children and Adolescents

Andrew Farb, MD
U.S. Food and Drug Administration, Washington, DC
Device Development for Cardiovascular Therapeutics: Concepts and Regulatory Implications

John D. Ferguson, MB ChB, MD
Associate Professor of Medicine, Cardiovascular Division, University of Virginia Health System, Charlottesville, Virginia
Pharmacologic Management of Supraventricular Tachycardias

Joseph T. Flynn, MD
Dr. Robert O. Hickman Endowed Chair in Pediatric Nephrology, Professor of Pediatrics, University of Washington School of Medicine, Seattle, Washington
Management of Hypertension in Children and Adolescents

Lisa W. Forbess, MD
Associate Professor of Medicine, Division of Cardiology, University of Texas Southwestern Medical Center, Dallas, Texas
Pharmacologic Options for Treating Cardiovascular Disease During Pregnancy

Keith A.A. Fox, MB ChB
Professor of Cardiology, Centre for Cardiovascular Research, University of Edinburgh, Edinburgh, United Kingdom
Stable Ischemic Heart Disease/Chronic Stable Angina

William H. Frishman, MD, MACP
Rosenthal Professor and Chairman, Department of Medicine, Professor of Pharmacology, New York Medical College; Director, Department of Medicine, Westchester Medical Center, Valhalla, New York
Pharmacologic Options for Treatment of Ischemic Disease

Victor F. Froelicher, MD
Professor of Medicine, Stanford University; Staff Cardiologist, Palo Alto VA Medical Center, Palo Alto, California
Rehabilitation of the Patient with Cardiovascular Disease

William H. Gaasch, MD
Senior Consultant in Cardiology, Lahey Clinic; Professor of Medicine, University of Massachusetts Medical School, Burlington, Massachusetts
Optimal Timing of Surgical and Mechanical Intervention in Native Valvular Heart Disease

Thomas A. Gaziano, MD, MSc
Assistant Professor, Harvard Medical School; Physician, Cardiovascular Medicine, Brigham and Women's Hospital, Boston, Massachusetts
Global Cardiovascular Therapy

Robert P. Giugliano, MD, SM
Senior Investigator, TIMI Study Group; Associate Physician, Cardiovascular Medicine, Brigham and Women's Hospital; Associate Professor of Medicine, Harvard Medical School, Boston, Massachusetts
Non–ST-Segment Elevation Acute Coronary Syndromes

Michael M. Givertz, MD
Medical Director, Heart Transplant and Circulatory Assist Program, Brigham and Women's Hospital; Associate Professor of Medicine, Harvard Medical School, Boston, Massachusetts
Pharmacologic Management of Heart Failure in the Ambulatory Setting
Strategies for Management of Acute Decompensated Heart Failure

Samuel Z. Goldhaber, MD
Director, Venous Thromboembolism Research Group; Professor of Medicine, Cardiovascular Division, Harvard Medical School, Boston, Massachusetts
Pulmonary Embolism and Deep Vein Thrombosis

Bruce R. Gordon, MD
Professor of Clinical Medicine and Surgery, Weill Medical College of Cornell University; Chief Operating Officer and Co-Director, Comprehensive Lipid Control Center, The Rogosin Institute; Attending Physician, New York-Presbyterian Hospital, New York, New York
Steps Beyond Diet and Drug Therapy for Severe Hypercholesterolemia

Christopher B. Granger, MD
Rosenthal Professor and Chairman, Department of Medicine, New York Medical College, Valhalla, New York
Systems of Health Care

Robert A. Harrington, MD
Arthur L. Bloomfield Professor of Medicine, Chair, Department of Medicine, Stanford University, Stanford, California
New Drug Development

Jennifer E. Ho, MD
Cardiology Research Fellow, Massachusetts General Hospital, Boston, Massachusetts
Manifestations, Mechanisms, and Treatment of HIV-Associated Cardiovascular Disease

Brian D. Hoit, MD
Professor of Medicine and Physiology and Biophysics, Case Western Reserve University; Director of Echocardiography, University Hospitals Case Medical Center, Cleveland, Ohio
Treatment of Pericardial Disease

Priscilla Y. Hsue, MD
Associate Professor of Medicine, University of California–San Francisco, San Francisco, California
Manifestations, Mechanisms, and Treatment of HIV-Associated Cardiovascular Disease

Lisa Cooper Hudgins, MD
Associate Professor of Pediatrics in Medicine and Pediatrics, Weill Medical College of Cornell University; Pediatric Program Director, Comprehensive Lipid Control Center, The Rogosin Institute; Associate Attending Physician, New York-Presbyterian Hospital, New York, New York
Steps Beyond Diet and Drug Therapy for Severe Hypercholesterolemia

Eric M. Isselbacher, MD
Co-Director, Thoracic Aortic Center, Associate Director, Heart Center, Massachusetts General Hospital; Associate Professor of Medicine, Harvard Medical School, Boston, Massachusetts
Aortic Disease

Michael R. Jaff, DO
Harvard Business School; Medical Director, Vascular Center, Massachusetts General Hospital, Boston, Massachusetts
Renal Artery Stenosis

Jan Kajstura, PhD
Departments of Anesthesia and Medicine, Division of Cardiovascular Medicine, Brigham and Women's Hospital, Harvard Medical School, Boston, Massachusetts
Regenerative Therapy for Heart Failure

S. Ananth Karumanchi, MD
Associate Professor of Medicine, Department of Medicine and Center for Vascular Biology, Harvard Medical School, Beth Israel Deaconess Medical Center, Boston, Massachusetts
Hypertension in Pregnancy

David F. Kong, AM, DMT
Associate Professor of Medicine, Department of Medicine; Co-Director, Cardiovascular Late Phase 3/Devices, Duke Clinical Research Institute, Duke University Medical Center, Research Triangle Park, North Carolina
New Drug Development

Daniel B. Kramer, MD
Cardiovascular Institute, Beth Israel Deaconess Medical Center; Instructor, Harvard Medical School, Boston, Massachusetts
Appendix: Cardiovascular Devices

Marc Z. Krichavsky, MD
Cardiac Specialists, Danbury, Connecticut
Peripheral Artery Disease

Marie Krousel-Wood, MD, MSPH
Professor of Clinical Epidemiology and of Clinical Family and Community Medicine, Tulane University Health Sciences; Director, Center for Health Research, Oschner Clinic Foundation, New Orleans, Louisiana
Initial Evaluation and Approach to the Patient with Hypertension

Frederick G. Kushner, MD
Clinical Professor of Medicine, Department of Medicine, Tulane University School of Medicine, New Orleans, Lousiana
ST-Segment Elevation Myocardial Infarction

Neal Lakdawala, MD, MSc
Instructor of Medicine, Harvard Medical School; Associate Physician, Cardiovascular Medicine, Brigham and Women's Hospital; VA Boston Healthcare System, Boston, Massachusetts
Hypertrophic, Restrictive, and Infiltrative Cardiomyopathies

Michael J. Landzberg, MD
Director, Boston Adult Congenital Heart (BACH) and Pulmonary Hypertension Group, Children's Hospital Boston, Brigham and Women's Hospital, Harvard Medical School, Boston, Massachusetts
Treatment of Pulmonary Arterial Hypertension
Care for Adults with Congenital Heart Disease

David C. Lange, MD
Chief Medical Resident, San Francisco VA Medical Center, University of California–San Francisco, San Francisco, California
Manifestations, Mechanisms, and Treatment of HIV-Associated Cardiovascular Disease

Annarosa Leri, MD
Departments of Anesthesia and Medicine, Division of Cardiovascular Medicine, Brigham and Women's Hospital, Harvard Medical School, Boston, Massachusetts
Regenerative Therapy for Heart Failure

J. Michael Mangrum, MD
Associate Professor of Medicine, Cardiovascular Division, University of Virginia Health System, Charlottesville, Virginia
Pharmacologic Management of Supraventricular Tachycardias

Jaimie Manlucu, MD
London Health Sciences Centre, London, Ontario, Canada
Implantable Devices for the Management of Heart Failure

Giuseppe J. Martucci, MD
Director, McGill Adult Unit for Congenital Heart Disease Excellence (MAUDE), McGill University Health Centre and Sir Mortimer B. Davis Jewish General Hospital, Faculty of Medicine, McGill University, Montreal, Quebec, Canada
Care for Adults with Congenital Heart Disease

Michael A. Mathier, MD
University of Pittsburgh, Pittsburgh, Pennsylvania
Cardiac Transplantation and Circulatory Support Devices

Laura Mauri, MD
Associate Professor of Medicine, Brigham and Women's Hospital, Harvard Medical School, Boston, Massachusetts
Advances in Coronary Revascularization

Kathy McManus, MS, RD
Director of Nutrition, Brigham and Women's Hospital, Boston, Massachusetts
Cardiovascular Disease and Lifestyle Modification

Jessica L. Mega, MD, MPH
Brigham and Women's Hospital, Boston, Massachusetts
Pharmacogenetics

Stephanie Mick, MD
Division of Cardiac Surgery, Brigham and Women's Hospital, Harvard Medical School, Boston, Massachusetts; Heart and Vascular Institute, Department of Thoracic and Cardiovascular Surgery, Cleveland Clinic, Cleveland, Ohio
Advances in Coronary Revascularization

Mary Mullen, MD, PhD
Director, Pulmonary Hypertension Service, Boston Adult
  Congenital Heart (BACH) Group, Children's Hospital, Brigham
  and Women's Hospital, Harvard Medical School, Boston,
  Massachusetts
Care for Adults with Congenital Heart Disease

Jonathan N. Myers, PhD
Clinical Professor, Department of Cardiology, VA Palo Alto
  Health Care System, Stanford University, Palo Alto, California
Rehabilitation of the Patient with Cardiovascular Disease

David E. Newby, PhD, BM DM
Professor of Cardiology, Centre for Cardiovascular Science,
  University of Edinburgh, Edinburgh, United Kingdom
Stable Ischemic Heart Disease/Chronic Stable Angina

Graham Nichol, MD, MPH
Medic One Foundation Endowed Chair in Prehospital
  Emergency Care, Director, University of Washington-
  Harborview Center for Prehospital Emergency Care; Medical
  Director, Resuscitation Outcome Consortium Clinical Trial
  Center; Professor of Medicine, University of Washington-
  Seattle, Seattle, Washington
Systems of Health Care

Suzanne Oparil, MD
Professor of Medicine and Physiology and Biophysics, Director,
  Vascular Biology & Hypertension Program; Department of
  Medicine, Division of Cardiovascular Disease, University of
  Alabama at Birmingham, Birmingham, Alabama
Initial Evaluation and Approach to the Patient with Hypertension

Alexander R. Opotowsky, MD, MPH
Boston Adult Congenital Heart (BACH) and Pulmonary
  Hypertension Group, Children's Hospital Boston, Brigham
  and Women's Hospital, Harvard Medical School, Boston,
  Massachusetts
Treatment of Pulmonary Arterial Hypertension

Neha J. Pagidipati, MD
Division of Women's Health, Brigham and Women's Hospital,
  Boston, Massachusetts
Global Cardiovascular Therapy

John D. Parker, MD
Program Medical Director, Heart & Circulation Program,
  University Health Network; Professor, University of
  Toronto, Toronto, Ontario, Canada
Pharmacologic Options for Treatment of Ischemic Disease

Joseph E. Parrillo, MD
Professor of Medicine, Robert Wood Johnson Medical School,
  University of Medicine and Dentistry of New Jersey; Chief,
  Department of Medicine, Edward D. Viner MD Chair, Director,
  Cooper Heart Institute, Cooper University Hospital, Camden,
  New Jersey
Treatment of Ventricular Tachycardia and Cardiac Arrest

Matthias Peltz, MD
Assistant Professor, Department of Cardiovascular and Thoracic
  Surgery, University of Texas Southwestern Medical Center,
  Dallas, Texas
Surgery for Valvular Heart Disease

Todd S. Perlstein, MD
Associate Physician, Cardiovascular Division, Brigham and
  Women's Hospital, Boston, Massachusetts
Peripheral Artery Disease

Gail E. Peterson, MD
University of Texas Southwestern Medical Center, Dallas, Texas
Prevention and Treatment of Infective Endocarditis

Gregory Piazza, MD
Staff Cardiologist, Cardiovascular Medicine Division, Brigham
  and Women's Hospital, Boston, Massachusetts
Pulmonary Embolism and Deep Vein Thrombosis

Sharon C. Reimold, MD
Professor of Medicine, Division of Cardiology, University of
  Texas Southwestern Medical Center, Dallas, Texas
*Pharmacologic Options for Treating Cardiovascular Disease
  During Pregnancy*

Klaus Romero, MD
Director of Clinical Research, Critical Path Institute, Tucson,
  Arizona
Clinical Pharmacology of Antiarrhythmic Drugs

Andrea M. Russo, MD
Professor of Medicine, Robert Wood Johnson Medical School,
  University of Medicine and Dentistry of New Jersey; Director,
  Cardiac Electrophysiology and Arrhythmia Services, Director,
  Clinical Electrophysiology Fellowship, Cooper University
  Hospital, Camden, New Jersey
Treatment of Ventricular Tachycardia and Cardiac Arrest

Marc S. Sabatine, MD, MPH
Chairman, TIMI Study Group, Brigham and Women's Hospital;
  Associate Professor of Medicine, Harvard Medical School,
  Boston, Massachusetts
Pharmacogenetics

Frank M. Sacks, MD
Professor of Cardiovascular Disease Prevention, Department of
  Nutrition, Harvard School of Public Health; Department of
  Medicine, Cardiovascular Division and Channing Laboratory,
  Brigham and Women's Hospital, Harvard Medical School,
  Boston, Massachusetts
Cardiovascular Disease and Lifestyle Modification

Joseph J. Saseen, PharmD
Professor of Clinical Pharmacy and Family Medicine,
  University of Colorado Anschutz Medical Campus, Skaggs
  School of Pharmacy and Pharmaceutical Sciences and
  School of Medicine; Professor of Family Medicine, University
  of Colorado School of Medicine, Aurora, Colorado
Pharmacologic Management of Hypertension

Frederick J. Schoen, MD, PhD
Executive Vice Chairman, Department of Pathology, Brigham
  and Women's Hospital; Professor of Pathology and Health
  Sciences and Technology, Harvard Medical School, Boston,
  Massachusetts
*Device Development for Cardiovascular Therapeutics: Concepts
  and Regulatory Implications*

John S. Schroeder, MD
Professor of Medicine, Department of Medicine, Stanford
  University, Stanford, California
Pharmacologic Options for Treatment of Ischemic Disease

Benjamin M. Scirica, MD, MPH
Investigator, TIMI Study Group; Associate Physician, Cardiovascular Division, Brigham and Women's Hospital; Assistant Professor of Medicine, Harvard Medical School, Boston, Massachusetts
Pharmacologic Options for Treatment of Ischemic Disease

Eric A. Secemsky, MD
Cardiovascular Fellow, Massachusetts General Hospital, Harvard Medical School, Boston, Massachusetts
Manifestations, Mechanisms, and Treatment of HIV-Associated Cardiovascular Disease

Ellen W. Seely, MD
Director of Clinical Research, Endocrinology, Diabetes, and Hypertension Division, Brigham and Women's Hospital; Professor of Medicine, Harvard Medical School, Boston, Massachusetts
Hypertension in Pregnancy

Prem S. Shekar, MD
Brigham and Women's Hospital, Boston, Massachusetts
Advances in Coronary Revascularization

Michael A. Shullo, PharmD
University of Pittsburgh, Pittsburgh, Pennsylvania
Cardiac Transplantation and Circulatory Support Devices

Piotr Sobieszczyk, MD
Cardiovascular Division, Vascular Medicine Section, Brigham and Women's Hospital, Harvard University Medical School, Boston, Massachusetts
Cerebrovascular Disease

Amy B. Stancoven, MD
Assistant Instructor, Internal Medicine, University of Texas Southwestern Medical Center, Dallas, Texas
Prevention and Treatment of Infective Endocarditis

Neil J. Stone, MD, MACP
Benow Professor of Medicine, Feinberg School of Medicine, Northwestern University; Medical Director, Vascular Center, Bluhm Cardiovascular Institute, Northwestern Memorial Hospital, Chicago, Illinois
Drugs for Elevated Low-Density Lipoprotein Cholesterol

Melanie S. Sulistio, MD
Assistant Professor, Division of Cardiology, Department of Internal Medicine, University of Texas Southwestern Medical Center, Dallas, Texas
Optimal Timing of Surgical and Mechanical Intervention in Native Valvular Heart Disease

Jeffrey Teuteberg, MD
Medical Director, Mechanical Circulatory Support, University of Pittsburgh, Pittsburgh, Pennsylvania
Cardiac Transplantation and Circulatory Support Devices

Raymond R. Townsend, MD
Department of Medicine, Perelman School of Medicine, University of Pennsylvania, Philadelphia, Pennsylvania
Hypertensive Crisis

Stephen Trzeciak, MD, MPH
Associate Professor of Medicine, Robert Wood Johnson Medical School, University of Medicine and Dentistry of New Jersey, Division of Critical Care Medicine, Department of Medicine and Department of Emergency Medicine, Cooper University Hospital, Camden, New Jersey
Treatment of Ventricular Tachycardia and Cardiac Arrest

Alice M. Wang, MD
Assistant Professor of Pediatrics, Boston University School of Medicine; Department of Pediatrics, Boston Medical Center, Boston, Massachusetts
Hypertension in Pregnancy

Ido Weinberg, MD, MSc, MHA
Department of Cardiology, Division of Vascular Medicine, Massachusetts General Hospital, Boston, Massachusetts
Renal Artery Stenosis

Stephen D. Wiviott, MD
Investigator, TIMI Study Group; Associate Physician, Cardiovascular Division, Brigham and Women's Hospital; Assistant Professor of Medicine, Harvard Medical School, Boston, Massachusetts
Non–ST-Segment Elevation Acute Coronary Syndromes

Mark A. Wood, MD
Professor of Medicine, Feinberg School of Medicine, Northwestern University, Chicago, Illinois
Role of Implantable Cardioverter-Defibrillators in Primary and Secondary Prevention of Sudden Cardiac Death

Christopher Woods, MD, PhD
Cardiology Fellow, Stanford University, Stanford, California
Pharmacologic Options for Treatment of Ischemic Disease

Raymond L. Woosley, MD, PhD
President Emeritus, Critical Path Institute; Professor of Medicine, Sarver Heart Center, University of Arizona College of Medicine, Tucson, Arizona
Clinical Pharmacology of Antiarrhythmic Drugs

Clyde W. Yancy, MD
Professor of Medicine, Department of Medicine, Stanford University School of Medicine, Stanford, California
Systems of Health Care

William F. Young Jr., MD, MSc
Chair, Division of Endocrinology, Diabetes, Metabolism, and Nutrition, Tyson Family Endocrinology Clinical Professor, Professor of Medicine, Mayo Clinic College of Medicine, Rochester, Minnesota
Endocrine Causes of Hypertension

Peter Zimetbaum, MD
Clinical Director of Cardiology, Beth Israel Deaconess Medical Center; Associate Professor of Medicine, Harvard Medical School, Boston, Massachusetts
Atrial Fibrillation

Bram D. Zuckerman, MD
U.S. Food and Drug Administration, Washington, DC
Device Development for Cardiovascular Therapeutics: Concepts and Regulatory Implications

FOREWORD

As recently as four decades ago, the treatment options available for patients with cardiovascular disease were quite limited. The major therapeutic measures included bed rest and warfarin for acute myocardial infarction; nitroglycerin for angina pectoris; dietary sodium restriction, bed rest, digitalis, and mercurial or thiazide diuretics for heart failure; quinidine or procainamide for tachyarrhythmia; large, clumsy pacemakers for complete heart block; sodium restriction and sympathetic blocking agents for severe hypertension; and palliative surgery for a limited number of complex congenital cardiac malformations. Mild or even moderate hypertension was not treated, nor were effective agents available to lower serum cholesterol in patients with coronary artery disease and hypercholesterolemia. Percutaneous coronary revascularization, implantable cardioverter-defibrillators, and modern pharmacotherapy of myocardial ischemia and fibrinolysis had not yet been developed. β-Adrenergic antagonists, angiotensin-converting enzyme inhibitors, and statins also were off in the future.

No aspect of medicine has undergone a more radical transformation in the past 40 years than has cardiovascular therapeutics, and the results have been truly spectacular. Overall mortality rates from heart disease have been steadily declining, and the rate of age-adjusted mortality secondary to coronary artery disease, the most common cause of cardiovascular deaths, has been falling at almost 1% per year. Effective treatment—albeit not cure—of almost all forms of heart disease is now possible, allowing a majority of patients with cardiovascular disease to live longer lives of high quality.

Drs. Antman and Sabatine and their associate editors—Drs. de Lemos, DiMarco, Givertz, Oparil, Sacks, Scirica, and Sobieszczyk—and a constellation of superb contributing authors should be congratulated on providing the most comprehensive modern text in cardiovascular therapeutics. Instead of focusing narrowly on a single therapeutic modality—drugs, interventional cardiology, devices, or surgery—this contemporary, authoritative, and eminently readable book deals with total patient management. The several types of therapy that can be offered for specific cardiovascular disorders are presented lucidly and in sufficient detail to serve as the basis for managing the vast majority of patients with cardiovascular disease. This excellent text will be of immense value not only to cardiologists but also to internists and primary care physicians, who are shouldering increasing responsibilities for the management of patients with cardiovascular disease.

This fourth edition of *Cardiovascular Therapeutics* is essentially a new book when compared with its predecessor. There are four new section editors and many new contributors. Thirteen of the 49 chapters are entirely new to this edition. The remainder have been carefully updated.

We are very proud that *Cardiovascular Therapeutics* is a companion to *Braunwald's Heart Disease: A Textbook of Cardiovascular Medicine*. We hope that the new edition, along with the other books now available as companion volumes to *Heart Disease*, will serve as an extensive cardiovascular information system.

Eugene Braunwald, MD
Robert O. Bonow, MD
Peter Libby, MD
Douglas Mann, MD
Douglas P. Zipes, MD

PREFACE

This fourth edition of *Cardiovascular Therapeutics*, a textbook originally proposed by the late Thomas Woodward Smith as a companion to *Braunwald's Heart Disease*, continues to emphasize an evidence-based approach to therapeutic recommendations for management of the patient with cardiovascular disease. We had the privilege of working with an experienced group of section editors, Dr. James de Lemos, Dr. John DiMarco, Dr. Michael Givertz, Dr. Suzanne Oparil, Dr. Frank Sacks, Dr. Benjamin Scirica, and Dr. Piotr Sobieszczyk, in producing the 49 chapters and the Appendix in this edition. The reader is provided with cutting-edge recommendations for treatment of patients with common problems such as ischemic heart disease, heart failure, dyslipidemia, dysrhythmias, hypertension, valvular heart disease, peripheral arterial disease, aortic syndromes, congenital heart disease, pericardial disease, cardiovascular disorders during pregnancy, and infective endocarditis.

Compared with the previous edition, 13 chapters are completely new and 36 chapters and the Appendix have been substantially revised. The introductory chapter on tools for understanding the evidence that drives guidelines recommendations has important new information from contemporary clinical trials. Critical chapters on emerging therapeutic approaches such as pharmacogenetics, regenerative therapy, and implantable devices for heart failure and arrhythmias have been added. To assist the clinician in understanding the details of the development and approval of cardiovascular devices, representatives from the Food and Drug Administration have contributed to an updated chapter.

Primary care physicians and cardiologists across a range of training and experience will find the fourth edition of *Cardiovascular Therapeutics* a critical resource for their practice. Once again, there are extensive cross-references to the ninth edition of *Braunwald's Heart Disease*, edited by Robert Bonow, Douglas Mann, Douglas Zipes, and Peter Libby. By using this edition of *Cardiovascular Therapeutics* along with *Braunwald's Heart Disease* and the other texts in the companion series in a synergistic fashion, clinicians will be able to make the most of an extraordinarily rich set of resources that have been rigorously prepared.

ACKNOWLEDGMENTS

A new edition of a text such as *Cardiovascular Therapeutics* provides an opportunity to acknowledge the contributions of many individuals. The continued training in rigorous scientific thinking, cardiovascular research, and clinical medicine provided by Eugene Braunwald is a treasured experience for which we are extremely grateful. The scientific and personal collaborations with Joseph Loscalzo have been an important asset in framing our thinking in preparing this edition. We wish also to acknowledge the generations of Cardiovascular Division Fellows and extraordinary faculty at the Brigham and Women's Hospital, under the leadership of Peter Libby, who provided the inspiration and professional environment for our work on *Cardiovascular Therapeutics*. A special note of gratitude is due to our colleagues in the TIMI Study Group, many of whom have contributed both directly and indirectly to this text. Sylvia Judd and Pamela Melhorn, our administrative assistants, were invaluable resources in countless ways related to the preparation and production of this book.

Finally, on behalf of all of the Section Editors and contributors, we wish to express appreciation for the efforts of the team at Elsevier who worked diligently to publish this text.

Elliott M. Antman, MD
Marc S. Sabatine, MD, MPH

CONTENTS

PART I DECISION MAKING AND THERAPEUTIC STRATEGIES IN CARDIOVASCULAR MEDICINE

CHAPTER 1 **Tools for Assessment of Cardiovascular Tests and Therapies** 1
Elliott M. Antman, Robert M. Califf, and Niteesh K. Choudhry

CHAPTER 2 **New Drug Development** 33
David F. Kong and Robert A. Harrington

CHAPTER 3 **Device Development for Cardiovascular Therapeutics: Concepts and Regulatory Implications** 41
Frederick J. Schoen, Bram D. Zuckerman, and Andrew Farb

CHAPTER 4 **Pharmacogenetics** 53
Janice Y. Chyou, Jessica L Mega, and Marc S. Sabatine

CHAPTER 5 **Systems of Health Care** 67
Clyde W. Yancy, Christopher B. Granger, and Graham Nichol

CHAPTER 6 **Global Cardiovascular Therapy** 75
Thomas A. Gaziano and Neha J. Pagidipati

PART II ISCHEMIC HEART DISEASE

CHAPTER 7 **Pharmacologic Options for Treatment of Ischemic Disease** 83
John S. Schroeder, William H. Frishman, John D. Parker, Dominick J. Angiolillo, Christopher Woods, and Benjamin M. Scirica

CHAPTER 8 **Stable Ischemic Heart Disease/ Chronic Stable Angina** 131
David E. Newby and Keith A.A. Fox

CHAPTER 9 **Non–ST-Segment Elevation Acute Coronary Syndromes** 153
Stephen D. Wiviott and Robert P. Giugliano

CHAPTER 10 **ST-Segment Elevation Myocardial Infarction** 178
Frederick G. Kushner and Eric R. Bates

CHAPTER 11 **Advances in Coronary Revascularization** 214
Suzanne J. Baron, Stephanie Mick, Prem S. Shekar, and Laura Mauri

PART III HEART FAILURE

CHAPTER 12 **Pharmacologic Management of Heart Failure in the Ambulatory Setting** 241
Michael M. Givertz and Jay N. Cohn

CHAPTER 13 **Implantable Devices for the Management of Heart Failure** 270
Jaimie Manlucu and William T. Abraham

CHAPTER 14 **Strategies for Management of Acute Decompensated Heart Failure** 281
Michael M. Givertz and Wilson S. Colucci

CHAPTER 15 **Cardiac Transplantation and Circulatory Support Devices** 307
Jeffrey Teuteberg, Michael A. Mathier, and Michael A. Shullo

CHAPTER 16 **Regenerative Therapy for Heart Failure** 322
Annarosa Leri, Jan Kajstura, and Piero Anversa

CHAPTER 17 **Hypertrophic, Restrictive, and Infiltrative Cardiomyopathies** 332
Neal Lakdawala and G. William Dec Jr.

PART IV ARRHYTHMIAS AND CONDUCTION DISTURBANCES

CHAPTER 18 **Clinical Pharmacology of Antiarrhythmic Drugs** 343
Klaus Romero and Raymond L. Woosley

CHAPTER 19 **Pharmacologic Management of Supraventricular Tachycardias** 365
John P. DiMarco, J. Michael Mangrum, and John D. Ferguson

CHAPTER 20 **Atrial Fibrillation** 372
Peter Zimetbaum and Rodney H. Falk

CHAPTER 21 **Nonpharmacologic Treatment of Tachyarrhythmias** 383
David J. Callans and Elad Anter

CHAPTER 22 **Role of Implantable Cardioverter-Defibrillators in Primary and Secondary Prevention of Sudden Cardiac Death** 396
Mark A. Wood and Kenneth A. Ellenbogen

CHAPTER 23 **Treatment of Ventricular Tachycardia and Cardiac Arrest** 408
Stephen Trzeciak, Andrea M. Russo, and Joseph E. Parillo

PART V DYSLIPOPROTEINEMIAS AND ATHEROSCLEROSIS

CHAPTER 24 **Drugs for Elevated Low-Density Lipoprotein Cholesterol** 421
Neil J. Stone

CHAPTER 25 **Therapy to Manage Low High-Density Lipoprotein Cholesterol and Elevated Triglycerides** 434
Michael H. Davidson

CHAPTER 26 **Cardiovascular Disease and Lifestyle Modification** 442
Frank M. Sacks and Kathy McManus

CHAPTER 27 **Steps Beyond Diet and Drug Therapy for Severe Hypercholesterolemia** 454
Bruce R. Gordon and Lisa Cooper Hudgins

PART VI HYPERTENSION

CHAPTER 28 **Initial Evaluation and Approach to the Patient with Hypertension** 463
Marie Krousel-Wood and Suzanne Oparil

CHAPTER 29 **Pharmacologic Management of Hypertension** 474
Joseph J. Saseen

CHAPTER 30 **Endocrine Causes of Hypertension** 490
William F. Young Jr.

CHAPTER 31 **Resistant Hypertension** 501
Maria Czarina Acelajado and David A. Calhoun

CHAPTER 32 **Hypertensive Crisis** 510
Brigitte M. Baumann and Raymond R. Townsend

CHAPTER 33 **Hypertension in Pregnancy** 521
Alice M. Wang, Ellen W. Seely, and S. Ananth Karumanchi

CHAPTER 34 **Management of Hypertension in Children and Adolescents** 529
Joseph T. Flynn and Bonita E. Falkner

PART VII OTHER VASCULAR CONDITIONS

CHAPTER 35 **Peripheral Artery Disease** 539
Todd S. Perlstein and Marc Z. Krichavsky

CHAPTER 36 **Cerebrovascular Disease** 553
Piotr Sobieszczyk

CHAPTER 37 **Renal Artery Stenosis** 571
Ido Weinberg and Michael R. Jaff

CHAPTER 38 **Pulmonary Embolism and Deep Vein Thrombosis** 580
Samuel Z. Goldhaber and Gregory Piazza

CHAPTER 39 **Treatment of Pulmonary Arterial Hypertension** 596
Alexander R. Opotowsky and Michael J. Landzberg

CHAPTER 40 **Aortic Disease** 606
Eric M. Isselbacher

PART VIII OTHER CARDIOVASCULAR CONDITIONS

CHAPTER 41 **Pharmacologic Options for Treating of Cardiovascular Disease During Pregnancy** 621
Sharon C. Reimold and Lisa W. Forbess

CHAPTER 42 **Care for Adults with Congenital Heart Disease** 632
Michael J. Landzberg, Giuseppe J. Martucci, and Mary Mullen

CHAPTER 43 **Prevention and Treatment of Infective Endocarditis** 652
Amy B. Stancoven and Gail E. Peterson

CHAPTER 44 **Treatment of Pericardial Disease** 667
Brian D. Hoit

CHAPTER 45 **Optimal Timing of Surgical and Mechanical Intervention in Native Valvular Heart Disease** 676
Melanie S. Sulistio, Edmund A. Bermudez, and William H. Gaasch

CHAPTER 46 **Surgery for Valvular Heart Disease** 691
Matthias Peltz

CHAPTER 47 **Percutaneous Treatment for Valvular Heart Disease** 714
Steven R. Bailey

CHAPTER 48 **Manifestations, Mechanisms, and Treatment of HIV-Associated Cardiovascular Disease** 728
David C. Lange, Eric A. Secemsky, Jennifer E. Ho, and Priscilla Y. Hsue

CHAPTER 49 **Rehabilitation of the Patient with Cardiovascular Disease** 738
Jonathan N. Myers and Victor F. Froelicher

PART IX   APPENDIX

Cardiovascular Devices 747
Daniel B. Kramer

Index 761

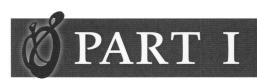

PART I

DECISION MAKING AND THERAPEUTIC STRATEGIES IN CARDIOVASCULAR MEDICINE

CHAPTER **1**

Tools for Assessment of Cardiovascular Tests and Therapies

Elliott M. Antman, Robert M. Califf, and Niteesh K. Choudhry

INTERPRETATION OF DIAGNOSTIC RESULTS, 1

CLINICAL TRIALS, 3

Need for Clinical Trials, 3
Clinical Trial Design, 4

HOW TO READ AND INTERPRET A CLINICAL TRIAL, 11

Missing Data, 12
Measures of Treatment Effect, 12
Detection of Treatment Effects in Clinical Trials, 13

META-ANALYSIS, 15

Principles of Pooling Studies, 16
Cumulative Meta-Analysis, 16
Meta-Regression, 17
Future Trends in Meta-Analysis, 18
How to Read and Interpret a Meta-Analysis, 18

COMPARATIVE EFFECTIVENESS RESEARCH, 19

Methods for Comparative Effectiveness Research, 20
Balancing Risks and Benefits, 22

COST-EFFECTIVENESS ANALYSIS, 23

Types of Economic Evaluation, 23
Methods for Performing a Cost-Effectiveness Analysis, 24
Other Methodologic Considerations, 26
Defining When a Therapy is Cost Effective, 29
How to Read an Economic Evaluation, 30

REFERENCES, 30

Cardiovascular disease continues to be a major health problem, estimated to be responsible for about 30% of all global deaths.[1] Currently, cardiovascular disease is the leading cause of death in the United States, and 17% of national health care expenditures are related to cardiovascular disease.[2] The direct medical costs related to cardiovascular disease in the United States are projected to increase from $272.5 billion in 2010 to $818.1 billion by 2030; the indirect costs (lost productivity) are projected to increase from $171.7 billion to $275.8 billion over the same time period.[2] Primary drivers for these increases in costs include the aging of the population, a growth in per capita medical spending, and the epidemic of such general medical problems as obesity and diabetes. Thus, selection of therapeutic strategies for patients with cardiovascular disease must be evidence based and requires consideration of comparative effectiveness, cost effectiveness, and involvement of the patient, when capable, in shared decision making.[3] The appropriate balance of evidence, cost, and patient involvement has not yet been vigorously established.[4-8] Furthermore, there is increasing recognition that although office practice remains valuable, the effective practitioner will use a variety of tools to create a "cardiovascular team" that can give the patient the best chance of avoiding disease progression and major cardiovascular events. This more complex environment, one that recognizes the value of teamwork in clinical care, creates a challenging but effective approach to improving decision making in cardiovascular care.

Therapeutic decision making in the office and hospital practice of cardiovascular medicine should proceed through an orderly sequence of events that begins with elicitation of the pertinent medical history and performance of a physical examination (Braunwald, Chapter 12). In the ideal situation, a variety of diagnostic tests are ordered, and the results are integrated into an assessment of the probability of a particular cardiac disease state. Based on this information and on an assessment of the evidence to support various treatments, a therapeutic strategy is formulated. In the arena of primary and secondary prevention, evidence points to the importance of reaching the patient at home or in the work environment by leveraging Internet-based technologies—such as e-mail, text messages, and so on—and mid-level providers. Despite the evolution in our understanding of these nontraditional settings, the fundamental structure by which evidence informs choices remains essential. The purpose of this chapter is to provide an overview of the quantitative tools used to interpret diagnostic tests, evaluate clinical trials, and assess comparative efficacy and cost effectiveness when selecting a treatment plan. The principles and techniques discussed here serve as a foundation for placing the remainder of the book in perspective, and they form the basis for the generation of guidelines for clinical practice.[9] Appropriate application of the therapeutic decision-making tools that are described and adherence to the guideline documents based on the tools translate into improved patient outcomes, an area where cardiovascular specialists have distinguished themselves among the various medical specialties.[10-12]

Interpretation of Diagnostic Tests

A useful starting point for interpreting a diagnostic test is the standard 2×2 table describing the presence or absence of disease, as determined by a gold standard, and the results of the test.[13] Even before the results of the test are known, clinicians should estimate the pretest likelihood of disease based on its prevalence in a population of patients with clinical characteristics similar to the patient being evaluated. Because no diagnostic test is perfect, a variety of quantitative terms are used to describe its operating characteristics, thereby enabling statistical inference about the value of the test (Figure 1-1). *Sensitivity* refers to the proportion of patients with the disease who have a positive test. *Specificity* is the proportion of patients without the disease who have a negative test. The probability that a test will be negative in the presence of disease is the *false-negative rate*, and the probability that a test will be positive in the absence of disease is the *false-positive rate*. Other useful terms are *positive predictive value*, which describes the probability that the disease is present if the test is positive, and *negative predictive value*, which describes the probability that the disease is absent when the test is negative. The Standards for Reporting of Diagnostic

Accuracy (STARD) initiative sets forth guidelines on how studies of reports on diagnostic accuracy should be prepared.[14]

Because the results of diagnostic tests are dependent on the profiles of patients being studied, the *likelihood ratio* has been introduced to express how many times more or less likely a test result is to be found in patients with disease compared with those without disease (see Figure 1-1; this is analogous to Bayes' rule, in which the prior probability of a disease state is updated based on the conditional probability of the observed test result to form a revised or posttest probability of a disease state).[15] By multiplying the pretest odds of disease by the likelihood ratio, clinicians can establish a posttest likelihood of disease and determine whether that likelihood crosses the threshold for treatment.[16] For example, in a patient with chest discomfort, the presence of ST-segment elevation on the 12-lead electrocardiogram—the diagnostic test—not only increases the probability that myocardial infarction (MI)—the disease state—is present, but also moves the decision-making process to the treatment threshold for reperfusion therapy without the necessity for further diagnostic testing. In the same patient, a nondiagnostic electrocardiogram does not appreciably alter the posttest likelihood of an MI. Additional tests (e.g., biomarkers of cardiac damage) are needed to establish the diagnosis of MI.

The example shown in Figure 1-1 is for a diagnostic test that produces dichotomous results, either positive or negative. Many tests in cardiology provide results on a continuous scale. Typically, diagnostic cutoffs are established based on tradeoffs between sensitivity and specificity made with knowledge of the goal of the testing. In the example shown in Figure 1-2, a diagnostic cutoff in the region of point A would have high sensitivity because it identifies the majority of patients with disease (true-positive results), but it does so at the expense of reduced specificity because it falsely declares the test to be abnormal in patients without disease. Using a range of diagnostic cutoffs for a positive test (e.g., see Figure 1-2, *A* to *C*), a receiver operating characteristic (ROC) curve can be plotted to illustrate the relation between sensitivity and specificity.[17] Better tests are those in which the ROC curve is positioned close to the top left corner. Comparison between two tests over a range of diagnostic cutoffs is accomplished by calculating the area under the ROC curve; the test with the larger area is generally considered to be superior, although at times the goal may be to optimize either sensitivity or specificity, even if one comes at the expense of the other.[16] In practice, it is difficult for many clinicians to apply the quantitative concepts illustrated in Figure 1-2 at the bedside. This has led many laboratories to provide annotated

FIGURE 1-1

Disease

		Present	Absent
Test	Positive	True Pos	False Pos
	Negative	False Neg	True Neg

Statistical Terms

Sens = TP / (TP + FN) = P (T+ if D+)

Spec = TN / (FP + TN) = P (T- if D-)

FNR = FN / (TP + FN) = P (T- if D+)

FPR = FP / (FP + TN) = P (T+ if D-)

PPV = TP / (TP + FP) = P (D+ if T+)

NPV = TN / (FN + TN) = P (D- if T-)

"Clinical" Terms

LR pos = Sens / FPR

LR neg = FNR / Spec

Pre Test odds of Dis.
LR = *Post Test odds of Dis.*

FIGURE 1-1 Interpretation of diagnostic tests. The standard 2 × 2 table (*top*) assigns patients into one of four cells based on the presence or absence of disease according to a gold standard and the results of a diagnostic test (positive or negative). Seven commonly used statistical abbreviations that describe the operating characteristics of the test are given (*bottom left*). A clinically useful term is *likelihood ratio* (*LR*), which expresses how many times a test result is more or less likely to be found in patients with disease compared with those without disease. This enables clinicians to update their pretest estimate of the odds of disease (*Dis*) and formulate a posttest odds of disease. The statistical terms can be interpreted along the lines of the following example: Sensitivity = probability (P) that the test is positive (T+) if the disease is present (D+). False Neg (FN), false negative; False Pos (FP), false positive; FNR, false-negative rate; FPR, false-positive rate; NPV, negative predictive value; PPV, positive predictive value; Sens, sensitivity; Spec, specificity; True Neg (TN), true negative; True Pos (TP) true positive.

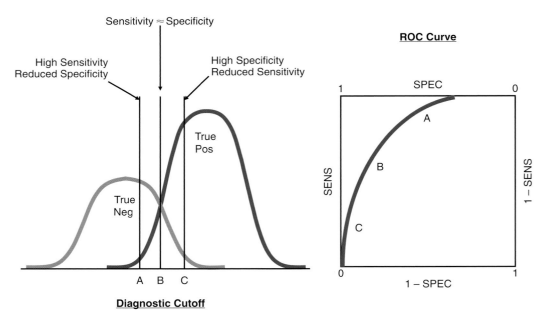

Diagnostic Cutoff

FIGURE 1-2 Influence of diagnostic cutoffs on interpretation of test performance. *Left,* Distributions of patients for whom the disease is present (*True Pos*) and absent (*True Neg*). Three different levels of a diagnostic cutoff (*A* to *C*) are shown for a test that is reported on a continuous scale. Diagnostic cutoff A has high sensitivity—that is, it identifies the majority of true-positive patients but at the expense of reduced specificity, and a large number of true-negative patients are classified as having disease. At the other extreme, diagnostic cutoff C has high specificity, so few true-negative patients are classified as having disease but at the expense of reduced specificity, so a large proportion of true-positive patients are not classified as having disease. *Right,* Typical receiver operator characteristic curve (ROC), illustrating the impact of cutoff levels *A* to *C* with respect to sensitivity (*SENS*) and specificity (*SPEC*).

reports to assist practitioners in forming a probabilistic estimate of the likelihood of a disease state being present.

Many diagnostic tests, risk scores, and models are used to predict future risk of events in patients who may or may not exhibit symptoms of cardiovascular risk. Important concepts when assessing the prognostic value of such tools include calibration, discrimination, and reclassification.[18]

Calibration refers to the ability of the prognostic test or risk score to correctly predict the proportion of subjects within a given group to experience events of interest. Calibration assesses the "goodness of fit" of the risk model and is evaluated statistically using the Hosmer-Lemeshow test. In contrast to the usual situation, for example, in a classical superiority trial, a low χ^2 value and corresponding high *P* values with the Hosmer-Lemeshow test are desirable, indicating little deviation of the observed data from the model and therefore a good fit.

Discrimination describes how well the model or risk score discriminates subjects at different degrees of risk. This is typically expressed mathematically with the C statistic, which literally ranks every pair of patients; it determines the proportion of pairs that have occurred with the predicted outcome in the person with the higher predicted probability from the test. In the case of a dichotomous outcome variable, this is equivalent to the area under the curve for an ROC curve. A test or model with no discrimination would have a C statistic of 0.50 because randomly choosing the patient more likely to have the outcome would be correct half the time, and a test that has perfect discrimination would have a C statistic of 1.0, indicating that every prediction correctly ranked the pairs.

Of particular interest to clinicians is a statement about the anticipated treatment effect of a therapeutic strategy stratified by a given risk score value. This is assessed via an interaction test. Given the large number of therapeutic options, burgeoning healthcare costs, and the emergence of an array of new risk markers, considerable efforts have been directed at refinement of the assessment of risk to provide treatments to those subjects at greatest risk. When new tests or models of risk are introduced, they are evaluated in terms of their ability to correctly reclassify subjects into higher or lower risk categories. Quantitative assessments of correct reclassifications are provided using the *net reclassification improvement* and *integrated with classification improvement* approaches.[18] A critical component of reclassification estimates is the understanding of risk thresholds that should prompt a different clinical decision, such as recommending more tests, admitting the patient to the intensive care unit, adding a medication, or performing an invasive procedure. As this field evolves, the imprecision of clinical practice comes into focus because different physicians and patients have different views of these thresholds.

Clinical Trials

Need for Clinical Trials

Uncontrolled observation studies of populations provide valuable insight into pathophysiology and serve as the source for important hypotheses regarding the potential value of particular interventions; however, medical therapy rarely has the dramatic effectiveness of penicillin for pneumococcal pneumonia, for example, for which epidemiologic data alone are sufficient for scientific acceptance and adoption into clinical practice. In view of the variability of the natural history of cardiovascular illnesses and the wide range of individual responses to interventions, clinical investigators, representatives of regulatory agencies, and practicing physicians have come to recognize the value of a rigorously performed clinical trial with a control group before widespread acceptance or rejection of a treatment (Braunwald, Chapter 6).[19]

A contemporary view of the clinical/translational spectrum of scientific investigations that result in therapeutic recommendations for various cardiovascular diseases is shown in Figure 1-3. Basic biomedical advances that have successfully progressed through the discovery and preclinical phases are ready to cross the threshold to human investigation. A series of translational blocks—labeled T_1, T_2, T_3, and T_4—must be overcome for the biomedical discovery to ultimately improve global health. T_1 refers to

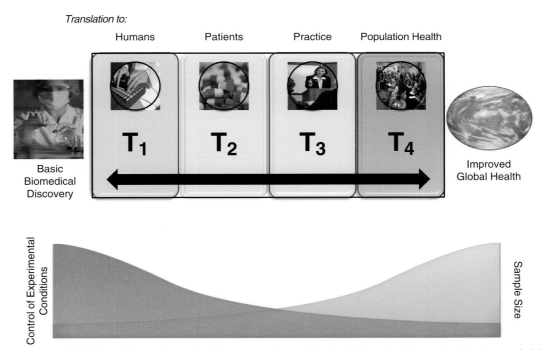

FIGURE 1-3 The spectrum of clinical/translational science. *Top,* The process of translating basic biomedical discoveries into improved global health involves overcoming a series of translational (*T*) blocks. T_1 = translation to human (first-in-human and proof-of-concept studies); T_2 = translation to patients with disease (randomized, controlled trials to establish efficacy); T_3 = translation to practice (control event rate plays an important role here); T_4 = translation of research findings on a population scale. *Bottom,* The concept that at the extreme left, investigators have a high degree of control over the experimental conditions and operate with a small sample size; moving to the right, approaching T_3 and T_4 research, the control over experimental conditions decreases and the sample size markedly increases.

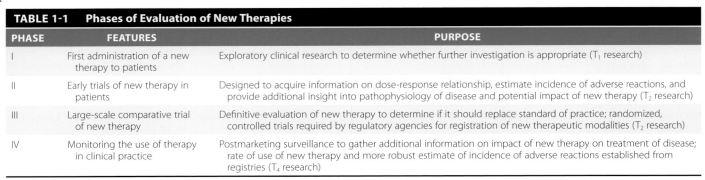

TABLE 1-1   Phases of Evaluation of New Therapies

PHASE	FEATURES	PURPOSE
I	First administration of a new therapy to patients	Exploratory clinical research to determine whether further investigation is appropriate (T_1 research)
II	Early trials of new therapy in patients	Designed to acquire information on dose-response relationship, estimate incidence of adverse reactions, and provide additional insight into pathophysiology of disease and potential impact of new therapy (T_2 research)
III	Large-scale comparative trial of new therapy	Definitive evaluation of new therapy to determine if it should replace standard of practice; randomized, controlled trials required by regulatory agencies for registration of new therapeutic modalities (T_2 research)
IV	Monitoring the use of therapy in clinical practice	Postmarketing surveillance to gather additional information on impact of new therapy on treatment of disease; rate of use of new therapy and more robust estimate of incidence of adverse reactions established from registries (T_4 research)

TABLE 1-2   Stages of a Clinical Trial

STAGE	ACTIVITIES DURING STAGE	EVENT MARKING END OF STAGE
Initial design	Formulation of scientific question, outcome measures established, sample size calculated	Initiation of funding
Protocol development	Trial protocol and manual of operations written, case report forms developed, data management systems and monitoring procedures established, training of clinical sites completed	Initiation of patient recruitment
Patient recruitment	Channels for patient referrals established; development of regular monitoring procedures of trial data for accuracy, patient eligibility, and site performance; preparation of periodic reports to DSMB for review of adverse or beneficial treatment effects	Completion of patient recruitment
Treatment and follow-up	Continued monitoring of patient recruitment, adverse effects, and site performance; updated trial materials sent to enrolling sites; reports sent to DSMB and recommendations reviewed; adverse event reports filed with regulatory agency; timetable for trial close-out procedures established	Initiation of close-out procedures
Patient/trial close-out	Identification of final data items that require clarification so database can be "cleaned and locked"; initiation of procedures for unblinding of treatment assignment, termination of study therapy, and monitoring of adverse events after discontinuation of treatment; preparation of final reports to DSMB; preparation of draft of final trial report	Completion of close-out procedures
Termination	Verify that all sites have completed close-out procedures, including disposal of unused study drugs; review final trial findings and submit manuscript for publication; submit final report to regulatory agency	Termination of funding for original trial
Posttrial follow-up (optional)	Recontact enrolling sites to acquire long-term follow-up on patients in trial; link follow-up data with initial trial data and prepare manuscript summarizing results	Termination of all follow-up

DSMB, Data safety monitoring board
Modified from Meinert C. *Clinical trials: design, conduct, and analysis.* New York, 1986, Oxford University Press.

research that yields knowledge about human physiology and the potential for intervention; it involves first-in-human and proof-of-concept experiments. T_2 research tests new interventions in patients with the disease under study to yield knowledge about the efficacy of interventions in optimal settings, such as phase II and many types of phase III trials (see Tables 1-1 and 1-2). T_3 research yields knowledge about the effectiveness of interventions in real-world practice settings. T_4 research focuses on factors and interventions that influence the health of populations.

Cardiovascular medicine has made a transition from practice based in large part on nonquantitative pathophysiologic reasoning to practice oriented around evidence-based medicine.[9] The importance of this concept has been reinforced by clinical trials that have demonstrated widely accepted concepts to be associated with a substantial adverse effect on mortality rates (Braunwald, Fig. 6-5). The initial major alert about this issue occurred in the Cardiac Arrhythmia Suppression Trial (CAST), when type I antiarrhythmic drugs, often prescribed because of frequent premature beats, were demonstrated to increase the risk of death.[20] Since then, the cardiovascular community continues to be surprised by the failure of therapies that seemed to be highly effective based on observation studies and selected small trials.

Despite current limitations, evidence-based therapeutic recommendations that involve drugs, devices, and procedures are in demand, with managed care, cost-saving measures, and guidelines

published by authoritative groups playing increasingly prominent roles in the fabric of clinical medicine.[21] Thus, the proper design, conduct, analysis, interpretation, and presentation of a clinical trial represent an "indispensable ordeal" for investigators.[8] Practitioners must also acquire the tools to critically read reports of clinical trials and, when appropriate, to translate the findings into clinical practice without the lengthy delays that occurred in the past (T_3 research). This is an especially important task for generalist physicians because of the increased emphasis on primary care physicians to control health care costs by managing chronic disease with appropriate testing and referral.

The sheer volume and broad range of clinical trials in cardiology are too large for even the most conscientious individual to digest on a regular basis. This has stimulated increased interest in biostatistical techniques to combine the findings from randomized controlled trials (RCTs) of the same intervention into a meta-analysis or an overview.[22]

Clinical Trial Design

When interpreting the evidence from a clinical trial, it is important to have a framework for dealing with a complex set of issues (Figures 1-4 and 1-5). Because of the importance of clinical trial findings, it is essential that investigators thoughtfully formulate the scientific question to be answered and have realistic estimates of the sample size required to show the expected difference in treatments. Trials that result in the conclusion that the difference between treatment A and treatment B is not statistically significant are often undersized and lack sufficient power to detect a difference when one truly exists. A well-coordinated organizational structure made up of experienced trialists, biostatisticians, and data analysts is important to prevent pitfalls in trial design, such as unrealistic assessments of the ease of patient recruitment and the timetable for completion of the trial (see Figures 1-4 and 1-5).

The stages of a clinical trial are summarized in Table 1-2. These should be viewed as a rough guide to the orderly sequence of events that characterizes the clinical trial process, as the dividing lines between stages are often indistinct. For example, sites at which patients are randomized may be brought into the trial in a rolling fashion such that some of the features of the protocol development stage may overlap with the patient recruitment phase. It is possible that some of the early sites that enroll patients

gain sufficient experience with the protocol to achieve different results than those sites that join the trial later, as demonstrated in the Valsartan in Acute Myocardial Infarction (VALIANT) trial,[23] which showed a clear learning curve characterized by a greater proportion of errors in trial protocol conduct in the initial phase of the trial. Evidence of this phenomenon is typically sought by performing a test for interaction between the enrolling site and treatment effect when the data are analyzed. The situation can rapidly become quite complex when international differences in treatment effect are observed, especially if benefit is noted predominantly in one international region and not in others.[24] Of note, even after a fully executed development sequence from phase I through phase III trials, important adverse consequences of a new treatment may not be apparent. Although in theory, postmarketing trials (phase IV; see Table 1-1) are supposed to catch such problems and identify treatments that should be withdrawn from clinical use, such trials are infrequently conducted, leaving several authorities to propose new methods for surveillance of the safety of marketed medical products.[25,26]

The term *control group* refers to participants in a clinical trial who receive the treatment against which the test intervention is being compared. Requirements for the control and test treatments are outlined in Box 1-1. *Randomized controlled trials* typically

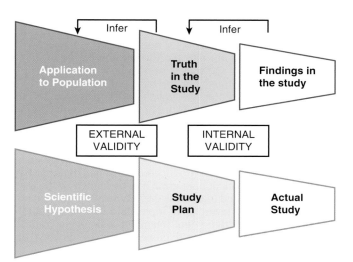

FIGURE 1-4 The six-step process for interpreting evidence from a clinical trial. The process begins at the bottom left, from formulation of the scientific process, and moves counterclockwise to the top left, to application of the findings of the trial to the broad population with the target disease of interest. *(From Antman EM. Evidence and education.* Circulation *2011;123:681-685.)*

Box 1-1 Requirements for the Control and Test Treatments

They must be distinguishable from one another.
They must be medically justifiable.
There must be an ethical base for use of either treatment.
Use of the treatments must be compatible with the health care needs of study patients.
Both treatments must be acceptable to study patients and to physicians administering the treatment.
A reasonable doubt must exist regarding the efficacy of the test treatment.
There should be reason to believe that the benefits will outweigh the risks of treatment.
The method of treatment administration must be compatible with the design needs of the trial (e.g., method of administration must be the same for all the treatments in a double-blind trial), and they should be as similar to real-world practice as possible.

From Meinert C. *Clinical trials: design, conduct, and analysis.* New York, 1986, Oxford University Press, p 469.

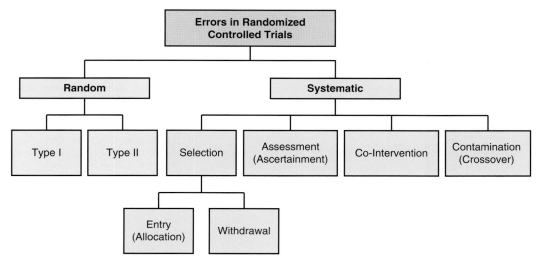

FIGURE 1-5 Errors that can affect interpretation of clinical trials. Random errors are considered at the design phase of a randomized controlled trial (RCT). They include a type 1 (α) error, typically set by regulatory authorities, and a type 2 (β) error selected by the investigators that determines the power ($1 - \beta$) of the study. A series of systematic errors must also be considered during the design, enrollment, follow-up, and analysis phase of an RCT. Selection, assessment, co-intervention, and crossover errors can lead to a bias in the profile of patients contributing data to the trial, and it may confound the ability of investigators to interpret the signal of a treatment effect of the test therapy. *(Modified from Keirse MJ, Hanssens M. Control of error in randomized clinical trials. Eur J Obstet Gynecol Reprod Biol 2000;92:67-74.)*

incorporate both test and control treatments and are considered the gold standard for the evaluation of new therapies. However, the previously noted definition of a control does not require that the treatment be a placebo, although frequently this is the case because new treatments may have to be compared with the current standard of practice to determine whether they are more efficacious (e.g., new antithrombin agents versus unfractionated heparin; see Chapters 9 and 10) or fall within a range of effectiveness deemed to be clinically not inferior (e.g., a bolus thrombolytic versus an accelerated infusion regimen of alteplase; see Chapters 9 and 10). This definition does not require that the control group be a collection of participants distinct from the treatment group studied contemporaneously and allocated by random assignment. Other possibilities include nonrandomized concurrent and historic controls; crossover designs and withdrawal trials, with each patient serving as a member of both the treatment and control groups; and group or cluster allocations, in which a group of participants or a treatment site is assigned as a block to either test or control (Braunwald, Fig. 6-3).

Two broad types of controlled trials exist: the *fixed sample size design*, in which the investigator specifies the necessary sample size before patient recruitment, and the *open* or *closed sequential design*, in which sequential pairs of patients are enrolled—one to test and one to control—only if the cumulative test-control difference from previous pairs of patients remains within prespecified boundaries.[27] The sequential trial design is usually less efficient than the fixed sample size design and is practical only when the outcome of interest can be determined soon after enrollment. In addition, trials with the fixed design can be organized such that randomization and/or follow-up continue until the requisite number of endpoints is reached. This "event-driven" trial design ensures that inadequate numbers of endpoints will not hamper the trial interpretation.

Case-control studies, which involve a comparison of people with a disease or outcome of interest (*cases*) with a suitable group of subjects without the disease or outcome (*matched controls*), are integral to epidemiologic research; however, they are not strictly clinical trials and are therefore not discussed in this chapter.[28]

RANDOMIZED CONTROLLED TRIALS

The RCT is the standard against which all other designs are compared, for several reasons.[8] In addition to the advantage of incorporating a control group, this type of trial centers around the process of randomization, which has the following three important influences:

1. It reduces the likelihood of patient selection bias that may occur either consciously or unconsciously in allocation of treatment.
2. It enhances the likelihood that differences between groups are random, so that comparable groups of subjects are compared, especially if the sample size is sufficiently large.
3. It validates the use of common statistical tests such as the χ^2 test for a comparison of proportions and Student t test for a comparison of means.[16]

Randomization may be fixed over the course of the trial, or it may be adaptive, based on the distribution of prior randomization assignments, baseline characteristic frequencies, or observed outcomes (Braunwald, Fig. 6-2).[29,30] Fixed randomization schemes are more common and are specified further according to the allocation ratio (uniform or nonuniform assignment to study groups), stratification levels, and block size (i.e., constraining the randomization of patients to ensure a balanced number of assignments to the study groups, especially if stratification is used in the trial). Ethical considerations related to randomization have been the subject of considerable discussion in clinical trial literature.[31]

Clinicians usually participate in an RCT if they are sufficiently uncertain about the potential advantages of the test treatment and can confidently convey this uncertainty to the research participants, who must provide informed consent.[31] It is important that clinicians realize that in the absence of rigorously obtained data, many therapeutic decisions believed to be in the best interest of the patient may be ineffective or even harmful. To identify the appropriate therapeutic strategies from a societal perspective, RCTs are needed.

A difficult philosophic dilemma arises when patients are enrolled in a trial, evidence is accumulating that tends to favor one study group over the other, and the degree of uncertainty about the likelihood of benefit or harm is constantly being updated. Because clinicians may feel uneasy about enrolling a patient who may be randomized to a treatment that the accumulating data suggest might be inferior, although that has not yet been proved statistically to be so with a conventional level of significance, the outcome data from the trial are not revealed to the investigators during the patient recruitment stage. The responsibility of safeguarding the welfare of patients enrolled in the trial rests with an external monitoring team known as a *data safety monitoring board* (DSMB) or *data safety monitoring committee* (DSMC).[32] Several prominent examples of the early termination of large RCTs because of compelling evidence of benefit or harm from one of the treatments under investigation are evidence that the DSMB has become an integral element of clinical trial research.[33]

When both the patient and the investigator are aware of the treatment assignment, the trial is said to be *unblinded*. Trials of this nature have the potential for bias, particularly during the process of data collection and patient assessment, if subjective measures are tabulated, such as the presence or absence of congestive heart failure (CHF). Because blinding of one or more of the treatment arms in an RCT can be challenging, investigators may use a prospective, randomized, open-label blinded endpoint (PROBE) design.[34] In an effort to reduce bias, progressively stricter degrees of blinding may be introduced. Single-blind trials mask the treatment from the patient but permit it to be known by the investigator, and double-blind trials mask the treatment assignment from both the patient and investigator. Triple-blind trials mask both of these and also mask the actual treatment assignment from the DSMB, and they provide data referenced only as "group A" and "group B."

The specialty of cardiology is replete with examples of RCTs. The recent requirement for most clinical trials pertinent to the United States to be registered in the National Institutes of Health (NIH) managed registry, ClinicalTrials.gov, has enabled researchers to assess the portfolio of trials according to specialties, which include cardiovascular medicine. In a review of more than 96,000 registered trials, 58% had fewer than 100 volunteers, and 96% had fewer than 1000 participants. Cardiovascular trials are larger on average than other trials and more often have DSMCs, but as with all specialties, major gaps in evidence are relative to the need to inform decision making.[35] An area particularly rich in this regard is the study of treatments for ST-segment elevation MI (see Chapter 10), in which multiple types of RCTs have been performed. However, in other areas, such as valvular and congenital heart disease, very few trials have been completed.

Efforts are under way to create an ontology to describe clinical research,[36] but until this work is completed, it is useful to broadly classify these trials into *minitrials* and *megatrials*. A further subdivision of the minitrials includes those that are of limited sample size and focus almost exclusively on mechanistic data, and those with a sample size an order of magnitude larger and hybrid goals that focus on mechanistic data as they relate to clinical outcomes, such as mortality. In trials of new cardiovascular therapies, because of the practical limitations of the very large sample size required when death is used as the primary endpoint and the fact that other outcomes are important to patients and their families and to health care systems, interest has arisen in the use of composite endpoints, such as the sum of death, nonfatal recurrent MI, and stroke as the primary endpoint.[24,37] Because most treatments have a modest effect (10% to 20%), it is important to be clear regarding the rationale for choice of endpoints; in some cases, such as treatment of angina and hypertension, endpoints other than death are essential. In acute treatment of

ST-segment–elevation MI, however, understanding of the effect of size on death is required.

NONRANDOMIZED CONCURRENT CONTROL STUDIES

Trials in which the investigator selects the subjects to be allocated to the control and treatment groups are *nonrandomized concurrent control studies*. The advantages of this simpler trial design are that clinicians do not leave to chance the assignment of treatment in each patient, and patients do not need to accept the concept of randomization. Implicit in this type of design is the assumption that the investigator can appropriately match subjects in the test and control groups for all relevant baseline characteristics. This is a difficult task, and it can produce a selection bias that may result in conclusions that differ in direction and magnitude from those obtained from RCTs (Braunwald, Fig. 6-3).

Observation analyses contain many of the same structural characteristics as randomized trials, except that the treatment is not randomized. These studies should use prospectively collected data with uniform definitions managed by a multidisciplinary group of investigators that includes clinicians, biostatisticians, and data analysts. Outcomes must be collected in a rigorous and unbiased fashion, just as in the randomized trial.

HISTORIC CONTROLS

Clinical trials that use historic controls compare a test intervention with data obtained earlier in a *nonconcurrent, nonrandomized control group* (Braunwald, Fig. 6-3).[39] Potential sources for historic controls include previously published medical literature and unpublished data banks of clinic populations. The use of historic controls allows clinicians to offer potentially beneficial therapies to all participants, thereby reducing the sample size for the study. Unfortunately, the capacity to understand the bias engendered in the selection of the control population is extremely limited, and failure of the historic controls to reflect contemporary diagnostic criteria and concurrent treatment regimens for the disease under study produces even more uncertainty. Thus, although historic controls are alluring, they should be used in the definitive assessment of a therapy only when a randomized trial is not feasible and a concurrent nonrandomized control is not available.

It should be noted, however, that prospectively recorded registry data may be more representative of actual clinical practice than the control groups in RCTs. Reports from such registries are useful for identifying gaps in translation into routine practice of therapies proven to be effective in clinical trials.[38] Accordingly, it seems appropriate to use RCTs to define the effectiveness of a treatment and then to fill in gaps by means of carefully conducted observation studies with a preference for the use of comprehensive clinical practice registries.

CROSSOVER DESIGN

The crossover design is a type of RCT in which each participant serves as his or her own control (Braunwald, Fig. 6-3).[39] A simple, two-period, crossover design randomly assigns each subject to either the test or control group in the first period and to the alternative in the second period. The appeal of this design lies in its ability to use the same subject for both test and control treatments, thereby diminishing the influence of interindividual variability and allowing a smaller sample size. However, important limitations to crossover design are the assumptions that the effects of the treatment assigned during the first period have no residual effect on the treatment assigned during the second period and that the patient's condition remains stable during both periods. The validity of these assumptions is often difficult to verify either clinically or statistically (e.g., testing for an interaction between period and intervention); this has led some authorities to discourage the use of crossover designs, although one possible use of the crossover trial design is for the preliminary evaluation of new

antianginal agents for patients with chronic, stable, exertional angina.[40]

WITHDRAWAL STUDIES

In withdrawal studies, patients with a chronic cardiovascular condition are either taken off therapy or undergo a reduction in dosage with the goal to evaluate the response to discontinuation of treatment or reduction in its intensity. An important limitation is that only patients who have tolerated the test intervention for a period of time are eligible for enrollment because those with incapacitating side effects would have been taken off the test intervention and would therefore not be available for withdrawal. This selection bias can overestimate benefit and underestimate toxicity associated with the test intervention. However, if the goal is to understand the duration of benefit of a treatment, or to assay a signal of efficacy without attempting to estimate the magnitude of the effect in a patient just beginning therapy, this design has an advantage.

In addition, changes in the natural history of the disease may influence the response to withdrawal of therapy. For example, if a therapeutic intervention is beneficial early after the onset of the disease but loses its benefit over time, the withdrawal of therapy late in the course of treatment might not result in deterioration of the patient's condition. A conclusion that the intervention was not helpful because its withdrawal during the chronic phase of treatment did not result in a worsening of the patient's condition provides no information about the potential benefit of treatment in the acute phase or subacute phase of the illness. Thus, withdrawal trials can provide clinically useful information, but they should be conducted with specific goals and with the same standards that are applied to controlled trials of prospective treatment, including randomization and blinding if possible.

One withdrawal trial in cardiology—the Randomized Assessment of Digoxin on Inhibitors of the Angiotensin-Converting Enzyme (RADIANCE)—illustrates many of the features previously discussed. Although digitalis has been used by physicians for more than 200 years, its benefits for the treatment of chronic CHF, particularly in patients with normal sinus rhythm, remain controversial. To assess the consequences of withdrawing digoxin from clinically stable patients with New York Heart Association functional class II to III CHF who are receiving angiotensin-converting enzyme inhibitors, investigators randomly allocated 178 patients in a double-blind manner to continue to receive digoxin or switch to a matched placebo.[41] Worsening heart failure that necessitated discontinuation from the study occurred in 23 patients who were switched to placebo but in only four patients who continued to receive digoxin ($P < .001$). The results of the RADIANCE trial seem to indicate that withdrawal of digoxin in patients with mild to moderate CHF as a result of systolic dysfunction is associated with adverse consequences, but it does not provide information on the potential mortality benefit of digoxin when *added* to a regimen of diuretics and angiotensin-converting enzyme inhibitors.[42] One classic RCT, the Digitalis Investigation Group (DIG) trial, showed that digoxin therapy was not associated with a mortality benefit but did provide symptomatic improvement in that it reduced the need for hospitalization for decompensated CHF.[43]

FACTORIAL DESIGN

When two or more therapies are tested in a clinical trial, investigators typically consider a *factorial design*, in which multiple treatments can be compared with controls through independent randomization within a single trial (Braunwald, Fig. 6-3).

Factorial design trials are more easily interpreted when there is believed to be no interaction between the various test treatments, as is often the case when drugs have unrelated mechanisms of action. If no interactions exist, multiple drug comparisons can be efficiently performed in a single, large trial that is smaller than the sum of two independent clinical trials. When interactions are detected, each intervention must be evaluated individually against a control and each of the other interventions in which an interaction exists.[44]

The factorial trial design has an important place in cardiology, in which multiple therapies are typically given to the same patient for important conditions such as MI, heart failure, and secondary prevention of atherosclerosis. Therefore, in practical terms, the factorial design is more reflective of actual clinical practice than trials in which only a single intervention is randomized. Clinicians need to know how much incremental value comes from the administration of one more drug to the patient, and whether any drug interactions exist. It is worth noting, however, that it is probably an insurmountable task to rule out the possibility of a drug interaction because of the imprecision with which interaction effects are estimated (i.e., wide confidence intervals), the poor power of tests for statistical significance of interactions between the test interventions, and the vast number of non–protocol-related drugs a patient may receive.[45]

TRIALS THAT TEST EQUIVALENCE OF THERAPIES

Advances in cardiovascular therapeutics have dramatically improved the treatment of various diseases, such that several therapies of proven efficacy may coexist for the same treatment. However, it may still be desirable to develop new therapies that are equally efficacious but have an important advantage, such as reduced toxicity, improved patient tolerability, a more favorable pharmacokinetic profile, fewer drug interactions, or lower cost.[8,39] Testing such new therapies using placebo-controlled trials poses problems on ethical grounds because half of the patients would be denied treatment when an accepted therapy of proven efficacy exists. This has led to a shift in clinical trial design to demonstrate the therapeutic equivalence of two treatments rather than the superiority of one of the treatments.

It is not possible to show two active therapies to be completely equivalent without a trial of infinite sample size. Instead, investigators resort to specifying a value (δ) and consider the test therapy to be equivalent to the standard therapy if the true difference in treatment effects is less than δ with a high degree of confidence (Figure 1-6, *A*).[46]

The nomenclature related to trials of tests of equivalence between two therapies can be confusing. In a classic equivalence trial, if the confidence intervals (CIs) for the estimate of the effects of the two treatments differ by more than the equivalence margin (δ) in either direction, then equivalence is said *not* to be present. For most clinical trials of new therapies, the objective is to establish that the new therapy is not worse than the standard therapy (active control) by more than δ. Such one-sided comparisons are referred to as *noninferiority trials*. The new therapy may satisfy the definition of *noninferiority* but, depending on the results, may or may not actually show superiority compared with the standard therapy.[34]

Specification of the appropriate margin, or δ, is often problematic. Clinicians prefer to set δ based on a clinical perception of a minimally important difference they believe would affect their practice. Regulatory authorities, who are bound by a legal mandate "to show that drugs work," assess the effect of the standard therapy based on prior trials, in which it was compared with placebo. Rather than specifying the point estimate for the full effect of the standard therapy over placebo, a more conservative approach is taken by selecting the lower bound of a CI for superiority of the standard therapy over placebo for setting the noninferiority margin.[46,47]

Figure 1-6, *B*, provides an example of the design of noninferiority trials and interpretation of six hypothetical trial results; the difference in events between the test drug and the standard drug is plotted along the horizontal axis. Based on trials against placebo, the standard drug provides a benefit over placebo at the +4 position, but the lower bound of its superiority over placebo is at the +2 position; thus, the noninferiority margin is set at +2. The six hypothetical trials (A to F) are shown, with the point estimate of the difference between the test drug and standard drug displayed

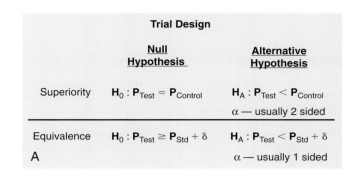

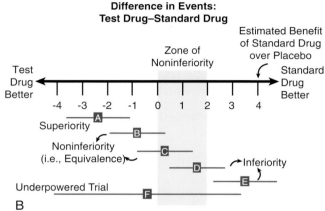

FIGURE 1-6 **A,** Statistical design of superiority and equivalence trials. In both superiority and equivalence trials, the investigators propose a null hypothesis (H_0) with the goal of the trial being to reject H_0 in favor of the alternative hypothesis (H_A). To determine whether the null hypothesis may be rejected, the type I (α) and type II (β) errors are specified before initiation of the trial. In superiority trials, α is usually two sided, whereas it is usually one sided in equivalence trials. The quantity ($1 - \chi$) is referred to as the *power of the trial* (not shown). **B,** Example of design and interpretation of noninferiority trials. The zone of inferiority is prespecified based on prior trials comparing the standard drug with placebo. Examples of hypothetical trials *A* to *F* are shown, some of which satisfy the definition of noninferiority. *Std,* Standard therapy. (*B, Modified from Antman EM: Clinical trials in cardiovascular medicine.* Circulation 2001;103[21]:E101-E104.)

as filled squares, and the width of the 95% CI for the difference is shown as blue horizontal lines.

The results of trial A fall entirely to the left of zero (i.e., the upper bound does not enter the zone of noninferiority); thus, it is possible to declare the test drug to be superior to the standard drug. In trials B and C, the upper bound falls within the zone of noninferiority, and in loose parlance, the test drug is declared to be "equivalent" to the standard drug. Note that in trials D and E, the noninferiority requirement is not satisfied—that is, the upper bound exceeds the margin in trial D, and the entire CI exceeds the margin in trial E—and the test drug is said to be inferior to the standard drug.

It is important to prespecify the noninferiority margin before starting the trial; if it is specified after the results are known, the trial could be criticized for a potential subjective bias. For example, if the results of trial D were known, and the noninferiority margin was set at +3, rather than +2, the test drug would satisfy the definition of noninferiority, but such an approach would be highly suspect. It is also important to have a sample size sufficient to draw meaningful conclusions. For example, although the point estimate for trial F is in favor of the test drug, the wide CIs are due to a small sample size. Trial F does not allow the investigators to claim superiority of the test drug compared with the standard drug, and it would be inappropriate to claim it to be "equivalent" to the standard drug, simply because superiority could not be demonstrated (note that the upper bound of trial F clearly exceeds the noninferiority margin).

Investigators can prespecify that a trial is being designed to test superiority and noninferiority simultaneously.[46] For a trial that is configured only as a noninferiority trial, it is acceptable to test for superiority at the conclusion of the trial. However, because of the subjective bias mentioned, the reverse is not true: trials configured for superiority cannot later test for noninferiority unless the margin was prespecified.[46]

An important commonality between superiority and noninferiority trials is that the clinical experts involved in trial design should consciously consider the minimally important clinical outcome difference. A common understanding of the difference between outcomes with two therapies forms the basis for providing the appropriate perspective on the interpretation of test statistics; in essence, the difference between "statistically significant" and "clinically important" is determined by the common view of the difference that would lead to a change in practice.[47]

Noninferiority trials, a more recent addition to the RCT repertoire, are prone to controversy, especially when disagreement exists over the noninferiority margin (i.e., the percentage of the treatment benefit of the gold standard therapy over placebo that would be retained by the new treatment and still be considered clinically equivalent).[46] The reporting of noninferiority trials in the medical literature is often deficient and fails to provide an adequate justification for the noninferiority margin or the sample size. In a fashion similar to that for reporting a superiority trial, the Consolidated Standards of Reporting Trials (CONSORT) Group has published recommendations for a checklist and visual display of the results of noninferiority trials.[48]

Of course, one of the most fragile assumptions in a noninferiority trial is the assumption of *constancy*, in which the trials that established the benefit of the gold standard over placebo are assumed to achieve the same result if the placebo-controlled trial were to be conducted in the era of the noninferiority trial. In essence, the statistical inference is based on a historic control, with all of the attendant issues previously discussed.

SELECTION OF ENDPOINT

A critical decision when designing a clinical trial is the selection of the outcome measure. In trials comparing two treatments in cardiovascular medicine, the outcome measure, or endpoint of the trial, characteristically is a clinical event. The characteristics of an ideal primary outcome measure are that it is easy to diagnose, free of measurement error, observable independent of treatment assignment, and clinically relevant, and it should be selected prior to the start of data collection for the trial.[39]

Improvements in cardiovascular treatments have, gratifyingly, led to a reduction in mortality rates and therefore a lower event rate in the control arm of clinical trials with an attendant increase in the required sample size. The desire to evaluate new therapeutic approaches in the face of rising costs to conduct large clinical trials has resulted in two primary approaches to the selection of endpoints. The first is to use a composite endpoint that combines mortality with one or more nonfatal negative outcomes, such as MI, stroke, recurrent ischemia, or hospitalization for heart failure. Trials with a logical grouping of composite endpoints that are likely to each be affected by the treatments being studied are clinically valuable and have been used to advance treatments for heart failure and acute coronary syndromes.[49] However, interpretation of composite endpoints becomes problematic when elements of a composite endpoint go in opposite directions in response to treatment (e.g., reduced mortality but increased nonfatal MI). To date, no consensus exists on an appropriate weighting scheme for composite endpoints.[49]

Another approach is to use a biomarker or putative surrogate endpoint as a substitute for clinical outcomes. A valid surrogate endpoint not only must be predictive of a clinical outcome, it must also evidence that modification of the surrogate endpoint captures the effect of a treatment on clinical outcomes because the surrogate is in the causal pathway of the disease process.[49] Few

biomarkers have met the high threshold for classification as a valid surrogate, but biomarkers remain highly valuable in developing therapies and therapeutic concepts. Examples of a successful surrogate endpoint and failed surrogate endpoints are schematically illustrated in Figure 1-7 (also see Braunwald, Fig. 6-5). Whether or not a surrogate endpoint is useful for determining whether a treatment is efficacious, a single surrogate cannot be used to develop a balanced view of risk and benefit, particularly compared with alternative therapies. This increasingly recognized critical element of therapeutic development and evaluation requires measurement of clinical outcomes in the relevant population over a relevant period of time.[50]

SAMPLE SIZE ESTIMATIONS AND SEQUENTIAL STOPPING BOUNDARIES

Estimation of the sample size for trials involves a statement of the scientific question in the form of a null hypothesis (H_0) and an alternative hypothesis (H_A).[13,39] For example, in the case of dichotomous variables (e.g., a primary outcome variable such as mortality), the null hypothesis states that the proportion of patients dying in the test group (PTest) is equal to that in the control group (PControl; see Figure 1-6,A), such that for

$$H_0 : P_{Test} - P_{Control} = 0$$

The alternative hypothesis is that for

$$H_A : P_{Test} - P_{Control} \neq 0$$

FALSE-POSITIVE AND FALSE-NEGATIVE ERROR RATES AND POWER OF CLINICAL TRIALS

To determine whether the null hypothesis may be rejected before initiation of the trial, the type I (α) and type II (β) errors, sometimes referred to as the *false-positive* and *false-negative rates*, are specified (see Figure 1-6,A). The conventional α of 5% indicates that the investigator is willing to accept a 5% likelihood that an observed difference as large as that projected in the sample size calculation occurred by chance and would lead to rejection of the null hypothesis when, in fact, the null hypothesis was correct (see Figure 1-5).[13,39] The β value reflects the likelihood that a specified difference might be missed or not found to be statistically significant because of an insufficient number of events in the trial at the time of analysis. The quantity $(1 - \beta)$ is referred to as the *power of the trial* and quantifies the ability of the trial to find true differences of a given magnitude between the groups (see Figure 1-5). The relations among estimated event rates, the prespecified α level, and the desired power of the trial determine the number of patients who must be randomized to detect the anticipated difference in outcomes according to standard formulas.[13,39] Similar concepts are applied to response variables that are not dichotomous but are measured on a continuous scale (e.g., blood pressure) or represent time to failure (e.g., Kaplan-Meier survival curves).[51,52]

Statistical methods are also available for monitoring a trial during the patient recruitment phase at certain prespecified intervals to determine whether the accumulated evidence strongly suggests an advantage of one treatment in the trial.[53,54] During such interim checks of the data, the differences between treatment groups, expressed as a standardized normal statistic (Z_i), are compared with boundaries such as those shown in Figure 1-8. If the Z_i statistic falls outside the boundaries at an ith interim look, the DSMB may seriously consider recommending termination of the trial. Typically, the data are arranged as *test: control*, so crossing of the upper boundary denotes statistically significant superiority of the test therapy over the control, and crossing of the lower boundary denotes superiority of the control therapy over the test therapy. Because of the considerable expense of large clinical trials, in some cases it may be desirable to discontinue a trial at an interim analysis if the accumulated data suggest that the probability of a positive result, if the trial proceeds to completion, has become

trial and were randomized with an allocation ratio of 1:1, so that 5000 patients received treatment A and 5000 received treatment B. Because only 600 primary outcome events occurred in group A (12% event rate) and 750 occurred in group B (15% event rate), it appears that treatment A is more effective than treatment B. Is this difference statistically significant, and is it clinically meaningful? When the data are arranged in a 2 × 2 table (see Figure 1-9), a χ^2 test or Fisher exact test can be readily performed according to standard formulas.[16]

Although the investigators of the trial will likely have analyzed the results using one of the methods illustrated in Figure 1-9, it is useful to have a measure of the precision of the findings and an impression of the potential impact of the results on clinical practice. Even a well-designed clinical trial can provide only an estimate of the treatment effect of the test intervention owing to random variation in the sample of subjects studied, who are selected from the entire population of patients with the same disease. The imprecision of the statement regarding treatment effect can be estimated and incorporated into the presentation of the trial results by calculating the 95% CIs around the observed treatment effect. If the 95% CIs are not reported in the trial, inspection of the P value may be useful to indicate whether the CI spans a null effect. Alternatively, the 95% CIs may be estimated as the treatment effect ± twice the standard error of the treatment effect (if reported), or it may be calculated directly.

Missing Data

Despite the best efforts at appropriate design and conduct of clinical trials, missing data occur for a variety of reasons. Trial subjects may not have a scheduled visit, or there may have been equipment failure that resulted in failure to ascertain data that might bear on a trial endpoint. Missing data are broadly classified based on the mechanism leading to their "missingness" (see Table 1-3). In general, when data are missing completely at random or missing at random, the impact on the assessment of the treatment effect is less than when the data are not missing at random.[62] Although in theory, data missing at random or completely missing at random are "ignorable" and data not missing at random are not, in practical terms, investigators usually cannot rigorously test the assumptions that distinguish the different classes of missing data, which have been a concern in outcomes research (patients are not randomized) but also are of concern to regulatory authorities when they assess the data from pivotal RCTs submitted for registration of a new cardiovascular therapeutic.[63,64] A report from the National Academies of Science on the prevention and treatment of missing data in clinical trials offers a series of recommendations that cover trial design, dropouts during the course of a trial, and sensitivity analyses that should take place at the data analysis phase.[65] Of course, the most important recommendation is to make every effort to design trials in ways that minimize missing data.

Measures of Treatment Effect

When the outcome is undesirable and the data are arranged as test group: control group comparison, a relative risk (RR) or odds ratio (OR) of less than 1 indicates benefit of the test treatment. The RR of 0.80 (95% CI, 0.72 to 0.88) and OR of 0.77 (95% CI, 0.69 to 0.87) in Figure 1-9 are indicative of benefit associated with treatment A. When the control rate is low, the OR will approximate the RR, and the OR may be thought of as an estimator of the RR. As the control rate increases, the OR deviates further from the RR, and clinicians should rely more on the latter. The *treatment effect*, expressed as an RR reduction in this example, is 20%, but its 95% CI ranges from 0.12 to 0.28. Such statements should be interpreted in the context of the absolute risk of the adverse outcome it is designed to prevent. The *absolute risk difference* (ARD) is even more meaningful if expressed as the number of patients who must be treated (= 1/ARD) to observe the beneficial effect, if it is as large as reported in the trial.[66]

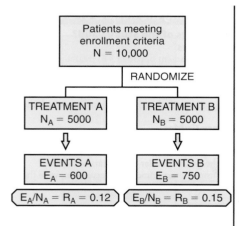

Randomized Controlled Trials
Summary Measures of Treatment Effect

	EVENT	NO EVENT	
A	$E_A = 600$	4400	5000
B	$E_B = 750$	4250	5000
	1350	8650	10,000

STATISTICAL TESTS OF Rx EFFECT

1. $\chi^2 = 19.268 \rightarrow P < .001$
2. Fisher Exact Test : $P < .001$
3. Comparison of Proportions: $Z = 4.360 \rightarrow P < .001$

STATEMENTS DESCRIBING Rx EFFECT

1. RELATIVE RISK = R_A/R_B = 0.80 *(0.72 – 0.88)*
2. RELATIVE RISK REDUCTION = [1 – RELATIVE RISK] = 0.20
3. ODDS RATIO = $\dfrac{R_A/(1 - R_A)}{R_B/(1 - R_B)}$ = 0.77 *(0.69 – 0.87)*
4. ABSOLUTE RISK DIFFERENCE = $(R_B - R_A)$ = ARD = 0.03
5. NUMBER NEEDED TO TREAT = [1/ABS. RISK DIFF] = 33

FIGURE 1-9 Evaluation of a randomized clinical trial (RCT). In this example, 10,000 patients meeting enrollment criteria for the RCT are randomized such that half receive treatment *(Rx)* A *(N$_A$)* and half receive treatment B *(N$_B$)*. Six hundred patients assigned to treatment A *(E$_A$)* had an event (e.g., death), yielding an event rate *(R$_A$)* of 12%, compared with 750 patients assigned to treatment B *(E$_B$)*, yielding an event rate *(R$_B$)* of 15%. The 2 × 2 table *(right)* is then constructed, and various statistical tests are performed to evaluate the significance of the difference in event rates between groups A and B. Common statements describing the treatment effect are the relative risk, the odds ratio, and the absolute risk difference *(ARD)* of events in treatment A versus treatment B using the formulas shown. A clinically useful method of expressing the results is to calculate the number of patients who need to be treated to prevent one event. *(Modified from Antman EM. Clinical trials in cardiovascular medicine. Circulation 2001;103[21]:E101-E104.)*

TABLE 1-3   **Mechanisms and Assumptions for Missing Data**

MECHANISM MISSING DATA	ASSUMPTION	EXAMPLE	ASSESSMENT OF ASSUMPTION
MCAR	Missing data are not related to observed and unobserved outcomes or covariates.	A box of CDs containing data are damaged because of a water leak.	Examine the difference in mean covariate values for observed variables between subjects with no missing data and subjects with missing data.
MAR	Missing data are not related to unobserved outcomes after adjustment for observed outcomes and observed covariates.	Older patients are more likely to have missing information on chest pain than younger patients.	Condition on as much data as possible.
NMAR	None of the above apply.	Because of side effects, some patients do not return for measurement, and side effect data are unavailable.	Not possible to use data to demonstrate; need to review literature to determine whether key confounders are missing and not related to measured confounders.

MCAR, missing completely at random; MAR, missing at random; NMAR, not missing at random.
Confounders are variables related to the probability of missing data and to the outcomes of interest.
From Normand SL. Some old and some new statistical tools for outcomes research. *Circulation* 2008;118:872-884.

If practitioners are given clinical trial results only in the form of RR reduction, they tend to perceive a greater effectiveness of the test intervention than if a more comprehensive statement is provided, including ARD and the number needed to treat.[67] Thus, in light of the baseline risk of 15% in the control group, a value that might represent the 1-month mortality rate of contemporary patients with MI not treated with fibrinolytic agents, the 12% event rate in the test group represents an ARD of 3%, which corresponds to 1/0.03, or approximately 33 patients who require treatment to prevent the occurrence of one adverse event. This statement is sometimes given as the number of lives saved per 1000 patients treated, or 30 lives in this example. Against this benefit must be weighed the risks associated with treatment (e.g., hemorrhagic stroke with fibrinolytic therapy for MI), which can be expressed as the *number needed to harm* (NNH = 1/ARI, where ARI is the absolute increase in events in the treatment group).[68] A composite term referred to as *net clinical benefit* has been introduced to incorporate both benefit and harm. In this example, if compared with treatment B, treatment A is associated with a 0.5% excess risk of an adverse outcome, such as stroke, then for every 1000 patients who receive treatment A, 30 lives would be saved at the expense of five strokes, for a net clinical benefit of 25 stroke-free lives saved.

These types of comparisons require the clinical community to make a judgment regarding the relative importance of various outcomes. How many deaths have to be prevented to offset one stroke? Another example is the possibility that some therapies (inotropic agents) may improve symptoms but at the same time may increase mortality rates, a scenario that may be acceptable to patients incapacitated by severe symptoms but not to patients with mild symptoms.[68] This issue can be addressed by decision analysis (see Cost-Effectiveness Analysis section).

The NNT is a complex concept that becomes even more difficult when the impact of therapies for chronic disease are considered. For acute therapies with only a short-term effect, such as thrombolytic therapy, the simple version of NNT is adequate. However, saving 10 lives per 100 patients treated in the first 30 days is quite different from the same effect over 5 years. In some therapies, the concept is even more complex because the more effective treatment may have an early hazard, leading to a reversal of the treatment effect over time.

When weighing the evidence from clinical trials for a treatment decision in an individual patient, physicians must consider more than the level of significance of the findings.[69] In addition to the rationale for a given treatment, practitioners need to know which patients to treat, what drug and dose to use, and when and where therapy should be initiated. Not all clinical trial reports provide all the information required to form a complete assessment of the validity, precision, and implications of the results, nor do they answer the questions previously noted. In addition, clinicians are cautioned against overinterpreting subgroup analyses from RCTs because most RCTs lack sufficient power to assess adequately the treatment effects in multiple subgroups. Repeated statistical testing across several subgroups can lead to false-positive findings by chance; it is therefore preferable to present subgroup results in a visual format that depicts the point estimate and CIs to illustrate the range of possible treatment effects (Braunwald, Fig. 6-7).[70] In an attempt to introduce consistency in the reporting of clinical trials in the biomedical literature, a checklist of information for trialists, journal editors, peer-review panels, and the general medical audience is available (Table 1-4).[71] The presentation of a minimal set of uniform information in clinical trial reports should assist clinicians in making treatment decisions.

Detection of Treatment Effects in Clinical Trials

The interplay of a variety of factors influences the ability of investigators to detect a treatment effect, either benefit or harm, in a clinical trial (Figure 1-10). Variables set by investigators during the design of a clinical trial include 1) the definition of events that constitute the trial endpoints (e.g., a hard endpoint, such as death, is infrequent and results in fewer events observed compared with a composite endpoint); 2) the duration of follow-up, because short-term follow-up limits the time during which events may occur and reduces the likelihood of detecting harm; and 3) sample size, because an inadequate sample size places investigators at the risk of a large type II error and failure to detect a treatment effect when one exists.[68]

Variables related to both the patient and the treatment being investigated influence the relative difference in events in the treatment groups and may minimize or magnify the signal of increased risk of events. These include 1) interactions with other treatments; 2) the risk of events in the control group, because the impact of the test treatment may be less evident in healthier subjects when relatively few events occur in the control group; and 3) the RR of events in the treatment group, which is related both to the intrinsic properties of the treatment being investigated and the choice of the comparator arm (e.g., a treatment effect is more easily detected if the comparator arm is placebo and less readily detected in trials with an active comparator). If the test treatment improves symptoms or biomarker measurements relative to control, the control group may be exposed to more counterbalancing beneficial therapies, a phenomenon described as *intensification*. Although this cannot be prevented ethically, consideration of this issue in trial design and monitoring during the study can minimize the impact of intensification.

To complicate the situation further, the interface of the patient and the treatment may change over the course of exposure to the treatment. For example, development of diabetes or worsening

TABLE 1-4   CONSORT 2010 Checklist of Information to Include When Reporting a Randomized Trial*

SECTION/TOPIC	ITEM NO.	CHECKLIST ITEM
Title and Abstract		
	1a	Identification as a randomized trial in the title
	1b	Structured summary of trial design, methods, results, and conclusions (for specific guidance, see CONSORT for abstracts)
Introduction		
Background and objectives	2a	Scientific background and explanation of rationale
	2b	Specific objectives or hypotheses
Methods		
Trial design	3a	Description of trial design (such as parallel, factorial), including allocation ratio
	3b	Important changes to methods after trial commencement, such as eligibility criteria, with reasons
Participants	4a	Eligibility criteria for participants
	4b	Settings and locations where the data were collected
Interventions	5	The interventions for each group with sufficient details to allow replication, including how and when they were actually administered
Outcomes	6a	Completely defined prespecified primary and secondary outcome measures, including how and when they were assessed
	6b	Any changes to trial outcomes after the trial commenced, with reasons
Sample size	7a	How sample size was determined
	7b	When applicable, explanation of any interim analyses and stopping guidelines
Randomization		
Sequence generation	8a	Method used to generate the random allocation sequence
	8b	Type of randomization; details of any restriction, such as blocking and block size
Allocation concealment mechanism	9	Mechanism used to implement the random allocation sequence, such as sequentially numbered containers, describing any steps taken to conceal the sequence until interventions were assigned
Implementation	10	Who generated the random allocation sequence, who enrolled participants, and who assigned participants to interventions
Blinding	11a	If done, who was blinded after assignment to interventions (e.g., participants, care providers, those assessing outcomes) and how
	11b	If relevant, description of the similarity of interventions
Statistical methods	12a	Statistical methods used to compare groups for primary and secondary outcomes
	12b	Methods for additional analyses, such as subgroup analyses and adjusted analyses
Results		
Participant flow (a diagram is strongly recommended)	13a	For each group, the numbers of participants who were randomly assigned, received intended treatment, and were analyzed for the primary outcome
	13b	For each group, losses and exclusions after randomization, together with reasons
Recruitment	14a	Dates defining the periods of recruitment and follow-up
	14b	Why the trial ended or was stopped
Baseline data	15	A table showing baseline demographic and clinical characteristics for each group
Numbers analyzed	16	For each group, number of participants (denominator) included in each analysis and whether the analysis was by original assigned groups
Outcomes and estimation	17a	For each primary and secondary outcome, results for each group and the estimated effect size and its precision (such as 95% confidence interval)
	17b	For binary outcomes, presentation of both absolute and relative effect sizes is recommended.
Ancillary analyses	18	Results of any other analyses performed, including subgroup analyses and adjusted analyses, distinguishing prespecified from exploratory
Harms	19	All important harms or unintended effects in each group (for specific guidance see CONSORT for harms)
Discussion		
Limitations	20	Trial limitations, addressing sources of potential bias, imprecision, and, if relevant, multiplicity of analyses
Generalizability	21	Generalizability (external validity and applicability) of the trial findings
Interpretation	22	Interpretation consistent with results, balancing benefits and harms, and considering other relevant evidence
Other Information		
Registration	23	Registration number and name of trial registry
Protocol	24	Where the full trial protocol can be accessed, if available
Funding	25	Sources of funding and other support (such as supply of drugs), role of funders

*We strongly recommend reading this statement in conjunction with the Consolidated Standards or Reporting (CONSORT) Group 2010 Explanation and Elaboration for important clarifications on all the items. If relevant, we also recommend reading CONSORT extensions for cluster randomized trials, noninferiority and equivalence trials, nonpharmacologic treatments, herbal interventions, and pragmatic trials. Additional extensions are forthcoming; for those and for up-to-date references relevant to this checklist, see www.consort-statement.org.
From Schulz KF, Altman DG, Moher D, for the CONSORT Group. CONSORT 2010 statement: updated guidelines for reporting parallel group randomised trials [Webappendix]. *Lancet* Published online March 24, 2010.

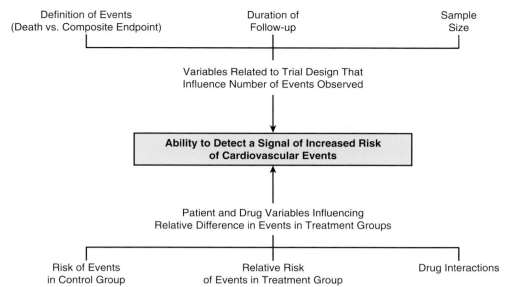

FIGURE 1-10 Detection of treatment effects in clinical trials. Factors related to trial design (*top*) and to the patient and drug being investigated (*bottom*) are shown. The interplay of these factors influences the ability to detect a treatment effect in a clinical trial. (*Modified from Antman EM, DeMets D, Loscalzo J. Cyclooxygenase inhibition and cardiovascular risk. Circulation 112:759-770, 2005.*)

of hypertension may culminate in disruption of a high-risk or vulnerable plaque with the development of a superimposed thrombus. As the acute situation evolves, the risk in the control arm and the RR associated with a drug may change—both in an adverse direction.

These considerations assume particular importance when assessing whether a signal of harm is present with a given treatment (e.g., the cardiovascular risks associated with coxib use).[68] The relations among the risk of events in the control group (control event rate [CER]), the RR of events with a particular drug (RR), and the NNH (critically related to the ability to detect a signal of harm) can be expressed by the following formula:

$$NNH = 1 / [(RR - 1) \times CER]$$

The surface shown in Figure 1-10 rises steeply to a high NNH (difficulty in detecting harm) with a low rate of events in the control group and/or low RR in the treatment group. The ability to detect harm improves as NNH drops, with increasing rates in the control arm and/or increasing RR in the treatment arm (see Figures 1-10 and 1-11).

When administering therapies that have a beneficial effect but are associated with serious potential for harm, the general goal is to operate on the steep portion of the surface in Figure 1-11, thereby minimizing patient risk. This can be accomplished by preferentially prescribing treatments (e.g., coxibs) only to patients at low risk of events, thereby moving to lower rates of events in the control group in Figure 1-11. Selecting drugs with a lower risk of harmful events and minimizing the dose and duration of treatment are also advisable (i.e., moving to a lower RR in Figure 1-11).

Meta-Analysis

Clinicians are frequently faced with many trials of a given treatment, some of which provide seemingly conflicting results. A method of summarizing the data is needed. Meta-analysis is a systematic, quantitative synthesis of data from multiple clinical sources that address a related question. Meta-analysis is a scientific and well-defined statistical discipline with established methods and standards. Synonymous terms encountered in the literature include *overview, pooling, data pooling, literature synthesis, research synthesis,* and *quantitative review*. Although the concept of data pooling has existed since the early 1900s, its introduction into

clinical literature has met with mixed reactions, ranging from exuberant support and in-depth analysis to overt skepticism. The large number of meta-analyses published in the field of cardiovascular medicine suggests that the technique is gaining in popularity and is likely to play an important role in the complex process of therapeutic decision making in the future, as well as in regulatory approval of new drugs and devices used in cardiology.[22] Authoritative bodies have begun to establish standards for improving the quality of reports of meta-analyses of clinical trials; these include PRISMA (Preferred Reporting Items for Systematic Reviews and Meta-Analyses; www.prisma-statement.org) and observation studies such as MOOSE (Meta-Analysis of Observational Studies in Epidemiology).[72] Meta-analysis software is available both commercially and on several public domain websites.[22] When pooling studies, it is important to locate all available trials and consider them for inclusion. Because investigators are more likely to report only positive findings, the issue of publication bias must also be considered when searching for trials to include in a meta-analysis.[22]

The fundamental principle of a meta-analysis is that the statistical power to estimate a treatment effect is enhanced because of an increase in sample size. An inherent assumption is that the available studies are sufficiently similar that pooling is appropriate. The various techniques of pooling construct a weighted average of the study outcomes; the selection of weighting techniques and the approach to handling between-study variability distinguish the different analytic methodologies.[22] Some authorities have proposed incorporating an adjustment for variations in the quality of individual trials when performing a meta-analysis, but this requires further research before formal recommendations can be made.[22]

Another important dimension of meta-analysis is the composite overview of therapies considered to be in the same "class." Particularly in the formulation of clinical practice guidelines, the general policy has been to review data for all members of the same class and then to make a recommendation about the class rather than about individual compounds or devices. In cardiovascular therapeutics, controversy has arisen concerning the antiplatelet agent, statin, low-molecular-weight heparin (LMWH), and β-blocker classes, and whether the risks and benefits of the many available agents are similar enough for them to be lumped together.[73]

LMWHs provide an excellent example of the difficulty involved in this issue. By combining all members of the class, the American

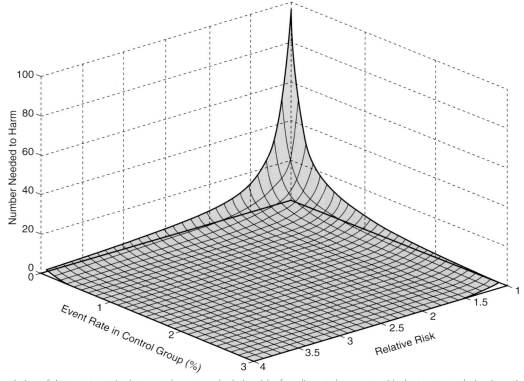

FIGURE 1-11 The relation of the event rate in the control group and relative risk of cardiovascular events with the treatment being investigated determines the number of patients who need to be treated with the drug to observe one cardiovascular event (Number Needed to Harm). The surface generated can be used to understand the relative ease or difficulty of detecting a signal of harm with a particular treatment (e.g., coxibs). *(Modified from Antman EM, DeMets D, Loscalzo J. Cyclooxygenase inhibition and cardiovascular risk.* Circulation *112:759-770, 2005.)*

College of Cardiology/American Heart Association Guidelines Committee on the Management of Patients with Unstable Angina was able to make a statement that LMWHs are superior to no antithrombin therapy.[73] However, when LMWHs are compared with unfractionated heparin, if all trials are pooled, no clear advantage is found for LMWHs compared with unfractionated heparin (Figure 1-12, *A*).[74] However, when data for the LMWH enoxaparin are separated from the remaining data, enoxaparin is seen to be significantly superior to unfractionated heparin (Figure 1-12, *B*).[73,74] Although testing for heterogeneity is a quantitative tool to guide investigators regarding the advisability of "lumping" versus "splitting," the test is not powerful, and additional tools are needed to sort out the development of quantitative estimates about class effect versus the attributes of individual therapies.[75]

Principles of Pooling Studies

The *fixed effects model* assumes that the trials are sampled from a homogeneous group. Under the homogeneity assumption, each trial provides an estimate of the single true treatment effect, and differences between the estimates from the various trials are the result only of experimental error (*within-trial variability*). The *random effects model* assumes that the trials are heterogeneous and that differences among the various estimates of the treatment effect are due to both experimental error (*within-trial variability*) and differences among the trials, such as trial design and characteristics of the patients enrolled (*between-trial variability*). The random effects model is generally favored because heterogeneity that cannot be explained by experimental error often exists among trials, and this model takes such heterogeneity into account in estimation and hypothesis testing, although this point is controversial.[22,76] Unless extreme heterogeneity is present among the trials, the point estimate of the treatment effect is similar using fixed and

random effects models, but the 95% CIs are generally wider with the random effects method because they incorporate the uncertainty present in the among-trial variation.

Cumulative Meta-Analysis

Some analysts have incorporated a Bayesian approach to synthesis of the results of RCTs.[76] In an effort to shorten the time delay between both the identification of an effective or ineffective therapy in clinical trials and translation of those findings into clinical practice, a related technique of continuously updating meta-analyses has been developed. This methodology, referred to as *cumulative meta-analysis*, updates the pooled estimate of the treatment effect each time the results of a new trial are published (Figures 1-13 and 1-14).

Cumulative meta-analysis is rooted in a Bayesian framework because it provides the history of the evolution of the posterior probability distribution of clinical trial results and allows quantification of changes in beliefs about treatment effects as the data accumulate.[77] When cumulative meta-analyses on RCTs of therapies for acute and secondary MI were compared with the textbook chapters and review articles, discrepancies were detected between the meta-analytic patterns of effectiveness and the recommendations of clinical experts.[78] The reasons for these discrepancies may be complex and include 1) a limited ability of authors of review articles to keep abreast of all the RCTs in a particular area, 2) failure to recognize the limited power of small, "negative" trials, 3) unfamiliarity or uncertainty about meta-analyses, and 4) a natural conservatism about recommending new therapies until extensive, large-scale clinical trials are completed. The use of cumulative meta-analysis in formulating therapeutic guidelines in the future requires additional methodologic study before its role can be properly defined. *Simulation studies* suggest that there may be

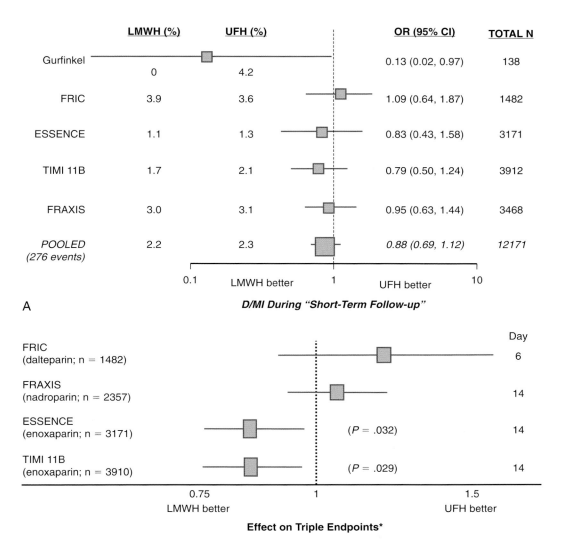

FIGURE 1-12 Examples of the complexity of pooling studies of multiple drugs within a class. Several different low-molecular-weight heparin *(LMWH)* preparations have been studied in patients with unstable angina/non–ST-segment elevation myocardial infarction *(MI)*. Although the consensus is that LMWHs are superior to placebo for reducing death and cardiac ischemia events, controversy exists when LMWHs are compared with unfractionated heparin *(UFH)*. **A,** Results of five trials of three different LMWHs versus UFH are plotted individually and then pooled under the assumption that they exhibit a class effect with little heterogeneity among the findings of the various trials. The pooled analysis shows a point estimate favoring LMWH for reducing death/MI during short-term follow-up, although the 95% confidence intervals *(CI)* are wide (owing to the low rate of events that occurred among the 12,171 patients at the time of ascertainment of the endpoint) and overlap unity. The authors found no evidence of the superiority of LMWHs over UFH. **B,** Four large phase III trials of three different LMWHs are plotted individually. Note that the endpoint analyzed is a composite of death *(D)*, MI, and recurrent ischemia without urgent revascularization and is ascertained at a later time point (6 to 14 days) than in **A**—two modifications that increase the power of the meta-analysis to discern differences among the LMWHs. Given the biochemical differences among the LMWHs and subtle but potentially important differences in trial design, the results were not pooled into a composite statement of LMWHs versus UFH. Two trials with enoxaparin show it to be significantly superior to UFH, whereas such a finding is not seen in the trials of dalteparin or nadroparin. ESSENCE, Efficacy and Safety of Subcutaneous Enoxaparin in Unstable Angina and Non–Q-Wave MI; FRAXIS, Fraxiparine in Ischemic Syndrome; FRIC, Fragmin in Unstable Coronary Artery Disease; OR, odds ratio; TIMI, Thrombolysis In Myocardial Infarction. *(Modified from Eikelboom JW, Anand SS, Malmberg K, et al. Unfractionated heparin and low-molecular-weight heparin in acute coronary syndrome without ST elevation: a meta-analysis.* Lancet *2000;355:1936-1942; and Braunwald E, Antman EM, Beasley JW, et al. ACC/AHA guidelines for the management of patients with unstable angina and non–ST-segment elevation myocardial infarction: a report of the American College of Cardiology/American Heart Association Task Force on Practice Guidelines [Committee on the Management of Patients with Unstable Angina].* J Am Coll Cardiol *2000;36:970-1062.)*

considerable sampling variation in the time when a cumulative meta-analysis is first significant.[79] Simulation methods can also estimate the type I error and power of a meta-analysis.[79] Because of the possibility in certain collections of trials of increasing risks of type I error, when multiple looks are taken at the accumulating data, more stringent statistical standards for the declaration of significance may be required.

Meta-Regression

The majority of meta-analyses in the cardiovascular literature report an average treatment effect estimated from the available studies. To move beyond the current methodology, investigators have proposed that estimates of the treatment effect be expressed as a function of study-specific features such as years of study,

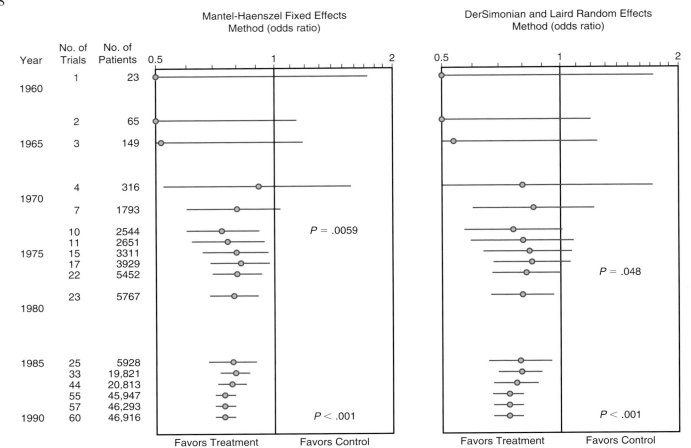

FIGURE 1-13 Cumulative meta-analyses of 60 trials of intravenous thrombolytic agents for myocardial infarction by the Mantel-Haenszel fixed effects method and DerSimonian and Laird random effects method. The odds ratios and 95% confidence intervals for a treatment effect on mortality rate are shown on a logarithmic scale. The statistical significance reached less than .05 in 1973 with the fixed effects method and in 1977 with the random effects method. *(Modified from Lau J, Antman EM, Jimenez-Silva J, et al. Cumulative meta-analysis of therapeutic trials for myocardial infarction.* N Engl J Med *1992;327:248-254.)*

drug dose, characteristics of patients enrolled (e.g., age, gender, race), or average mortality rate in the control group. Adjustments for covariates in clinical trials can be accomplished with the use of regression techniques; thus the term *meta-regression* has been introduced.[80] Meta-regression is useful for identifying sources of heterogeneity among clinical trials and for establishing clinically important relationships, such as the dose-response relationship, and changes in the incidence of outcome variables between studies conducted in the distant past and those conducted later.

Future Trends in Meta-Analysis

The previous discussion on meta-analysis treats the individual RCT as the unit of analysis. The difference between the aggregate result for the test and control groups for each trial is calculated and then pooled with the observed differences in other trials. Ideally, the individual patients in each trial should be the unit of analysis to assess whether the treatment effect is modified by certain patient characteristics. Collaborative efforts of trialists studying antiplatelet therapy for a wide range of cardiovascular conditions, direct thrombin inhibitor therapy for acute coronary syndromes,[81] fibrinolytic therapy for suspected MI, and coronary artery bypass surgery (CABG) versus medical therapy for coronary heart disease, and the Cholesterol Treatment Trialists' Collaboration illustrate the power of pooling individual patient-level data to provide estimates of the treatment effect stratified by various clinical profiles (e.g., age, gender, ventricular function, history of infarction or stroke; Figures 1-15 and 1-16).[82-85] The success of these efforts is likely to

inspire other investigators to plan prospectively for pooling of case reports from information across related trials.

This issue of the prospective pooling of data has many rapidly evolving aspects. The requirement to report trial results in the ClinicalTrials.gov registry now means that primary and key secondary outcomes, as well as adverse event totals, will be available to the public, and this situation will engender ad hoc overviews. In addition, the new Food and Drug Administration regulations regarding adverse event reporting are focused on aggregate data for the lifetime of the development of a drug, which is distinct from the previous focus on isolated individual reports. These trends point to the imperative for planning to pool data and to take advantage of such capabilities by using individual participant data to avoid erroneous conclusions from well-intentioned analysts who do not have access to these data. An interesting byproduct of this work will be the need to develop rules for interim analysis of accumulating information from ongoing disparate trials, both for efficacy and safety endpoints. This becomes even more urgent with the possibility of adding in nonrandomized data from ongoing surveillance activities that include the sentinel network in the United States, with plans to aggregate 100 million electronic health records, and similar efforts in Europe.

How to Read and Interpret a Meta-Analysis

A series of practical questions that readers should ask when assessing a meta-analysis are shown in Box 1-3. The same standards should apply whether the physician is reading an overview of a therapeutic modality, the results of a diagnostic test for a medical

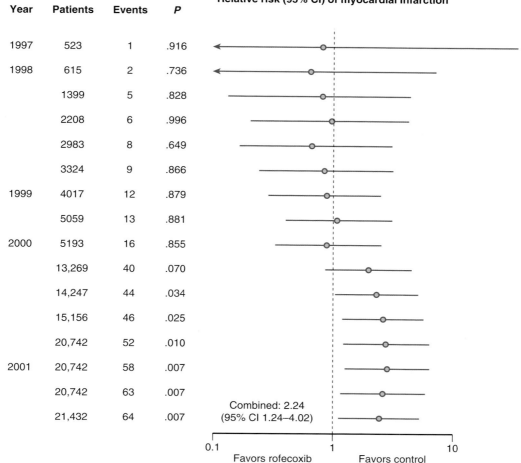

Relative risk (95% CI) of myocardial Infarction

Year	Patients	Events	P
1997	523	1	.916
1998	615	2	.736
	1399	5	.828
	2208	6	.996
	2983	8	.649
	3324	9	.866
1999	4017	12	.879
	5059	13	.881
2000	5193	16	.855
	13,269	40	.070
	14,247	44	.034
	15,156	46	.025
	20,742	52	.010
2001	20,742	58	.007
	20,742	63	.007
	21,432	64	.007

Combined: 2.24
(95% CI 1.24–4.02)

0.1   1   10
Favors rofecoxib   Favors control

FIGURE 1-14 Cumulative meta-analysis of 16 randomized clinical trials comparing rofecoxib versus control. By 2000, an increased risk of myocardial infarction was already evident, when 14,247 patients had been randomized, and a total of 44 events had occurred. Subsequent trials increased the number of patients to 21,432 and the number of events to 64. The 95% confidence intervals (CI) were narrowed as subsequent trials were reported, but the point estimate still favored control therapy. *(Redrawn with permission from Juni P, Nartey L, Reichenbach S, et al. Risk of cardiovascular events and rofecoxib: cumulative meta-analysis.* Lancet *2004;364:2021-2029.)*

condition,[86] or an assessment of the interventions in health care systems. Readers must be convinced that the authors attempted to answer a focused question of clinical importance, that all relevant studies were included, and that an attempt was made to assess the data for evidence of heterogeneity and to explain any between-trial variability if it is present. As with individual clinical trial reports, an overview should include a statement of the pooled treatment effect that incorporates both RR reduction and ARD and conveys the information in a clinically practical fashion (e.g., number to treat and number of lives saved per 1000 patients treated).

When attempting to apply the findings of an RCT or an overview of multiple RCTs to an individual patient, the clinician must determine whether his or her patient is similar to those enrolled in the trials. Although it may be tempting to focus on subgroup information from the meta-analysis to determine whether a given patient is likely to experience more or less than the average benefit of the treatment, this can be misleading (Braunwald, Fig. 6-7). Subgroup analyses are more reliable if the treatment difference is highly significant, if they represent hypotheses established before trial initiation, if they are consistent across studies, and if they are biologically plausible. The potential risks of the therapeutic intervention should be considered and discussed with the patient to ensure that the treatment decision is consistent with his or her concerns about quality of life.[87]

Comparative Effectiveness Research

The literature evaluating diagnostic and therapeutic interventions for cardiovascular disease is vast and full of rigorously performed studies. However, the majority of these compare a given test or treatment to a placebo or nonactive comparator.[88] Even studies that compare active agents—such as a direct thrombin inhibitor to warfarin, or different statins of equivalent potency—are performed in highly monitored settings, apply strict eligibility criteria that by design maximize internal validity over generalizability, are of relatively short duration, and frequently rely on surrogate measures rather than clinical endpoints. In other words, there is a relative absence of high quality empirical data to precisely guide many of the decisions that physicians and their patients face every day in actual practice.

CER is intended to fill this void. The Institute of Medicine defines CER as "the generation and synthesis of evidence that compares the benefits and harms of alternative methods to prevent, diagnose, treat, and monitor a clinical condition or to improve the delivery of care."[88] By intent, the scope of CER is extremely broad and reflects the diversity of issues relevant to patients with cardiovascular disease (Table 1-5). In 2009, the American Recovery and Reinvestment Act set aside $1.1 billion in funding for CER based on the belief that this information can "assist consumers, clinicians, purchasers, and policymakers to make informed

Presentation features	Percent of patients dead		Stratified statistics		Odds ratio and CIs		χ^2 test of odds ratios in different patient categories	
	Fibrinolytic	Control	O–E	Variance	Fibrinolytic better	Control better	Heterogeneity	Trend
ECG								
BBB	18.7%	23.6%	−24.5	83.3				
ST elev, anterior	13.2%	16.9%	−122.0	420.6				
ST elev, interior	7.5%	8.4%	−27.1	237.4				
ST elev, other	10.6%	13.4%	−42.1	159.6			21.28 on 6 df	
ST depression	15.2%	13.8%	12.9	108.7			(P < .01)	
Other abnormality	5.2%	5.8%	−9.6	103.2				
Normal	3.0%	2.3%	3.4	12.9				
Hours from onset								
0–1	9.5%	13.0%	−29.3	83.3				
2–3	8.2%	10.7%	−100.2	354.8			9.69 on 4 df	9.55 on 1 df
4–6	9.7%	11.5%	−78.5	387.6			(P < .05)	(2P < .002)
7–12	11.1%	12.7%	−51.5	336.7				
13–24	10.0%	10.5%	−11.1	212.6				
Age (years)								
<55	3.4%	4.6%	−45.9	155.6				
55–64	7.2%	8.9%	−86.3	360.0			8.27 on 3 df	6.58 on 1 df
65–74	13.5%	16.1%	−113.7	533.0			(P < .05)	(2P < .01)
75 +	24.3%	25.3%	−12.6	266.6				
Gender								
Male	8.2%	10.1%	−208.1	928.0			1.99 on 1 df	
Female	14.1%	16.0%	−62.2	436.8			(NS)	
Systolic BP (mm Hg)								
<100	28.9%	35.1%	−38.7	132.2				
100–149	9.6%	11.5%	−168.9	850.0			1.31 on 3 df	0.68 on 1 df
150–174	7.2%	8.7%	−59.2	290.0			(NS)	(NS)
175 +	7.2%	8.2%	−10.8	74.1				
Heart rate (beats/min)								
<80	7.2%	8.5%	−83.2	464.9				
80–99	9.2%	11.3%	−65.8	287.2			0.51 on 2 df	0.31 on 1 df
100 +	17.4%	20.7%	−51.7	238.6			(NS)	(NS)
Prior MI								
Yes	12.5%	14.1%	−43.7	322.4			2.09 on 1 df	
No	8.9%	10.9%	−228.5	1001.9			(NS)	
Diabetes								
Yes	13.6%	17.3%	−41.4	145.7			1.57 on 1 df	
No	8.7%	10.2%	−142.6	830.4			(NS)	
ALL PATIENTS 2820 / 29,315 3357 / 29,285	9.6%	11.5%	−269.5	1377.4			18% SD 2 odds reduction 2P < .00001	

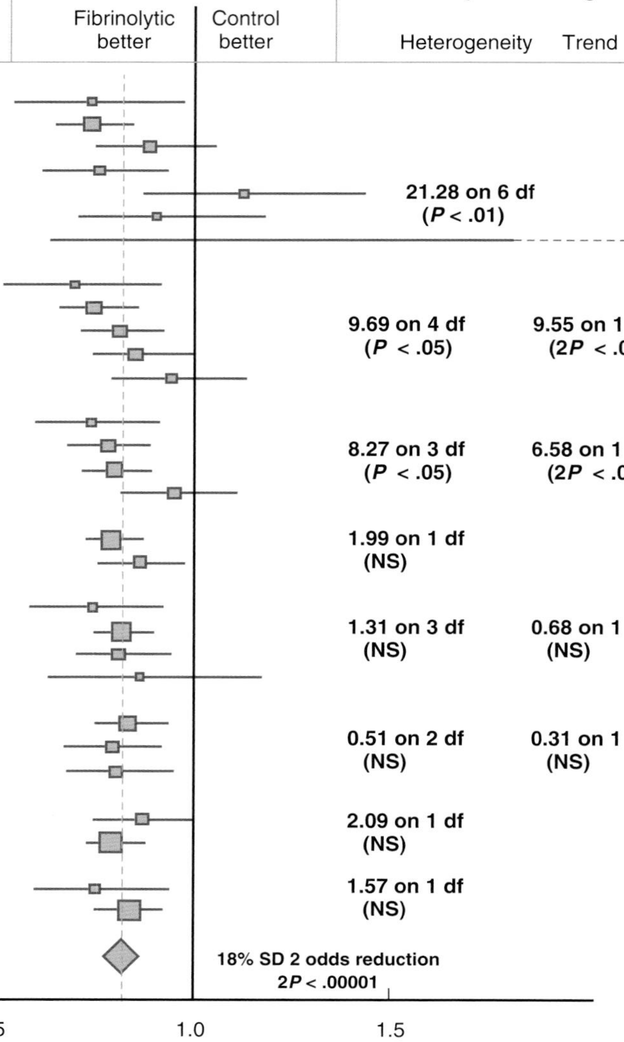

0.5   1.0   1.5

FIGURE 1-15 Proportional effects of fibrinolytic therapy on mortality rate during days 0 to 35 subdivided by presentation features. An *observed minus expected (O–E)* number of events among fibrinolytic-allocated patients and its variance is given for subdivisions of presentation features, stratified by trial. This is used to calculate odds ratios of death among patients allocated to fibrinolytic therapy to those allocated to control. The *solid squares* are odds ratios, with areas proportional to the amount of "statistical information" contributed by the trials, plotted with their 99% confidence intervals *(CIs)* as *horizontal lines*. *Squares* to left of the solid vertical line correspond to benefit (significant at two-tailed *P* < .01, only where the entire CI is to the left of the vertical line). Overall result and 95% CIs are represented by the *diamond*, with overall proportional reduction in the odds of death and statistical significance given alongside. The χ^2 tests are also given for evidence of heterogeneity of, or trends in, the size of odds ratios in subdivisions of each presentation feature. BBB, bundle branch block; BP, blood pressure; df, degrees of frequency; ECG, electrocardiogram; MI, myocardial infarction; NS, not significant; SD, standard deviation. *(Modified from Fibrinolytic Therapy Trialists' [FTT] Collaborative Group. Indications for fibrinolytic therapy.* Lancet *1994;343:311-322.)*

decisions that will improve health care at both the individual and population levels."[88]

Methods for Comparative Effectiveness Research

The methods used to evaluate whether a therapy or diagnostic test is superior to placebo can, with modification, also be used to answer questions of comparative effectiveness and safety (see Table 1-6). For example, many contemporary cardiovascular trials directly compare an investigative agent with an alternative drug that represents the standard of care. As such, they provide information on the comparative value of therapeutic options. However, these trials usually evaluate the impact of an intervention under ideal circumstances (*efficacy*) rather than its impact in real-world settings (*effectiveness*). Characteristics of randomized trials that are specifically intended to answer questions of comparative effectiveness include (1) the enrollment of populations that are representative of typical practice, including patients with common comorbid conditions; (2) the involvement of providers in nonacademic settings; (3) the use of study designs, such as adaptive randomization, that allow maximum efficiency; and (4) the explicit evaluation of subgroups of patients, such as the elderly.[89]

Meta-analyses and pooled analyses of patient-level data from RCTs are important techniques in comparative effectiveness research. As previously described, these methods enhance statistical power. They also facilitate analyses of important patient subgroups and secondary endpoints that individual trials may have been underpowered to evaluate. However, because active

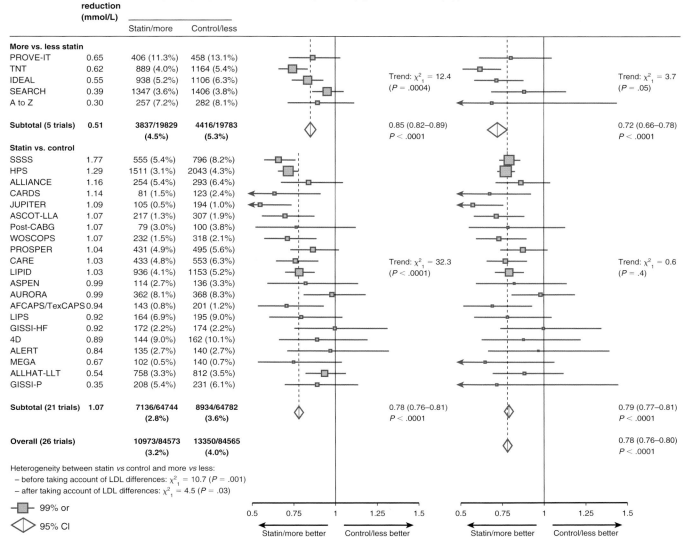

	LDL-C reduction (mmol/L)	Events (% per year) Statin/more	Events (% per year) Control/less	Unweighted RR (CI)	RR (CI) per 1 mmol/L reduction in LDL-C
More vs. less statin					
PROVE-IT	0.65	406 (11.3%)	458 (13.1%)		
TNT	0.62	889 (4.0%)	1164 (5.4%)	Trend: $\chi^2_1 = 12.4$	Trend: $\chi^2_1 = 3.7$
IDEAL	0.55	938 (5.2%)	1106 (6.3%)	$(P = .0004)$	$(P = .05)$
SEARCH	0.39	1347 (3.6%)	1406 (3.8%)		
A to Z	0.30	257 (7.2%)	282 (8.1%)		
Subtotal (5 trials)	**0.51**	**3837/19829** (4.5%)	**4416/19783** (5.3%)	0.85 (0.82–0.89) $P < .0001$	0.72 (0.66–0.78) $P < .0001$
Statin vs. control					
SSSS	1.77	555 (5.4%)	796 (8.2%)		
HPS	1.29	1511 (3.1%)	2043 (4.3%)		
ALLIANCE	1.16	254 (5.4%)	293 (6.4%)		
CARDS	1.14	81 (1.5%)	123 (2.4%)		
JUPITER	1.09	105 (0.5%)	194 (1.0%)		
ASCOT-LLA	1.07	217 (1.3%)	307 (1.9%)		
Post-CABG	1.07	79 (3.0%)	100 (3.8%)		
WOSCOPS	1.07	232 (1.5%)	318 (2.1%)		
PROSPER	1.04	431 (4.9%)	495 (5.6%)		
CARE	1.03	433 (4.8%)	553 (6.3%)	Trend: $\chi^2_1 = 32.3$	Trend: $\chi^2_1 = 0.6$
LIPID	1.03	936 (4.1%)	1153 (5.2%)	$(P < .0001)$	$(P = .4)$
ASPEN	0.99	114 (2.7%)	136 (3.3%)		
AURORA	0.99	362 (8.1%)	368 (8.3%)		
AFCAPS/TexCAPS	0.94	143 (0.8%)	201 (1.2%)		
LIPS	0.92	164 (6.9%)	195 (9.0%)		
GISSI-HF	0.92	172 (2.2%)	174 (2.2%)		
4D	0.89	144 (9.0%)	162 (10.1%)		
ALERT	0.84	135 (2.7%)	140 (2.7%)		
MEGA	0.67	102 (0.5%)	140 (0.7%)		
ALLHAT-LLT	0.54	758 (3.3%)	812 (3.5%)		
GISSI-P	0.35	208 (5.4%)	231 (6.1%)		
Subtotal (21 trials)	**1.07**	**7136/64744** (2.8%)	**8934/64782** (3.6%)	0.78 (0.76–0.81) $P < .0001$	0.79 (0.77–0.81) $P < .0001$
Overall (26 trials)		**10973/84573** (3.2%)	**13350/84565** (4.0%)		0.78 (0.76–0.80) $P < .0001$

Heterogeneity between statin *vs* control and more *vs* less:
– before taking account of LDL differences: $\chi^2_1 = 10.7$ $(P = .001)$
– after taking account of LDL differences: $\chi^2_1 = 4.5$ $(P = .03)$

99% or
95% CI

0.5   0.75   1   1.25   1.5   0.5   0.75   1   1.25   1.5

Statin/more better   Control/less better   Statin/more better   Control/less better

FIGURE 1-16 Effects on any major vascular event in each study. At *left*, unweighted rate ratios *(RR)* for each trial comparing first event rates between randomly allocated treatment groups are plotted along with 99% confidence intervals *(CIs)*. Trials are ordered according to the absolute reduction in low-density lipoprotein cholesterol *(LDL-C)* at 1 year within each type of trial comparison (more vs. less statin and statin vs. control). At *right*, RRs are weighted per 1 mmol/LDL-C difference at 1 year. Subtotals and totals with 95% CIs are shown by *open diamonds. (From Cholesterol Treatment Trialists' [CTT] Collaboration. Efficacy and safety of more intensive lowering of LDL cholesterol meta-analysis of data from 170,000 participants in 26 randomised trials. Lancet 2010;376:1670-168.)*

Box 1-3   How to Use Review Articles

What Are the Results?
Were the results similar from study to study?
What are the overall results of the review?
How precise were the results?

Are the Results Valid?
Did the review include explicit and appropriate eligibility criteria?
Was biased selection and reporting of studies unlikely?
Were the primary studies of high methodologic quality?
Were assessments of studies reproducible?

How Can I Apply the Results to Patient Care?
Were all patients-important outcomes considered?
Are any postulated subgroup effects credible?
What is the overall quality of the evidence?
Are the benefits worth the costs and potential risks?

From Guyatt G, Jaeschke R, Prasad K, Cook DJ. Summarizing the evidence. In Guyatt G, Rennie D, Meade MO, Cook DJ, editors: *Users' guides to the medical literature: a manual for evidence-based clinical practice,* 2nd ed, New York, 2008, McGraw-Hill, p 527.

comparator trials are rare, systematic reviews of these types of studies are often not possible. *Indirect meta-analyses* may overcome such limitations by estimating the relative value of two or more interventions that have been independently compared with placebo or another common comparator.[90] In other words, the effectiveness of interventions can be indirectly compared based on their relative effectiveness with a third intervention.

Much attention in comparative effectiveness research focuses on the use of nonrandomized observation studies. These evaluations represent actual use by patients with a broad range of clinical and demographic characteristics who receive care in real-world settings. Such studies frequently have sample sizes that are orders of magnitude larger than many clinical trials; thus they allow for precise estimates of outcomes, especially in important patient subgroups. Of course, to be evaluated with an observation study, the interventions being compared must have been approved for use in routine practice. These studies are also confronted by numerous methodological challenges and assumptions. For example, observation studies rely on the assumption that treatment choices are,

TABLE 1-5   Comparative Effectiveness Research in Cardiovascular Research

RESEARCH AREA	CONDITION	EXAMPLE
Cardiology-specific questions	Atrial fibrillation	Treatment strategies for atrial fibrillation, including surgery, catheter ablation, and pharmacologic treatment
	CAD	Aggressive medical management vs. percutaneous coronary interventions in treating stable disease for patients of different ages with various comorbidities
	CHF	Various innovative treatment strategies (e.g., cardiac resynchronization, remote physiologic monitoring, pharmacologic treatment, novel agents such as CRF-2 receptors)
	Venous thromboembolism	Various anticoagulant therapies (e.g., low-intensity warfarin, aspirin, injectable anticoagulants) for patients undergoing hip or knee arthroplasty surgery
General research areas relevant to cardiology	Health care delivery	Effectiveness of different techniques (e.g., audio, visual, written) for informing patients about proposed treatments during the process of informed consent / Strategies for enhancing patients' adherence to medication regimens
	Health disparities	Effectiveness of interventions (e.g., community-based, multilevel interventions, simple health education, usual care) to reduce health disparities
	Drug dependence	Effectiveness of smoking cessation strategies (e.g., medication, individual or quitline counseling, combinations of these)

CAD, coronary artery disease; CHF, congestive heart failure; CRF-2, corticotropic releasing factor 2.
Modified from the Institute of Medicine. *Initial national priorities for comparative effectiveness research.* Washington, DC, 2009, Institute of Medicine.

TABLE 1-6   Methodologies Frequently Used in Comparative Effectiveness Research

RESEARCH DESIGN	IDEAL FEATURES FOR COMPARATIVE EFFECTIVENESS	LIMITATIONS OF PUBLISHED STUDIES	EXAMPLE
Randomized trials	Enroll patients with common comorbidities cared for in typical care settings / Use adaptive randomization designs to maximize enrollment in efficiency / Use a priori evaluation of important patient subgroups (e.g., elderly)	Evaluates surrogate measures rather than health outcomes / Short duration / Insufficiently powered to evaluate important subgroups or assess adverse events	DOSE trial: bolus vs. continuous and high-dose vs. low-dose diuretic regimens for decompensated congestive heart failure[121]
Meta-analyses and pooled analyses from clinical trials	Maximize statistical power by combining data from multiple studies / Allow assessment of important subgroups that may not be possible in some trials / Perform indirect meta-analyses (i.e., based on studies of two therapies, each to placebo) to allow comparative assessments when direct comparisons have not been made	Rely on estimates from trials that assess efficacy rather than effectiveness / Few head-to-head trials of alternative therapies that evaluate clinically meaningful endpoints, leaving few data to pool	Meta-analysis of trials comparing angiotensin-converting enzyme inhibitors and angiotensin receptor blockers for essential hypertension[122]
Observational studies	Evaluate patients in actual practice, including those often excluded from randomized trials / Studies may have extremely large sample sizes	May be hard to address confounding by indication and other important biases / Can only evaluate interventions used in routine practice (i.e., cannot evaluate investigational agents)	Retrospective cohort study of post–myocardial infarction patients comparing mortality rates for patients prescribed different angiotensin-converting enzyme inhibitors[123]

DOSE, Diuretic Optimization Strategies Evaluation.

for the most part, made randomly; however, in actual practice, choices between treatments with different safety or effectiveness profiles are often based on patient characteristics that are associated with the outcomes of interest.[91] This can give rise to incorrect inferences about treatment effectiveness or safety. For example, an observation study comparing rates of MI in patients receiving different classes of oral hypoglycemics may erroneously conclude that rosiglitazone use is associated with a reduced rate of cardiovascular events if, in actual practice, this agent were preferentially given to lower risk patients. In other words, the apparent association between treatment and outcome may actually be the result of *confounding by indication.* These and other important biases can be minimized through design, such as by studying "new" users, ensuring that outcomes are evaluated after exposure has been determined, and using a variety of advanced analytic methods (e.g., propensity scores and instrumental variables).[91] However, the internal validity of observational treatment comparisons remains a matter of debate, because unmeasured confounders are challenging to control without randomization.

Balancing Risks and Benefits

Comparative effectiveness research provides estimates of both the comparative benefits and the comparative risks of interventions. In situations where one treatment is more effective but also more risky than another, determining which is superior can be challenging. For example, for patients with acute coronary syndrome undergoing percutaneous coronary intervention, prasugrel appears to be more effective than clopidogrel but also has a higher risk of bleeding.[37]

The most straightforward approach to balancing benefits and risks is to determine, when compared with the standard care, whether the number of outcomes (e.g., MIs and strokes) prevented by a novel therapy is larger than the number of adverse events that it causes (e.g., intracranial and gastrointestinal bleeding). This can also be done by comparing NNTs and NNHs, as described in the Measures of Treatment section above; a *superior treatment* may be defined as one for which the NNT is smaller than the NNH—that is, fewer patients need to be treated for one patient to benefit than the number of patients who need to be treated for one patient to be harmed. A third strategy involves the evaluation of composite outcomes that incorporate both risks and benefits. With respect to prasugrel and clopidogrel, such an outcome could include thrombotic and hemorrhagic events that would provide a global comparison of the two treatment strategies.

None of these methods account for the fact that patients consider some clinical outcomes to be more undesirable than others. For example, many patients would rather risk experiencing a gastrointestinal hemorrhage than an MI, and thus one-to-one trade-offs of these events may not accurately represent patient preference. This limitation can be overcome by converting outcome events into a "common currency" with the aid of *utilities*, which measure a patient's strength of preference for a given health state under situations of uncertainty.

Utilities range from 0 to 1, corresponding to death and perfect health, respectively, with all other health states assigned a value in between these extremes. For example, in an analysis comparing dabigatran with warfarin for patients with atrial fibrillation, stroke with a major residual deficit was assigned a utility of 0.39, whereas major gastrointestinal hemorrhage had a utility of 0.8.[92] Utilities can be elicited directly from patients using choice-based methods, such as the standard gamble or time trade-off, or using scaling methods, such as a rating or visual analog scale.[93] Utilities may also be calculated from surveys that measure health status by applying validated point scores.[93]

To facilitate the comparison of benefits and risks, utilities can be used to weight survival. One common metric is the *quality-adjusted life-year* (QALY), which is widely used in cost-effectiveness analysis; it is calculated by multiplying life expectancy by utility. Interventions with a different balance of benefits and risks will have different numbers of QALYs; the option that maximizes QALYs is considered superior from the perspective of comparative effectiveness. Because patients face the risk of many different outcomes that include stroke, CHF, and bleeding, and because patients may experience these risks at different times, decision analytic techniques, described in the following sections, are necessary to calculate QALYs and to compare interventions using this methodology.

One alternative to the QALY for measuring health-adjusted life years[94] is the *disability life year* (DALY), used by the World Health Organization (WHO). The DALY measures the gap between population health and a hypothetical ideal for health achievement. DALYs rate health-related quality of life on a scale from 0 to 1, where 0 represents perfect health. In contrast to QALYs, the weights in DALYs are based on assessments of experts, rather than individuals, to standardize scores across societies.[94]

Cost-Effectiveness Analysis

Compared with existing treatments, new and effective therapies generally increase health spending, even when considering the downstream savings from events that they avert. Our ability to afford all health care interventions that provide added health benefit is increasingly limited; therefore techniques to assess the *value* of medical and health care interventions—that is, to examine their benefits and risks in relation to their cost—are of great importance, especially in the practice of cardiology. Cost-effectiveness analysis provides such a methodology.

Types of Economic Evaluation

Cost-effectiveness analysis is part of a large family of methods for economic evaluation, all of which seek to compare "alternative courses of action in terms of both the cost and consequences"[93] (Table 1-7). Strategies differ in the assumptions they make about effectiveness and the way they quantify it.

Cost-minimization analysis aims to identify the therapeutic option that is least costly based on the assumption that evaluated interventions are equally effective. For example, based on the assumed equivalence of different antihypertensive classes, a cost-minimization analysis found diuretic-based regimens to be less costly than other treatment options for the management of isolated systolic hypertension in the elderly.[95] Because the assumption of equivalent effectiveness and safety is unusual, cost-minimization analyses rarely appear in the medical literature.

Cost-benefit analysis seeks to identify interventions with net benefits greater than their costs (i.e., benefits – cost > 0), because such interventions are, by definition, worth adopting. In such analyses, *costs* are those expenses attributable to the intervention itself (e.g., the added cost of a new medication) and all other resources that are consumed (e.g., testing, hospitalization, surgical costs). The benefits of intervention are the monetary savings from events that are averted—that is, those costs that are *not* expended as a result of a new intervention—plus the value of the resulting health improvements. In cost-benefit analysis, health value is expressed in monetary terms, or in other words, rates of clinical events are converted from their natural units, such as lives saved, into measures of economic value (e.g., dollars). This can be done using methods that estimate the value of a treatment in terms of the present value of future earnings that would be gained from the treatment, known as the *human capital approach*, or that assess or infer how much someone would be willing to pay to avoid a given condition.[93] By monetizing health, cost–benefit analysis can facilitate the comparison of health care interventions with those from other sectors of the economy, such as housing or education. However, quantifying life is fraught with practical and ethical challenges; therefore, these types of analyses rarely appear in the published medical literature.

The most widely used strategies for evaluating the value of a health care intervention are *cost-effectiveness* and *cost-utility analyses*. The objective of these methods is to identify the treatment alternative that provides the greatest health for a given level of expenditure, or, equivalently, that has the lowest cost for a given level of health. Thus, they are most relevant when treatments differ with respect to both cost or effectiveness. These methods

TABLE 1-7	Major Methods of Economic Evaluation				
		Units of Measure			
TYPE OF ANALYSIS	GOALS AND KEY ASSUMPTIONS	COSTS	EFFECTIVENESS	METRIC	
Cost minimization	Identify the lowest cost alternative; assumes options are equally effective	Monetary units	NA	Cost of new intervention minus cost of comparator	
Cost benefit	Identify alternative that maximizes net benefit	Monetary units	Monetary units	Incremental cost of new intervention vs. incremental benefit of new intervention	
Cost effectiveness	Identify alternative that maximizes "health" subject to budget limit	Monetary units	Natural units (e.g., life-years gained)	Incremental cost per incremental unit of health (e.g., dollars per life-year gained)	
Cost utility	Identify alternative that maximizes "utility" subject to budget limits	Monetary units	Health status (e.g., QALY)	Incremental cost per incremental unit of health status (e.g., dollars per QALY gained)	

NA, not applicable; QALY, quality-adjusted life-year.

TABLE 1-8   Cost-Effectiveness and Cost-Utility Analysis of hs-CRP Testing and Rosuvastatin Treatment for Patients with Levels >2 mg/L for Men ≥50 Years and Women ≥60 Years with LDL Cholesterol Levels <130 mg/dL and No Known Cardiovascular Disease

OUTCOME	Treatment Arm		DIFFERENCE
	USUAL CARE	hs-CRP SCREENING AND ROSUVASTATIN TREATMENT IF ELEVATED	
Costs ($US)			
Screening and treatment	1032	11,366	10,334
Vascular events	12,241	8077	−4164
Adverse events	6444	8173	1729
Total	19,717	27,616	7899
Effectiveness			
Life-years gained	12.38	12.75	0.36
QALYs	10.29	10.61	0.31
Cost-Effectiveness			
Incremental cost-effectiveness ratio ($/life-years gained)	—	—	$22,160
Incremental cost-utility ratio ($/QALY)	—	—	$25,198

All future costs and QALYs were discounted at a rate of 3% per year.
hs-CRP, C-reactive protein; QALY, quality-adjusted life-year.
From Choudhry NK, Patrick AR, Glynn RJ, Avorn J. The cost-effectiveness of C-reactive protein testing and rosuvastatin treatment for patients with normal cholesterol levels. *J Am Coll Cardiol* 2011;57(7):784-791.

differ only in the manner in which they quantify health; therefore they differ in the summary estimates they generate (see Table 1-8). Although their results have different interpretations, in practice, the general term *cost-effectiveness analysis* is used to refer to both.

The relevant costs in a cost-effectiveness analysis include those of the interventions themselves and costs that occur *downstream* as a result of clinical events that are caused or averted by treatment.[3] For example, a comparison of the cost-effectiveness of dabigatran and warfarin for the treatment of atrial fibrillation would consider the costs of the drugs, monitoring, and care of patients who suffer an ischemic or hemorrhagic stroke.[92]

Cost-effectiveness analysis compares the *incremental* (or *added*) *cost* from a new intervention with its *incremental benefits*. Benefits, which include risks, are quantified in natural units of health, such as life years gained, cases prevented, or percent reduction in LDL cholesterol. The summary estimate of cost-effectiveness analysis is an *incremental cost-effectiveness ratio* (ICER):

$$\frac{\text{Cost}_{\text{New Treatment}} - \text{Cost}_{\text{Old Treatment}}}{\text{Effect}_{\text{New Treatment}} - \text{Effect}_{\text{Old Treatment}}} = \frac{\Delta \text{Cost}}{\Delta \text{Health Effect}}$$

Interventions with lower ICERs are considered to be more cost-effective (i.e., the cost is less per added unit of health). Cost-utility analysis quantifies health in utilities, most commonly with QALYs, and on this basis it calculates an *incremental cost/utility ratio* (ICUR):

$$\frac{\text{Cost}_{\text{New Treatment}} - \text{Cost}_{\text{Old Treatment}}}{\text{Utility}_{\text{New Treatment}} - \text{Utility}_{\text{Old Treatment}}} = \frac{\Delta \text{Cost}}{\Delta \text{Utility}}$$

Although the units in cost-effectiveness analysis are easily interpretable, cost-utility analysis has the advantage of facilitating comparisons between treatments that are intended for completely different conditions or those that have substantially different effects on quantity and quality of life. For example, the value of implantable cardioverter defibrillators, statins for primary prevention, and hemodialysis in end-stage renal disease can all be compared from estimates of their incremental cost-utility relative to the standard of care.

Methods for Performing a Cost-Effectiveness Analysis

Cost-effectiveness analyses can be performed as part of a clinical trial by using decision modeling or as a combination of the two.

TRIAL-BASED ANALYSES

Trial-based analyses collect economic data prospectively along with the information necessary for the evaluation of an intervention's effectiveness and safety. Trial-based economic evaluations have numerous strengths. They exploit the methodologic advantages of this research design (e.g., random allocation), evaluate costs and effects in the same patient populations, and require few of the many assumptions that are often made with performing cost-effectiveness modeling (discussed in more detail below).[96] In contrast, trial-based analyses do not incorporate information from other important sources, such as other trials of similar interventions. In addition, they may evaluate populations of patients selected to maximize the trial's internal validity and may capture costs that are specifically mandated by the trial protocol but that do not reflect care in typical settings and, as with the trials themselves, occur in only a relatively short period of follow-up.[97] Variance is often much greater around high-cost items, such as hospitalization, than around clinical event rates; thus estimates from trials may be underpowered to generate robust economic estimates.[98]

Ideally, prospectively collected economic information includes the actual *costs* that are incurred during the course of the trial. For multicenter trials, costs may vary substantially from country to country, or even from center to center within a given country; thus local costing data are necessary. The use of *charges* based on bills submitted by physicians, hospitals, pharmacies, and other providers to payers such as Medicare represents a simplified approach for capturing prospective data, especially in the United States.[99] Their use may be acceptable for establishing the relative impact of two interventions, but charges for many services are set well above their actual price to ensure reimbursement at all levels of payment. Charges can be deflated to actual costs using published *cost-to-charge ratios*.[100]

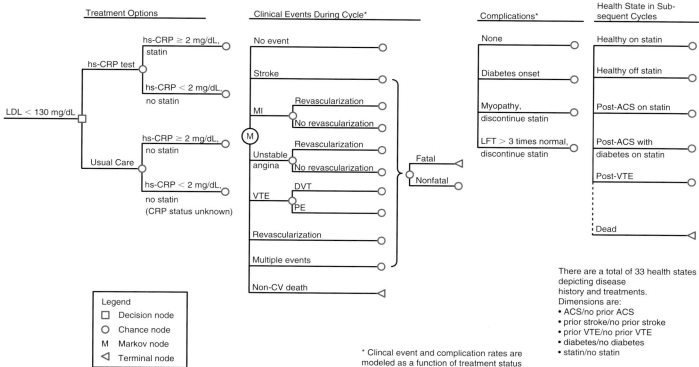

FIGURE 1-17 Cost-effectiveness model structure comparing the strategy of C-reactive protein (hs-CRP) testing—and rosuvastatin treatment, if hs-CRP is elevated—and usual care for men aged 50 years and older and women aged 60 years and older with low-density lipoprotein *(LDL)* cholesterol levels below 130 mg/dL and no known cardiovascular disease. The model simulates a cohort of patients with an age, gender, and Framingham risk score distribution based on the JUPITER trial participants. In each 1-year cycle, patients may have eight possible clinical events, resulting in survival or death, and one or more complications. Based on their status at the end of the cycle, patients begin the next 1-year cycle in one of 33 possible health states. ACS, acute coronary syndrome; CV, cardiovascular; DVT, deep venous thrombosis; LFT, liver function test; MI, myocardial infarction; PE, pulmonary embolism; VTE, venous thromboembolism. *(Modified from Choudhry NK, Patrick AR, Glynn RJ, Avorn J. The cost-effectiveness of C-reactive protein testing and rosuvastatin treatment for patients with normal cholesterol levels. J Am Coll Cardiol 2011;57[7]:784-791.)*

If explicit cost or charge data cannot be collected, a common alternative is to quantify all of the major resources consumed in the course of a patient's care and multiply each of these by their cost. In this case, costs are usually based on published sources, such as the Medicare reimbursement rates. For example, an in-trial economic evaluation of the Trial to Assess Improvement in Therapeutic Outcomes by Optimizing Platelet Inhibition with Prasugrel-Thrombolysis in Myocardial Infarction (TRITON-TIMI) 38 trial comparing prasugrel and clopidogrel for patients with acute coronary syndrome measured rates of hospitalizations, physician services, procedures, and medications for trial participants in eight prespecified countries and multiplied these by price weights derived from comparable populations of U.S. patients.[101]

MODELING APPROACHES

Modeled analyses use decision analytic techniques, most notably Markov modeling, to estimate the clinical and economic consequences of an intervention and its comparators. These models seek to distill a complex clinical situation into its component parts with the use of a *decision tree*. The tree lays out pathways that represent all probable outcomes, along with their clinical and economic consequences, for patients facing a decision between two or more alternative courses of action, such as a new medication or the standard of care.[93]

The most frequently used models for cost-effectiveness analysis incorporate both whether and when an event occurs. These dynamic state-transition models, called *Markov models*, evaluate a hypothetical cohort of patients as they move through health states that simulate the natural history of disease over time (e.g., from being healthy to MI to post-MI to CHF and ultimately death).

The model is based on set time periods, called *cycles*, which can be days, months, years, decades, or any other period of time that may be relevant to the research. In each cycle, some patients change health states and others remain the same. The likelihood of patients changing health states is based on transitional probabilities that are influenced by patient demographics, comorbidities, treatment, and other clinical factors. The model calculates the time spent in each health state to yield estimates of average life expectancy or average quality-adjusted life expectancy and average lifetime costs. The model is run separately for each intervention being evaluated, and this process generates the information necessary to calculate incremental costs and effects.

For example, Figure 1-17 presents a Markov model used to evaluate the cost-effectiveness of a treatment strategy based on the Justification for the Use of Statins in Prevention: An Intervention Trial Evaluating Rosuvastatin (JUPITER) trial of rosuvastatin treatment for patients with elevated levels of C-reactive protein (hs-CRP).[102] The model begins with a choice between a "test-and-treat" strategy and usual care for men aged 50 years and older and women aged 60 years and older with LDL cholesterol levels below 130 mg/dL and no known cardiovascular disease. In each 1-year cycle, patients may have one or more complications and eight possible clinical events, resulting in survival or death. Based on their status at the end of the cycle, patients begin the next 1-year cycle in one of 33 possible health states.

Data for cost-effectiveness models come from a variety of sources, including meta-analyses of randomized trials, representative cohort studies, natural history studies (the Framingham trial is frequently used),[103] population-based life tables, and U.S. Vital Statistics. Contemporary and clinically realistic models, such as that presented in Figure 1-17, are extremely complex, require many decisions about appropriate data sources, and incorporate numerous assumptions about treatment outcomes, especially when appropriate data do not exist. Although the impact of these choices can be evaluated in sensitivity analyses (detailed below), adequately evaluating the validity of these models can be complex, and it limits their transparency for nonexpert readers.

HYBRID APPROACHES

Whereas randomized trials provide results with high internal validity, they typically evaluate treatments over a relatively short period of time and include highly selected patient populations. In contrast, many cardiovascular therapies, such as statins, are used indefinitely, have long-term effects, and are prescribed to patients with comorbid conditions or other characteristics that would have excluded them from trial enrollment. Decision modeling can be used to extend the results of trial-based analyses to address these deficiencies. For example, in a classic cost-effectiveness study comparing thrombolytic strategies for acute MI, 1-year survival observed in the Global Use of Strategies to Open Coronary Arteries (GUSTO) trial was extended using cohort data from the Duke Cardiovascular Disease Database and a Gompertz survival function (Figure 1-18).[104]

Other Methodologic Considerations

SENSITIVITY ANALYSIS

Because of uncertainties surrounding estimates included in cost-effectiveness analyses, sensitivity analyses are used to evaluate the robustness of the results against the assumptions made in the primary or *base case analysis*. Potentially influential variables are initially varied one at a time in *one-way sensitivity analyses* across a broad range of plausible values. These values can be generated, for example, from 95% CIs from the point estimates used in the base case analysis, the ranges observed in the literature, or estimates from content experts. For example, Figure 1-19 presents the impact of varying the improvements in the amount of time that patients with atrial fibrillation spend in their target international

normalized ratio (INR) range as a result of using genotypic information to guide warfarin dosing.[105] This parameter was varied from 0%, or no improvement, to 30%, or perfect INR control. Because of the large number of variables that are subjected to one-way analyses, a *tornado diagram* or *tornado plot* can demonstrate which variables most influence a study's results (Figure 1-20).[102]

Two-way sensitivity analyses alter two potentially influential variables at the same time. These analyses may be represented as a

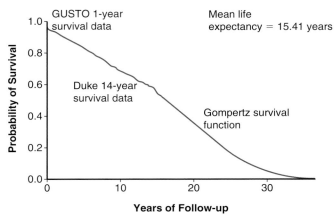

FIGURE 1-18 Probability of survival for patients treated with tissue plasminogen activator used in a cost-effectiveness analysis comparing thrombolytic strategies for acute myocardial infarction. The curve consists of three parts: the survival pattern in the first year after treatment in the Global Utilization of Streptokinase and Tissue Plasminogen Activator for Occluded Coronary Arteries *(GUSTO)* study, data for an additional 14 years on survivors of myocardial infarction in the Duke Cardiovascular Disease Database, and a Gompertz parametric survival function adjusted to agree with the empirical survival data at the 10- and 15-year follow-up points. *(From Mark DB, Hlatky MA, Califf RM, et al. Cost effectiveness of thrombolytic therapy with tissue plasminogen activator as compared with streptokinase for acute myocardial infarction. N Engl J Med 1995;332:1418-1424.)*

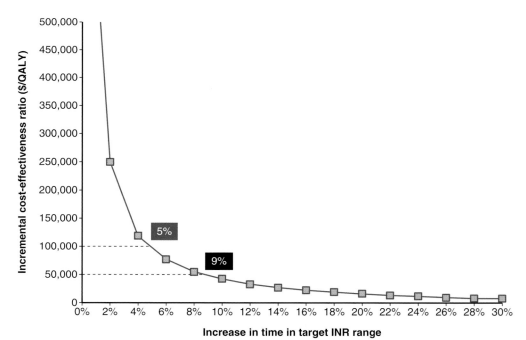

FIGURE 1-19 One-way sensitivity analysis of the impact of improvements in anticoagulation control using genotypic warfarin dosing on the cost effectiveness of this treatment strategy compared with algorithm-based warfarin dosing. The x axis presents the added amount of time patients spend in their target international normalized ration *(INR)* range as a result of genotyping. The y axis presents the incremental cost-effectiveness ratio of the strategy. As time in target range increases, cost effectiveness improves. For cost-effectiveness thresholds of $50,000 and $100,000 per quality-adjusted life-year *(QALY)*, genetically guided dosing would be cost effective if it increased the proportion of time that patients spend in the target INR range by 9 or more percentage points and added 5 or more percentage points, respectively. *(Modified from Patrick AR, Avorn J, Choudhry NK. Cost-effectiveness of genotype-guided warfarin dosing for patients with atrial fibrillation. Circ Cardiovasc Qual Outcomes 2009;2:429-436.)*

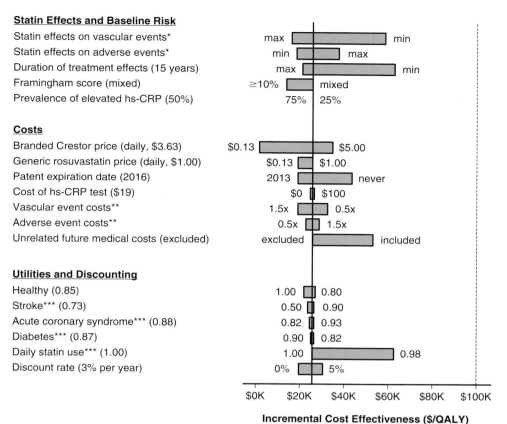

FIGURE 1-20 One-way sensitivity analyses of variables included in a cost-effectiveness model of C-reactive protein *(hs-CRP)* testing and rosuvastatin treatment for patients with elevated levels ("test and treat") based on the Justification for the Use of Statins in Prevention: An Intervention Trial Evaluating Rosuvastatin *(JUPITER)* trial results. Each bar represents the incremental cost-effectiveness ratio of the test-and-treat strategy for different assumptions concerning the parameter listed. The *vertical line* depicts the scenario in which all parameters are set at their base case values, listed in parentheses. *For statin effects, "min" and "max" represent the weakest and strongest effects based on the 95% confidence interval of the point estimates observed in JUPITER. For the duration of treatment effects, "min" represents the scenario in which the statin effects from JUPITER were assumed to persist for 5 years only, and the "max" scenario, full treatment effects, were assumed to persist for 25 years and then taper off over the subsequent 10 years. **Values represent multiples of base case values. ***Utilities were calculated by multiplying utilities for the specific event with age-specific utilities for healthy individuals. QALY, quality-adjusted life-year. *(Modified from Choudhry NK, Patrick AR, Glynn RJ, Avorn J. The cost-effectiveness of C-reactive protein testing and rosuvastatin treatment for patients with normal cholesterol levels. J Am Coll Cardiol 2011;57[7]:784-791.)*

family of one-way analyses. For example, in the cost-effectiveness model presented in Figure 1-17, a two-way analysis could simultaneously vary treatment efficacy and baseline patient risk (Figure 1-21).[102] Alternatively, two-way sensitivity analyses can be presented as a plane of possible values in which the *x* and *y* axes may represent the ranges tested for each of the two variables being evaluated, with shading that indicates the preferred strategies for a given pairing of parameter values (Figure 1-22).[106]

Probabilistic sensitivity analysis, also known as *Monte Carlo simulations,* varies multiple parameters at the same time. Ranges and distributions are assigned to each influential variable in an analysis. Typically, such analyses run 1000 to 10,000 simulations in which a different value for each parameter is drawn from its particular distribution. Based on this, the mean cost-effectiveness value and 95% CI for all simulations can be calculated. The incremental cost and incremental effectiveness estimate derived from each simulation can be displayed visually (Figure 1-23).[102] Cost-effectiveness thresholds can be added to such plots, and the number of simulations that fall below the assigned value can be estimated.

PERSPECTIVE

Numerous entities, such as hospitals, health maintenance organizations, providers, patients, or society as a whole, may derive benefits or incur costs from an intervention. Each may view costs from the perspective of its own particular "silo," and thus interests may

clash. For example, a shortened hospital length of stay of a patient benefits the hospital because payments from insurance companies are prospective (via diagnosis-related groups) and similar regardless of the length of stay. For the patient, it may be economically advantageous to stay in the hospital, because many out-of-pocket costs are thereby avoided, including the costs of any home care. Although an individual entity may find cost-effectiveness analysis very useful in making rational allocations of resources from its own perspective, the broader societal perspective is generally recommended to ensure comparability between analyses.[107]

DISCOUNTING

Discounting is a method used to equalize present and future costs.[108-111] In both economics and life, future benefits and adversities are not valued in the same manner as those of the present. In general, money spent now for benefits is worth more than money spent in the future. The method used for equalizing time is *discounting* both future costs and effectiveness. A 3% per year discount of future items is recommended (a reflection of average yield in public investments), although many past analyses have used 5% per year. Because the timing of cost and benefits of a particular intervention varies, the impact of discounting also varies. In the case of long-term drug treatment (e.g., for hypertension), costs are relatively uniform over time (e.g., drug costs, intermittent diagnostic testing, complications), and benefits are delayed. For surgical or procedural interventions the initial cost is large,

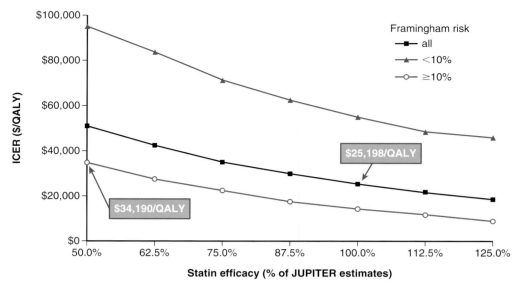

FIGURE 1-21 Impact of statin efficacy and baseline patient risk (i.e., Framingham risk) on the cost effectiveness of C-reactive protein *(hs-CRP)* testing and rosuvastatin treatment if hs-CRP is elevated for men aged 50 years and older and women aged 60 years and older with low-density lipoprotein cholesterol levels of 130 mg/dL or lower and no known cardiovascular disease. *Black squares* represent the impact of varying statin efficacy for the entire study population (based on the Justification for the Use of Statins in Prevention: An Intervention Trial Evaluating Rosuvastatin *[JUPITER]* trial). *Circles* and *diamonds* represent the impact of changing both the treatment effect and the targeted population. ICER, incremental cost-effectiveness ratio; QALY, quality-adjusted life-year. *(Modified from Choudhry NK, Patrick AR, Glynn RJ, Avorn J. The cost-effectiveness of C-reactive protein testing and rosuvastatin treatment for patients with normal cholesterol levels. J Am Coll Cardiol 2011;57[7]:784-791.)*

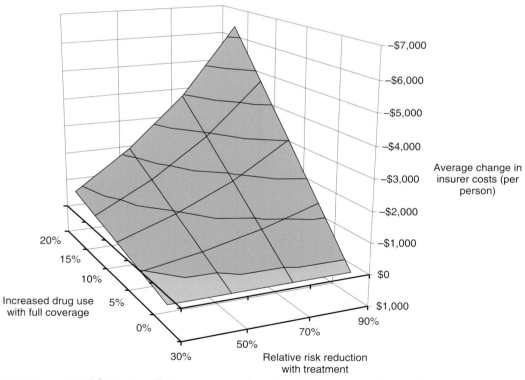

FIGURE 1-22 Two-way sensitivity graph from a cost-effectiveness analysis of providing full drug coverage for secondary prevention medications to patients after myocardial infarction. The analysis estimates the impact on insurer costs of simultaneously varying the estimated treatment effect of drug therapy on event rates (i.e., the relative reduction with treatment) and the incremental change in drug utilization that may result from full coverage. The *green area* represents the set of values for which a full, compared with usual, coverage strategy results in cost savings. *(Modified from Choudhry NK, Avorn J, Antman EM, et al. Should patients receive secondary prevention medications for free after a myocardial infarction? An economic analysis. Health Aff (Millwood) 2007;26:186-194.)*

with much more modest long-term costs, and benefit starts immediately. With this method, the initial investment pays returns over time. Although the overall cost effectiveness of these two types of medical interventions may be comparable, a higher discount rate has more of an impact in devaluing the benefits of prevention because these benefits occur more in the future.

TIME HORIZON

The time horizon of a cost-effectiveness analysis refers to the length of time during which benefits and costs are evaluated. A model should extend far enough into the future to capture all of the major effects of an intervention, both intended and unintended.[112] In the case of cardiovascular disease, this often means that patients may be monitored until their deaths, an analysis that uses a *lifetime time horizon*. Choice of time horizon, which is distinct from the assumed duration of treatment effect, can substantially influence estimates of cost effectiveness (Figure 1-24).[113] However, when a positive discount rate is used, the impact of extending a time horizon beyond a certain point will make little difference in a study's results because health effects and costs far into the future will have little present value.[112] In some cases, or

from certain perspectives, short-term horizons may be extremely relevant. For example, when considering the impact of a change in the generosity of insurance coverage for cardiovascular medications, a short (3-year) time horizon may be of interest from the perspective of private insurance companies in the United States because of the frequency with which patients change insurance coverage.[106,114]

Defining When a Therapy Is Cost Effective

The goal of cost-effectiveness analysis is to inform decisions about whether a new intervention represents a good value for the money and whether it should therefore be adopted into practice. In principle, an analysis of two interventions that differ with respect to both effectiveness and cost can have four possible results (Table 1-9). If the new intervention is both more effective and less costly than the standard of care—that is, it improves health and reduces spending—it is referred to as a *dominant* strategy and should almost always be adopted. If, in contrast, the new treatment increases costs and achieves worse outcomes, it is considered to be a *dominated* strategy and should be abandoned. In Western societies, interventions that provide lower quality health are seldom considered worthwhile, even if they reduce costs.

The majority of new technologies provide added health at added expense (see Table 1-9). Defining what level of added expense represents cost-effective care has been extensively debated for decades and generally relates to a given society's *cost-effectiveness threshold*. This threshold likely varies from setting to setting and is influenced by the role of the decision maker (e.g., a patient, an insurance company, or society as a whole),[3] their values and perceptions of risk,[115] and their respective budgetary constraints.

A threshold of $50,000 to $100,000 per QALY is extensively quoted in the literature but actually has little theoretical basis.[116] This level is thought to reflect the cost effectiveness of dialysis several decades ago, which is thought to be more than $120,000 per QALY when inflated to current levels.[3] In the United States, most modern health care interventions appear to have cost-utility ratios of between $109,000 and $297,000 per QALY.[117] In the United Kingdom, where cost effectiveness is one of the factors explicitly

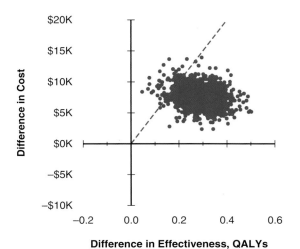

FIGURE 1-23 Probabilistic analysis based on the cost-effectiveness model presented in Figure 1-17. Each point represents the incremental cost and effectiveness of a test-and-treat strategy versus usual care for one simulation that samples the values for each variable in the model from a defined sensitivity range. In this analysis, 94% of the simulations produced cost-effectiveness rates below a willingness-to-pay threshold of $50,000 per quality-adjusted life-year (QALY), depicted by the *red dashed line*. (*Modified from Choudhry NK, Patrick AR, Glynn RJ, Avorn J. The cost-effectiveness of C-reactive protein testing and rosuvastatin treatment for patients with normal cholesterol levels. J Am Coll Cardiol 2011;57[7]:784-791.*)

TOOLS FOR ASSESSMENT OF CARDIOVASCULAR TESTS AND THERAPIES

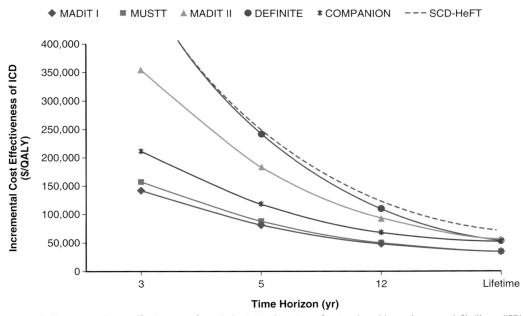

FIGURE 1-24 Variation in the incremental cost effectiveness of prophylactic implantation of an implantable cardioverter-defibrillator *(ICD)* with changes in the time horizon of ICD effectiveness in preventing sudden death. Shown are results from six trials in which the ICD was found to be efficacious. The *x* axis shows the time horizon of the analysis, which is also the duration of ICD-related reduction in mortality, after which there is no benefit; the *y* axis shows cost effectiveness. COMPANION, Comparison of Medical Therapy, Pacing, and Defibrillation in Heart Failure trial; DEFINITE, Defibrillators in Non-Ischemic Cardiomyopathy Treatment Evaluation trial; MADIT, Multicenter Automatic Defibrillator Implantation Trial; MUSTT, Multicenter Unsustained Tachycardia Trial; SCD-HeFT, Sudden Cardiac Death in Heart Failure Trial. (*Modified from Sanders GD, Hlatky MA, Owens DK. Cost-effectiveness of implantable cardioverter defibrillators. N Engl J Med 2005;353:1471-1480.*)

TABLE 1-9	Thresholds for Determining Whether a New Treatment Represents Good Value and Should Be Adopted Relative to an Existing Treatment		
COMPARED WITH EXISTING TREATMENTS	IMPROVED OUTCOMES	WORSE OUTCOMES
Reduces cost	Yes (dominant strategy)	Probably not
Increases cost	Maybe (based on cost-effectiveness/ utility ratio)	No (dominated strategy)

Box 1-4 How to Use an Economic Analysis

Are the results valid?
Did the recommendations consider all relevant patient groups, management options, and possible outcomes?
- Did investigators adopt a sufficiently broad viewpoint?
- Are results reported separately for relevant patient subgroups?
Is there a systematic review and summary of evidence linking options to outcomes for each relevant question?
- Were costs measured accurately?
- Did investigators consider the timing of costs and consequences?
How can I apply the results to patient care?
Are the treatment benefits worth the risks and costs?
Can I expect similar costs in my setting?
What are the results?
What were the incremental costs and effects of each strategy?
Do incremental costs and effects differ between subgroups?
How much does allowance for uncertainty change the results?

From Drummond M, Goeree R, Moayyedi P, Levine M. Economic analysis. In Guyatt G, Rennie D, Meade MO, Cook DJ, editors: *Users' Guides to the Medical Literature: A Manual for Evidence-Based Clinical Practice,* 2nd ed, New York, 2008, McGraw-Hill, p. 627.

evaluated when making coverage decisions, a threshold of $20,000 to $30,000 per QALY is generally considered to represent good value.[97] The WHO recommends a cutoff that corresponds to three times a country's gross domestic product, which results in thresholds of $5000 to $120,000 per QALY.[118]

How to Read an Economic Evaluation

A series of practical questions that readers should ask when assessing a cost-effectiveness analysis is presented in Box 1-4.[119] To determine whether the analysis provides a valid assessment of the value of an intervention, the reader must first be convinced that all relevant clinical strategies were evaluated and that the analysis considered an appropriate viewpoint or perspective, often that of society at large. All relevant clinical and economic outcomes must have been identified, including, for example, the costs of lost productivity, if this is relevant and appropriately estimated.[119] The results should present estimates of the incremental costs and the incremental effects of the interventions being considered and, in the case of cost-effectiveness and cost-utility analysis, the ratio of these two. Results should also be presented for important patient subgroups. Appropriate sensitivity analyses must have been conducted and presented to allow for the identification of factors that may have influenced the results.[120]

Determining whether the results apply to the decision maker's practice setting should be based on whether clinical outcomes similar to those found in the analysis could reasonably be expected and whether estimates of absolute and relative costs are largely comparable.[120] Finally, as discussed in the previous section, comparing the results to an appropriate cost-effectiveness threshold will help determine whether the added treatment benefits are worth the incremental harms and costs.

REFERENCES

1. World Health Organization. Web site. Accessed Feb 7, 2011 at www.who.int/en.
2. Heidenreich PA, Trogdon JG, Khavjou OA, et al. Forecasting the future of cardiovascular disease in the United States: a policy statement from the American Heart Association. *Circulation* 2011;123(8):933-944.
3. Owens DK, Qaseem A, Chou R, Shekelle P. High-value, cost-conscious health care: concepts for clinicians to evaluate the benefits, harms, and costs of medical interventions. *Ann Intern Med* 2011;154(3):174-180.
4. Sox HC. Comparative effectiveness research: a progress report. *Ann Intern Med* 2010;153(7):469-472.
5. Wong JB, Mulrow C, Sox HC. Health policy and cost-effectiveness analysis: yes we can. Yes we must. *Ann Intern Med* 2009;150(4):274-275.
6. Gibbons RJ, Gardner TJ, Anderson JL, et al. The American Heart Association's principles for comparative effectiveness research: a policy statement from the American Heart Association. *Circulation* 2009;119(22):2955-2962.
7. Wilensky GR. Cost-effectiveness information: yes, it's important, but keep it separate, please! *Ann Intern Med* 2008;148(12):967-968.
8. Antman EM. Evidence and education. *Circulation* 2011;123:681-685.
9. Gibbons RJ, Smith S, Antman E. American College of Cardiology/American Heart Association clinical practice guidelines: Part I: where do they come from? *Circulation* 2003;107(23):2979-2986.
10. Jong P, Gong Y, Liu PP, et al. Care and outcomes of patients newly hospitalized for heart failure in the community treated by cardiologists compared with other specialists. *Circulation* 2003;108(2):184-191.
11. Cook NL, Ayanian JZ, Orav EJ, Hicks LS. Differences in specialist consultations for cardiovascular disease by race, ethnicity, gender, insurance status, and site of primary care. *Circulation* 2009;119(18):2463-2470.
12. Williams SC, Schmaltz SP, Morton DJ, Koss RG, Loeb JM. Quality of care in U.S. hospitals as reflected by standardized measures, 2002-2004. *N Engl J Med* 2005;353(3):255-264.
13. Gauvreau K. Hypothesis testing: proportions. *Circulation* 2006;114(14):1545-1548.
14. Vandenbroucke JP. STREGA, STROBE, STARD, SQUIRE, MOOSE, PRISMA, GNOSIS, TREND, ORION, COREQ, QUOROM, REMARK ... and CONSORT: for whom does the guideline toll? *J Clin Epidemiol* 2009;62(6):594-596.
15. Grimes DA, Schulz KF. Refining clinical diagnosis with likelihood ratios. *Lancet* 2005;365(9469):1500-1505.
16. Rosner B. *Fundamentals of biostatistics,* 7th ed. Pacific Grove, CA, 2010, Duxbury Press.
17. Cook NR. Use and misuse of the receiver operating characteristic curve in risk prediction. *Circulation* 2007;115(7):928-935.
18. Greenland P, Alpert JS, Beller GA, et al. 2010 ACCF/AHA guideline for assessment of cardiovascular risk in asymptomatic adults: a report of the American College of Cardiology Foundation/American Heart Association Task Force on Practice Guidelines. *Circulation* 2010;122(25):e584-e636.
19. Antman EM. Design and conduct of clinical trials. In Bonow RO, Libby P, Mann DL, Zipes DP, editors: *Braunwald's heart disease: a textbook of cardiovascular medicine,* 9th ed. Philadelphia, 2011, Saunders Elsevier.
20. Cardiac Arrhythmia Suppression Trial Investigators. Preliminary report: effect of encainide and flecainide on mortality in a randomized trial of arrhythmia suppression after myocardial infarction. The CAST Investigators. *N Engl J Med* 1989;321:406-412.
21. Gibbons RJ, Smith SC Jr, Antman E. American College of Cardiology/American Heart Association clinical practice guidelines. Part II: evolutionary changes in a continuous quality improvement project. *Circulation* 2003;107(24):3101-3107.
22. Cleophas TJ, Zwinderman AH. Meta-analysis. *Circulation* 2007;115(22):2870-2875.
23. Taekman JM, Stafford-Smith M, Velazquez EJ, et al. Departures from the protocol during conduct of a clinical trial: a pattern from the data record consistent with a learning curve. *Qual Saf Health Care* 2010;19(5):405-410.
24. Wallentin L, Becker RC, Budaj A, et al. Ticagrelor versus clopidogrel in patients with acute coronary syndromes. *N Engl J Med* 2009;361(11):1045-1057.
25. Behrman RE, Benner JS, Brown JS, et al. Developing the sentinel system—a national resource for evidence development. *N Engl J Med* 2011;364:498-499.
26. Hamburg MA. Shattuck lecture: innovation, regulation, and the FDA. *N Engl J Med* 2010;363(23):2228-2232.
27. Friedman LM, Furberg CD, DeMets DL. *Fundamentals of clinical trials,* 4th ed. New York, 2010, Springer.
28. Clarke GM, Anderson CA, Pettersson FH, et al. Basic statistical analysis in genetic case-control studies. *Nat Protoc* 2011;6(2):121-133.
29. US Department of Health and Human Services, Food and Drug Administration, Center for Drug Evaluation and Research (CDER), Center for Biologics Evaluation and Research (CBER). Guidance for Industry: Adaptive Design Clinical Trials for Drugs and Biologics. 2010. Available at http://www.fda.gov/Drugs/GuidanceComplianceRegulatoryInformation/Guidances/ucm201790.pdf. Accessed Feb 7, 2011.
30. Mehta C, Gao P, Bhatt DL, et al. Optimizing trial design: sequential, adaptive, and enrichment strategies. *Circulation* 2009;119(4):597-605.
31. Miller FG, Joffe S. Equipoise and the dilemma of randomized clinical trials. *N Engl J Med* 2011;364(5):476-480.
32. DAMOCLES Study Group. A proposed charter for clinical trial data monitoring committees: helping them to do their job well. *Lancet* 2005;365(9460):711-722.
33. DeMets DL, Pocock SJ, Julian DG. The agonising negative trend in monitoring of clinical trials. *Lancet* 1999;354(9194):1983-1988.
34. Connolly SJ, Ezekowitz MD, Yusuf S, et al. Dabigatran versus warfarin in patients with atrial fibrillation. *N Engl J Med* 2009;361(12):1139-1151.
35. Tricoci P, Allen JM, Kramer JM, Califf RM, Smith SC Jr. Scientific evidence underlying the ACC/AHA clinical practice guidelines. *JAMA* 2009;301(8):831-841.
36. Sim I, Carini S, Tu S, et al. The human studies database project: federating human studies design data using the ontology of clinical research. *AMIA Summits Transl Sci Proc* 2010;Mar 1:51-55.

37. Wiviott SD, Braunwald E, McCabe CH, et al. Prasugrel versus clopidogrel in patients with acute coronary syndromes. *N Engl J Med* 2007;357(20):2001-2015.

38. Matlock DD, Peterson PN, Heidenreich PA, et al. Regional variation in the use of implantable cardioverter-defibrillators for primary prevention: results from the national cardiovascular data registry. *Circ Cardiovasc Qual Outcomes* 2011;4(1):114-121.

39. Stanley K. Design of randomized controlled trials. *Circulation* 2007;115(9):1164-1169.

40. Cole P, Beamer A, McGowan N, et al. Efficacy and safety of perhexiline maleate in refractory angina: a double-blind placebo-controlled clinical trial of a novel antianginal agent. *Circulation* 1990;81:1260-1270.

41. Packer M, Gheorghiade M, Young JB, et al. Withdrawal of digoxin from patients with chronic heart failure treated with angiotensin-converting-enzyme inhibitors. RADIANCE Study. *N Engl J Med* 1993;329(1):1-7.

42. Smith T. Digoxin in heart failure. *N Engl J Med* 1993;329:51-53.

43. The Digitalis Investigation Group. The effect of digoxin on mortality and morbidity in patients with heart failure. *N Engl J Med* 1997;336(8):525-533.

44. Mehta SR, Bassand JP, Chrolavicius S, et al. Design and rationale of CURRENT-OASIS 7: a randomized, 2 x 2 factorial trial evaluating optimal dosing strategies for clopidogrel and aspirin in patients with ST and non–ST-elevation acute coronary syndromes managed with an early invasive strategy. *Am Heart J* 2008;156(6):1080-1088, e1081.

45. Fuster V. Fine-tuning therapy for acute coronary syndromes. *N Engl J Med* 2010;363(10):976-977.

46. US Department of Health and Human Services, Food and Drug Administration, Center for Drug Evaluation and Research (CDER), Center for Biologics Evaluation and Research (CBER). Guidance for Industry: Non-Inferiority Clinical Trials, 2010. Available at http://www.fda.gov/downloads/Drugs/GuidanceComplianceRegulatoryInformation/Guidances/UCM202140.pdf. Accessed Feb 7, 2011.

47. Fleming TR. Current issues in non-inferiority trials. *Stat Med* 2008;27(3):317-332.

48. Piaggio G, Elbourne DR, Altman DG, et al. Reporting of noninferiority and equivalence randomized trials: an extension of the CONSORT statement. *JAMA* 2006;295(10):1152-1160.

49. DeMets DL, Califf RM. Lessons learned from recent cardiovascular clinical trials: part I. *Circulation* 2002;106(6):746-751.

50. Micheel CM, Ball JR, eds. *Evaluation of Surrogate Endpoints and Biomarkers in Chronic Disease*. Institute of Medicine Consensus Report. Washington, DC, 2010, National Academies Press.

51. Davis RB, Mukamal KJ. Hypothesis testing: means. *Circulation* 2006;114(10):1078-1082.

52. Rao SR, Schoenfeld DA. Survival methods. *Circulation* 2007;115(1):109-113.

53. US Department of Health and Human Services, Food and Drug Administration, Center for Biologics Evaluation and Research (CBER), Center for Drug Evaluation and Research (CDER), Center for Devices and Radiological Health (CDRH). Guidance for Clinical Trial Sponsors: Establishment and Operation of Clinical Trial Data Monitoring Committees, 2006. Available at http://www.fda.gov/OHRMS/DOCKETS/98fr/01d-0489-gdl0003.pdf. Accessed Feb 7, 2011.

54. US Department of Health and Human Services, Food and Drug Administration, Center for Drug Evaluation and Research (CDER), Center for Biologics Evaluation and Research (CBER). Guidance for Industry: E9 Statistical Principles for Clinical Trials, 1998. Available at http://www.fda.gov/downloads/Drugs/GuidanceComplianceRegulatoryInformation/Guidances/ucm073137.pdf. Accessed Feb 7, 2011.

55. Ware J, Muller J, Braunwald E. The futility index: an approach to the cost-effective termination of randomized clinical trials. *Am J Med* 1985;78:635-643.

56. Ellenberg SS, Fleming TR, DeMets DL. *Responsibilities of the Data Monitoring Committee and motivating illustrations. Data monitoring committees in clinical trials: a practical perspective*. Chichester, UK, 2002, John Wiley & Sons, pp 19-43.

57. DeMets DL, Furberg CD, Friedman LM. *Data monitoring in clinical trials: a case studies approach*. New York, 2006, Springer.

58. Pocock SJ. When (not) to stop a clinical trial for benefit. *JAMA* 2005;294(17):2228-2230.

59. Montori VM, Devereaux PJ, Adhikari NK, et al. Randomized trials stopped early for benefit: a systematic review. *JAMA* 2005;294(17):2203-2209.

60. Bassler D, Montori VM, Briel M, Glasziou P, Guyatt G. Early stopping of randomized clinical trials for overt efficacy is problematic. *J Clin Epidemiol* 2008;61(3):241-246.

61. Jones HE, Ohlssen DI, Neuenschwander B, Racine A, Branson M. Bayesian models for subgroup analysis in clinical trials. *Clin Trials* 2011;8(2):129-143.

62. Normand SL. Some old and some new statistical tools for outcomes research. *Circulation* 2008;118(8):872-884.

63. US Department of Health and Human Services, Food and Drug Administration, Office of the Commissioner (OC), Good Clinical Practice Program (GCPP). Guidance for Sponsors, Clinical Investigators, and IRBs: Data Retention When Subjects Withdraw from FDA-Regulated Clinical Trials, 2008. Available at http://www.fda.gov/downloads/regulatoryinformation/guidances/ucm126489.pdf. Accessed Feb 7, 2011.

64. Fleming TR. Addressing missing data in clinical trials. *Ann Intern Med* 2011;154(2):113-117.

65. National Research Council, Panel on Handling Missing Data in Clinical Trials. *The Prevention and Treatment of Missing Data in Clinical Trials*. Washington, DC, 2010, National Academies Press.

66. Kassai B, Gueyffier F, Boissel JP, et al. Absolute benefit, number needed to treat and gain in life expectancy: which efficacy indices for measuring the treatment benefit? *J Clin Epidemiol* 2003;56(10):977-982.

67. Bucher H, Weinbacher M, Gyr K. Influence of method of reporting study results on decision of physicians to prescribe drugs to lower cholesterol concentration. *Br Med J* 1994;309:761-764.

68. Antman EM, DeMets DL, Loscalzo J. Cyclooxygenase inhibition and cardiovascular risk. *Circulation* 2005;112:759-770.

69. Rothwell PM, Mehta Z, Howard SC, et al. Treating individuals 3: from subgroups to individuals: general principles and the example of carotid endarterectomy. *Lancet* 2005;365(9455):256-265.

70. Lagakos SW. The challenge of subgroup analyses—reporting without distorting. *N Engl J Med* 2006;354(16):1667-1669.

71. Schulz KF, Altman DG, Moher D, for the CONSORT Group. CONSORT 2010 statement: updated guidelines for reporting parallel group randomised trials. *PLoS Med* 7(3):31000251, 2010.

72. Stroup DF, Berlin JA, Morton SC, et al. Meta-analysis of observational studies in epidemiology: a proposal for reporting. Meta-analysis Of Observational Studies in Epidemiology (MOOSE) group. *JAMA* 2000;283(15):2008-2012.

73. Braunwald E, Antman E, Beasley J, et al. ACC/AHA 2002 guideline update for the management of patients with unstable angina and non–ST-segment elevation myocardial infarction: summary article: a report of the American College of Cardiology/American Heart Association Task Force on Practice Guidelines (Committee on the Management of Patients with Unstable Angina). *Circulation* 2002;106:1893-1900.

74. Eikelboom JW, Anand SS, Malmberg K, et al. Unfractionated heparin and low-molecular-weight heparin in acute coronary syndrome without ST elevation: a meta-analysis. *Lancet* 2000;355(9219):1936-1942.

75. Salanti G, Ades AE, Ioannidis JP. Graphical methods and numerical summaries for presenting results from multiple-treatment meta-analysis: an overview and tutorial. *J Clin Epidemiol* 2011;64(2):163-171.

76. Knottnerus JA, Tugwell P. Ongoing innovation in meta-analysis. *J Clin Epidemiol* 2011;64(2):117-118.

77. Bagos PG, Nikolopoulos GK. Generalized least squares for assessing trends in cumulative meta-analysis with applications in genetic epidemiology. *J Clin Epidemiol* 2009; 62(10):1037-1044.

78. Antman EM, Lau J, Kupelnick B, Mosteller F, Chalmers TC. A comparison of results of meta-analyses of randomized control trials and recommendations of clinical experts: treatments for myocardial infarction. *JAMA* 1992;268(2):240-248.

79. Berkey CS, Mosteller F, Lau J, Antman EM. Uncertainty of the time of first significance in random effects cumulative meta-analysis. *Control Clin Trials* 1996;17(5):357-371.

80. Morton SC, Adams JL, Suttorp MJ, Shekelle PG. *Meta-regression Approaches: What, Why, When, and How?* Technical Review 8 (Prepared by Southern California-RAND Evidence-based Practice Center under Contract No 290-97-0001). AHRQ Publication No. 04-0033. Rockville, MD, 2004, Agency for Healthcare Research and Quality.

81. Yusuf S, Mehta SR, Chrolavicius S, et al. Effects of fondaparinux on mortality and reinfarction in patients with acute ST-segment elevation myocardial infarction: the OASIS-6 randomized trial. *JAMA* 2006;295(13):1519-1530.

82. Antithrombotic Trialists' Collaboration. Collaborative meta-analysis of randomised trials of antiplatelet therapy for prevention of death, myocardial infarction, and stroke in high risk patients. *Br Med J* 2002;324(7329):71-86.

83. Fibrinolytic Therapy Trialists' Collaborative Group. Indications for fibrinolytic therapy in suspected acute myocardial infarction: collaborative overview of mortality and major morbidity results from all randomised trials of more than 1000 patients. FTT Collaborative Group. *Lancet* 1994;343:311-322.

84. Yusuf S, Zucker D, Peduzzi P, et al. Effect of coronary artery bypass graft surgery on survival: an overview of 10-year results from randomised trials by the Coronary Artery Bypass Graft Surgery Trialists Collaboration. *Lancet* 1994;344:563-570.

85. Cholesterol Treatment Trialists' Collaboration (CTT). Available at http://www.ctsu.ox.ac.uk/projects/ctt. Accessed Feb 7, 2011.

86. Lewin S, Lavis JN, Oxman AD, et al. Supporting the delivery of cost-effective interventions in primary health-care systems in low-income and middle-income countries: an overview of systematic reviews. *Lancet* 2008;372(9642):928-939.

87. Keirns CC, Goold SD. Patient-centered care and preference-sensitive decision making. *JAMA* 2009;302(16):1805-1806.

88. Institute of Medicine. *Initial National Priorities for Comparative Effectiveness Research*. Washington, DC, 2009, Institute of Medicine.

89. Luce BR, Kramer JM, Goodman SN, et al. Rethinking randomized clinical trials for comparative effectiveness research: the need for transformational change. *Ann Intern Med* 2009;151(3):206-209.

90. Song F, Altman DG, Glenny AM, Deeks JJ. Validity of indirect comparison for estimating efficacy of competing interventions: empirical evidence from published meta-analyses. *Br Med J* 2003;326(7387):472.

91. Schneeweiss S. Developments in post-marketing comparative effectiveness research. *Clin Pharmacol Ther* 2007;82(2):143-156.

92. Freeman JV, Zhu RP, Owens DK, et al. Cost-effectiveness of dabigatran compared with warfarin for stroke prevention in atrial fibrillation. *Ann Intern Med* 2011;154(1):1-11.

93. Drummond MF, O'Brien BJ, Stoddart GL, Torrance GW. *Methods for the economic evaluation of health care programs*. Oxford, UK, 1997, Oxford University Press.

94. Gold MR, Stevenson D, Fryback DG. HALYs and QALYs and DALYs, oh my: similarities and differences in summary measures of population health. *Annu Rev Public Health* 2002;23:115-134.

95. Chen GJ, Ferrucci L, Moran WP, Pahor M. A cost-minimization analysis of diuretic-based antihypertensive therapy reducing cardiovascular events in older adults with isolated systolic hypertension. *Cost Eff Resour Alloc* 2005;3(1):2.

96. Mark DB, Hlatky MA. Medical economics and the assessment of value in cardiovascular medicine: part I. *Circulation* 2002;106(4):516-520.

97. Appleby J, Devlin N, Parkin D. NICE's cost effectiveness threshold. *Br Med J* 2007;335(7616):358-359.

98. Drummond MF, Davies L. Economic analysis alongside clinical trials: revisiting the methodological issues. *Int J Technol Assess Health Care* 1991;7(4):561-573.

99. Finkler SA. The distinction between cost and charges. *Ann Intern Med* 1982;96(1):102-109.

100. Heidenreich PA, Masoudi FA, Maini B, et al. Echocardiography in patients with suspected endocarditis: a cost-effectiveness analysis. *Am J Med* 1999;107(3):198-208.

101. Mahoney EM, Wang K, Arnold SV, et al. Cost-effectiveness of prasugrel versus clopidogrel in patients with acute coronary syndromes and planned percutaneous coronary intervention: results from the trial to assess improvement in therapeutic outcomes by optimizing platelet inhibition with prasugrel-thrombolysis in myocardial infarction TRITON-TIMI 38. *Circulation* 2010;121(1):71-79.

102. Choudhry NK, Patrick AR, Glynn RJ, Avorn J. The cost-effectiveness of C-reactive protein testing and rosuvastatin treatment for patients with normal cholesterol levels. *J Am Coll Cardiol* 2011;57(7):784-791.

103. Weintraub WS, Mahoney EM, Lamy A, et al. Long-term cost-effectiveness of clopidogrel given for up to one year in patients with acute coronary syndromes without ST-segment elevation. *J Am Coll Cardiol* 2005;45(6):838-845.

104. Mark DB, Hlatky MA, Califf RM, et al. Cost-effectiveness of thrombolytic therapy with tissue plasminogen activator as compared with streptokinase for acute myocardial infarction. *N Engl J Med* 1995;332(21):1418-1424.

105. Patrick AR, Avorn J, Choudhry NK. Cost-effectiveness of genotype-guided warfarin dosing for patients with atrial fibrillation. *Circ Cardiovasc Qual Outcomes* 2009; 2(5):429-436.

106. Choudhry NK, Avorn J, Antman EM, Schneeweiss S, Shrank WH. Should patients receive secondary prevention medications for free after a myocardial infarction? An economic analysis. *Health Aff (Millwood)* 2007;26(1):186-194.

107. Russell LB, Gold MR, Siegel JE, Daniels N, Weinstein MC. The role of cost-effectiveness analysis in health and medicine. Panel on Cost-Effectiveness in Health and Medicine. *JAMA* 1996;276(14):1172-1177.

108. Kupersmith J, Holmes-Rovner M, Hogan A, Rovner D, Gardiner J. Cost-effectiveness analysis in heart disease, Part I: general principles. *Prog Cardiovasc Dis* 1994;37(3): 161-184.

109. Detsky AS, Naglie IG. A clinician's guide to cost-effectiveness analysis. *Ann Intern Med* 1990;113(2):147-154.

110. Sox HC, Blatt MA, Higgins MC, et al. *Medical decision making.* Stoneham, MA, 1988, Butterworth.

111. Kuntz KM, Tsevat J, Weinstein MC, Goldman L. Expert panel vs decision-analysis recommendations for postdischarge coronary angiography after myocardial infarction. *JAMA* 1999;282(23):2246-2251.

112. Gold MR, Siegel JE, Russel L, Weinstein MC. *Cost-effectiveness in health and medicine.* Oxford, UK, 1996, Oxford University Press.

113. Sanders GD, Hlatky MA, Owens DK. Cost-effectiveness of implantable cardioverter-defibrillators. *N Engl J Med* 2005;353(14):1471-1480.

114. Choudhry NK, Patrick AR, Antman EM, Avorn J, Shrank WH. Cost-effectiveness of providing full drug coverage to increase medication adherence in post-myocardial infarction Medicare beneficiaries. *Circulation* 2008;117(10):1261-1268.

115. Garber AM, Phelps CE. Economic foundations of cost-effectiveness analysis. *J Health Econ* 1997;16(1):1-31.

116. Ubel PA, Hirth RA, Chernew ME, Fendrick AM. What is the price of life and why doesn't it increase at the rate of inflation? *Arch Intern Med* 2003;163(14):1637-1641.

117. Braithwaite RS, Meltzer DO, King JT Jr, Leslie D, Roberts MS. What does the value of modern medicine say about the $50,000 per quality-adjusted life-year decision rule? *Med Care* 2008;46(4):349-356.

118. World Health Organization. *Choosing Interventions that are cost effective (WHO-CHOICE).* Available at www.who.int/choice/en. Accessed March 22, 2011.

119. Drummond MF, Richardson WS, O'Brien BJ, Levine M, Heyland D. Users' guides to the medical literature. XIII. How to use an article on economic analysis of clinical practice. A. Are the results of the study valid? Evidence-Based Medicine Working Group. *JAMA* 1997;277(19):1552-1557.

120. O'Brien BJ, Heyland D, Richardson WS, Levine M, Drummond MF. Users' guides to the medical literature. XIII. How to use an article on economic analysis of clinical practice. B. What are the results and will they help me in caring for my patients? Evidence-Based Medicine Working Group. *JAMA* 1997;277(22):1802-1806.

121. Felker GM, Lee KL, Bull DA, et al. Diuretic strategies in patients with acute decompensated heart failure. *N Engl J Med* 2011;364(9):797-805.

122. Matchar DB, McCrory DC, Orlando LA, et al. Systematic review: comparative effectiveness of angiotensin-converting enzyme inhibitors and angiotensin II receptor blockers for treating essential hypertension. *Ann Intern Med* 2008;148(1):16-29.

123. Pilote L, Abrahamowicz M, Rodrigues E, Eisenberg MJ, Rahme E. Mortality rates in elderly patients who take different angiotensin-converting enzyme inhibitors after acute myocardial infarction: a class effect? *Ann Intern Med* 2004;141(2):102-112.

CHAPTER 2

New Drug Development

David F. Kong and Robert A. Harrington

OVERVIEW OF THE DRUG DEVELOPMENT PROCESS, 33

Phase I to IV Paradigm, 33
Cycle of New Therapeutic Development, 33
Regulation of New Drugs: Prototypical Interface with the Food
   and Drug Administration, 34
Advisory Panels, 35
Labeling, 35
Postmarketing Surveillance, 35
Exemptions from Investigational New Drug Application and
   Practice of Medicine, 36
CDER Versus CBER: Key Differences for Biologics, 36

INTERNATIONAL DRUG DEVELOPMENT OVERVIEW, 36

Ethics of Drug Development in Developing Countries, 37

ANATOMY OF A CLINICAL TRIAL: OPERATIONS, 37

Protocol Development, 37
Site Management, 38
Data Management, 38
Statistics, 38
Safety Surveillance, 38
Clinical Events Adjudication, 38

ECONOMICS OF NEW DRUG DEVELOPMENT, 38

Prescription Drug User Fee Act, 38
National Institutes of Health Roadmap Program, 39
Patent Considerations, 39

SUMMARY, 39

REFERENCES, 39

Cardiovascular medicine has been in the vanguard of new therapeutic development since 1955, when President Dwight Eisenhower's myocardial infarction (MI) in office captured worldwide attention.[1] Many forces contribute to this positioning of cardiovascular medicine among specialties, including the alignment of patient care needs, multidisciplinary translational research, market forces, industrial production, and public health priorities. Another enabling feature is a regulatory environment that is rapidly becoming more harmonized as the process of development of new therapeutics becomes a more global endeavor. However, despite advances in translational discoveries and enormous investment in development programs, the number of new compounds that receive regulatory approval has slowly declined. A thorough understanding of new cardiovascular therapeutic development is essential for navigating an increasingly complex economic and regulatory environment and for managing the forces that contribute to challenges in development programs.

Overview of the Drug Development Process

Phase I to IV Paradigm

For a promising candidate drug to become commercially available, the developer must demonstrate efficacy and safety.[2] Although some preliminary assessments can be performed in the preclinical setting, the principal purpose of preclinical laboratory and animal model studies is to provide data showing that the new drug will not expose human subjects to unreasonable risks when used in limited, early-stage clinical studies. (Investigation of the effects of a drug in human subjects is governed by rules that fall within the oversight responsibility of the U.S. Food and Drug Administration [FDA] and are discussed in the next section.)

Additional safety and pharmacokinetic information is gathered during phase I development. In this phase, the new compound is administered to healthy human volunteers. Rates of elimination and pharmacodynamic measurements are often obtained to provide information about absorption, bioavailability, half-life, elimination, and other biomarkers. In addition, there is close monitoring for safety signals and major toxicity.

Based on the preliminary measures of effect observed in phase I, the new drug is administered to affected subjects in phase II, which provides information on dosing as a prelude to establishing both effectiveness and safety. Several potential phase II designs may be used, including dose-escalation, "drop-the-loser," and parallel-group studies. At the end of phase II, the goal is to have determined the preferred dose for use in larger phase III trials. The penalty for using the wrong dose, or for not identifying the correct dose, can have substantial implications for later phases.[3,4]

In phase III, the new drug is administered to a large number of patients in a manner similar to its intended use in an attempt to demonstrate safety and effectiveness. The high prevalence of cardiovascular disease (approximately 1.25 million new and recurrent acute coronary syndromes are diagnosed annually in the United States[5]) allows most phase III trials to demonstrate efficacy using conventional statistics. New treatments that offer only modest improvements over existing therapy may require more complex statistical methods, prompting the FDA to develop guidance documents for adaptive and noninferiority clinical trial designs.[6,7] The information compiled in phases I through III is then submitted for evaluation by a regulatory authority and forms the basis for marketing approval. Once approved, the drug can be marketed commercially.

Often interest continues in refining the precision of estimates of a particular drug's safety and effectiveness, even after initial regulatory approval. Phase IV trials may seek to refine dosing, expand the drug indication to additional populations that were less well represented in earlier development work, or provide ongoing safety surveillance. Overall, the resources required to sustain this pipeline are considerable. Between 1994 and 2003, annual biomedical research funding in the United States increased from $37.1 billion to $94.3 billion, yet FDA approvals dropped from 36 to 23 new molecular entities per year.[8] Thousands of candidate molecules are scanned in the drug discovery process, yet only 8% of new molecular entities will successfully emerge from preclinical assessments to a commercial launch. The process of discovering and developing a new molecular entity on average requires approximately 13.5 years, not including the time required to identify the drug target (Figure 2-1).[9]

Cycle of New Therapeutic Development

Beyond phase I through IV trials, which provide key evidence to support or repudiate a new therapy, other aspects to the product life cycle exist (Figure 2-2). In the cycle of clinical therapeutic development, new concepts resulting from discovery and translational research advance through the phase I through IV paradigm to create evidence that supports clinical decision making. The overall evidence, which compares the efficacy and safety of different therapeutic strategies against one another, not just against placebo, forms the basis for clinical practice guidelines. Implementation of the guidelines is subject to their acceptance by the clinical community and to societal willingness to accept the nonclinical consequences of new treatment paradigms, such as cost. Key performance indicators provide education and feedback for the guidelines and help identify critical needs for additional therapeutic strategies. Assessments of performance and outcomes drive subsequent rounds of evidence synthesis and therapeutic innovation.

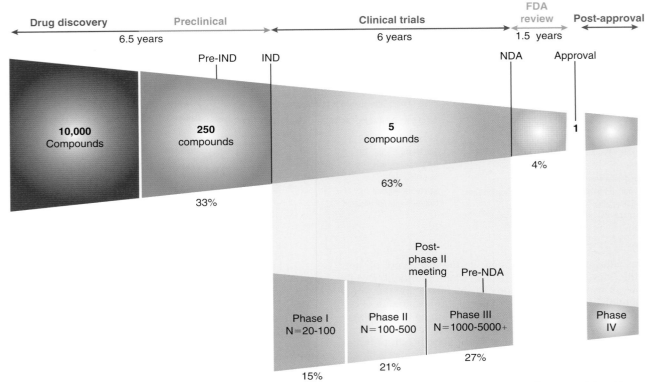

FIGURE 2-1 A typical drug development pipeline. More than 10,000 candidate compounds may be evaluated to launch a single approved drug. Key regulatory meetings and milestones are indicated. The relative costs of the preclinical phase (phases I through III) and regulatory submission to the development program are shown as percentages. These proportions exclude the costs of drug discovery and postapproval (phase IV) activities. FDA, Food and Drug Administration; NDA, New Drug Application. *(Modified from Robertson D, Williams G (eds).* Clinical and translational science: principles of human research. *Waltham, MA, 2008, Academic Press; Paul SM, Mytelka DS, Dunwiddie CT, et al. How to improve R&D productivity: the pharmaceutical industry's grand challenge.* Nat Rev Drug Discov *9:203-214, 2010; and U.S. Food and Drug Administration. Guidances. Available at* http://www.fda.gov/opacom/morechoices/industry/guidedc.htm.)

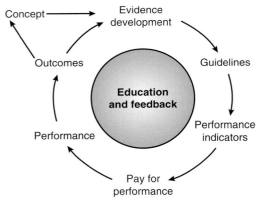

FIGURE 2-2 The cycle of clinical therapeutics. *(Modified from Califf RM, Peterson ED, Gibbons RJ, et al. Integrating quality into the cycle of therapeutic development.* J Am Coll Cardiol *2002;40:1895-1901.)*

Regulation of New Drugs: Prototypical Interface with the Food and Drug Administration

In the United States, new cardiovascular therapies are regulated by the FDA, which has three main centers: the Center for Drug Evaluation and Research (CDER), which oversees chemical drugs; the Center for Biologics Evaluation and Research (CBER), which oversees biologics; and the Center for Devices and Radiological Health, which governs medical devices. The regulatory process for devices

is outlined in Chapter 3. Rules that govern the regulatory processes for investigation and approval of new therapeutics in the United States are found in the Code of Federal Regulations (CFR), which is divided into 50 titles. FDA-regulated research is described in Title 21, and general rules for protection of human subjects are found in title 45. For drugs, the key regulations are found in 21 CFR 312.[10]

A new drug's eligibility for interstate commerce, including shipment across state lines for distribution to clinical research sites, depends on an approved marketing application from the FDA. When a new therapeutic compound moves from the preclinical arena (bench or animal testing) to clinical development (testing in humans), it becomes a drug subject to specific federal regulations. To be exempted from the requirements for marketing approval, the sponsor must obtain an exemption from the FDA in the form of an Investigational New Drug (IND) Application.[11]

BEFORE THE INVESTIGATIONAL NEW DRUG APPLICATION

The FDA encourages sponsors to communicate with the agency to obtain guidance on the data necessary to support an IND submission. Most cardiovascular therapeutic evaluations are assigned to the Division of Cardiovascular and Renal Products (cardio-renal), although some anticoagulant products have been reviewed by the Division of Hematology Products. Pre-IND advice may be requested for many issues related to initial drug development plans, regulatory requirements for demonstrating safety and efficacy, and data requirements for an IND. These include the data needed to support the rationale for testing a drug in humans and the design of nonclinical pharmacology, toxicology, and drug activity studies, including treatment studies in animal models. Pre-IND interactions are considered preliminary communications based on early development information and generally take the form of written comments that may be supplemented by teleconferences or meetings. Additions or modifications to these communications may arise as information becomes available during follow-up, pre-IND interactions, or when an IND is established.

TYPES OF INVESTIGATIONAL NEW DRUG APPLICATION

Broadly defined, there are three different types of INDs. An *investigator IND* is submitted by a physician, who both initiates and conducts an investigation and under whose immediate direction the investigational drug is administered or dispensed. A physician might submit an investigator IND to propose studying an unapproved drug or an approved product for a new indication or in a new patient population. An *emergency use IND* allows the FDA to authorize use of an experimental drug in an emergency situation that does not allow time for submission of the typical IND. It is also used for patients who do not meet the criteria of an existing study protocol or when an approved study protocol does not exist. A *treatment IND* is submitted for experimental drugs showing promise in clinical testing for serious or immediately life-threatening conditions while the final clinical work is conducted and the FDA review takes place.

IND applications provide information to the FDA about animal studies, manufacturing information, and clinical development protocols. Sponsors must submit sufficient preclinical data to establish that the new compound is reasonably safe to begin initial testing in humans.[12,13] Any previous experience with the compound in humans, often from data collected outside the United States, must also be included in the application. Detailed manufacturing data describing the drug's composition, its manufacturer, its stability, and the controls used for manufacturing the new drug are reviewed to ensure that the company can adequately produce and supply consistent batches of the new drug.

Of greatest importance to clinical investigators, the IND includes detailed protocols for the anticipated clinical studies, which allow the FDA to ascertain the risks to participants in the initial trials. The IND also includes assurances that study leaders will adhere to the pertinent regulations regarding clinical trial conduct and human subject protection, including informed consent and institutional review board evaluation.

Once the IND is submitted, the sponsor must wait 30 calendar days before initiating any clinical trials. During this time, the FDA has an opportunity to review the IND for safety to ensure that research participants will not be subjected to unreasonable risk.

Advisory Panels

Ultimately, the FDA is responsible for evaluating IND applications that propose the marketing of new drugs or the expansion of indications for previously approved drugs. A new drug that confers substantial benefit with minimal toxicity or other risks poses no major problems for FDA regulators. In many cases, however, the risk/benefit ratio is less certain, and the pharmaceutical sponsor and the FDA may differ in their evaluations of these issues.

Since 1972, the FDA has called on panels of experts to provide advice in such situations. For cardiovascular drugs, this advice is offered by the Cardiovascular and Renal Drugs Advisory Committee (CRAC).[14,15] The advisory panels do not actually decide whether drugs should be approved; rather, they provide recommendations to the FDA, which holds the legal authority to grant or deny approval. The FDA is not obliged to accept recommendations made by its advisory panels.

Labeling

Once the FDA has determined that a new therapeutic compound is potentially approvable, much attention is given to how the product is labeled to ensure truth and accuracy. The drug label directly affects the statements that can be made by the sponsor in future claims, promotions, and advertisements for the new drug. In general, labels must summarize the essential scientific information required for safe and effective use of the drug and must be based on as much supporting human experience data as possible. By regulation, all express or implied claims in labeling must be supported by substantial evidence (21 CFR 201.56[a][3]).[16] As a consequence, the dosing and indications described in the label usually reflect the doses and populations that were used in the phase III clinical trials submitted for regulatory approval.

In some instances, certain statements about a drug or class of drugs are required by regulation to be included in the label. For example, 21 CFR 310.517 mandates that labeling for sulfonylurea class oral hypoglycemics must include specific warnings.[17] In other instances, labels for all drugs within a class contain identical statements (class labeling) to describe a risk or effect that is typically associated with the class based on the pharmacology or chemistry of the drug class. For example, the boxed warning about the risk of using an angiotensin-converting enzyme inhibitor during the second and third trimesters of pregnancy is uniformly presented in all labeling for this class of drugs.[18]

CASE STUDY: ANTIHYPERTENSIVES. Until recently, the labeling for antihypertensive products included only the information that the drugs were indicated to reduce blood pressure; it did not include information on the clinical benefits related to cardiovascular outcomes expected from blood pressure reductions. In 2005, CRAC discussed class labeling for cardiovascular outcome claims for drugs indicated to treat hypertension. The committee voiced a broad consensus in favor of antihypertensive agent labeling changes that would describe the cardiovascular outcome benefits expected from lowering blood pressure. Subsequently, in 2008, the FDA formulated a drug-labeling industry guidance for cardiovascular outcome claims for drugs indicated for hypertension.[19]

CASE STUDY: ORAL HYPOGLYCEMIC AGENTS. Sitagliptin was the first in a class of diabetic drugs (dipeptidyl peptidase-4 inhibitors) designed to increase endogenous insulin secretion and suppress glucagon release. In October 2006, the FDA approved sitagliptin based on clinical studies showing that the drug reduced glycated hemoglobin A1c levels compared with placebo. At that time, hemoglobin A1c was regarded as the primary efficacy endpoint for glucose reduction. In 2007, cardiovascular events associated with rosiglitazone prompted additional discussion at the FDA regarding the types of evidence required for new diabetes drugs to obtain approval. In July 2008, the Endocrinologic and Metabolic Drugs Advisory Committee was asked whether sponsors of a drug or biologic should conduct a long-term cardiovascular trial or provide equivalent evidence to exclude unacceptable cardiovascular risks, even in the absence of a cardiovascular safety signal during phase II and phase III development. Of the 16 voting members, 14 voted yes.[20] In December 2008, the FDA issued guidance regarding the evaluation of cardiovascular risk for diabetes therapies.[21] The guidance asks manufacturers to demonstrate that new therapies for type 2 diabetes do not unacceptably increase cardiovascular risk. The subsequent reviews of saxagliptin and liraglutide were evaluated closely for cardiovascular safety outcomes and exemplify the regulatory shift from sole evaluation of surrogate biomarkers, such as hemoglobin A1c, to a broader evaluation of clinical safety events.

Postmarketing Surveillance

Although phase III pivotal studies may evaluate the safety of a new compound in thousands of patients, additional adverse effects may remain undetected at the time of initial regulatory approval. Consequently, postmarketing surveillance and risk-assessment programs are essential for identifying safety signals that are not apparent before approval. The FDA uses the data from postmarketing surveillance to update drug labeling and, on rare occasions, to reevaluate the approval or marketing decision (21 CFR 314.80).[22,23]

The Adverse Event Reporting System (AERS) is a computerized database designed to support the FDA's postmarketing safety surveillance program. AERS includes voluntary reports submitted by health professionals and the public through the MedWatch program, as well as reports from manufacturers that are required by regulation. Reports in AERS are evaluated by the Center for Drug Evaluation and Research Office of Surveillance and Epidemiology to detect safety signals. These analyses may prompt the FDA to improve product safety by taking regulatory action, such as by updating a product's labeling information, sending out a notification ("Dear Health Care Professional") letter,[24,25] or reevaluating an approval decision.

CASE STUDY: DRONEDARONE. Dronedarone is an antiarrhythmic agent similar to amiodarone, often used for suppression of atrial fibrillation. Few direct comparisons of dronedarone and amiodarone exist, although each drug has been evaluated extensively against placebo. The safety profile of dronedarone led to regulatory approval by the FDA and other regulatory authorities, although indirect analyses suggested that dronedarone was less effective for the prevention of atrial fibrillation compared with amiodarone.[26] The FDA approval included a risk evaluation and mitigation strategy, as well as additional requirements for postmarketing drug safety surveillance.[27] After approval, the FDA received several case reports of hepatic failure in patients treated with dronedarone, including two postmarketing reports of acute hepatic failure requiring transplantation. A notification letter was issued by the manufacturer to communicate these additional risks to clinicians, and the labeling was subsequently revised.[28]

Exemptions from Investigational New Drug Application and Practice of Medicine

In the practice of medicine, it is not uncommon for some therapeutic agents to become de facto standards of care on an empirical basis before there is a labeled indication for that particular use. The government has long permitted physicians to prescribe or administer any legally marketed product within the practice of medicine, which is generally regulated by state laws. If physicians use a drug for an indication not in the approved labeling, they should base their decision on sound scientific evidence as part of good medical practice.

The FDA may consider some research studies exempt from specific regulations governing new therapeutic agents. In general, research protocols may be eligible for exemption from the IND requirements by evaluating drugs 1) that are already approved by the FDA, 2) that do not significantly increase the risk or decrease the acceptability of risk to study subjects, 3) that use the drugs in a manner consistent with their approved labeling, and 4) that are not intended to be reported to the FDA in support of a labeling or advertising change.

INVESTIGATOR-INITIATED INVESTIGATIONAL NEW DRUG APPLICATION

Many research protocols involving new drugs, or new uses for existing drugs, do not meet the criteria for exemption from regulation and therefore require investigator-initiated INDs. Changes to established dosing, drug delivery systems, routes of administration, or concomitant therapy (such as a new combination product) may result in the need for an IND. An investigator IND is submitted by a physician who both initiates and conducts an investigation and under whose immediate direction the investigational drug is administered or dispensed. Investigator-initiated research comprises a much larger share of INDs than pharmaceutical company–sponsored research. Academic institutions and individual practitioners submitted approximately 3.5 INDs for every commercial IND submitted between 1986 and 2005.[29] If the investigator also assumes the role of sponsor for a new drug, additional documentation and reporting to the FDA are required. These include safety and adverse event reports within the required timeframes and an annual report within 60 days of the anniversary date on which the IND went into effect. The sponsor is also expected to select qualified investigators, perform ongoing monitoring, and ensure compliance. If the investigator is using a commercially manufactured drug and secures permission from the manufacturer, it is possible to reference the existing Drug Master File at the FDA for details of the manufacturing data.

CDER Versus CBER: Key Differences for Biologics

The FDA regulates biologic products—blood components and products made from blood, such as clotting factors, gene therapy, tissues for transplantation, and vaccines—through CBER. Biologic products introduced into interstate commerce are regulated under 21 CFR 600-680. Since its inception in 1987, CBER has been closely tied with CDER, and the two centers have weathered several rounds of reorganization over the ensuing decades. Most recently, the oversight for biopharmaceuticals—proteins extracted from animals or microorganisms that are intended for therapeutic use, including recombinant versions of these products, except clotting factors—was transferred from CBER to CDER.[30] Biopharmaceutical development often has different challenges compared with that of traditional chemical drugs, including variations in potency, less correlation between animal and human models, and unique uncertainties with regard to mechanisms of action and potential risks to human subjects. As the development of biopharmaceuticals has become more common, the regulatory practices of CDER and CBER have become remarkably harmonized, in part due to active efforts between the two centers to share regulatory decisions and standardize review processes. Consequently, future regulation of biologics is likely to resemble traditional pharmaceutical development more closely. An evolving area of interest concerns biosimilar compounds, for which the factors of identity and potency are still less certain than those for generic chemical drugs.[31]

When regulatory pathways were well defined and agents from both centers were developed in parallel, CDER and CBER regulatory standards did not differ. CDER's regulatory requirements for bivalirudin, a direct thrombin inhibitor for the treatment of postinfarction angina with angioplasty, were nearly identical to those used by CBER for abciximab, a biopharmaceutical glycoprotein IIb/IIIa inhibitor seeking the same indication.[32,33]

International Drug Development Overview

As cardiovascular therapeutic development becomes increasingly global, the processes for regulatory approval of new cardiovascular drugs to be used outside the United States become vital to the global pharmaceutical industry. Since 2002, the number of FDA-regulated investigators based outside the United States has grown by 15%, while the number of U.S.-based investigators has declined by 5.5%. Of 300 clinical trials published in the *New England Journal of Medicine*, the *Journal of the American Medical Association*, and the *Lancet* between 1995 and 2005, the number of non-U.S. trial sites more than doubled, whereas the proportion of trials in the United States decreased.[34] Ideally, clinical research performed in one country should inform regulatory decisions made in another; however, for many years this ideal was removed from reality as individual regulatory authorities applied their own unique standards for efficacy and safety.

Frequent concerns with data collected in a different country or region include the potential for differences to exist in practice guidelines, standards of care, or use of adjunct therapies. Most regulatory authorities desire studies to be conducted in populations that include the types of patients who would be exposed to the drug if it were to become commercially available. Quality of study conduct, adherence to study protocol, and loss of subjects to follow-up are also common concerns. Furthermore, rapid advances in pharmaceutical development in the 1960s and 1970s led to a broad divergence in regulations and technical requirements among different companies, adding expense and complexity to global therapeutic development programs.[35]

CASE STUDY: ACCOUNTING FOR REGIONAL VARIATION IN GLOBAL THERAPEUTIC DEVELOPMENT PROGRAMS. Ticagrelor, a P2Y12 platelet inhibitor, was compared with clopidogrel in a large randomized clinical trial of more than 18,000 patients. Although ticagrelor was globally superior to clopidogrel for preventing the composite of cardiovascular death, MI, and stroke, a prespecified subgroup analysis showed a significant interaction between treatment and region, with less effect of ticagrelor in North America than in the rest of the world.[36] The regional interaction could arise from chance alone or could reflect an underlying statistical interaction with concomitant aspirin dosing. The European Medicines Agency approved ticagrelor on December 6, 2010, but U.S. regulators grappled with the subgroup analysis, eventually leading to approval in July 2011 with a warning that use of ticagrelor with aspirin doses greater than 100 mg daily decreases the drug's effectiveness. Conversely, the initial evaluation of eptifibatide, a glycoprotein IIb/IIIa receptor antagonist, had regional differences, with point estimates of relative treatment effect greater in North America than in Eastern Europe.[37] These circumstances led to U.S. approval in May 1998 but delayed European approval until July 1999.

Many of these differences are rapidly resolving through harmonization efforts. The European Union (EU) maintains an agency, the European Medicines Agency (EMA), which is responsible for the scientific evaluation of medicines for use in the EU. Since 1995, the EMA has maintained a centralized authorization procedure for human and veterinary medicinal products, and it regulates marketing, manufacture, and distribution. Current priorities for the EMA include stimulating drug development in areas of unmet medical need, facilitating new approaches to medicine development, addressing the high attrition rate of therapeutics during pharmacologic development, and strengthening postauthorization evidence bases.[38]

The World Trade Organization has been a driving force for harmonization of regulatory review in China, with central regulation of drug approvals in place since 1985. In India, the central government regulates new drug approvals, clinical trials, and importation of drugs, and regulation of the manufacture, sale, and distribution of pharmaceuticals is decentralized to state authorities. Japanese drug development is regulated by the Pharmaceuticals and Medical Devices Agency (PMDA), which has separate offices for new drugs, biologics, and medical devices. The PMDA was established in 2004 through the integration of two earlier centers, and it handles all consultation and review from the preclinical stage to approval and postmarketing surveillance.[39] In Latin America, Brazil and Mexico have mature regulatory systems, with emerging regulatory environments elsewhere. MERCOSUR (Common Market of the South) and Andean member countries tend to harmonize with Brazil, whereas Mexico has a structure more similar to its North American allies that parallels the FDA in the United States.

Much of the adaptation occurring among the regulatory systems in the United States, Europe, and Japan is a result of the International Conference on Harmonisation of Technical Requirements for Registration of Pharmaceuticals for Human Use (ICH). Established in 1990, the ICH has convened the regulatory authorities and pharmaceutical industries of Europe, Japan, and the United States to discuss scientific and technical aspects of drug registration with a mission to achieve greater harmonization to ensure that safe, effective, quality medicines are developed and registered in the most resource-efficient manner. ICH guidelines establish a globally harmonized consensus for 1) GMP (Good Manufacturing Practices) and pharmaceutical quality; 2) the design, conduct, safety, and reporting of clinical trials of pharmaceuticals and biologics; 3) detection of safety signals for carcinogenicity and toxicity; and 4) multidisciplinary work in data standards, medical terminology, and technical standards.[40] Unlike clinical practice guidelines, which provide broad consensus perspectives for the practice of medicine but are not universally binding, the ICH guidelines are formally incorporated into national and regional internal regulatory procedures. In the United States, FDA regulations for clinical trials address both Good Clinical Practice (GCP) and human subject protection (HSP). Adherence to the principles of GCP, including adequate HSP, is universally recognized as a critical requirement for the conduct of research involving human subjects. Clinical trials that do not adhere to ICH GCP are not considered suitable evidence for regulatory submissions. It is this end effect that accounts for much of the success behind these global harmonization efforts.

Ethics of Drug Development in Developing Countries

Some studies indicate that regulatory efforts in developing countries are being imperfectly executed[41] and have identified trials with unethical designs that were part of approved EU marketing applications. Clinical trials that would be considered unethical in the United States or Western Europe are sometimes approved by the local ethics committees outside these regions. Once officially approved by a local ethics committee, no obstacles prevent inclusion of the trial in the technical dossier of a marketing application. Ensuring good clinical trial conduct, resolution of conflicts of interest, and adequate protection for human subjects remain priorities for international regulators, industry, and research organizations.[34]

Anatomy of a Clinical Trial: Operations

The design, execution, and dissemination of results from a global cardiovascular drug development program constitute a major undertaking (see Chapter 1 and Braunwald, Chapter 6). Current estimates suggest that the overall cost of developing a new pharmaceutical, including capital investment and the costs of drug failures, is now approaching $1 billion.[42] The implementation of large-scale clinical trials requires a clinical research infrastructure, which until recently was engineered separately for each individual development program. Few commercial sponsors have the resources to construct and maintain these complex systems for clinical research, particularly smaller companies pursuing novel compounds early in their product life cycles. Academic research organizations (AROs) and contract research organizations (CROs) provide opportunities for companies to outsource activities required of sponsors. These activities may include protocol design, selection or monitoring of research sites, data collection, statistical analysis, and preparation of materials to be submitted to the FDA.[43] By outsourcing, a pharmaceutical company can convert the fixed costs of maintaining the clinical research infrastructure into variable costs and can obtain specialized knowledge for a particular disease state, patient population, or global region that would be challenging and often impractical to develop internally. The ARO model further leverages the collective experience of an academic institution's faculty to provide essential knowledge in key domains.[44]

To understand the magnitude of the services required for a successful clinical development program, it is helpful to divide trial operations into key functional components. Individual AROs and CROs may offer all these components ("full service") or may provide a subset of these services. It is not unusual for a large phase III clinical trial to require close collaboration between the sponsor and several academic and contract research organizations to coordinate these activities on a global scale.

Protocol Development

The clinical trial protocol explicitly describes the scientific background, rationale, design, conduct, and endpoints of the study.

Clinical trial protocols intended for the United States, Europe, and Japan generally follow the specifications enumerated in the ICH GCP guidance.[45] The critical elements of protocol design lie in the document's content rather than its form. Adequate procedures for screening and enrollment, including inclusion and exclusion criteria; endpoint definition and assessment; randomization; and operational oversight are crucial for trial success. Unanticipated shortcomings in any of these areas of the protocol can result in a noninformative investigation. Although protocol amendments can remedy some of these problems, excessive or frequent changes to the study design are inefficient and costly.

Site Management

Clinical research sites span a broad range of practice settings with varying degrees of sophistication, from community-based primary care settings to university-based quaternary care settings. Some sites may be limited to individual investigators, but others may represent institutions that enroll hundreds of study subjects annually. Matching a particular study protocol to clinical research sites that both serve the intended study population and have the facilities needed to conduct the study interventions and assessments requires specialized knowledge and thorough oversight. A site-management portfolio of services may include identification and selection of local site investigators, training of study sites in protocol-specific procedures, monitoring of clinical trial enrollment, and ensuring compliance with ICH GCP and applicable regulations. Compliance with the protocol and regulations is often accomplished through on-site monitoring, although the implementation of electronic systems for patient enrollment and data collection has reduced the overall demand for routine on-site monitoring in favor of "for cause" or "triggered" monitoring visits.

Data Management

Design, implementation, and maintenance of information systems for clinical trial operations are essential for preserving data integrity and satisfying the needs of regulatory agencies responsible for evaluation of new therapeutics. Although small clinical trials may still use paper case report forms, which require subsequent dedicated data entry, the vast majority of therapeutic-based clinical trials have moved to electronic data-capture systems. Electronic data management facilitates rapid ascertainment of data integrity and derivation of study status metrics. By reducing errors at the time of data acquisition, the need to send subsequent queries to sites for additional information is reduced, and the time required to finalize the databases for analysis and regulatory submissions is shortened. Electronic data collection systems can also be tied to electronic source data from other information systems, such as electrocardiogram archives, pacemaker databases, and hemodynamic monitoring systems. The FDA has endorsed several electronic data standards (e.g., Clinical Data Interchange Standards Consortium Study Data Tabulation Model) for regulatory submissions in the United States, which has facilitated the design and interoperability of clinical database management systems.[46] At the conclusion of the trial, an analysis dataset is extracted from the raw clinical trial data management system and forwarded to statisticians for analysis.

Statistics

Clinical trials planning, implementation, operations, and analyses rely heavily on collaborations between biostatisticians and clinical experts. The need for statistical services is most critical in the design phase, when sample size estimates, interim analyses, and stopping rules are formulated as part of protocol development. The trial start-up phase requires statistical involvement for creation of the randomization scheme, as well as design and validation of the analysis databases. Monitoring for data quality throughout the time course of a study is critical, and statistical demands hit another peak as the trial concludes, when interim and final trial results must be prepared for incorporation into regulatory submissions and publications.

Safety Surveillance

Every new drug and biologic can be expected to have adverse effects. Serious or unanticipated adverse events encountered during a clinical investigation incur mandatory reporting to the sponsor, institutional review boards, and the FDA. Standards for the timeliness of these reports are outlined in the regulations.[47] The collection, review, and follow-up of serious adverse events usually require an additional database dedicated to safety surveillance. Each adverse event in the database is coded using a harmonized dictionary, often the Medical Dictionary for Regulatory Activities (MedDRA) developed by the ICH. The safety surveillance staff oversees the preparation of the clinical narratives that accompany adverse event descriptions in final study reports and conducts reconciliation of the safety database and the clinical databases.

Clinical Events Adjudication

Although some clinical endpoints, such as all-cause mortality, can be readily determined by local site investigators, the use of investigator-adjudicated endpoints assumes the risk of ascertainment bias.[48,49] As endpoint definitions become increasingly complex, particularly for bleeding and MI, uniform application of the definitions becomes increasingly important. Central events adjudication committees provide the means by which events may be assessed by multiple reviewers blinded to treatment assignment. Typically, sites are asked to report any possible endpoint event, even if the local investigator believes that it is unlikely to be a true event, thus reducing false negatives. This reporting process leads to collection of more spurious events, but the central adjudication process is intended to remove those from consideration, thereby reducing false positives. This process ensures the best overall data reporting for the trial. Rates of rejection by the committee depend on the chosen endpoint definitions. A "softer" endpoint, such as recurrent angina, typically has a much larger rejection rate than a "harder" endpoint, such as intracranial hemorrhage. Central committees also allow events to be reviewed by relevant specialist experts. In typical cardiology multicenter trials, 20% to 30% of stroke endpoints are rejected by central neurology adjudicators.[50]

Although extremely valuable for reducing bias in superiority trial designs, the use of independent blinded adjudication may not prevent bias in noninferiority studies. In the noninferiority setting, sensitive application of endpoint definitions, even by a blinded committee, may inflate the overall event rate in both arms, making the arms appear more similar and therefore potentially not inferior to one another.

Economics of New Drug Development

Prescription Drug User Fee Act

Enacted by Congress in 1992, the Prescription Drug User Fee Act (PDUFA) allowed the FDA to offset the costs of reviewing new drug approvals by collecting New Drug Application (NDA) fees from sponsors.[51] Congress amended and extended PDUFA in 1997 (PDUFA II),[52] 2002 (PDUFA III),[53] and 2007 (PDUFA IV).[54] These extensions authorized the FDA to use revenue from application fees for postapproval surveillance and monitoring of direct-to-consumer advertising. PDUFA IV also extended the ability of the FDA to require postapproval surveillance from sponsors and to mandate label changes in response to new safety information for previously approved drugs. Under PDUFA IV, application fees, establishment fees, and product fees each contribute one third of the total fee revenues in a fiscal year. Fees collected and appropriated but not spent by the end of a fiscal year continue to remain available for the FDA to spend in future fiscal years. In FY 2009, the FDA obligated $512 million from PDUFA fee revenues. This accounted for about 60% of all funds obligated by the FDA from all sources in support of the review of human drug applications, which represented a total expenditure by the FDA of over $855 million.[55] Although the PDUFA fees represent a substantial commitment of resources for FDA review, the approach has been generally successful for maintaining satisfactory timelines for regulatory review in the United States, despite the increasing trend toward manufacturing and clinical trial operations documentation being submitted from abroad in support of NDA applications.

National Institutes of Health Roadmap Program

A key driver of the clinical research enterprise is the continuing discovery of chemical and biopharmaceutical entities that make up the substrate for new cardiovascular therapeutics. The translational research pipeline carrying these developments from the bench to the bedside depends on support from both industry and government. High-risk ideas or therapies for uncommon disorders frequently do not attract private sector investment, and public resources are required to bridge the gap. The National Institutes of Health (NIH) Roadmap for Medical Research facilitates translational research through the Clinical and Translational Science Awards (CTSA).[56] Launched in October 2006, the CTSA consortium originated with 12 academic health centers. When fully implemented in 2012, the CTSA will incorporate approximately 60 institutions to provide a national resource for clinical and translational science.[57,58] Members of the CTSA consortium are expected to integrate basic, translational, and clinical investigators, professional societies, and industry to facilitate the development of new research programs that blend the domains of translational research and clinical investigation.

Patent Considerations

A new therapeutic drug is usually protected by several patents covering its structure, called a *composition of matter* patent, and the manufacturing process or methods used to synthesize the drug. The expiration of these patents may occur at varying points in the product life cycle, depending on the total time required to bring the drug to market. Patent law is not globally harmonized, resulting in the various patents for a drug expiring at different times in different regions. In general, a new drug is protected from generic competition as long as its patents are enforceable. The FDA also recognizes a 5-year exclusivity period for new drugs that have not been previously approved, during which no generic applications can be submitted. These protections allow the original manufacturer to recoup the costs of developing the drug. A generic manufacturer generally incurs less cost to test and develop a generic formulation of a chemical drug because the composition and synthesis of the drug are already known, and some prior information is available regarding the drug's safety and effectiveness. The development of generic drugs is regulated through the Abbreviated New Drug Application (ANDA) process.[59] The Drug Price Competition and Patent Term Restoration Act of 1984, also known as the *Hatch-Waxman Act*,[60] expedites the development of generic drugs by using standards for strength, quality, purity, and identity (*bioequivalence*) as a basis for approval as an alternative to duplicative clinical trials. Under the Hatch-Waxman Act, a generic manufacturer must also certify in its ANDA that the generic drug does not infringe on the patents protecting the original drug. This provision allows pioneer manufacturers to delay approval of generic alternatives by litigating patent infringement suits against generic developers, during which time the derived profits from the patented drug outweigh the litigation costs.[61]

For biologics and biopharmaceuticals, the degree of similarity of a generic version may be uncertain, as it may vary considerably, depending on the complexity of the parent biologic compound. For this reason, many use the term *biosimilar* to describe these follow-on compounds and reserve the term *generic* to describe follow-on chemical drugs. The development of biologic compounds is generally more expensive than the development of their generic chemical counterparts, because of the need to address the uncertainties surrounding potential safety and effectiveness concerns. Enacted in 2010, the Patient Protection and Affordable Care Act authorizes the FDA to approve biosimilar drugs and grants biologics manufacturers 12 years of exclusive use before applications for competing biosimilar drugs can be submitted.[62]

Summary

The field of cardiovascular therapeutics uniquely spans a multitude of frontiers in translational science, corporate strategy, and federal regulation. Advances in the understanding of disease states and pharmacologic mechanisms have driven investigators and industry to seek rapid and efficient methods to deliver innovative drugs and biologics to the bedside. Simultaneously, the excitement surrounding new therapies must be tempered by responsible protection of the public health by reasonable assurances of safety and effectiveness. The clinical and academic communities help establish these thresholds and inform regulatory decision making through clinical practice guidelines and FDA advisory committees. This collaborative implementation of the "cycle of clinical therapeutics" constitutes a robust development model for other specialties, while continually evolving to accommodate innovative technologies.

REFERENCES

1. Lasby CG. *Eisenhower's heart attack: how Ike beat heart disease and held on to the presidency*. Lawrence, KS, 1997, University Press of Kansas.
2. Federal Food Drug and Cosmetic Act. Section 505 [21 USC §355 (b)(1)(A)]. Available at http://www.fda.gov/regulatoryinformation/legislation/FederalFoodDrugandCosmeticAct FDCAct/FDCActChapterVDrugsandDevices/ucm108125.htm. Updated April 30, 2009. Accessed August 30, 2011.
3. Integrilin [package insert]. Kenilworth, NJ, 2009, Schering-Plough.
4. Aggrastat [package insert]. Whitehouse Station, NJ, 2003, Merck.
5. Roger VL, Go AS, Lloyd-Jones DM, et al. American Heart Association Statistics Committee and Stroke Statistics Subcommittee. Heart disease and stroke statistics—2011 update: a report from the American Heart Association. *Circulation* 2011;123:e18-e209.
6. U.S. Department of Health and Human Services, Food and Drug Administration, Center for Drug Evaluation and Research, Center for Biologics Evaluation and Research. Guidance for industry: adaptive design clinical trials for drugs and biologics. Available at http://www.fda.gov/downloads/Drugs/GuidanceComplianceRegulatoryInformation/Guidances/UCM201790.pdf. February 2010. Accessed August 30, 2011.
7. U.S. Department of Health and Human Services, Food and Drug Administration, Center for Drug Evaluation and Research, Center for Biologics Evaluation and Research. Guidance for industry: non-inferiority clinical trials. Available at http://www.fda.gov/downloads/Drugs/GuidanceComplianceRegulatoryInformation/Guidances/UCM202140.pdf. March 2010. Accessed August 30, 2011.
8. Eisenstein EL, Collins R, Cracknell BS, et al. Sensible approaches for reducing clinical trial costs. *Clin Trials* 2008;5:75-84.
9. Paul SM, Mytelka DS, Dunwiddie CT, et al. How to improve R&D productivity: the pharmaceutical industry's grand challenge. *Nat Rev Drug Discov* 2010;9:203-214.
10. Investigational New Drug Application. 21 CFR 312. Available at http://www.accessdata.fda.gov/scripts/cdrh/cfdocs/cfcfr/cfrsearch.cfm?cfrpart=312. Updated April 1, 2011. Accessed August 30, 2011.
11. U.S. Food and Drug Administration. Investigational New Drug (IND) Application. Available at http://www.fda.gov/Drugs/DevelopmentApprovalProcess/HowDrugsareDevelopedandApproved/ApprovalApplications/InvestigationalNewDrugINDApplication/default.htm. Updated June 6, 2011. Accessed August 30, 2011.
12. U.S. Department of Health and Human Services, Food and Drug Administration, Center for Drug Evaluation and Research. Guidance for industry, investigators, and reviewers: exploratory IND studies. Available at http://www.fda.gov/downloads/Drugs/GuidanceComplianceRegulatoryInformation/Guidances/UCM078933.pdf. January 2006. Accessed August 30, 2011
13. Center for Drug Evaluation and Research, Center for Biologics Evaluation and Research. Guidance for industry: content and format of investigational new drug applications (INDs) for phase I studies of drugs, including well-characterized, therapeutic, biotechnology-derived products. Available at http://www.fda.gov/downloads/Drugs/GuidanceComplianceRegulatoryInformation/Guidances/UCM074980.pdf. November 1995. Accessed August 30, 2011.
14. Roden DM, Temple R. The U.S. Food and Drug Administration Cardio-renal Advisory Panel and the drug approval process. *Circulation* 2005;111:1697-1702.
15. U.S. Food and Drug Administration. Cardiovascular and Renal Drugs Advisory Committee. Available at http://www.fda.gov/AdvisoryCommittees/CommitteesMeetingMaterials/Drugs/

CardiovascularandRenalDrugsAdvisoryCommittee/default.htm. Updated July 15, 2011. Accessed August 30, 2011.

16. U.S. Department of Health and Human Services, Food and Drug Administration, Center for Drug Evaluation and Research, Center for Biologics Evaluation and Research. Guidance for industry: clinical studies section of labeling for human prescription drug and biological products: content and format. Available at http://www.fda.gov/downloads/Drugs/GuidanceComplianceRegulatoryInformation/Guidances/ucm075059.pdf. January 2006. Accessed February 8, 2011

17. Labeling for oral hypoglycemic drugs of the sulfonylurea class. *Fed Regist* 1984;49:14331.

18. U.S. Department of Health and Human Services, Food and Drug Administration, Center for Drug Evaluation and Research, Center for Biologics Evaluation and Research. Guidance for industry: labeling for human prescription drug and biological products —implementing the new content and format requirements. Available at http://www.fda.gov/downloads/Drugs/GuidanceComplianceRegulatoryInformation/Guidances/ucm075082.pdf. January 2006. Accessed February 7, 2011.

19. U.S. Department of Health and Human Services, Food and Drug Administration, Center for Drug Evaluation and Research. Guidance for industry: hypertension indication— drug labeling for cardiovascular outcome claims. Available at http://www.fda.gov/downloads/Drugs/GuidanceComplianceRegulatoryInformation/Guidances/ucm075072.pdf. March 2008. Accessed February 7, 2011.

20. U.S. Food and Drug Administration. Official transcript: Endocrinologic and Metabolic Drugs Advisory Committee meeting, April 1, 2009. Available at http://www.fda.gov/downloads/AdvisoryCommittees/CommitteesMeetingMaterials/Drugs/EndocrinologicandMetabolicDrugsAdvisoryCommittee/UCM151169.pdf. Accessed September 21, 2011.

21. U.S. Department of Health and Human Services, Food and Drug Administration, Center for Drug Evaluation and Research. Guidance for industry: diabetes mellitus—evaluating cardiovascular risk in new anti-diabetic therapies to treat type 2 diabetes. Available at http://www.fda.gov/downloads/Drugs/GuidanceComplianceRegulatoryInformation/Guidances/ucm071627.pdf. December 2008. Accessed September 21, 2011.

22. Postmarketing reporting of adverse drug experiences. 21 CFR 314.80. Available at http://www.accessdata.fda.gov/scripts/cdrh/cfdocs/cfcfr/CFRSearch.cfm?fr=314.80. Revised April 20, 2010. Accessed February 8, 2011.

23. U.S. Food and Drug Administration. Regulations and policies and procedures for postmarketing surveillance programs. Available at http://www.fda.gov/Drugs/GuidanceComplianceRegulatoryInformation/Surveillance/ucm090394.htm. Accessed February 7, 2011.

24. U.S. Department of Health and Human Services, Food and Drug Administration, Center for Drug Evaluation and Research, Center for Biologics Evaluation and Research. Guidance for industry and FDA staff: "dear health care provider" letters: improving communication of important safety information. Available at http://www.fda.gov/downloads/Drugs/GuidanceComplianceRegulatoryInformation/Guidances/UCM233769.pdf. November 2010. Accessed August 30, 2011.

25. Center for Drug Evaluation and Research. Manual of policies and procedures (6020.10): NDAs—"dear heath care providers" letters. Available at http://www.fda.gov/downloads/AboutFDA/CentersOffices/CDER/ManualofPoliciesProcedures/ucm082012.pdf. July 2, 2003. Accessed August 31, 2011.

26. Piccini JP, Hasselblad V, Peterson ED, et al. Comparative efficacy of dronedarone and amiodarone for the maintenance of sinus rhythm in patients with atrial fibrillation. *J Am Coll Cardiol* 2009;54:1089-1095.

27. Temple R. NDA approval letter to Sanofi-Aventis for dronedarone. Available at http://www.accessdata.fda.gov/drugsatfda_docs/appletter/2009/022425s000ltr.pdf. July 1, 2009. Accessed August 30, 2011.

28. Southworth MR. Supplemental NDA approval letter to Sanofi-Aventis for dronedarone. Available at http://www.accessdata.fda.gov/drugsatfda_docs/appletter/2011/022425s005ltr.pdf. February 11, 2011. Accessed August 30, 2011.

29. Arbit HM. Investigator-initiated research: the IND and IDE processes. *SoCRA Source* August 2007:19-24.

30. Schwieterman WD. Regulating biopharmaceuticals under CDER versus CBER: an insider's perspective. *Drug Discov Today* 2006;11:945-951.

31. Kozlowski S, Woodcock J, Midthun K, Sherman RB. Developing the nation's biosimilars program. *N Engl J Med* 2011;365:385-388.

32. Angiomax [package insert]. Parsippany, NJ, 2005, The Medicines Company.

33. ReoPro [package insert]. Indianapolis, IN, 2005, Eli Lilly & Company.

34. Glickman SW, McHutchison JG, Peterson ED, et al. Ethical and scientific implications of the globalization of clinical research. *N Engl J Med* 2009;360:816-823.

35. Califf RM, Harrington RA. American industry and the U.S. Cardiovascular Clinical Research Enterprise: an appropriate analogy? *J Am Coll Cardiol* 2011;58:677-680.

36. Mahaffey KW, Wojdyla DM, Carroll K, et al. Ticagrelor compared with clopidogrel by geographic region in the Platelet Inhibition and Patient Outcomes (PLATO) trial. *Circulation* 2011;124:544-554.

37. Akkerhuis KM, Deckers JW, Boersma E, et al. Geographic variability in outcomes within an international trial of glycoprotein IIb/IIIa inhibition in patients with acute coronary syndromes: results from PURSUIT. *Eur Heart J* 2000; 21:371-381.

38. European Medicines Agency. The European Medicines Agency road map to 2015: the agency's contribution to science, medicines, health. Available at http://www.ema.europa.eu/docs/en_GB/document_library/Report/2010/01/WC500067952.pdf. January 26, 2010. Accessed February 7, 2011.

39. Japan Pharmaceutical Manufacturers Association. Pharmaceutical administration and regulations in Japan. Available at http://www.jp/english/parj/pdf/2012.pdf. March 2012. Accessed April.

40. International Conference on Harmonisation of Technical Requirements for Registration of Pharmaceuticals for Human Use. ICH guidelines. Available at http://www.ich.org/products/guidelines.html. Accessed February 7, 2011.

41. Schipper I. Clinical Trials in Developing Countries: How to Protect People against Unethical Practices? Brussels, Belgium: European Parliament, 2009. Available at http://www.edctp.org/fileadmin/documents/ethics/Clinical_Trials_in_Developing_Countries_How_to_Protect_Peoples_Against_Unethical_Practices.pdf. Accessed February 7, 2011.

42. Adams CP, Brantner VV. Spending on new drug development. *Health Econ* 2010; 19:130-141.

43. Investigational new drug application: definitions and interpretations. 21 CFR 312.3(b). Available at http://www.accessdata.fda.gov/scripts/cdrh/cfdocs/cfcfr/CFRSearch.cfm?fr=312.3. Revised April 2, 2010. Accessed February 8, 2011.

44. Califf RM, Armstrong PW, Granger CB, et al, for the Virtual Coordination Centre for Global Collaborative Cardiovascuoar Research (VIGOUR) organization. Towards a new order in cardiovascular medicine: re-engineering through global collaboration. *Eur Heart J* 2010;31:911-917.

45. International Conference on Harmonisation of Technical Requirements for Registration of Pharmaceuticals for Human Use. Guideline for good clinical practice E6(R1). Available at http://www.ich.org/fileadmin/Public_Web_Site/ICH_Products/Guidelines/Efficacy/E6_R1/Step4/E6_R1_Guideline.pdf. June 10, 1996. Accessed February 8, 2011.

46. McCourt B, Harrington RA, Fox K, et al. Data standards: at the intersection of sites, clinical research networks, and standards development initiatives. *Drug Inf J* 2007;41:393-404.

47. Records and reports concerning adverse drug experiences on marketed prescription drugs for human use without approved new drug applications. 21 CFR 310.305. Available at http://www.accessdata.fda.gov/scripts/cdrh/cfdocs/cfcfr/CFRSearch.cfm?fr=310.305. Revised April 2, 2010. Accessed February 8, 2011.

48. Mahaffey KW, Harrington RA, Akkerhuis M, et al. Systematic adjudication of myocardial infarction endpoints in an international clinical trial. *Curr Control Trials Cardiovasc Med* 2001;2:180-186.

49. Kirwan BA, Lubsen J, de Brouwer S, et al. Diagnostic criteria and adjudication process both determine published event rates: the ACTION trial experience. *Contemp Clin Trials* 2007;28:720-729.

50. Kerr DR, Nasco E. Value of central event adjudication. *Stroke* 2009;40:e638.

51. U.S. Food and Drug Administration. Prescription Drug User Fee Act (PDUFA) of 1992. Available at http://www.fda.gov/RegulatoryInformation/Legislation/FederalFoodDrugandCosmeticActFDCAct/SignificantAmendmentstotheFDCAct/ucm147983.htm. Updated May 20, 2009. Accessed February 8, 2011.

52. U.S. Food and Drug Administration. Food and Drug Administration Modernization Act (FDAMA) of 1997. Available at http://www.fda.gov/RegulatoryInformation/Legislation/FederalFoodDrugandCosmeticActFDCAct/SignificantAmendmentstotheFDCAct/FDAMA/FullTextofFDAMAlaw/default.htm. Updated October 22, 2009. Accessed February 8, 2011.

53. U.S. Food and Drug Administration. Prescription Drug User Fee Amendments of 2002. Available at http://www.fda.gov/ForIndustry/UserFees/PrescriptionDrugUserFee/ucm118851.htm. Updated April 30, 2009. Accessed February 8, 2011.

54. U.S. Food and Drug Administration. Food and Drug Administration Amendments Act (FDAAA) of 2007. Available at http://www.fda.gov/RegulatoryInformation/Legislation/FederalFoodDrugandCosmeticActFDCAct/SignificantAmendmentstotheFDCAct/FoodandDrugAdministrationAmendmentsActof2007/FullTextofFDAAALaw/default.htm. Updated August 17, 2009. Accessed February 8, 2011.

55. U.S. Food and Drug Administration. Executive summary: FY 2009 PDUFA financial report. Available at http://www.fda.gov/AboutFDA/ReportsManualsForms/Reports/UserFeeReports/FinancialReports/PDUFA/ucm226680.htm. Updated October 5, 2010. Accessed February 8, 2011.

56. Clinical and Translational Science Awards. Available at http://www.CTSAcentral.org. Accessed August 30, 2011.

57. National Center for Research Resources. Fact sheet: Clinical and Translational Science Awards. Available at http://www.ncrr.nih.gov/publications/pdf/ctsa_factsheet.pdf. Summer 2011. Accessed August 30, 2011.

58. NIH Common Fund. Translational research. Available at http://commonfund.nih.gov/clinicalresearch/overview-translational.aspx. Accessed August 30, 2011.

59. U.S. Food and Drug Administration. Abbreviated New Drug Application (ANDA): generics. Available at http://www.fda.gov/drugs/developmentapprovalprocess/howdrugsaredevelopedandapproved/approvalapplications/abbreviatednewdrugapplicationandagenerics/default.htm. Updated March 21, 2011. Accessed August 30, 2011.

60. Drug Price Competition and Patent Term Restoration Act of 1984, P. L. 98–417, 98 Stat. 1585 (1984) (codified as amended 21 U.S.C. §355 [1994]).

61. Eurek SE. Hatch-Waxman reform and accelerated market entry of generic drugs: is faster necessarily better? *Duke Law Technol Rev* 2003;rev 0018.

62. U.S. Food and Drug Administration. Biosimilars. Available at http://www.fda.gov/Drugs/DevelopmentApprovalProcess/HowDrugsareDevelopedandApproved/ApprovalApplications/TherapeuticBiologicApplications/Biosimilars/default.htm. Updated August 17, 2011. Accessed August 30, 2011.

Device Development for Cardiovascular Therapeutics: Concepts and Regulatory Implications

Frederick J. Schoen, Bram D. Zuckerman, and Andrew Farb*

OVERVIEW, 41

MEDICAL DEVICE DEVELOPMENT AND DIFFERENCES FROM DRUGS, 41

Development and Implementation of Cardiovascular Medical Devices: An Overview, 41
Differences Between Devices and Drugs and Associated Regulatory Implications, 42

REGULATORY FUNDAMENTALS, 42

History of Device Regulation and the Medical Device Classification System, 42
Pathways for Regulatory Review of Cardiovascular Devices, 43

CONTEMPORARY REGULATORY ISSUES, 44

Randomized Versus Nonrandomized Studies in Medical Device Evalution, 44
Endpoints and Surrogate Endpoints in Cardiovascular Device Trials, 45
Study Blinding in Cardiovascular Device Trials, 46
Use of Foreign Data for U.S. Product Approval, 46
Independent Oversight of Cardiovascular Device Trials, 46
Labeling and Off-Label Use of Cardiovascular Devices, 46

RISK, BENEFIT, AND THE PRODUCT LIFE CYCLE, 47

Total Product Life Cycle Approach, 47
Device Safety and Failure Concepts, 47

ENSURING THE SAFETY OF MARKETED DEVICES, 48

Postmarket Safety Assessment Tools, 48
Cardiologists' Role in Ensuring Device Safety and Performance, 50
Product Recall and Center for Devices and Radiological Health, 50

OTHER KEY REGULATORY TOPICS, 50

Combination Products, 50
Role of the Advisory Panel, 51
CDRH Interactions with External Stakeholders and Government Partners, 51

REFERENCES, 51

Overview

Over the past 50 years, new medical devices and related innovations have contributed greatly to the decrease in deaths from cardiovascular causes. Indeed, cardiovascular device development has advanced dramatically over the past several decades, yielding a remarkable increase in the variety and complexity of available devices and diagnostic tests for cardiac illnesses. In ischemic, valvular, myocardial, cardiac rhythm, and peripheral vascular disease, the clinical benefits have been substantial.

Catheter-based endovascular stents emerged in the 1990s. Initially composed of bare-metal wires and later with drug-eluting coatings, stents have revolutionized the percutaneous treatment of severe coronary atherosclerosis.[1] Metallic stents have been approved as a percutaneous alternative to surgical carotid endarterectomy. In valve disease, a singular advance was surgical valve replacement, which began in the 1960s.[2] In contrast to a *mortality* rate of 50% at 2 to 3 years in patients with critical aortic stenosis, *survival* following surgical valve replacement with contemporary mechanical or bioprosthetic devices is 50% to 70% at 10 to 15 years.[3] A new approach to valve replacement is transcatheter aortic and pulmonary valve implantation, less invasive interventions currently at varying stages of development, clinical study, and clinical use.[4]

Devices that aid or replace the heart's pumping function, including ventricular assist devices (VADs) and total implantable artificial hearts, are used less frequently than stents or valves, but their implantation enables survival of some patients who would otherwise succumb without profound cardiac support.[5] Pacemakers, implantable cardioverter-defibrillators (ICDs), radiofrequency catheters, and cryoablation catheters have substantially improved the prognosis of patients with life-limiting and life-threatening cardiac arrhythmias.[6] Synthetic vascular grafts and stent grafts provide effective repair of stenotic peripheral arteries and aneurysmal disease of the thoracic and abdominal aorta.[7] Vascular grafts have also enabled long-term vascular access for hemodialysis treatment in patients with renal failure who lack suitable veins for arteriovenous (AV) fistulas.[8]

Most permanently implanted cardiovascular devices are designed to treat underlying medical conditions or provide enhanced function. Nevertheless, device failure and/or other tissue-biomaterial interactions may cause complications that necessitate reoperation or cause morbidity or death. In some cases, deleterious outcomes occur after many years of uneventful patient benefit (Figure 3-1).

Assessment of the safety and effectiveness of new cardiovascular products, and the ongoing evaluation of approved products, is challenging. The Food and Drug Administration (FDA) Center for Devices and Radiological Health (CDRH) plays an essential role in promoting and protecting the public health by ensuring that medical devices marketed in the United States provide a reasonable assurance of safety and effectiveness and confer a favorable risk/benefit profile for their intended use population.

This chapter discusses the process of cardiovascular medical device development, validation, and regulatory review and describes differences in the regulation of devices versus drugs; it also covers special topics of interest to the practicing physician, including off-label use and the responsibilities of cardiologists to ensure safe and effective use of devices.

Medical Device Development and Differences from Drugs

Development and Implementation of Cardiovascular Medical Devices: An Overview

The medical device development process has become increasingly complex in recent years as a result of the advent of new technologies, regulatory requirements, and the increased importance of reimbursement decisions for successful device commercialization.[9] The entire process requires strategic planning,

---

*This work represents the professional opinion of the authors and is not an official document, agency guidance, or policy of the U.S. Government, the Department of Health and Human Services, or the Food and Drug Administration, nor should any official endorsement be inferred.

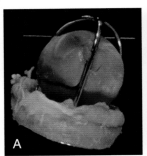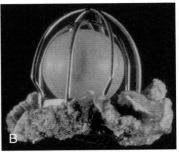

FIGURE 3-1 Late failure of prosthetic heart valves. **A,** Ball variance (absorption of blood lipids with resulting swelling, cracking, and occluder immobilization) 19 years following implantation of a caged-ball heart valve. **B,** Infective endocarditis 22 years following implantation of a caged-ball heart valve.

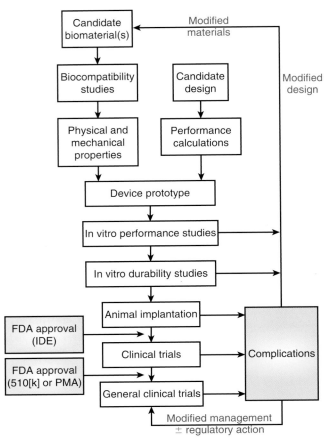

FIGURE 3-2 Development and validation of a cardiovascular medical device. Points at which problems can arise are indicated, and potential generic strategies for solving those problems are indicated. Junctures for regulatory action are also shown. *FDA,* Food and Drug Administration; *IDE,* Investigational Device Exemption; *PMA,* premarket approval application.

coordinated decisions, and consistent, rigorous scientific and business methods. Development and clinical use of a medical device comprise a complicated process, progressive but not entirely linear, that includes concept generation, prototype development, intellectual property development, regulatory requirements, reimbursement issues, business models, research and development (including the scientific and engineering work required to transition from an early-stage concept to a user-ready and validated final device), clinical trials, marketing and stakeholder considerations, quality and process management, manufacturing, and sales and distribution.[10] From a technical perspective, key considerations of the development of a design concept responsive to a clinical need include selection and evaluation of suitable biomaterials and incorporation of the materials into a device prototype to evaluate functionality and anticipated potential complications via bench testing and in animal models (Figure 3-2). After FDA approval of an *Investigational Device Exemption* (IDE), for a significant risk investigational device, a human clinical study of the device may be conducted under carefully monitored clinical trial conditions. All preclinical and clinical data undergo regulatory evaluation prior to market entry via the premarket notification, 510(k), or the premarket approval application (PMA) regulatory pathway (see below). At any point in the development and use of an investigational device, untoward results and subsequent analysis, which frequently includes implant retrieval and pathologic evaluation, may necessitate reassessment of the device concept, modification of biomaterial or design, and adjustments in the management of patients who have received the device. Any of these changes will affect regulatory review.

Differences Between Devices and Drugs and Associated Regulatory Implications

Medical devices and drugs differ in both their development and regulatory pathways; the latter are set forth in the statutory mandate given to the FDA by the U.S. Congress. *Drugs* are chemical entities that may be metabolized either before or after their intended action. They have a measurable half-life and are ultimately metabolized and/or excreted. Drugs solve a biochemical problem; their action is systemic and cannot be seen directly, and their mechanism of action is often not well understood. In contrast, medical devices predominantly solve a mechanical or other physical problem; their intended action is generally local, and their mechanism can typically be directly or indirectly observed. Furthermore, although drugs are metabolized and/or excreted with a measurable half-life and can be redosed or discontinued with ease, devices are often permanent implants; their removal may have important clinical implications. Therefore, device interactions with the patient are frequently ongoing, and the risks of potential adverse effects can be prolonged for many years. Moreover, unlike a drug regimen, nonadherence with an implanted medical device

is not an option; however, nonadherence with adjunctive drug regimens, such as anticoagulants or antiplatelet agents, can cause significant problems.

Surgeons and interventionalists are often involved in the development and evaluation of devices, and operator technique, expertise, and thus the extent of experience with a particular device type, can play a critical role in the successful use of a device. Phase III drug trials often recruit thousands of patients over a relatively short time, but the number of patients available for pivotal clinical trials of new or modified medical devices is typically smaller. Moreover, double-blind, randomized, controlled trials (RCTs) are often not feasible for evaluation of medical devices. Large companies dominate the pharmaceutical industry, but smaller companies are often intimately involved in medical device development from concept through market entry, and the early stages in the process may be marked by iterative innovation in device design and biomaterials.[11]

Table 3-1 summarizes key features of devices and drugs that influence development and regulatory review; they include device-related and population-related factors. Contemporary publications have amplified these differences.[12,13]

Regulatory Fundamentals

History of Device Regulation and the Medical Device Classification System

The 1976 Medical Device Amendments created a system for the FDA review process for medical devices. Three separate

TABLE 3-1	Comparison of Drug and Device Development	
DEVELOPMENTAL FEATURE	**DEVICE**	**DRUG**
Rate of technology change	Fast	Slow
Mode of action	Physical effect	Chemical effect
Duration	Long	Short
Potential adherence issues	No	Yes
Learning curve	Yes	No
Ease of in vitro assessment	High	Low
Ability to blind treatments	Difficult	Easy
Ability to recruit large patient groups	Difficult	Easy

classification levels were designated based on the device's level of clinical risk. *Class I devices* include minimal risk devices such as bandages, examination gloves, and certain manual, handheld surgical instruments. The majority of class I devices are exempt from premarket notification and FDA clearance before marketing. These devices are subject to General Controls—the basic requirements of the Food, Drug and Cosmetic Act (as amended) that apply to all medical devices—which include product registration and listing requirements, Good Manufacturing Practices, labeling requirements, banning provisions, and medical device reporting (MDR) requirements.

Class II devices represent intermediate risk, and most require submission of a 510(k) application to the FDA before the device can be cleared for marketing. Examples of class II cardiovascular devices include guidewires, guide catheters, introducer sheaths, hemostasis devices, and computerized electrocardiographic devices. In addition to General Controls, class II devices must also comply with Special Controls, which include device-specific labeling requirements, performance standards, and postmarket surveillance.

The highest risk devices are categorized as *class III devices,* which are used in supporting or sustaining human life, are of substantial importance in preventing impairment of human health, or present a potential unreasonable risk of illness or injury (21 C.F.R., Part 814).[14] In most cases, Class III devices require the submission and FDA approval of a PMA prior to marketing. Any device in commercial distribution prior to the passage of the 1976 Medical Device Amendments was considered a *preamendment* device and was effectively grandfathered; that is, it was allowed to stay on the market without additional FDA review, unless the FDA had taken a specific regulatory action to require a PMA. These devices were assigned to the least-regulated class that allowed a reasonable assurance of safety and effectiveness. A device marketed for the first time after 1976 must follow the regulatory requirements for its particular device classification.

Pathways for Regulatory Review of Cardiovascular Devices

The first step in the device evaluation process is to determine the device's classification level to determine the regulatory requirements. Based on the device classification, a medical device manufacturer would usually take either of two key regulatory pathways: the 510(k) premarket notification submission or submission of a PMA (Figure 3-3).

510(k) PREMARKET NOTIFICATION

The 1976 Medical Device Amendments added a premarket notification provision to Section 510(k) of the Food, Drug and Cosmetic Act, requiring that each firm register their manufacturing facility with the FDA. For those devices that require a 510(k) submission prior to marketing, the application should include a description

of device design, function, and principles of operation; reference to performance standards if available; a bibliography of all published and unpublished reports; proposed labeling; and manufacturing information. The manufacturer must demonstrate that the new device is "substantially equivalent" to one or more legally marketed devices, known as *predicate devices*, in terms of the intended use, technology, and performance. If the new device has different technological characteristics, the differences must not raise new safety or effectiveness concerns, and the manufacturer must demonstrate that the new device is at least as safe and effective as the predicate. The FDA has a statutory requirement of 90 days to review and make a marketing clearance determination. A manufacturer must receive a clearance letter from the FDA allowing it to market the device prior to its commercial distribution in the United States.

The majority of medical devices the FDA has approved for the U.S. market have entered via the 510(k) premarket notification process; most are cleared after FDA review of comprehensive nonclinical testing (bench studies and animal testing, when necessary). For example, percutaneous transluminal coronary angioplasty (PTCA) catheters are considered class II devices. A new PTCA catheter would generally require bench testing alone; however, a new clinical study would be warranted if the indications for use were significantly different, or if the technology raised safety or effectiveness concerns that could only be addressed with a clinical study. Approximately 10% to 15% of 510(k) submissions contain data from clinical trials. For example, an intravascular embolic protection device is a class II device that typically requires clinical data for a determination of substantial equivalence.

PREMARKET APPROVAL APPLICATION

As a condition for FDA approval of a PMA, a manufacturer must demonstrate reasonable assurance of the *safety* and *effectiveness* of a device for its indications for use. For class III cardiovascular devices—such as heart valves, pacemakers, intracoronary stents, and circulatory support devices—a demonstration of device safety and effectiveness almost always requires clinical data to form the basis of product approval. In determining the safety and effectiveness of a class III device, some of the factors considered by the FDA include the intended use of the device, the population for which the device is intended, device reliability, and the risk of device use compared with the likely benefit of using the device. To make a determination of a reasonable assurance of safety and effectiveness, the FDA relies on *valid scientific evidence*.[15]* A hierarchy of the types of data that comprise valid scientific evidence exists, from RCTs, partially controlled studies, studies without matched controls, and well-documented case histories conducted by qualified experts to reports of significant human experience with a marketed device.

The main goal of FDA device review is to assess the clinical utility of the device, based on its risk/benefit profile, to determine product safety and effectiveness. The FDA's interpretation of valid scientific evidence for medical device approval has become more rigorous for cardiovascular devices over the past decade, incorporating greater use of randomized, controlled, and even blinded studies when applicable.

INVESTIGATIONAL DEVICE EXEMPTION

Clinical studies performed in the United States using investigational devices that present a significant risk to human subjects

---

*21 C.F.R. § 860.7(c)(2) Valid scientific evidence is defined as "evidence from well-controlled investigations, partially controlled studies, studies and objective trials without matched controls, well-documented case histories conducted by qualified experts, and reports of significant human experience with a marketed device, from which it can be fairly and reasonably concluded by qualified experts that there is a reasonable assurance of the safety and effectiveness of a device under its conditions of use."

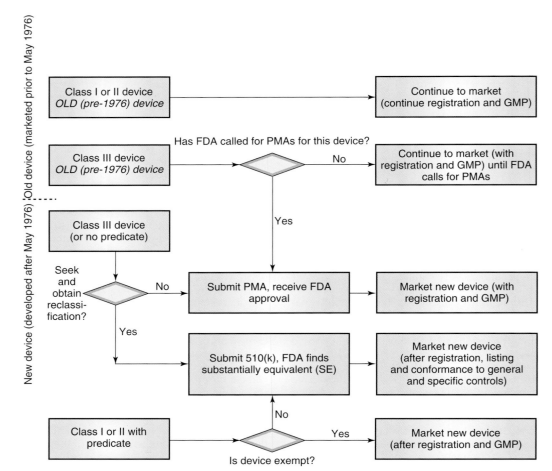

FIGURE 3-3 Pathways for regulatory marketing clearance and approval. *FDA,* Food and Drug Administration; *GMP,* good manufacturing practice; *PMA,* premarket approval application.

(some class II devices and all class III devices) are performed under an IDE application approved by the FDA. IDE applications typically provide a detailed device description; proposed indications for use; a report of prior investigations, including all nonclinical studies (bench and animal); previous clinical experience; a summary of the manufacturing process and quality systems; the proposed investigational plan; proposed labeling; and an informed consent document to be used in the study. FDA approval of an IDE gives permission to a manufacturer or clinical investigator to conduct a study of an investigational device, or of an approved device for nonapproved indications, on patients in the United States to generate data in support of the device's safety and effectiveness. The purpose of an IDE is to "encourage…the discovery and development of useful devices intended for human use," while at the same time protecting the public health and ensuring that clinical investigations are performed in a safe and ethical manner (21 C.F.R. §812.1[a]). To maintain optimum freedom for scientific investigators in the pursuit of device development, the statutory time requirement for the FDA to complete its review of an IDE application is 30 calendar days. After reviewing the IDE application, the FDA may grant 1) full approval to begin the clinical trial; 2) conditional approval, which indicates that the FDA deems the trial sufficiently safe to commence, but there remain some outstanding issues that need to be addressed by the sponsor prior to full approval; or 3) disapproval. Clinical data obtained from a study under an approved IDE can then be used to support a 510(k) or PMA, depending on the pathway necessary for marketing.

HUMANITARIAN DEVICE EXEMPTION

A Humanitarian device exemption (HDE) application is an option for devices intended for use in a very small patient population (<4000 individuals per year) for an uncommon clinical condition. An HDE application is similar in both form and content to a PMA and has the same safety requirements. However, in contrast to a PMA, in which the devices must provide a reasonable assurance of safety and effectiveness, an HDE application must demonstrate that the device is safe and provides *probable benefit* to the patient.

Contemporary Regulatory Issues

Randomized Versus Nonrandomized Studies in Medical Device Evaluation

Determination of what constitutes an appropriate level of *valid scientific evidence* depends on the type of technology used and the risk posed by the device. The FDA considers data from RCTs to be the highest level of scientific data and therefore encourages use of RCTs in cardiovascular device studies. However, the use of an RCT design may be challenging with some cardiovascular devices because of sample size issues or ethical dilemmas. Low adverse-event rates associated with mature device technologies, such as surgical prosthetic heart valves, would require an unfeasible sample size to demonstrate either superiority or noninferiority of the new device compared with the control. For disease entities in which there is either no standard of care, or the standard of care is known to be suboptimal, lack of clinical equipoise can create ethical dilemmas by mandating that patients be randomized to a study arm that may be perceived by clinicians and/or patients to be an inferior treatment. Thus, a proper assessment of device technology must balance the competing demands of maximizing scientific validity against the practical realities of performing (and effectively completing) clinical studies. For this reason, nonrandomized clinical studies may be acceptable in certain situations in support of a marketing application.[16,17]

For surgical heart valves, a mature technology with well-defined performance profiles and complication rates, the FDA took the approach that a rigorously evaluated historic control dataset could be used in single-arm trials of new heart valves to define acceptable rates of the most frequent complications. In 1993, in consultation with a committee of experts from industry and academia, the FDA developed objective performance criteria (OPC) derived from patient-level data from studies of FDA-approved surgical heart valves, representing a sample size of 800 valve years.[18,19] This OPC approach is an efficient method to evaluate new surgical heart valves submitted for FDA approval.[20]

Moreover, incremental design changes to an existing cardiovascular device, such as an electrophysiologic ablation catheter well characterized with engineering and animal testing data, may be evaluated for safety and effectiveness with a single-arm clinical study in some circumstances; however, use of a nonrandomized study design must include the careful selection of a suitable historic control (see Chapter 1). In addition, a detailed statistical analysis plan should be developed that accounts for differences in baseline clinical covariates and other time-related improvements in cardiovascular disease management that could bias against historic control data. Statistical methodologies such as propensity score analysis are useful to balance measured covariates among nonrandomized treatment arms.[21] However, it must be recognized that all nonrandomized studies are subject to bias, and despite the rigor with which they are applied, propensity score analyses and other methods of statistical adjustment have important limitations. Moreover, because operator technique and expertise can greatly influence clinical outcomes, many studies of novel devices include a "roll-in" phase to account for a physician learning curve.

Endpoints and Surrogate Endpoints in Cardiovascular Device Trials

Ideally, clinical trial endpoints should be objective, readily assessable, clinically important, meaningful to patients, interpretable by physicians, and assessable in a trial of reasonable size. To make a determination of a device's safety and effectiveness, thorough consideration must be given to select the most informative and relevant endpoints for clinical studies. For most cardiovascular devices, clinical outcome parameters, such as death, myocardial infarction (MI), stroke, and congestive heart failure admission, are used. Composite endpoints representing combinations of clinically important parameters, such as major adverse cardiac events (death, MI, and target lesion revascularization) and target vessel failure (cardiac death, target vessel MI, and target vessel revascularization), are frequently used. Composite endpoints are best suited for well-characterized disease states, when there is consensus that all individual components are clinically important, and for which there is an expectation that all individual components would be affected in the same direction (e.g., trends for reduced rates of death, MI, and stroke).

The main advantages of composite endpoints are amplification of treatment benefits and an increase in the overall number of events so that sample size may be reduced; however, potential limitations on the interpretability of composite endpoint data are evident. For example, in most cases, equal weight applied to

components assumes equal importance, which may not be justified, and it may be difficult to find consensus on an acceptable weighting scheme among individual components. There is a chance that the outcomes of individual components could trend in opposite directions (e.g., lower repeat revascularization rates but higher MI rates). Finally, the outcome difference between the new intervention and the control may be driven by the clinically *least* important component of the composite.

With some cardiovascular devices, successive improvements in device technology have led to decreased rates of adverse events. Improvement in patient outcome is clearly desirable, but it has the effect of making comparative analysis in trials of next-generation devices more difficult. Coronary drug-eluting stent (DES) technology provides one example.* The first two devices to be approved, the Cypher sirolimus-eluting coronary stent (Cordis Corporation, Warren, NJ) and the Taxus paclitaxel-eluting coronary stent (Boston Scientific, Natick, MA), were tested against bare-metal stent controls in their pivotal trials; they demonstrated a reduction in major cardiac adverse-event rates, driven by a dramatic reduction in repeat revascularization rates.[22,23] In a trial of one DES versus another, low event rates require larger numbers of study patients to demonstrate either superiority or noninferiority of the new device compared with the control stent. One potential approach to designing feasible trials is to enroll a more enriched population that includes higher risk subjects (e.g., non–ST-elevation MI patients) or more complex lesions (long lesions or small vessels) that would be associated with higher event rates.

A *surrogate endpoint* is a marker that is intended to substitute for a clinical endpoint and is expected to predict clinical outcomes based on epidemiologic, therapeutic, pathophysiologic, or other scientific evidence. A surrogate endpoint must fulfill two critical criteria to be considered valid: first, the surrogate must be highly predictive of the clinical outcome, and second, it must fully reflect the treatment effect, both positive and negative, on the clinical outcome (see Chapter 1).[24] In cardiovascular drug trials, blood pressure reduction and lipid lowering have been used as physiologic and biochemical surrogate endpoints for coronary heart disease and stroke, respectively. Surrogate endpoints have been suggested as alternate outcome measures for technologies such as DESs and devices designed to reduce myocardial infarct size.

Percent-diameter stenosis and late lumen loss are potential surrogate markers for clinical effectiveness endpoints for coronary stent trials. Several studies show that these angiographic outcome measures serve as a surrogate for the need for repeat revascularization procedures in the treatment of noncomplex coronary lesions. As a result, percent-diameter stenosis and late lumen loss have the advantage of providing quantitative data for comparisons of different stent implantation strategies. Consequently, they have the potential for increasing the effect size difference between treatments, which requires fewer patients to be studied.

Multiple issues are associated with the exclusive use of imaging-based surrogate endpoints. Angiographic endpoints require optimal image quality, consistent views from the index procedure to follow-up, and standardized core lab protocols and software. By definition, angiographic surrogate endpoints entail a high degree of subject compliance with follow-up angiography. Given the expected low event rates, patients may be reluctant to undergo a protocol-driven, rather than symptom-driven, repeat invasive imaging study. The acceptability of study results could be compromised because of data loss secondary to a substantial subject dropout. In addition, it is uncertain whether imaging-based

---

*It should be noted that coronary DESs are officially classified by the FDA as combination drug-device products, with features of drug as well as device therapies. Based on the FDA's official designation, CDRH has served as the lead review center for DES, with the Center for Drug Evaluation and Research serving a consultative role. Hence, the clinical testing pathway for DESs has followed the PMA pathway for device approval. Considerations for combination devices are discussed later in this chapter.

surrogate endpoint models would apply to more complicated patient and lesion subsets. Finally, although the use of a valid surrogate may result in a reduced sample size to demonstrate device effectiveness, this approach is often inadequate to assess device safety. Alternative trial design strategies that combine conventional clinical outcome measures with a validated surrogate parameter, potentially as co-primary endpoints, may be considered. Because of these considerations, surrogate endpoints may be most useful as primary effectiveness endpoints for second and/or later generation devices (i.e., iterative changes in an approved device). Continued exploration of scientifically valid surrogate endpoints and innovative trial designs may aid in the development of helpful strategies in the assessment of novel technologies.[25]

Study Blinding in Cardiovascular Device Trials

The use of blinding reinforces the integrity of the treatment effect of patient assignment in RCTs. For example, the pivotal studies conducted for the Cypher and Taxus DESs used double-blind study designs, given that the products were visually and radiographically identical in appearance. However, for most cardiovascular device trials, designing a double-blind study cannot be done because of the physical characteristics and/or mode of action of the device, as in the case of a trial of two different DESs in which the operator and catheterization laboratory staff are aware of treatment assignment based on the unique physical properties of each product. Further, neither patient nor operator blinding is possible in a treatment strategy trial such as percutaneous coronary intervention (PCI) versus bypass surgery. Thus, device trials frequently cannot accommodate blinding of both patients and implanting physicians. For example, in the Randomized Evaulation of Mechanical Assistance for the Treatment of Congestive Heart Failure (REMATCH) trial, in which end-stage heart failure patients were randomized to left ventricular assist device therapy or optimal medical management arms, the study could not be blinded.[26] Randomized but unblinded studies have also been used for comparing surgical and interventional therapies for coronary artery obstructions,[27] different types of heart valve prostheses (mechanical vs. biologic substitutes),[28] and open versus transcatheter valve replacement.[29]

Given these limitations on study blinding, it must be recognized that investigator and/or patient bias introduced by the knowledge of treatment assignment may possibly confound clinical study outcomes and diminish the scientific validity of a study. Study designs should therefore incorporate blinding to the maximum extent possible, maintaining the blinding for patients, investigators, and study personnel who conduct follow-up clinical assessments. In addition, the use of objective, rather than subjective, study endpoints and analytical tools to evaluate the potential effect of bias on study outcome augments the scientific validity of the study results.

Use of Foreign Data for U.S. Product Approval

A potential advantage in collecting data from different geographies, in either a single global study or several individual studies, is the ability to evaluate device performance across a more diverse population than can be achieved by a single geographic population alone. Study results could thus be more generalizable to a broader population of patients. Furthermore, demonstration of comparable device performance across different geographies can provide a more robust conclusion of product safety and effectiveness.

Increasingly, studies for cardiovascular devices are conducted in centers outside the United States, and the FDA will consider data obtained from sites outside the United States as supportive evidence for U.S. product approval (21 CFR § 814.15). However, such data must be demonstrated to be *applicable to the U.S. population and practice of medicine*. Unless consideration of the potential differences in patient populations and study characteristics is made prior to initiating studies outside the United States, the data from such trials might have limited applicability.

A key consideration when assessing data from outside the United States is the generalizability to the U.S. patient population. Important factors include patient demographic and clinical characteristics, geographic differences in medical practice, and differences in study protocols, especially the extent to which patients are monitored for clinical events and long-term follow-up. Prespecified statistical analyses are recommended to evaluate data comparability by testing the homogeneity of demographic and procedural covariates across centers and geographical regions, as well as testing for interactions between treatment and region.

Independent Oversight of Cardiovascular Device Trials

Many cardiovascular device studies evaluate breakthrough technologies that have novel uses and potential unforeseen risks to patients enrolled in clinical trials. To ensure adequate protection of patient safety, the FDA often recommends the use of independent data safety and monitoring boards (DSMBs). Study DSMBs should have monitoring plans to ensure that patients are not subjected to undue risk. In cases where cardiovascular devices are evaluated in multiple, concurrent trials, it may be appropriate to use the same DSMB to streamline safety monitoring from a global perspective.[30] The FDA also strongly recommends the use of independent core labs for imaging and pathology, with clinical events adjudicated by an independent clinical events committee. These independent monitoring bodies complement the role of the study DSMB, reinforce study integrity, and reduce issues of bias and conflict of interest.

Labeling and Off-Label Use of Cardiovascular Devices

One of the most important aspects of the device approval process is the development of understandable and accurate instructions for the use of a product, and the FDA works closely with device manufacturers to craft the product label. Labeling is defined as a "display of written, printed, or graphic matter upon the immediate container of any article," and it includes "all labels and other written, printed, or graphic matter" (Sections 201[k] and [m] of the Federal Food, Drug, and Cosmetic Act). Device labeling is a means to communicate to physicians and patients a description of the device, how and in whom the device should be used, when it should be used with caution or not used, and the safety and effectiveness outcomes associated with use of the device in one or more clinical studies. The "indication for use" statement identifies the target population, a significant portion of whom have demonstrated through sufficient, valid scientific evidence that use of the device as labeled will provide clinically significant results, and, at the same time, it will not present an unreasonable risk of illness or injury. The label also includes details regarding the clinical studies performed in support of the product's approval, including the specific populations tested.

Despite specific language in labeling, a physician can use a device in a manner different from the labeled indication because of expectations that the beneficial effects seen in clinical trials may transfer to relatively untested patient subgroups; this is known as *off-label use,* and it is a means by which a legally marketed device may be used as a physician deems appropriate to benefit an individual patient as part of the practice of medicine. However, both the physician using a device in this way and the patient on whom the device is used should understand that the off-label use may not have been tested sufficiently to establish its full risk/benefit profile, and that the clinical evidence needed to generalize safety and effectiveness expectations to a broader patient population may not be available.

Although off-label use by a physician in the routine practice of medicine is not within the FDA's regulatory purview, off-label device use diminishes the incentive for a manufacturer to study or seek FDA approval for the indication for which the product is being used off-label. In addition, inadequate safety and effectiveness data to evaluate device performance in important patient subsets limit the ability of a clinician to decide whether a specific product is appropriate for the patient. This lack greatly hinders the process of appropriately informing patients of the risks and benefits of such therapy.

If physicians use a device for an indication beyond the approved labeling, they have the responsibility to be well informed about the product, to base the product's use on sound scientific rationale, and to maintain records of the product's use and effectiveness. Specific language introduced by the FDA Modernization Act of 1997 addressed "practice of medicine" (21 U.S.C. 396 § 906, see also Food and Drug Modernization Act of 1997 § 214), stating that "nothing in this act shall be construed to limit or interfere with the authority of a health care practitioner to prescribe or administer any legally marketed device to a patient for any condition or disease within a legitimate health care practitioner-patient relationship." However, the act did make clear that promotion of medical devices falls under the FDA's purview, and therefore promotional activity for medical devices must be consistent with the device's approved labeling.

Risk, Benefit, and the Product Life Cycle

The regulatory mandate given by Congress to the FDA was to ensure a *reasonable assurance* of a device's safety and effectiveness before allowing the device to be marketed. The requirement of reasonable assurance reflected the understanding that there was no regulatory mechanism that would guarantee *absolute* safety and effectiveness of a medical device. Implicit in the requirement for reasonable assurance of a device's safety and effectiveness is an understanding of the underlying illness being treated. In other words, effective medical devices may have the capacity to do harm, and an assessment of a device's safety and effectiveness should take into account the device's risk weighed against the potential benefit in terms of clinical utility. Although the reasonable assurance mandate allows the FDA to rely on prudent risk-benefit assessments in its decision-making process, this requirement adds to the complexity of the FDA's task in determining the appropriate level of information needed before allowing a product to be marketed, given that there is no "one size fits all" approach for medical devices. Throughout a device's life cycle, ongoing risk-benefit assessments must be made by the FDA to protect and promote public health.

Total Product Life Cycle Approach

All medical devices have a finite product life cycle, from the concept phase through product obsolescence (Figure 3-4). The FDA views device development in terms of a continuum of development phases in which product risk and benefit evaluation must take place across all stages of the product life cycle. The product life cycle from concept through obsolescence for most cardiovascular devices is much shorter compared with the average drug. The optimal regulatory strategy must take into account the rapid product life cycle of cardiovascular devices. Novel approaches are necessary to evaluate serial iterations of existing technologies, so that a product is not confined to obsolescence after completion of a clinical trial designed to test the first-generation device. Allowing manufacturers to submit supplements to already-approved PMAs is one approach to streamline the regulatory review process for incremental device changes. In addition, the practice of device regulation views the product life cycle in its entirety; preclinical development, clinical testing, marketing, and postmarket surveillance of a device are not divided phases but represent a continuing spectrum of development.

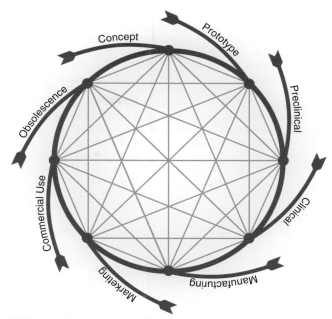

FIGURE 3-4 The total product life cycle.

Device Safety and Failure Concepts

The design, biomaterials, and developmental and implementation testing programs used for clinical implants and other medical devices are intended to minimize the severity and likelihood of failures. The majority of approved medical devices serve their patients well, alleviating pain and disability, enhancing quality of life, and increasing survival. Nevertheless, some medical devices fail, often following extended intervals of satisfactory function. Problems involving medical device technology are often called *medical device errors*.[31] Unraveling a cause of failure in an individual case usually requires systematic integration of clinical and laboratory information pertaining to the patient and pathologic analyses of the device, often called *failure mode analysis*. When possible, this should occur in the relevant anatomic and pathophysiologic context. Analysis of a cohort of failed devices can involve many such cases and sometimes additional investigation, such as review of corporate quality assurance or other documents. Regardless of implant site or desired function of the device, the overwhelming majority of clinical complications produced by implanted cardiovascular devices fall into several well-defined categories that include 1) thrombosis and thromboembolism; 2) device-associated infection; 3) exuberant or defective healing; 4) degeneration, fracture, or other biomaterial failure; 5) adverse local tissue interaction, such as toxicity; and 6) adverse systemic effects, such as distant migration of biomaterials or hypersensitivity. The clinical manifestations and relative frequencies of these problems vary among different device types, and some problems are unique to specific applications and models.

Medical device failures have some features in common with medical errors in general, in that they result from an alignment of "windows of opportunity" in a system's defenses.[32,33] Thus, conditions that relate to demographic, structural, functional, or physiologic conditions in the patient—age, implant site anatomy, patient activity level, genetic predisposition to thrombosis, allergies—and the implantation procedure—implant type, technical procedural aspects, potential damage to the implant—are superimposed on *latent* conditions related to the design, biomaterials, device fabrication, and postmanufacture conditions that provide vulnerabilities to particular failure modes. Indeed, device failure in the clinical setting often involves multiple contributing factors. For example, a tendency toward thrombosis with a new design of prosthetic heart valve may become important only in a patient whose level of anticoagulation drops below a critical point, or in a patient who has a genetic hypercoagulability disorder or local blood stasis owing to atrial fibrillation. The process of pathologic analysis called *implant retrieval and evaluation* is often an important feature in determining the causes and contributory mechanisms of failure in implants and other devices.[34,35]

The fundamental objective of incident investigation is to identify the *root cause* of an incident and eliminate or decrease the risk of recurrence based on the probability and severity.[36] The results of implant failure analysis have several potential implications for quality care in individual patients or cohorts of prior and potential recipients; thus the FDA's MDR regulations require investigation and reporting of certain device-related incidents.[37] Analysis of an isolated failed implant or of multiple implants that have exhibited a consistent failure mode can provide important information for individual patient care. Such information can:

- Have an impact on implant selection and patient-prosthesis matching.
- Mandate altered management of a specific patient, such as for selection of the type or dose of anticoagulant therapy or serial echocardiographic assessments of an at-risk type of heart valve replacement.
- Reveal a vulnerability of a cohort of patients with a specific prosthesis to a particular mode or mechanism of device failure, which can lead to closer scrutiny of patients with this device already implanted or can stimulate the need for a change in design, materials selection, processing or fabrication, management of this group of patients, or potential action by regulatory agencies, such as further testing or withdrawal from the market.

For example, information derived from many studies of the pathologic evaluation of replacement heart valves has 1) established the rates, morphology, and mechanisms of prosthesis-associated complications; 2) elucidated the structural basis of favorable device performance; 3) predicted the effects of developmental modifications on safety and efficacy; and 4) enhanced our understanding of patient-prosthesis and blood-tissue interactions.

Mechanical failure of biomaterials and adverse tissue-biomaterial interactions are often implicated as the key factors in a device failure. A device or implant can fail simply because the component biomaterials did not have the requisite physical, chemical, or biologic properties for the intended application. Some important mechanisms of tissue-biomaterial interaction are similar across device types, and thus several generic types of device-related complications can occur in recipients of nearly all cardiovascular implants; however, some complications are seen only in some cohorts of specific device types with a particular design or specific materials. Generic complications of cardiovascular devices (e.g., thrombus formation), those specific to particular models, and those specific to a particular device type and model are illustrated in Figure 3-5.

Device design is critical to performance. The design of a heart valve affects the pattern of blood flow and associated platelet damage and the presence of regions of blood stasis, all of which contribute to the risk of thrombosis.[38] However, redesigning a medical device to eliminate one complication can have unintended, potentially serious consequences. When a widely used tilting-disk heart valve was redesigned to allow more complete opening and thereby enhance its hemodynamic function and reduce the incidence of thrombosis, a large number of mechanical failures occurred (Figure 3-6).[39,40] Device failures that directly lead, or could potentially lead, to patient injury require comprehensive root analyses and prompt reporting to the FDA for regulatory action, which could lead to product recall.

Ensuring the Safety of Marketed Devices

One of the most complex tasks faced by the FDA for class III devices is finding the proper balance between ensuring product safety and effectiveness while making beneficial therapies available to the public as quickly as possible. To achieve the appropriate balance, the FDA considers multiple factors across all stages of the product development life cycle. For example, initiation of a clinical study requires an adequate determination of safety based on preclinical laboratory, engineering, and animal testing. Subsequently, approval of class III devices, and regulatory clearance of some class II devices, in turn requires a determination of safety and effectiveness based on data generated from clinical testing. Risk and benefit evaluation continue in the postapproval setting and include a review of device use in lesions and in patients not assessed in the premarket testing for product approval. The optimal balance of preapproval/postapproval requirements for device safety and effectiveness information must weigh the appropriate level of testing to permit marketing against potential delays in the availability of potentially life-saving or life-enhancing products for patients.

Although preclinical and clinical testing of cardiovascular devices provides invaluable information on safety and effectiveness in a select population, data are typically incomplete regarding device performance in populations not included in premarket clinical trials ("real world" use) and over many years after implantation. Furthermore, preclinical and clinical studies performed for device approval may not be adequate to detect rare yet catastrophic adverse events. Such low-occurrence events might be detected only in large patient populations and over longer follow-up periods, making it necessary to gather information after a product is available for general clinical use. Hence, the need arises for continued device evaluation after a product is allowed on the market.

Postmarket Safety Assessment Tools

Postapproval surveillance of medical devices provides a means to collect data regarding real-world use, long-term reliability, usefulness of training programs, subgroup evaluation within and beyond the approved patient population, and rare adverse events over a longer period of follow-up than is typically achievable in the premarketing phase. Several methods are used to collect postapproval clinical information for devices, and each is subject to various levels of scientific rigor, ranging from RCTs to qualitative, adjunct forms of data collection (Box 3-1). Under current MDR regulations, as specified in the Safe Medical Devices Act of 1990 (PL 101-629), the FDA requires device manufacturers and health care institutions to report within 10 days all device-related deaths and serious illnesses or injuries. Data from pathologic studies of surgically retrieved implants and autopsy studies augment clinical data; however, given the absence of denominator information (the total number of devices actually used), assessment of adverse-event rates is not possible via this mechanism. Accurate determination of adverse-event rates requires a prospective study with a defined sample size and follow-up period.

The increased rate of technology turnover, shorter product life cycles, and obstacles to conducting large, randomized clinical

---

Box 3-1 Examples of Post-Approval Data Collection Methods

- Randomized, blinded controlled clinical trial
- Randomized, nonblinded clinical trial
- Comparative and noncomparative cohort clinical study
- Case-control study
- Registry study
- Survey
- Active surveillance
- Passive surveillance via Medical Device Reporting (MDR) system, Medical Device Safety Network (MedSun), and International Vigilance

Examples ranked in order of level of scientific rigor, starting from the most scientifically valid method of data collection to purely descriptive and potentially more-biased forms of obtaining data.

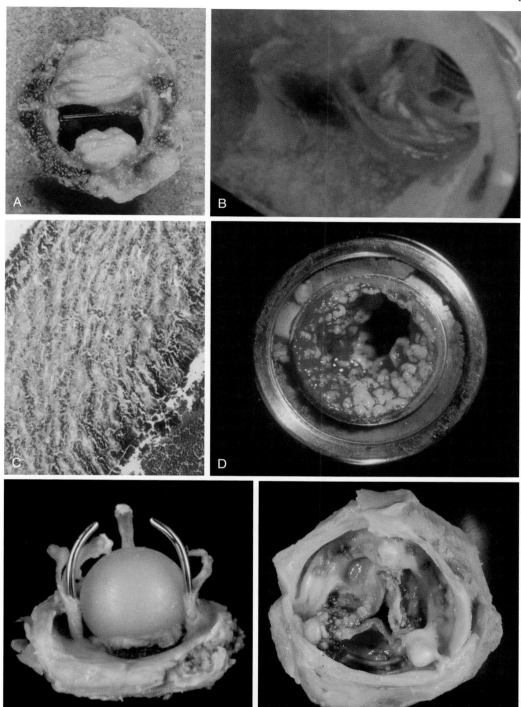

FIGURE 3-5 Common cardiovascular medical device complications: thrombus, infection, and durability limitations. **A,** Thrombus on a mechanical heart valve. **B,** Thrombus in a left ventricular assist device (LVAD). **C,** Infection associated with a synthetic vascular graft. Photomicrograph showing dark blue bacteria and acute inflammatory cells (hematoxylin and eosin; x40). **D,** Fungal infection in an LVAD conduit. **E,** Cloth wear on a cloth-covered ball-in-cage valve. **F,** Calcification of a bioprosthetic heart valve. (*B, From Fyfe B, Schoen FJ: Pathologic analysis of 34 explanted Symbion ventricular assist devices and 10 explanted Jarvik-7 total artificial hearts. Cardiovasc Pathol 1993;2:187-197. D, From Schoen FJ, Edwards WD: Pathology of cardiovascular interventions, including endovascular therapies, revascularization, vascular replacement, cardiac assist/replacement, arrhythmia control and repaired congenital heart disease. In Silver MD, Gotlieb AI, Schoen FJ (eds): Cardiovascular pathology, 3rd ed. Philadelphia, 2001, WB Saunders, p 678.*)

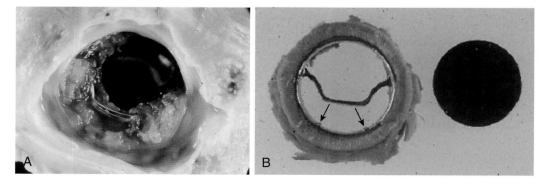

FIGURE 3-6 Bjork-Shiley valve models and associated complications. **A,** Thrombosis of the standard valve. **B,** Strut fracture of the redesigned convexo-concave valve. The *arrows* designate the sites of fracture of the struts localized to the welded joints. (*From Schoen FJ, Levy RJ, Piehler HR: Pathological considerations in replacement cardiac valves. Cardiovasc Pathol 1992;1:29-52.*)

trials for every medical device iteration underscore the importance of postapproval surveillance studies to evaluate long-term device performance. Postapproval studies can reveal unanticipated problems associated with product manufacturing changes, device modifications, or human factors such as changes in operator technique. Over the past 5 years, the FDA has frequently required postapproval studies for high-risk devices as a condition of approval. These studies often consist of registries designed to enroll a consecutive series of patients at multiple clinical sites to provide critical information on the safety and effectiveness of the device in general use. Importantly, the sample sizes of these postapproval registries need to be large enough to provide the rates of uncommon serious adverse events with sufficient precision.

Effective postapproval device assessment relies on active collaboration among device manufacturers, regulatory bodies, health care facilities, and physicians to detect and report device-related injuries and other adverse events. Postmarket surveillance is particularly relevant to the field of cardiovascular devices in view of the rapidity of technology advancement and shortened product life cycles. Extended follow-up of subjects enrolled in feasibility and pivotal preapproval studies (typically through 5 years for EDSs and other high-risk permanent implants) and postapproval studies are therefore critical to confirm long-term device safety and effectiveness. For new devices that are rapidly adopted by physicians for use in patients, it is imperative that postapproval surveillance studies initiate enrollment at the time of PMA approval. The intended use and indications for use of an approved device are clearly described in the product's labeling and instructions for use; however, it is expected that postapproval studies will include more complex patient and lesion subsets than were present in preapproval trials. An appreciation of the true rate of rare but serious adverse events may emerge from the expanded database provided by these postapproval studies. These data can greatly enhance clinical decision making by individual physicians by providing a better informed balance of the risks and benefits of device use versus alternative therapies.

A vexing issue that illustrates the need for large datasets from preapproval and postapproval studies and monitoring of off-label use is DES thrombosis and the optimal duration of dual antiplatelet therapy. Stent thrombosis that occurs after either bare-metal or DES placement is often a catastrophic event leading to acute MI or sudden death. Preapproval studies of first-generation DESs used in noncomplex lesions demonstrated a potential safety signal of late stent thrombosis emerging more than 1 year after implantation. The FDA-required postapproval DES studies played a critical role in amplifying this safety signal by showing higher rates of late stent thrombosis in more complex lesion and patient subsets. These clinical data were consistent with preclinical studies, which suggested that DESs were associated with delayed arterial healing, leading to a longer duration of stent thrombosis risk for drug-eluting versus bare-metal stents.

On the issue of late stent thrombosis, basic science, premarket clinical trials, and postapproval study data led directly to 1) the detection of an important clinical problem, 2) a recommendation for longer treatment with dual antiplatelet therapy in patients implanted with DESs, and 3) the design and initiation of the Dual Antiplatelet Therapy (DAPT) study to evaluate the optimal duration of such therapy.[41]

Cardiologists' Role in Ensuring Device Safety and Performance

The FDA uses a variety of regulatory tools, applied both before and after commencing product marketing, to assist in the assessment of device safety and effectiveness. Clinicians also play a vital role in this process by knowing the clinical indications of the devices they use, understanding and documenting the potential adverse effects they encounter, and informing patients about benefits and risks. It is important for all physicians to review a

product's instructions for use, usually an insert within the device's packaging, regarding the populations tested in supportive clinical studies and to be thoroughly familiar with the approved indications and proper use of the product. It is equally important that clinicians and health care facilities be familiar with the FDA's MDR system for product-related adverse events, and that they report such events expeditiously. (Adverse events can be reported online at www.fda.gov/cdrh/mdr.) Resources for reporting medical device–related adverse events can be found at www.fda.gov/MedicalDevices/Safety/ReportaProblem/default.htm.

Product Recall and Center for Devices and Radiological Health

CDRH is responsible for managing medical device recalls. A *recall* is an action that is taken to address a problem with a medical device when the problem violates an FDA regulation. A device is termed *violative* and is subject to recall when it is defective or when it poses a risk to public health. Recalls are subject to FDA oversight to ensure that the actions taken by the recalling company are appropriate to protect the public health. This may include audits and follow-up with the company to ensure that the recall is completed in a timely manner to minimize the likelihood of a recurrence of the problem.

A recall does not necessarily imply that the device can no longer be used or that it must be returned to the responsible manufacturer. In some instances, a recall simply indicates that the device must be checked or repaired or that the labeling must be changed or replaced to ensure the continued safe operation of the device. Implanted devices, such as pacemakers and heart valves, may or may not need to be replaced, depending on the nature of the defect or risk. On occasion, a recall can be completed by notifying the public of the situation, so that individuals affected by the recall can contact their physicians for appropriate follow-up. A recall may be either a *correction*, in which the problem can be addressed with the device in place, or a *removal*, in which the device must be physically removed from the place where it is used or sold.

Recalls are classified based on the potential risk to public health imposed by the device problem. Class I recalls represent the highest risk, class II recalls pose a less serious risk, and class III recalls represent the lowest risk. Classification of the recall informs the public about the seriousness of the problem and also determines the nature and extent of audits and other regulatory follow-up actions. More information on recalls and the relationship among the FDA, industry, and the public in the event of a recall can be found online at www.fda.gov/cdrh/recalls/learn.htm.

Other Key Regulatory Topics
Combination Products

A combination product consists of two or more regulated products—device, drug, or biologic—either combined physically or chemically (e.g., DESs or hormone-releasing skin patches), packaged together in a single unit (e.g., an asthma inhaler plus cartridge), or packaged separately but labeled such that both products, either approved or investigational, are needed to achieve the intended effect.

As the FDA has historically been divided into separate centers for device, drug, and biologic products, defining a consistent and appropriate process for the review of a combination product containing both a drug and device, drug and biologic, or biologic and device has been challenging. In response to the substantial growth in the number of combination products, the Medical Device User Fee and Modernization Act of 2002 established an FDA Office of Combination Products (OCP). The OCP has several functions: 1) it assigns primary jurisdiction to an FDA center for review of a combination product; 2) it ensures timely and effective premarket review by overseeing reviews involving more than one center; 3) it ensures the consistency and appropriateness of postmarket regulation of combination products; and 4) it updates agreements, guidance documents, and practices specific to the assignment of combination products.

In the case of DESs, the FDA's approach was directed through the request for designation process, which determined that the primary mode of action was the mechanical support of the vessel wall provided by the stent, with the drug acting to enhance its action by potentially reducing restenosis. Because the device component was found to be primarily responsible for the therapeutic effect of the product, CDRH was named the lead center, with significant consultation to be provided by the FDA's Center for Drug Evaluation and Research.

Assessment of combination products poses numerous challenges for both premarket and postmarket evaluation. The premarket review requires the participation of numerous scientific experts from multiple centers, and testing recommendations may differ between centers. Furthermore, analysis of adverse events can also be challenging; it may not be clear whether a single component or the combination of components is responsible for the event. For example, in the small number of reports of hypersensitivity reactions associated with DESs, it is difficult to discern whether the reactions were due to the metal stent, the polymer coating, the drug in the coating, or adjunctive medications.

Role of the Advisory Panel

The FDA employs scientists, engineers, and clinicians to review marketing applications, but for first-of-a-kind technologies or for controversial applications, an advisory panel of external experts may also be consulted for a recommendation regarding device approval. Advisory panels usually consist of physicians, statisticians, ethicists, biomedical engineers, patient advocates, and an industry representative. Panel members have expertise relevant to the application being considered and no financial and/or intellectual conflicts of interest with either the subject device or competing devices. To be considered for participation as an advisory panel member, an expert must have the training and experience necessary to evaluate information objectively and to interpret its significance. The panel is considered to be advisory only; the FDA has responsibility for making final decisions on marketing applications.

CDRH Interactions with External Stakeholders and Government Partners

Active interaction among industry, investigators, the clinical community, and regulatory agencies is essential to maximize efficiency and expedite the advancement of new technologies across all stages of the product development life cycle. In recent years, the CDRH has undertaken a concerted effort to increase contact and cooperation with a wide variety of stakeholders. Effective communication with the medical device industry, academic investigators, and government bodies within the Department of Health and Human Services has always been a key element in the center's mission to protect and promote public health. Although the CDRH does not specify the exact parameters of device development protocols, in most cases, it works constructively with industry sponsors with the goal of promoting well-designed nonclinical and clinical studies that can lead to innovative and successful products reaching the market in a timely fashion. Moreover, the CDRH has collaborated with industry trade groups to develop topics for FDA guidance documents, increase educational opportunities, and cosponsor public workshops on key issues such as premarket evaluation, postmarket surveillance, and risk communication.

One of the major challenges confronting medical device developers is reimbursement for procedures that use innovative devices.

Traditionally, there has been a separation between the FDA's premarket assessment and regulation of devices versus reimbursement of medical procedures as established by the Centers for Medicare and Medicaid Services (CMS). Although both the FDA and CMS reside within HHS, their missions are both complementary and significantly different. The mission of the CDRH is to ensure that medical devices are safe and effective, whereas CMS is charged with developing and overseeing coverage policies based on a determination that procedures and products are reasonable and necessary to serve the health care needs of their beneficiaries. As a consequence, medical device developers have typically been required to interact first with the FDA and then separately with CMS. In an effort to facilitate the introduction of beneficial innovative devices and medical procedures that are important to the public health, the FDA and CMS have begun to work together in selected areas to explore the implications of new medical technologies, particularly with regard to identification of appropriate target patient populations and opportunities for data sharing.

REFERENCES

1. Daemen J, Serruys PW. Drug-eluting stent update 2007: part I. A survey of current and future generation drug-eluting stents: meaningful advances or more of the same? *Circulation* 2007;116:316-28.
2. Chaikoff EL. The development of prosthetic heart valves—lessons in form and function. *N Engl J Med* 2007;357:1368-1371.
3. Rahimtoola SH. Choice of prosthetic heart valve for adult patients: an update. *J Am Coll Cardiol* 2010;55:2413-2426.
4. Ye J, Cheumg A, Lichtenstein SV, et al. Transapical transcatheter aortic valve implantation: 1-year outcome in 26 patients. *J Thorac Cardiovasc Surg* 2009;137:167-173.
5. Joyce LD, Noon GP, Joyce DL, DeBakey ME. Mechanical circulatory support—a historical review. *ASAIO J.* 2004;50:10-12.
6. DiMarco JP. Implantable cardioverter-defibrillators. *N Engl J Med* 2003;349:1836-1847.
7. Greenhalgh RM, Powell JT. Endovascular repair of abdominal aortic aneurysm. *N Engl J Med* 2008;358:494-501.
8. Scott EC, Glickman MH. Conduits for hemodialysis access. *Semin Vasc Surg* 2007;20:158-163.
9. Pietsch JB, Shluzas LA, Pate-Cornell, et al. Stage-gate process for the development of medical devices. *J Med Dev* 2009;30:2104-1–02104-16.
10. Zenios S, Makower J, Yock P. *Biodesign: the process of innovating medical technologies,* Cambridge, UK, 2010, Cambridge University Press.
11. Ergina PL, Cook JA, Blazeby JM, et al. Challenges in evaluating surgical innovation. *Lancet* 2009;374:1097-1104.
12. Muni NI, Zuckerman BD. The process of regulatory review for new cardiovascular devices. In Antman EM (ed): *Cardiovascular therapeutics: a companion to Braunwald's heart disease,* 3rd ed. Philadelphia, 2007, Saunders Elsevier, pp 67-75.
13. Li H, Yue LQ. Statistical and regulatory issues in nonrandomized medical device clinical studies. *J Biopharm Stat* 2008;18:20-30.
14. Muni NI, Ho C, Mallis EJ. Regulatory issues for computerized electrocardiographic devices. *J Electrocardiol* 2004;37:74-77.
15. U.S. Department of Health and Human Services, U.S. Food and Drug Administration, Center for Devices and Radiological Health. CDRH FY 2004 annual report, June 24, 2005. Available at http://www.fda.gov/cdrh/annual/fy2004.
16. Sapirstein W, Zuckerman B, Dillard J. FDA approval of coronary artery brachytherapy. *N Engl J Med* 2001;344:297-299.
17. Kramer DB, Mallis E, Zuckerman BD, et al. Premarket clinical evaluation of novel cardiovascular devices: quality analysis of premarket clinical studies submitted to the Food and Drug Administration 2000-2007. *Am J Therapeut* 2010;17:2-7.
18. Grunkemeier GL, Starr A, Rahimtoola SH. Prosthetic heart valve performance: long-term follow-up. *Curr Probl Cardiol* 1992;17:329-406.
19. Wheatley DJ. Clinical evaluation: statistical considerations and how to meet them in clinical practice. *J Heart Valve Dis* 2004;13:S11-S13.
20. Grunkemeier GL, Johnson DM, Naftel DC. Sample size requirements for evaluating heart valves with constant risk events. *J Heart Valve Dis* 1994;3:53-58.
21. Grunkemeier GL, Payne N, Jin R, et al. Propensity score analysis of stroke after off-pump coronary artery bypass grafting. *Ann Thorac Surg* 2002;74:301-305.
22. Moses JW, Leon MB, Popma JJ, et al. Sirolimus-eluting stents versus standard stents in patients with stenosis in a native coronary artery. *N Engl J Med* 2003;349:1315-1323.
23. Stone GW, Ellis SG, Cox DA, et al. A polymer-based, paclitaxel-eluting stent in patients with coronary artery disease. *N Engl J Med* 2004;350:221-231.
24. Fleming TR. Surrogate endpoints and FDA's accelerated approval process. *Health Affairs* 2011;24:67-78.
25. DeGruttola VG, Clax P, DeMets DL, et al. Considerations in the evaluation of surrogate endpoints in clinical trials: summary of a National Institutes of Health workshop. *Controlled Clin Trials* 2001;22:485-502.
26. Dembitsky WP, Tector AJ, Park S, et al. Left ventricular assist device performance with long-term circulatory support: lessons from the REMATCH trial. *Ann Thorac Surg* 2004;78:2123-2129.
27. Park SJ, Kim YH, Park DW, et al. Randomized trial of stents versus bypass surgery for left main coronary artery disease. *N Engl J Med* 2011;364:1718-1727.

CH
3

DEVICE DEVELOPMENT FOR CARDIOVASCULAR THERAPEUTICS: CONCEPTS AND REGULATORY IMPLICATIONS

28. Hammermeister K, Sethi GK, Henderson WG, et al: Outcomes 15 years after valve replacement with a mechanical versus a bioprosthetic valve: final report of the Veterans Affairs randomized trial. *J Am Coll Cardiol* 2000;36:1152-1158.

29. Leon MB, Smith CR, Mack M, et al. Transcatheter aortic-valve implantation for aortic stenosis in patients who cannot undergo surgery. *N Engl J Med* 2010;363:1597-1607.

30. U.S. Food and Drug Administration. Guidance for clinical trial sponsors on the establishment and operation of clinical trial data monitoring committees, 2001. Available at http://www.fda.gov/cber/gdlns/clindatmon.htm.

31. Goodman GR. Medical device error. *Crit Care Nurs Clin North Am* 2002;14:407-416.

32. Carthey J, de Leval MR, Reason JT. The human factor in cardiac surgery: errors and near misses in a high technology medical domain. *Ann Thorac Surg* 2001;72:300-305.

33. Reason J. Human error: models and management. *Br Med J* 2000;320:768-770.

34. Anderson JM, Schoen FJ, Brown SA, Merritt K. Implant retrieval and evaluation. In Ratner BD, Hoffman AS, Schoen FJ, Lemons JE (eds): *Biomaterials science: an introduction to materials in medicine*, 2nd ed. Philadelphia, 2004, Saunders Elsevier, pp 771-782.

35. Schoen FJ, Hoffman AS. Implant and device failure. In Ratner BD, Hoffman AS, Schoen FJ, Lemons JE (eds): *Biomaterials science: an introduction to materials in medicine*, 2nd ed. Philadelphia, 2004, Saunders Elsevier, pp 760-765.

36. Baretich MF. Medical device incident investigation. *Biomed Sci Instrum* 2007;43: 302-305.

37. Shepherd M. SMDA '90 (Safe Medical Devices Act of 1990): user facility requirements of the final medical device reporting regulation. *J Clin Eng* 1996;21:114-148.

38. Yoganathan AP, Corcoran WH, Harrison EC, Carl JR. The Bjork-Shiley aortic prosthesis: flow characteristics, thrombus formation and tissue overgrowth. *Circulation* 1978; 58:70-76.

39. Walker AM, Funch DP, Sulsky SI, Dreyer NA. Patient factors associated with strut fracture in Bjork-Shiley 60 convexo-concave heart valves. *Circulation* 1995;92:3235-3239.

40. Blot WJ, Ibrahim MA, Ivey TD, et al. Twenty-five–year experience with the Björk-Shiley Convexoconcave heart valve: a continuing clinical concern. *Circulation* 2006;iii:2850-2857.

41. Mauri L, Kereiakes DJ, Normand SL, et al. Rationale and design of the dual antiplatelet therapy study: a prospective multicenter, randomized, double-blind trial to assess the effectiveness and safety of 12 versus 30 months of dual antiplatelet therapy in subjects undergoing percutaneous coronary intervention with either drug-eluting stent or bare metal stent placement for the treatment of coronary artery lesions. *Am Heart J* 2010;160:1035-1041.

CHAPTER 4

Pharmacogenetics

Janice Y. Chyou, Jessica L. Mega, and Marc S. Sabatine

CLOPIDOGREL, 53

Drug, Indications, Mechanism of Action, and
 Pharmacology, 53
Drug Interactions, 53
Pharmacogenetics of Clopidogrel Therapy, 53
Therapeutic Modifications, 56
Future Directions, 57

WARFARIN, 57

Drug, Indications, Mechanism of Action, and
 Pharmacology, 57
Drug Interactions, 57
Pharmacogenetics of Warfarin Therapy, 57
Therapeutic Implications, 59
Future Directions, 60

STATINS, 60

Drug, Indications, Mechanism of Action, and Pharmacology, 60
Drug Interactions, 60
Pharmacogenetics of Statin Therapy, 61
Therapeutic Implications, 63
Future Directions, 63

REFERENCES, 63

Interindividual variability of drug response has been well documented. In addition to drug-drug and drug-environment interactions, genetic factors have emerged as contributors to variability in response to several cardiovascular medications. *Pharmacogenetics* is the study of genetic determinants of drug response. Polymorphisms of genes encoding for proteins involved in the drug pathway, from absorption to activation (if administered as a prodrug) to action, and to elimination, may contribute to drug response (Table 4-1). Genetic variants can contribute to altered pharmacokinetics and pharmacodynamics and subsequently affect a drug's efficacy and safety profile (Table 4-2).

The study of pharmacogenetics may be particularly illuminating when 1) compromised medication efficacy can be serious or fatal; 2) the therapeutic window is very narrow; or 3) the predictive value of specific genetic variants for serious or fatal drug-associated side effects has been firmly established, and timely testing may prevent development of serious side effects by therapeutic modifications. These considerations have driven explorations into the pharmacogenetics of clopidogrel, warfarin, and statin therapy.

Incorporation of pharmacogenetic testing more broadly into cardiovascular therapeutics will require the availability of cost-effective pharmacogenetic assays, evidence that pharmacogenetic-guided therapy improves care, and effective evidence-based therapeutic modifications based on pharmacogenetic testing.

Clopidogrel

Drug, Indications, Mechanism of Action, and Pharmacology

Clopidogrel is an irreversible oral thienopyridine. As part of dual antiplatelet therapy in combination with aspirin, clopidogrel is indicated in the management of acute coronary syndromes (ACS) with or without percutaneous coronary interventions (PCI).[1-6] The optimal dosage and duration of dual antiplatelet therapy is an area of active research.[7-9]

Clopidogrel is ingested as a prodrug. Its absorption limited by intestinal efflux transporter P-glycoprotein.[10] Upon absorption, 85% of the prodrug is hydrolyzed by esterases into an inactive carboxylic acid derivative. The remaining 15% of the prodrug is metabolized by the hepatic cytochrome P450 (CYP450) system, especially the CYP2C19 enzyme, into active thiol metabolites. Peak plasma concentrations of the active metabolites are reached within several hours with increased peak concentrations after administration of 600 mg versus 300 mg of clopidogrel as a loading dose.[11] The active thiol metabolites irreversibly bind the $P2Y_{12}$ component of the adenosine diphosphate (ADP) receptors on the platelet surface, inducing inhibition of ADP-dependent platelet activation and aggregation that persists for the lifetime of the platelet.

Drug Interactions

Variable platelet inhibition with clopidogrel therapy has been observed and approximates a bell-shaped distribution (Figure 4-1). Drug-drug interactions have been investigated as potential contributors to variable clopidogrel response, and interactions of clopidogrel with statins and proton-pump inhibitors (PPIs) have been particularly explored. Concomitant statin therapy has been shown to attenuate platelet inhibition by clopidogrel in a dose-dependent manner without an increase in clinical cardiovascular events.[12]

PPIs are inhibitors of the CYP2C19 enzyme, an important enzyme involved in clopidogrel metabolism. Initial observational data raised concerns about the potential association of concurrent PPI (especially omeprazole) and clopidogrel therapy with increased cardiovascular events and mortality.[13] However, a subgroup analysis of Trial to Assess Improvement in Therapeutic Outcomes by Optimizing Platelet Inhibition with Prasugrel–Thrombolysis in Myocardial Infarction (TRITON-TIMI) 38 and Prasugrel in Comparison to Clopidogrel for Inhibition of Platelet Activation and Aggregation–Thrombolysis in Myocardial Infarction (PRINCIPLE-TIMI) 44 found no association of concurrent PPI and thienopyridine therapy with adverse clinical outcomes, although an attenuation in in vitro platelet inhibition was noted in patients on concomitant PPI therapy.[14] The prospective, randomized controlled Clopidogrel and the Optimization of Gastrointestinal Events (COGENT) trial reported no difference in the primary cardiovascular safety endpoint—defined as the composite of death from cardiovascular causes, nonfatal myocardial infraction (MI) coronary revascularization, or ischemic stroke—and a benefit in reduction of gastrointestinal (GI) bleeding in patients concomitantly taking a PPI and clopidogrel compared with those taking clopidogrel alone.[15] The totality of data led to a 2010 Expert Consensus Document that recommended that "PPIs are appropriate in patients with multiple risk factors for GI bleeding who require antiplatelet therapy. Routine use of either a PPI or an histamine 2–receptor antagonist (H2RA) is not recommended for patients at lower risk of upper GI bleeding."[16] A subsequent analysis of the French Registry of Acute ST-Elevation and Non–ST-Elevation Myocardial Infarction (FAST-MI) registry, published after the release of the Expert Consensus Document, also found no association between concurrent PPI therapy and increased cardiovascular events and mortality.[17] Further studies focusing on PPI use will continue to help guide decisions about PPI therapy among clopidogrel-treated patients, weighing the GI bleeding versus the cardiovascular risks.

Pharmacogenetics of Clopidogrel Therapy

Polymorphisms of genes involved in clopidogrel's absorption (*ABCB1*), metabolism (*CYP2C19*), and action (*P2RY12*) have been investigated for potential association with clopidogrel response

(Figure 4-2, Table 4-3). Of these, the association between polymorphisms in the *CYP2C19* gene and clopidogrel response has been most consistently replicated, and variants in the *CYP2C19* gene were the only significant polymorphisms noted in a genome-wide association study (GWAS) that specifically examined the genetic influence of clopidogrel pharmacologic response.[18]

CYP2C19

The *CYP2C19* gene is highly polymorphic, with known reduced-function and enhanced-function variants. The *CYP2C19* gene encodes for the CYP450 2C19 enzyme involved in both steps of hepatic activation of clopidogrel to its active metabolite (see Figure 4-2). Among the reduced-function variants—such as the *2, *3, *4, *5, *6, *7, and *8 variants—the *2 variant is the most common.[19-21] The *2 variant (rs4244285) involves a single base-pair mutation of G→A at position 681, which creates an aberrant splice site, resulting in downstream synthesis of a truncated, nonfunctional CYP2C19 protein.

Subgroup analyses of clinical trials and registry databases, as well as a GWA study and a meta-analysis, have identified reduced-function *CYP2C19* variants to be independently associated with diminished inhibition of ADP-induced platelet aggregation[18,22-25] and with increased risk of death and ischemic events in the setting of clopidogrel therapy.[18,21,26-31] Compared with noncarriers, carriers of at least one copy of a reduced-function *CYP2C19* allele have approximately 30% lower levels of active clopidogrel metabolite and approximately 25% relatively less platelet inhibition with clopidogrel.[26] Carriers of both one and two *CYP2C19* reduced-function alleles appear to be at increased risk for adverse cardiovascular outcomes: meta-analyses of patients treated with clopidogrel predominantly for PCI found carriers of one and two reduced-function *CYP2C19* alleles to have about a 1.5-fold increase in the risk of cardiovascular death, MI, or stroke and a threefold increase in the risk for stent thrombosis compared with noncarriers.[21,30]

Genetic studies of patients receiving clopidogrel predominantly *not* for PCI yielded different results. The Clopidogrel for High Atherothrombotic Risk and Ischemic Stabilization, Management, and Avoidance (CHARISMA) genomics substudy, which involved patients with stable atherothrombotic diseases, found patients homozygous but not heterozygous for *CYP2C19*2 to have an increased risk of ischemic events and decreased risk of bleeding with dual antiplatelet therapy.[32] Genetic analysis of the Clopidogrel in Unstable Angina to Prevent Recurrent Events (CURE) trial, which studied patients with non–ST-elevation ACS managed predominantly without PCI, found that carrier status of *CYP2C19* reduced-function alleles did not affect clopidogrel efficacy.[33]

TABLE 4-1	Key Genes Along the Drug Pathway of Clopidogrel, Warfarin, and Statin		
	CLOPIDOGREL	**WARFARIN**	**STATIN**
Absorption	*ABCB1*		*ABCB1*
Metabolism	*CYP2C19* *CYP3A4* *CYP3A5*	*CYP2C9*	*CYP3A4* *CYP3A5* *CYP2C9* *CYP2D6* *SLCO1B1*
Action	*P2RY12*	*VKORC1*	*APOB* *APOE* *CETP* *HMGCR* *LDLR*

TABLE 4-2	Contributions of Genetic Polymorphism to the Efficacy and Safety Profile of Clopidogrel, Warfarin, and Statin Therapy	
	Genetic Implications	
	OF DRUG EFFICACY	**OF DRUG-RELATED ADVERSE EVENTS**
Clopidogrel	↓ Efficacy: *CYP2C19*2	↑ Adverse events (↑ bleed): *CYP2C19*17
Warfarin	Time to therapeutic threshold: *VKORC1* haplotype A	↑ Bleed: *CYP2C9*2 and *3, especially *3
Statin	LDL cholesterol lowering: *APOE, PCSK9, ?CETP*	Myopathy: *SLCO1B1*

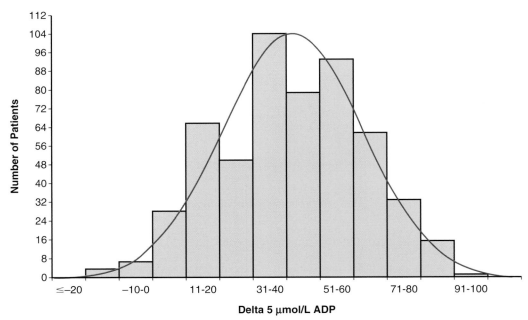

FIGURE 4-1 A total of 544 patients receiving clopidogrel were studied. By light-transmittance aggregometry and 5 μmol of adenosine diphosphate (*ADP*) as the agonist, change in platelet aggregation from baseline after the initiation of clopidogrel therapy was analyzed. Mean change in aggregation was 41.9%, with a standard deviation of 20.8%. Histogram of change in platelet aggregation from baseline after initiation of clopidogrel therapy of the study population resembled a bell-shaped distribution. (*From Serebruany VL, Steinhubl SR, Berger PB et al. Variability in platelet responsiveness to clopidogrel among 544 individuals.* J Am Coll Cardiol 45:246-251.)

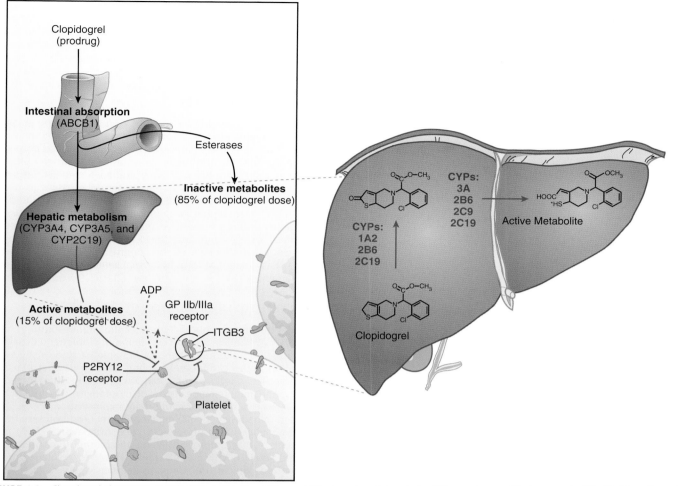

FIGURE 4-2 Clopidogrel absorption, metabolism, and action pathway. ADP, adenosine diphosphate; CYP, cytochrome; GP, glycoprotein. *(Modified from Simon T, Verstuyft C, Mary-Krause M, et al. Genetic determinants of response to clopidogrel and cardiovascular events. N Engl J Med 2009;360:363-375.)*

TABLE 4-3	Key Clopidogrel Pharmacogenetic Variants			
GENE (LOCATION)	**ENCODES FOR**	**VARIANT STUDIED (EFFECT ON PROTEIN)**	**FREQUENCY OF ALLELE***	**ASSOCIATED DISEASE PHENOTYPE AND RELATIVE RISK**
ABCB1 (7q21.1)	P-glycoprotein drug efflux transporter, involved in intestinal absorption of clopidogrel	C3435T (rs1045642)	T allele: • European: 57.1% • Asian: 41.7%-45.9% • Sub-Saharan African: 11.1%	*Biochemical:* lower levels of the active metabolite with TT genotype[10] *Clinical:* higher rate of cardiovascular events with TT genotype FAST-MI and TRITON-TIMI 38 genetic studies[26,35] but with CC genotype in PLATO genetic study[36]
CYP2C19 (10q24.1-q24.3)	Eponymous protein essential in the two-step CYP450 hepatic metabolism of clopidogrel prodrug	*2 (rs4244285, G681A) (reduced function)	A allele: • European: 15.5% • Asian: 25.6%-28.4% • Sub-Saharan African: 14.4%	*Biochemical:* relative reduction of 32.4% in plasma exposure to the active metabolite and 25% in platelet inhibition[25] *Clinical:* 1.5 times increased risk of cardiovascular events and three times increased risk of stent thrombosis in patients undergoing PCI[30]
		*3 (rs4986893) (reduced function)	A allele: • White: 0% • Pacific Rim heritage: 8.7% • African: 2.1%	
		*17 (rs12248560, *C806T*) (enhanced function)	T allele: • European: 21.7% • Asian: 0%-2.2% • Sub-Saharan African: 27.5%	*Biochemical:* enhanced inhibition of ADP-induced platelet aggregation[34] *Clinical:* increased risk of bleeding without significant influence on stent thrombosis in the initial study[34]; a subsequent study found enhanced clopidogrel efficacy (decreased cardiovascular events in ACS) without increase in major bleeding[33] Gene-dose-dependent biochemical and clinical phenotypic effects[34]

*Allele frequency is per HapMap phase 2[139] except otherwise noted.

ACS, acute coronary syndromes; ADP, adenosine diphosphate; FAST-MI, French Registry of Acute ST-Elevation and Non–ST-Elevation Myocardial Infarction; PCI, percutaneous coronary intervention; PLATO, Platelet Inhibition and Patient Outcomes; TRITON-TIMI, Trial to Assess Improvement in Therapeutic Outcomes by Optimizing Platelet Inhibition with Prasugrel–Thrombolysis in Myocardial Infarction.

Differences in the patient populations (stable atherothrombotic disease vs. acute coronary syndrome) and exposure to PCI may in part explain the differential findings of the CHARISMA and CURE genetic studies versus those based on trials predominantly involving patients with ACS for PCI.

The enhanced-function *CYP2C19*17* variant has also been reported to influence clopidogrel therapy and involves a single base-pair mutation of C→T at position 808. It has been associated with increased transcriptional activity of the CYP2C19 enzyme, extensive clopidogrel metabolism with enhanced production of active clopidogrel metabolites, greater inhibition of ADP-induced platelet aggregation, and increased risk of bleeding in a gene–dose-dependent fashion without significant impact on stent thrombosis, combined 30-day ischemic endpoint of death or MI, or urgent target vessel revascularization.[34] Genetic analysis of the CURE study found carrier status of the *CYP2C19*17* allele to be associated with more pronounced reductions of cardiovascular events with clopidogrel therapy.[33]

ABCB1

The *ABCB1* gene, also known as *MDR1*, encodes for the xenobiotic efflux P-glycoprotein pump involved in the intestinal absorption of clopidogrel. The C3435T polymorphism has been variably associated with clopidogrel response, and the 3435TT genotype has been associated with decreased peak plasma concentrations of clopidogrel and its active metabolites.[10] In the FAST-MI registry, carriers of TT and CT genotypes, compared with carriers of the wild-type genotype, had an increase in cardiovascular events in the setting of treatment with clopidogrel therapy after an acute MI.[26] Likewise, in the setting of treatment with clopidogrel in TRITON–TIMI 38, *ABCB1* 3435TT homozygotes experienced a 72% increased risk of adverse cardiovascular events compared with CT/CC individuals.[35] Data from the Platelet Inhibition and Patient Outcomes (PLATO) trial provided contrasting results with an association between 3435CC genotype and higher rates of ischemic events.[36]

PON1

The *PON1* gene encodes for paraoxonase-1, an esterase synthesized in the liver and associated with high-density lipoprotein (HDL) in the blood. Using in vitro metabolomic profiling followed by subsequent analyses of a case-cohort study and an independent replication study, another study identified *PON1* Q192R polymorphism to affect variability in clopidogrel efficacy and to confer increased risks for definite stent thrombosis.[37] The impact of the *PON1* Q192R polymorphism on clopidogrel treatment effect was thought to be mediated by the role of paraoxonase-1 in bioactivation of clopidogrel from the intermediate product formed by the cytochromes in the liver to the active metabolite in the bloodstream.[37] However, *PON1* Q192R was not associated with clopidogrel treatment effect in a previously published GWAS of clopidogrel pharmacogenomics,[18] and the study that identified this novel *PON1* Q192R polymorphism was unable to reproduce the well-replicated effect of *CYP2C19* loss-of-function alleles on clopidogrel therapy. A larger study, which specifically investigated the impact of *PON1* Q192R genotype in parallel to that of *CYP2C19*2* on clopidogrel response and stent thrombosis, found no association of *PON1* Q192R with platelet response to clopidogrel and risk of stent thrombosis, although it confirmed the effect of *CYP2C19*2* on clopidogrel antiplatelet response and risks for stent thrombosis.[38]

Therapeutic Implications

In March 2010, the U.S. Food and Drug Administration (FDA) approved a new label for clopidogrel with the addition of a boxed warning regarding pharmacogenetics, noting diminished effectiveness of therapy in poor metabolizers (defined as having two loss-of-function *CYP2C19* alleles). The boxed warning further states that "tests are available to identify a patient's *CYP2C19* genotype and can be used as an aid in determining therapeutic safety [and to] consider alternative treatment or treatment strategies in patients identified as *CYP2C19* poor metabolizers."[39]

PHARMACOGENETIC TESTING IN CLOPIDOGREL THERAPY

Although tests to identify a patient's *CYP2C19* genotype are available, clopidogrel pharmacogenetic testing is not routinely performed.[40] Local "point of care" assays have been piloted at specific institutions. The role and predictive value of clopidogrel pharmacogenetic testing are being actively studied. Key questions under investigations include 1) determining the best assays to use to guide clopidogrel therapy (e.g., which platelet function assays, if any, *CYP2C19* genotyping, or a combination of the two); 2) assessing whether testing and therapies guided by testing results improve outcomes; and 3) estimating the cost effectiveness of testing to tailor clopidogrel therapy (to be generic in the United States in 2012) versus treating with nongeneric therapies with less interpatient variability.

THERAPEUTIC MODIFICATIONS

Potential therapeutic modifications for individuals found to carry the *CYP2C19*2* allele include escalation of clopidogrel dosage or switching to an alternate agent. Earlier smaller studies suggested that tailoring the clopidogrel loading dose to platelet reactivity may improve cardiovascular outcome[41,42] and that increased loading and maintenance doses of clopidogrel (up to 1200 mg loading dose and up to 150 mg daily maintenance dose),[43,44] or repeated reloading with 600 mg clopidogrel based on serial vasodilator-stimulated phosphoprotein phosphorylation (VASP) measurements,[45] may improve platelet inhibition in carriers of a reduced-function *CYP2C19*2* allele. However, results from the randomized clinical trial Gauging Responsiveness with a VerifyNow Assay–Impact on Thrombosis and Safety (GRAVITAS) study, which enrolled 2796 mostly stable angina patients for elective PCI, did not suggest a benefit in cardiovascular outcomes or stent thrombosis with doubling the dose of clopidogrel (from 75 mg to 150 mg after reloading with another 600 mg) in clopidogrel nonresponders identified by high residual platelet activity.[46] Nonetheless, findings from the GRAVITAS study did not definitively rule out the use of tailoring thienopyridine therapy based on platelet function testing; further studies are warranted. The ELEVATE-TIMI 56 study found that among patients with stable cardiovascular disease, tripling the maintenance dose of clopidogrel to 225 mg/day in *CYP2C19*2* heterozygotes achieved levels of platelet reactivity similar to those seen with the standard 75-mg dose in noncarriers. However, doses as high as 300 mg/day did not result in comparable degrees of platelet inhibition in *CYP2C19*2* homozygotes.[46a]

Alternate therapeutic options for patients requiring dual antiplatelet therapy for ACS and PCI are available. Prasugrel is a third-generation thienopyridine that irreversibly binds the platelet $P2Y_{12}$ receptor to inhibit ADP-induced platelet aggregation.[47] The TRITON-TIMI 38 trial found prasugrel to have superior efficacy compared with clopidogrel in reducing all-cause mortality or vascular complications, including stent thrombosis, but with an increased risk of bleeding.[48] The FDA approved prasugrel for use in PCI for ACS in July 2009. A genetic analysis within the TRITON-TIMI 38 trial found that polymorphisms in several genes, including *CYP2C19*, did not affect active metabolite levels, platelet aggregation inhibition, or clinical cardiovascular event rates in individuals treated with prasugrel.[19] The impact of *CYP2C19* polymorphisms on clopidogrel compared with that on prasugrel is likely mediated by differential involvement of esterases and the CYP450 system in the activation of clopidogrel and prasugrel. For clopidogrel, esterases shunt the majority of ingested clopidogrel to a dead-end inactive pathway with the remaining prodrug requiring a two-step CYP-dependent oxidation to produce active clopidogrel metabolites; for prasugrel, esterases are part of the activation pathway, and activation of prasugrel requires only a single CYP-dependent oxidative step.[19] The *ABCB1* C3435T polymorphism, which has inconsistently been reported to influence clopidogrel therapy in some studies, was also found not to affect clinical or pharmacologic outcomes in patients treated with prasugrel.[35]

Another therapeutic option for patients is ticagrelor, an oral reversible antagonist of the platelet ADP P2Y$_{12}$ receptor, approved for use in Europe and the United States. Superior efficacy of ticagrelor to clopidogrel in ACS was established by the PLATO trial, which found ticagrelor (180 mg loading dose, 90 mg twice daily maintenance dose) to be superior to clopidogrel (300 to 600 mg loading dose, 75 mg daily maintenance dose) in reduction of vascular death, MI, or stroke but with an increase in the rate of non–procedure-related bleeding.[49] Ticagrelor is an active compound and not a prodrug, and thus it does not require hepatic CYP450-mediated activation. Pharmacogenetic analysis of the Randomized Double-Blind Assessment of the Onset and Offset of the Antiplately Effects of Ticagrelor Versus Clopidogrel in Patients with Stable Coronary Artery Disease (ONSET/OFFSET and RESPOND) confirmed that the antiplatelet effect of ticagrelor was consistently superior to clopidogrel irrespective of *CYP2C19* genotype, including the *2 poor metabolizer and *17 ultrametabolizer.[50] A genetic analysis within the PLATO trial found ticagrelor superior to clopidogrel in treatment of ACS irrespective of *CYP2C19* polymorphism, although the magnitude of benefit tended to be greater in carriers of loss-of-function alleles.[36]

COST EFFECTIVENESS OF CLOPIDOGREL PHARMACOGENETICS TESTING

Universal reimbursement policies for pharmacogenetic testing or platelet function testing for clopidogrel remain to be defined. Although cost may compromise the feasibility and utility of current commercial clopidogrel pharmacogenetic testing, the availability of clopidogrel in generic form in the near future may offset the cost of testing. Furthermore, technological advances and increased availability of testing may shorten the turnaround time, making it easier for test results to be incorporated into clinical decision making. Currently, inexpensive and rapid point-of-care testing has been locally developed and pioneered at several institutions. Formal cost-effectiveness analyses of clopidogrel pharmacogenetic testing will continue to provide useful data.

Future Directions

Prospective clinical trials will be helpful to further evaluate whether genetic testing indeed improves outcome in the setting of antiplatelet therapy, whether pharmacogenetic and platelet function testing are complementary, and whether testing of all patients versus only the high-risk population is most feasible. Several clinical trials are ongoing to further investigate the impact of antiplatelet therapy for PCI guided by platelet function testing (ARCTIC, NCT00827411) or genotyping (GIANT NCT01134380; TARGET-PCI, NCT01177592; Genotype Guided Comparison of Clopidogrel and Prasugrel Outcomes Study, NCT00995514). These studies will assist in determining the optimal way to use pharmacogenetic testing to select among different antiplatelet regimens.

Warfarin

Drug, Indications, Mechanism of Action, and Pharmacology

Warfarin is an oral anticoagulant used for treatment of venous thromboembolism and for perioperative prevention of venous thromboembolism, anticoagulation for mechanical heart valves, and prevention of stroke in patients with atrial fibrillation. Warfarin exerts its anticoagulant effects by antagonizing vitamin K.

Warfarin is ingested as a combination of active R- and S-warfarin enantiomers, with the S-enantiomer about three to five times more potent than the R-enantiomer. Warfarin is rapidly absorbed with near complete bioavailability. It circulates primarily bound to albumin with a mean plasma half-life of 40 hours. Warfarin interrupts hepatic vitamin K recycling by inhibiting vitamin K epoxide reductase and vitamin K quinine reductase (Braunwald, Fig. 87-13). Depletion of vitamin K reserve compromises the vitamin K–dependent gamma-carboxylation necessary for production of coagulation factors II, VII, IX, and X and anticoagulant proteins C and S. Full anticoagulation effects of warfarin are observed at least 24 to 72 hours after initiation of therapy, when clotting factors previously synthesized have been depleted. S-warfarin is inactivated by CYP2C9-mediated hydrolysis; the less active R-enantiomer is metabolized by CYP1A2 and CYP3A4 enzymes.

Patients treated with warfarin are routinely monitored for their International Normalized Ratio (INR), with an INR target of 2 to 3, except for those patients with a mechanical mitral valve, in whom the INR target range is 2.5 to 3.5. Excessive anticoagulation by warfarin and preoperative reversal of warfarin effects are managed with administration of vitamin K and, when acute reversal is indicated, with additional repletion of clotting factors via infusion of fresh frozen plasma.

Drug Interactions

Warfarin is well known for its narrow therapeutic window and extensive drug-drug and drug-diet interactions, which make the titration of warfarin dosage challenging. Increase in total-body vitamin K reserve through ingestion of vitamin K–rich foods or a decrease in vitamin K reserve during antibiotic therapy as a result of reduced GI tract production of vitamin K, respectively, attenuates or accentuates warfarin's anticoagulant effects. Concomitant therapy with CYP2C9 inducers or inhibitors, respectively, accelerates or reduces metabolism of the active S-warfarin enantiomer. CYP1A2 and CYP3A4, which metabolize the R-warfarin enantiomer, can also be inhibited by quinolone and macrolides, respectively, and both may be inhibited by azoles. Concurrent therapy with other anticoagulants or antiplatelet agents may potentiate bleeding risk.[51] Other cardiovascular medications, including amiodarone and statins, may also interact with warfarin. Amiodarone and its major metabolites inhibit CYP2C9, thereby potentiating the anticoagulant effects and bleeding risks of warfarin. Small retrospective studies, case series, and case reports suggest that fluvastatin, lovastatin, simvastatin, and rosuvastatin may accentuate warfarin's effect, potentially via inhibition of CYP2C9, CYP3A4, or both.[51]

Pharmacogenetics of Warfarin Therapy

Genetic polymorphisms along the warfarin pathway have been explored. GWASs have confirmed the association between genetic polymorphisms in *VKORC1*, *CYP2C9*, and *CYP4F2* genetic polymorphisms and warfarin dosing variability.[52,53] Polymorphisms of these three genes have been reported to account for about 20% to 30%, about 12%, and 1% to 4%, respectively, of variability in warfarin dosage.[52,55a,55b]

VKORC1

The *VKORC1* gene on chromosome 16 encodes for the vitamin K epoxide reductase complex 1 that is the molecular target of warfarin (Figure 4-3). *VKORC1* haplotypes were noted to stratify patients into groups with differing warfarin maintenance dose requirements.[55] Specifically, haplotype A (more prevalent in Asian populations) was associated with a lower warfarin requirement,

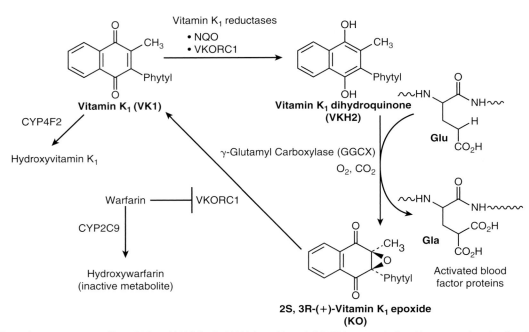

FIGURE 4-3 Warfarin pharmacogenetics. *(From McDonald MG, Rieder MJ, Nakano M, et al. CYP4F2 is a vitamin K1 oxidase: an explanation for altered warfarin dose in carriers of the V433M variant. Mol Pharmacol 2009;75:1337)*

TABLE 4-4	Key Warfarin Pharmacogenetic Variants				
GENE (LOCATION)	**ENCODES FOR**	**VARIANT STUDIED (EFFECT ON PROTEIN)**	**MINOR ALLELE FREQUENCY***	**ASSOCIATED DISEASE PHENOTYPE**	**THERAPEUTIC IMPLICATIONS**
VKORC1 (16p11.2)	VK epoxide reductase complex 1, site of warfarin action[55]	rs9923231, in LD with rs9934438	T allele: • European: 39.8% • Asian: 90.1%-94.2% • Sub-Saharan African: 2.2%	*Biochemical:* twofold reduction in VKORC1 mRNA level in human liver[60] *Clinical:* Reduced warfarin maintenance dose requirement Shorter time to first therapeutic INR[66] (as part of *VKORC1* haplotype A)	Warfarin-sensitivity: need less warfarin
		rs9934438, in LD with rs9923231	A allele: • European: 39.8% • Asian: 90.1%-94.2% • Sub-Saharan African: 2.2%		
CYP2C9 (10q24)	Eponymous protein involved in metabolizing the active warfarin (S-warfarin)	*2, rs1799853 (reduced function)	T allele: • European: 10.4% • Asian: 0% • Sub-Saharan African: 0%	*Biochemical:* decreased clearance of S-warfarin, increased plasma S- to R-warfarin ratio *Clinical:* Reduced warfarin maintenance dose requirement[64] Increased risk of major hemorrhage[64,65]	Decreased warfarin metabolism: need less warfarin
		*3, rs1057910 (reduced function)	C allele: • European: 5.8% • Asian: 3.3%-4.4% • Sub-Saharan African: 0%		
CYP4F2 (19p13)	Eponymous protein involved in metabolism of active VK	rs2108622 (reduced function)	T allele: • European: 23.3% • Asian: 23.3%-26.7% • Sub-Saharan African: 5.8%	*Biochemical:* decreased metabolism of VK1[69] *Clinical:* May potentially need increased warfarin dose[53,54,55a,71]	May need more warfarin

*Allele frequency per HapMap phase 2[139] except otherwise noted.
INR, international normalized ratio; LD, linkage disequilibrium; VK, vitamin K.

and haplotype B (more prevalent in African populations) was associated with higher warfarin maintenance dose requirement. Haplotype combinations of A/A, A/B, and B/B, respectively, confer low-, intermediate-, and high-maintenance dose requirements of warfarin.[55] Two noncoding single-nucleotide polymorphisms (SNPs) from haplotype A rs9923231 (−1639G>A, also known as *VKORC1**2) and rs9934438 (1173C>T), which are in linkage disequilibrium (LD), have consistently been associated with a lowered warfarin dosage requirement.[52,56-61] The minor allelic frequency of rs9923231 and rs9934438 both vary among racial groups (Table 4-4).[56] However, the presence of the rs9923231 or rs9934438 variants, irrespective of race, was consistently associated with a decrease in warfarin dosage requirement in all three of the racial groups—Asians, whites, and blacks—specifically studied in the International Warfarin Pharmacogenetics Consortium (IWPC) cohort.[56]

A different variant, rs61742245 (D36Y), has been associated with a higher warfarin dosage requirement.[62,63] The D36Y variant denotes a missense mutation in *VKORC1*, noted only in the background of −1639G/G with minor allele frequency of 0.043 in

Ashkenazi Jews and 0.006 in Sephardic Jews, and has been reported to contribute to additional warfarin dosage variability.[62] However, the association between warfarin dosage variability and rs61742245 (D36Y) was not noted in GWASs of genetic determinants of warfarin dose based on Swedish and American cohorts.[52,53]

CYP2C9

The *CYP2C9* gene on chromosome 10 encodes for the CYP2C9 protein crucial for inactivation of potent S-warfarin (see Figure 4-3). Two nonsynonymous exonic variants of *CYP2C9* have repeatedly been associated with variability in warfarin response.[52,53,58] The *2 variant involves substitution of cysteine for arginine at amino acid 144; the *3 variant involves substitution of leucine for isoleucine at residue 359. Both variants lead to production of reduced-function CYP2C9 protein and impaired warfarin metabolism. As such, *CYP2C9*2 and *CYP2C9*3 variants have been associated with a decreased warfarin maintenance dose requirement[64] and increased hemorrhage risk.[64,65]

The respective roles of VKORC1 and CYP2C9 proteins in warfarin's action (pharmacodynamics) and metabolism (pharmacokinetics) likely underscore the differential influences of their genetic polymorphisms. The *VKORC1* genetic polymorphism, but not *CYP2C9* genetic polymorphism, affects time to first therapeutic INR; in particular, *VKORC1* haplotype A has been associated with accelerated achievement of first therapeutic INR.[66-68] Both the *CYP2C9* (*2, *3) and the *VKORC1* (haplotype A,[67] rs9923221[68]) polymorphisms were associated with overanticoagulation, defined as INR above 4.[67,68] However, *CYP2C9* poor-metabolizer variants, but not *VKORC1* polymorphisms, were associated with an increased risk of major hemorrhage with persistently increased risk after stabilization of warfarin therapy.[65]

CYP4F2

The *CYP4F2* gene on chromosome 19 encodes for the CYP4F2 protein, which has been shown to catalyze hydroxylation of vitamin K_1 (VK1) into its hydroxylated form as a "siphoning" pathway for excess VK1 (see Figure 4-3).[69] The *CYP4F2* rs2108622 variant, which involves a V433M missense mutation with downstream reduced CYP4F2 activity and reduced VK1 metabolism,[69] has been associated with an increased warfarin dose requirement,[52-54,55a,55b,69] presumably because of elevated levels of active vitamin K, thereby necessitating higher warfarin dosage to elicit an anticoagulant response.[69] In addition, rs2108622 has been reported to account for a modest additional 1% to 4% of warfarin dosage variability.[52,54,55a,55b]

Although CYP4F2's role in metabolizing VK1 offers a biologically plausible explanation for the potential association between rs2108622 and an increased warfarin dosing requirement, this association has not been consistently replicated.[73] A prospective candidate gene study from the United Kingdom found no association between rs2108622 and warfarin dosage variability but noted another *CYP4F2* variant, rs2189784 (in strong LD with rs2108622), to be associated with lengthened time to therapeutic INR.[73] Available data on *CYP4F2* and warfarin dosage so far suggest a possible association between these *CYP4F2* variants and the potential need for an increased warfarin requirement, whether as maintenance or to achieve therapeutic INR; however, further studies are needed to elucidate this potential relationship.

Therapeutic Implications

Clinical factors such as age, gender, body surface area, and target INR account for about 15% to 17% of variability in therapeutic warfarin dose.[52,54] *CYP2C9* and *VKORC1* genotype information account for an additional 40% of variability in warfarin dosing; together with clinical factors, about 55% of variability in warfarin dosing can be explained,[52,54,68] and *CYP4F2* genotype information may contribute an additional 2% of variability.[54] In 2007, the FDA updated the warfarin label with mention that *VKORC1* and *CYP2C9*

variants may influence warfarin dosage requirement. In 2010, the label was further updated with inclusion of a pharmacogenetic-guided dosing scheme for initiation of warfarin therapy that factored in the presence or absence of *VKORC1*-1369 G→A and *CYP2C9*2 or *CYP2C9*3.

PHARMACOGENETIC TESTING IN WARFARIN THERAPY

Algorithms incorporating a patient's genotype, demographic factors, and comedications have been developed in an attempt to improve prediction of initial warfarin dosing.[68,74,75] These algorithms most greatly benefit patients needing extremes of warfarin dosage (≤21 mg/week or ≥49 mg/week).[75]

Early relatively small prospective randomized trials comparing clinical efficacy of genotype-based versus standard warfarin dosing have generated inconsistent results. Whereas one study compared algorithms that incorporated the *CYP2C9* genotype versus the standard warfarin dose-initiation algorithm and noted the genotype-based algorithm to be associated with a statistically significant reduction in time to first therapeutic INR and time outside therapeutic INR range,[76] other prospective randomized studies that incorporated the *CYP2C9* genotype[77] or *CYP2C9* and *VKORC1* genotype data[78,79] could not replicate these findings. More recently, a nonrandomized prospective study comparing a genotype-guided warfarin algorithm with clinical algorithms using clinical factors and INR response available after 2 to 3 days of warfarin therapy found genotype-guided warfarin adjustment to result in more time spent in the therapeutic INR range and fewer laboratory or clinical adverse events.[80] The Mayo-Medco study also reported a statistically significant 31% reduction in all-cause hospitalization and a 28% reduction in hospitalization for bleeding or thromboembolism during a 6-month follow-up period in the genotyped cohort (genotyped for *CYP2C9* and *VKORC1* with 11- to 60-day turnaround time for receipt of genotype data) compared with the control group.[81] Although prospective, the Mayo-Medco study was nonrandomized and therefore susceptible to confounding. The benefit of adding genotype information to clinical features requires assessment in prospective randomized trials, which are ongoing.

COST EFFECTIVENESS OF WARFARIN PHARMACOGENETICS TESTING

By cost-effectiveness analyses, genotype-guided warfarin dosing for patients with atrial fibrillation would be cost effective if restricted to patients at high risk of hemorrhage (HEMORR$_2$HAGES score of 1 to 2)[82]; if testing turnaround time is less than 24 hours and cost less than $200; if genotype-guided therapy can prevent more than 32% of major bleeding events[82]; or if genotype-guided therapy increases the time spent in the therapeutic INR range by 9% points.[83] Cost effectiveness of warfarin pharmacogenetic testing is currently limited by the average cost of testing; however, the costs and ease of the testing are improving greatly. In addition, there is a need for large-scale randomized prospective studies to determine whether genotype-guided therapy indeed improves clinical outcomes. At present, pharmacogenetic testing for warfarin is not covered by Medicare except within the confines of a clinical trial specifically designed to demonstrate the clinical effects of warfarin pharmacogenetics testing.[84]

THERAPEUTIC MODIFICATIONS

For carriers of *VKORC1* and/or *CYP2C9* polymorphisms indicated for warfarin therapy, potential therapeutic modifications include 1) consideration for pharmacogenetic-guided warfarin therapy as described above, or 2) consideration of alternate anticoagulant therapy. Several novel oral anticoagulants that do not require routine monitoring and titration now exist as therapeutic alternatives to warfarin. Novel oral anticoagulants with published data, such as reversible oral direct thrombin inhibitors (dabigatran) and reversible oral Xa inhibitors (rivaroxaban, edoxaban, and apixaban) have been studied for a variety of conditions, including prophylaxis[85-97] and treatment[98] of venothromboembolism and anticoagulation for atrial fibrillation.[99-102] Importantly, although the above studies establishing efficacy and cost effectiveness of novel anticoagulants in stroke prophylaxis for patients with atrial fibrillation were conducted against warfarin therapy, studies establishing efficacy and cost effectiveness of novel anticoagulants in VTE prophylaxis were conducted against low-molecular-weight heparin, not against warfarin therapy. No outpatient oral therapeutic alternates to warfarin currently exist for anticoagulation for mechanical valves.

Future Directions

Several large-scale prospective studies (NCT00162435, NCT00927862, NCT00904293, NCT00654823), including the Clarification of Optimal Anticoagulation through Genetics (COAG) trial,[103] funded by the National Heart, Lung, and Blood Institute, are under way to further elucidate whether genotype-guided algorithms improve clinical outcomes. Novel anticoagulants that include dabigatran, rivaroxaban, apixaban, and edoxoban appear to be promising alternatives to warfarin. Substudies of landmark trials and additional trials are under way to further define the indication, duration, potential interactions, and selection consideration of these novel anticoagulants. Future directions include research that directly compares the efficacy and safety of novel anticoagulants with a pharmacogenetic-guided warfarin regimen and the relative cost effectiveness of each. Investigation on pharmacogenetics of novel anticoagulants may also be important; however, considering that there is less interpatient variability with the new agents, the impact of genetic polymorphisms would presumably be less apparent.

Statins

Drug, Indications, Mechanism of Action, and Pharmacology

Statins (β-hydroxy-β-methylglutaryl coenzyme A [HMG-CoA] reductase inhibitors) exert their effects primarily through two mechanisms. First, statins act as lipid-lowering agents by interfering with synthesis of cholesterol and lipid intermediate molecules. Statins inhibit HMG-CoA reductase, thwarting the formation of the rate-limiting mevalonate; consequently, plasma low-density lipoprotein (LDL) clearance is increased, and hepatic very-low-density lipoprotein (VLDL) and LDL production is decreased. Second, statins have antiinflammatory effects (see Chapter 24 and Braunwald, Chapter 47). Statins have been used in the management of dyslipidemia, coronary artery disease, stroke, peripheral artery disease, and perioperative risk reduction; statins have also been investigated for immunomodulation for heart failure (Braunwald, Chapter 33) and for prevention of venous thromboembolism.[104]

Pharmacodynamics and pharmacokinetics of commonly used statins are summarized in Table 4-5. Notably, atorvastatin, simvastatin, and lovastatin are heavily metabolized by CYP3A4, fluvastatin is metabolized by CYP2C9, and rosuvastatin is partially metabolized by CYP2C9 and CYP2C19 but is largely excreted as the parent compound. Pravastatin metabolism is predominantly unaffected by the hepatic cytochrome system and is partially degraded in the stomach and metabolized by non-CYP enzymes via sulfation; it is then excreted as the parent compound into feces and urine. Differences in the metabolism of the different statins affect potential drug-drug and drug-dietary interactions and safety profiles.

Drug Interactions

Drug-drug interactions of CYP3A4-dependent simvastatin, lovastatin, and atorvastatin with medications that affect the CYP3A4 enzymes are well established. CYP3A4 inhibitors such as azole antifungal medications, macrolide antibiotics (e.g., azithromycin, erythromycin, clarithromycin), verapamil and diltiazem, imatinib, and HIV protease inhibitors increase plasma statin concentrations and elevate the potential risk for rhabdomyolysis. Grapefruit and pomegranate juice contribute to diet-drug interaction through CYP3A4 inhibition. Phenytoin, rifampin, and carbamazepine are CYP3A4 inducers and may accelerate clearance of simvastatin, atorvastatin, and lovastatin.

Amiodarone is thought to interact with statins via CYP3A4 inhibition—affecting simvastatin, lovastatin, and atorvastatin most significantly—and via CYP2C9 inhibition, affecting fluvastatin. The FDA has issued a warning to avoid concomitant therapy of amiodarone with more than 20 mg of simvastatin.[105] Cyclosporine, a potent inhibitor of the OATP1B1 transporter, can increase plasma

TABLE 4-5	Clinical Pharmacodynamics and Pharmacokinetics of HMG-CoA Reductase Inhibitors*					
	SIMVASTATIN	**LOVASTATIN**	**ATORVASTATIN**	**FLUVASTATIN**	**ROSUVASTATIN**	**PRAVASTATIN**
T_{max} (h)	1.3-2.4	2-4	2-3	0.5-1	3	0.9-1.6
C_{max} (ng/mL)	10-34	10-20	27-66	448	37	45-55
Bioavailability (%)	5	5	12	19-29	20	18
Lipophilicity	Yes	Yes	Yes	Yes	No	No
Administered as	Lipophilic lactone prodrug	Lipophilic lactone prodrug	Active statin acid	Active statin acid	Active statin acid	Active statin acid
Protein binding (%)	94-98	>95	80-90	>99	88	43-55
Metabolism	CYP3A4	CYP3A4	CYP3A4	CYP2C9	CYP2C9, 2C19 (minor) Excreted mainly unchanged	Sulfation
Metabolites	Active	Active	Active	Inactive	Active (minor)	Inactive
Transporter protein substrates	Yes	Yes	Yes	No	Yes	Yes/no
$T_{1/2}$ (h)	2-3	2.9	15-30	0.5-2.3	20.8	1.3-2.8
Urinary excretion (%)	13	10	2	6	10	20
Fecal excretion (%)	58	83	70	90	90	71

*Based on a 40-mg oral dose, with the exception of fluvastatin XL (80 mg).
HMG-CoA, β-hydroxy-β-methylglutaryl coenzyme A.
Modified from Bellosta S, Rodolfo P, Corsini A. Safety of statins: focus on clinical pharmacokinetics and drug interactions. *Circulation* 2004;109:50.

concentrations of pravastatin, rosuvastatin, and simvastatin. The addition of gemfibrozil, which affects glucoronidation of statins, to cerivastatin therapy resulted in a higher statin concentration and a higher incidence of rhabdomyolysis; this contributed to the removal of cerivastatin from the market and led to the recommendation of fenofibrate as the fibrate of choice when needed in addition to a statin for lipid control. Statins may also alter the plasma levels of other medications; for example, they increase digoxin levels by inhibiting P-glycoprotein transport. Simvastatin, fluvastatin, and rosuvastatin have also been noted to potentiate the effect of warfarin.

Pharmacogenetics of Statin Therapy

Genetic polymorphisms of several genes encoding for proteins along the statin pathway (Tables 4-6 and 4-7) have been explored. To date, two GWAS have been published on statin pharmacogenetics, one with an emphasis on statin response[106] and the other with an emphasis on statin-induced myopathy.[107]

KEY GENETIC VARIANTS AFFECTING STATIN EFFICACY

APOE

The APOE polymorphisms have been most consistently shown to modulate statin response. APOE encodes for apolipoprotein E, which functions as a ligand that mediates uptake of chylomicrons, very-low-density lipoprotein (VLDL), and high-density lipoprotein (HDL) from the bloodstream into the liver by lipoprotein receptors. An early meta-analysis found statin response to be increased in carriers of the APOE*2 variant but decreased in carriers of the APOE*4 variant[108]; these findings were also seen in the Pravastatin or Atorvastatin Evaluation and Infection Therapy–Thrombolysis in Myocardial Infarction (PROVE IT-TIMI) 22 study[109] and the Genetics of Diabetes Audit and Research (Go-DARTS) diabetic cohort.[110] The specific association between enhanced LDL cholesterol lowering with statin therapy in carriers of the APOE*2 variant has been replicated by many studies[111,112] with statistical significance even at the genome-wide level.[111] The Scandinavian Simvastatin Survival Study (4S) further noted in a follow-up substudy that MI survivors with the APOE*4 variant have excess mortality, but that mortality can be mitigated by treatment with simvastatin.[113]

PCSK9

A robust and biologically plausible association between PCSK9 polymorphisms and statin response has also been reported. PCSK9 encodes for the proprotein convertase subtilisin/kexin 9 protein that guides the LDL receptor to proteolysis. Proteolysis of the LDL receptor decreases cholesterol uptake into the hepatocyte, leading to increased cholesterol in the bloodstream and decreased hepatic availability of cholesterol susceptible to statin-mediated inhibition of cholesterol synthesis and recycling. Thus, a gain-of-function PCSK9 mutation would be expected to increase LDL cholesterol concentration and reduce susceptibility to statin therapy, whereas a loss-of-function PCSK9 mutation would be expected to decrease plasma LDL cholesterol concentration and increase susceptibility to statin therapy. PCSK9 rs11591147 involves a missense arg46-to-leu (R46L) mutation, leading to reduced-function PCSK9 protein, which has been associated with a reduction in the plasma level of total cholesterol and LDL cholesterol[114] and with a reduction in coronary artery events.[114,115] Combined whole-genome analysis of the Treating to New Targets (TNT) cohort found a significant association between PCSK9 rs11591147 with statin response at the genome-wide level.[111]

HMGCR

HMGCR encodes for the HMG Co-A reductase that is the rate-limiting step of cholesterol biosynthesis and the molecular target of statins. The HMGCR H7 haplotype,[116] defined by the presence of three intronic SNPs—rs17244841, rs17238540, and rs3846662—has been associated with reduced LDL cholesterol lowering in response to statin therapy in candidate gene studies.[116-119] The rs3846662 variant has been associated with variation in the proportion of HMGCR mRNA that is alternatively spliced; this variation in alternative splicing has been postulated to modify HMG-CoA reductase activity and statin-binding ability.[120] In studies exclusively involving atorvastatin therapy, rs10464433, rs17671591, and rs6453131—but not the previously discussed rs17244841, rs17238540, or rs3846662—were modestly associated with statin response.[111,112]

CETP

CETP encodes for cholesteryl ester transfer protein, which transfers cholesteryl esters from HDL to apolipoprotein B–containing particles in exchange for triglyceride, thereby reducing the concentration of HDL. Statin has been noted to decrease CETP protein concentration and CETP-related activity. The two most notable CETP variants are the B1 variant (biochemical phenotype of high CETP concentration, low HDL) and the B2 variant (biochemical phenotype of low CETP concentration, high HDL). The effect of CETP genotype on statin therapy is not clear. Although the initial study suggested preferential angiographic response to statin

TABLE 4-6	Key Genes and Proteins in the Statin Pathway	
ROLE IN STATIN PATHWAY	**GENES**	**PROTEIN**
Absorption	ABCB1/MDR1	P-glycoprotein drug efflux transporter
Uptake into hepatocytes	SCLO1B1/OATP1B1	Organic anion transporter
Action	HMGCR	HMG-CoA reductase, rate-limiting step of cholesterol synthesis and molecular target of statin
	CETP	Cholesteryl ester transfer protein, which transfers cholesteryl esters from HDL to ApoB-containing particles in exchange for triglyceride, thereby reducing the concentration of HDL
	LDLR	Receptor for plasma LDL
	APOE	ApoE, major binding protein for VLDL/IDL cholesterol
	PCSK9	Proprotein convertase subtilisin kexin 9 protein that guides the LDL receptor to proteolysis
Metabolism	CYP3A4	Eponymous cytochrome 450 protein involved in metabolism of simvastatin, lovastatin, atorvastatin
	CYP3A5	Eponymous cytochrome 450 protein involved in metabolism of atorvastatin
	CYP2C9	Eponymous cytochrome 450 protein involved in metabolism of fluvastatin
	CYP2D6	Eponymous cytochrome 450 protein
Others genes studied	KIF6	Kinesin-family 6
	CLMN	Calmin, highly expressed in liver and adipose tissue but exact role in cholesterol or lipoprotein metabolism unknown
	APOC1	Apoprotein C1, in strong LD with ApoE

Apo, apolipoprotein; HDL, high-density lipoprotein; HMG-CoA, β-hydroxy-β-methylglutaryl coenzyme A; LD, linkage disequilibrium; LDL, low-density lipoprotein; VLDL, very-low-density lipoprotein; IDL, intermediate-density lipoprotein.

TABLE 4-7　Key Statin Pharmacogenetic Variants

GENE (LOCATION)	ENCODES FOR	VARIANT STUDIED (EFFECT ON PROTEIN)	MINOR ALLELE FREQUENCY*	ASSOCIATED DISEASE PHENOTYPE
APOE (19q13.2)	Apolipoprotein E	*2 (e2), rs7412 Arg176Cys	T allele: • European: 5.5%[111†] • Asian: 5.4%-9.5% • Sub-Saharan African: 9.5%	Greater LDL cholesterol lowering with statin therapy, strongly associated with statin response[111,112]
		*4 (e4), rs429358 Cys130Arg	C allele: • European: 16.2%[111†] • Asian: 0%-1.1% • Sub-Saharan African:1.7%	Decreased LDL cholesterol lowering with statin therapy, increased risk of mortality in myocardial infarction survivor, but risk abolished with statin therapy[113]
KIF6 (6p21)	Kinesin-like family protein-6	rs20455 Trp719Arg in strong LD with rs9462535, rs9471077	C allele: • European: 37.2% • Asian: 47.7%-57.0% • Sub-Saharan African: 90.4%	Previously reported association with increased CAD risks (OR 1.1-1.5)[126-128] not replicated in GWAS[129-133] Enhanced reduction of coronary events with statin therapy (37%-50% relative reduction of risk)[126,140-142]
PCSK9 (1p34.1-p32)	Proprotein convertase subtilisin kexin 9 protein	rs11591147 Arg46Leu	T allele: • European: 2.8% • Asian: 0% • Sub-Saharan African: 0%	Lower baseline total cholesterol and LDL cholesterol concentration[114] Reduced risk of coronary events[114,115]
CLMN (14q32.13)	Calmin	rs8014194	A allele: • European: 19.8% • Asian: 10%-16.3% • Sub-Saharan African: 56.2%	Association with statin-mediated change in total cholesterol and LDL cholesterol concentrations[106]
APOC1 (19q13.2)	Apoprotein C1	rs4420638	G allele: • European: 18.3% • Asian: 6.5%-11.6% • Sub-Saharan African: 13.1%	Association with statin-mediated change in total cholesterol and LDL cholesterol concentrations[106]
SLCO1B1 (12p12)	Organic anion transporter	rs4363657 T>C, intronic In LD with rs4149056	C allele: • European: 16.4% • Asian: 37.8%-54.7% • Sub-Saharan African: 14.2%	Associated with statin-induced myopathy by GWAS, OR 4.3 per C allele[107]
		*5, rs4149056 Val174Ala	C allele: • European: 15.0% • Asian: 11.1%-15.1% • Sub-Saharan African: 0.9%	Increased risk of statin-induced myopathy (OR 4.5-4.7 per C allele) with simvastatin 80 mg/day (OR 2.6 per C allele) with simvastatin 40 mg/day regimen[107] Highest attributable risk for myopathy in first year of statin therapy[107] Twofold increase in myopathy and myalgia with and without CK increase[138]
		rs2306283 Asn130Asp	T allele: • European: 59.7% • Asian: 16.3%-34.9% • Sub-Saharan African: 19.0%	Lower statin concentration[107] Lower risk of myopathy in SEARCH[107]
		*15 (defined by rs4149056 + rs2306283; Val174Ala and Asn130Asp)	Japanese: 15%[143]	Slow response to pravastatin[144]

*Allele frequency per HapMap phase 2[139] except otherwise noted.
†Allele frequency data not available via HapMap phase 2.
CAD, cardiac artery disease; CK, creatine kinase; GWAS, genome-wide association study; LDL, low-density lipoprotein; OR, odds ratio; SEARCH, Study of the Effectiveness of Additional Reductions in Cholesterol and Homocysteine.

therapy with the B1 but not with the B2 variant,[121] a later study noted enhanced statin benefit and decreased event rates in B2 alleles upon statin therapy,[122] yet other studies reported increased cardiovascular events[123] and mortality rates[123,124] in B2 allele carriers receiving statin therapy. A meta-analysis of 13,677 subjects from a total of seven large studies found no interaction between CETP genotype and pravastatin therapy.[125]

LDLR

LDLR encodes for the LDL receptor involved in the uptake of LDL cholesterol into hepatocytes. The LDLR L5 haplotype has been associated with lessened simvastatin-induced reduction of LDL cholesterol, total cholesterol, non-HDL, and apolipoprotein, but this has not been consistently replicated in larger studies.[118]

KIF6

KIF6 encodes for the kinesin-like family protein-6. Initial reports noted KIF6 Trp719Arg carriers to be at modestly increased risk for coronary artery disease (odds ratio [OR], 1.1 to 1.5).[126-128] Moreover, the benefit of statin therapy appeared to be greater in those harboring the KIF6 719Arg variant; however, subsequent studies have not been able to replicate the association between KIF6 Trp719Arg and increased coronary artery risk.[129-134] In the Justification for the Use of Statins in Prevention: An Intervention Trial Evaluating Rosuvastatin (JUPITER), KIF Trp719Arg polymorphism did not affect the efficacy of rosuvastatin 20 mg/day on the reduction of LDL cholesterol or primary cardiovascular endpoint.[135] Results from a study involving two meta-analyses (inclusive of data from JUPITER) and a meta-regression analysis provided a biologically plausible explanation for these conflicting findings. KIP6 719Arg allele appears to increase vulnerability to LDL cholesterol. This genetically mediated differential vulnerability to LDL cholesterol thereby modifies the expected clinical benefit from therapies that lower serum LDL cholesterol levels.[135a]

GENOME-WIDE ASSOCIATION STUDIES OF STATIN RESPONSE

A large GWAS pooling the Pravastatin Inflammation/CRP Evaluation (PRINCE), Cholesterol and Pharmacogenetic Study (CAP), and TNT cohorts reported SNP rs8014194 in the CLMN gene and SNP rs4420638 in APOC1 near APOE to be the only SNPs associated with LDL cholesterol change at the genome-wide significance level. Also, rs4420638 is a polymorphism of the APOC1 gene that is adjacent to, coinherited, and in strong LD with APOE; association between rs4420638 and statin-mediated reduction in LDL cholesterol may be explained by APOC1's strong LD with APOE, as well as ApoC1 protein's previously reported role in cholesterol metabolism with inhibition of CETP, inhibition of lipoprotein particle clearance via VLDL receptor, and yet with preserved binding of the ApoC1-enriched lipoprotein to the LDL receptor.[106] The GWAS also revealed an association between a novel intronic polymorphism of the CLMN gene (rs8014194) and statin-mediated change in total cholesterol and LDL concentrations. The calmin protein sequence contains a calponin-like binding domain with expected actin-binding activity. Calmin is highly expressed in liver and adipose tissue, but the exact role of calmin in cholesterol or lipoprotein metabolism is unknown.[106] Further studies are needed to replicate the finding of the CLMN gene and to understand the functional significance of this new candidate gene.

KEY GENETIC VARIANTS AFFECTING STATIN ADVERSE EFFECTS

Recognized adverse effects of statin therapy include muscle toxicity and elevation of liver enzymes. Asymptomatic mild elevation of liver enzymes has been reported with all statins; the rate of liver failure has been reported to be about 1 per million person-years of statin use.[136] Muscle toxicity ranges from myalgia without elevation of creatinine kinase (CK), mild myopathy with mild CK elevation (11 per 100,000 person-years), to rhabdomyolysis with CK elevation and renal failure (3.4 per 100,000 person-years).[136] Myopathy risks are increased with the simvastatin 80-mg regimen,[107] which has led to restriction of this high-dose simvastatin regimen by the FDA[137]; it is also increased in the female gender and[138] in drug-drug interactions, especially with concomitant use of statins dependent on CYP3A4 metabolism (lovastatin, simvastatin, atorvastatin), with potent CYP3A4 inhibitors, or with amiodarone or calcium antagonists.[105,107] Additionally, some genetic variants, such as those in SLCO1B1, influence the side-effect profile of some statins.

SLCO1B1

Polymorphisms in the SLCO1B1 gene have been associated with myopathy, ranging from mild myalgia without CK elevation to mild myopathy with mild CK elevation to rhabdomyolysis.[107,138] The SLCO1B1 gene encodes for the organic anion transport polypeptide OATP1B1, which facilitates active uptake of statins from the bloodstream into hepatocytes. Variants in the SCLO1B1 gene were the only genetic polymorphisms significantly associated with simvastatin-induced myopathy in a GWAS.[107] In the Study of the Effectiveness of Additional Reductions in Cholesterol and Homocysteine (SEARCH) study, both noncoding rs4363657 and nonsynonymous rs4149056, which are in near complete LD with each other, were found to be strongly associated with statin-induced myopathy (OR of 4.5 and 4.7, respectively). Cumulative risks for myopathy with simvastatin 80 mg therapy were noted to be 18% for individuals with the CC genotype (homozygous for at-risk

alleles), 3% for the CT genotype, and 0.6% for the TT wild-type genotype.[107] More than 60% of myopathies in simvastatin 80-mg therapy were attributable to the rs4149056 C variant in SLCO1B1 in the SEARCH trial.[107]

In a candidate gene study that specifically tested the association among polymorphisms of SLCO1B1, CYP3A4, CYP2C8, CYP2C9, CYP2D6, and statin-induced side effects, variants in SLCO1B1 were once again found to be associated with statin side effects.[138] In the Statin Response Examined by Genetic Haplotype Marker (STRENGTH) study, carriers of the *5 allele (rs4149056) of SLCO1B1 were found to have a twofold increase in risk for experiencing composite adverse events, defined as premature continuation of the study drug for any side effect or myalgia, irrespective of CK values, or CK elevation greater than three times the upper limit of normal irrespective of symptoms.[138] As with the SEARCH results,[107] a gene-dose effect was also observed in the STRENGTH population in that the proportion of individuals with an adverse event increased with increasing numbers of the at-risk *5 allele.[138]

This gene-statin interaction (of increased adverse events in carriers compared with noncarriers of SLCO1B1*5 allele upon statin therapy) was seen with simvastatin and atorvastatin therapy but not with pravastatin therapy.[138]

Therapeutic Implications

Although genetic variants have been associated with statin efficacy and adverse effects, pharmacogenetic testing is not part of the standard of care for statin therapy. Variants in several genes—such as APOE and PCSK9—have been variably associated with altered lipid-lowering properties in the setting of statin therapy. Future studies will help determine whether testing these variants offers clinical utility; nonetheless, the biologic insights generated from genetic association studies can be particularly informative. For example, PCSK9 inhibitors have been developed and are being tested for treatment of dyslipidemia. Given the strong association between SLCO1B1 polymorphism and simvastatin-induced myopathy, future developments of testing for the SLCO1B1 polymorphism may help identify patients at risk for simvastatin-induced myopathy and guide the choice of statin for therapy to minimize side effects, promote adherence, and balance costs.

Future Directions

Randomized clinical trials are under way to investigate the pharmacogenetics of rosuvastatin therapy (NCT00934258) as well as the impact of SLCO1B1 polymorphism on rosuvastatin therapy (NCT01218347) and on the interaction between pravastatin and darunavir/ritonavir (NCT00630734).

REFERENCES

1. King SB 3rd, Smith SC Jr, Hirshfeld JW Jr, et al. 2007 focused update of the ACC/AHA/SCAI 2005 guideline update for percutaneous coronary intervention. J Am Coll Cardiol 2008;51:172-209.

2. Sabatine MS, Cannon CP, Gibson CM, et al. Addition of clopidogrel to aspirin and fibrinolytic therapy for myocardial infarction with ST-segment elevation. N Engl J Med 2005;352:1179-1189.

3. Chen ZM, Jiang LX, Chen YP, et al. Addition of clopidogrel to aspirin in 45,852 patients with acute myocardial infarction: randomised placebo-controlled trial. Lancet 2005; 366:1607-1621.

4. Sabatine MS, Cannon CP, Gibson CM, et al. Effect of clopidogrel pretreatment before percutaneous coronary intervention in patients with ST-elevation myocardial infarction treated with fibrinolytics: the PCI-CLARITY study. JAMA 2005;294:1224-1232.

5. Anderson JL, Adams CD, Antman EM, et al. ACC/AHA 2007 guidelines for the management of patients with unstable angina/non ST-elevation myocardial infarction. Circulation 2007;116:e148-e308.

6. Kushner FG, Hand M, Smith SC Jr, et al. 2009 focused updates: ACC/AHA guidelines for the management of patients with ST-elevation myocardial infarction. Circulation 2009; 120:2271-2306.

7. Mehta SR, Tanguay JF, Eikelboom JW, et al. Double-dose versus standard-dose clopidogrel and high-dose versus low-dose aspirin in individuals undergoing percutaneous coronary intervention for acute coronary syndromes (CURRENT-OASIS 7): a randomised factorial trial. Lancet 2010;376:1233-1243.

8. Mehta SR, Bassand JP, Chrolavicius S, et al and the CURRENT-OASIS 7 Investigators. Dose comparisons of clopidogrel and aspirin in acute coronary syndromes. *N Engl J Med* 2010;363:930-942.

9. Mauri L, Kereiakes DJ, Normand SL, et al. Rationale and design of the dual antiplatelet therapy study, a prospective, multicenter, randomized, double-blind trial to assess the effectiveness and safety of 12 versus 30 months of dual antiplatelet therapy in subjects undergoing percutaneous coronary intervention with either drug-eluting stent or bare metal stent placement for the treatment of coronary artery lesions. *Am Heart J* 2010;160:1035-1041.

10. Taubert D, von Beckerath N, Grimberg G, et al. Impact of P-glycoprotein on clopidogrel absorption. *Clin Pharmacol Ther* 2006;80:486-501.

11. von Beckerath N, Taubert D, Pogatsa-Murray G, et al. Absorption, metabolization, and antiplatelet effects of 300-, 600-, and 900-mg loading doses of clopidogrel: results of the ISAR-CHOICE (Intracoronary Stenting and Antithrombotic Regimen: Choose between 3 High Oral doses for Immediate Clopidogrel Effect) trial. *Circulation* 2005;112:2946-2950.

12. Saw J, Brennan DM, Steinhubl SR, et al. Lack of evidence of a clopidogrel-statin interaction in the CHARISMA trial. *J Am Coll Cardiol* 2007;50:291-295.

13. Ho PM, Maddox TM, Wang L, et al. Risk of adverse outcomes associated with concomitant use of clopidogrel and proton pump inhibitors following acute coronary syndrome. *JAMA* 2009;301:937-944.

14. O'Donoghue ML, Braunwald E, Antman EM, et al. Pharmacodynamic effect and clinical efficacy of clopidogrel and prasugrel with or without a proton-pump inhibitor: an analysis of two randomised trials. *Lancet* 2009;374:989-997.

15. Bhatt DL, Cryer BL, Contant CF, et al. Clopidogrel with or without omeprazole in coronary heart disease. *N Engl J Med* 2010;363:1909-1917.

16. Abraham NS, Hlatky MA, Antman EM, et al. ACCF/ACG/AHA 2010 expert consensus document on the concomitant use of proton pump inhibitors and thienopyridines: a focused update of the ACCF/ACG/AHA 2008 expert consensus document on reducing the gastrointestinal risks of antiplatelet therapy and NSAID use. *Circulation* 2010;122:2619-2633.

17. Simon T, Steg PG, Gilard M, et al. Clinical events as a function of proton pump inhibitor use, clopidogrel use, and cytochrome P450 2C19 genotype in a large nationwide cohort of acute myocardial infarction: results from the French Registry of Acute ST-Elevation and Non-ST-Elevation Myocardial Infarction (FAST-MI) Registry. *Circulation* 2011;123:474-482.

18. Shuldiner AR, O'Connell JR, Bliden KP, et al. Association of cytochrome P450 2C19 genotype with the antiplatelet effect and clinical efficacy of clopidogrel therapy. *JAMA* 2009;302:849-857.

19. Mega JL, Close SL, Wiviott SD, et al. Cytochrome P450 genetic polymorphisms and the response to prasugrel: relationship to pharmacokinetic, pharmacodynamic, and clinical outcomes. *Circulation* 2009;119:2553-2560.

20. Sibbing D, Stegherr J, Latz W, et al. Cytochrome P450 2C19 loss-of-function polymorphism and stent thrombosis following percutaneous coronary intervention. *Eur Heart J* 2009;30:916-922.

21. Hulot JS, Collet JP, Silvain J, et al. Cardiovascular risk in clopidogrel-treated patients according to cytochrome P450 2C19*2 loss-of-function allele or proton pump inhibitor coadministration: a systematic meta-analysis. *J Am Coll Cardiol* 2010;56:134-143.

22. Trenk D, Hochholzer W, Fromm MF, et al. Cytochrome P450 2C19 681G>A polymorphism and high on-clopidogrel platelet reactivity associated with adverse 1-year clinical outcome of elective percutaneous coronary intervention with drug-eluting or bare-metal stents. *J Am Coll Cardiol* 2008;51:1925-1934.

23. Hulot JS, Bura A, Villard E, et al. Cytochrome P450 2C19 loss-of-function polymorphism is a major determinant of clopidogrel responsiveness in healthy subjects. *Blood* 2006;108:2244-2247.

24. Brandt JT, Close SL, Iturria SJ, et al. Common polymorphisms of CYP2C19 and CYP2C9 affect the pharmacokinetic and pharmacodynamic response to clopidogrel but not prasugrel. *J Thromb Haemost* 2007;5:2429-2436.

25. Mega JL, Close SL, Wiviott SD, et al. Cytochrome P-450 polymorphisms and response to clopidogrel. *N Engl J Med* 2009;360:354-362.

26. Simon T, Verstuyft C, Mary-Krause M, et al. Genetic determinants of response to clopidogrel and cardiovascular events. *N Engl J Med* 2009;360:363-375.

27. Reference deleted in proofs.

28. Reference deleted in proofs.

29. Collet JP, Hulot JS, Pena A, et al. Cytochrome P450 2C19 polymorphism in young patients treated with clopidogrel after myocardial infarction: a cohort study. *Lancet* 2009;373:309-317.

30. Mega JL, Simon T, Collet JP, et al. Reduced-function CYP2C19 genotype and risk of adverse clinical outcomes among patients treated with clopidogrel predominantly for PCI: a meta-analysis. *JAMA* 2010;304:1821-1830.

31. Giusti B, Gori AM, Marcucci R, et al. Relation of cytochrome P450 2C19 loss-of-function polymorphism to occurrence of drug-eluting coronary stent thrombosis. *Am J Cardiol* 2009;103:806-811.

32. Bhatt DL, Simonsen KL, Emison ES, et al. *CHARISMA genomics substudy: evaluation of the CYP2C19 polymorphism in a prospective, randomized, placebo-controlled trial of chronic clopidogrel use for primary and secondary prevention.* Presented at the Transcatheter Cardiovascular Therapeutics Conferences, San Francisco, CA, 2009.

33. Pare G, Mehta SR, Yusuf S, et al. Effects of CYP2C19 genotype on outcomes of clopidogrel treatment. *N Engl J Med* 2010;363:1704-1714.

34. Sibbing D, Koch W, Gebhard D, et al. Cytochrome 2C19*17 allelic variant, platelet aggregation, bleeding events, and stent thrombosis in clopidogrel-treated patients with coronary stent placement. *Circulation* 2010;121:512-518.

35. Mega JL, Close SL, Wiviott SD, et al. Genetic variants in ABCB1 and CYP2C19 and cardiovascular outcomes after treatment with clopidogrel and prasugrel in the TRITON-TIMI 38 trial: a pharmacogenetic analysis. *Lancet* 2010;376:1312-1319.

36. Wallentin L, James S, Storey RF, et al. Effect of CYP2C19 and ABCB1 single nucleotide polymorphisms on outcomes of treatment with ticagrelor versus clopidogrel for acute coronary syndromes: a genetic substudy of the PLATO trial. *Lancet* 2010;376:1320-1328.

37. Bouman HJ, Schömig E, van Werkum JW, et al. Paraoxonase-1 is a major determinant of clopidogrel efficacy. *Nat Med* 2011;17:110-116.

38. Sibbing D, Koch W, Massberg S, et al. No association of paraoxonase-1 Q192R genotypes with platelet response to clopidogrel and risk of stent thrombosis after coronary stenting. *Eur Heart J* 2011;32:1605-1613.

39. Plavix (clopidogrel bisulfate) tablets prescribing information, 2009. Accessed December 10, 2010 at http://products.sanofi-aventis.us/PLAVIX/PLAVIX.html.

40. Holmes DR Jr, Dehmer GJ, Kaul S. ACCF/AHA clopidogrel clinical alert: approaches to the FDA "boxed warning." A report of the American College of Cardiology Foundation Task Force on Clinical Expert Consensus Documents and the American Heart Association. *Circulation* 2010;56:321-341.

41. Bonello L, Camoin-Jau L, Arques S, et al. Adjusted clopidogrel loading doses according to vasodilator-stimulated phosphoprotein phosphorylation index decrease rate of major adverse cardiovascular events in patients with clopidogrel resistance: a multicenter randomized prospective study. *J Am Coll Cardiol* 2008;51:1404-1411.

42. Bonello L, Camoin-Jau L, Armero S, et al. Tailored clopidogrel loading dose according to platelet reactivity monitoring to prevent acute and subacute stent thrombosis. *Am J Cardiol* 2009;103:5-10.

43. Gladding P, Webster M, Zeng I, et al. The pharmacogenetics and pharmacodynamics of clopidogrel response: an analysis from the PRINC (Plavix Response in Coronary Intervention) trial. *JACC Cardiovasc Interv* 2008;1:620-627.

44. Gladding P, White H, Voss J, et al. Pharmacogenetic testing for clopidogrel using the rapid INFINITI analyzer: a dose-escalation study. *JACC Cardiovasc Interv* 2009;2:1095-1101.

45. Bonello L, Armero S, Ait Mokhtar O, et al. Clopidogrel loading dose adjustment according to platelet reactivity monitoring in patients carrying the 2C19*2 loss of function polymorphism. *J Am Coll Cardiol* 2010;56:1630-1636.

46. Price MJ, Berger PB, Teirstein PS, et al. Standard- vs high-dose clopidogrel based on platelet function testing after percutaneous coronary intervention: the GRAVITAS randomized trial. *JAMA* 2011;305:1097-1105.

46a. Mega JL, Hochholzer W, Frelinger AL 3rd, et al. Dosing clopidogrel based on CYP2C19 genotype and the effect on platelet reactivity in patients with stable cardiovascular disease. *JAMA* 2011;306(20):2221-2228.

47. Niitsu Y, Jakubowski JA, Sugidachi A, et al. Pharmacology of CS-747 (prasugrel, LY640315), a novel, potent antiplatelet agent with in vivo P2Y12 receptor antagonist activity. *Semin Thromb Hemost* 2005;31:184-194.

48. Wiviott SD, Braunwald E, McCabe CH, et al. Prasugrel versus clopidogrel in patients with acute coronary syndromes. *N Engl J Med* 2007;357:2001-2015.

49. Wallentin L, Becker RC, Budaj A, et al. Ticagrelor versus clopidogrel in patients with acute coronary syndromes. *N Engl J Med* 2009;361:1045-1057.

50. Tantry US, Bliden KP, Wei C, et al. First analysis of the relation between CYP2C19 genotype and pharmacodynamics in patients treated with ticagrelor versus clopidogrel: the ONSET/OFFSET and RESPOND genotype studies. *Cir Cardiovsasc Genet* 2010;3:556-566.

51. Holbrook AM, Pereira JA, Labiris R, et al. Systematic overview of warfarin and its drug and food interactions. *Arch Intern Med* 2005;165:1095-1106.

52. Takeuchi F, McGinnis R, Bourgeois S, et al. A genome-wide association study confirms VKORC1, CYP2C9, and CYP4F2 as principal genetic determinants of warfarin dose. *PLoS Genet* 2009;5:e1000433.

53. Cooper GM, Johnson JA, Langaee TY, et al. A genome-wide scan for common genetic variants with a large influence on warfarin maintenance dose. *Blood* 2008;112:1022-1027.

54. Caldwell MD, Awad T, Johnson JA, et al. CYP4F2 genetic variant alters required warfarin dose. *Blood* 2008;111:4106-4112.

55. Rieder MJ, Reiner AP, Gage BF, et al. Effect of VKORC1 haplotypes on transcriptional regulation and warfarin dose. *N Engl J Med* 2005;352:2285-2293.

55a. Pautas E, Moreau C, Gouin-Thibault I, et al. Genetic factors (VKORC1, CYP2C9, EPHX1, and CYP4F2) are predictor variables for warfarin response in very elderly, frail inpatients. *Clin Pharmacol Ther* 2010;87:57-64.

55b. Sagreiya H, Berube C, Wen A, et al. Extending and evaluating a warfarin dosing algorithm that includes CYP4F2 and pooled rare variants of CYP2C9. *Pharmacogenet Genomics* 2010;20:407-413.

56. Limdi NA, Wadelius M, Cavallari L, et al. Warfarin pharmacogenetics: a single VKORC1 polymorphism is predictive of dose across 3 racial groups. *Blood* 2010;115:3827-3834.

57. D'Andrea G, D'Ambrosio R, Di Perna P, et al. A polymorphism in the VKORC1 gene is associated with an interindividual variability in the dose-anticoagulant effect of warfarin. *Blood* 2005;105:645-649.

58. Wadelius M, Chen L, Eriksson N, et al. Association of warfarin dose with genes involved in its action and metabolism. *Hum Genet* 2007;121:23-24.

59. Sconce EA, Khan TI, Wynne HA, et al. The impact of CYP2C9 and VKORC1 genetic polymorphism and patient characteristics upon warfarin dose requirements: proposal for a new dosing regimen. *Blood* 2005;106:2329-2333.

60. Wang D, Chen H, Momary KM, et al. Regulatory polymorphism in vitamin K epoxide reductase complex subunit 1 (VKORC1) affects gene expression and warfarin dose requirement. *Blood* 2008;112:1013-1021.

61. Geisen C, Watzka M, Sittinger K, et al. VKORC1 haplotypes and their impact on the inter-individual and inter-ethnical variability of oral anticoagulation. *Thromb Haemost* 2005;94:773-779.

62. Scott SA, Edelmann L, Kornreich R, et al. Warfarin pharmacogenetics: CYP2C9 and VKORC1 genotypes predict different sensitivity and resistance frequencies in the Ashkenazi and Sephardi Jewish populations. *Am J Hum Genet* 2008;82:495-500.

63. Loebstein R, Dvoskin I, Halkin H, et al. A coding VKORC1 Asp36Tyr polymorphism predisposes to warfarin resistance. *Blood* 2007;109:2477-2480.

64. Sanderson S, Emery J, Higgins J. CYP2C9 gene variants, drug dose, and bleeding risk in warfarin-treated patients: a HuGEnet systematic review and meta-analysis. *Genet Med* 2005;7:97-104.

65. Limdi NA, McGwin G, Goldstein JA, et al. Influence of CYP2C9 and VKORC1 1173C/T genotype on the risk of hemorrhagic complications in African-American and European-American patients on warfarin. *Clin Pharmacol Ther* 2008;83:312-321.
66. Li C, Schwarz UI, Ritchie MD, et al. Relative contribution of CYP2C9 and VKORC1 genotypes and early INR response to the prediction of warfarin sensitivity during initiation of therapy. *Blood* 2009;113:3925-3930.
67. Schwarz UI, Ritchie MD, Bradford Y, et al. Genetic determinants of response to warfarin during initial anticoagulation. *N Engl J Med* 2008;358:999-1008.
68. Wadelius M, Chen LY, Lindh JD, et al. The largest prospective warfarin-treated cohort supports genetic forecasting. *Blood* 2009;113:784-792.
69. McDonald MG, Rieder MJ, Nakano M, et al. CYP4F2 is a vitamin K1 oxidase: an explanation for altered warfarin dose in carriers of the V433M variant. *Mol Pharmacol* 2009; 75:1337-1346.
70. Reference deleted in proofs.
71. Borgiani P, Ciccacci C, Forte V, et al. CYP4F2 genetic variant (rs2108622) significantly contributes to warfarin dosing variability in the Italian population. *Pharmacogenomics* 2009;10:261-266.
72. Reference deleted in proofs.
73. Zhang JE, Jorgensen AL, Alfirevic A, et al. Effects of CYP4F2 genetic polymorphisms and haplotypes on clinical outcomes in patients initiated on warfarin therapy. *Pharmacogenet Genomics* 2009;19:781-789.
74. Gage BF, Eby C, Johnson JA, et al. Use of pharmacogenetic and clinical factors to predict the therapeutic dose of warfarin. *Clin Pharmacol Ther* 2008;84:326-331.
75. Consortium, International Warfarin Pharmacogenetics. Improved warfarin dosing with a global pharmacogenetics algorithm. *N Engl J Med* 2009;360:753-764.
76. Caraco Y, Blotnick S, Muszkat M. CYP2C9 genotype-guided warfarin prescribing enhances the efficacy and safety of anticoagulation: a prospective randomized controlled study. *Clin Pharmacol Ther* 2008;83:460-470.
77. Hillman MA, Wilke RA, Yale SH, et al. A prospective, randomized pilot trial of model-based warfarin dose initiation using CYP2C9 genotype and clinical data. *Clin Med Res* 2005;3:137-145.
78. Anderson JL, Horne BD, Stevens SM, et al. Randomized trial of genotype-guided versus standard warfarin dosing in patients initiating oral anticoagulation. *Circulation* 2007;116:2563-2570.
79. McMillin GA, Melis R, Wilson A, et al. Gene-based warfarin dosing compared with standard of care practices in an orthopedic surgery population: a prospective, parallel cohort study. *Ther Drug Monit* 2010;32:338-345.
80. Lenzini PA, Grice GR, Milligan PE, et al. Laboratory and clinical outcomes of pharmacogenetic vs. clinical protocols for warfarin initiation in orthopedic patients. *J Thromb Haemost* 2008;6:1655-1662.
81. Epstein RS, Moyer TP, Aubert RE, et al. Warfarin genotyping reduces hospitalization rates results from the MM-WES (Medco-Mayo Warfarin Effectiveness study). *J Am Coll Cardiol* 2010;55:2804-2812.
82. Eckman MH, Rosand J, Greenberg SM, et al. Cost-effectiveness of using pharmacogenetic information in warfarin dosing for patients with nonvalvular atrial fibrillation. *Ann Intern Med* 2009;150:73-83.
83. Patrick AR, Avorn J, Choudhry NK. Cost-effectiveness of genotype-guided warfarin dosing for patients with atrial fibrillation. *Circ Cardiovasc Qual Outcomes* 2009;2: 402-403.
84. Centers for Medicare and Medicaid Services. *Proposed decision memo for pharmacogenomic testing for warfarin response (CAG-00400 N)*, 2009.
85. Friedman RJ, Dahl OE, Rosencher N, et al. Dabigatran versus enoxaparin for prevention of venous thromboembolism after hip or knee arthroplasty: a pooled analysis of three trials. *Thromb Res* 2010;126:175-182.
86. Eriksson BI, Dahl OE, Rosencher N, et al. Dabigatran etexilate versus enoxaparin for prevention of venous thromboembolism after total hip replacement: a randomised, double-blind, non-inferiority trial. *Lancet* 2007;370:949-956.
87. Eriksson BI, Dahl OE, Rosencher N, et al. Oral dabigatran etexilate vs. subcutaneous enoxaparin for the prevention of venous thromboembolism after total knee replacement: the RE-MODEL randomized trial. *J Thromb Haemost* 2007;5:2178-2185.
88. Eriksson BI, Borris LC, Friedman RJ, et al. Rivaroxaban versus enoxaparin for thromboprophylaxis after hip arthroplasty. *N Engl J Med* 2008;358:2765-2775.
89. Lassen MR, Ageno W, Borris LC, et al. Rivaroxaban versus enoxaparin for thromboprophylaxis after total knee arthroplasty. *N Engl J Med* 2008;358:2776-2786.
90. Kakkar AK, Brenner B, Dahl OE, et al. Extended duration rivaroxaban versus short-term enoxaparin for the prevention of venous thromboembolism after total hip arthroplasty: a double-blind, randomised controlled trial. *Lancet* 2008;372:31-39.
91. Turpie AG, Lassen MR, Davidson BL, et al. Rivaroxaban versus enoxaparin for thromboprophylaxis after total knee arthroplasty (RECORD4): a randomised trial. *Lancet* 2009; 373:1673-1680.
92. Diamantopoulos A, Lees M, Wells PS, et al. Cost-effectiveness of rivaroxaban versus enoxaparin for the prevention of postsurgical venous thromboembolism in Canada. *Thromb Haemost* 2010;104:760-770.
93. Stevenson M, Scope A, Holmes M, et al. Rivaroxaban for the prevention of venous thromboembolism: a single technology appraisal. *Health Technol Assess* 2009;13:43-48.
94. Treasure T, Hill J. NICE guidance on reducing the risk of venous thromboembolism in patients admitted to hospital. *J R Soc Med* 2010;103:210-212.
95. Raskob G, Cohen AT, Eriksson BI, et al. Oral direct factor Xa inhibition with edoxaban for thromboprophylaxis after elective total hip replacement: a randomised double-blind dose-response study. *Thromb Haemost* 2010;104:642-649.
96. Lassen MR, Raskob GE, Gallus A, et al. Apixaban versus enoxaparin for thromboprophylaxis after knee replacement (ADVANCE-2): a randomised double-blind trial. *Lancet* 2010;375:807-815.
97. Lassen MR, Raskob GE, Gallus A, et al. Apixaban or enoxaparin for thromboprophylaxis after knee replacement. *N Engl J Med* 2009;361:594-604.
98. Bauersachs R, Berkowitz SD, et al, for the EINSTEIN investigators. Oral rivaroxaban for symptomatic venous thromboembolism. *N Engl J Med* 2010;363:2499-2510.
99. Connolly SJ, Ezekowitz MD, Yusuf S, et al. Dabigatran versus warfarin in patients with atrial fibrillation. *N Engl J Med* 2009;361:1139-1151.
100. Freeman JV, Zhu RP, Owens DK, et al. Cost-effectiveness of dabigatran compared with warfarin for stroke prevention in atrial fibrillation. *Ann Intern Med* 2011;154:1-11.
101. ROCKET AF Study. Rivaroxaban-once daily, oral, direct factor Xa inhibition compared with vitamin K antagonism for prevention of stroke and Embolism Trial in Atrial Fibrillation: rationale and design of the ROCKET AF study. *Am Heart J* 2010; 159:340-347.
102. Eikelboom JW, O'Donnell M, Yusuf S, et al. Rationale and design of AVERROES: apixaban versus acetylsalicylic acid to prevent stroke in atrial fibrillation patients who have failed or are unsuitable for vitamin K antagonist treatment. *Am Heart J* 2010;159:348-353.
103. COAG (Clarification of Optimal Anticoagulation through Genetics) Investigators. Statistical design of personalized medicine interventions: the Clarification of Optimal Anticoagulation through Genetics (COAG) trial. *Trials* 2010;11:108.
104. Glynn RJ, Danielson E, Fonseca FA, et al. A randomized trial of rosuvastatin in the prevention of venous thromboembolism. *N Engl J Med* 2009;360:1851-1861.
105. Food and Drug Administration. Information for healthcare professionals: simvastatin (marketed as Zocor and generics), ezetimibe/simvastat (marketed as Vytorin), niacin extended-release/simvastatin (marketed as Simcor), used with amiodarone (Cordarone, Pacerone), 2008.
106. Barber MJ, Mangravite LM, Hyde CL, et al. Genome-wide association of lipid-lowering response to statins in combined study populations. *PloS One* 2010;5:e9763.
107. The SEARCH Collaborative Group. SLCO1B1 variants and statin-induced myopathy—a genomewide study. *N Engl J Med* 2008;359:789-799.
108. Ordovas JM, Lopez-Miranda J, Perez-Jimenez F, et al. Effect of apolipoprotein E and A-IV phenotypes on the low density lipoprotein response to HMG CoA reductase inhibitor therapy. *Atherosclerosis* 1995;113:157-166.
109. Mega JL, Morrow DA, Brown A, et al. Identification of genetic variants associated with response to statin therapy. *Arterioscler Thromb Vasc Biol* 2009;29:1310-1315.
110. Donnelly LA, Palmer CN, Whitley AL, et al. Apolipoprotein E genotypes are associated with lipid-lowering responses to statin treatment in diabetes: a Go-DARTS study. *Pharmacogenet Genomics* 2008;18:279-287.
111. Thompson JF, Hyde CL, Wood LS, et al. Comprehensive whole-genome and candidate gene analysis for response to statin therapy in the Treating to New Targets (TNT) cohort. *Circ Cardiovasc Genet* 2009;2:173-181.
112. Thompson JF, Man M, Johnson KJ, et al. An association study of 43 SNPs in 16 candidate genes with atorvastatin response. *Pharmacogenomics* 2005;5:352-358.
113. Gerdes LU, Gerdes C, Kervinen K, et al. The apolipoprotein epsilon4 allele determines prognosis and the effect on prognosis of simvastatin in survivors of myocardial infarction: a substudy of the Scandinavian simvastatin survival study. *Circulation* 2000; 101:1366-1371.
114. Cohen JC, Boerwinkle E, Mosley TH Jr, et al. Sequence variations in PCSK9, low LDL, and protection against coronary heart disease. *N Engl J Med* 2006;354:1264-1272.
115. Kathiresan S, Myocardial Infarction Genetics Consortium. A PCSK9 missense variant associated with a reduced risk of early-onset myocardial infarction. *N Engl J Med* 2008;358:2299-2300.
116. Krauss RM, Mangravite LM, Smith JD, et al. Variation in the 3-hydroxyl-3-methylglutaryl coenzyme A reductase gene is associated with racial differences in low-density lipoprotein cholesterol response to simvastatin treatment. *Circulation* 2008;117:1537-1544.
117. Chasman DI, Posada D, Subrahmanyan L, et al. Pharmacogenetic study of statin therapy and cholesterol reduction. *JAMA* 2004;291:2821-2827.
118. Mangravite LM, Medina MW, Cui J, et al. Combined influence of LDLR and HMGCR sequence variation on lipid-lowering response to simvastatin. *Arterioscler Thromb Vasc Biol* 2010;30:1485-1492.
119. Donnelly LA, Doney AS, Dannfald J, et al. A paucimorphic variant in the HMG-CoA reductase gene is associated with lipid-lowering response to statin treatment in diabetes: a GoDARTS study. *Pharmacogenet Genomics* 2008;18:1021-1026.
120. Medina MW, Gao F, Ruan W, et al. Alternative splicing of 3-hydroxy-3-methylglutaryl coenzyme A reductase is associated with plasma low-density lipoprotein cholesterol response to simvastatin. *Circulation* 2008;118:355-362.
121. Kuivenhoven JA, Jukema JW, Zwinderman AH, et al. The role of a common variant of the cholesteryl ester transfer protein gene in the progression of coronary atherosclerosis. The Regression Growth Evaluation Statin Study Group. *N Engl J Med* 1998;338:86-93.
122. Carlquist JF, Muhlestein JB, Horne BD, et al. The cholesteryl ester transfer protein Taq1B gene polymorphism predicts clinical benefit of statin therapy in patients with significant coronary artery disease. *Am Heart J* 2003;146:1007-1014.
123. Mohrschladt MF, van der Sman-de Beer F, Hofman MK, et al. TaqIB polymorphism in CETP gene: the influence on incidence of cardiovascular disease in statin-treated patients with familial hypercholesterolemia. *Eur J Hum Genet* 2005;13:877-882.
124. Regieli JJ, Jukema JW, Grobbee DE, et al. CETP genotype predicts increased mortality in statin-treated men with proven cardiovascular disease: an adverse pharmacogenetic interaction. *Eur Heart J* 2008;29:2792-2799.
125. Boekholdt SM, Sacks FM, Jukema JW, et al. Cholesteryl ester transfer protein TaqIB variant, high-density lipoprotein cholesterol levels, cardiovascular risk, and efficacy of pravastatin treatment: individual patient meta-analysis of 13,677 subjects. *Circulation* 2005;111:278-287.
126. Iakoubova OA, Sabatine MS, Rowland CM, et al. Polymorphism in KIF6 gene and benefit from statins after acute coronary syndromes: results from the PROVE IT-TIMI 22 study. *J Am Coll Cardiol* 2008;51:449-455.
127. Iakoubova OA, Tong CH, Rowland CM, et al. Association of the Trp719Arg polymorphism in kinesin-like protein 6 with myocardial infarction and coronary heart disease in two prospective trials: the CARE and WOSCOPS trials. *J Am Coll Cardiol* 2008; 51:435-443.
128. Shiffman D, Chasman DI, Zee RY, et al. A kinesin family member 6 variant is associated with coronary heart disease in the Women's Health Study. *J Am Coll Cardiol* 2008;51:444-448.
129. Samani NJ, Erdmann J, Hall AS, et al. Genomewide association analysis of coronary artery disease. *N Engl J Med* 2007;357:443-453.

130. McPherson R, Pertsemlidis A, Kavaslar N, et al. A common allele on chromosome 9 associated with coronary heart disease. *Science* 2007;316:488-491.

131. Helgadottir A, Thorleifsson G, Manolescu A, et al. A common variant on chromosome 9p21 affects the risk of myocardial infarction. *Science* 2007;316:1491-1493.

132. Wellcome Trust Case Control Consortium. Genome-wide association study of 14,000 cases of seven common diseases and 3,000 shared controls. *Nature* 2007;447: 661-678.

133. Kathiresan S, Voight BF, Purcell S, et al. Genome-wide association of early-onset myocardial infarction with single nucleotide polymorphisms and copy number variants. *Nat Genet* 2009;41:334-341.

134. Assimes TL, Hólm H, Kathiresan S, et al. Lack of association between the Trp719Arg polymorphism in kinesin-like protein-6 and coronary artery disease in 19 case-control studies. *J Am Coll Cardiol* 2010;56:1552-1563.

135. Ridker PM, Macfadyen JG, Glynn RJ, et al. Kinesin-like protein 6 (KIF6) polymorphism and the efficacy of rosuvastatin in primary prevention. *Circ Cardiovasc Genet* 2011;4: 312-317.

135a. Ference BA, Yoo W, Flack JM, et al. A common KIF6 polymorphism increases vulnerability to low-density lipoprotein cholesterol: two meta-analyses and a meta-regression analysis. *PloS One* 2011;6(12):e28834.

136. Law M, Rudnicka AR. Statin safety: a systematic review. *Am J Cardiol* 2006;97:52C-60C.

137. Food and Drug Administration. *FDA drug safety communication: new restrictions, contraindications, and dose limitations for Zocor (simvastatin) to reduce the risk of muscle injury,* 2011.

138. Voora D, Shah SH, Spasojevic I, et al. The SLCO1B1*5 genetic variant is associated with statin-induced side effects. *J Am Coll Cardiol* 2009;54:1609-1616.

139. The International HapMap Consortium. A second generation human haplotype map of over 3.1 million SNPs. *Nature* 2007;449:851-861.

140. Li Y, Sabatine MS, Tong CH, et al. Genetic variants in the KIF6 region and coronary event reduction from statin therapy. *Hum Genet* 2011;129:17-23.

141. Shiffman D, Sabatine MS, Louie JZ, et al. Effect of pravastatin therapy on coronary events in carriers of the KIF6 719Arg allele from the cholesterol and recurrent events trial. *Am J Cardiol* 2010;105:1300-1305.

142. Li Y, Iakoubova OA, Shiffman D, et al. KIF6 polymorphism as a predictor of risk of coronary events and of clinical event reduction by statin therapy. *Am J Cardiol* 2010;106:994-996.

143. Nishizato Y, Ieiri I, Suzuki H, et al. Polymorphisms of OATP-C (SLC21A6) and OAT3 (SLC22A8) genes: consequences for pravastatin pharmacokinetics. *Clin Pharmacol Ther* 2003;73:553-565.

144. Takane H, Miyata M, Burioka N, et al. Pharmacogenetic determinants of variability in lipid-lowering response to pravastatin therapy. *J Hum Genet* 2006;51:822-826.

CH
4

Systems of Health Care

Clyde W. Yancy, Christopher B. Granger, and Graham Nichol

SYSTEMS THEORY, 67

WHY SYSTEMS OF CARE ARE NEEDED, 67

EXPERIENCE TO DATE WITH CARDIOVASCULAR SYSTEMS OF CARE, 68

ST-Segment Elevation Myocardial Infarction, 68
Heart Failure, 69
Cardiac Arrest, 70

QUALITY IMPROVEMENT THEORY, 70

EXPERIENCE TO DATE WITH CARDIOVASCULAR QUALITY IMPROVEMENT, 71

ST-Segment Elevation Myocardial Infarction, 71
Heart Failure, 72
Out-of-Hospital Cardiac Arrest, 72

LESSONS LEARNED, 72

REFERENCES, 72

A *system* is an interconnected set of elements organized to achieve a function or purpose.[1] A *system of care* is an interconnected care delivery system, usually in a geographically contiguous region, organized to provide the opportunity to improve processes and outcomes of care.[2] A critical element of any effective system of care is ongoing measurement and response to the quality of care. This chapter describes systems theory, experience with cardiovascular systems of care, quality improvement theory, experience with cardiovascular quality improvement programs, and lessons learned from these efforts about how further improvements and optimization of cardiovascular care can be achieved.

Systems Theory

Systems theory is the interdisciplinary study of systems, with the goal of elucidating common principles that can be applied to diverse systems. The founding of systems theory is attributed to multiple individuals. The origin of systems theory has been attributed to the Industrial Revolution, when the relationships among structure, function, and output of manufacturing processes were evaluated with science, logic, and reductionism.[1] Albert Einstein promulgated the concept that multiple perspectives exist, with differing levels of behavior and knowledge that are interlinked to observe, understand, and change phenomena.

Systems thinking is the process of understanding how factors influence one another within a whole. In nature, examples of systems include ecosystems, in which various elements—such as air, water, movement, plants, and animals—work together to ensure that organisms within the system survive; without such cooperation, they would perish. In organizations, systems consist of people, processes, and structures that work together to make an organization healthy or unhealthy. Structures may consist of a physical plant or devices.

For systems of care, improvements in process may include increased use of effective drugs, devices, or procedures; decreased use of ineffective interventions; delivery of the same interventions with fewer resources; or improved organizational culture. Systems of care are distinct from health systems and are intended to meet the health care needs of patients with one or more specific clinical disorders (e.g., out-of-hospital cardiac arrest [OHCA], ST-elevation myocardial infarction [STEMI], heart failure, stroke, or trauma). According to the World Health Organization, health care systems meet the health care needs of a target population by providing 1) a financing mechanism, 2) a well-trained and adequately paid workforce, 3) reliable information on which to base decisions and policies, and 4) well-maintained facilities and logistics to deliver quality medicines and technologies.

Why Systems of Care Are Needed

Significant and important regional variations are found in process and outcome for a variety of cardiovascular conditions including cardiac arrest,[3] STEMI,[4-6] and heart failure.[7] Moreover, patients with coronary artery disease (CAD) receive the recommended quality of care only 68% of the time.[8] These differences in quality of care received mainly reflect disparities in access to or use of quality health care by demography or geography rather than differences in patient choice or risk. Some of these differences are associated with the characteristics of the hospital, such as urban location,[9] teaching status,[6,10] or safety net status.[11] However, variations in outcome tend not to be associated with large differences in protocols or processes of care, such as the use of rapid response teams, hospitalists, clinical guidelines, and medication checks.[12] Instead, hospitals in the top or bottom tier of risk-standardized mortality rates after myocardial infarction (MI) have been shown to differ substantially in terms of their organizational goals and values, senior management involvement, staff presence and expertise in care for patients with the condition of interest, communication and coordination among relevant groups, and problem solving and learning. A particular challenge in health care in the United States is the fragmented nature of our overall health care system. Overcoming this fragmentation is a theme that is the focus of much of health care reform,[13] and it is a key element of the rationale for implementing and maintaining systems of care.

Interestingly, research showing that a given therapy is effective does not directly result in the use of that therapy in practice.[14] *Dissemination* is the transfer of research results to decision makers to change the behavior of patients or providers so as to improve health. Effective implementation must include the identification of barriers to use of evidence and includes a strategy to actively overcome them. Dissemination and implementation interventions used to date have had variable degrees of success in various clinical conditions.[15-18]

Patients who have an acute cardiovascular event in the out-of-hospital setting are transported to multiple physical locations for treatment delivered by diverse health care providers. These patients require time-sensitive interventions that must be continuously available so they can be quickly delivered to an eligible patient. Few hospitals are able to provide primary percutaneous coronary intervention (PCI) 24 hours a day, 7 days a week for STEMI or OHCA. In addition, hospital-based providers often infrequently treat patients who have an acute cardiovascular event such as OHCA—given the low rates of occurrence in areas with low population density, as well as low initial field resuscitation in their communities—so systems of care to address such events are rarely optimized. Identification that a patient has had an acute cardiovascular event outside of the hospital can improve both processes and outcomes of care by triaging a patient to a facility capable of providing quality care and by notifying the receiving facility immediately, so they can begin to prepare to provide timely care even before the patient has arrived.

Multiple examples may be found throughout the field of medicine of the positive correlation between greater provider experience or greater procedure volume and better patient outcome. These include the care of patients with conditions that require time-sensitive intervention, including in-hospital and out-of-hospital cardiac arrest,[19] OHCA alone,[20] and traumatic injury[21]; it also includes patients hospitalized with STEMI[22,23] and those with STEMI who undergo primary angioplasty.[24] However, the relationship between volume and outcome is a complex one. Procedural volume appears to be a surrogate marker for multiple patient, physician, and health care factors that have an impact on outcome but are difficult to quantify individually. Transferring patients from institutions with limited facilities to those able to provide time-sensitive interventions may have a salutary effect on outcomes by increasing the volume of patients treated by the receiving physicians and hospital.

Experience to Date with Cardiovascular Systems of Care

ST-Segment Elevation Myocardial Infarction

Survival following MI can be improved by reperfusion therapies that open the occluded infarct-related coronary artery. The earlier reperfusion is achieved, the greater the survival benefit. Moreover, reperfusion by primary PCI, as long as it is done in a timely fashioned by experienced centers, is more effective than fibrinolytic therapy to open occluded coronary arteries and improve survival. In some countries, time has been saved by providing fibrinolytic therapy in the ambulance, at least for patients who called emergency medical services (EMS) for assistance. Moreover, simply obtaining a 12-lead electrocardiogram (ECG) in the prehospital setting by EMS can result in an earlier diagnosis and faster treatment once the patient arrives at the hospital.[25] Multiple randomized trials conducted mainly in Europe have demonstrated that outcome can be improved among patients who come to a non-PCI center in need of coronary intervention by transferring them to a PCI center for primary PCI, as long as it is done in an organized and rapid fashion.[26-31]

Although only an estimated 1500 of more than 5000 acute care hospitals in the United States have primary PCI capability, the majority of the population lives within 60 minutes of a PCI-capable

hospital,[32] and many non-PCI hospitals are within a 30- to 60-minute transfer time to a PCI center. Between 30% and 50% of patients with STEMI arrive at hospitals via EMS, and traditionally patients have been taken to the nearest hospital irrespective of PCI capability. Therefore, coordination of how patients flow through EMS, non-PCI centers, and PCI centers is crucial to optimize delivery of efficient care (Figure 5-1).

These developments—early fibrinolytic therapy, primary PCI, prehospital diagnosis, and interhospital transfer for primary PCI—established the need for regional systems of care to ensure that all eligible patients receive reperfusion in the form of primary PCI, if it can be done in a timely fashion by an experienced center. Opportunities to develop systems of care that address each element of the care process with multidisciplinary stakeholders were addressed in a conference organized by the American Heart Association (AHA) and summarized in manuscripts that included an executive summary.[33] Development of regional systems of coordinated care between EMS and networks of hospitals has become a strong (class I) recommendation in the 2009 American College of Cardiology (ACC)/AHA STEMI guideline update.[34] Several experiences, summarized below, illustrate opportunities to improve care of STEMI through systems development and improvement (Table 5-1).

PREHOSPITAL DIAGNOSIS, CATHETERIZATION LABORATORY ACTIVATION, AND TRANSPORT TO PRIMARY PERCUTANEOUS CORONARY INTERVENTION CENTERS

Integrated EMS and hospital care enables treatment to be "moved forward," such that the initial diagnosis and initiation of the reperfusion process can occur in the prehospital setting by trained EMS providers. Experience was reported in 10 regions, including Los Angeles, where prehospital ECG diagnosis was used to activate cardiac catheterization laboratories.[35] Door-to-balloon (D2B) times were approximately 60 minutes, and first-medical-contact-to-device times averaged less than 90 minutes, an achievement that demonstrated what an integrated system can accomplish. A similar

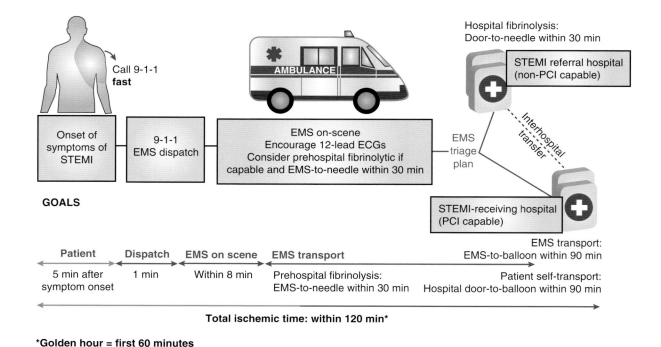

FIGURE 5-1 *ECG*, electrocardiogram; *EMS*, emergency medical systems; *PCI*, percutaneous coronary intervention. *(From Antman EM, et al. 2007 focused update of the American College of Cardiology/American Heart Association guidelines for the management of patients with ST elevation myocardial infarction guidelines.* Circulation *2008;117:296-329.)*

TABLE 5-1   Selected Programs Developing Systems of Care for STEMI

PROGRAM (REFERENCE)	TYPE	PARTICIPANTS	ELEMENTS	LESSONS
STEMI Receiving Center Networks[35]	EMS triage to PCI centers	10 U.S. regions	Prehospital ECGs, prehospital diagnosis, use prehospital diagnosis to activate the catheterization lab, and direct transport to primary PCI center	Linking EMS diagnosis and triage to PCI centers can result in excellent D2B and first medical contact to device times
Primary PCI Network[36]	EMS triage to PCI center	University of Ottawa Heart Institute and surrounding EMS and hospitals	Prehospital ECGs, prehospital diagnosis, use prehospital diagnosis to activate the catheterization lab, and direct transport to primary PCI center	EMS triage to primary PCI center results in much faster overall care than interhospital transfer
MHI Level 1 Protocol[38]	Regional transfer network	Minneapolis Heart Institute and 30 non-PCI centers within 210-mile radius	Non-PCI centers, ambulance and helicopter transport systems, primary PCI center	Transfer for primary PCI can be done in 90 to 100 minutes first-door-to-device in hospitals out to 60 miles, and within about 120 minutes (with initial treatment with half-dose fibrinolytic therapy) out to 210 miles, with excellent clinical outcomes.
Mayo Clinic Protocol[37]	Regional transfer network	St. Mary's Primary PCI Center and 28 non-PCI centers up to 150 miles away	Non-PCI centers, ambulance and helicopter transport systems, primary PCI center	Transfer first-door-to-device was achieved at a median of 116 minutes with initial use of fibrinolytic therapy for patients within 3 hours of symptom onset, with excellent outcomes
RACE program[39]	Statewide STEMI systems	Five regions across North Carolina, including EMS, 10 primary PCI centers, 55 non-PCI centers	EMS, non-PCI centers, primary PCI centers	All times (including door to needle, D2B, transfer first door to device) substantially improved, with median of 106 minutes first door-to-device for centers routinely transferring

D2B, door-to-balloon; ECG, electrocardiogram; EMS, emergency medical services; MHI, Minneapolis Heart Institute; PCI, percutaneous coronary intervention; RACE, Reperfusion of Acute Myocardial Infarction in North Carolina Emergency Departments; STEMI, ST-segment elevation myocardial infarction.

program in Ottawa, Canada, has shown impressive reductions in time to reperfusion with prehospital diagnosis and direct transfer to a PCI center.[36]

REGIONAL TRANSFER PROTOCOLS

Although randomized controlled trials (RCTs) have shown that transferring patients from non-PCI centers for primary PCI, rather than administering fibrinolytic therapy, can improve outcomes, it has been difficult to accomplish a door-to-device time of less than 120 minutes, as was achieved in the trials. Using standardized protocols with data collection and feedback, efficient transfer for primary PCI for hospitals in a 60-mile radius was achieved in the regions of Minneapolis and Olmsted County, Minnesota, with door-to-device times in the 90- to 100-minute range and excellent clinical outcomes.[37,38] Similar protocols have been successfully implemented in other communities.

STATE SYSTEMS FOR ST-SEGMENT ELEVATION MYOCARDIAL INFARCTION CARE

A statewide system in which each hospital (PCI and non-PCI) and EMS system has a standardized protocol for STEMI care has resulted in substantial improvements in care in North Carolina in the Reperfusion of Acute MI in Carolina Emergency Departments (RACE) program.[39] The state used a single data collection tool (ACTION Registry—Get With The Guidelines) and common protocols, which have enabled communities to receive standardized, quality care. Support by professional societies, including the ACC, and sponsorship by the AHA have been powerful tools to coordinate care in communities with more than one primary PCI center, where competition has been a barrier to collaboration. Nearly 90% of patients brought by EMS to PCI centers have prehospital ECGs, and EMS frequently takes patients to the nearest PCI center, rather than to closer, non-PCI centers. As is happening in many STEMI systems of care, coordination of cardiac arrest care is being incorporated into the system.

MISSION: LIFELINE PROGRAM TO IMPROVE ST-SEGMENT ELEVATION MYOCARDIAL INFARCTION CARE

Mission: Lifeline is an AHA program designed to improve STEMI outcomes through integration of regional systems of care (see www.heart.org/HEARTORG/HealthcareProfessional/Mission-Lifeline-Home-Page_UCM_305495_SubHomePage.jsp). Using elements from the demonstration projects above, it has established criteria based on evidence of best care to guide development and improvement of STEMI systems of care. With nearly 600 systems registered in 2011, and more than half the U.S. population covered by Mission: Lifeline systems, this national program has become the standard for development of regional systems of STEMI care. Many hospitals now have received recognition for their accomplishments, and an accreditation plan is being implemented. The impact of participation in Mission: Lifeline on processes of care or patient outcome remains to be determined.

Heart Failure

Compliance with recommended processes of care is low and variable among patients with heart failure in an outpatient setting.[40] Hospitalization for heart failure is frequent, debilitating, and costly.[41] Readmission after hospitalization for heart failure also occurs frequently. To date, no published evidence exists for or against the effectiveness of an interconnected care delivery system for patients with heart failure in a geographically contiguous region. But multiple randomized trials and other observational experiences have assessed interconnected strategies to reduce rates of initial admission or readmission for heart failure and to reduce mortality rates. Because of the heterogeneous nature of these interventions, it is infeasible either to pool the results of the trials or to tease out which component of the intervention was effective.[42] Nonetheless, these trials demonstrated that interventions that use follow-up by a specialized multidisciplinary team in a clinic or nonclinic setting reduce heart failure hospitalizations, all-cause hospitalizations, and mortality rate. Interventions used enhanced patient self-care activities to reduce heart failure hospitalizations and all-cause hospitalizations but not mortality rate. Interventions that used automated telephone contact only, with advice to see a primary care physician in the event of deterioration, failed to reduce heart failure hospitalizations, all-cause hospitalizations, or mortality rate.

Cardiac Arrest

As of February 2011, a few regions of the United States have implemented cardiac resuscitation systems of care to improve outcomes after OHCA (e.g., Arizona, Maryland, parts of Minnesota, New York, Ohio, Texas, and Virginia). Those that exist usually developed ad hoc, without comprehensive evidence-based criteria, common standards, or dedicated reimbursement. Some institutions have designated themselves as resuscitation centers of excellence that may or may not be part of a regional system. Some regions have attempted to create a system of care by transporting patients resuscitated in the field from OHCA only to hospitals capable of inducing hypothermia,[43] but other regions have been unable to do so.[44] EMS providers and physicians have recently begun to work collaboratively in Arizona, Minnesota, North Carolina, Pennsylvania, and Washington to improve processes and outcomes after OHCA by sharing knowledge, tools, and techniques as part of the Heart Rescue Project. Some of these cardiac resuscitation systems link to STEMI systems of care. To date, there is no published evidence for or against the effectiveness of such programmatic interventions on the structure, process, or outcome of cardiac resuscitation, because regional systems of care for OHCA have not been evaluated formally. Therefore, we summarize evidence of the effectiveness of interconnected field and hospital-based interventions for OHCA.

Several cities have implemented multiple interconnected changes to EMS care for patients with OHCA, and most have reported improved outcomes compared with historical controls.[45-47] Because of the observational nature of these studies, it is not possible to ascertain which component of the intervention was effective. Components that may be important include 1) emphasis on improved chest compressions; 2) reduced pauses for rhythm analysis; 3) use of a single, rather than stacked, shock sequence; or 4) use of devices intended to improve venous return.

Moreover, several groups have implemented multiple interconnected changes to hospital care for patients resuscitated from OHCA.[2] All have reported improved outcomes compared with historical controls. Again, due to the observational nature of these studies, it is not possible to ascertain which component of the intervention was effective. Components that may be important include 1) delivery of therapeutic hypothermia to selected comatose patients, 2) coronary angiography when there is a high degree of suspicion of an acute ischemic trigger, 3) early hemodynamic stabilization of the patient with the ability to effectively treat rearrest, 4) reliable prognostication, and 5) cardiac electrophysiologic assessment and treatment before discharge.

If patients resuscitated from cardiac arrest are to be preferentially transported to designated receiving hospitals, an interesting issue is how outcomes are related to the distance or duration of transport. Multiple observational studies in the pre-hypothermia and post-hypothermia eras demonstrate that transport time to the hospital was not significantly associated with survival to hospital discharge after OHCA.[48-50] Interpretation of some of these studies is limited by their high rate of missing transport time data or low overall survival. In another multicenter observational study of patients with OHCA in North America, survival to discharge tended to be lower among those taken to the closest hospital compared with those transported to distant hospitals.[51] But this study did not measure which hospital-based interventions patients received, although the distant hospitals were more likely to have PCI facilities, electrophysiology laboratories, more beds, higher patient volumes, and teaching hospital status. Collectively these studies suggest that it is feasible to bypass a less capable hospital after the patient's circulation has been restored. No current studies define a safe journey time, the use of different modes of transport, or the role of secondary transfer to a regional center after initial care at a local hospital.

Quality Improvement Theory

Systems-based interventions make extensive use of feedback to providers. The development of the theory of providing feedback to workers to improve process and outcomes is attributed to W.E. Deming,[52] Joseph Juran,[53] and Armand Feigenbum.[53] The underlying principle is that individuals reflect on their performance to encourage change in their behavior or in the system. Small incremental changes are applied throughout the work process.[54] A strong dose-response association has been found between adherence to guidelines or performance measures and outcomes.[55]

Multiple methods are used to improve personnel performance, work processes, and products in business or health care settings.[56-58] These include total quality management, reengineering, rightsizing, restructuring, cultural change, turnaround, disruption and lean management, and other methods. None of these methods is consistently better than the others, and each of these improvement processes goes through a series of phases that usually requires time to achieve the intended change in process and outcome. Skipping steps creates the illusion of speed, but it does not lead to a satisfying result. Mistakes in any of the phases can reduce impact, momentum, and hard-won gains. Measurement of processes of care is necessary but not sufficient to achieving improved outcomes.

Four key barriers stand in the way of implementing change to improve processes and outcomes in an organization.[59] The first barrier is lack of understanding that change is needed. For EMS agencies and hospitals that treat patients who have acute cardiovascular events, this need for change is driven by the large regional, intrahospital, and interhospital disparity in outcomes. The second barrier is resource limitations, which force organizations to change resource allocations. The third barrier is a lack of desire among individuals to make changes. A final barrier can be institutional politics.

A tipping-point approach to implementing change can be considered.[59] Initial efforts to change should focus on local opinion leaders who have a disproportionate influence in the organization. For EMS agencies, such a leader could be the medical director, shift supervisor, or person responsible for training or quality assurance. Once such an individual is committed to change, that person's achievements should be highlighted to encourage others to change also. In the unlikely event that individuals are not committed to change, consideration can be given to reassigning their duties. Lecturing on the need for change is unlikely to succeed, so the organization should seek to continuously experience the realities that make change necessary. For organizations responsible for care of patients with acute cardiovascular events, this includes monitoring survival to discharge and performing functional measures before or after discharge (e.g., ejection fraction for patients with STEMI, Minnesota Living with Heart Failure questionnaire for patients with heart failure, neurologic status based on modified Rankin score for patients resuscitated from cardiac arrest). Resources can be redistributed from activities that are high effort and low yield to those that are low effort and high yield. For resuscitation organizations, this might include shifting away from training and equipping field providers to obtain intravenous access to training providers and the public to deliver effective chest compressions. For hospitals, this might include shifting away from routine use of pulmonary artery catheters to improving organizational culture or training providers to counsel patients on daily weight measurement and to see their primary care physician in the event of clinical deterioration. Each organization will have different activities that require redistribution. Finally, a resuscitation organization should appoint a mentor who is highly respected, knowledgeable about those who support change and those who resist it, and able to devise strategies and build the coalitions necessary for change. The mentor can advise the change leader of what is happening at lower levels of the organization.

Process improvements are unlikely to be sustained without evidence that outcomes are also improved. This is especially true when financial resources are involved. The duration of the measurement period will vary with the process variable. A reasonable approach is periodic examination of process data (e.g., quarterly) and outcomes data (e.g., annually). During the measurement period, relevant providers should be given timely feedback on both process variables and outcomes. If process variables were not affected by the intervention, efforts should be made to determine why, and alternative approaches should be identified and implemented. If the intervention was successful, and benchmarks were achieved, the next weakest link should be addressed. A structured approach can be used to identify which links are weak and what leverage points can be modified to address them.[60] Collectively, application of these theories and methods can be used to achieve sustained and important improvements in the process, outcome, and quality of cardiovascular care.

Experience to Date with Cardiovascular Quality Improvement

ST-Segment Elevation Myocardial Infarction

According to data from a multicenter observational study, fewer than half of patients with STEMI are treated within guideline-recommended D2B times.[61] A high rate of noncompliance/nonadherence with guideline-recommended prescription of medications is seen for patients who come to medical attention with MI.[62] Moreover, a high rate of noncompliance/nonadherence is also found with guideline-recommended prescription of medications at discharge for patients with MI.[63]

Multiple groups have implemented and evaluated strategies to try to improve the quality of care for patients with acute MI. The Cooperative Cardiovascular Project was a before/after study of data review and feedback by peer review organizations. Included were all Medicare patients in multiple states throughout the country who had a principal diagnosis of acute infarction. Quality indicators were derived from current ACC/AHA guidelines. Data were abstracted from the clinical record and provided to the practitioners, with encouragement to initiate quality improvement activities for the treatment of MI. Prescription of aspirin during hospitalization, prescription of β-blockers at discharge, and mortality rate at 30 days improved significantly.

The Guidelines Applied in Practice (GAP) initiative was a before/after study intended to improve adherence to evidence-based therapies for patients with acute MI.[64] Included were a random sample of Medicare and non-Medicare patients at 10 centers treated for confirmed MI. The intervention included a kickoff presentation, creation of customized guideline-oriented tools that were intended to facilitate compliance/adherence to key quality indicators, recruitment of local opinion leaders, grand rounds, site visits, and data measurement and feedback. Significant increases in adherence to prescription of aspirin and β-blockers on admission and smoking-cessation counseling were observed. Nonsignificant but favorable improvements in compliance/adherence to other treatment goals were observed. The impact of the intervention on mortality was not reported.

The EFFECT study was a cluster randomized trial of a public release of report cards on hospital performance.[65] Included were 86 hospitals with patients admitted for acute infarction or heart failure. The intervention was early (January 2004) or delayed (September 2005) feedback of a public report card on baseline performance (between 1999 and 2001) on process of care indicators. Public release of hospital-specific quality indicators did not significantly improve process of care indicators or mortality.

AMERICAN COLLEGE OF CARDIOLOGY DOOR-TO-BALLOON ALLIANCE

The Door-to-Balloon Alliance was a national quality campaign sponsored by the ACC to increase the proportion of patients who receive primary PCI for STEMI treated within 90 minutes of hospital presentation.[66] The program identified hospital features associated with faster D2B times and coupled this with a comprehensive program to implement change that included EMS, emergency medicine, cardiology, and hospital administration. By March 2008, the program succeeded in achieving over 75% D2B within 90 minutes (compared with about 50% in 2005); however, reduction in D2B time alone is insufficient to decrease mortality rates.[67]

CRUSADE INITIATIVE

The Can Rapid Risk Stratification of Unstable Angina Patients Suppress Adverse Outcomes with Early Implementation of the ACC/AHA Guidelines (CRUSADE) initiative was a multidisciplinary quality improvement effort; it included a registry, assessment of compliance/adherence with recommended initial hospital management of patients with non–ST-elevation acute coronary syndromes, feedback of institutional treatment patterns to practitioners with comparison to national norms, and educational efforts by the CRUSADE steering committee.[68] Adherence/compliance to practice guideline recommendations improved over the duration of the program.[69] Better compliance/adherence to practice guideline recommendations was associated with significantly reduced mortality.[70]

GET WITH THE GUIDELINES—CORONARY ARTERY DISEASE PROGRAM

The AHA Get with the Guidelines—Coronary Artery Disease program (GWTG-CAD) was a national quality campaign to improve compliance/adherence to guidelines for patients with CAD.[71] The GWTG-CAD program used a patient management tool, education, and benchmarked quality reports to improve adherence. The GWTG program has expanded over time to include modules for in-hospital cardiac arrest (GWTG-Resuscitation, formerly the AHA National Registry for Cardiopulmonary Resuscitation), heart failure (Target: Heart Failure), stroke (Target: Stroke), and outpatient care (Guideline Advantage) as a comprehensive approach to improve quality of care for patients with cardiovascular disease.

Greater adherence to guidelines was observed among hospitals that participated in GWTG-CAD compared with those that did not and also among hospitals with a larger volume of patients with acute MI, geographic location in the Northeast, and teaching hospital status.[72] For each participating hospital, D2B time among patients with acute MI undergoing primary PCI decreased over time.[73] These measures were not significantly correlated with changes in the CMS Joint Commission on Accreditation of Health Care Organizations core measure of performance or in-hospital mortality rate. These results demonstrate that holistic approaches are needed to improve the quality of care rather than putting the focus on a single process measure.

ACUTE CORONARY TREATMENT AND INTERVENTION OUTCOMES NETWORK

The American Heart Association's GWTG-CAD program joined the Acute Coronary Treatment and Intervention Outcomes Network to create the National Cardiovascular Data Registry ACTION-Get with the Guidelines (AR-G) in June 2008 in recognition of the need for a national unified registry to measure and improve processes and outcomes for patients with acute MI.[74] This ongoing program includes efforts to ensure data quality, provide quarterly performance feedback, provide quality improvement tools, and to enable periodic user group meetings. AR-G is the only national registry to focus on process and outcome measures for systems of care for STEMI, and as such it provides a key foundation for the Mission: Lifeline program. Data from AR-G form the basis for recognition of quality improvement efforts and accomplishment in Mission: Lifeline, such as achievement of first medical contact to device time of less than 90 minutes in at least 75% of cases, which requires integrating systems care with EMS and PCI hospitals.

Heart Failure

Hospitals that have received the highest quality awards for heart failure care within the GWTG program show better outcomes, and those hospitals that have achieved better than national average outcomes within the CMS database compare favorably with those centers rewarded for best processes of care. Outpatient quality improvement initiatives show that adherence to evidence-based quality measures can be substantially improved by process improvement interventions. Though laudable, adherence is not sufficient, because outcomes must be favorably influenced. Data now demonstrate in theoretical models that even with conservative estimates, a considerable number of lives can be saved over the intermediate term in heart failure. Thus, having a good process leads to good outcomes, and having good outcomes points to having had a good process.

Out-of-Hospital Cardiac Arrest

Physicians associated with the Seattle Fire Department pioneered the application of audit and feedback to improve outcomes after field resuscitation of cardiac arrest in 1969.[75-81] A few years later, other physicians implemented similar processes in surrounding King County. As of February 2011, few EMS agencies give such feedback to their providers. As evidence of the effectiveness of care accumulates, stakeholders decide which practices are defined as necessary care.[82] Care is then audited to ensure compliance with these performance measures, and information is fed back to providers periodically. Whether because of these ongoing quality improvement efforts or other factors, such as quantity of EMS provider training or experience, Seattle and surrounding King County now report a higher rate of survival compared with most other communities after EMS-treated OHCA or subgroups with a favorable prognosis such as those with witnessed ventricular fibrillation.[3] Moreover, such differences in survival are not explained by differences in patient characteristics[83] or EMS processes of care.[84]

The synergies for quality improvement for cardiovascular emergencies—including STEMI, OHCA, and stroke—are readily apparent. Efforts to coordinate features across systems for different emergencies are under way, including those of the AHA. These include data collection and feedback, integration of EMS and networks of hospitals, teams involved with quality improvement across cardiovascular emergencies, and opportunities to recognize and accredit hospitals for excellence in systems development.

Lessons Learned

Large regional variations are seen in processes of care, compliance with guideline recommendations, and patient outcome. Systems of care and quality improvement programs are intended to improve processes of care and patient outcome. Two key elements are *audit* of processes of care and *feedback* to providers.

To date, most successful efforts have been grassroots regional programs with passionate leaders who have convinced hospitals to invest in the infrastructure needed to develop systems. Expansion of these regional efforts to become the national standard is a substantial challenge. A part of the challenge is the limited resources of many hospitals that participate in systems of care or quality improvement programs. Some registries have merged in recognition of hospitals' limited willingness or ability to support duplicate data entry. Experts have recommended that participants receive reimbursement to support quality improvement activities.[3] Thus, the temptation to collect all possible information as opposed to a finite set of essential variables is a barrier to broad participation. In recognition of these limits, some quality improvement programs have made limited data entry options available in an attempt to increase participation.

Another challenge is that the distinction between quality improvement and research is sometimes unclear.[85] In the United States, experts have recommended clarification of regulations related to research and patient consent so as to facilitate ongoing efforts to collect and collate data to improve care.[86] A common but not universal approach is to consider local data collection as a quality improvement activity and to deidentify these data before they are collated centrally. Another approach is to collect a finite dataset with waiver of documented written consent under minimal risk criteria.[87]

A final challenge is that simply knowing what to change is not sufficient; the change must be implemented. And to be successfully implemented, a standardized and systematic approach is needed. Those practitioners who value physician independence in decision making must realize that it is just such reasoning that has resulted in highly varied outcomes. Adopting best practices that have been proven safe and effective enhances practitioner efficiency, optimizes patient outcomes, and preserves more resources within the system to support needed care throughout. As for broadly implementing systems of care, with quality improvement programs to improve processes and outcomes for patients with heart disease, the time is now.

REFERENCES

1. Meadows DH. *Thinking in systems: a primer.* White River Junction, VT, 2008, Chelsea Green Publishing.
2. Nichol G, Aufderheide TP, Eigel B, et al. Regional systems of care for out-of-hospital cardiac arrest: a policy statement from the American Heart Association. *Circulation* 2010; 121(5):709-729.
3. Nichol G, Thomas E, Callaway CW, et al. Regional variation in out-of-hospital cardiac arrest incidence and outcome. *JAMA* 2008;300(12):1423-1431.
4. Krumholz HM, Chen J, Rathore SS, et al. Regional variation in the treatment and outcomes of myocardial infarction: investigating New England's advantage. *Am Heart J* 2003;146(2):242-249.
5. Normand ST, Glickman ME, Sharma RG, McNeil BJ. Using admission characteristics to predict short-term mortality from myocardial infarction in elderly patients: results from the Cooperative Cardiovascular Project. *JAMA* 1996;275(17):1322-1328.
6. Krumholz HM, Merrill AR, Schone EM, et al. Patterns of hospital performance in acute myocardial infarction and heart failure 30-day mortality and readmission. *Circ Cardiovasc Qual Outcomes* 2009;2(5):407-413.
7. Zhang W, Watanabe-Galloway S. Ten-year secular trends for congestive heart failure hospitalizations: an analysis of regional differences in the United States. *Congest Heart Fail* 2008;14(5):266-271.
8. Asch SM, Kerr EA, Keesey J, et al. Who is at greatest risk for receiving poor quality health care? *N Engl J Med* 2006;354:1147-1156.
9. Baldwin LM, MacLehose RF, Hart LG, et al. Quality of care for acute myocardial infarction in rural and urban US hospitals. *J Rural Health* 2004;20(2):99-108.
10. Allison JJ, Kiefe CI, Weissman NW, et al. Relationship of hospital teaching status with quality of care and mortality for Medicare patients with acute MI. *JAMA* 2000; 284(10):1256-1262.
11. Ross JS, Cha SS, Epstein AJ, et al. Quality of care for acute myocardial infarction at urban safety-net hospitals. *Health Aff (Millwood)* 2007;26(1):238-248.
12. Curry LA, Spatz E, Cherlin E, et al. What distinguishes top-performing hospitals in acute myocardial infarction mortality rates? A qualitative study. *Ann Intern Med* 2011;154(6):384-390.
13. Berwick DM. Launching accountable care organizations—the proposed rule for the Medicare Shared Savings Program. *N Engl J Med* 2011;364(16):e32.
14. Siegel D. The gap between knowledge and practice in the treatment and prevention of cardiovascular disease. *Prev Cardiol* 2000;3(4):167-171.
15. Continuing education meetings and workshops: effects on professional practice and health care outcomes. *Cochrane Database Syst Rev* 2009;(2):CD003030.
16. Zwarenstein M, Goldman J, Reeves S. Interprofessional collaboration: effects of practice-based interventions on professional practice and healthcare outcomes. *Cochrane Database Syst Rev* 2009;(3):CD000072.
17. Tailored interventions to overcome identified barriers to change: effects on professional practice and health care outcomes. *Cochrane Database Syst Rev* 2010;(3):CD005470.
18. Doumit G, Gattellari M, Grimshaw J. Local opinion leaders: effects on professional practice and health care outcomes. *Cochrane Database Syst Rev* 2007;(1):CD000125.

19. Carr BG, Kahn JM, Merchant RM, et al. Inter-hospital variability in post-cardiac arrest mortality. *Resuscitation* 2009;80(1):30-34.

20. Callaway CW, Schmicker R, Kampmeyer M, et al. Receiving hospital characteristics associated with survival after out-of-hospital cardiac arrest. *Resuscitation* 2010;81(5):524-529.

21. Nathens AB, Jurkovich GJ, Maier RV, et al. Relationship between trauma center volume and outcomes. *JAMA* 2001;285(9):1164-1171.

22. Ross JS, Normand SL, Wang Y, et al. Hospital volume and 30-day mortality for three common medical conditions. *N Engl J Med* 2010;362(12):1110-1118.

23. Thiemann DR, Coresh J, Oetgen WJ, Powe NR. The association between hospital volume and survival after acute myocardial infarction in elderly patients. *N Engl J Med* 1999;340(21):1640-1648.

24. Canto JG, Every NR, Magid DJ, et al. The volume of primary angioplasty procedures and survival after acute myocardial infarction. National Registry of Myocardial Infarction 2 Investigators. *N Engl J Med* 2000;342(21):1573-1580.

25. Ting HH, Krumholz HM, Bradley EH, et al. Implementation and integration of prehospital ECGs into systems of care for acute coronary syndrome: a scientific statement from the American Heart Association Interdisciplinary Council on Quality of Care and Outcomes Research, Emergency Cardiovascular Care Committee, Council on Cardiovascular Nursing, and Council on Clinical Cardiology. *Circulation* 2008;118(10):1066-1079.

26. Vermeer F, Oude Ophuis AJ, van Berg EJ, et al. Prospective randomised comparison between thrombolysis, rescue PTCA, and primary PTCA in patients with extensive myocardial infarction admitted to a hospital without PTCA facilities: a safety and feasibility study. *Heart* 1999;82(4):426-431.

27. Widimsky P, Groch L, Zelizko M, et al. Multicentre randomized trial comparing transport to primary angioplasty vs immediate thrombolysis vs combined strategy for patients with acute myocardial infarction presenting to a community hospital without a catheterization laboratory. The PRAGUE study. *Eur Heart J* 2000;21(10):823-831.

28. Bonnefoy E, Lapostolle F, Leizorovicz A, et al. Primary angioplasty versus prehospital fibrinolysis in acute myocardial infarction: a randomised study. *Lancet* 2002;360(9336):825-829.

29. Grines CL, Westerhausen DR Jr, Grines LL, et al. A randomized trial of transfer for primary angioplasty versus on-site thrombolysis in patients with high-risk myocardial infarction: the Air Primary Angioplasty in Myocardial Infarction study. *J Am Coll Cardiol* 2002;39(11):1713-1719.

30. Widimsky P, Budesinsky T, Vorac D, et al. Long distance transport for primary angioplasty vs immediate thrombolysis in acute myocardial infarction. Final results of the randomized national multicentre trial—PRAGUE-2. *Eur Heart J* 2003;24(1):94-104.

31. Andersen HR, Nielsen TT, Rasmussen K, et al. A comparison of coronary angioplasty with fibrinolytic therapy in acute myocardial infarction. *N Engl J Med* 2003;349(8):733-742.

32. Nallamothu BK, Bates ER, Wang Y, et al. Driving times and distances to hospitals with percutaneous coronary intervention in the United States: implications for prehospital triage of patients with ST-elevation myocardial infarction. *Circulation* 2006;113(9):1189-1195.

33. Jacobs AK, Antman EM, Faxon DP, et al. Development of systems of care for ST-elevation myocardial infarction patients: executive summary. *Circulation* 2007;116(2):217-230.

34. Kushner FG, Hand M, Smith SC Jr, et al. 2009 Focused Updates: ACC/AHA Guidelines for the Management of Patients with ST-Elevation Myocardial Infarction (updating the 2004 Guideline and 2007 Focused Update) and ACC/AHA/SCAI Guidelines on Percutaneous Coronary Intervention (updating the 2005 Guideline and 2007 Focused Update): a report of the American College of Cardiology Foundation/American Heart Association Task Force on Practice Guidelines. *Circulation* 2009;120(22):2271-2306.

35. Rokos IC, French WJ, Koenig WJ, et al. Integration of pre-hospital electrocardiograms and ST-elevation myocardial infarction receiving center (SRC) networks: impact on door-to-balloon times across 10 independent regions. *JACC Cardiovasc Interv* 2009;2(4):339-346.

36. Le May MR, So DY, Dionne R, et al. A citywide protocol for primary PCI in ST-segment elevation myocardial infarction. *N Engl J Med* 2008;358(3):231-240.

37. Ting HH, Rihal CS, Gersh BJ, et al. Regional systems of care to optimize timeliness of reperfusion therapy for ST-elevation myocardial infarction: the Mayo Clinic STEMI Protocol. *Circulation* 2007;116(7):729-736.

38. Henry TD, Sharkey SW, Burke MN, et al. A regional system to provide timely access to percutaneous coronary intervention for ST-elevation myocardial infarction. *Circulation* 2007;116(7):721-728.

39. Jollis JG, Roettig ML, Aluko AO, et al. Implementation of a statewide system for coronary reperfusion for ST-segment elevation myocardial infarction. *JAMA* 2007;298(20):2371-2380.

40. Chan PS, Oetgen WJ, Buchanan D, et al. Cardiac performance measure compliance in outpatients: the American College of Cardiology and National Cardiovascular Data Registry's PINNACLE (Practice Innovation And Clinical Excellence) program. *J Am Coll Cardiol* 2010;56(1):8-14.

41. Roger VL, Go AS, Lloyd-Jones DM, et al. Heart disease and stroke statistics—2011 update: a report from the American Heart Association. *Circulation* 2011;123(4):e18-e209.

42. McAlister FA, Stewart S, Ferrua S, McMurray JJ. Multidisciplinary strategies for the management of heart failure patients at high risk for admission: a systematic review of randomized trials. *J Am Coll Cardiol* 2004;44(4):810-819.

43. Hartocollis A. City pushes cooling therapy for cardiac arrest. *New York Times,* December 4, 2008.

44. Spector H. MetroHealth, Cleveland EMS don't back regional approach for cardiac arrest therapy. MetroHealth, EMS: not enough evidence to alter treatment. *Plain Dealer* March 23, 2009.

45. Rea TD, Helbock M, Perry S, et al. Increasing use of cardiopulmonary resuscitation during out-of-hospital ventricular fibrillation arrest: survival implications of guideline changes. *Circulation* 2006;114(25):2760-2765.

46. Hinchey PR, Myers JB, Lewis R, et al. Improved out-of-hospital cardiac arrest survival after the sequential implementation of 2005 AHA guidelines for compressions, ventilations, and induced hypothermia: the Wake County experience. *Ann Emerg Med* 2010;56(4):348-357.

47. Lick CJ, Aufderheide TP, Niskanen RA, et al. Take Heart America: a comprehensive, community-wide, systems-based approach to the treatment of cardiac arrest. *Crit Care Med* 2011;39(1):26-33.

48. Davis DP, Fisher R, Aguilar S, et al. The feasibility of a regional cardiac arrest receiving system. *Resuscitation* 2007;74(1):44-51.

49. Spaite DW, Bobrow BJ, Vadeboncoeur TF, et al. The impact of prehospital transport interval on survival in out-of-hospital cardiac arrest: implications for regionalization of post-resuscitation care. *Resuscitation* 2008;79(1):61-66.

50. Spaite DW, Stiell IG, Bobrow BJ, et al. Effect of transport interval on out-of-hospital cardiac arrest survival in the OPALS study: implications for triaging patients to specialized cardiac arrest centers. *Ann Emerg Med* 2009;54(2):248-255.

51. Cudnik MT, Schmicker RH, Vaillancourt C, et al. A geospatial assessment of transport distance and survival to discharge in out of hospital cardiac arrest patients: implications for resuscitation centers. *Resuscitation* 2010;81(5):518-523.

52. Deming WE. *Elementary principles of the statistical control of quality.* Tokyo, 1950, Nippon Kagaku.

53. Juran J. *Quality control handbook.* New York, 1951, McGraw-Hill.

54. Berwick DM. Continuous improvement as an ideal in health care. *N Engl J Med* 1989;320:53-56.

55. Mehta RH, Peterson ED, Califf RM. Performance measures have a major effect on cardiovascular outcomes: a review. *Am J Med* 2007;120(5):398-402.

56. Kotter JP. *Leading change.* Boston, 1996, Harvard Business School Press.

57. Christensen J, Grossman JH, Hwang J. *The innovator's prescription: a disruptive solution for health care.* New York, 2009, McGraw-Hill.

58. Shook J. *Managing to learn: using the A3 management process.* Cambridge, MA, 2008, Lean Enterprise Institute.

59. Kim W, Mauborgne R. *Blue ocean strategy: how to create uncontested market space and make the competition irrelevant.* Boston, 2005, Harvard Business School Press.

60. Meadows DH. *Leverage points: places to intervene in a system.* Hartland, VT, 1999, Sustainability Institute.

61. Bradley EH, Curry LA, Webster TR, et al. Achieving rapid door-to-balloon times: how top hospitals improve complex clinical systems. *Circulation* 2006;113(8):1079-1085.

62. McGlynn EA, Asch SM, Adams J, et al. The quality of health care delivered to adults in the United States. *N Engl J Med* 2003;348(26):2635-2645.

63. Lappe JM, Muhlestein JB, Lappe DL, et al. Improvements in 1-year cardiovascular clinical outcomes associated with a hospital-based discharge medication program. *Ann Intern Med* 2004;141(6):446-453.

64. Mehta RH, Montoye CK, Gallogly M, et al. Improving quality of care for acute myocardial infarction: the Guidelines Applied in Practice (GAP) initiative. *JAMA* 2002;287(10):1269-1276.

65. Tu JV, Donovan LR, Lee DS, et al. Effectiveness of public report cards for improving the quality of cardiac care: the EFFECT study: a randomized trial. *JAMA* 2009;302(21):2330-2337.

66. Bradley EH, Nallamothu BK, Herrin J, et al. National efforts to improve door-to-balloon time results from the Door-to-Balloon Alliance. *J Am Coll Cardiol* 2009;54(25):2423-2429.

67. Flynn A, Moscucci M, Share D, et al. Trends in door-to-balloon time and mortality in patients with ST-elevation myocardial infarction undergoing primary percutaneous coronary intervention. *Arch Intern Med* 2010;170(20):1842-1849.

68. Roe MT, Ohman EM, Pollack CV Jr, et al. Changing the model of care for patients with acute coronary syndromes. *Am Heart J* 2003;146(4):605-612.

69. Mehta RH, Roe MT, Chen AY, et al. Recent trends in the care of patients with non–ST-segment elevation acute coronary syndromes: insights from the CRUSADE initiative. *Arch Intern Med* 2006;166(18):2027-2034.

70. Mehta RH, Chen AY, Ohman EM, et al. Influence of transfer-in rates on quality of care and outcomes at receiving hospitals in patients with non–ST-segment elevation myocardial infarction. *Am Heart J* 2010;160(3):405-411.

71. LaBresh KA, Fonarow GC, Smith SC Jr, et al. Improved treatment of hospitalized coronary artery disease patients with the Get With The Guidelines program. *Crit Path Cardiol* 2007;6(3):98-105.

72. Lewis WR, Peterson ED, Cannon CP, et al. An organized approach to improvement in guideline adherence for acute myocardial infarction: results with the Get With The Guidelines quality improvement program. *Arch Intern Med* 2008;168(16):1813-1819.

73. Wang TY, Fonarow GC, Hernandez AF, et al. The dissociation between door-to-balloon time improvement and improvements in other acute myocardial infarction care processes and patient outcomes. *Arch Intern Med* 2009;169(15):1411-1419.

74. Peterson ED, Roe MT, Rumsfeld JS, et al. A call to ACTION (Acute Coronary Treatment and Intervention Outcomes Network): a national effort to promote timely clinical feedback and support continuous quality improvement for acute myocardial infarction. *Circ Cardiovasc Qual Outcomes* 2009;2(5):491-499.

75. Schaffer WA, Cobb LA. Recurrent ventricular fibrillation and modes of death in survivors of out-of-hospital ventricular fibrillation. *N Engl J Med* 1975;293(6):259-262.

76. Cobb LA, Baum RS, Alvarez H 3rd, Schaffer WA. Resuscitation from out-of-hospital ventricular fibrillation: 4 years follow-up. *Circulation* 1975;52(6 Suppl):III223-235.

77. Baum RS, Alvarez H 3rd, Cobb LA. Survival after resuscitation from out-of-hospital ventricular fibrillation. *Circulation* 1974;50(6):1231-1235.

78. Cobb LA, Alvarez H 3rd, Copass MK. A rapid response system for out-of-hospital cardiac emergencies. *Med Clin North Am* 1976;60(2):283-293.

79. Cobb LA, Weaver WD, Hallstrom AP, Copass MK. Cardiac resuscitation in the community: the Seattle experience. *Cardiologia* 1990;35(1 Suppl):85-90.

80. Cobb LA, Weaver WD, Fahrenbruch CE, et al. Community-based interventions for sudden cardiac death: impact, limitations, and changes. *Circulation* 1992;85(1 Suppl):198-202.

81. Cobb LA. Data collection and retrieval to document the outcomes of cardiopulmonary resuscitation. *New Horiz* 1997;5(2):164-166.

82. Committee on Quality of Health Care in America. *Crossing the quality chasm: a new health system for the 21st century.* Washington, DC, 2001, Institute of Medicine.

83. Rea TD, Cook AJ, Stiell IG, et al. Predicting survival after out-of-hospital cardiac arrest: role of the Utstein data elements. *Ann Emerg Med* 2010;55(3):249-257.

84. Zive D, Koprowicz K, Schmidt T, et al. Variation in out-of-hospital cardiac arrest resuscitation and transport practices in the Resuscitation Outcomes Consortium: ROC Epistry–Cardiac Arrest. *Resuscitation* 2011;82(3):277-284.

85. Casarett D, Karlawish JH, Sugarman J. Determining when quality improvement initiatives should be considered research: proposed criteria and potential implications. *JAMA* 2000;283(17):2275-2280.

86. Bufalino VJ, Masoudi FA, Stranne SK, et al. The American Heart Association's recommendations for expanding the applications of existing and future clinical registries: a policy statement from the American Heart Association. *Circulation* 2011;123(19): 2167-2179.

87. Morrison LJ, Nichol G, Rea TD, et al. Rationale, development and implementation of the Resuscitation Outcomes Consortium Epistry-Cardiac Arrest. *Resuscitation* 2008; 78(2):161-169.

CHAPTER 6

Global Cardiovascular Therapy

Thomas A. Gaziano and Neha J. Pagidipati

INTRODUCTION TO GLOBAL CHALLENGES
IN CARDIOVASCULAR DISEASE
THERAPY, 75

BURDEN OF CARDIOVASCULAR
DISEASE, 75

CURRENT TRENDS AND CHALLENGES, 75

Acute Management and Secondary Prevention, 75
Challenges to Therapeutic Usage, 77
Primary Prevention, 79
Polypill, 79

POPULATION STRATEGIES, 80

Risk Factors for Cardiovascular Disease, 80

SUMMARY, 81

REFERENCES, 81

Introduction to Global Challenges in Cardiovascular Disease Therapy

Cardiovascular disease (CVD) has become the single greatest cause of death worldwide. In 2004, CVD caused an estimated 17 million deaths and led to 151 million disability-adjusted life-years (DALYs) lost—approximately 30% of all deaths and 14% of all DALYs lost that year.[1] This chapter reviews the variable pattern and burden of CVD, current trends for therapies at the individual level, the diverse challenges for instituting therapeutic medications in low-income countries, and population or public health strategies aimed at the major risk factors for CVD. The cost effectiveness of various interventions to reduce the burden is reviewed in each of the relevant sections.

Burden of Cardiovascular Disease

Examination of regional variations is helpful in understanding global trends in the burden of disease, particularly CVD. Even as age-adjusted rates fall in high-income countries, CVD rates are accelerating worldwide because most low- and middle-income countries are entering the second and third phases of the epidemiologic transition, marked by rising CVD rates. Because 85% of the world's population lives in low- and middle-income countries, rates in these countries largely drive global rates of CVD, which is the leading cause of death in all developing regions, with the exception of sub-Saharan Africa. However, vast differences in the burden of CVD are seen (Figure 6-1), with CVD death rates as high as 60% in Eastern Europe and as low as 10% in sub-Saharan Africa. These numbers compare with a CVD death rate of 38% in high-income countries.

The World Health Organization (WHO) predicts that by 2030, 33% of all deaths worldwide will be caused by CVD—approximately 24.2 million.[2] CVD tends to strike at an earlier age in developing countries: nearly 80% of deaths in high-income countries occur among those older than 60 years compared with 42% in low- and middle-income countries.[1] In addition, case fatality rates tend to be higher in the lower income countries.[4]

Finally, the economic impact of CVD is enormous. Over the next decade or so, countries such as China, India, and Russia could lose between $200 billion and $550 billion in national income as a result of heart disease, stroke, and diabetes.[5] The costs attributable to nonoptimal levels of blood pressure as mediated through stroke and MI were evaluated for all regions of the world recently. Globally, health care costs of elevated blood pressure were estimated at $370 billion (U.S. dollars) for the year 2001.[6] This amount represented approximately 10% of all global health care expenditures for that year.

In developing countries, a much higher proportion of CVD burden occurs earlier among adults of working age. Under current projections, in developing countries such as South Africa, CVD will strike 40% of adults between the ages of 35 and 64 years compared with 10% in the United States.[7] India and China will have death rates in the same age group that are two and three times that of

most developed countries. Given the large populations in these two rapidly growing economies, this trend could have profound economic effects, as workers in their prime succumb to CVD.

Three complementary types of interventions were developed chronologically and can be used to address the global burden of CVD, just as they have been used to address CVD in developed countries. One strategy, referred to as *secondary prevention*, targets those with acute or established CVD; *primary prevention* entails risk assessment to target those at high risk as a result of multiple risk factors for intervention before their first CVD event. The third strategy, called *primordial prevention*, uses mass education or policy interventions directed at the entire population to reduce the overall level of risk. The following sections address these three strategies in the context of efforts to reduce global CVD.

Current Trends and Challenges

Acute Management and Secondary Prevention

ACUTE CORONARY SYNDROME

The use of fibrinolytic therapy for acute coronary syndrome (ACS) varies by region. Though this therapy is used more frequently in countries with low gross national income (GNI), the time to initiation of fibrinolysis takes longer than it does in their high-GNI counterparts (4.3 vs. 2.8 hours).[8] In the Global Registry of Acute Coronary Events (GRACE) registry, which included 14 countries in North and South America, Europe, Australia, and New Zealand, streptokinase was the lytic therapy used most often in patients with ST-segment elevation myocardial infarction (STEMI), followed by tissue plasminogen activator and recombinant plasminogen activator.[9] Streptokinase is used most routinely in developing nations because its cost is one tenth that of tissue plasminogen activator.[10]

Fibrinolysis with streptokinase is cost effective in developing nations according to WHO standards.[11] Investigators found that the incremental cost in U.S. dollars per DALY averted was $634 to $734 for aspirin, atenolol, and streptokinase and slightly less than $16,000 for aspirin, atenolol, and tissue plasminogen activator. Secondary analysis further showed that streptokinase given sooner than 6 hours following onset of MI reduces the incremental cost per DALY to less than $440 compared with more than $1300 if given after 6 hours.

As of 2002, the majority of patients with ACS in multiple regions of the world did not undergo any type of revascularization procedure. Rates of percutaneous coronary intervention (PCI) were highest in the United States and were particularly low in Eastern Europe.[12,13] Unsurprisingly, PCI use was significantly associated with GNI; only 1.3% of STEMI patients in low-GNI countries received PCI compared with 22.7% of STEMI patients in high-GNI countries (Figure 6-2).[8] Reinfarction following fibrinolysis was also much less commonly treated with PCI in non-Western countries, particularly in Russia and Eastern Europe.[14]

Several studies in the past decade have begun to elucidate the use of evidence-based medications for ACS in various parts of the world. The GRACE study found that across the 14 countries

CH
6

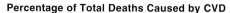

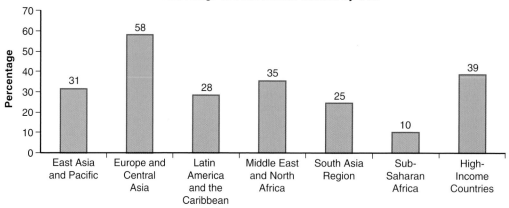

Percentage of Total Deaths Caused by CVD

FIGURE 6-1 Percentage of total deaths caused by cardiovascular disease *(CVD)* by World Bank region. *(Data from Lopez AD, Mathers CD, Ezzati M, et al (eds).* Global burden of disease and risk factors. *New York, 2006, Oxford University Press.)*

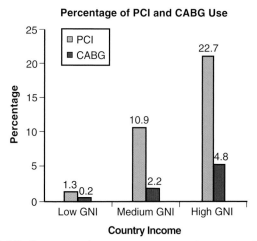

FIGURE 6-2 Percentage of percutaneous coronary intervention *(PCI)* and cardiac artery bypass graft *(CABG)* use across country income. GNI, gross national income. *(Data from Orlandini A, Diaz R, Wojdyla D, et al. Outcomes of patients in clinical trials with ST-segment elevation myocardial infarction among countries with different gross national incomes.* Eur Heart J *2006;27:527-533.)*

included in North and South America, Europe, Australia, and New Zealand, aspirin was used on average in 91% of registered ACS patients. When looked at more closely, however, it was found that countries in Eastern Europe on average used aspirin in only 75% of patients with ACS. A more current study, which stratified countries based on GNI, found that aspirin usage in STEMI patients was actually slightly higher in low-GNI countries compared with high-GNI countries (99.3% vs. 95.4%; $P < .0001$).[8] Conversely, β-blocker use was lower in low-GNI countries, likely related to higher rates of heart failure. Glycoprotein (GP) IIb/IIIa inhibitors were used as adjunctive therapy to PCI in 39% of patients undergoing PCI in the United States but only in 1% of patients in Eastern Europe and in 4% of patients in Latin America undergoing PCI.[12] The availability of catheterization facilities was associated with an increased use of these agents. However, more up-to-date data on the current trends in GP IIb/IIIa usage globally are lacking.

Angiotensin-converting enzyme (ACE) inhibitors were given to patients with ACS more frequently in Latin America, Eastern Europe, and Asia than in Western countries, presumably because of the higher rates of heart failure in these regions.[13] This finding was supported by Orlandini et al (2006), who confirmed that ACE inhibitors were used more frequently in low-GNI countries.[8]

Lipid-lowering agents, as described below, have only recently been added to the WHO Essential Drug List, and therefore data about their use are minimal.

Although it is tempting to ascribe many of the variations in treatment to the high cost of medications and lack of access in developing nations, economics alone cannot explain all of the regional variations seen. For example, Eastern Europe has a high usage rate of ACE inhibitors, which is a relatively expensive medication. However, it has the lowest use of aspirin, which is very inexpensive.[13] Clearly, factors other than cost are contributing to the different prescribing practices seen across the globe.

Data on the number of cardiac surgeries performed internationally and on their outcomes are sparse. In the GRACE study, cardiac artery bypass grafting (CABG) was performed in 4% of patients with STEMI, 10% of those with non-STEMI, and 5% of those with unstable angina, although it is unclear how these percentages differed in developed versus developing countries.[9] Cardiac surgeries are undertaken much less frequently in developing countries compared with their developed counterparts; for example, it was only in 2007 that open-heart surgeries with cardiopulmonary bypass were first performed in Uganda.[15] Groups in some developing nations have decided to evaluate the mortality rate associated with cardiac surgery in their countries,[16] but no global database or systematic method exists by which all countries can collect and submit such data. Such an international database could help identify key areas for improvement and focus efforts by surgeons in developed countries.[17]

SECONDARY PREVENTION

It has been estimated that treatment of patients with ischemic heart disease with aspirin, β-blockers, ACE inhibitors, or lipid-lowering drugs can each independently lower the risk of future vascular events by about one fourth; when taken in combination, a reduction in vascular events by two thirds to three fourths can be expected.[18] Multidrug regimens for secondary prevention in low- and middle-income countries are cost effective according to WHO standards, meaning that the intervention would cost less than three times the GNI of these countries.[19]

Despite the clear efficacy of the above medications in the secondary prevention of ischemic heart disease, their use in developing countries is alarmingly low. The WHO study on Prevention of Recurrences of Myocardial Infarction and Stroke (PREMISE), published in 2005, was a cross-sectional survey of 10,000 patients with coronary heart disease and/or cerebrovascular disease in three low-income and seven middle-income countries.[20] It found that in patients with coronary heart disease, 18.8% did not receive aspirin,

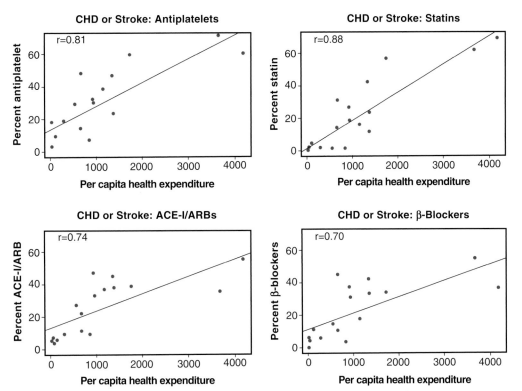

FIGURE 6-3 Percentage of the use of medications versus per capita health expenditures. CHD, congestive heart disease; ACE-I, angiotensin-converting enzyme inhibitor; ARB, angiotensin receptor blocker. *(Data from Yusuf S, Islam S, Chow K, et al. Use of secondary prevention drugs for cardiovascular disease in the community in high-income, middle-income, and low-income countries (the PURE Study): a prospective epidemiological survey.* Lancet *2011;378[9798]:1231-1243.)*

51.9% did not receive β-blockers, 60.2% did not receive ACE inhibitors, and 79.2% did not receive statins. Of particular concern is the fact that one tenth of patients with coronary heart disease in the PREMISE study were not on any medications for their heart disease at all. This is in comparison to the European Action on Secondary Prevention by Intervention to Reduce Events (EUROASPIRE II) study, in which 66.4% of patients were on a β-blocker (compared with 48.1% in PREMISE), and 57.7% were on a statin (compared with 20.8% in PREMISE).[21] A similar percentage of patients, however, were on aspirin and ACE inhibitors.

More recently, the Prospective Urban Rural Epidemiology (PURE) study examined the global usage of efficacious medications for secondary prevention of ischemic heart disease.[22] This study was conducted in communities in 17 countries of varying economic status from January 2003 through December 2009. The investigators found that the use of medications—antiplatelet drugs including aspirin, β-blockers, ACE inhibitors or angiotensin receptor blockers (ARBs), and statins—for secondary prevention decreased as country income level decreased (Figure 6-3). Most strikingly, they found that although 11.2% of patients in high-income countries received no medications at all, this percentage increased to 45.1% in upper middle-income countries, 69.3% in lower middle-income countries, and 80.2% in low-income countries. Country-level factors such as economic status influenced the rates of usage more than did individual-level factors such as age, sex, education, smoking status, body mass index (BMI), and hypertension and diabetes status. These estimates are far more grim than those reported in the WHO-PREMISE study and may have to do with the fact that the WHO-PREMISE study included patients who were already accessing hospital-level care and who therefore may have had greater access to medications as well.

Two countries in which the issue of secondary prevention has been more closely studied are India and China, where the prevalence of coronary artery disease (CAD) is very high. A 2009 study of physician prescribing practices at different levels of Indian health care found that among patients with stable known coronary

heart disease, aspirin was prescribed in 90.6% of cases, β-blockers in 68.7%, ACE inhibitors or ARBs in 82.5%, statins in 68.8%, and other lipid-lowering drugs were prescribed in 13.5% of patients.[23] Although these rates seem fairly high, only 35.5% of patients were prescribed drugs in all four classes. Interestingly, a trend of decreased use of each of the above agents was evident, and it continued at the primary and secondary levels of health care compared with the tertiary level, indicating a likely slow transition of knowledge in secondary prevention strategies to the community level. This is significant because the majority of patients in India receive their chronic disease care from the primary and secondary levels (12.6% at primary level, 57.2% at secondary level, 30.1% at tertiary level). Gupta et al (2009) confirmed the above finding of low rates of secondary prevention in the primary care setting and further found that women in particular were less likely to receive aspirin or any combination of drugs for secondary prevention than were their male counterparts.[24] In China, the Clinical Pathways for Acute Coronary Syndromes (CPACS) trial was conducted as a prospective study in nearly 3000 patients with suspected ACS. It found that less than 50% of patients were discharged from the hospital on a four-drug regimen of aspirin, β-blocker, ACE inhibitor/ARB, and statin, and the rate of use of these medications was even lower (41%) at 1-year follow-up.[25]

Challenges to Therapeutic Usage

CURRENT STATE OF CARDIOVASCULAR DISEASE DRUG AVAILABILITY AND AFFORDABILITY IN LOW- AND MIDDLE-INCOME COUNTRIES

A clear barrier to the prevention and treatment of CVD in developing countries is the low availability and affordability of medications. Investigators conducted a survey of 32 medications used to treat chronic diseases such as CVD in three low-income countries—Bangladesh, Malawi, and Nepal—and three low-middle income countries—Brazil, Pakistan, and Sri Lanka.[26] The authors found

78

CH
6

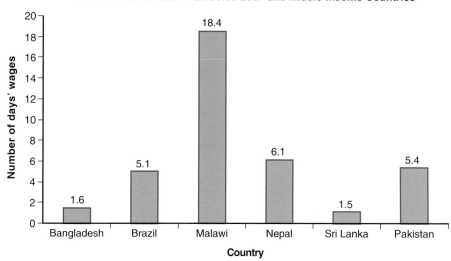

Affordability of Standard Treatment for Coronary Heart Disease in the Private Sector in Selected Low- and Middle-Income Countries

FIGURE 6-4 Affordability of standard treatment for coronary heart disease in the private sector in selected low- and middle-income countries. *Affordability* is defined as the number of days' wages it would take the lowest paid government worker to buy a 1-month supply of generic aspirin (100 mg daily), an angiotensin-converting enzyme inhibitor (10 mg daily), atenolol (100 mg daily), and a statin (20 mg daily). *(Data from Mendis S, Fukino K, Cameron A, et al. The availability and affordability of selected essential medicines for chronic diseases in six low- and middle-income countries.* Bull World Health Organ *2007;85[4]:279-288.)*

that the availability of cardiovascular medications was poor in the public sector. For example, hydrochlorothiazide was available in brand or generic form in only 5% of public outlets surveyed in Bangladesh; however, it was available in 85% of private outlets surveyed. Similarly, lovastatin was not available in any public outlets surveyed in Brazil but was present in 75% of private outlets.

Equally as striking is the low level of affordability of these drugs in developing countries. The above study found that a month of combination therapy with the lowest-priced generic version of aspirin, a β-blocker, and an ACE inhibitor cost 1.5 days' wages of the lowest level government worker in Sri Lanka; more than 5 days' wages in Brazil, Nepal, and Pakistan; and more than 18 days' wages in Malawi (Figure 6-4).[26] Actual affordability is likely worse because many people in developing countries earn less than the lowest paid government worker. Medications in the private sector in the above study were generally more expensive than in the public sector and were reflective of wholesale and retail markups. Specifically, add-on costs to the manufacturer's price ranged from 18% in Pakistan to more than 90% in countries such as Malawi, where there are no regulatory policies.

A large study of five antihypertensive medications in 36 countries of varying levels of income confirmed the stark reality of the availability and affordability of cardiovascular medicines.[27] Investigators showed that the overall availability of the antihypertensive medicines was poor (mean of 26.3% in the public sector for lowest priced generic, 57.3% in the private sector). Further, the lowest priced generic was in all cases more affordable than the brand product in both the public and private sectors. In fact, buying a brand product cost 4.2 times as much as buying the lowest priced generic.

ROLE OF THE WORLD HEALTH ORGANIZATION ESSENTIAL DRUG LIST

One of the challenges to improving access is ensuring adequate listing of effective CVD medications on the WHO Essential Drug List (EDL), which is a compilation of medications that the WHO believes are necessary to satisfy the health needs of any population.[28,29] Since its initial publication in 1977, the list has become a global standard that guides nations in how to allocate health care spending. This is particularly important for developing nations, which spend 25% to 66% of total public and private health spending on pharmaceuticals compared with less than 20% in developed countries. In addition, many international organizations such

as the United Nations Children's Fund (UNICEF), along with non-profit organizations and supply agencies, base their medicine supply system on the EDL.

Medications are chosen on the basis of disease prevalence, evidence of efficacy and safety, and cost effectiveness. The list is revised every 2 years by the WHO Expert Committee. The addition of a statin in 2007 provides an important case study of how medications can take some time to be added to the EDL.[30] Trials dating back to the mid-1990s had shown that statin therapy leads to improved cardiovascular outcomes in both primary and secondary prevention. In addition, it had been shown by 2003 that statins were cost effective for prevention of CVD in developing countries by WHO standards. However, when the WHO Expert Committee considered statins for inclusion in the EDL in 2005, they concluded that "since no single drug has been shown to be significantly more effective or less expensive than others in the group, none is included in the Model List; the choice of drug for use in patients at highest risk should be decided at the national level."[31] Subsequently, simvastatin became generic in 2006, leading to a significant reduction in price. Given this new development, two medical students in the United States[30] submitted an application to the Expert Committee in the Fall of 2006, and it was approved in April 2007 for inclusion in the 2007 EDL.[32]

HUMAN RESOURCES SHORTAGES

Although drug access may contribute to the low treatment rates for CVD, one of the most important contributing factors is the shortage of human resources (Figure 6-5). Although attempts have been made to increase education opportunities and train more doctors and nurses, developing countries continue to lose large numbers of trained professionals, as many newly graduated doctors and nurses in developing nations leave to find greater opportunity and better financial compensation in more developed economies. For example, of all the medical graduates produced by the University of Witwatersrand in South Africa in the past 35 years, more than 45%—approximately 2000 physicians—have left the country. In addition, increasing numbers of physicians and nurses seek employment in private industry for better compensation and benefits. To address health care worker shortages in low- and middle-income countries, the WHO has promoted *task shifting*, which is the process through which tasks are delegated, when appropriate, to less specialized health workers such as nurses. Limited studies have shown that nurses can effectively initiate and manage hypertension treatment.[33]

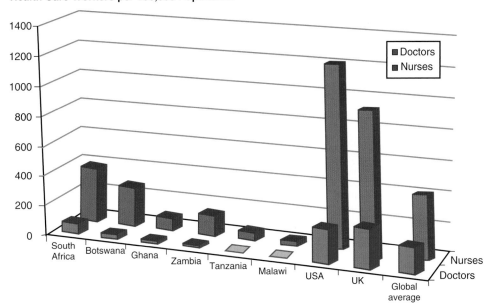

Health Care Workers per 100,000 Population

FIGURE 6-5 Health care workers per 100,000 population. *(Data from the World Health Organization.* Working together for health: the World Health Report. *Geneva, 2006, World Health Organization.)*

Primary Prevention

Primary prevention is paramount for the large number of individuals who are at high risk for CVD. In particular, a significant amount of the reduction in CVD mortality has come from control of risk factors.[34] However, control rates for the major risk factors remain poor globally. For example, several Western European countries have hypertension control rates (<140/90 mm Hg) of less than 10%, with Spain having a control rate of less than 5%.[35] Control rates for lipids are likely even worse because many countries do not have the facilities to measure lipids, and statins have become available only recently in low-income regions. Low control rates reflect low detection rates in addition to poor drug availability.

Given the limited resources, finding low-cost prevention strategies is a top priority. Using prediction rules or risk scores to identify those at higher risk in order to target specific behavioral or drug interventions is a well-established primary prevention strategy and has proven to be cost effective in developing countries.[19,36] Most studies include age, sex, hypertension, smoking status, diabetes mellitus, and lipid values; others also include family history.[37-40] Many investigators have been attempting to see whether additional laboratory-based risk factors can add to predictive discrimination of the risk factors used in the Framingham Heart Study Risk Score. Analyses in the Atherosclerosis Risk in Communities (ARIC) study[42] and the Framingham Offspring study[43,44] suggested that little additional information was gained when other blood-based novel risk factors were added to traditional risk factors. Although the Reynolds Risk Score[45] for women—which added family history, C-reactive protein (hsCRP), and hemoglobin A1c levels—had only a marginally higher C-statistic (0.808) than the Framingham covariates (0.791), it correctly reclassified many individuals at intermediate risk. Women who were otherwise thought to have been low risk by the Framingham Risk Score were reclassified as intermediate or high risk according to the Reynolds Risk Score and thus would have been eligible for more aggressive management. Those women who initially were at high risk according to the Framingham Score were reclassified as lower risk and thus would not have needed treatment.

More attention is now focused on developing risk scores that would be easier to use in clinical practice without loss of predictive discrimination in resource-poor countries. In high-income countries, a prediction rule that requires a laboratory test is an inconvenience; but in low-income countries with limited testing facilities, it may be too expensive for widespread screening, or its use may be precluded altogether. In response to this real concern, the WHO released risk-prediction charts for the different regions of the world with and without cholesterol testing.[46] A study based on the U.S. National Health and Nutrition Examination Survey (NHANES) follow-up cohort demonstrated that a non–lab-based risk tool that uses information obtained in a single encounter—age, systolic blood pressure, BMI, diabetes status, and smoking status—can predict CVD outcomes as well as one that requires laboratory testing, with C-statistics of 0.79 for men and 0.83 for women, similar to the Framingham-based risk tool.[47] Furthermore, the results of the goodness-of-fit tests suggest that the non–lab-based model is well calibrated across a wide range of absolute risk levels, without changes in classification of risk, and has been validated in another cohort.[48]

Polypill

One solution to affordability and availability has been the idea of combining generic medications into one pill. In 2003, Wald and Law published a landmark paper in the *British Medical Journal* introducing the concept of the "polypill" in CVD prevention.[49] They proposed that all individuals aged 55 years and all those with known CVD at any age be treated with a combination pill composed of a statin, three blood pressure–lowering drugs, folic acid, and aspirin. The authors estimated that this single intervention could reduce ischemic heart disease events by 88% and strokes by 80%.

The novel concept of primary prevention without assessment of individual risk factor levels or monitoring of biochemical safety parameters sparked a great deal of controversy and excitement, especially in developing countries, where resources are limited. The potential advantages of a polypill for primary prevention include reducing the need for dose titrations, improved adherence, and use of inexpensive generics in a single formulation.[50] However, these potential advantages, while seemingly intuitive, are as yet unproven.

Disadvantages to the polypill approach to primary prevention based on age alone include the possibility that some people will receive therapy without significant benefit, garnering only side effects from the medications, and others at higher risk for CVD may not receive sufficient therapy.[51] Other disadvantages include the possibility that a side effect to any one of the components of the polypill might cause patients to discontinue the pill altogether. The desire of clinicians to titrate the dose of one or more components of a polypill is also a logistical challenge.

Given the above pros and cons, it is clear that a large-scale study of the efficacy of the polypill in primary prevention of CVD is necessary. At the time of this writing, no such study with CVD endpoints has been published, although several are currently under way.[50,52,53] In the meantime, several trials have investigated the safety of various polypill formulations and their effects on risk factor levels. The first to be published is the Indian Polycap Study (TIPS), which showed that a polypill could safely and effectively lower risk factor levels in asymptomatic individuals at moderate risk for CVD.[54] Other trials on the effects of the polypill on risk factor levels are ongoing or are yet to be published.

The use of a polypill in secondary prevention is less controversial because even though no trial has proven its efficacy in this setting, multiple trials show that the individual component drugs—aspirin, statins, β-blockers, and blockers of the renin-angiotensin system—improve outcomes in patients with known CVD or high risk factor levels.[50] In addition, a large case-control analysis of 13,029 patients with ischemic heart disease in the United Kingdom indicated that combinations of drugs—statin, aspirin, and β-blockers—rather than single agents, decrease mortality rates in patients with known CVD.[55] Finally, the use of combination therapy was shown to be cost effective for low- and middle-income countries for both primary and secondary prevention, with the best cost-effectiveness ratio for secondary prevention and acceptable but increasing cost per QALY ratios as the absolute CVD risk declined in primary prevention.[19]

Just as the appropriate use of the polypill in primary versus secondary prevention has been debated, so too has its ideal formulation. Wald and Law initially proposed the inclusion of a statin, three blood pressure–lowering medications at half the standard dose, folic acid, and low-dose aspirin.[49] Since then, it has been shown that folic acid does not improve CVD outcomes.[56] In addition, the benefit of reducing CVD events using low-dose aspirin as primary prevention in low-risk patients must be weighed against the possibility of increased major bleeds.[57] Blood pressure–lowering medications and statins have clear efficacy in both primary and secondary prevention. However, in the TIPS trial—which used low-dose aspirin, simvastatin 20 mg, ramipril 5 mg, hydrochlorothiazide 12.5 mg, and atenolol 50 mg—blood pressure and cholesterol reduction rates were less than those predicted by Wald and Law.[49,54] This raises the possibility that full doses of blood pressure–lowering drugs and a higher dose or more potent form of statin should be used, all of which may also increase adverse effects of the polypill.[50,58] The Indian Polycap-K Trial (TIPS-K) is currently under way to evaluate the effect of doubling the dose of the Polycap used in the TIPS trial (Cadila Pharmaceuticals Ltd; Ahmedabad, India), with or without potassium, on risk factor levels and safety profile. Other areas of uncertainty include whether an ARB should be used instead of an ACE inhibitor to decrease the risk of cough and increase adherence.[50] It is also unclear whether different strengths of the polypill should be made to titrate the β-blocker—for instance, in patients with asthma—or the statin in patients with known CVD who require lower low-density lipoprotein (LDL) targets[50]; however, this would necessitate dose titration, which would likely interfere with the simplicity of the regimen, currently one of its biggest advantages.

Other issues regarding the polypill that also need to be resolved include 1) whether the polypill will improve medication adherence, 2) whether physicians and patients will accept this new paradigm of CVD prevention, 3) whether the polypill will be safe in the long term, 4) whether people in the poorest regions will be able to afford it, and 5) whether a role exists for over-the-counter distribution.[58]

Overall, the concept of a polypill for CVD prevention is one that holds great promise, especially in the developing world, where resources are sparse, but CVD burden is on the rise. However, the exact formulation of the pill, the population in which it is used, the cost, the manner in which it is delivered, the side effects of the drug, and long-term outcomes of its use need to be more fully investigated before its use can become widespread.

Population Strategies

Risk Factors for Cardiovascular Disease

TOBACCO

By many accounts, tobacco use is the most preventable cause of death in the world. Overall, one in six noncommunicable disease deaths is attributable to tobacco. More than 1.3 billion people use tobacco worldwide; more than 1 billion of them smoke,[59] and the rest use oral or nasal tobacco. More than 80% of tobacco use occurs in low- and middle-income countries, and if current trends continue unabated, more than 1 billion deaths will be due to tobacco during the twenty-first century.[60] Smoking-related CHD deaths in the developing world totaled 360,000 in 2000, compared with 200,000 cerebrovascular deaths that year.[61]

Tobacco control can be conceptualized in terms of strategies that reduce the supply of, or demand for, tobacco. Most public health and clinical strategies to date focus on reducing demand through economic disincentives (taxes), health promotion through media efforts and packaging warnings, restricted access to advertising and tobacco consumption, creation of smoke-free areas (work and public), or clinical assistance for cessation. The WHO effort to catalyze the creation of a global treaty against tobacco use was a key milestone. In May 2003, the WHO World Health Assembly unanimously adopted the WHO Framework Convention in Tobacco Control (FCTC), which is the first global tobacco treaty.[60] The FCTC had been ratified by 174 countries as of January 2012, making it one of the most widely embraced treaties of the United Nations.[60] The FCTC has spurred efforts for tobacco control across the globe by providing both rich and poor nations with a common framework of evidence-based legislation and implementation strategies known to reduce tobacco use. Supply-side measures supported in the FCTC include control of illicit, mostly cross-border trade. Fully implementing four of the FCTC strategies for reducing demand could lead to 5.5 million fewer deaths in 23 countries that bear nearly 75% of the CVD burden.[62]

Furthermore, these strategies are quite cost effective. Jha and colleagues presented a landmark analysis in 2006 of tobacco control cost effectiveness.[63] They calculated the reductions in future tobacco deaths that would follow a range of tax, treatment, and non-price interventions among smokers alive in 2000. They found that a 33% price increase would result in a reduction of between 19.7 and 56.8 million (5.4% to 15.9% of total) deaths in smokers from the developing world who were alive in 2000.[63] A range of non-price interventions—such as advertising bans, health warnings, and smoke-free laws—would reduce deaths by between 5.7 and 28.6 million (1.6% to 7.9% of total) in that cohort.[63] These reductions would translate into developing world cost-effectiveness values of between $3 and $42 dollars per QALY saved for tax increases (not including tax revenue), $55 to $761 per QALY for nicotine replacement therapies, and $54 to $674 per QALY for non-price measures.[63]

BLOOD PRESSURE

The population-based intervention most touted as an effective means to lower blood pressure is reduction of salt intake. In the United States, reducing salt intake by 3 g/day could reduce systolic blood pressure by 3.6 to 5.61 mm Hg in patients with hypertension; in all other patients, the effect was 1.8 to 3.51 mm Hg.[64] Meta-analyses of randomized, controlled trials (RCTs) that examine the long-term effects of salt reduction in people with and without hypertension have shown that reductions in salt intake can reduce absolute systolic blood pressure by a small but important amount.[62]

The effect of salt reduction on blood pressure reduction was found to be linear over the range of 0 to 3 g/day, for an approximate 1:1 ratio in reduction in salt intake (g/day) and decrease in mean systolic blood pressure. Reducing population-wide salt consumption by only 15%, through mass media campaigns and reformulation of food products by industry, would avert more than 8.5 million deaths in 23 high-burden countries over a 10-year period.[62]

The cost-effectiveness analyses on salt reduction as a result of public education are quite favorable. The intervention ranges from being cost saving to averting $200 per DALY.[64] However, a contemporary study found a positive association of a 1.71 mm Hg increase in systolic blood pressure per 100-mmol increase in sodium excretion but found an inverse relationship between sodium excretion and CVD mortality[65]; other studies have seen reductions in mortality rates with reductions in sodium intake.[66,67] Further studies to evaluate the direction and magnitude of this effect need to be conducted. The WHO goal is to reduce sodium intake to 2 g/day.

LIPIDS

Worldwide, high cholesterol levels are estimated to cause 56% of ischemic heart disease and 18% of strokes, amounting to 4.4 million deaths annually. Unfortunately, most developing countries have limited data on cholesterol levels and often only total cholesterol values are collected. In the high-income countries, mean population cholesterol levels are generally falling, but in the low- and middle-income countries, a wide variation in these levels is seen. In general, the Eastern Europe and Central Asian regions have the highest levels, with the East Asian and sub-Saharan African regions having the lowest levels.[68] As countries move through the epidemiologic transition, mean population plasma cholesterol levels tend to rise. This shift is largely driven by greater consumption of dietary fats, primarily from animal products and processed vegetable oils, and decreased physical activity.

Efforts to reduce saturated fats could be cost effective based on prior estimates of the effect of a campaign for reducing saturated fat and replacing it with polyunsaturated fat.[69] A 3% decline in saturated fat and a $6 per capita education cost resulted in a cost as low as $1800 per DALY averted in the South Asian region and up to $4000 per DALY averted in the Middle East and North Africa region. The educational plan could be cost saving if the reduction were to be achieved for less than $0.50 per capita, which may be possible in areas where media use is much less expensive.

Furthermore, studies show that replacing 2% of energy from trans fats with polyunsaturated fats was estimated to reduce CHD by 7% to 8%, assuming changes in LDL cholesterol (LDL-c) only, and up to a 40% CHD reduction, assuming benefits beyond LDL-c reduction, such as changes in triglycerides, endothelial function, and inflammatory markers.[70] In 2003, Denmark became the first country to virtually outlaw trans fats by placing a limit of 2% of fats from this source on foods destined for human consumption. Switzerland followed with a similar ban in 2008. In the United States, cities such as New York have banned trans fats in restaurants. Because such changes can occur through voluntary action by industry or by regulation, these initiatives can be achieved without a large media campaign or high costs. According to the U.S. Food and Drug Administration, this is achievable for less than $0.50 per capita. Using this figure and the conservative estimate of an 8% reduction in CHD, the intervention is highly cost effective at $25 to $75 per DALY averted across the developing world. Assuming a greater reduction of 40% reduction in CHD, the intervention becomes cost saving.

OBESITY

According to the latest WHO data, approximately 1.1 billion adults in the world are overweight, with 115 million of them in the developing world known to be living with obesity-related problems.[71] A 2005 compilation of population-based surveys revised this number to approximately 1.3 billion and estimated that 23% of adults older than 20 years are overweight (BMI >25), and an additional 10% are obese (BMI >30).[72] In developing countries such as Egypt, Mexico, and Thailand, rates of overweight are increasing at two to five times those in the United States. In China, over an 8-year period, the prevalence of the population with a BMI greater than 25 increased more than 50% in both men and women.

Consensus has not been reached, however, on the single ideal dietary approach to weight reduction. Some agree that physical activity in addition to dietary means is more likely to be successful. Other approaches include dietary advice, exercise, behavior modification, drug therapy, and bariatric surgery. These interventions are difficult to adhere to and may be expensive. Furthermore, few interventions have been conducted for a long duration or with long-term reductions in major outcomes, such as CVD among previously healthy individuals.[73] Without precise estimates of the benefit, and with substantial variability in the intervention strategy, estimating the cost/benefit ratio of weight-loss programs or interventions has been challenging. Beyond the interventions mentioned above, population-based education programs regarding improved diet, increased physical activity, and reduction of blood glucose levels are promoted by many nonprofit organizations in programs such as the AHA's Simple Seven Program.[74]

Summary

The burden of CVD throughout the world is large and growing. Most of the increasing burden is now being felt in low- and middle-income countries, which have limited resources to combat the enormous health and economic consequences of CVD. Individual treatments and population-based strategies to reduce the burden exist and are cost effective; however, significant challenges persist in identifying and treating those at high risk. These challenges include limited public health system infrastructure, decreased affordability and availability of essential medicines, and the scarcity of human resources.

REFERENCES

1. Lopez AD, Mathers CD, Ezzati M, et al (eds). *Global burden of disease and risk factors: Disease Control Priorities Project.* New York, 2006, The World Bank and Oxford University Press, p 552.
2. Alwan A (ed). *Global status report on noncommunicable diseases 2010.* Geneva, 2011, World Health Organization.
3. Reference deleted in proofs.
4. Xavier D, Pais P, Devereaux PJ, et al. Treatment and outcomes of acute coronary syndromes in India (CREATE): a prospective analysis of registry data. *Lancet* 2008;371(9622): 1435-1442.
5. World Health Organization. Preventing chronic diseases: a vital investment. WHO global report. Geneva, 2005, World Health Organization.
6. Gaziano TA, Bitton A, Anand S, et al. The global cost of nonoptimal blood pressure. *J Hypertens* 2009;27(7):1472-1477.
7. Leeder S, et al. *A race against time: the challenge of cardiovascular disease in developing countries.* New York, 2004, Columbia University.
8. Orlandini A, Diaz R, Wojdyla D, et al. Outcomes of patients in clinical trials with ST-segment elevation myocardial infarction among countries with different gross national incomes. *Eur Heart J* 2006;27(5):527-533.
9. Steg PG, Goldberg RJ, Gore JM, et al. Baseline characteristics, management practices, and in-hospital outcomes of patients hospitalized with acute coronary syndromes in the Global Registry of Acute Coronary Events (GRACE). *Am J Cardiol* 2002;90(4):358-363.
10. Sikri N, Bardia A. A history of streptokinase use in acute myocardial infarction. *Tex Heart Inst J* 2007;34(3):318-327.
11. Gaziano TA. Cardiovascular disease in the developing world and its cost-effective management. *Circulation* 2005;112(23):3547-3553.
12. Giugliano RP, Llevadot J, Wilcox RG, et al. Geographic variation in patient and hospital characteristics, management, and clinical outcomes in ST-elevation myocardial infarction treated with fibrinolysis: results from InTIME-II. *Eur Heart J* 2001;22(18):1702-1715.
13. Kramer JM, Newby LK, Chang WC, et al. International variation in the use of evidence-based medicines for acute coronary syndromes. *Eur Heart J* 2003;24(23):2133-2141.
14. Edmond JJ, French JK, Aylward PE, et al. Variations in the use of emergency PCI for the treatment of re-infarction following intravenous fibrinolytic therapy: impact on outcomes in HERO-2. *Eur Heart J* 2007;28(12):1418-1424.
15. Akomea-Agyin C, Galukande M, Mwambu T, et al: Pioneer human open heart surgery using cardiopulmonary by pass in Uganda. *Afr Health Sci* 2008;8(4):259-260.
16. Ribeiro AL, Gagliardi SP, Nogueira JL, et al. Mortality related to cardiac surgery in Brazil, 2000-2003. *J Thorac Cardiovasc Surg* 2006;131(4):907-909.
17. Pezzella AT. Global statistics/outcomes. *J Thorac Cardiovasc Surg* 2006;132(3):726.
18. Yusuf S. Two decades of progress in preventing vascular disease. *Lancet* 2002; 360(9326):2-3.

19. Gaziano TA, Opie LH, Weinstein MC. Cardiovascular disease prevention with a multidrug regimen in the developing world: a cost-effectiveness analysis. *Lancet* 2006;368(9536): 679-686.

20. Mendis S, Abegunde E, Yusuf S, et al. WHO study on Prevention of REcurrences of Myocardial Infarction and StrokE (WHO-PREMISE). *Bull World Health Organ* 2005;83(11): 820-829.

21. EUROASPIRE I and II Group and European Action on Secondary Prevention by Intervention to Reduce Events. Clinical reality of coronary prevention guidelines: a comparison of EUROASPIRE I and II in nine countries. *Lancet* 2001;357(9261):995-1001.

22. Yusuf, S, Islam S, Chow CK, et al. Use of secondary prevention drugs for cardiovascular disease in the community in high-income, middle-income, and low-income countries (the PURE study): a prospective epidemiological survey. *Lancet* 2011;378(9798):1231-1243.

23. Sharma KK, Gupta R, Agrawal A, et al. Low use of statins and other coronary secondary prevention therapies in primary and secondary care in India. *Vasc Health Risk Manag* 2009;5:1007-1014.

24. Gupta R. Secondary prevention of coronary artery disease in urban Indian primary care. *Int J Cardiol* 2009;135(2):184-186.

25. Bi Y, Gao R, Patel A, et al. Evidence-based medication use among Chinese patients with acute coronary syndromes at the time of hospital discharge and 1 year after hospitalization: results from the Clinical Pathways for Acute Coronary Syndromes in China (CPACS) study. *Am Heart J* 2009;157(3):509-516.e1.

26. Mendis S, Fukino K, Cameron A, et al. The availability and affordability of selected essential medicines for chronic diseases in six low- and middle-income countries. *Bull World Health Organ* 2007;85(4):279-288.

27. van Mourik MS, Cameron A, Ewen M, Laing RO. Availability, price and affordability of cardiovascular medicines: a comparison across 36 countries using WHO/HAI data. *BMC Cardiovasc Disord* 2010;10:25.

28. Califf RM, Harrington RA, Madre LK, et al. Curbing the cardiovascular disease epidemic: aligning industry, government, payers, and academics. *Health Aff (Millwood)* 2007; 26(1):62-74.

29. World Health Organization. *World Health Organization Essential Medicines*. Available at www.who.int/medicines/services/essmedicines_def/en/index.html. Accessed April 6, 2011.

30. Kishore SP, Herbstman BJ. Adding a medicine to the WHO model list of essential medicines. *Clin Pharmacol Ther* 2009;85(3):237-239.

31. Committee WE. *WHO Model List (revised March 2005): explanatory notes*. Available at http://whqlibdoc.who.int/hq/2005/a87017_eng.pdf. Accessed April 7, 2011.

32. World Health Organization. *Proposal for the inclusion of a statin for the secondary prevention of cardiovascular disease in the WHO Model List of Essential Medicines, 2006*. Available at http://archives.who.int/eml/expcom/expcom15/applications/newmed/statins/Statins.pdf. Accessed April 7, 2011.

33. Fezeu L, Kengne AP, Balkau B, et al. Ten-years' change in blood pressure levels and prevalence of hypertension in urban and rural Cameroon. *J Epidemiol Community Health* 2010;64(4):360-366.

34. Ford ES, Capewell S. Proportion of the decline in cardiovascular mortality disease due to prevention versus treatment: public health versus clinical care. *Annu Rev Public Health* 2011;32:5-22.

35. Wolf-Maier K, Cooper RS, Kramer H, et al. Hypertension treatment and control in five European countries, Canada, and the United States. *Hypertension* 2004;43(1):10-17.

36. Gaziano TA, Steyn K, Cohen DJ, et al. Cost-effectiveness analysis of hypertension guidelines in South Africa: absolute risk versus blood pressure level. *Circulation* 2005;112(23): 3569-3576.

37. Wilson PW, D'Agostino RB, Levy D, et al. Prediction of coronary heart disease using risk factor categories. *Circulation* 1998;97(18):1837-1847.

38. Assmann G, Cullen P, Schulte H. Simple scoring scheme for calculating the risk of acute coronary events based on the 10-year follow-up of the prospective cardiovascular Munster (PROCAM) study. *Circulation* 2002;105(3):310-315. Erratum *Circulation* 2002; 105(7):900.

39. Conroy RM, Pyörälä K, Fitzgerald AP, et al. Estimation of ten-year risk of fatal cardiovascular disease in Europe: the SCORE project. *Eur Heart J* 2003;24(11):987-1003.

40. Ferrario M, Chiodini P, Chambless LE, et al. Prediction of coronary events in a low incidence population: assessing accuracy of the CUORE cohort study prediction equation. *Int J Epidemiol* 2005;34(2):413-421.

41. Reference deleted in proofs.

42. Folsom AR, Chambless LE, Ballantyne CM, et al. An assessment of incremental coronary risk prediction using C-reactive protein and other novel risk markers: the Atherosclerosis Risk in Communities Study. *Arch Intern Med* 2006;166(13):1368-1373.

43. Wang TJ, Gona P, Larson MG, et al. Multiple biomarkers for the prediction of first major cardiovascular events and death. *N Engl J Med* 2006;355(25):2631-2639.

44. Ware JH. The limitations of risk factors as prognostic tools. *N Engl J Med* 2006; 355(25):2615-2617.

45. Ridker PM, Buring AG, Rifai N, Cook NR. Development and validation of improved algorithms for the assessment of global cardiovascular risk in women: the Reynolds Risk Score. *JAMA* 2007;297(6):611-619.

46. Mendis S, Lindholm LH, Mancia G, et al. World Health Organization (WHO) and International Society of Hypertension (ISH) risk prediction charts: assessment of cardiovascular risk for prevention and control of cardiovascular disease in low and middle-income countries. *J Hypertens* 2007;25(8):1578-1582.

47. Gaziano TA, Young CR, Fitzmaurice G, et al. Laboratory-based versus non–laboratory-based method for assessment of cardiovascular disease risk: the NHANES I follow-up study cohort. *Lancet* 2008;371(9616):923-931.

48. Pandya A, Weinstein MC, Gaziano TA. A comparative assessment of non–laboratory-based versus commonly used laboratory-based cardiovascular disease risk scores in the NHANES III population. *PLoS One* 2011;6(5):e20416.

49. Wald NJ, Law MR. A strategy to reduce cardiovascular disease by more than 80%. *Br Med J* 2003;326(7404):1419.

50. Lonn E, Bosch J, Teo KK, et al. The polypill in the prevention of cardiovascular diseases: key concepts, current status, challenges, and future directions. *Circulation* 2010;122(20): 2078-2088.

51. Combination Pharmacotherapy and Public Health Research Working Group, Heart Outcomes Prevention Evaluation-3 [Clinical Trial #NCT00468923]. Available at http://clinicaltrials.gov/ct2/show/NCT00468923.

52. Yusuf S, Pais P, Xavier D. The Indian Polycap Study (TIPS): authors' reply. *Lancet* 2009;374: 782.

53. Heart Outcomes Prevention Evaluation-3 (HOPE-3). Availale at http://clinicaltrials.gov/ct2/show/NCT00468923?term=NCT00468923&rank=1. Accessed March 28, 2011.

54. Yusuf S, Pais P, Afzal R, et al, for the Indian Polycap Study (TIPS). Effects of a polypill (Polycap) on risk factors in middle-aged individuals without cardiovascular disease (TIPS): a phase II, double-blind, randomised trial. *Lancet* 2009;373(9672):1341-1351.

55. Hippisley-Cox J, Coupland C. Effect of combinations of drugs on all cause mortality in patients with ischaemic heart disease: nested case-control analysis. *Br Med J* 2005;330(7499):1059-1063.

56. Clarke R, Halsey J, Lewington S, et al. Effects of lowering homocysteine levels with B vitamins on cardiovascular disease, cancer, and cause-specific mortality: meta-analysis of 8 randomized trials involving 37 485 individuals. *Arch Intern Med* 2010;170(18): 1622-1631.

57. Baigent C, Blackwell L, Collins R, et al, for the Antithrombotic Trialists' (ATT) Collaboration. Aspirin in the primary and secondary prevention of vascular disease: collaborative meta-analysis of individual participant data from randomised trials. *Lancet* 2009;373(9678): 1849-1860.

58. Lonn E, Yusuf S. Polypill: the evidence and the promise. *Curr Opin Lipidol* 2009;20(6):453-459.

59. Shafey O, et al. *The tobacco atlas*, 3rd ed. Atlanta, 2009, American Cancer Society.

60. Parties to the WHO Framework Convention on Tobacco Control. *WHO framework convention on tobacco control*. Available at http://www.who.int/fctc/signatories_parties/en/index.html. Accessed April 6, 2012.

61. Ezzati M, Henley SJ, Thun MJ, Lopez AD. Role of smoking in global and regional cardiovascular mortality. *Circulation* 2005;112(4):489-497.

62. Asaria P, Chisolm L, Mathers C, et al. Chronic disease prevention: health effects and financial costs of strategies to reduce salt intake and control tobacco use. *Lancet* 2007;370(9604):2044-2053.

63. Jha P, et al. Tobacco addiction. In *Disease control priorities in developing countries*, 2nd ed. New York, 2006, Oxford University Press.

64. Bibbins-Domingo K, Chertow GM, Coxson PG, et al. Projected effect of dietary salt reductions on future cardiovascular disease. *N Engl J Med* 2010;362(7):590-599.

65. Stolarz-Skrzypek K, Kuznetsova T, Thijs L, et al. Fatal and nonfatal outcomes, incidence of hypertension, and blood pressure changes in relation to urinary sodium excretion. *JAMA* 2011;305(17):1777-1785.

66. Cook NR, Cutler JA, Obarzanek E, et al. Long term effects of dietary sodium reduction on cardiovascular disease outcomes: observational follow-up of the trials of hypertension prevention (TOHP). *Br Med J* 2007;334(7599):885-888.

67. Strazzullo P, D'Elia L, Kandala MB, Cappuccio FP. Salt intake, stroke, and cardiovascular disease: meta-analysis of prospective studies. *Br Med J* 2009;339:b4567.

68. Ezzati M, et al. Comparative quantification of mortality and burden of disease attributable to selected risk factors. In Lopez AD, Ezzati M, Jamieson DT, Murray CJL (eds): *Global burden of disease and risk factors*. New York, 2006, Oxford University Press, pp 241-396.

69. Gaziano TA, Galea G, Reddy KS. Chronic disease 2: scaling up interventions for chronic disease prevention: the evidence. *Lancet* 2007;370(9603):1939-1946.

70. Mozaffarian D, Katan MB, Ascherio A, et al. Trans fatty acids and cardiovascular disease. *N Engl J Med* 2006;354(15):1601-1613.

71. Misra A, Khurana L. Obesity and the metabolic syndrome in developing countries. *J Clin Endocrinol Metab* 2008;93(11 Suppl 1):S9-S30.

72. Kelly T, Yang W, Chen CS, et al. Global burden of obesity in 2005 and projections to 2030. *Int J Obes (Lond)* 2008;32(9):1431-1437.

73. Gregg EW, Cheng YJ, Caldwell BL, et al. Secular trends in cardiovascular disease risk factors according to body mass index in US adults. *JAMA* 2005;293(15):1868-1874.

74. American Heart Association. My life check: live better with life's simple 7. Available at http://mylifecheck.heart.org/Default.aspx. Accessed September 14, 2011.

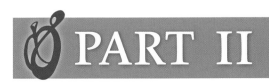

PART II

ISCHEMIC HEART DISEASE

CHAPTER **7**

Pharmacologic Options for Treatment of Ischemic Disease

John S. Schroeder, William H. Frishman, John D. Parker, Dominick J. Angiolillo, Christopher Woods, and Benjamin M. Scirica

ORGANIC NITRATES, 83

Overview, 83
Mechanisms of Action, 83
Pharmacokinetics, 84
Pharmacodynamic Effects, 84
Side Effects of Organic Nitrates, 84
Clinical Efficacy of Organic Nitrates, 85
Nitrate Tolerance, 87
Nonhemodynamic Effects of Organic Nitrates, 88
Current Perspectives on Therapy with Organic Nitrates, 89

CALCIUM CHANNEL BLOCKERS, 89

Fundamental Mechanisms of Calcium Channel Blockers, 89
Calcium Channels: L and T Types, 90
Pharmacologic Properties of Calcium Channel Blockers, 90
Classification of Calcium Channel Blockers, 91
Vascular Selectivity, 91
Noncardiovascular Effects, 91
Pharmacokinetics, 91
Major Indications for Calcium Channel Blockers, 92

Specific Calcium Channel Blockers, 92
Drug Interactions of Calcium Channel Blockers, 94
Calcium Channel Blockers: The "Safety" Controversy, 94

β-ADRENERGIC BLOCKERS, 96

β-Adrenergic Receptors, 96
Effects in Angina Pectoris, 97
Comparison with Other Antianginal Therapies, 97
Angina at Rest and Vasospastic Angina, 97
Combined Use of β-Blockers with Other Antianginal Therapies in Angina Pectoris, 99
Conditions Associated with Angina Pectoris, 99
Other Cardiovascular Conditions Associated with Angina Pectoris, 100
Perioperative Therapy in High-Risk Patients with Ischemic Heart Disease, 100
Pharmacologic Differences Among β-Adrenergic Receptor–Blocking Drugs, 101
Adverse Effects of β-Adrenergic Receptor Blockers, 103
Contraindications to β-Adrenergic Receptor Blockers, 104

Overdosage, 104
β-Adrenergic Receptor Blocker Withdrawal, 104
Drug-Drug Interactions, 104

NEWER OPTIONS FOR TREATMENT OF CHRONIC ANGINA, 104

Nicorandil, 104
Ivabradine, 104
Ranolazine, 105
Trimetazidine, 106

THROMBOSIS AND ISCHEMIC CARDIOVASCULAR HEART DISEASE, 107

Antiplatelet Therapy, 107
Novel Antiplatelet Agents, 115
Anticoagulant Therapy, 115
Factor Xa Inhibitors, 121
Oral Anticoagulants, 121

REFERENCES, 124

Organic Nitrates

Overview

Nitroglycerin (glyceryl trinitrate [GTN]) was first synthesized in 1847 by Ascanio Sobrero, who described a "violent headache" upon self-administration of a "minute quantity" of the drug.[1] A number of reports of the therapeutic effects of GTN in the latter half of the nineteenth century included those of Field, Brunton, and Murrell.[2-4] Although sublingual GTN has been commonly used for more than a century to treat acute attacks of angina, the development of organic nitrates with sustained activity was limited by their poor oral bioavailability. Eventually, this difficulty was overcome with transdermal formulations of GTN and the development of long-acting oral nitrate preparations, including isosorbide dinitrate, isosorbide-5-mononitrate, erythrityl tetranitrate, and pentaerythritol tetranitrate. Today, the organic nitrates continue to play an important role in the management of both angina and congestive heart failure (CHF).

Mechanisms of Action

Organic nitrates are prodrugs that must undergo enzymatic denitrification to mediate their pharmacodynamic effects (Figures 7-1 and 7-2). In 1977, Murad first suggested that nitric oxide (NO) mediated the effects of GTN.[5] Since that time, it has generally been

accepted that all the organic nitrates exert their effects via release of NO or some NO-containing moiety. As the understanding of NO biology grew and the importance of decreased NO bioavailability in cardiovascular (CV) disease was recognized, it was postulated that the organic nitrates could supplement endogenous NO with favorable biologic effects. Despite its appeal, this hypothesis has never been formerly tested, and no available evidence suggests that exogenous NO donors favorably modify the natural history of CV disease.

The exact mechanism of nitrate biotransformation (denitrification) was the subject of debate for several decades. Multiple enzymatic candidates were proposed, including cytochrome P450 (CYP), endothelial NO synthase, and glutathione transferase.[6-9] Interest in defining the denitrification pathway was intense because it was believed that the development of abnormalities in this process might explain the loss of nitrate effects during sustained therapy, a phenomenon termed *nitrate tolerance*. More recent studies have proposed a role for mitochondrial aldehyde dehydrogenase type 2 (mALDH-2) in the biotransformation of GTN.[10] The role of this enzyme in the activation of GTN supported the dependence of GTN-induced cyclic guanosine monophosphate (cGMP) production, based on the presence of this enzyme and the fact that specific antagonists of mALDH-2 inhibit the vasoactive actions of GTN.[10-12] The relevance of this biotransformation pathway in humans is supported by observations of reduced hemodynamic responses to GTN in Asian subjects, who are

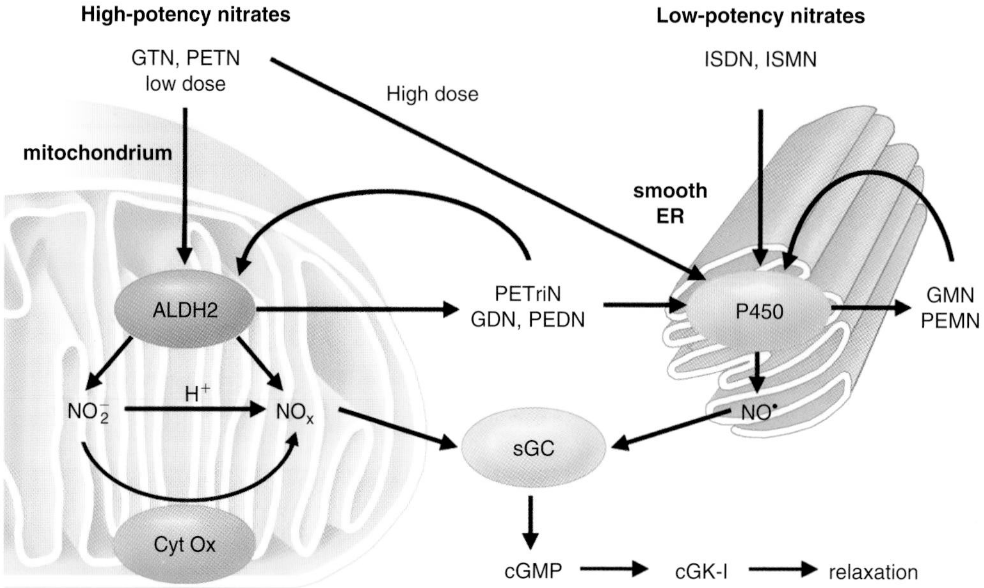

84

CH
7

FIGURE 7-1 Pathways of organic nitrate bioactivation in vascular cells. ALDH2, aldehyde dehydrogenase 2; cGMP, cyclic guanosine monophosphate; cGK-I, cGMP dependent protein kinase-I; Cyt Ox, cytochrome oxidase; ER, endoplasmic reticulum; GDN, glycerol dinitrate; GMN, glycerol mononitrate; GTN, glyceril trinitrate (nitroglycerin); ISDN, isosorbide dinitrate; ISMN, isosorbide mononitrate; NO, nitric oxide; PEDN, pentaerythrityl dinitrate; PEMN, pentaerythrityl mononitrate; PETN, pentaerythrityl tetranitrate; PETriN, pentaerythrityl trinitate; sGC, soluble guanylate cyclase.

genetically deficient in the enzyme aldehyde dehydrogenase.[13,14] Importantly, the function of this biotransformation pathway is consistent with a number of observations concerning nitrate tolerance (see the discussion below). Although the discovery of the mALDH-2 biotransformation pathway provided important new insights concerning the actions of GTN, many unanswered questions remain. Most importantly, the denitrification of other organic nitrates, including isosorbide dinitrate and isosorbide-5-mononitrate, does not depend on mALDH-2.[15] These observations emphasize that our knowledge of these processes remains incomplete.

Following organic nitrate bioactivation, and despite uncertainties concerning the exact nature of the NO moiety derived, there is activation of soluble guanylate cyclase and increased cGMP synthesis. The subsequent increase in the bioavailability of cGMP triggers a molecular cascade that mediates vasorelaxation through multiple pathways, which lead to a reduction in intracellular Ca^{2+} concentrations, including activation of protein kinases involved in the regulation of intracellular Ca^{2+} levels, such as the sarcoplasmic Ca^{2+}-ATPase.[16,17] NO donors, as with endogenous NO, appear to have multiple biologic effects, including thiol modification, regulation of mitochondrial respiration, modulation of K^+ channel activity, and protein nitration, although less evidence is available concerning the therapeutic relevance of these effects.[18-21] As discussed below, these diverse biochemical responses to the organic nitrates appears to be responsible for their recently described nonhemodynamic effects.[22]

Pharmacokinetics

Organic nitrates are available in a variety of formulations with differing routes of administration. GTN undergoes hepatic and intravascular metabolism with a half-life of approximately 1 to 4 minutes with biologically active dinitrate metabolites that have a half-life of approximately 40 minutes. GTN is very effective when given by the sublingual and transdermal routes. Transdermal administration of GTN is the only method of administration that provides a clinically effective long-acting form of GTN. When given orally, first-pass metabolism of GTN is extensive. Oral GTN is available for the therapy of angina, but no evidence of clinical efficacy exists.

Although it provides hemodynamic and antianginal effects, isosorbide dinitrate is rapidly metabolized, with a plasma half-life of approximately 40 minutes. Its major metabolites, isosorbide-2-mononitrate and isosorbide-5-mononitrate, are both biologically active, with half-lives of approximately 2 and 4 hours, respectively. Isosorbide-5-mononitrate does not undergo first-pass hepatic metabolism and is completely bioavailable. Both of these nitrates are available in sustained-release preparations; the sustained, phasic-release form of isosorbide-5-monitrate is the most popular, with once-daily dosing and favorable pharmacokinetics that avoid tolerance. Although not prescribed in North America, both erythrityl tetranitrate and pentaerythritol tetranitrate are used in certain parts of the world for the treatment of angina.

Pharmacodynamic Effects

The organic nitrates are potent vasodilators, whose vascular effects vary widely in different distributions of the vasculature (Figure 7-3).[23] They have potent effects in the venous capacitance bed and reduce ventricular volume and preload. They also dilate conduit arteries, and at the doses used clinically, they have no effect on peripheral vascular resistance. The nitrates dilate epicardial coronary arteries but have little or no effect on the coronary resistance vessels.[24] In patients with coronary artery disease (CAD), nitrates can dilate coronary stenoses and collateral vessels, which can improve and redistribute coronary blood flow.[25] Because they do not reduce coronary vascular resistance, nitrates avoid the risk myocardial ischemia because of coronary steal, which can occur with arteriolar dilators, such as dipyridamole and short-acting dihydropyridines (DHPs), in which coronary blood flow is diverted away from areas of ongoing ischemia. Therefore, the nitrates possess a unique combination of vascular effects that can favorably affect the mismatch between myocardial oxygen supply and demand in patients with CAD.

Side Effects of Organic Nitrates

Headaches are common during nitrate therapy and are generally most pronounced early after initiation of therapy (Table 7-1). In

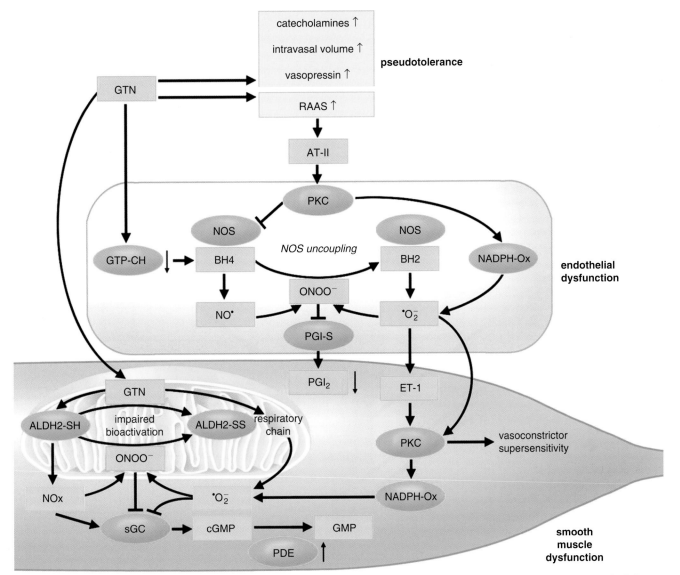

FIGURE 7-2 Molecular mechanisms of nitrate tolerance. ALDH2, aldehyde dehydrogenase; AT-II, angiotensin II; BH2, dihydrobiopterin; BH4, tetrahydrobiopterin; cGMP, cyclic guanosine monophosphate; ET-1, endothelin-1; GMP, guanosine monophosphate; GTN, glyceril trinitrate (nitroglycerin); GTP-CH, guanosine triphosphate cyclohydrolase; NOS, nitric oxide synthetase; PDE, phosphodiesterase; PGI, prostacyclin; PKC, protein kinase C; RAAS, renin-angiotensin-aldosterone system; NADPH-Ox, nicotinamide adenine dinucleotide phosphate oxidase; sGC, soluble guanylate cyclase.

some patients, the headache diminishes over a few days, but not uncommonly, the nitrate must be discontinued. Hypotension can occur with all nitrates but is more common when nitrates with a rapid onset of action are used, such as sublingual GTN or short-acting isosorbide dinitrates. Many patients experience dizziness, presyncope, or even syncope on initial exposure to sublingual GTN or initial doses of isosorbide dinitrate. Symptomatic hypotension is less common after transdermal GTN administration. In general, patients taking their first dose of nitrates should sit or lie down during administration if necessary. In the case of isosorbide dinitrate, the dose should be uptitrated over several days, starting with the 10-mg dose. Reduction in dose or a change of agent should be considered when such symptomatic hypotension occurs. Other side effects are uncommon. With transdermal GTN, some patients develop marked erythema and some local edema at the site of the application of the transdermal preparation. This likely represents a marked response to local hyperemia, but in some patients, it may represent a local allergic reaction to the preparation itself. In some this reaction is troublesome enough that the transdermal preparation must be discontinued. Although rare, methemoglobinemia has been reported after high-dose intravenous GTN therapy.[26,27]

Clinical Efficacy of Organic Nitrates

SUBLINGUAL NITRATES

Sublingual GTN represents a classic therapy for the treatment of acute attacks of angina (Table 7-2; also see Figure 7-3). Whether given as a tablet or spray, it has a rapid onset of action that offers prompt symptomatic relief. Historically, sublingual GTN was often prescribed as a prophylactic therapy, taken by the patient before activity that would generally lead to anginal symptoms. Given in this manner, it significantly increases exercise capacity, a finding that has now been confirmed in clinical trials.[28] In select patients, this can be a very effective way to improve symptoms and quality of life, when other approaches to the prevention of angina are not effective. Sublingual isosorbide dinitrate is also available. Although not commonly used, it can both treat and prevent angina in select patients.

LONG-ACTING NITRATES

A classic pharmacodynamic characteristic of the organic nitrates is the phenomenon of tolerance. It has been repeatedly demonstrated

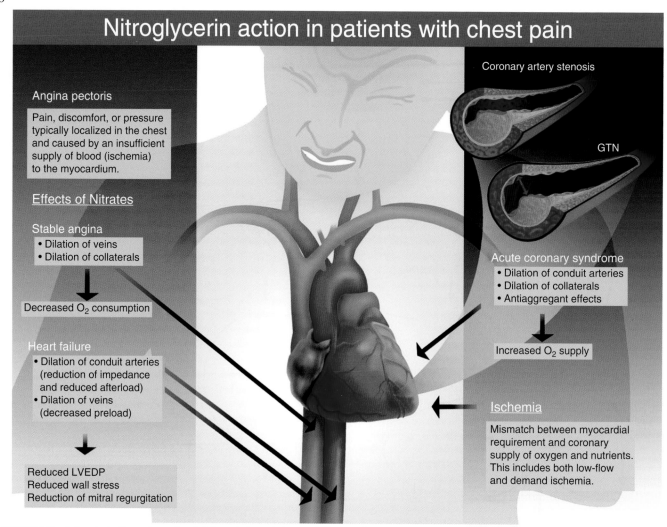

Nitroglycerin action in patients with chest pain

Coronary artery stenosis

GTN

Angina pectoris

Pain, discomfort, or pressure typically localized in the chest and caused by an insufficient supply of blood (ischemia) to the myocardium.

Effects of Nitrates

Stable angina
- Dilation of veins
- Dilation of collaterals

Decreased O₂ consumption

Acute coronary syndrome
- Dilation of conduit arteries
- Dilation of collaterals
- Antiaggregant effects

Increased O₂ supply

Heart failure
- Dilation of conduit arteries (reduction of impedance and reduced afterload)
- Dilation of veins (decreased preload)

Ischemia

Mismatch between myocardial requirement and coronary supply of oxygen and nutrients. This includes both low-flow and demand ischemia.

Reduced LVEDP
Reduced wall stress
Reduction of mitral regurgitation

FIGURE 7-3 Antianginal effects of acutely administered glyceryl trinitrate (*GTN*; nitroglycerin). LVEDP, left ventricular end-diastolic pressure.

TABLE 7-1   Nitrate Preparations, Routes of Administration, and Dosing Strategies

DRUG	ROUTE	DOSE RANGE	FREQUENCY
Treatment of Anginal Attacks			
Nitroglycerin tablets	Sublingual	0.3-0.6 mg	1-3 times
Nitroglycerin spray	Sublingual	0.4-0.8 mg	1-3 times
Nitroglycerin buccal tablets	Buccal	1-3 mg	Once
Prevention of Anginal Attacks			
Nitroglycerin tablets	Sublingual	0.3-0.6 mg	2-5 minutes before activity
Nitroglycerin spray	Sublingual	0.4-0.8 mg	
Nitroglycerin buccal tablets	Buccal	1-3 mg	2-5 minutes before activity or three times daily; tablet is removed overnight
Nitroglycerin SR	Oral	2.6-10.4 mg	Two to three times daily
Nitroglycerin patch	Transdermal	0.2-0.8 mg/h	Once daily, 12-h patch-free interval
Isosorbide dinitrate SF	Sublingual	2.5-10 mg	5-10 min before activity
Isosorbide dinitrate SF	Oral	10-45 mg	3 times daily, 14-h tablet-free interval
Isosorbide dinitrate SR	Oral	20-80 mg	Once or twice daily
Isosorbide-5-mononitrate SF	Oral	10-20 mg	Twice daily, 7 h between doses
Isosorbide-5-mononitrate SR	Oral	30-240 mg	Once daily

SF, standard formulation; SR, sustained-release formulation that provides therapeutic plasma concentrations for 12 hours.

TABLE 7-2   Side Effects of Organic Nitrates

DRUG	ROUTE	SIDE EFFECTS	COMMENTS
Nitroglycerin Isosorbide dinitrate	Sublingual	Headache Postural hypotension Syncope	Dose reduction may be required
Nitroglycerin Isosorbide dinitrate Isosorbide-5-mononitrate Erythrityl tetranitrate Pentaerythritol tetranitrate	Oral	Headache Postural hypotension Syncope Nausea	Headache and postural lightheadedness often resolve after several days of therapy Resolution of headache does not necessarily mean loss of efficacy
Nitroglycerin	Transdermal	Same as for oral nitrates Skin erythema and inflammation at site of patch application	Initiate treatment with small doses and increase as necessary Vary application site

that long-acting nitrates are effective in angina, improving exercise duration and reducing the frequency of anginal attacks if given using dosing intervals or formulations that allow for a low or nitrate-free period during the day.[29-31] Isosorbide-5-mononitrate in a phasic-release formulation that provides effective plasma concentrations during the day but low concentrations during the night is effective in the therapy of exertional angina.[32] In some countries, the organic nitrate pentaerythritol tetranitrate is also prescribed for the therapy of angina. This nitrate appears to have some unique biochemical properties that make is less susceptible to tolerance.[33-35] Unfortunately, few data are available to document its antianginal effects.

CONGESTIVE HEART FAILURE

The administration of nitrates in patients with CHF has potent and favorable hemodynamic effects. When given acutely, nitrates can dramatically lower filling pressure without adverse effects on systemic blood pressure.[36,37] In acutely ill patients with markedly elevated filling pressures, sublingual or intravenous GTN can be particularly useful. Although they have not been clearly demonstrated to improve clinical outcome, organic nitrates are generally believed to be safe and effective in the relief of symptoms in patients with acute decompensated heart failure. In patients with acute heart failure and active ischemia, organic nitrates can be the therapy of choice. They are also effective in the therapy of chronic heart failure.

Approximately 25 years ago, the combination of isosorbide dinitrate and hydralazine was the first drug regimen shown to reduce mortality rate in chronic CHF.[38] In 2004, the African-American Heart Failure trial (A-HeFT) documented a favorable effect of this drug combination in African Americans using a twice-daily dosing formulation that combined isosorbide dinitrate and hydralazine.[39] This combination is indicated therapy in African Americans with chronic heart failure as a result of systolic dysfunction, and it is useful as an adjunct therapy in other populations with chronic CHF.

OTHER NITRATE INDICATIONS

Nitrates are also useful in the management of unstable angina and acute myocardial infarction (MI). In patients with acute symptomatic ischemia, nitrates can be extremely effective. Sublingual GTN is often used, but intravenous (IV) and transdermal formulations also have a role. In this setting, beyond their effects on loading conditions, their mechanism of action likely includes their ability to dilate and prevent constriction of epicardial coronary arteries, thus improving coronary blood flow. Furthermore, the potential antiplatelet effects of GTN may play a role in this situation. The question of tolerance in this setting is controversial, although recent evidence suggests that tolerance may not develop to conduit artery dilation[40,41] and may not develop as rapidly in this situation compared with other clinical settings.

Nitrate Tolerance

When given acutely, nitrates have potent hemodynamic and therapeutic effects. As long-acting nitrates were developed for clinical use, questions arose concerning their potency. Early investigations questioned the efficacy of the oral isosorbide dinitrate, as first-pass metabolism was felt to be complete, because portal vein administration in animals had no hemodynamic effects.[42] Subsequent studies in patients with CAD refuted these findings because oral isosorbide dinitrate clearly produced significant hemodynamic and antianginal effects.[43-45] However, later investigations confirmed that the clinical effects of nitrates were lost rapidly during sustained therapy, documenting that the phenomenon of nitrate tolerance is a significant clinical problem.[44,46] Tolerance develops in response to all nitrates, although evidence suggests that it is not as prominent with pentaerythritol tetranitrate.[19] When nitrates are administered using dosing regimens that lead to significant plasma concentrations throughout a 24-hour period, their hemodynamic and symptomatic effects are almost completely lost. Tolerance develops early, within 24 hours of the initiation of therapy, and it cannot be overcome with the administration of higher doses.[47,48] This loss of therapeutic effect in the face of continued therapeutic plasma concentrations has led to more than three decades of intense investigation concerning the etiology of tolerance, a controversy that continues to this day. Shortly after the initial description of tolerance, it was recognized that nitrate effects could be maintained using dosing regimens that allowed for a nitrate-free or low-nitrate concentration for several hours each day. This observation led to the adoption of intermittent or eccentric dosing regimens that now represent the standard of care, particularly in the setting of stable exertional angina. The mechanisms of nitrate tolerance have been the subject of extensive investigation for decades. Several hypotheses have been proposed, although agreement concerning a single unifying hypothesis has never been obtained. A brief overview of approaches to this classic pharmacologic question is outlined below.

BIOTRANSFORMATION HYPOTHESIS

The observation that nitrate concentrations remained at therapeutic levels in the setting of tolerance ruled out a pharmacokinetic etiology and suggested that the loss of their effect was secondary to a decrease in their bioactivation. Although the role of nitrates as NO donors was not yet understood, it was known that nitrate effects were based on enzymatic biotransformation. Initial hypothesis concerning the etiology of nitrate tolerance suggested it was secondary to impaired biotransformation during sustained therapy. Classic investigations by Needleman et al demonstrated that nitrate biotransformation was dependent on reduced sulfhydryl groups and that depletion of these as substrate or cofactors led to loss of nitrate effects.[49] This sulfhydryl depletion hypothesis spawned a series of investigations that attempted to prevent or reverse nitrate tolerance using thiol donors such as N-acetylcysteine.[37,50] Although substantial in vitro data supported this view, the use of thiol donors to prevent nitrate tolerance was never adopted into clinical practice. In general, early investigations of reduced nitrate biotransformation as the basis of nitrate tolerance were inconclusive, hindered by the fact that the enzyme responsible for the biotransformation process had not been identified. In 2002, two decades after Needleman proposed the sulfhydryl depletion hypothesis, the importance of abnormalities of biotransformation in the setting of tolerance was confirmed by Chen and colleagues with their description of mALDH-2 as the responsible enzyme.[10] This finding has greatly improved the understanding of the phenomenon of nitrate tolerance and is closely linked to the free radical hypothesis of tolerance, which is presented in more detail below.

NEUROHORMONAL HYPOTHESIS

In the late 1980s, a number of investigators proposed the neurohormonal hypothesis, which states that the loss of nitrate effects is mediated by reflex activation of the renin-angiotensin and sympathetic nervous systems secondary to the acute effects of nitrates on loading conditions.[51,52] This hypothesis was supported by observations that nitrate therapy was associated with evidence of neurohormonal activation along with evidence of plasma volume expansion.[53] Further studies suggested that tolerance could be prevented with concurrent use of angiotensin-converting enzyme (ACE) inhibitors[54] or diuretics,[55] although other observations did not confirm these findings.[56] Overall, the neurohormonal hypothesis did not lead to a clinical solution to the problem of nitrate tolerance, but it did remind investigators that powerful vasoactive agents, such as the organic nitrates, could induce counterregulatory responses, probably at multiple levels.

FREE RADICAL HYPOTHESIS

In 1995, Münzel and colleagues reported an observation that had great impact on the field of nitrate pharmacology.[57] They demonstrated that sustained exposure to GTN was associated with increased vascular free radical production and that the endothelium was the source of these free radicals. They also documented that tolerance was reversed by exposure to the antioxidant liposomal superoxide dismutase, which restored responses to GTN and to the endothelium-dependent vasodilator acetylcholine. Based on these findings, the authors proposed the *free radical hypothesis* of nitrate tolerance, in which a nitrate-induced increase in free radical production limits nitrate responsiveness. The mechanism of the nitrate-induced free radical production has been extensively explored in both animal and human models. Multiple enzymatic sources have been suggested, including membrane-bound nicotinamide adenine dinucleotide phosphate (NADPH) oxidase, xanthine oxidase, and endothelial NO synthase itself.[19] Animal investigations have documented an important role for angiotensin II in this process.[58] Although the inciting cause was not clear, GTN therapy increased angiotensin II production, increasing NADPH production of superoxide anion. The concurrent administration of an angiotensin II receptor inhibitor prevented the increase in superoxide anion production, maintaining nitrate responsiveness.[58] This pathway deserves emphasis because it is known that hydralazine has antioxidant activity that inhibits NADPH-mediated production of superoxide anion[59] and provides a potential explanation for the beneficial effect of hydralazine in combination with isosorbide dinitrate in CHF.[38,39]

How an increase in vascular free radical production leads to a decrease in nitrate responsiveness is unclear. Possibilities include 1) abnormalities in nitrate biotransformation secondary to the oxidative state, 2) a decrease in net NO bioavailability secondary to free radical quenching of NO, and 3) free radical–induced changes in signal transduction. Discovery and investigation of the central role of mALDH-2 in GTN biotransformation provided a unifying hypothesis concerning the mechanism of nitrate biotransformation and the development of tolerance. This enzyme is essential to the bioactivity of GTN at therapeutic concentrations, but prolonged exposure to GTN is associated with oxidative inhibition of its function.[10-12,60] This oxidative inhibition of mALDH-2 activity provides a mechanism linking nitrate-induced free-radical production with inhibition of nitrate biotransformation with tolerance. What is not clear is what triggers the initial increase in reactive oxygen species. Of note, recent evidence suggests that increased superoxide formation may result directly from GTN mALDH-2 biotransformation,[61] although other potential sources have been suggested.[19]

Despite the importance of mALDH-2 as a mechanism of nitrate biotransformation and tolerance, it is clear that other mechanisms are involved. Münzel and colleagues recently summarized the complexity of this area,[19] but a full description is beyond the scope of this chapter. Important highlights include the observation that mALDH-2 does not mediate the biotransformation of isosorbide dinitrate and isosorbide-5-mononitrate.[15] These nitrates, as well as high concentrations of GTN, are biotransformed by other enzyme systems that may include glutathione-S-transferases, xanthine oxidoreductase, and CYP. Furthermore, tolerance develops in response to all nitrates, emphasizing that this phenomenon must also be more than abnormalities in mALDH-2 function. The alternative mechanisms of tolerance remain poorly defined, but it appears that a decrease in NO bioavailability from increased free radical production may be a feature common to all nitrates. Furthermore, the same increase in free radicals may lead to oxidative inhibition of other nitrate biotransformation enzymes, as well as those involved in NO signal transduction, such as guanylate cyclase. Finally, the fact that therapy with GTN causes abnormalities in endothelial NO synthase function is noteworthy, emphasizing the potential of organic nitrates to have quite unexpected biologic effects.[62,63] In normal volunteers, transdermal GTN causes abnormalities in NO synthase function, markedly inhibiting their responses to the NO synthase inhibitor L-NMMA.[64] This response appears to be secondary to reduction of tetrahydrobiopterin, which is oxidized by GTN-induced increases in peroxynitrite. This in turn leads to the phenomenon of NO synthase uncoupling, with the result that this enzyme yields superoxide anion rather than NO. The resulting increase in superoxide leads to further dysfunction of NO synthase in a positive feedback mechanism.[20,21]

Nonhemodynamic Effects of Organic Nitrates

A number of studies have documented that the organic nitrates can inhibit platelet aggregation. Platelets produce NO, which acts to inhibit granule release and aggregation. GTN has been shown to inhibit platelet aggregation both in vitro and in a number of human experiments.[65-67] Whether tolerance develops to this antiplatelet effect is controversial, and in general, the clinical relevance of this effect is unclear; however, it has been postulated that this effect may be particularly important in the setting of acute coronary syndromes (ACS), although the efficacy of GTNs in this situation remains only hypothetical.[68]

Another impact of the organic nitrates unrelated to their hemodynamic effects is their ability to precondition. GTN has been shown to have important preconditioning effects in a number of animal models.[69-71] In humans, short-term exposure to a GTN leads to decreased evidence of ischemia during percutaneous coronary intervention (PCI)[72,73] and in the setting of exercise-induced ischemia. Human models have documented that development of the preconditioned phenotype is inhibited by the administration of an antioxidant during exposure to GTN.[74,75] Little information is available concerning the ability of other organic nitrates to precondition, but one human study found that protection from ischemia and reperfusion was not found after administration of isosorbide-5-mononitrate.[74]

The observation that mALDH-2 plays a critical role in the development of ischemic preconditioning draws an interesting link between the biotransformation of GTN, the subsequent increase in free radical bioavailability, and the preconditioning phenotype.[76] To date, this capacity of the GTN to precondition has not found any meaningful clinical application. Of note, a recent report on normal volunteers suggested that the acute preconditioning effects of a single short-term exposure (2 hours) to transdermal GTN were lost during sustained daily exposure to GTN, suggesting that tolerance develops to the preconditioning effect.[77]

As the importance of NO bioavailability in CV disease became clear, it was believed that NO donors, such as the organic nitrates, would have a beneficial effect as supplemental sources of NO. Although this benefit remained a matter of conjecture, it was never believed that organic nitrates could have adverse effects on vascular function. Given this background, the demonstration that animals exposed to GTN developed significant abnormalities of endothelial function was unexpected.[57] GTN has long been considered a non–endothelium-dependent vasodilator with actions confined to vascular smooth muscle cells. Nevertheless, these observations in animals were followed by human experiments, which confirmed that sustained nitrate exposure causes significant and surprising abnormalities of vascular function. In patients with CAD, 48 hours of intravenous GTN increased the sensitivity of the arterial resistance vessels to angiotensin II and phenylephrine.[78] Further studies revealed that continuous GTN therapy also caused important abnormalities in endothelial function in normal volunteers[64] and worsened endothelial function in those with CAD.[79] Similar abnormalities of vascular function have also been documented during both intermittent transdermal[80] GTN and once-daily administration of isosorbide-5-mononitrate.[81]

The importance of NO biology in the function of the sympathetic nervous system has been recognized.[82] Nitric oxide and NO donors have been shown to have inhibitory effects on sympathetic outflow at multiple sites, both peripheral and central.[83-87] When given acutely, the pronounced hemodynamic effects of these drugs causes reflex stimulation of the sympathetic nervous system, which complicates experimental observations in this area. Animal observations suggest that sustained nitrate therapy might be associated with an increase in sympathetic outflow.[88] Interestingly, in a human model, continuous transdermal GTN caused a reduction in tonic and reflex modulation of heart rate, leading to a relatively greater sympathetic influence.[89] The overall effect was a blunting of spontaneous baroreflex function, an abnormality usually associated with specific CV diseases. The clinical implications of this are not clear but are an example of a "nitrate effect" associated with abnormalities that generally are believed to have a negative effect on prognosis.

Current Perspectives on Therapy with Organic Nitrates

Despite approximately 150 years of clinical use, many biologic effects of the organic nitrates remain poorly understood. Given the current state of knowledge, it appears that these drugs can have both beneficial and potentially harmful effects, depending on how they are prescribed and for what indication. The understanding of the potential for harm is limited, but it warrants both attention and further study.

In terms of benefits, the effectiveness of organic nitrates in the relief of episodes of angina is unquestioned. Although their use in ACS and acute decompensated heart failure has not been evaluated in large-scale clinical trials, their utility is these settings is widely accepted. They are effective in the treatment of chronic angina, although the development of tolerance is a limitation, and their impact in long-term clinical outcome has never been tested in this population. The clear beneficial role of nitrates in combination with hydralazine in the treatment of chronic CHF was previously discussed. Of note, it has yet to be documented that a nitrate alone can benefit long-term outcome in this patient population. It is now known the GTN has preconditioning effects that limit the

adverse effects of ischemia and reperfusion; however, as with other preconditioning approaches, a clearly beneficial application of this biologic effect of nitrates has yet to be defined.

With respect to adverse effects, the finding that sustained nitrate therapy is associated with increased free radical production and evidence of endothelial dysfunction suggests the possibility that these drugs could have harmful effects during chronic therapy. Although these nitrate-induced abnormalities in vascular function have been documented for more than a decade, they have not yet modified the clinical utilization of nitrate therapy. The clinical implications of these findings are unclear, serving to highlight the paucity of clinical data available with respect to clinical outcome during sustained administration with nitrates. Nitrates have been tested in relatively large numbers of patients in the early postinfarction period[90,91]; however, the treatment and follow-up periods of these trials were too short to examine the question of safety. Of note, two retrospective analyses of post-MI patients have suggested that long-acting nitrate therapy is associated with an increased mortality rate. Although studies in heart failure (discussed above) have documented a beneficial effect of isosorbide-5-mononitrate when given in combination with hydralazine, the safety and efficacy of a nitrate alone in the setting of chronic heart failure has never been examined. Although it is unclear whether clinical outcome studies will ever be completed, it can be stated that there should be no assumption of clinical safety when these drugs are used as long-term therapy.

It is also important to recall that almost all available information concerning the development of tolerance and/or endothelial dysfunction during nitrate therapy was obtained in normal volunteers or patients not taking other cardiac medications. Of note are both animal and human studies in which tolerance is prevented by concurrent therapy with 3-hydroxy-3-methylglutaryl coenzyme A (HMG Co-A) reductase inhibitors as well as agents that inhibit the renin-angiotensin system.[54,92,93] In the absence of concurrent therapy with either of these classes of medications, studies were carried out in patients with stable angina; these represent the classic human model of tolerance to the symptomatic benefit of nitrates. A recent study in humans demonstrated that atorvastatin given concomitantly with continuous GTN completely prevented the development of both tolerance and abnormalities of endothelial dysfunction during sustained therapy.[94] Given this background, it can be said that some historic models of nitrate tolerance should be revisited in the current era of pharmacotherapy.

Calcium Channel Blockers

Calcium channel blockers (CCBs) are agents that inhibit several specific calcium-dependent functions in the cardiovascular system. By decreasing vascular smooth muscle contraction and tone they produce peripheral and coronary vasodilation. The non-DHPs (NDHPs) have a negative inotropic effect, which is an undesired action if it becomes excessive. Certain CCBs (e.g., verapamil, diltiazem) inhibit calcium-dependent sinoatrial (SA) and atrioventricular (AV) nodal conduction. The CCBs are approved for use in hypertension, angina pectoris, and acute supraventricular tachycardias. In the United States, the most commonly used available CCBs are diltiazem, verapamil, nifedipine, amlodipine, and felodipine. Bepridil, isradipine, and nicardipine are available but are used relatively infrequently; nimodipine is usually used only for subarachnoid hemorrhage or ruptured cerebral aneurysm.

Fundamental Mechanisms of Calcium Channel Blockers

CALCIUM CHANNEL AS SITE OF ACTION

CCBs interfere with the entry of Ca^{2+} into cells through voltage-dependent L- and T-type calcium channels.[95] The major cardiovascular sites of action are 1) vascular smooth muscle cells, 2) cardiac myocytes, and 3) SA and AV nodal cells. By binding to

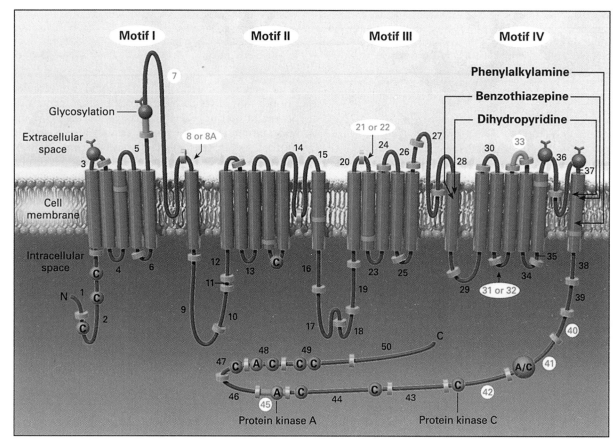

FIGURE 7-4 Proposed arrangement of the polypeptide chain of the channel forming a 12 subunit of the L-type calcium channel in humans. Four motifs—I, II, III, and IV—are repetitive, and each consists of six putative transmembrane segments. Both the N terminal and the C terminal point to the cytoplasm. Rings separate the segments encoded by numbered exons. The transmembrane segments encoded by alternative exons 8 or 8A, 21, or 22, and 31 or 32 are shown. Sequences encoded by invariant exons 7, 33, and 45, which are subject to constitutive splicing, are also shown. Exons 40, 41, and 42 are subject to alternative splicing. Putative sites of glycosylation and of phosphorylation involving protein kinase C (C) and protein kinase A (A) are shown, as are the discrete binding areas of the three types of calcium antagonists—phenylalkylamine (verapamil-like), benzothiazepine (diltiazem-like), and dihydropyridine (nifedipine-like). *(From Abernethy DR, Schwartz JB. Calcium-antagonist drugs.* N Engl J Med *1999;341:1448.)*

specific sites in the proteins of the calcium channel known as *subunits*, these agents are able to diminish the degree to which the calcium channel pores open in response to voltage depolarization (Figure 7-4).

Molecular Structure

The calcium channel consists of four high-molecular-weight subunits: $\alpha1, \alpha2, \beta$, and γ. Of these, the $\alpha1$ subunit contains the calcium channel pores and the binding sites for CCBs. The subunits have a complex structure with four major domains (see Figure 7-4), each with six transmembrane units.[96] The calcium channel pores exist between the fifth and sixth units, and the voltage sensor is located near the fourth transmembrane unit of each domain.

Two regulatory aspects of calcium channel blockade are important. First, when cyclic adenosine monophosphate (cAMP) activates protein kinase A to phosphorylate the calcium channel, a number of phosphorylation sites are available on the COOH-terminal portion of each of the $\alpha1$ subunits. Such phosphorylation allows the channel to persist in a more open state. Second, the β subunit binds to the cytoplasmic link between domains I and II of the $\gamma1$ subunit and thereby enhances calcium channel opening.[95]

Drug Binding Sites

At least three binding sites exist for these drugs, commonly identified by the prototype agents verapamil, nifedipine, and diltiazem, respectively; these are known as the *V-*, or *phenylalkylamine-*; *N-*, or *DHP-*; and *D-*, or *benzothiazepine-*, binding sites. The N-binding site is also termed the *DHP site*, to which all DHPs are thought to bind. Each of the different agents binds to specified sites on various

domains, and none binds to all of the pores in all of the domains. Thus, calcium channel blockade can never be complete.

Calcium Channels: L and T Types

The most important property of the CCBs is to selectively inhibit the inward flow of charge-bearing Ca^{2+} when the calcium channel becomes permeable, or "open." At least two types of calcium channels are relevant to the treatment of CV disorders: the L and T types. The major calcium channel related to pharmacologic antagonism, the voltage-gated L-type (long-acting, slowly activating) channel, is blocked by all available CCBs. The function of the L-type channel is to allow entry of sufficient Ca^{2+} for initiation of contraction by calcium-induced intracellular calcium release from the sarcoplasmic reticulum.

The T-type (transient) channel appears at more negative potentials than the L type and probably plays an important role in the initial depolarization of SA and AV nodal tissue. The L-type calcium channel is found in vascular smooth muscle, in nonvascular smooth muscle in many tissues, and in a number of noncontractile tissues. Blockade of the L-type channel is responsible for the pharmacologic actions of the available CCBs.

Pharmacologic Properties of Calcium Channel Blockers

PHARMACODYNAMIC EFFECTS

Despite their structural diversity and binding differences, CCBs display many common important pharmacologic actions; however,

TABLE 7-3 Vasodilator Potency and Inotropic, Chronotropic, and Dromotropic Effects of Calcium Channel Blockers

	AMLODIPINE	DILTIAZEM	NIFEDIPINE	VERAPAMIL
Heart rate	↑/–	↓	↓	↓
Sinoatrial node conduction	–	↓	–	↓
Atrioventricular node conduction	–	↓	–	↓
Myocardial contractility	↓/–	↓	↓/–	↓↓
Neurohormonal activation	↑/–	↑	↑	↑
Vascular dilation	↑↑	↑	↑↑	↑
Coronary flow	↑	↑	↑	↑

↓, decrease; –, no change; ↑, increase
Modified from Abernethy DR. Pharmacologic and pharmacokinetic profile of mibefradil, a T- and L-type calcium channel antagonist. *Am J Cardiol* 1997;80:4c-11c.

there are significant differences between the sites of action of the DHPs and NDHPs (Table 7-3).

MAJOR CARDIOVASCULAR ACTIONS OF CALCIUM CHANNEL BLOCKERS

1. *Vasodilation* is more marked in arterial and arteriolar vessels than on veins and includes the coronary vasculature; veins do not appreciably dilate with CCBs.
2. *Negative chronotropic and dromotropic effects* are seen on the SA and AV nodal conducting tissue (NDHP agents only).
3. *Negative inotropic effects* are seen on myocardial cells; in the case of DHPs, this effect may be offset by reflex adrenergic stimulation after peripheral vasodilation.

Classification of Calcium Channel Blockers

The differing pharmacodynamic effects of various CCBs accounts for their classification. All the DHPs bind to the same sites on the α1 subunit and exert a greater Ca^{2+} inhibitory effect on vascular smooth muscle than on the myocardium, which explains their common property of vascular selectivity; thus their major hemodynamic and therapeutic effect is peripheral and coronary vasodilation.

Nifedipine is the prototypical DHP. The fast-acting capsular form produces rapid vasodilation, alleviates hypertension, and terminates attacks of coronary spasm. However, the brisk peripheral vasodilation produced by this formulation may result in significant hypotension and reflex adrenergic activation that often causes tachycardia and stimulation of the sympathetic and renin-angiotensin systems. The introduction of truly long-acting DHP compounds—such as amlodipine or sustained-release formulations of nifedipine, felodipine, or isradipine—has resulted in substantially fewer symptoms from the vasodilatory side effects. It is a commonly held belief that the short-acting DHPs, particularly nifedipine, account for the majority of presumed negative or adverse clinical results in many older trials.[95,97] The second-generation DHPs are distinguished by a longer half-life, as in the case of amlodipine, or by a greater vascular selectivity.

Although each binds to a different site on the α1 subunit, the NDHPs verapamil and diltiazem have many properties in common. Both act on nodal (SA and AV) tissue and are therapeutically effective in supraventricular tachycardias. Both decrease the sinus discharge rate. These drugs inhibit myocardial contractility more than the DHPs; in effect, they are less vascularly selective. Both verapamil and diltiazem have greater effects on the AV node than on the SA node, and the explanation for this may relate to frequency dependence; thus there is better access to the binding sites when the calcium channel pore is open. During supraventricular tachycardia, the calcium channel of the AV node opens more frequently, so the CCB binds more avidly, hence it more specifically inhibits the AV node to interrupt the reentry circuit.

Regarding side effects, because NDHPs are less active on vascular smooth muscle, they produce fewer vasodilatory adverse reactions than the DHPs. Sinus tachycardia is uncommon, in part because of the inhibitory effects on the SA node. High-degree AV block is a risk with preexisting AV nodal disease or during cotherapy with other AV node–depressant drugs, such as β-blockers. NDHPs have a more marked depressive effect on ventricular function than DHPs. In addition, constipation occurs as a side effect with verapamil but seldom with diltiazem, although the latter may cause peripheral edema.

Vascular Selectivity

The cellular mechanism of vascular smooth muscle contraction differs from that of the myocardium. Although smooth muscle contraction is ultimately calcium dependent, it is the myosin light-chain kinase that is activated by calcium calmodulin. In the human myocardium, Godfraind and associates[98] proposed that the ratios of vasodilation to negative inotropy for the prototype CCBs were 10:1 for nifedipine, 1:1 for diltiazem, and 1:1 for verapamil. Other DHP compounds have even greater vascular selectivity, up to 1000:1. In terms of clinical use, these observations provide the basis for considering a clinical division of the CCBs into two groups: *DHPs*, which include nifedipine and its analogs, and *NDHPs*, such as verapamil, diltiazem, and their derivatives.

Noncardiovascular Effects

Although highly active on vascular smooth muscle, CCBs have little or no effect on other smooth muscle throughout the body, such as that of the bronchi, gut, or genitourinary tract. These agents may relax uterine smooth muscle and have been used in therapy for preterm contractions, although it is generally recommended that they be stopped before delivery. This action probably reflects variations between tissues in either the structure or function of their calcium channels. Also crucial to the therapeutic applicability of CCBs is the fact that skeletal muscle does not respond to conventional CCBs. As a result, skeletal muscle weakness is not a side effect of calcium channel blockade. In skeletal muscle, depolarization-activated calcium release from the sarcoplasmic reticulum is the principal source of the myoplasmic calcium rise. Thus only the myocardium, not skeletal muscle, responds to calcium entry through the voltage-dependent calcium channels; and the myocardium, not skeletal muscle, has its rise in contractile calcium inhibited by CCBs.

Pharmacokinetics

From the point of view of drug interactions, all of the CCBs are metabolized in the liver by an enzyme system that is inhibited by cimetidine, azole antifungals, and hepatic dysfunction; CCBs are increased in activity by phenytoin and phenobarbital.

Major Indications for Calcium Channel Blockers

SYSTEMIC HYPERTENSION

The various CCBs act on peripheral arterioles. They are effective antihypertensive agents in all ethnicities and age groups. All DHPs decrease peripheral vascular resistance and appear to have an additional ill-understood diuretic effect. Verapamil and diltiazem are less powerful vasodilators, and some believe that their negative inotropic effect may contribute to their antihypertensive mechanism. Table 7-4 lists some major hypertension trials that used CCBs.

ANGINA PECTORIS

Although the antianginal mechanisms of the different types of CCBs differ somewhat, these drugs share some properties, including 1) coronary vasodilation, especially in relation to exercise-induced coronary constriction, and 2) afterload reduction as a result of decreased blood pressure. In the case of verapamil and diltiazem, it is possible that slowing of the sinus node, with a decrease in nonmaximal exercise heart rate and the negative inotropic effect, may contribute to decreased myocardial work.

As coronary dilators, the CCBs have a site of action on the coronary tree different from that of the nitrates. The CCBs act more specifically on the smaller coronary resistance vessels, where the tone is higher, and the calcium inhibitory effect is more marked. CCBs are particularly effective in those types of angina caused by or exacerbated by coronary spasm or constriction, such as Prinzmetal angina or cold-induced angina. An overview of a large number of angina drug trials concluded that the CCBs have a very similar clinical efficacy to β-blockers.[99]

SUPRAVENTRICULAR TACHYCARDIA

Through their inhibitory effect on the AV node, verapamil and diltiazem interrupt the reentry circuit in supraventricular tachycardias and are useful in terminating those arrhythmias. They are also effective in slowing the ventricular response in atrial fibrillation (AF) and may be used in chronic AF; the DHPs are ineffective for these arrhythmias because of minimal effects on the SA and AV nodes.

POSTINFARCT PROTECTION

Verapamil is licensed in Scandinavian countries for postinfarct protection for patients in whom β-blockers are contraindicated. In the Danish Verapamil Infarction Trials (DAVIT-1 and DAVIT-2), a modest protective benefit against death and cardiac ischemic events in post-MI subjects was documented in subjects without a history of heart failure.[100] Diltiazem has been shown to be beneficial in post-MI subjects with relatively normal left ventricular (LV) function and no heart failure.[101] A short-term (2-week) study in non–Q-wave MI patients with high-dose diltiazem reduced the rates of recurrent ischemia and infarction.[101]

Specific Calcium Channel Blockers

VERAPAMIL

After peripheral vasodilation induced by verapamil, the cardiac output and LV ejection fraction do not increase as much as they do with the DHPs, probably owing to the negative inotropic effect and depression of contractility of verapamil.

Pharmacokinetics

The elimination half-life of standard verapamil tablets is usually 3 to 7 hours, but it increases significantly during long-term administration and in patients with liver or renal insufficiency. In significant hepatic dysfunction, the dose of verapamil should be decreased by 50% to 75%. In significant renal dysfunction, such as a creatinine clearance of less than 30 mL/min, the dose should be reduced by 50%. Bioavailability is only 10% to 20% (high first-pass liver metabolism). The parent compound and the active hepatic metabolite, norverapamil, are excreted 75% by the kidneys and 25% by the gastrointestinal (GI) tract. Verapamil is 87% to 93% protein bound.

TABLE 7-4	Selected Characteristics of Trials of Calcium Channel Blockers		
STUDY	**AGENTS USED**	**PATIENTS ENROLLED**	**PATIENT CHARACTERISTICS**
ALLHAT	Amlodipine vs. chlorthalidone vs. lisinopril	33,357	Hypertension and one risk factor for coronary artery disease
INVEST	Verapamil slow-release ± trandolapril ± hydrochlorothiazide vs. atenolol ± hydrochlorothiazide ± trandolapril	22,576	Hypertension and coronary artery disease
CONVINCE	Extended-release verapamil vs. atenolol or hydrochlorothiazide	16,602	Hypertension and one risk factor for coronary artery disease
NORDIL	Diltiazem vs. diuretics + β-blockers	10,881	Hypertension
STOP-2	Felodipine or isradipine vs. conventional antihypertensive agents	6614	Hypertension
INSIGHT	Nifedipine gastrointestinal therapeutic system vs. hydrochlorothiazide + amiloride	6321	Hypertension and one risk factor for coronary artery disease
VHAS	Verapamil vs. chlorothiazide	1414	Hypertension
MIDAS	Isradipine vs. hydrochlorothiazide	883	Hypertension
ABCD	Nisoldipine vs. enalapril	470	Hypertension and diabetes mellitus
NICS-EH	Nicardipine vs. trichloromethiazide	429	Hypertension and age >60 years
FACET	Amlodipine vs. fosinopril	380	Hypertension and diabetes mellitus
CASTEL	Nifedipine vs. clonidine or atenolol + chlorthalidone	351	Hypertension and age >65 years

ABCD, Appropriate Blood Pressure Control in Diabetes; ALLHAT, Antihypertensive and Lipid-Lowering Treatment to Prevent Heart Attack trial; CASTEL, Cardiovascular Study in the Elderly; CONVINCE, Controlled Onset Verapamil Investigation of Cardiovascular Endpoints; FACET, Fosinopril versus Amlodipine Cardiovascular Events Trial; INSIGHT, International Nifedipine Gastrointestinal Therapeutic System Study–Intervention as a Goal in Hypertension Treatment; INVEST, International Verapamil Slow-Release/Trandolapril Study; MIDAS, Multicenter Isradipine Diuretic Atherosclerosis Study; NICS-EH, National Intervention Cooperative Study in Elderly Hypertensives; NORDIL, Nordic Diltiazem; STOP, Swedish Trial in Old Patients with Hypertension; VHAS, Verapamil in Hypertension and Atherosclerosis Study.

Modified from Eisenberg MJ, Brox A, Bestauwros AN. Calcium channel blockers: an update. *Am J Med* 2004;116:35-43.

Dose
ORAL PREPARATIONS

The usual dosage of the standard preparation is 80 to 120 mg three times daily. During long-term oral dosing, less frequent daily doses are needed (norverapamil metabolites). Slow-release preparations (240 to 480 mg/day) are available and are the usual regimen.

INTRAVENOUS USE

For supraventricular reentry tachycardias, a bolus of 5 to 10 mg (0.1 to 0.15 mg/kg) can be administered over 2 minutes and repeated 15 to 20 minutes later if needed. After successful administration, the dose may be stopped or continued at 0.005 mg/kg/min for approximately 30 to 60 minutes, decreasing thereafter. When used for control of the ventricular rate in AF, verapamil may be administered at 0.005 mg/kg/min, increasing as needed, or as an IV bolus of 5 mg, followed by a second bolus of 10 mg if needed. In the presence of myocardial disease or interacting drugs, a very low dosage (0.0001 mg/kg/min) may be infused and titrated upward against the ventricular response. However, safer AV-slowing agents, such as digoxin and adenosine, are available for patients with impaired LV systolic function.

Side Effects

Side effects include headaches, facial flushing, dizziness, and ankle edema—all lower in frequency than with DHPs. Constipation occurs in up to one third of patients who receive verapamil, and the negative inotropic effect of verapamil may precipitate or exacerbate CHF. When IV verapamil is used, the risk of hypotension is increased if the patient is receiving β-blockers or other vasodilators or has depressed cardiac function.

Contraindications

Sick sinus syndrome and preexisting AV nodal disease are relative contraindications to IV and oral verapamil. The effective use of oral verapamil preparations in these conditions may require a pacemaker. In Wolff-Parkinson-White syndrome with AF, IV verapamil may promote antegrade conduction of impulses down the bypass tract, with a risk of very rapid AF and even ventricular fibrillation. In a wide–QRS complex ventricular tachycardia, verapamil is contraindicated because the combined negative inotropic and peripheral vasodilatory effects can be fatal. Furthermore, verapamil is unlikely to terminate a ventricular arrhythmia and should not be used in the setting of moderate or severe LV dysfunction or severe hypotension.

PREGNANCY

Category C specifies use only if potential benefit justifies the potential risk to fetus; no well-controlled trials are available.

DILTIAZEM

Diltiazem is used for the same spectrum of CV disease as verapamil: hypertension, angina pectoris, prevention of AV nodal reentry, tachycardia, and rate control in acute and chronic AF. The side-effect profile is similar, except that constipation is much less common.

Pharmacokinetics

More than 90% of oral diltiazem is absorbed, with approximately 45% bioavailability (first-pass hepatic metabolism). The onset of action is within 15 to 30 minutes, and peak effects occur at 1 to 2 hours. The elimination half-life is 4 to 7 hours, and protein binding is 80% to 90%. Diltiazem is acetylated in the liver to the active metabolite desacetyl diltiazem (40% of the activity of the parent compound), which accumulates during long-term therapy. Only 35% of diltiazem is excreted by the kidneys; the rest is excreted by the GI tract.

Dose

The standard oral dose of short-acting diltiazem is 120 to 360 mg daily in three or four divided daily doses. The slow-release preparations are administered once or twice daily. IV diltiazem (approved for arrhythmias) is administered as 0.25 mg/kg over 2 minutes with electrocardiographic (ECG) and blood pressure monitoring; if the response is inadequate, the dose is repeated as 0.35 mg/kg in 15 to 20 minutes. Acute loading therapy may be followed by an infusion of 5 to 15 mg/h.

Side Effects

Side effects are few and are limited to headaches, dizziness, and ankle edema in 6% to 10% of patients. The extended or slow-release preparations appear to have a side-effect profile similar to that of placebo. Sinus bradycardia and first-degree or higher AV nodal block may be produced by diltiazem. It is important to avoid or reduce dosing in subjects with SA or AV nodal disease. In heart failure with significant LV dysfunction (e.g., ejection fraction <35%), this drug can be hazardous. Exfoliative dermatitis and skin rash occasionally occur, and the side effects of IV diltiazem resemble those of IV verapamil.

Contraindications

Contraindications are similar to those of verapamil: preexisting depression of the SA or AV node, hypotension, low ejection fraction, heart failure, and AF associated with Wolff-Parkinson-White syndrome. LV failure ejection fraction of less than 40% after MI is a clear contraindication.[99]

PREGNANCY

Category C specifies use only if potential benefit justifies the potential risk to the fetus; no well-controlled trials are available.

DIHYDROPYRIDINES

The major therapeutic action of the DHPs is arterial and arteriolar dilation, which is responsible for their efficacy in hypertension and angina pectoris as well as in Prinzmetal or variant angina and Raynaud phenomenon. Direct negative inotropic effects of DHPs are minimal. Amlodipine is the CCB of choice in patients with severely depressed LV function, because it does not decrease LV contractility at standard doses. No clinically significant evidence is available showing the effect of DHP on either the SA or the AV node; these agents are not effective in supraventricular arrhythmias; however, they may be more readily combined with β-blockers in hypertension or angina pectoris than the rate-slowing CCBs, with less concern about depression of the SA and AV nodes.

First-Generation Dihydropyridines

Oral nifedipine is the prototypical DHP. It is rapidly absorbed with peak blood levels in 20 to 45 minutes and a duration of action of 4 to 8 hours. Because of its short half-life and difficulty controlling the degree of blood pressure lowering, it is rarely used in its short-acting form. Slow-release forms are currently available and are preferred by most physicians. The dose for the slow-release form is 30 to 90 mg once a day.

Contraindications and Cautions

The short-acting forms are generally contraindicated because of their rapid hypotensive effect in some patients.

Side Effects

Because DHPs have no SA or AV effects, reflex tachycardia may occur if excessive blood pressure lowering occurs. Headache can occur with any of the CCBs, but they occur more frequently with the first-generation DHPs.

PREGNANCY

Category C specifies use only if potential benefit justifies the potential risk to the fetus; no well-controlled trials are available.

SECOND-GENERATION CALCIUM CHANNEL BLOCKERS

Theoretically, the more vascular-selective DHPs—such as felodipine, isradipine, amlodipine, and nicardipine—should be safer than nifedipine in the management of angina or hypertension, particularly when LV function is impaired. These drugs may produce adverse effects in patients with CHF, although felodipine and amlodipine appear to be quite safe in patients with depressed LV function.[102,103] In fact, amlodipine has been shown to have no adverse effect and no benefit compared with placebo in the Prospective Randomized Amlodipine Survival Evaluation (PRAISE) and PRAISE-2 heart failure trials. These compounds are the DHPs of choice in subjects with decreased LV function or a history of heart failure, and they are also popular because of their once-daily dosing schedule.

Although amlodipine is no more vascularly selective than nifedipine, it has unusual pharmacokinetics, including slow onset and offset of binding to the calcium channel site and a prolonged elimination half-life.[104] Based on these pharmacokinetic characteristics and new extensive experience with this agent in both angina and antihypertensive studies, amlodipine has become the DHP of choice for most physicians in the Western Hemisphere.

Drug Interactions of Calcium Channel Blockers

β-BLOCKERS

Verapamil and diltiazem contribute to SA or AV nodal and myocardial depression; in addition, they may interact via hepatic mechanisms with β-blockers metabolized by the liver, such as propranolol and metoprolol. Although these drugs have been successfully combined with β-blockade in the therapy of angina and hypertension, clinicians should monitor patients for possible serious adverse effects when a rate-slowing CCB is combined with a β-blocker.

DIGOXIN

Verapamil increases blood digoxin levels by decreasing the renal excretion of digoxin. Enhancement of AV nodal block can be serious and even fatal when IV verapamil is administered to patients with digitalis intoxication.

DILTIAZEM

In general, drug interactions with diltiazem are similar to those of verapamil, but diltiazem has a slight or negligible effect on blood digoxin levels. Although it may be cautiously combined with β-blockade, the combination appears to be no more effective in some studies than high-dose diltiazem alone. Cimetidine may increase diltiazem bioavailability and result in a 50% to 60% increase in plasma diltiazem levels.

DIHYDROPYRIDINES

The combination of DHPs with β-blockers is safer than that with NDHP CCBs. When LV depression is present, the added negative inotropic effects of a β-blocker and DHP may precipitate overt heart failure, but this is unusual; amlodipine or felodipine is the CCB of choice in such individuals.

Calcium Channel Blockers: The "Safety" Controversy

Beginning in 1995, a question about the safety of all CCBs was raised when a retrospective analysis of the short-acting form of nifedipine appeared to increase heart attacks in ACS patients, but the data were grouped with all CCBs. As prospective trials did not confirm these fears, and as physicians gained experience with the slow-release NDHPs and long-acting DHPs such as amlodipine, this issue gradually died. In fact, several antihypertensive trials have established the safety and benefit of these agents.[95,97]

There has been a burst of data on the use of CCBs in the past decade, which offers important and reassuring safety data regarding CCB use in patients with ischemic heart disease. The Antihypertensive and Lipid-Lowering Treatment to Prevent Heart Attack Trial (ALLHAT) was a study of 33,357 patients aged older than 55 years with hypertension and at least one other common heart disease risk factor. The patients were randomized to one of four antihypertensive regimens: chlorthalidone, a diuretic; doxasin, an α-blocker; amlodipine, a CCB; and lisinopril, an ACE inhibitor.[105] The doxasin arm was terminated early because of an increased CV risk; however, no differences were evident in the diuretic, CCB, or ACE-inhibitor arms in terms of the primary outcome of combined fatal CHD and nonfatal MI or all-cause mortality.

A second trial, the Valsartan Antihypertensive Long-term Use Evaluating (VALUE) trial, was designed specifically to test the hypothesis that the angiotensin receptor blocker valsartan would be superior to amlodipine for the same blood pressure (BP) control.[106] A total of 15,245 patients older than 50 years were followed for a mean of 4.2 years, until 1450 events had accumulated.[107] BP was reduced by both treatments, but the amlodipine-based therapies were more effective in BP control, particularly early in the study, achieving 4.0/2.1 mm Hg lower pressure compared with the valsartan group at 1 month, and achieving 1.5/1.3 mm Hg lower pressure at 1 year. Most importantly, no evidence of harm was found in the patient population, and a nonstatistically significant slightly lower overall event rate occurred in the amlodipine group: 810 patients in the valsartan group (25.5 per 1000 patient-years) and 789 in the amlodipine group (24.7 per 1000 patient-years). In addition, of the secondary outcomes, MI occurred more frequently ($P = .02$) in the valsartan group compared with the amlodipine group (Figure 7-5). The authors hypothesized that the lower BPs in the calcium channel group may explain the lack of superiority of the angiotensin receptor blocker, but it seems unlikely that it could also explain the statistically significantly lower infarction rate.

The Comparison of Amlodipine Versus Enlapril to Limit Occurrences of Thrombosis (CAMELOT) trial randomized 1992 patients with angiographically proven CAD who were *normotensive* at baseline (mean BP, 129/78 mm Hg for both arms) to amlodipine or enalapril versus placebo.[108] The incidence of CV events was 23% in the placebo arm, 20% with enalapril, and 17% with amlodipine, with similar BP results in the two active treatment arms that were significantly lower than the placebo; this reduction was driven solely by coronary revascularization and angina, not hard endpoints, although a nonsignificant trend was observed toward benefit in hard CV endpoints for both treatment arms compared with placebo. Importantly, given data from Action to Control Cardiovascular Risk in Diabetes (ACCORD)—which suggests that aggressive therapy in high-risk diabetic patients to a systolic BP less than 120 mm Hg may not be beneficial compared with a goal of less than 140 mm Hg[109]—the mean systolic BP after therapy dropped by only 4.5 mm Hg, meaning that BPs in the treatment arm were still higher than the goal in the ACCORD trial.

As is commonly found in clinical practice, combination therapy to reach target BP is often required, which limits the generalizability of prior trials that tested single-agent regimens. More recent trials have attempted to address this concern by comparing predefined combination therapies. One of these trials to assess the prevention of CV events with an antihypertensive regimen of amlodipine, adding perindopril as required, versus atenolol, adding bendroflumethiazide as required, was the Anglo-Scandinavian Cardiac Outcomes Trial–Blood Pressure Lowering Arm (ASCOT-BPLA). It examined of the efficacy of CCBs or β-blockers as first-line therapy, in combination with a renin-angiotensin-aldosterone system (RAAS) inhibitor, versus diuretic in 19,257 patients with hypertension who were 40 to 79 years old and at high CV risk.[110] The primary outcome was a combined endpoint of fatal coronary events and nonfatal MI. In the CCB arm, 39% of patients were concomitantly on an RAAS inhibitor, and in the β-blocker arm, 49% were concomitantly on a diuretic. The trial was stopped early because of increased CV events in the β-blocker arm. Patients in the CCB arm had fewer CV events (27.4 vs. 32.8 per 1000 patient-years; relative risk [RR], 0.84), a lower all-cause mortality (13.9% vs.

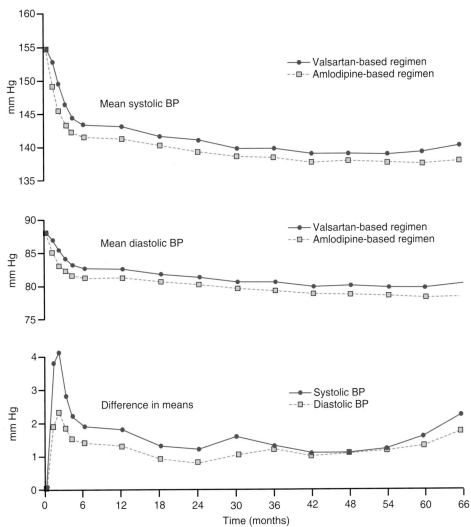

FIGURE 7-5 Systolic and diastolic blood pressure (*BP*) and differences (valsartan and amlodipine) in BP between treatment groups during follow-up. BP difference between the two groups in the Valsartan Antihypertensive Long-Term Use Evaluating (VALUE) trial was significant (*P* < .0001) at every time point, favoring the amlodipine-based regimen. Overall differences in systolic BP were 2.23 mm Hg (standard error, 0.18); overall differences in diastolic BP were 1.59 mm Hg (standard error, 0.11). (*Modified from Julius S, Kjeldsen V, Weber M, et al, for the VALUE trial group. Outcomes in hypertensive patients at high cardiovascular risk treated with regimens based on valsartan or amlodipine: the VALUE randomised trial.* Lancet 2004;363:2024.)

15.5%; RR, 0.89), and although not a primary endpoint, less incidence of diabetes, the latter reflecting known side effects of both β-blocker and thiazide diuretics. In contrast to the beneficial finding of NDHP in the ASCOT trial, another large trial of DHP CCBs did not demonstrate any benefit compared with RAAS inhibition. The International Verapamil-Trandolapril Study (INVEST)[111] randomized 22,576 patients with CAD to verapamil or trandolarpril and found no difference in either arm in terms of the primary endpoint of first occurrence of all-cause death, nonfatal MI, or nonfatal stroke.

An important question addressed partially in ASCOT is what to do when multiple agents need to be started in patients at high CV risk. In particular, it is uncertain which agent to add to RAAS inhibition, which is often already indicated in patients with diabetes, in post-MI patients, and in those with established CV disease. The largest trial to address this question is the Avoiding Cardiovascular Events through Combination Therapy in Patients Living with Systolic Hypertension (ACCOMPLISH) trial,[112] which randomized 11,506 patients to a two-drug regimen. Both arms included benazepril, and the trial compared the addition of the CCB amlodipine versus diuretic therapy with hydrochlorthiazide. The primary outcome of the trial was the composite of death from CV causes, nonfatal MI, nonfatal stroke, hospitalization for angina, resuscitation after sudden cardiac arrest, and coronary revascularization. BP goals were achieved in both arms, yet the combination with the CCB had a 2.2% absolute risk reduction in the primary endpoint compared with the diuretic regimen (hazard ratio [HR], 0.80; 95% confidence interval [CI], 0.72 to 0.90; *P* < .001; Figure 7-6).

There is a theoretical concern that DHP CCBs may worsen renal function, in particular in patients with diabetes. In contrast to the effect of RAAS inhibitors, CCB may preferentially vasodilate the afferent arteriole and thereby worsen renal function. This was specifically evaluated in the Gauging Albuminuria Reduction with Lotrel in Diabetic Patients with Hypertension (GUARD) trial,[113] which randomized 332 patients with hypertension and albuminuric type 2 diabetes to benazepril, with either hydrochlorthiazide or amlodipine, and followed them for 1 year. This was a noninferiority trial, and the primary endpoint was urinary creatinine ratio as a measure of albuminuria. Both arms demonstrated a regression in proteinuria that likely reflected improved BP control. However, a near 30% change favored the combination of RAAS inhibitor and diuretic, although these findings should be tempered by the more rapid decline in estimated glomerular filtration rate (GFR) in the diuretic arm, which may have biased the results. The results of the GUARD and ACCOMPLISH trials together make tailoring combined therapy more challenging for the physician, in that GUARD

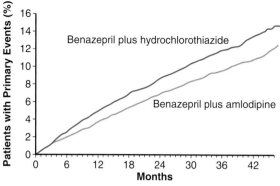

FIGURE 7-6 Cardiovascular morbidity and mortality with combination therapy. Primary outcomes in the Avoiding Cardiovascular Events through Combination Therapy in Patients Living with Systolic Hypertension (ACCOMPLISH) trial were significantly different and favored the use of benazepril-amlodipine to amlodipine-hydrochlorothiazide. The relative risk reduction was 20% (hazard ratio, 0.80; 95% confidence interval, 0.72 to 0.90; P < .001). *(From Jamerson K, Weber MA, Bakris GL, et al, for the ACCOMPLISH trial investigators. Benazepril plus amlodipine or hydrochlorothiazide for hypertension in high-risk patients.* N Engl J Med *2008;359[23]:2417-2428.)*

suggests that a trade-off may exist such that reducing CV risk may come at the cost of proteinuria when using a combined DHP and CCB. Given the small size of the trial and the confounding progression in kidney disease, this issue requires further investigation.

Regarding the particular issue of whether to use a DHP instead of an NDHP CCB for the treatment of essential hypertension, concern has been raised over the use of a short-acting DHP (nifedipine) and NDHP (verapamil, diltiazem) in patients at high risk for MI. This concern came from an observational study conducted in the 1990s.[114] In this case-control study, patients treated with nifedipine, diltiazem, or verapamil had an increased risk for MI that was not seen with other antihypertensives, particularly when these drugs were used at high doses. However, this finding was likely confounded by the fact that the use of calcium channel blockade is much higher in patients with symptomatic CAD given the potent role these agents have as antianginal medications.[115] It is important to note that no concern has been reported for the long-acting DHP CCBs and any increased risk of MI in patients treated for essential hypertension in multiple trials. The INVEST investigators specifically examined the risk of CV outcomes between long-acting verapamil versus atenolol in a subgroup of patients with prior MI and found no difference between treatment arms.[116] Although results of substudies must be interpreted with caution, these data in the context of other studies suggest that NDHPs are at least as effective as β-blocker therapy.

In summary, based on the trials above, convincing evidence suggests that DHP CCBs are safe and efficacious for most patients with high CV risk who require further BP control or angina treatment, and that in particular, these are useful in combination therapy. Concerns initially raised about the risks observed in studies of short-acting CCBs are not seen in contemporary trials of long-acting CCBs. In a meta-analysis that included 27 trials and 175,634 patients, the authors examined DHP CCBs versus others agents or placebo in patients with hypertension who also had other high-risk features and found that although the odds ratio (OR) for a heart failure was increased (and may reflect the side effect of pedal edema), the OR was 0.96 (P = .026) for all-cause death *favoring* DHP CCBs, with no increase in MI in the subgroup of patients with CAD.

β-Adrenergic Blockers

As a major pharmacotherapeutic advance,[117,118] β-blockers were initially conceived for the treatment of patients with angina pectoris and arrhythmias; however, they also have therapeutic effects in many other clinical disorders, including systemic hypertension, hypertrophic cardiomyopathy, congestive cardiomyopathy,[119] mitral valve prolapse, aortic dissection, silent myocardial ischemia, migraine, glaucoma, essential tremor, and thyrotoxicosis.[117] β-Blockers have been effective in treating unstable angina and in

reducing the risks of CV death and nonfatal reinfarction in patients who have survived an acute MI.[120] β-Adrenergic receptor blockade is also a potential treatment modality, with and without fibrinolytic therapy, to reduce the extent of myocardial injury and death during the hyperacute phase of MI.

β-Adrenergic Receptors

The effects of an endogenous hormone or exogenous drug ultimately depend on physiochemical interactions with macromolecular structures of cells called *receptors*. Agonists interact with a receptor and elicit a response; antagonists interact with receptors and prevent the action of agonists.

In the case of catecholamine action, the circulating hormone or drug ("first messenger") interacts with its specific receptor on the external surface of the target cells. The drug hormone/receptor complex, mediated by the G protein (Gs), activates the adenyl cyclase enzyme on the internal surface of the plasma membrane of the target cell, which accelerates the intracellular formation of cAMP, whereupon cAMP-dependent protein kinases ("second messengers") then stimulate or inhibit various metabolic or physiologic processes.[117,121,122] Catecholamine-induced increases in intracellular cAMP are usually associated with the stimulation of β-adrenergic receptors, whereas α-adrenergic receptor stimulation is mediated by glycoprotein Gi and is associated with lower concentrations of cAMP and possibly increased amounts of GMP in the cell. These different receptor effects may result in the production of opposing physiologic actions from catecholamines, depending on which adrenergic receptor system is activated.

Most research on receptor action previously bypassed the initial binding step and the intermediate steps and examined either the accumulation of cAMP or the end step, the physiologic effect. Radioactive agonists or antagonists (radioligands) that attach to and label the receptors have been used to study binding and hormone action.[123] The cloning of adrenergic receptors has also revealed important clues about receptor function.[124] The crystal structure of the human β-adrenergic receptor has also been identified.[125]

In contrast to the older concept of adrenergic receptors as static entities in cells that simply initiate the chain of events, newer theories hold that the adrenergic receptors are subject to a wide variety of controlling influences that result in dynamic regulation of adrenergic receptor sites or their sensitivity to catecholamines or both.[126] Changes in tissue concentration of receptor sites are probably involved in mediating important fluctuations in tissue sensitivity to drug action.[123,127] These principles may have significant clinical and therapeutic implications. For example, an apparent increase in the number of β-adrenergic receptors, and thus a supersensitivity to agonists, may be induced by long-term exposure to antagonists.[123,127] With prolonged adrenergic receptor blocker therapy, receptor occupancy by catecholamines can be diminished, and the number of available receptors can be increased.[127] When the β-adrenergic receptor blocker is suddenly withdrawn, an increased pool of sensitive receptors is available for endogenous catecholamine stimulation. The resultant adrenergic stimulation may precipitate unstable angina pectoris, an MI, or both.[128] Specific gene polymorphisms of both the β1 and β2 receptors may also influence the pharmacologic response to β-blocking agents.[129]

Effects in Angina Pectoris

Ahlquist[130] demonstrated that sympathetic innervation of the heart causes the release of norepinephrine, activating β-adrenergic receptors in myocardial cells. This adrenergic stimulation causes an increment in heart rate, isometric contractile force, and maximal velocity of muscle-fiber shortening, all of which lead to an increase in cardiac work and myocardial oxygen consumption.[121] The decrease in intraventricular pressure and volume caused by the sympathetic-mediated enhancement of cardiac contractility tends to reduce myocardial oxygen consumption by reducing myocardial wall tension (LaPlace's law).[131] Although there is a net increase in myocardial oxygen demand, this is normally balanced by an increase in coronary blood flow. Angina pectoris is believed to occur when oxygen demand exceeds supply (i.e., when coronary blood flow is restricted by coronary atherosclerosis).[132] Because the conditions that precipitate anginal attacks—exercise, emotional stress, food—cause an increase in sympathetic cardiac activity, it might be expected that blockade of cardiac β-adrenergic receptors would relieve anginal symptoms. It is on this basis that the early clinical studies with β-blocking drugs in patients with angina pectoris were initiated.[117]

Three main factors contribute to the myocardial oxygen requirements of the LV: *heart rate, ventricular systolic pressure*, and *size of the LV*. Of these, heart rate and systolic pressure appear to be important, and the product of heart rate multiplied by the systolic BP is a reliable index for predicting the precipitation of angina in a given patient[133]; however, myocardial contractility may be even more important.[134]

The reduction in heart rate effected by β-blockade has two favorable consequences: a decrease in blood pressure, thus reducing myocardial oxygen needs, and a longer diastolic filling time associated with a slower heart rate, allowing for increased coronary perfusion.[134] β-Blockade also reduces exercise-induced BP increments, the velocity of cardiac contraction, and oxygen consumption at any patient's workload (Box 7-1).[133] After treatment, a reduced heart rate variability, a marker for abnormal autonomic control of the heart, or low exercise tolerance may predict those patients who will respond best to treatment with β-blockade.[134] Despite the favorable effects on heart rate, the

Box 7-1 Possible Mechanisms by Which β-Adrenergic–Blocking Agents Protect the Ischemic Myocardium

Reduction in myocardial consumption, heart rate, blood pressure, and myocardial contractility
Augmentation of coronary blood flow, increase in diastolic perfusion time by heart rate reduction, augmentation of collateral blood flow, and redistribution of blood flow to ischemic areas
Prevention or attenuation of atherosclerotic plaque rupture and subsequent coronary thrombosis
Alterations in myocardial substrate utilization
Decrease in microvascular damage
Stabilization of cell and lysosomal membranes
Shift of oxyhemoglobin dissociation curve to the right
Inhibition of platelet aggregation
Inhibition of myocardial apoptosis, which allows natural cell regeneration to occur

From Frishman WH. Alpha- and beta-adrenergic blocking drugs. In Frishman WH, Sonnenblick EH, Sica DA, editors: *Cardiovascular pharmacotherapeutics*, 2nd ed. New York, 2003, McGraw-Hill, pp 67-97.

blunting of myocardial contractility with β-blockers may be the primary mechanism of their antianginal benefit.[134,135] In normal human coronary arteries, β2-adrenergic receptor–mediated vasodilation enhances coronary perfusion, an effect that is impaired by severe atherosclerosis.[136]

Studies in dogs have shown that propranolol causes a decrease in coronary blood flow.[137] However, subsequent experimental animal studies have demonstrated that β-blocker–induced shunting occurs in the coronary circulation, maintaining blood flow to ischemic areas, especially in the subendocardial region.[138] In humans, concomitant with the decrease in myocardial oxygen consumption, β-blockers can cause a reduction in coronary blood flow and an increase in coronary vascular resistance.[133] On the basis of coronary autoregulation, the overall reduction in myocardial oxygen needs with β-blockers may be sufficient cause for this clinically tolerated decrease in coronary blood flow.[133]

Virtually all β-blockers produce some degree of increased work capacity without pain in patients with angina pectoris, regardless of whether they have partial agonist activity, α-adrenergic receptor–blocking effects, direct vasodilating effects, membrane-stabilizing activity, or general or selective β-blocking properties. Therefore, it must be concluded that this results from their common property: blockade of cardiac β-adrenergic receptors (Table 7-5). Both d- and l-propranolol have membrane-stabilizing activity, but only l-propranolol has significant β-blocking activity. The racemic mixture (d,l-propranolol) causes decreases in both heart rate and force of contraction in dogs, whereas the d-isomer has hardly any β-adrenergic receptor–blocking effect. In humans, d-propranolol, which has "membrane" activity but no β-blocking properties, has been found to be ineffective in relieving angina pectoris even at very high doses.[139]

Although exercise tolerance improves with β-blockade, the increments in heart rate and BP with exercise are blunted, and the rate/pressure product (systolic BP multiplied by heart rate) achieved when pain occurs is lower than that reached during a control run.[140] The depressed rate/pressure product at the onset of pain, about 20% reduction from control, is reported to occur with various β-blockers, probably related to decreased cardiac output and possibly to a decrease in coronary perfusion. Thus, although exercise tolerance is increased with β-blockade, patients exercise less than might be expected. This may also relate to the action of β-blockers in increasing LV size, causing increased LV wall tension and an increase in oxygen consumption at a given BP.

Comparison with Other Antianginal Therapies

In a meta-analysis of clinical trial experience over 20 years that compared β-blockers, CCBs, and nitrates in patients who had stable angina pectoris, it was demonstrated that β-blockers provide an equivalent reduction in angina and lead to similar or reduced rates of adverse experiences compared with either CCBs or long-acting nitrates.[68,140] The rates of cardiac death and MI were not significantly different for β-blockers than for CCBs.

Angina at Rest and Vasospastic Angina

Unstable angina pectoris can be caused by multiple mechanisms, including coronary vasospasm, myocardial bridging, and thrombosis, which appear to be responsible for ischemia in a significant proportion of patients with unstable angina and angina at rest.[68,117,133-142] Therefore, because β-blockers primarily reduce myocardial oxygen consumption but fail to exert vasodilating effects on coronary vasculature, they may not be totally effective in patients whose angina is caused or increased by dynamic alterations in coronary luminal diameter.[133] Despite potential dangers in rest and vasospastic angina, β-blockers have been used successfully as monotherapy and in combination with vasodilating antianginal agents in the majority of patients. In addition, there is evidence that β-blockers can reduce C-reactive protein levels, an inflammatory marker of increased CV morbidity and mortality.[143]

CH
7

TABLE 7-5 Pharmacodynamic Properties and Cardiac Effects of β-Adrenergic–Blocking Drugs

DRUG	RELATIVE β1 SELECTIVITY*	ISA	MSA	RESTING HEART RATE	EXERCISE HEART RATE	RESTING MYOCARDIAL CONTRACTILITY	RESTING BLOOD PRESSURE	EXERCISE BLOOD PRESSURE	RESTING AV CONDUCTION	ANTIARRHYTHMIC EFFECT
Acebutolol	+	+	+	↓	↓	↓	↓	↓	↓	+
Atenolol	++	0	0	↓	↓	↓	↓	↓	↓	+
Betaxolol	++	0	+	↓	↓	↓	↓	↓	↓	+
Bisoprolol†	++	0	0	↓	↓	↓	↓	↓	↓	+
Carteolol	0	+	0	↓	↓	↓	↓	↓	↓	+
Carvedilol‡	0	0	++	↓	↓	↓	↓	↓	↓	+
Esmolol	++	0	0	↓	↓	↓	↓	↓	↓	+
Labetalol§	0	+	0	↓	↓	↓	↓	↓↓	↓	+
Metoprolol	++	0	0	↓	↓	↓	↓	↓	↓	+
Nadolol	0	0	0	↓	↓	↓	↓	↓	↓	+
Nebivolol¶	++	0	0	↓	↓	↓	↓	↓	↓	+
Oxprenolol	0	+	+	↓	↓	↓	↓	↓	↓	+
Penbutolol	0	+	0	↓	↓	↓	↓	↓	↓	+
Pindolol	0	++	+	↓	↓	↓	↓	↓	↓	+
Propranolol	0	0	++	↓	↓	↓	↓	↓	↓	+
Isomer-d-propranolol¶	0	0	++	–	–	–	–	–	–	+
Sotalol	0	0	0	↓	↓	↓	↓	↓	↓	+
Timolol	0	0	0	↓	↓	↓	↓	↓	↓	+

*β1 selectivity is seen only with low therapeutic drug concentrations. With higher concentrations, β1 selectivity is not seen.
†Bisoprolol is also approved as a first-line antihypertensive therapy in combination with a very-low-dose diuretic.
‡Carvedilol has peripheral vasodilating activity and additional α1-adrenergic–blocking activity.
§Labetalol has additional α1-adrenergic–blocking activity and direct vasodilatory activity.
¶Nebivolol has additional actions to increase endothelium-dependent vasodilation by increasing the activity of nitric oxide.
¶Effects of d-propranolol with doses in humans well above the therapeutic level; the isomer also lacks β-blocking activity.
AV, atrioventricular; ISA, intrinsic sympathomimetic activity; MSA, membrane stabilizing activity; ++, strong effect; +, modest effect; 0, absent effect; ↓, reduction; –, no change.
Modified from Frishman WH. Clinical pharmacology of the β-adrenoceptor blocking drugs, ed 2, Norwalk, CT, 1984, Appleton-Century-Crofts, p 15.

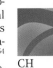

Combined Use of β-Blockers with Other Antianginal Therapies in Angina Pectoris

NITRATES

As noted earlier, combined therapy with nitrates and β-blockers may be more efficacious for the treatment of angina pectoris than the use of either drug alone.[117,142] The primary effects of β-blockers are to cause a reduction in both resting heart rate and the response of heart rate to exercise. Because nitrates produce a reflex increase in heart rate and contractility from a reduction in arterial pressure, concomitant β-blocker therapy is extremely effective because it blocks this reflex increment in the heart rate. Similarly, the preservation of diastolic coronary blood flow with a reduced heart rate will also be beneficial.[117] In patients with a propensity for myocardial failure who may have a slight increase in heart size with the β-blockers, the nitrates will counteract this tendency by reducing heart size as a result of its peripheral venodilator effects. During the administration of nitrates, the reflex increase in contractility mediated through the sympathetic nervous system will be blunted by the presence of β-blockers. Similarly, the increase in coronary resistance associated with β-blocker administration can be ameliorated by the administration of nitrates.[117,142]

CALCIUM CHANNEL BLOCKERS

Some CCBs (diltiazem, verapamil) also slow the heart rate and inhibit AV nodal conduction. Combined therapy with β-blockers and CCBs can provide clinical benefits for patients with angina pectoris who remain symptomatic with the use of either agent alone.[144,145] Because adverse CV effects can also occur with combination treatment, such as heart block and excessive myocardial depression, patients being considered for such treatment must be carefully selected and observed.[144,145]

Hemodynamically, these two types of agents have different effects on the circulation (see Tables 7-3 and 7-5), leading to the possibility of therapeutic combination. Of the combinations, β-blockade plus a DHP such as nifedipine is likely to be simplest. The DHPs do not inhibit the SA or AV node and therefore can be more readily combined with a β-blocker than can the NDHPs, such as verapamil and diltiazem. Because the tendency to produce tachycardia with the DHPs is antagonized by the β-blocker, there are no additive effects on the SA or AV node. Through vasodilation, including coronary vasodilation, the DHPs can contribute to the antianginal effect. β-Blockade should be combined with the NDHPs, such as verapamil and diltiazem, only after consideration of the risks and after plans are in place for patient monitoring. With NDHP CCBs comes the risk of extreme bradycardia, AV nodal block, or a marked negative inotropic effect. Second-generation CCBs—such as the DHPs amlodipine, felodipine, isradipine, and nicardipine—can also be readily combined with β-blockade.

RANOLAZINE

Ranolazine is a piperazine derivative that is approved in an extended-release tablet as a first-line treatment for chronic angina pectoris.[146] The drug can also be combined with β-blockers to provide additional antianginal relief,[147] but it is not approved for use in unstable angina.

Conditions Associated with Angina Pectoris

ARRHYTHMIAS

β-Blockers are an important treatment modality for various cardiac arrhythmias, especially in patients with ischemic heart disease. Although it was initially believed that β-blockers were more effective in treating supraventricular arrhythmias than ventricular arrhythmias, subsequent studies suggest that this may not be the case.[148] β-Blockers can be quite useful in the prevention and treatment of ventricular tachyarrhythmias in the setting of myocardial ischemia, mitral valve prolapse, the hereditary QT-interval prolongation syndrome, and other CV conditions, such as cardiomyopathy.[148-153] β-Blockers can be combined with amiodarone with relative safety and synergy of antiarrhythmic action[154] and with implantable cardioverter-defibrillators to reduce the frequency of shocks.[155]

HYPERTENSION

The mechanism of the antihypertensive effect of β-blockade is still under dispute,[156] but its effect on overall CV mortality appears to be similar to other classes of antihypertensive drugs.[157] Initially, β-blockers decrease the heart rate and cardiac output falls by about 20%, yet the BP does not fall because the arteriolar resistance reflexively increases. Within 24 hours of the start of β-blocker treatment, the peripheral resistance starts to fall, so arterial pressure declines. The mechanism of this delayed hypotensive effect is unclear, but it is thought to involve inhibition of prejunctional β-adrenergic receptors.[156] Alternatively, inhibition of the renin-angiotensin system may account for the delayed vasodilation.[156] Additional antihypertensive mechanisms may involve a central action and decreased renin release.

SURVIVORS OF ACUTE MYOCARDIAL INFARCTION

β-Blockers have beneficial effects on many determinants of myocardial ischemia (see Box 7-1 and Chapters 9 and 10).[120,133,158] The results of placebo-controlled, long-term treatment trials with some β-blockers in survivors of acute MI demonstrated a favorable effect on total mortality rates; CV mortality rates, including sudden and nonsudden cardiac deaths; and the incidence of nonfatal reinfarction. Patients in these studies included those who had relative contraindications to β-blockade but still appeared to benefit[159] and in patients with diabetes, who also responded favorably to treatment.[160] The beneficial results of β-blocker therapy can be explained by both the antiarrhythmic and antiischemic effects of these drugs.[133,161] It has also been proposed that β-blockers reduce the risk of atherosclerotic plaque fissure and subsequent thrombosis.[162] Two nonselective β-blockers, propranolol and timolol, are approved for use in reducing the risk of death in MI survivors when started 5 to 28 days after an MI. Metoprolol and atenolol, two β1-selective blockers, are approved for the same indication, and both can be used intravenously in the hyperacute phase of an MI. β-Blockers have also been suggested as a treatment to reduce the extent of myocardial injury[163] and deaths during the hyperacute phase of MI.[164,165] The α-/β-blocker carvedilol is indicated to reduce CV mortality in clinically stable patients who have survived the acute phase of MI and have an LV ejection fraction of less than 40% with or without symptomatic heart failure.[166] IV and oral atenolol have been shown to be effective in causing a modest reduction in early mortality rates when administered during the hyperacute phase of acute MI.[164] Atenolol and metoprolol reduce early infarct mortality rates by 15%,[164,165] an effect that may be improved when β-blockade is combined with thrombolytic therapy.[167] Despite all of the evidence showing that β-blockers are beneficial in patients who survive MI,[163] they are still considerably underused in clinical practice.[168] β-Blockers should not be administered in patients who come to medical attention with MI and have evidence of heart failure, low cardiac output, or increased risk of cardiogenic shock.

"SILENT" MYOCARDIAL ISCHEMIA

Investigators have observed that not all myocardial ischemic episodes detected on ECG are associated with detectable symptoms.[169] Positron emission imaging techniques have validated the theory that these silent ischemic episodes are indicative of true myocardial ischemia.[170] Compared with symptomatic ischemia, the prognostic importance of silent myocardial ischemia that occurs at rest or during exercise has not been determined.

β-Blockers are as successful in reducing the frequency and timing of silent ischemic episodes detected by ambulatory ECG monitoring as they are in reducing the frequency of painful ischemic events.[170-173]

Other Cardiovascular Conditions Associated with Angina Pectoris

Although β-blockers have been studied extensively in patients with angina pectoris, arrhythmias, and hypertension, they have also been shown to be safe for other CV conditions associated with angina pectoris.

HYPERTROPHIC CARDIOMYOPATHY

β-Blockers without partial agonist activity have been proven effective for patients with hypertrophic cardiomyopathy.[117,174,175] These drugs are useful for reducing dyspnea, angina, and syncope.[158,176] β-Blockers have also been shown to lower the intraventricular pressure gradient both at rest and with exercise.

The outflow pressure gradient is not the only abnormality in hypertrophic cardiomyopathy; more important is the loss of ventricular compliance, which impedes normal LV function. It has been shown through both invasive and noninvasive methods that propranolol can improve LV function in this condition.[177] The drug also produces favorable changes in ventricular compliance while it relieves symptoms. Propranolol has been approved for this condition and may be combined with the CCB verapamil or disopyramide in patients who do not respond to the β-blocker alone.

The salutary hemodynamic and symptomatic effects produced by β-blockers derive from their inhibition of sympathetic stimulation of the heart.[178] No evidence suggests that the drug alters the primary cardiomyopathic process; many patients remain in or return to their severely symptomatic state, and some patients die despite β-blocker administration.[174,175]

CONGESTIVE CARDIOMYOPATHY

The ability of IV sympathomimetic amines to effect an acute increase in myocardial contractility through stimulation of the β-adrenergic receptor had prompted the hope that the use of oral catecholamine analogs could provide long-term benefit for patients with severe heart failure. However, observations concerning the regulation of the myocardial adrenergic receptor and abnormalities of β-adrenergic receptor–mediated stimulation of the failing myocardium have caused a critical reappraisal of the scientific validity of sustained β-adrenergic receptor stimulation.[179] Evidence suggests that β-adrenergic receptor blockade, when tolerated, may have a favorable effect on the underlying cardiomyopathic process.[119,180]

Enhanced sympathetic activation is seen consistently in patients with CHF and is associated with decreased exercise tolerance,[181] hemodynamic abnormalities,[182] and increased mortality rates.[183] Increases in sympathetic tone can potentiate the renin-angiotensin system in patients and lead to increased salt and water retention, arterial and venous constriction, and increments in ventricular preload and afterload.[180] Elevated levels of catecholamines can increase heart rate and cause coronary vasoconstriction,[133] adversely influence myocardial contractility on the cellular level,[184] and cause myocyte hypertrophy[185] and vascular remodeling. Catecholamines can stimulate growth and provoke oxidative stress in terminally differentiated cardiac cells; these two factors can trigger the process of programmed cell death known as *apoptosis*.[186] Finally, excess catecholamines can increase the risk of sudden death in patients with CHF by adversely influencing the electrophysiologic properties of the failing heart.[187]

Controlled trials with several β-blockers in patients with either ischemic or nonischemic cardiomyopathy showed that these drugs improve symptoms, ventricular function, and functional capacity while reducing the need for hospitalization.[119,188] A series of placebo-controlled clinical trials with the α-/β-blocker carvedilol[119] and the β1-selective agents bisoprolol and metoprolol[189-191] have shown a mortality benefit in patients with New York Heart Association (NYHA) functional class II to IV heart failure, when the drug was used in addition to diuretics, ACE inhibitors, and digoxin. For patients with class II to III heart failure, initial treatment with a β-blocker followed by an ACE inhibitor was found to be at least as effective as beginning with an ACE inhibitor.[192]

The mechanisms of benefit with β-blocker use are not yet known. Possible mechanisms for β-blocker benefit in chronic heart failure include the upregulation of impaired β-adrenergic receptor expression in the heart[167,193] and an improvement in impaired baroreceptor functioning, an effect that can inhibit excess sympathetic outflow.[180] It has been suggested that long-term therapy with β-blockers improves the left atrial contribution to LV filling[194] while increasing the levels of cardiac natriuretic peptides.[195,196]

MITRAL VALVE PROLAPSE

Atypical chest pain, malignant arrhythmias, and nonspecific ST- and T-wave abnormalities have been observed with this condition. By decreasing sympathetic tone, β-blockers have been shown to be useful for relieving the chest pains and palpitations that many of these patients experience and for reducing the incidence of life-threatening arrhythmias and other ECG abnormalities.[197]

DISSECTING ANEURYSMS

β-Blockade plays a major role in the treatment of patients with acute aortic dissection. During the hyperacute phase, β-blockers reduce the force and velocity of myocardial contraction (dP/dT) and hence slow the progression of the dissecting hematoma.[198] Moreover, β-blockade should be initiated simultaneously with the institution of other antihypertensive therapy (e.g., sodium nitroprusside) that may cause reflex tachycardia and increases in cardiac output, factors that can aggravate the dissection process. β-Blockade is administered intravenously to reduce the heart rate to less than 60 beats/min. Once a patient is stabilized—that is, once adequate control of heart rate and BP has been achieved and no further pain from dissection is apparent—and long-term medical management is contemplated, the patient should be maintained on oral β-blocker therapy to prevent the recurrence of dissection.[194]

EHLERS-DANLOS SYNDROME

In a placebo-controlled study, the long-term use of a β-blocker has been shown to reduce the risk of spontaneous rupture of the aorta in the vascular subtype of Ehlers-Danlos syndrome.[199]

SYNDROME X

A dysfunction of small coronary arterial vessels has been hypothesized to be responsible for syndrome X, a chest pain syndrome that often occurs without evidence of large-vessel CAD. The treatment of syndrome X, however, remains largely empiric and is often unsatisfactory. Some investigators found that β-blockers, rather than CCBs and nitrates, were useful in relieving symptoms,[200] suggesting that they may be the preferred drugs when starting pharmacologic treatment for syndrome X.

Perioperative Therapy in High-Risk Patients with Ischemic Heart Disease

β-Adrenergic drugs will reduce the risk of perioperative ischemia[201,202] and arrhythmias.[203] Based on these studies, several national organizations have endorsed the perioperative use of β-blockers as a best practice.[204] However, some recent evidence would suggest that the routine use of β-blockers may actually cause harm in some patients.[205] Currently, the best available evidence supports their use in two patient groups: 1) those undergoing vascular surgery who have known ischemic heart disease or multiple risk factors for it and 2) those undergoing vascular surgery who are already receiving β-blockers for cardiovascular conditions.[117,206,207] When feasible, β-blockers should be started 1 month before cardiac surgery, with the dose titrated to achieve a heart rate of 60 beats/min, and should be continued for 1 month after surgery.[117]

Pharmacologic Differences Among β-Adrenergic Receptor–Blocking Drugs

More than 100 β-blockers have been synthesized, and more than 30 are available worldwide for clinical use.[117] Selectivity for two subgroups of the β-adrenergic–receptor population has been prominent in the development of β-blockers: β1-adrenergic receptors in the heart and β2-adrenergic receptors in the peripheral circulation and bronchi.[208] More controversial has been the introduction of β-blockers with α-adrenergic receptor–blocking actions, varying amounts of selective and nonselective intrinsic sympathomimetic activity (partial agonist activity), CCB activity, nitric oxide potentiating action, and nonspecific membrane-stabilizing effects (Table 7-6).[176] Pharmacokinetic differences also exist among β-blockers that may be of clinical importance.[208]

Sixteen β-blockers are marketed in the United States for CV disorders: *propranolol* for angina pectoris, arrhythmias, systemic hypertension, migraine prophylaxis, essential tremor, hypertrophic cardiomyopathy, and reduction in the risk of CV death in survivors of an acute MI; *nadolol* for hypertension and angina pectoris; *timolol* for hypertension and to reduce the risk of CV death and nonfatal reinfarction in survivors of MI and for a topical form for glaucoma; *atenolol* and *metoprolol* for hypertension and angina and in IV and oral formulations to reduce the risk of CV death in survivors of MI; *penbutolol, bisoprolol, nebivolol, pindolol,* and *carvedilol* for hypertension; *betaxolol* and *carteolol* for hypertension and in a topical form for glaucoma; *acebutolol* for hypertension and ventricular arrhythmias; IV *esmolol* for supraventricular arrhythmias; *sotalol* for atrial and ventricular arrhythmias; and *labetalol* for hypertension and in an IV form for hypertensive emergencies.[167,168,176,209-213] Carvedilol, metoprolol, and bisoprolol are approved for clinical use in the treatment of CHF.

Despite extensive experience with β-blockers in clinical practice, no studies have been done that suggest any of these agents provides major advantages or disadvantages compared with the others for the treatment of many CV diseases. When any available β-blocker is titrated properly, it can be effective in patients with arrhythmia, hypertension, or angina pectoris (see Table 7-6).[176,208-212,214] However, one agent may be more effective than other agents in reducing adverse reactions in some patients and in managing specific situations.[117]

POTENCY

β-Blockers are competitive inhibitors of catecholamine binding at β-adrenergic receptor sites. The dose-response curve of the catecholamine is shifted to the right; that is, a given tissue response requires a higher concentration of agonist in the presence of β-blockers.[158] β1-Blocking potency can be assessed by the inhibition of tachycardia produced by isoproterenol or exercise (the more reliable method in the intact organism), and potency varies among compounds.[158] These differences in potency are of no therapeutic relevance, but they do explain the different drug doses needed to achieve effective β-blockade when initiating therapy in patients or when switching from one agent to another.[208,215]

β1 SELECTIVITY

β-Blockers may be classified as *selective* or *nonselective* based on their relative ability to antagonize the actions of sympathomimetic amines in some tissues at lower doses than those required in other tissues.[208,214,215] When used in low doses, β1-selective blockers such as acebutolol, betaxolol, bisoprolol, esmolol, atenolol, and metoprolol inhibit cardiac β1-adrenergic receptors but have less influence on bronchial and vascular β-adrenergic receptors (β2). In higher doses, however, β1-selective blockers also block β2-adrenergic receptors. Accordingly, β1-selective agents may be safer than nonselective agents in patients with obstructive pulmonary disease, because β2-adrenergic receptors remain available to mediate adrenergic bronchodilation.[216] Even relatively selective β-blockers may aggravate bronchospasm in certain patients, so these drugs should generally not be used in patients with active bronchospastic disease.

A second theoretical advantage is that, unlike nonselective β-blockers, β1-selective blockers in low doses may not block the β2-adrenergic receptors that mediate the dilation of arterioles. During the infusion of epinephrine, nonselective β-blockers can cause a pressor response by blocking β2-adrenergic receptor–mediated vasodilation, because β-adrenergic vasoconstrictor receptors are still operative. Selective β1-blockers may not induce this pressor effect in the presence of epinephrine and may lessen the impairment of peripheral blood flow. It is possible that leaving the β2-adrenergic receptors unblocked and responsive to epinephrine may be functionally important in some patients with asthma, hypoglycemia, hypertension, or peripheral vascular disease when they are treated with β-blockers.[176,208,214]

INTRINSIC SYMPATHOMIMETIC ACTIVITY (PARTIAL AGONIST ACTIVITY)

Certain β-blockers have an intrinsic sympathomimetic activity (partial agonist activity) at β1-adrenergic receptor sites, β2-adrenergic receptor sites, or both. In a β-blocker, this property is identified as a slight cardiac stimulation that can be blocked by propranolol.[176,208,211] The β-blockers with this property partially activate the β-adrenergic receptor in addition to preventing the access of natural or synthetic catecholamines to the receptor. Dichloroisoprenaline, the first β-adrenergic receptor-blocking drug to be synthesized, exerted such marked partial agonist activity that it was unsuitable for clinical use.[118] However, compounds with less partial agonist activity are effective β-blockers. The partial agonist effects of β-blockers such as pindolol differ from those of agonists epinephrine and isoproterenol in that the maximum pharmacologic response that can be obtained is low, although the affinity for the receptor is high. In the treatment of patients with arrhythmias, angina pectoris of effort, and hypertension, drugs with mild to moderate partial agonist activity appear to be as efficacious as β-blockers that lack this property. It is still debated whether the presence of partial agonist activity in a β-blocker constitutes an overall advantage or disadvantage in cardiac therapy.[211] Drugs with partial agonist activity cause less slowing of the heart rate at rest than do propranolol and metoprolol, although the increments in heart rate with exercise are similarly blunted. These β-blockers reduce peripheral vascular resistance and may cause less depression or AV conduction than drugs that lack these properties.[211,217] Some investigators claim that partial agonist activity in a β-blocker protects against myocardial depression, adverse lipid changes, bronchial asthma, and peripheral vascular complications, such as those caused by propranolol.[211,217]

The evidence to support these claims is not conclusive, and more definitive clinical trials will be necessary to resolve these issues.

α-ADRENERGIC ACTIVITY

Labetalol is a β-blocker with antagonistic properties at both α- and β-adrenergic receptors, and it has direct vasodilator activity.[158,176,218] Labetalol has been shown to be 6 to 10 times less potent than phentolamine at α-adrenergic receptors, 1.5 to 4 times less potent than propranolol at β-adrenergic receptors, and is itself 4 to 16 times less potent at α- than at β-adrenergic receptors.[158,176,218] Like

TABLE 7-6 Properties of Various β-Adrenoceptor Antagonist Agents: Noncardioselective vs. Cardioselective and Vasodilatory Agents

DRUG	ISA	PLASMA HALF-LIFE (HOURS)	LIPID SOLUBILITY*	FIRST-PASS EFFECT	LOSS BY LIVER/ KIDNEY	PLASMA PROTEIN BINDING (%)	USUAL DOSE FOR ANGINA (OTHER INDICATIONS)	USUAL DOSE AS SOLE THERAPY FOR MILD/ MODERATE HYPERTENSION
Noncardioselective								
Propranolol (Inderal, Innopran)†‡	–	1-6	+++	++	Liver	90	80 mg bid usually adequate (may give 160 mg bid)	Start with 10 to 40 mg bid, mean 160 to 320 mg/day, 1 or 2 doses
Inderal LA	–	8-11	+++	++	Liver	90	80-320 mg qd	80-320 mg daily
Innopran XL	–	8-11	+++	++	Liver	90	Not indicated	80-120 mg at bedtime
Carteolol (Cartrol)†	+	5-6	0/+	0	Kidney	20-30	Not evaluated	2.5-10 mg single dose
Nadolol (Corgard)†‡	–	20-24	0	0	Kidney	30	40-80 mg qd up to 240 mg	40-80 mg/day up to 320 mg
Penbutolol (Levatol)†	+	20-25	+++	++	Liver	98	Not studied	10-20 mg/day
Sotalol (Betapace, Betapace AF)§	–	7-18, mean 12	0	0	Kidney	5	80-240 mg bid in 2 doses for serious ventricular arrhythmias; up to 160 mg bid for atrial fibrillation, flutter	80-320 mg/day, mean 190 mg/day
Timolol (Blocadren)†	–	4-5	+	+	Liver, kidney	60	10 mg bid after MI	10-20 mg bid
Cardioselective								
Acebutolol (Sectral)†	++	8-13	0	0	Liver, kidney	15	400-1200 mg/day in 2 doses for PVCs	400-200 mg/day; can be given as a single dose
Atenolol (Tenormin)†‡	–	6-7	0	0	Kidney	10	50-200 mg qd	50-100 mg/day
Betaxolol (Kerlone)†	–	14-22	++	++	Liver, kidney	50	–	10-20 mg/day
Bisoprolol (Zebeta)†	–	9-12	+	0	Liver, kidney	30	10 mg qd (not in the United States)	2.5-40 mg/day
Metoprolol (Lopressor, Toprol)†‡	–	3-7	+	++	Liver	12	50-200 mg bid	100-400 mg/day in 1 or 2 doses
Toprol-XL		Slow release	+	++	Liver	12	100-400 mg qd	As above, 1 dose
Vasodilatory β-Blockers								
Noncardioselective								
Labetalol (Trandate, Normodyne)†	–	6-8	+++	++	Liver, some kidney	90	As for hypertension	300-600 mg/day in 3 doses; top dose 2400 mg/day
Pindolol (Visken)†	β1, β2	4	+	+	Liver, kidney	55	2.5-7.5 mg tid (not in the United States)	5-30 mg in 2 daily doses
Carvedilol (Coreg)†¶	–	6	+	++	Liver	95	In the United States and United Kingdom, licensed for heart failure up to 25 mg bid; start with low dose	12.5-25 mg bid
Cardioselective								
Nebivolol (Bystolic)	–	6-10	++	++	Liver, kidney	98	2.5-10 mg qd	2.5-10 mg qd

*Octanol-water distribution coefficient (pH 7.4, 37° C), where 0 is ≤0.5, + is 0.5 to 2, ++ is 2 to 10, and +++ is ≥10.
†Approved by the FDA for hypertension.
‡Approved by the FDA for angina pectoris.
§Approved by the FDA for life-threatening ventricular tachyarrhythmias.
¶Approved by the FDA for heart failure.
ISA, intrinsic sympathomimetic activity; MI, myocardial infarction; PVC, premature ventricular contraction; +++, very strong effect; ++, strong effect; +, modest effect; 0, absent effect; –, negative effect.
Modified from Opie LH, Yusuf S. Beta-blocking agents. In Opie LH, Gersh BJ, editors: *Drugs for the heart*, 5th ed. Philadelphia, 2001, WB Saunders, pp 1-32.

other β-blockers, it is useful in the treatment of hypertension and angina pectoris.[158,219] Unlike most β-blockers, however, the additional α-adrenergic receptor–blocking actions of labetalol lead to a reduction in peripheral vascular resistance that may maintain cardiac output.[158,218] Whether concomitant α-adrenergic receptor–blocking activity is actually advantageous in a β-blocker remains to be determined.

Carvedilol is another β-blocker with additional β-adrenergic receptor–blocking activity, with an α1- to β-blockade ratio of 1:10. On a milligram/milligram basis, carvedilol is about 2 to 4 times more potent than propranolol as a β-blocker.[119] In addition, carvedilol may have antioxidant and antiproliferative activities,[119] it has been used for the treatment of hypertension and angina pectoris, and it is approved as a treatment for hypertension and for patients with symptomatic heart failure.[119,220]

NITRIC OXIDE POTENTIATING EFFECT

A novel aspect of the pharmacology of the β1-selective antagonist nebivolol is its ability to produce endothelium-dependent vasodilation through a nitric oxide pathway. Nebivolol produces vasodilation by acting as a β3-receptor agonist, which increases the activity of nitric oxide.[213] Nitric oxide activity is also augmented by nebivolol through the prevention of nitric oxide deactivation.[213] The nitric oxide–mediated vasodilatory effects of nebivolol occur primarily in the small arteries and contribute to the effect of the drug on arterial BP.[213]

PHARMACOKINETICS

Although the β-blockers as a group have similar therapeutic effects, their pharmacokinetic properties are markedly different.[176,215,221] Their varied aromatic ring structures lead to differences in completeness of GI absorption, amount of first-pass hepatic metabolism, lipid solubility, protein binding, extent of distribution in the body, penetration into the brain, concentration in the heart, rate of hepatic biotransformation, pharmacologic activity of metabolites, and renal clearance of a drug and its metabolites, which may influence the clinical usefulness of these drugs in some patients.[176,208,215,221] The desirable pharmacokinetic characteristics of β-blockers in general are a lack of major individual differences in bioavailability and in metabolic clearance of the drug and a rate of removal from active tissue sites that is slow enough to allow longer dosing intervals.[176,208]

The β-blockers can be divided by their pharmacokinetic properties into two broad categories: those eliminated via hepatic metabolism, which tend to have relatively short plasma half-lives, and those eliminated unchanged by the kidney, which tend to have longer half-lives.[176] Propranolol and metoprolol are both lipid soluble, are almost completely absorbed by the small intestine, and are largely metabolized by the liver. They tend to have more variable bioavailability and relatively short plasma half-lives.[176,214,215,221] A lack of correlation between the duration of clinical pharmacologic effect and plasma half-life may allow these drugs to be administered once or twice daily.[208]

In contrast, agents such as atenolol and nadolol are more water soluble, are incompletely absorbed through the gut, and are eliminated unchanged by the kidney.[209,210] They tend to have less variable bioavailability in patients with normal renal function in addition to longer half-lives, which allows once-a-day dosing.[209,210] The longer half-lives may be useful in patients who find compliance with frequent β-blocker dosing problematic.[209]

Long-acting sustained-release preparations of propranolol and metoprolol are available. Studies have shown that long-acting propranolol and metoprolol can provide a much smoother curve of daily plasma levels than can be comparable to divided doses of conventional immediate-release formulations.[222,223] In addition, a delayed-release/sustained-release formulation of propranolol is available that is designed to target early morning elevations in BP and heart rate related to circadian rhythms.[224]

The specific pharmacokinetic properties of individual β-blockers—first-pass metabolism, active metabolites, lipid solubility, and protein binding—may be clinically important.[158] When drugs with extensive first-pass metabolism are taken by mouth, they undergo so much hepatic biotransformation that relatively little drug reaches the systemic circulation.[176,208,215] Depending on the extent of first-pass effect, an oral dose of β-blocker must be larger than an IV dose to produce the same clinical effects.[214,215] Some β-blockers are transformed into pharmacologically active compounds (e.g., acebutolol) rather than inactive metabolites.[221] The total pharmacologic effect depends on the amount of the drug administered and its active metabolites.[221] Characteristics of lipid solubility in a β-blocker have been associated with the ability of the drug to concentrate in the brain,[176,208] and many side effects of these drugs—such as lethargy, mental depression, and hallucinations—that have not been clearly related to β-blockers may result from their actions on the central nervous system.[208,210] However, it is still uncertain whether drugs that are less lipid soluble cause fewer of these adverse reactions.[209,210,225,226] Some genetic polymorphisms can influence the metabolism of various β-blockers, including propranolol, metoprolol, timolol, and carvedilol.[227] A one-codon difference of CYP 2D6 may explain a significant proportion of interindividual variation in the pharmacokinetics of propranolol in Chinese subjects.[227] In addition, exercise has not been shown to have any effect on the pharmacokinetics of propranolol.[228]

Adverse Effects of β-Adrenergic Receptor Blockers

An evaluation of adverse effects is complex because of the use of different definitions of side effects, the kinds of patients studied, study design features, and different methods of ascertaining and reporting adverse side effects among studies.[229,230] Overall, the types and frequencies of adverse effects attributed to various β-blocker compounds appear similar.[229,230] The side-effect profiles resemble those seen with concurrent placebo treatments, attesting to the remarkable safety margin of β-blockers.

Adverse effects of β-blockers are an exaggeration of the normal cardiac therapeutic effects, resulting in excess bradycardia, AV nodal block, and excess negative inotropic effect. All β-blockers tend to promote bronchospasm, with low doses of β1-selective agents being the least harmful. Cold extremities occur with both selective and nonselective agents,[231] yet agents with intrinsic sympathomimetic activity may provide a slightly better skin temperature than propranolol, at least during an acute study.[232] The adverse effects of all β-blockers on the peripheral circulation may be less marked than previously thought.[233]

Fatigue is a frequent side effect, again found particularly with propranolol, with less of an effect when a β1-selective or vasodilatory blocker is used, so both central and peripheral hemodynamic mechanisms may be involved.[234] Although one double-blind study shows no difference between the effects of the β1-selective agent atenolol and placebo,[231] exercise physiologists find that some impairment in peak exercise occurs with all β-blockers.

Impotence is often reported by patients who receive β-blockers, usually middle-aged men with atherosclerotic arterial disease.[235] In one study, erectile dysfunction occurred in 11% of patients administered a β-blocker for hypertension compared with 26% of these patients administered a diuretic and 3% of placebo-treated patients.[236]

An impaired quality of life found especially with propranolol[237] is theoretically ascribed to its lipid solubility and brain penetration. Yet a variety of β-blockers other than propranolol, and with different pharmacologic properties, preserve quality of life in hypertensive patients.[238] Central effects of β-blockers are often subtle and are not always explicable by the lipid-penetration hypothesis.[239]

β-Blockers have effects on various metabolic parameters, including blood glucose and blood lipids. In a prospective cohort study of 12,550 nondiabetic individuals with hypertension, β-blockers were shown to increase the risk of developing type 2 diabetes, a finding not observed with thiazide diuretics, ACE inhibitors, or CCBs.[240] This increased risk of diabetes must be weighed against the proven benefits of β-blockers in reducing the risk of CV events in patients with ischemic heart disease. Studies are needed to determine whether the use of ACE inhibitors in conjunction with β-blockers might counteract the adverse effects of β-blockers with respect to glucose tolerance.[241] Carvedilol has been shown not to affect glycemic control, and it improves some components of the metabolic syndrome relative to metoprolol in diabetic patients.[220] Similarly, β-blockers without intrinsic sympathomimetic activity have been shown in hypertensive patients to decrease high-density lipoprotein cholesterol concentrations by 7% to 10% and to raise triglyceride concentrations by 10% to 20%.[242] These small changes in lipids induced by β-blockers do not appear to diminish the beneficial effects of BP lowering on morbidity and mortality rates from coronary heart disease and stroke.

Contraindications to β-Adrenergic Receptor Blockers

Several absolute contraindications exist, which include CV contra-indications such as severe bradycardia (heart rate <40 beats/min); preexisting high-degree AV nodal block (PR interval of >0.24 seconds without a functioning pacemaker); overt LV failure, except when the β-blocker is administered initially at low doses and under supervision to patients already receiving diuretics, digoxin, and an ACE inhibitor; and active peripheral vascular disease with rest ischemia. Severe bronchospasm is an absolute contraindication, even to β-selective agents; severe psychological depression is an important relative contraindication, particularly for propranolol.[225]

Overdosage

Suicide attempts and accidental overdosing with β-blockers are being described with increasing frequency. Because β-blockers are competitive pharmacologic antagonists, their life-threatening effects—bradycardia, myocardial failure, and ventilatory failure—can be overcome with an immediate infusion of a β-agonist agent such as isoproterenol or dobutamine.[243] When catecholamines are not effective, IV glucagon, amrinone, or milrinone has been used.[243] There are no published recommended doses of IV catecholamines or phosphodiesterase inhibitors to treat β-blocker overdose; such agents should be used in their usual pharmacologic concentration until it is certain that reversal of β-blocker toxicity—reversal of heart blocks, excessive bradycardia, and myocardial depression—has occurred.

Monitoring of cardiorespiratory function is necessary for at least 24 hours in an intensive care unit after the patient responds to treatment of the β-blocker overdose. Patients who recover usually have no long-term sequelae; however, they should be observed for the cardiac signs of sudden β-blocker withdrawal.[243]

β-Adrenergic Receptor Blocker Withdrawal

After abrupt cessation of long-term β-blocker therapy, exacerbation of angina pectoris and, in some cases, acute MI and death have been reported.[128] Observations made in multiple double-blind ran-domized trials have confirmed the reality of a propranolol with-drawal reaction.[128,244] The mechanism for this reaction is unclear, but some evidence suggests that the withdrawal phenomenon may be due to the generation of additional β-adrenergic receptors during the period of β-blockade. When the β-blocker is then with-drawn, the increased β-adrenergic receptor population readily results in excessive β-adrenergic receptor stimulation, which is clinically important when the delivery and use of oxygen are finely balanced, as occurs in ischemic heart disease. Other suggested

mechanisms for the withdrawal reaction include heightened plate-let aggregability, an elevation in thyroid hormone activity, and an increase in circulating catecholamines.[128] Similar withdrawal prob-lems have been seen with β-blocker discontinuation in patients with heart failure previously responsive to treatment.[245]

Drug-Drug Interactions

β-Blockers are commonly used with other cardiovascular and non-cardiovascular drugs, and the list of drugs with which they interact is extensive (Table 7-7).[230] The majority of the reported interactions have been associated with propranolol, the best-studied β-blocker, and such findings may not necessarily apply to other drugs in this class.

Newer Options for Treatment of Chronic Angina

Several new antianginal agents—ivabradine, nicorandil, trimetazi-dine, and ranolazine—have been extensively evaluated in clinical studies over the past decade; they offer novel approaches to alter-ing the ischemia supply/demand mismatch in stable ischemic heart disease and to reducing anginal symptoms. Ranolazine is approved in the United States to treat angina, and ivabradine, trimetazidine, and nicorandil are widely available in other regions of the world. Each agent alters the fundamental balance of oxygen supply and demand via novel mechanisms of action; therefore these may offer complementary antiischemic activity in addition to traditional antianginal agents of nitrates, β-blockers, and CCBs.

Nicorandil

Nicorandil may improve ischemia by two proposed mechanisms of action. The first is by activating adenosine triphosphate (ATP)-dependent potassium channels, which directly dilates peripheral and coronary arteries. Like nitrates, nicorandil also promotes smooth muscle cell relaxation and vasodilation via increased cGMP activity through a nitrate moiety. In the Impact of Nicorandil in Angina (IONA) trial of 5126 patients with stable angina, treat-ment with nicorandil resulted in a significant 17% reduction in the primary endpoint of coronary heart disease death, MI, or unplanned hospitalization for chest pain compared with placebo (13.1% vs. 15.5%; HR, 0.83; 95% CI, 0.72 to 0.97; $P = .014$), although no differ-ence in overall mortality rate was noted (Figure 7-7).[246] As with nitrates, long-term therapy may promote tachyphylaxis, but toler-ance does not cross-react with nitrates, so they can be used together.

Ivabradine

Ivabradine, an inhibitor of the I_f current in the sinoatrial cells, reduces resting and exercise heart rate in patients in sinus rhythm but has no significant hemodynamic effects. In several smaller studies of patients with chronic angina, ivabradine was shown to prolong the symptom-free interval of ST-segment depression on exercise stress test compared with placebo[247] and resulted in similar reductions in anginal symptoms and nitroglycerin use com-pared with atenolol.[248] In the Morbidity-Mortality Evaluation of the I_f Inhibitor Ivabradine in Patients with Coronary Disease and Left Ventricular Dysfunction (BEAUTIFUL) trial, almost 11,000 patients with CAD and reduced LV function were studied.[249] Compared with placebo, ivabradine reduced the average resting heart rate by 6 beats/min but had no overall benefit in terms of the primary endpoint of CV death, MI, or admission for new or worsening heart failure (HR, 1.00; 95% CI, 0.91 to 1.1; $P = .94$). In a prespecified subgroup of patients with a resting heart rate of at least 70 beats/min, ivabradine did reduce MI (HR, 0.64; 95% CI, 0.49 to 0.84; $P = .001$) and coronary revascularization (HR, 0.70; 95% CI, 0.52 to 0.93; $P = .016$). A greater number of patients assigned to ivabradine

TABLE 7-7	**Drug Interactions of β-Adrenergic–Blocking Agents**			
CARDIAC DRUGS	**INTERACTING DRUGS**	**MECHANISM**	**CONSEQUENCE**	**PROPHYLAXIS**
Hemodynamic Interactions				
All β-blockers	Calcium antagonists, especially nifedipine	Added hypotension	Risk of myocardial ischemia	BP control, adjust doses
	Verapamil or diltiazem	Added negative inotropic effect	Risk of myocardial failure	Check for CHF, adjust doses
	Flecainide	Hypotension	Check LV function, flecainide levels	
	Sympathomimetics	Opposing effects	Loss of clinical benefit	Avoid sympathomimetics
Electrophysiologic Interactions				
All β-blockers	Verapamil	Added inhibition of SA and AV nodes	Bradycardia, asystole, complete heart block	Exclude "sick sinus" syndrome, AV nodal disease; adjust dose; exclude prodrug LV failure
	Diltiazem	Added negative inotropic effect	Excess hypotension	
Hepatic Interactions				
Propranolol	Cimetidine	Cimetidine decreases propranolol metabolism	Excess propranolol effects	Reduce both drug doses
	Lidocaine	Low hepatic blood flow	Excess lidocaine effects	Reduce lidocaine dose
Metoprolol	Verapamil	Verapamil decreases metoprolol metabolism	Excess metoprolol effects	Reduce metoprolol dose
	Cimetidine	Cimetidine decreases metoprolol metabolism	Excess metoprolol effects	Reduce both drug doses
Labetolol	Cimetidine	Cimetidine decreases labetolol metabolism	Excess labetolol and cimetidine effects	Reduce both drug doses
Carvedilol	Cimetidine	Cimetidine decreases carvedilol metabolism	Excess carvedilol effects	Reduce both drug doses
Antihypertensive Interactions				
All β-blockers	Indomethacin, other NSAIDs	Indomethacin inhibits vasodilatory prostaglandins	Decreased antihypertensive effect	Omit indomethacin; use alternative drugs
Immune-Interacting Drugs				
Acebutolol	Other drugs altering immune status; procainamide, hydralazine, captopril	Theoretical risk of additive immune effects	Theoretical risk of lupus or neutropenia	Check antinuclear factors and neutrophils; low doses during cotherapy

AV, atrioventricular; BP, blood pressure; CHF, congestive heart failure; LV, left ventricular; NSAIDs, nonsteroidal antiinflammatory drugs; SA, sinoatrial.
From Frishman WH, Opie LH, Sica DA. Adverse cardiovascular drug interactions and complications. In Fuster V, Alexander RW, O'Rourke RA, editors: *Hurst's the heart,* 11th ed. New York, 2004, McGraw-Hill, pp 2169-2188.

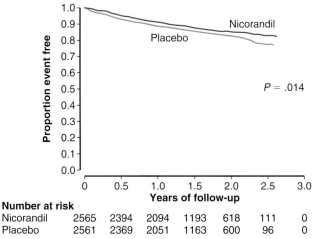

Number at risk

Nicorandil	2565	2394	2094	1193	618	111	0
Placebo	2561	2369	2051	1163	600	96	0

FIGURE 7-7 Reduction in coronary heart disease death, nonfatal myocardial infarction, or unplanned hospital admission with nicorandil compared with placebo among patients with stable angina in the Impact of Nicorandil in Angina (IONA) trial.

discontinued the study drug because of bradycardia compared with placebo (13% vs. 2%), although only 21% of those cases were symptomatic.

Ivabradine was studied in 6558 patients with symptomatic heart failure or LV ejection fraction less than 35% and a resting heart rate greater than 70 beats/min. Patients were randomized to placebo or ivabradine and uptitrated to a maximum of 7.5 mg twice daily. Over a 23-month follow-up, ivabradine reduced the rate of the primary endpoint, CV death or hospitalization for heart failure (24% vs. 29%; HR, 0.82; 95% CI, 0.75 to 0.90; $P < .0001$). A total of 5% of patients taking ivabradine had symptomatic bradycardia compared with 1% of the placebo group ($P < .0001$).[250]

In addition to bradycardia, the other most common side effects are luminous phenomena (phosphenes), which are described as a transient enhanced visual brightness, headaches, and blurred vision. Ivabradine should not be used in patients with second-degree AV block or in those with a resting heart rate less than 50 beats/min. Ivabradine is approved in Europe for the treatment of chronic stable angina in patients in normal sinus rhythm who have a contraindication or intolerance to β-blockers. The recommended starting dose is 5 mg twice daily, which can be increased to 7.5 mg twice daily. The dose should be reduced, or therapy stopped, for persistent bradycardia less than 50 beats/min or signs and symptoms of hypotension.

Ranolazine

MECHANISM OF ACTION

Ranolazine is a piperazine derivative first believed to inhibit partial fatty acid oxidation and thereby to preferentially shunt cardiac metabolism to a more metabolically favorable glucose pathway. Subsequent cellular and animal experimental models indicate that at clinically relevant levels, ranolazine does not significantly inhibit partial fatty acid oxidation, but rather it inhibits the late phase of the sodium current (late I_{Na}).

Under normal physiologic conditions, late I_{Na} contributes a relatively small proportion of the total sodium influx during cardiac repolarization. In several disease states, such as ischemia and heart failure, late I_{Na} is augmented, which leads to increased concentrations of cytosolic sodium and then calcium via the sodium-calcium exchanger.[251] Dysregulation of sodium and calcium homeostasis leads to cytosolic calcium overload, impaired diastolic relaxation, increased wall tension, and decreased coronary blood flow.[252] In experimental models of induced ischemia, heart failure, or increased reactive oxygen species in single myocardial cells and isolated hearts, ranolazine has been shown to preferentially inhibit late I_{Na} to reduce intracellular sodium and calcium overload and thereby improve diastolic function.[253-255]

The extended-release formulation of ranolazine was approved for the treatment of stable angina based on the results of three studies in patients with chronic stable angina. The Monotherapy Assessment of Ranolazine in Stable Angina (MARISA)[256] and Combination Assessment of Ranolazine in Stable Angina (CARISA) trials examined the effect of several doses of ranolazine on treadmill exercise test parameters in patients with chronic angina and documented ST-segment depression and angina at low workloads.[256] In the CARISA trial, 823 patients on a background therapy of atenolol, amlodipine, or diltiazem were randomized to ranolazine (750 mg or 1000 mg twice daily) or placebo. Treatment with ranolazine increased total exercise duration compared with placebo at trough plasma concentrations by 24 seconds ($P = .01$) and increased time to ischemia and ST-segment depression. Moreover, patients assigned to ranolazine reported fewer angina attacks and required fewer sublingual nitroglycerin tablets over the course of the 12-week study (Figure 7-8).[257] No meaningful difference was noted in heart rate or BP between patients assigned to ranolazine versus those assigned to placebo. A third stable angina study, Efficacy of Ranolazine in Chronic Angina (ERICA), assigned 565 patients with chronic angina to ranolazine (1000 mg twice daily) or placebo in addition to amlodipine (10 mg/day). Compared with placebo, ranolazine significantly, although modestly, reduced the frequency of angina episodes (2.88 ± 0.19 episodes/

week on ranolazine vs. 3.31 ± 0.22 on placebo; $P = .028$) and weekly nitroglycerin use (2.03 ± 0.20 on ranolazine vs. 2.68 ± 0.22; $P = .014$).[258]

The efficacy and safety of ranolazine were examined in a broader and more clinically unstable population in the Metabolic Efficiency with Ranolazine for Less Ischemia in Non–ST-Elevation Acute Cardiac Syndrome–Thrombolysis in Myocardial Infarction (MERLIN-TIMI 36) trial, which randomized 6560 patients with moderate- to high-risk non–ST-elevation acute cardiac syndrome (NSTE-ACS) to either ranolazine or placebo in addition to standard care. Overall, treatment with ranolazine did not reduce the primary endpoint of CV death, new or recurrent MI, or recurrent ischemia. Specifically, similar to other antianginals such as nitrates and calcium antagonists, ranolazine had no effect on CV death or recurrent MI (12.9% vs. 13.7%; HR, 0.99; 95% CI, 0.85 to 1.15; $P = .87$), but it did reduce recurrent ischemia (17.3% vs. 20.0%; HR, 0.87; 95% CI, 0.76 to 0.99).[259] Among the more than 3500 patients with prior angina enrolled in the trial, ranolazine resulted in a significant reduction in recurrent ischemia (HR, 0.78; 95% CI, 0.67 to 0.91), which included worsening angina (HR, 0.77; 95% CI, 0.59 to 1.00) and prolonged exercise duration at 8 months (514 vs. 482 seconds; $P = .002$).[260]

OTHER POTENTIAL USES OF RANOLAZINE

Several additional intriguing effects of ranolazine remain under investigation. A statistically significant 0.7% absolute reduction was observed in hemoglobin A1c levels in patients in the CARISA trial treated with 1000 mg of ranolazine ($P = .002$),[261] a finding confirmed in the MERLIN-TIMI 36 trial, in which patients with diabetes treated with ranolazine demonstrated an HbA1c decline of approximately 0.6% ($P < .001$).[262] The mechanism of this reduction is not fully understood but may be related to I_{Na} inhibition in the pancreas.

Growing evidence suggests ranolazine also exerts antiarrhythmic actions despite a small prolongation of the QTc interval. In experimental models, ranolazine suppresses early afterdepolarization and reduces dispersion of transmyocardial repolarization and other proarrhythmic electrophysiologic phenomena.[263,264] Among the 6300 patients in the MERLIN-TIMI 36 trial who had 7-day continuous ECG monitoring at the time of randomization, patients treated with ranolazine had fewer episodes of ventricular tachycardia lasting at least 8 beats (5.3% vs. 8.3%; $P < .001$), supraventricular tachycardia (44.7% v. 55.0%; $P < .001$), new-onset AF (1.7% vs. 2.4%; $P = .08$), or ventricular pauses lasting at least 3 seconds (3.1% vs. 4.3%; $P = .01$).[265] However, the potential antiarrhythmic actions of ranolazine require further validation in prospective clinical studies.

Trimetazidine

Trimetazidine is believed to improve myocardial metabolism during ischemia by inhibiting partial fatty acid oxidation and enhancing utilization of glucose-dependent oxidation, which generates ATP more efficiently in a low-oxygen environment. In clinical trials of patients with angina, trimetazidine has been shown to reduce weekly symptomatic episodes and prolong the interval before ST depression on exercise testing, even in patients on maximal amounts of traditional antianginal agents.[266]

Trimetazidine was studied in patients brought to medical attention with acute MI in the European Myocardial Infarct Project–Free Radicals (EMIP-FR) trial. More than 19,000 subjects were randomized to bolus IV trimetazidine followed by 48-hour infusion or placebo. The overall results demonstrated no difference in short- or long-term mortality rates, although opposing trends were observed when the results were stratified by whether thrombolysis was administered; thrombolysed patients showed a tendency toward more deaths over the short term with trimetazidine compared with placebo (11.3% vs. 10.5%; $P = .15$), but nonthrombolysed patients demonstrated a trend toward a benefit (14.0% vs. 15.1%; $P = .14$).[267]

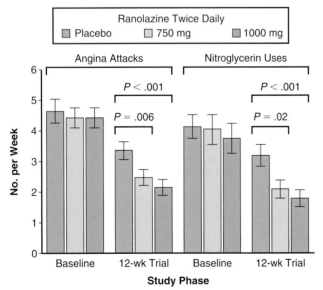

FIGURE 7-8 Reduction in weekly angina attacks frequency and nitroglycerin use in the Combination Assessment of Ranolazine in Stable Angina (CARISA) trial, which compared ranolazine versus placebo in patients with chronic angina on a background therapy of atenolol 50 mg/day, amlodipine 5 mg/day, or diltiazem 180 mg/day.

Thrombosis and Ischemic Cardiovascular Heart Disease

The hemostatic process strikes a fine balance between prothrombotic and antithrombotic factors in the vasculature. Although normal hemostasis prevents hemorrhage, these same processes can lead to pathologic thrombosis and vessel occlusion.[268] Arterial thrombosis is typically highly dependent on platelet-mediated processes on the vessel wall.[269] In particular, in the coronary artery, rupture of an atheromatous plaque and subsequent thrombus formation underlie the majority of ACS. Plaque rupture or erosion exposes subendothelial collagen, which allows platelet adhesion at the site of vessel injury; this is followed by activation and aggregation of platelets (Figure 7-9).[268,269] Vascular injury is also associated with release of tissue factor, which activates the extrinsic pathway of the coagulation cascade that ultimately favors thrombin generation and fibrin deposition.[268] Fibrinogen forms bridges between activated platelets and contributes to thrombus stabilization; thrombus in acute atherothrombotic events can be either partially or completely occlusive.[270,271] Fibrinogen is composed primarily of platelet aggregates, and thrombus is composed of platelet aggregates and a fibrin-rich clot generated by the coagulation cascade. Platelet-rich white thrombi are typically not completely occlusive and are often associated with NSTE-ACS. Progression to completely occlusive thrombus mediated by the coagulation cascade involves the formation of a fibrin-rich red clot superimposed on the underlying, platelet-rich white thrombus, and it is usually found in ST-segment elevation MI (STEMI) patients.[270,271] Advances in the understanding of the mechanisms regulating thrombosis have been pivotal for the development of antithrombotic therapies that inhibit platelets (*antiplatelet therapies*) and coagulation factors (*anticoagulant therapies*) used for the prevention of recurrent atherothrombotic events.[268]

Antiplatelet Therapy

Currently, three classes of antiplatelet agents are approved for the treatment and/or prevention of recurrent events in patients with CAD. These include cyclooxygenase (COX)-1 inhibitors, adenosine diphosphate (ADP) $P2Y_{12}$ receptor antagonists, and glycoprotein (GP) IIb/IIIa inhibitors. Indeed, other categories of agents have antiplatelet properties, such as phosphodiesterase inhibitors (e.g., cilostazol, dipyridamole, pentoxifylline), which do not have a clinical indication for prevention of recurrent events in CAD patients, although they may have a role in other atherothrombotic disease processes (e.g., peripheral vascular disease, cerebrovascular disease; see Chapters 35 and 36). Details of the mechanism of action, indications for use, dosage, side effects, and contraindications of antiplatelet agents approved for prevention of ischemic events in patients with CAD manifestations are provided in this section.

ASPIRIN

Mechanisms of Action

Aspirin is rapidly absorbed in the upper GI tract and is associated with detectable platelet inhibition within 60 minutes.[272,273] The plasma half-life of aspirin is approximately 20 minutes, and peak plasma levels are achieved within 30 to 40 minutes. Enteric-coated aspirin delays absorption, and peak plasma levels are achieved 3 to 4 hours after ingestion. Aspirin exerts its effects by irreversibly inactivating COX activity of prostaglandin H (PGH) synthases 1 and 2, also referred to as *COX-1* and *COX-2*, respectively.[272,273] These isozymes catalyze the conversion of arachidonic acid to PGH_2, which serves as substrate for the generation of several prostanoids, including thromboxane A_2 (TXA_2) and prostacyclin (PGI_2; Figure 7-10). To exert its effects, aspirin diffuses through the cell membrane and enters a narrow, hydrophobic channel that connects the cell membrane to the catalytic pocket of the COX enzyme. Aspirin acetylates a serine residue (serine 529 in human COX-1 and serine 516 in human COX-2) that impedes arachidonic acid from gaining access to the catalytic site of the COX enzyme (Figure 7-11). Only high doses of aspirin can inhibit COX-2, which has antiinflammatory and analgesic effects; low doses of aspirin are sufficient to inhibit COX-1 activity and lead to antiplatelet effects.[272,273] Vascular endothelial cells and newly formed platelets (8% to 10% of circulating platelets) express both COX-1 and COX-2, but mature platelets express only COX-1. Importantly, TXA_2, an amplifier of platelet activation and a vasoconstrictor, is mainly derived from platelet

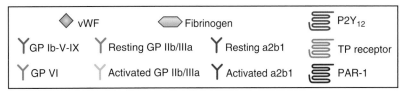

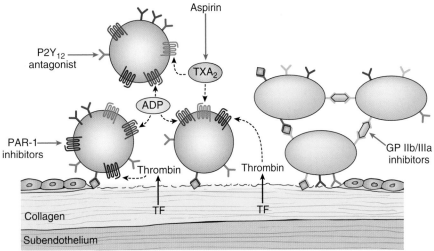

FIGURE 7-9 Platelet-mediated thrombosis. The interaction between glycoprotein *(GP)* Ib and von Willebrand factor *(vWF)* mediates platelet tethering that enables subsequent interaction between GP VI and collagen. This triggers the shift of integrins to a high-affinity state and initiates the release of adenosine diphosphate *(ADP)* and thromboxane A_2 *(TXA$_2$)*, which bind to the $P2Y_{12}$ and thrombo receptors, respectively. Tissue factor *(TF)* locally triggers thrombin formation, which contributes to platelet activation via binding to the platelet protease–activated receptor *(PAR-1)*. (From Angiolillo DJ, Ueno M, Goto S. Basic principles of platelet biology and clinical implications. Circ J 2010;74:597-607.)

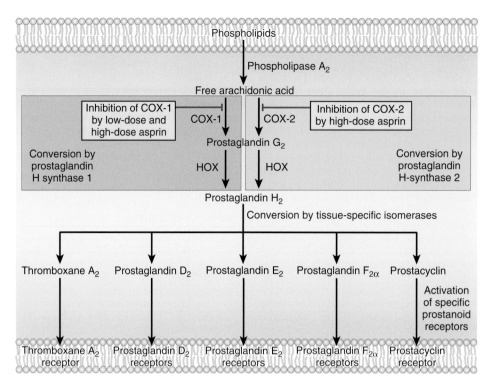

FIGURE 7-10 Mechanism of action of aspirin. Arachidonic acid, a 20-carbon fatty acid containing four double bonds, is released from membrane phospholipids by several forms of phospholipase A_2, which are activated by diverse stimuli. Arachidonic acid is converted by cytosolic prostaglandin H synthases, which have both cyclooxygenase and hydroperoxidase *(HOX)* activity, to the unstable intermediates prostaglandin G_2 and prostaglandin H_2, respectively. The synthases are also termed *cyclooxygenases* and exist in two forms, *cyclooxygenase-1 (COX-1)* and *cyclooxygenase-2 (COX-2)*. Low-dose aspirin selectively inhibits COX-1, whereas high-dose aspirin inhibits both COX-1 and COX-2. Prostaglandin H_2 is converted by tissue-specific isomerases to multiple prostanoids. These bioactive lipids activate specific cell-membrane receptors of the superfamily of G-protein–coupled receptors, such as the thromboxane receptor, the prostaglandin D_2 receptors, the prostaglandin E_2 receptors, the prostaglandin F_{2a} receptors, and the prostacyclin receptor. *(From Patrono C, Garcia Rodríguez LA, Landolfi R, Baigent C. Low-dose aspirin for the prevention of atherothrombosis.* N Engl J Med *2005;353:2373-2383.)*

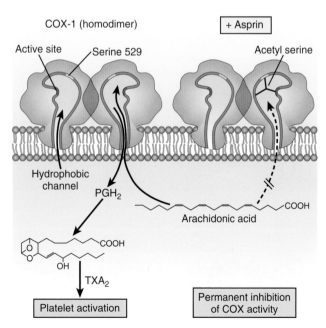

FIGURE 7-11 Mechanism of aspirin inhibition of cyclooxygenase. The target enzyme is platelet cyclooxygenase 1 (COX-1). The substrate of COX-1, arachidonic acid, is converted to prostaglandin H_2 *(PGH2)*, which is consequently converted to thromboxane A_2 *(TXA2)* by thromboxane synthase. Aspirin irreversibly inhibits COX-1 through acetylation of a serine residue at position 529 and obstructs the COX-1 channel just below the catalytic pocket. *(From Sweeny JM, Gorog DA, Fuster V. Antiplatelet drug resistance. Part 1: mechanisms and clinical measurements.* Nat Rev Cardiol *2009;6:273-282.)*

COX-1 and is highly sensitive to inhibition by aspirin; vascular PGI_2, a platelet inhibitor and a vasodilator, is derived largely from COX-2 and is less susceptible to inhibition by low doses of aspirin. Therefore, low-dose aspirin ultimately blocks platelet formation of TXA_2 preferentially and diminishes platelet activation and aggregation processes mediated by thromboxane (TP) receptor pathways. Because 1) platelets have minimal capacity for protein synthesis and 2) COX-1 blockade induced by aspirin is irreversible, COX-mediated TXA_2 synthesis is prevented for the entire life span of the platelet (approximately 7 to 10 days).[272,273]

Aspirin may also influence hemostasis and CV disease by mechanisms independent of prostaglandin production. Although less clearly defined, the non–prostaglandin-mediated effects of aspirin on hemostasis are thought to be dose dependent and unrelated to COX-1 activity. These effects include vitamin K antagonism, decreased platelet production of thrombin, and acetylation of one or more clotting factors.[274] In addition to its direct platelet effects, aspirin may alter the pathogenesis of CV disease by protecting low-density lipoprotein (LDL) from oxidative modification, improving endothelial dysfunction in atherosclerotic patients, and by attenuating the inflammatory response by acting as an antioxidant.[275]

Indication

Aspirin is an effective antiplatelet agent with proven benefit in the prevention of atherothrombotic complications of CV disease. Clinical trials and expert consensus statements evaluating the use of aspirin for primary prevention of CV events have been controversial, and description of such use goes beyond the scope of this chapter.[276-278] On the contrary, aspirin is still the antiplatelet drug of choice for secondary prevention of recurrent ischemic events in patients with various clinical manifestations of CAD, including stable CAD and ACS (unstable angina [UA], non-STEMI [NSTEMI]), and those undergoing coronary revascularization, either percutaneous or surgical.[276-278] In high-risk patients, particularly those with ACS or those undergoing PCI, aspirin should be given as promptly as possible at an initial dose of 162 to 325 mg followed by a daily dose of 75 to 162 mg.[279,280] Despite the established benefit, the absolute risk of recurrent vascular events among patients taking aspirin remains relatively high: an estimated 8% to 18% after 2 years.[281] Therapeutic resistance to aspirin might explain a portion of this risk, although the mechanisms remain uncertain; a combination of clinical, biologic, and genetic properties affect platelet function, and the redundancy of platelet activation pathways and receptors may contribute to recurrent atherothrombotic events despite the use of aspirin.[281]

Dosages

The optimal dose of aspirin for prevention of CV events has been the subject of controversy. Pharmacodynamic and in vitro studies have shown that aspirin may be effective in inhibiting COX-1 activity at doses as low as 30 mg/day.[272,273] The Antiplatelet Trialists' Collaboration demonstrated that oral aspirin doses of 75 to 150 mg/day are as effective as higher doses for long-term prevention of ischemic events. Aspirin doses less than 75 mg have been less widely assessed in clinical trials and thus are not recommended.[276-278] Importantly, higher doses of aspirin (>150 mg) do not offer greater protection from recurrent ischemic events.[276-278] This is also supported by the recently reported Clopidogrel Optimal Loading Dose Usage to Reduce Recurrent Events–Organization to Assess Strategies in Ischemic Syndromes (CURRENT-OASIS)-7 trial,[282] a large-scale prospective, randomized study that compared high- versus low-dose aspirin therapy in patients with ACS (n = 25,087) scheduled to undergo angiography. The study had a 2 × 2 factorial design, and patients were randomized in a double-blind fashion to high or standard doses of clopidogrel for 30 days. The study also included an open-label randomization to a high dose (300 to 325 mg/day) versus a low dose (75 to 100 mg/day) of aspirin. The trial did not show significant differences in efficacy between high- and low-dose aspirin. Although no differences were noted in major bleeds between the two aspirin doses, a trend toward an increased rate of GI bleeds in the high-dose group (0.38% vs. 0.24%; P = .051) was observed.

Based on earlier randomized trial protocols and clinical experience, the initial dose for the acute management of patients presenting with ACS should be between 162 and 325 mg.[279,280] However, given the results of biochemical studies on its mechanism of action, the lack of dose-response relationship in clinical studies evaluating its antithrombotic effects, and the dose dependence of its side effects, low-dose aspirin (75 to 162 mg) should be the preferred long-term treatment regimen.[279,280] This is also the case when aspirin is used in combination with other antiplatelet or anticoagulant medications. In fact, when given in combination with clopidogrel, the standard of care for patients with ACS, a post-hoc analysis from the Clopidogrel in Unstable Angina to Prevent Recurrent Events (CURE) study showed similar efficacy but less major bleeding with low-dose (<100 mg) compared with high-dose (>200 mg) aspirin.[283] Similarly, low-dose (<100 mg) aspirin should be considered in patients who require concomitant treatment with an anticoagulant (e.g., vitamin K antagonists).

Side Effects and Contraindications

The side effects of aspirin are primarily gastrointestinal and dose related and are ameliorated by using low doses (75 to 162 mg/day). Aspirin use can lead to gastric erosions, hemorrhage, and ulcers that can contribute to anemia.[274] In the Antithrombotic Trialists' Collaboration meta-analysis,[276-278] an approximate 60% increase in risk of a major extracranial bleed was reported with antiplatelet therapy. The proportional increase in fatal bleeds was not significantly different from that for nonfatal bleeds; however, only the excess of nonfatal bleeds was significant.[276-278] The risk of bleeding

complications with aspirin is reduced with low-dose regimens.[274] Use of aspirin is associated with a small increase in the incidence of hemorrhagic stroke in healthy men, but in secondary prevention trials, aspirin reduces the overall incidence of stroke. In one small study, aspirin (75 to 325 mg/day) was associated with a significant decrease in creatinine clearance and a decrease in uric acid excretion after 2 weeks of therapy in elderly patients.[284] The risk of bleeding is increased in subjects with coagulopathies and in those who are being treated with other anticoagulants (e.g., warfarin).[274] Concerns have emerged that some nonsteroidal antiinflammatory drugs (NSAIDs) may interfere with the action of aspirin by competing for the COX-1 active site when administered concomitantly, resulting in attenuation of aspirin's antiplatelet effects.[274] This may contribute to the increased risk of ischemic events in patients treated with NSAIDs, underscoring the need for careful consideration when prescribing NSAIDs to patients using aspirin.

Three types of aspirin sensitivity have been described: *respiratory sensitivity* (asthma and/or rhinitis), *cutaneous sensitivity* (urticaria and/or angioedema), and *systemic sensitivity* (anaphylactoid reaction).[274] The prevalence of aspirin-exacerbated respiratory tract disease is approximately 10%; for aspirin-induced urticaria, the prevalence varies from 0.07% to 0.2% in the general population.[285] In patients with CAD who come to medical attention with allergy or intolerance to aspirin, clopidogrel is the treatment of choice.[279] Desensitization using escalating doses of oral aspirin is also a therapeutic option.[286]

P2Y₁₂ RECEPTOR ANTAGONISTS

Mechanisms of Action

Platelet ADP-signaling pathways mediated by the $P2Y_1$ and $P2Y_{12}$ receptors play a key role in platelet activation and aggregation processes.[287-289] The $P2Y_1$ and $P2Y_{12}$ receptors are G-coupled, and both are required for aggregation. However, ADP-stimulated effects are mediated mainly by $P2Y_{12}$ receptor activation, which leads to sustained platelet aggregation and stabilization of the platelet aggregate; $P2Y_1$ is responsible for an initial weak and transient phase of platelet aggregation and change in platelet shape.[287-289] The $P2Y_{12}$ receptor is coupled to a G_i protein, which regulates activation of phosphoinositide-3-kinase and inhibition of adenylyl cyclase. Phosphoinositide-3-kinase activation leads to GP IIb/IIIa activation through activation of intraplatelet kinases, and inhibition of adenylyl cyclase decreases cAMP levels. Reduction of cAMP levels modulates the activity of cAMP-dependent protein kinases, reducing cAMP-mediated phosphorylation (P) of vasodilator-stimulated phosphoprotein (VASP) and eliminating its protective effect on GP IIb/IIIa receptor activation (Figure 7-12).[287-289]

Several families of $P2Y_{12}$ inhibitors have been developed (Table 7-8). Thienopyridine derivatives (ticlopidine, clopidogrel, prasugrel) are indirect, orally administered, and irreversible $P2Y_{12}$ receptor inhibitors that selectively and irreversibly inhibit the $P2Y_{12}$ ADP receptor subtype.[290] When given in combination with aspirin, thienopyridines have a synergistic effect and therefore achieve greater platelet inhibition than either agent alone.[291] The inhibition of platelet aggregation by thienopyridines is concentration dependent. However, thienopyridines are prodrugs and are thus inactive in vitro and need to be metabolized by the hepatic CYP system to give origin to an active metabolite, which selectively inhibits the $P2Y_{12}$ receptor.[290] Because blockade of $P2Y_{12}$ is irreversible, platelet inhibitory effects induced by thienopyridines lasts for the entire life span of the platelet.

Ticlopidine was the first thienopyridine to be developed, and it achieves significant inhibition after 2 to 3 days of therapy at the approved dosage of 250 mg twice daily.[287-289] Ticlopidine showed its superiority in combination with aspirin when compared with aspirin alone or with anticoagulation in combination with aspirin in trials for prevention of recurrent ischemic events in patients undergoing coronary stenting.[292-295] However, because of safety concerns, in particular neutropenia, ticlopidine has been largely

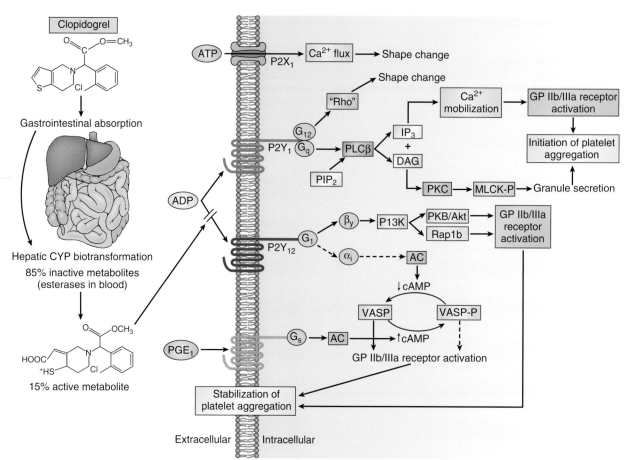

FIGURE 7-12 P2 receptors and mechanism of action of clopidogrel. Clopidogrel is a prodrug administered orally. Approximately 85% of the prodrug is hydrolyzed by esterases in the blood to an inactive carboxylic acid derivative, and only 15% of the prodrug is metabolized by the cytochrome P450 *(CYP)* system in the liver to generate an active metabolite. The active metabolite irreversibly inhibits the adenosine diphosphate *(ADP)* P2Y$_{12}$ receptor. Activation of the P2X$_1$ and P2Y$_1$ receptors leads to alteration in shape and initiates a weak and transient phase of platelet aggregation. P2X$_1$ mediates extracellular calcium influx and uses adenosine triphosphate *(ATP)* as an agonist. The binding of ADP to the G$_q$-coupled P2Y$_1$ receptor leads to activation of phospholipase C *(PLC)*, which generates diacylglycerol *(DAG)* and inositol triphosphate *(IP$_3$)* from phosphatidylinositol bisphosphate *(PIP$_2$)*. DAG activates protein kinase C *(PKC)*, leading to phosphorylation of myosin light-chain kinase *(MLCK-P)*; IP$_3$ leads to mobilization of intracellular calcium. The P2Y$_1$ receptor is coupled to another glycoprotein, which can lead to change in platelet shape. The binding of ADP to the G$_i$-coupled P2Y$_{12}$ receptor liberates the G$_i$ protein subunits α$_i$ and β$_γ$ and results in stabilization of platelet aggregation. The α$_i$ subunit leads to inhibition of adenylyl cyclase *(AC)*, which reduces cyclic adenosine monophosphate *(cAMP)* levels. This in turn diminishes cAMP-mediated phosphorylation of vasodilator-stimulated phosphoprotein *(VASP-P)*. The status of VASP-P modulates glycoprotein *(GP)* IIb/IIIa receptor activation. The subunit β$_γ$ activates the phosphatidylinositol 3-kinase *(PI3K)*, which leads to GPIIb/IIIa receptor activation through activation of kinases. Prostaglandin E$_1$ *(PGE$_1$)* activates AC, which increases cAMP levels and status of VASP-P. *Solid arrows* indicate activation. *Dashed arrows* indicate inhibition. *(From Angiolillo DJ, Fernandez-Ortiz A, Barnardo E, et al. Variability in individual responsiveness to clopidogrel: clinical implications, management, and future perspectives. J Am Coll Cardiol 2007;49:1505-1516.)*

TABLE 7-8	Current and Emgerging P2Y$_{12}$ ADP Receptor Antagonists				
AGENT	**CLASS**	**MECHANISM OF ACTION**	**MODE OF ADMINISTRATION**	**FREQUENCY OF ADMINISTRATION**	**APPROVAL STATUS**
Ticlodipine	Thienopyridine (first generation)	Prodrug; irreversible	Oral	Daily	Approved 1991
Clopidogrel	Thienopyridine (second generation)	Prodrug; irreversible	Oral	Daily	Approved 1997
Prasugrel	Thienopyridine (third generation)	Prodrug; irreversible	Oral	Daily	Approved 2009
Ticagrelor (AZD6140)	Cyclopentyltriazolopyrimidine	Direct acting; reversible	Oral	Twice daily	Phase III PLATO trial completed in 2009
Cangrelor	ATP analog	Direct acting; reversible	IV	NA	Phase III CHAMPION-PLATFORM and CHAMPION-PCI trials completed in 2009; additional trials ongoing
Elinogrel (PRT060128)	Quinazolinedione	Direct acting; reversible	IV and oral	Twice daily	Phase II trials completed in 2009

ADP, adenosine diphosphate; ATP, adenosine triphosphate; CHAMPION-PCI, A Clinical trial to Demonstrate the Efficacy of Cangrelor; CHAMPION-PLATFORM, Cangrelor Versus Standard Therapy to Achieve Optimal Management of Platelet Inhibition; IV, intravenous; NA, not applicable; PLATO, A Comparison of Ticagrelor (AZD6140) and Clopidogrel in Patients with Acute Coronary Syndrome.
From Angiolillo DJ, Ueno M, Goto S. Basic principles of platelet biology and clinical implications. *Circ J* 2010;74:597-607.

replaced by clopidogrel because of its superior safety profile; clopidogrel is currently the most broadly used $P2Y_{12}$ receptor antagonist.

Clopidogrel, a second-generation thienopyridine, differs structurally from ticlopidine by the addition of a carboxymethyl group.[287-291] The inhibition of platelet activation and aggregation processes by clopidogrel is concentration dependent. Clopidogrel is an inactive prodrug that requires a two-step oxidation by the hepatic CYP system to generate an active metabolite. However, approximately 85% of the prodrug is hydrolyzed by esterases to an inactive carboxylic acid derivative, and only 15% of the prodrug is metabolized by the CYP system into an active metabolite. CYP3A4, CYP3A5, CYP2C9, and CYP1A2 are involved in one oxidation step; CYP2B6 and CYP2C19 are involved in both steps.[290] The reactive thiol group of the active metabolite of clopidogrel forms a disulfide bridge between one or more cysteine residues of the $P2Y_{12}$ receptor, resulting in its irreversible blockade. Although clopidogrel has a half-life of only 8 hours, it has an irreversible effect on platelets that lasts from 7 to 10 days. Unlike ticlopidine, clopidogrel can be delivered in a loading dose, which allows antiplatelet effects to be achieved within hours of administration.

The approved loading and maintenance doses of clopidogrel are 300 mg and 75 mg, respectively.[279,280] However, numerous pharmacodynamic studies have shown a broad variability in levels of platelet inhibition in patients treated with clopidogrel.[296,297] A multitude of factors—some clinical (diabetes mellitus, ACS, obesity, smoking, drug interaction), some cellular (platelet turnover rates), and some genetic (CYP polymorphisms)—have been implied in this phenomenon.[296,297] Importantly, several studies have shown that reduced levels of platelet inhibition in clopidogrel-treated patients are associated with an increased rate of recurrent atherothrombotic events.[296,297] This has led some to investigate the effects of clopidogrel at higher doses. Studies conducted mostly in patients undergoing PCI have shown that regimens that use a high loading dose ($\geq$600 mg) can achieve more rapid and potent platelet inhibition compared with a lower 300-mg dose.[296,297] A high loading dose has also been associated with a reduction in periprocedural MI in patients undergoing PCI.[298-300] Although regimens that use a high maintenance dose (150 mg) also increase platelet inhibition, less evidence supports any meaningful clinical benefit with this dosing regimen.[301] These observations have also prompted further investigation in the field to identify $P2Y_{12}$ receptor antagonists with more potent and reliable platelet inhibitory effects, such as prasugrel and ticagrelor.[302] Although platelet function tests have been advocated to monitor the effects in patients treated with clopidogrel, to date limited evidence is available to support routine testing, as strategies aimed to optimize platelet inhibition using platelet-function assays have not shown improved outcomes in large-scale studies.[303] Several ongoing studies are evaluating the safety and efficacy of platelet function and genetic testing to guide oral antiplatelet therapy.[303]

Prasugrel is a third-generation thienopyridine that has been recently approved for clinical use in ACS patients undergoing PCI.[304] It is orally administered and, similar to other thienopyridines, it requires hepatic metabolism to give origin to its active metabolite, which irreversibly inhibits the $P2Y_{12}$ receptor. However, unlike other thienopyridines, prasugrel is more rapidly and effectively converted to an active metabolite[290] through a process involving hydrolysis by carboxyesterases, mainly in the intestine, followed by only a single hepatic CYP-dependent step that involves CYP3A, CYP2B6, CYP2C9, and CYP2C19 isoforms. This more favorable pharmacokinetic profile translates into better pharmacodynamic effects with more potent platelet inhibition, lower interindividual variability in platelet response, and a faster onset of activity compared with clopidogrel, even if used at high loading and maintenance doses.[305,306] A 60-mg loading dose of prasugrel achieves 50% platelet inhibition by 30 minutes and 80% to 90% inhibition by 1 to 2 hours.

Ticagrelor is a nonthienopyridine that forms part of a new class of $P2Y_{12}$ inhibitors called *cyclopentyltriazolopyrimidines* (CPTPs).[307]

Ticagrelor is a first-in-class CPTP. It is orally administered and differs in its mechanism of action from thienopyridines because of its direct (no metabolism required) and reversible inhibitory effects on the $P2Y_{12}$ receptor.[307] Ticagrelor is rapidly absorbed and has a half-life of 7 to 12 hours, thus requiring twice-daily dosing. Compared with clopidogrel, ticagrelor exhibits a higher degree of platelet inhibition, which is achieved more rapidly and with less interpatient variability.[308-310]

Indication

Clopidogrel is the antiplatelet treatment of choice for secondary prevention in patients with intolerance or allergy to aspirin. This indication is based on the Clopidogrel Versus Aspirin in Patients at Risk of Ischemic Events (CAPRIE) trial, which evaluated the efficacy of clopidogrel (75 mg daily) versus aspirin (325 mg daily) in reducing the risk of ischemic outcomes in patients with a history of recent MI, recent ischemic stroke, or established peripheral artery disease.[311] The trial showed a marginal, albeit significant, lower annual rate of the composite endpoint—vascular death, MI, or ischemic stroke—with clopidogrel (5.32% vs. 5.83%; $P = .043$). In patients with symptomatic atherosclerotic peripheral arterial disease, clopidogrel was even more effective than aspirin at reducing the incidence of vascular ischemic events.

Adding clopidogrel to aspirin has been shown to be particularly beneficial in the setting of PCI and across the spectrum of ACS manifestations. Table 7-9 summarizes the pivotal PCI and ACS trials that have compared dual antiplatelet therapy with aspirin and clopidogrel versus aspirin alone. In summary, the CURE, PCI-CURE, and Clopidogrel for the Reduction of Events During Observation (CREDO) trials all reported the long-term benefit of dual antiplatelet therapy (9 to 12 months) over single antiplatelet therapy.[312-314] The benefit of clopidogrel has also been demonstrated in patients with STEMI in the Clopidogrel and Metoprolol in Myocardial Infarction (COMMIT) and Clopidogrel as Adjunctive Reperfusion Therapy (CLARITY)-TIMI 28 trials when given in addition to aspirin or to aspirin plus fibrinolytic therapy.[315-317] In contrast to the positive results of these ACS/PCI trials, the Clopidogrel for High Atherothrombotic Risk and Ischemic Stabilization, Management, and Avoidance (CHARISMA) trial showed that after 28 months, addition of clopidogrel to aspirin was not better than aspirin alone in reducing the primary composite endpoint—CV death, MI, or stroke—in patients with CV disease or multiple CV risk factors (see Table 7-9).[318] In the subgroup of patients with clinically evident atherothrombosis, a significant reduction was seen in event rates with clopidogrel.[319] However, increased bleeding and higher mortality rates were reported in patients with multiple risk factors alone. Overall, the results of the clinical trial experience with clopidogrel suggest that dual antiplatelet therapy is useful in high-risk settings, such as in patients with various clinical manifestations of ACS or in those undergoing PCI; it is not beneficial, rather it is potentially harmful, in lower-risk patients.

Most recently, the CURRENT-OASIS 7 trial evaluated the efficacy and safety of double-dose clopidogrel in patients with ACS.[282] In this trial, double-dose clopidogrel was defined as a 600-mg loading dose and 150 mg once daily for 7 days, followed by 75 mg once daily. Standard-dose clopidogrel was defined as a 300-mg loading dose followed by 75 mg once daily. Patients were also randomized to receive low-dose (75 to 100 mg/day) or high-dose (300 to 325 mg/day) aspirin. In the overall study population, no significant difference was noted in the primary endpoint—composite of CV death, MI, or stroke—at 30 days between patients receiving double-dose clopidogrel versus those receiving the standard dose. However, in patients who underwent PCI, double-dose clopidogrel was associated with a significant reduction in the primary endpoint and in rates of stent thrombosis compared with the standard-dose regimen.[320]

Prasugrel is currently indicated to reduce the rate of thrombotic CV events, including stent thrombosis, in patients with acute ACS who are to be managed with PCI.[279,280] This indication derives from the Trial to Assess Improvement in Therapeutic Outcomes by

TABLE 7-9 Phase III Trials of Clopidogrel Therapy for Acute Coronary Sydrome, Percutaneous Coronary Intervention, and Secondary Prevention of Atherothrombotic Disease

TRIAL	N	PATIENTS	TREATMENT*	PRIMARY ENDPOINT	EVENT RATE (TREATMENT VS. CONTROL)	P VALUE
CAPRIE	19,185	Previous stroke or MI or symptomatic PAD	Clopidogrel vs. ASA	Ischemic stroke, MI, or vascular death at 1 year	5.3% vs. 5.8%	.043
CURE	12,562	NSTE ACS, unstable angina	Clopidogrel + ASA vs. ASA	CV death, nonfatal MI, and stroke at 1 year	9.3% vs. 11.4%	<.001
CREDO	2116	ACS with PCI	Clopidogrel + ASA vs. ASA	CV death, MI, or stroke at 1 year	8.5% vs. 11.5%	.02
PCI-CURE	2658	NSTE ACS with PCI	Clopidogrel + ASA vs. ASA	CV death, MI, or revascularization within 30 days	4.5% vs. 6.4%	.03
CLARITY-TIMI 28	3491	STEMI	Clopidogrel + ASA + FA vs. ASA + FA	Occluded infarct-related artery, death, or recurrent MI before angiography	15.0% vs. 21.7%	<.001
COMMIT	45,852	STEMI	Clopidogrel + ASA vs. ASA	CV death, reinfarction, or stroke at 28 days	9.2% vs. 10.1%	.002
CHARISMA	15,603	CVD or multiple risk factors	Clopidogrel + ASA vs. ASA	MI, stroke, or CV death at 28 months	6.8% vs. 7.3%	.22
CURRENT-OASIS 7	25,087	ACS with planned early invasive management with intended PCI	Double-dose clopidogrel + ASA vs. low-dose clopidogrel + ASA	CV death, MI, or stroke at 30 days	4.2% vs. 4.4% (overall cohort)	.37

*Clopidogrel was given as a loading dose of 300 mg then 75 mg daily in CURE, CREDO, PCI-CURE, CLARITY, COMMIT, and CHARISMA. Clopidogrel 75 mg daily was administered in CAPRIE. In CURRENT-OASIS 7, double-dose clopidogrel was defined as a 600-mg loading dose and 150 mg once daily for 7 days followed by 75 mg once daily. Standard-dose clopidogrel was defined as a 300-mg loading dose followed by 75 mg once daily. Patients were also randomized to receive low-dose (75-100 mg/day) or high-dose (300-325 mg/day) aspirin.

ACS, acute coronary syndrome; CAPRIE, Clopidogrel versus Aspirin in Patients at Risk of Ischemic Events; CHARISMA, Clopidogrel for High Atherothrombotic Risk and Ischemic Stabilization, Management, and Avoidance; CLARITY, Clopidogrel as Adjunctive Reperfusion Therapy; COMMIT, Clopidogrel and Metoprolol in Myocardial Infarction; CREDO, Clopidogrel for the Reduction of Events During Observation; CURE, Clopidogrel in Unstable Angina to Prevent Recurrent Events; CURRENT-OASIS-7, Clopidogrel Optimal Loading Dose Usage to Reduce Recurrent Events/ Optimal Antiplatelet Strategy for Intervention trial. STEMI, ST-elevation myocardial infarction; TIMI, Thrombolysis in Myocardial Infarction; ASA, aspirin; CVD, cardiovascular disease; CV, cardiovascular; FA, fibrinolytic agent; MI, myocardial infarction; NSTE, non–ST-segment elevation; PAD, peripheral artery disease; PCI, percutaneous coronary intervention.
From Angiolillo DJ, Ueno M, Goto S. Basic principles of platelet biology and clinical implications. *Circ J* 2010;74:597-607.

Optimizing Platelet Inhibition with Prasugrel (TRITON)-TIMI 38, which showed that prasugrel (60-mg loading dose, 10-mg maintenance dose) plus aspirin was significantly more effective than clopidogrel (300-mg loading dose, 75-mg maintenance dose) plus aspirin in preventing short- and long-term (up to 15 months) ischemic events in moderate- to high-risk ACS patients, with and without ST-segment elevation, undergoing PCI.[321] These events were mainly driven by a reduction in MI, but a marked reduction was also seen in stent thrombosis rates with prasugrel therapy. However, prasugrel was also associated with a significantly higher risk for major bleeding, including life-threatening bleeding, compared with clopidogrel. The increased risk of bleeding was greater in certain subgroups, which limited the net clinical benefit of prasugrel. Patients with prior stroke or transient ischemic attack (TIA) had net clinical harm from prasugrel, and it should be avoided in these patients. Patients aged 75 years and older and weighing less than 60 kg had no net benefit from prasugrel. In contrast, the net clinical benefit from prasugrel was greater in patients with diabetes and in patients undergoing PCI for STEMI, in whom there was no excess in major bleeding.[322,323] Based on TRITON-TIMI 38 data, prasugrel appears to be most appropriate for use in patients younger than 75 years who weigh at least 60 kg with ACS managed with PCI and no history of TIA or stroke.

Ticagrelor is approved in Europe and the United States for reduction of recurrent ischemic events based on the results of the Platelet Inhibition and Outcomes (PLATO) trial, which assessed the efficacy and safety of 1-year treatment with ticagrelor plus aspirin versus clopidogrel plus aspirin. It was recently reported in patients with and without ST-segment elevation ACS,[58,59] which included patients undergoing PCI and coronary artery bypass graft (CABG) surgery and medically managed patients. Subjects were randomized to treatment with either a ticagrelor 180-mg loading dose followed by 90 mg twice daily or a clopidogrel 300- or 600-mg loading dose followed by 75 mg daily for up to 12 months. Ticagrelor showed better short- and long-term outcomes (composite of CV death, nonfatal MI, or nonfatal stroke). Of note, the rate of all-cause mortality was 22% lower with ticagrelor versus clopidogrel. No significant difference in the rates of major bleeding was found using study definition criteria between the ticagrelor and clopidogrel groups, but ticagrelor was associated with a higher rate of major bleeding not related to CABG, including more instances of fatal intracranial bleeding.[324] Of interest, a predefined subgroup analysis of patients enrolled in the PLATO trial showed a borderline significant interaction with enrollment geographic area ($P = .05$), driven by a trend toward more efficacy of clopidogrel, rather than ticagrelor, among patients recruited in North America.

Dosages

The standard dosage of ticlopidine is 250 mg twice daily when used as an antithrombotic agent in patients with claudication, unstable angina, peripheral artery bypass surgery, and cerebrovascular disease. However, because of clopidogrel's superior safety profile, it has largely replaced ticlopidine.[325] The approved loading and maintenance doses of clopidogrel are 300 mg and 75 mg, respectively. In the setting of PCI, the recommended loading dose of clopidogrel is 300 to 600 mg.[279,280] A 300-mg loading dose of clopidogrel should be given to patients younger than 75 years, with STEMI treated with fibrinolytic therapy. This should be followed by a maintenance dose of 75 mg daily. No dosage adjustment is necessary for patients with renal impairment, including patients with end-stage renal disease.

In patients presenting with and ACS or in those undergoing PCI, a clopidogrel loading dose should be given as early as possible.[279,280] Pretreatment with clopidogrel prior to PCI improves 30-day outcomes compared with those not pretreated.[313,314] In a meta-analysis of the results of three randomized trials, clopidogrel pretreatment before PCI was found to be beneficial and safe regardless of whether a GP IIb/IIIa inhibitor is used at the time of PCI.[326] To achieve the pretreatment benefit of early clopidogrel, patients must be treated from 6 to 12 hours prior to PCI.[327] Use of a 600-mg clopidogrel load may allow a reduction in the pretreatment period to as little as 2 hours prior to PCI.[328] In patients coming to medical attention with an ACS, clopidogrel 75 mg daily should be given for at least 12 months irrespective of treatment management (medical, PCI, or CABG).[279] In patients undergoing PCI, 75-mg daily doses should be given for at least 12 months irrespective of whether the patient was treated with a bare-metal stent (BMS) or drug-eluting stent (DES).[279,280] Premature discontinuation of antiplatelet therapy, particularly in patients treated with a DES, is associated with a marked increase in the risk of stent thrombosis.[279,280] If the risk of morbidity because of bleeding outweighs the anticipated benefit afforded by thienopyridine therapy, earlier discontinuation should be considered. In patients undergoing DES placement, continuation of clopidogrel beyond 1 year may also be considered on an individualized basis.[279,280] In patients taking clopidogrel for whom CABG is planned and can be delayed, it is recommended that the drug be discontinued to allow for dissipation of the antiplatelet effect. The period of withdrawal should be at least 5 days in patients receiving clopidogrel.[279,280]

Prasugrel is currently indicated to reduce the rate of thrombotic CV events, including stent thrombosis, in patients with acute ACS who are to be managed with PCI.[279,280] These indications include patients with UA/NSTEMI and patients with STEMI managed with primary or delayed PCI. Treatment with prasugrel should be initiated with a single 60-mg oral loading dose, continued at 10 mg orally once daily. Lowering the maintenance dose to 5 mg in patients who weigh less than 60 kg may be considered, although the effectiveness and safety of the 5-mg dose has not been prospectively studied. Treatment is recommended for up to 15 months, although earlier discontinuation should be considered if clinically indicated, for example if bleeding occurs. In patients taking prasugrel, for those in whom CABG is planned and can be delayed, it is recommended that the drug be discontinued for at least 7 days to allow for dissipation of the antiplatelet effect.[279,280]

Ticagrelor is indicated for the prevention of atherothrombotic events in adult patients with ACS—UA, NSTEMI, or STEMI—including those managed medically and those who are managed with PCI or CABG.[329,330] Treatment should be initiated with a single 180-mg loading dose, continued at 90 mg twice daily. Treatment is recommended for up to 12 months. Earlier discontinuation should be considered if clinically indicated, for example if bleeding should occur. In patients taking ticagrelor, for those in whom CABG is planned and can be delayed, it is recommended that the drug be discontinued for at least 5 days to allow for dissipation of the antiplatelet effect.

Side Effects and Contraindications

Treatment with ticlopidine is associated with a high incidence of neutropenia (1.3% to 2.1%), which is usually reversible on discontinuation of treatment; however, in a few cases, it is irreversible and potentially fatal.[325] Patients must be monitored every 2 weeks, especially in the first 3 months of treatment, to detect this serious complication. Other rare but potentially life-threatening complications of ticlopidine therapy are bone marrow aplasia and thrombotic thrombocytopenia purpura (TTP). Other adverse effects include diarrhea, nausea, and vomiting, which are common with ticlopidine and may occur in up to 30% to 50% of patients,[331] and skin rash, which occurs rarely.[332] Clopidogrel represents an advance in antiplatelet therapy because its use is very rarely complicated by neutropenia (0.1%). In the Clopidogrel Aspirin Stent International Cooperative Study (CLASSICS), major peripheral or bleeding complications were similar between clopidogrel (1.3%) and ticlopidine (1.2%).[325] In the CAPRIE trial, GI hemorrhage occurred at a rate of 2.0% and 2.7% in patients treated with clopidogrel and aspirin, respectively.[311] The incidence of intracranial hemorrhage

was 0.4% for clopidogrel compared with 0.5% for aspirin. TTP is very rare with clopidogrel but is potentially fatal.[325] The additional bleeding risk of thienopyridines appears to depend on the clinical setting. The risk of major bleeding has been shown to be increased among patients treated with clopidogrel in the CURE trial, primarily GI bleeding.[312] However, in that trial, the risk of bleeding was increased in patients using higher doses of aspirin.[283] The incidence of intracranial hemorrhage (0.1%) and fatal bleeding (0.2%) was the same in both groups. In CREDO, CLARITY-TIMI 28, and COMMIT, no significant differences were seen in major bleeding associated with adjunctive clopidogrel therapy.[314-317] Much of the debate centers on the increased bleeding noted among patients treated with clopidogrel who subsequently require surgery. In the CURE trial, the overall benefits of starting clopidogrel on admission appear to outweigh the risks, even among those who proceed to bypass surgery during the initial hospitalization.[312] However, it is well demonstrated that preoperative clopidogrel exposure increases the risk of reoperation and the requirements for blood and blood product transfusion during and after CABG.[312] Drug regulating agencies have recently prompted a boxed warning based on the presence of a pharmacodynamic interaction between proton-pump inhibitors (PPIs) and clopidogrel that limits its antiplatelet effects.[333,334] This applies for PPIs that interfere with the activity of CYP2C19, such as omeprazole and esomeprazole, but not pantoprazole. A boxed warning was also issued for homozygote carriers of loss-of-function alleles of the *CYP2C19* gene, known as *poor metabolizers;* this condition affects approximately 3% of whites, 5% of African Americans, and 12% of Asians. These subjects should consider high clopidogrel dosing regimens or alternative treatment strategies not influenced by *CYP2C19* genotypes (e.g., prasugrel, ticagrelor). Overall, allergic or hematologic reactions occur in approximately 1% of patients taking clopidogrel, which is the thienopyridine of choice. Limited information on switching thienopyridines in patients with adverse reactions is available,[335] and desensitization protocols using escalating doses of oral clopidogrel have been proposed in allergic patients.[336]

Important safety information must be considered to minimize the risks associated with prasugrel.[279,280] Prasugrel should not be used in patients with active pathologic bleeding (e.g., peptic ulcer) or a history of TIA or stroke. Patients who have a stroke or TIA while taking prasugrel generally should have therapy discontinued. In patients aged 75 years and older, prasugrel is generally not recommended because of the increased risk of fatal and intracranial bleeding and uncertain benefit, except in high-risk situations—such as in patients with diabetes or a history of prior MI, in whom its effect appears to be greater—for which its use may be considered. Prasugrel should not be started in patients likely to undergo urgent CABG, and it should be discontinued at least 7 days before any surgery to minimize the risk of bleeding. TTP is rare with prasugrel, but it can be potentially fatal. Drug compatibility studies have shown that prasugrel can be administered with drugs that are inducers or inhibitors of CYP enzymes, including statins and PPIs (e.g., omeprazole), which have been shown not to interfere with its pharmacodynamic properties. Because of the potential for increased risk of bleeding, prasugrel should be used with caution when coadministering with vitamin K antagonists or NSAIDs used long term. No dosage adjustment is necessary for patients with renal impairment, including those with end-stage renal disease. Limited data are available on rates of cross-reactivity when switching to prasugrel in patients with allergic reactions to other thienopyridines.

Similar to prasugrel, the more potent antiplatelet effects associated with ticagrelor therapy give cause for caution with use in patients with active pathologic bleeding or propensity to bleed.[329,330] Ticagrelor therapy is associated with a higher rate of major bleeding not related to CABG, including more instances of fatal intracranial bleeding. Ticagrelor is contraindicated in patients with a history of intracranial hemorrhage, in those with moderate and severe hepatic impairment, and in patients treated with strong CYP3A4 inhibitors. Ticagrelor should be discontinued at least 5 days prior to CABG to minimize the risk of bleeding. Rates of other nonbleeding adverse events have been shown to be higher with ticagrelor versus clopidogrel, including dyspnea, syncope, ventricular pauses of 3 seconds or greater, and increases in serum uric acid and serum creatinine, which have been associated with high rates of treatment discontinuation. Ticagrelor should not be used in patients with marked bradycardia or sick sinus syndrome in the absence of a pacemaker. In addition, ticagrelor should be used with caution in patients with moderate to severe renal impairment and those receiving concomitant treatment with an ARB, a history of hyperuricemia or gouty arthritis, and a history of asthma or chronic obstructive pulmonary disease. Statins and PPIs (e.g., omeprazole) do not interfere with the pharmacodynamic properties of ticagrelor, although because of the potential for increased risk of bleeding, ticagrelor should be used with caution when coadministering with vitamin K antagonists or NSAIDs used chronically. No dosage adjustment is necessary for patients with renal impairment. Based on a relationship observed in the PLATO trial between maintenance aspirin dose and relative efficacy of ticagrelor compared with clopidogrel, coadministration of ticagrelor and a high maintenance dose of aspirin (>300 mg) is not recommended.

GLYCOPROTEIN IIB/IIIA RECEPTOR ANTAGONISTS

Mechanisms of Action

The GP IIb/IIIa receptor is an integrin, a heterodimer consisting of noncovalently associated α and β subunits; the GP IIb/IIIa receptor consists of the $\alpha 2b$ and $\beta 3$ subunits.[337,338] By competing with fibrinogen and von Willebrand factor (vWF) for GP IIb/IIIa binding, GP IIb/IIIa antagonists interfere with platelet cross-linking and platelet-derived thrombus formation. Because the GP IIb/IIIa receptor represents the final common pathway leading to platelet aggregation, these agents are very potent platelet inhibitors. Investigations of oral GP IIb/IIIa inhibitors have been stopped because of their lack of benefit and increased mortality rate in patients with ACS and in those undergoing PCI.[339] The reasons for these negative outcomes remain unknown. Currently, only parenteral GP IIb/IIIa inhibitors are approved for clinical use and recommended for patients with ACS undergoing PCI. Although GP IIb/IIIa inhibitors have been shown to reduce major adverse cardiac events—death, MI, and urgent revascularization—by 35% to 50% in patients undergoing PCI, their use has been limited because they are associated with an increased risk of bleeding, and other antithrombotic agents with a more favorable safety profile are now available.[340]

Three parenteral GP IIb/IIIa antagonists are approved for clinical use: *abciximab, eptifibatide,* and *tirofiban.* Abciximab is a large chimeric monoclonal antibody that has a high binding affinity that results in a prolonged pharmacologic effect.[341,342] In particular, it is a monoclonal antibody that is a fragment antigen–binding (Fab) fragment of a chimeric human-mouse genetic reconstruction of 7E3.[341,342] The Fc portion of the antibody was removed to decrease immunogenicity, and the Fab portion was attached to the constant regions of a human immunoglobulin. Abciximab binding is specific for the $\beta 3$ subunit and explains its ability to bind other $\beta 3$ receptors, such as vitronectin (αV $\beta 3$). Unlike the small-molecule GP IIb/III inhibitors eptifibatide and tirofiban, abciximab interacts with the GP IIb/IIIa receptor at sites distinct from the ligand-binding RGD sequence site (tripeptide Arg-Gly-Asp), and it exerts its inhibitory effect through a noncompetitive mechanism. Its plasma half-life is biphasic, with an initial half-life of less than 10 minutes and a second-phase half-life of about 30 minutes. However, because of its high affinity for the GP IIb/IIIa receptor, it has a biologic half-life of 12 to 24 hours. Because of its slow clearance from the body, it has a functional half-life of up to 7 days and platelet-associated abciximab can be detected for more than 14 days after treatment discontinuation.

The *small-molecule agents* eptifibatide and tirofiban do not induce immune response and have lower affinity for the GP IIb/IIIa receptor. Eptifibatide is a reversible and highly selective

heptapeptide with a rapid onset and a short plasma half-life of 2 to 2.5 hours.[343,344] Its molecular design is based on barbourin, a member of the disintegrin family that contains a novel Lys-Gly-Asp (KGD) sequence, making it highly specific for the GP IIb/IIIa receptor. Recovery of platelet aggregation occurs within 4 hours of infusion discontinuation.

Tirofiban is a tyrosine-derived nonpeptide inhibitor that functions as a mimic of the RGD sequence and is highly specific for the GP IIb/IIIa receptor.[345,346] Tirofiban is associated with a rapid onset and short duration of action, with a plasma half-life of approximately 2 hours. Like eptifibatide, substantial recovery of platelet aggregation is present within 4 hours of completion of infusion.

Indications

Evidence supports the use of GP IIb/IIIa antagonists in patients with UA/NSTEMI undergoing PCI.[347] American College of Cardiology (ACC) and American Hospital Association (AHA) guidelines advise that high-risk patients, especially troponin-positive patients, should receive a GP IIb/IIIa antagonist.[279,280] The small-molecule agents, eptifibatide and tirofiban, may be started 1 to 2 days before and continued during the procedure. However, recent clinical trial data do not support the routine use of upstream compared with ad hoc GP IIb/IIIa inhibition in ACS patients undergoing PCI.[348] Any of the GP IIb/IIIa antagonists may be started immediately before or during the procedure; however, none of the GP IIb/IIIa antagonists appears to be effective in the routine management of low-risk, troponin-negative patients in whom early coronary intervention is not planned.

The use of GP IIb/IIIa inhibitors, in particular abciximab, in STEMI patients undergoing primary PCI is supported by a meta-analysis of 11 randomized trials involving a total 27,115 patients that found that the administration of abciximab was associated with a significant reduction in the rate of reinfarction, as well as death, at 30 days.[349] However, most studies were conducted in patients who had not been pretreated with a $P2Y_{12}$ receptor inhibitor, and more recent data argue against routine use of upstream GP IIb/IIIa inhibitors in pretreated patients undergoing primary PCI.

The guidelines for use of GP IIb/IIIa inhibitors in patients not undergoing PCI are less clear. The small-molecule GP IIb/IIIa antagonists eptifibatide and tirofiban appear to reduce modestly the combined endpoint of death or MI with some increase in bleeding.[350] As shown by a meta-analysis, patients who underwent early revascularization appeared to derive the greatest benefit. The use of abciximab in patients with UA/NSTEMI in whom intervention is not planned is not indicated, based on the results of the Global Utilization of Strategies to Open Occluded Coronary Arteries (GUSTO) IV ACS trial.[351]

Dosages

The dosage of GP IIb/IIIa antagonist depends on the specific agent being used. The recommended dosage for abciximab is a bolus dose of 0.25 mg/kg followed by a 12-hour infusion at 0.125 µg/kg/min (to a maximum of 10 µg/min) for patients undergoing PCI.[347] No renal adjustments are required. In UA/NSTEMI prior to cardiac catheterization, a bolus of 0.25 mg/kg 18 to 24 hours before the procedure, followed by a continuous infusion of 10 µg/min until 1 hour after the procedure, has also been used.[352]

In the setting of PCI, a double bolus (10 minutes apart) and infusion regimen of eptifibatide is recommended (180-µg/kg followed by a second 180-µg/kg bolus followed by 2-µg/kg/min for a minimum of 12 hours); peak plasma levels are established shortly after the bolus dose, and a slightly lower concentration is subsequently maintained throughout the infusion period. Because eptifibatide is mostly eliminated through renal mechanisms, a lower infusion dose (1 µg/kg/min) is recommended in patients with creatinine clearance less than 50 mL/min. In UA/NSTEMI prior to cardiac catheterization, a 180-µg/kg bolus of eptifibatide is used followed by a 2-µg/kg/min infusion.[353] The infusion rate should be decreased by 50% in patients with a creatinine clearance of less than 50 mL/min.

Tirofiban has not been approved by the Food and Drug Administration (FDA) for PCI, although it is both approved and widely used throughout Europe for this indication (bolus of 10 µg/kg followed by infused 0.15 µg/kg/min for 18 to 24 hours). Several studies have documented that this approved bolus-and-infusion regimen for tirofiban achieves suboptimal levels of platelet inhibition for up to 4 to 6 hours that likely accounted for inferior clinical results in the PCI setting.[346] For this reason, a high-dose bolus regimen (25 µg/kg) to achieve more optimal platelet inhibition has been suggested.[354,355] Because tirofiban is mostly eliminated through renal mechanisms, the dose should be reduced by 50%, and adjustment is required for patients with renal insufficiency (creatinine clearance of <30 mL/min). In UA/NSTEMI prior to cardiac catheterization, tirofiban is used in a bolus of 0.4 µg/kg/min over 30 minutes followed by an infusion of 0.1 µg/kg/min.

Side Effects and Contraindications

The primary adverse reactions to GP IIb/IIIa receptor antagonists are bleeding and thrombocytopenia. Immune mechanisms responsible for the thrombocytopenia have been identified.[356] Although the overall incidence is relatively low, the effects may be life threatening. Thrombocytopenia with abciximab, as defined by a platelet count less than 100,000/L, occurs in 2.5% to 6% of patients; severe thrombocytopenia, a platelet count less than 50,000/L, occurs in 0.4% to 1.6% of patients in reported clinical trials. Severe thrombocytopenia requires immediate cessation of therapy, but thrombocytopenia is less common with eptifibatide and tirofiban. Thrombocytopenia in patients undergoing PCI is associated with more ischemic events, bleeding complications, and transfusions.[357] The platelet count typically falls within hours of GP IIb/IIIa administration. Readministration of abciximab, but not eptifibatide and tirofiban, is associated with a slightly increased risk of thrombocytopenia.[358] It is important to note that treatment with GP IIb/IIIa inhibitors can also cause pseudothrombocytopenia, which occurs as a result of artifactual platelet clumping in vitro, yielding a falsely decreased platelet count. This observation may be dependent on the use of specific anticoagulants for the assays that include citrate, ethylenediaminetetraacetic acid (EDTA), or nonchelating anticoagulants. The incidence of pseudothrombocytopenia may be as high as 2.1% with the use of abciximab. A smear to directly examine for the presence of clumped platelets may be required.

Novel Antiplatelet Agents

Several agents that inhibit different targets that mediate platelet activation and aggregation processes are under clinical development (Figure 7-13).[359] The P2Y$_{12}$ receptor has represented the platelet target subject to most of the clinical development in antiplatelet strategies over the most recent years, as highlighted above. All the currently available P2Y$_{12}$ receptor antagonists are administered orally, and agents for parenteral use are under clinical investigation. Cangrelor is a stable ATP analog and a highly selective reversible P2Y$_{12}$ receptor antagonist administered intravenously with a very short half-life.[360] Therefore, cangrelor achieves potent platelet inhibition very rapidly (>90% inhibition in a few minutes) with complete restoration of baseline platelet function within 60 minutes after treatment discontinuation. However, cangrelor failed to show any clinical benefit in two large-scale phase III trials of patients undergoing PCI.[361,362] This may have been attributed to limitations in trial design. Cangrelor is currently being evaluated in another large-scale phase III clinical trial of patients undergoing PCI and as a strategy to bridge patients to CABG, when discontinuation of oral P2Y$_{12}$ receptor therapy can be associated with an increased risk of ischemic events. Elinogrel is another P2Y$_{12}$ receptor antagonist that is the only agent available in both oral and IV formulations; it has recently completed phase II investigation.[363]

Another family of emerging antiplatelet agents is directed toward inhibition of the platelet thrombin receptor or protease activated receptors (PARs).[364] This pathway is of key importance because thrombin is considered to be the most potent activator of

platelets. PAR-1 is the principal thrombin receptor on human platelets; PAR-1 antagonists block the binding of thrombin to its receptor, thus inhibiting thrombin-induced activation and aggregation of platelets. Preclinical observations have shown that inhibition of the platelet PAR-1 receptor selectively interferes with thrombin-induced platelet activation but not with thrombin-mediated fibrin generation and coagulation that is essential for hemostasis.[364] PAR-1 antagonists may therefore have the potential for offering more comprehensive platelet inhibition without the liability of increased bleeding when used with current standard-of-care dual antiplatelet therapy. Two PAR-1 antagonists are currently being tested in clinical trials for the prevention of arterial thrombosis: atopaxar (E5555) and vorapaxar (SCH530348). Encouraging data have been shown in phase II clinical trials with both drugs.[364] However, the large-scale phase III trials raise concern over increased risk of bleeding. The Thrombin Receptor Antagonist for Clinical Event Reduction in Acute Coronary Syndrome (TRACER) trial compared vorapaxar with placebo in 12,944 patients who had ACS without ST-segment elevation. The trial was stopped prematurely for safety concerns, specifically because of increased rates of moderate and severe bleeding in the vorapaxar group and 5.2% in the placebo group (7.2% vs. 5.3%; $P < .001$) and intracranial hemorrhage rates (1.1% and 0.2%; $P < .001$). A trend was seen toward reduced ischemic events among patients receiving vorapaxar (2-year rate of cardiovascular death, MI, stroke, recurrent ischemia with rehospitalization, or urgent coronary revascularization of 18.5% vs. 19.9%; $P = .07$).[365]

Other agents are targeted to inhibit TXA$_2$-induced platelet activation mediated by thromboxan receptors.[366] The rationale for the development of TP receptor antagonists (e.g., terutroban) is that platelets may continue to be exposed to TXA$_2$ despite complete COX-1 blockade with aspirin. Preclinical and clinical studies are currently ongoing for this family of platelet inhibitors, as well as for other targets, including serotonin and collagen receptors.

Anticoagulant Therapy

The role of anticoagulant therapies is to block the activity of coagulation factors. The understanding of the role of coagulation factors in thrombotic processes has led to the development of anticoagulant agents that target specific markers, which in turn has also led to anticoagulant agents with more favorable safety (less bleeding) and efficacy (less thrombosis) profiles. Factors IIa and Xa are two serine proteases with central roles in the coagulation cascade that have been the targets in the development of numerous anticoagulant therapies. Anticoagulants are classified according to the target coagulation enzyme being inhibited: anti–factor IIa or antithrombins, anti–factor Xa, and so on. They are further categorized based on whether inhibitory effects are direct or indirect, warranting a cofactor.

UNFRACTIONATED HEPARIN

Mechanisms of Action

Unfractionated heparin (UFH) is a heterogeneous mixture of variable molecular weight (2000 to 30,000 Da) polysaccharide molecules. UFH has two structural components that are pivotal to determine its function: 1) a unique pentasaccharide sequence, mainly responsible for factor Xa inhibition, and 2) saccharide chain lengths greater than 18 units long needed to achieve thrombin inhibition. The pentasaccharide sequence is required for binding UFH to antithrombin (AT), thereby increasing the potency of AT by up to 1000-fold (Figure 7-14). This UFH-AT complex inactivates multiple proteases that include factors IIa, Xa, IXa, XIa, and XIIa. Factor IIa, or thrombin, and factor Xa are the most sensitive to activated AT, but thrombin is about 10 times more susceptible than factor Xa.[367] The pentasaccharide binding to AT causes a conformational change that converts AT from a slow to a very rapid thrombin inhibitor.[367,368] However, the UFH chain lengths must be sufficiently long to bridge between AT and thrombin to form a

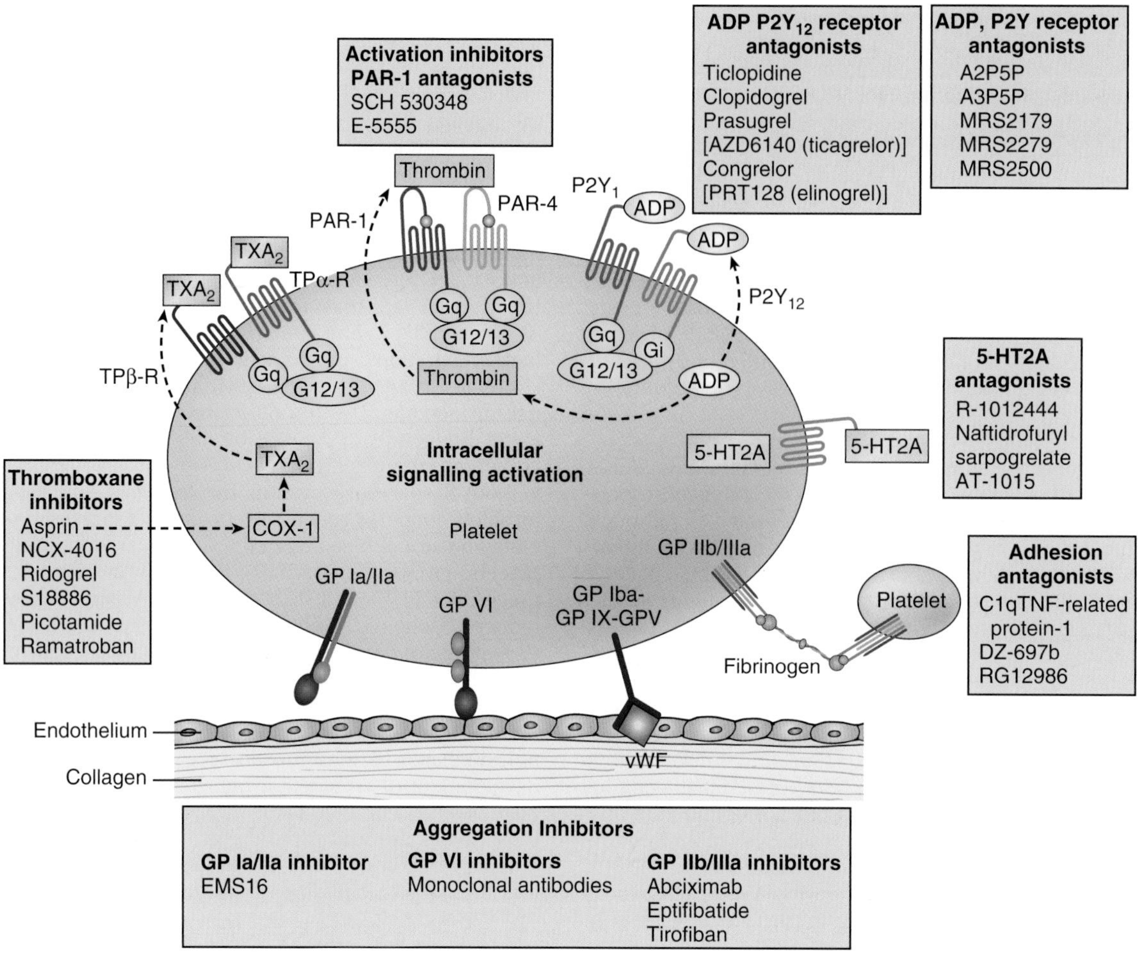

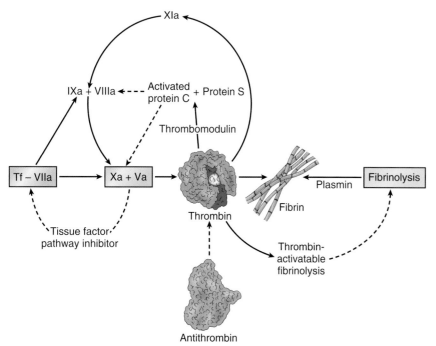

Activation inhibitors
PAR-1 antagonists
SCH 530348
E-5555

ADP P2Y₁₂ receptor antagonists
Ticlopidine
Clopidogrel
Prasugrel
[AZD6140 (ticagrelor)]
Congrelor
[PRT128 (elinogrel)]

ADP, P2Y receptor antagonists
A2P5P
A3P5P
MRS2179
MRS2279
MRS2500

Thrombin
PAR-1
PAR-4
P2Y₁
ADP
ADP
TXA₂
TXA₂
TPα-R
Gq
Gq
G12/13
Thrombin
Gq
Gi
P2Y₁₂
TPβ-R
Gq
G12/13
ADP

5-HT2A antagonists
R-1012444
Naftidrofuryl
sarpogrelate
AT-1015

Thromboxane inhibitors
Asprin
NCX-4016
Ridogrel
S18886
Picotamide
Ramatroban

TXA₂
COX-1
Intracellular signalling activation
Platelet
5-HT2A
5-HT2A
GP IIb/IIIa

Adhesion antagonists
C1qTNF-related protein-1
DZ-697b
RG12986

GP Ia/IIa
GP VI
GP Iba-GP IX-GPV
Platelet
Fibrinogen

Endothelium
Collagen
vWF

Aggregation Inhibitors

GP Ia/IIa inhibitor	GP VI inhibitors	GP IIb/IIIa inhibitors
EMS16	Monoclonal antibodies	Abciximab Eptifibatide Tirofiban

FIGURE 7-13 Sites of action of current and emerging antithrombotic drugs and antiplatelet agents. Platelet adherence to the endothelium occurs at sites of vascular injury through the binding of glycoprotein *(GP)* receptors to exposed extracellular matrix proteins (collagen and von Willebrand factor *[vWF]*). Platelet activation occurs via complex intracellular signaling processes and causes the production and release of multiple agonists, including thromboxane A₂ *(TXA₂)* and adenosine diphosphate *(ADP)*, and local production of thrombin. These factors bind to their respective G-protein–coupled receptors, mediating paracrine and autocrine platelet activation. Further, they potentiate each other's actions (P2Y₁₂ receptor signaling modulates thrombin generation). The major platelet integrin GP IIb/IIIa mediates the final common step of platelet activation by undergoing a conformational shape change and binding fibrinogen and vWF, which leads to platelet aggregation. The net result of these interactions is thrombus formation mediated by platelet-platelet interactions with fibrin. Current and emerging therapies inhibiting platelet receptors, integrins, and proteins involved in platelet activation include the thromboxane inhibitors, the ADP receptor antagonists, the GP IIb/IIIa inhibitors, and the novel protease activated receptor antagonists and adhesion antagonists. Reversible-acting agents are indicated by *brackets*. TP, thromboxane receptor; 5-HT2A, 5-hydroxytryptamine 2A receptor. *(From Angiolillo DJ, Capodanno D, Goto S. Platelet thrombin receptor antagonism and atherothrombosis. Eur Heart J 2010;31:17-28.)*

XIa
IXa + VIIIa
Activated protein C
+ Protein S
Thrombomodulin
Tf – VIIa
Xa + Va
Thrombin
Fibrin
Plasmin
Fibrinolysis
Tissue factor pathway inhibitor
Thrombin-activatable fibrinolysis
Antithrombin

FIGURE 7-14 Mechanism of thrombin generation. The activation of coagulation proceeds through a stepwise activation of proteases that eventually results in the fibrin framework. After vascular injury, tissue factor expression by endothelial cells is a critical step in the initial formation of fibrin, whereas the activation of factors XI, IX, and VIII is important to continue the formation of fibrin. The molecule of thrombin plays a central role within the coagulation cascade. The formation of the clot is highly regulated by natural anticoagulant mechanisms that confine the hemostatic process to the site of the injury to the vessel. Most of these natural anticoagulants are directed against the generation or action of thrombin and include antithrombin and the protein C system. *Solid lines* denote activation pathways, and *dashed lines* denote inhibitory pathways. *(From Di Nisio M, Middledorp S, Büller HR. Direct thrombin inhibitors. N Engl J Med 2005;353:1028-1040.)*

ternary complex to inhibit thrombin.[367,368] Once formed, this ternary complex inhibits thrombin to a greater degree than factor Xa. UFH chains fewer than 18 saccharide units are unable to form this ternary complex (UFH-AT–thrombin); therefore they primarily inhibit factor Xa via AT over thrombin, as described in the section on low-molecular-weight heparins (LMWHs).

Clearance of UFH occurs via two distinct processes: 1) the primary elimination pathway is by a rapid but saturable depolymerization process, in which UFH binds to endothelial cells and macrophages[369]; and 2) the slower, first-order mechanism of clearance occurs via nonsaturable renal clearance, which occurs mostly with supraclinical doses of UFH.[370] These kinetics make the anticoagulant response to heparin nonlinear at therapeutic doses, with both the intensity and duration of effect rising disproportionately with increasing dose. Thus the apparent biologic half-life of heparin increases from 30 minutes after an IV bolus of 25 U/kg to 60 minutes with an IV bolus of 100 U/kg and 150 minutes with a bolus of 400 U/kg.[371] Given the relatively rapid clearance, the anticoagulant effect of UFH is lost within a few hours after withdrawal, which can lead to a risk of reactivation of the coagulation process, known as *heparin rebound,* and thereby a transiently increased risk of thrombosis.[372]

UFH has anticoagulant activity and a variety of other biologic effects that result from its heterogeneous binding properties to a variety of cells and proteins. The most clinically significant nonanticoagulant effect of UFH is its potential to induce immune-mediated platelet activation, known as *heparin-induced thrombocytopenia* (HIT).[371]

Indications

UFH has been used in the management of UA/NSTEMI for many years, and its benefit when added to platelet inhibitors has been clearly established.[279,280] In addition, many of the platelet inhibitor trials have been conducted with the coadministration of heparin, which has established it as a class IA therapy when used with platelet inhibitors. The use of heparin as an adjuvant with fibrinolysis has also been examined in clinical trials. The use of subcutaneous (SC) or IV heparin as an adjunct to streptokinase remains controversial; however, heparin is recommended in streptokinase-treated patients at high risk of thrombosis.[279,280] Patients with STEMI who are receiving tissue plasminogen activator (tPA) should also be given heparin as a 60-U/kg IV bolus (maximum 4000 U at initiation of the tPA infusion, with an initial maintenance infusion of 12 U/kg/h at a maximum of 1000 U/h to maintain the activated partial thromboplastin time [aPTT] at 1.5 to 2 times the control rate).[280] A 48-hour infusion is likely to be sufficient if aspirin is being given, and IV heparin therapy should be sustained only if a high risk of systemic embolism is apparent, such as a large anterior MI, CHF, previous systemic embolus, or AF. Otherwise, only low-dose heparin therapy (7500 U/12 hours SC) is indicated as temporary prophylaxis against venous thrombosis, although it has been suggested that a similar approach may be used for patients who have received reteplase or tenecteplase (TNK).[280]

Dosages

In patients with ACS, the dose of UFH is usually adjusted to maintain aPTT at an intensity equivalent to a heparin level of 0.2 to 0.4 U/mL as measured by protamine titration or by an anti–factor Xa level of 0.30 to 0.7 U/mL. For many aPTT reagents, this is equivalent to a ratio of 1.5:2.5 (patient/control aPTT).[279,280] Treatment with UFH is usually initiated at clinical presentation in a patient with ACS. For UA/NSTEMI, an initial IV bolus of 60 to 70 U/kg (maximum 4000 U) followed by continuous infusion of 12 to 15 U/kg/h (maximum 1000 U/h).[279,280] For STEMI patients receiving non-streptokinase fibrinolytic therapy regimens, the dosing of UFH is at the lower end of this range, with an initial IV bolus of 60 U/kg (maximum 4000 U) followed by continuous infusion of 12 U/kg/h (maximum 1000 U/h), adjusted to maintain the aPTT at 1.5 to 2.0 times control (~50 to 70 seconds). Monitoring of aPTT should be performed 6 hours after any dosing change or if there is a

significant change in the patient's condition. The duration of UFH infusion after fibrinolytic therapy should generally not exceed 48 hours. Low body weight, older age, and female sex have been associated with higher aPTT responses to UFH, factors that should be considered in dosing decisions. Reversal of the anticoagulant effect of UFH can be achieved rapidly with an IV bolus of protamine using 1 mg of protamine to neutralize 100 U of UFH. Smoking and diabetes have been associated with an attenuated response to UFH. *Heparin resistance* describes the phenomenon of inadequate response to UFH, which necessitates higher than usual doses of UFH to achieve the desired anticoagulant effect.[373]

Side Effects and Contraindications

The primary side effect associated with the use of UFH is bleeding. The risk of bleeding with IV unfractionated heparin is less than 3% in recent trials.[374] The bleeding risk increases with higher heparin dosages, concomitant use of antiplatelet drugs or oral anticoagulants, and increasing age (>70 years).[374] Another problem associated with heparin is the development of HIT, usually between 5 and 15 days after the initiation of heparin therapy. A more rapid-onset form may occur in patients who have previously been exposed to heparin. HIT occurs when heparin binds to platelets, leading to platelet activation and the release of platelet factor IV.[375-377] Antibodies are generated against the heparin–platelet factor IV complex. The thrombotic processes associated with HIT may be due to immune-mediated platelet activation and microparticle formation. In the setting of HIT, an alternative antithrombin drug must be selected. Less commonly, long-term use of heparin can be associated with the development of osteoporosis and rare allergic reactions.

LOW-MOLECULAR-WEIGHT HEPARIN

Mechanisms of Action

The use of UFH has several limitations that include nonspecific binding, the production of antiheparin antibodies that may induce thrombocytopenia, the need for continuous IV infusion, and the need for frequent monitoring. Because of the many known limitations associated with the use of UFH, LMWHs have been developed. Issues such as the need for continuous IV infusion and frequent monitoring are not problems normally encountered with the use of LMWHs, which are potent inhibitors of both thrombin (anti-IIa effects) and factor Xa.[378] LMWHs can be given by subcutaneous administration and do not require monitoring because of their more rapid and predictable absorption. The LMWHs also produce fewer platelet agonist effects and are less often associated with HIT. Following SC injection, LMWHs have a more predictable anticoagulant response and greater than 90% bioavailability. Anti-Xa levels peak 3 to 5 hours after an SC dose of LMWH.[348,380] The elimination half-life of LMWHs is largely dose independent and occurs 3 to 6 hours following an SC dose. However, LMWHs are cleared by the kidney, leading to a prolonged anti-Xa effect and linear accumulation of anti-Xa activity in patients with a creatinine clearance below 30 mL/min.

LMWHs are produced through depolymerization of the polysaccharide chains of UFH, producing fragments ranging from 2000 to 10,000 Da.[348,380] These shorter chain lengths contain the unique pentasaccharide sequence necessary to bind to AT but are too short (<18 saccharides) to form the ternary complex crosslinking AT and thrombin. Therefore, the primary effect of LMWHs is limited to AT-dependent factor Xa inhibition. Compared with UFH, in which the ratio of factor Xa to thrombin inhibition is 1:1, LMWHs result in a factor Xa to thrombin inhibition ratio ranging from 2:1 to 4:1.[381] LMWHs also have reduced binding to plasma proteins and cells compared to UFH, thereby providing a more favorable and predictable pharmacokinetic profile.

Although many different LMWH preparations have been developed, enoxaparin is the most studied in clinical trials of UA/NSTEMI, STEMI, and PCI. The primary difference between the LMWHs is their molecular weight and therefore the relative anti-Xa/

anti-IIa ratio: enoxaparin has a mean molecular weight of 4200 Da with an anti-Xa/anti-IIa ratio of 3.8; dalteparin, with a mean molecular weight of 6000 Da, has an anti-Xa/anti-IIa ratio of 2.7.

Indications

The safety and efficacy of LMWHs have been established in patients with UA/NSTEMI and STEMI and in those undergoing PCI.[279,280,381] A meta-analysis by Petersen et al that pooled the data from six trials of enoxaparin in UA/NSTEMI showed significant reductions in death/MI by 30 days, especially in patients who had not received any antithrombin before randomization.[383] In contrast, the observations with other LMWHs, including dalteparin and fraxiparine, have been less encouraging. This may be due to enoxaparin's greater anti-Xa/anti-IIa ratio when compared with dalteparin, the greater severity of illness in the patients enrolled in the reported studies, and the extension of its antithrombotic actions to include inhibition of platelet aggregation by suppression of the release of vWF.[384] The largest and most recent trial to compare enoxaparin to UFH randomized 10,027 high-risk patients with UA/NSTEMI intended for an early invasive strategy using guideline-recommended aspirin, clopidogrel, and GP IIb/IIIa inhibitors.[385] At 30 days, the primary composite endpoint of death or MI was no different between enoxaparin and UFH. Thrombolysis in Myocardial Infarction (TIMI)-grade major bleeding was significantly higher with enoxaparin compared with UFH, which was largely attributed to anticoagulant switching effects as a result of prerandomization anticoagulant use. The ACC/AHA guidelines suggest that enoxaparin, but not the other LMWHs, is preferred over UFH for the medical management of UA/NSTEMI.[279,280] Patients with elevated troponin values may derive the greatest benefit.

The safety and efficacy of enoxaparin versus UFH as adjunctive pharmacotherapy for STEMI patients receiving fibrinolytics has been evaluated. When compared with UFH, enoxaparin added to fibrinolytic therapy reduced the risk of in-hospital reinfarction or refractory ischemia but increased the rate of intracranial hemorrhage among patients older than 75 years.[386,387] The ExTRACT-TIMI 25 trial investigators randomized 20,506 STEMI patients receiving thrombolytic therapy to enoxaparin or UFH for at least 48 hours.[388] Importantly, a lower dose of enoxaparin was given to patients older than 75 years (no bolus was given, and the SC dose was reduced to 0.75 mg/kg twice daily) and to those with impaired renal function defined as estimated creatinine clearance greater than 30 mL/min (1 mg/kg SC once daily). Enoxaparin treatment was associated with a significant reduction in the risk of death and reinfarction at 30 days when compared with UFH (9.9% vs. 12%; $P = .001$). TIMI major bleeding was significantly increased within the enoxaparin group (2.1% vs. 1.4% with UFH). The net clinical benefit—absence of death, nonfatal infarction, or intracranial hemorrhage—favored enoxaparin and was observed regardless of the type of fibrinolytic agent or age of the patient.[389,390]

Dosages

Anticoagulant therapy should be added to antiplatelet therapy in UA/NSTEMI patients as soon as possible upon arrival at the care center.[279,280] For patients in whom an invasive strategy is selected, enoxaparin (1 mg/kg SC twice daily) has established efficacy for patients in whom an invasive or conservative strategy is selected. Careful attention is needed to appropriately adjust the LMWH dosage in patients with renal insufficiency (1 mg/kg SC q24h for patients with an estimated creatinine clearance of less than 30 mL/min). If LMWH has been started as the upstream anticoagulant, it should be continued without stacking of UFH. If patients undergo PCI, enoxaparin can be administered in several ways. The first dosing option is 1 mg/kg SC twice daily; when this route is taken, it is important to ensure that the last dose of subcutaneous LMWH is administered within 8 hours of the procedure, and that at least two SC doses of LMWH are given before the procedure to ensure steady state. In the second dosing option, if the last dose of enoxaparin was given 8 to 12 hours before PCI, a 0.3-mg/kg bolus of IV

enoxaparin is recommended at the time of PCI. The third dosing regimen option is 1 mg/kg enoxaparin intravenously, if no GP IIb/IIIa inhibitor is used, or 0.75 mg/kg if a GP IIb/IIIa inhibitor is used at the time of PCI.[279,280] For elective PCI, an IV dose of 0.5 mg/kg was found to be safe in the Safety and Efficacy of Enoxaparin in PCI Patients, an International Randomized Evaluation (STEEPLE) study.[391]

In patients with STEMI treated with fibrinolysis in the presence of preserved renal function, the recommended dosing for enoxaparin is a 30-mg IV bolus followed by 1 mg/kg SC q12h (maximum of 100 mg for the first two SC doses) for patients younger than 75 years; for those older than 75 years, no IV bolus, 0.75 mg/kg SC q12h (maximum of 75 mg for the first two SC doses). Enoxaparin is preferred over UFH and should be given before fibrinolytic administration. Typically, the enoxaparin regimen is maintained for the duration of the hospitalization or through day 8, whichever comes first. Continuing therapy after discharge has not shown benefit.[280]

Side Effects and Contraindications

As with UFH, LMWH should not be given to patients with contraindications to anticoagulant therapy that include active bleeding, significant thrombocytopenia, recent neurosurgery, intracranial bleed, or ocular surgery. Caution should be exercised in patients with bleeding diathesis, brain metastases, recent major trauma, endocarditis, and severe hypertension. LMWH is associated with less major bleeding compared with UFH in acute venous thromboembolism. UFH and LMWH are not associated with an increase in major bleeding in ischemic coronary syndromes but are associated with an increase in major bleeding in ischemic stroke.[392] Bleeding complications are increased in patients with renal dysfunction, who should have their dose of enoxaparin appropriately titrated. If hemorrhagic complications occur as a result of LMWH, protamine sulfate may be administered to neutralize the anti-IIa effect of LMWH; however, the degree to which the anti-Xa activity of LMWH is neutralized by protamine is variable and uncertain. Patients treated with LMWH can develop HIT; therefore these drugs are not recommended for use in patients with documented or suspected HIT.

DIRECT THROMBIN INHIBITORS

Direct thrombin inhibitors (DTIs) currently available and approved for use include leprudin, argatroban, and bivalirudin.[393] All DTIs exert their anticoagulant effects by direct binding to thrombin (Figure 7-15). In turn, this inhibits thrombin activity and thrombin-mediated activation of other coagulation factors (e.g., fibrin from fibrinogen) as well as thrombin-induced platelet aggregation.[393] DTIs inhibit clot-bound and free thrombin, thereby providing a potential rationale for clinical use in the setting of ACS and PCI.

HIRUDIN (LEPIRUDIN)

Mechanisms of Action

Hirudin is a polypeptide found in the salivary glands of the leech *Hirudo medicinalis*, and it is among the most potent of the natural thrombin inhibitors. Various biochemical and molecular biologic techniques have been used to study the specific nature of the hirudin-thrombin interaction. The amino-terminal region of hirudin binds via a hydrophobic interaction with the apolar binding site of thrombin. The carboxy-terminal region appears to bind ionically to the anion binding exosite of thrombin. Direct interaction of hirudin with both the catalytic site and the anion binding exosite of thrombin probably accounts for its potent inhibition of all thrombin-mediated reactions, and this inhibition is equipotent toward free and fibrin-bound thrombin. The most commonly used measures for the anticoagulant activity of hirudin are the thrombin time (TT) and the aPTT. Hirudin does not have direct effects on platelet aggregation or secretion, and the bleeding time is not significantly altered.

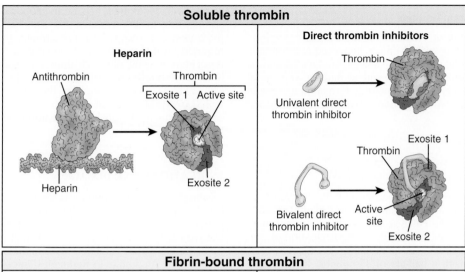

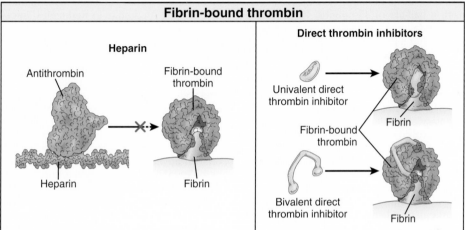

FIGURE 7-15 Mechanism of action of direct thrombin inhibitors compared with heparin. In the absence of heparin, the rate of thrombin inactivation by antithrombin is relatively low, but after conformational change induced by heparin, antithrombin irreversibly binds to and inhibits the active site of thrombin. Thus, the anticoagulant activity of heparin originates from its ability to generate a ternary heparin-thrombin-antithrombin complex. The activity of direct thrombin inhibitors (DTIs) is independent of the presence of antithrombin and is related to the direct interaction of these drugs with the thrombin molecule. Although bivalent DTIs simultaneously bind the exosite 1 and the active site, the univalent drugs in this class interact only with an active site of the enzyme. In the lower panel, the heparin-antithrombin complex cannot bind fibrin-bound thrombin, whereas given their mechanism of action, DTIs can bind to and inhibit the activity of not only soluble thrombin but also thrombin bound to fibrin, as is the case in a blood clot. *(From Di Nisio M, Middledorp S, Büller HR. Direct thrombin inhibitors.* N Engl J Med *2005;353:1028-1040.)*

Indications and Dosages

Both the TIMI 9 and the Global Utilization of Strategies to Open Occluded Coronary Arteries (GUSTO) II trials compared a single dose of heparin with a single dose of hirudin.[394,395] Both trials initially used high doses of hirudin (0.6-mg/kg bolus followed by 0.2 mg/kg/h) and weight-adjusted heparin, and both trials were terminated prematurely because of an unacceptably high rate of intracerebral hemorrhage in both treatment arms. These trials were continued as TIMI 9b and GUSTO IIb, using lower doses of both hirudin (0.1 mg/kg bolus followed by 0.1 mg/kg/h) and heparin (not weight adjusted). Results from the TIMI 9b trial showed heparin and hirudin to be equally effective as adjunctive therapies for streptokinase or tPA in individuals with acute Q-wave MI, without a difference in bleeding events. Results of the GUSTO IIb trial showed a marginally significant benefit of hirudin over heparin early after infarction in individuals with both Q-wave and non–Q-wave MI; however, this effect lessened over time.[396] Results from the Organisation to Assess Strategies for Ischemic Syndromes (OASIS)-2 trial suggest that recombinant hirudin may be useful when compared with heparin in preventing CV death, MI, and refractory angina with an acceptable safety profile in patients who have UA/NSTEMI and who receive aspirin.[397] In this study, 10,141 patients were randomly assigned heparin or hirudin for 72 hours.

At 7 days, 4.2% of patients in the heparin group and 3.6% in the hirudin group had experienced CV death or new MI (RR, 0.84; 95% CI, 0.69 to 1.02; $P = .077$).[397]

An approved clinical application for recombinant hirudin (lepirudin) is in the treatment of HIT. When compared with historic controls, lepirudin-treated patients had consistently lower incidences of combined endpoints primarily because of a reduced risk for new thromboembolic complications.[393] It is given as a 0.4-mg/kg bolus, followed by a 0.15 mg/kg/h infusion for 72 hours to maintain the aPTT between 60 and 100 seconds. It has a narrow therapeutic window and requires monitoring. During treatment with lepirudin, aPTT ratios of 1.5:2.5 produce optimal clinical efficacy with a moderate risk for bleeding, aPTT ratios lower than 1.5 are subtherapeutic, and aPTT levels greater than 2.5 are associated with high bleeding risk. The plasma half-life of hirudin is 60 minutes following IV injection.[398] Clearance occurs primarily through the kidneys, necessitating dose reduction in even mild renal impairment.[398] Bleeding events that require transfusion were significantly more frequent in patients taking lepirudin than in historic control patients. Lepirudin has also been used for anticoagulation in patients treated with extracorporeal circulation during open heart surgery; however, comprehensive data on this group of patients are lacking.

Side Effects and Contraindications

Hirudin should not be used when anticoagulation is contraindicated. The risk of bleeding with hirudin is increased in the setting of concomitant anticoagulation or platelet inhibitors. Hirudin is renally cleared and should not be used in patients with renal dysfunction. Lepirudin can induce antibody formation to hirudin in up to 40% of patients, who may then experience anaphylaxis if reexposed.

ARGATROBAN

Mechanisms of Action

Argatroban is a synthetic direct thrombin inhibitor derived from L-arginine.[393] This compound is a synthetic N2-substituted arginine derivative that binds to the catalytic site of thrombin with high affinity. It binds rapidly and reversibly to both clot-bound and soluble thrombin. Argatroban is metabolized via the CYP 3A4 pathway in the liver with a half-life of 45 minutes. Its reversible binding allows for rapid restoration of normal hemostasis on cessation of therapy. Argatroban has a predictable dose response that correlates with changes in anticoagulant parameters.

Indications

Studies with argatroban primarily have assessed its use as adjunctive therapy with fibrinolytics, in the treatment of HIT, and in patients undergoing coronary angioplasty.[279,280] Data with argatroban are limited; thus it is approved only for use in HIT. Argatroban causes a dose-dependent increase in aPTT and TT. The half-life of the anticoagulant effect is approximately 25 minutes when argatroban is used alone. For patients with HIT who are administered IV argatroban, benefit is noted as compared with historic controls. In HIT patients, argatroban therapy improves outcomes compared with historic controls, particularly relative to new thrombosis and death caused by thrombosis.[399]

Dosages

In individuals with unstable angina, argatroban (0.5 to 5.0 μg/kg/min for 4 hours) is administered. For patients with HIT, argatroban at 2 μg/kg/min is adjusted to maintain the aPTT at 1.5 to 3 times the baseline value for a mean of 5 to 7 days. Argatroban is not excreted by the kidneys, so dose adjustment with renal impairment is unnecessary.

Side Effects and Contraindications

Patients who have contraindications to anticoagulant therapy should avoid using argatroban because it is metabolized by the liver. In patients with hepatic impairment, the maximum concentration and half-life of argatroban are increased approximately twofold to threefold, and clearance is one fourth that of healthy volunteers.

BIVALIRUDIN (HIRULOG)

Mechanisms of Action

Hirudin-derived thrombin inhibitors known as *hirulogs* are synthetic peptides that contain the two distinct domains of hirudin with antithrombin activity. Subtle modifications of hirulogs can increase their affinity for thrombin to a level equal to that of native hirudin. Bivalirudin (hirulog-1) is a 20–amino acid polypeptide and is a synthetic version of hirudin. Its amino-terminal D-Phe-Pro-Arg-Pro domain, which interacts with the active site of thrombin, is linked via 4 Gly residues to a dodecapeptide analog of the carboxy-terminal of hirudin (thrombin exosite; see Figure 7-15).[400] Bivalirudin forms a 1:1 stoichiometric complex with thrombin, but once bound, the amino terminal of bivalirudin is cleaved by thrombin, thereby restoring thrombin activity.[401] Bivalirudin has a half-life of 25 min with proteolysis, hepatic metabolism, and renal excretion contributing to its clearance.[402,403] The half-life of bivalirudin is prolonged with severe renal impairment, and dose adjustment is required for dialysis patients.[404] In contrast to hirudin, bivalirudin is not immunogenic, although antibodies against hirudin can cross-react with bivalirudin with unknown clinical consequences.[393] Clinical trial experience supports the use of bivalirudin in patients with UA/NSTEMI,[405] in patients with STEMI undergoing primary PCI as an alternative to UFH plus GP IIb/IIIa inhibitor,[406] in patients undergoing CABG,[407] and in HIT.[408]

INDICATIONS AND DOSAGE

Bivalirudin is currently approved for use during PCI as an alternative to UFH. The benefit of bivalirudin as an anticoagulant in patients undergoing PCI has been demonstrated across the spectrum of CAD manifestations—stable CAD, UA/NSTEMI, and STEMI. In the Randomized Evaluation in Percutaneous Coronary Intervention Linking Angiomax to Reduced Clinical Events (REPLACE)-2 study, patients (n = 6010) undergoing urgent or elective PCI were randomized to receive bivalirudin with provisional GP IIb/IIIa inhibition or UFH with planned GP IIb/IIIa inhibition.[409] The study demonstrated that bivalirudin was noninferior to UFH plus GP IIb/IIIa inhibition with regard to ischemic endpoints and was associated with significantly less major and minor bleeding. In the Acute Catheterization and Urgent Intervention Triage Strategy (ACUITY) study, patients with UA/NSTEMI (n = 13,189) were randomized to one of three antithrombotic regimens: 1) UFH or enoxaparin plus GP IIb/IIIa inhibitor, 2) ivalirudin plus GP IIb/IIIa inhibitor, or 3) bivalirudin alone.[405] Bivalirudin alone was noninferior with respect to the combined ischemic endpoint, and it was superior in regard to bleeding (3.0% vs. 5.7% for UFH/enoxaparin plus GP IIb/IIIa; P < .001), leading to superior net clinical benefit with bivalirudin alone (10.1% vs. 11.7%; P = .02). Importantly, prerandomization treatment with UFH or enoxaparin did not abrogate the net clinical benefit of bivalirudin.

In the Harmonizing Outcomes with Revascularization and Stents in Acute Myocardial Infarctions (HORIZONS-AMI) trial,[406] STEMI patients (n = 3602) who presented within 12 hours after onset of symptoms were randomized to UFH plus GP IIb/IIIa inhibition or to treatment with bivalirudin alone for primary PCI. At 30 days, the bivalirudin-alone group demonstrated lower rates of death (2.1% vs. 3.1%; P = .047) and major bleeding (4.9% vs. 8.3%; P < .001) compared with the heparin plus GP IIb/IIIa group, leading to a significantly lower rate of net adverse clinical events (9.2% vs. 12.1%; P = .005). A 1% absolute excess rate of acute stent thrombosis occurred with bivalirudin alone, likely indicating the importance of clopidogrel or prasugrel preloading. After 1 year, the rates of cardiac mortality (2.1% vs. 3.8%; HR, 0.57; CI 0.38 to 0.84; P = .005) and all-cause mortality (3.5% vs. 4.8%; HR, 0.71; CI 0.51 to 0.98; P = .037) were significantly lower in the bivalirudin-alone treatment group.[410]

The current recommended dosage of bivalirudin in the setting of PCI is an IV bolus of 0.75 mg/kg followed by an infusion of 1.75 mg/kg/h for the duration of the procedure. Five minutes after the bolus, activated clotting time should be measured, and an additional 0.3 mg/kg should be given by IV as needed. Bivalirudin requires dosage adjustment in patients with renal dysfunction, except that no reduction in the bolus dose is needed for any degree of renal impairment; the infusion dose of bivalirudin may need to be reduced, and anticoagulant status monitored, in patients with renal impairment. Patients with moderate renal impairment (30 to 59 mL/min) should receive an infusion of 1.75 mg/kg/h. If the creatinine clearance is less than 30 mL/min, reduction of the infusion rate to 1 mg/kg/h should be considered. If a patient is on hemodialysis, the infusion rate should be reduced to 0.25 mg/kg/h, and the infusion may be continued for 4 hours after the procedure at the discretion of the operator.

Factor Xa Inhibitors

FONDAPARINUX

Mechanisms of Action

Fondaparinux is a synthetic analog of the AT-binding pentasaccharide sequence found in UFH. Fondaparinux is a selective factor Xa inhibitor that binds reversibly to AT to produce an irreversible conformational change at the reactive site of AT that enhances its reactivity with factor Xa.[411] Once released from AT, fondaparinux is available to activate additional AT molecules, and it has been shown to have 100% bioavailability after SC injection with rapid absorption, achieving a steady state after three to four daily doses.[411,412] The elimination half-life is 17 hours with clearance that occurs primarily via the kidney; it is therefore contraindicated in patients with severe renal impairment. Fondaparinux produces a predictable anticoagulant response and exhibits linear pharmacokinetics when given in SC doses of 2 to 8 mg or in IV doses ranging from 2 to 20 mg that result in anti-Xa activity that is approximately seven times that of LMWHs.[411,412] The anticoagulant effect of fondaparinux can be measured in anti–factor Xa units, although monitoring is not required. Fondaparinux does not affect other parameters of anticoagulation, including aPTT, activated clotting time, or prothrombin time.[411,412] It has minimal nonspecific binding to plasma proteins,[413] does not induce the formation of UFH–platelet factor IV complexes, and does not cross-react with HIT antibodies, making HIT unlikely to occur.[414]

Indications and Dosages

The efficacy and safety of fondaparinux (2.5 mg SC daily) compared with enoxaparin (1 mg/kg SC twice daily) in patients with UA/NSTEMI was evaluated in the OASIS-5 trial,[415] which showed that the primary outcome of noninferiority of combined death, MI, or refractory ischemia at 9 days was achieved with significantly lower major bleeding with fondaparinux, resulting in superior net clinical benefit with fondaparinux compared with enoxaparin. Importantly, mortality rate at 6 months was also reduced with fondaparinux compared with enoxaparin. However, in the group of patients who underwent PCI, more catheter-related thrombus formation was evident with fondaparinux, indicating that anticoagulation with fondaparinux alone is insufficient for PCI and adjunctive UFH should be used.[415,416]

In patients with STEMI, fondaparinux was evaluated as an alternative to standard adjunctive anticoagulation in the OASIS-6 trial.[417] Fondaparinux was administered 2.5 mg SC daily for 8 days and compared with either no UFH (stratum I) or UFH infusion (stratum II) for 48 hours. Primary PCI was performed in approximately 25% of patients; thrombolytic therapy was administered to approximately half the patients, 73% of whom received streptokinase. The primary outcome of 30-day death or MI was significantly reduced in patients who received fondaparinux, although this was driven by patients in stratum I only. Patients who either underwent primary PCI or were in stratum II had no significant benefit with fondaparinux. Of concern, patients who underwent primary PCI with fondaparinux had more catheter-related thrombi, more coronary complications, and a trend toward higher rates of death and MI compared with UFH. It is important to note that despite guideline recommendations for the use of fondaparinux in ACS, it is not approved for such use by the FDA in the United States.

Based on a dose-ranging study of fondaparinux versus enoxaparin in the setting of UA/NSTEMI, fondaparinux 2.5 mg daily was shown to have the best efficacy and safety profile when compared with 4-, 8-, and 12-mg doses of fondaparinux and with enoxaparin 1 mg/kg twice daily.[418] In patients with moderate renal impairment (30 to 50 mL/min), the dose of fondaparinux should be reduced by half.[393] Coagulation monitoring is not recommended. Fondaparinux is recommended for UA/NSTEMI ACS patients in whom an early conservative or a delayed invasive strategy of management is considered. For patients treated with upstream fondaparinux who are undergoing PCI, additional IV boluses of UFH should be given at the time of the procedure, along with additional IV doses of fondaparinux (2.5 mg if the patient is also receiving a GP IIb/IIIa inhibitor, 5 mg if not). For patients with acute STEMI who are not receiving reperfusion therapy, the recommended dosing for fondaparinux is 2.5 mg IV for the first dose and then SC once daily for up to 9 days. For patients with acute STEMI receiving fibrinolytic therapy, fondaparinux (2.5 mg IV for the first dose, SC once daily for up to 9 days) could be used as an alternative to heparin, but it should not be used in patients with acute STEMI who are undergoing primary PCI.[279,280]

Oral Anticoagulants

WARFARIN

Mechanisms of Action

Warfarin and coumarin derivatives are vitamin K antagonists that prevent the cyclic interconversion of vitamin K and its 2,3-epoxide. Vitamin K is a cofactor for posttranslational carboxylation of glutamic acid residues that are on the amino terminus of vitamin K–dependent coagulation factors—including factors II, VII, IX, and X—and anticoagulant proteins C and S. The antithrombotic properties of coumarin derivatives are delayed for 72 to 96 hours.

Indications

Although standard for the treatment and prevention of venous thrombosis, oral anticoagulant therapy has also been investigated in patients with ischemic heart disease. Warfarin, in combination with aspirin or given alone, was superior to aspirin alone in reducing the incidence of composite events after an acute MI but was associated with a higher risk of bleeding.[419] In the Warfarin-Aspirin Reinfaction Study (WARIS II), the combination therapy targeted an international normalized ratio (INR) of 2 to 2.5, and the warfarin-alone group had a target INR of 2.8 to 4.2. Using a fixed, low dose of warfarin added to aspirin in the long term after MI did not demonstrate reduction in the combined risk of CV death, reinfarction, or stroke. A fixed, low dose of warfarin added to aspirin reduced the risk of stroke, but this was a secondary endpoint. The combination of aspirin and warfarin was also associated with an increased risk of bleeding.[420] Although the studies have been mixed, current available data based on nearly 20,000 patients participating in randomized clinical trials demonstrate that, when given in adequate doses, oral anticoagulants reduce the rates of reinfarction and thromboembolic stroke, but they do so at the cost of increased rates of hemorrhagic events.[421] However, the use of warfarin, even in controlled trials, is fraught with difficulties, as in the WARIS II study, in which the INR was below target in about one third of patients, and those older than 75 years were excluded.[421]

Dosages

Dosages of warfarin should be adjusted based on the INR, which in turn is based on the use of an International Sensitivity Index (ISI) assigned to each thromboplastin reagent so as to standardize the dose.

Side Effects and Contraindications

Oral anticoagulants have a narrow therapeutic window and a highly variable dose-response relation. The most frequent complication of warfarin therapy is bleeding. The major determinants of vitamin K-antagonist–induced bleeding are the intensity of the anticoagulant effect, underlying patient characteristics, and the length of therapy. Good evidence shows that vitamin K antagonist therapy with a targeted INR of 2.5 (range, 2.0 to 3.0) is associated with a lower risk of bleeding than is therapy targeted at an INR above 3.0.[392] A rare complication of warfarin therapy is skin necrosis. Warfarin-induced skin necrosis usually develops soon after initiation of therapy and is more frequent in patients with protein

C or S deficiency. Patients with known protein C or S deficiencies should be started on warfarin only after therapeutic doses of heparin have been initiated. Warfarin is also teratogenic, and its use should be avoided during pregnancy, although the use of oral anticoagulants versus UFH/LMWH during pregnancy is an ongoing area of investigation.

NOVEL ANTICOAGULANT AGENTS

Warfarin has limitations that are well established; these include a narrow therapeutic index, the need for impeccable dose management, and interactions with other drugs, foods, and comorbid conditions. Oral factor IIa and Xa inhibitors are currently under intense clinical investigation for deep venous thrombosis (DVT), AF, and ACS, with the hopes of replacing the coumarins for the long-term treatment of thromboembolic disorders (Figure 7-16).[422] Ximelagatran was a direct oral antithrombin agent thought to be promising because of its rapid absorption, low protein binding, lack of drug interactions, and fixed dose. However, ximelagatran failed to receive FDA approval because of the potential for hepatotoxicity.[423] Dabigatran is a direct oral thrombin inhibitor that has been recently approved for clinical use as a replacement for warfarin in patients with AF in the Randomized Evaluation of Long-Term Anticoagulant Therapy (RE-LY) trial.[424] Dabigatran has a half-life of 12 to 17 hours and is administered twice daily without need for monitoring. Dabigatran administered at a dose of 150 mg twice daily was associated with lower rates of stroke and systemic embolism, but rates of major hemorrhage as compared with warfarin were similar; at a dose of 110 mg twice daily, rates of stroke and systemic embolism were similar, but rates of major hemorrhage were lower. The efficacy and safety of dabigatran in ACS is under investigation. Apixiban, an oral anti-Xa inhibitor, was evaluated in ACS in the Apixaban for Prevention of Acute Ischemic and Safety Events (APPRAISE) trial, which randomized 1715 patients to four doses of apixiban—2.5 mg twice daily, 5 mg twice daily, 10 mg daily, and 10 mg twice daily—versus placebo. The two 10-mg doses were stopped early because of excess bleeding. An increase in bleeding was also observed at the lower doses, although a reduction was evident in ischemic events compared with placebo.[425] APPRAISE 2, the large phase III trial, was terminated prematurely after 7392 patients were enrolled because of increased bleeding without any clear counterbalance in reduction in ischemic events. The risk of TIMI major bleeding was more than twofold higher among patients receiving the 5-mg dose twice daily of apixiban.[426]

Rivaroxaban was evaluated in a large phase II trial[427] and in the 15,526 patients in the Anti-Xa Therapy to Lower Cardiovascular Events in Addition to Standard Therapy in Subjects with Acute Coronary Syndrome–TIMI 51 (ATLAS ACS 2-TIMI 51) trial.[428] In that trial, both the 2.5-mg dose twice daily and the 5-mg dose twice daily reduced the risk of CV death, MI, and stroke (9.1% vs. 10.7%; $P = .02$; 8.8% vs. 10.7%; $P = .03$). The 2.5 mg twice-daily dose reduced the rates of death from CV causes (2.7% vs. 4.1%; $P = .002$) and from any cause (2.9% vs. 4.5%; $P = .002$), a survival benefit that was not seen with the 5-mg dose. Compared with placebo, rivaroxaban increased the rates of non-CABG major bleeding (2.1% vs. 0.6%; $P < .001$) and intracranial hemorrhage (0.6% vs. 0.2%; $P = .009$), without a significant increase in fatal bleeding (0.3% vs. 0.2%; $P = .66$). Thus, even when used together with aspirin and clopidogrel, a very low dose of rivaroxaban reduced the risk of adverse ischemic events, including death.

Other novel anticoagulant strategies are under investigation that use recombinant proteins directed at the initiation of coagulation, targeting tissue factor or factor VII.[429,430] Another novel anticoagulant approach involves using RNA aptamer technology to target coagulation factors, such as factor IXa.[431] The advantage of this approach is in the ability to initiate rapid anticoagulation that can be reversed immediately with a complementary RNA strand.

FIBRINOLYTICS

Fibrinolytic drugs have been incorporated into the standard management of STEMI. With these therapies, short-term mortality rate gains are accompanied by an improvement in ventricular function and a reduction in major CV complications. Follow-up studies have demonstrated that these short-term gains, after a single fibrinolytic administration, are sustained for at least 8 years. Of note, only about 50% of patients achieve normal epicardial coronary artery flow (TIMI 3) within 90 minutes of administration of tPA or TNK.

Mechanisms of Action

Plasminogen is a proenzyme that is converted to the active enzyme plasmin by plasminogen activators. Plasmin degrades fibrin into soluble degradation products. Plasminogen activators cause thrombus dissolution by initiating this cascade, a process inhibited by plasminogen activator inhibitors that prevent excessive plasminogen activation by tPA and urokinase-type plasminogen activator (uPA).

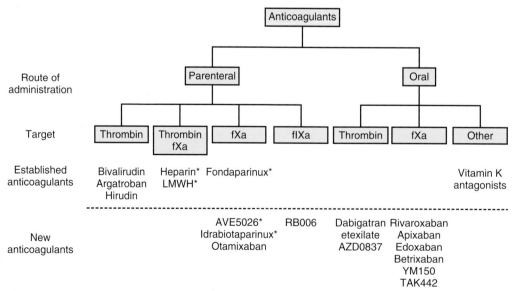

FIGURE 7-16 Classification of established anticoagulants and new anticoagulants. fIXa, factor IXa. *Indirectly inhibits coagulation by interacting with antithrombin. AVE5026 is an ultralow-molecular-weight heparin that primarily inhibits fXa and has minimal activity against thrombin. (*From Eikelboom JW, Weitz JI. New anticoagulants. Circulation 2010;121:1523-1532.*)

TABLE 7-10   Properties of Fibrinolytic Therapies

CHARACTERISTIC	SK	tPA	rPA	nPA	TNK
Mode of administration	Infusion over 30-60 min	Bolus + infusion over 90 min	Double bolus 30 min apart	Single bolus	Single bolus
Dose	1.5 × 106 U	≤100 mg*	10 U + 10 U	120 ku/kg	30-50 mg/kg
Weight-adjusted dosing	No	Yes	No	Yes	Yes
Antigenicity	++	—	—	—	—
Plasma half-life, mean (SD)	30 min	3.5 (1.4) min	14 (6) min	47 (13) min	17 (7) min
Plasma clearance (mL/min), mean (SD)	—	572 (132)	283 (101)	57 (19)	151 (55)
Excretion	Hepatic	Hepatic	Renal/hepatic	Hepatic	Hepatic
Fibrin specificity†	—	++	+	+	++++
90-min patency	++	+++	++++	+++/++++	+++/++++
Mortality rate reduction	+	++	++	+++	++
Hemorrhagic stroke	++	++	++	+++	++
Cost‡	+	+++	+++	NA	+++

*Bolus, 15 mg; infusion, 0.75 mg/kg, not to exceed 50 mg/30 min; 0.5 mg/kg, not to exceed 35 mg/h.
†Semiquantitative scale based on depletion of fibrinogen and other measures of systemic anticoagulation.
‡Based on average wholesale price listings in *Drug Topics Red Book 2000* and November Update (Tenecteplase [TNKase] for thrombolysis. *Med Lett Drugs Ther* 2000;42:106.
NA, not applicable (nPA is not commercially available); nPA, lanoteplase; rPA, reteplase; SD, standard deviation; SK, streptokinase; TNK, tenecteplase; tPA, tissue plasminogen activator (alteplase).
Modified from Antman EM, Anbe DT, Armstrong PW, et al. ACC/AHA guidelines for the management of patients with ST-elevation myocardial infarction: a report of the American College of Cardiology/American HeartAssociation Task Force on Practice Guidelines (Committee to Revise the 1999 Guidelines for the Management of Patients with Acute Myocardial Infarction). *J Am Coll Cardiol* 2004;44(3):E1-E211; and Llevadot J, Giugliano RP, Antman EM, et al. Bolus fibrinolytic therapy in acute myocardial infarction. *JAMA* 2001;286(4):442-449.

Indications

Fibrinolytic therapy has been used in patients who have had at least 30 minutes of ischemic chest pain and either 1-mm ST-segment elevation in at least two adjacent limb leads, 2-mm ST-segment elevation in at least two adjacent precordial leads, or complete left bundle branch block (Table 7-10).[432] Patients should be treated within 12 hours of the onset of symptoms. Most important in terms of survival advantage is the time from the onset of symptoms to the initiation of therapy, with the greatest benefit achieved by treatment within the first hour. The mortality rate benefit is greater in the setting of anterior STEMI. No benefit is seen when fibrinolytic therapy is used for unstable coronary syndromes not associated with ST-segment elevation.[433]

Dosages

Streptokinase (SK) is a bacterial protein that consists of three plasminogen-binding domains, although none can activate plasminogen independently. SK is usually administered as an IV infusion of 1.5 million U over 30 to 60 minutes. Once bound to plasminogen, this activator complex of SK-plasminogen converts plasminogen to the active enzyme, plasmin, which cleaves fibrin. Plasmin generation by SK is not fibrin specific, and treatment with SK leads to proteolysis of fibrinogen, factor V, and factor III and to depletion of clotting factors that may result in increased bleeding. SK is highly immunogenic and neutralizing antibody formation generally precludes readministration. With IV administration, peak plasma levels occur rapidly, with maximal fibrinolytic effect after 30 minutes. The plasma half-life is 30 to 40 minutes with hepatic-mediated clearance.[434,435] SK remains the most frequently administered fibrinolytic agent worldwide.

Second-generation agents were designed for bolus administration, enhanced potency, and plasminogen activator inhibitor (PAI)-1 resistance to enhance the efficiency of reperfusion.[436] The relative fibrin specificity of a thrombolytic agent may play an important role in its efficacy and safety profile, although clinical data are controversial. Recombinant tPA is relatively fibrin selective. The most commonly used dosage of tPA is a 15-mg bolus over 3 minutes, followed by a 0.75-mg/kg infusion (not to exceed 50 mg) over 30 minutes, and then 0.5 mg/kg (not to exceed 35 mg/kg) over an additional 60 minutes.

Reteplase is a truncated form of tPA that lacks the first Kringle domain. It has a longer half-life compared with tPA but has not shown superiority over accelerated tPA. It is administered as two IV boluses of 10 U given 30 min apart with each bolus administered over 2 min.

Tenecteplase is a mutated form of tPA that has an extended half-life and greater fibrin specificity. It is equivalent to accelerated tPA and can be given in a single bolus (5 to 10 seconds) in a dose according to body weight: 30 mg to patients weighing less than 60 kg; 35 mg to patients weighing 60 to 69.9 kg; 40 mg to patients weighing 70.0 to 79.9 kg; 45 mg to patients weighing 80.0 to 89.9 kg; and 50 mg to patients weighing 90 kg or more.[437]

Recent clinical trials of fibrinolytic agents have focused on adjunctive pharmacotherapy with antiplatelet and anticoagulant agents to improve efficacy and safety. The Enoxaparin and Thrombolysis Reperfusion for Acute Myocardial Infarction Treatment (ExTRACT) TIMI 25 trial randomized STEMI patients treated with fibrinolysis (20% SK) to receive enoxaparin throughout the index hospitalization or weight-based UFH for at least 48 hours.[388] Major bleeding occurred more frequently with enoxaparin in the first 30 days, but the rate of intracranial hemorrhage was similar despite the longer duration of enoxaparin therapy. Net clinical benefit favored enoxaparin over UFH. Clopidogrel therapy (75 mg daily) with or without a 300-mg loading dose was shown to improve infarct-related artery patency when added to thrombolytic therapy in STEMI patients.[315,316] Importantly, the 36% relative reduction in the combined endpoint of TIMI 0/1 flow, death, or recurrent MI before angiography was seen regardless of the type of thrombolytic agent used.[316]

Side Effects and Contraindications

Bleeding is the major adverse side effect common to fibrinolytic agents. The risk of intracranial hemorrhage averages 0.5% with the relatively fibrin-specific agents; rates of intracranial hemmorhage rise to 1% to 2% with increasing patient age. SK is known to cause allergic reactions in approximately 5% of patients, but anaphylaxis is rare. Absolute and relative contraindications to fibrinolytic therapy are listed in Box 7-2.

Box 7-2 Absolute and Relative Contraindications for Fibrinolysis in STEMI

Absolute Contraindications

- Any prior ICH
- Known structural cerebrovascular lesion (e.g., arteriovenous malformation)
- Known malignant intracranial neoplasm, primary or metastatic
- Ischemic stroke within 3 months, except acute ischemic stroke within 3 hours
- Suspected aortic dissection
- Active bleeding or bleeding diathesis (excluding menses)
- Significant closed-head or facial trauma within 3 months

Relative Contraindications

- History of chronic, severe, poorly controlled hypertension
- Severe uncontrolled hypertension on arrival (systolic BP >180 mm Hg or diastolic BP >110 mm Hg)
- History of ischemic stroke more than 3 months prior, known intracranial pathology not covered in contraindications, or dementia
- Traumatic or prolonged (>10 min) cardiopulmonary resuscitation or major surgery in the previous 3 weeks
- Internal bleeding within the previous 2-4 weeks
- Noncompressible vascular punctures
- For streptokinase/anistreplase: exposure >5 days prior or any prior allergic reaction to these agents
- Pregnancy
- Active peptic ulcer
- Current use of vitamin K antagonists: the higher the international normalized ratio, the higher the risk of bleeding

BP, blood pressure; ICH, intracranial hemmorhage; STEMI, ST-segment myocardial infarction.
Modified from Antman EM, Anbe DT, Armstrong PW, et al. ACC/AHA guidelines for the management of patients with ST elevation myocardial infarction: a report of the American College of Cardiology/American Heart Association Task Force on Practice Guidelines (Committee to Revise the 1999 Guidelines for the Management of patients with acute myocardial infarction). *J Am Coll Cardiol* 2004;44(3):E1-E211.

REFERENCES

1. Marsh N, Marsh A. A short history of nitroglycerine and nitric oxide in pharmacology and physiology. *Clin Exp Pharmacol Physiol* 2000;27:313-319.
2. Field A. On the toxicol and medicinal properties of nitrate of oxyd of glycl. *Med Times Gazette* 1858;16:291.
3. Murrell W. Nitro-glycerine as a remedy for angina pectoris. *Lancet* 1879;1:80-81.
4. Brunton TL. Use of nitrate of amyl in angina pectoris. *Lancet* 1867;2:97-98.
5. Arnold WP, Mittal CK, Katsuki S, Murad F. Nitric oxide activates guanylate cyclase and increases guanosine 3′:5′-cyclic monophosphate levels in various tissue preparations. *Proc Natl Acad Sci U S A* 1977;74:3203-3207.
6. Bredt DS, Hwang PM, Glatt CE, et al. Cloned and expressed nitric oxide synthase structurally resembles cytochrome p-450 reductase. *Nature* 1991;351:714-718.
7. McDonald BJ, Bennett BM. Cytochrome p-450 mediated biotransformation of organic nitrates. *Can J Physiol Pharmacol* 1990;68:1552-1557.
8. Minamiyama Y, Imaoka S, Takemura S, et al. Escape from tolerance of organic nitrate by induction of cytochrome p450. *Free Radic Biol Med* 2001;31:1498-1508.
9. Ratz JD, McGuire JJ, Anderson DJ, Bennett BM. Effects of the flavoprotein inhibitor, diphenyleneiodonium sulfate, on ex vivo organic nitrate tolerance in the rat. *J Pharmacol Exp Ther* 2000;293:569-577.
10. Chen Z, Zhang J, Stamler JS. Identification of the enzymatic mechanism of nitroglycerin bioactivation. *Proc Natl Acad Sci U S A* 2002;99:8306-8311.
11. Chen Z, Foster MW, Zhang J, et al. An essential role for mitochondrial aldehyde dehydrogenase in nitroglycerin bioactivation. *Proc Natl Acad Sci U S A* 2005;102:12159-12164.
12. Zhang J, Chen Z, Cobb FR, Stamler JS. Role of mitochondrial aldehyde dehydrogenase in nitroglycerin-induced vasodilation of coronary and systemic vessels: an intact canine model. *Circulation* 2004;110:750-755.
13. Mackenzie IS, Maki-Petaja KM, McEniery CM, et al. Aldehyde dehydrogenase 2 plays a role in the bioactivation of nitroglycerin in humans. *Arterioscler Thromb Vasc Biol* 2005;25:1891-1895.
14. Li Y, Zhang D, Jin W, et al. Mitochondrial aldehyde dehydrogenase-2 (aldh2) glu504lys polymorphism contributes to the variation in efficacy of sublingual nitroglycerin. *J Clin Invest* 2006;116:506-511.
15. Wenzel P, Hink U, Oelze M, et al. Number of nitrate groups determines reactivity and potency of organic nitrates: a proof of concept study in aldh-2−/− mice. *Br J Pharmacol* 2007;150:526-533.
16. Lincoln TM, Cornwell TL, Taylor AE. cGMP-dependent protein kinase mediates the reduction of Ca2+ by cAMP in vascular smooth muscle cells. *Am J Physiol* 1990;258:C399-407.
17. Lincoln TM, Dey N, Sellak H. Invited review: cGMP-dependent protein kinase signaling mechanisms in smooth muscle: from the regulation of tone to gene expression. *J Appl Physiol* 2001;91:1421-1430.
18. Bolotina VM, Najibi S, Palacino JJ, et al. Nitric oxide directly activates calcium-dependent potassium channels in vascular smooth muscle. *Nature* 1994;368:850-853.
19. Munzel T, Daiber A, Gori T. Nitrate therapy: new aspects concerning molecular action and tolerance. *Circulation* 2011;123:2132-2144.
20. Gori T, Parker JD. Nitrate tolerance: a unifying hypothesis. *Circulation* 2002;106:2510-2513.
21. Gori T, Parker JD. The puzzle of nitrate tolerance: Pieces smaller than we thought? *Circulation* 2002;106:2404-2408.
22. Gori T, Parker JD. Nitrate-induced toxicity and preconditioning: a rationale for reconsidering the use of these drugs. *J Am Coll Cardiol* 2008;52:251-254.
23. Bassenge E, Stewart DJ. Effects of nitrates in various vascular sections and regions. *Z Kardiol* 1986;3:1-7.
24. Harrison DG, Bates JN. The nitrovasodilators: new ideas about old drugs. *Circulation* 1993;87:1461-1467.
25. Brown BG, Bolson E, Petersen RB, et al. The mechanisms of nitroglycerin action: stenosis vasodilatation as a major component of the drug response. *Circulation* 1981;64:1089-1097.
26. Gibson GR, Hunter JB, Raabe DS Jr, et al. Methemoglobinemia produced by high-dose intravenous nitroglycerin. *Ann Intern Med* 1982;96:615-616.
27. Marshall JB, Ecklund RE. Methemoglobinemia from overdose of nitroglycerin. *JAMA* 1980;244:330.
28. Parker JO, VanKoughnett KA, Farrell B. Nitroglycerin lingual spray: clinical efficacy and dose-response relation. *Am J Cardiol* 1986;57:1-5.
29. Parker J, Farrell B, Lahey K, Moe G. Effect of intervals between doses on the development of tolerance to isosorbide dinitrate. *N Engl J Med* 1987;316:1440-1444.
30. Parker JO, Amies MH, Hawkinson RW, et al. Intermittent transdermal nitroglycerin therapy in angina pectoris: clinically effective without tolerance or rebound. Minitran efficacy study group. *Circulation* 1995;91:1368-1374.
31. DeMots H, Glasser SP. Intermittent transdermal nitroglycerin therapy in the treatment of chronic stable angina. *J Am Coll Card* 1989;13:786-788.
32. Chrysant SG, Glasser SP, Bittar N, et al. Efficacy and safety of extended-release isosorbide mononitrate for stable effort angina pectoris. *Am J Cardiol* 1993;72:1249-1256.
33. Mollnau H, Wenzel P, Oelze M, et al. Mitochondrial oxidative stress and nitrate tolerance–comparison of nitroglycerin and pentaerithrityl tetranitrate in Mn-SOD+/− mice. *BMC Cardiovasc Disord* 2006;6:44.
34. Wenzel P, Oelze M, Coldewey M, et al. Heme oxygenase-1: a novel key player in the development of tolerance in response to organic nitrates. *Arterioscler Thromb Vasc Biol* 2007;27:1729-1735.
35. Daiber A, Munzel T. Characterization of the antioxidant properties of pentaerithrityl tetranitrate (PETN)-induction of the intrinsic antioxidative system heme oxygenase-1 (HO-1). *Methods Mol Biol* 2010;594:311-326.
36. Leier CV, Huss P, Magorien RD, Unverferth DV. Improved exercise capacity and differing arterial and venous tolerance during chronic isosorbide dinitrate therapy for congestive heart failure. *Circulation* 1983;67:817-822.
37. Packer M, Lee WH, Kessler PD, et al. Prevention and reversal of nitrate tolerance in patients with congestive heart failure. *N Engl J Med* 1987;317:799-804.
38. Cohn JN, Archibals DG, Zeische S, et al. Effect of vasodilator therapy on mortality in chronic congestive heart failure. Results of a Veterans Administration cooperative study. *N Engl J Med* 1986;314:1547-1552.
39. Taylor AL, Ziesche S, Yancy C, et al. Combination of isosorbide dinitrate and hydralazine in blacks with heart failure. *N Engl J Med* 2004;351:2049-2057.
40. Jeserich M, Münzel T, Pape L, et al. Absence of vascular tolerance in conductance vessels after 48 hours of intravenous nitroglycerin in patients with coronary artery disease. *J Am Coll Cardiol* 1995;26:50-56.
41. Gori T, Harvey P, Floras JS, Parker JD. Continuous therapy with nitroglycerin impairs endothelium-dependent vasodilation but does not cause tolerance in conductance arteries: a human in vivo study. *J Cardiovasc Pharmacol* 2004;44:601-606.
42. Needleman P, Land S, Johnson EMJ. Organic nitrates: relationship between biotransformation and rational angina pectoris therapy. *J Pharmacol Exp Ther* 1972;181:489-497.
43. Glancy DL, Richter MA, Ellis EV, Johnson W. Effect of swallowed isosorbide dinitrate on blood pressure, heart rate and exercise capacity in patients with coronary artery disease. *Am J Med* 1977;62:39-46.
44. Thadani U, Fung H-L, Dark AC, Parker JO. Oral isosorbide dinitrate in angina pectoris: comparison of duration of action and dose response relation during acute and sustained therapy. *Am J Cardiol* 1982;89:1074-1080.
45. Thadani U, Fung H-L, Darke AC, Parker JO. Oral isosorbide dinitrate in the treatment of angina pectoris: dose response relationship and duration of action during acute therapy. *Circulation* 1980;62:591-602.
46. Dalal JJ, Parker JO. Nitrate cross-tolerance: effect of sublingual isosorbide dinitrate and nitroglycerin during sustained nitrate therapy. *Am J Cardiol* 1984;54:286-288.
47. Acute and chronic antianginal efficacy of continuous twenty-four-hour application of transdermal nitroglycerin. Steering Committee, Transdermal Nitroglycerin Cooperative Study. *Am J Cardiol* 1992;68:1263-1273.
48. Thadani U, Hamilton SF, Olsen E, et al. Transdermal nitroglycerin patches in angina pectoris: dose titration, duration of effect and rapid tolerance. *Ann Intern Med* 1986;105:485-492.
49. Needleman P, Johnson EM Jr. Mechanism of tolerance development to organic nitrates. *J Pharmacol Exp Ther* 1973;184:709-715.
50. Horowitz JD, Antman EM, Lorell BH, et al. Potentiation of the cardiovascular effects of nitroglycerin by N-acetylcysteine. *Circulation* 1983;68:1247-1253.
51. Parker JO, Parker JD. Neurohormonal activation during nitrate therapy: a possible mechanism for tolerance. *Am J Cardiol* 1992;70:93B-97B.
52. Munzel T, Daiber A, Mulsch A. Explaining the phenomenon of nitrate tolerance. *Circ Res* 2005;97:618-628.
53. Parker JD, Farrell B, Fenton T, et al. Counter-regulatory responses to continuous and intermittent therapy with nitroglycerin. *Circulation* 1991;84:2336-2345.

54. Katz RJ, Levy WS, Buff L, Wasserman AG. Prevention of nitrate tolerance with angiotension converting enzyme inhibitors. *Circulation* 1991;83:1271-1277.

55. Sussex BA, Campbell NRC, Raju MK, McKay DW. The antianginal efficacy of isosorbide dinitrate therapy is maintained during diuretic treatment. *Clin Pharmacol Ther* 1994; 56:229-234.

56. Parker JD, Parker JO. Effect of therapy with an angiotensin-converting enzyme inhibitor on hemodynamic and counterregulatory responses during continuous therapy with nitroglycerin. *J Am Coll Cardiol* 1993;21:1445-1453.

57. Munzel T, Sayegh H, Freeman BA, et al. Evidence for enhanced vascular superoxide anion production in nitrate tolerance: a novel mechanism underlying tolerance and cross-tolerance. *J Clin Invest* 1995;95:187-194.

58. Kurz S, Münzel T, Harrison D. A role for angiotensin II in nitrate tolerance: chronic AT-1 receptor blockade prevents the development of tolerance and cross tolerance. *Circulation* 1995;92(Suppl 1):1-392.

59. Münzel T, Kurz S, Rajagopalan S, Harrison DG. Hydralazine prevents nitroglycerin tolerance by inhibiting vascular superoxide production. *Circulation* 1995;92(Suppl 1):1-4.

60. Sydow K, Daiber A, Oelze M, et al. Central role of mitochondrial aldehyde dehydrogenase and reactive oxygen species in nitroglycerin tolerance and cross-tolerance. *J Clin Invest* 2004;113:482-489.

61. Wenzl MV, Beretta M, Gorren AC, et al. Role of the general base Glu-268 in nitroglycerin bioactivation and superoxide formation by aldehyde dehydrogenase-2. *J Biol Chem* 2009;284:19878-19886.

62. Munzel T, Li H, Mollnau H, et al. Effects of long-term nitroglycerin treatment on endothelial nitric oxide synthase (NOS III) gene expression, NOS III–mediated superoxide production, and vascular NO bioavailability. *Circ Res* 2000;86:E7-E12.

63. Knorr M, Hausding M, Kroller-Schuhmacher S, et al. Nitroglycerin-induced endothelial dysfunction and tolerance involve adverse phosphorylation and S-glutathionylation of endothelial nitric oxide synthase: beneficial effects of therapy with the AT1 receptor blocker telmisartan. *Arterioscler Thromb Vasc Biol* 2011;31:2223-2231.

64. Gori T, Mak SS, Kelly S, Parker JD. Evidence supporting abnormalities in nitric oxide synthase function induced by nitroglycerin in humans. *J Am Coll Cardiol* 2001; 38:1096-1101.

65. Lam JY, Chesebro JH, Fuster V. Platelets, vasoconstriction, and nitroglycerin during arterial wall injury: a new antithrombotic role for an old drug. *Circulation* 1988;78: 712-716.

66. Folts JD, Stamler J, Loscalzo J. Intravenous nitroglycerin infusion inhibits cyclic blood flow responses caused by periodic platelet thrombus formation in stenosed canine coronary arteries. *Circulation* 1991;83:2122-2127.

67. Diodati JG, Cannon RO 3rd, Hussain N, Quyyumi AA. Inhibitory effect of nitroglycerin and sodium nitroprusside on platelet activation across the coronary circulation in stable angina pectoris. *Am J Cardiol* 1995;75:443-448.

68. Horowitz JD. Role of nitrates in unstable angina pectoris. *Am J Cardiol* 1992;70:64B-71B.

69. Ramamurthy S, Mehan V, Kaufmann U, et al. Effect of pre-treatment with transdermal glyceryl trinitrate on myocardial ischaemia during coronary angioplasty. *Heart* 1996;76: 471-476.

70. Banerjee S, Tang XL, Qiu Y, et al. Nitroglycerin induces late preconditioning against myocardial stunning via a PKC-dependent pathway. *Am J Physiol* 1999;277:H2488-H2494.

71. Hill M, Takano H, Tang XL, et al. Nitroglycerin induces late preconditioning against myocardial infarction in conscious rabbits despite development of nitrate tolerance. *Circulation* 2001;104:694-699.

72. Leesar MA, Stoddard MF, Dawn B, et al. Delayed preconditioning-mimetic action of nitroglycerin in patients undergoing coronary angioplasty. *Circulation* 2001;103: 2935-2941.

73. Jneid H, Chandra M, Alshaher M, et al. Delayed preconditioning-mimetic actions of nitroglycerin in patients undergoing exercise tolerance tests. *Circulation* 2005;111: 2565-2571.

74. Dragoni S, Gori T, Lisi M, et al. Pentaerythrityl tetranitrate and nitroglycerin, but not isosorbide mononitrate, prevent endothelial dysfunction induced by ischemia and reperfusion. *Arterioscler Thromb Vasc Biol* 2007;27:1955-1959.

75. Gori T, Di Stolfo G, Sicuro S, et al. Nitroglycerin protects the endothelium from ischaemia and reperfusion: human mechanistic insight. *Br J Clin Pharmacol* 2007;64:145-150.

76. Chen CH, Budas GR, Churchill EN, et al. Activation of aldehyde dehydrogenase-2 reduces ischemic damage to the heart. *Science* 2008;321:1493-1495.

77. Gori T, Dragoni S, Di Stolfo G, et al. Tolerance to nitroglycerin-induced preconditioning of the endothelium: a human in vivo study. *Am J Physiol Heart Circ Physiol* 2010; 298:H340-H345.

78. Heitzer T, Just H, Brockhoff C, et al. Long-term nitroglycerin treatment is associated with supersensitivity to vasoconstrictors in men with stable coronary artery disease: prevention by concomitant treatment with captopril. *J Am Coll Cardiol* 1998;31:83-88.

79. Caramori P, Adelman A, Azevedo E, et al. Therapy with nitroglycerin increases coronary vasoconstriction in response to acetylcholine. *J Am Coll Card* 1998;32:1969-1974.

80. Azevedo ER, Schofield AM, Kelly S, Parker JD. Nitroglycerin withdrawal increases endothelium-dependent vasomotor response to acetylcholine. *J Am Coll Cardiol* 2001;37:505-509.

81. Thomas GR, DiFabio JM, Gori T, Parker JD. Once daily therapy with isosorbide-5-mononitrate causes endothelial dysfunction in humans: evidence of a free-radical–mediated mechanism. *J Am Coll Cardiol* 2007;49:1289-1295.

82. Ma SX, Schmid PG Jr, Long JP. Noradrenergic mechanisms and the cardiovascular actions of nitroglycerin. *Life Sci* 1994;55:1595-1603.

83. Chowdhary S, Vaile JC, Fletcher J, et al. Nitric oxide and cardiac autonomic control in humans. *Hypertension* 2000;36:264-269.

84. Chowdhary S, Nuttall SL, Coote JH, Townend JN. L-arginine augments cardiac vagal control in healthy human subjects. *Hypertension* 2002;39:51-56.

85. Chowdhary S, Ng GA, Nuttall SL, et al. Nitric oxide and cardiac parasympathetic control in human heart failure. *Clin Sci (Lond)* 2002;102:397-402.

86. Wecht JM, Weir JP, Goldstein DS, et al. Direct and reflexive effects of nitric oxide synthase inhibition on blood pressure. *Am J Physiol Heart Circ Physiol* 2008;294:H190-H197.

87. Schwarz P, Diem R, Dun NJ, Forstermann U. Endogenous and exogenous nitric oxide inhibits norepinephrine release from rat heart sympathetic nerves. *Circ Res* 1995; 77:841-848.

88. Zanzinger J, Czachurski J, Seller H. Impaired modulation of sympathetic excitability by nitric oxide after long-term administration of organic nitrates in pigs. *Circulation* 1998;97:2352-2358.

89. Gori T, Floras JS, Parker JD. Effects of nitroglycerin treatment on baroreflex sensitivity and short-term heart rate variability in humans. *J Am Coll Cardiol* 2002;40:2000-2005.

90. GISSI-3: effects of lisinopril and transdermal glyceryl trinitrate singly and together on 6-week mortality and ventricular function after acute myocardial infarction. Gruppo Italiano per lo Studio della Sopravvivenza nell'infarto Miocardico [see comments]. *Lancet* 1994;343:1115-1122.

91. Group I-FISoISC. Isis-4: a randomised factorial trial assessing early oral captopril, oral mononitrate, and intravenous magnesium sulphate in 58,050 patients with suspected acute myocardial infarction. ISIS-4 (Fourth International Study of Infarct Survival) Collaborative Group [see comments]. *Lancet* 1995;345:669-685.

92. Otto A, Fontaine J, Tschirhart E, et al. Rosuvastatin treatment protects against nitrate-induced oxidative stress in enos knockout mice: implication of the NAD(P)H oxidase pathway. *Br J Pharmacol* 2006;148:544-552.

93. Otto A, Fontaine D, Fontaine J, Berkenboom G. Rosuvastatin treatment protects against nitrate-induced oxidative stress. *J Cardiovasc Pharmacol* 2005;46:177-184.

94. Liuni A, Luca MC, Di Stolfo G, et al. Coadministration of atorvastatin prevents nitroglycerin-induced endothelial dysfunction and nitrate tolerance in healthy humans. *J Am Coll Cardiol* 2011;57:93-98.

95. Eisenberg MJ, Brox A, Bestawros AN. Calcium channel blockers: an update. *Am J Med* 2004;116:35-43.

96. Abernethy DR, Schwartz JB. Calcium-antagonist drugs. *N Engl J Med* 1999;341: 1447-1457.

97. Doggrell SA. Has the controversy over the use of calcium channel blockers in coronary artery disease been resolved? *Expert Opin Pharmacother* 2005;6:831-834.

98. Godfraind T, Salomone S, Dessy C, et al. Selectivity scale of calcium antagonists in the human cardiovascular system based on in vitro studies. *J Cardiovasc Pharmacol* 1992; 20:S34-S41.

99. Heidenreich PA, McDonald KM, Hastie T, et al. Meta-analysis of trials comparing beta-blockers, calcium antagonists, and nitrates for stable angina. *JAMA* 1999;281: 1927-1936.

100. The Danish Verapamil Infarction Trial II—DAVIT II. Effect of verapamil on mortality and major events after acute myocardial infarction. *Am J Cardiol* 1990;66:779-785.

101. The Multicenter Diltiazem Postinfarction Trial Research Group. The effect of diltiazem on mortality and reinfarction after myocardial infarction. *N Engl J Med* 1988;319: 385-392.

102. Cohn JN, Ziesche S, Smith R, et al. Effect of the calcium antagonist felodipine as supplementary vasodilator therapy in patients with chronic heart failure treated with enalapril: V-HeFT III. Vasodilator-Heart Failure Trial (V-HeFT) Study Group. *Circulation* 1997;96: 856-863.

103. Packer M, O'Connor CM, Ghali JK, et al. Effect of amlodipine on morbidity and mortality in severe chronic heart failure. Prospective Randomized Amlodipine Survival Evaluation Study Group. *N Engl J Med* 1996;335:1107-1114.

104. Van Zwieten PA. Amlodipine: an overview of its pharmacodynamic and pharmacokinetic properties. *Clin Cardiol* 1994;17:1113-1116.

105. Messerli FH. Case-control study, meta-analysis, and bouillabaisse: putting the calcium antagonist scare into context. *Ann Intern Med* 1995;123:888-889.

106. Jezek T, Balazovjech I. The Valsartan Antihypertensive Long-term Use Evaluation (VALUE) trial in Slovakia. *Bratisl Lek Listy* 2003;104:19-26.

107. Julius S, Kjeldsen SE, Weber M, et al. Outcomes in hypertensive patients at high cardiovascular risk treated with regimens based on valsartan or amlodipine: the VALUE randomized trial. *Lancet* 2004;363:2022-2031.

108. Nissen SE, Tuzcu EM, Libby P, et al. Effect of antihypertensive agents on cardiovascular events in patients with coronary disease and normal blood pressure: the CAMELOT study: a randomized controlled trial. *JAMA* 2004;292:2217-2225.

109. Cushman WC, Evans GW, Byington RP, et al. Effects of intensive blood-pressure control in type 2 diabetes mellitus. *N Engl J Med* 2010;362:1575-1585.

110. Dahlof B, Sever PS, Poulter NR, et al. Prevention of cardiovascular events with an antihypertensive regimen of amlodipine adding perindopril as required versus atenolol adding bendroflumethiazide as required, in the Anglo-Scandinavian Cardiac Outcomes Trial-Blood Pressure Lowering Arm (ASCOT-BPLA): a multicentre randomised controlled trial. *Lancet* 2005;366:895-906.

111. Pepine CJ, Handberg EM, Cooper-DeHoff RM, et al. A calcium antagonist vs a non-calcium antagonist hypertension treatment strategy for patients with coronary artery disease. The International Verapamil-Trandolapril Study (INVEST): a randomized controlled trial. *JAMA* 2003;290:2805-2816.

112. Jamerson K, Weber MA, Bakris GL, et al. Benazepril plus amlodipine or hydrochlorothiazide for hypertension in high-risk patients. *N Engl J Med* 2008;359:2417-2428.

113. Bakris GL, Toto RD, McCullough PA. Rationale and design of a study comparing two fixed-dose combination regimens to reduce albuminuria in patients with type II diabetes and hypertension. *J Hum Hypertens* 2005;19:139-144.

114. Psaty BM, Heckbert SR, Koepsell TD, et al. The risk of myocardial infarction associated with antihypertensive drug therapies. *JAMA* 1995;274:620-625.

115. Leader S, Mallick R, Roht L. Using medication history to measure confounding by indication in assessing calcium channel blockers and other antihypertensive therapy. *J Hum Hypertens* 2001;15:153-159.

116. Bangalore S, Messerli FH, Cohen JD, et al. Verapamil-sustained release-based treatment strategy is equivalent to atenolol-based treatment strategy at reducing cardiovascular events in patients with prior myocardial infarction: an INternational VErapamil SR-Trandolapril (INVEST) substudy. *Am Heart J* 2008;156:241-247.

117. Frishman WH. β-Adrenergic blockers: a 50-year historical perspective. *Am J Therap* 2008; 15:565-576.

118. Frishman WH. Fifty years of beta-adrenergic blockade: a golden era in clinical medicine and molecular pharmacology. *Am J Med* 2008;121:933-934.
119. Frishman WH. Carvedilol. *N Engl J Med* 1998;339:1759-1765.
120. Ellison KE, Gandhi G. Optimising the use of beta-adrenoceptor antagonists in coronary artery disease. *Drugs* 2005;65:787-797.
121. Sonnenblick EH, Ross J Jr, Braunwald E. Oxygen consumption of the heart: newer concepts of its multifactorial determination. *Am J Cardiol* 1968;22:328-336.
122. Lefkowitz RJ. The superfamily of heptahelical receptors. *Nat Cell Biol* 2000;2:E133-E136.
123. Benovic JL, Bouvier M, Caron MG, Lefkowitz RJ. Regulation of adenylyl cyclase–coupled beta-adrenergic receptors. *Annu Rev Cell Biol* 1988;4:405-428.
124. Lefkowitz RJ. Seven transmembrane receptors: something old, something new. *Acta Physiol* 2007;190:9-19.
125. Rasmussen SGE, Choi H-J, Rosenbaum DM, et al. Crystal structure of the human β2-adrenergic G-protein-coupled receptor. *Nature* 2007;450:383-388.
126. Lefkowitz RJ, Rockman HA, Koch WJ. Catecholamines, cardiac beta-adrenergic receptors, and heart failure. *Circulation* 2000;101:1634-1637.
127. Glaubiger G, Lefkowitz RJ. Elevated beta-adrenergic receptor number after chronic propranolol treatment. *Biochem Biophys Res Commun* 1977;78:720-725.
128. Frishman WH. Beta-adrenergic blocker withdrawal. *Am J Cardiol* 1987;59:26F-32F.
129. Johnson JA, Liggett SB. Cardiovascular pharmacogenomics of adrenergic receptor signaling: clinical implications and future directions. *Clin Pharmacol Ther* 2011;89:366-378.
130. Ahlquist RP. Study of the adrenotropic receptors. *Am J Physiol* 1948;153:486.
131. Sonnenblick EH, Skelton CL. Myocardial energetics: basic principles and clinical implications. *N Engl J Med* 1971;285:668-675.
132. Steg P. Stable angina: pathophysiology, diagnosis and treatment. *Am J Cardiovasc Drugs* 2003;3:1-10.
133. Frishman WH. Multifactorial actions of beta-adrenergic blocking drugs in ischemic heart disease: current concepts. *Circulation* 1983;67:I11-I18.
134. Frishman WH, Gabor R, Pepine C, Cavusoglu E. Heart rate reduction in the treatment of chronic stable angina pectoris: experiences with a sinus node inhibitor. *Am Heart J* 1996;131:204-210.
135. Frishman WH, Pepine CJ, Weiss RJ, Baiker WM. Addition of zatebradine, a direct sinus node inhibitor, provides no greater exercise tolerance benefit in patients with angina taking extended-release nifedipine: results of a multicenter, randomized, double-blind, placebo-controlled, parallel-group study. The Zatebradine Study Group. *J Am Coll Cardiol* 1995;26:305-312.
136. Barbato E, Piscione F, Bartunek J, et al. Role of beta2 adrenergic receptors in human atherosclerotic coronary arteries. *Circulation* 2005;111:288-294.
137. Parratt JR, Grayson J. Myocardial vascular reactivity after beta-adrenergic blockade. *Lancet* 1966;1:338-340.
138. Becker LC, Fortuin NJ, Pitt B. Effect of ischemia and antianginal drugs on the distribution of radioactive microspheres in the canine left ventricle. *Circ Res* 1971;28:263-269.
139. Bjorntorp P. Treatment of angina pectoris with beta-receptor blockade, mode of action. *Acta Med Scand* 1968;184:259-262.
140. Frishman WH, Smithen C, Befler B, et al. Noninvasive assessment of clinical response to oral propranolol therapy. *Am J Cardiol* 1975;35:635-644.
141. Fraker TD Jr, Fihn SD. Focused update of the 2002 ACC/AHA 2002 guideline for the management of patients with chronic stable angina: a report of the American College of Cardiology/American Heart Association Task Force on practice guidelines writing group to develop a focused update of the 2002 guidelines. *J Am Coll Cardiol* 2007;50:2264-2274.
142. Packer M. Drug therapy: combined beta-adrenergic and calcium-entry blockade in angina pectoris. *N Engl J Med* 1989;320:709-718.
143. Jenkins NP, Keevil BG, Hutchinson IV, Brooks NH. Beta-blockers are associated with lower C-reactive protein concentrations in patients with coronary artery disease. *Am J Med* 2002;112:269-274.
144. Frishman WH, Sica DA. Calcium channel-blockers. In Frishman WH, Sonnenblick EH, Sica DA, editors: *Cardiovascular pharmacotherapeutics*, 2nd ed. New York, 2003, McGraw-Hill, pp 105-130.
145. Weiner DA, Klein MD. Calcium antagonists for the treatment of angina pectoris. In Weiner DA, Frishman WH, editors: *Therapy of angina pectoris*. New York, 1986, Marcel Dekker, pp 145-204.
146. Chaitman BR. Ranolazine for the treatment of chronic angina and potential use in other cardiovascular conditions. *Circulation* 2006;113:2462-2472.
147. Chaitman BR, Pepine CJ, Parker JO, et al. Effects of ranolazine with atenolol, amlodipine, or diltiazem on exercise tolerance and angina frequency in patients with severe chronic angina: a randomized controlled trial. *JAMA* 2004;291:309-316.
148. Antz M, Cappato R, Kuck KH. Metoprolol versus sotalol in the treatment of sustained ventricular tachycardia. *J Cardiovasc Pharmacol* 1995;26:627-635.
149. Tisdale JE, Sun H, Zhao H, et al. Antifibrillatory effect of esmolol alone and in combination with lidocaine. *J Cardiovasc Pharmacol* 1996;27:376-382.
150. Cavusoglu E, Frishman WH. Sotalol: a new beta-adrenergic blocker for ventricular arrhythmias. *Prog Cardiovasc Dis* 1995;37:423-440.
151. Kennedy HL, Brooks MM, Barker AH, et al. Beta-blocker therapy in the Cardiac Arrhythmia Suppression Trial. CAST Investigators. *Am J Cardiol* 1994;74:674-680.
152. Steinbeck G, Andresen D, Bach P, et al. A comparison of electrophysiologically guided antiarrhythmic drug therapy with beta-blocker therapy in patients with symptomatic, sustained ventricular tachyarrhythmias. *N Engl J Med* 1992;327:987-992.
153. Ellison KE, Hafley GE, Hickey K, et al. Effect of beta-blocking therapy on outcome in the Multicenter UnSustained Tachycardia Trial (MUSTT). *Circulation* 2002;106:2694-2699.
154. Boutitie F, Boissel JP, Connolly SJ, et al. Amiodarone interaction with beta-blockers: analysis of the merged EMIAT (European Myocardial Infarct Amiodarone Trial) and CAMIAT (Canadian Amiodarone Myocardial Infarction Trial) databases. The EMIAT and CAMIAT Investigators. *Circulation* 1999;99:2268-2275.
155. Pacifico A, Hohnloser SH, Williams JH, et al. Prevention of implantable-defibrillator shocks by treatment with sotalol. d,l-Sotalol Implantable Cardioverter-Defibrillator Study Group. *N Engl J Med* 1999;340:1855-1862.
156. Frishman WH, Sica DA. β-Adrenergic blockers. In Izzo JL Jr, Sica DA, Black HR, editors: *Hypertension primer*, 4th ed. Dallas, 2008, American Heart Association, pp 446-450.
157. Turnbull F. Effects of different blood-pressure-lowering regimens on major cardiovascular events: results of prospectively designed overviews of randomised trials. *Lancet* 2003;362:1527-1535.
158. Frishman WH. *Clinical pharmacology of the β-adrenoceptor blocking drugs*, 2nd ed. Norwalk, 1984, Appleton-Century-Crofts.
159. Gottlieb SS, McCarter RJ, Vogel RA. Effect of beta-blockade on mortality among high-risk and low-risk patients after myocardial infarction. *N Engl J Med* 1998;339:489-497.
160. Chen J, Marciniak TA, Radford MJ, et al. Beta-blocker therapy for secondary prevention of myocardial infarction in elderly diabetic patients. Results from the National Cooperative Cardiovascular Project. *J Am Coll Cardiol* 1999;34:1388-1394.
161. Furberg CD, Hawkins CM, Lichstein E. Effect of propranolol in postinfarction patients with mechanical or electrical complications. *Circulation* 1984;69:761-765.
162. Frishman WH, Lazar EJ. Reduction of mortality, sudden death and non-fatal reinfarction with beta-adrenergic blockers in survivors of acute myocardial infarction: a new hypothesis regarding the cardioprotective action of beta-adrenergic blockade. *Am J Cardiol* 1990;66:66G-70G.
163. Frishman WH, Furberg CD, Friedewald WT. Beta-adrenergic blockade for survivors of acute myocardial infarction. *N Engl J Med* 1984;310:830-837.
164. ISIS-I Collaborative Group. Randomised trial of intravenous atenolol among 16,027 cases of suspected acute myocardial infarction: ISIS-1. First International Study of Infarct Survival Collaborative Group. *Lancet* 1986;2:57-66.
165. MIAMI Trial Research Group. Metoprolol in Acute Myocardial Infarction (MIAMI): a randomised placebo-controlled international trial. *Eur Heart J* 1985;6:199-226.
166. Dargie HJ. Effect of carvedilol on outcome after myocardial infarction in patients with left-ventricular dysfunction: the CAPRICORN randomised trial. *Lancet* 2001;357:1385-1390.
167. Pfisterer M, Cox JL, Granger CB, et al. Atenolol use and clinical outcomes after thrombolysis for acute myocardial infarction: the GUSTO-I experience. Global Utilization of Streptokinase and TPA (alteplase) for Occluded Coronary Arteries. *J Am Coll Cardiol* 1998;32:634-640.
168. Radford MJ, Krumholz HM. Beta-blockers after myocardial infarction—for few patients, or many? *N Engl J Med* 1998;339:551-553.
169. Frishman WH, Teicher M. Antianginal drug therapy for silent myocardial ischemia. *Med Clin North Am* 1988;72:185-196.
170. Andrews TC, Fenton T, Toyosaki N, et al. Subsets of ambulatory myocardial ischemia based on heart rate activity: circadian distribution and response to anti-ischemic medication. The Angina and Silent Ischemia Study Group (ASIS). *Circulation* 1993;88:92-100.
171. Rogers WJ, Bourassa MG, Andrews TC, et al. Asymptomatic Cardiac Ischemia Pilot (ACIP) study: Outcome at 1 year for patients with asymptomatic cardiac ischemia randomized to medical therapy or revascularization. The ACIP Investigators. *J Am Coll Cardiol* 1995;26:594-605.
172. Pepine CJ, Cohn PF, Deedwania PC, et al. Effects of treatment on outcome in mildly symptomatic patients with ischemia during daily life: the Atenolol Silent Ischemia Study (ASIST). *Circulation* 1994;90:762-768.
173. Frishman WH, Glasser S, Stone P, et al. Comparison of controlled-onset, extended-release verapamil with amlodipine and amlodipine plus atenolol on exercise performance and ambulatory ischemia in patients with chronic stable angina pectoris. *Am J Cardiol* 1999;83:507-514.
174. Cohen LS, Braunwald E. Amelioration of angina pectoris in idiopathic hypertrophic subaortic stenosis with beta-adrenergic blockade. *Circulation* 1967;35:847-851.
175. Swan DA, Bell B, Oakley CM, Goodwin J. Analysis of symptomatic course and prognosis and treatment of hypertrophic obstructive cardiomyopathy. *Br Heart J* 1971;33:671-685.
176. Frishman WH. Beta-adrenergic blockers. *Med Clin North Am* 1988;72:37-81.
177. Hubner PJ, Ziady GM, Lane GK, et al. Double-blind trial of propranolol and practolol in hypertrophic cardiomyopathy. *Br Heart J* 1973;35:1116-1123.
178. Epstein SE. Asymmetric septal hypertrophy. *Ann Intern Med* 1974;81:650-680.
179. Engelhardt S, Bohm M, Erdmann E, Lohse MJ. Analysis of beta-adrenergic receptor mRNA levels in human ventricular biopsy specimens by quantitative polymerase chain reactions: progressive reduction of beta 1-adrenergic receptor mRNA in heart failure. *J Am Coll Cardiol* 1996;27:146-154.
180. Sackner-Bernstein JD, Mancini DM. Rationale for treatment of patients with chronic heart failure with adrenergic blockade. *JAMA* 1995;274:1462-1467.
181. Francis GS, Goldsmith SR, Cohn JN. Relationship of exercise capacity to resting left ventricular performance and basal plasma norepinephrine levels in patients with congestive heart failure. *Am Heart J* 1982;104:725-731.
182. Viquerat CE, Daly P, Swedberg K, et al. Endogenous catecholamine levels in chronic heart failure: relation to the severity of hemodynamic abnormalities. *Am J Med* 1985;78:455-460.
183. Cohn JN, Levine TB, Olivari MT, et al. Plasma norepinephrine as a guide to prognosis in patients with chronic congestive heart failure. *N Engl J Med* 1984;311:819-823.
184. Daly PA, Sole MJ. Myocardial catecholamines and the pathophysiology of heart failure. *Circulation* 1990;82:I35-I43.
185. Pauletto P, Vescove G, Scannapieco G, et al. Cardioprotection by beta blockers: molecular and structural aspects in experimental hypertension. *Drugs Exp Clin Res* 1990;3:1055.
186. Shizukuda Y, Buttrick PM, Geenen DL, et al. β-Adrenergic stimulation causes cardiocyte apoptosis: influence of tachycardia and hypertrophy. *Am J Physiol* 1998;275:H961-H968.
187. Podrid PJ, Fuchs T, Candinas R. Role of the sympathetic nervous system in the genesis of ventricular arrhythmia. *Circulation* 1990;82:I103-I113.
188. Brophy JM, Joseph L, Rouleau JL. Beta-blockers in congestive heart failure: a Bayesian meta-analysis. *Ann Intern Med* 2001;134:550-560.
189. MERIT-HF Study Group. Effect of metoprolol CR/XL in chronic heart failure: metoprolol CR/XL Randomised Intervention Trial in Congestive Heart Failure (MERIT-HF). *Lancet* 1999;353:2001-2007.

190. CIBIS II Investigators and Committee. The Cardiac Insufficiency Bisoprolol Study II (CIBIS-II): a randomised trial. *Lancet* 1999;353:9-13.

191. Poole-Wilson PA, Swedberg K, Cleland JG, et al. Comparison of carvedilol and metoprolol on clinical outcomes in patients with chronic heart failure in the Carvedilol or Metoprolol European Trial (COMET): randomised controlled trial. *Lancet* 2003;362:7-13.

192. Willenheimer R, van Veldhuisen DJ, Silke B, et al. Effect on survival and hospitalization of initiating treatment for chronic heart failure with bisoprolol followed by enalapril, as compared with the opposite sequence: results of the randomized Cardiac Insufficiency Bisoprolol Study (CIBIS) III. *Circulation* 2005;112:2426-2435.

193. Whyte K, Jones CR, Howie CA, et al. Haemodynamic, metabolic, and lymphocyte beta 2-adrenoceptor changes following chronic beta-adrenoceptor antagonism. *Eur Heart J* 1987;32:237-243.

194. Shimoyama H, Sabbah HN, Rosman H, et al. Effect of beta-blockade on left atrial contribution to ventricular filling in dogs with moderate heart failure. *Am Heart J* 1996;131: 772-777.

195. Luchner A, Burnett JC Jr, Jougasaki M, et al. Augmentation of the cardiac natriuretic peptides by beta-receptor antagonism: evidence from a population-based study. *J Am Coll Cardiol* 1998;32:1839-1844.

196. Frishman WH. Alpha and beta-adrenergic blocking drugs. In Frishman WH, Sonnenblick EH, Sica DA, editors: *Cardiovascular pharmacotherapeutics manual*, 2nd ed. New York, 2004, McGraw–Hill, pp 19-57.

197. Winkle RA, Lopes MG, Goodman DJ, et al. Propranolol for patients with mitral valve prolapse. *Am Heart J* 1977;93:422-427.

198. Mukherjee D, Eagle KA. Aortic dissection—an update. *Curr Probl Cardiol* 2005; 30:287-325.

199. Ong K-T, Perdu J, DeBacker J, et al. Effect of celiprolol on prevention of cardiovascular events in vascular Ehlers-Danlos syndrome: a prospective randomised, open, blinded-endpoints trial. *Lancet* 2010;376:1476-1484.

200. Lanza GA, Colonna G, Pasceri V, Maseri A. Atenolol versus amlodipine versus isosorbide-5-mononitrate on anginal symptoms in syndrome X. *Am J Cardiol* 1999;84:854-856.

201. Mangano DT, Layug EL, Wallace A, Tateo I. Effect of atenolol on mortality and cardiovascular morbidity after noncardiac surgery: multicenter study of perioperative ischemia research group. *N Engl J Med* 1996;335:1713-1720.

202. Poldermans D, Boersma E, Bax JJ, et al for the Dutch Echocardiographic Cardiac Risk Evaluation Applying Stress Echocardiography Study Group. The effect of bisoprolol on peri-operative mortality and myocardial infarction in high-risk patients undergoing vascular surgery. *N Engl J Med* 1999;341:1789-1794.

203. Salazar C, Frishman W, Friedman S, et al. Beta blockade therapy for supraventricular tachyarrhythmias after coronary surgery: a propranolol withdrawal syndrome? *Angiology* 1979;30:816-819.

204. National Quality Forum. *Safe practices for better healthcare—2006 update.* Washington, DC, 2006, National Quality Forum.

205. POISE Study Group, et al. Effects of extended-release metoprolol succinate in patients undergoing non-cardiac surgery (POISE trial): a randomized, controlled trial. *Lancet* 2008;371;1839-1841.

206. Harte B, Jaffer AK. Perioperative beta-blockers in noncardiac surgery: evolution of the evidence. *Cleveland Clinic J Med* 2008;75:513-519.

207. Fleisher LA, Beckman JA, Buller CE, et al. 2009 ACCF/AHA focused update on perioperative beta blockade: a report of the American College of Cardiology Foundation/American Heart Association Task Force on Practice Guidelines. *J Am Coll Cardiol* 2009;54:e13.

208. Koch-Weser J, Frishman WH. Beta-adrenoceptor antagonists: new drugs and new indications. *N Engl J Med* 1981;305:500-506.

209. Frishman WH. Atenolol and timolol: two new systemic beta-adrenoceptor antagonists. *N Engl J Med* 1982;306:1456-1462.

210. Frishman WH. Nadolol: a new beta-adrenoceptor antagonist. *N Engl J Med* 1981;305: 678-682.

211. Frishman WH. Pindolol: a new beta-adrenoceptor antagonist with partial agonist activity. *N Engl J Med* 1983;308:940-944.

212. Frishman WH, Cheng-Lai A, Nawarskas J. *Current cardiovascular drugs*, 4th ed. Philadelphia, 2005, Current Medicine, p 152.

213. Sule SS, Frishman W. Nebivolol: new therapy update. *Cardiol Rev* 2006;14(6):259-265.

214. Koch-Weser J. Metoprolol. *N Engl J Med* 1979;301:698-703.

215. Frishman WH, Alwarshetty M. Beta-adrenergic blockers in systemic hypertension: pharmacokinetic considerations related to the current guidelines. *Clin Pharmacokinet* 2002;41:505-516.

216. Salpeter SR, Ormiston TM, Salpeter EE. Cardioselective beta-blockers in patients with reactive airway disease: a meta-analysis. *Ann Intern Med* 2002;137:715-725.

217. Frishman WH. Clinical perspective on celiprolol: cardioprotective potential. *Am Heart J* 1991;121:724-729.

218. Frishman WH, Halprin S. Clinical pharmacology of the new beta-adrenergic blocking drugs. Part 7. New horizons in beta-adrenoceptor blockade therapy: labetalol. *Am Heart J* 1979; 98:660-665.

219. Frishman WH, Strom JA, Kirschner M, et al. Labetalol therapy in patients with systemic hypertension and angina pectoris: effects of combined alpha and beta adrenoceptor blockade. *Am J Cardiol* 1981;48:917-928.

220. Bakris GL, Fonseca V, Katholi RE, et al. Metabolic effects of carvedilol vs metoprolol in patients with type 2 diabetes mellitus and hypertension: a randomized controlled trial. *JAMA* 2004;292:2227-2236.

221. Frishman WH, Lazar EJ, Gorodokin G. Pharmacokinetic optimisation of therapy with beta-adrenergic blocking agents. *Clin Pharmacokinet* 1991;20:311-318.

222. Halkin H, Vered I, Saginer A, Rabinowitz B. Once daily administration of sustained release propranolol capsules in the treatment of angina pectoris. *Eur J Clin Pharmacol* 1979;16: 387-391.

223. Sandberg A, Blomqvist I, Jonsson UE, Lundborg P. Pharmacokinetic and pharmacodynamic properties of a new controlled-release formulation of metoprolol: a comparison with conventional tablets. *Eur J Clin Pharmacol* 1988;33:S9-S14.

224. Sica D, Frishman WH, Manowitz N. Pharmacokinetics of propranolol after single and multiple dosing with sustained release propranolol or propranolol CR (innopran XL), a new chronotherapeutic formulation. *Heart Dis* 2003;5:176-181.

225. Keller S, Frishman WH. Neuropsychiatric effects of cardiovascular drug therapy. *Cardiol Rev* 2003;11:73-93.

226. Kostis JB, Rosen RC. Central nervous system effects of beta-adrenergic-blocking drugs: the role of ancillary properties. *Circulation* 1987;75:204-212.

227. Ward SA, Walle T, Walle UK, et al. Propranolol's metabolism is determined by both mephenytoin and debrisoquin hydroxylase activities. *Clin Pharmacol Ther* 1989;45:72-79.

228. Panton LB, Guillen GJ, Williams L, et al. The lack of effect of aerobic exercise training on propranolol pharmacokinetics in young and elderly adults. *J Clin Pharmacol* 1995;35:885-894.

229. Frishman W, Silverman R, Strom J, et al. Clinical pharmacology of the new beta-adrenergic blocking drugs. Part 4. Adverse effects: choosing a beta-adrenoreceptor blocker. *Am Heart J* 1979;98:256-262.

230. Frishman WH, Opie LH, Sica DA. Adverse cardiovascular drug interactions and complications. In Fuster V, Alexander RW, O'Rourke RA, editors: *Hurst's the heart*, 11th ed. New York, 2004, McGraw–Hill, pp 2169-2188.

231. Simpson WT. Nature and incidence of unwanted effects with atenolol. *Postgrad Med J* 1997;53:162-167.

232. Vandenburg MJ, Conlon C, Ledingham JM. A comparison of the effects of propranolol and oxprenolol on forearm blood flow and skin temperature. *Br J Clin Pharmacol* 1981;11:485-490.

233. Thadani U, Whitsett TL. Beta-adrenergic blockers and intermittent claudication: time for reappraisal. *Arch Intern Med* 1991;151:1705-1707.

234. Ko DT, Hebert PR, Coffey CS, et al. Beta-blocker therapy and symptoms of depression, fatigue, and sexual dysfunction. *JAMA* 2002;288:351-357.

235. Dusing R. Sexual dysfunction in male patients with hypertension: influence of antihypertensive drugs. *Drugs* 2005;65:773-786.

236. Wassertheil-Smoller S, Oberman A, Blaufox MD, et al. The Trial of Antihypertensive Interventions and Management (TAIM) study: final results with regard to blood pressure, cardiovascular risk, and quality of life. *Am J Hypertens* 1992;5:37-44.

237. Croog SH, Levine S, Testa MA, et al. The effects of antihypertensive therapy on the quality of life. *N Engl J Med* 1986;314:1657-1664.

238. Beto JA, Bansal VK. Quality of life in treatment of hypertension: a meta-analysis of clinical trials. *Am J Hypertens* 1992;5:125-133.

239. Streufert S, DePadova A, McGlynn T, et al. Impact of beta-blockade on complex cognitive functioning. *Am Heart J* 1988; 116:311-315.

240. Gress TW, Nieto FJ, Shahar E, et al. Hypertension and antihypertensive therapy as risk factors for type 2 diabetes mellitus: Atherosclerosis Risk in Communities study. *N Engl J Med* 2000;342:905-912.

241. Sowers JR, Bakris GL. Antihypertensive therapy and the risk of type 2 diabetes mellitus. *N Engl J Med* 2000;342:969-970.

242. Fogari R, Zoppi A, Corradi L, et al. Beta blocker effects on plasma lipids during prolonged treatment of hypertensive patients with hypercholesterolemia. *J Cardiovasc Pharmacol* 1999; 33:534-539.

243. Frishman W, Jacob H, Eisenberg E, Ribner H. Clinical pharmacology of the new beta-adrenergic blocking drugs. Part 8. Self-poisoning with beta-adrenoceptor blocking agents: recognition and management. *Am Heart J* 1979;98:798-811.

244. Frishman WH, Klein N, Strom J, et al. Comparative effects of abrupt withdrawal of propranolol and verapamil in angina pectoris. *Am J Cardiol* 1982;50:1191-1195.

245. Morimoto S, Shimizu K, Yamada K, et al. Can beta-blocker therapy be withdrawn from patients with dilated cardiomyopathy? *Am Heart J* 1999;138:456-459.

246. IONA Study Group. Effect of nicorandil on coronary events in patients with stable angina: the Impact of Nicorandil in Angina (IONA) randomised trial. *Lancet* 2002;359: 1269-1275.

247. Borer JS, Fox K, Jaillon P, Lerebours G. Antianginal and antiischemic effects of ivabradine, an I(f) inhibitor, in stable angina: a randomized, double-blind, multicentered, placebo-controlled trial. *Circulation* 2003;107:817-823.

248. Tardif JC, Ford I, Tendera M, et al. Efficacy of ivabradine, a new selective I(f) inhibitor, compared with atenolol in patients with chronic stable angina. *Eur Heart J* 2005; 26:2529-2536.

249. Fox K, Ford I, Steg PG, et al. Ivabradine for patients with stable coronary artery disease and left-ventricular systolic dysfunction (BEAUTIFUL): a randomised, double-blind, placebo-controlled trial. *Lancet* 2008;372:807-816.

250. Swedberg K, Komajda M, Bohm M, et al. Ivabradine and outcomes in chronic heart failure (SHIFT): a randomised placebo-controlled study. *Lancet* 2010;376:875-885.

251. Zaza A, Belardinelli L, Shryock JC. Pathophysiology and pharmacology of the cardiac "late sodium current." *Pharmacol Ther* 2008;119:326-339.

252. Belardinelli L, Shryock JC, Fraser H. Inhibition of the late sodium current as a potential cardioprotective principle: effects of the late sodium current inhibitor ranolazine. *Heart* 2006;92(Suppl 4):iv6-iv14.

253. Undrovinas AI, Belardinelli L, Undrovinas NA, Sabbah HN. Ranolazine improves abnormal repolarization and contraction in left ventricular myocytes of dogs with heart failure by inhibiting late sodium current. *J Cardiovasc Electrophysiol* 2006;17(Suppl 1):S169-S177.

254. Fraser H, Belardinelli L, Wang L, et al. Ranolazine decreases diastolic calcium accumulation caused by ATX-II or ischemia in rat hearts. *J Mol Cell Cardiol* 2006;41:1031-1038.

255. Sossalla S, Wagner S, Rasenack EC, et al. Ranolazine improves diastolic dysfunction in isolated myocardium from failing human hearts: role of late sodium current and intracellular ion accumulation. *J Mol Cell Cardiol* 2008;45:32-43.

256. Chaitman BR, Skettino SL, Parker JO, et al. Anti-ischemic effects and long-term survival during ranolazine monotherapy in patients with chronic severe angina. *J Am Coll Cardiol* 2004;43:1375-1382.

257. Chaitman BR, Pepine CJ, Parker JO, et al. Effects of ranolazine with atenolol, amlodipine, or diltiazem on exercise tolerance and angina frequency in patients with severe chronic angina: a randomized controlled trial. *JAMA* 2004;291:309-316.

PHARMACOLOGIC OPTIONS FOR TREATMENT OF ISCHEMIC DISEASE

CH 7

258. Stone PH, Gratsiansky NA, Blokhin A, et al. Antianginal efficacy of ranolazine when added to treatment with amlodipine: the ERICA (Efficacy of Ranolazine in Chronic Angina) trial. J Am Coll Cardiol 2006;48:566-575.

259. Morrow DA, Scirica BM, Karwatowska-Prokopczuk E, et al. Effects of ranolazine on recurrent cardiovascular events in patients with non–ST-elevation acute coronary syndromes: the MERLIN-TIMI 36 randomized trial. JAMA 2007;297:1775-1783.

260. Wilson SR, Scirica BM, Braunwald E, et al. Efficacy of ranolazine in patients with chronic angina observations from the randomized, double-blind, placebo-controlled MERLIN-TIMI (Metabolic Efficiency with Ranolazine for Less Ischemia in Non–ST-Segment Elevation Acute Coronary Syndromes) 36 trial. J Am Coll Cardiol 2009;53:1510-1516.

261. Timmis AD, Chaitman BR, Crager M. Effects of ranolazine on exercise tolerance and HbA1c in patients with chronic angina and diabetes. Eur Heart J 2006;27:42-48.

262. Morrow DA, Scirica BM, Chaitman BR, et al. Effect of ranolazine on hemoglobin A1c in the MERLIN-TIMI 36 randomized controlled trial. Circulation 2007;116:II_539-c-540.

263. Antzelevitch C, Belardinelli L, Zygmunt AC, et al. Electrophysiological effects of ranolazine, a novel antianginal agent with antiarrhythmic properties. Circulation 2004;110: 904-910.

264. Song Y, Shryock JC, Belardinelli L. An increase of late sodium current induces delayed afterdepolarizations and sustained triggered activity in atrial myocytes. Am J Physiol Heart Circ Physiol 2008;294:H2031-H2039.

265. Scirica BM, Morrow DA, Hod H, et al. Effect of ranolazine, an antianginal agent with novel electrophysiological properties, on the incidence of arrhythmias in patients with non ST-segment elevation acute coronary syndrome: results from the Metabolic Efficiency with Ranolazine for Less Ischemia in Non ST-Elevation Acute Coronary Syndrome Thrombolysis in Myocardial Infarction 36 (MERLIN-TIMI 36) randomized controlled trial. Circulation 2007;116:1647-1652.

266. Marzilli M, Klein WW. Efficacy and tolerability of trimetazidine in stable angina: a meta-analysis of randomized, double-blind, controlled trials. Coron Artery Dis 2003;14: 171-179.

267. The EMIP-FR group. Effect of 48-h intravenous trimetazidine on short- and long-term outcomes of patients with acute myocardial infarction, with and without thrombolytic therapy: a double-blind, placebo-controlled, randomized trial. European Myocardial Infarction Project—Free Radicals. Eur Heart J 2000;21:1537-1546.

268. Angiolillo DJ, Ueno M, Goto S. Basic principles of platelet biology and clinical implications. Circ J 2010;74:597-607.

269. Freedman JE. Molecular regulation of platelet-dependent thrombosis. Circulation 2005;112:2725-2734.

270. Davì G, Patrono C. Platelet activation and atherothrombosis. N Engl J Med 2007;357:2482-2494.

271. Libby P, Theroux P. Pathophysiology of coronary artery disease. Circulation 2005; 111:3481-3488.

272. Patrono C. Aspirin as an antiplatelet drug. N Engl J Med 1994;330:1287-1294.

273. Patrono C, García Rodríguez LA, Landolfi R, Baigent C. Low-dose aspirin for the prevention of atherothrombosis. N Engl J Med 2005;353:2373-2383.

274. Patrono C, Coller B, Dalen JE, et al. Platelet-active drugs: the relationships among dose, effectiveness, and side effects. Chest 2001;119:39S-63S.

275. Cipollone F, Rocca B, Patrono C. Cyclooxygenase-2 expression and inhibition in atherothrombosis. Arterioscler Thromb Vasc Biol 2004;24:246-255.

276. Antiplatelet Trialists' Collaboration. Collaborative overview of randomised trials of antiplatelet therapy—I: Prevention of death, myocardial infarction, and stroke by prolonged antiplatelet therapy in various categories of patients. Br Med J 1994;308:81-106.

277. Antithrombotic Trialists' Collaboration. Collaborative meta-analysis of randomised trials of antiplatelet therapy for prevention of death, myocardial infarction, and stroke in high risk patients. Br Med J 2002;324:71-86.

278. Baigent C, Blackwell L, Collins R, et al; Antithrombotic Trialists' (ATT) Collaboration. Aspirin in the primary and secondary prevention of vascular disease: collaborative meta-analysis of individual participant data from randomised trials. Lancet 2009;373:1849-1860.

279. Wright RS, Anderson JL, Adams CD, et al. 2011 ACCF/AHA focused update of the guidelines for the management of patients with unstable angina/non-ST-elevation myocardial infarction (updating the 2007 guideline): a report of the American College of Cardiology Foundation/American Heart Association Task Force on Practice Guidelines Developed in Collaboration With the American College of Emergency Physicians, Society for Cardiovascular Angiography and Interventions, and Society of Thoracic Surgeons. J Am Coll Cardiol 2011;57:1920-1959.

280. Kushner FG, Hand M, Smith SC Jr, et al. 2009 focused updates: ACC/AHA guidelines for the management of patients with ST-elevation myocardial infarction (updating the 2004 guideline and 2007 focused update) and ACC/AHA/SCAI guidelines on percutaneous coronary intervention (updating the 2005 guideline and 2007 focused update) a report of the American College of Cardiology Foundation/American Heart Association Task Force on Practice Guidelines. J Am Coll Cardiol 2009;54:2205-2241.

281. Angiolillo DJ. Variability in responsiveness to oral antiplatelet therapy. Am J Cardiol 2009;103(3 Suppl):27A-34A.

282. Mehta SR, Bassand JP, Chrolavicius S, et al; CURRENT-OASIS 7 Investigators. Dose comparisons of clopidogrel and aspirin in acute coronary syndromes. N Engl J Med 2010;363:930-942.

283. Peters RJ, Mehta SR, Fox KA, et al; Clopidogrel in Unstable Angina to Prevent Recurrent Events (CURE) Trial Investigators. Effects of aspirin dose when used alone or in combination with clopidogrel in patients with acute coronary syndromes: observations from the Clopidogrel in Unstable angina to prevent Recurrent Events (CURE) study. Circulation 2003;108:1682-1687.

284. Segal R, Lubart E, Leibovitz A, et al. Early and late effects of low-dose aspirin on renal function in elderly patients. Am J Med 2003;115:462-466.

285. Gollapudi RR, Teirstein PS, Stevenson DD, Simon RA. Aspirin sensitivity: implications for patients with coronary artery disease. JAMA 2004;292:3017-3023.

286. Rossini R, Angiolillo DJ, Musumeci G, et al. Aspirin desensitization in patients undergoing percutaneous coronary interventions with stent implantation. Am J Cardiol 2008;101: 786-789.

287. Gachet C. ADP receptors of platelets and their inhibition. Thromb Haemost 2001;86:222-232.

288. Hollopeter G, Jantzen HM, Vincent D, et al. Identification of the platelet ADP receptor targeted by antithrombotic drugs. Nature 2001;409:202-207.

289. Turner NA, Moake JL, McIntire LV. Blockade of adenosine diphosphate receptors P2Y(12) and P2Y(1) is required to inhibit platelet aggregation in whole blood under flow. Blood 2001;98:3340-3345.

290. Farid NA, Kurihara A, Wrighton SA. Metabolism and disposition of the thienopyridine antiplatelet drugs ticlopidine, clopidogrel, and prasugrel in humans. J Clin Pharmacol 2010;50:126-142.

291. Cadroy Y, Bossavy JP, Thalamas C, et al. Early potent antithrombotic effect with combined aspirin and a loading dose of clopidogrel on experimental arterial thrombogenesis in humans. Circulation 2000;101:2823-2828.

292. Schömig A, Neumann FJ, Kastrati A, et al. A randomized comparison of antiplatelet and anticoagulant therapy after the placement of coronary-artery stents. N Engl J Med 1996;334:1084-1089.

293. Leon MB, Baim DS, Popma JJ, et al. A clinical trial comparing three antithrombotic drug regimens after coronary-artery stenting. Stent Anticoagulation Restenosis Study Investigators. N Engl J Med 1998;339:1665-1671.

294. Bertrand ME, Legrand V, Boland J, et al. Randomized multicenter comparison of conventional anticoagulation versus antiplatelet therapy in unplanned and elective coronary stenting: the Full Anticoagulation versus Aspirin and Ticlopidine (FANTASTIC) study. Circulation 1998;98:1597-1603.

295. Urban P, Macaya C, Rupprecht HJ, et al. Randomized evaluation of anticoagulation versus antiplatelet therapy after coronary stent implantation in high-risk patients: the multicenter aspirin and ticlopidine trial after intracoronary stenting (MATTIS). Circulation 1998;98:2126-2132.

296. Angiolillo DJ, Fernandez-Ortiz A, Bernardo E, et al. Variability in individual responsiveness to clopidogrel: clinical implications, management, and future perspectives. J Am Coll Cardiol 2007;49:1505-1516.

297. Ferreiro JL, Angiolillo DJ. Clopidogrel response variability: current status and future directions. Thromb Haemost 2009;102:7-14.

298. Cuisset T, Frere C, Quilici J, et al. Benefit of a 600-mg loading dose of clopidogrel on platelet reactivity and clinical outcomes in patients with non–ST-segment elevation acute coronary syndrome undergoing coronary stenting. J Am Coll Cardiol 2006;48: 1339-1345.

299. Patti G, Colonna G, Pasceri V, et al. Randomized trial of high loading dose of clopidogrel for reduction of periprocedural myocardial infarction in patients undergoing coronary intervention: results from the ARMYDA-2 (Antiplatelet Therapy for Reduction of Myocardial Damage during Angioplasty) study. Circulation 2005;111:2099-2106.

300. Lotrionte M, Biondi-Zoccai GG, Agostoni P, et al. Meta-analysis appraising high clopidogrel loading in patients undergoing percutaneous coronary intervention. Am J Cardiol 2007;100:1199-1206.

301. Angiolillo DJ, Shoemaker SB, Desai B, et al. Randomized comparison of a high clopidogrel maintenance dose in patients with diabetes mellitus and coronary artery disease: results of the Optimizing Antiplatelet Therapy in Diabetes Mellitus (OPTIMUS) study. Circulation 2007;115:708-716.

302. Vivas D, Angiolillo DJ. Platelet P2Y12 receptor inhibition: an update on clinical drug development. Am J Cardiovasc Drugs 2010;10:217-226.

303. Bonello L, Tantry US, Marcucci R, et al; Working Group on High On-Treatment Platelet Reactivity. Consensus and future directions on the definition of high on-treatment platelet reactivity to adenosine diphosphate. J Am Coll Cardiol 2010;56:919-933.

304. Angiolillo DJ, Suryadevara S, Capranzano P, Bass TA. Prasugrel: a novel platelet ADP P2Y12 receptor antagonist: a review on its mechanism of action and clinical development. Expert Opin Pharmacother 2008;9:2893-2900.

305. Wiviott SD, Trenk D, Frelinger AL, et al; PRINCIPLE-TIMI 44 Investigators. Prasugrel compared with high loading- and maintenance-dose clopidogrel in patients with planned percutaneous coronary intervention: the Prasugrel in Comparison to Clopidogrel for Inhibition of Platelet Activation and Aggregation-Thrombolysis in Myocardial Infarction 44 trial. Circulation 2007;116:2923-2932.

306. Angiolillo DJ, Badimon JJ, Saucedo JF, et al. A pharmacodynamic comparison of prasugrel vs. high-dose clopidogrel in patients with type 2 diabetes mellitus and coronary artery disease: results of the Optimizing Anti-Platelet Therapy in diabetes Mellitus (OPTIMUS)-3 trial. Eur Heart J 2011;32:838-846.

307. Capodanno D, Dharmashankar K, Angiolillo DJ. Mechanism of action and clinical development of ticagrelor, a novel platelet ADP P2Y12 receptor antagonist. Expert Rev Cardiovasc Ther 2010;8:151-158.

308. Gurbel PA, Bliden KP, Butler K, et al. Randomized double-blind assessment of the ONSET and OFFSET of the antiplatelet effects of ticagrelor versus clopidogrel in patients with stable coronary artery disease: the ONSET/OFFSET study. Circulation 2009;120: 2577-2585.

309. Storey RF, Angiolillo DJ, Patil SB, et al. Inhibitory effects of ticagrelor compared with clopidogrel on platelet function in patients with acute coronary syndromes: the PLATO (PLATelet inhibition and patient Outcomes) PLATELET substudy. J Am Coll Cardiol 2010;56:1456-1462.

310. Husted S, Emanuelsson H, Heptinstall S, et al. Pharmacodynamics, pharmacokinetics, and safety of the oral reversible P2Y12 antagonist AZD6140 with aspirin in patients with atherosclerosis: a double-blind comparison to clopidogrel with aspirin. Eur Heart J 2006;27:1038-1047.

311. CAPRIE Steering Committee. A randomised, blinded, trial of clopidogrel versus aspirin in patients at risk of ischaemic events (CAPRIE). Lancet 1996;348:1329-1339.

312. Yusuf S, Zhao F, Mehta SR, et al; Clopidogrel in Unstable Angina to Prevent Recurrent Events Trial Investigators. Effects of clopidogrel in addition to aspirin in patients with acute coronary syndromes without ST-segment elevation. N Engl J Med 2001;345: 494-502.

313. Mehta SR, Yusuf S, Peters RJ, et al; Clopidogrel in Unstable angina to prevent Recurrent Events trial (CURE) Investigators. Effects of pretreatment with clopidogrel and aspirin

followed by long-term therapy in patients undergoing percutaneous coronary intervention: the PCI-CURE study. *Lancet* 2001;358:527-533.

314. Steinhubl SR, Berger PB, Mann JT 3rd, et al; CREDO Investigators. Clopidogrel for the Reduction of Events During Observation: early and sustained dual oral antiplatelet therapy following percutaneous coronary intervention: a randomized controlled trial. *JAMA* 2002;288:2411-2420.

315. Chen ZM, Jiang LX, Chen YP, et al; COMMIT (Clopidogrel and Metoprolol in Myocardial Infarction Trial) collaborative group. Addition of clopidogrel to aspirin in 45,852 patients with acute myocardial infarction: randomised placebo-controlled trial. *Lancet* 2005; 366:1607-1621.

316. Sabatine MS, Cannon CP, Gibson CM, et al; CLARITY-TIMI 28 Investigators. Addition of clopidogrel to aspirin and fibrinolytic therapy for myocardial infarction with ST-segment elevation. *N Engl J Med* 2005;352:1179-1189.

317. Sabatine MS, Cannon CP, Gibson CM, et al; Clopidogrel as Adjunctive Reperfusion Therapy (CLARITY)-Thrombolysis in Myocardial Infarction (TIMI) 28 Investigators. Effect of clopidogrel pretreatment before percutaneous coronary intervention in patients with ST-elevation myocardial infarction treated with fibrinolytics: the PCI-CLARITY study. *JAMA* 2005;294:1224-1232.

318. Bhatt DL, Fox KA, Hacke W, et al; CHARISMA Investigators. Clopidogrel and aspirin versus aspirin alone for the prevention of atherothrombotic events. *N Engl J Med* 2006; 354:1706-1717.

319. Bhatt DL, Flather MD, Hacke W, et al; CHARISMA Investigators. Patients with prior myocardial infarction, stroke, or symptomatic peripheral arterial disease in the CHARISMA trial. *J Am Coll Cardiol* 2007;49:1982-1988.

320. Mehta SR, Tanguay JF, Eikelboom JW, et al; CURRENT-OASIS 7 trial investigators. Double-dose versus standard-dose clopidogrel and high-dose versus low-dose aspirin in individuals undergoing percutaneous coronary intervention for acute coronary syndromes (CURRENT-OASIS 7): a randomised factorial trial. *Lancet* 2010;376:1233-1243.

321. Wiviott SD, Braunwald E, McCabe CH, et al; TRITON-TIMI 38 Investigators. Prasugrel versus clopidogrel in patients with acute coronary syndromes. *N Engl J Med* 2007;357:2001-2015.

322. Wiviott SD, Braunwald E, Angiolillo DJ, et al; TRITON-TIMI 38 Investigators. Greater clinical benefit of more intensive oral antiplatelet therapy with prasugrel in patients with diabetes mellitus in the trial to assess improvement in therapeutic outcomes by optimizing platelet inhibition with prasugrel–thrombolysis in myocardial infarction 38. *Circulation* 2008;118:1626-1636.

323. Montalescot G, Wiviott SD, Braunwald E, et al; TRITON-TIMI 38 investigators. Prasugrel compared with clopidogrel in patients undergoing percutaneous coronary intervention for ST-elevation myocardial infarction (TRITON-TIMI 38): double-blind, randomised controlled trial. *Lancet* 2009;373:723-731.

324. ema.europa.eu/Find medicine/Human medicines/European Public Assessment Reports.

325. Bertrand ME, Rupprecht HJ, Urban P, Gershlick AH; CLASSICS Investigators. Double-blind study of the safety of clopidogrel with and without a loading dose in combination with aspirin compared with ticlopidine in combination with aspirin after coronary stenting: the Clopidogrel Aspirin Stent International Cooperative Study (CLASSICS). *Circulation* 2000;102:624-629.

326. Sabatine MS, Hamdalla HN, Mehta SR, et al. Efficacy and safety of clopidogrel pretreatment before percutaneous coronary intervention with and without glycoprotein IIb/IIIa inhibitor use. *Am Heart J* 2008;155:910-917.

327. Steinhubl SR, Berger PB, Brennan DM, Topol EJ, for the CREDO Investigators. Optimal timing for the initiation of pre-treatment with 300 mg clopidogrel before percutaneous coronary intervention. *J Am Coll Cardiol* 2006;47:939-943.

328. Kandzari DE, Berger PB, Kastrati A, et al; ISAR-REACT Study Investigators. Influence of treatment duration with a 600-mg dose of clopidogrel before percutaneous coronary revascularization. *J Am Coll Cardiol* 2004;44:2133-2136.

329. Wallentin L, Becker RC, Budaj A, et al. Ticagrelor versus clopidogrel in patients with acute coronary syndromes. *N Engl J Med* 2009;361:1045-1057.

330. Wijns W, Kolh P, Danchin N, et al; European Association for Percutaneous Cardiovascular Interventions. Guidelines on myocardial revascularization: the Task Force on Myocardial Revascularization of the European Society of Cardiology (ESC) and the European Association for Cardio-Thoracic Surgery (EACTS). *Eur Heart J* 2010;31:2501-2555.

331. Quinn MJ, Fitzgerald DJ. Ticlopidine and clopidogrel. *Circulation* 1999;100:1667-1672.

332. Whetsel TR, Bell DM. Rash in patients receiving ticlopidine after intracoronary stent placement. *Pharmacotherapy* 1999;19:228-231.

333. Angiolillo DJ, Gibson CM, Cheng S, et al. Differential effects of omeprazole and pantoprazole on the pharmacodynamics and pharmacokinetics of clopidogrel in healthy subjects: randomized, placebo-controlled, crossover comparison studies. *Clin Pharmacol Ther* 2011;89:65-74.

334. Holmes DR Jr, Dehmer GJ, Kaul S, et al. ACCF/AHA clopidogrel clinical alert: approaches to the FDA "boxed warning": a report of the American College of Cardiology Foundation Task Force on clinical expert consensus documents and the American Heart Association, endorsed by the Society for Cardiovascular Angiography and Interventions and the Society of Thoracic Surgeons. *J Am Coll Cardiol* 2010;56:321-341.

335. Lokhandwala JO, Best PJM, Butterfield JH, et al. Frequency of allergic or hematologic adverse reactions to ticlopidine among patients with allergic or hematologic adverse reactions to clopidogrel. *Circ Cardiovasc Intervent* 2009;2:348-351.

336. von Tiehl KF, Price MJ, Valencia R, et al. Clopidogrel desensitization after drug-eluting stent placement. *J Am Coll Cardiol* 2007;50:2039-2043.

337. Wagner CL, Mascelli MA, Neblock DS, et al. Analysis of GPIIb/IIIa receptor number by quantification of 7E3 binding to human platelets. *Blood* 1996;88:907-914.

338. Pytela R, Pierschbacher MD, Ginsberg MH, et al. Platelet membrane glycoprotein IIb/IIIa: member of a family of Arg-Gly-Asp–specific adhesion receptors. *Science* 1986;231:1559-1562.

339. Chew DP, Bhatt DL, Sapp S, Topol EJ. Increased mortality with oral platelet glycoprotein IIb/IIIa antagonists: a meta-analysis of phase III multicenter randomized trials. *Circulation* 2001;103:201-206.

340. Bhatt DL, Topol EJ. Current role of platelet glycoprotein IIb/IIIa inhibitors in acute coronary syndromes. *JAMA* 2000;284:1549-1558.

341. Coller BS, Peerschke EI, Scudder LE, Sullivan CA. A murine monoclonal antibody that completely blocks the binding of fibrinogen to platelets produces a thrombasthenic-like state in normal platelets and binds to glycoproteins IIb and/or IIIa. *J Clin Invest* 1983;72:325-338.

342. Coller BS. A new murine monoclonal antibody reports an activation-dependent change in the conformation and/or microenvironment of the platelet glycoprotein IIb/IIIa complex. *J Clin Invest* 1985;76:101-108.

343. Granada JF, Kleiman NS. Therapeutic use of intravenous eptifibatide in patients undergoing percutaneous coronary intervention: acute coronary syndromes and elective stenting. *Am J Cardiovasc Drugs* 2004;4:31-41.

344. Scarborough RM, Naughton MA, Teng W, et al. Design of potent and specific integrin antagonists: peptide antagonists with high specificity for glycoprotein IIb-IIIa. *J Biol Chem* 1993;268:1066-1073.

345. Topol EJ, Byzova TV, Plow EF. Platelet GPIIb-IIIa blockers. *Lancet* 1999;353:227-231.

346. Schneider DJ, Herrmann HC, Lakkis N, et al. Increased concentrations of tirofiban in blood and their correlation with inhibition of platelet aggregation after greater bolus doses of tirofiban. *Am J Cardiol* 2003;91:334-336.

347. Kastrati A, Mehilli J, Neumann FJ, et al. Abciximab in patients with acute coronary syndromes undergoing percutaneous coronary intervention after clopidogrel pretreatment: the ISAR-REACT 2 randomized trial. *JAMA* 2006;295:1531-1538.

348. Giugliano RP, White JA, Bode C, et al; EARLY ACS Investigators. Early versus delayed, provisional eptifibatide in acute coronary syndromes. *N Engl J Med* 2009;360:2176-2190.

349. De Luca G, Suryapranata H, Stone GW, et al. Abciximab as adjunctive therapy to reperfusion in acute ST-segment elevation myocardial infarction: a meta-analysis of randomized trials. *JAMA* 2005;293:1759-1765.

350. Boersma E, Harrington RA, Moliterno DJ, et al. Platelet glycoprotein IIb/IIIa inhibitors in acute coronary syndromes: a meta-analysis of all major randomised clinical trials. *Lancet* 2002;359:189-198.

351. Simoons ML. Effect of glycoprotein IIb/IIIa receptor blocker abciximab on outcome in patients with acute coronary syndromes without early coronary revascularization: the GUSTO IV-ACS randomised trial. *Lancet* 2001;357:1915-1924.

352. CAPTURE Investigators. Randomised placebo-controlled trial of abciximab before and during coronary intervention in refractory unstable angina: the CAPTURE study. *Lancet* 1997;349:1429-1435.

353. Inhibition of the platelet glycoprotein IIb/IIIa receptor with tirofiban in unstable angina and non–Q-wave myocardial infarction. Platelet Receptor Inhibition in Ischemic Syndrome Management in Patients Limited by Unstable Signs and Symptoms (PRISM-PLUS) study Investigators. *N Engl J Med* 1998;338:1488-1497.

354. Valgimigli M, Percoco G, Barbieri D, et al. The additive value of tirofiban administered with the high-dose bolus in the prevention of ischemic complications during high-risk coronary angioplasty: the ADVANCE Trial. *J Am Coll Cardiol* 2004;44:14-19.

355. Valgimigli M, Biondi-Zoccai G, Tebaldi M, et al. Tirofiban as adjunctive therapy for acute coronary syndromes and percutaneous coronary intervention: a meta-analysis of randomized trials. *Eur Heart J* 2010;31:35-49.

356. Dasgupta H, Blankenship JC, Wood GC, et al. Thrombocytopenia complicating treatment with intravenous glycoprotein IIb/IIIa receptor inhibitors: a pooled analysis. *Am Heart J* 2000;140:206-211.

357. Merlini PA, Rossi M, Menozzi A, et al. Thrombocytopenia caused by abciximab or tirofiban and its association with clinical outcome in patients undergoing coronary stenting. *Circulation* 2004;109:2203-2206.

358. Tcheng JE, Kereiakes DJ, Lincoff AM, et al. Abciximab readministration: results of the ReoPro Readministration Registry. *Circulation* 2001;104:870-875.

359. Angiolillo DJ, Bhatt DL, Gurbel PA, Jennings LK. Advances in antiplatelet therapy: agents in clinical development. *Am J Cardiol* 2009;103(3 Suppl):40A-51A.

360. Ferreiro JL, Ueno M, Angiolillo DJ. Cangrelor: a review on its mechanism of action and clinical development. *Expert Rev Cardiovasc Ther* 2009;7:1195-1201.

361. Harrington RA, Stone GW, McNulty S, et al. Platelet inhibition with cangrelor in patients undergoing PCI. *N Engl J Med* 2009;361:2318-2329.

362. Bhatt DL, Lincoff AM, Gibson CM, et al; CHAMPION PLATFORM Investigators. Intravenous platelet blockade with cangrelor during PCI. *N Engl J Med* 2009;361:2330-2341.

363. Ueno M, Rao SV, Angiolillo DJ. Elinogrel: pharmacological principles, preclinical and early phase clinical testing. *Future Cardiol* 2010;6:445-453.

364. Angiolillo DJ, Capodanno D, Goto S. Platelet thrombin receptor antagonism and atherothrombosis. *Eur Heart J* 2010;31:17-28.

365. Tricoci P, Huang Z, Held C, et al; TRACER Investigators. Thrombin-receptor antagonist vorapaxar in acute coronary syndromes. *N Engl J Med* 2012;366:20-33.

366. Chamorro A. TP receptor antagonism: a new concept in atherothrombosis and stroke prevention. *Cerebrovasc Dis* 2009;27(Suppl 3):20-27.

367. Bjork I, Lindahl U. Mechanism of the anticoagulant action of heparin. *Mol Cell Biochem* 1982;48:161-182.

368. Casu B, Oreste P, Torri G, et al. The structure of heparin –oligosaccharide fragments with high anti–factor Xa activity containing the minimal antithrombin III–binding sequence: chemical and 13C nuclear-magnetic-resonance studies. *Biochem J* 1981;197:599-609.

369. Dawes J, Papper DS. Catabolism of low-dose heparin in man. *Thromb Res* 1979;14:845-860.

370. de Swart CA, Nijmeyer B, Roelofs JM, Sixma JJ. Kinetics of intravenously administered heparin in normal humans. *Blood* 1982;60:1251-1258.

371. Hirsh J. Heparin. *N Engl J Med* 1991;324:1565-1574.

372. Granger CB, Miller JM, Bovill EG, et al. Rebound increase in thrombin generation and activity after cessation of intravenous heparin in patients with acute coronary syndromes. *Circulation* 1995;91:1929-1935.

373. Young E, Prins M, Levine MN, Hirsh J. Heparin binding to plasma proteins, an important mechanism for heparin resistance. *Thromb Haemost* 1992;67:639-643.

374. Hirsh J, Anand SS, Halperin JL, Fuster V. Mechanism of action and pharmacology of unfractionated heparin. *Arterioscler Thromb Vasc Biol* 2001;21:1094-1096.

375. Visentin GP, Ford SE, Scott JP, Aster RH. Antibodies from patients with heparin-induced thrombocytopenia/thrombosis are specific for platelet factor IV complexed with heparin or bound to endothelial cells. *J Clin Invest* 1994;93:81-88.

376. Greinacher A, Liebenhoff U, Kiefel V, et al. Heparin-associated thrombocytopenia: the effects of various intravenous IgG preparations on antibody mediated platelet activation—a possible new indication for high dose i.v. IgG. *Thromb Haemost* 1994;71(5):641-645.

377. Arepally GM, Ortel TL. Clinical practice: heparin-induced thrombocytopenia. *N Engl J Med* 2006;355:809-817.

378. Hirsh J, Warkentin TE, Raschke R, et al. Heparin and low-molecular weight heparin: mechanisms of action, pharmacokinetics, dosing considerations, monitoring, efficacy, and safety. *Chest* 1998;114(5 Suppl):489S-510S.

379. Reference deleted in proofs.

380. Weitz JI. Low-molecular-weight heparins. *N Engl J Med* 1997;337:688-698.

381. Choay J, Petitou M, Lormeau JC, et al. Structure-activity relationship in heparin: a synthetic pentasaccharide with high affinity for antithrombin III and eliciting high anti–factor Xa activity. *Biochem Biophys Res Commun* 1983;116:492-499.

382. Reference deleted in proofs.

383. Petersen JL, Mahaffey KW, Hasselblad V, et al. Efficacy and bleeding complications among patients randomized to enoxaparin or unfractionated heparin for antithrombin therapy in non–ST-segment elevation acute coronary syndromes: a systematic overview. *JAMA* 2004;292:89-96.

384. Antman EM. The search for replacements for unfractionated heparin. *Circulation* 2001;103:2310-2314.

385. Ferguson JJ, Califf RM, Antman EM, et al. Enoxaparin vs unfractionated heparin in high-risk patients with non–ST-segment elevation acute coronary syndromes managed with an intended early invasive strategy: primary results of the SYNERGY randomized trial. *JAMA* 2004;292:45-54.

386. Efficacy and safety of tenecteplase in combination with enoxaparin, abciximab, or unfractionated heparin: the ASSENT-3 randomised trial in acute myocardial infarction. *Lancet* 2001;358:605-613.

387. Wallentin L, Goldstein P, Armstrong PW, et al. Efficacy and safety of tenecteplase in combination with the low-molecular-weight heparin enoxaparin or unfractionated heparin in the prehospital setting: the Assessment of the Safety and Efficacy of a New Thrombolytic Regimen (ASSENT)-3 PLUS randomized trial in acute myocardial infarction. *Circulation* 2003;108:135-142.

388. Antman EM, Morrow DA, McCabe CH, et al. Enoxaparin versus unfractionated heparin with fibrinolysis for ST-elevation myocardial infarction. *N Engl J Med* 2006;354:1477-1488.

389. Giraldez RR, Nicolau JC, Corbalan R, et al. Enoxaparin is superior to unfractionated heparin in patients with ST elevation myocardial infarction undergoing fibrinolysis regardless of the choice of lytic: an ExTRACT-TIMI 25 analysis. *Eur Heart J* 2007;28:1566-1573.

390. White HD, Braunwald E, Murphy SA, et al. Enoxaparin vs. unfractionated heparin with fibrinolysis for ST-elevation myocardial infarction in elderly and younger patients: results from ExTRACT-TIMI 25. *Eur Heart J* 2007;28:1066-1071.

391. Montalescot G, White HD, Gallo R, et al; STEEPLE Investigators. Enoxaparin versus unfractionated heparin in elective percutaneous coronary intervention. *N Engl J Med* 2006;355:1058-1060.

392. Levine MN, Raskob G, Beyth RJ, et al. Hemorrhagic complications of anticoagulant treatment: the Seventh ACCP Conference on Antithrombotic and Thrombolytic Therapy. *Chest* 2004;126:287S-310S.

393. Di Nisio M, Middeldorp S, Büller HR. Direct thrombin inhibitors. *N Engl J Med* 2005;353:1028-1040.

394. The Global Use of Strategies to Open Occluded Coronary Arteries (GUSTO) IIa Investigators. Randomized trial of intravenous heparin versus recombinant hirudin for acute coronary syndromes. *Circulation* 1994;90:1631-1637.

395. Antman EM. Hirudin in acute myocardial infarction: thrombolysis and thrombin inhibition in myocardial infarction (TIMI) 9B trial. *Circulation* 1996;94:911-921.

396. GUSTO IIb Investigators. A comparison of recombinant hirudin with heparin for the treatment of acute coronary syndromes. *N Engl J Med* 1996;335:775-782.

397. OASIS-2 Investigators. Effects of recombinant hirudin (lepirudin) compared with heparin on death, myocardial infarction, refractory angina, and revascularisation procedures in patients with acute myocardial ischaemia without ST elevation: a randomised trial. *Lancet* 1999;353:429-438.

398. Lefevre G, Duval M, Gauron S, et al. Effect of renal impairment on the pharmacokinetics and pharmacodynamics of desirudin. *Clin Pharmacol Ther* 1997;62:50-59.

399. Lewis BE, Wallis DE, Leya F, et al, for the Argatroban-915 Investigators. Argatroban anticoagulation in patients with heparin-induced thrombocytopenia. *Arch Intern Med* 2003;163:1849-1856.

400. Skrzypczak-Jankun E, Carperos VE, Ravichandran KG, et al. Structure of the hirugen and hirulog 1 complexes of alpha-thrombin. *J Mol Biol* 1991;221:1379-1393.

401. Witting JI, Bourdon P, Brezniak DV, et al. Thrombin-specific inhibition by and slow cleavage of hirulog-1. *Biochem J* 1992;283 (Pt 3):737-743.

402. Fox I, Dawson A, Loynds P, et al. Anticoagulant activity of Hirulog, a direct thrombin inhibitor, in humans. *Thromb Haemost* 1993;69:157-163.

403. Robson R, White H, Aylward P, Frampton C. Bivalirudin pharmacokinetics and pharmacodynamics: effect of renal function, dose, and gender. *Clin Pharmacol Ther* 2002;71:433-439.

404. Chew DP, Bhatt DL, Kimball W, et al. Bivalirudin provides increasing benefit with decreasing renal function: a meta-analysis of randomized trials. *Am J Cardiol* 2003;92:919-923.

405. Stone GW, McLaurin BT, Cox DA, et al; ACUITY Investigators. Bivalirudin for patients with acute coronary syndromes. *N Engl J Med* 2006;355:2203-2216.

406. Stone GW, Witzenbichler B, Guagliumi G, et al. Bivalirudin during primary PCI in acute myocardial infarction. *N Engl J Med* 2008;358:2218-2230.

407. Wasowicz M, Vegas A, Borger MA, Harwood S. Bivalirudin anticoagulation for cardiopulmonary bypass in a patient with heparin-induced thrombocytopenia. *Can J Anaesth* 2005;52:1093-1098.

408. Mahaffey KW, Lewis BE, Wildermann NM, et al. The anticoagulant therapy with bivalirudin to assist in the performance of percutaneous coronary intervention in patients with heparin-induced thrombocytopenia (ATBAT) study: main results. *J Invasive Cardiol* 2003;15:611-616.

409. Lincoff AM, Bittl JA, Harrington RA, et al. Bivalirudin and provisional glycoprotein IIb/IIIa blockade compared with heparin and planned glycoprotein IIb/IIIa blockade during percutaneous coronary intervention: REPLACE-2 randomized trial. *JAMA* 2003;289:853-863.

410. Mehran R, Lansky AJ, Witzenbichler B, et al. Bivalirudin in patients undergoing primary angioplasty for acute myocardial infarction (HORIZONS-AMI): 1-year results of a randomised controlled trial. *Lancet* 2009;374:1149-1159.

411. Donat F, Duret JP, Santoni A, et al. The pharmacokinetics of fondaparinux sodium in healthy volunteers. *Clin Pharmacokinet* 2002;41(Suppl 2):1-9.

412. Lieu C, Shi J, Donat F, et al. Fondaparinux sodium is not metabolised in mammalian liver fractions and does not inhibit cytochrome P450-mediated metabolism of concomitant drugs. *Clin Pharmacokinet* 2002;41(Suppl 2):19-26.

413. Paolucci F, Clavies MC, Donat F, Necciari J. Fondaparinux sodium mechanism of action: identification of specific binding to purified and human plasma–derived proteins. *Clin Pharmacokinet* 2002;41(Suppl 2):11-18.

414. Savi P, Chong BH, Greinacher A, et al. Effect of fondaparinux on platelet activation in the presence of heparin-dependent antibodies: a blinded comparative multicenter study with unfractionated heparin. *Blood* 2005;105:139-144.

415. Yusuf S, Mehta SR, Chrolavicius S, et al. Comparison of fondaparinux and enoxaparin in acute coronary syndromes. *N Engl J Med* 2006;354:1464-1476.

416. Steg PG, Jolly SS, Mehta SR, et al; FUTURA/OASIS-8 Trial Group. Low-dose vs standard-dose unfractionated heparin for percutaneous coronary intervention in acute coronary syndromes treated with fondaparinux: the FUTURA/OASIS-8 randomized trial. *JAMA* 2010;304:1339-1349.

417. Yusuf S, Mehta SR, Chrolavicius S, et al. Effects of fondaparinux on mortality and reinfarction in patients with acute ST-segment elevation myocardial infarction: the OASIS-6 randomized trial. *JAMA* 2006;295:1519-1530.

418. Simoons ML, Bobbink IW, Boland J, et al. A dose-finding study of fondaparinux in patients with non–ST-segment elevation acute coronary syndromes: the Pentasaccharide in Unstable Angina (PENTUA) Study. *J Am Coll Cardiol* 2004;43:2183-2190.

419. Hurlen M, Abdelnoor M, Smith P, et al. Warfarin, aspirin, or both after myocardial infarction. *N Engl J Med* 2002;347:969-974.

420. Herlitz J, Holm J, Peterson M, et al. Effect of fixed low-dose warfarin added to aspirin in the long term after acute myocardial infarction: the LoWASA Study. *Eur Heart J* 2004;25:232-239.

421. Becker RC. Antithrombotic therapy after myocardial infarction. *N Engl J Med* 2002;347:1019-1022.

422. Eikelboom JW, Weitz JI. New anticoagulants. *Circulation* 2010;121:1523-1532.

423. Albers GW, Diener HC, Frison L, et al; SPORTIF Executive Steering Committee for the SPORTIF V Investigators. Ximelagatran vs warfarin for stroke prevention in patients with nonvalvular atrial fibrillation: a randomized trial. *JAMA* 2005;293:690-698.

424. Connolly SJ, Ezekowitz MD, Yusuf S, et al. Dabigatran versus warfarin in patients with atrial fibrillation. *N Engl J Med* 2009;361:1139-1151.

425. Alexander JH, Becker RC, Bhatt DL, et al. Apixaban, an oral, direct, selective factor Xa inhibitor, in combination with antiplatelet therapy after acute coronary syndrome: results of the Apixaban for Prevention of Acute Ischemic and Safety Events (APPRAISE) trial. *Circulation* 2009;119:2877-2885.

426. Alexander JH, Lopes RD, James S, et al, for the APPRAISE-2 Investigators. Apixaban with antiplatelet therapy after acute coronary syndrome. *N Engl J Med* 2011 Aug 25;365(8):699-708.

427. Mega JL, Braunwald E, Mohanavelu S, et al. Rivaroxaban versus placebo in patients with acute coronary syndromes (ATLAS ACS-TIMI 46): a randomised, double-blind, phase II trial. *Lancet* 2009;374:29-38.

428. Mega JL, Braunwald E, Wiviott SD, et al; ATLAS ACS 2–TIMI 51 Investigators. Rivaroxaban in patients with a recent acute coronary syndrome. *N Engl J Med* 2012:366:9-19.

429. Bergum PW, Cruikshank A, Maki SL, et al. Role of zymogen and activated factor X as scaffolds for the inhibition of the blood coagulation factor VIIa-tissue factor complex by recombinant nematode anticoagulant protein c2. *J Biol Chem* 2001;276:10063-10071.

430. Giugliano RP, Wiviott SD, Stone PH, et al. Recombinant nematode anticoagulant protein c2 in patients with non–ST-segment elevation acute coronary syndrome: the ANTHEM-TIMI-32 trial. *J Am Coll Cardiol* 2007;49:2398-2407.

431. Dyke CK, Steinhubl SR, Kleiman NS, et al. First-in-human experience of an antidote ontrolled anticoagulant using RNA aptamer technology: a phase 1a pharmacodynamic evaluation of a drug-antidote pair for the controlled regulation of factor IXa activity. *Circulation* 2006;114:2490-2497.

432. Ridker PM, O'Donnell C, Marder VJ, Hennekens CH. Large-scale trials of thrombolytic therapy for acute myocardial infarction: GISSI-2, ISIS-3, and GUSTO-1. *Ann Intern Med* 1993;119:530-532.

433. TIMI IIIB Investigators. Effects of tissue plasminogen activator and a comparison of early and invasive strategies in unstable angina and non–Q-wave myocardial infarction: results of the TIMI IIIb trial. *Circulation* 1994;89:1545-1556.

434. Brogden RN, Speight TM, Avery GS. Streptokinase: a review of its clinical pharmacology, mechanism of action and therapeutic uses. *Drugs* 1973;5:357-445.

435. Gonias SL, Einarsson M, Pizzo SV. Catabolic pathways for streptokinase, plasmin, and streptokinase activator complex in mice: in vivo reaction of plasminogen activator with alpha 2-macroglobulin. *J Clin Invest* 1982;70:412-423.

436. Llevadot J, Giugliano RP, Antman EM. Bolus fibrinolytic therapy in acute myocardial infarction. *JAMA* 2001;286:442-449.

437. ASSENT-2 Investigators. Single-bolus tenecteplase compared with front-loaded alteplase in acute myocardial infarction: the ASSENT-2 double-blind randomised trial. *Lancet* 1999;354:716-722.

CHAPTER 8

Stable Ischemic Heart Disease/ Chronic Stable Angina

David E. Newby and Keith A.A. Fox

EPIDEMIOLOGY, 131

NATURAL HISTORY, 131

ASSESSMENT AND INVESTIGATION, 131

Clinical Assessment, 131
Risk Stratification, 131

THERAPEUTIC INTERVENTIONS, 137

Lifestyle and Risk Factor Modifications, 137
Symptomatic Therapy, 140
Prevention of Coronary Events, 144

POTENTIAL FUTURE THERAPIES, 149

Cholesteryl Ester Transfer Protein Inhibitors, 149
Novel Antiplatelet Therapies, 149

REFERENCES, 149

Stable or predictable angina on effort predominantly occurs in the setting of a fixed atherosclerotic stenosis of the coronary artery. Similar symptoms can also arise in other conditions, such as aortic stenosis and hypertrophic cardiomyopathy. Conversely, obstructive coronary heart disease can occur in the absence of typical angina of effort or, indeed, without any symptoms at all. This chapter discusses chronic stable angina in relation to obstructive coronary atheroma, although other forms of angina exist (Table 8-1) and vasospasm associated with nonobstructive atheromatous plaques can occur.

Epidemiology

Coronary atherosclerosis is associated with many risk factors, such as cigarette smoking, hyperlipidemia, family history, hypertension, and diabetes mellitus (see Chapters 24 through 29).[1] The prevalence and extent of both coronary atheroma and angina pectoris increase with age and have a male preponderance.[2] Distribution among ethnic groups is unequal, with higher rates in Indo-Asians and lower rates in East Asians and Afro-Caribbeans compared with whites.[3]

The epidemiology of coronary heart disease (CHD) and angina pectoris is changing. In some regions of the world—such as North America, Western Europe, Japan, and Australia—the incidence, mortality rates, and in-hospital case fatalities are declining,[4] although the overall prevalence of CHD is still rising, in keeping with an aging population. However, Eastern Europe in particular is experiencing escalating rates of CHD and associated mortality, with age-adjusted death rates also rising in many of the developing economies. The World Health Organization (WHO) estimates that the global number of deaths from CHD will have risen from approximately 7 million in 2002 to 11 million by 2020.

Natural History

Angina pectoris results in substantial morbidity. In two thirds of patients, angina limits the ability to work and to undertake recreational, sexual, and other daily activities. On average, a patient with angina pectoris will consult a primary health care professional two or three times each year. The complications of angina pectoris in part relate to the extent and severity of CHD and include myocardial infarction (MI), congestive heart failure, dysrhythmias, and sudden cardiac death. In general, patients with stable angina pectoris have a 2.5% to 5% risk of death or nonfatal MI each year.[5,6] In middle-aged men, the annual event rate is 2.4% for a major CHD event, 0.6% for stroke, and 3.0% for death.[7]

The likelihood of sustaining an acute MI increases with the severity and extent of atheromatous involvement of the coronary arteries (Figure 8-1). In addition, left ventricular (LV) function and the frequency and severity of angina (Figures 8-2 and 8-3), as well as demographics such as age and gender, all influence the risk of MI.[8,9] There is a 10-fold range in risk of death, MI, or stroke according to baseline characteristics.[10]

Assessment and Investigation

Clinical Assessment

In patients with chronic stable angina, episodes of angina are usually initiated at consistent levels of physical stress and promptly disappear with cessation of activity (Box 8-1). Worsening angina provoked by progressively less exertion over a short period of time, often culminating in pain at rest, is indicative of an acute coronary syndrome (ACS; see Chapters 9 and 10).

The likelihood of CHD being the cause is increased by the presence of established risk factors. Beyond stigmata of hyperlipidemia (rare) or signs of peripheral atheromatous vascular disease, no physical signs of angina are usually present. However, patients should be examined for signs of other possible causes of anginal chest pain, such as aortic stenosis and hypertrophic obstructive cardiomyopathy.

Risk Stratification

CLINICAL INDICATORS

A number of clinical indicators identify patients at relatively high risk for clinical events (Box 8-2 and Figure 8-4). The threshold for the consideration of invasive coronary angiography should be lower in high-risk patients than in those being considered purely on the basis of their symptoms. The list of high-risk indicators in Box 8-2 is not comprehensive but incorporates the principal factors that determine risk.

NONINVASIVE EVALUATION

Electrocardiogram

A resting electrocardiogram (ECG) should always be recorded as part of the diagnostic evaluation of patients with chronic stable angina. The resting ECG may also be useful for adjusting medical therapy, such as for titration of β-blocker therapy. Although the sensitivity of the ECG is low for the diagnosis of CHD—in fact, it appears normal in almost one half of patients who come to medical attention with the disease[11]—it does provide prognostic information. Resting ST-segment depression predicts an increased likelihood of subsequent MI and death.[12] Patients with evidence of previous MI or ST-T–wave abnormalities without transmural Q-wave MI have a reduced survival rate.[13,14]

TABLE 8-1	Causes of Anginal Chest Pain not Attributable to Fixed Atheromatous Stenosis of the Coronary Artery
VASCULAR DISORDERS	**CARDIAC DISORDERS**
Variant angina	Hypertrophic cardiomyopathy
Atheroma-associated vasospasm	Aortic stenosis
Microvascular angina or syndrome X	Hypertensive heart disease and left ventricular hypertrophy Mitral valve prolapse Severe pulmonary hypertension and right ventricular hypertrophy

Exercise ECG testing is usually performed for two principal reasons: the diagnosis of angina as a result of CHD and as an assessment of prognosis. However, exercise ECG is an inappropriate screening test for CHD when used in isolation. In a population with a low prevalence of CHD, the false-positive rate is high, particularly in the absence of symptoms (Figure 8-5). The false-positive rate is also higher in younger individuals and in women. Conversely, the negative predictive value for CHD is poor, and the exercise ECG is therefore an inappropriate test to exclude its presence.

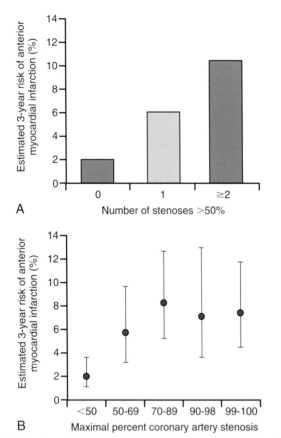

FIGURE 8-1 Three-year risk of anterior myocardial infarction according to the number (**A**) and severity (**B**) (mean ± 95% confidence interval) of coronary artery stenoses in the left anterior descending coronary artery. *(Data from Ellis S, Alderman E, Cain K, et al. Prediction of risk of anterior myocardial infarction by lesion severity and measurement method of stenoses in the left anterior descending coronary distribution: a CASS Registry study. J Am Coll Cardiol 1988;11:908.)*

Box 8-1 Canadian Cardiovascular Society Functional Classification of Stable Angina Pectoris

Class 1
Ordinary physical activity, such as walking and climbing stairs, does not cause angina. Angina comes with strenuous or rapid or prolonged exertion at work or during recreation.

Class 2
Slight limitation of ordinary activity occurs walking or climbing stairs rapidly, walking uphill, walking or stair climbing after meals, in cold, in wind, or when under emotional stress, or only during the few hours after awakening. Walking more than two blocks on level ground and climbing more than one flight of ordinary stairs at a normal pace and in normal conditions triggers angina.

Class 3
Marked limitation of ordinary physical activity occurs walking one to two blocks on level ground and climbing more than one flight of stairs under normal conditions.

Class 4
Patient is unable to carry on any physical activity without discomfort; anginal syndrome may be present at rest.

From Cox J, Naylor CD. The Canadian Cardiovascular Society grading scale for angina pectoris: Is it time for refinements? *Ann Intern Med* 1992;117:677.

Box 8-2 Clinical Indicators of Adverse Prognosis in Patients with Chronic Stable Angina

- Previous myocardial infarction
- Recent episode of unstable angina or new-onset stable angina
- Coexisting heart failure or evidence of left ventricular dysfunction
- Coexisting risk factors for coronary artery disease, such as hypertension and diabetes mellitus
- Age (the likelihood of death or nonfatal ischemic event increases with age)
- Family history, an independent predictor of death
- Pattern of anginal symptoms (quiescent angina is associated with a reduced risk of death and cardiac ischemic events)

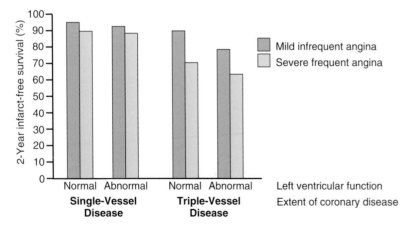

FIGURE 8-2 Two-year infarction-free survival rate of patients with angina pectoris according to angina frequency, extent of coronary artery disease, and left ventricular function (ejection fraction: normal, ≥50%; abnormal, <50%). *(Data from Califf RM, Mark DB, Harrell FE, et al. Importance of clinical measures of ischemia in the prognosis of patients with documented coronary artery disease. J Am Coll Cardiol 1988;11:20.)*

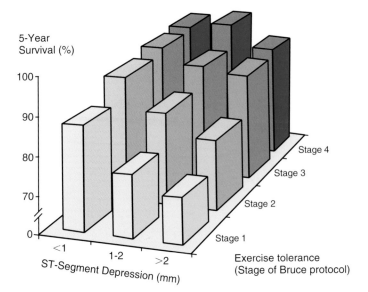

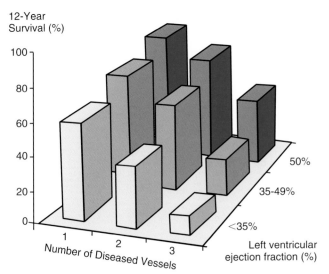

FIGURE 8-3 The 5- and 12-year survival rates of medically treated patients according to exercise tolerance, exercise-induced ST-segment depression, number of diseased vessels, and left ventricular function. *(Data from Emond M, Mock MB, David KB, et al. Long-term survival of medically treated patients in the Coronary Artery Surgery Study (CASS) Registry. Circulation 1994;90:2645; and Weiner DA, Ryan TJ, McCabe CH, et al. Prognostic importance of a clinical profile and exercise test in medically treated patients with coronary artery disease. J Am Coll Cardiol 1984;3:772.)*

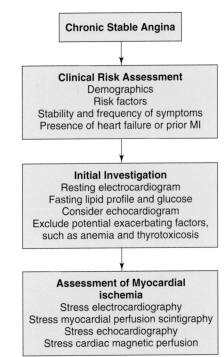

FIGURE 8-4 *Schema for the initial assessment and investigation of patients with chronic stable angina. When assessing the patient for provocable ischemia, clinicians should select one of the methods shown; do not perform all four. MI, myocardial infarction.*

Box 8-3 Features on Exercise Electrocardiogram Associated with a Poor Prognosis and Indicative of Severe Disease

- Poor maximal exercise capacity (less than stage 3 on the Bruce protocol)
- ≥1 mm ST-segment depression during stage 2 or less (Bruce protocol)
- ≥2 mm ST-segment depression at any time
- Limited blood pressure response (fall or no rise from baseline)

The clinical context, associated symptoms, and overall cardiovascular (CV) response to exercise can be as important as the ECG response to exercise (Box 8-3). Exercise testing is easily performed and, when used appropriately, is a method of risk stratification in patients with stable angina.[8,15-17] It is a particularly useful method of identifying individuals at highest risk and those who would benefit from further and potentially more invasive investigation and intervention.

Echocardiography

Echocardiography is used to assess cardiac function at rest and during pharmacologic or physical stress. LV dysfunction at rest or with exercise identifies patients with a poor prognosis.[8,18]

As with myocardial scintigraphy, stress echocardiography can be used to identify patients with CHD[19,20] and those with LV dysfunction and hibernating myocardium who would potentially benefit from coronary revascularization. Stress echocardiography

has some advantages and disadvantages over standard approaches to stress testing. Because of the problems associated with movement, pharmacologic stress echocardiography is sometimes the preferred approach; positive inotropes and chronotropes, such as dobutamine and arbutamine, are given as a continuous intravenous infusion, sometimes augmented by atropine to increase the heart rate further. The contractile performance of the heart is then assessed in multiple views, incorporating the 16 segments of the heart, both at rest and during graded stress. Stress echocardiography is therefore a demanding technique that requires a rigorous and skilled approach by highly trained operators.

Stress echocardiography is directed mainly at assessing the development of, or improvement in, myocardial wall motion abnormalities during stress. Deteriorating regional wall motion during increasing stress suggests the development of myocardial ischemia and underlying coronary artery disease (CAD). Alternatively, previously akinetic or hypokinetic areas of myocardium can improve during dobutamine stress and may indicate the presence of "stunned" myocardium, in which a recent period of profound ischemia has led to a temporary reduction in contractile function. A combination of features may also exist, where the contractile function initially improves with low-dose dobutamine infusion, only to deteriorate at higher doses. This suggests the presence of

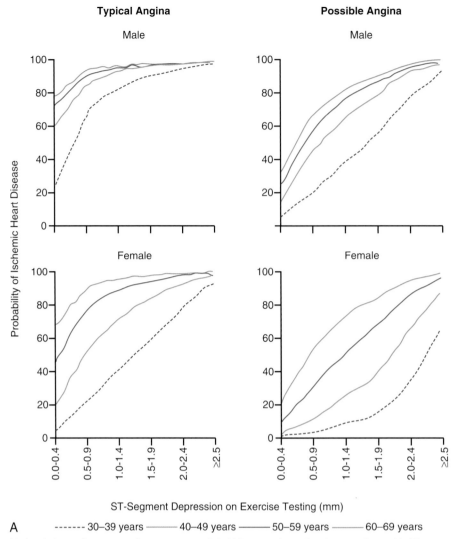

FIGURE 8-5 Probability of ischemic heart disease according to age, sex, clinical history, and exercise electrocardiographic ST-segment depression. **A,** Probability of ischemic heart disease in patients presenting with either typical or possible angina (stratified by gender and age).

Continued

"hibernating" myocardium, in which a critical coronary artery stenosis causes contractile dysfunction at rest, but the myocardium retains the ability to develop short-lived improvement in contractile function with inotropic stimulation before subsequent ischemic deterioration occurs at higher workloads. A completely unresponsive akinetic segment indicates an area of infarcted myocardium.

Cardiac Magnetic Resonance Imaging

Magnetic resonance coronary angiography has been reported but does require long acquisition times, cooperative subjects, and high field-strength scanners. Because of this, it is not sufficiently robust for routine clinical use. In contrast, magnetic resonance (MR) first-pass myocardial perfusion imaging is an established noninvasive method to detect myocardial perfusion defects and to quantify infarct size without the need for ionizing radiation.[21,22] MR imaging has excellent spatial and temporal resolution, and with the small addition of further imaging sequences, it can also provide quantification of myocardial fibrosis and infarct volumes. Several studies have demonstrated that perfusion cardiac magnetic resonance imaging (MRI) has high sensitivity (89%), specificity (81%), and accuracy (86%) for detection of CHD.[21-24] Cardiac MRI perfusion also has prognostic value in the assessment of patients with CAD[25]

and is now a well-established noninvasive standard for assessment of CHD.[26]

Myocardial Perfusion Scintigraphy

Stress myocardial perfusion imaging or scintigraphy has greater accuracy for diagnosing CHD than does exercise testing,[27] with a sensitivity of 80% versus 68% and a specificity of 92% versus 84%, respectively. However, stress myocardial scintigraphy adds little additional information for patients already identified as high risk through the use of conventional exercise testing. It is particularly helpful in individuals who have equivocal exercise ECG changes, an abnormal resting ECG, suspected false-positive or false-negative exercise ECG results, or submaximal exercise tolerance. It may also prove useful in identifying the territory of ischemia in patients with multivessel disease, in whom selective revascularization strategies, such as culprit lesion angioplasty, are being considered. The identification of hibernating myocardium may be of particular benefit in patients with LV dysfunction who have the most to gain from coronary revascularization.

Normal stress myocardial scintigraphy is associated with an excellent prognosis of less than 1% annual risk of a major adverse cardiac event, even in patients with CHD.[28,29] However, severe and extensive perfusion defects identify patients at high risk for future cardiac events and point to a poor prognosis (Box 8-4).[30]

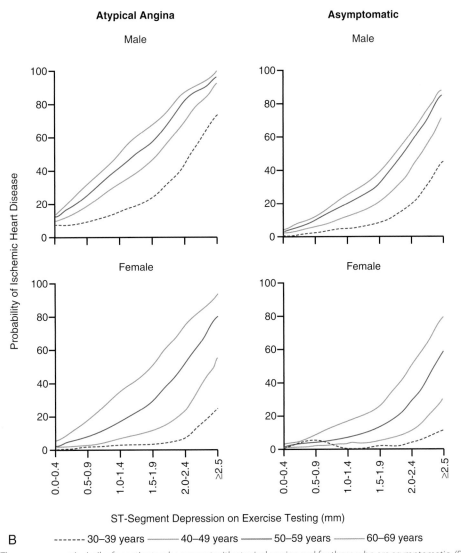

Atypical Angina

Male

Female

Asymptomatic

Male

Female

ST-Segment Depression on Exercise Testing (mm)

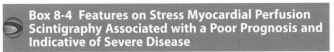

B · · · · · · 30–39 years ——— 40–49 years ——— 50–59 years ——— 60–69 years

FIGURE 8-5, cont'd   B, The arrangement is similar for patients who present with atypical angina and for those who are asymptomatic. *(Data from European Society of Cardiology Working Group on Exercise Physiology, Physiopathology and Electrocardiography. Guidelines for cardiac exercise testing.* Eur Heart J *1993;14:969.)*

Box 8-4 Features on Stress Myocardial Perfusion Scintigraphy Associated with a Poor Prognosis and Indicative of Severe Disease

- Reversible radionuclide perfusion defect in more than one territory
- Reduced radionuclide ejection fraction with exercise
- Increased lung uptake of radionuclide

The use of scintigraphy is likely to decline further with the greater availability, and similar or superior performance, of other techniques such as cardiac MR, echocardiography, and computed tomography (CT).

Computed Tomography

All of the noninvasive techniques above use surrogate measures—such as ST-segment shift, myocardial contraction, and tissue perfusion—to diagnose CHD. However, these techniques identify the functional significance, rather than the presence, of CAD, which underlies the relative lack of specificity and sensitivity in diagnosing the presence of epicardial CAD. In contrast, CT coronary angiography can directly identify the presence of CAD and also

provides information regarding the extent of atherosclerotic plaque burden that even invasive coronary angiography cannot. The potential weakness of CT coronary angiography lies in its inability to determine whether a lesion limits flow.

CORONARY CALCIUM SCORE

Coronary artery calcification is an independent risk factor for CHD, with even low coronary calcium scores doubling the risk of coronary events.[31] The relative risk associated with coronary calcification is similar to that associated with established factors such as smoking, hypertension, and diabetes mellitus. Progression of coronary artery calcification is associated with a higher incidence of coronary events even in those people who are asymptomatic at the time of initial scanning.[32] Thus, the presence of coronary artery calcification is indicative of not only atheromatous plaque disease, but also its progression may correspond with CV event rates.

The degree of calcification correlates with atherosclerotic burden, but it does not identify soft plaque and may not predict the response to medical interventions.[33,34] The presence of coronary artery calcification does not in itself predict the presence of obstructive atheroma. Calcification can therefore be used as a surrogate marker of the extent of coronary atherosclerotic disease rather than as a measure of luminal stenosis.[35]

COMPUTED TOMOGRAPHY CORONARY ANGIOGRAPHY

Major advances in scanning technology have now led to the establishment of noninvasive coronary angiography by multidetector CT (Figure 8-6). Indeed, coronary angiography performed by modern multidetector CT scanners has a very good agreement with invasive coronary angiography[36] and intravascular ultrasound.[37] The temporal and spatial resolution of modern scanners allows quantification of luminal stenoses and identification of uncalcified, "soft" atherosclerotic plaque.[37]

Pooled analysis of more than 800 patients indicates a sensitivity of 89% (95% confidence interval [CI], 87% to 90%) and specificity of 96% (95% CI, 96% to 97%) for 64-row multidetector CT in comparison with invasive coronary angiography.[38] The major strength is in the negative predictive value of 98% (95% CI, 98% to 99%). The major limitations have been the poor image quality in those with arrhythmia or fast heart rates and the high radiation dose of the examination (approximately 20 mSv).[38] Pulsed sequences, dual-source systems, and dynamic volume scanners with greater detector numbers are now overcoming these limitations. Thus, the current evolution of scanning technology has led to greater spatial and temporal resolution with lower radiation doses (2 to 4 mSv). This translates into a highly effective and safe imaging strategy. The most promising application is in the evaluation of stable patients with possible CHD[39] and the exclusion of coronary atherosclerosis. However, despite the high sensitivity, the specificity for the identification of obstructive CAD is low because of "blooming" artifacts from coronary calcification. This is particularly an issue in populations with a high prevalence of coronary calcification, such as those with stable angina and CHD.

With the advent of large (256 to 320) rows of detectors, dynamic volume CT scanning is now possible. Here, the entire heart is encompassed within the field of view, and extra images can be obtained during the transit of contrast through the myocardium (see Figure 8-6). This enables stress CT perfusion to be performed that has very high spatial resolution, which is superior to radionuclide techniques and, to a certain degree, MR techniques.

Selection and Frequency of Noninvasive Stress Testing

There are advantages and disadvantages with each of the four main noninvasive modalities of stress testing (Table 8-2). Exercise ECG testing is easily performed, has been extensively validated, and remains the noninvasive test of choice for many patients. However, the sensitivity and specificity of exercise ECG are suboptimal and can lead to significant misclassification. This also applies to the other noninvasive forms of stress testing. For the diagnosis of CHD, CT coronary angiography is increasingly likely to play a major role.

No clear guidelines exist as to how frequently noninvasive testing should be undertaken in patients with chronic stable angina.[40] After the initial prognostic assessment, recurrent testing is unlikely to be helpful unless new symptoms arise or other symptoms change, vocational requirements change, or the patient has undergone, or is being considered for, an intervention such as coronary revascularization or major noncardiac surgery.[40]

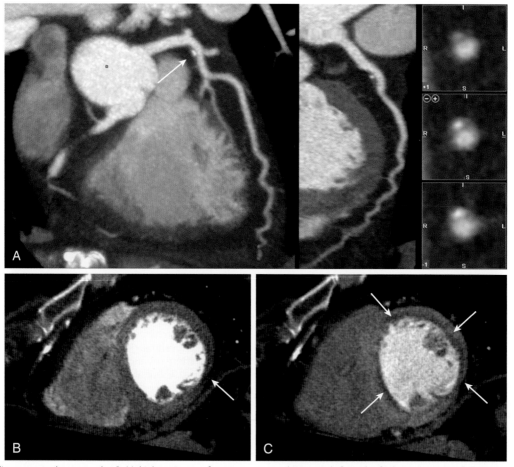

FIGURE 8-6 Cardiac computed tomography. **A,** Multiplanar image of a coronary artery showing calcific and soft plaque (*arrow*) with cross-sectional images shown in the three right panels. **B,** Myocardial perfusion at rest, showing resting perfusion defect and wall thinning consistent with infarction (*arrow*). **C,** During stress, showing widespread subendocardial perfusion defects (*arrows*) indicative of triple-vessel coronary artery disease.

TABLE 8-2   Relative Advantages and Disadvantages of the Four Main Noninvasive Stress Testing Methods

	STRESS ELECTROCARDIOGRAPHY	MYOCARDIAL PERFUSION SCINTIGRAPHY	STRESS ECHOCARDIOGRAPHY	CARDIAC MAGNETIC RESONANCE PERFUSION
Technical difficulty	+	++	+++	+++
Ease of interpretation	+++	++	+++	++
Diagnostic sensitivity (%)	50-80	65-90	65-90	70-90
Diagnostic specificity (%)	80-95	90-95	90-95	90-95
Risk stratification	++	++	++	+
Identification of hibernating myocardium	–	++	+++	+++
Identification of ischemic territory	+	++	++	+++
Limitations	Conduction or repolarization anomalies	Radiation exposure	Diagnostic images not possible in all patients	Claustrophobia and incompatibility with devices
Cost	+	+++	++	+++

Plus signs denote relative strength or magnitude of each modality.

Box 8-5 Indications for Coronary Angiography

Severe or Disabling Angina
The severity of symptoms indicating the need for coronary angiography will vary depending on the patient's, and the physician's, perception of the illness. However, most experts agree that despite optimal medical therapy, patients with symptoms in Canadian Cardiovascular Society class 3 or 4 may benefit symptomatically from coronary artery bypass graft surgery or percutaneous coronary intervention.

Clinical Indicators and Noninvasive Testing Suggestive of Adverse Prognosis

Continuing Chest Pain with Inconclusive or Negative Noninvasive Tests
In this context, a normal coronary angiogram can be very helpful in excluding obstructive coronary artery disease, removing uncertainty about the diagnosis, reassuring the patient, and thereby reducing their use of health care resources. This will be of particular concern when the symptoms limit the lifestyle of the patient, or when a diagnosis of coronary artery disease will have occupational ramifications.

INVASIVE EVALUATION

Invasive coronary angiography is used to aid the diagnosis and management of known or suspected CHD and is considered when either medical therapy has failed to provide effective symptomatic control or clinical and noninvasive tests suggest that the patient may be at high risk or may otherwise benefit from intervention. This can be further complemented by the functional assessment of coronary stenoses using the pressure-wire assessment of fractional flow reserve. This can guide the appropriate management and revascularization of patients with CHD (Box 8-5).[41]

OVERALL ASSESSMENT OF RISK

A number of scoring systems have been developed that incorporate both clinical characteristics and noninvasive investigations in the determination of risk.[8,16,17,42-44] These models provide a more comprehensive assessment of risk and prognosis in patients with stable angina. Coronary angiography is appropriate in patients whose clinical characteristics or noninvasive investigations suggest they have an adverse prognosis and may therefore benefit prognostically from coronary artery bypass graft surgery (CABG; Figure 8-7).

The hazards of any intervention are more likely to outweigh the potential symptomatic and prognostic benefits in patients at low risk. In contrast, patients at high risk have the most to gain from interventions such as revascularization. Risk stratification is

therefore an essential part of the initial assessment of a patient with stable angina. The main determinants of risk are patient characteristics such as age; diabetes mellitus; hypertension; and the results of clinical investigations, such as exercise or other forms of stress testing, the extent of coronary disease (the number and type of vessels affected), and LV function (see Figures 8-1 to 8-3).

Therapeutic Interventions

The treatment of patients with chronic stable angina pectoris should be directed toward both the alleviation of symptoms and an improvement in prognosis. This involves several approaches that include lifestyle modification, management of risk factors, pharmacologic therapy, and coronary revascularization. All forms of intervention present certain hazards and should be instituted only if the perceived benefits, in terms of improved symptoms and prognosis, are likely to outweigh the associated risks. Such judgments are best made in the context of an overall treatment strategy that seeks to minimize the impact of the disease throughout the remainder of the patient's life. Figure 8-4 and Figures 8-7 through 8-10 provide a general guide to the initial investigation and management of patients with chronic stable angina.

Lifestyle and Risk Factor Modifications

Lifestyle and risk factor modifications are integral parts of, and complementary to, the treatment of patients with chronic stable angina because they may provide both symptomatic and prognostic benefits. The benefits of exercise and exercise programs and the management of hyperlipidemia are discussed later in this chapter. The treatment and management of hypertension are discussed in Chapters 28 through 34.

SMOKING

Cigarette smoking is a major risk factor for the development of fatal and nonfatal MI.[45] Cessation of smoking is associated with major benefits, and repeated brief and supportive advice should be given to all patients.[46,47] Short-term nicotine replacement therapy should be offered to individuals who are heavy consumers of tobacco (>10 cigarettes per day) because it is associated with up to a ninefold increased likelihood of success.[48,49] The antidepressants bupropion and nortriptyline also aid long-term smoking cessation, but selective serotonin reuptake inhibitors, such as fluoxetine, do not.[50] This suggests that these agents produce their beneficial effects independent of an antidepressant effect. The partial nicotine receptor agonist, varenicline, increases the likelihood of smoking cessation twofold to threefold and appears to be more

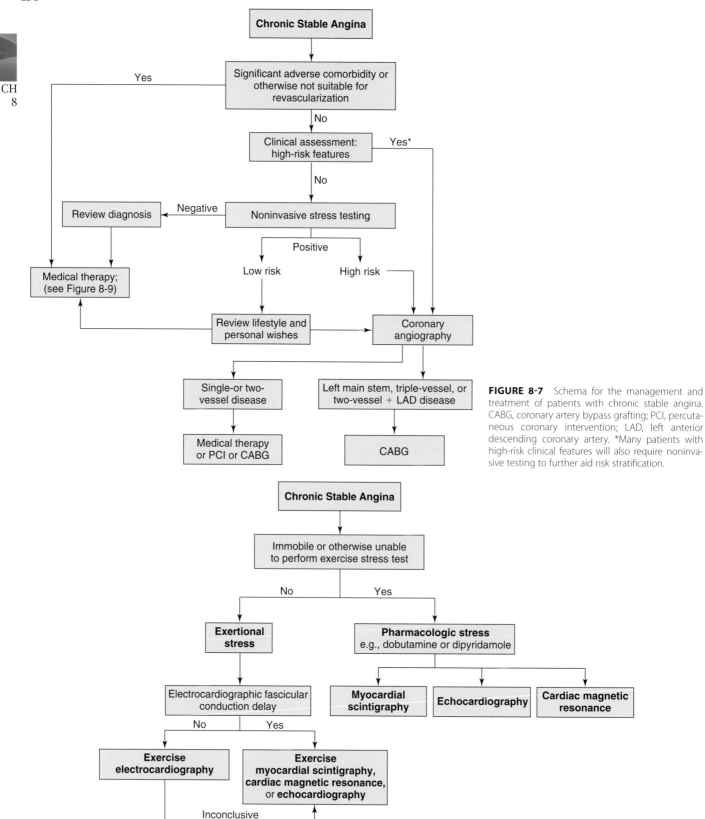

FIGURE 8-7 Schema for the management and treatment of patients with chronic stable angina. CABG, coronary artery bypass grafting; PCI, percutaneous coronary intervention; LAD, left anterior descending coronary artery. *Many patients with high-risk clinical features will also require noninvasive testing to further aid risk stratification.

FIGURE 8-8 Schema for the selection of noninvasive stress testing for patients with chronic stable angina.

effective than bupropion.[51] Although no previous specific treatment strategy has been able to prevent relapses,[52] varenicline does appear to sustain smoking cessation and prevent subsequent relapses.[51] Some reports have linked varenicline with serious adverse events that include a depressed mood, agitation, and suicidal thoughts, but these are so far unsubstantiated.

DIETARY INTERVENTION

Dietary intervention clearly complements the use of lipid-lowering therapy. Although a low-fat diet reduces serum cholesterol concentrations by an average of only 5%[53] even in motivated individuals,[54] dietary modification may provide additional preventive benefits,

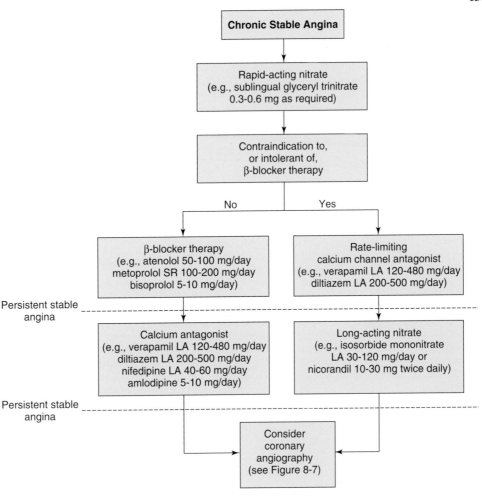

FIGURE 8-9 Schema for the symptomatic medical management of patients with chronic stable angina. The specific drug and dosage recommendations shown are not arranged in preferred sequence based on clinical trials and are not meant to exclude other drugs within the same class. Instead, they are examples of therapeutic suggestions based on the experience of the authors. LA, long-acting; SR, sustained-release.

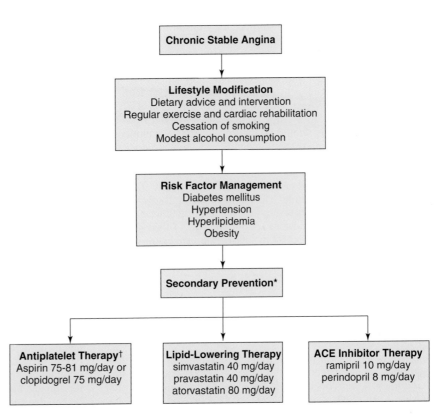

FIGURE 8-10 Schema for secondary prevention in patients with chronic stable angina. *If the patient is high risk, consider coronary angiography if the patient is suitable for revascularization. †Aspirin is preferred over clopidogrel as antiplatelet monotherapy. In patients who have undergone stent implantation, dual antiplatelet therapy is prescribed. The specific drug and dosage recommendations shown are not arranged in preferred sequence based on clinical trials and are not meant to exclude other drugs within the same class. Instead, they are examples of therapeutic suggestions based on the experience of the authors. ACE, angiotensin-converting enzyme.

such as those obtained from a Mediterranean-type diet[55] or those high in polyunsaturated (n-3) fatty acids of fish oils.[56,57] Observational studies[58,59] and randomized trials[60] have suggested that the consumption of fruits and vegetables containing high levels of antioxidant vitamins or supplementation with vitamin E[61,62] is protective against the development of coronary events. However, three large-scale (6000 to 30,000) multicenter, randomized, controlled trials (RCTs) demonstrated that low- or high-dose vitamin E supplementation has no effect on CV outcomes.[57,63,64] Modest alcohol consumption is associated with a reduced risk of CHD and should be limited to 21 to 28 U/week (1 U = 8 g of absolute alcohol) for men and 14 to 21 U/week for women.[65]

OBESITY

A significant and independent association has been found between body mass index (BMI) and the risk of CV events.[66] Despite the high prevalence of obesity, no interventional trials have been done to show that weight reduction in obese patients with chronic stable angina or CHD improves symptoms or outcome. However, it is reasonable to assume that weight reduction would reduce the frequency of anginal episodes and potentially improve prognosis.

Currently escalating levels of obesity, particularly in Western societies, are associated with the development of *metabolic syndrome,* which is characterized by obesity, insulin resistance, hypertension, hyperuricemia, and dyslipidemia. This has raised concerns about the incidence and prevalence of CV disease in the future. Novel therapeutic strategies, such as the endocannabinoid receptor antagonis rimonabant, may be able to reduce obesity and the associated metabolic abnormalities. However, in an RCT of nearly 20,000 at-risk subjects,[67] rimonabant had no effect on adverse CV outcomes but was associated with increased general and serious neuropsychiatric problems, including suicide.

DIABETES MELLITUS

Good glycemic control is essential in all patients with diabetes mellitus because of the reduced risk of long-term complications, including CHD. Although no specific trials of diabetic control in patients with chronic stable angina have been done, primary prevention trials[68,69] and secondary prevention trials in patients after MI[70] indicate that CV morbidity and mortality rates are reduced with intensive hypoglycemic therapy regimens. Moreover, poor glycemic control at the time of presentation with MI is a poor prognostic sign.[71] Although previous studies[72] had suggested that sulfonylureas, tolbutamide in particular, are associated with an increased risk of CV death, this was not confirmed in the U.K. Prospective Diabetes Study (UKPDS) trial.[73] That trial did, however, suggest that metformin should be the first-line agent of choice in overweight patients with diabetes mellitus because it is associated with a decreased risk of diabetes-related endpoints, less weight gain, and fewer hypoglycemic episodes.

The control of hyperglycemia is important, but overly strict glycemic control can be harmful. The application of intensive blood glucose control in patients with type 2 diabetes mellitus is associated with an increase in adverse CV outcomes.[74,75] This is likely to arise from the harmful effects of hypoglycemia, especially in those with concurrent CHD; therefore a balance must be struck between avoidance of prolonged hyperglycemia and invocation of adverse hypoglycemic episodes.

Symptomatic Therapy

CARDIAC REHABILITATION

Cardiac rehabilitation involves a multidisciplinary approach that addresses needs related to medical and psychosocial care that include exercise, education, secondary prevention, and vocational advice.[76] Although predominantly applied to the immediate post-MI or postoperative period (after CABG), it is equally applicable to patients with chronic stable angina. The rehabilitation process encompasses the following three main components: 1) explanation and understanding; 2) specific intervention, such as secondary prevention, exercise training, and psychological support; and 3) long-term adaptation and education.

Patients with stable angina who attend a regular exercise and rehabilitation program have less angina and may have fewer recurrent MIs, and they have better cardiorespiratory fitness and vocational status.[77,78] Exercise programs improve patient confidence and functional capacity, and although such programs are labor intensive, they are an efficacious and potentially cost-effective approach to the treatment of patients with stable angina (see Chapter 49).[79] Indeed, an RCT suggested that an exercise program produced a better improvement in exercise capacity, was associated with fewer adverse cardiac events, and was more cost-effective than percutaneous coronary intervention (PCI).[80]

PHARMACOLOGIC THERAPY

No single class of drug has been shown to be superior to another in the reduction of anginal episodes. However, because of the inferred secondary preventive benefits, β-blockers should be the first-line agents of choice (see Figure 8-9). Moreover, a meta-analysis suggests that β-blockers are better tolerated and may be more efficacious than CCBs in the treatment of chronic stable angina.[105]

If monotherapy does not control anginal symptoms, the introduction of a second antianginal agent provides significant but modest additional benefits (see Figure 8-9). The combination of β-blockade and rate-limiting calcium channel blockade may cause excessive bradycardia or heart block. However, this interaction is uncommon, and if there is concern, a long-acting dihydropyridine-type CCB should also be prescribed. No definitive evidence is available to suggest that triple or quadruple antianginal therapy produces further benefit beyond dual therapy. Two large-scale RCTs (n = 5126 and n = 7665) of the addition of nicorandil[6] or nifedipine[5] to one or more antianginal medications, predominantly β-blocker therapies, demonstrated no major change in anginal symptoms, although nifedipine use was associated with a modest reduction in the need for coronary angiography (absolute reduction of 1.23% per year) and coronary artery bypass surgery (absolute reduction of 0.44% per year). Once-daily and sustained-release preparations should be used whenever possible to aid compliance.

β-Blockers

β-Blockers inhibit the β-adrenergic receptors of the myocardium to produce negative chronotropism and negative inotropism of the heart. The attenuation of the heart rate response to exercise and stress reduces the myocardial oxygen demand and severity of ischemia. It also prolongs diastole, a major determinant of myocardial perfusion time. RCTs[81,82] have demonstrated that β-blocker therapy is efficacious in reducing symptoms of angina and episodes of ischemia and in improving exercise capacity.

No evidence supports the suggestion that one type of β-blocker is superior to another. The highly selective β-blockers, such as celiprolol or bisoprolol—or those with combined vasodilation and antioxidant properties, such as carvedilol—have no proven benefits above conventional β-blockers such as atenolol or metoprolol. However, the secondary preventive benefits of β-blockers may be lost when agents have intrinsic sympathomimetic action,[83] and the use of such agents should be avoided.

True side effects from β-blocker therapy are uncommon and occur in less than 10% of patients but include symptoms such as fatigue and lethargy, commonly reported on routine inquiry. A causative association should be established before permanent discontinuation of β-blocker therapy. Because of β-adrenergic receptor upregulation in the presence of β-blockade, patients should not be rapidly withdrawn from therapy, as this can cause an acute withdrawal syndrome; also, it has been suggested that this may even precipitate acute MI.[84]

Calcium Channel Blockers

Patients who are intolerant of a β-blocker should be considered for a rate-limiting calcium channel blocker (CCB) such as diltiazem or verapamil. In the second Danish Verapamil Infarction Trial (DAVIT II), a post hoc analysis suggested that verapamil may be beneficial after MI in the absence of heart failure.[85] However, other CCBs[86] and classes of antianginal agents[87-89] are equally effective in relieving symptoms. The addition of nifedipine to other antianginal therapies does appear to reduce the need for further invasive investigation and revascularization.[5]

Controversy exists as to whether CCBs can be used safely in patients with heart failure.[90] Amlodipine has been shown to have a neutral effect on mortality rates in patients with heart failure and is an appropriate choice in patients with angina and significant LV dysfunction.[91]

Nitrates

Nitrates were the first form of antianginal drug therapy to be discovered and used. Their mechanism of action is exerted through the release of nitric oxide (NO) either indirectly—as with glyceryl trinitrate (GTN) and reactions with sulfhydryl groups, such as methionine or cysteine—or directly (sodium nitroprusside), by interaction with plasma or cell membranes. The liberated NO causes endothelium-independent relaxation of vascular smooth muscle by increasing intracellular cyclic guanidine monophosphate (cGMP; see Chapter 7).

RCTs[87,92] have demonstrated that nitrates are effective in reducing the frequency of anginal symptoms and in improving exercise capacity. However, as with CCBs, their use in severe aortic stenosis and hypertrophic obstructive cardiomyopathy should be avoided because of the potential to compromise coronary perfusion through peripheral vasodilation and systemic arterial hypotension.

ACUTE RELIEF OF ANGINA

Sublingual or buccal nitrates produce rapid and effective relief of acute anginal episodes. All patients should be provided with a sublingual nitrate preparation. Buccal preparations provide a more protracted release of nitrate, which is appropriate for prolonged activities that may provoke episodes of angina.

PREVENTION OF ANGINAL EPISODES

Long-acting nitrates, either oral or transdermal, provide effective relief of angina. Nitrates undergo extensive first-pass metabolism through hepatic glutathione reductases; however, topical and transdermal nitrate preparations are able to bypass such metabolism, and consequently, the overall dosage can be reduced. Alternatively, some nitrate preparations, such as isosorbide mononitrate, undergo less extensive hepatic metabolism and have better bioavailability and more prolonged action.

One of the main limitations of prophylactic nitrate use is the development of tolerance (see Chapter 7). This phenomenon requires a daily nitrate-free period,[93,94] usually nocturnal, to prevent the loss of efficacy—a problem with all of the established nitrate preparations. The mechanism of nitrate tolerance appears, at least in part, to be due to the depletion of sulfhydryl groups.[95] The development of S-nitrosothiols potentially heralds a novel class of nitrates that may be devoid of nitrate tolerance[96] and may have additional antiplatelet actions.[97]

Potassium Channel Agonists

This class of antianginal agents has vasodilatory and potential cardioprotective actions. Potassium channel openers act on the ion channels of the vascular smooth muscle cell and cardiac myocyte. Consequently, they may have a role in enhancing ischemic preconditioning[98] and improving the myocardial response to an ischemic insult.[99]

Nicorandil is the only preparation of this class in clinical use. It is effective in the treatment of angina and has both nitrate and potassium channel–opening properties. However, no evidence suggests that potassium channel openers are superior to other classes of antianginal agents, and their addition to preexisting antianginal therapy does not appear to improve symptoms.[6] The Impact of Nicorandil in Angina (IONA) trial[6] in 5126 patients with stable angina did demonstrate that nicorandil 20 mg twice daily was associated with a modest 17% relative risk reduction in its primary endpoint of CHD death, nonfatal MI, or unplanned hospitalization. However, the trial failed to demonstrate a difference in the secondary endpoint of CHD death and MI.

Miscellaneous Medical Therapies

Ivabradine is an inhibitor of I_f, the so-called *funny ion channel* found in the sinoatrial (SA) node, and it reduces heart rate in patients who are in sinus rhythm. This heart rate–lowering effect is associated with antianginal effects that are comparable[100] and additive[101] to other antianginal therapies. Ivabradine is particularly useful in those patients who are intolerant of β-blockers and who also have a high resting heart rate.

Ranolazine is a novel antianginal therapy that does not have a clearly understood mechanism of action, but it appears to modulate the metabolism of ischemic myocardial cells and improve the efficiency of oxygen use. It also appears to provide additional antianginal benefits when added to other therapies.[102,103] Ranolazine has also been shown to safely reduce ischemia in patients following ACS.[104]

CORONARY REVASCULARIZATION

Both CABG and PCI carry measurable early morbidity and mortality risks. As indicated, all interventions should be instituted only if the perceived benefits, in terms of improved symptoms and prognosis, are likely to outweigh the associated risks. This is particularly important when the therapy is targeted at symptomatic, rather than prognostic, benefits such as with PCI or CABG for single-vessel disease.

Selection of the appropriateness and type of revascularization procedure will be heavily influenced by technical aspects of the coronary anatomy and by factors such as comorbidity and patient preference. What is considered to be an acceptable level of symptoms, optimal medical therapy, and tolerable drug side effects may vary greatly from patient to patient. Thus the need for and type of coronary revascularization should take into account both objective clinical criteria and the patient's symptoms (see Chapter 11).

Several factors must be considered when evaluating the applicability and evidence of the clinical usefulness of coronary revascularization strategies. First, the major randomized trials are based on highly selected patient groups and may not reflect the broad mix of patients who present to the clinic. For example, the Angioplasty Compared with Medicine (ACME) trial[106] recruited only 212 patients of the nearly 5000 who were screened. Second, most trials have not exclusively selected patients with chronic stable angina pectoris. Third, many datasets reported in the literature are outdated. Medical therapy has improved and has become more effective; similarly, the surgical results do not take into account the improvements in techniques and the increasing use of arterial conduits (Figure 8-11). Indeed, the initial failure and restenosis rate in PCI has been reduced by the introduction of coronary artery stent deployment (Figure 8-12), drug-eluting stents, and adjuvant therapy with antiplatelet agents.[107]

Percutaneous Coronary Intervention

The success and complication rate of PCI are influenced by many factors that include age, gender, clinical presentation, LV function, comorbidity (e.g., diabetes mellitus), and the experience of the operator.[108,109] However, the most important determinant of outcome is the nature of the target lesion. A short, discrete, soft lesion on a straight segment of artery that does not compromise a major branch is ideal for PCI. Lesions less suitable for PCI include

CH
8

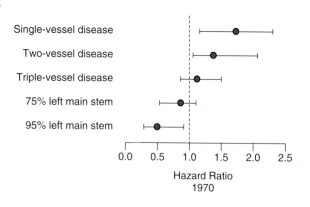

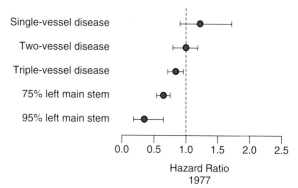

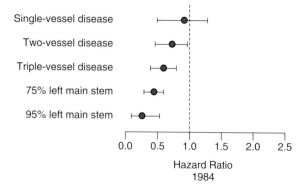

FIGURE 8-11 Improvements in survival with coronary artery bypass graft surgery (to left of *dashed lines*) during a 14-year period. *(Data from Califf RM, Harrell FE, Lee KL, et al. The evolution of medical and surgical therapy for coronary artery disease: a 15-year perspective. JAMA 1989;261:2077.)*

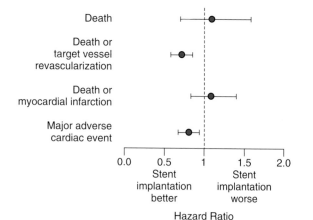

FIGURE 8-12 Improvements in 1-year clinical outcome with the introduction of coronary stenting. *(Data from Rankin JM, Spinelli JJ, Carere RG, et al. Improved clinical outcome after widespread use of coronary artery stenting in Canada. N Engl J Med 1999;341:1957.)*

chronic total occlusions, long lesions, calcifications, lesions that lie on tortuous segments or flexures, and lesions that involve branch vessels. PCI has a high success rate and low complication rate for ideal lesions but a low success rate and high complication rate for complex lesions.

INDICATIONS: PERCUTANEOUS CORONARY INTERVENTION VERSUS
MEDICAL TREATMENT

The first RCT to assess the usefulness of PCI in comparison with medical therapy was the ACME trial.[106] This study recruited patients with single-vessel disease, the majority of whom (>90%) had stable angina pectoris. It demonstrated that PCI is associated with superior subjective and objective improvements in anginal symptoms at 6 months.[106,110] However, concern was raised that PCI was associated with a higher incidence of complications, particularly recurrent revascularization procedures.

The subsequent Randomised Intervention Treatment of Angina (RITA-2) trial[111] was a larger RCT (n = 1018) designed to compare the effects of balloon angioplasty with medical therapy in patients with angina and single-vessel (60%) or multivessel (40%) disease. However, the study population included patients who had quiescent angina with no symptoms (20%) or recent (7 to 90 days before randomization) unstable angina (10%). Consistent with the ACME trial,[106] an initial strategy of angioplasty was associated with less angina for at least 2 years after the procedure compared with medical treatment. This reduction in anginal symptoms was associated with a diminished requirement for antianginal drug therapy, an increase in exercise capacity, and an overall improvement in quality of life.[111,112] However, reflecting the low-risk population of patients recruited into this trial, angioplasty was associated with nearly twice the risk of death or nonfatal MI (6.3% vs. 3.3% at 2.7 years; *P* = .02), which occurred predominantly in the first 3 months after randomization. It should also be noted that one fourth of patients randomized to medical treatment required a revascularization procedure during follow-up for worsening symptoms.

The symptomatic benefits of angioplasty in the RITA-2 trial appeared to be most marked in the patients with severe symptoms or limited exercise tolerance; therefore it may be necessary to accept a small, initial, procedure-related hazard from angioplasty to gain relief from severe or limiting anginal symptoms. However, improved imaging and stent technologies combined with better antiplatelet therapies, such as the thienopyridines and glycoprotein (GP) IIb/IIIa receptor antagonists, mean that the hazards identified in RITA-2 have been overestimated in the current era. Thus, PCI is an appropriate intervention in patients with suitable coronary anatomy who have chronic stable angina with limiting symptoms despite medical treatment (see Figure 8-7). Indeed, the more contemporary Clinical Outcomes Utilizing Revascularization and Aggressive Drug Evaluation (COURAGE) trial[113] was a study of 2287 patients with stable CHD who were randomized to PCI with optimal medical therapy or optimal medical therapy alone. PCI was again associated with improved symptoms, and modest but significantly greater proportions of patients were rendered free of angina at 1 year (66% vs. 58% angina free; *P* < .001) and 3 years (72% vs. 66%; *P* < .02) but not at 5 years. This was achieved without any increase in adverse events, with similar rates of death and nonfatal MI out to 5 years.

PERCUTANOUS CORONARY INTERVENTION VERSUS CORONARY ARTERY
BYPASS GRAFTING

A meta-analysis of eight large RCTs that compared PCI (n = 1710) with CABG (n = 1661) in patients with predominantly stable angina (80%) has shown no significant difference in survival between the two revascularization strategies during a mean follow-up of 2.7 years.[114] However, a significant difference was evident in the subsequent need for additional revascularization, with 17.8% of patients randomized to PCI requiring CABG within 1 year, and about 2% per year requiring CABG in subsequent years. The prevalence of angina at 1 year was considerably higher in the PCI group (1.5-fold to twofold), but at 3 years, this difference was no longer significant.[114]

The Bypass Angioplasty Revascularization Investigation (BARI) trial[115] was published after the meta-analysis by Pocock and colleagues[114] and is the largest study to compare PCI with CABG, although only 40% of patients recruited into this trial had stable angina. The BARI trial also showed no difference in survival or risk of MI between PCI and CABG patients; however, PCI was again associated with a higher rate of subsequent revascularization procedures (8% for CABG vs. 54% for PCI at 5 years). This excess of additional procedures for PCI was again seen predominantly in the first year. However, in the Arterial Revascularisation Therapy Study (ARTS)[116] and Stent or Surgery (SOS) trials,[117] the introduction of elective coronary artery stenting reduced the apparent need for recurrent revascularization procedures in patients with multivessel disease (4% to 6% for CABG vs. 17% to 21% for PCI at 1 to 2 years).

The Synergy Between Percutaneous Coronary Intervention with Taxus and Cardiac Surgery (SYNTAX) trial[118] randomized 1800 patients with three-vessel or left main stem disease to either PCI with drug-eluting stents or CABG.[118] Approximately 60% of enrolled patients came to medical attention with angina. At 1 year, no difference was seen in the combined endpoint of death, MI, or stroke (7.7% vs. 7.6%; $P = .99$), but PCI was associated with a greater need for repeat revascularization (13.5% vs. 5.9%; $P < .001$), whereas CABG was associated with an increased risk of stroke (2.2% vs. 0.6%; $P = .003$).

The Duke University database (n = 9263) describes a single-center prospective experience of the outcomes in patients with ischemic heart disease (20% of patients had stable angina) who were managed with medical therapy, PCI, or CABG. These data suggested that patients with one-vessel disease or two-vessel disease without involvement of the proximal left anterior descending (LAD) coronary artery experience better clinical outcomes with PCI than with CABG.[119,120] This contrasts with the findings of the Pocock and colleagues[114] meta-analysis, in which the combined endpoint of death or MI in one-vessel disease appeared to be less frequent with CABG than with PCI (4.5% vs. 7.2%). However, the subgroup analysis reported by Pocock and colleagues encompassed only three trials with small numbers (n = 350 for each group), and the authors question the reliability of the finding.[119] In contrast to the Duke University database, the patients in these randomized trials were highly selected populations; for example, the RITA trial[121] recruited only 3% of patients undergoing an angiogram.

It would appear that PCI is an appropriate alternative to CABG in patients with symptom-limiting chronic stable angina despite medical treatment, especially those with one- or two-vessel disease without a significant proximal LAD stenosis. It would also appear that in patients with multivessel disease, those with a lesion having a fractional flow reserve less than 0.8 benefit most from PCI.[41]

CULPRIT LESION PERCUTANEOUS CORONARY INTERVENTION
When the main objective of revascularization is the relief of angina, it may be advisable to consider PCI of the lesion believed to be responsible for the patient's symptoms, even when multivessel disease is evident that might otherwise be treated with CABG. This strategy, known as *culprit lesion PCI*, is often appropriate in symptomatic patients with multivessel CHD who have a single, exceptionally severe stenosis and many minor lesions; it is also beneficial in patients who are unsuitable for CABG because of comorbid conditions such as cerebrovascular disease or chronic obstructive airway disease.[122] Culprit lesion PCI is also a reasonable option when surgical revascularization with CABG would be incomplete, in which case it may not confer prognostic benefit.

PERCUTANEOUS CORONARY INTERVENTION AFTER CORONARY ARTERY BYPASS GRAFTING
Five years after undergoing CABG, 50% of patients will have redeveloped angina,[40] and by 12 years 30% will have undergone repeat revascularization.[123] Repeat CABG is associated with a higher risk and a lower likelihood of benefit than the initial intervention. In an analysis of 632 nonrandomized patients with previous CABG who required either elective repeat CABG or PCI,

complete revascularization was achieved in 38% of patients who underwent PCI compared with 92% of patients who underwent CABG; however, complications were significantly lower with PCI (0.3% vs. 7.3%), and survival was similar at 1- and 6-year follow-up. Both procedures resulted in similar event-free survival from death, MI, and angina, but by 6 years, further revascularization with either repeat PCI or CABG was significantly higher with PCI (64% vs. 8%).[124]

These findings were confirmed in a larger cohort of 4174 patients who underwent coronary revascularization (nonrandomized PCI or CABG) after previous CABG.[125] Repeat CABG was associated with a higher in-hospital mortality rate (6.8%) than PCI (1.2%), but mortality rates were similar at 1, 5, and 10 years. PCI was again associated with an increased risk of recurrent angina and additional procedures.

When technically feasible, we prefer an initial strategy of PCI rather than repeat CABG in chronic stable angina patients with limiting angina despite previous CABG and medical therapy.

STENTS
Intracoronary stents were initially used for the management of serious complications arising from PCI, such as acute or threatened vessel occlusion, a so-called *bailout stent implantation*. This provided an extremely useful way of maintaining vessel patency and led to a reduction in the need for emergency CABG after PCI.[126] Observational studies[126-129] and initial RCTs have confirmed the clear usefulness of the technique in the management of acute vessel closure.

Several RCTs have assessed the efficacy of elective intracoronary stenting. Some of the studies have methodological limitations, such as control patients who did not receive matched anticoagulation regimens (the Stent Restenosis Study [STRESS])[130] or investigators who were not fully blinded (the Belgian Netherlands Stent [BENESTENT] and Stenting in Chronic Coronary Occlusion [SICCO] trials).[131-133] However, all trials report consistent findings: elective stenting is associated with improved procedural and clinical outcomes and a reduction in the need for subsequent revascularization procedures. The clearest evidence has come from PCI procedures for higher risk lesions, namely chronically occluded arteries,[133-135] saphenous vein grafts,[136] proximal LAD stenoses,[137] and restenosis after prior PCI.[138,139] Stent implantation is also appropriate when conventional PCI has produced a suboptimal result.[140]

In the BENESTENT study,[131] the effect of elective stenting of all lesions was compared with the use of PCI alone in patients with stable angina and a single new lesion. No procedure-related deaths occurred in this trial, and stenting was associated with improved clinical and angiographic outcomes. The subsequent BENESTENT II study[141] included patients with unstable angina (40%) and confirmed the benefits of elective stent implantation using heparin-coated stents. However, a more selective approach of stent implantation for high-risk lesions or suboptimal angiographic results may confer similar benefits and may be more appropriate.[142]

Observational studies[126,127,143] and RCTs[130-132,144] indicate that after stent implantation, patients have less restenosis and greater event-free survival from MI and repeated coronary intervention. Subsequent to the widespread use of stents in Canada, evidence of improved clinical outcome, particularly a reduced need for recurrent coronary intervention, was observed (see Figure 8-12).[127]

Stents are now available that have agents impregnated into their polymer coating (see Chapter 11). One of the first to be used was a heparin-coated stent. This was used to reduce the incidence of stent thrombosis and restenosis; however, these heparin-coated stents had limited benefits above bare-metal stents. There has been major interest in the use of drug-eluting stents that contain antiproliferative agents. Sirolimus is a macrolide antibiotic with antifungal, immunosuppressive, and antimitotic properties that has been used in the prevention of renal transplant rejection. Sirolimus-coated stents are associated with a dramatic reduction in the incidence of in-stent restenosis, with failure of target vessel revascularization falling from 21.0% to 8.6% in the Sirolimus-Eluting Stent in Coronary Lesions (SIRIUS) study of 1058 patients with CHD.[145] Paclitaxel is a microtubule-stabilizing agent with potent antitumor activity that has also been successfully used in stent coatings with similar reductions of in-stent restenosis. Stent platforms continue to improve, and newer stent platforms and eluting drugs, such as everolimus and zotarolimus, continue to show substantial improvements and excellent outcomes.[146]

ANTIPLATELET THERAPY

All patients with CHD should be maintained on aspirin therapy, which is discussed later (see Figure 8-10).[147] Aspirin therapy is associated with a 53% reduction in the rate of vascular occlusion after PCI (2.7% vs. 5.5%).[147] The combination of ticlopidine (250 mg twice daily) and aspirin (100 mg twice daily) compared with conventional anticoagulant therapy reduces both cardiac events and the associated hemorrhagic and vascular complications after PCI and stent deployment.[148] Indeed, the combination of aspirin and ticlopidine is superior to the use of aspirin either alone or in combination with warfarin.[149] Observational data[150] indicate that clopidogrel (75 mg/day) is as efficacious as ticlopidine in the prevention of stent thrombosis.[151] However, newer and more potent antiplatelet agents, such as prasugrel and ticagrelor, are associated with lower stent thrombosis rates in comparison with clopidogrel.[152,153]

More potent platelet antagonists have become available that inhibit the platelet GP IIb/IIIa receptors (see Chapter 7). A meta-analysis[154] of 16 RCTs incorporating 32,135 patients confirms the modest beneficial effects of platelet GP IIb/IIIa antagonists in patients during PCI or ACS. The Intracoronary Stenting and Anti-thrombotic Regimen: Rapid Early Action for Coronary Treatment (ISAR-REACT) trial has brought into question the role of GP IIb/IIIa receptor antagonists in elective PCI.[155] When all patients are pretreated with a large oral loading dose (600 mg) of clopidogrel, there appears to be no additional benefit of a GP IIb/IIIa receptor antagonist, although appropriately powered trials with a broad spectrum of patients at different degrees of risk of events need to be performed.

COMPLICATIONS

The most common serious complication of PCI is acute occlusion of the dilated vessel as a result of dissection or thrombosis. Other complications include vascular damage; thromboembolism, including stroke; and hemorrhage resulting from anticoagulant therapy. Although the risks are greatest with ACS,[108,156] elective PCI is associated with overall angiographic success rates of greater than 95% and a very low complication rate (transmural MI, 0.08%; stroke, 0.02%), emergency coronary bypass surgery rates of 0.4%, and in-hospital mortality rates of 0.1%.[157]

The reported risk of angiographic restenosis for isolated balloon angioplasty is 25% to 40%.[158-160] Restenosis occurs predominantly within the first 3 to 6 months,[159,160] does not always lead to recurrent symptoms, and has been dramatically reduced by the widespread use of intracoronary stents,[127,131,158,161] particularly drug-eluting stents. Indeed, isolated balloon angioplasty without stent implantation is now unusual and is considered only when treating small-caliber vessels or adverse anatomy. Current rates of restenosis with drug-eluting stents are low (approximately 5%).[145]

Coronary Artery Bypass Graft Surgery

INDICATIONS: CORONARY ARTERY BYPASS GRAFTING VERSUS MEDICAL TREATMENT

The three major RCTs that compared CABG with medical therapy are the Coronary Artery Surgery Study (CASS),[162] the Veterans Affairs (VA) Cooperative Study,[13,163] and the European Coronary Surgery Study (ECSS).[14,164] These studies form the basis of the meta-analysis by Yusuf and colleagues[165] that compares CABG with medical therapy in patients with chronic stable angina. In comparison with medical therapy, CABG significantly improves exercise capacity and symptoms of angina and reduces the need for antianginal therapy.[162] After CABG, more than 70% of patients are free of angina at 1 year, and 50% are free at 5 years.[162,164] Patients

experience a better quality of life after CABG,[162,166,167] and they report less limitation in physical activity.[162] A reported 73% are working 1 year after CABG.[167]

CABG is an appropriate intervention in patients who have suitable coronary anatomy with chronic stable and symptom-limiting angina despite medical treatment (see additional discussion in Chapter 11).

COMPLICATIONS

When contemplating revascularization surgery in patients with chronic stable angina, it should be recalled that CABG is a safe operation with an elective surgical mortality rate frequently reported at around 2% to 4%, depending on the case mix.[168] Various factors that influence surgical mortality rates include age, gender, degree of LV impairment, and the presence of other comorbid conditions such as diabetes mellitus, obesity, and hypertension (Figure 8-13).[168]

ARTERIAL CONDUITS

As a consequence of graft vasculopathy, saphenous vein bypass grafts have an accelerated failure rate that is particularly evident beyond the fifth year. Arterial conduits are being used increasingly in an attempt to improve graft survival. The internal mammary arteries are the principal conduits that have been assessed, although other conduits, such as the radial and gastroepiploic arteries, may also be used (see Chapter 11).

Fifteen years after CABG, 88% of left internal mammary artery grafts remain patent compared with only 32% of saphenous vein grafts.[169] Observational and quasi-experimental studies have shown that this improved patency rate is associated with better long-term survival rates and a reduction in the risk of angina, hospitalization, MI, and repeat operation.[170-172] Overall, patients who undergo CABG with saphenous vein grafts have only a 1.6-fold greater risk of death over 10 years compared with those who receive an internal mammary artery graft.[170] Given the chronic nature of ischemic heart disease, where technically feasible, CABG surgery should incorporate the use of arterial conduits, such as one or both of the internal mammary arteries.

Prevention of Coronary Events

Looking beyond symptomatic relief, many approaches have been taken to improve the prognosis of patients with CHD (see Figure 8-10). Some therapeutic interventions are associated with marked benefits, whereas others remain unproven or have neutral effects (Figure 8-14). As in the case of coronary revascularization, it may be necessary to accept a small initial risk to improve the patient's symptoms and quality of life.

CARDIAC REHABILITATION

The majority of RCTs of cardiac rehabilitation have been conducted in patients who have sustained a recent MI and indicate that significant morbidity and mortality benefits can be achieved.[173] Although the benefits appear to be most prominent in the first 2 years, the secondary preventive effects appear to be sustained during a 10-year period.[174] Although these benefits have not been definitively demonstrated in populations of patients with chronic stable angina in the absence of MI, the referral of such patients to a cardiac rehabilitation program is appropriate (see Chapter 49).

ANTIPLATELET THERAPY

Although aspirin is a weak inhibitor of platelet aggregation, it is a simple and effective treatment in patients with chronic stable angina. The Antithrombotic Trialists' Collaboration performed a meta-analysis that demonstrated a morbidity and mortality benefit (33% relative risk reduction) with long-term aspirin therapy in patients with chronic stable angina,[147] especially in those who had undergone coronary revascularization (Figure 8-15).[147] Because of this proven reduction in the risk of death and MI, all patients with stable angina pectoris should be maintained on regular

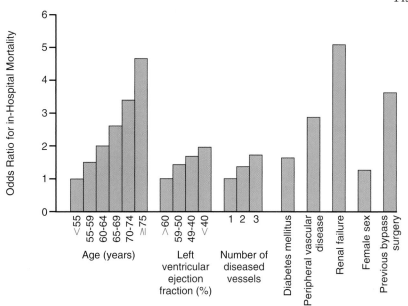

FIGURE 8-13 Odds ratio for in-hospital mortality rate for a selection of patient characteristics. Patients with chronic stable angina make up 40% of the study population. *(Data from O'Connor GT, Morton JR, Diehl MJ, for the Northern New England Cardiovascular Disease Study Group. Differences between men and women in hospital mortality associated with coronary artery bypass graft surgery. Circulation 1993;88:2104.)*

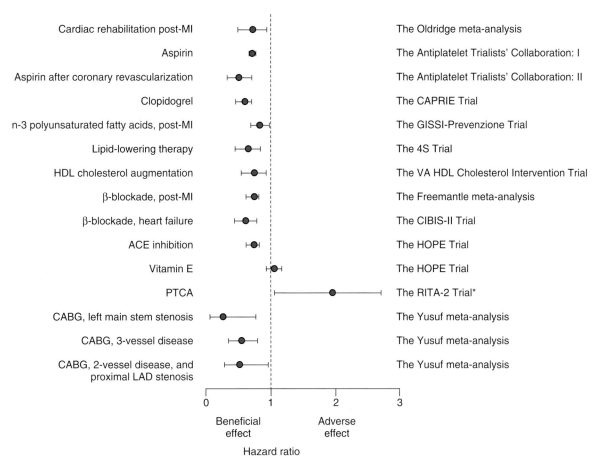

FIGURE 8-14 Proportionate benefits of a range of potential secondary preventive therapies. *The second Randomized Intervention Treatment of Angina (RITA-2) trial predominantly recruited patients at low cardiovascular risk. ACE, angiotensin-converting enzyme; CABG, coronary artery bypass grafting; HDL, high-density lipoprotein; LAD, left anterior descending artery; MI, myocardial infarction; PTCA, percutaneous transluminal coronary angioplasty. See text for expansion of trial names. *(From the RITA-2 Trial Participants. Coronary angioplasty versus medical therapy for angina: the second Randomized Intervention Treatment of Angina (RITA-2) Trial. Lancet 1997;350:461.)*

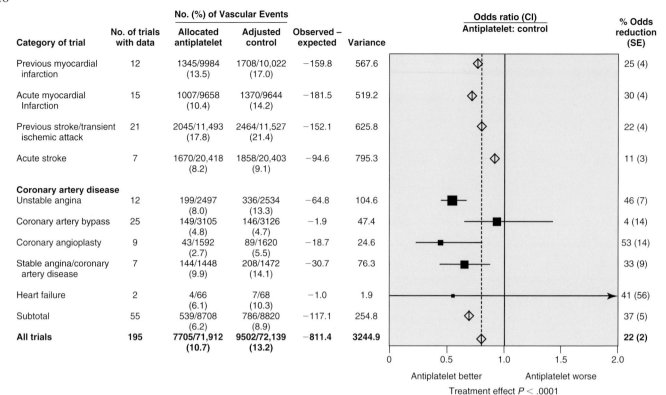

Category of trial	No. of trials with data	No. (%) of Vascular Events Allocated antiplatelet	Adjusted control	Observed – expected	Variance	Odds ratio (CI) Antiplatelet: control	% Odds reduction (SE)
Previous myocardial infarction	12	1345/9984 (13.5)	1708/10,022 (17.0)	−159.8	567.6		25 (4)
Acute myocardial Infarction	15	1007/9658 (10.4)	1370/9644 (14.2)	−181.5	519.2		30 (4)
Previous stroke/transient ischemic attack	21	2045/11,493 (17.8)	2464/11,527 (21.4)	−152.1	625.8		22 (4)
Acute stroke	7	1670/20,418 (8.2)	1858/20,403 (9.1)	−94.6	795.3		11 (3)
Coronary artery disease							
Unstable angina	12	199/2497 (8.0)	336/2534 (13.3)	−64.8	104.6		46 (7)
Coronary artery bypass	25	149/3105 (4.8)	146/3126 (4.7)	−1.9	47.4		4 (14)
Coronary angioplasty	9	43/1592 (2.7)	89/1620 (5.5)	−18.7	24.6		53 (14)
Stable angina/coronary artery disease	7	144/1448 (9.9)	208/1472 (14.1)	−30.7	76.3		33 (9)
Heart failure	2	4/66 (6.1)	7/68 (10.3)	−1.0	1.9		41 (56)
Subtotal	55	539/8708 (6.2)	786/8820 (8.9)	−117.1	254.8		37 (5)
All trials	**195**	**7705/71,912 (10.7)**	**9502/72,139 (13.2)**	**−811.4**	**3244.9**		**22 (2)**

Antiplatelet better   Antiplatelet worse
Treatment effect *P* < .0001

FIGURE 8-15 Benefits of aspirin therapy in patients with, or at risk of, cardiovascular disease. CI, confidence interval; SE, standard error. *(From the Antithrombotic Trialists' Collaboration. Collaborative meta-analysis of randomised trials of antiplatelet therapy for prevention of death, myocardial infarction, and stroke in high risk patients.* Br Med J *2002;324:71.)*

aspirin therapy. Similar benefits of aspirin therapy are seen at all doses, whereas bleeding risks increase in a dose-dependent manner. It would appear that 75 to 81 mg daily is the preferred aspirin dose for long-term secondary prevention. If the risk of peptic ulceration and gastrointestinal bleeding is a concern, coadministration of a proton-pump inhibitor (PPI) is appropriate.[175]

The weak antiplatelet action of aspirin has led to the search for other, more potent antiplatelet agents. In the Clopidogrel Versus Aspirin in Patients at Risk of Ischemic Events (CAPRIE) trial,[176] long-term clopidogrel treatment (75 mg/day) is at least as efficacious as aspirin in the prevention of ischemic stroke, MI, or vascular death in patients with atherosclerotic vascular disease. Although the overall secondary preventive benefits of clopidogrel statistically exceeded those of aspirin, the relative benefits were modest (relative risk reduction, 8.7%; *P* = .04); because of significant study population heterogeneity (*P* = .04), it may not confer superior benefit to aspirin in patients with stable CHD. Clopidogrel is beneficial when used in combination with aspirin in patients with ACS (see Chapters 9 and 10) and is indicated as an alternative to aspirin, particularly in patients with aspirin sensitivity. Combination therapy with aspirin and clopidogrel is of minimal benefit in patients with chronic stable angina and cannot be recommended for long-term secondary prevention. Indeed, the Clopidogrel for High Atherothrombotic Risk and Ischemic Stabilization, Management, and Avoidance (CHARISMA) trial of 15,603 patients demonstrated no benefit of dual antiplatelet therapy with clopidogrel and aspirin compared with aspirin alone.[177] The long-term secondary preventative benefits of the addition of prasugrel or ticagrelor to aspirin therapy are currently unknown.

LIPID-LOWERING THERAPY

Serum cholesterol concentrations should be assessed in all patients with chronic stable angina to detect hypercholesterolemia and should be treated with a hydroxy-3-methyl glutaryl coenzyme

A reductase inhibitor (a statin) irrespective of the serum cholesterol concentration (see Chapter 24). Several large-scale RCTs have addressed the issue of lipid-lowering therapy in patients with CHD. The Scandinavian Simvastatin Survival Study (4S) trial[151] was the first to demonstrate an improvement (relative risk reduction of 30%) in mortality rates with the use of statins in patients with CHD and a serum cholesterol concentration of more than 210 mg/dL (>5.5 mmol/L). These mortality benefits have been demonstrated with both simvastatin and pravastatin,[178] and the goal of therapy appears to be suppression of the serum total cholesterol concentration to at least below 190 mg/dL (<5.0 mmol/L). The Cholesterol and Recurrent Events (CARE) study[178] has, in addition, suggested that patients with average cholesterol concentrations (low-density lipoprotein [LDL] cholesterol 120 to 150 mg/dL, 3.2 to 3.9 mmol/L) should also be considered for lipid-lowering therapy because it is associated with a similar 26% relative risk reduction in future adverse cardiac events. However, the absolute risk of a subsequent cardiac event is proportionally lower in patients with such normal concentrations, especially in patients with only chronic stable angina. In contrast, more aggressive lipid lowering appears to have substantial additional benefits in patients who have undergone saphenous vein bypass grafting,[179] and under such circumstances, target LDL cholesterol (LDL-c) concentrations should be below 100 mg/dL (<2.6 mmol/L).

The 4S trial[180] has been the only large-scale mortality study to specifically recruit patients with chronic stable angina. However, the benefits of lipid-lowering therapy in chronic stable angina were also demonstrated in the Atorvastatin Versus Revascularization Treatment (AVERT) study.[181] During an 18-month follow-up period, this trial was able to demonstrate that in patients with chronic stable angina, atorvastatin reduced the number of acute ischemic events—hospitalization for worsening angina or coronary revascularization procedures—compared with intervention with PCI (13% vs. 21%, respectively). However, PCI was associated with a greater improvement in chronic anginal symptoms than atorvastatin (54%

vs. 41%, respectively), and a large part of the effect seen is likely to reflect the RITA-2 trial observations,[111] that PCI improves chronic symptoms at the cost of a small but significant increase in short-term ischemic events.

In the initial secondary prevention trials, patients were predominantly recruited if serum total cholesterol concentrations were above a certain threshold, usually around 190 mg/dL. A threshold effect apparent in the CARE trial[178] suggested no merit in reducing serum LDL-c concentrations to below 120 mg/dL. The subsequent Heart Protection Study[182] has now definitively established that all patients with CHD should receive statin therapy; it is the overall absolute risk that is important rather than the cholesterol concentration per se. Patients at high risk will benefit from cholesterol reduction irrespective of cholesterol concentrations (i.e., no threshold effect is evident for the benefits of statin therapy). For example, in the Heart Protection Study,[182] patients with a total cholesterol concentration of less than 190 mg/dL had a 5-year event rate of 22.1% that was reduced to 16.9% by simvastatin 40 mg daily. Thus, a patient with chronic stable angina, diabetes mellitus, or peripheral vascular disease will merit having statin therapy, even if his or her total cholesterol concentration is 136 mg/dL. A meta-analysis[183] of 14 major statin trials that incorporated 90,056 individuals has reaffirmed these benefits and suggests that event reduction is proportional to LDL-c reduction (Figure 8-16).

How low should the serum cholesterol concentration be in patients with chronic stable angina? The Pravastatin or Atorvastatin Evaluation and Infection Therapy (PROVE-IT)[184] and Treating to New Targets (TNT)[185] trials have assessed, respectively, whether more intensive lipid-lowering therapy is associated with better outcomes in patients with recent unstable or chronic stable CHD. Both trials show a consistent benefit in reducing serum LDL-c concentrations below contemporary guidelines (to a mean of 62 to 77 mg/dL). In the TNT trial,[185] 30 patients treated with atorvastatin 80 mg daily for 5 years will avoid one major CV event compared with those receiving atorvastatin 10 mg daily. The Incremental Decrease in Clinical Endpoints Through Aggressive Lipid Lowering (IDEAL) trial compared atorvastatin 80 mg daily with simvastatin 20 mg daily as secondary prevention in patients with a previous MI.[186] The achieved LDL-c was 81 mg/dL compared with 104 mg/dL in the simvastatin group. The composite primary endpoint of coronary death, nonfatal MI, or resuscitated cardiac arrest tended to be lower in the high-dose atorvastatin group (HR, 0.89; 95% CI, 0.78 to 1.01; $P = .07$); nonfatal MI was significantly reduced with high-dose atorvastatin (HR, 0.83; 95% CI, 0.71 to 0.98; $P = .02$) over a median follow-up of 4.8 years.

Other classes of drugs—such as fibrates, binding agents, niacin, and ezetimibe—also lower serum lipid concentrations, but although it is inferred, they have not been shown to clearly reduce mortality rates in RCTs. One exception to this is the VA trial of gemfibrozil, which demonstrated significant secondary preventive benefits of elevating reduced high-density lipoprotein cholesterol (HDL-c) concentrations.[187] Patients with CHD, including patients with chronic stable angina, and a normal LDL-c concentration (≤140 mg/dL) but a reduced HDL-c concentration (≤40 mg/dL) benefited from 1.2 g/day gemfibrozil, which elevated HDL-c concentrations by 6% and reduced total cholesterol and triglyceride concentrations by 4% and 31% respectively, without altering LDL-c concentrations. Fibrates should therefore be considered in patients with normal LDL-c but low HDL-c concentrations.

β-BLOCKERS

No RCTs have demonstrated β-blocker therapy to improve survival in patients with chronic stable angina. However, post-MI,[83,188] hypertension, and case-control[189] studies have shown that patients maintained on β-blockers are less likely to have a vascular event and have a reduced mortality rate if they subsequently experience an MI. For these reasons, we believe β-blockers should be the first-line agents of choice for patients with chronic stable angina. Furthermore, despite claims to the contrary, hypertension[190] and angina[82,105]

trials indicate that β-blockers are better tolerated and have fewer side effects than calcium channel antagonists. Concerns are unfounded that β-blocker therapy is associated with reduced peripheral perfusion as a result of unopposed α-adrenergic vasoconstriction and blockade of β-2 vascular receptors,[191] even in patients with peripheral vascular disease. β-Blockers may have significant secondary preventive benefits in patients with peripheral vascular disease, as suggested by the marked reductions in perioperative mortality and MI rates in such patients undergoing major vascular surgery.[192]

Because of the common risk factor of smoking, many patients with angina have chronic obstructive pulmonary disease (COPD) and are denied β-blocker therapy because of the concern of provoking bronchospasm. However, a large body of observation data demonstrates that patients with obstructive pulmonary disease derive similar mortality benefits (40% relative risk reduction) after MI with β-blocker therapy.[188] Therefore, such patients should be given a trial of β-blockade because the majority tolerate therapy well. If genuine concern of clinically significant reversible bronchospasm is an issue, formal spirometry in the presence and absence of a β₂ agonist, such as 5 mg nebulized salbutamol, should be performed.

Patients with chronic stable angina and coexistent heart failure are particularly at risk and should also be given β-blocker therapy as the agent of choice. Several large-scale RCTs have demonstrated major mortality and morbidity benefits in patients with mild to severe heart failure[193,194] who were maintained on β-blocker therapy. Although cautious dose uptitration and close clinical observation for cardiac decompensation are necessary, the withdrawal rates of patients with heart failure from β-blocker therapy are modest (15%) and equivalent to those for placebo.[194] Moreover, rates of rehospitalization are reduced and symptoms of heart failure are improved with β-blocker therapy.[194]

ANGIOTENSIN-CONVERTING ENZYME INHIBITION

The major morbidity and mortality benefits of angiotensin-converting enzyme (ACE) inhibitor therapy on ischemic events were first demonstrated in patients with heart failure.[195,196] These benefits are likely to reflect an antiischemic action of ACE inhibition, particularly given the evidence from the Heart Outcomes Prevention Evaluation (HOPE)[197] and the European Trial on Reduction of Cardiac Events with Perindopril in Stable Coronary Heart Disease (EUROPA) studies.[198] The HOPE study[197] was a large-scale RCT of 9297 high-risk patients with vascular disease (55% with chronic stable angina) in the absence of documented heart failure. During the 4.5 years of follow-up, ramipril was associated with reductions in all-cause mortality, MI, and stroke.[197] These beneficial effects appeared to be independent of the associated reductions in blood pressure and were particularly marked in patients with diabetes mellitus.[199] These findings have been subsequently confirmed in the EUROPA trial of 13,655 patients with stable CHD.[198] Perindopril 8 mg daily was associated with a 20% relative risk reduction in the likelihood of CV death, MI, or cardiac arrest, and 50 patients needed to be treated for 4 years to avoid one event. Findings of the Prevention of Events with Angiotensin Converting Enzyme Inhibition (PEACE) trial[200] are in contrast to the HOPE[197] and EUROPA[198] trials because PEACE failed to demonstrate a benefit of trandolapril in 8290 patients with stable CHD. However, the event rate in this trial was unexpectedly low and less than the rate in the treatment arms of both the HOPE and EUROPA trials.[197,198]

All patients with chronic stable angina with a predicted 10-year event rate greater than 15% should be maintained on long-term ACE inhibitor therapy because of the associated major secondary preventive benefits.

CORONARY REVASCULARIZATION

No RCTs have demonstrated that PCI improves long-term prognosis and survival in patients with chronic stable angina. Indeed,

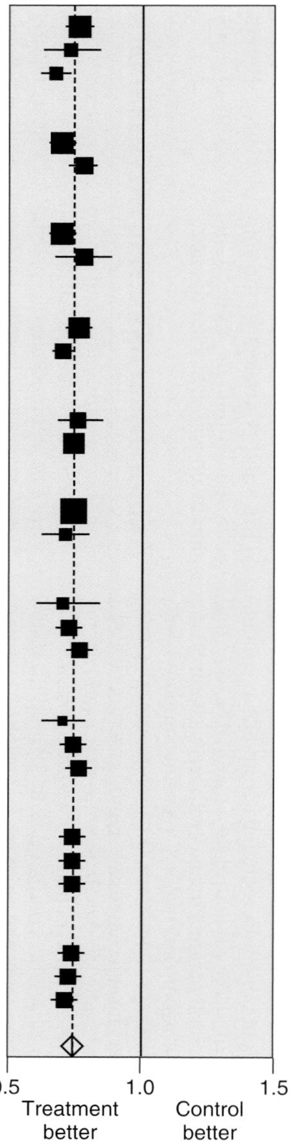

Global test for heterogeneity: χ^2_{15} –15.1; $P = .4$

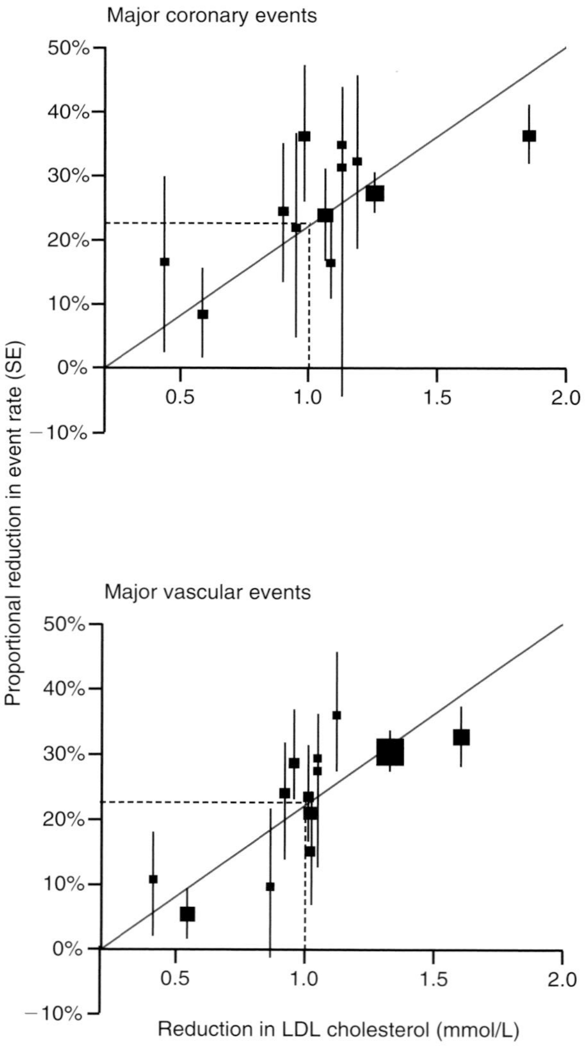

Treatment effect $P < .0001$

FIGURE 8-16 Benefits of statin therapy in subgroups of at-risk populations (*left panel*) are proportional to reductions in low-density lipoprotein (*LDL*) cholesterol concentrations (*right panel*). Cholesterol concentration conversion: 1 mmol/L = 38 mg/dL. *HDL*, high-density lipoprotein; *LDL*, low-density lipoprotein; *SE*, standard error. (*From the Cholesterol Treatment Trialists' (CTT) Collaboration. Baigent C, Keetch A, Kearney PM, and the CTT Collaborators. Efficacy and safety of cholesterol-lowering treatment: prospective meta-analysis of data from 90,056 participants in 14 randomised trials of statins. Lancet 2005;366:1267.*)

several studies indicated that PCI is associated with a worse medium-term prognosis than medical therapy.[111,181] In contrast, in selected groups, CABG is associated with major reductions in mortality rates compared with medical therapy. Comparisons of the prognostic benefits of PCI and CABG demonstrated no statistically significant differences between the two approaches,[114,115] but this does not establish equivalence. Indeed, this is underlined by the SYNTAX trial, in which PCI failed to achieve noninferiority when compared with CABG.[118] In the context of chronic stable angina, PCI remains an important treatment to relieve symptoms, but it is associated with a small early risk.

Coronary Artery Bypass Graft Surgery

In comparison with medical therapy, CABG improves long-term (10-year) survival in patients with stable angina. Subgroup analysis demonstrates that patients with greater than 50% left main stem stenosis had the greatest survival benefit with CABG.[14,165,201] Survival benefits are also seen in patients with three-vessel disease or two-vessel disease that includes proximal LAD stenosis.[14,165] However, patients with one-vessel disease or those with two-vessel disease without proximal LAD stenosis do not derive any survival advantage from CABG. Patients with abnormal LV function or strongly positive exercise tests results derive greater absolute survival benefit from CABG than from medical therapy.

The survival benefit for coronary artery surgery is related to the severity of the CHD. Those with the most severe disease have the most to gain from coronary artery surgery, and the benefits are greatest in those with left main stem disease, followed by those with three-vessel disease and then by those with one- or two-vessel disease (see Figures 8-11 and 8-14). Further observational evidence from the Duke University database supports the observation that patients with two-vessel disease that involves the proximal LAD and those with three-vessel disease have a lower hazard ratio (for mortality) with CABG than do those who receive medical treatment.[119]

It is important to note that in the trials cited earlier, a significant number of patients with three-vessel disease who were initially randomized to medical therapy crossed over to surgery (41% at 10 years). These studies are therefore not a sole comparison of surgery and medical therapy but rather a comparison of initial surgical versus initial medical treatment. This factor has diluted the observed benefits of CABG because a high proportion of the patients initially randomized to medical therapy may have gained a survival benefit from surgery. In the meta-analysis of Yusuf and colleagues,[165] only 9.9% of patients received an internal mammary artery graft, and only 25% of the patients who underwent CABG were receiving antiplatelet agents. These RCTs may have underestimated the benefits of CABG and do not take into account improvements in surgical techniques (see Figure 8-11).[202]

Potential Future Therapies

Cholesteryl Ester Transfer Protein Inhibitors

Together with aspirin, lipid-lowering therapy has been a major advance in the prevention of CHD. However, incident and recurrent CV events remain a major problem despite these advances, and despite claims to the contrary, coronary atherosclerosis continues to progress despite the most intensive lipid-lowering regimes. A recent approach has been to assess the impact of raising the plasma concentrations of the cardioprotective HDL-c particles. This can be achieved by the inhibition of cholesteryl ester transfer proteins (CETPs), and several agents have been shown to increase plasma HDL-c concentrations by 30% to 60%. In the first major RCT of a CETP inhibitor, the Investigation of Lipid Level Management to Understand its Impact in Atherosclerotic Events (ILLUMINATE) trial, torcetrapib increased plasma HDL-c concentrations by 72% and reduced LDL-c by 25% in 15,067 at-risk subjects; however, its use was associated with a substantial and unexpected increased risk of CV events that caused early termination of the trial and discontinuation of the torcetrapib development program.[203] It has been suggested that this may reflect an off-target effect on blood pressure rather than a failure of the CETP-inhibitor therapeutic strategy. Indeed, early safety studies of other CETP inhibitors, such as anacetrapib, have not seen the hypertensive effects described for torcetrapib.[204] Major RCTs are ongoing of at least two CETP inhibitors, anacetrapib and dalcetrapib, that will determine whether this therapeutic approach can truly reduce CV events further.

Novel Antiplatelet Therapies

Despite major advances in antiplatelet therapies, recurrent CV events remain high after ACS. Furthermore, incremental benefits achieved in the reduction of atherothrombotic events has almost always been at the expense of hemorrhagic side effects. Thrombin is the most potent platelet-activating factor known, and it makes important interactions with the endothelium and vascular smooth muscle with proinflammatory, proatherogenic effects. Distinct from its activity within the coagulation cascade, thrombin mediates these effects via protease-activated receptor (PAR)-1. Interest has been piqued recently in the use of PAR-1 antagonists because they may provide important antiatherothrombotic effects without attendant bleeding complications and could represent a major breakthrough for the treatment of CV diseases. Recently, the first large-scale randomized, controlled trial of PAR-1 inhibition has been reported after 3 years of follow-up in 26,449 stable patients with cardiovascular disease.[205] In this trial, the PAR-1 antagonist vorapaxar significantly reduced the risk of cardiovascular death, myocardial infarction, or stroke by 13% but also increased the risk of major bleeding by 66% and doubled the rate of intracranial hemorrhage. Patients with prior stroke had a particularly high risk of intracranial hemorrhage, and treatment was stopped early in this subgroup. Thus, future consideration of vorapaxar will require careful patient selection.

REFERENCES

1. Davies M. The pathophysiology of acute coronary syndromes. *Heart* 2000;83:361.
2. Gandhi MM, Lampe F, Wood DA. Incidence of stable angina pectoris. *Eur Heart J* 1992;13:181.
3. Balarajan R. Ethnic differences in mortality from ischaemic heart disease in England and Wales. *Br Med J* 1991;302:500.
4. Sytkowski P, Kannel W, D'Agostino R. Changes in risk factors and the decline in mortality from cardiovascular disease. *N Engl J Med* 1990;322:1635.
5. Poole-Wilson PA, Lubsen J, Kirwan BA, et al; Coronary Disease Trial Investigating Outcome with Nifedipine Gastrointestinal Therapeutic System Investigators. Effect of long-acting nifedipine on mortality and cardiovascular morbidity in patients with stable angina requiring treatment (ACTION trial): randomised controlled trial. *Lancet* 2004;364:849.
6. IONA Study Group. Effect of nicorandil on coronary events in patients with stable angina: the Impact of Nicorandil in Angina (IONA) randomised trial. *Lancet* 2002;359:1269.
7. Lampe FC, Whincup PH, Wannamethee SG, et al. The natural history of prevalent ischaemic heart disease in middle-aged men. *Eur Heart J* 2000;21:1052-1062.
8. Califf RM, Mark DB, Harrell FE, et al. Importance of clinical measures of ischemia in the prognosis of patients with documented coronary artery disease. *J Am Coll Cardiol* 1988;11:20.
9. Kannel WB, Feinleib M. Natural history of angina pectoris in the Framingham Study: prognosis and survival. *Am J Cardiol* 1972;29:154.
10. Clayton TC, Lubsen J, Pocock SJ, et al. Risk score for predicting death, myocardial infarction, and stroke in patients with stable angina, based on a large randomised trial cohort of patients. *Br Med J* 2005;331:869.
11. Norell M, Lythall D, Coghlan G, et al. Limited value of the resting electrocardiogram in assessing patients with recent onset chest pain: lessons from a chest pain clinic. *Br Heart J* 1992;67:53.
12. Miranda CP, Lehmann KG, Froelicher VF. Correlation between resting segment depression, exercise testing, coronary angiography and long-term prognosis. *Am Heart J* 1991;122:1617.
13. The Veterans Administration Coronary Artery Bypass Surgery Cooperative Study Group. Eleven-year survival in the Veterans Administration randomized trial of coronary bypass surgery for stable angina. *N Engl J Med* 1984;311:1333.
14. The European Coronary Surgery Study Group. Long-term results of prospective randomised study of coronary artery bypass surgery in stable angina pectoris. *Lancet* 1982;2:1173.
15. Fletcher GF, Balady G, Froelicher VF, et al. Exercise standards: a statement for healthcare professionals from the American Heart Association. *Circulation* 1995;91:580.
16. Mark DB, Shaw L, Harrell FE, et al. Prognostic value of a treadmill exercise score in outpatients with suspected coronary artery disease. *N Engl J Med* 1991;325:849.

17. Weiner DA, Ryan TJ, McCabe CH, et al. Value of exercise testing in determining the risk classification and the response to coronary artery bypass grafting in three-vessel coronary artery disease: a report from the Coronary Artery Surgery Study (CASS) registry. *Am J Cardiol* 1987;60:262.
18. Myers WO, Schaff HV, Gersh BJ, et al. Improved survival of surgically treated patients with triple vessel coronary artery disease and severe angina pectoris: a report from the Coronary Artery Surgery Study (CASS) registry. *J Thorac Cardiovasc Surg* 1989;97:487.
19. O'Keefe JH, Barnhart CSS, Bateman TM. Comparison of stress echocardiography and myocardial perfusion scintigraphy for diagnosing coronary artery disease and assessing its severity. *Am J Cardiol* 1995;75:1D.
20. Krivocavitch J, Child JS, Gerber RS, et al. Prognostic usefulness of positive or negative stress echocardiography for predicting cardiac events in ensuing 12 months. *Am J Cardiol* 1993;71:641.
21. Wolff SD, Schwitter J, Coulden R, et al. Myocardial first-pass perfusion magnetic resonance imaging: a multicenter dose-ranging study. *Circulation* 2004;110:732-737.
22. Schwitter J, Wacker CM, van Rossum AC, et al. MR-IMPACT: comparison of perfusion-cardiac magnetic resonance with single-photon emission computed tomography for the detection of coronary artery disease in a multicentre, multivendor, randomized trial. *Eur Heart J* 2008;29:480-489.
23. Plein S, Radjenovic A, Ridgway JP, et al. Coronary artery disease: myocardial perfusion MR imaging with sensitivity encoding versus conventional angiography. *Radiology* 2010;235:423-430.
24. Klem I, Heitner JF, Shah DJ, et al. Improved detection of coronary artery disease by stress perfusion cardiovascular magnetic resonance with the use of delayed enhancement infarction imaging. *J Am Coll Cardiol* 2006;47:1630-1638.
25. Jahnke C, Nagel E, Gebker R, et al. Prognostic value of cardiac magnetic resonance stress tests: adenosine stress perfusion and dobutamine stress wall motion imaging. *Circulation* 2007;115:1769-1776.
26. Hundley WG, Bluemke DA, Finn JP, et al. ACCF/ACR/AHA/NASCI/SCMR 2010 expert consensus document on cardiovascular magnetic resonance: a report of the American College of Cardiology Foundation Task Force on Expert Consensus Documents. *J Am Coll Cardiol* 2010;55:2614-2662.
27. Morise AP, Detrano R, Bobbio M, et al. Development and derivation of a logistic regression derived algorithm for estimating the incremental probability of coronary artery disease before and after exercise testing. *J Am Coll Cardiol* 1992;20:1187.
28. Brown KA. Prognostic value of thallium-201 myocardial perfusion imaging: a diagnostic tool comes of age. *Circulation* 1991;83:363.
29. Ladenheim ML, Pollock BH, Rosanski A, et al. Extent and severity of myocardial hypoperfusion as predictors of prognosis in patients with suspected coronary artery disease. *J Am Coll Cardiol* 1986;7:464.
30. Travin MI, Boucher CA, Newell JB, et al. Variables associated with a poor prognosis in patients with an ischemic thallium-201 exercise test. *Am Heart J* 1993;125:335.
31. Pletcher MJ, Tice JA, Pignone M, Browner WS. Using the coronary artery calcium score to predict coronary heart disease events: a systematic review and meta-analysis. *Arch Intern Med* 2004;164:1285.
32. Raggi P, Cooil B, Shaw LJ, et al. Progression of coronary calcium on serial electron beam tomographic scanning is greater in patients with future myocardial infarction. *Am J Cardiol* 2003;92:827.
33. Nicholls SJ, Tuzcu EM, Wolski K, et al. Coronary artery calcification and changes in atheroma burden in response to established medical therapies. *J Am Coll Cardiol* 2007;49:263-270.
34. Houslay E, Cowell SJ, Northridge DB, et al. Progression of coronary calcification despite intensive lipid-lowering therapy: a randomized controlled trial. *Heart* 2006;92: 1207-1212.
35. Rubinshtein R, Gaspar T, Halon DA, et al. Prevalence and extent of obstructive coronary artery disease in patients with zero or low calcium score undergoing 64-slice cardiac multidetector computed tomography for evaluation of a chest pain syndrome. *Am J Cardiol* 2007;99:472-475.
36. Kopp AF, Schroeder S, Kuettner A, et al. Non-invasive coronary angiography with high resolution multidetector-row computed tomography: results in 102 patients. *Eur Heart J* 2002;23:1714-1725.
37. Leber AW, Becker A, Knez A, et al. Accuracy of 64-slice computed tomography to classify and quantify plaque volumes in the proximal coronary system: a comparative study using intravascular ultrasound. *J Am Coll Cardiol* 2006;47:672-677.
38. Schroeder S, Achenbach S, Bengel F, et al. Cardiac computed tomography: indications, applications, limitations, and training requirements: report of a writing group deployed by the Working Group Nuclear Cardiology and Cardiac CT of the European Society of Cardiology and the European Council of Nuclear Cardiology. *Eur Heart J* 2008;29:531-536.
39. Achenbach S. Computed tomography coronary angiography. *J Am Coll Cardiol* 2006;48:1919-1928.
40. Gibbons RJ, Balady GJ, Beasley JW, et al. ACC/AHA guidelines for exercise testing. *J Am Coll Cardiol* 1997;30:260.
41. Tonino PA, De Bruyne B, Pijls NH, et al; FAME Study Investigators. Fractional flow reserve versus angiography for guiding percutaneous coronary intervention. *N Engl J Med* 2009;360:213-224.
42. Califf RM, Phillips HR, Hindman MC, et al. Prognostic value of a coronary artery jeopardy score. *J Am Coll Cardiol* 1985;5:1055.
43. Proudfit WJ, Bruschke AV, MacMillan JP, et al. Fifteen year survival study of patients with obstructive coronary artery disease. *Circulation* 1983;68:986.
44. Pocock SJ, McCormack V, Gueyffier F, et al. A score for predicting risk of death from cardiovascular disease in adults with raised blood pressure, based on individual patient data from randomised controlled trials. *Br Med J* 2001;323:75.
45. Håheim LL, Holme I, Hjermann I, et al. The predictability of risk factors with respect to incidence and mortality of myocardial infarction and total mortality: a 12-year follow-up of the Oslo Study, Norway. *J Intern Med* 1993;234:17.
46. Jorenby DE. Smoking cessation strategies for the 21st century. *Circulation* 2001; 104:e51-e52.
47. Kottke TE, Battista RN, DeFriese GH, et al. Attributes of successful smoking cessation interventions in medical practice: a meta-analysis of 39 controlled trials. *JAMA* 1988; 259:2883.
48. Silagy C, Mant D, Fowler G, et al. Nicotine replacement therapy for smoking cessation (Cochrane Review). *Cochrane Library, Issue 2*. Oxford, UK, 1997, Update Software.
49. Miller N, Frieden TR, Liu SY, et al. Effectiveness of a large-scale distribution programme of free nicotine patches: a prospective evaluation. *Lancet* 2005;365:1849.
50. Hughes J, Stead L, Lancaster T. Antidepressants for smoking cessation. *Cochrane Database Syst Rev* 2004;(4):CD000031.
51. Cahill K, Stead LF, Lancaster T. Nicotine receptor partial agonists for smoking cessation. *Cochrane Database Syst Rev* 2011;(2):CD006103.
52. Hajek P, Stead LF, West R, Jarvis M. Relapse prevention interventions for smoking cessation. *Cochrane Database Syst Rev* 2005;(1):CD003999.
53. Tang JL, Armitage JM, Lancaster T, et al. Systematic review of dietary intervention trials to lower blood total cholesterol in free-living subjects. *Br Med J* 1998;316:1213.
54. Acquilani R, Tramarin R, Pedretti RFE, et al. Despite good compliance, very low fat diet alone does not achieve recommended cholesterol goals in outpatients with coronary heart disease. *Eur Heart J* 1999;20:1020.
55. de Lorgeril M, Renaud S, Mamelle N, et al. Mediterranean alpha-linoleic acid–rich diet in the secondary prevention of coronary heart disease. *Lancet* 1994;343:1454.
56. Burr ML, Fehily AM, Gilbert JF, et al. Effects of changes in fat, fish and fibre intakes on death and myocardial reinfarction: diet and reinfarction trial. *Lancet* 1994;343: 1454.
57. The GISSI-Prevenzione Trial. Dietary supplementation with n-3 polyunsaturated fatty acids and vitamin E after myocardial infarction: results of the GISSI-Prevenzione Trial. *Lancet* 1999; 354:447.
58. Knekt P, Reunanen A, Jarvinen R, et al. Antioxidant vitamin intake and coronary mortality in a longitudinal population study. *Am J Epidemiol* 1994;139:1180.
59. Kushi LH, Folsom AR, Prineas RJ, et al. Dietary antioxidant vitamins and death from coronary heart disease in post-menopausal women. *N Engl J Med* 1996;334:1156.
60. Singh RB, Rastogi SS, Verma R, et al. Randomised controlled trial of cardioprotective diet in patients with recent acute myocardial infarction: results of one year follow up. *Br Med J* 1992;304:1015.
61. Stampfer MJ, Hennekens CH, Manson JE, et al. Vitamin E consumption and the risk of coronary heart disease in women. *N Engl J Med* 1993;328:1444.
62. Rimm EB, Stampfer MJ, Ascherio A, et al. Vitamin E consumption and the risk of coronary heart disease in men. *N Engl J Med* 1993;328:1450.
63. The Alpha-Tocopherol, β-Carotene Cancer Prevention Study Group. The effect of vitamin E and β carotene on the incidence of lung cancer and other cancers in male smokers. *N Engl J Med* 1994;330:1029.
64. The Heart Outcomes Prevention Evaluation Study Investigators. Vitamin E supplementation and cardiovascular events in high-risk patients. *N Engl J Med* 2000;342:154.
65. Gaziano JM, Buring JE, Breslow JL, et al. Moderate alcohol intake increased levels of high-density lipoprotein and its subfractions, and decreased risk of myocardial infarction. *N Engl J Med* 1993;329:1829.
66. Calle EE, Thun MJ, Petrelli JM, et al. Body-mass index and mortality in a prospective cohort of U.S. adults. *N Engl J Med* 1999;341:1097.
67. Topol EJ, Bousser MG, Fox KA, et al; the CRESCENDO Investigators. Rimonabant for prevention of cardiovascular events (CRESCENDO): a randomised, multicentre, placebo-controlled trial. *Lancet* 2010;376:517-523.
68. The UK Prospective Diabetes Study (UKPDS) Group. Effect of intensive blood-glucose control with metformin on complications in overweight patients with type 2 diabetes (UKPDS 34). *Lancet* 1998;352:854.
69. The Diabetes Control and Complications Trial Research Group. The effect of intensive treatment of diabetes on the development and progression of long-term complications in insulin-dependent diabetes mellitus. *N Engl J Med* 1993;329:977.
70. Malmberg K. Prospective randomised study of intensive insulin treatment on long-term survival after acute myocardial infarction in patients with diabetes mellitus. DIGAMI (Diabetes Mellitus, Insulin Glucose Infusion in Acute Myocardial Infarction) Study Group. *Br Med J* 1997;314:1512.
71. Malmberg K, Norhammar A, Wedel H, et al. Glycometabolic state at admission: important risk marker of mortality in conventionally treated patients with diabetes mellitus and acute myocardial infarction: long-term results from the Diabetes and Insulin-Glucose Infusion in Acute Myocardial Infarction (DIGAMI) study. *Circulation* 1999;99:2626.
72. The University Group Diabetes Program. A study of the effects of hypoglycemic agents on vascular complications in patients with adult-onset diabetes: diabetes 1976, regression analysis. *Br Med J* 1999;318:1730.
73. The UK Prospective Diabetes Study (UKPDS) Group. Intensive blood-glucose control with sulphonylureas or insulin compared with conventional treatment and risk of complications in patients with type 2 diabetes (UKPDS 33). *Lancet* 1998; 352:837.
74. The Action to Control Cardiovascular Risk in Diabetes Study Group. Effects of intensive glucose lowering in type 2 diabetes. *N Engl J Med* 2008;358:2545-2559.
75. The ADVANCE Collaborative Group. Intensive blood glucose control and vascular outcomes in patients with type 2 diabetes. *N Engl J Med* 2008;358:2560-2572.
76. Thompson DR, Bowman GS, Kitson AL, et al. Cardiac rehabilitation in the United Kingdom: guidelines and audit standards. *Heart* 1996;75:89.
77. Dugmore LD, Tipson RJ, Phillips MH, et al. Changes in cardiorespiratory fitness, psychological well being, quality of life, and vocational status following a 12 month cardiac exercise rehabilitation program. *Heart* 1999;81:359.
78. Todd IC, Ballantyne D. Effect of exercise training on the total ischaemic burden as assessed by 24 hour ambulatory electrocardiographic monitoring. *Br Heart J* 1992;68:560.
79. Chua TP, Lipkin DP. Cardiac rehabilitation should be available to all who would benefit. *Br Med J* 1993;306:731.
80. Hambrecht R, Walther C, Mobius-Winkler S, et al. Percutaneous coronary angioplasty compared with exercise training in patients with stable coronary artery disease: a randomized trial. *Circulation* 2004;109:1371.

81. Stone PH, Gibson RS, Glasser SP, et al. Comparison of propranolol, diltiazem and nifedipine in the treatment of ambulatory ischemia in patients with stable angina. *Circulation* 1990;82:1962.

82. Dargie HJ, Ford I, Fox KM. Total Ischaemic Burden European Trial (TIBET): effects of ischaemia and treatment with atenolol, nifedipine SR and their combination on outcome in patients with chronic stable angina. *Eur Heart J* 1996;7:104.

83. Freemantle N, Cleland J, Young P, et al. beta-Blockade after myocardial infarction: systematic review and meta regression analysis. *Br Med J* 1999;318:1730.

84. Psaty BM, Koepsell TD, Wagner EH, et al. The relative risk of incident coronary heart disease associated with recently stopping the use of beta-blockers. *JAMA* 1990;263:1653.

85. The Danish Study Group on Verapamil in Myocardial Infarction. Effect of verapamil on mortality and major events after acute myocardial infarction (The Danish Verapamil Infarction Trial-DAVIT II). *Am J Cardiol* 1990; 66:779.

86. Rodrigues EA, Kohli RS, Hains ADB, et al. Comparison of nicardipine and verapamil in the management of chronic stable angina. *Int J Cardiol* 1988;18:357.

87. Friedensohn A, Meshulam R, Schlesinger Z. Randomised double-blind comparison of the effects of isosorbide dinitrate retard, verapamil sustained-release, and their combination on myocardial ischaemic episodes. *Cardiology* 1991;79(Suppl 2):31.

88. Steffensen R, Grande P, Pedersen F, et al. Effects of atenolol and diltiazem on exercise tolerance and ambulatory ischaemia. *Int J Cardiol* 1993;40:143.

89. van der Does R, Eberhardt R, Derr I, et al. Treatment of chronic stable angina with carvedilol in comparison with nifedipine slow release. *Eur Heart J* 1991;12:60.

90. Elkayam U, Amin J, Mehra A, et al. A prospective, randomised, double-blind, crossover study to compare the efficacy and safety of chronic nifedipine therapy with that of isosorbide dinitrate and their combination in the treatment of chronic congestive heart failure. *Circulation* 1990;82:1954.

91. Packer M, O'Connor CM, Ghali JK, et al. Effect of amlodipine on mortality and morbidity in severe chronic heart failure. Prospective Randomized Amlodipine Survival Evaluation Study Group. *N Engl J Med* 1996;335:1107.

92. Chrysant SG, Glasser SP, Bittar N, et al. Efficacy and safety of extended release isosorbide mononitrate for stable effort angina pectoris. *Am J Cardiol* 1993;72:1249.

93. Parker JO, Farrell B, Lahey KA, et al. Effect of intervals between doses on the development of tolerance to isosorbide dinitrate. *N Engl J Med* 1987;316:1440.

94. DeMots H, Glasser SP. Intermittent transdermal nitroglycerin therapy in the treatment of chronic stable angina. *J Am Coll Cardiol* 1989;13:786.

95. Levy WS, Katz RJ, Wasserman AG. Methionine restores the venodilative response to nitroglycerin after the development of tolerance. *J Am Coll Cardiol* 1991;17:474.

96. Bauer JA, Fung HL. Differential hemodynamic effects and tolerance properties of nitroglycerin and an S-nitrosothiol in experimental heart failure. *J Pharmacol Exp Ther* 1991;256:249.

97. Langford EJ, Brown AS, Wainwright RJ, et al. Inhibition of platelet activity by S-nitrosoglutathione during coronary angioplasty. *Lancet* 1994;344:1458.

98. Matsubara T, Minatoguchi S, Matsuo H, et al. Three minute, but not one minute, ischemia and nicorandil have a preconditioning effect in patients with coronary artery disease. *J Am Coll Cardiol* 2000;35:345.

99. Patel DJ, Purcell HJ, Fox KM. Cardioprotection by opening of the K(ATP) channel in unstable angina. *Eur Heart J* 1999;20:51.

100. Tardif JC, Ford I, Tendera M, et al; INITIATIVE Investigators. Efficacy of ivabradine, a new selective I(f) inhibitor, compared with atenolol in patients with chronic stable angina. *Eur Heart J* 2005;26:2529-2536.

101. Tardif JC, Ponikowski P, Kahan T, et al, for the ASSOCIATE Study Investigators. Efficacy of the I(f) current inhibitor ivabradine in patients with chronic stable angina receiving β-blocker therapy: a 4-month, randomized, placebo-controlled trial. *Eur Heart J* 2009;30:540-548.

102. Chaitman BR, Pepine CJ, Parker JO, et al; Combination Assessment of Ranolazine In Stable Angina (CARISA) Investigators. Effects of ranolazine with atenolol, amlodipine, or diltiazem on exercise tolerance and angina frequency in patients with severe chronic angina: a randomized controlled trial. *JAMA* 2004;291:309-316.

103. Stone PH, Gratsiansky NA, Blokhin A, et al, for the ERICA Investigators. Antianginal efficacy of ranolazine when added to treatment with amlodipine: the ERICA (Efficacy of Ranolazine in Chronic Angina) trial. *J Am Coll Cardiol* 2006;48:566-575.

104. Morrow DA, Scirica BM, Karwatowska-Prokopczuk E, et al. Effects of ranolazine on recurrent cardiovascular events in patients with non-ST–elevation acute coronary syndromes: the MERLIN-TIMI 36 randomized trial. *JAMA* 2007;297:1775-1783.

105. Heidenreich PA, McDonald KM, Hastie T, et al. Meta-analysis of trails comparing β-blockers, calcium antagonists and nitrates for stable angina. *J Am Coll Cardiol* 1999;281:1927.

106. Parisi AF, Folland ED, Hartigan P. A comparison of angioplasty with medical therapy in the treatment of single-vessel coronary artery disease. Veterans Affairs ACME Investigators. *N Engl J Med* 1992;326:10.

107. The EPISTENT Investigators. Randomised placebo-controlled and balloon-angioplasty–controlled trial to assess safety of coronary stenting with the use of platelet glycoprotein IIb/IIIa blockade. *Lancet* 1998;352:87.

108. Ellis SG, Weintraub W, Holmes D, et al. Relation of operator volume and experience to procedural outcome of percutaneous coronary revascularization at hospitals with high interventional volumes. *Circulation* 1997;95:2479.

109. Ellis SG, Vandormael MG, Cowley MJ, et al. Coronary morphologic and clinical determinants of procedural outcome with angioplasty for multivessel coronary disease. Multivessel Angioplasty Prognosis Study Group. *Circulation* 1990;82:1193.

110. Strauss WE, Fortin T, Hartigan P, et al. A comparison of quality of life scores in patients with angina pectoris after angioplasty compared with after medical therapy: outcomes of a randomized clinical trial. Veterans Affairs Study of Angioplasty Compared to Medical Therapy Investigators. *Circulation* 1995;92:1710.

111. The RITA-2 Trial Participants. Coronary angioplasty versus medical therapy for angina: the second Randomised Intervention Treatment of Angina (RITA-2) trial. *Lancet* 1997;350:461.

112. Pocock SJ, Henderson RA, Clayton T, et al. Quality of life after coronary angioplasty or continued medical treatment for angina: three-year follow-up in the RITA-2 trial. Randomized Intervention Treatment of Angina. *J Am Coll Cardiol* 2000;35:907.

113. Boden WE, O'Rourke RA, Teo KK, et al. Optimal medical therapy with or without PCI for stable coronary disease. COURAGE Trial Research Group. *N Engl J Med* 2007; 356:1503-1516.

114. Pocock SJ, Henderson RA, Rickards AF, et al. Meta-analysis of randomised trials comparing coronary angioplasty with bypass surgery. *Lancet* 1995;346:1184.

115. The Bypass Angioplasty Revascularization Investigation (BARI) Investigators. Comparison of coronary bypass surgery with angioplasty in patients with multivessel disease. *N Engl J Med* 1996;335:217.

116. Serruys PW, Unger F, Sousa JE, et al. Comparison of coronary-artery bypass surgery and stenting for the treatment of multivessel disease. *N Engl J Med* 2001;344:1117.

117. The Stent or Surgery Trial Investigators. Coronary artery bypass surgery versus percutaneous coronary intervention with stent implantation in patients with multivessel coronary artery disease: a randomised controlled trial. *Lancet* 2002;360:965.

118. Serruys PW, Morice MC, Kappetein AP, et al, for the SYNTAX investigators. Percutaneous coronary intervention versus coronary artery bypass grafting for severe coronary artery disease. *N Engl J Med* 2009;360:961-972.

119. Mark DB, Nelson CL, Califf RM, et al. Continuing evolution of therapy for coronary artery disease: initial results from the era of coronary angioplasty. *Circulation* 1994; 89:2015.

120. Jones RH, Kesler K, Phillips HR, et al. Long-term survival benefits of coronary artery bypass grafting and percutaneous transluminal angioplasty in patients with coronary artery disease. *J Thorac Cardiovasc Surg* 1996;111:1013.

121. The RITA Trial Participants. Coronary angioplasty versus coronary artery bypass surgery: the Randomized Intervention Treatment of Angina (RITA) trial. *Lancet* 1993;341:573.

122. Ryan TJ, Bauman WB, Kennedy JW, et al. Guidelines for percutaneous transluminal coronary angioplasty: a report of the American College of Cardiology/American Heart Association Task Force on Assessment of Diagnostic and Therapeutic Cardiovascular Procedures (Committee on Percutaneous Transluminal Coronary Angioplasty). *J Am Coll Cardiol* 1993;22:2033.

123. Weintraub WS, Jones EL, Craver JM, et al. Frequency of repeat coronary bypass or coronary angioplasty after coronary artery bypass surgery using saphenous vein grafts. *Am J Cardiol* 1994;73:103.

124. Stephan WJ, O'Keefe JH, Piehler JM, et al. Coronary angioplasty versus repeat coronary bypass grafting for patients with previous bypass surgery. *J Am Coll Cardiol* 1996;28:1140.

125. Weintraub WS, Jones EL, Morris DC, et al. Outcome of reoperative coronary bypass surgery versus coronary angioplasty after previous bypass surgery. *Circulation* 1997;95:868.

126. Altmann DB, Racz M, Battleman DS, et al. Reduction in angioplasty complications after the introduction of coronary stents: results from a consecutive series of 2242 patients. *Am Heart J* 1996;132:503.

127. Rankin JM, Spinelli JJ, Carere RG, et al. Improved clinical outcome after widespread use of coronary artery stenting in Canada. *N Engl J Med* 1999;341:1957.

128. Sigwart U, Puel J, Mirkovitch V, et al. Intravascular stents to prevent occlusion and restenosis after transluminal angioplasty. *N Engl J Med* 1987;316:701.

129. Roubin GS, Cannon AD, Agrawal SK, et al. Intracoronary stenting for acute and threatened closure complicating percutaneous transluminal coronary angioplasty. *Circulation* 1992;85:916.

130. Fischman DL, Leon MB, Baim DS, et al. A randomized comparison of coronary-stent placement and balloon angioplasty in the treatment of coronary artery disease. Stent Restenosis Study Investigators. *N Engl J Med* 1994;331:496.

131. Serruys PW, de Jaegere P, Kiemeneij F, et al. A comparison of balloon-expandable-stent implantation with balloon angioplasty in patients with coronary artery disease. Benestent Study Group. *N Engl J Med* 1994;331:489.

132. Macaya C, Serruys PW, Ruygrok P, et al. Continued benefit of coronary stenting versus balloon angioplasty: one-year clinical follow-up of Benestent trial. Benestent Study Group. *J Am Coll Cardiol* 1996;27:255.

133. Sirnes PA, Golf S, Myreng Y, et al. Stenting In Chronic Coronary Occlusion (SICCO): a randomised controlled trial of adding stent implantation after successful angioplasty. *J Am Coll Cardiol* 1996;28:1444.

134. Rubartelli P, Niccoli L, Verna E, et al. Stent implantation versus balloon angioplasty in chronic coronary occlusion: results for the GISSOC trial. *J Am Coll Cardiol* 1998;32:90.

135. Hoher M, Wohrle J, Grebe OC, et al. A randomized trial of elective stenting after balloon recanalization of chronic total occlusions. *J Am Coll Cardiol* 1999;34:722.

136. Savage MP, Douglas JS, Fischman DL, et al. Stent placement compared with balloon angioplasty for obstructed coronary bypass grafts. Saphenous Vein De Novo Trial Investigators. *N Engl J Med* 1997;337:740.

137. Versaci F, Gaspardone A, Tomai F, et al. A comparison of coronary-artery stenting with angioplasty for isolated stenosis of the proximal left anterior descending coronary artery. *N Engl J Med* 1997;336:817.

138. Colombo A, Ferraro M, Itoh A, et al. Results of coronary stenting for restenosis. *J Am Coll Cardiol* 1996;28:830.

139. Erbel R, Haude M, Hopp HW, et al. Coronary-artery stenting compared with balloon angioplasty for restenosis after initial balloon angioplasty. Restenosis Stent Study Group. *N Engl J Med* 1998;339:1672.

140. Knight CJ, Curzen NP, Groves PH, et al. Stenting implantation reduces restenosis in patients with suboptimal results following coronary angioplasty. *Eur Heart J* 1999;20:1783.

141. Serruys PW, van Hout B, Bonnier H, et al. Randomised comparison of implantation of heparin-coated stents with balloon angioplasty in selected patients with coronary artery disease. *Lancet* 1998;352:673.

142. Rodriguez A, Ayala F, Bernardi V, et al. Optimal coronary balloon angioplasty with provisional stenting versus primary stent (OCBAS): immediate and long-term follow-up results. *J Am Coll Cardiol* 1998;32:1351.

143. Kimura T, Yokoi H, Nakagawa Y, et al. Three-year follow-up after implantation of metallic coronary-artery stents. *N Engl J Med* 1996;334:561.
144. Betriu A, Masotti M, Serra A, et al. Randomized comparison of coronary stent implantation and balloon angioplasty in the treatment of de novo coronary artery lesions (START): a four year follow-up. *J Am Coll Cardiol* 1999;34:1498.
145. Moses JW, Leon MB, Popma JJ, et al. SIRIUS Investigators. Sirolimus-eluting stents versus standard stents in patients with stenosis in a native coronary artery. *N Engl J Med* 2003;349:1315.
146. Silber S, Windecker S, Vranckx P, et al, for the RESOLUTE All Comers investigators. Unrestricted randomised use of two new generation drug-eluting coronary stents: 2-year patient-related versus stent-related outcomes from the RESOLUTE All Comers trial. *Lancet* 2011;377:1241-1247.
147. Antithrombotic Trialists' Collaboration. Collaborative meta-analysis of randomised trials of antiplatelet therapy for prevention of death, myocardial infarction, and stroke in high risk patients. *Br Med J* 2002;324:71.
148. Schömig A, Neumann FJ, Kastrati A, et al. A randomized comparison of antiplatelet and anticoagulant therapy after the placement of coronary-artery stents. *N Engl J Med* 1996;334:1084.
149. Leon MB, Baim DS, Popma JJ, et al. A clinical trial comparing three antithrombotic-drug regimens after coronary-artery stenting. Stent Anticoagulation Restenosis Study Investigators. *N Engl J Med* 1998;339:1665.
150. Berger PB, Bell MR, Rihal CS, et al. Clopidogrel versus ticlopidine after intracoronary stent placement. *J Am Coll Cardiol* 1999;34:1891.
151. Brookes CIO, Sigwart U. Taming platelets in coronary stenting: ticlopidine out, clopidogrel in? *Heart* 1999;82:651.
152. Wallentin L, Becker RC, Budaj A, et al. Ticagrelor versus clopidogrel in patients with acute coronary syndromes. *N Engl J Med* 2009;361:1045-1057.
153. Wiviott SD, Braunwald E, McCabe CH, et al. TRITON-TIMI 38 Investigators. Prasugrel versus clopidogrel in patients with acute coronary syndromes. *N Engl J Med* 2007;357: 2001-2015.
154. Kong DF, Califf RM, Miller DP, et al. Clinical outcomes of therapeutic agents that block the glycoprotein IIb/IIIa integrin in ischemic heart disease. *Circulation* 1998;98:2829.
155. Kastrati A, Mehilli J, Schuhlen H, et al. A clinical trial of abciximab in elective percutaneous coronary intervention after pretreatment with clopidogrel. Intracoronary Stenting and Antithrombotic Regimen-Rapid Early Action for Coronary Treatment Study Investigators. *N Engl J Med* 2004;350:232.
156. Jollis JG, Peterson ED, DeLong ER, et al. The relation between the volume of coronary angioplasty procedures at hospitals treating Medicare beneficiaries and short-term mortality. *N Engl J Med* 1994;331:1625.
157. British Cardiovascular Intervention Society audit 2009. Available at www.bcis.org.uk/resources/BCIS_Audit_2009_data_version_08-10-2010_for_web.pdf.
158. Gruentzig AR, King SB, Schlumpf M, Siegenthaler W. Long-term follow-up after percutaneous transluminal coronary angioplasty: the early Zurich experience. *N Engl J Med* 1987;316:1127.
159. Nobuyoshi M, Kimura T, Nosaka H, et al. Restenosis after successful percutaneous transluminal coronary angioplasty: serial angiographic follow-up of 229 patients. *J Am Coll Cardiol* 1988;12:616.
160. Topol EJ, Califf RM, Weisman HF, et al. Randomised trial of coronary intervention with antibody against platelet IIb/IIIa integrin for reduction of clinical restenosis: results at six months. The EPIC Investigators. *Lancet* 1994;343:881.
161. Serruys PW, Emannuelsson H, van der Giessen W, et al. Heparin-coated Palmaz-Schatz stents in human coronary arteries: early outcome of the Benestent-II Pilot Study. *Circulation* 1996;93:412.
162. The Coronary Artery Surgery Study (CASS). A randomized trial of coronary artery bypass surgery: quality of life in patients randomly assigned to treatment groups. *Circulation* 1983;68:951.
163. The Veterans Affairs Coronary Artery Bypass Surgery Cooperative Study Group. Eighteen-year follow-up in the Veterans Affairs Cooperative Study of Coronary Artery Bypass Surgery for stable angina. *Circulation* 1992;86:121.
164. The European Coronary Surgery Study Group. Prospective randomised study of coronary artery bypass surgery in stable angina pectoris: second interim report by the European Coronary Surgery Study Group. *Lancet* 1980;ii:491.
165. Yusuf S, Zucker D, Peduzzi P, et al. Effect of coronary artery bypass graft surgery on survival: overview of 10-year results from randomised trials by the Coronary Artery Bypass Graft Surgery Trialists Collaboration. *Lancet* 1994;344:563.
166. Sjoland H, Wiklund I, Caidahl K, et al. Improvement in quality of life and exercise capacity after coronary bypass surgery. *Arch Intern Med* 1996;156:265.
167. Caine N, Harrison SCW, Sharples LD, et al. Prospective study of quality of life before and after coronary artery bypass grafting. *Br Med J* 1991;302:511.
168. O'Connor GT, Morton JR, Diehl MJ, et al. Differences between men and women in hospital mortality associated with coronary artery bypass graft surgery. Northern New England Cardiovascular Disease Study Group. *Circulation* 1993;88:2104.
169. Tatoulis J, Buxton BF, Fuller JA. Patencies of 2127 arterial to coronary conduits over 15 years. *Ann Thorac Surg* 2004;77:93.
170. Loop FD, Lytle BW, Cosgrove DM, et al. Influence of the internal-mammary-artery graft on 10-year survival and other cardiac events. *N Engl J Med* 1986;314:1.
171. Zacharias A, Habib RH, Schwann TA, et al. Improved survival with radial artery versus vein conduits in coronary bypass surgery with left internal thoracic artery to left anterior descending artery grafting. *Circulation* 2004;109:1489.
172. Boylan MJ, Lytle BW, Loop FD, et al. Surgical treatment of isolated left anterior descending coronary stenosis: comparison of left internal mammary artery and venous autograft at 18 to 20 years of follow-up. *J Thorac Cardiovasc Surg* 1994;107:657.
173. Linden W, Stossel C, Maurice J. Psychosocial interventions for patients with coronary artery disease: a meta-analysis. *Arch Intern Med* 1996;156:745.
174. Hedbäck B, Perk J, Wodlin P. Long-term reduction of cardiac mortality after myocardial infarction: 10-year results of a comprehensive rehabilitation programme. *Eur Heart J* 1993;14:831.
175. Leontiadis GI, Sharma VK, Howden CW. Systematic review and meta-analysis of proton pump inhibitor therapy in peptic ulcer bleeding. *Br Med J* 2005;330:568.
176. The CAPRIE Steering Committee. A randomised, blinded trial of clopidogrel versus aspirin in patients at risk of ischaemic events. *Lancet* 1996;348:1329.
177. Bhatt DL, Fox KA, Hacke W, et al. Clopidogrel and aspirin versus aspirin alone for the prevention of atherothrombotic events. CHARISMA Investigators. *N Engl J Med* 2006;354:1706-1717.
178. Sacks FM, Pfeffer MA, Moye LA, et al. The effect of pravastatin on coronary events after myocardial infarction in patients with average cholesterol levels. *N Engl J Med* 1996;335:1001.
179. The Post Coronary Artery Bypass Graft Trial Investigators. The effect of aggressive lowering of low-density lipoprotein cholesterol levels and low-dose anticoagulation on obstructive changes in saphenous-vein coronary-artery bypass grafts. *N Engl J Med* 1997;336:153.
180. The Scandinavian Simvastatin Survival Study Group. Randomised trial of cholesterol lowering in 4,444 patients with coronary heart disease: the Scandinavian Simvastatin Survival Study (4S). *Lancet* 1994;344:1383.
181. Pitt B, Waters D, Brown WV, et al. Aggressive lipid-lowering therapy compared with angioplasty in stable coronary artery disease. Atorvastatin versus Revascularization Treatment Investigators. *N Engl J Med* 1999;341:70.
182. Heart Protection Study Collaborative Group. MRC/BHF Heart Protection Study of cholesterol lowering with simvastatin in 20,536 high-risk individuals: a randomised placebo-controlled trial. *Lancet* 2002;360:7.
183. Cholesterol Treatment Trialists' (CTT) Collaborators. Efficacy and safety of cholesterol-lowering treatment: prospective meta-analysis of data from 90,056 participants in 14 randomised trials of statins. *Lancet* 2005;366:1267.
184. Cannon CP, Braunwald E, McCabe CH, et al. Intensive versus moderate lipid lowering with statins after acute coronary syndromes. *N Engl J Med* 2004;350:1495.
185. LaRosa JC, Grundy SM, Waters DD, et al. Treating to New Targets (TNT) Investigators. Intensive lipid lowering with atorvastatin in patients with stable coronary disease. *N Engl J Med* 2005;352:1425.
186. Pederson TR, Faergeman O, Kastelein JJ, et al. High-dose atorvastatin vs. usual-dose simvastatin for secondary prevention after myocardial infarction: the IDEAL study. A randomized controlled trial. *JAMA* 2005;294:2437.
187. Bloomfield Rubins H, Robins SJ, Collins D, et al. Gemfibrozil for the secondary prevention of coronary heart disease in men with low levels of high-density lipoprotein cholesterol. Veterans Affairs High-Density Lipoprotein Cholesterol Intervention Trial Study Group. *N Engl J Med* 1999;341:410.
188. Gottlieb SS, McCarter RJ, Vogel RA. Effect of beta-blockade on mortality among high risk and low risk patients after myocardial infarction. *N Engl J Med* 1998;339:489.
189. Nidorf SM, Thompson PL, Jamrozik KD, Hobbs MST. Reduced risk of death at 28 days in patients taking beta-blocker before admission to hospital with myocardial infarction. *Br Med J* 1990;300:71.
190. Philipp T, Anlauf M, Distler A, et al. Randomised, double blind, multicentre comparison of hydrochlorothiazide, atenolol, nitrendipine, and enalapril in antihypertensive treatment: results of the HANE study. HANE Trial Research Group. *Br Med J* 1997;315:154.
191. Mimran A, Ducailar G. Systemic and regional haemodynamic profile of diuretics and alpha- and beta-blockers. *Drugs* 1988;35(Suppl 6):60.
192. Poldermans D, Boersma E, Bax JJ, et al. The effect of bisoprolol on perioperative mortality and myocardial infarction in high-risk patients undergoing vascular surgery. Dutch Echocardiographic Cardiac Risk Evaluation Applying Stress Echocardiography (DECREASE) Study Group. *N Engl J Med* 1999;341:1789.
193. Packer M, Bristow MR, Cohn JN, et al. The effect of carvedilol on morbidity and mortality in patients with chronic heart failure. U.S. Carvedilol Heart Failure Study Group. *N Engl J Med* 1996;334:1349.
194. The CIBIS II Investigators and Committees. The Cardiac Insufficiency Bisoprolol Study II (CIBIS II): a randomised trial. *Lancet* 1999;353:9.
195. The CONSENSUS Trial Study Group. Effects of enalapril on mortality in severe congestive heart failure: results of the Cooperative North Scandinavian Enalapril Survival Study (CONSENSUS). *N Engl J Med* 1987;316:1429.
196. The SOLVD Investigators. Effect of enalapril on survival in patients with reduced left ventricular ejection fractions and congestive heart failure. *N Engl J Med* 1991; 325:293.
197. The Heart Outcomes Prevention Evaluation Study Investigators. Effects of an angiotensin-converting enzyme inhibitor, ramipril, on cardiovascular events in high-risk patients. *N Engl J Med* 2000;342:145.
198. Fox KM, European Trial on Reduction of Cardiac Events with Perindopril in Stable Coronary Artery Disease Investigators. Efficacy of perindopril in reduction of cardiovascular events among patients with stable coronary artery disease: randomised, double-blind, placebo-controlled, multicentre trial (the EUROPA study). *Lancet* 2003;362:782.
199. The Heart Outcomes Prevention Evaluation Study Investigators. Effects of ramipril on cardiovascular and microvascular outcomes in people with diabetes mellitus: results of the HOPE study and MICRO-HOPE substudy. *Lancet* 2000;355:253.
200. Braunwald E, Domanski MJ, Fowler SE, et al. Angiotensin-converting-enzyme inhibition in stable coronary artery disease. *N Engl J Med* 2004;351:2058.
201. Cox J, Naylor CD. The Canadian Cardiovascular Society grading scale for angina pectoris: Is it time for refinements? *Ann Intern Med* 1992;117:677.
202. Califf RM, Harrell FE, Lee KL, et al. The evolution of medical and surgical therapy for coronary artery disease: a 15-year perspective. *JAMA* 1989;261:2077.
203. Barter PJ, Caulfield M, Eriksson M, et al. Effects of torcetrapib in patients at high risk for coronary events. ILLUMINATE Investigators. *N Engl J Med* 2007;357:2109-2122.
204. Cannon CP, Shah S, Dansky HM, et al. Safety of anacetrapib in patients with or at high risk for coronary heart disease. Determining the Efficacy and Tolerability Investigators. *N Engl J Med* 2010;363:2406-2415.
205. Morrow DA, Braunwald E, Bonaca MP, et al, for the TRA 2P–TIMI 50 Steering Committee and Investigators. Vorapaxar in the secondary prevention of atherothrombotic events. *N Engl J Med* 2012;366:1404-1413.

CHAPTER 9

Non–ST-Segment Elevation Acute Coronary Syndromes

Stephen D. Wiviott and Robert P. Giugliano

ANTIISCHEMIC MEDICATIONS, 153

Nitrates, 153
β-Adrenergic Receptor Blockers, 154
Calcium Channel Antagonists, 154
Ranolazine, 155

ANTIPLATELET AGENTS, 155

Aspirin, 155
P2Y$_{12}$ Antagonists, 156
Clopidogrel, 156
Prasurgel, 156
Ticagrelor, 157
Duration of Therapy, 157

PLATELET FUNCTION TESTING AND GENETICS, 157

Intravenous Platelet Inhibitors, 158
Conclusions, 159

ANTICOAGULANTS, 159

Unfractionated Heparin and Low-Molecular-Weight
    Heparin, 159
Direct Thrombin Inhibitors, 161
Factor Xa Inhibitors, 162
Other Anticoagulants, 163
Summary on Anticoagulant Selection, 163

INVASIVE VERSUS CONSERVATIVE STRATEGY FOR
CARDIAC CATHETERIZATION, 163

HOSPITAL DISCHARGE AND POSTDISCHARGE CARE, 165

Antiplatelet Therapy, Anticoagulation, Angiotensin-Converting
    Enzyme Inhibitors, and Angiotensin Receptor Blockade, 166
β-Blockade and Blood Pressure Control, 167
Cholesterol Treatment and Cigarette Smoking Cessation, 167
Diabetes Management and Diet, 168

Exercise, 168
Influenza Vaccine, 168
Cardiac Syndrome X, 168
Cocaine and Methamphetamines, 169
Diabetes Mellitus, 170
The Elderly, 171
Women, 171
Chronic Kidney Disease, 172

REFERENCES, 172

In this chapter, we have drawn from evidence-based guidelines, adopted the standard classification schemas used to grade the level of recommendation and strength of supportive evidence, and provided updated information from the literature on non–ST-elevation acute coronary syndrome (NSTE-ACS).[1,2] A recurring theme is the need for integrative risk assessment to allow tailoring of therapy based on a patient's probability of adverse outcomes. Efforts have been made to incorporate physiologic, laboratory, and demographic characteristics of patients into risk scores such as the Thrombolysis in Myocardial Infarction (TIMI) risk score for unstable angina/non–ST-segment elevation myocardial infarction (UA/NSTEMI). Other scores derived from clinical trials[3,4] and registries[5-7] were developed to assess the risk of patients with NSTE-ACS and to help identify patients most likely to benefit from aggressive therapy. An analysis comparing three risk scores—TIMI, Platelet Glycoprotein IIb/IIIa in Unstable Angina: Receptor Suppression Using Integrilin Therapy (PURSUIT), and Global Registry of Acute Coronary Events (GRACE) scores (Table 9-1)—concluded that all three demonstrated good predictive accuracy for death or MI.[8] The TIMI UA/NSTEMI Risk Score has been found to be useful in the prediction of angiographic severity and extent of coronary artery disease (CAD),[9] including the prediction of greater intracoronary thrombus burden and impaired flow.[10] Patients with higher TIMI risk scores derive greater benefit from aggressive antithrombotic strategies[11,12] and an early invasive strategy of angiography and coronary intervention.[13]

Antiischemic Medications

Management of UA/NSTEMI should be directed toward the dual goals of relief of the symptoms of myocardial ischemia and prevention of the severe short- and long-term sequelae, which include recurrent myocardial infarction (MI), congestive heart failure (CHF), and death. Therapeutic efforts should be focused intensely on therapies that achieve both of these goals, and a multifaceted and continuously updated approach to the management of patients with NSTE-ACS may be necessary. For instance, a medication such as nitroglycerin, which may be used on first encounter with a patient with ongoing ischemic chest pain to provide symptomatic relief, may be replaced with agents such as angiotensin-converting enzyme (ACE) inhibitors, which are expected to modify long-term risk. Patients for whom initial intensive pharmacologic

therapy does not produce relief of ischemic symptoms should be considered as candidates for early cardiac catheterization and revascularization or for ischemic relief with mechanical therapies, such as intraaortic balloon counterpulsation. For the majority of patients with NSTE-ACS, relief of ischemic symptoms can be achieved by pharmacologic measures.

Myocardial ischemia is a consequence of an imbalance in myocardial oxygen supply and demand. In most cases of UA/NSTEMI, the principal cause of this imbalance is abrupt reduction of blood flow resulting from nonocclusive coronary thrombosis.[14] For this reason, mainstays of therapy for UA/NSTEMI include antithrombotic and antiplatelet therapies and coronary revascularization.[15] Revascularization may not always be immediately available, practical, safe or appropriate, and pharmacologic management of myocardial oxygen demand (MVO$_2$)—and, to a lesser extent, supply—may result in relief of symptoms. The principal components of MVO$_2$ are heart rate, myocardial contractility, and wall stress.[16] Controlling and reducing these factors helps improve the balance and relieve angina. Major classes of antianginal therapy include nitrates, β-adrenergic receptor antagonists (β-blockers), and calcium channel blockers (CCBs). Morphine sulfate has mixed effects that reduce oxygen demand and angina.

Nitrates

The use of nitrates in NSTE-ACS is based on physiologic principles and expert consensus.[15] Nitroglycerin should be used in UA/NSTEMI for the rapid relief of ischemia and ischemia-related symptoms, including angina and CHF (Figure 9-1). In suitable patients, nitrate administration should begin with sublingual administration of 0.4 mg (tablets or spray) given at 5-minute intervals, up to three doses. Intravenous (IV) nitroglycerin treatment may be initiated in patients with refractory symptoms and without hypotension despite adequate doses of β-blocker.[15] IV nitroglycerin is initiated at 5 to 10 μg/min of continuous infusion and may be titrated upward at 3- to 5-minute intervals, until 20 μg/min is reached. If this dose is tolerated without hypotension and anginal symptoms persist, larger titration steps of 20 μg/min are usually well tolerated. Titration should cease when symptom relief is achieved, when hypotension ensues, or when a maximum dose of approximately 200 to 300 μg/min is reached. Tolerance to the antiischemic effects of nitrates may develop within 12 to 24 hours and can be

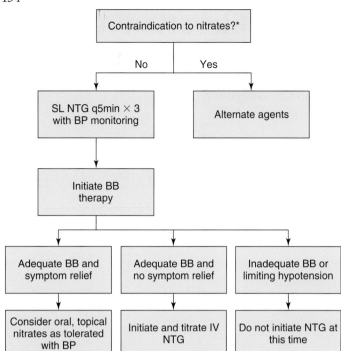

FIGURE 9-1 Schematic for early use of nitrates in acute coronary syndrome. *Use of phosphodiesterase-5 inhibitor within 24 hours, severe aortic stenosis, hypotension, hypertrophic cardiomyopathy, right ventricular infarction with hypotension, hemodynamically significant pulmonary embolism. BB, β-blocker; BP, blood pressure; IV, intravenous; NTG, nitroglycerin; SL, sublingual.

TABLE 9-1	Integrative Clinical Risk Scores for Unstable Angina/Non–ST-Segment Elevation Myocardial Infarction	
SCORE	**FEATURES**	**COMMENTS**
TIMI	Age ≥65 years or older, ≥3 cardiac risk factors, aspirin use in last 7 days, known CAD (previous stenosis ≥50%), recurrent angina in last 24 hours, ST-segment deviation, elevated markers of necrosis	Sum of number of features (1 point each)
PURSUIT	Age by decade, sex, worst CCS class in previous 6 weeks, signs of heart failure, ST-segment depression	Weighted score based on different point total (range, 0-14) for each feature
GRACE	Age, heart rate, systolic BP, creatinine level, Killip class, cardiac arrest, elevated markers, ST-segment deviation	Weighted score based on different point total (range, 0-91) for each feature

BP, blood pressure; CAD, coronary artery disease; CCS class, Canadian Cardiovascular Society anginal class; GRACE, Global Registry of Acute Coronary Events; PURSUIT, Platelet Glycoprotein IIb/IIIa in Unstable Angina: Receptor Suppression Using Integrilin Therapy; TIMI, Thrombolysis in Myocardial Infarction.

ameliorated by nitrate-free intervals. If symptoms do not allow for nitrate-free intervals, increasing the dose may be effective. Despite tolerance, abrupt removal of nitrates may result in recurrent ischemia[17] and discontinuation of high-dose IV nitrates should be performed by stepped-down titration.

The pharmacologic effects of nitrates, predominantly the venodilation and reduction of ventricular preload, may be detrimental to patients who are highly dependent on ventricular preload for the maintenance of cardiac output, and it can result in substantial hypotension. Nitrates should generally be avoided, or used with considerable caution, in patients with right ventricular infarction, severe aortic stenosis, hypertrophic cardiomyopathy, or pulmonary embolism. Nitrates are contraindicated for patients who have used phosphodiesterase-5 (PDE-5) inhibitors—sildenafil, tadalafil, or vardenafil—within the preceding 24 to 48 hours[15] because of exaggeration and prolongation of nitrate effects from the inhibition of the breakdown of cyclic guanosine monophosphate (cGMP), which modulates the vasodilator effects of nitrates. The combination of PDE-5 inhibitors and nitrates has been associated with severe hypotension, myocardial ischemia, and death.[18,19]

β-Adrenergic Receptor Blockers

Clinical trial data for the use of β-blockers are sparse, specifically in UA/NSTEMI. A systematic review of the accumulated trial data suggests that β-blockers reduce the risk of progression to MI in NSTE-ACS.[20] In contrast, a large body of randomized, controlled trial data suggests benefits in reducing recurrent MI and death by early use of β-blocker therapy in STEMI.[21-23] Therefore the evidence for the use of β-blockers in NSTE-ACS results largely from extrapolation from STEMI trials and physiologic principles.

Based on these data, β-blockers should be initiated in the treatment of UA/NSTEMI as early as possible for patients without contraindications. IV β-blockers should be used with particular caution in patients with CHF on arrival at the care center, based on results from the Clopidogrel and Metoprolol in Myocardial Infarction Trial (COMMIT); use in patients with STEMI shows adverse outcomes in this population.[24] However, oral β-blockers are strongly recommended for patients who have stabilized CHF or reduced left ventricular (LV) function before discharge.[25] β-Blockers should be used cautiously or avoided in patients with significant first-degree atrioventricular (AV) block, and they should be withheld in patients with severe bradycardia or second- or third-degree AV block without a pacemaker. Selective β-blockade should be used in patients for whom NSTE-ACS is secondary to profound catecholamine excess, such as with pheochromocytoma or cocaine use. For patients with reactive airway disease, the use of a cardioselective (β1) agent is recommended. Initial therapy for patients with evidence of ongoing ischemia should be an IV β-blocker, such as metoprolol, 5 mg every 5 minutes up to three doses as tolerated by heart rate and blood pressure. After initial IV dosing, oral β-blocker therapy should be initiated early to avoid a rebound effect between the offset of the IV agent and the onset of the oral agent.

Calcium Channel Antagonists

Dihydropyridine CCBs have predominantly peripheral vasodilatory actions, whereas nondihydropyridine CCBs have significant sinoatrial (SA) and AV node depressant effects and possible myocardial depressant effects with lesser amounts of peripheral vasodilation. Coronary vasodilation appears to be similar among various agents.[15] The predominant clinical role for CCBs has been in the control of hypertension; however, the physiologic properties of arterial vasodilation, heart rate slowing, and contractility reduction favorably alter myocardial oxygen balance. Because of these differences in properties, the two types of CCBs are discussed separately.

The dihydropyridine CCBs cause a reflex tachycardia in the absence of adequate β-blocker therapy, a mechanism that may underlie apparent adverse effects of these agents on patients with NSTE-ACS.[26,27] In contrast to the dihydropyridines, diltiazem and verapamil are heart rate–slowing agents and appear to not increase rates of ischemic events in patients with UA/NSTEMI. However, concerns have been raised that myocardial depressant effects may increase the risk of heart failure. The relationship of the nondihydropyridine CCBs to CHF is somewhat controversial. In retrospective analyses of CCB trials, evidence was found for increased rates of CHF and an increase in the mortality rate in patients with diminished ejection fraction.[28,29] These findings, however, are counterbalanced by studies that show beneficial effects of CCBs in patients with heart failure who are treated concurrently with ACE inhibitors.[30]

In summary, CCBs reduce symptomatic ischemia. Short-acting dihydropyridine CCBs have not been shown to improve cardiac outcomes and may result in worse outcomes in the absence of β-blockers. Newer, longer acting dihydropyridine CCBs have not been studied in NSTE-ACS. Nondihydropyridine CCBs are antianginal, do not result in harm, and may improve outcomes in patients with NSTE-ACS, especially those patients without LV dysfunction; therefore nondihydropyridine CCBs can be considered for use in patients who cannot tolerate β-blockers.[15]

Ranolazine

Ranolazine is an antianginal agent that exerts its effects uniquely, without alteration of heart rate or blood pressure. The mechanism of the antianginal effects is thought to arise from inhibition of the late phase of the sodium current, which is pathologically increased during ischemia.[31] Ranolazine has been demonstrated to be effective in the reduction of chronic stable angina as monotherapy and in combination with a CCB or β-blocker.[31] When evaluated in a broad population of patients with NSTE-ACS in the Metabolic Efficiency with Ranolazine for Less Ischemia in Non–ST-Elevation Coronary Syndromes (MERLIN)-TIMI 36 trial, ranolazine did not affect the primary outcome of cardiovascular (CV) death, MI, or recurrent ischemia, but it did reduce recurrent ischemia alone.[32] No increase was seen in CV death or arrhythmia; therefore ranolazine can be administered safely for angina relief but does not appear to alter the disease process.

Antiplatelet Agents

Antiplatelet agents represent the cornerstone of therapy for patients with NSTE-ACS. Pharmacologic inhibition of platelet function can be achieved by interfering with a number of processes: inhibition of cyclooxygenase (COX), phosphodiesterase, adenosine diphosphate (ADP), thromboxane, serotonin, platelet adhesion, and platelet aggregation. This has led to the development of numerous platelet inhibitors (Box 9-1), of which aspirin, the $P2Y_{12}$ ADP receptor blockers, and the intravenous glycoprotein (GP) IIb/IIIa inhibitors have been studied most extensively.

Aspirin

Several small- to medium-sized clinical trials to compare aspirin with placebo in NSTE-ACS demonstrated an approximate 50% reduction in death or MI (Figure 9-2). These data support the class I indication in the 2007 American College of Cardiology (ACC) and American Heart Association (AHA) UA/NSTEMI guidelines to begin aspirin immediately and to treat indefinitely upon establishment of the diagnosis of NSTE-ACS.[25] Because aspirin is one of the most inexpensive drugs available, and with a known safety profile, it is unlikely that future placebo-controlled studies will be undertaken. Thus aspirin is likely to remain the first-line antiplatelet agent in NSTE-ACS for the foreseeable future.

Despite its long history, the optimal dose of aspirin remains to be definitively established. Increased doses have been associated with more bleeding, yet the relationship of the dose with efficacy is less clear.[31] A dose of 40 mg was found to achieve maximal inhibition once steady state has been achieved, although doses greater than 160 mg are needed to produce a rapid clinical antithrombotic effect, and doses of less than 75 mg daily have not been well studied in clinical trials.[32-35] A meta-analysis by the Antiplatelet Trialists' Collaboration demonstrated no increase in benefit of aspirin across maintenance doses ranging from 75 mg to 1500 mg daily, whereas gastrointestinal (GI) bleeding was increased at doses above 300 mg daily.[31] Two nonrandomized subgroup analyses[36,37] compared different doses of aspirin and confirmed that higher doses were associated with an increased risk of bleeding and no apparent reduction in ischemic complications. A random effects multivariate regression model concluded that efficacy of aspirin did not increase at higher doses; in fact, the point estimates suggest less benefit at higher doses.[38]

The largest clinical trial of aspirin dosing in ACS is the Clopidogrel and Aspirin Optimal Dose Usage to Reduce Recurrent Events–Seventh Organization to Assess Strategies in Ischemic Syndromes (CURRENT-OASIS 7) trial.[33,34] This trial was a 2 × 2 factorial study of standard versus higher dose clopidogrel and also of low- versus high-dose aspirin—a dose of 75 to 100 mg/day (low dose) compared with 300 to 325 mg/day (high dose) for 30 days. The aspirin comparison in this trial demonstrated no difference in either the primary outcome of CV death, MI, or stroke (4.2% vs. 4.4%; hazard ratio [HR], 0.97; 95% confidence interval [CI], 0.86 to 1.09; $P = .61$) or in major bleeding (2.3% vs. 2.3%; HR, 0.99; 95% CI, 0.84 to 1.17; $P = .90$); however, the higher dose aspirin group had slightly higher rates of study-defined minor bleeding. These data allow only for

---

Box 9-1 Classification Scheme of Selected Antiplatelet Agents

Arachidonic Acid Inhibitors
COX Inhibitors: aspirin, indobufen, triflusal, nonsteroidal antiinflammatory agents, sulfinpyrazone
Non-COX inhibition of arachidonic acid; phosphodiesterase inhibitors: dipyridamole, pentoxifylline, cilostazol, trapidil
Other: omega-3 fatty acids, eicosanoids (prostacyclin, prostaglandin analogues)

$P2Y_{12}$ ADP Receptor Inhibitors
Thienopyridines (ADP antagonists): ticlopidine, clopidogrel, prasugrel
ATP derivatives: cangrelor
CPTPs: ticagrelor
Elinogril

Thrombin Protease-Activated Receptor-1 Inhibitors
Vorapaxar, E-5555

Platelet Glycoprotein IIb/IIIa Receptor Blockers
Intravenous: abciximab, tirofiban, eptifibatide

Drugs with Secondary Antiplatelet Activity
Direct thrombin inhibitors, heparin, nitrates, fibrates, calcium channel antagonists, others

ADP, adenosine diphosphate; ATP, adenosine triphosphate; COX, cyclooxygenase; CPTPs, cyclopentyltriazolopyrimidines.

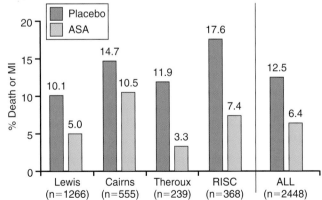

FIGURE 9-2 Placebo-controlled trials with aspirin (ASA) in patients with non–ST-segment elevation acute coronary syndrome. Aspirin was associated with a 50% reduction in death or myocardial infarction (MI) compared with placebo. (From Braunwald E, Antman EM, Beasley JW, et al. ACC/AHA guideline update for the management of patients with unstable angina and non–ST-segment elevation myocardial infarction—2002. Summary article: a report of the American College of Cardiology/American Heart Association Task Force on Practice Guidelines [Committee on the Management of Patients with Unstable Angina]. Circulation 2002;106[14]:1893-1900.)

CH
9

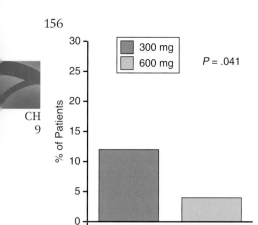

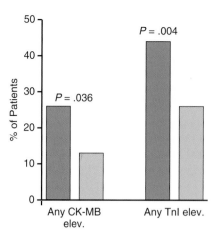

FIGURE 9-3 Main results of the ARMYDA-2 trial. ARMYDA-2 compared 600 mg clopidogrel with 300 mg administered 4 to 8 hours before percutaneous coronary intervention (PCI) in 255 patients with known coronary artery disease. The rate of the primary composite endpoint of death, myocardial infarction (MI), or target vessel revascularization up to 30 days after PCI, as well as the rates of elevated biomarkers of myonecrosis after PCI, were reduced with clopidogrel 600 mg. The rate of MI following PCI with 300 mg was unexpectedly higher than has been reported in similar studies. CK-MB elev., creatine kinase–myocardial band elevation; TnI elev., Troponin I elevation. *(From Patti G, Colonna G, Pasceri V, et al. Randomized trial of high loading dose of clopidogrel for reduction of periprocedural myocardial infarction in patients undergoing coronary intervention: results from the ARMYDA-2 (Antiplatelet Therapy for Reduction of Myocardial Damage during Angioplasty) study. Circulation 2005;111:2099-2106.)*

assessment of the effects of early aspirin dosing, but they are consistent with meta-analyses and are supportive of the concept of low-dose aspirin therapy.

Guidelines for patients with NSTE-ACS or for those undergoing percutaneous coronary intervention (PCI) recommend an initial dose of 162 mg to 325 mg.[2] After stenting, the recommended dose has been 325 mg for at least 1 month (bare-metal stent), 3 months (sirolimus-coated stent), or 6 months (paclitaxel-coated stent). To decrease the risk of bleeding, the aspirin dose may be reduced to 81 mg to 162 mg.[2] However, recent PCI-based guidelines allow for the long-term use of 81 mg daily in place of a higher dose.[1]

P2Y₁₂ Antagonists

Management of ACS involves dual antiplatelet therapy with aspirin and a P2Y₁₂ antagonist such as clopidogrel or prasugrel, which are thienopyridines, or ticagrelor, a member of a different chemical class. Three currently available thienopyridines include ticlopidine, clopidogrel, and prasugrel. Thienopyridines act by irreversibly blocking the P2Y₁₂ ADP receptor on the platelet surface, thereby interrupting platelet activation and aggregation. When administered at the currently approved doses, clopidogrel 75 mg daily and ticlopidine 250 mg twice daily achieve at steady state a moderate level of median platelet inhibition (20% to 35%)[35,36] as assessed by using 20 μmol/L ADP as the agonist. Prasugrel at 10 mg achieves a level of inhibition of approximately 60% to the same agonist.[37,38] An earlier effect on platelet function occurs with administration of a loading dose, although the absolute degree of platelet inhibition is marginally increased with higher doses once steady state is achieved. The thienopyridines also have a number of other effects that are not fully characterized on platelet function beyond inhibition of ADP-induced aggregation, such as inhibition of platelet activation, reduction in fibrinogen levels and blood viscosity, and less erythrocyte deformability and aggregability. If rapid onset of platelet inhibition is required (e.g., at the time of intracoronary stenting), a loading dose should be administered.

Clopidogrel

The combination of aspirin plus clopidogrel was compared with aspirin alone in the Clopidogrel in Unstable Angina to Prevent Recurrent Events (CURE) trial of 12,562 patients with NSTE-ACS treated for 3 to 12 months.[39,40] Clopidogrel reduced the composite of death, MI, and stroke by 20% compared with placebo, with benefit evident both in the first 30 days and over the ensuing average follow-up of up to 9 months. In addition, a 38% increase was seen in the rate of bleeding overall, with patients who underwent coronary artery bypass graft (CABG) within 5 days of the discontinuation of clopidogrel at particular risk (53% increased rate). In a secondary analysis (PCI-CURE) of patients in the CURE trial who underwent PCI, patients pretreated with clopidogrel for

a median of 10 days had a reduction in both early (30 day) and long-term CV events.[39,40] ACC/AHA UA/NSTEMI guidelines consider the use of clopidogrel in addition to aspirin to have a class I indication for patients with NSTE-ACS who are undergoing an early noninterventional or interventional approach and who are not at risk for major bleeding.[2] For patients with planned elective CABG, the drug should be withheld for 5 to 7 days to reduce the risk of perioperative bleeding and transfusion.

Several important issues regarding treatment with clopidogrel remain controversial: the optimal loading dose, duration of therapy, and clinical relevance of genetic differences and clopidogrel resistance. Without a loading dose, clopidogrel achieves steady-state levels of platelet inhibition in 4 to 7 days. Administration of various loading doses has been studied, with reductions in the time to steady state of 12 to 48 hours (for 300 mg) to 2 to 6 hours (for 600 to 900 mg). Data from the Clopidogrel for the Reduction of Events During Observation (CREDO) trial suggested that a minimum of 12 to 15 hours between the loading dose and PCI was required for a 300-mg load to demonstrate clinical benefit compared with no load,[41] whereas the Antiplatelet Therapy for Reduction of Myocardial Damage During Angioplasty (ARMYDA)-2 study showed better outcomes with 600 mg versus 300 mg when clopidogrel was initiated 4 to 8 hours before PCI (Figure 9-3).[42] The CURRENT-OASIS 7 trial compared a high-dose (600-mg load followed by 150 mg/day for 7 days) to a standard dose (300-mg load followed by 75 mg/day) clopidogrel strategy in patients with ACS and planned PCI. More than 25,000 subjects were randomized in the trial. Overall, no difference was found in the primary outcome of CV death, MI, or stroke (4.2% vs. 4.4%; HR, 0.94; 95% CI, 0.83 to 1.06; $P = .30$); however, study-defined major bleeding was higher (2.5% vs. 2.0%; HR, 1.24; 95% CI, 1.05 to 1.46; $P = .01$).[34] These data do not formally support the use of higher dose clopidogrel following ACS. However, in the more than 17,000 patients who underwent PCI during the trial, a 15% relative reduction in the primary endpoint was observed.[43] Current ACS and PCI guidelines allow for loading doses of 300 to 600 mg, followed by 75 mg daily in patients with ACS.

Prasugrel

Prasugrel is a thienopyridine, which compared with clopidogrel has 1) faster onset of action for more efficient metabolism, 2) a higher degree of ex vivo platelet inhibition, and 3) less intrapatient variability.[38] In pharmacodynamic studies, prasugrel had fewer poor responders compared with a standard or higher dose of clopidogrel.[37] Prasugrel (60-mg loading dose followed by 10 mg/day) was compared with clopidogrel (300-mg loading dose followed by 75 mg/day) for up to 15 months in patients with ACS and planned PCI in the Trial to Assess Improvement in Therapeutic Outcomes by Optimizing Platelet Inhibition with Prasugrel (TRITON)–Thrombolysis in Myocardial Infarction TIMI 38.[44,45] More than 13,500 subjects were randomized to prasugrel or clopidogrel in combination with aspirin. Prasugrel treatment resulted in a reduction in the primary endpoint of CV death, MI, or stroke (9.9% vs. 12.1%; HR, 0.81; 95% CI, 0.73 to 0.90; $P < .001$). The difference in the outcomes was largely related to a 24% reduction in MI.[46] Rates of stent thrombosis were also significantly reduced with prasugrel,[47] and prasugrel treatment also resulted in an increase in the primary safety assessment of non–coronary bypass–associated TIMI major bleeding with 1.8% versus 2.4% of subjects (HR, 1.32; 95% CI, 1.03 to 1.68; $P = .03$). The most severe bleeding events, including fatal bleeding, were also increased. An analysis of the data from this study identified patients with prior stroke or transient ischemic attack (TIA) as a subgroup that did not benefit from more intensive antiplatelet therapy with prasugrel compared with clopidogrel.[45] In addition, patients who were older than 75 years or who weighed less than 60 kg were subgroups for whom the benefit did not clearly exceed the risk. As a result of these data, prasugrel was approved for use in patients with ACS and planned PCI. Based on trial design, in patients with NSTE-ACS, prasugrel should be given once it is known that PCI is planned; it should not be given in a broad ACS population, such as that studied in the CURE trial. Higher rates of CABG-related bleeding were also observed.

In the 2011 UA/NSTEMI ACC/AHA guideline update, prasugrel is given a class I indication for patients with ACS in whom PCI is planned but a class III recommendation (not recommended) in patients with a prior stroke or TIA.[1,2] In patients for whom CABG is planned, it is recommended that prasugrel be withheld for 7 days prior to the procedure whenever possible.

Ticagrelor

Ticagrelor is an oral antiplatelet agent that is the first member of a new class of $P2Y_{12}$ receptor antagonists known as the *cyclopentyltriazolopyrimidines* (CPTPs).[48] Ticagrelor is a direct-acting antiplatelet agent that does not require metabolism for its effect, distinct from the thienopyridines.[48] In addition, it does not bind irreversibly to the $P2Y_{12}$ receptor. Ticagrelor results in more rapid onset of antiplatelet effect, more potent antiplatelet effect, and fewer poor responders than standard-dose clopidogrel.[49,50] Although ticagrelor is pharmacologically reversible because of the higher level of platelet inhibition even after discontinuation, compared with clopidogrel, higher levels of platelet inhibition remain for approximately 4 days.[50] Ticagrelor (180-mg loading dose followed by 90 mg twice daily) was compared with clopidogrel (300- to 600-mg loading dose followed by 75 mg/day) in the Platelet Inhibition and Patient Outcomes (PLATO) trial.[51,52] More than 18,500 subjects with ACS were randomized to be treated medically, surgically, or with PCI. Overall, ticagrelor treatment resulted in a reduction in the primary endpoint of CV death, MI, or stroke of 9.8% versus 11.7% with clopidogrel (HR, 0.84; 95% CI, 0.77 to 0.92; $P < .001$). The difference in primary outcome was driven by significant reductions in CV death (21%) and MI (16%). Rates of stent thrombosis were also reduced with ticagrelor, and it was not associated with an increase in total study-defined major bleeding episodes. However, study-defined non–CABG-related major bleeding was increased by 19%, and CABG-related bleeding was similar between groups.[53] Consistent reductions in major efficacy events were seen across broad subgroups of patients, and no specific subgroups at risk were identified. No benefit was observed in patients who were treated long term with high-dose aspirin (predominantly in the United States), although no plausible mechanism of action to explain these results in known.[54] Patients were more likely to experience dyspnea, which tended to be self-limited[55,56] and was not demonstrated to be associated with CV or pulmonary pathology. As a result of these data, ticagrelor was approved for use across the spectrum of ACS; however, the U.S. Food and Drug Administration (FDA) has issued a warning that ticagrelor should be used in combination with low-dose aspirin (<100 mg) and should be withheld from patients undergoing CABG for 5 days prior whenever possible.[1]

Duration of Therapy

The duration of treatment with antiplatelet therapy is an important clinical issue because the drug is costly to administer and is associated with an increased risk of bleeding. The major antiplatelet therapy trials in ACS had treatment durations of 9 to 15 months.[45,52,57] Some data suggest increased risk of stent thrombosis in patients with drug-eluting stents when antiplatelet therapy is discontinued even beyond 1 year.[58-60] In ACS patients who are not at high risk for bleeding complications, dual antiplatelet therapy is recommended for at least 1 year.[2] After PCI, the optimal duration of clopidogrel therapy depends on the risk of subsequent thrombosis, which itself is related to the type of intervention, use of an intracoronary stent, and the type of drug-eluting stent placed, if any. These recommendations are based largely on observational data and randomized trial protocols, as opposed to randomized comparisons; further studies are awaited, including the definitive Dual Antiplatelet Therapy (DAPT) study.[61] Other observational data have identified a strong link between the interruption of antiplatelet therapy after ACS and an increased risk of adverse outcomes, including stent thrombosis.[62] Thus, the threshold to hold or terminate antiplatelet therapy early should be high (e.g., life-threatening bleeding or need for high-risk emergency surgery).

The Clopidogrel for High Atherothrombotic Risk, Ischemic Stabilization, Management, and Avoidance (CHARISMA) trial evaluated the usefulness of clopidogrel in addition to aspirin for a median of 28 months in high-risk patients with stable CV disease across a wide range of patients.[63,64] Although no difference was noted in the primary endpoint of CV death, MI, or stroke between the clopidogrel plus aspirin group (6.8%) and the placebo plus aspirin group (7.3%; $P = .22$), the secondary endpoint, which also included rehospitalization for ischemic events, was reduced by 8% ($P = .04$) with dual antiplatelet therapy.[63] The secondary prevention subgroup—approximately 80% of patients enrolled had documented preexisting CV disease—had a 12% ($P = .046$) lower incidence of the primary composite, whereas the remainder of asymptomatic patients (primary prevention) had a 20% excess ($P = .20$), including a higher rate of CV death (3.9% vs. 2.2%; $P = .01$).[63] The greatest benefit appeared to be in patients with prior MI.[65] In the overall study population, severe bleeding tended to be more frequent in the clopidogrel group (1.7% vs. 1.3%; $P = .09$). Thus, longer term clopidogrel, in addition to aspirin, appeared beneficial in secondary prevention of ischemic complications among patients with established CV disease, with a trend toward more severe bleeding, but it was not useful and was found to be potentially harmful in asymptomatic patients (primary prevention).

Platelet Function Testing and Genetics

Several studies of platelet function have documented the variable pharmacologic response to standard dose clopidogrel among groups of individuals. Depending on the method, timing, and definition of "resistance," between 5% and 30% of patients do not achieve the expected pharmacologic response to clopidogrel.[36,66] Failure of clopidogrel to achieve the desired pharmacologic effect is associated with increased rates of CV events, including stent thrombosis and death.[66] Several studies have demonstrated that increasing doses of clopidogrel can partly overcome this variability in subjects who respond poorly to standard doses.[67,68] The largest study to date to examine modification of clopidogrel based on platelet function testing—Gauging Responsiveness with a Verify Now Assay: Impact on Thrombosis and Safety (GRAVITAS)—confirmed that low response to clopidogrel was associated with worse outcomes, but it failed to demonstrate that increasing doses could improve clinical outcomes.[69,70] Both prasugrel and ticagrelor are associated with higher levels of platelet inhibition and lower rates of poor response. So the major results of TRITON-TIMI 38[45] and PLATO,[52] showing lower ischemic event rates, support the hypothesis that targeting higher levels of platelet inhibition reduces recurrent thrombosis.

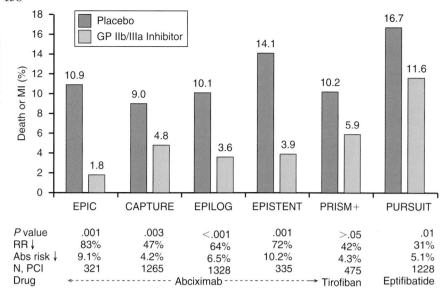

FIGURE 9-4 Intravenous glycoprotein *(GP)* IIb/IIIa inhibitors in patients with non–ST-segment acute coronary syndrome undergoing percutaneous coronary intervention. The outcome of death or myocardial infarction *(MI)* in six clinical trials of intravenous GP IIb/IIIa inhibitors that involve more than 10,000 patients is shown. Abs, absolute; PCI, percutaneous coronary intervention; RR, relative risk. *(From Braunwald E, Antman EM, Beasley JW, et al. ACC/AHA guideline update for the management of patients with unstable angina and non–ST-segment elevation myocardial infarction—2002: summary article: a report of the American College of Cardiology/ American Heart Association Task Force on Practice Guidelines (Committee on the Management of Patients With Unstable Angina). Circulation 2002;106:1893-1900.)*

It is believed that this variable response is due in large part to genetic polymorphisms in cytochrome (CY) P450 enzymes responsible for metabolism of clopidogrel to its active metabolite.[71] Approximately 25% to 30% of Western patients are carriers of at least one reduced-function allele of CYP 2C19. Multiple studies in patients treated with clopidogrel have demonstrated that carriers of one or more reduced-function alleles for this enzyme are associated with increased rates of ischemic events, particularly stent thrombosis.[72-74] Like platelet function testing, some uncertainty remains regarding the clinical role of genetic testing. Prasugrel[75] and ticagrelor[76] have not been demonstrated to have worse outcomes in CYP 2C19 reduced-function carriers. The utility of altering therapy for clinical outcomes is uncertain, however; one study demonstrated that increasing the clopidogrel maintenance dose could in part overcome low platelet response in carriers of one CYP 2C19 reduced-function allele.[68]

Intravenous Platelet Inhibitors

Glycoprotein (GP) IIb/IIIa blockers inhibit the final common pathway of platelet aggregation, namely, the binding of fibrinogen or von Willebrand factor (vWF) to the membrane GP IIb/IIIa integrin receptor. Thus they remain the most potent platelet inhibitors developed to date. Of the three agents commercially available, one is an irreversible monoclonal antibody (abciximab); the other two, eptifibatide and tirofiban, are reversible small-molecule inhibitors. The development of oral GP IIb/IIIa blockers was halted after five consecutive phase III studies demonstrated an associated increase in the mortality rate.[77,78]

Initially introduced as adjuncts to PCI,[79] the intravenous GP IIb/IIIa blockers were also studied in other populations, including patients with ACS managed medically,[80] those about to undergo PCI,[81] and those undergoing primary PCI for STEMI,[82] albeit with mixed results when administered outside the catheterization laboratory. In six large, placebo-controlled trials of patients with NSTE-ACS who were undergoing PCI, the relative risks of death or MI at 30 days were reduced by 31% to 83% with the addition of IV GP IIb/IIIa inhibitors (Figure 9-4).[83] Although a meta-analysis suggested that addition of IV GP IIb/IIIa antagonists to aspirin may reduce mortality rate by one third across a wide range of patients undergoing PCI[84] compared with those receiving single antiplatelet therapy with aspirin, the role for GP IIb/IIIa inhibitors in the era of dual oral antiplatelet inhibition is less clear.

On a background of aspirin (varying dose) and clopidogrel (600 mg), abciximab reduced the composite of death, MI, or urgent target vessel revascularization within 30 days compared with placebo by 25% (*P* = .003) in 2022 patients with NSTE-ACS enrolled

in the Intracoronary Stenting and Antithrombotic Regimen: Rapid Early Action for Coronary Treatment (ISAR-REACT) 2 trial.[85] However, the benefit of abciximab was restricted to those patients with an elevated baseline troponin level (relative risk [RR], 0.71) because those with a normal baseline troponin level demonstrated no benefit (RR, 0.99; *P* interaction = .07). No similar randomized studies have been performed on a background of the more potent oral P2Y$_{12}$ inhibitors that have been recently approved for use.

Two randomized trials[86,87] did not demonstrate a benefit with routine early administration of IV GP IIb/IIIa antagonists prior to PCI compared with delayed provisional use at PCI in patients with NSTE-ACS. In a meta-analysis of these two large trials plus three smaller studies, routine upstream administration before PCI was associated with a 9% reduction in the odds of death or MI at 30 days of borderline statistical significance and no difference in mortality rate (odds ratio [OR], 1.00), at a cost of increases in major bleeding (OR, 1.34) and transfusion (OR, 1.31).[88]

Among patients with NSTE-ACS who are not routinely scheduled to undergo coronary revascularization, a meta-analysis involving 31,402 patients demonstrated a smaller reduction in the odds of death or MI (9%; 95% CI, 0.02 to 0.16; *P* = .015) with addition of IV GP IIb/IIIa inhibitor therapy.[89] However, evidence was found for heterogeneity by drug because the largest trial[80] with abciximab, which does not sustain a high degree of platelet inhibition beyond 12 hours, showed a directionally negative effect, whereas trials with the small-molecule intravenous GP IIb/IIIa blockers revealed modest benefits. Furthermore, post-hoc analyses demonstrated greater benefit among patients at higher risk at baseline, as identified by an elevated baseline troponin level[89] or higher TIMI risk score.[90]

More recently, among 2022 patients with NSTE-ACS undergoing PCI, all of whom were preloaded with 600 mg of clopidogrel at least 2 hours before, the GP IIb/IIIa inhibitor abciximab reduced ischemic complications by 25% in the ISAR-REACT 2 trial.[85] However, the benefit was seen only in patients with an elevated troponin level at baseline. An excess of thrombocytopenia was observed, but no difference in clinically important bleeding was seen among patients treated with abciximab.

Two other potent IV platelet inhibitors, cangrelor and elinogrel, are in late stages of clinical testing. Cangrelor is an IV inhibitor of the P2Y$_{12}$ receptor with a rapid action and quick onset and offset. It is more potent than clopidogrel, achieving 90% inhibition of platelet aggregation within minutes of administration of an IV infusion between 1 and 4 µg/kg/min.[91] In the Cangrelor Versus Standard Therapy to Achieve Optimal Management of Platelet Inhibition (CHAMPION) PLATFORM[92] and CHAMPION-PCI[93] trials conducted in patients undergoing PCI, the majority of whom had ACS, no

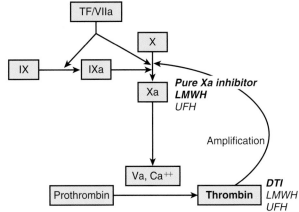

FIGURE 9-5 Activation of the coagulation cascade and platelet aggregation in patients with acute coronary syndromes. After disruption of a vulnerable plaque, tissue factor *(TF)* is exposed, complexes with factor VIIa, and initiates the coagulation cascade. Factor X is activated and leads to the production of thrombin through its interaction with the prothrombinase complex (factor Va, factor Xa, calcium ion [*Ca++*]) on the membrane of activated platelets. Platelets may be activated via a number of pathways: two of the more potent agonists are thrombin and adenosine 5′-diphosphate. The final common step to platelet activation is fibrinogen binding, which mediates platelet-platelet interaction. Unfractionated heparin *(UFH)* inhibits factor Xa and thrombin to a similar degree, and low-molecular-weight heparin *(LMWH)* exerts a proportionally greater effect on factor Xa; direct thrombin inhibitors *(DTIs)* act predominantly on thrombin. Boldface indicates a qualitatively greater effect. *(Modified from Antman EM. The search for replacements for unfractionated heparin. Circulation 2001;103:2310-2314.)*

statistically significant reduction was noted in the primary composite endpoint of death, MI, or ischemia-driven revascularization (OR, 0.97; *P* = .68) in a pooled analysis. However, secondary composite endpoints that included new Q-wave MI and stent thrombosis showed large, statistically significant benefits of 39% to 45%. An ongoing study, a Clinical Trial Comparing Cangrelor to Clopidogrel Standard of Care Therapy in Subjects who Require Percutaneous Coronary Intervention (CHAMPION-PHOENIX), is evaluating cangrelor in more than 10,000 patients with stable and unstable ACS undergoing PCI who are thienopyridine naïve; it is expected to complete in late 2012.

Elinogrel is a reversible competitive P2Y$_{12}$ receptor antagonist that is direct acting and available for both IV and oral administration. It achieves immediate and near-maximal platelet inhibition intravenously and has a half-life of 12 hours. It has been studied in a pilot trial in patients undergoing primary PCI for STEMI[94] and in patients undergoing nonurgent PCI,[95] but large studies in patients with ACS are pending.

Conclusions

The current role of IV GP IIb/IIIa blockers in patients with NSTE-ACS is more restricted in the 2011 guidelines (Box 9-2),[2] with the strongest support as an adjunct in high-risk patients undergoing PCI or to manage thrombotic complications during PCI.[1] A policy of routine early "upstream" administration of GP IIb/IIIa blockers is of marginal benefit, if any, and is associated with more bleeding and transfusion. Newer, potent IV inhibitors of the P2Y$_{12}$ receptor are being developed.

Anticoagulants

Beginning with the expression of tissue factor and ending with the production of thrombin, the biologic complexity of the coagulation cascade has yielded a number of promising targets for anticoagulation therapy (Figure 9-5).[96] Agents that inhibit the earlier portion of the cascade—tissue factor (TF) antibodies, TF/factor VIIa complex inhibitors, factor Xa inhibitors—are potent inhibitors of thrombin generation, whereas those that target more distally, such as direct thrombin inhibitors (DTIs), derive most of their pharmacologic effect by inhibiting preexisting thrombin and are important inhibitors of the contact pathway (Table 9-2). Because of biologic redundancies and multiple feedback loops in the coagulation system, inhibition at one level of the cascade can have complex effects that make it difficult to predict the clinical response to these drugs.

Unfractionated heparin (UFH) had been the standard anticoagulant for decades, although extensive study over the past 2 decades with low-molecular-weight heparins (LMWHs), DTIs, and inhibitors of factor Xa are leading to updates of practice guidelines (see Chapter 8).[2,25]

Unfractionated Heparin and Low-Molecular-Weight Heparin

The optimal dose of unfractionated heparin (UFH) has not been rigorously established; however, several studies support a lower, weight-based dosing regimen to improve the safety profile without apparent loss of efficacy (Table 9-3).[6] In the ISAR-REACT 3A trial,[97] patients with symptoms of unstable angina and negative initial biomarkers were randomized to a lower, single bolus of UFH (100 U/kg) and compared with the standard UFH bolus used in Germany (140 U/kg). All patients received aspirin and clopidogrel prior to PCI. In these low-risk patients, the lower dose UFH was found to be very similar to higher dose heparin in suppressing ischemia and reducing bleeding. Even lower doses of UFH (e.g., 30 to 60 U/kg), particularly in combination with GP IIb/IIIa inhibitors, have been proposed and tested in small studies.[98] Nevertheless, the presence of a number of limitations of UFH (Table 9-4) have led to the search for a replacement anticoagulant.[96]

Unlike UFH, the LMWHs have a number of other advantages that include less nonspecific binding to proteins and platelets, less

TABLE 9-2   Pharmacokinetic and Pharmacodynamics of Five Novel Oral Anticoagulants

	DABIGATRAN (PRADAXA)	RIVAROXABAN (XARELTO)	APIXABAN (ELIQUIS)	EDOXABAN (LIXIANA)	BETRIXABAN (PRT054021)
Target	IIa (thrombin)	Xa	Xa	Xa	Xa
Hours to C_{max}	2	2-4	1-3	1-2	NR
CYP metabolism	None	32%	15%	<4%	None
Bioavailability	7%	80%	66%	>45%	34%-47%
Transporters	P-gp	P-gp/BCRP	P-gp	P-gp	P-gp
Protein binding	35%	>90%	87%	55%	NR
Half-life	12-14 h	9-13 h	8-15 h	8-10 h	19-20 h
Renal elimination	80%	66%*	25%	35%	<5%
Linear PK	Yes	No	Yes	Yes	Yes

BCRP, breast cancer resistance protein; CYP, cytochrome P450; NR, not reported; P-gp, P-glycoprotein; PK, pharmacokinetics.
*33% unchanged, 33% inactive metabolite.
Modified from Ruff CR, Giugliano RP. New oral antithrombotic strategies. *Hot Topics in Cardiology* 2010;4:7-14; Ericksson BI, Quinlan DJ, Weitz JI. Comparative pharmacodynamics and pharmacokinetics of oral direct thrombin and factor Xa inhibitors in development. *Clin Pharmacokinet* 2009;48:1-22; and Ruff CR, Giugliano RP, Antman EM, et al. Evaluation of the novel factor Xa inhibitor edoxaban compared with warfarin in patients with atrial fibrillation: design and rationale for the Effective aNticoaGulation with factor xA next GEneration in Atrial Fibrillation–Thrombolysis In Myocardial Infarction study 48 (ENGAGE AF-TIMI 48). *Am Heart J* 2010;160:635-641.

TABLE 9-3   Dosing of Antithrombotic Agents in Patients with Non–ST-Segment Elevation ACS

	INITIAL MEDICAL THERAPY	During PCI		POST PCI
		IF RECEIVED PRIOR TO PCI	NO PRE-PCI THERAPY	
Bivalirudin	Bolus: 0.1 mg/kg IV Inf: 0.25 mg/kg/h	Bolus: 0.5 mg/kg IV Inf: 1.75 mg/kg/h	Bolus: 0.75 mg/kg IV Inf: 1.75 mg/kg/h	None or continue for up to 4 h
Dalteparin	120 IU/kg SC q12h*	Add UFH to target ACT; dose depends on use of GP IIb/IIIa and device‖	Add UFH; dose depends on use of GP IIb/IIIa**	None
Enoxaparin	Bolus (optional): 30 U IV 1 mg/kg SC q12h†	Last SC dose <8 h: none Last SC dose >8 h: 0.3 mg/kg IV	0.5-0.75 mg/kg IV	None
Fondaparinux	2.5 mg SC q24h	Add UFH: 50-60 U/kg	Add UFH: 50-60 U/kg	None
UFH	Bolus: 60 U/kg‡ Inf: 12 U/kg/h¶	Target ACT depending on use of GP IIb/IIIa§	Dose depends on use of GP IIb/IIIa**	None
Rivaroxaban	2.5 mg PO twice daily	Not applicable	Not applicable	2.5 mg PO q12h

*10,000 IU maximum.
†q24h dosing if creatinine clearance <30 mL/min.
‡4000 U maximum.
¶1000 U/h maximum initial infusion, thereafter titrated to aPTT 1.5 to 2.5 times control.
§If GP IIb/IIIa inhibitor: target ACT 200 sec. If no GP IIb/IIIa inhibitor, target ACT 250-300 sec for HemoTec, 300-350 sec for Hemochron.
‖If GP IIb/IIIa inhibitor: target ACT 200 sec using UFH. If no GP IIb/IIIa inhibitor, target ACT 250-300 sec for HemoTec, 300-350 sec for Hemochron.
**If GP IIb/IIIa inhibitor: UFH 60-70 U/kg. If no GP IIb/IIIa inhibitor, UFH 100-140 U/kg.
ACS, acute coronary syndrome; ACT, activated clotting time; aPTT, activated partial thromboplastin time; GP, glycoprotein; Inf., infusion; IV, intravenous; PCI, percutaneous coronary intervention; PO, oral; UFH, unfractionated heparin; SC, subcutaneous.
Modified from Anderson JL, Adams CD, Antman EM, et al. 2011 ACCF/AHA focused update incorporated into the ACC/AHA 2007 guidelines for the management of patients with unstable angina/non–ST-elevation myocardial infarction: a report of the American College of Cardiology Foundation/American Heart Association Task Force on Practice Guidelines. *Circulation* 2011;123:e426-e579.

depletion of TF pathway inhibitor, and greater inhibition of vWF. Furthermore, the better bioavailability and longer half-life permits subcutaneous dosing, thereby improving the ease of administration both in and out of the hospital (see Table 9-4). Although more than a dozen different LMWH preparations have been developed, only two—enoxaparin and dalteparin—have been widely studied in patients with ACS.[99] Enoxaparin has a lower molecular weight (4200 vs. 6000 Da), slightly higher anti-Xa/anti-IIa ratio (3.8:1 vs. 2.7:1), and greater inhibition of vWF compared with dalteparin. Both drugs are administered subcutaneously in a weight-based fashion in their maintenance dosing, whereas an IV bolus dose of 30 mg enoxaparin has also been studied in NSTE-ACS and as an adjunct to fibrinolysis in STEMI (see Table 9-3).[100] In the only randomized clinical trial that compared two LMWHs head to head, enoxaparin was more efficacious than tinzaparin.[101]

A meta-analysis of four trials composed of 999 patients demonstrated a large reduction (5.5% to 2.6%; P = .018) in death or MI

with the addition of UFH to aspirin compared with aspirin monotherapy.[83] Similarly, the Fragmin During Instability in Coronary Artery Disease (FRISC) trial demonstrated a 63% reduction in death or MI at 7 days with dalteparin plus aspirin compared with aspirin monotherapy (4.8% vs. 1.8%; P = .001).[102]

Several randomized trials have compared LMWH with UFH on a background of aspirin.[83] Dalteparin and fraxiparin did not improve outcomes compared with UFH in the Fragmin in Unstable Coronary Artery Disease (FRIC)[103] and Fraxaparin in Ischaemic Syndrome (FRAX.I.S)[104] trials, respectively. However, several trials comparing enoxaparin with UFH have demonstrated either superiority of enoxaparin or, at worst, noninferiority compared to UFH with regard to prevention of ischemic complications. In a meta-analysis of six trials in more than 22,000 patients conducted over the past 15 years, enoxaparin was associated with a 9% reduction in the rate of death or MI with no increase in the rates of major bleeding or transfusions (Figure 9-6).[105] This robust dataset with

TABLE 9-4 Limitations of UFH and Comparison with Other Anticoagulants

PROPERTIES OF UFH	PHARMACOLOGIC CONSEQUENCES	CLINICAL CONSEQUENCES	Comparator Anticoagulants		
			LMWH	DTI	FXA INHIBITOR
Thrombin-Dependent Properties					
Nonspecific protein binding	Less drug binding to thrombin	Variable anticoagulation levels; requires frequent monitoring	+	0	0
		Sensitivity to inactivation by PF4 and histidine-rich glycoprotein	+	0	0
Depletion of TFPI	↓ Attenuation of TF/factor VIIa complex	Rebound hypercoaguability	0	++	0
Relative inability to inhibit fibrin-bound thrombin	Thrombin generation after clot lysis at therapeutic levels	Rebound thrombosis during and after therapy	++	0	?
Requires co-factor (AT III) to optimally bind thrombin	↓ Thrombin-inhibition if AT III not available	Cannot be used in patients with AT III deficiency	0	0	++
Thrombin-Independent Properties					
↑ Binding to platelets	Immunogenicity	↑ Potential for bleeding, HITTS, or thrombosis	+	0	0
	↑ Platelet activation/adhesion		+	0	0
Inability to blunt the increase in vWF levels	↑ vWF levels	↑ Potential for thrombosis	0	+	?
Primarily excreted renally	↓ Drug clearance, ↑ blood levels with renal insufficiency	↑ Potential for bleeding in renal insufficiency	++	*	*

*Dependent on the specific drug.
AT, antithrombin; DTI, direct thrombin inhibitor; LMWH, low-molecular-weight heparin; UFH, unfractionated heparin; HITTS, heparin-induced thrombosis-thrombocytopenia syndrome; PF4, platelet factor IV; TF, tissue factor; TFPI, tissue factor pathway inhibitor; vWF, von Willebrand factor; ↑, increased; ↓, decreased.
Modified from Antman EM. The search for replacements for unfractionated heparin. *Circulation* 2001;103:2310-2314.

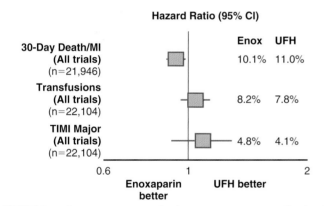

FIGURE 9-6 Systematic overview of trials comparing enoxaparin *(Enox)* with unfractionated heparin *(UFH)* in non–ST-segment acute coronary sydrome (NSTE-ACS). Enoxaparin reduced the rate of death or new myocardial infarction *(MI)* at 30 days by 0.9% (9% relative risk reduction) in an analysis of six trials in 21,946 patients with NSTE-ACS. No statistical difference was found between the treatments in the rates of transfusion or major bleeding. CI, confidence interval; TIMI, Thrombolysis in Myocardial Infarction.

enoxaparin has led to both major guidelines endorsing enoxaparin as a class I recommendation in patients with NSTE-ACS, whether managed conservatively or with plans for early angiography.[2,106]

In the Superior Yield of the new Strategy of Enoxaparin, Revasculization and Glycoprotein IIb/IIIa Inibitors (SYNERGY) trial comparing UFH with enoxaparin, patients who received an antithrombin before randomization experienced higher absolute rates of bleeding after randomization.[107] This finding was confirmed in the Stack-on to Enoxaparin (STACKENOX) trial[108] in which a 70 U/kg bolus of UFH 4 to 10 hours after the last dose of enoxaparin (1 mg/kg) resulted in excess peri- and post-PCI bleeding in the setting of supratherapeutic anti-Xa and anti-IIa levels. Furthermore, inhibition of thrombin generation was complete despite an activated clotting time less than 270 seconds. Thus, the practice of switching between antithrombins in the same patient in the course of a single hospitalization should be avoided whenever possible.

Given similar or slightly better efficacy with enoxaparin compared with UFH in patients and other practical conveniences—twice-daily subcutaneous injections, absence of the need for routine monitoring, and simple weight-based dosing—the use of enoxaparin should generally be preferred over UFH in most patients with NSTE-ACS (class IIa recommendation).[2]

Direct Thrombin Inhibitors

Three parenteral DTIs—hirudin, bivalirudin, and argatroban—are currently available for clinical use in the United States.[109-111] They are termed *direct* because they do not require a cofactor, as do the heparins, and they directly inhibit existing thrombin but have minimal effects on the proximal portions of the coagulation cascade (see Figure 9-5).

A meta-analysis[112] of five trials involving 20,570 patients with NSTE-ACS randomized to a DTI versus UFH concluded that DTI reduced death or MI by 20% (OR, 0.80; 95% CI, 0.70 to 0.92) from 4.6% to 3.7% with similar effects on death (OR, 0.82) and MI (OR, 0.78) individually. DTIs were associated with a near doubling in the rate of major bleeding (1.0% vs. 0.5%; OR, 1.79; 95% CI, 1.29 to 2.50); however, heterogeneity in the applied definitions and observed results, both among different agents and across studies with the same agent, limits the precision of this estimate. In addition, the reductions in ischemic events were inconsistent across different DTIs, with no evidence of benefit with monovalent agents (inogatran, effegatran). Thus, in patients with a history of heparin-induced thrombocytopenia (HIT) or heparin-induced thrombocytopenia and thrombosis syndrome (HITTS), hirudin, argatroban, and bivalirudin are reasonable alternatives to LMWHs and UFH.

More contemporary data are now available on the use of DTIs in patients who are treated with more modern adjuncts that include the thienopyridines, IV GP IIb/IIIa inhibitors, and drug-eluting stents. In the Randomized Evaluation in PCI Linking Angiomax to Reduced Clinical Events (REPLACE-2) trial of 6010 patients who were undergoing urgent or elective PCI, bivalirudin (with provisional use of an IV GP IIb/IIIa blocker in 7% of patients) was not inferior to the combination of UFH and an IV GP IIb/IIIa blocker, as assessed by the quadruple composite endpoint of

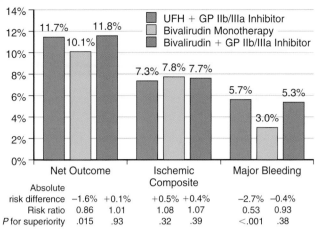

FIGURE 9-7 Major findings at 30 days in the Acute Catheterization and Urgent Intervention Triage Strategy (ACUITY) trial. In this trial, 13,819 patients were randomized to either bivalirudin monotherapy, bivalirudin plus a glycoprotein (GP) IIb/IIIa inhibitor, or heparin (unfractionated heparin [UFH] or enoxaparin) plus a GP IIb/IIIa inhibitor. Bivalirudin reduced the net clinical outcome (composite ischemia or major bleeding) compared with either arm with a GP IIb/IIIa inhibitor, a difference primarily driven by the reduction in ACUITY major bleeding. No difference was found in the composite ischemic endpoint among the three groups. (From Stone GW, McLaurin BT, Cox DA, et al. Bivalirudin for patients with acute coronary syndromes. N Engl J Med 2006;355:2203-2216.)

death, MI, urgent target vessel revascularization, and major bleeding.[113] No differences emerged in long-term efficacy relative to death, MI, or repeat revascularization.

The Acute Catheterization and Urgent Intervention Triage Strategy (ACUITY) trial was a three-arm trial that compared bivalirudin with or without GP IIb/IIIa inhibition with heparin plus GP IIb/IIa inhibition in 13,819 patients with ACS managed with an early invasive strategy.[114] The principal finding was that treatment with bivalirudin alone reduced the net clinical composite endpoint—death, reinfarction, unplanned revascularization for ischemia, major bleeding—at 30 days compared with either arm that included a GP IIb/IIIa blocker, although the results were primarily driven by a reduction in bleeding (Figure 9-7). In addition, bivalirudin alone was noninferior (25% boundary) to UFH/enoxaparin plus a GP IIb/IIIa inhibitor for the triple ischemic endpoint of death, reinfarction, and unplanned revascularization for ischemia. The combination of bivalirudin plus a GP IIb/IIIa inhibitor did not appear to offer any additional ischemic benefit and was associated with more bleeding compared with bivalirudin monotherapy. In other analyses from the ACUITY trial, switching to bivalirudin monotherapy, either before[115] or at the time of PCI,[116] was as safe and effective as UFH plus a GP IIb/IIIa blocker.

Results at 1 year were consistent with the 30-day results, and no difference in mortality rate was found among the three groups through 1 year, despite the early reduction in bleeding observed with bivalirudin.[117] An economic analysis concluded that despite higher drug costs associated with bivalirudin-based strategies, the aggregate costs through 30 days were lowest with bivalirudin monotherapy compared with several alternative strategies that included GP IIb/IIIa inhibitors, whether administered routinely early or selectively at the time of PCI, with heparin.[118] If bivalirudin monotherapy is selected, to avoid early stent thrombosis it is important to initiate early and potent oral dual antiplatelet therapy, such as aspirin plus 600 mg clopidogrel or one of the newer, more potent P2Y₁₂ inhibitors.

In ISAR-REACT 3,[119] 4570 patients with stable or unstable angina pretreated with clopidogrel 600 mg at least 2 hours prior to PCI were randomized to bivalirudin or UFH 140 U/kg (no GP IIb/IIIa inhibitors). Similar rates of the net clinical composite, ischemia plus bleeding, occurred (8.3% vs. 8.7%; P = .57). Although fewer

major bleeds occurred with bivalirudin, this was offset by a numeric excess in ischemic complications (5.9% vs. 5.0%). Of note, the dose of UFH used is higher than what is typically used in North America and higher than the dose recommended in current guidelines.[2]

In the ISAR-REACT 4 trial, 1721 patients with NSTEMI were randomized to abciximab plus UFH 70 U/kg or bivalirudin monotherapy.[120] No differences were seen in either the primary (death, large MI, urgent target-vessel revascularization, or major bleeding) or secondary (above minus bleeding) composite endpoints at 30 days between the groups. Major bleeding occurred less frequently with bivalirudin monotherapy (2.6% vs. 4.6%; P = .02).

Oral DTIs have also been developed and could potentially have a role during or after NSTE-ACS.[121] In a dose-ranging trial after MI, ximelagatran was more effective than placebo at reducing ischemic complications, although an excess in asymptomatic elevation of liver function tests was noted with ximelagatran.[122] Furthermore, in larger studies to prevent venothromboembolism and to prevent embolic stroke in atrial fibrillation, rare but serious clinical hepatotoxicity was observed with ximelagatran,[123] and an FDA advisory panel has recommended against its approval.

In summary, use of bivalirudin without a GP IIb/IIIa blocker compared with heparin, either UFH or enoxaparin, reduces bleeding and offers similar to slightly less effective protection against ischemic events. This makes bivalirudin an excellent choice as an anticoagulant in patients undergoing an early invasive approach who are at high risk for bleeding.[2,106]

Factor Xa Inhibitors

Several parenteral[124] pure inhibitors of factor Xa have been developed, and one synthetic parenteral pentasaccharide, fondaparinux,[125] is approved for use in the prevention and treatment of venothromboembolism in the United States. Fondaparinux has also been approved for use in ACS on the basis of the OASIS-5 trial, but notably not in the United States.[126] This study compared fondaparinux 2.5 mg administered once daily subcutaneously (SC) with enoxaparin (1 mg/kg SC q12h) in 20,078 patients with NSTE-ACS. Fondaparinux was not inferior to enoxaparin with respect to the primary efficacy triple composite of death, MI, or recurrent ischemia through 9 days (5.8% vs. 5.7%; HR, 1.01 [0.90 to 1.13]). Fondaparinux was associated with approximately half the number of major bleeding events (2.2% vs. 4.1%; HR, 0.52; P < .001) and 25% fewer transfusions. Fondaparinux achieved significantly lower intensity and less variability of anticoagulation than enoxaparin,[127] although the dosing of enoxaparin—particularly around the time of coronary angiography and PCI, when UFH was added in addition to enoxaparin—may not have been optimal. The mortality rates at 30 days (P = .02) and 6 months (P = .05) were lower with fondaparinux, although the explanation for the mortality reduction is not clear. An economic analysis from OASIS-5 estimated that fondaparinux during hospitalization for NSTE-ACS would save an average of $547 per patient over a 6-month period, and it increased the number of quality-adjusted life years (QALYs) under most scenarios.[128] The European Society of Cardiology (ESC) now endorses fondaparinux as the preferred anticoagulant in patients with NSTE-ACS.[106]

It should be noted that a higher rate of catheter-related thrombosis was seen in OASIS-5[126] as well as in patients undergoing primary PCI for STEMI in OASIS-6,[129] and has limited the acceptance of fondaparinux, particularly among interventionalists. Because fondaparinux does not directly inhibit factor IIa, and is consequently less effective at blocking the contact pathway, the addition of UFH during PCI was studied. A low-dose UFH regimen of 50 U/kg to support PCI in patients treated upstream with fondaparinux 2.5 mg daily was found to be as safe and effective as standard-dose UFH in the Fondaparinux Trial with Unfractionated Heparin During Revascularization in Acute Coronary Syndromes (FUTURA)-OASIS 8 trial.[130] Therefore in patients with NSTE-ACS who are treated with fondaparinux and require PCI, the addition of low-dose UFH is recommended to reduce the risk of catheter-related thrombosis.

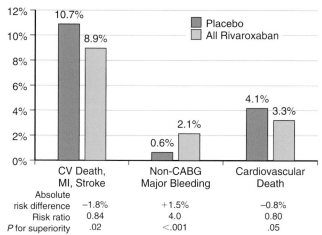

FIGURE 9-8 Primary efficacy and safety outcomes in Anti-Xa Therapy to Lower Cardiovascular Events in Addition to Standard Therapy in Subjects with Acute Coronary Syndromes (ATLAS-ACS) Thrombolysis in Myocardial Infarction (TIMI) 51. Rivaroxaban (2.5 mg and 5.0 mg twice daily, dose groups pooled) reduced the primary efficacy composite of cardiovascular *(CV)* death, myocardial infarction *(MI)*, or stroke by 1.8% absolute compared with placebo in the intention-to-treat analysis in 15,526 patients after acute coronary syndrome. A 1.5% absolute increase was seen in non–coronary artery bypass graft *(CABG)* Thrombolysis in Myocardial Infarction major bleeding, but CV mortality rate was reduced by 0.8% with rivaroxaban. *(From Mega JL, Braunwald E, Wiviott SD, et al. Rivaroxaban in patients with a recent acute coronary syndrome. N Engl J Med 2012;366:9-19.)*

TABLE 9-5	Anticoagulant Recommendations in the 2011 ACCF/AHA and ESC Practice Guidelines		
	ACCF/AHA	**ESC**	**COMMENTS**
UFH	IA	IC	ACCF/AHA: Enoxaparin or fondaparinux preferred if conservative management (IIaB) ESC: Only if fondaparinux and enoxaparin are not available
Enoxaparin	IA	IB	ESC: If fondaparinux is not available
Bivalirudin	IB	IB	Only if an early invasive approach
Fondaparinux	IB	IA	ACCF/AHA: Preferable if increased bleeding risk and conservative management ESC: Favors as first line

Recommendations are shown as the grade of recommendation (I, IIa, IIb, or III), and the level of evidence (A, B, or C).
ACCF, American College of Cardiology Foundation; AHA, American Heart Association; ESC, European Society of Cardiology.

From Anderson JL, Adams CD, Antman EM, et al. 2011 ACCF/AHA focused update incorporated into the ACC/AHA 2007 guidelines for the management of patients with unstable angina/non–ST-elevation myocardial infarction: a report of the American College of Cardiology Foundation/American Heart Association Task Force on Practice Guidelines. *Circulation* 2011;123:e426-e579; and Hamm CW, Bassand JP, Agewall S, et al. ESC guidelines for the management of acute coronary syndromes in patients presenting without persistent ST-segment elevation: the Task Force for the Management of Acute Coronary Syndromes (ACS) in Patients Presenting without Persistent ST-Segment Elevation. European Society of Cardiology (ESC). *Eur Heart J* 2011;32:2999-3054.

A second parenteral and direct factor Xa inhibitor, otamixaban, that does not appear to increase catheter-related thrombosis is in late stage development.[131] In the Otamixaban for the Treatment of Patients with Non–ST-Elevation Acute Coronary Syndromes (SEPIA-ACS1-TIMI) 42 trial, IV infusions of otamixaban of 0.105 and 0.140 mg/kg/h reduced ischemic complications and had a similar bleeding profile to UFH plus eptifibatide. The Randomized, Double-Blind, Triple-Dummy Trial to Compare the Efficacy of Otamixaban with UFH Plus Eptifibatide in Patients with Unstable Angina/NSTEMI Scheduled to Undergo an Early Invasive Strategy (TAO), a large phase III trial with otamixaban in patients with NSTE-ACS, is well under way.

A number of oral factor Xa inhibitors have been developed (see Table 9-2), and two have been studied in large phase III trials. Apixiban (5 mg twice daily) was investigated in the Apixaban for Prevention of Acute Ischemic Events (APPRAISE)-2 trial in combination with aspirin plus clopidogrel.[132] The trial was prematurely terminated by an independent data safety monitoring board because of an unacceptably high rate of bleeding without demonstration of efficacy. Meanwhile, in the Anti-Xa Therapy to Lower Cardiovascular Events in Addition to Standard Therapy in Subjects with Acute Coronary Syndrome–Thrombolysis in MI (ATLAS AC2-TIMI) 51 trial, low doses of rivaroxaban (2.5 mg bid and 5.0 mg bid, which are 25% and 50% of the approved dose, respectively, for patients with atrial fibrillation) reduced the primary composite of death, MI, or stroke by 16% (8.9% and 10.7%, respectively; *P* = .008) compared with standard antiplatelet therapy alone without an anticoagulant in 15,527 patients following ACS (Figure 9-8).[133] In addition, substantial reductions were also noted in the overall mortality and stent thrombosis rates with rivaroxaban, although an excess of bleeding, including intracranial bleeding, was observed.

Other Anticoagulants

Drugs with proximal targets in the coagulation cascade, such as TF antibodies,[134] TF pathway inhibitors,[135] TF/factor VIIa complex inhibitors,[136] and factor XIIa inhibitors,[137] are in earlier stages of clinical development. A monoclonal antibody to the TF/factor VIIa complex derived from the hookworm, rNAPc2, was studied in 253 patients with NSTE-ACS and effectively suppressed new thrombin generation as determined by serial assessment of prothrombin

factor F1.2.[136] In addition, higher doses of rNAPc2 reduced ischemia on continuous electrocardiographic (ECG) monitoring over the first week after NSTE-ACS. However, similar to fondaparinux, some heparin appears necessary in addition to rNAPc2 to inhibit thrombus formation on catheters and other foreign materials during instrumentation in the catheterization laboratory.

A reversible, direct factor IXa inhibitor, the RNA aptamer RB006, and its matching aptamer pair reversal agent, RB007, were studied in patients undergoing PCI and were found to be simple to use, safe, and effective.[138] A factor XIIa inhibitor, recombinant human albumin infestin-4, prolonged the activated partial thromboplastin time (aPTT) in vitro with human plasma and abolished occlusive arterial thrombus in animal models.[137] Of note, the factor XII–induced coagulation pathway is essential for pathologic thrombus formation but is dispensable for hemostasis. Because of the complexity and biologic redundancy of the coagulation system, it is difficult to predict from ex vivo mechanistic studies which, if any, of these strategies will be most useful in clinical practice, although clinical studies are ongoing with several of these compounds.

Summary on Anticoagulant Selection

Data from randomized clinical trials support drugs from each of the four major anticoagulant classes—UFHs, LMWHs, DTIs, and factor Xa inhibitors—in patients with NSTE-ACS. Because of important differences in pharmacokinetic and pharmacodynamic effects, which have translated to clinically important differences in randomized studies, the selection of anticoagulant should be made according to the individual patient characteristics and the clinical scenario. The most recent ACC/AHA[2] and ESC[106] guideline recommendations are given in Table 9-5.

Invasive Versus Conservative Strategy for Cardiac Catheterization

In addition to the pharmacologic measures used to treat patients with UA/NSTEMI, one of the most important decisions during hospitalization is the early strategy of care regarding coronary angiography and resultant revascularization. The goals of coronary

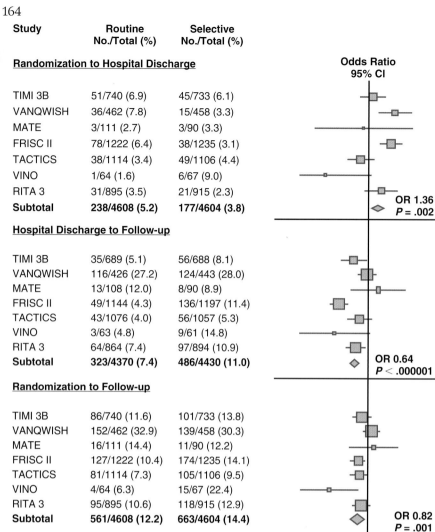

Study	Routine No./Total (%)	Selective No./Total (%)
Randomization to Hospital Discharge		
TIMI 3B	51/740 (6.9)	45/733 (6.1)
VANQWISH	36/462 (7.8)	15/458 (3.3)
MATE	3/111 (2.7)	3/90 (3.3)
FRISC II	78/1222 (6.4)	38/1235 (3.1)
TACTICS	38/1114 (3.4)	49/1106 (4.4)
VINO	1/64 (1.6)	6/67 (9.0)
RITA 3	31/895 (3.5)	21/915 (2.3)
Subtotal	**238/4608 (5.2)**	**177/4604 (3.8)**
Hospital Discharge to Follow-up		
TIMI 3B	35/689 (5.1)	56/688 (8.1)
VANQWISH	116/426 (27.2)	124/443 (28.0)
MATE	13/108 (12.0)	8/90 (8.9)
FRISC II	49/1144 (4.3)	136/1197 (11.4)
TACTICS	43/1076 (4.0)	56/1057 (5.3)
VINO	3/63 (4.8)	9/61 (14.8)
RITA 3	64/864 (7.4)	97/894 (10.9)
Subtotal	**323/4370 (7.4)**	**486/4430 (11.0)**
Randomization to Follow-up		
TIMI 3B	86/740 (11.6)	101/733 (13.8)
VANQWISH	152/462 (32.9)	139/458 (30.3)
MATE	16/111 (14.4)	11/90 (12.2)
FRISC II	127/1222 (10.4)	174/1235 (14.1)
TACTICS	81/1114 (7.3)	105/1106 (9.5)
VINO	4/64 (6.3)	15/67 (22.4)
RITA 3	95/895 (10.6)	118/915 (12.9)
Subtotal	**561/4608 (12.2)**	**663/4604 (14.4)**

Odds Ratio
95% CI

OR 1.36
P = .002

OR 0.64
P < .000001

OR 0.82
P = .001

0.1 0.2 0.5 1 2 5 10
Favors routine — Favors selective

FIGURE 9-9 Composite of death or myocardial infarction (MI) in the hospital, after discharge, and overall in trials of routine (early invasive) versus selective (early conservative) management of acute coronary syndrome. Tests for heterogeneity: death or MI from randomization to hospital discharge, P = .001; death or MI after hospital discharge to follow-up, P = .001; death or MI from randomization to follow-up, P = .06. Random effects model results: death or MI from randomization to hospital discharge, relative risk (RR), 1.31; 95% confidence interval (CI), 0.85 to 2.01. Death or MI after hospital discharge to follow-up: RR, 0.65; 95% CI, 0.46 to 0.91. Death or MI from randomization to follow-up: RR, 0.82; 95% CI, 0.68 to 0.99. OR, odds ratio. *(From Kastrati A, Neumann FJ, Mehilli J, et al. Bivalirudin versus unfractionated heparin during percutaneous coronary intervention. N Engl J Med 2008;359:688-696.)*

angiography are to provide information about prognosis based on location and extent of coronary atherosclerosis and to identify patients who will derive clinical benefit from revascularization, either percutaneous or surgical. An early conservative strategy refers to medical management of patients, reserving the use of coronary angiography and revascularization for evidence of recurrent ischemia at rest, or with minimal activity, or a strongly positive predischarge stress test. An early invasive strategy refers to the routine recommendation for coronary angiography and revascularization (within 12 to 48 hours of presentation) in patients without contraindications.

Several clinical trials have been performed to evaluate which strategy is superior in the treatment of patients with UA/NSTEMI. Early trials such as TIMI 3B[139] and Veterans Affairs Non–Q-Wave Infarct Strategies in Hospital (VANQWISH)[140] study showed similar clinical outcomes regardless of treatment strategy. However, subsequent trials that used more modern antiplatelet, antithrombotic, and catheterization techniques—including FRISC II[141] and Treat Angina with Aggrastat and Determine Cost of Therapy with an Invasive or Conservative Strategy (TACTICS)-TIMI[18,142]—have shown a significant benefit from pursuing an early invasive strategy, especially in patients who have indicators of high risk.

To reconcile the differences in clinical trials of invasive versus conservative strategies, three meta-analyses were performed. Each of the three meta-analyses[143-145] demonstrated a benefit for an early invasive strategy compared with an early conservative strategy. A meta-analysis by Mehta and colleagues[143] that included TIMI 3B, VANQWISH, FRISC II, TACTICS, and others concluded that a routine invasive strategy was associated with a significant reduction in death or MI, a nonsignificant trend toward fewer deaths, and a significant relative reduction in MI alone through the end of follow-up, with an early increase in events outweighed by a later reduction (Figure 9-9). A meta-regression analysis[144] showed that the most significant predictors of the benefits of an early invasive strategy were the use of aggressive antiplatelet treatment, defined as use of an intravenous GP IIb/IIIa blocker or thienopyridine in addition to aspirin, and intracoronary stenting in the early invasive group, a conclusion supported by a direct comparison of two trials performed before (TIMI 3B) and after (TACTICS-TIMI)[18] these agents were routinely available.[146] Controversy has arisen over the relative benefit of an invasive versus conservative strategy in women in particular. A meta-analysis directly examined this question and demonstrated a similar, 19% reduction in CV events in favor of invasive therapy in women and 27% in men.[147] Of particular interest, women who had elevated cardiac biomarkers had a significant 33% reduction in CV events.

One study stands in contrast to the data that favor an early invasive strategy. In the Invasive Versus Conservative Treatment in

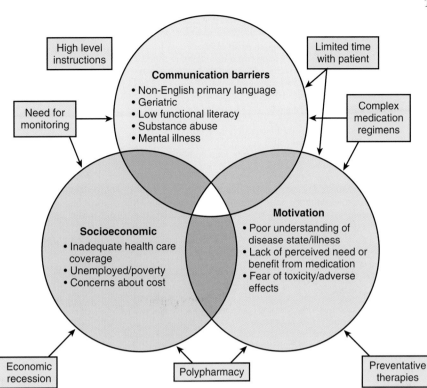

FIGURE 9-10 Barriers to patient compliance with medications. Major challenges that reduce patient compliance with the prescribed medical regimen include communication barriers, socioeconomic issues, and lack of patient motivation. *(From Baroletti S, Dell'Orfano H. Medication adherence in cardiovascular disease.* Circulation *2010;121:1455-1458.)*

NON–ST-SEGMENT ELEVATION ACUTE CORONARY SYNDROMES

Unstable Coronary Syndromes (ICTUS) trial of 1200 patients with NSTE-ACS, an elevated troponin T level, and either ischemic ECG changes or a documented history of CAD, randomization to an early invasive versus a selective invasive strategy found similar rates of death, MI, and rehospitalization for ACS at 1 year.[148] Potential explanations for the lack of benefit with an early invasive approach include the high rate of catheterization and revascularization in the conservative arm and a relatively short follow-up period compared with other studies.[149]

In summary, the majority of data suggest a benefit for patients with NSTE-ACS who are treated with an early invasive strategy. This benefit appears to be particularly strong in patients with high-risk indicators, with the strongest benefit for those with ST-segment deviation and elevated cardiac troponins. It should be noted, however, that patients treated conservatively should be managed invasively if they develop high-risk indicators or have a strongly positive stress test prior to discharge. Once an invasive strategy is undertaken, the decision for revascularization is based on the results of coronary angiography and is similar to the indications for revascularization in patients with chronic stable angina,[150] with a stronger indication for some form of revascularization because of the severity of initial symptoms.

Hospital Discharge and Postdischarge Care

After the initial stabilization of an episode of NSTE-ACS with medical therapy and/or revascularization, patients remain at increased risk for major CV events for at least 1 to 3 months before reverting to a risk profile that approximates that of patients with chronic stable CAD. Thus, institution of an effective comprehensive discharge plan is crucial to prevent early recurrent ischemic events. Critical pathways, discharge tools, and participation in quality improvement initiatives[151] are useful to increase adherence with treatment guidelines and have been associated with improved clinical outcomes.[152,153]

Unfortunately, optimal therapy is the exception rather than the rule, as was seen in a Canadian registry that concluded only 23% of patients received the guideline-recommended therapies after NSTE-ACS.[154] Even when secondary preventive medications were provided free of charge in the Myocardial Infarction Free Rx Event and Economic Evaluation (MI-FREE) trial, only a 4% absolute increase (from 39% to 44%) in complete adherence was seen.[155] Multiple barriers to patient compliance with medications clearly exist (Figure 9-10), and more research is needed to better understand the root causes and to provide more effective solutions. Patients with NSTE-ACS who have no or only low-level troponin elevation,[156] renal insufficiency,[157] or multiple comorbidities[158] have an increased chance of being suboptimally treated. Promising novel approaches include the application of a systematic, standardized collection of information on drug exposure directly from patients[159] and pharmacist-based interventions targeting patients with low literacy in CV disease.[160] On the way to the ultimate goal of *ideal CV health*, defined as ideal health behaviors and health factors, the AHA has set a target to improve the CV health of all Americans by 20% by 2020, while reducing deaths from CV disease and stroke by 20%.[161]

Most patients can be discharged within 24 hours after a normal or low-risk noninvasive evaluation or within 24 hours after uncomplicated PCI.[2,106] Patients who are managed with CABG and have no major postoperative issues can generally be targeted for discharge to home or to a short-stay rehabilitation facility on the fifth through seventh postoperative days.[2,106] Three important goals in the discharge period include 1) evaluation and patient education regarding NSTE-ACS, the procedures performed, secondary risk-factor reduction, and discharge medications, diet, and exercise; 2) instructions regarding the appropriate level of activity and plans to resume usual activities in the near future; and 3) confirmation of long-term medical follow-up.

A multidisciplinary approach that involves physicians, their assistants, nurses, pharmacists, dietitians, and rehabilitation specialists can help achieve these goals. Gluckman and colleagues[162] developed an "ABCDE" approach (Box 9-3) for the management of NSTE-ACS that provides a practical and systematic means to implement evidence-based medicine, including both medication (Box 9-4) and lifestyle modification (Table 9-6) into clinical practice.

Box 9-3 ABCDE Approach to Postdischarge Care

A: **A**ntiplatelet therapy, **A**nticoagulation, **A**CEI, **A**RB
  ■ Antiplatelets: aspirin ≥75 mg daily, continue indefinitely, and $P2Y_{12}$ inhibitor (clopidogrel, prasugrel, or ticagrelor); duration dependent on management strategy and type of stent placed
  ■ Anticoagulation: atrial fibrillation, LV thrombus, severe wall motion abnormalities
  ■ ACEI: congestive heart failure, LV ejection fraction <40%, hypertension, diabetes (substitute ARB if intolerant to ACEI)
B: **B**-Blockade, **B**lood pressure control
  ■ β-Blockade: all patients without absolute contraindications
  ■ Blood pressure control: goal <130/85 mm Hg using lifestyle modifications and medications as needed
C: **C**holesterol treatment, **C**igarette smoking cessation
  ■ Cholesterol: low–saturated fat (<7% total calories), low-cholesterol (<200 mg/day) diet rich in fish with omega-3 fatty acids or supplemented by omega-3 supplements of 1 g/day, with a goal LDL of less than 100 mg/dL (optional target <70 mg/dL)
  ■ Cigarettes: Ask, advise cessation, avoid secondhand exposure
D: **D**iabetes management, **D**iet
  ■ Diabetes: goal glycosylated hemoglobin <7%, treat other risk factors
  ■ Diet: low in saturated fat and cholesterol, rich in omega-3 fatty fish, fresh vegetables, whole grains; goal body mass index 18.5 to 24.9 kg/m²; routinely measure waist circumference to goal of <40 inches (men) or <35 inches (women)
E: **E**xercise: Ideally 30 minutes or more daily, supplemented by an active lifestyle; refer to cardiac rehabilitation/secondary prevention for patients with multiple risk factors, or if supervised exercise program is required because of high-risk status

ACEI, angiotensin-converting enzyme inhibitor; ARB, angiotensin receptor blocker; LDL, low-density lipoprotein; LV, left ventricular.
Modified from Gluckman TJ, Sachdev M, Schulman SP, Blumenthal RS. A simplified approach to the management of non–ST-segment elevation acute coronary syndromes. *JAMA* 2005;293:349-357.

Box 9-4 Discharge Medications for Patients with NSTE-ACS

1. Aspirin 75 to 325 mg/day or, if intolerant to aspirin (e.g., hypersensitive), clopidogrel 75 mg/day
2. Clopidogrel 75 mg/day, prasugrel 10 mg/day, or ticagrelor 90 mg twice daily or in addition to aspirin for up to 9 months
3. β-Blocker in the absence of absolute contraindications
4. Lipid-lowering agent and diet management in patients with LDL-c >130 mg/dL or LDL-c >100 mg/dL after diet therapy
5. ACEI, or ARB if intolerant to ACEI, for patients with congestive heart failure, left ventricular dysfunction (ejection fraction <40%), hypertension, or diabetes mellitus
6. Sublingual or spray nitroglycerin with instructions on proper use

ACEI, angiotensin-converting enzyme inhibitor; ARB, angiotensin receptor blocker; LDL-c, low-density lipoprotein cholesterol; NSTE-ACS, Non–ST-elevation acute cardiac syndrome.
Modified from Braunwald E, Antman EM, Beasley JW, et al. ACC/AHA 2002 guideline update for the management of patients with unstable angina and non–ST-segment elevation myocardial infarction: a report of the American College of Cardiology/American Heart Association Task Force on Practice Guidelines (Committee on the Management of Patients With Unstable Angina). *Circulation* 2002;106:1893-1900.

Antiplatelet Therapy, Anticoagulation, Angiotensin-Converting Enzyme Inhibitors, and Angiotensin Receptor Blockade

All patients without an absolute contraindication should be discharged on aspirin indefinitely and on a second antiplatelet agent—clopidogrel, prasugrel, or ticagrelor—the duration of which depends on the clinical scenario (see the antiplatelet section above).[2,106] The high cost, and in some areas, the need for prior approval of $P2Y_{12}$ inhibitors, have been barriers to use. For example, in Ontario, Canada, only 35% of patients prescribed clopidogrel after stenting filled the prescription in the first 30 days (on average

TABLE 9-6 Lifestyle Modifications

RISK FACTOR	GOAL/TARGET
Smoking cessation	Complete cessation, avoidance of secondary exposure
Weight control	Body mass index 18.5-24.9 kg/m² ; waist circumference <40 inches (men), <35 inches (women)
Exercise	Daily aerobic exercise for ≥30 minutes, minimum three to four times weekly*
Diet	7% or fewer calories from saturated fat, ≤200 mg/day cholesterol
	Increase fresh vegetables and fruit, fish rich in omega-3 fatty acids, whole grains, soluble fiber
Cholesterol management	LDL-c substantially <100 mg/dL, non–HDL-c substantially <130 mg/dL, triglycerides <200 mg/dL
Blood pressure control	<130/85 mm Hg (<130/80 mm Hg if diabetes or chronic kidney disease), modest sodium restriction
Diabetes management	Glycosylated hemoglobin <7%
Depression/anxiety	Assessment of psychosocial status, appropriate referral for support and/or therapy

Modified from Braunwald E, Antman EM, Beasley JW, et al. ACC/AHA 2002 guideline update for the management of patients with unstable angina and non-ST-segment elevation myocardial infarction: a report of the American College of Cardiology/American Heart Association Task Force on Practice Guidelines (Committee on the Management of Patients With Unstable Angina). 2002. Available at http://www.acc.org/clinical/guidelines/unstable/unstable/pdf.
LDL-c, Low-density lipoprotein cholesterol; HDL-c, High-density lipoprotein cholesterol
*Optimally daily

at day 9 postdischarge), when a prior authorization was required.[163] This improved dramatically to 88% (on average at day 0) when the approval process was rescinded. Both the lack of use of dual antiplatelet therapy[164] and late initiation[165] (seen in 1 in 6 patients in a U.S. analysis) have been associated with adverse outcomes. Indeed, follow-up of the Ontario experience demonstrated a reduction in the adjusted composite rates of death, reinfarction, PCI, and CABG from 15% to 11% ($P = .02$).[163] With generic versions of clopidogrel expected to be available in many countries by 2012, it is hoped that compliance will improve globally.

Oral anticoagulation therapy at discharge is recommended for patients who have atrial fibrillation or LV thrombus, and it is reasonable in patients with LV dysfunction and extensive regional wall motion abnormalities.[2,106] More frequent monitoring of the patient is advised when combining warfarin with antiplatelet therapy. The 2011 focus update of the ACCF/AHA now specifically draws attention to the increased risk of bleeding in patients on warfarin plus dual antiplatelet therapy and suggests that patients and clinicians monitor patients closely for signs and symptoms of bleeding, especially GI bleeding, with a low threshold to seek medical evaluation if bleeding is present.[166] In an attempt to mitigate the risk of bleeding, use of low-dose aspirin (75 to 81 mg/day) in combination with warfarin titrated to an international normalized ratio (INR) of 2.0 to 2.5 appears a preferable alternative to higher doses of both, particularly when a second antiplatelet agent is necessary (e.g., poststenting).

ACE inhibitors should be given and continued indefinitely in patients after NSTE-ACS with CHF, LV ejection fraction less than 40%, hypertension, or diabetes, unless there is a contraindication.[2,106] For patients intolerant of ACE inhibitors, an angiotensin receptor blocker (ARB) may be substituted. Long-term aldosterone receptor blockade is recommended in patients with creatinine clearance greater than 30 mL/min and normal potassium who are already on an ACE inhibitor or ARB and one of the clinical factors listed above applies.[2]

The role for both ACE inhibitiors and ARBs is less clear, although current guidelines note that such a combination may be considered in patients with persistent symptomatic heart failure with LV dysfunction that is refractory to conventional therapy that includes one of these agents.[2]

β-Blockade and Blood Pressure Control

β-Blockers are recommended for all patients in the absence of absolute contraindications (see Antiischemic Medications above).[2,106] The dose should be adjusted as needed to manage angina and blood pressure, with a target blood pressure of less than 130/80 mm Hg. Research indicates that physicians frequently fail to titrate β-blockers to the recommended targets,[167] thus limiting their effectiveness. In patients with moderate or severe LV failure, the dose should be gradually titrated up to avoid worsening of heart failure.[2]

Cholesterol Treatment and Cigarette Smoking Cessation

The primary goal of cholesterol management in patients after ACS should be a target low-density lipoprotein cholesterol (LDL-c) substantially less than 100 mg/dL, with an optimal target of less than 70 mg/dL.[168] Two studies of aggressive lipid lowering demonstrated regression of CAD using intravascular ultrasound following ACS when an LDL below 70 mg/dL was achieved.[169,170] Statins initiated before discharge are preferred as first-line agents to lower LDL-c in patients with an LDL-c less than 100 mg/dL, whereas statins in combination with other lipid-lowering drugs (e.g., ezetimibe 10 mg/day, bile acid sequestrants, or niacin) may be necessary in patients whose LDL-c is above 100 mg/dL. An additional key goal is to reduce the non–high-density lipoprotein (HDL)-c—that is, the total cholesterol minus HDL cholesterol—to substantially less than 130 mg/dL.[171] If the triglycerides are 200 to 499 mg/dL after initiating LDL-c–lowering therapy, then a fibrate or niacin may be added. For patients with higher triglyceride levels (i.e., fasting levels >500 mg/dL), fibrate or niacin should be considered before initiating LDL-c–lowering therapy.

Although physicians have widely embraced the use of lipid-lowering agents early after ACS—89% of patients in the Medications Applied and Sustained over Time (MAINTAIN) registry were discharged on a lipid-lowering drug[172]—the doses are generally too low and do not achieve the more stringent goals recommended for post-ACS patients. For example, data from the Can Rapid Risk Stratification of Unstable Angina Patients Suppress Adverse Outcomes with Early Implementation (CRUSADE) and Acute Coronary Treatment and Intervention Outcomes Network (ACTION) registries showed that only 37% of patients with an LDL-c above 100 mg/dL had an uptitration of the statin dose by the time of discharge, and the vast majority (70%) of all patients were not achieving the more stringent LDL-c target of less than 70 mg/dL.[172] An important step toward achieving these goals is represented by the more frequent use of higher potency regimens (e.g., atorvastatin 40 to 80 mg, rosuvastatin 20 to 40 mg, or combination of a statin plus ezetimibe daily), which were prescribed for only 38% of patients admitted with ACS in an analysis from the Get With the Guidelines CAD registry.[173]

Strong support for intensive statin therapy after ACS is derived from the Pravastatin or Atorvastatin Evaluation and Infection Therapy (PROVE-IT)-TIMI 22 trial,[174] in which 4162 patients hospitalized with ACS were randomized within 10 days to either pravastatin 40 mg or atorvastatin 80 mg daily and followed for a mean of 24 months. Atorvastatin 80 mg reduced the median LDL-c further (62 mg/dL vs. 95 mg/dL; $P < .001$), and 16% of patients experienced major CV events or died over the following 2 years ($P = .005$). Interestingly, the reduction in clinical events became apparent quite early, within 30 days after the initiation of therapy,[175] and reductions were also seen in heart failure independent of reductions in reinfarction.[176] Even patients with baseline LDL-c as low as 66 mg/dL appeared to benefit from intensive statin therapy after ACS.[177]

An important corollary observed in PROVE-IT TIMI 22 was that acute antiinflammatory effects were associated with better clinical outcomes, and such a pleiotropic effect may partially explain the early and non–ischemia-mediated benefits describe above. In a retrospective analysis, patients who achieved a C-reactive protein (CRP) level below 2 mg/L had lower event rates than those who had higher CRP levels, regardless of the LDL-c achieved (Figure 9-11).[178] Prospective confirmation of the relationship between the achievement of the dual goals and improved clinical outcomes is under way in ongoing studies, such as the Improved Reduction of Outcomes: Vitorin Efficacy International Trial (IMPROVE IT),[179] which is comparing the combination of simvastatin plus ezetimibe with simvastatin monotherapy in 18,057 patients stabilized within 10 days after admission for ACS. This study will provide important information on the safety and efficacy of ezetimibe and the utility of reducing LDL even further, to 50 to 55 mg/dL; this is more than had been achieved in prior large, post-ACS studies.

A meta-analysis of 13 trials involving 17,963 patients within 14 days of hospitalization for ACS demonstrated a 16% reduction in the risk of CV events that began within 4 months after initiation of early, intensive statin therapy (Figure 9-12).[180] The mechanism of the early benefit remains to be elucidated; however, a favorable rapid effect on immunomodulation—specifically, reductions in tumor necrosis factor-α and interferon-γ production in stimulated T lymphocytes within 72 hours after treatment with rosuvastatin 20 mg[181]—may partially explain the benefit.

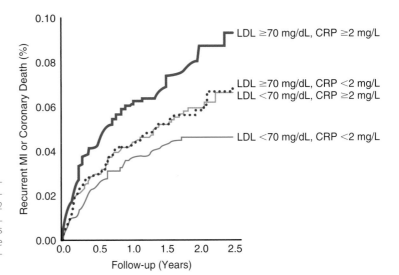

FIGURE 9-11 Achieved low-density lipoprotein *(LDL)* and hs–C-reactive protein *(CRP)* in the Pravastatin or Atorvastatin Evaluation and Infection Therapy (PROVE-IT)-Thrombolysis in Myocardial Infarction (TIMI) 22 trial.[178] The achieved LDL and hs-CRP, stratified at cutpoints of 70 mg/dL and 2 mg/L, respectively, identified four groups of patients. Event rates were highest in the group with "high" LDL and "high" hs-CRP; they were lowest in the group with "low" LDL and "low" hs-CRP; hs, high sensitivity; MI, myocardial infarction.

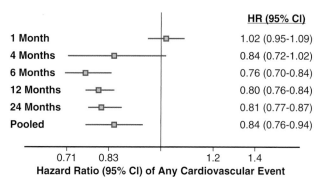

Meta-Analysis of Intensive Statin Therapy in ACS

	HR (95% CI)
1 Month	1.02 (0.95-1.09)
4 Months	0.84 (0.72-1.02)
6 Months	0.76 (0.70-0.84)
12 Months	0.80 (0.76-0.84)
24 Months	0.81 (0.77-0.87)
Pooled	0.84 (0.76-0.94)

Hazard Ratio (95% CI) of Any Cardiovascular Event

FIGURE 9-12 Meta-analysis of early intensive statin therapy in acute coronary sydrome (ACS). By 4 months, the use of an early intensive statin regimen compared with placebo or low-dose statin reduced the risk of overall cardiovascular events in an analysis of 17,963 patients from 13 trials of patients hospitalized within 14 days after an ACS. Estimates to the left of the line of unity favor intensive statin therapy; those to the right favor control. CI, confidence interval; HR, hazard ratio. (*From Giugliano RP, Braunwald E. The year in non–ST-segment elevation acute coronary syndrome. J Am Coll Cardiol 2007;50:1386-1395.*)

The letter C (for cigarettes) in the ABCDE mnemonic also reminds the health care provider to ask the patient about his or her tobacco status. Smoke-free legislation appears to have been successful in reducing hospitalizations for ACS[182]; thus patients and family members should be strongly encouraged to stop. Avoidance of exposure to environmental tobacco smoke at work and home should be urged; even exposure to secondhand smoke can trigger ACS.[183] Practical measures that can be taken by all physicians include assessment of the patient's willingness to quit, counseling and developing a plan for quitting, considering pharmacologic therapy (e.g., nicotine replacement, buproprion), and referral to specialized programs. A stepwise plan known as the *Five A Strategy—Ask, Advise, Assess, Assist,* and *Arrange*—is recommended by the ACCF/AHA.[2]

Diabetes Management and Diet

The goal of diabetes management is a glycosylated hemoglobin level below 7% (further recommendations in patients with diabetes are provided later in this chapter). A diet that limits saturated fats and dietary cholesterol but is rich in omega-3 fatty fish, vegetables, and whole grains is recommended to achieve a goal body mass index (BMI) of 18.5 to 24.9 kg body weight/m^2 height.[83] The waist circumference should be measured as part of the evaluation, and increased values (>40 in for men, >35 in for women) should trigger lifestyle changes and consideration of treatment strategies for metabolic syndrome. On each patient visit, health care providers should consistently encourage weight maintenance or reduction through a balance of physical activity, restriction of calories, and formal behavioral programs as appropriate for the individual patient. The initial goal of weight loss should be a 10% reduction from baseline; once achieved, additional weight loss can be attempted if indicated after further assessment. Unfortunately, adherence to behavioral advice is poor after ACS regarding diet, exercise, and smoking cessation, and fewer than one third of patients comply with all three of the recommendations.[184]

Exercise

All patients ideally should exercise 30 to 60 minutes per day, preferably 7 days per week, but at a minimum of at least 5 days per week. Such activity should be supplemented by an increase in daily lifestyle activities such as walking during work breaks, gardening, and doing household work.[2] Referral to cardiac rehabilitation or secondary prevention programs is recommended for patients with multiple modifiable risk factors and for patients at higher risk for whom a supervised exercise training program is indicated. The low rate (56%) of referral for cardiac rehabilitation seen in a large U.S. survey[185] underscores the need for greater attention to this class I recommendation.[2]

Influenza Vaccine

Modification of the mnemonic above to include an "F" for "flu" (influenza) vaccine allows incorporation of one the newer post-ACS guideline recommendations. Administration of the influenza vaccine is now widely endorsed following demonstration of a reduction in CV events after ACS using this practice.[186]

Cardiac Syndrome X

The term *cardiac syndrome X*, or more simply *syndrome X*, was introduced in 1973 by Kemp[187] in an editorial commenting on a study that investigated ECG and hemodynamic responses to atrial pacing in patients with chest pain and normal coronary angiograms.[188] One interesting subgroup of patients, labeled group X, had normal LV performance function despite typical ischemic ECG changes and increased myocardial lactate production consistent with myocardial ischemia. The three characteristic features of this clinical entity include 1) anginal discomfort with exertion, 2) ST-segment depression on exercise treadmill testing, and 3) absence of obstructive CAD, including no evidence of spontaneous or inducible spasm.[189,190] Nearly 25% of patients with ACS in the Clopidogrel and Acetyl Salicylic Acid in Bypass Surgery for Peripheral Arterial Disease (CASPAR) study[191] did not have a culprit lesion identified, yet almost half of these patients developed ischemic ST abnormalities following intracoronary acetylcholine, suggesting that endothelial dysfunction, as well as coronary morphologic abnormalities, can play an important role in causing ACS.

Although consensus is lacking in regard to the specific definition of cardiac syndrome X (e.g., some definitions do not require the presence of ischemic ECG changes during exercise), and the pathogenic mechanisms responsible for this condition appear to be multiple, we include cardiac syndrome X in this chapter because up to 15% of patients with ACS do not have hemodynamically significant evidence of CAD by conventional angiography.[192] Importantly, cardiac syndrome X must not be confused with *metabolic syndrome X*, defined as the condition in which patients meet at least three of the following five criteria: 1) increased waist circumference, 2) elevated triglycerides, 3) high blood pressure, 4) elevated fasting glucose, or 5) depressed HDL.[139] A small number of patients may show evidence of both syndromes.

The two major pathogenic mechanisms believed to be responsible for cardiac syndrome X are coronary microvascular dysfunction[193] and abnormal cardiac pain sensitivity; either or both may be present in any one individual.[194] The presence of microvascular dysfunction is supported by studies that have demonstrated impairment of endothelial-dependent arterial vasodilation, including coronary artery hyperreactivity and spasm in some patients; abnormal levels of metabolic/hormonal mediators of vascular tone (decreased nitric oxide production, estrogen deficiency, release of the endogenous peptides neuropeptide Y and endothelin-1); increased sensitivity to sympathetic stimulation with increased sympathetic tone; and prearteriolar constriction and/or coronary vasoconstriction in response to exercise that may be due in part to increased platelet aggregability.[195,196] The observations that CRP levels are elevated in cardiac syndrome X[197] and that CRP has been related to endothelial dysfunction[198] are more evidence of the importance of coronary microvascular dysfunction as a potential mechanism.

Abnormal cardiac pain sensitivity is a nonischemic mechanism that also appears to be operative in a substantial proportion of patients with cardiac syndrome X. Studies have demonstrated enhanced pain perception,[199] exaggerated pain response to adenosine, abnormal release of interstitial potassium, and activation of the right anterior insula cortex that may result in abnormal

> ### Box 9-5 Treatment Recommendations for Cardiac Syndrome X
>
> #### Class I
> 1. Risk factor modification
> 2. Medical therapy with nitrates, β-blockers, and calcium channel blockers, either alone or in combination (LOE B)
>
> #### Class IIb (If Symptoms Persist Despite Implementation of Class I Recommendations)
> 1. Imipramine or aminophylline may be considered (LOE C).
> 2. TENS may be considered (LOE B).
> 3. SCS may be considered (LOE B).
>
> LOE, level of evidence; SCS, spinal cord stimulation; TENS, transcutaneous electrical nerve stimulation.
> Modified from Anderson JL, Adams CD, Antman EM, et al. 2011 ACCF/AHA focused update incorporated into the ACC/AHA 2007 guidelines for the management of patients with unstable angina/non–ST-elevation myocardial infarction: a report of the American College of Cardiology Foundation/American Heart Association Task Force on Practice Guidelines. *Circulation* 2011;123:e426-e579.

neural function.[200] It has also been postulated that both microvascular dysfunction and abnormal pain perception are operative as independent abnormalities, and that in some patients, cardiac syndrome X becomes manifest only because of the presence of coronary microvascular dysfunction in patients with increased cardiac pain perception.[196]

Reassurance regarding the overall excellent intermediate-term prognosis historically has been an important first step in the treatment plan. However, more recent data from the Women's Ischemia Syndrome Evaluation (WISE) trial challenged the assertion of a benign prognosis in women with cardiac syndrome X, repeating a 4-year rate of CV death or nonfatal MI of 9.4% despite the presence of nonobstructive CAD.[201] Furthermore, the lifetime treatment costs approach that of women with three-vessel CAD because of the need for long-term, intensive therapy.[202]

Therapies to prevent angina generally fall into one of four major categories: 1) antiischemics, 2) agents that improve endothelial function, 3) analgesics, and 4) lifestyle or behavioral approaches.[203] Box 9-5 summarizes the therapies recommended in the 2011 update to the ACC/AHA UA/NSTEMI guideline.[2] The most extensive data support the use of β-blockers as first-line therapy, with studies demonstrating a reduction in chest pain, reduction in exercise-induced ST-segment depression, fewer episodes of silent ischemia by continuous ECG monitoring, improvement in microcirculation, and better quality of life. Data from clinical trials have also (inconsistently) supported a role for nitrates and CCBs, particularly to reduce exercise-induced angina and ischemic ST changes. Nicorandil,[204] an adenosine triphosphate (ATP)-sensitive potassium channel opener that also has nitratelike effects, and trimetazidine,[205] an inhibitor of oxidative phosphorylation that shifts energy production from free fatty acid to glucose oxidation, have also been associated with improvements in exercise tolerance, whereas α-blockers and aminophylline appear to have a more limited role in selected patients.

Because impairment in normal endothelial function of the coronary microvasculature that results in inadequate flow reserve appears to play an important role in some patients with cardiac syndrome X, therapies aiming to improve endothelial function have been tried with modest success. In a placebo-controlled trial, pravastatin 40 mg/day improved brachial artery flow-mediated dilation, exercise duration, and time to ischemia in patients with cardiac syndrome X.[206] A study combining ACE inhibition with statin therapy suggested that these agents can improve endothelial function and quality of life in cardiac syndrome X and may work by reducing oxidative stress, as determined by superoxide dismutase activity, in the vascular wall.[207] Although it improves endothelium-dependent coronary vasomotion in some postmenopausal women with cardiac syndrome X, estrogen therapy is controversial, particularly in light of randomized trials of hormonal replacement that demonstrate an increase risk of CV events.[208]

When antiischemic drugs and statins prove ineffective at controlling symptoms, a trial of analgesic-based therapies is recommended, given the evidence of altered somatic and visceral pain perception in some patients with cardiac syndrome X. Imipramine reduced chest pain in placebo-controlled trials, including studies with[209] and without[210] concomitant background antiischemic therapy. Monitoring of side effects—dizziness, dry mouth, and constipation—is necessary because these can have an adverse impact on quality of life.[209] Electrostimulation techniques, such as transcutaneous electrical nerve stimulation[211] and spinal cord stimulation,[212] reduced symptoms in studies of patients with angina and normal coronary angiograms. Thus, such therapy may be considered for patients with angina refractory to multiple drug therapies. Physical training improves exercise capacity and delays the onset of exercise-induced angina, particularly among patients who are deconditioned.[213] Structured cognitive behavioral approaches, particularly if instituted early after diagnosis, may be helpful to reduce chest pain and the psychologic morbidity associated with cardiac syndrome X.[214-217]

Because of heterogeneity among patients diagnosed with cardiac syndrome X, an individualized patient-based approach that attempts to achieve optimal symptom control is recommended, using multiple disciplines if necessary. A sympathetic physician's appreciation of the adverse impact on quality of life that patients often experience is important. A stepwise and largely empiric approach is described in Figure 9-13, pending additional data from randomized studies.

Cocaine and Methamphetamines

Cocaine use results in a marked increase in sympathetic tone by blocking the reuptake of norepinephrine from synapses by preganglionic neurons. The use of cocaine increases myocardial ischemia and the risk of infarction through several mechanisms, including increases in myocardial oxygen demand, decreases in myocardial oxygen supply, and accelerated atherosclerosis and thrombosis.[218] Oxygen demand is increased as a result of tachycardia, greater myocardial contractility, and increased wall stress (β-adrenergic effects), whereas supply is limited by vasoconstriction (α-adrenergic effects), resulting in a large mismatch between supply and demand. However, the CV toxicity is not limited to these dynamic effects. Cocaine also produces endothelial damage, enhanced platelet activation and aggregation, and decreases in plasminogen activator inhibitor.[218] Although the risk of events is highest when concentrations of cocaine in the blood are maximal and heart rate and blood pressure effects are apparent, these alternate pathophysiologic mechanisms may help explain why patients using cocaine continue to be at risk for increased cardiac ischemic events after cocaine levels have decreased. Because the pathophysiology and clinical presentation are similar following methamphetamine use, the therapeutic recommendations in the current guidelines are the same following ingestion of either of these two stimulants (Box 9-6).

The common use of cocaine among patients who come to emergency departments with chest pain and the differences in treatment between cocaine-induced coronary ischemia and that in patients who do not use cocaine mandate that the health care provider be vigilant to the possibility of use among all patients. Use of selective β-adrenergic receptor blockers can exacerbate coronary vasoconstriction in users of cocaine by creating a relative excess of β-adrenergic stimulation. Therefore the use of selective β-blockers, as opposed to mixed α- and β-blockers, as first-line agents for cocaine-related myocardial ischemia is discouraged.[218]

Cocaine-related vasospasm can be reversed by verapamil, nitroglycerin, and α-adrenergic blockers such as phentolamine. Nitrates and CCBs and benzodiazepines are generally considered first-line treatment for cocaine-related ischemia.[83] The clinician should remember, however, that coronary thrombosis is not infrequent with cocaine use, and aspirin and other antithrombotic measures should be taken. In the presence of refractory ischemia,

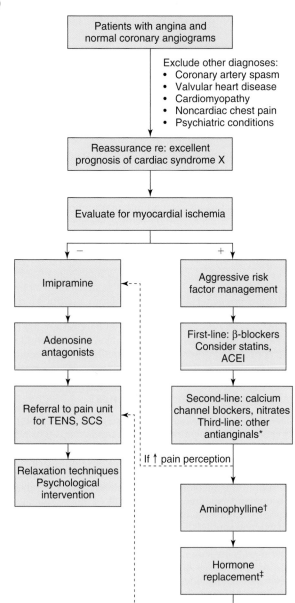

FIGURE 9-13 Stepwise approach to the diagnosis and management of patients with syndrome X. *Nicorandil, trimetazidine. †Especially with concomitant chronic obstructive pulmonary disease, asthma, or unexplained dyspnea. ‡Consider only in postmenopausal women if no contraindications exist; need to balance potential for increased risk of thrombotic complications. ACEI, angiotensin-converting enzyme inhibitor; SCS, spinal cord stimulation; TENS, transcutaneous electrical nerve stimulation.

 Box 9-6 Treatment Recommendations for Patients with Ischemic Chest Discomfort After Cocaine or Methamphetamine Use

Class I: Patients with ST-Segment Elevation or Depression
Sublingual or intravenous nitroglycerin (LOE C)
Intravenous or oral calcium channel blockers (LOE C)

Class IIa: Patients with Normal ECGs or with Minimal ST-Segment Depression
Nitroglycerin (LOE C)
Oral calcium channel blockers (LOE C)

Class IIb
Combination α- and β-blocker agents (e.g., labetalol) may be administered in patients with hypertension or tachycardia if nitroglycerin and/or a calcium channel blocker have been given within the prior hour (LOE C).

ECG, electrocardiogram; LOE, level of evidence.
Modified from Anderson JL, Adams CD, Antman EM, et al. 2011 ACCF/AHA focused update incorporated into the ACC/AHA 2007 guidelines for the management of patients with unstable angina/non-ST-elevation myocardial infarction: a report of the American College of Cardiology Foundation/American Heart Association Task Force on Practice Guidelines. *Circulation* 2011;123:e426-e579.

screen are important, particularly in younger patients who come to medical attention with ACS.

Diabetes Mellitus

Death as a result of heart disease among adults with diabetes are twofold to fourfold higher than in adults without diabetes.[220] Because nearly two thirds of all diabetics die of some form of heart or blood vessel disease,[220] focused attention on the evaluation and management of diabetic patients with NSTE-ACS is warranted.

In the Global Registry of Acute Coronary Events (GRACE), more than one fourth of patients with NSTE-ACS had diabetes.[221] Patients with diabetes tend to have a greater number of comorbidities, such as advanced age, prior CAD, hypertension, obesity, and history of heart failure—but they are less likely to smoke. Nevertheless, after multivariate adjustment, diabetes itself confers a 20% to 30% increased risk of death or ischemic complications.[222] This finding was confirmed in a more recent comprehensive analysis from the TIMI trials.[223] Even milder forms of impaired glucose metabolism have been linked to increased CV risk. Metabolic syndrome was present in 25% of patients admitted with ACS in an Israeli national survey, and these patients had a twofold higher adjusted mortality rate through 1 year.[224]

Established medical therapies for NSTE-ACS should be administered to patients with diabetes as they are to nondiabetic patients, with additional attention directed toward control of blood glucose. Four key recommendations from an AHA scientific statement on the management of hyperglycemia in patients with ACS[225] are summarized in Box 9-7. Most importantly, the target glucose range has been changed (preprandial goal <110 mg/dL, maximum glucose <180 mg/dL), and the latest guideline recommendations specifically mention to avoid hypoglycemia because of its association with increased mortality.[166]

Patients with diabetes had a similar benefit with an early invasive strategy as did nondiabetic patients in the FRISC II[226] and TACTICS-TIMI 18 trials.[227] Thus the 2011 writing group for the ACCF/AHA focused update[2] added diabetes to the list of characteristics for which an early invasive strategy is generally preferred. Patients with diabetes have a worse long-term outcome after revascularization compared with nondiabetic patients, in particular after PCI,[228] because they are at a higher risk for restenosis and disease progression of nonculprit lesions. Use of GP IIb/IIIa inhibitors and intracoronary stents appears to be of particular benefit in diabetic patients who undergo PCI.[229] In particular, more potent platelet inhibitors may be warranted in diabetes with elevated baseline

particularly if accompanied by persistent ST-segment elevation despite nitrates and calcium channel blockade, cardiac catheterization with percutaneous intervention is recommended.[83] Coronary angiography is not recommended in patients with chest pain after cocaine or methamphetamine use if the ECG, including stress testing, and cardiac biomarkers are normal.

In an 8-year prospective analysis of ACS patients admitted to a coronary care unit of a university hospital in Barcelona, Spain, 12% of patients had a history of cocaine use with an increasing prevalence over time from 7% in 2001 to 22% in 2008 (P = .04).[219] In patients younger than 30 years, the rates of prior cocaine use and positive light cocaine use at presentation were more than fourfold higher than those seen in older patients. Cocaine use was associated with larger infarcts, lower ejection fractions, and a 10-fold increase in hospital mortality (8.3% vs. 0.8%; P = .03); therefore a careful medical history and a low threshold for a urine toxicology

---

Box 9-7 Recommendations for Management of Hyperglycemia

1. Measure plasma glucose concentrations in all patients with suspected ACS.
2. Monitor glucose closely, and consider intensive glucose control with intravenous insulin in patients with glucose levels >180 mg/dL in the ICU.
3. Maintain glucose concentrations <180 mg dL with subcutaneous insulin in the non-ICU setting.
4. Determine the severity of the metabolic derangement after discharge in patients with no prior history of diabetes mellitus who demonstrated hyperglycemia during hospitalization after an ACS.

ACS, acute coronary syndrome; ICU, intensive care unit.
Modified from Deedwania P, Kosiborod M, Barrett E, et al. Hyperglycemia and acute coronary syndrome: a scientific statement from the American Heart Association Diabetes Committee of the Council on Nutrition, Physical Activity, and Metabolism. *Circulation* 2008;117:1610-1619.

---

glucose levels because these patients have more severe platelet dysfunction.[230]

With regard to revascularization, use of the left internal mammary artery as a bypass conduit for CABG is preferred over PCI in diabetic patients with multivessel disease,[231] although additional studies are needed with newer therapies (e.g., drug-eluting stents, thienopyridines) to determine the optimal role for multivessel PCI in diabetics. PCI is considered a reasonable revascularization strategy in patients with single-vessel disease and inducible ischemia.

Unfortunately, nearly one third of diabetic patients who are admitted with NSTE-ACS do not have hemoglobin A1c measured during the hospitalization.[232] Furthermore, of those who are assessed, at least 60% demonstrate suboptimal control (i.e., hemoglobin A1c >7.0%). A significant opportunity exists to improve the care of ACS patients with diabetes.

The Elderly

Prevalent CAD increases with aging. As a result, elderly patients are overrepresented among patients with coronary disease. It has been reported that 35% of patients with UA/NSTEMI are older than 75 years, and 11% are older than 85 years.[233] Despite the burden of risk in elderly patients, evidence-based therapies are underused in this age group.[234-236]

More frequent medical and cardiac comorbidities affect all aspects of the diagnosis and management of elderly patients with NSTE-ACS. Risk factors and physiologic differences also manifest in the care of older patients with NSTE-ACS. Elderly patients are more likely to come to medical attention with atypical symptoms of ACS, including dyspnea and confusion,[237] and they are more likely than younger patients to have noncoronary causes of NSTE-ACS, such as hypertension, myocardial hypertrophy, and diastolic dysfunctions.[238] Reduced hepatic and renal function also results in impaired metabolism and decreased clearance of medication, so elderly patients tend to have decreased arterial compliance that results in increased cardiac afterload and diminished β-sympathetic response.[239] These factors, combined with polypharmacy, increase the risk of drug-drug interactions and side effects in the elderly. In addition, elderly patients are more likely to present with atypical symptoms of UA/NSTEMI, such as shortness of breath or CHF, resulting from exaggerated increases in ventricular pressures[240]; therefore a high index of suspicion must be maintained for diagnosis of UA/NSTEMI in the elderly.

General recommendations for the pharmacologic treatment of UA/NSTEMI in the elderly is to follow the accepted treatment for younger patients, recognizing and anticipating increased side-effect profiles of therapeutics in the elderly population.[241] However, greater caution regarding dosing and monitoring of side effects is necessary. For instance, older patients are more prone to the exaggerated hypotensive effects of nitroglycerin.[242] Elderly patients also have diminished responsiveness to adrenergic stimuli and

decreased AV nodal conduction; thus the response to β-blockers may not be predictable. Of particular importance, the prevalence of reduced renal function in the elderly is high, even in the setting of seemingly normal serum creatinine. Specific calculation of creatinine clearance or glomerular filtration rate should be performed in the elderly to guide therapy and to dose medications cleared by the kidney, particularly LMWHs and GP IIb/IIIa inhibitors, as overdosing of these agents is more common in the elderly.[243]

Decisions regarding whether to undertake invasive or conservative management must also be considered in the context of the age of the patient. Elderly patients are more likely to have severe CAD that could benefit from invasive management, but they are also more likely to have medical comorbidities that can result in adverse outcomes. Observational studies have shown that elderly patients are much less likely than younger patients to undergo coronary angiography and revascularization.[236,244] Studies have shown results similar to younger patients in carefully chosen subjects[245]; however, some studies show decreased procedural success rates and increased complications at extremes of age,[246,247] including an increase in periprocedural MI.[248]

Most clinical trials have not specifically addressed the issue of invasive versus conservative management of the elderly. The Trial of Invasive Versus Medical Therapy in Elderly Patients (TIME), one prospective, randomized trial of invasive versus conservative therapy in patients older than 75 years with chronic CAD, has been published.[249] Patients undergoing revascularization had a lower rate of major adverse cardiac events at 6 months and improvement in symptomatic status compared with patients who had an initial conservative management strategy. In an analysis of the TACTICS-TIMI 18 trial,[250] a larger clinical benefit was seen in elderly patients undergoing an invasive strategy than in younger patients, but this was somewhat offset by an increased rate of hemorrhage in elderly patients. A similar pattern of risk and benefit was observed in the FRISC II trial, with the majority of the benefit of early invasive therapy seen in patients older than 65 years.[141]

As with other treatments, the rates of important adverse events after CABG, including cerebrovascular events, is significantly increased in elderly patients[251]; however, observational studies have shown improved clinical outcomes among octogenarians who underwent CABG compared with patients with similarly severe CAD who did not undergo CABG.[83]

An approach to the care of an elderly patient with NSTE-ACS should focus on factors similar to those relative to the management of younger patients. Because of physiologic and psychosocial differences, and because of more frequent polypharmacy and medical comorbidities, each therapy should be considered specifically for its possible adverse effects and interactions. Particular attention should be given to renal function and impaired clearance of medications and to consideration of appropriate dose adjustment. The practitioner should attempt to identify the signs and symptoms of depression in the elderly and to provide treatment. In addition, the importance of physical therapy and rehabilitation to maintain mobility and enhance recovery is magnified in the elderly.[252]

In summary, data suggest that well-chosen elderly patients are likely to derive an important benefit from proven strategies. Barring medical comorbidities that provide contraindications, advanced age should be considered an indication for comprehensive treatment of NSTE-ACS, not a contraindication to it.

Women

Although CHD has traditionally been considered a disease of middle-aged men, approximately 43% of patients discharged with ACS from a U.S. hospital in 2003 were female.[253] In general, women diagnosed with NSTE-ACS should be managed in a manner similar to men, despite an underrepresentation of women in published trial literature that serves as the primary evidence for treatment guidelines. A number of key observations that pertain to women (on average) should be kept in mind. Women with NSTE-ACS tend to be older than men, with an incidence of CHD that lags by approximately a decade until the seventh decade.[254] The "typical" presentation of ACS based on prior studies, predominantly in men, differs from the "typical" presentation in women, which is more complex and multifactorial.[255] Nonatherosclerotic etiologies of angina, such as microvascular dysfunction,[256] are more frequent in women than in men.

Evaluation of women with biomarkers, ECG, noninvasive testing, and coronary angiography should be similar to an evaluation in men, although a few points deserve to be highlighted. Repolarization abnormalities on resting ECG are strong independent predictors of CHD events, death, and CHF in postmenopausal women.[257,258] Exercise ECG testing is less specific in women, and addition of an imaging study to the stress ECG improves diagnostic accuracy.[259,260] Because women have a more complex, multifactorial etiology of NSTE-ACS and are subject to greater diagnostic uncertainty, assessment of additional information—such as evaluation of plaque burden, vascular reactivity,[261] and functional capacity[262]—may be of relatively greater importance in women.[255] Similar to men, women with a high-risk indicator or with high-risk noninvasive test results should be referred for coronary angiogram with the understanding that women are at higher risk for bleeding complications, in part because of older age, lower body weight, and impaired renal function. As with elderly patients, women tend to be of lower body weight, may have impaired renal function, and are at particular risk of overdosing on medications with renal clearance, such as LMWHs or GP IIb/IIIa inhibitors.[243]

The reasons why women tend to be treated less intensively than men are likely complex and multifactorial.[263] Nonetheless, the underutilization of proven therapies in NSTE-ACS that have a high risk/benefit ratio (e.g., aspirin, statins) indicates the presence of a gender bias in treatment[264] that persists despite publication of numerous treatment guidelines over the past decade.[265] Women with CAD are referred less frequently for coronary angiography and revascularization,[265] in part because of the presence of less extensive epicardial CAD. Recent studies have challenged the concept that women fare less well than men following invasive therapy.[147,266] Targeting obesity and physical inactivity may be especially important after NSTE-ACS because these factors contribute independently to congestive heart disease morbidity and mortality in women.[267]

In summary, according to guidelines, women with UA/NSTEMI should be managed similarly to men in respect to diagnostic workup, pharmacotherapy, and evaluation for invasive therapy.[2] Particular attention should be paid to medication dosing to avoid excess dosing of anticoagulants. Women with high-risk features have similar recommendations for invasive management as men.

Chronic Kidney Disease

Chronic renal impairment, or chronic kidney disease (CKD), is associated with more frequent development of CAD[268] and is associated with worse outcomes following ACS.[269] CKD represents an independent risk factor for death and recurrent CV events following ACS, with particularly high risk associated with patients undergoing hemodialysis.[2] Most major CV clinical trials exclude patients with moderate or severe CKD; therefore the evidence basis for treatment recommendations is limited. Patients with CKD tend to have impaired platelet function and are more likely to be overdosed with anticoagulant medications[243]; therefore they are at high risk for bleeding complications. In addition, patients with CKD, but not end-stage renal disease, are at high risk for contrast nephropathy and acute kidney injury, which may be reduced with isoosmolar contrast agents. Thus, recognizing the presence of CKD is important in the management of patients with UA/NSTEMI to allow for proper dosing of medications and appropriate risk assessment and management during invasive procedures.[2]

REFERENCES

1. Levine GN, Bates ER, Blankenship JC, et al. 2011 ACCF/AHA/SCAI guideline for percutaneous coronary intervention: a report of the American College of Cardiology Foundation/American Heart Association Task Force on Practice Guidelines and the Society for Cardiovascular Angiography and Interventions. *Circulation* 2011;124:e574-e651.
2. Anderson JL, Adams CD, Antman EM, et al. 2011 ACCF/AHA focused update incorporated into the ACC/AHA 2007 guidelines for the management of patients with unstable angina/non–ST-elevation myocardial infarction: a report of the American College of Cardiology Foundation/American Heart Association Task Force on Practice Guidelines. *Circulation* 2011;123:e426-e579.
3. Antman EM, Cohen M, Bernink PJ, et al. The TIMI risk score for unstable angina/non–ST-elevation MI: a method for prognostication and therapeutic decision making. *JAMA* 2000;284:835-842.
4. Boersma E, Pieper KS, Steyerberg EW, et al. Predictors of outcome in patients with acute coronary syndromes without persistent ST-segment elevation: results from an international trial of 9461 patients. The PURSUIT Investigators. *Circulation* 2000;101:2557-2567.
5. Jacobs DR Jr, Kroenke C, Crow R, et al. PREDICT: a simple risk score for clinical severity and long-term prognosis after hospitalization for acute myocardial infarction or unstable angina: the Minnesota heart survey. *Circulation* 1999;100:599-607.
6. Calvin JE, Klein LW, VandenBerg EJ, et al. Validated risk stratification model accurately predicts low risk in patients with unstable angina. *J Am Coll Cardiol* 2000;36:1803-1808.
7. Granger CB, Goldberg RJ, Dabbous O, et al. Predictors of hospital mortality in the global registry of acute coronary events. *Arch Intern Med* 2003;163:2345-2353.
8. Goncalves PD, Ferreira J, Aguiar C, Seabra-Gomes R. TIMI, PURSUIT, and GRACE risk scores: sustained prognostic value and interaction with revascularization in NSTEACS. *Eur Heart J* 2005;865-872.
9. Garcia S, Canoniero M, Peter A, de Marchena E, Ferreira A. Correlation of TIMI risk score with angiographic severity and extent of coronary artery disease in patients with non–ST-elevation acute coronary syndromes. *Am J Cardiol* 2004;93:813-816.
10. Mega JL, Morrow DA, Sabatine MS, et al. Correlation between the TIMI risk score and high-risk angiographic findings in non–ST-elevation acute coronary syndromes. *Am Heart J* 2005;149:846-850.
11. Cohen M, Demers C, Gurfinkel EP, et al. A comparison of low-molecular-weight heparin with unfractionated heparin for unstable coronary artery disease. Efficacy and Safety of Subcutaneous Enoxaparin in Non–Q-Wave Coronary Events Study Group. *N Engl J Med* 1997;337:447-452.
12. Morrow DA, Antman EM, Snapinn SM, et al. An integrated clinical approach to predicting the benefit of tirofiban in non–ST elevation acute coronary syndromes: application of the TIMI Risk Score for UA/NSTEMI in PRISM-PLUS. *Eur Heart J* 2002;23:223-229.
13. Cannon CP, Weintraub WS, Demopoulos LA, et al. Comparison of early invasive and conservative strategies in patients with unstable coronary syndromes treated with the glycoprotein IIb/IIIa inhibitor tirofiban. *N Engl J Med* 2001;344:1879-1887.
14. Braunwald E. Unstable angina: a classification. *Circulation* 1989;80:410-414.
15. Braunwald E, Antman EM, Beasley JW, et al. ACC/AHA 2002 guideline update for the management of patients with unstable angina and non–ST-segment elevation myocardial infarction: a report of the American College of Cardiology/American Heart Association Task Force on Practice Guidelines (Committee on the Management of Patients With Unstable Angina). 2002. Available at http://www.acc.org/clinical/guidelines/unstable/unstable/.pdf.
16. Braunwald E. 50th anniversary historical article. Myocardial oxygen consumption: the quest for its determinants and some clinical fallout. *J Am Coll Cardiol* 2000;35:45B-48B.
17. Figueras J, Lidon R, Cortadellas J. Rebound myocardial ischaemia following abrupt interruption of intravenous nitroglycerin infusion in patients with unstable angina at rest. *Eur Heart J* 1991;12:405-411.
18. Cheitlin MD, Hutter AM Jr, Brindis RG, et al. Use of sildenafil (Viagra) in patients with cardiovascular disease. Technology and Practice Executive Committee. *Circulation* 1999;99:168-177.
19. Cheitlin MD, Hutter AM Jr, Brindis RG, et al. ACC/AHA expert consensus document: use of sildenafil (Viagra) in patients with cardiovascular disease. American College of Cardiology/American Heart Association. *J Am Coll Cardiol* 1999;33:273-282.
20. Yusuf S, Wittes J, Friedman L. Overview of results of randomized clinical trials in heart disease. II. Unstable angina, heart failure, primary prevention with aspirin, and risk factor modification. *JAMA* 1988;260:2259-2263.
21. Randomised trial of intravenous atenolol among 16 027 cases of suspected acute myocardial infarction: ISIS-1. First International Study of Infarct Survival Collaborative Group. *Lancet* 1986;2:57-66.
22. Metoprolol in acute myocardial infarction (MIAMI): a randomised placebo-controlled international trial. The MIAMI Trial Research Group. *Eur Heart J* 1985;6:199-226.
23. Roberts R, Rogers WJ, Mueller HS, et al. Immediate versus deferred β-blockade following thrombolytic therapy in patients with acute myocardial infarction: results of the Thrombolysis in Myocardial Infarction (TIMI) II-B study. *Circulation* 1991;83:422-437.
24. Chen ZM, Pan HC, Chen YP, et al. Early intravenous then oral metoprolol in 45,852 patients with acute myocardial infarction: randomised placebo-controlled trial. *Lancet* 2005;366:1622-1632.
25. Anderson JL, Adams CD, Antman EM, et al. ACC/AHA 2007 guidelines for the management of patients with unstable angina/non–ST-elevation myocardial infarction: a report of the American College of Cardiology/American Heart Association Task Force on Practice Guidelines (Writing Committee to Revise the 2002 Guidelines for the Management of Patients With Unstable Angina/Non–ST-Elevation Myocardial Infarction): developed in collaboration with the American College of Emergency Physicians, the Society for Cardiovascular Angiography and Interventions, and the Society of Thoracic Surgeons. Endorsed by the American Association of Cardiovascular and Pulmonary Rehabilitation and the Society for Academic Emergency Medicine. *Circulation* 2007;116:e148-e304.
26. Tijssen JG, Lubsen J. Early treatment of unstable angina with nifedipine and metoprolol—the HINT trial. *J Cardiovasc Pharmacol* 1988;12:S71-S77.

27. The Holland Interuniversity Nifedipine/Metoprolol Trial (HINT) Research Group. Early treatment of unstable angina in the coronary care unit: a randomised, double blind, placebo controlled comparison of recurrent ischaemia in patients treated with nifedipine or metoprolol or both. *Br Heart J* 1986;56:400-413.
28. Hansen JF, Hagerup L, Sigurd B, et al; Danish Verapamil Infarction Trial (DAVIT) Study Group. Cardiac event rates after acute myocardial infarction in patients treated with verapamil and trandolapril versus trandolapril alone. *Am J Cardiol* 1997;79:738-741.
29. Gibson RS, Boden WE, Theroux P, et al. Diltiazem and reinfarction in patients with non–Q-wave myocardial infarction: results of a double-blind, randomized, multicenter trial. *N Engl J Med* 1986;315:423-429.
30. Hansen JF, Tingsted L, Rasmussen V, et al. Verapamil and angiotensin-converting enzyme inhibitors in patients with coronary artery disease and reduced left ventricular ejection fraction. *Am J Cardiol* 1996;77:16D-21D.
31. Chaitman BR. Ranolazine for the treatment of chronic angina and potential use in other cardiovascular conditions. *Circulation* 2006;113:2462-2472.
32. Morrow DA, Scirica BM, Karwatowska-Prokopczuk E, et al. Effects of ranolazine on recurrent cardiovascular events in patients with non–ST-elevation acute coronary syndromes: the MERLIN-TIMI 36 randomized trial. *JAMA* 2007;297:1775-1783.
33. Mehta SR, Bassand JP, Chrolavicius S, et al. Design and rationale of CURRENT-OASIS 7: a randomized, 2 x 2 factorial trial evaluating optimal dosing strategies for clopidogrel and aspirin in patients with ST and non–ST-elevation acute coronary syndromes managed with an early invasive strategy. *Am Heart J* 2008;156:1080-1088, e1081.
34. Mehta SR, Bassand JP, Chrolavicius S, et al. Dose comparisons of clopidogrel and aspirin in acute coronary syndromes. *N Engl J Med* 2010;363:930-942.
35. Kleiman NS, Grazeiadei N, Maresh K, et al. Abciximab, ticlopidine, and concomitant abciximab-ticlopidine therapy: ex vivo platelet aggregation inhibition profiles in patients undergoing percutaneous coronary interventions. *Am Heart J* 2000;140:492-501.
36. Gurbel PA, Bliden KP, Hiatt BL, O'Connor CM. Clopidogrel for coronary stenting: response variability, drug resistance, and the effect of pretreatment platelet reactivity. *Circulation* 2003;107:2908-2913.
37. Wiviott SD, Trenk D, Frelinger AL, et al. Prasugrel compared with high loading- and maintenance-dose clopidogrel in patients with planned percutaneous coronary intervention: the Prasugrel in Comparison to Clopidogrel for Inhibition of Platelet Activation and Aggregation–Thrombolysis in Myocardial Infarction 44 trial. *Circulation* 2007;116:2923-2932.
38. Wiviott SD, Antman EM, Braunwald E. Prasugrel. *Circulation* 2010;122:394-403.
39. Mehta SR, Yusuf S, Peters RJ, et al. Effects of pretreatment with clopidogrel and aspirin followed by long-term therapy in patients undergoing percutaneous coronary intervention: the PCI-CURE study. *Lancet* 2001;358:527-533.
40. Yusuf S, Zhao F, Mehta SR, et al. Effects of clopidogrel in addition to aspirin in patients with acute coronary syndromes without ST-segment elevation. *N Engl J Med* 2001;345:494-502.
41. Steinhubl SR, Darrah S, Brennan D, et al. Optimal duration of pretreatment with clopidogrel prior to PCI: data from the CREDO trial [abstract]. *Circulation* 2003;108(Suppl): IV-374.
42. Patti G, Colonna G, Pasceri V, et al. Randomized trial of high loading dose of clopidogrel for reduction of periprocedural myocardial infarction in patients undergoing coronary intervention: results from the ARMYDA-2 (Antiplatelet Therapy for Reduction of Myocardial Damage during Angioplasty) study. *Circulation* 2005;111:2099-2106.
43. Mehta SR, Tanguay JF, Eikelboom JW, et al. Double-dose versus standard-dose clopidogrel and high-dose versus low-dose aspirin in individuals undergoing percutaneous coronary intervention for acute coronary syndromes (CURRENT-OASIS 7): a randomised factorial trial. *Lancet* 2010;376:1233-1243.
44. Wiviott SD, Antman EM, Winters KJ, et al. A randomized comparison of prasugrel (CS-747, LY640315), a novel thienopyridine P2Y12 antagonist, to clopidogrel in percutaneous coronary intervention: results of the Joint Utilization of Medications to Block Platelets Optimally (JUMBO)–TIMI 26 trial. *Circulation* 2005;111:3366-3373.
45. Wiviott SD, Braunwald E, McCabe CH, et al. Prasugrel versus clopidogrel in patients with acute coronary syndromes. *N Engl J Med* 2007;357:2001-2015.
46. Morrow DA, Wiviott SD, White HD, et al. Effect of the novel thienopyridine prasugrel compared with clopidogrel on spontaneous and procedural myocardial infarction in the Trial to Assess Improvement in Therapeutic Outcomes by Optimizing Platelet Inhibition with Prasugrel–Thrombolysis in Myocardial Infarction 38: an application of the classification system from the universal definition of myocardial infarction. *Circulation* 2009;119:2758-2764.
47. Wiviott SD, Braunwald E, McCabe CH, et al. Intensive oral antiplatelet therapy for reduction of ischaemic events including stent thrombosis in patients with acute coronary syndromes treated with percutaneous coronary intervention and stenting in the TRITON-TIMI 38 trial: a subanalysis of a randomised trial. *Lancet* 2008;371:1353-1363.
48. Husted S, van Giezen JJ. Ticagrelor: the first reversibly binding oral P2Y12 receptor antagonist. *Cardiovasc Ther* 2009;27:259-274.
49. Gurbel PA, Bliden KP, Butler K, et al. Response to ticagrelor in clopidogrel nonresponders and responders and effect of switching therapies: the RESPOND study. *Circulation* 2010;121:1188-1199.
50. Gurbel PA, Bliden KP, Butler K, et al. Randomized double-blind assessment of the ONSET and OFFSET of the antiplatelet effects of ticagrelor versus clopidogrel in patients with stable coronary artery disease: the ONSET/OFFSET study. *Circulation* 2009;120: 2577-2585.
51. James S, Akerblom A, Cannon CP, et al. Comparison of ticagrelor, the first reversible oral P2Y(12) receptor antagonist, with clopidogrel in patients with acute coronary syndromes: rationale, design, and baseline characteristics of the PLATelet inhibition and patient Outcomes (PLATO) trial. *Am Heart J* 2009;157:599-605.
52. Wallentin L, Becker RC, Budaj A, et al. Ticagrelor versus clopidogrel in patients with acute coronary syndromes. *N Engl J Med* 2009;361:1045-1057.
53. Held C, Asenblad N, Bassand JP, et al. Ticagrelor versus clopidogrel in patients with acute coronary syndromes undergoing coronary artery bypass surgery: results from the PLATO (Platelet Inhibition and Patient Outcomes) trial. *J Am Coll Cardiol* 2011;57:672-684.
54. Mahaffey KW, Wojdyla DM, Carroll K, et al. Ticagrelor compared with clopidogrel by geographic region in the Platelet Inhibition and Patient Outcomes (PLATO) trial. *Circulation* 2011;124:544-554.
55. Storey RF, Becker RC, Harrington RA, et al. Characterization of dyspnoea in PLATO study patients treated with ticagrelor or clopidogrel and its association with clinical outcomes. *Eur Heart J* 2011;32:2945-2953.
56. Storey RF, Becker RC, Harrington RA, et al. Pulmonary function in patients with acute coronary syndrome treated with ticagrelor or clopidogrel (from the Platelet Inhibition and Patient Outcomes [PLATO] Pulmonary Function Substudy). *Am J Cardiol* 2011;108: 1542-1546.
57. Yusuf S, Zhao F, Mehta SR, et al. Effects of clopidogrel in addition to aspirin in patients with acute coronary syndromes without ST-segment elevation. *N Engl J Med* 2001;345: 494-502.
58. Serruys PW, Kukreja N. Late stent thrombosis in drug-eluting stents: return of the 'VB syndrome.' *Nat Clin Pract Cardiovasc Med* 2006;3:637.
59. Webster MW, Ormiston JA. Drug-eluting stents and late stent thrombosis. *Lancet* 2007;370:914-915.
60. Windecker S, Meier B. Late coronary stent thrombosis. *Circulation* 2007;116:1952-1965.
61. Mauri L, Kereiakes DJ, Normand SL, et al. Rationale and design of the dual antiplatelet therapy study, a prospective, multicenter, randomized, double-blind trial to assess the effectiveness and safety of 12 versus 30 months of dual antiplatelet therapy in subjects undergoing percutaneous coronary intervention with either drug-eluting stent or bare metal stent placement for the treatment of coronary artery lesions. *Am Heart J* 2010;160:1035-1041, e1031.
62. Palmerini T, Dangas G, Mehran R, et al. Predictors and implications of stent thrombosis in non–ST-segment elevation acute coronary syndromes: the ACUITY trial. *Circ Cardiovasc Interv* 2011;4(6):577-584.
63. Bhatt DL, Fox KA, Hacke W, et al. Clopidogrel and aspirin versus aspirin alone for the prevention of atherothrombotic events. *N Engl J Med* 2006;354:1706-1717.
64. Bhatt DL, Topol EJ. Clopidogrel added to aspirin versus aspirin alone in secondary prevention and high-risk primary prevention: rationale and design of the Clopidogrel for High Atherothrombotic Risk and Ischemic Stabilization, Management, and Avoidance (CHARISMA) trial. *Am Heart J* 2004;148:263-268.
65. Bhatt DL, Flather MD, Hacke W, et al. Patients with prior myocardial infarction, stroke, or symptomatic peripheral arterial disease in the CHARISMA trial. *J Am Coll Cardiol* 2007;49:1982-1988.
66. Bonello L, Tantry US, Marcucci R, et al. Consensus and future directions on the definition of high on-treatment platelet reactivity to adenosine diphosphate. *J Am Coll Cardiol* 2010;56:919-933.
67. Bonello L, Armero S, Ait Mokhtar O, et al. Clopidogrel loading dose adjustment according to platelet reactivity monitoring in patients carrying the 2C19*2 loss of function polymorphism. *J Am Coll Cardiol* 2010;56:1630-1636.
68. Mega JL, Hochholzer W, Frelinger AL 3rd, et al. Dosing clopidogrel based on CYP2C19 genotype and the effect on platelet reactivity in patients with stable cardiovascular disease. *JAMA* 2011;306:2221-2228.
69. Price MJ, Berger PB, Teirstein PS, et al. Standard- vs high-dose clopidogrel based on platelet function testing after percutaneous coronary intervention: the GRAVITAS randomized trial. *JAMA* 2011;305:1097-1105.
70. Price MJ, Angiolillo DJ, Teirstein PS, et al. Platelet reactivity and cardiovascular outcomes after percutaneous coronary intervention: a time-dependent analysis of the Gauging Responsiveness with a VerifyNow P2Y12 assay: Impact on Thrombosis and Safety (GRAVITAS) trial. *Circulation* 2011;124:1132-1137.
71. Shuldiner AR, O'Connell JR, Bliden KP, et al. Association of cytochrome P450 2C19 genotype with the antiplatelet effect and clinical efficacy of clopidogrel therapy. *JAMA* 2009;302:849-857.
72. Pare G, Mehta SR, Yusuf S, et al. Effects of CYP2C19 genotype on outcomes of clopidogrel treatment. *N Engl J Med* 2010;363:1704-1714.
73. Mega JL, Simon T, Collet JP, et al. Reduced-function CYP2C19 genotype and risk of adverse clinical outcomes among patients treated with clopidogrel predominantly for PCI: a meta-analysis. *JAMA* 2010;304:1821-1830.
74. Mega JL, Close SL, Wiviott SD, et al. Cytochrome p-450 polymorphisms and response to clopidogrel. *N Engl J Med* 2009;360:354-362.
75. Mega JL, Close SL, Wiviott SD, et al. Cytochrome P450 genetic polymorphisms and the response to prasugrel: relationship to pharmacokinetic, pharmacodynamic, and clinical outcomes. *Circulation* 2009;119:2553-2560.
76. Wallentin L, James S, Storey RF, et al. Effect of CYP2C19 and ABCB1 single nucleotide polymorphisms on outcomes of treatment with ticagrelor versus clopidogrel for acute coronary syndromes: a genetic substudy of the PLATO trial. *Lancet* 2010;376:1320-1328.
77. Topol EJ, Easton D, Harrington RA, et al. Randomized, double-blind, placebo-controlled, international trial of the oral IIb/IIIa antagonist lotrafiban in coronary and cerebrovascular disease. *Circulation* 2003;108:399-406.
78. Chew DP, Bhatt DL, Sapp S, Topol EJ. Increased mortality with oral platelet glycoprotein IIb/IIIa antagonists: a meta-analysis of phase III multicenter randomized trials. *Circulation* 2001;103:201-206.
79. Use of a monoclonal antibody directed against the platelet glycoprotein IIb/IIIa receptor in high-risk coronary angioplasty: the EPIC Investigation [see comments]. *N Engl J Med* 1994;330:956-961.
80. Effect of glycoprotein IIb/IIIa receptor blocker abciximab on outcome in patients with acute coronary syndromes without early coronary revascularisation: the GUSTO IV-ACS randomised trial. *Lancet* 2001;2001:1915-1924.
81. Boersma E, Akkerhuis KM, Theroux P, et al. Platelet glycoprotein IIb/IIIa receptor inhibition in non–ST-elevation acute coronary syndromes: early benefit during medical treatment only, with additional protection during percutaneous coronary intervention. *Circulation* 1999;100:2045-2048.
82. Montalescot G, Borentain M, Payot L, et al. Early vs late administration of glycoprotein IIb/IIIa inhibitors in primary percutaneous coronary intervention of acute ST-segment elevation myocardial infarction: a meta-analysis. *JAMA* 2004;292:362-366.

83. Braunwald E, Antman EM, Beasley JW, et al. ACC/AHA guideline update for the management of patients with unstable angina and non–ST-segment elevation myocardial infarction—2002: summary article: a report of the American College of Cardiology/American Heart Association Task Force on Practice Guidelines (Committee on the Management of Patients With Unstable Angina). *Circulation* 2002;106:1893-1900.
84. Karvouni E, Katritsis DG, Ioannidis JP. Intravenous glycoprotein IIb/IIIa receptor antagonists reduce mortality after percutaneous coronary interventions. *J Am Coll Cardiol* 2003;41:26-32.
85. Kastrati A, Mehilli J, Neumann FJ, et al. Abciximab in patients with acute coronary syndromes undergoing percutaneous coronary intervention after clopidogrel pretreatment: the ISAR-REACT 2 randomized trial. *JAMA* 2006;295:1531-1538.
86. Stone GW, Bertrand ME, Moses JW, et al. Routine upstream initiation vs deferred selective use of glycoprotein IIb/IIIa inhibitors in acute coronary syndromes: the ACUITY Timing trial. *JAMA* 2007;297:591-602.
87. Giugliano RP, White JA, Bode C, et al. Early versus delayed, provisional eptifibatide in acute coronary syndromes. *N Engl J Med* 2009;360:2176-2190.
88. Tricoci P, Newby LK, Hasselblad V, et al. Upstream use of small-molecule glycoprotein IIb/IIIa inhibitors in patients with non–ST-segment elevation acute coronary syndromes: a systematic overview of randomized clinical trials. *Circ Cardiovasc Qual Outcomes* 2011;4:448-458.
89. Boersma E, Harrington RA, Moliterno DJ, et al. Platelet glycoprotein IIb/IIIa inhibitors in acute coronary syndromes: a meta-analysis of all major randomised clinical trials. *Lancet* 2002;359:189-198.
90. Morrow DA, Sabatine MS, Antman EM, et al. Usefulness of tirofiban among patients treated without percutaneous coronary intervention (TIMI high-risk patients in PRISM-PLUS). *Am J Cardiol* 2004;94:774-776.
91. Meadows TA, Bhatt DL. Clinical aspects of platelet inhibitors and thrombus formation. *Circ Res* 2007;100:1261-1275.
92. Harrington RA, Stone GW, McNulty S, et al. Platelet inhibition with cangrelor in patients undergoing PCI. *N Engl J Med* 2009;361:2318-2329.
93. Bhatt DL, Lincoff AM, Gibson CM, et al. Intravenous platelet blockade with cangrelor during PCI. *N Engl J Med* 2009;361:2330-2341.
94. Berger JS, Melloni C, Wang TY, et al. Reporting and representation of race/ethnicity in published randomized trials. *Am Heart J* 2009;158:742-747.
95. Leonardi S, Rao SV, Harrington RA, et al. Rationale and design of the randomized, double-blind trial testing INtraveNous and Oral administration of elinogrel, a selective and reversible P2Y(12)-receptor inhibitor, versus clopidogrel to eVAluate Tolerability and Efficacy in nonurgent Percutaneous Coronary Interventions patients (INNOVATE-PCI). *Am Heart J* 2010;160:65-72.
96. Antman EM. The search for replacements for unfractionated heparin. *Circulation* 2001;103:2310-2314.
97. Schulz S, Mehilli J, Neumann FJ, et al. ISAR-REACT 3A: a study of reduced dose of unfractionated heparin in biomarker negative patients undergoing percutaneous coronary intervention. *Eur Heart J* 2010;31:2482-2491.
98. Le May M, Kurdi M, Labinaz M, et al. Safety of coronary stenting with eptifibatide and ultra-low-dose heparin. *Am J Cardiol* 2005;95:630-632.
99. Eikelboom JW, Anand SS, Malmberg K, et al. Unfractionated heparin and low-molecular-weight heparin in acute coronary syndrome without ST elevation: a meta-analysis [see comments]. *Lancet* 2000;355:1936-1942.
100. Antman EM, McCabe CH, Gurfinkel EP, et al. Enoxaparin prevents death and cardiac ischemic events in unstable angina/non–Q-wave myocardial infarction: results of the thrombolysis in myocardial infarction (TIMI) 11B trial [see comments]. *Circulation* 1999;100:1593-1601.
101. Katsouras C, Michalis LK, Papamichael N, et al. Enoxaparin versus tinzaparin in non–ST-segment elevation acute coronary syndromes: results of the enoxaparin versus tinzaparin (EVET) trial at 6 months. *Am Heart J* 2005;150:385-391.
102. Low-molecular-weight heparin during instability in coronary artery disease. Fragmin during Instability in Coronary Artery Disease (FRISC) study group. *Lancet* 1996;347: 561-568.
103. Klein W, Buchwald A, Hillis SE, et al. Comparison of low-molecular-weight heparin with unfractionated heparin acutely and with placebo for 6 weeks in the management of unstable coronary artery disease. Fragmin in unstable coronary artery disease study (FRIC) [see comments; published erratum appears in Circulation 1998 Feb 3;97(4):413]. *Circulation* 1997;96:61-68.
104. Comparison of two treatment durations (6 days and 14 days) of a low molecular weight heparin with a 6-day treatment of unfractionated heparin in the initial management of unstable angina or non–Q wave myocardial infarction: FRAX.I.S. (FRAxiparine in Ischaemic Syndrome) [see comments]. *Eur Heart J* 1999;20:1553-1562.
105. Petersen JL, Mahaffey KW, Hasselblad V, et al. Efficacy and bleeding complications among patients randomized to enoxaparin or unfractionated heparin for antithrombin therapy in non–ST-Segment elevation acute coronary syndromes: a systematic overview. *JAMA* 2004;292:89-96.
106. Hamm CW, Bassand JP, Agewall S, et al. ESC guidelines for the management of acute coronary syndromes in patients presenting without persistent ST-segment elevation: the Task Force for the Management of Acute Coronary Syndromes (ACS) in Patients Presenting without Persistent ST-Segment Elevation. European Society of Cardiology (ESC). *Eur Heart J* 2011;32:2999-3054.
107. Ferguson JJ, Califf RM, Antman EM, et al. Enoxaparin vs unfractionated heparin in high-risk patients with non–ST-segment elevation acute coronary syndromes managed with an intended early invasive strategy: primary results of the SYNERGY randomized trial. *JAMA* 2004;292:45-54.
108. Drouet L, Bal dit Sollier C, Martin J. Adding intravenous unfractionated heparin to standard enoxaparin causes excessive anticoagulation not detected by activated clotting time: results of the STACK-on to ENOXaparin (STACKENOX) study. *Am Heart J* 2009;158:177-184.
109. Chesebro JH. Direct thrombin inhibitor therapy in the cardiovascular patient. *Am J Health Syst Pharm* 2003;60(Suppl 5):S19-S26.
110. Direct thrombin inhibitors in acute coronary syndromes and during percutaneous coronary intervention: design of a meta-analysis based on individual patient data. Direct Thrombin Inhibitor Trialists' Collaborative Group. *Am Heart J* 2001;141:E2.
111. Gladwell TD. Bivalirudin: a direct thrombin inhibitor. *Clin Ther* 2002;24:38-58.
112. Direct thrombin inhibitors in acute coronary syndromes: principal results of a meta-analysis based on individual patients' data. *Lancet* 2002;359:294-302.
113. Lincoff AM, Bittl JA, Harrington RA, et al. Bivalirudin and provisional glycoprotein IIb/IIIa blockade compared with heparin and planned glycoprotein IIb/IIIa blockade during percutaneous coronary intervention: REPLACE-2 randomized trial. *JAMA* 2003;289:853-863.
114. Stone GW, McLaurin BT, Cox DA, et al. Bivalirudin for patients with acute coronary syndromes. *N Engl J Med* 2006;355:2203-2216.
115. White HD, Chew DP, Hoekstra JW, et al. Safety and efficacy of switching from either unfractionated heparin or enoxaparin to bivalirudin in patients with non–ST-segment elevation acute coronary syndromes managed with an invasive strategy: results from the ACUITY (Acute Catheterization and Urgent Intervention Triage strategY) trial. *J Am Coll Cardiol* 2008;51:1734-1741.
116. Gibson CM, Ten Y, Murphy SA, et al. Association of prerandomization anticoagulant switching with bleeding in the setting of percutaneous coronary intervention (a REPLACE-2 analysis). *Am J Cardiol* 2007;99:1687-1690.
117. White HD, Ohman EM, Lincoff AM, et al. Safety and efficacy of bivalirudin with and without glycoprotein IIb/IIIa inhibitors in patients with acute coronary syndromes undergoing percutaneous coronary intervention: 1-year results from the ACUITY (Acute Catheterization and Urgent Intervention Triage strategY) trial. *J Am Coll Cardiol* 2008;52: 807-814.
118. Pinto DS, Stone GW, Shi C, et al. Economic evaluation of bivalirudin with or without glycoprotein IIb/IIIa inhibition versus heparin with routine glycoprotein IIb/IIIa inhibition for early invasive management of acute coronary syndromes. *J Am Coll Cardiol* 2008;52:1758-1768.
119. Kastrati A, Neumann FJ, Mehilli J, et al. Bivalirudin versus unfractionated heparin during percutaneous coronary intervention. *N Engl J Med* 2008;359:688-696.
120. Kastrati A, Neumann FJ, Schulz S, et al. Abciximab and heparin versus bivalirudin for non–ST-elevation myocardial infarction. *N Engl J Med* 2011;365:1980-1989.
121. Gustafsson D. Oral direct thrombin inhibitors in clinical development. *J Intern Med* 2003;254:322-334.
122. Wallentin L, Wilcox RG, Weaver WD, et al. Oral ximelagatran for secondary prophylaxis after myocardial infarction: the ESTEEM randomised controlled trial. *Lancet* 2003;362:789-797.
123. Lee WM, Larrey D, Olsson R, et al. Hepatic findings in long-term clinical trials of ximelagatran. *Drug Saf* 2005;28:351-370.
124. Bauer KA. Fondaparinux sodium: a selective inhibitor of factor Xa. *Am J Health Syst Pharm* 2001;58(Suppl 2):S14-S17.
125. Turpie AG. Fondaparinux: a factor Xa inhibitor for antithrombotic therapy. *Expert Opin Pharmacother* 2004;5:1373-1384.
126. Yusuf S, Mehta SR, Chrolavicius S, et al. Comparison of fondaparinux and enoxaparin in acute coronary syndromes. *N Engl J Med* 2006;354:1464-1476.
127. Anderson JA, Hirsh J, Yusuf S, et al. Comparison of the anticoagulant intensities of fondaparinux and enoxaparin in the Organization to Assess Strategies in Acute Ischemic Syndromes (OASIS)-5 trial. *J Thromb Haemost* 2010;8:243-249.
128. Sculpher MJ, Lozano-Ortega G, Sambrook J, et al. Fondaparinux versus enoxaparin in non–ST-elevation acute coronary syndromes: short-term cost and long-term cost-effectiveness using data from the Fifth Organization to Assess Strategies in Acute Ischemic Syndromes Investigators (OASIS-5) trial. *Am Heart J* 2009;157:845-852.
129. Yusuf S, Mehta SR, Chrolavicius S, et al. Effects of fondaparinux on mortality and reinfarction in patients with acute ST-segment elevation myocardial infarction: the OASIS-6 randomized trial. *JAMA* 2006;295:1519-1530.
130. Steg PG, Jolly SS, Mehta SR, et al. Low-dose vs standard-dose unfractionated heparin for percutaneous coronary intervention in acute coronary syndromes treated with fondaparinux: the FUTURA/OASIS-8 randomized trial. *JAMA* 2010;304:1339-1349.
131. Sabatine MS, Antman EM, Widimsky P, et al. Otamixaban for the treatment of patients with non–ST-elevation acute coronary syndromes (SEPIA-ACS1 TIMI 42): a randomised, double-blind, active-controlled, phase 2 trial. *Lancet* 2009;374:787-795.
132. Alexander JH, Lopes RD, James S, et al. Apixaban with antiplatelet therapy after acute coronary syndrome. *N Engl J Med* 2011;365:699-708.
133. Mega JL, Braunwald E, Wiviott SD, et al. Rivaroxaban in patients with a recent acute coronary syndrome. *N Engl J Med* 2012;366:9-19.
134. Morrow DA, Antman EM, Murphy SA, et al. The Risk Score Profile: a novel approach to characterising the risk of populations enrolled in clinical studies. *Eur Heart J* 2004;25:1139-1145.
135. Weitz JI, Bates SM. New anticoagulants. *J Thromb Haemost* 2005;3:1843-1853.
136. Giugliano RP, Wiviott SD, Stone PH, et al. Recombinant nematode anticoagulant protein c2 in patients with non–ST-segment elevation acute coronary syndrome: the ANTHEM-TIMI-32 trial. *J Am Coll Cardiol* 2007;49:2398-2407.
137. Hagedorn I, Schmidbauer S, Pleines I, et al. Factor XIIa inhibitor recombinant human albumin Infestin-4 abolishes occlusive arterial thrombus formation without affecting bleeding. *Circulation* 2010;121:1510-1517.
138. Cohen MG, Purdy DA, Rossi JS, et al. First clinical application of an actively reversible direct factor IXa inhibitor as an anticoagulation strategy in patients undergoing percutaneous coronary intervention. *Circulation* 2010;122:614-622.
139. Effects of tissue plasminogen activator and a comparison of early invasive and conservative strategies in unstable angina and non–Q-wave myocardial infarction: results of the TIMI IIIB Trial. Thrombolysis in Myocardial Ischemia. *Circulation* 1994;89: 1545-1556.
140. Boden WE, O'Rourke RA, Crawford MH, et al. Outcomes in patients with acute non–Q-wave myocardial infarction randomly assigned to an invasive as compared with a conservative management strategy. Veterans Affairs Non–Q-Wave Infarction Strategies in Hospital (VANQWISH) Trial Investigators. *N Engl J Med* 1998;338: 1785-1792.

141. Invasive compared with non-invasive treatment in unstable coronary-artery disease: FRISC II prospective randomised multicentre study. FRagmin and Fast Revascularisation during InStability in Coronary artery disease Investigators. *Lancet* 1999;354:708-715.
142. Cannon CP, McCabe CH, Borzak S, et al; TIMI 12 Investigators. Randomized trial of an oral platelet glycoprotein IIb/IIIa antagonist, sibrafiban, in patients after an acute coronary syndrome: results of the TIMI 12 trial. *Circulation* 1998;97:340-349.
143. Mehta SR, Cannon CP, Fox KA, et al. Routine versus selective invasive strategies in patients with acute coronary syndromes: a collaborative meta-analysis of the randomized trials. *JAMA* 2005;293:2908-2917.
144. Biondi-Zoccai GG, Abbate A, Agostoni P, et al. Long-term benefits of an early invasive management in acute coronary syndromes depend on intracoronary stenting and aggressive antiplatelet treatment: a metaregression. *Am Heart J* 2005;149:504-511.
145. Bavry AA, Kumbhani DJ, Quiroz R, et al. Invasive therapy along with glycoprotein IIb/IIIa inhibitors and intracoronary stents improves survival in non–ST-segment elevation acute coronary syndromes: a meta-analysis and review of the literature. *Am J Cardiol* 2004;93:830-835.
146. Sabatine MS, Morrow DA, Giugliano RP, et al. Implications of upstream glycoprotein IIb/IIIa inhibition and coronary artery stenting in the invasive management of unstable angina/non–ST-elevation myocardial infarction: a comparison of the Thrombolysis In Myocardial Infarction (TIMI) IIIB trial and the Treat angina with Aggrastat and determine Cost of Therapy with Invasive or Conservative Strategy (TACTICS)-TIMI 18 trial. *Circulation* 2004;109:874-880.
147. O'Donoghue M, Boden WE, Braunwald E, et al. Early invasive vs conservative treatment strategies in women and men with unstable angina and non–ST-segment elevation myocardial infarction: a meta-analysis. *JAMA* 2008;300:71-80.
148. Schellekens S, Verheugt FW. Hotline sessions of the 26th European Congress of Cardiology. *Eur Heart J* 2004;25:2164-2166.
149. Fox KA, Poole-Wilson P, Clayton TC, et al. 5-year outcome of an interventional strategy in non–ST-elevation acute coronary syndrome: the British Heart Foundation RITA 3 randomised trial. *Lancet* 2005;366:914-920.
150. Gibbons RJ, Abrams J, Chatterjee K, et al. ACC/AHA 2002 guideline update for the management of patients with chronic stable angina—summary article: a report of the American College of Cardiology/American Heart Association Task Force on practice guidelines (Committee on the Management of Patients with Chronic Stable Angina). *J Am Coll Cardiol* 2003;41:159-168.
151. Glickman SW, Boulding W, Staelin R, et al. A framework for quality improvement: an analysis of factors responsible for improvement at hospitals participating in the Can Rapid Risk Stratification of Unstable Angina Patients Suppress Adverse Outcomes with Early Implementation of the ACC/AHA Guidelines (CRUSADE) quality improvement initiative. *Am Heart J* 2007;154:1206-1220.
152. Giugliano RP, Camargo CA Jr, Lloyd-Jones DM, et al. Elderly patients receive less aggressive medical and invasive management of unstable angina: potential impact of practice guidelines. *Arch Intern Med* 1998;158:1113-1120.
153. Yan AT, Yan RT, Tan M, et al. Optimal medical therapy at discharge in patients with acute coronary syndromes: temporal changes, characteristics, and 1-year outcome. *Am Heart J* 2007;154:1108-1115.
154. Bagnall AJ, Yan AT, Yan RT, et al. Optimal medical therapy for non–ST-segment-elevation acute coronary syndromes: exploring why physicians do not prescribe evidence-based treatment and why patients discontinue medications after discharge. *Circ Cardiovasc Qual Outcomes* 2010;3:530-537.
155. Choudhry NK, Avorn J, Glynn RJ, et al. Full coverage for preventive medications after myocardial infarction. *N Engl J Med* 2011;365:2088-2097.
156. Halim SA, Mulgund J, Chen AY, et al. Use of guidelines-recommended management and outcomes among women and men with low-level troponin elevation: insights from CRUSADE. *Circ Cardiovasc Qual Outcomes* 2009;2:199-206.
157. Patel UD, Ou FS, Ohman EM, et al. Hospital performance and differences by kidney function in the use of recommended therapies after non–ST-elevation acute coronary syndromes. *Am J Kidney Dis* 2009;53:426-437.
158. Joynt KE, Huynh L, Amerena JV, et al. Impact of acute and chronic risk factors on use of evidence-based treatments in patients in Australia with acute coronary syndromes. *Heart* 2009;95:1442-1448.
159. Grimaldi-Bensouda L, Rossignol M, Aubrun E, et al. Agreement between patients' self-report and physicians' prescriptions on cardiovascular drug exposure: the PGRx database experience. *Pharmacoepidemiol Drug Saf* 2010;19:591-595.
160. Schnipper JL, Roumie CL, Cawthon C, et al. Rationale and design of the Pharmacist Intervention for Low Literacy in Cardiovascular Disease (PILL-CVD) study. *Circ Cardiovasc Qual Outcomes* 2010;3:212-219.
161. Lloyd-Jones DM, Hong Y, Labarthe D, et al. Defining and setting national goals for cardiovascular health promotion and disease reduction: the American Heart Association's strategic Impact Goal through 2020 and beyond. *Circulation* 2010;121:586-613.
162. Gluckman TJ, Sachdev M, Schulman SP, Blumenthal RS. A simplified approach to the management of non–ST-segment elevation acute coronary syndromes. *JAMA* 2005;293:349-357.
163. Jackevicius CA, Tu JV, Demers V, et al. Cardiovascular outcomes after a change in prescription policy for clopidogrel. *N Engl J Med* 2008;359:1802-1810.
164. Ho PM, Tsai TT, Wang TY, et al. Adverse events after stopping clopidogrel in post-acute coronary syndrome patients: insights from a large integrated healthcare delivery system. *Circ Cardiovasc Qual Outcomes* 2010;3:303-308.
165. Ho PM, Tsai TT, Maddox TM, et al. Delays in filling clopidogrel prescription after hospital discharge and adverse outcomes after drug-eluting stent implantation: implications for transitions of care. *Circ Cardiovasc Qual Outcomes* 2010;3:261-266.
166. Wright RS, Anderson JL, Adams CD, et al. 2011 ACCF/AHA focused update of the guidelines for the management of patients with unstable angina/ non–ST-elevation myocardial infarction (updating the 2007 guideline): a report of the American College of Cardiology Foundation/American Heart Association Task Force on Practice Guidelines. *Circulation* 2011;123:2022-2060.
167. Herman M, Donovan J, Tran M, et al. Use of β-blockers and effects on heart rate and blood pressure post-acute coronary syndromes: are we on target? *Am Heart J* 2009;158:378-385.
168. Grundy SM, Cleeman JI, Merz CN, et al. Implications of recent clinical trials for the National Cholesterol Education Program Adult Treatment Panel III guidelines. *Circulation* 2004;110:227-239.
169. Arai AE, Kimura T, Morimoto T, et al. Effect of early intensive statin therapy on regression of coronary atherosclerosis in patients with acute coronary syndrome: rationale for lower cholesterol target in diabetic patients: subanalysis of JAPAN-ACS Study. *J Am Coll Cardiol* 2009;Suppl A:A330.
170. Bae JH, Kwon TG, Kim K, et al. Rationale of decreasing LDL-cholesterol level <70 mg/dL in patients with coronary artery disease: intravascular ultrasound–virtual histology study. *JACC* 2009;Suppl A:A318.
171. Executive Summary of the Third Report of the National Cholesterol Education Program (NCEP) Expert Panel on Detection, Evaluation, and Treatment of High Blood Cholesterol in Adults (Adult Treatment Panel III). *JAMA* 2001;285:2486-2497.
172. Melloni C, Shah BR, Ou FS, et al. Lipid-lowering intensification and low-density lipoprotein cholesterol achievement from hospital admission to 1-year follow-up after an acute coronary syndrome event: results from the Medications ApplIed aNd SusTAINed Over Time (MAINTAIN) registry. *Am Heart J* 2010;160:1121-1129, e1121.
173. Javed U, Deedwania PC, Bhatt DL, et al. Use of intensive lipid-lowering therapy in patients hospitalized with acute coronary syndrome: an analysis of 65,396 hospitalizations from 344 hospitals participating in Get With The Guidelines (GWTG). *Am Heart J* 2010;160:1130-1136, e1131-1133.
174. Cannon CP, Braunwald E, McCabe CH, et al. Intensive versus moderate lipid lowering with statins after acute coronary syndromes. *N Engl J Med* 2004;350:1495-1504.
175. Ray KK, Cannon CP, McCabe CH, et al. Early and late benefits of high-dose atorvastatin in patients with acute coronary syndromes: results from the PROVE IT-TIMI 22 trial. *J Am Coll Cardiol* 2005;46:1405-1410.
176. Scirica BM, Morrow DA, Cannon CP, et al. Intensive statin therapy and the risk of hospitalization for heart failure after an acute coronary syndrome in the PROVE IT-TIMI 22 study. *J Am Coll Cardiol* 2006;47:2326-2331.
177. Giraldez RR, Giugliano RP, Mohanavelu S, et al. Baseline low-density lipoprotein cholesterol is an important predictor of the benefit of intensive lipid-lowering therapy: a PROVE IT-TIMI 22 (Pravastatin or Atorvastatin Evaluation and Infection Therapy-Thrombolysis In Myocardial Infarction 22) analysis. *J Am Coll Cardiol* 2008;52:914-920.
178. Ridker PM, Cannon CP, Morrow D, et al. C-reactive protein levels and outcomes after statin therapy. *N Engl J Med* 2005;352:20-28.
179. Cannon CP, Giugliano RP, Blazing MA, et al. Rationale and design of IMPROVE-IT (IMProved Reduction of Outcomes: Vytorin Efficacy International Trial): comparison of ezetimbe/simvastatin versus simvastatin monotherapy on cardiovascular outcomes in patients with acute coronary syndromes. *Am Heart J* 2008;156:826-832.
180. Hulten E, Jackson JL, Douglas K, et al. The effect of early, intensive statin therapy on acute coronary syndrome: a meta-analysis of randomized controlled trials. *Arch Intern Med* 2006;166:1814-1821.
181. Link A, Ayadhi T, Bohm M, Nickenig G. Rapid immunomodulation by rosuvastatin in patients with acute coronary syndrome. *Eur Heart J* 2006;27:2945-2955.
182. Pell JP, Haw S, Cobbe S, et al. Smoke-free legislation and hospitalizations for acute coronary syndrome. *N Engl J Med* 2008;359:482-491.
183. Pope CA 3rd, Burnett RT, Krewski D, et al. Cardiovascular mortality and exposure to airborne fine particulate matter and cigarette smoke: shape of the exposure-response relationship. *Circulation* 2009;120:941-948.
184. Chow CK, Jolly S, Rao-Melacini P, et al. Association of diet, exercise, and smoking modification with risk of early cardiovascular events after acute coronary syndromes. *Circulation* 2010;121:750-758.
185. Brown TM, Hernandez AF, Bittner V, et al. Predictors of cardiac rehabilitation referral in coronary artery disease patients: findings from the American Heart Association's Get With The Guidelines program. *J Am Coll Cardiol* 2009;54:515-521.
186. Phrommintikul A, Kuanprasert S, Wongcharoen W, et al. Influenza vaccination reduces cardiovascular events in patients with acute coronary syndrome. *Eur Heart J* 2011;32:1730-1735.
187. Kemp HG, Jr. Left ventricular function in patients with the anginal syndrome and normal coronary arteriograms. *Am J Cardiol* 1973;32:375-376.
188. Arbogast R, Bourassa MG. Myocardial function during atrial pacing in patients with angina pectoris and normal coronary arteriograms: comparison with patients having significant coronary artery disease. *Am J Cardiol* 1973;32:257-263.
189. Kaski JC. Pathophysiology and management of patients with chest pain and normal coronary arteriograms (cardiac syndrome X). *Circulation* 2004;109:568-572.
190. Kaski JC, Aldama G, Cosin-Sales J. Cardiac syndrome X: diagnosis, pathogenesis and management. *Am J Cardiovasc Drugs* 2004;4:179-194.
191. Ong P, Athanasiadis A, Hill S, et al. Coronary artery spasm as a frequent cause of acute coronary syndrome: the CASPAR (Coronary Artery Spasm in Patients with Acute Coronary Syndrome) study. *J Am Coll Cardiol* 2008;52:523-527.
192. Diver DJ, Bier JD, Ferreira PE, et al. Clinical and arteriographic characterization of patients with unstable angina without critical coronary arterial narrowing (from the TIMI-IIIA Trial). *Am J Cardiol* 1994;74:531-537.
193. Cannon RO 3rd, Epstein SE. "Microvascular angina" as a cause of chest pain with angiographically normal coronary arteries. *Am J Cardiol* 1988;61:1338-1343.
194. Turiel M, Galassi AR, Glazier JJ, et al. Pain threshold and tolerance in women with syndrome X and women with stable angina pectoris. *Am J Cardiol* 1987;60:503-507.
195. Crea F, Lanza GA. Angina pectoris and normal coronary arteries: cardiac syndrome X. *Heart* 2004;90:457-463.
196. Kaski JC, Russo G. Cardiac syndrome X: an overview. *Hosp Pract (Off Ed)* 2000;35:75-76, 79-82, 85-78 passim.
197. Cosin-Sales J, Pizzi C, Brown S, Kaski JC. C-reactive protein, clinical presentation, and ischemic activity in patients with chest pain and normal coronary angiograms. *J Am Coll Cardiol* 2003;41:1468-1474.

198. Pasceri V, Willerson JT, Yeh ET. Direct proinflammatory effect of C-reactive protein on human endothelial cells. *Circulation* 2000;102:2165-2168.

199. Valeriani M, Sestito A, Le Pera D, et al. Abnormal cortical pain processing in patients with cardiac syndrome X. *Eur Heart J* 2005;26:975-982.

200. Rosen SD, Paulesu E, Wise RJ, Camici PG. Central neural contribution to the perception of chest pain in cardiac syndrome X. *Heart* 2002;87:513-519.

201. Bugiardini R, Bairey Merz CN. Angina with "normal" coronary arteries: a changing philosophy. *JAMA* 2005;293:477-484.

202. Shaw LJ, Merz CN, Pepine CJ, et al. The economic burden of angina in women with suspected ischemic heart disease: results from the National Institutes of Health—National Heart, Lung, and Blood Institute–sponsored Women's Ischemia Syndrome Evaluation. *Circulation* 2006;114:894-904.

203. Kaski JC, Valenzuela Garcia LF. Therapeutic options for the management of patients with cardiac syndrome X. *Eur Heart J* 2001;22:283-293.

204. Chen JW, Lee WL, Hsu NW, et al. Effects of short-term treatment of nicorandil on exercise-induced myocardial ischemia and abnormal cardiac autonomic activity in microvascular angina. *Am J Cardiol* 1997;80:32-38.

205. Nalbantgil S, Altintig A, Yilmaz H, et al. The effect of trimetazidine in the treatment of microvascular angina. *Int J Angiol* 1999;8:40-43.

206. Kayikcioglu M, Payzin S, Yavuzgil O, et al. Benefits of statin treatment in cardiac syndrome-X1. *Eur Heart J* 2003;24:1999-2005.

207. Pizzi C, Manfrini O, Fontana F, Bugiardini R. Angiotensin-converting enzyme inhibitors and 3-hydroxy-3-methylglutaryl coenzyme A reductase in cardiac syndrome X: role of superoxide dismutase activity. *Circulation* 2004;109:53-58.

208. Manson JE, Hsia J, Johnson KC, et al. Estrogen plus progestin and the risk of coronary heart disease. *N Engl J Med* 2003;349:523-534.

209. Cox ID, Hann CM, Kaski JC. Low dose imipramine improves chest pain but not quality of life in patients with angina and normal coronary angiograms. *Eur Heart J* 1998;19:250-254.

210. Cannon RO 3rd, Quyyumi AA, Mincemoyer R, et al. Imipramine in patients with chest pain despite normal coronary angiograms. *N Engl J Med* 1994;330:1411-1417.

211. Sanderson JE, Woo KS, Chung HK, et al. The effect of transcutaneous electrical nerve stimulation on coronary and systemic haemodynamics in syndrome X. *Coron Artery Dis* 1996;7:547-552.

212. Eliasson T, Albertsson P, Hardhammar P, et al. Spinal cord stimulation in angina pectoris with normal coronary arteriograms. *Coron Artery Dis* 1993;4:819-827.

213. Eriksson BE, Tyni-Lenne R, Svedenhag J, et al. Physical training in syndrome X: physical training counteracts deconditioning and pain in syndrome X. *J Am Coll Cardiol* 2000;36:1619-1625.

214. Klimes I, Mayou RA, Pearce MJ, et al. Psychological treatment for atypical non-cardiac chest pain: a controlled evaluation. *Psychol Med* 1990;20:605-611.

215. Mayou RA, Bryant BM, Sanders D, et al. A controlled trial of cognitive behavioural therapy for non-cardiac chest pain. *Psychol Med* 1997;27:1021-1031.

216. van Peski-Oosterbaan AS, Spinhoven P, van Rood Y, et al. Cognitive-behavioral therapy for noncardiac chest pain: a randomized trial. *Am J Med* 1999;106:424-429.

217. Potts SG, Lewin R, Fox KA, Johnstone EC. Group psychological treatment for chest pain with normal coronary arteries. *QJM* 1999;92:81-86.

218. Lange RA, Hillis LD. Cardiovascular complications of cocaine use. *N Engl J Med* 2001;345:351-358.

219. Carrillo X, Curos A, Muga R, et al. Acute coronary syndrome and cocaine use: 8-year prevalence and inhospital outcomes. *Eur Heart J* 2011;32:1244-1250.

220. Diabetes data & trends: Available at http://apps.nccd.cdc.gov/DDTSTRS/default.aspx.

221. Franklin K, Goldberg RJ, Spencer F, et al. Implications of diabetes in patients with acute coronary syndromes. The Global Registry of Acute Coronary Events. *Arch Intern Med* 2004;164:1457-1463.

222. McGuire DK, Newby LK, Bhapkar MV, et al. Association of diabetes mellitus and glycemic control strategies with clinical outcomes after acute coronary syndromes. *Am Heart J* 2004;147:246-252.

223. Donahoe SM, Stewart GC, McCabe CH, et al. Diabetes and mortality following acute coronary syndromes. *JAMA* 2007;298:765-775.

224. Feinberg MS, Schwartz R, Tanne D, et al. Impact of the metabolic syndrome on the clinical outcomes of non-clinically diagnosed diabetic patients with acute coronary syndrome. *Am J Cardiol* 2007;99:667-672.

225. Deedwania P, Kosiborod M, Barrett E, et al. Hyperglycemia and acute coronary syndrome: a scientific statement from the American Heart Association Diabetes Committee of the Council on Nutrition, Physical Activity, and Metabolism. *Circulation* 2008;117:1610-1619.

226. Invasive compared with non-invasive treatment in unstable coronary-artery disease: FRISC II prospective randomised multicentre study. FRagmin and Fast Revascularisation during InStability in Coronary artery disease Investigators [see comments]. *Lancet* 1999;354:708-715.

227. Januzzi JL, Cannon CP, DiBattiste PM, et al. Effects of renal insufficiency on early invasive management in patients with acute coronary syndromes (The TACTICS-TIMI 18 Trial). *Am J Cardiol* 2002;90:1246-1249.

228. Kip KE, Faxon DP, Detre KM, et al. Coronary angioplasty in diabetic patients: the National Heart, Lung, and Blood Institute Percutaneous Transluminal Coronary Angioplasty Registry. *Circulation* 1996;94:1818-1825.

229. Lincoff AM, Califf RM, Moliterno DJ, et al. Complementary clinical benefits of coronary-artery stenting and blockade of platelet glycoprotein IIb/IIIa receptors: Evaluation of Platelet IIb/IIIa Inhibition in Stenting Investigators. *N Engl J Med* 1999;341:319-327.

230. Worthley MI, Holmes AS, Willoughby SR, et al. The deleterious effects of hyperglycemia on platelet function in diabetic patients with acute coronary syndromes mediation by superoxide production, resolution with intensive insulin administration. *J Am Coll Cardiol* 2007;49:304-310.

231. Influence of diabetes on 5-year mortality and morbidity in a randomized trial comparing CABG and PTCA in patients with multivessel disease: the Bypass Angioplasty Revascularization Investigation (BARI). *Circulation* 1997;96:1761-1769.

232. Green Conaway DL, Enriquez JR, Barberena JE, et al. Assessment of and physician response to glycemic control in diabetic patients presenting with an acute coronary syndrome. *Am Heart J* 2006;152:1022-1027.

233. Alexander KP, Roe MT, Chen AY, et al. Evolution in cardiovascular care for elderly patients with non–ST-segment elevation acute coronary syndromes: results from the CRUSADE National Quality Improvement Initiative. *J Am Coll Cardiol* 2005;46:1479-1487.

234. Krumholz HM, Radford MJ, Ellerbeck EF, et al. Aspirin in the treatment of acute myocardial infarction in elderly Medicare beneficiaries: patterns of use and outcomes. *Circulation* 1995;92:2841-2847.

235. Krumholz HM, Radford MJ, Wang Y, et al. National use and effectiveness of β-blockers for the treatment of elderly patients after acute myocardial infarction: National Cooperative Cardiovascular Project. *JAMA* 1998;280:623-629.

236. Stone PH, Thompson B, Anderson HV, et al. Influence of race, sex, and age on management of unstable angina and non–Q-wave myocardial infarction: the TIMI III registry. *JAMA* 1996;275:1104-1112.

237. Nadelmann J, Frishman WH, Ooi WL, et al. Prevalence, incidence and prognosis of recognized and unrecognized myocardial infarction in persons aged 75 years or older: the Bronx Aging Study. *Am J Cardiol* 1990;66:533-537.

238. Lakatta E, Gerstenblith G, Weisfeldt M. The aging heart: structure, function and disease. In Braunwald E, editor: *Heart disease*. Philadelphia, 1997, WB Saunders, pp 1687-1673.

239. Gerstenblith G. *Cardiovascular disease in the elderly*. Totowa, NJ, 2005, Humana Press.

240. Lernfelt B, Wikstrand J, Svanborg A, Landahl S. Aging and left ventricular function in elderly healthy people. *Am J Cardiol* 1991;68:547-549.

241. Patel MR, Roe MT. Pharmacological treatment of elderly patients with acute coronary syndromes without persistent ST segment elevation. *Drugs Aging* 2002;19:633-646.

242. Cahalan MK, Hashimoto Y, Aizawa K, et al. Elderly, conscious patients have an accentuated hypotensive response to nitroglycerin. *Anesthesiology* 1992;77:646-655.

243. Alexander KP, Chen AY, Roe MT, et al. Excess dosing of antiplatelet and antithrombin agents in the treatment of non–ST-segment elevation acute coronary syndromes. *JAMA* 2005;294:3108-3116.

244. Collinson J, Flather MD, Fox KA, et al. Clinical outcomes, risk stratification and practice patterns of unstable angina and myocardial infarction without ST elevation: Prospective Registry of Acute Ischaemic Syndromes in the UK (PRAIS-UK). *Eur Heart J* 2000;21:1450-1457.

245. Nasser TK, Fry ET, Annan K, et al. Comparison of six-month outcome of coronary artery stenting in patients < 65, 65–75, and > 75 years of age. *Am J Cardiol* 1997;80:998-1001.

246. Weyrens FJ, Goldenberg I, Mooney JF, et al. Percutaneous transluminal coronary angioplasty in patients aged > or = 90 years. *Am J Cardiol* 1994;74:397-398.

247. Morrison DA, Bies RD, Sacks J. Coronary angioplasty for elderly patients with "high risk" unstable angina: short-term outcomes and long-term survival. *J Am Coll Cardiol* 1997;29:339-344.

248. Thompson RC, Holmes DR Jr, Gersh BJ, et al. Percutaneous transluminal coronary angioplasty in the elderly: early and long-term results. *J Am Coll Cardiol* 1991;17:1245-1250.

249. Trial of invasive versus medical therapy in elderly patients with chronic symptomatic coronary-artery disease (TIME): a randomised trial. *Lancet* 2001;358:951-957.

250. Bach RG, Cannon CP, DiBattiste PM, et al. Enhanced benefit of early invasive management of acute coronary syndromes in the elderly: results from TACTICS-TIMI 18. *Circulation* 2001;104:548.

251. Peterson ED, Jollis JG, Bebchuk JD, et al. Changes in mortality after myocardial revascularization in the elderly: the national Medicare experience. *Ann Intern Med* 1994;121:919-927.

252. Williams MA, Fleg JL, Ades PA, et al. Secondary prevention of coronary heart disease in the elderly (with emphasis on patients > or = 75 years of age): an American Heart Association scientific statement from the Council on Clinical Cardiology Subcommittee on Exercise, Cardiac Rehabilitation, and Prevention. *Circulation* 2002;105:1735-1743.

253. Thom T, Hasse N, Rosamond W, et al. Heart disease and stroke statistics—2006 update. *Circulation* 2006;113:e85-e151.

254. Lerner DJ, Kannel WB. Patterns of coronary heart disease morbidity and mortality in the sexes: a 26-year follow-up of the Framingham population. *Am Heart J* 1986;111:383-390.

255. Bairey Merz CN, Shaw LJ, Reis SE, et al. Insights from the NHLBI-sponsored Women's Ischemia Syndrome Evaluation (WISE) study. Part II: gender differences in presentation, diagnosis, and outcome with regard to gender-based pathophysiology of atherosclerosis and macrovascular and microvascular coronary disease. *J Am Coll Cardiol* 2006;47:S21-S29.

256. Pepine CJ, Kerensky RA, Lambert CR, et al. Some thoughts on the vasculopathy of women with ischemic heart disease. *J Am Coll Cardiol* 2006;47:S30-S35.

257. Rautaharju PM, Kooperberg C, Larson JC, LaCroix A. Electrocardiographic abnormalities that predict coronary heart disease events and mortality in postmenopausal women: the Women's Health Initiative. *Circulation* 2006;113:473-480.

258. Rautaharju PM, Kooperberg C, Larson JC, LaCroix A. Electrocardiographic predictors of incident congestive heart failure and all-cause mortality in postmenopausal women: the Women's Health Initiative. *Circulation* 2006;113:481-489.

259. Morise AP, Diamond GA. Comparison of the sensitivity and specificity of exercise electrocardiography in biased and unbiased populations of men and women. *Am Heart J* 1995;130:741-747.

260. Morise AP, Diamond GA, Detrano R, Bobbio M. Incremental value of exercise electrocardiography and thallium-201 testing in men and women for the presence and extent of coronary artery disease. *Am Heart J* 1995;130:267-276.

261. Handberg E, Johnson BD, Arant CB, et al. Impaired coronary vascular reactivity and functional capacity in women: results from the NHLBI Women's Ischemia Syndrome Evaluation (WISE) study. *J Am Coll Cardiol* 2006;47:S44-S49.

262. Shaw LJ, Olson MB, Kip K, et al. The value of estimated functional capacity in estimating outcome: results from the NHBLI-sponsored Women's Ischemia Syndrome Evaluation (WISE) study. *J Am Coll Cardiol* 2006;47:S36-S43.

263. Shaw LJ, Miller DD, Romeis JC, et al. Gender differences in the noninvasive evaluation and management of patients with suspected coronary artery disease. *Ann Intern Med* 1994;120:559-566.

264. Hochman JS, McCabe CH, Stone PH, et al. Outcome and profile of women and men presenting with acute coronary syndromes: a report from TIMI IIIB. TIMI Investigators. Thrombolysis in Myocardial Infarction. *J Am Coll Cardiol* 1997;30:141-148.

265. Daly C, Clemens F, Lopez Sendon JL, et al. Gender differences in the management and clinical outcome of stable angina. *Circulation* 2006;113:490-498.

266. Jacobs AK, Kelsey SF, Brooks MM, et al. Better outcome for women compared with men undergoing coronary revascularization: a report from the bypass angioplasty revascularization investigation (BARI). *Circulation* 1998;98:1279-1285.

267. Li TY, Rana JS, Manson JE, et al. Obesity as compared with physical activity in predicting risk of coronary heart disease in women. *Circulation* 2006;113:499-506.

268. Brosius FC 3rd, Hostetter TH, Kelepouris E, et al. Detection of chronic kidney disease in patients with or at increased risk of cardiovascular disease: a science advisory from the American Heart Association Kidney and Cardiovascular Disease Council; the Councils on High Blood Pressure Research, Cardiovascular Disease in the Young, and Epidemiology and Prevention; and the Quality of Care and Outcomes Research Interdisciplinary Working Group: developed in collaboration with the National Kidney Foundation. *Circulation* 2006;114:1083-1087.

269. Fox CS, Muntner P, Chen AY, et al. Use of evidence-based therapies in short-term outcomes of ST-segment elevation myocardial infarction and non–ST-segment elevation myocardial infarction in patients with chronic kidney disease: a report from the National Cardiovascular Data Acute Coronary Treatment and Intervention Outcomes Network registry. *Circulation* 2010;121:357-365.

CH
9

NON–ST-SEGMENT ELEVATION ACUTE CORONARY SYNDROMES

ST-Segment Elevation Myocardial Infarction

Frederick G. Kushner and Eric R. Bates

OVERVIEW, 178

PRE–ST-SEGMENT ELEVATION MYOCARDIAL
INFARCTION MANAGEMENT, 178

PREHOSPITAL MANAGEMENT, 178

Symptom Recognition, 178
Out-of-Hospital Arrest, 179
Emergency Medical Services and Systems of Care, 179
Prehospital Fibrinolysis, 179
Prehospital Destination Protocols, 179

EMERGENCY DEPARTMENT MANAGEMENT, 179

Patient Triage, 179
Patient Evaluation, 180

EARLY RISK ASSESSMENT, 181

Medications Used in the Acute Phase, 181
Reperfusion Therapy, 184

HOSPITAL MANAGEMENT, 190

Location, 190
Routine Measures, 192
Medications, 192
Hemodynamic Disturbances, 193
Mechanical Complications, 196
Arrhythmias, 198
Recurrent Chest Pain, 199

Other Complications, 200
Hemorrhagic Complications, 201
Coronary Artery Bypass Surgery, 202
Risk Stratification, 202

LONG-TERM MANAGEMENT, 204

Risk Factor Control, 204
Medications, 206
Functional Status, 207

REFERENCES, 207

Overview

ST-segment elevation myocardial infarction (STEMI) is a significant health problem in industrialized countries and is becoming an increasingly significant problem in developing countries. STEMI is a clinical syndrome defined by characteristic symptoms of myocardial ischemia in association with electrocardiographic (ECG) ST-segment changes (usually elevation) indicative of the occlusion of a major epicardial coronary artery. The incidence of STEMI varies according to the database examined (Table 10-1).[1] STEMI comprised approximately 40% of all MI presentations in the first two quarters of 2009 at hospitals participating in the Acute Coronary Treatment and Intervention Outcomes Network Registry (ACTION)–Get With the Guidelines (GWTG). One third of patients will die within the first 24 hours of presentation, many by sudden death. In the past few decades, the mortality rate from STEMI has steadily declined, but the rate of decline appears to have slowed. This appears to be due to both a fall in the incidence of STEMI and a reduction in the case fatality rate.[1-5] A significant increase in the use of evidence-based treatments from 1996 to 2007 in the Swedish registry of 61,238 patients with STEMI was associated with significantly improved in-hospital, 30-day, and 1-year mortality rates that was maintained after multivariate adjustment.[6] A progressive increase in the proportion of patients who present with non-STEMI has also occurred. This chapter follows the clinical course of the STEMI patient from before STEMI to management in the prehospital setting, the emergency department (ED), the hospital, and after hospital discharge.

Pre—ST-Segment Elevation Myocardial Infarction Management

Primary and secondary prevention interventions aimed at the risk factors associated with coronary heart disease (CHD) reduce the risk of STEMI.[7] These include smoking cessation,[8] diet, exercise, lipid management,[9] blood pressure (BP) control,[10] and diabetes management. Primary care providers should evaluate the presence and control of major risk factors in each patient every 3 to 5 years. The 10-year risk of developing symptomatic CHD should be calculated for all patients who have two or more major risk factors to assess the need for primary prevention strategies.[7] Patients with established CHD should be identified for secondary prevention, and patients with a CHD risk equivalent (e.g., diabetes mellitus, chronic kidney disease, peripheral vascular disease, 10-year risk >20% as calculated by the Framingham equations) should receive equally intensive risk factor intervention as those with clinically apparent CHD.[11]

Morbidity and mortality from STEMI can be reduced if patients and bystanders are taught to recognize symptoms early and activate emergency medical services (EMS). Patients with symptoms of STEMI should be transported to the nearest appropriate hospital by ambulance so they can receive cardiopulmonary resuscitation (CPR) and defibrillation, if necessary, as well as early reperfusion therapy. One in every 300 patients with chest pain transported to the ED by private vehicle goes into cardiac arrest en route.[12-16]

Although the traditional recommendation is for patients to take one sublingual nitroglycerin dose up to three doses, 5 minutes apart, before calling EMS, this recommendation has been modified to encourage earlier EMS contact.[17] If symptoms suggestive of STEMI are unimproved or worsen 5 minutes after one nitroglycerin dose, patients should immediately call 911.

Prehospital Management

Symptom Recognition

Early recognition of symptoms is the first step in the Chain of Survival.[14] Although most people recognize chest pain as a presenting symptom of STEMI, many are unaware of associated symptoms, such as arm pain, lower jaw pain, shortness of breath, and diaphoresis or anginal equivalents.[15] For a variety of reasons, the average patient does not seek medical attention for at least 1.5 hours after symptom onset.[16,17] Longer delay times occur among non-Hispanic blacks, older patients, Medicaid patients, and women.[18,19] Fully one third of patients with confirmed STEMI may present to the hospital with symptoms other than chest discomfort, and as many as half of all STEMI events are clinically silent or unrecognized by the patient.[20] A high index of suspicion for STEMI should be maintained when evaluating women, diabetics, older patients, and those with a history of heart failure, as well as patients complaining of chest discomfort but who have a permanent pacemaker or bundle branch block that may confound the recognition of STEMI on ECG.[21]

TABLE 10-1	Estimates of the Proportion of Patients with STEMI*	
MI REGISTRY		**% STEMI**
National Registry of Myocardial Infarction (NRMI-4)		29%
AHA Get with the Guidelines		32%
Global Registry of Acute Coronary Events (GRACE)		38%

*Primary and secondary diagnoses. Approximate 570,000 with non-STEMI and 540,000 with unstable angina.
AHA, American Heart Association; MI, myocardial infarction; STEMI, ST-segment elevation myocardial infarction.
Data from Heart Disease and Stroke Statistics 2009 update. *Circulation* 2009;119;e21-e181.

Out-of-Hospital Arrest

The majority of deaths from STEMI occur in the first 1 to 2 hours after symptom onset, usually from ventricular fibrillation (VF). Every minute the patient spends in VF decreases the chance of survival by 7% to 10%.[14] Key elements of the Chain of Survival include early activation of the EMS system, early CPR and defibrillation for those who need it, and advanced cardiac life support protocols.[14,22] Survival was doubled in the National Institutes of Health sponsored Public Access Defibrillation (PAD) trial by training lay volunteers to use an automatic external defibrillator (AED) in high-risk public settings.[23] Largely through the educational initiatives of the American Heart Association (AHA), 60% of Americans say they are familiar with CPR, 98% understand what an AED does, and 31.4% of out-of-hospital cardiac arrests receive bystander CPR.[1] With this in mind, family members of STEMI patients should be advised to take CPR and AED training. Because of the high prevalence of acute coronary artery occlusion in out-of-hospital cardiac arrest patients who are successfully resuscitated, especially those whose initial rhythm is VF in the setting of STEMI, the AHA 2010 CPR/emergency cardiovascular care guideline[24,25] recommends emergent coronary angiography with prompt primary percutaneous coronary intervention (PCI). Therapeutic hypothermia should be started as soon as possible in patients with STEMI and anoxic encephalopathy who survive out-of-hospital cardiac arrest.[26,27]

Emergency Medical Services and Systems of Care

The AHA and the American College of Cardiology (ACC) have worked together to promote systems of care for STEMI patients.[28] The AHA "Mission Lifeline" program recommendations include a multifaceted community-wide approach involving patient education, improvements in EMS and ED care, establishment of networks of referral (non-PCI capable) and receiving (PCI capable) hospitals, and coordinated advocacy efforts to work with payers and policymakers to implement these changes. Information about the initiative is available at the AHA website (www.americanheart.org). In 2006, the ACC launched its Door-to-Balloon (D2B; www.d2b.acc.org) and ACTION-GWTG registry through the National Cardiovascular Data Registry[29] to help participating hospitals reach the recommended time for primary PCI (P-PCI) within 90 minutes of first medical contact and implement guideline-recommended therapies. In addition, the American College of Cardiology Foundation (ACCF)/AHA Task Force for Practice Guidelines and the ACC/AHA Performance Measures have updated clinical practice guidelines and quality metrics. It is now recommended that each community develop a STEMI system of care that includes prehospital identification of STEMI patients and catheterization laboratory activation, destination protocols for STEMI receiving centers, and transfer protocols for high-risk STEMI patients who are P-PCI candidates, are fibrinolytic ineligible, or are in cardiogenic shock.[30] To minimize time to treatment, particularly for cardiopulmonary arrest, many communities allow volunteers and/or firefighters and other first-aid providers to function as first responders, providing CPR and early defibrillation with an AED until EMS arrives. The EMS ambulance response is a tiered system. The basic EMT level includes first aid and early defibrillation with AEDs. Other units are staffed by paramedics or other intermediate-level EMTs who can give basic care, start intravenous (IV) lines, intubate, and administer medications. In some systems, the advanced providers can also perform a 12-lead ECG, provide external pacing for symptomatic bradycardia, and use other techniques. Some high-performance EMS systems have only advanced life support–staffed ambulances.

Prehospital EMS providers should administer 162 to 325 mg of chewable aspirin, unless contraindicated, to patients suspected to be having an STEMI. The use of 12-lead ECGs by paramedics to evaluate all patients with possible ischemic chest discomfort in the prehospital setting is strongly encouraged.[31] For patients with ECG evidence for STEMI, a reperfusion checklist may be relayed along with the ECG to a predetermined medical control facility or hospital.

Prehospital Fibrinolysis

Randomized, controlled trials have demonstrated the benefit of initiating fibrinolytic therapy as early as possible after the onset of STEMI.[32] Prehospital administration allows half of patients to be treated within 2 hours of symptom onset, when the greatest treatment benefit can be expected.[33] A French national registry has demonstrated lower 1-year mortality rates with prehospital fibrinolytic therapy than with in-hospital fibrinolysis or P-PCI (Figure 10-1).[34] However, a prehospital fibrinolytic program requires either a physician in the ambulance or a highly organized program with well-trained paramedics who can transmit the ECG to a medical command center with a medical director.

Prehospital Destination Protocols

Every community should have a written protocol that guides EMS personnel in determining where to take patients with suspected or confirmed STEMI (Figure 10-2).[30] In general, patients with suspected STEMI should be taken to the nearest PCI-capable hospital if the anticipated first medical contact to balloon or device time is within 90 minutes.[35] Patients with STEMI who present to, or are transported to, hospitals without PCI capability should be transported secondarily to a PCI-capable hospital if the anticipated first medical contact to balloon or device time is less that 120 minutes, especially patients with high-risk features who are candidates for P-PCI.[36,37] For patients presenting to a hospital without PCI capability, if the first medical contact to device time is anticipated to be greater than 120 minutes and there are no contraindications, fibrinolysis should be administered within 30 minutes of first medical contact. Secondary transport to a PCI-capable hospital—urgently after fibrinolysis for evidence of reperfusion failure or reocclusion[38] or within 3 to 24 hours as part of an invasive strategy—can then occur.[39]

Emergency Department Management

Patient Triage

The effectiveness of a variety of treatment options diminishes rapidly within the first several hours after symptom onset, so rapid triage is important.[40-42] The traditional ED evaluation of patients with chest pain relies heavily on the patient's history, physical examination, and ECG. All patients presenting to the ED with chest discomfort or other symptoms suggestive of STEMI should immediately be placed on a cardiac monitor with emergency resuscitation equipment nearby, including a defibrillator. An IV line should be started for rapid delivery of medications. An ECG should be performed and shown to an experienced emergency medicine physician within 10 minutes of ED arrival if one has not

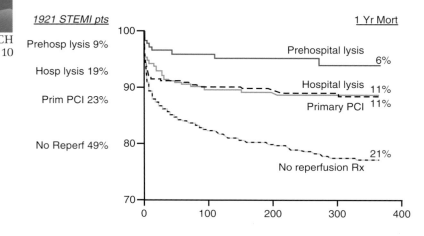

Impact of Prehospital Fibrinolysis on
in-Hospital and 1-Yr Outcome after STEMI:
French USIC 2000 Survey – 83% CCUs in Nov 2000

FIGURE 10-1 Age-adjusted Kaplan-Meier 1-year survival according to reperfusion strategy in the French USIC 2000 survey of 83% of coronary care units in November 2000. After adjustment by Cox multivariable analysis, prehospital fibrinolysis remained associated with improved survival. CCUs, coronary care units; Mort, mortality; PCI, percutaneous coronary intervention; Prim, primary; Reperf, reperfusion; Rx, pharmacologic therapy; STEMI, ST-segment elevation myocardial infarction. *(Reproduced from Danchin N, Blanchard D, Steg PG, et al. Impact of prehospital thrombolysis for acute myocardial infarction on 1-year outcome: Results from the French Nationwide USIC 2000 Registry. Circulation 2004;110:1909-15.)*

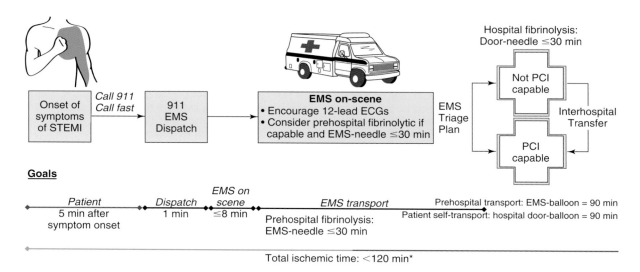

FIGURE 10-2 Options for transportation of patients with ST-segment elevation myocardial infarction (*STEMI*) and initial reperfusion treatment. Patients should call 911 to activate the emergency medical services (*EMS*) system. The goal is to keep total ischemic time less than 120 minutes from first medical contact to reperfusion. For patients transported to a hospital without percutaneous coronary intervention (*PCI*) capability, a decision should be made regarding transfer to a PCI-capable hospital for primary PCI. This is desirable when the first medical contact to balloon or device time is anticipated to be ≤120 minutes. If the time for transfer and PCI is >120 minutes, immediate fibrinolysis should be performed with a door-to-needle time ≤30 minutes. Transfer from a non–PCI-capable hospital to a PCI-capable hospital for angiography and reperfusion should be initiated for patients with cardiogenic shock, hemodynamic instability, continuing ischemia, or evidence of failed reperfusion or following fibrinolysis for routine angiography and PCI between 3 and 24 hours after the onset of ischemic symptoms. For patients presenting to, or transported to a PCI-capable hospital, the first medical contact to reperfusion by PCI should be ≤90 minutes. ECG, electrocardiogram. *(Modified from Armstrong PW, Collen D, Antman E. Fibrinolysis for acute myocardial infarction: The future is here and now. Circulation 2003;107:2533-2537.)*

already been sent from the ambulance. Advanced directives should be clarified, especially in elderly patients, to prevent treatment contrary to the patient's wishes. If STEMI is present, the decision whether the patient will be treated with fibrinolytic therapy or P-PCI should be made within the next 10 minutes. The goal should be to achieve a door-to-needle time within 30 minutes or a door-to-balloon time within 90 minutes, or interhospital transport with first medical contact to device time less that 120 minutes. If the initial ECG is not diagnostic, the patient remains symptomatic, and there is a high clinical suspicion for STEMI, serial ECGs at 5- to 10-minute intervals or continuous ST-segment monitoring should be performed. The choice of initial STEMI treatment should be made by the emergency medicine physician based on a predetermined, institution-specific, written protocol. If the

initial diagnosis and treatment plan are not clear, immediate cardiology consultation should be obtained.

Patient Evaluation

A targeted history should ascertain whether the patient has had prior stable or unstable angina, MI, coronary artery bypass graft (CABG) surgery, or PCI. Evaluation of the patient's symptoms should focus on chest discomfort, associated symptoms, sex- and age-related differences in presentation, hypertension, diabetes mellitus, possibility of aortic dissection, risk of bleeding, and clinical cerebrovascular disease (e.g., amaurosis fugax, facial/limb weakness or clumsiness, sensory loss, ataxia, or vertigo). A brief targeted physical examination should focus on potential complications of STEMI, such as CHF, cardiogenic shock, ventricular septal defect (VSD), or ischemic mitral regurgitation (MR). A differential diagnosis should be reviewed to exclude other conditions that may mimic STEMI, such as aortic dissection, pulmonary embolism, pericarditis, or cocaine ingestion.

The 12-lead ECG in the ED is at the center of the therapeutic decision pathway. The risk of death increases with the number of ECG leads that show ST-segment elevation, the sum of ST-segment deviation in 12 leads, and the presence of Q waves on presentation.[43,44] Important predictors of death include anterior location and left bundle branch block (LBBB). Patients with inferior STEMI should have right-sided leads obtained to screen for ST elevation suggestive of right ventricular (RV) infarction. Although patients without ST elevation should not be treated with fibrinolytic therapy, it may be used appropriately when there is marked ST-segment depression confined to leads V1 through V4 and accompanied by tall R waves in the right precordial leads and upright T waves indicative of a true posterior injury current.[45] Patients with new or presumed new LBBB and signs and symptoms of STEMI should also be considered for reperfusion therapy. LBBB with concordant ST-segment elevation of 0.1 mV or greater toward the major QRS deflection in at least one lead, or concordant ST-segment depression (with a dominant S wave) of 0.1 mV or greater in anterior precordial leads V1, V2, or V3, or discordant ST-segment elevation of 0.5 mV or greater in leads with a negative QRS suggest STEMI.[46] ST-segment elevation in lead aVR or V1 of 0.1 mV or greater when accompanied by ST-segment depression of 0.1 mV or greater in eight or more leads may indicate left main or multivessel obstruction.[47,48] ECG abnormalities that may mimic STEMI, such as hyperkalemia, pericarditis, acute cerebral hemorrhage, Brugada syndrome, left ventricular (LV) hypertrophy, tako-tsubo syndrome, Prinzmetal angina, or cocaine ingestion should be distinguished from STEMI by ECG changes, history, and physical examination.[45,49]

Laboratory measurements should include serial cardiac biomarkers (MB fraction of creatine kinase [CK-MB], troponins) for cardiac damage, complete blood count, platelet count, international normalized ratio (INR), activated partial thromboplastin time (aPTT), electrolytes, magnesium, blood urea nitrogen, creatinine, glucose, and serum lipids. Therapeutic decisions should not be delayed until these results are returned. Cardiac biomarkers are useful for confirming the diagnosis of STEMI, assessing the success of fibrinolytic therapy, estimating infarct size, and providing prognostic information.

Several imaging tests can be used to evaluate chest pain. Portable chest radiography should be performed but should not delay initiation of reperfusion therapy. Transthoracic and/or transesophageal echocardiography is quite useful for evaluating ventricular function and diagnosing mechanical complications. Contrast chest computed tomography (CT) may be required to exclude aortic dissection. CT angiography and magnetic resonance imaging are not indicated in patients with suspected STEMI. Radionuclide imaging is not indicated in the acute setting.

Early Risk Assessment

Assessing global risk allows the physician to integrate patient-specific characteristics into a semiquantitative score that can provide an estimate of a patient's prognosis, dictate the acuity and intensity of care needed, and triage to the appropriate location of care. Some examples of independent predictors for early death from STEMI include advanced age, higher Killip class, cardiac arrest, tachycardia, hypotension, anterior infarct location, prior infarction, diabetes, renal insufficiency, and positive initial cardiac markers and Q waves. The Thrombolysis in Myocardial Infarction (TIMI) risk score for STEMI (www.mdcalc.com/timi-risk-score-for-stemi) uses a combined clinical endpoint that includes death, stroke, and recurrent ischemia. Risk assessment should be a continuous process, repeated throughout the index hospitalization.

Medications Used in the Acute Phase

OXYGEN

Supplemental oxygen is appropriate for patients with STEMI who are hypoxemic (oxygen saturation <90%) and may have a salutary, albeit placebo, effect in others.[50] In patients with severe CHF, pulmonary edema, or mechanical complications, endotracheal intubation and mechanical ventilation may be required.

NITROGLYCERIN

Nitrates are indicated to relieve ischemic pain and control hypertension and as a vasodilator in patients with LV failure or coronary spasm. Clinical trial results have suggested only a modest benefit from nitroglycerin therapy. A pooled analysis of more than 60,000 patients treated with nitrate-like preparations intravenously or orally in 22 trials revealed a mortality rate of 7.7% in the control group and 7.4% in the nitrate group. These data are consistent with a possible small treatment effect of nitrates on mortality rates (three to four fewer deaths for every 1000 patients treated).[51]

Nitrates should be avoided in patients with initial systolic BP less than 90 mm Hg, marked bradycardia or tachycardia, and known or suspected RV infarction.[52] Phosphodiesterase inhibitors potentiate the hypotensive effects of nitrates by releasing nitric oxide.[53] Therefore, nitrates should not be administered to patients who have used a phosphodiesterase inhibitor for erectile dysfunction in the prior 24 to 48 hours.

Patients with ongoing ischemic discomfort should receive sublingual nitroglycerin (0.4 mg) every 5 minutes for a total of three doses, after which an assessment should be made about the need for IV administration. A useful IV regimen uses an initial infusion rate of 5 to 10 µg/min with increases of 5 to 20 µg/min until symptoms are relieved, or mean arterial BP is reduced by 10% of its baseline level in normotensive patients and up to 30% in hypertensive patients. In no case should the systolic pressure be brought below 90 mm Hg or drop 30 mm Hg below baseline. In view of their marginal treatment benefits, nitrates should not be used if hypotension limits the administration of β-blockers or angiotensin-converting enzyme (ACE) inhibitors, which have more powerful salutary effects.

ANALGESIA

The clinician should focus on two aspects of pain management: acute relief of the symptoms of ongoing myocardial ischemia and necrosis, and the general relief of anxiety and apprehension that frequently exacerbate pain. Pain, which may be severe in the acute phase of STEMI, contributes to the hyperadrenergic state that has been implicated as having a role in plaque fissuring and thrombus propagation, and in reducing the threshold for VF.

The tendency to underdose patients should be avoided. Control of cardiac pain typically is accomplished with a combination of nitrates, opiate analgesic agents, oxygen, and β-blockers. Morphine sulfate has remained the analgesic agent of choice for STEMI patients. The dose required varies in relation to age and body size as well as BP and heart rate. Morphine sulfate (2 to 4 mg intravenously with increments of 2 to 8 mg repeated at 5- to 15-minute intervals) may be given to a total dose of 10 to 30 mg as necessary. Morphine administration is particularly helpful in acute pulmonary edema, for which it may promote peripheral arterial and venous dilation. An important consideration when using IV nitrates is not to lower BP to a level that would preclude adequate dosing of morphine.

Side effects of morphine administration, such as hypotension, can be minimized by keeping the patient supine and elevating the lower extremities if systolic pressure drops below 100 mm Hg. The concomitant use of atropine in 0.5-mg doses intravenously may be helpful in reducing the excessive vagomimetic effects of morphine if significant bradycardia or hypotension occurs. Although respiratory depression is relatively uncommon, the respiration rate should be monitored, particularly as cardiovascular status improves. The narcotic-reversing agent naloxone, 0.4 to 2 mg intravenously every 3 minutes up to 10 mg, can reverse the effects of morphine if respiratory compromise occurs. Nausea and vomiting, which are potential side effects of large doses of morphine, may be treated with a phenothiazine. The use of nonsteroidal antiinflammatory drugs (NSAIDs), both nonselective as well as cyclooxygenase-2–selective agents, except for aspirin, should not be administered during hospitalization for STEMI because of the increased risk of death, reinfarction, hypertension, heart failure, and myocardial rupture.[54]

ANTIPLATELET AGENTS

Aspirin

In the Second International Study of Infarct Survival (ISIS-2),[55] aspirin reduced 35-day mortality rate by 23%. When aspirin was combined with streptokinase, the relative reduction in mortality rate was 42%. A meta-analysis demonstrated that aspirin reduced coronary reocclusion and recurrent ischemic events after fibrinolytic therapy with either streptokinase or alteplase.[56] The initial dose should be 162 to 325 mg (325 mg preferred for P-PCI). A maintenance dose of 81 mg daily should be continued indefinitely. This dose has been found to be as effective as higher doses and with less toxicity.[57,58] Aspirin suppositories (300 mg) can be used safely for patients with severe nausea and vomiting or severe upper gastrointestinal problems. In patients with true aspirin hypersensitivity (e.g., hives, nasal polyps, bronchospasm, anaphylaxis), clopidogrel may be substituted with at least equal effectiveness if desensitization is not pursued.[59] The use of ibuprofen or other NSAIDs may limit the cardioprotective effect of aspirin.

Clopidogrel

The Clopidogrel and Metoprolol in Myocardial Infarction Trial (COMMIT)/Second Chinese Cardiac Study (CCS-2) demonstrated a 13% reduction in death, MI, and stroke in medically managed patients treated within 12 hours of symptom onset with clopidogrel 75 mg daily.[60] The Clopidogrel as Adjunctive Reperfusion Therapy (CLARITY)-TIMI 28 trial demonstrated a 20% reduction in death, MI, and urgent revascularization in medically managed patients treated with a 300-mg loading dose of clopidogrel and a 75-mg daily maintenance dose as part of an early invasive strategy in patients younger than 75 years (Figure 10-3).[61] Neither trial showed an increase in major bleeding or intracranial hemorrhage (ICH). Therefore, for patients receiving fibrinolysis or no reperfusion therapy, dual antiplatelet therapy with aspirin and clopidogrel (with a loading dose of 300 mg in patients <75 years) is recommended. A loading dose of 600 mg is recommended for P-PCI.[62] For patients on clopidogrel in whom CABG is planned, the drug should be withheld for at least 5 days (preferably 7 days) unless the urgent need for revascularization outweighs the risk of excess bleeding.[63]

Prasugrel

Prasugrel, a thienopyridine that achieves faster and greater platelet inhibition with less variability than clopidogrel, was superior to clopidogrel in STEMI patients in the Trial to Assess Improvement in Therapeutic Outcomes by Optimizing Platelet Inhibition with Prasugrel (TRITON)-TIMI 38 trial. All patients had planned PCI.[64,65] The difference in the primary endpoint was due to fewer nonfatal MIs. In a post hoc analysis,[65] patients with anterior MI seemed to benefit more from prasugrel. Patients 75 years or older, with body weight less than 60 kg or a history of stroke or transient ischemic attack, should not receive prasugrel. Prasugrel should be withheld if possible for 7 days before CABG or other major surgery.[30] Prasugrel has not been studied in the setting of fibrinolysis.

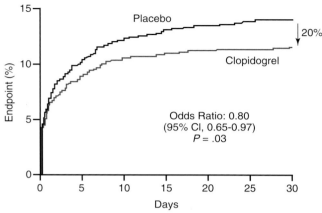

FIGURE 10-3 Cumulative incidence of the endpoint of death from cardiovascular causes, recurrent myocardial infarction (*MI*), or recurrent ischemia leading to the need for urgent revascularization. The odds ratio for this endpoint was significantly lower in the clopidogrel group than in the placebo group at 30 days (11.6% vs. 14.1%; odds ratio, 0.80; 95% confidence interval, 0.65 to 0.97; *P* = .03). (*Modified from Sabatine MS, Cannon CP, Gibson CM, et al: Addition of clopidogrel to aspirin and fibrinolytic therapy for myocardial infarction with ST segment elevation. N Engl J Med 2005;352:1179-1189.*)

Ticagrelor

Ticagrelor is a new non-thienopyridine-reversible $P2Y_{12}$ receptor antagonist that can be given orally and does not require hepatic metabolic conversion to an active form. In the Platelet Inhibition and Patient Outcomes (PLATO) trial, a 180-mg oral loading dose of ticagrelor followed by 90 mg twice daily was superior to clopidogrel, including a decrease in mortality rate.[66] Compared with clopidogrel, non-CABG bleeding rates were increased, but there was no significant difference in CABG related bleeding. Therefore, ticagrelor should be discontinued for at least 5 days before elective CABG.

Glycoprotein IIb/IIIa Inhibitors

Abciximab in combination with fibrinolytic therapy did not improve survival in two trials.[67,68] It did reduce reinfarction rates in patients younger than 75 years with anterior STEMI, but it increased ICH rates in older patients. IV glycoprotein (GP) IIb/IIIa receptor inhibitors have also been studied as supportive antiplatelet therapy in patients undergoing PCI. However, much of the evidence was accumulated prior to the era of combined dual antiplatelet and anticoagulant therapy. A number of trials have evaluated GP IIb/IIIa antagonists as adjuncts to oral antiplatelet therapy in P-PCI for STEMI.[69-75] These studies also looked at the timing of their administration. In light of the results of these and other trials, the current ACC/AHA guidelines have made the use of GP IIb/IIIa receptor antagonists (abciximab, high-dose tirofiban, and double-bolus eptifibatide) a class IIa recommendation if given at the time of P-PCI with or without stenting in selected patients with STEMI. It was suggested that the benefit would accrue more to patients with a large thrombus burden or patients who have not received adequate P2Y12 inhibitor loading.[30] Studies comparing the intracoronary and IV delivery of the agents have been performed, and additional trials are ongoing.[76,77]

ANTICOAGULANT AGENTS

Antithrombins

Unfractionated heparin (UFH) and low-molecular-weight heparin (LMWH) are antithrombins. They decrease the rates of infarct artery reocclusion, deep venous thrombosis, pulmonary embolism, LV mural thrombus formation, and cerebral embolization.

Effect of UFH in MI Trials

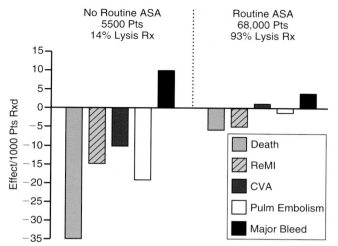

FIGURE 10-4 Effect of unfractionated heparin (*UFH*) in ST-segment elevation myocardial infarction (*MI*) trials. The treatment effect of UFH/1000 patients is shown for trials without routine aspirin (*ASA*) on the *left* and with routine ASA on the *right*. Benefits of UFH are plotted below the horizontal line and harm is plotted above the line. CVA, cerebrovascular accident; Pulm, pulmonary; ReMI, recurrent myocardial infarction; Rxd, treated. (*Modified from Collins R, Peto R, Baigent C, Sleight P: Aspirin, heparin, and fibrinolytic therapy in suspected acute myocardial infarction. N Engl J Med 1997;336:847-860.*)

Anticoagulation is recommended in patients not receiving reperfusion therapy because data from the prethrombolytic era demonstrated benefit in the absence of other interventions.[78]

Because streptokinase produces a systemic coagulopathy, additional antithrombin therapy with UFH offers the small advantage of only five lives saved per 1000 patients treated at a cost of one to two hemorrhagic strokes and three to five systemic bleeds (Figure 10-4).[78] Therapy is most useful in patients at high risk for systemic embolism, including patients with large or anterior MI, atrial fibrillation (AF), previous embolism, or known LV thrombus. With fibrin-specific agents (alteplase, reteplase, tenecteplase), UFH should be given intravenously with an aPTT target of 1.5 to 2.0 times control (50 to 70 seconds). A 60-U/kg bolus followed by a maintenance infusion of 12 U/kg/h (with a maximum of 4000 U bolus and 1000-U/h initial infusion) is recommended. During PCI for patients who did not receive prior UFH or fibrinolysis, a bolus dose of 70 to 100 U/kg with a target activated clotting time (ACT) of 250 to 300 seconds is recommended if no IV GP IIb/IIIa is used. If IV GP IIb/IIIa is used, the dose is reduced to a 50- to 70-U/kg bolus to achieve an ACT of 200 to 250 seconds. If the patients have received prior treatment with UFH, additional boluses should be given as needed during P-PCI to achieve the above goals. All patients should receive aspirin and an antiplatelet agent in addition to UFH.[30,78] Prolonged treatment with UFH beyond 48 hours may result in heparin-induced thrombocytopenia (HIT).

LMWH can be considered an acceptable alternative to UFH as ancillary therapy for patients younger than 75 years who are receiving fibrinolytic therapy, provided significant renal dysfunction (serum creatinine >2.5 mg/dL in men or >2.0 mg/dL in women) is not present. Enoxaparin (30 mg IV bolus followed 15 minutes later by 1.0 mg/kg subcutaneously [SC] every 12 hours until hospital discharge) used in combination with full-dose tenecteplase is the most comprehensively studied regimen in patients younger than 75 years (Figure 10-5).[79] However, older patients have an unacceptable excess rate of ICH with this dose.[79] In those patients, the initial IV bolus is eliminated and the SC dose is reduced to 0.75 mg/kg every 12 hours. When combined with clopidogrel, LMWH is associated with significantly improved rates of infarct artery patency and lower rates of death/MI compared with UFH.[80] Major bleeding occurred in 2.1% and 1.4% in the

LMWH vs. UFH arms, respectively.[80-82] Regardless of age, if the creatinine clearance is estimated to be less than 30 mL/min, the SC regimen is 1.0 mg/kg every 24 hours. For prior treatment with enoxaparin, if the last SC dose was administered at least 8 to 12 hours before planned PCI, an IV dose of 0.3 mg/kg should be given. If the last SC dose was administered within the prior 8 hours before PCI, no additional enoxaparin should be given.[68,83] Maintenance dosing with enoxaparin should be continued for the duration of the hospitalization or until revascularization. The use of enoxaparin in the setting of P-PCI was recently shown to be superior to UFH in terms of reducing ischemic events, with comparable rates of bleeding.[84] In a nonrandomized substudy of the Facilitated Intervention with Enhanced Reperfusion Speed to Stop Events (FINESSE) trial, enoxaparin seemed to be associated with a lower risk of adverse cardiovascular outcomes compared with UFH.[85]

Direct Thrombin Inhibitors

Direct thrombin inhibitors such as bivalirudin bind to the substrate recognition and the catalytic sites of thrombin. In doing so, they directly block the formation of fibrin from fibrinogen and inhibit the thrombin-induced component of platelet aggregation. In the Harmonizing Outcomes with Revascularization and Stents in Acute Myocardial Infarction (HORIZONS-AMI) trial, major adverse cardiac event rates were identical in the bivalirudin monotherapy and UFH plus GP IIb/IIIa arms, but there was a decrease in major bleeding and all-cause mortality with bivalirudin (3.4% vs. 4.8%; *P* = .03).[72] Concerns about the trial include its open label design, the administration of UFH before randomization in 66% of the patients in the bivalirudin arm, its definition of major bleeding, which included hematomas of 5 cm, and the composite primary endpoint of efficacy and safety. The occurrence of an increase in early stent thrombosis in the bivalirudin arm and the excess bleeding with UFH and GP IIb/IIIa inhibitors may have been related to the degree of platelet inhibition and the antithrombin activity associated with these treatments. Bivalirudin is an acceptable alternative to UFH and GP IIb/IIIa receptor blockers to support P-PCI with or without prior treatment with UFH, especially when there is an increased risk of bleeding complications.[30]

Bivalirudin is useful in patients with HIT and/or at a high risk of bleeding.[30,86] For patients who have received UFH, wait 30 minutes, then give a 0.75-mg/kg bolus, then 1.75 mg/kg/h infusion (reduce dose to 1 mg/kg/h in patients with creatine clearance of <30 mL/min) with aspirin and 600 mg clopidogrel. If no heparin was given, proceed immediately with the bolus and infusion.

Fondaparinux

Fondaparinux, a pentasaccharide indirect factor Xa inhibitor that is rarely used in the United States, was evaluated in the Sixth Organization to Assess Strategies in Acute Ischemic Syndromes (OASIS 6) trial.[87] The benefits of fondaparinux were confined to those receiving fibrinolytic therapy or not undergoing reperfusion therapy, for which there was less bleeding. No benefit and a trend toward harm were seen in patients undergoing P-PCI. The dose is 2.5 mg initially IV with subsequent SC injections of 2.5 mg once daily for the duration of the hospitalization (with serum creatinine <3.0 mg/dL).

β-BLOCKERS

β-Blockers diminish myocardial oxygen demand by reducing heart rate, systemic arterial pressure, and myocardial contractility. Reduction in heart rate prolongs the diastolic period and may augment perfusion to the subendocardium. In patients not receiving fibrinolytic therapy, early trials suggested reduction in infarct size[88] and mortality rate.[89] In patients receiving fibrinolytic therapy, recent trials have not found a mortality rate reduction,[90,91] although recurrent ischemia and reinfarction rates were reduced. It has also been suggested that β-blockers decrease ventricular arrhythmias and decrease the risk of intracerebral hemorrhage with lytic therapy. The evidence base for β-blocker therapy was

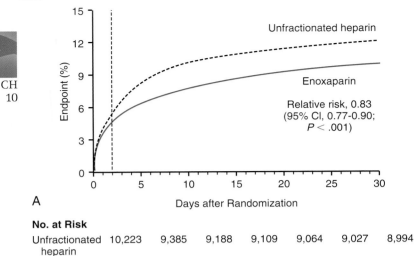

No. at Risk

Unfractionated heparin	10,223	9,385	9,188	9,109	9,064	9,027	8,994
Enoxaparin	10,256	9,595	9,460	9,362	9,301	9,263	9,234

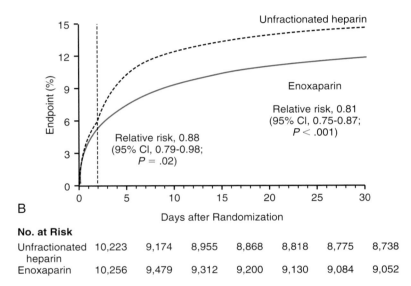

No. at Risk

Unfractionated heparin	10,223	9,174	8,955	8,868	8,818	8,775	8,738
Enoxaparin	10,256	9,479	9,312	9,200	9,130	9,084	9,052

FIGURE 10-5 Cumulative incidence of the primary endpoint (death or nonfatal myocardial infarction) and secondary endpoint (death, nonfatal myocardial infarction, or urgent revascularization). In **A,** the rate of the primary endpoint at 30 days was significantly lower in the enoxaparin group than in the unfractionated heparin group (9.9% vs. 12.0%; P < .001 by the log-rank test). The *dashed vertical line* indicates the comparison at day 2 (direct pharmacologic comparison), at which time a trend in favor of enoxaparin was seen. In **B,** the rate of the main secondary endpoint at 30 days was significantly lower in the enoxaparin group than in the unfractionated heparin group (11.7% vs. 14.5%; P < .001 by the log-rank test). The difference was already significant at 48 hours (6.1% in the unfractionated heparin group vs. 5.3% in the enoxaparin group; P = .02 by the log-rank test). The interval shown is the time (in 24-hour intervals) from randomization to an event or the last follow-up visit. CI, confidence interval. (*Modified from Antman EM, Morrow DA, McCabe CH, et al, for the ExTRACT-TIMI 25 Investigators: Enoxaparin versus unfractionated heparin with fibrinolysis for ST-elevated myocardial infarction. N Engl J Med 2006;354:1477-1488.*)

developed more than 25 years ago in a treatment environment that differs from contemporary practice. COMMIT/CCS-2 underscored the potential risk of administering IV β-blockers to patients with severe heart failure or cardiogenic shock.[92] The use of IV β-blockers is reasonable in patients who are hypertensive at the time of presentation and who do not have signs of heart failure, evidence of a low output state, or risk for the development of cardiogenic shock (age >70 years, systolic BP <120 mm Hg, sinus tachycardia >110 beats/min, heart rate <60 beats/min) or other relative contraindications, such as marked first-degree atrioventricular (AV) block, second- or third-degree AV block, or active asthma or reactive airway disease. Otherwise, oral β-blockers should be initiated in the first 24 hours, unless there are contraindications, and titrated as tolerated for the duration of the index hospitalization. Patients who cannot tolerate β-blockade in the first 24 hours (those with moderate or severe LV failure) should be reevaluated for therapy as secondary prevention. It is prudent to begin with metoprolol 25 to 50 mg (or its equivalent) every 6 hours, transitioning to a maximal dose of 200 mg/day orally, or the maximum tolerated dose. If bradycardia or hypotension occurs with therapy, isoproterenol 1 to 5 μg/min can be administered.

Reperfusion Therapy

GENERAL CONCEPTS

All STEMI patients should undergo rapid evaluation for reperfusion therapy and have a reperfusion strategy promptly implemented after contact with the medical system. Although rapid spontaneous reperfusion of the occluded infarct artery may occur, restoration of flow usually requires either fibrinolytic therapy or P-PCI. A system plan for triage and transfer should be in place (see Figure 10-2). Early, complete, and sustained infarct artery patency is a key determinant of both short- and long-term prognosis regardless of whether reperfusion is accomplished by fibrinolysis[33] or P-PCI.[93] Reperfusion therapy should be administered to patients with STEMI with symptom onset within the previous 12 hours and perhaps within 12 to 24 hours with clinical evidence of ongoing ischemia. P-PCI is the preferred method of reperfusion when it can be performed in a timely fashion by experienced operators. Every effort should be made to shorten the time from symptom onset to contact with the medical system and to implement a reperfusion strategy with the concept of medical system goals. These include a first medical contact-to-needle (or EMS-to-needle) time for fibrinolytic therapy within 30 minutes or a first medical contact-to-balloon (or EMS-to-balloon) time for P-PCI within 90 minutes in at least 75% of nontransferred patients with STEMI. These goals should not be understood as "ideal" times, but rather the longest times that should be considered acceptable in every appropriate patient unless there is a good reason for delay, such as uncertainty about the diagnosis, need for the evaluation and treatment of other life-threatening conditions (e.g., respiratory failure), or delays associated with the patient's informed choice to consider therapy. Transfer from a non–PCI-capable hospital to a PCI-capable hospital for angiography and P-PCI is preferred if it can be accomplished consistently with a first medical contact to balloon or device time of less than 120 minutes. Fibrinolytic therapy should be administered in the absence of contraindications if the anticipated first medical contact-to-device time exceeds 120 minutes.[36] For those presenting to a non–PCI-capable hospital, rapid assessment of 1) the time from onset of symptoms, 2) the mortality risk of STEMI based on patient characteristics and infarct location, 3) the risk of bleeding, and 4) the time required for transfer and the interval from first medical contact to balloon or device must all be considered.

Even when fibrinolysis or P-PCI is successful in restoring infarct artery flow, perfusion of the infarct zone may still be compromised by a combination of microvascular damage and reperfusion injury.[94]

Time from Symptom Onset

Fibrinolytic therapy administered within the first 2 (especially the first) hours can occasionally abort MI and dramatically reduces mortality rates.[32,33] Prehospital fibrinolysis reduces treatment delays by up to 1 hour, allowing the majority of patients to be treated within 2 hours of symptom onset, and reduces mortality rates by 17% compared with therapy initiated in the hospital.[95] However, the efficacy of fibrinolytic agents in lysing thrombus diminishes with increasing treatment delays.[96] In contrast, P-PCI can seldom be performed within 2 hours of symptom onset, but reperfusion rates are superior to fibrinolytic therapy and independent of time. Although the Comparison of Angioplasty and Prehospital Thrombolysis in Acute Myocardial Infarction (CAPTIM)[97] and Primary Angioplasty in Patients Transferred from General Community Hospitals to Specialized PTCA [percutaneous transluminal coronary angioplasty] Units with or Without Emergency Thrombolysis (PRAGUE)-2[98] studies reached different conclusions about the overall superiority of P-PCI over fibrinolysis, similar results were seen in time-to-treatment subset analyses. Patients treated within 2 hours of symptom onset in CAPTIM had improved outcomes with prehospital tissue plasminogen activator versus transfer for P-PCI.[99] Patients treated within 3 hours of symptom onset in PRAGUE-2 had equivalent mortality rate whether treated with streptokinase or transferred for P-PCI.[98] Conversely, both studies showed superior outcomes with P-PCI in patients with symptom duration greater than 3 hours.

Risk Stratification in ST-Segment Elevation Myocardial Infarction

Different risk stratification tools are available to quantify risk (Figure 10-6).[100-102] Patients with low mortality risk have similar outcomes with fibrinolysis or P-PCI.[103,104] Patients with anterior STEMI,[103,104] older age, congestive heart failure,[105] or cardiogenic shock[106] have better outcomes with P-PCI. The point of equipoise between strategies is an estimated 30-day mortality risk of 3%.[107]

Risk of Bleeding

The higher the risk of bleeding with fibrinolytic therapy, the more P-PCI would be favored as the reperfusion strategy. The increased risk for ICH in the elderly is a strong factor that favors P-PCI in this subgroup.

Predicted Transfer and Door-to-Balloon Time

P-PCI is superior to fibrinolytic therapy when it can be performed expeditiously by experienced teams in high-volume hospitals.[108]

The benefit noted in the randomized, clinical trials (Figure 10-7)[109-113] was strongly influenced by a reduction of nonfatal recurrent MI. Several trials have suggested a benefit from transferring patients from a non–PCI-capable hospital to a PCI-capable hospital for P-PCI.[36,114] In the United States, only 25% of hospitals are capable of performing P-PCI. Although several trials have suggested a benefit to transferring patients, transfer times remain unreasonably long. In the National Cardiovascular Data Registry,[115] only 9.9% of transferred patients were treated with P-PCI within 90 minutes, and approximately 30% had door-to-balloon times greater than 3 hours. When the anticipated time from first medical contact to device exceeds 120 minutes, fibrinolysis should be administered in the absence of contraindications.

FIBRINOLYTIC THERAPY

Indications and Contraindications

In the absence of contraindications, and when there is a delay to P-PCI, fibrinolytic therapy should be administered to STEMI patients with symptom onset within the prior 12 hours and ST-segment elevation greater than 0.1 mV in at least two contiguous leads, or new, or presumably new, LBBB. Patients with true posterior MI and patients with symptom duration for 12 to 24 hours and ST-segment elevation are also reasonable candidates. Contraindications and cautions for using fibrinolytic therapy are shown in Box 10-1. Hemorrhage is the most critical risk, especially ICH, which is fatal in more than half of patients. Several models for estimating the risk of ICH after fibrinolysis have been developed.[116-118] Patients with more than 4% risk of ICH should be treated with P-PCI rather than fibrinolytic therapy. Streptokinase without heparin has the lowest ICH rate.

Mortality Benefit

Placebo-controlled trials have demonstrated the survival benefit associated with fibrinolytic therapy.[55,119-121] Mortality reduction is greatest within the first few hours of symptoms, especially the first hour, because of salvage of ischemic myocardium with reduced infarct size. The mortality benefit seen with later treatment depends more on improved infarct healing and myocardial remodeling, reduced electrical heterogeneity, and potential for life-threatening ventricular arrhythmias. Patients with LBBB, anterior MI, hypotension, and tachycardia have higher risk from STEMI and achieve greater therapeutic benefit.[32] The patient risk and potential therapeutic benefit in inferior MI is increased with RV involvement, precordial ST-segment depression, or complete heart block.[122] The number of ECG leads involved and the extent of ST-segment deviation is an excellent predictor of potential STEMI risk.[43] Although patients older than 75 years might better be treated with PCI, the absolute number of lives saved per 1000 patients treated with fibrinolytic therapy compared with placebo is actually greater than in younger patients (34 vs. 28).[123]

Effect on Left Ventricular Function

Successful early reperfusion reduces infarct size, preserves regional wall motion, decreases ventricular dilation, and maintains global LV function, an important predictor of survival. Restoration of normal infarct artery flow does not reflect microvascular reperfusion, which is better evaluated by myocardial blush on angiography, contrast perfusion on echocardiography, or prompt resolution of ST-segment elevation on ECG. Poor microvascular reperfusion is associated with increased infarct size, morbidity, and death.

Complications

The major complication of fibrinolytic therapy is hemorrhage, which may or may not require transfusion. Risk factors include older age, female gender, lower body weight, and hypertension. ICH encompasses parenchymal hemorrhage, intraventricular hemorrhage, subarachnoid hemorrhage, subdural hematoma, and epidural hematoma. Typical presenting features include an

	GRACE Risk Score	TIMI Risk Score STEMI
Population	All ACS	STEMI
Outcome	Death	Death
Key Elements	9	8
Age	X	X
Gender		
Prior MI/CAD	X	X*
DM, CRFs		X
Pace of sx		
Weight		X
HR	X	X
SBP	X	X
CHF	X	X
ECG	X	X
CKMB/cTn	X	
Serum Cr	X	
In-hosp PCI	X	
Rx Delay		X
Possible max score	263	14
c-statistic	0.81	0.78

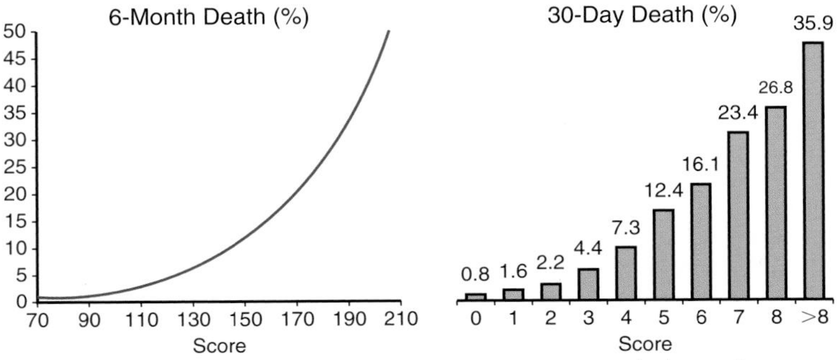

Web access — www.outcomes-umassmed.org/grace/ — www.mdcalc.com/timi-risk-score-for-stemi

FIGURE 10-6 Summary of clinical risk scores for ST-segment elevation myocardial infarction (*STEMI*). The reported c-statistics are from the derivation set. ACS, acute coronary syndrome; CAD, coronary artery disease; CHF, congestive heart failure; CKMB, MB fraction of creatine kinase; Cr, creatinine; CRFs, cardiac risk factors; cTn, cardiac troponin; DM, diabetes mellitus; ECG, electrocardiogram; GRACE, Global Registry of Acute Coronary Events; HR, heart rate; In-hosp, in hospital; max, maximum; MI, myocardial infarction; PCI, percutaneous coronary intervention; Rx, treatment; SBP, systolic blood pressure; sx, symptoms. *(From Morrow DA. Cardiovascular risk prediction in patients with stable and unstable coronary heart disease. Circulation 2010;121:2681-2691.)*

acute change in level of consciousness, unifocal or multifocal neurologic signs, coma, headache, nausea, vomiting, and seizures. The occurrence of a change in neurologic status during or after reperfusion therapy, particularly within the first 24 hours after initiation of treatment, is considered to be caused by ICH until proven otherwise (Figure 10-8). Fibrinolytic, antiplatelet, and anticoagulant therapies should be discontinued until a brain imaging scan shows no evidence of ICH. Neurology and/or neurosurgery consults should be obtained as dictated by clinical circumstances. Immediate measures to reduce intracranial pressure include mannitol infusion, elevation of the head of the bed to 30 degrees, endotracheal intubation, and hyperventilation to achieve a pCO_2 of 25 to 30 mm Hg. Cryoprecipitate (10 U) will increase the fibrinogen level by approximately 0.70 g/L and the factor VIII level by approximately 30% in a 70-kg adult. Fresh frozen plasma restores levels of factors V and VIII. Protamine (1 mg/100 U of UFH given in the preceding 4 hours) reverses heparin anticoagulation. Platelet transfusions (6 to 8 U) can be given if the bleeding time is abnormal. BP and blood glucose levels should be optimized. Neurosurgical evacuation of ICH may be required in selected patients.[124]

Comparison of Fibrinolytic Agents

Fibrinolytic agents are plasminogen activators. Plasmin dissolves the fibrin mesh that holds red blood cells and platelets together as a thrombus. The four approved IV agents are compared in Table 10-2. Alteplase is superior to streptokinase in reducing morbidity and mortality but is more expensive and confers a slightly higher risk of ICH.[125] Bolus dosing with reteplase[126] or tenecteplase[127] produces equivalent results compared with alteplase. The cost/benefit ratio is more favorable for the expensive agents in patients with a large myocardial area of risk and a low risk of ICH. Streptokinase is used by some clinicians when predicted infarct size is small or ICH risk is higher, but should not be reused because of the high prevalence of neutralizing antibody titers.

PERCUTANEOUS CORONARY INTERVENTION

Primary

More than 90% of STEMI patients are candidates for P-PCI. Patency rates greater than 90% and TIMI-3 flow rates of 70% to 90% have been reported. If immediately available, P-PCI should be performed

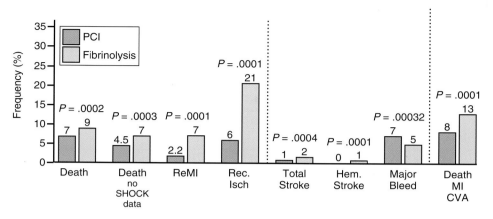

PCI vs. Fibrinolysis:
Short-Term Clinical Outcomes

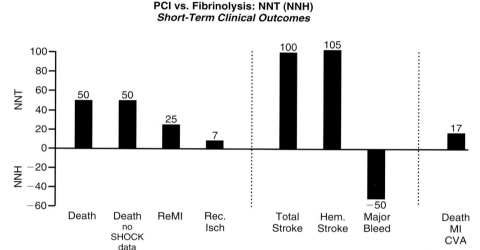

PCI vs. Fibrinolysis: NNT (NNH)
Short-Term Clinical Outcomes

FIGURE 10-7 Percutaneous coronary intervention (*PCI*) versus fibrinolysis for ST-elevation myocardial infarction (STEMI). The short-term (4 to 6 weeks, *top left*) and long-term (*top right*) outcomes for the various endpoints shown are plotted for patients with STEMI randomized to PCI or fibrinolysis for reperfusion in 23 trials (N = 7739). Based on the frequency of events for each endpoint in the two treatment groups, the number needed to treat (*NNT*) or number needed to harm (*NNH*) is shown for the short-term (*bottom left*) and long-term (*bottom right*) outcomes. The magnitude of the treatment differences for death, nonfatal reinfarction, and stroke vary depending on whether PCI is compared with streptokinase or a fibrin-specific lytic. For example, when primary PCI is compared with alteplase and the Should We Emergently Revascularize Occluded Coronaries for Cardiogenic Shock (*SHOCK*) trial is excluded, the mortality rate is 5.5% vs. 6.7% (odds ratio, 0.81; 95% confidence interval, 0.64 to 1.03, *P* = .081). CVA, cerebrovascular accident; Hem., hemorrhagic; MI, myocardial infarction; Rec. Isch, recurrent ischemia; ReMI, recurrent myocardial infarction. (*Modified from Keeley EC, Boura JA, Grines CL: Primary angioplasty versus intravenous thrombolytic therapy for acute myocardial infarction: A quantitative review of 23 randomised trials. Lancet 2003;361:13-20.*)

Box 10-1 Contraindications and Cautions for Fibrinolysis in STEMI*

Absolute Contraindications
- Any prior ICH
- Known structural cerebral vascular lesion (e.g., atrioventricular malformation)
- Known malignant intracranial neoplasm (primary or metastatic)
- Ischemic stroke within 3 months EXCEPT acute ischemic stroke within 3 hours
- Suspected aortic dissection
- Active bleeding or bleeding diathesis (excluding menses)
- Significant closed head or facial trauma within 3 months

Relative Contraindications
- History of chronic, severe, poorly controlled hypertension
- Severe uncontrolled hypertension on presentation (SBP > 180 or DBP > 110 mm Hg)†
- History of prior ischemic stroke >3 months, dementia, or known intracranial pathology not covered in contraindications
- Traumatic or prolonged (>10 minutes) CPR or major surgery (<3 weeks)
- Recent (within 2-4 weeks) internal bleeding
- Noncompressible vascular punctures
- For streptokinase/anistreplase: prior exposure or prior allergic reaction to these agents
- Pregnancy
- Active peptic ulcer
- Current use of anticoagulants: the higher the INR, the higher the risk of bleeding

*Viewed as advisory for clinical decision making and may not be all inclusive or definitive.
†Could be an absolute contraindication in low-risk patients with myocardial infarction.
CPR, cardiopulmonary resuscitation; DBP, diastolic blood pressure; ICH, intracranial hemorrhage; INR, international normalized ratio; SBP, systolic blood pressure; STEMI, ST-segment elevation myocardial infarction.
Modified from Antman EM, Anbe DT, Armstrong PW, et al: ACC/AHA guidelines for the management of patients with ST-elevation myocardial infarction: A report of the American College of Cardiology/American Heart Association Task Force on Practice Guidelines (Committee to revise the 1999 Guidelines for the Management of Patients with Acute Myocardial Infarction). Circulation 2004;588-636.

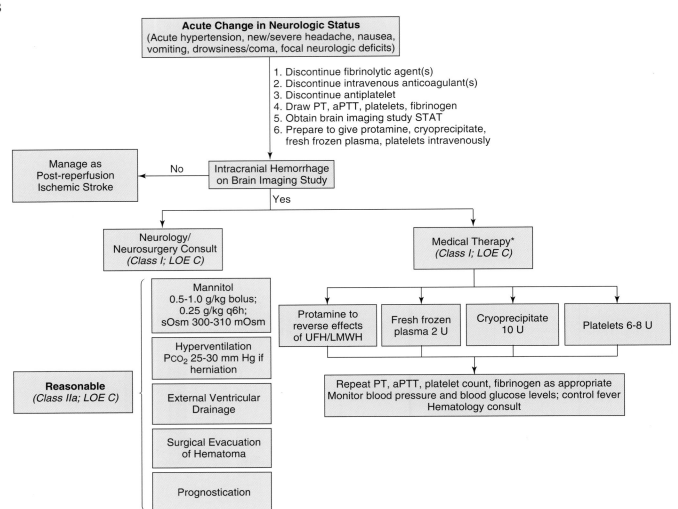

FIGURE 10-8 Algorithm for evaluation of intracranial hemorrhage complicating fibrinolytic therapy for ST-elevation myocardial infarction. *As dictated by clinical circumstances. aPTT, activated partial thromboplastin time; LMWH, low-molecular-weight heparin; LOE, level of evidence; PT, prothrombin time; sOsm, serum osmolality; UFH, unfractionated heparin. *(Modified from The National Institute of Neurological Disorders and Stroke (NINDS) rt-PA Stroke Study Group: A systems approach to immediate evaluation and management of hyperacute stroke: Experience at eight centers and implications for community practice and patient care. Stroke 1997;28:1530-40.)*

TABLE 10-2	Comparison of Approved Fibrinolytic Agents			
	STREPTOKINASE	**ALTEPLASE**	**RETEPLASE**	**TENECTEPLASE**
Dose	1.5 MU over 30-60 min	Up to 100 mg in 90 min (based on weight)*	10 U × 2, each over 2 min	30-50 mg (based on weight)
Bolus administration	No	No	Yes	Yes
Antigenic	Yes	No	No	No
Allergic reactions (hypotension most common)	Yes	No	No	No
Systemic fibrinogen depletion	Marked	Mild	Moderate	Minimal
90-min patency rates (approximate %)	50	75	75	75
TIMI grade 3 flow (%)	32	54	60	63
Cost (in dollars) per dose	$613	$2974	$2750	$2833 for 50 mg

*Bolus 15 mg, infusion 0.75 mg/kg over 30 min (maximum, 50 mg), then 0.5 mg/kg not to exceed 35 mg over the next 60 min to an overall maximum of 100 mg.
†30 mg for weight <60 kg; 35 mg for 60-69 kg; 40 mg for 70-79 kg; 45 mg for 80-89 kg; 50 mg for ≥90 kg.
MU, million units; TIMI, Thrombolysis In Myocardial Infarction.
Modified from Antman EM, Anbe DT, Armstrong PW, et al: ACC/AHA guidelines for the management of patients with ST-elevation myocardial infarction: A report of the American College of Cardiology/American Heart Association Task Force on Practice Guidelines (Committee to revise the 1999 Guidelines for the Management of Patients with Acute Myocardial Infarction). Circulation 2004;110:588-636.

in patients with STEMI (including true posterior MI) or MI with new, or presumably new, LBBB who can undergo PCI of the infarct artery within 12 hours of symptom onset (or >12 hours if ischemic symptoms persist), if performed in a timely fashion (balloon inflation within 90 minutes of presentation) by persons skilled in the procedure (individuals who perform more than 75 PCI procedures per year). The procedure should be supported by experienced personnel in an appropriate laboratory environment (that performs more than 400 PCI procedures per year, of which at least 36 are P-PCI for STEMI, and has cardiac surgery capability).[128]

Randomized clinical trials performed in selected patients by experienced providers demonstrated that PCI-treated patients experience lower short-term mortality rates (5.0% vs. 7.0%; relative risk [RR], 0.70; 95% confidence interval [CI], 0.58 to 0.85; P = .0002), less nonfatal reinfarction (3.0% vs. 7.0%; RR, 0.35; 95% CI, 0.27 to 0.45; P = .0003), and less hemorrhagic stroke (0.05% vs. 1.0%; RR, 0.05; 95% CI, 0.006 to 0.35; P = .0001) than those treated by fibrinolysis, but with an increased risk for major bleeding (7.0% vs. 5.0%; RR, 1.3; CI, 1.02 to 1.65; P = .032) (see Figure 10-7).[109] The efficacy differences are smaller when PCI is compared with alteplase, the invasive strategy is allowed after fibrinolytic therapy, patients are treated by less-experienced operators or in low-volume facilities, or door-to-balloon times are excessively prolonged.

The survival benefit with P-PCI is time dependent (Figure 10-9). To reproduce the outcomes in the randomized trials in which P-PCI was performed by experienced operators with an additional mean treatment delay of 40 minutes for P-PCI instead of fibrinolytic therapy, strict performance criteria must be followed. These include door-to-balloon times less than 90 minutes, TIMI 2/3 flow rates in more than 90% of patients, emergency bypass surgery rates less than 2%, and performance of P-PCI in more than 85% of patients brought to the laboratory. Risk-adjusted hospital mortality rates should be less than 7% in patients without cardiogenic shock, which would be comparable to that reported for fibrinolytic therapy[109] and consistent with previously reported registry results for which mortality rates were not different between treatment strategies.[34,129-131] If the performance criteria stated above cannot be met, fibrinolytic therapy should be considered unless it is contraindicated.

P-PCI has its greatest mortality benefit in high-risk patients. P-PCI has been associated with an absolute 9% reduction in 30-day mortality rate in cardiogenic shock[106] and a 33% relative risk reduction (vs. 9% with fibrinolytic therapy) in congestive heart failure.[111] Compared with fibrinolytic therapy, P-PCI reduces mortality rates

in patients with anterior MI, but there is no difference in patients with nonanterior MI.[109,110] Reocclusion rates are 15% after percutaneous transluminal coronary angioplasty (PTCA) and 5% after stenting compared with 30% after fibrinolytic therapy.[132] Potential complications include problems with the arterial access site; adverse reactions to volume loading, contrast medium, and antithrombotic medications; technical complications; and reperfusion events.

Recommended adjunctive antiplatelet and antithrombotic therapy to support perfusion with P-PCI is presented in Tables 10-3 and 10-4.

TABLE 10-3	Adjunctive Antiplatelet Therapy to Support Reperfusion with Primary PCI	
ANTIPLATELET THERAPY	**CLASS**	**LEVEL OF EVIDENCE**
Aspirin		
Preprocedure: 325 mg	I	A
Postprocedure: 81-160 mg/day indefinitely	I	A
Maintenance: 81 mg/day	IIa	B
P2Y12 Inhibitors		
Loading Dose		
Clopidogrel: 600 mg as early as possible before or at the time of PCI	I	B
Prasugrel: 60 mg at PCI	I	B
Ticagrelor: 180 mg at PCI	I	B
Maintenance Dose with DES ≤1 Year		
Clopidogrel: 75 mg/day	I	C
Prasugrel: 10 mg/day	I	B
Ticagrelor: 90 mg bid†	I	B
Duration of Therapy ≥1 year	IIb	C
Maintenance Dose with BMS or Balloon Angioplasty Only*		
Clopidogrel: 75 mg/day	I	B
Prasugrel: 10 mg/day	I	B
Prasugrel in STEMI patients with prior stroke/TIA, weight <60 kg, or age ≥75 years or greater	III	B
Ticagrelor: 90 mg bid	I	B
GP IIb/IIIa Receptor Antagonists (in Conjunction with UFH) in Patients with Large Thrombus Burden		
Abciximab: 0.25 mg/kg IV bolus, then 0.125 µg/kg/min (maximum 10 µg/min) up to 12 hours	IIa	A
Abciximab: 0.25 mg IC bolus	IIb	B
Eptifibatide (double bolus): 180 µg/kg IV bolus, then 2 µg/kg/min; a second 180 µg/kg bolus is administered 10 min after the first bolus	IIa	B
In patients with CrCl <50 mL/min (Cockcroft-Gault formula), give single bolus and reduce infusion by 50%	IIa	B
Tirofiban (high bolus dose): 25 µg/kg IV bolus, then 0.15 µg/kg/min	IIa	B
In patients with CrCl <50 mL/min (Cockcroft-Gault formula), reduce infusion by 50%	IIa	B
GP IIb/IIIa inhibitors in conjunction with bivalirudin	IIb	B

*Continue for at least 1 month up to 1 year.
†The recommended maintenance dose of aspirin to be used with ticagrelor is 81 mg.
CrCl, creatine clearance; BMS, bare-metal stent; DES, drug-eluting stent; GP, glycoprotein; IC, intracoronary; IV, intravenous; PCI, percutaneous coronary intervention; STEMI, ST-segment elevation myocardial infarction; TIA, transient ischemic attack; UFH, unfractionated heparin.

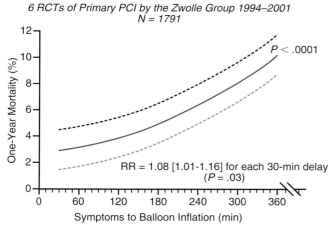

6 RCTs of Primary PCI by the Zwolle Group 1994–2001
N = 1791

P < .0001

RR = 1.08 [1.01-1.16] for each 30-min delay
(P = .03)

One-Year Mortality (%) — Symptoms to Balloon Inflation (min)

FIGURE 10-9 Symptoms to balloon time and mortality in primary percutaneous coronary intervention (*PCI*) for ST-elevation myocardial infarction. The relationship between time to treatment and death at 1 year, as continuous functions, was assessed by using a quadratic regression model. The dotted lines represent 95% confidence intervals of the predicted mortality rate. RCTs, randomized, controlled trials; RR, relative risk. (*Modified from De Luca G, Suryapranata H, Ottervanger JP, Antman EM: Time delay to treatment and mortality in primary angioplasty for acute myocardial infarction: Every minute of delay counts. Circulation 2004;109:1223-1225.*)

TABLE 10-4	Adjunctive Anticoagulant Therapy to Support Reperfusion with Primary PCI		
ANTICOAGULANT THERAPY		**CLASS**	**LEVEL OF EVIDENCE**
UFH to maintain ACT			
With GP IIb/IIIa receptor antagonist planned: 50-70 U/kg bolus IV to achieve ACT of 200-250 sec		I	C
No GP IIb/IIIa receptor antagonist planned: 70-100 U/kg bolus to achieve ACT of 250-300 sec for HemoTec, 300-350 sec for Hemochron		I	C
Bivalirudin			
0.75 mg/kg IV bolus, then 1.75 mg/kg/h infusion, with or without prior treatment with UFH, to achieve therapeutic ACT for the duration of the procedure; an additional bolus of 0.3 mg/kg may be given if needed		I	B
Reduce infusion to 1 mg/kg/h with estimated CrCl <30 mL/min		IIa	B
Preferred over UFH with GP IIb/IIIa receptor antagonists or LMWH with GP IIb/IIIa receptor antagonists in patients at high risk of bleeding		IIa	B
Fondaparinux: not recommended as sole anticoagulant for primary PCI		III	B

ACT, activated clotting time; CrCl, creatine clearance; GP, glycoprotein; IV, intravenous; LMWH, low-molecular-weight heparin; PCI, percutaneous coronary intervention; UFH, unfractionated heparin.

Use of Stents

Compared with PTCA, intracoronary stents achieve a better immediate angiographic result with a larger arterial lumen, less reocclusion and restenosis of the infarct artery, and fewer subsequent ischemic events, but there are no differences in mortality or reinfarction rates.[133] Studies comparing bare-metal stents (BMS) with drug-eluting stents (DES) in STEMI show no differences in mortality rate, MI rate, or stent thrombosis risk. The major advantage of DES over BMS in this setting is a small reduction in target vessel revascularization rates.[134-139] The greatest challenge in selecting patients for DES implantation during STEMI, however, is determining in an emergency situation whether the patient is a candidate for prolonged dual antiplatelet therapy. Financial barriers and social barriers that may limit patient compliance, or medical issues that involve bleeding risks or the need for invasive or surgical procedures in the following year that would interrupt antiplatelet therapy, must be considered.

Thrombus Aspiration

Two small trials and a meta-analysis support the use of aspiration thrombectomy for STEMI.[140-143] The concept is to minimize athero-thrombotic debris, limit microvascular obstruction, and maximize myocardial salvage. It is reasonable to perform aspiration thrombectomy in patients undergoing P-PCI and in patients with short ischemic times and large thrombus burdens.

Pharmacoinvasive Management

P-PCI is the preferred choice of treatment for STEMI if it can be performed in a timely manner by experienced operators. Unfortunately, only 25% of hospitals in the United States are capable of performing P-PCI, and transfer times from non–PCI-capable to PCI-capable hospitals are often unreasonably long. IV fibrinolytic therapy fails to restore infarct artery patency in 25% to 50% of patients. The REACT trial showed a benefit of PCI performed in patients with moderate to high risk with failed reperfusion following fibrinolytic therapy versus repeat fibrinolysis.[144] Several

strategies have been developed to test whether a pharmaco-invasive strategy could accomplish the goal of timely reperfusion, especially for patients presenting at a non–PCI-capable hospital. Different combinations of antithrombotic regimens (full- or half-dose fibrinolytic agents, antithrombins, GP IIb/IIIa receptor blockers, dual antiplatelet therapy) prior to P-PCI have been compared with standard P-PCI without significant clinical benefit.[145,146] Six trials and a meta-analysis[147-151] have shown promise for the early transfer strategy: fibrinolytic therapy at a non–PCI-capable hospital followed by transfer to a PCI-capable hospital for routine angiography and probable PCI within 24 hours following STEMI for high-risk patients. This is in contrast to the "ischemia-driven" approach, in which only those who show signs of hemodynamic instability or failed reperfusion are sent for angiography.

Patients best suited for transfer for PCI are STEMI patients who present with high-risk features, those with a high risk of bleeding, and patients presenting late (more than 4 hours after onset of symptoms). Patients best suited for fibrinolytic therapy present early after symptom onset with low bleeding risk. After fibrinolytic therapy, if the patient is not at high risk, transfer to a PCI-capable facility may be considered, especially if symptoms persist and failure to reperfuse is suspected.

The Occluded Artery Trial (OAT) demonstrated that routine PCI for total occlusions 1 to 28 days after STEMI in stable patients did not reduce the composite of death, reinfarction, or class IV heart failure provided the patients received optimal medical therapy.[152] Patients who were in New York Heart Association (NYHA) class III or IV, had rest angina or inducible ischemia, had a creatinine level greater than 2.5 mg/dL, were clinically unstable, or had main left or triple-vessel disease were excluded.

Hospitals Without on-Site Cardiac Surgery

Whereas hospitals with onsite cardiac surgery can offer immediate access to a PCI laboratory, hospitals without this resource must establish more complicated treatment protocols that include inter-hospital transfer agreements. Fibrinolytic therapy will usually be the primary reperfusion strategy. However, many patients are ineligible for fibrinolytic therapy because of bleeding risk and should be considered for transfer for P-PCI.[153] Patients who do not respond to fibrinolysis and are candidates for rescue PCI should also be transferred, as should patients with congestive heart failure or cardiogenic shock.

Some hospitals with cardiac catheterization laboratories are able to offer P-PCI without on-site cardiac surgery. Several performance criteria must be met for this strategy to reproduce the favorable results in published reports (Box 10-2).[154,155] The operators must be experienced interventionalists (performing at least 75 interventions per year), the lab must perform at least 36 procedures per year, and the nursing and technical staff must be fully trained. The full range of PCI equipment must be available, and intraaortic balloon counterpulsation expertise is required. Appropriate case selection and continuous quality improvement are important components (Box 10-3). High-risk patients should be transferred to a hospital with on-site surgery for P-PCI.

Hospital Management

Location

Patients should be admitted to the coronary care unit (CCU) or monitored step-down unit with immediate access to defibrillators. Initial patient evaluation includes assessment of vital signs, pulse oximetry, cardiac rhythm and ST segments, and symptoms of acute cardiac ischemia. Outstanding (and abnormal) results should be followed up, and standard admitting orders should be implemented (Box 10-4). Intraarterial and pulmonary artery pressure monitoring should be available for hypotensive patients. Intra-aortic balloon pumps (IABPs) or other ventricular assist devices should be available for treatment of cardiogenic shock. Oral β-blocker therapy should be administered in an adequate dose to

Box 10-2 Criteria for the Performance of Primary PCI at Hospitals Without on-Site Cardiac Surgery

- The operators must be experienced interventionalists who regularly perform elective PCI at a surgical center (at least 75 cases/year). The catheterization laboratory must perform a minimum of 36 primary PCI procedures per year.
- The nursing and technical catheterization laboratory staff must be experienced in handling acutely ill patients and be comfortable with interventional equipment. They must have acquired experience in dedicated interventional laboratories at a surgical center and participate in a 24-hour, 365-day call schedule.
- The catheterization laboratory itself must be well equipped, with optimal imaging systems, resuscitation equipment, IABP support, and a broad array of interventional equipment.
- The cardiac care unit nurses must be adept in hemodynamic monitoring and IABP management.
- The hospital administration must fully support the program and enable the fulfillment of the above institutional requirements.
- Formalized written protocols must be in place for immediate and efficient transfer of patients to the nearest cardiac surgical facility that are reviewed/tested on a regular (quarterly) basis.
- Primary PCI must be performed routinely as the treatment of choice for a large proportion of patients with STEMI to ensure streamlined care paths with increased case volumes.
- Case selection for the performance of primary PCI must be rigorous. Criteria for the types of lesions appropriate for primary PCI and for the selection for transfer for emergent aortocoronary bypass surgery are shown in Table 11-5.
- An ongoing program of outcomes analysis and formalized periodic case review must be in place.
- Institutions should participate in a 3- to 6-month period of implementation during which time development of a formalized primary PCI program is instituted that includes establishing standards, training staff, detailed logistic development, and creation of a quality assessment and error management system.

IABP, intraaortic balloon pump; PCI, percutaneous coronary intervention; STEMI, ST-segment elevation myocardial infarction.
Modified from Antman EM, Anbe DT, Armstrong PW, et al: ACC/AHA guidelines for the management of patients with ST-elevation myocardial infarction: A report of the American College of Cardiology/American Heart Association Task Force on Practice Guidelines (Committee to revise the 1999 Guidelines for the Management of Patients with Acute Myocardial Infarction). Circulation 2004;110:588-636.

Box 10-3 Patient Selection for Primary PCI and Emergent Aortocoronary Bypass at Hospitals Without on-Site Cardiac Surgery

Avoid Intervention in Hemodynamically Stable Patients with:

- Significant (≥60%) stenosis of an unprotected left main coronary artery upstream from an acute occlusion in the left coronary system that might be disrupted by the angioplasty catheter
- Extremely long or angulated infarct-related lesions with TIMI grade 3 flow
- Infarct-related lesions with TIMI grade 3 flow in stable patients with triple-vessel disease
- Infarct-related lesions of small or secondary vessels
- Hemodynamically significant lesions in other than the infarct artery

Transfer Patients for Emergency Aortocoronary Bypass Surgery

- After primary PCI of occluded vessels if high-grade residual left main or multivessel coronary disease with clinical or hemodynamic instability is present (preferably with intraaortic balloon pump support)

PCI, percutaneous coronary intervention; TIMI, Thrombolysis In Myocardial Infarction.
Modified from Antman EM, Anbe DT, Armstrong PW, et al: ACC/AHA guidelines for the management of patients with ST-elevation myocardial infarction: A report of the American College of Cardiology/American Heart Association Task Force on Practice Guidelines (Committee to revise the 1999 Guidelines for the Management of Patients with Acute Myocardial Infarction). Circulation 2004;110:588-636.

Box 10-4 Sample Admitting Orders for the Patient with STEMI

- Condition: Serious
  - IV: Normal saline or 5% dextrose in water to keep vein open. Start a second IV if IV medication is being given. This may be a heparin lock.
  - Vital signs: Every 30 minutes until stable, then every 4 hours as needed. Notify physician if heart rate is <60 beats/min or >100 beats/min, SBP is <100 mm Hg or >150 mm Hg, respiratory rate is <8 breaths/min or >22 breaths/min.
  - Monitor: Continuous ECG monitoring for arrhythmia and ST-segment deviation.
  - Diet: NPO except for sips of water until stable. Then start sodium 2 g/day, low saturated fat (<7% of total calories/day) and low-cholesterol (<200 mg/day) diet, such as Therapeutic Lifestyle Changes diet.
  - Activity: Bed rest and bedside commode and light activity when stable.
  - Oxygen: Continuous oximetry monitoring. Nasal cannula at 2 L/min. When stable for 6 hours, discontinue oxygen and assess for oxygen need (i.e., <90% saturation), and consider discontinuing oxygen.

Medications
NTG
- Use sublingual NTG 0.4 mg q5min as needed for chest discomfort
- IV NTG for CHF, hypertension, or persistent ischemia

ASA
- If ASA not given in the ED, chew non-enteric-coated ASA 162-325 mg.†
- If ASA has been given, start daily maintenance of 75-162 mg. May use enteric-coated ASA for gastrointestinal protection.

β-Blocker
- If not given in the ED, assess for contraindications (i.e., bradycardia and hypotension). Continue daily assessment to ascertain eligibility for β-blocker.
- If given in the ED, continue daily dose and optimize as dictated by HR and BP.

ACE Inhibitor
- Start ACE inhibitor orally in patients with anterior infarction, pulmonary congestion, or LVEF <40% if the following are absent: hypotension (SBP <100 mm Hg or <30 mm Hg below baseline) or known contraindications to this class of medications.

ARB
- Start ARB orally in patients who are intolerant of ACE inhibitors and who have either clinical or radiologic signs of heart failure or LVEF <40%.

Pain medication
- IV morphine sulfate 2-4 mg with increments of 2-8 mg at 5- to 15-minute intervals as needed to control pain.

Anxiolytics (based on a nursing assessment)
Daily stool softener

Laboratory Tests
- Serum biomarkers for cardiac damage,* CBC with platelet count, INR, aPTT, electrolytes, magnesium, BUN, creatinine, glucose, serum lipids

*Do not wait for results before implementing reperfusion strategy.
†Although some trials have used enteric-coated aspirin for initial dosing, more rapid buccal absorption occurs with non-enteric-coated formulations.
ACE, angiotensin-converting enzyme; ARB, angiotensin-receptor blocker; aPTT, activated partial thromboplastin time; ASA, aspirin; BP, blood pressure; BUN, blood urea nitrogen; CBC, complete blood count; CHF, congestive heart failure; ECG, electrocardiogram; ED, emergency department; HR, heart rate; INR, international normalized ratio; IV, intravenous; LVEF, left ventricular ejection fraction; NPO, nothing by mouth; NTG, nitroglycerin; SBP, systolic blood pressure; STEMI, ST-segment elevation myocardial infarction.
Modified from Antman EM, Anbe DT, Armstrong PW, et al: ACC/AHA guidelines for the management of patients with ST-elevation myocardial infarction: A report of the American College of Cardiology/American Heart Association Task Force on Practice Guidelines (Committee to revise the 1999 Guidelines for the Management of Patients with Acute Myocardial Infarction). Circulation 2004;110:588-636.

control heart rate. IV nitroglycerin is useful for control of angina, hypertension, or acute heart failure. Oxygen can be discontinued if the oxygen saturation is greater than 90%.

Nursing care should be provided by individuals certified in critical care, with staffing based on the specific needs of patients and provider competencies as well as organizational priorities. Patients should be monitored for the development of heart failure, serious arrhythmias, or recurrent ischemia. Medications such as stool softeners and antianxiety agents should be given based on nursing judgment.

Patients typically are transferred to a monitored bed in a step-down unit after 12 to 24 hours of clinical stability. Similarly, low-risk patients who have undergone successful PCI can be directly admitted to the step-down unit for post-PCI care rather than to the CCU. Pulse oximetry, ECG monitoring, and defibrillation equipment should be available. The nursing staff should have a skill set similar to CCU nurses so they may evaluate and respond to any clinical complications.

Routine Measures

Bed rest should be limited to 12 to 24 hours because of the concern about physical deconditioning and orthostatic hypotension. Patients should have no oral intake before a procedure, but otherwise should be prescribed the National Cholesterol Education Program's Adult Treatment Panel III Therapeutic Lifestyle Changes diet focusing on reduced intake of fats and cholesterol, less than 7% of total calories as saturated fats, less than 200 mg/day of cholesterol, increased consumption of omega-3 fatty acids, and appropriate caloric intake for energy needs. Diabetic patients need an appropriate diet, and sodium intake should be restricted in patients with hypertension or heart failure. Patient counseling regarding risk factor modification, including smoking cessation, medication compliance, diet, and exercise should be part of every patient encounter.

It is reasonable to use anxiolytic medications to alleviate short-term anxiety. Withdrawal of caffeine is associated with headache and increases in heart rate. One to two cups of coffee a day, enough to avert caffeine withdrawal, has not been associated with BP increases or ventricular arrhythmias. Smokers may experience symptoms of nicotine withdrawal, including anxiety, insomnia, depression, difficulty concentrating, irritability, anger, restlessness, and slowed heart rate. Anxiolytics, bupropion, and nicotine replacement therapy are treatment options. IV haloperidol is a rapidly acting neuroleptic that can be given to cardiac patients with agitation. Communication with the patient and family, liberalized visiting rules, psychological support, and counseling can decrease anxiety and depression for both the patient and the family members.

Medications

NITROGLYCERIN

IV nitroglycerin is indicated in the first 48 hours after STEMI for treatment of persistent ischemia that responds to nitrate therapy, CHF, or hypertension. Intravenous, oral, or topical nitrates are useful beyond the first 48 hours after STEMI for treatment of recurrent angina or persistent CHF if their use does not preclude therapy with β-blockers or ACE inhibitors. The continued use of nitrate therapy beyond the first 24 to 48 hours in the absence of symptoms is not well established in current practice. If sustained nitrate therapy is planned, a nitrate-free interval during daily dosing is important to avoid nitrate tolerance.

ANTITHROMBOTIC AGENTS

Aspirin should be continued indefinitely unless aspirin allergy exists.[57] Low-dose aspirin (81 mg/day) is preferred for long-term treatment because of a dose-dependent increase in bleeding risk.

A thienopyridine should be substituted for aspirin when aspirin is contraindicated because of hypersensitivity or major gastrointestinal intolerance. Gastric side effects may be reduced by administration of proton pump inhibitors, H2 antagonists, antacids, or use of enteric-coated aspirin. Available data suggest that dual antiplatelet therapy with both aspirin and either clopidogrel, prasugrel, or ticagrelor should be continued for at least 1 year in all patients.[30]

IV UFH should be used for up to 48 hours in patients not undergoing P-PCI. Similarly, enoxaparin and fondaparinux should be continued for the duration of the hospitalization up to 8 days or until revascularization. Anticoagulants are discontinued in patients at the conclusion of P-PCI so that the vascular sheaths can be removed. Deep venous thrombosis prophylaxis with SC LMWH (dosed appropriately for specific agent) or with SC UFH (7500 to 12,500 U twice daily) until the patient is completely ambulatory may be useful, but the effectiveness of such a strategy is not well established in the contemporary era of routine aspirin use and early mobilization.

An aPTT measurement and dose adjustment should be made 3 hours after starting IV UFH therapy and repeated 6 hours after each dose adjustment and daily thereafter. Rather than abruptly stopping therapy, reducing UFH infusions in a gradual fashion (e.g., by half within 6 hours, then discontinuing over the subsequent 12 hours) may decrease the risk of hypercoagulability from heparin rebound. Platelet counts should be monitored daily because of the 3% risk of HIT.

β-BLOCKERS

Meta-analysis of trials from the pre-fibrinolytic era involving more than 24,000 patients who received β-blockers in the convalescent phase has shown a reduction in acute ischemic events and a 23% reduction in long-term mortality rate.[156] The risk is a 3% incidence of provocation of congestive heart failure or complete heart block and a 2% incidence of cardiogenic shock. β-Blockers are especially beneficial in patients with persistent or recurrent ischemia, evidence for infarct extension, or tachyarrhythmias. Initiation of therapy can be undertaken within 24 to 48 hours of freedom from relative contraindications that include bradycardia and congestive heart failure. Commonly used β-blockers are metoprolol tartrate 25 to 50 mg every 6 to 12 hours orally, then transitioning to twice-daily dosing for metoprolol tartrate or daily dosing of metoprolol succinate titrated to a dose of 200 mg as tolerated, or carvedilol beginning with 3.125 to 6.25 mg twice daily, titrated to 25 mg twice daily as tolerated.

INHIBITION OF THE RENIN-ANGIOTENSIN-ALDOSTERONE SYSTEM

An ACE inhibitor should be administered orally during convalescence in patients who tolerate this class of medication. ACE inhibitors should not be used if systolic BP is less than 100 mm Hg or less than 30 mm Hg below baseline in the presence of clinically relevant renal failure, a history of bilateral renal artery stenosis, or known allergy to ACE inhibitors. The proportional benefit of ACE inhibitor therapy is largest in higher risk subgroups: patients with previous MI, heart failure, depressed LV ejection fraction (LVEF), or tachycardia. These patients should receive long-term therapy.[157-159] Survival benefit for the elderly and low-risk subgroups is less robust. Treatment can be initiated with captopril or an equivalent, 6.25 to 12.5 mg three times daily, and titrated to 50 mg three times daily. If tolerated, a once- or twice-daily ACE inhibitor (lisinopril 2.5 to 5 mg daily titrated to 10 mg daily as tolerated, or ramipril 2.5 mg twice daily titrated to 5 mg twice daily as tolerated) can be substituted.

An angiotensin receptor blocker should be administered to STEMI patients who are intolerant of ACE inhibitors and with either clinical or radiologic signs of heart failure or LVEF of 40% or less.[160] Valsartan (beginning with 20 mg twice daily for a target dose

80 mg twice daily) and candesartan (beginning with 4 mg daily for a target dose 32 mg daily)[160,161] have demonstrated efficacy for this recommendation.

Long-term aldosterone blockade should be prescribed for patients without significant renal dysfunction (creatinine ≤2.5 mg/dL in men and ≤2.0 mg/dL in women) or hyperkalemia (potassium ≥5.0 mEq/L) who are already receiving therapeutic doses of an ACE inhibitor, have an LVEF less than 40%, and have either symptomatic heart failure or diabetes.[162,163] The Randomized Aldactone Evaluation Study treated patients with NYHA class III to IV heart failure with either spironolactone (25 to 50 mg daily) or placebo.[162] Over 24 months of follow-up, spironolactone treatment was associated with an 11% absolute and a 24% relative risk reduction in all-cause mortality. The Eplerenone Post-Acute Myocardial Infarction Heart Failure Efficacy and Survival Study (EPHESUS) randomized 6632 patients after MI with an LVEF of 40% or less and heart failure or diabetes to receive eplerenone (target dose, 50 mg daily) or placebo in conjunction with routinely indicated cardiac medications.[163] There was a significant reduction in overall mortality, cardiovascular mortality, and cardiac hospitalizations.

GLYCEMIC CONTROL

Although hyperglycemia is associated with adverse outcomes after AMI, it is not clear that intensive glycemic control is associated with improved outcomes.[164-168] Therefore, treatment for hyperglycemia greater than 180 mg/dL is recommended, while avoiding hypoglycemia.

CALCIUM CHANNEL BLOCKERS

It is reasonable to give verapamil or diltiazem to patients for whom β-blockers are ineffective or contraindicated (e.g., bronchospastic disease) for relief of ongoing ischemia or control of a rapid ventricular response with AF or flutter after STEMI in the absence of CHF, LV dysfunction, or AV block.[169,170] There are no current data, however, to suggest that these agents decrease cardiac events. Nifedipine (immediate release) is generally contraindicated in the treatment of STEMI because of the reflex sympathetic activation, tachycardia, and hypotension associated with its use.[171]

Hemodynamic Disturbances

HEMODYNAMIC ASSESSMENT

Use of a pulmonary artery catheter to measure hemodynamics in patients developing progressive CHF or hypotension may permit the early diagnosis of a preshock state in which aggressive pharmacologic support can prevent the onset of cardiogenic shock.[172] Before PCI is performed for cardiogenic shock, the interventional cardiologist should insert a pulmonary artery catheter to maximize the hemodynamic status of the patient and to diagnose unrecognized mechanical complications. After reperfusion therapy, the pulmonary artery catheter may be used to guide diuretic, inotropic, and vasopressor agents in hemodynamically unstable patients while the stunned myocardium is recovering. Although no randomized clinical trial has tested whether hemodynamic monitoring alters clinical outcome in STEMI, one would expect that revascularization of ischemic myocardium would be required for outcomes to be improved.

Complications of pulmonary artery catheterization include ventricular tachyarrhythmias (during manipulation), pulmonary hemorrhage or infarction, and transient right bundle branch block, which can lead to heart block in those with preexisting LBBB. The catheter should not be inserted if the patient quickly responds to other interventions or if treatment is expected to be futile. The catheter should be expeditiously removed when it is no longer needed to monitor therapy or before 4 to 5 days because of risk of infection.

HYPOTENSION

Hypotension (systolic BP pressure <90 mm Hg or 30 points below previous mean arterial pressure) can result from hypovolemia, arrhythmias, RV or LV failure, mechanical complications of MI, or superimposed complications such as sepsis or pulmonary embolism. Hypovolemia is a common occurrence and may be due to inadequate intake, diaphoresis and vomiting, overdiuresis, excessive use of vasodilators, or inappropriate reflex peripheral vasodilation. Hemorrhage is an increasingly common problem associated with the use of invasive procedures, fibrinolytics, antiplatelet agents, and anticoagulant agents. Therefore, rapid volume loading is recommended as an initial therapeutic strategy for all patients without clinical evidence for volume overload (Figure 10-10). Persistent hypotension should be evaluated by echocardiogram to define the cardiac anatomy and a hemoglobin measurement. Correction or control of rhythm disturbances or conduction abnormalities often reverses hypotension. In patients with inotropic failure, vasopressors and inotropic agents are required. Dopamine or norepinephrine may be required for marked hypotension. There may be more arrhythmic events with dopamine than with norepinephrine. Once arterial pressure is brought to at least 90 mm Hg, IV dobutamine may be given simultaneously in an attempt to reduce the rate of the dopamine infusion. In addition, consideration should be given to initiating IABP counterpulsation or inserting an LV assist device.

LOW-OUTPUT STATE

A preshock state of hypoperfusion with normal BP may develop before circulatory collapse and is manifested by cold extremities, cyanosis, oliguria, or decreased mentation.[172] Hospital mortality rate is high, so these patients should be aggressively diagnosed and treated as if they had cardiogenic shock (Figure 10-11). Dobutamine infusion is the initial pharmacologic intervention. IABP therapy or LV assist devices may be required to improve coronary artery perfusion pressure if hypotension is present. If the BP permits, afterload-reducing agents should be added to decrease cardiac work and pulmonary congestion. Coronary artery revascularization of ischemic myocardium with either PCI or CABG has been shown to decrease mortality rate in patients with cardiogenic shock and is strongly recommended for suitable candidates.[106,173] Likewise, patients with ventricular septal rupture, papillary muscle rupture, or pericardial tamponade may benefit from emergency surgical repair.

PULMONARY CONGESTION

LV filling pressures may rapidly rise after acute coronary occlusion. This leads to rapid redistribution of fluid from the intravascular space into the lung interstitium and alveoli. The etiology of pulmonary edema (systolic, diastolic, MR, or ventricular septal rupture) should be rapidly assessed with a two-dimensional echocardiogram with color-flow Doppler. Pulmonary congestion increases the risk of death and pulmonary edema and is associated with a 20% to 40% 30-day mortality rate even in the reperfusion era.[174,175]

Oxygen supplementation should be administered to maintain the arterial saturation greater than 90%. Management includes the use of agents that acutely reduce preload—nitrates, morphine sulfate, and diuretics (see Figure 10-10)—and avoidance of acute administration of negative inotropic agents (e.g., β-blockers, calcium channel antagonists). A 10- to 20-μg nitroglycerin bolus should be administered, followed by a 10-μg/min infusion, increased by 5 to 10 μg/min every 5 to 10 minutes until dyspnea is relieved, the mean arterial pressure is lowered by 10% in normotensive patients or by 30% in hypertensive patients, or until the heart rate increases by more than 10 beats/min. Loop diuretics (furosemide, torsemide, bumetanide) should be initiated in low to intermediate doses in patients with associated hypervolemia.

CH
10

Emergency Management of Complicated STEMI

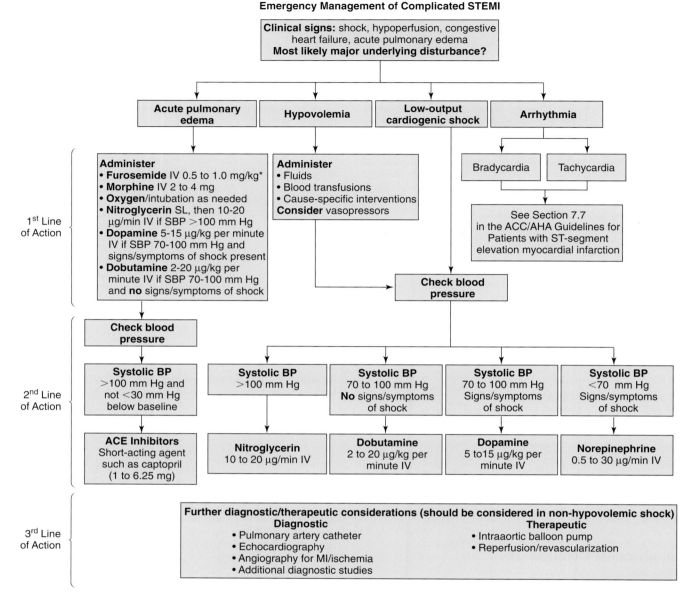

FIGURE 10-10 Emergency management of complicated ST-elevation myocardial infarction (*STEMI*). The emergency management of patients with cardiogenic shock, acute pulmonary edema, or both, is shown. *Furosemide <0.5 mg/kg for new-onset acute pulmonary edema without hypovolemia; 1 mg/kg for acute or chronic volume overload, renal insufficiency. Nesiritide has not been studied adequately in patients with STEMI. Combinations of medications (e.g., dobutamine and dopamine) may be used. ACC, American College of Cardiology; ACE, angiotensin-converting enzyme; AHA, American Heart Association; BP, blood pressure; IV, intravenously; MI, myocardial infarction; SBP, systolic blood pressure; SL, sublingual. (*Modified from ECC Guidelines: part 7: the era of reperfusion; section 1: acute coronary syndromes [acute myocardial infarction]. Circulation 2000;102:I-172-203.)*

Oral ACE inhibitors, preferably a short-acting agent such as captopril, beginning with 1 to 6.25 mg, should be instituted early in normotensive or hypertensive patients. The dosage may be doubled with each subsequent dose, as tolerated, up to 25 to 50 mg every 8 hours, then changed to a long-acting agent. For patients who presented with CHF complicating MI, ramipril administration between days 3 and 10 significantly reduces 30-day mortality rate.[176] Therefore, ACE inhibitors are preferred if BP limits the use of vasodilators. IV sodium nitroprusside substantially reduces afterload as well as preload; however, its use has been associated with coronary steal. Digitalis has no role in the management of pulmonary edema that complicates STEMI unless rapid AF is present.

Eplerenone, an aldosterone antagonist, prevented death and recurrent hospitalization in patients 3 to 14 days after MI with congestive heart failure and an LVEF less than 40%.[163] Spironolactone improved survival in a population of patients with chronic CHF, which includes those with remote MI,[162] and is generic.

In contrast to the recommendation to avoid β-blockade during pulmonary edema, β-blockers are strongly recommended before hospital discharge for secondary prevention of cardiac events.[177] The initial dose and titration should be based on clinical heart failure status and LVEF.

Mechanical ventilation may be required. It may be reasonable to consider mechanical support when pulmonary congestion is refractory. Analyses from the Global Use of Strategies to Open Occluded Coronary Arteries in Acute Coronary Syndromes (GUSTO IIb) trial[178] and the National Registry for Myocardial Infarction[119] showed a marked benefit of PCI compared with fibrinolytic therapy for patients with CHF. Coronary angiography and revascularization, based on the anatomy, should be performed when late CHF complicates the hospital course.

CARDIOGENIC SHOCK

Fewer than 1% of patients with STEMI present to the hospital in cardiogenic shock, and approximately 7% develop shock after hospital admission. A useful definition of cardiogenic shock is clinical evidence of systemic hypoperfusion with systolic BP less than 90 mm Hg for at least 30 minutes (or the need for supportive measures to maintain systolic BP >90 mm Hg), cardiac index less than 2.2 L/min/m^2, and pulmonary capillary wedge pressure of at least 15 mm Hg.

Cardiogenic shock is caused by extensive LV dysfunction in 75% of patients. Other causes include acute severe MR, ventricular septal rupture, subacute free wall rupture with tamponade, and RV infarction. Aortic dissection and hemorrhagic shock may mimic cardiogenic shock and must be excluded. Echocardiography with color-flow Doppler should be used to define the etiology of shock.

Patients with cardiogenic shock secondary to myocardial ischemia and infarction should be resuscitated as quickly as possible. Restoration of sinus rhythm, adequate ventilation, correction of acid-base abnormalities, and inotropic and vasopressor therapy to support tissue perfusion are important interventions. Patients should be treated with reperfusion therapy unless further care is deemed futile (see Figure 10-11). However, reperfusion rates with fibrinolytic therapy are reduced in cardiogenic shock because of low cardiac output, and it is not clear that survival rates are improved. In contrast, more than 20 observational studies have suggested that reperfusion with PCI or CABG improves survival rates.[175]

The results of the Should We Emergently Revascularize Occluded Coronaries for Cardiogenic Shock (SHOCK) trial[106,173] and registry and the Swiss Multicenter Trial of Angioplasty for Shock (SMASH)[179] have proven that appropriate candidates with cardiogenic shock complicating acute MI should be referred for coronary angiography and emergent revascularization unless contraindications exist. These include life-shortening illnesses, previously defined coronary anatomy unsuitable for revascularization, anoxic brain damage, and patients for whom further therapy appears to be futile.

Triple-vessel disease (60%) and left main artery disease (20%) are often present when shock complicates STEMI. Among the emergency revascularization groups in the SHOCK trial, 60% received PCI and 40% had CABG. The 30-day mortality rates were 45% and 42%, respectively, despite more severe coronary artery disease (CAD) and twice the frequency of diabetes in patients treated with CABG. This was in contrast to the 69% in-hospital mortality rate reported for those with triple-vessel CAD who underwent PCI. Although CABG is an option for some patients, most are treated with PCI of the infarct artery. Surviving patients with multivessel disease can subsequently be considered for additional PCI or CABG to achieve more complete revascularization.

The only subgroup of patients that did not receive a treatment benefit in the SHOCK trial included the 56 patients who were 75 years or older. However, analysis of the 44 elderly patients in the SHOCK trial registry[180] selected for early revascularization showed a significantly lower mortality rate than that of the 233 patients who did not undergo revascularization (48% vs. 81%; P = .0002). Other reports[181,182] also support the use of P-PCI in carefully selected older patients with cardiogenic shock complicating MI, so age alone should not be an exclusion criterion for selecting patients for cardiac catheterization.

Fibrinolytic therapy should be administered to those who are not candidates for early revascularization and who do not have contraindications for lytic therapy. Patients who present to hospitals without revascularization capability should be transferred to a hospital with revascularization capability. IABP placement prior to transport may help stabilize the patient. If the patient presents in shock within 3 to 6 hours of MI onset and delays in transport and intervention are anticipated, both fibrinolytic therapy and IABP counterpulsation may be initiated.[183]

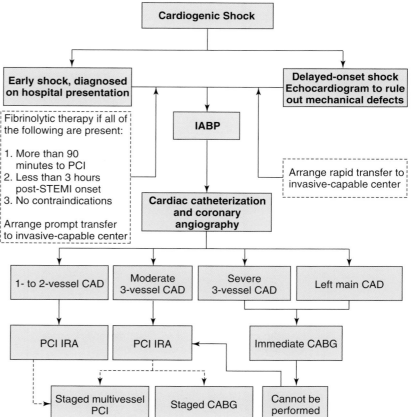

FIGURE 10-11 Recommendations for initial reperfusion therapy when cardiogenic shock complicates ST-segment elevation myocardial infarction (*STEMI*). Early mechanical revascularization with percutaneous coronary intervention (PCI)/coronary artery bypass grafting (CABG) is a class I recommendation for candidates <75 years with ST-segment elevation or left bundle branch block who develop shock <36 hours from STEMI and in whom revascularization can be performed within 18 hours of shock, and a class IIa recommendation for patients ≥75 years with the same criteria. Eighty-five percent of shock cases are diagnosed after initial therapy for STEMI, but shock develops in most patients within 24 hours. An intraaortic balloon pump (*IABP*) is recommended when shock is not quickly reversed with pharmacologic therapy as a stabilizing measure for patients who are candidates for further invasive care. *Dashed lines* indicate that the procedure should be performed in patients with specific indications only. CAD, coronary artery disease; IRA, infarct-related artery. (*Modified from Hochman JS: Cardiogenic shock complicating acute myocardial infarction: expanding the paradigm. Circulation 2003;107:2998-3002.*)

RIGHT VENTRICULAR INFARCTION

RV ischemia can be demonstrated in up to half of patients with inferior STEMI, although only 10% to 15% show the classic hemodynamic abnormalities of clinically significant RV infarction.[122,184] These patients represent a high-risk subgroup of patients with a 25% to 30% mortality rate.[185] In the SHOCK trial registry, patients with predominant RV infarction and cardiogenic shock had a mortality rate similar to patients with LV shock (53% vs. 61%).[186]

The right coronary artery usually supplies most of the RV myocardium. Occlusion of this artery proximal to the RV branches leads to RV ischemia. Most survivors demonstrate a return of normal RV function over a period of weeks to months, suggesting that RV stunning, rather than irreversible necrosis, has occurred. Pathophysiologic reasons for this phenomenon include lower oxygen demand because of lower myocardial mass than in the LV,[187] coronary perfusion during both diastole and systole,[188] and more favorable oxygen supply than in the LV because of more extensive collateral supply.[189]

The extent of RV dysfunction, the restraining effect of the surrounding pericardium, and interventricular dependence related to the shared interventricular septum determine the hemodynamic effect of RV ischemia. The ischemic RV dilates, increasing intrapericardial pressure because of the restraining forces of the pericardium. Consequently, RV systolic pressure and output are reduced, LV preload is decreased, LV end-diastolic dimension and stroke volume are decreased, and the interventricular septum shifts toward the LV.[190] The pressure gradient between the right and left atria becomes an important driving force for pulmonary perfusion. Factors that reduce preload (volume depletion, diuretics, morphine, nitrates) or diminish augmented right atrial contraction (atrial infarction, loss of AV synchrony, AF), or factors that increase RV afterload (LV dysfunction), can have profound adverse hemodynamic effects.[191,192] Paradoxic interventricular septal motion that bulges in pistonlike fashion into the RV, is important in generating systolic force, which improves pulmonary perfusion.[193] Concomitant septal infarction may result in the loss of this compensatory mechanism.

All patients with inferior STEMI should be evaluated for possible RV ischemia or infarction. The clinical triad of hypotension, clear lung fields, and elevated jugular venous pressure in the setting of impending MI is specific but has a sensitivity of less than 25%.[194] Distended neck veins alone or the presence of the Kussmaul sign (distention of the jugular vein on inspiration) are both sensitive and specific[195] unless the patient is volume depleted. All patients with inferior STEMI should be screened for RV MI with right-sided ECG recordings at the time of admission (Figure 10-12). Demonstration of 1-mm ST-segment elevation in lead V1 and in the right precordial lead V4R is the most predictive ECG finding in patients with RV ischemia[196] but may resolve within 10 hours of symptom onset.[197] Echocardiography can show RV dilation and asynergy or abnormal interventricular and interatrial septal motion. Right-to-left shunting through a patent foramen ovale should be suspected when persistent hypoxia is not responsive to supplemental oxygen and can be documented with the color-flow Doppler exam.[198] Pulmonary artery catheterization may be helpful in diagnosing RV ischemia or infarction. A right atrial pressure of 10 mm Hg or greater and more than 80% of pulmonary wedge pressure is a relatively sensitive and specific finding.

Successful reperfusion therapy can prevent or reverse the hemodynamic complications of RV MI. PCI is particularly useful in patients with hypotension or shock because RV ischemic dysfunction resolves quickly with successful reperfusion. The medical treatment of patients with RV ischemic dysfunction is different, and often diametrically opposed to, management of LV dysfunction. The first goal is to maintain RV preload. Nitrates, morphine, and diuretics are routinely used in LV MI but should be avoided in RV MI because they may reduce RV preload, cardiac output, and BP. Volume loading with normal saline can improve cardiac output and BP, but it should not be excessive because RV dilation shifts the interventricular septum into the LV, decreasing LV output.[199] The second goal is to provide inotropic support for the ischemic RV with dobutamine. The third goal is to maintain AV synchrony. High-degree AV block may occur in as many as half of these patients.[200] AV sequential pacing may restore normal BP when ventricular pacing alone has been unsuccessful.[201] AF may occur in up to one third of patients and should be treated with cardioversion if hemodynamic compromise is present. The fourth goal is to decrease RV afterload in the setting of LV failure. This can be accomplished with pulmonary vasodilators.

Mechanical Complications

MITRAL REGURGITATION

Patients with mild MR after STEMI have a worse prognosis than patients without MR.[202] Severe MR may be due to either posterior papillary muscle infarction or be secondary to extensive infarction (Table 10-5). Initial management should include afterload

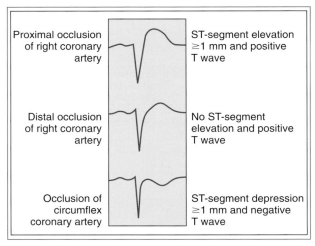

Clinical findings:
Shock with clear lungs, elevated JVP, Kussmaul sign

Hemodynamics:
Increased RA pressure (prominent y descent)
Square root sign in RV tracing

ECG:
ST elevation in R-sided leads

Echo:
Depressed RV function

Management:
Maintain RV preload
Lower RV afterload (PA-PCW)
Restore AV synchrony
Inotropic support
Reperfusion

V₄R

FIGURE 10-12 Electrocardiographic tracings of right ventricular infarction. AV, atrioventricular; ECG, electrocardiogram; JVP, jugular venous pressure; PA, pulmonary artery; PCW, pulmonary capillary wedge; RA, right atrial; RV, right ventricular. (*Modified from Wellens HJ: The value of the right precordial leads of the electrocardiogram. N Engl J Med 1999;340:381-383.*)

TABLE 10-5	Characteristics of Ventricular Septal Rupture, Rupture of the Ventricular Free Wall, and Papillary Muscle Rupture		
CHARACTERISTIC	**VENTRICULAR SEPTAL RUPTURE**	**RUPTURE OF VENTRICULAR FREE WALL**	**PAPILLARY MUSCLE RUPTURE**
Incidence	1%-3% without reperfusion therapy, 0.2%-0.34% with fibrinolytic therapy, 3.9% in patients with cardiogenic shock	0.8%-6.2%; fibrinolytic therapy does not reduce risk; primary PTCA seems to reduce risk	Approximately 1% (posteromedial more frequent than anterolateral papillary muscle)
Time course	Bimodal peak; within 24 hours and 3-5 days; range, 1-14 days	Bimodal peak; within 24 hours and 3-5 days; range, 1-14 days	Bimodal peak; within 24 hours and 3-5 days; range, 1-14 days
Clinical manifestations	Chest pain, shortness of breath, hypotension	Anginal, pleuritic, or pericardial chest pain; syncope; hypotension; arrhythmia; nausea; restlessness; hypotension; sudden death	Abrupt onset of shortness of breath and pulmonary edema; hypotension
Physical findings	Harsh holosystolic murmur, thrill (+), S3, accentuated second heart sound, pulmonary edema, RV and LV failure, cardiogenic shock	JVD (29% of patients), pulsus paradoxus (47%), electromechanical dissociation, cardiogenic shock	A soft murmur in some cases, no thrill, varying signs of RV overload, severe pulmonary edema, cardiogenic shock
Echocardiographic findings	Ventricular septal rupture, left-to-right shunt on color-flow Doppler echocardiography through the ventricular septum, pattern of RV overload	>5 mm pericardial effusion not visualized in all cases; layered, high-acoustic echoes within the pericardium (blood clot); direct visualization of tear, signs of tamponade	Hypercontractile LV, torn papillary muscle or chordae tendineae, flail leaflet, severe mitral regurgitation on color-flow Doppler echocardiography
Right heart catheterization	Increase in oxygen saturation from the RA to RV, large V waves*	Ventriculography insensitive, classic signs of tamponade not always present (equalization of diastolic pressures among the cardiac chambers)	No increase in oxygen saturation from the RA to RV, large V waves,* very high pulmonary capillary wedge pressures

*Large V waves are from the pulmonary capillary wedge pressure.
JVD, jugular venous distention; LV, left ventricle; PTCA, percutaneous transluminal coronary angioplasty; RA, right atrium; RV, right ventricle.
Modified from Antman EM, Anbe DT, Armstrong PW, et al: ACC/AHA guidelines for the management of patients with ST-elevation myocardial infarction: A report of the American College of Cardiology/American Heart Association Task Force on Practice Guidelines (Committee to revise the 1999 Guidelines for the Management of Patients with Acute Myocardial Infarction). Circulation 2004;110:588-636.

reduction and possible IABP or LV assist device. If the MR does not improve over several days or if surgery is required because of critical coronary anatomy or ongoing ischemia, transesophageal echocardiography should be performed to help determine whether valve replacement or annuloplasty is indicated. Mitral valve surgery, usually annuloplasty, should be performed at the same time as CABG for patients with moderately severe ischemic MR.[203]

The presence of pulmonary edema or cardiogenic shock suggests the possibility of acute papillary muscle rupture. If acute papillary muscle rupture is confirmed by echocardiography, urgent surgery should be pursued because delay increases the risk of further myocardial injury, other organ injury, and death.[204] These patients should be stabilized with afterload reduction, inotropic support, and an IABP and should undergo coronary angiography before surgery. In the SHOCK trial registry,[205] 8% of patients with shock presented with severe MR and had an overall hospital mortality rate of 55%. Mortality rate with medical treatment was 71% compared with 40% treated with surgery.

VENTRICULAR SEPTAL RUPTURE

The frequency of acute ventricular septal rupture appears to have declined in the era of prompt reperfusion. The diagnosis can be confirmed by color-flow Doppler echocardiography or by a step up in oxygen saturation from the right atrium to the pulmonary artery (see Table 10-5). Similar to acute severe MR, management includes inotropic and vasodilator therapy, intraaortic balloon counterpulsation, and immediate surgical repair. The usual operation involves excision of all necrotic tissue, patch repair of the septal rupture, and CABG. In the GUSTO-1 trial,[206] the mortality rates for surgical or medically treated patients with ventricular septal rupture were 47% and 94%, respectively. In patients with cardiogenic shock enrolled in the SHOCK registry,[207] mortality rates for surgical and medically treated patients were 81% and 96%, respectively. Percutaneous VSD closure is a less-invasive option than surgery. Even partial closure of the VSD with this technique may stabilize a severely compromised patient and serve as a bridge to surgery. Therefore, if possible, hemodynamically stable patients should undergo treatment with emergency surgery or percutaneous VSD closure[208] before the onset of shock. Future multicenter, randomized trials are needed to identify patients who are best suited to surgical or interventional closure.

LEFT VENTRICULAR FREE WALL RUPTURE

Cardiac rupture occurs in 1% to 6% of patients and accounts for 15% of in-hospital deaths (see Table 10-5).[209] Early reperfusion and the presence of collateral circulation decrease the risk of free wall rupture. Risk factors include advanced age, female gender, first infarction, large infarction, and delivery of fibrinolytic therapy more than 14 hours after onset of symptoms.[207,210] Many patients rapidly die with irreversible electromechanical dissociation, but others develop hypotension and pericardial tamponade. The diagnosis of tamponade or pseudoaneurysm can be made quickly by echocardiography. Rapid volume administration and transfer to the operating room without cardiac catheterization for emergency surgery is recommended. The surgical mortality rate is approximately 60%.[211,212]

LEFT VENTRICULAR ANEURYSM AND LEFT VENTRICULAR THROMBUS

Ventricular aneurysm formation usually occurs in association with left anterior descending artery occlusion and a wide area of infarction. Clinical complications include angina pectoris, CHF, thromboembolism, and ventricular arrhythmias. Successful reperfusion therapy decreases the risk of aneurysm formation. Surgery is rarely required to control heart failure or intractable ventricular arrhythmias unresponsive to conventional therapy. Surgical techniques include plication, excision with linear repair, and ventricular reconstruction with endoventricular patches to maintain better physiologic function.[213] LV size and function determine prognosis. Surgical mortality rates are 3% to 7%. Systemic embolization from a mural thrombus generally occurs in the first few days after STEMI. A meta-analysis of several studies suggests that systemic anticoagulation appears to reduce the risk of embolization.[214] Because most episodes of embolization occur in the first 3 months following STEMI, warfarin can be limited to that time period.

MECHANICAL SUPPORT DEVICES

IABP counterpulsation improves diastolic coronary blood flow and reduces myocardial work by afterload reduction. It should be used in patients with hypotension (systolic BP <90 mm Hg or 30 points below previous mean arterial pressure) that does not respond to other interventions, low output syndrome, or cardiogenic shock. It also is useful for patients with recurrent ischemic-type chest discomfort and signs of hemodynamic instability, poor LV function, or a large area of myocardium at risk to stabilize them for cardiac catheterization and possible revascularization. Intra-aortic balloon counterpulsation may also be a reasonable intervention in the management of refractory polymorphic ventricular tachycardia (VT) or refractory congestive heart failure. Novel percutaneous LV assist devices are now available to aid patients in cardiogenic shock. Several small trials have tested these devices, showing improved hemodynamics but no change in mortality rate.[215,216] It is reasonable to use these devices if IABP fails to improve hemodynamics in patients with cardiogenic shock. Survivors may become elective cardiac transplantation candidates.

Arrhythmias

BRADYARRHYTHMIAS

Bradyarrhythmias may be due to overstimulation of vagal afferent receptors and resulting cholinergic stimulation or to ischemic injury of conducting tissue. Sinus bradycardia is frequent, especially in the first hours of inferior STEMI, with reperfusion of the right coronary artery (Bezold-Jarisch reflex), or after the use of β-blocker or calcium antagonist medications. Intraventricular conduction delay has been reported in 10% to 20% of patients, and heart block may develop in 6% to 14% of patients (Table 10-6). Both are associated with an increased mortality risk because they are generally related to a larger ischemia/infarct zone.[32]

Symptomatic Mobitz I AV block, symptomatic sinus bradycardia, sinus pauses greater than 3 seconds, and sinus bradycardia with a heart rate less than 40 beats/min associated with hypotension or signs of systemic hemodynamic compromise should be treated with an IV bolus of atropine 0.6 to 1.0 mg. Isoproterenol and aminophylline are not recommended because they are arrhythmogenic and increase myocardial oxygen demand. Glucagon has been used to treat bradycardia caused by toxic doses of β-blockers and calcium channel blockers.[217] If bradycardia is persistent, and maximal doses (2 mg) of atropine have been used, transcutaneous or transvenous temporary pacing should be instituted. When there is infranodal AV block, atropine may increase the sinus rate without affecting infranodal conduction, so the effective ratio of conduction may decrease and ventricular rate may decrease. Therefore, temporary pacing should be used instead of pharmacologic therapy.

Ventricular asystole may be caused either by failure of the sinus node to generate a cardiac impulse or by the development of complete heart block, with concurrent failure of the usual underlying atrial, junctional, or ventricular escape mechanisms. Treatment of the acute event requires prompt institution of chest compressions, atropine, vasopressin (40 IU), epinephrine, and transcutaneous

TABLE 10-6	Features of Atrioventricular Conduction Disturbances in Acute Myocardial Infarction	
	Location of AV Conduction Disturbance	
FEATURE	**PROXIMAL**	**DISTAL**
Site of block	Intranodal	Infranodal
Site of infarction	Inferoposterior	Anteroseptal
Compromised arterial supply	90% RCA, 10% LCx	Septal perforators of LAD
Pathogenesis	Ischemia, necrosis, hydropic cell swelling, excess parasympathetic activity	Ischemia, necrosis, hydropic cell swelling
Predominant type of AV nodal block	First degree (PR >200 ms), Mobitz type I second degree	Mobitz type II second degree
Common promontory features of third-degree AV block or escape following third-degree block:	First-second degree Mobitz type I pattern	Third degree
Location	Proximal conduction system (His bundle)	Distal conduction system (bundle branches)
QRS width	<0.12 sec*	>0.12 sec*
Rate of escape rhythm	45-60/min but may be as low as 30/min	Often <30/min
Stability of escape rhythm	Rate usually stable; asystole uncommon	Rate often unstable with moderate to high risk of ventricular asystole
Duration of high-grade AV block	Usually transient (2-3 days)	Usually transient, but some form of AV conduction disturbances and/or intraventricular defect may persist
Associated mortality rate	Low unless associated with hypotension and/or congestive heart failure	High because of extensive infarction associated with power failure or ventricular arrhythmias
Pacemaker therapy		
Temporary	Rarely required; may be considered for bradycardia associated with left ventricular power failure, syncope, or angina	Indicated in patients with anteroseptal infarction and acute bifascicular block
Permanent	Almost never indicated because conduction defect is usually transient	Indicated for patients with high-grade AV block with block in His-Purkinje systems and those with transient advanced AV block and associated bundle branch block

*Some studies suggest that a wide QRS escape rhythm (>0.12 sec) after high-grade AV block in inferior infarction is associated with a worse prognosis.
AV, atrioventricular; LAD, left anterior descending artery; LCx, left circumflex artery; RCA, right coronary artery.
Modified from Antman EM, Anbe DT, Armstrong PW, et al: ACC/AHA guidelines for the management of patients with ST-elevation myocardial infarction: A report of the American College of Cardiology/American Heart Association Task Force on Practice Guidelines (Committee to revise the 1999 Guidelines for the Management of Patients with Acute Myocardial Infarction). Circulation 2004;110:588-636.

pacing. It is important to address the underlying cause and discontinue medications that suppress electrical activity.

The decision to implant a permanent pacemaker for sinus node dysfunction or Mobitz I second-degree AV block should be delayed several days because the conduction abnormality usually resolves and does not affect long-term prognosis.[218] Permanent ventricular pacing is indicated for persistent second- or third-degree AV block or transient second- or third-degree infranodal AV block associated with bilateral bundle branch block. Patients who have permanent AF or flutter should receive a ventricular pacing system. Patients who are in sinus rhythm should receive a permanent dual-chamber pacemaker. Patients with heart failure may be candidates for resynchronization therapy with biventricular pacing. Patients who have severe LV dysfunction and an indication for permanent pacing should be evaluated for implantable cardioverter-defibrillator (ICD) indications.

SUPRAVENTRICULAR ARRHYTHMIA

AF can occur in as many as 20% of patients in high-risk subgroups. Precipitating factors for AF and atrial flutter include excessive sympathetic stimulation, atrial stretch due to LV or RV dysfunction, atrial infarction due to circumflex or right coronary artery lesions, pericarditis, hypokalemia, underlying chronic lung disease, and hypoxia. AF predicts a worse in-hospital and long-term outcome.[219,220] Systemic embolization is more frequent in patients with paroxysmal AF (1.7%) compared with those without (0.6%), with half of embolic events occurring on the first day of hospitalization and more than 90% occurring by the fourth day.[221] Patients with AF or atrial flutter must be considered for cardioversion, rate control, and anticoagulation therapy.

Synchronized cardioversion should be performed if the patient has persistent ischemic pain or is unstable because of tachycardia, hypotension, or heart failure. Brief general anesthesia or conscious sedation should precede an initial monophasic shock of 200 J for AF and 50 J for atrial flutter. Successive shocks, if required, should increase in increments of 100 J. The interval between two consecutive shocks should not be less than 1 minute to avoid myocardial damage.[222]

Rate control can be achieved with IV β-blocker therapy, IV diltiazem (20 mg [0.25 mg/kg]) over 2 minutes followed by an infusion of 10 mg/h, or IV verapamil (2.5 to 10 mg over 2 minutes; may repeat after 15 to 30 minutes). If these agents are contraindicated because of CHF or severe pulmonary disease, amiodarone is effective and well tolerated. If anticoagulation is required, either UFH or LMWH may be used.

Reentrant paroxysmal supraventricular tachycardia, because of its rapid rate, should be treated with the following in sequence: carotid sinus massage, IV adenosine (6 mg over 1 to 2 seconds; if no response, 12 mg over 1 to 2 seconds), IV β-adrenergic blockade, intravenous diltiazem, and IV digoxin. Both paroxysmal supraventricular tachycardia and atrial flutter can be terminated with atrial pacing.

VENTRICULAR ARRHYTHMIAS

The mechanisms for ventricular tachyarrhythmias include loss of transmembrane resting potential, reentrant mechanisms due to dispersion of refractoriness in the border zones between infarcted and nonischemic tissues, and the development of foci of enhanced automaticity. Reperfusion arrhythmias appear to involve washout of toxic metabolites and various ions, such as lactate and potassium. Important contributing factors include heightened adrenergic tone, hypokalemia, hypomagnesemia, intracellular hypercalcemia, acidosis, free fatty acid production from lipolysis, and free radical production from reperfusion of ischemic myocardium.

Treatment of isolated ventricular premature beats, couplets, nonsustained VT, and accelerated idioventricular rhythm is not indicated. Electrolytes and pH should be normalized. The majority of

episodes of VT and VF after STEMI occur within the first 48 hours.[223] Sustained VT or VF that occurs more than 48 hours after STEMI may denote an arrhythmic substrate that deserves further evaluation by electrophysiologic testing.

Immediate cardioversion generally is not needed for sustained VT rates less than 150 beats/min unless hemodynamic compromise is present. Sustained monomorphic VT not associated with angina, pulmonary edema, or hypotension (BP <90 mm Hg) should be treated with amiodarone 150 mg infused over 10 minutes (alternative dose, 5 mg/kg) and repeated 150 mg every 10 to 15 minutes as needed. An alternative infusion is 360 mg over 6 hours (1 mg/min), then 540 mg over the next 18 hours (0.5 mg/min). The total cumulative dose, including additional doses given during cardiac arrest, must not exceed 2.2 g over 24 hours. A procainamide bolus and infusion is another option. Synchronized electrical cardioversion starting at monophasic energies of 50 J can also be performed. Sustained VT (>30 seconds or causing hemodynamic collapse) should immediately be treated with a synchronized electric shock of 200 J. Increasing energies may be used if the initial shock is not successful.

Sustained polymorphic VT should be considered in a similar fashion to VF and managed with an unsynchronized electric shock starting at 200 J. Uncontrolled ischemia and increased sympathetic tone are best treated by IV β-blockade, IABP, or emergency revascularization. IV magnesium may be needed to increase serum magnesium to a level greater than 2.0 mg/dL, and serum potassium level should be greater than 4.0 mEq/L. If the patient has a heart rate of less than 60 beats/min or a long QTc interval, temporary pacing at a higher rate may be instituted.

Primary VF is more prevalent in patients older than 75 years,[224] and the incidence is highest (3% to 5%) in the first 4 hours of STEMI.[223] Current early therapeutic interventions appear to have decreased the incidence of primary VF,[225] and the case fatality rate appears to be declining.[226] Primary VF increases hospital mortality but not long-term prognosis in survivors.[227] Current data do not support prophylactic antiarrhythmic therapy.[228,229] However, IV β-blockade and normalization of potassium and magnesium levels may decrease the risk of primary VF.[230] VF or pulseless VT should be treated with an unsynchronized electric shock with an initial monophasic shock energy of 200 J, progressing to 200 J, 300 J, and 360 J, if necessary. For patients with VF not easily converted by defibrillation, vasopressin 40 U IV push may be substituted for epinephrine 1 mg.[231] VF or pulseless VT refractory to electrical shock can be treated with amiodarone (300 mg or 5 mg/kg, IV bolus) followed by a repeat unsynchronized electric shock.

An ICD is indicated for patients with VF or sustained VT more than 48 hours after STEMI (Figure 10-13).[232-234] Prophylactic ICD implantation is also indicated for patients with a reduced LVEF (≤30%) at least 40 days after STEMI and 3 months after coronary artery revascularization.[235-238] For patients with an LVEF between 31% and 40% and evidence for nonsustained VT, an electrophysiology study is indicated to determine the need for ICD implantation. If inducible VF or VT is found, an ICD is indicated.

Recurrent Chest Pain

RECURRENT ISCHEMIA OR INFARCTION

Chest pain similar to the initial ischemic-type chest discomfort can occur at rest or with limited activity during hospitalization. This may or may not be associated with reelevation of the CK-MB, ST-segment depression or elevation, or pseudonormalization of inverted T waves. Reinfarction occurs in 4% to 5% of patients after fibrinolytic therapy and aspirin. Diagnosis should be based on recurrence of severe ischemic-type chest discomfort that lasts at least 30 minutes, recurrent ST-segment elevation, and reelevation of CK-MB to more than the upper limit of normal or increased by at least 50% over the previous value. Complications include severe CHF, cardiogenic shock, arrhythmias, cardiac arrest, and death.[125,239]

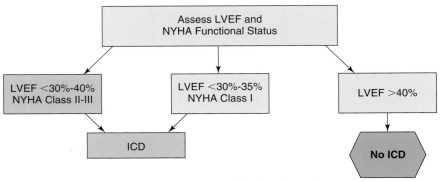

ICD Implantation After STEMI
At Least 40 days After STEMI;
No Spontaneous VT or VF 48 hours post STEMI

FIGURE 10-13 Algorithm for assessment of need for an implantable cardioverter-defibrillator (*ICD*). The appropriate management is selected based on measurement of left ventricular ejection fraction and assessment of the New York Heart Association (*NYHA*) functional class. Patients with depressed left ventricular function at least 40 days after ST-segment elevation myocardial infarction (STEMI) are referred for insertion of an ICD if the left ventricular ejection fraction (*LVEF*) is less than 30% to 40% and they are in NYHA class II to III or if the LVEF is less than 30% to 35% and they are in NYHA class I. Patients with preserved LV function (LVEF >40%) do not receive an ICD regardless of NYHA functional class. All patients are treated with medical therapy after STEMI. VF, ventricular fibrillation; VT, ventricular tachycardia. (*Modified from data contained in Zipes DP, Camm AJ, et al. ACC/AHA/ESC 2006 guidelines for management of patients with ventricular arrhythmias and the prevention of sudden cardiac death; a report of the American College of Cardiology/American Heart Association Task Force and the European Society of Cardiology Committee for Practice Guidelines [Writing Committee to Develop Guidelines for Management of Patients with Ventricular Arrhythmias and the Prevention of Sudden Cardiac Death]. J Am Coll Cardiol 2006;48:1064-1108.*)

Recurrent MI after fibrinolysis increases the risk of death, but most of the deaths occur in the hospital with little additional risk of death occurring between the time of the index hospitalization and 2 years.[240]

Nitrate and β-blocker therapy should be optimized, and therapeutic anticoagulation should be achieved. Secondary causes of recurrent ischemia (poorly controlled heart failure, anemia, and arrhythmias) should be corrected. Coronary arteriography can clarify the cause of chest discomfort and facilitate PCI or CABG if indicated. Readministration of fibrinolytic therapy may be reasonable for patients who are not considered candidates for revascularization or for whom coronary angiography and PCI cannot be rapidly implemented.

PERICARDITIS

Pericarditis can complicate transmural STEMI and is associated with larger infarcts, a lower LVEF, and a higher incidence of CHF.[241,242] Pericarditis may appear up to several weeks after STEMI and can be confused with recurrent ischemia. However, pericardial pain is usually pleuritic and/or positional and radiates to the left shoulder, scapula, or trapezius muscle. Detection of a three-component rub is diagnostic of pericarditis. The ECG may demonstrate J-point elevation with concave upward ST-segment elevation and PR depression. A small pericardial effusion on an echocardiogram is not diagnostic of pericarditis. The incidence of pericarditis has decreased in the reperfusion era, and Dressler syndrome (a post-MI syndrome), an autoimmune-type carditis, is quite rare.[243]

Aspirin (160 to 325 mg/day) is the treatment of choice, but high doses (650 mg every 4 to 6 hours) may be required.[244] Colchicine 0.6 mg orally every 12 hours or acetaminophen 500 mg orally every 12 hours can be used if episodes are not controlled with aspirin.[245] NSAIDs should not be used because they can decrease aspirin efficacy and increase the risk of myocardial scar thinning and infarct expansion. Corticosteroids should not be used except as a last resort because they have been associated with scar thinning and myocardial rupture.[246] Antithrombotic therapy can usually be continued safely but requires added vigilance for the detection of enlarging pericardial effusion or signs of hemodynamic instability.[247]

Other Complications

ISCHEMIC STROKE

Acute stroke complicates 0.75% to 1.2% of STEMIs and has a greater than 40% mortality rate.[248] Prior stroke, hypertension, old age, decreased EF, multiple ulcerated plaques, and AF are the major risk factors for embolic stroke after STEMI.[249] Embolic stroke after STEMI originates from LV thrombus or from the left atrium in the setting of AF and occurs even in patients treated with fibrinolysis. Most ischemic cerebral infarctions after fibrinolytic therapy occur more than 48 hours after treatment.[250] The highest risk period is the first 28 days after STEMI,[251] but risk is elevated for at least up to 1 year. Compared with ICH, patients with ischemic cerebral infarction present more commonly with focal neurologic deficits and less commonly with a depressed level of consciousness. Headache, vomiting, and coma are uncommon.[252]

An algorithm for evaluation and antithrombotic therapy for ischemic stroke is shown in Figure 10-14. Ischemic cerebral dysfunction may be presumed with the sudden onset of a focal neurologic deficit, an initial CT scan negative for blood or mass effect, and the absence of a severe metabolic disorder, seizures, autoimmune disease, or cancer. Neurologic consultation is recommended for neurovascular evaluation and management issues. The location and nature of the ischemic brain lesion should be defined with repeat CT or magnetic resonance scanning. Vascular lesions should be evaluated with noninvasive techniques, such as carotid duplex sonography, transcranial Doppler, magnetic resonance angiography, CT angiography, or transesophageal echocardiography. For carotid territory symptoms and signs, evidence for more than 50% stenosis should be sought.

Both aspirin[55] and clopidogrel[253] reduce the occurrence of ischemic stroke. Patients with cardiogenic sources of embolism, such as AF, LV mural thrombi or akinetic segment of the LV myocardium should receive moderate-intensity warfarin anticoagulation (INR, 2 to 2.5) in combination dual antiplatelet therapy[254] to minimize the risk of hemorrhagic complications. In general, STEMI patients with LV mural thrombus should receive 3 months of warfarin therapy. Ischemic stroke patients with preexisting or persistent AF require lifelong warfarin therapy. A significant

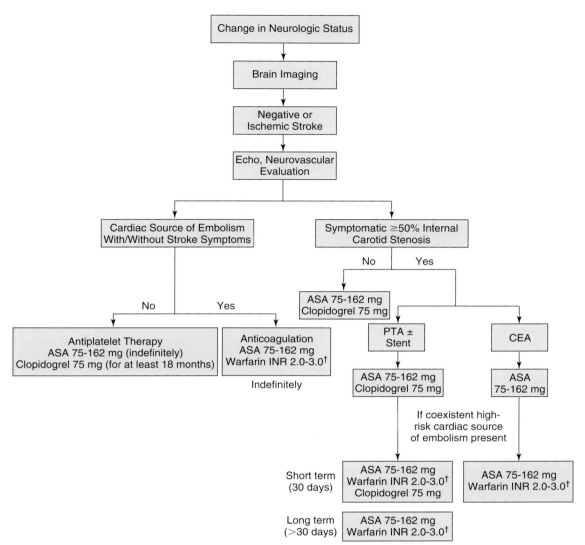

FIGURE 10-14 Algorithm for postreperfusion ischemic stroke treatment. Daily doses of antithrombotic therapy are shown in the algorithm. *An international normalized ratio (INR) of 2.0 to 3.0 is acceptable with tight control, but the lower end of the range is preferable. The combination of antiplatelet therapy and warfarin may be considered in patients <75 years with low bleeding risk and who can be reliably monitored. ASA, aspirin; CEA, carotid endarterectomy; PTA, percutaneous transluminal angioplasty (carotid). (*Modified from Antman EM, Anbe DT, Armstrong PW, et al: ACC/AHA guidelines for the management of patients with ST-elevation myocardial infarction: A report of the American College of Cardiology/American Heart Association Task Force on Practice Guidelines [Committee to revise the 1999 Guidelines for the Management of Patients with Acute Myocardial Infarction]. Circulation 2004;110:588-636.)*

carotid artery stenosis may require treatment either with carotid stenting or carotid endarterectomy.

DEEP VENOUS THROMBOSIS AND PULMONARY EMBOLISM

Deep venous thrombosis and pulmonary embolism occur infrequently. Low-dose heparin prophylaxis, preferably with an LMWH, should be given to patients with CHF who are unable to ambulate or who are considered at high risk for deep venous thrombosis.[255] Most patients with deep venous thrombosis or pulmonary embolism should be anticoagulated with LMWH.[256] Warfarin should be initiated concurrently with LMWH, and LMWH should be continued until INR reaches the therapeutic range of 2 to 2.5. Warfarin should be continued for a duration specific to the individual patient's risk profile.[257]

Hemorrhagic Complications

Bleeding that complicates acute coronary syndromes is associated with recurrent MI, stroke, and death.[258] The magnitude of hazard

approaches that for recurrent MI. Risk factors include age, history of bleeding, renal insufficiency, hypertension, and the antithrombotic regimen chosen (Box 10-5). For example, bivalirudin has been associated with less bleeding than heparin plus GP IIb/IIIa receptor inhibitors in acute coronary syndromes, whereas prasugrel has been associated with increased bleeding compared with clopidogrel in patients who weigh less that 60 kg or are older than 75 years.[30]

To minimize the risk of bleeding, therapies should be chosen that take into account patient specific risk factors. For instance, patients who are at risk for intracranial hemorrhage (elderly, female, history of stroke, low body weight) should receive PCI instead of fibrinolysis. The selection of BMSs versus DESs may be influenced by a history of significant gastrointestinal bleeding or the threat of impending major surgery.[259] Aspirin 81 mg daily should be given daily for life. For those who also require warfarin for AF or cardioembolic events, or who have mechanical heart valves, the INR should be tightly controlled.[254] The risk of periprocedural bleeding may be minimized by meticulous care of the femoral artery site, radial artery access, the use of bivalirudin instead of heparin, and possibly the use of vascular closure

Advanced age (>75 years)
Female gender
History of GI bleeding
Presentation with STEMI or non-STEMI (vs. UAP)
Severe renal dysfunction (CrCl <30 mL/min)
Elevated white blood cell count
Anemia
Fibrinolytic therapy
Invasive strategy
Inappropriate dosing of antithrombotic medications
Bivalirudin monotherapy (protective)

ACS, acute coronary syndromes; CrCl, creatine clearance; GI, gastrointestinal; STEMI, ST-segment elevation myocardial infarction; UAP, unstable angina pectoris.
Data from Mehran R, Popcock SJ, Nikolsky E, et al. A risk score to predict bleeding in patients with acute coronary syndromes. J Am Coll Cardiol 2010;55:2556-2566; Schulman S, Beyth RJ, Kearon C, et al. Hemorrhagic complications of anticoagulant and thrombolytic treatment: American College of Chest Physicians Evidence-Based Clinical Practice Guidelines (8th edition). Chest 2008;133:257S-298S; and Alexander KP, Chen AY, Roe MT, et al. Excess dosing of antiplatelet and antithrombin agents in the treatment of non-ST-segment elevation acute coronary syndromes. JAMA 2005;294:3108-3116.

devices.[260,261] Unexpected postprocedural hypotension and bradycardia should raise suspicion of a retroperitoneal bleed. CT or ultrasound can be confirmatory. Conservative management is usually adequate but vascular consultation should be sought if conservative measures fail. The optimal threshold for transfusion is not known but should probably be less than 8 mg/dL.[262-264]

Coronary Artery Bypass Surgery

Surgery after STEMI may carry substantial risk, particularly in unstable patients with Q-wave infarction and decreased LV function. Prior CABG, female sex, comorbidities, and advanced age are factors that considerably compound this risk.[265] Patients who have mechanical complications of myocardial infarction, such as ventricular septal rupture or papillary muscle rupture, or who have ongoing ischemia that has been unresponsive to other medical therapy and have vessels suitable for CABG, should undergo emergency surgery. Stable patients should have surgery delayed for 3 to 7 days to allow myocardial recovery to occur.

An internal mammary artery graft to a significantly stenosed left anterior descending artery should be used whenever possible because of better long-term survival. Unstable patients undergoing CABG shortly after fibrinolytic therapy, primarily for continuing myocardial ischemia, have a higher operative mortality rate (13% to 17%) and increased use of blood products.[266] CABG should be considered when recurrent ischemia occurs in patients whose coronary artery anatomy is not suitable for PCI. Contemporary modifications of standard on-pump cross-clamped CABG and improvements in anesthetic management and perioperative care have contributed to decreasing mortality rates.[267,268] Elective CABG should improve survival relative to medical therapy in patients with MI who have 1) left main coronary artery stenosis; 2) left main equivalent disease (significant ≥70% stenosis of the proximal left anterior descending and proximal left circumflex arteries); 3) triple-vessel disease, particularly with decreased LV function; 4) two-vessel disease with significant proximal left anterior descending stenosis, not amenable to PCI, and either EF less than 50% or demonstrable ischemia on noninvasive testing; and 5) one- or two-vessel disease, not amenable to PCI, without proximal left anterior descending stenosis but with a large area of viable myocardium at risk and high-risk criteria on noninvasive testing.[269] Aspirin should not be withheld before surgery, but if possible, clopidogrel should be withheld for 5 to 7 days, prasugrel for 7 days, and ticagrelor for 5 to 7 days[30,63,269] unless urgent or emergent CABG is necessary. Platelet aggregation returns to normal 4 hours

after discontinuing eptifibatide or tirofiban. Platelet transfusions may need to be given to restore platelet function if surgery is performed within 24 hours of receiving abciximab because of its prolonged effect.

Risk Stratification

The purpose of risk stratification testing is to determine which patients are at increased risk for recurrent ischemic events, congestive heart failure, or sudden death. Major management decisions include whether to refer a patient for cardiac catheterization (Figure 10-15) or for placement of an ICD (see Figure 10-13).

EXERCISE TESTING

Exercise testing may be performed to 1) predict the likelihood of a subsequent cardiac event, 2) establish exercise parameters for cardiac rehabilitation, 3) assess functional capacity and the patient's ability to perform tasks at home and at work, 4) evaluate recurrent chest pain, and 5) evaluate the efficacy of the patient's current medical regimen.[270]

Two different protocols have been used. Low-level exercise testing appears to be safe if patients have had no symptoms of angina or heart failure and have a stable baseline ECG 48 to 72 hours before the exercise test. The traditional submaximal exercise test is stopped when one of the following endpoints is reached: peak heart rate of 120 to 130 beats/min or 70% of maximal predicted for age, peak work level of 5 metabolic equivalents (METS), clinical or ECG endpoints of mild angina or dyspnea, ST-segment depression greater than 2 mm, exertional hypotension, or three or more consecutive premature ventricular contractions. The second protocol is performance of a symptom-limited exercise test in low-risk patients days to weeks after STEMI. Although this will result in a higher frequency of abnormal exercise tests, the prognostic value of ST-segment depression occurring at higher work levels in deconditioned patients is uncertain. The results of a symptom-limited test can also be used to establish intensity and target heart rate during cardiac rehabilitation. The duration of exercise is also known to be an important predictor of outcome. The ability to perform at least 5 METS of exercise without ST-segment depression and with a normal rise in BP has negative predictive power and is reassuring. STEMI patients without complications who have not undergone coronary angiography, and who are potential candidates for revascularization, should undergo exercise ECG before or within a few weeks after discharge.

Baseline abnormalities that compromise ECG interpretation include greater than 1-mm ST-segment depression on the resting tracing, LBBB, LV hypertrophy with strain, ventricular preexcitation, and ventricular pacing. If exercise testing is performed in the presence of these abnormalities, echocardiography or myocardial perfusion imaging should be added. Exercise testing should not be performed within 2 to 3 days of STEMI in patients who have not undergone successful reperfusion. Exercise testing should not be performed to evaluate patients with STEMI who have unstable postinfarction angina, decompensated CHF, life-threatening cardiac arrhythmias, noncardiac conditions that severely limit the ability to exercise, or other absolute contraindications to exercise testing.

ECHOCARDIOGRAPHY

Echocardiography should be used to assess both global and regional ventricular function in patients not undergoing contrast left ventriculography. It should also be used to evaluate suspected complications, including RV infarction, acute MR, ventricular septal rupture, cardiogenic shock, infarct expansion, intracardiac thrombus, and pericardial effusion.[271,272]

The incremental value of exercise echocardiography over regular exercising testing after STEMI has not been established.

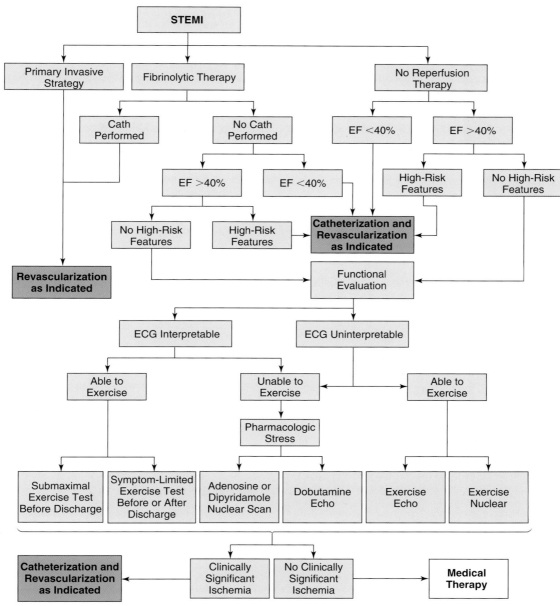

FIGURE 10-15 Evidence-based approach to need for catheterization (*Cath*) and revascularization after ST-segment elevation myocardial infarction (*STEMI*). The algorithm shows treatment paths for patients who initially undergo a primary invasive strategy, receive fibrinolytic therapy, or do not undergo reperfusion therapy for STEMI. Patients who have not undergone a primary invasive strategy and have no high-risk features should undergo functional evaluation with one of the non-invasive tests shown. When clinically significant ischemia is detected, patients should undergo catheterization and revascularization as indicated; if no clinically significant ischemia is detected, medical therapy is prescribed after STEMI. ECG, electrocardiogram; EF, ejection fraction. *(Modified from Antman EM, Anbe DT, Armstrong PW, et al: ACC/AHA guidelines for the management of patients with ST-elevation myocardial infarction: A report of the American College of Cardiology/American Heart Association Task Force on Practice Guidelines [Committee to revise the 1999 Guidelines for the Management of Patients with Acute Myocardial Infarction]. Circulation 2004;588-636.)*

However, echocardiography or perfusion imaging should be added to exercise testing whenever baseline abnormalities are expected to compromise ECG interpretation. Pharmacologic stress echocardiography with a graded protocol beginning at low doses of dobutamine can be substituted for exercise in predischarge functional testing for ischemia in patients with limited exercise capacity and can help in assessing myocardial viability early after STEMI.

MYOCARDIAL PERFUSION IMAGING

When baseline abnormalities are expected to compromise ECG exercise test interpretation, myocardial perfusion imaging or echocardiography should be added. An advantage for nuclear scintigraphy is the quantitative measurement of LVEF. Dipyridamole, adenosine, or regadenosine stress perfusion nuclear scintigraphy for patients who are unable to exercise or who have baseline ECG abnormalities is safe and can be used for early (48 to 72 hours) risk stratification.[273,274]

LEFT VENTRICULAR FUNCTION

Assessment of LV function after STEMI has been shown to be one of the most accurate predictors of future cardiac events.[275] The assessment can include such basic factors as clinical estimates based on the patient's symptoms (exertional dyspnea, functional status) and physical findings (rales, murmurs, elevated jugular venous pressure, cardiomegaly, S3 gallop). Measurement of LVEF by contrast ventriculography, radionuclide ventriculography, and two-dimensional echocardiography has important prognostic value. Because of the dynamic nature of LV function recovery after STEMI, the timing of the imaging study must be considered. An LVEF less than 40% is an indication for ACE inhibitor therapy and less than 30% is an indication for an ICD. Postinfarction LV dilation, demonstrated by increased end-systolic volume greater than 130 mL, may be a better predictor of death after MI than an LVEF less than 40% or increased end-diastolic volume.[276]

MYOCARDIAL VIABILITY

In some patients, viable but dysfunctional myocardium contributes to LV dysfunction and may be significantly reversible with revascularization. Processes of myocardial hibernation (chronic low-flow states associated with depressed myocardial function)[277] and stunning (depression of ventricular function after acute ischemia despite adequate restoration of blood flow)[278] contribute to the potential reversibility of ventricular function. Radionuclide imaging and dobutamine echocardiography can identify patients most likely to benefit from revascularization.[279] Positron emission tomography[280] and contrast-enhanced magnetic resonance imaging[281,282] are promising experimental techniques. However, more conclusive diagnostic efficacy studies are needed to demonstrate patient benefit from viability testing before it becomes standard testing.

INVASIVE EVALUATION

All survivors of STEMI who are candidates for revascularization therapy with spontaneous ischemia, intermediate- or high-risk findings on noninvasive testing, hemodynamic or electrical instability, mechanical defects, prior revascularization, or high-risk clinical features should be considered for coronary arteriography. PCI or CABG may be considered in these patients if they are found to have significant obstructive coronary artery disease. Previous randomized trials testing a strategy of routine catheterization after fibrinolytic therapy suggested that such an approach was deleterious.[283-287] However, those trials were conducted in an era when aspirin was inconsistently administered, high doses of UFH without ACT monitoring were used, and the interventional catheters, radiographic imaging equipment, and supportive antiplatelet agents were suboptimal. Subsequent data suggest that the early invasive strategy is associated with a lower risk of recurrent MI and death.[147,149]

Multivessel CAD is present in 40% to 65% of patients presenting with STEMI who undergo P-PCI and is associated with adverse prognosis.[288,289] PCI of an angiographically significant stenosis in a patent infarct artery more than 24 hours after STEMI, whether or not the patient received reperfusion therapy, may be considered as part of an invasive strategy to preserve long-term patency or relieve ischemia.[290-292] Adequate randomized trial data to evaluate the benefit of staged PCI of the noninfarct artery after STEMI are lacking. Consensus and observational data support delayed PCI of a nonculprit stenosis if there is evidence of spontaneous or provoked ischemia, or intermediate- or high-risk findings on noninvasive testing. Patients with a low risk of complications may be candidates for early discharge.[293]

ASSESSMENT OF ELECTRICAL SUBSTRATE

The two most important predictors for arrhythmic death after STEMI are LV dysfunction and the severity and timing of ventricular arrhythmias. If LVEF is reduced during the acute hospital phase, it should be reassessed 40 days after MI or 3 months after revascularization. If the LVEF remains 35% or less and the patient has signs or symptoms of class II or III NYHA CHF, or if the LVEF

is 30% or less an ICD is indicated.[294,295] For patients with an LVEF of 35% or less and a QRS duration of 120 ms or more, cardiac resynchronization therapy along with an ICD is recommended for patients with NYHA class III or IV CHF along with optimal medical therapy (see Figure 10-13).[296] Sustained VT or VF within the first 24 to 48 hours of STEMI is associated with increased in-hospital mortality rate but not necessarily with long-term mortality. Late sustained VT/VF however, in the absence of a reversible cause and associated with significant LV dysfunction, carries an increased risk of late sudden death and is an indication for ICD implantation. The presence of nonsustained VT on telemetry or by Holter monitoring within 6 to 40 days of STEMI did not predict or improve overall survival with early ICD implantation.[297] A number of other noninvasive strategies have been used to try to identify patients at high risk for arrhythmic events. Signal-averaged ECG identifies delayed, fragmented conduction in the infarct zone in the form of late potentials at the terminus of the QRS complex and represents an anatomic substrate that predisposes the patient to reentrant VT.[298] Heart rate variability, an analysis of the beat-to-beat variation in cycle length, largely reflects the sympathovagal interaction regulating heart rate. Low heart rate variability, indicative of decreased vagal tone, is a predictor of increased mortality risk, including sudden death, in patients after MI.[299] Baroreceptor sensitivity also quantifies the influence of parasympathetic tone on the heart. It is measured as the slope of a regression line that relates beat-to-beat heart rate change in response to a change in BP, often accomplished by giving a small bolus of phenylephrine.[300] Abnormalities in ventricular repolarization are detectable by microvolt alterations of T-wave amplitude, or T-wave alternans, and have been shown to be associated with inducible ventricular arrhythmias during programmed ventricular stimulation and spontaneous arrhythmic events.[301] The clinical importance of these tests has yet to be determined.

Long-Term Management
Risk Factor Control

Secondary prevention therapies are an essential part of the management of all patients with STEMI (Table 10-7).[302] Because atherosclerotic vascular disease is frequently found in multiple vascular beds, the physician should also search for symptoms or signs of peripheral vascular disease or cerebrovascular disease in patients with STEMI. Approximately 70% of CHD deaths and 50% of MIs occur in patients who have previously established coronary artery disease.[303] It is estimated that the likelihood of fatal and nonfatal MI is four to six times higher in patients with apparent coronary disease. Within 6 years of a recognized MI, 18% of men and 35% of women will have another[303]; most episodes of cardiac arrest occur within 18 months after hospital discharge for STEMI.[304] Therefore, the institution of secondary prevention therapies and risk reduction strategies in patients recovering from STEMI represent major opportunities to reduce the toll of cardiovascular disease.

WEIGHT MANAGEMENT

Obesity is a recognized major risk factor for cardiovascular disease and an important component of metabolic syndrome. The diagnosis of metabolic syndrome includes three of the following: waist circumference greater than 40 inches in men or more than 35 inches in women; triglyceride levels of 150 mg/dL or higher; high-density lipoprotein (HDL) levels less than 40 mg/dL in men or less than 50 mg/dL in women; BP greater than 130/85 mm Hg; and fasting blood glucose level of 100 mg/dL or higher. The primary treatment strategies are calorie control and physical activity. A desirable body mass index range is 18.5 to 24.9 kg/m^2. Weight loss should be part of the cardiac rehabilitation program after STEMI with a goal of losing 10% of body weight over 6 months at a rate of 1 to 2 lb/week.

TABLE 10-7 Secondary Prevention for Patients with STEMI

FACTOR	GOAL	INTERVENTION RECOMMENDATION
Risk Factors		
Smoking	Complete cessation	Assess tobacco use. Strongly encourage patient and family to stop smoking and to avoid secondhand smoke. Provide counseling, pharmacologic therapy (including nicotine replacement and bupropion) and formal smoking cessation programs as appropriate.
Blood pressure control	<140/90 mm Hg <130/80 mm Hg with CKD or diabetes	If blood pressure ≥120/80 mm Hg: Initiate lifestyle modification (weight control; physical activity; alcohol moderation; moderate sodium restriction; emphasis on fruits, vegetables, and low-fat dairy products) in all patients. Add blood pressure-reducing medications, emphasizing the use of β-blockers and inhibitors of the renin-angiotensin-aldosterone system.
Lipid management (TG <200 mg/dL)	LDL-C substantially <100 mg/dL, preferably ≤70 mg/dL	Start dietary therapy in all patients (<7% of total calories as saturated fat and <200 mg/day cholesterol). Promote physical activity and weight management. Encourage increased consumption of omega-3 fatty acids. Assess fasting lipid profile, preferably within 24 hours of STEMI. Add drug therapy as follows: • LDL-C <100 mg/dL (baseline or on-treatment): use statins to lower LDL-C • LDL-C ≥100 mg/dL (baseline or on-treatment): intensify LDL-C-lowering therapy with drug treatment, preferably with statins
Lipid management (TG ≥200 mg/dL)	Non-HDL-C* <130 mg/dL	TG ≥150 mg/dL or HDL-C <40 mg/dL: emphasize weight management and physical activity; advise smoking cessation TG 200-499 mg/dL: after LDL-lowering therapy,† consider adding fibrate or niacin‡ TG is ≥500 mg/dL: consider fibrate or niacin‡ before LDL-C-lowering therapy† and omega-3 fatty acids as adjunct
Physical activity	Minimum: 30 min 3-4 days/wk	Assess risk, preferably with exercise test, to guide prescription. Encourage minimum of 30-60 min activity, preferably daily, or at least 3 or 4 times weekly (walking, jogging, cycling, other aerobic activity) supplemented by an increase in daily lifestyle activities (walking breaks at work, gardening, household work). Cardiac rehabilitation programs are recommended for patients with STEMI, particularly those with multiple modifiable risk factors and/or moderate- to high-risk patients in whom supervised exercise training is warranted.
Weight management	BMI 18.5-24.9 kg/m² Waist circumference: Women: <35 in Men: <40 in	Calculate BMI and measure waist circumference as part of evaluation. Monitor response of BMI and waist circumference to therapy. Start weight management and physical activity as appropriate. If waist circumference is ≥35 inches in women or ≥40 inches in men, initiate lifestyle changes and treatment strategies for metabolic syndrome.
Diabetes management	HbA1c <7%	Appropriate hypoglycemic therapy to achieve near-normal fasting plasma glucose. Treatment of other risk factors (physical activity, weight management, blood pressure, and cholesterol management).
Pharmacologic Treatment		
Antiplatelet agents/anticoagulants		Start, and continue indefinitely, aspirin 81 mg/day if not contraindicated. For STEMI patients with a stent: • If patient received a loading dose of clopidogrel, continue at 75 mg/day for at least 1 year. • If patient received a loading dose of prasugrel, continue at 10 mg/day for at least 1 year. • If patient received a loading dose of ticagrelor, continue at 90 mg bid for at least 1 year. Manage warfarin to INR 2.0-2.5 when indicated in post-STEMI patients on dual antiplatelet therapy.
Renin-angiotensin-aldosterone system blockers		ACE inhibitors in all patients indefinitely; start early in stable high-risk patients (anterior MI, previous MI, Killip class ≥II [S3 gallop, rales, radiographic CHF], LVEF <40%). ARBs in patients intolerant to ACE inhibitors and either clinical or radiologic signs of CHF or LVEF <40%. Aldosterone blockade in patients without significant renal dysfunction§ or hyperkalemia‖ who are already receiving therapeutic doses of an ACE inhibitor, have LVEF 40%, and either diabetes or heart failure.
β-Blockers		Start in all patients. Continue indefinitely. Observe usual contraindications.

*Non-HDL-C = Total cholesterol − HDL-C.
†Treat to a goal of non-HDL-C substantially <130 mg/dL.
‡Dietary supplement niacin must not be used as a substitute for prescription niacin; over-the-counter niacin should be used only if approved and monitored by a physician.
§Creatinine should be ≤2.5 mg/dL in men or ≤2.0 mg/dL in women.
‖Potassium should be <5.0 mEq/L.
ACE, angiotensin-converting enzyme; ARBs, angiotensin receptor blockers; BMI, body mass index; CHF, congestive heart failure; HbA1c, hemoglobin A1c; HDL-C, high-density lipoprotein cholesterol; INR, international normalized ratio; LDL-C, low-density lipoprotein cholesterol; LVEF, left ventricular ejection fraction; MI, myocardial infarction; STEMI, ST-elevation myocardial infarction; TG, triglycerides.
Modified from Smith SC, Benjamin EJ, Bonow RO, et al. AHA/ACCF secondary prevention and risk reduction therapy for patients with coronary and other atherosclerotic vascular disease: 2011 update. J Am Coll Cardiol 2011;58(23):2432-2446; and Levine GN, Bates ER, Blankenship JC, et al. 2011 ACCF/AHA/SCAI guideline for percutaneous coronary intervention: executive summary. Circulation 2011;124:2574-2609.

SMOKING CESSATION

Smoking increases coronary vasomotor tone, reduces the antiischemic effects of β-adrenoceptor blockers, and doubles mortality risk after STEMI.[305] Smoking cessation reduces rates of reinfarction and death within 1 year of quitting, but one third to one half of patients relapse within 6 to 12 months.[306] Family members who live in the same household should also be encouraged to quit smoking to help reinforce the patient's effort and decrease the risk of second-hand smoke exposure. The most effective pharmacologic adjuncts for treating nicotine dependence are nicotine replacement therapy (gums and patches), bupropion, and other pharmacologic approaches combined with behavioral counseling.[307]

LIPID MANAGEMENT

A diet low in saturated fat and cholesterol (<7% of total calories as saturated fat and <200 mg/day cholesterol) should be started after recovery from STEMI. Patients should increase consumption of omega-3 fatty acids, fruits, vegetables, soluble (viscous) fiber, and whole grains. The Heart Protection Study[304] and the Pravastatin or Atorvastatin Evaluation and Infection Therapy (PROVE IT)-TIMI 22 trial,[308] among others,[309] suggests that the goal for statin therapy in these patients should be to lower low-density lipoprotein (LDL) cholesterol to 70 mg/dL. Approximately 25% of patients who have recovered from STEMI demonstrate desirable total cholesterol values but a low HDL level. Low HDL is an independent risk factor for the development for CAD.[310] Patients with non-HDL cholesterol levels less than 130 mg/dL who have HDL levels less than 40 mg/dL should receive special emphasis on nonpharmacologic therapy (i.e., exercise, weight loss) to increase HDL. Those who do not respond may be started on fibrates or niacin. It is reasonable to add either niacin or fibrates to the diet regardless of LDL and HDL levels when triglyceride levels are greater than 500 mg/dL. In this setting, non-HDL cholesterol (goal <130 mg/dL) should be the cholesterol target rather than LDL. Diet and drug treatment are also effective in the elderly.[311] Patients started on lipid-lowering therapy before hospital discharge are three times more likely to be taking medication at 6 months than those who start therapy after discharge.[312]

BLOOD PRESSURE CONTROL

Lifestyle modifications for patients with BP of 140/90 mm Hg or higher include weight reduction if overweight or obese, consumption of a diet rich in fruits and vegetables and low in total fat and saturated fat, and reduction of sodium to no more than 2.4 g/day. A diet rich in potassium and calcium is also recommended for those with normal renal function. After STEMI, patients should be treated with β-blockers, ACE inhibitors (or angiotensin receptor blockers if ACE inhibitors are not tolerated), and, if necessary, aldosterone antagonists to a target BP of less than 140/90 mm Hg. Patients with chronic kidney disease or diabetes should be treated to a target less than 130/80 mm Hg.[302,313] Most patients require two or more drugs to reach goal, and when the BP is greater than 20/10 mm Hg above goal, two drugs should typically be used from the outset. Thiazides or long-acting calcium channel blockers may be used if other agents are not tolerated or are not sufficient to reach BP goal. Short-acting calcium antagonists should not be used.

DIABETES MANAGEMENT

Tight glucose control (hemoglobin A1c <7.0%) in diabetics during and after STEMI has been shown to lower short-term and 1-year mortality rates.[314] Pioglitazone may be used as monotherapy or in combination with other oral hypoglycemic agents, insulin, and diet for control of diabetes. Pioglitazone may also be associated with fluid retention and an increase in LV preload[315] resistant to diuretics, so it should not be used in patients recovering from STEMI who have NYHA class III or IV heart failure.[316]

Medications

ANTIPLATELET AGENTS

The Antiplatelet Trialists' Collaboration reported a 25% reduction in the risk of recurrent infarction, stroke, or vascular death in patients who received prolonged antiplatelet therapy (36 fewer events for every 1000 patients treated).[57] No antiplatelet therapy has proved superior to aspirin, and a daily dose of 81 mg aspirin should be continued indefinitely. The salutary effect of aspirin may be diminished by the concomitant use of ibuprofen or other NSAIDs and should be discouraged.[317,318] Clopidogrel is the best alternative to aspirin in patients who have a true aspirin allergy.[319] Dual antiplatelet therapy should ideally be continued for 1 year in patients who are not treated with PCI and for at least 1 year or longer in patients who receive PCI.[30,60,61]

β-BLOCKERS

The benefits of β-blocker therapy in patients without contraindications are historically established with or without reperfusion therapy and in all age groups. The greatest mortality benefit is seen in patients with impaired LV function, ventricular arrhythmias, and occluded infarct arteries. The benefit is less in low-risk patients, but β-blockers may still minimize the likelihood of recurrent ischemic symptoms and control heart rate and BP during exertion. In patients with moderate or severe LV failure, β-blocker therapy should be administered on a gradual titration scheme.[320] Even when relative contraindications exist (mild asthma not currently active, insulin-dependent diabetes, chronic obstructive pulmonary disease, peripheral vascular disease, PR interval >0.24 seconds, moderate LV failure), the benefit in reducing mortality rate and reinfarction with β-blocker therapy may outweigh the risks. Data from large trials suggest that therapy should be continued for at least 2 to 3 years and probably should be continued indefinitely.

STATINS

Statin therapy reduces the risk of MI, stroke, and death in all subgroups.[308,321-333] Benefit has been shown at all levels of LDL, although the greatest benefit was seen with LDL greater than 125 mg/dL. A strong argument can be made for starting all patients on statin therapy regardless of LDL level. The treatment goal should be an LDL level of 70 mg/dL or less.[308]

INHIBITION OF THE RENIN-ANGIOTENSIN-ALDOSTERONE SYSTEM

ACE inhibitors inhibit ventricular remodeling and dilation after STEMI and should be prescribed at discharge for all patients without contraindications to decrease the risk of MI, CHF, and death.[324-327] Although the largest benefit appears to be in those with an EF less than 40% and with anterior MI, other trials have shown benefit in patients without known LV dysfunction or CHF.[328,329]

Angiotensin receptor blockers should be prescribed for those STEMI patients who are intolerant of ACE inhibitors and have either clinical or radiologic signs of heart failure and an LVEF less than 40%. Valsartan may be initiated at 20 mg/day and titrated to a maximum of 160 mg twice a day.[330] Candesartan can be initiated at 4 to 8 mg daily and titrated to 32 mg daily.[331]

An aldosterone inhibitor (spironolactone, at a target dose of 50 mg, or eplerenone, at a target dose of 50 mg) should be added to an ACE inhibitor or angiotensin receptor blocker in patients with LVEF of 40% or less and CHF or diabetes, provided the serum creatinine is 2.5 mg/dL or less in men or 2.0 mg/dL or less in women, and the serum potassium is 5.0 mEq/L or less.[162,163]

WARFARIN

The indications for long-term anticoagulation after STEMI are controversial and evolving. Markers of thrombin generation remain elevated after STEMI, and recurrent ischemic events occur even in the presence of aspirin and clopidogrel. In the Antithrombotics in the Prevention of Reocclusion in Coronary Thrombolysis (APRICOT) study,[332] the use of medium-intensity warfarin (INR, 2 to 3) plus aspirin resulted in less infarct artery reocclusion after fibrinolytic therapy and a significant reduction in the combined endpoints of death, MI, and revascularization compared with aspirin alone. The Warfarin, Aspirin, or Both After Myocardial Infarction (WARIS II) trial[333] compared high-intensity warfarin alone (INR, 2.8 to 4.2), medium-intensity warfarin (INR, 2 to 2.5) plus 81 mg aspirin, and 160 mg aspirin alone. There was a significant reduction in nonfatal MI and nonfatal thromboembolic stroke with warfarin, but bleeding was more common and a significant number of patients discontinued therapy. Patients older than 75 years have not been adequately studied.

Warfarin should be used in STEMI patients with persistent or paroxysmal AF. It should be prescribed for LV thrombus noted on an imaging study for at least 3 months and may be useful when extensive regional wall motion abnormalities are present. When the combination of warfarin and dual antiplatelet therapy is required, clopidogrel should be stopped as soon as possible,[334,335] and the INR kept as close to 2 to 2.5 as possible.

HORMONE REPLACEMENT THERAPY

Postmenopausal women should not receive combination estrogen and progestin therapy for secondary prevention.[336,337] It is recommended to discontinue use of hormone therapy for women who have STEMI.[338] Women who are 1 to 2 years past initiation of hormone therapy and want to continue it should weigh the risks and benefits, recognizing a greater risk of cardiovascular events. Hormone therapy should not be continued while patients are on bed rest in the hospital because of the increased risk for venous thromboembolic events.

Functional Status

PHYSICAL ACTIVITY

Walking can be encouraged immediately after discharge. In stable uncomplicated patients, sexual activity with the usual partner can be resumed within 1 week to 10 days. Driving can begin 1 week after discharge if the patient is judged to be in compliance with individual state laws. Air travel within the first 2 weeks of STEMI should be undertaken only in the absence of angina or dyspnea at rest. Based on assessment of risk, ideally with an exercise test to guide the prescription, all patients recovering from STEMI should be encouraged to exercise for a minimum of 30 minutes, preferably daily, but at least five times per week (walking, jogging, cycling, or other aerobic activity). The 30 minutes can be spread out over two or three segments during the day. This should be supplemented by an increase in daily lifestyle activities (e.g., walking breaks at work, gardening, household work). Patients also require specific instruction on strenuous activities (e.g., heavy lifting, climbing stairs, yard work, household activities) that are permissible and those they should avoid. In addition to aerobic training, mild to moderate resistance training is also recommended. This can be started 2 to 4 weeks after aerobic training has begun.[302,339]

CARDIAC REHABILITATION

Comprehensive cardiac rehabilitation services include long-term programs that involve medical evaluation, prescribed exercise, cardiac risk factor modification, education, and counseling.[340] These programs are designed to limit the physiologic and psychological effects of cardiac illness, reduce the risk for sudden death or reinfarction, control cardiac symptoms, stabilize or reverse the atherosclerotic process, and enhance the psychosocial and vocational status of selected patients. Enrollment in a cardiac rehabilitation program after discharge may enhance patient education and compliance with the medical regimen as well as assist with the implementation of a regular exercise program. A cardiac rehabilitation program is recommended for all patients, particularly those with multiple modifiable risk factors and moderate- to high-risk patients in whom supervised exercise training is warranted.

PSYCHOSOCIAL IMPACT

Major depression may occur in 15% to 20% of patients and minor depression in as many as 50%.[341] These patients are more likely to be rehospitalized within 1 year and have a decreased long-term survival. They are also less likely to complete cardiac rehabilitation, comply with lifestyle changes and medication prescriptions, return to work, or resume a normal quality of life. Therefore, the psychosocial status of the patient should be evaluated, including inquiries regarding symptoms of depression, anxiety, or sleep disorders, as well as social support environment. Treatment of depression with combined cognitive behavioral therapy and selective serotonin reuptake inhibitors improves outcome in terms of depressive symptoms and social function.[342]

FOLLOW-UP VISIT

A caring and supportive doctor-patient relationship is vital to the well-being of survivors and their families. It is common practice to see these patients 3 to 6 weeks after hospital discharge to assess their progress. A number of issues should be addressed. 1) The presence or absence of cardiovascular symptoms and the functional state of the patient should be delineated. 2) The list of current medications should be verified and reevaluated. Doses of β-blockers, ACE inhibitors, and statins should be titrated when appropriate. 3) The risk assessment workup should be completed and reviewed. This should include a check of LV function for patients whose early post-STEMI EF was 30% to 40% or lower regarding possible ICD use. 4) The physician should review the principles of secondary prevention with the patient and family. 5) The psychosocial status of the patient should be evaluated, including inquiries regarding symptoms of depression, anxiety, sleep disorders, and the social support environment. Cognitive behavioral therapy and antidepressants should be initiated if indicated. 6) The resumption of physical activity, return to work, resumption of sexual activity, and travel should be discussed. 7) Patients and their families should be asked if they are interested in CPR and AED training. 8) The physician should review with the patient the risk of reinfarction, symptoms of angina and STEMI, and the advisability of calling 911 if symptoms are unimproved or worsen 5 minutes after a sublingual nitroglycerin tablet. 9) Cardiac rehabilitation programs where available and appropriate should be recommended.

RETURN TO WORK AND DISABILITY

Return to work rates and disability rates are influenced by multiple factors. Besides the cardiac functional status of the patient, factors such as age, depressive symptoms, job security, job satisfaction, financial stability, and company policies all influence the ability and decision to return to work.

REFERENCES

1. Executive summary: heart disease and stroke statistics. 2010 update. *Circulation* 121:948-954, 2010.
2. Fang J, Alderman MH, Keenan NL, et al: Acute myocardial infarction hospitalization in the United States, 1979 to 2005. *Am J Med* 123:259-266, 2010.

3. Chen J, et al: Recent declines in hospitalizations for acute myocardial infarction for Medicare fee-for-service beneficiaries. *Circulation* 121:1322-1328, 2010.
4. Roger V, et al: Trends in incidence, severity, and outcome of hospitalized myocardial infarction. *Circulation* 121:863-869, 2010.
5. Myerson M, et al: Declining severity of myocardial infarction 1987 to 2002.The Atherosclerosis Risk in Communities (ARIC) study. *Circulation* 119:503-514, 2009.
6. Jenberg J, Johanson P, Held C, et al: Association between adoption of evidence based treatment and survival for patients with ST-elevation myocardial infarction. *JAMA* 305:1677-1684, 2011.
7. Pearson TA, Blair SN, Daniels SR, et al: AHA Guideline for primary prevention of cardiovascular diseases and stroke: 2002 update: consensus panel guide to comprehensive risk reduction for adult patients without coronary or other atherosclerotic vascular diseases. American Heart Association Science Advisory and Coordinating Committee. *Circulation* 2002;106:388-391.
8. Schroeder SA: What to do with a patient who smokes. *JAMA* 2005;294:482-487.
9. Executive summary of the third report of the National Detection, Evaluation, and Treatment of High Blood Cholesterol in Adults (Adult Treatment Panel III). *JAMA* 2001;285:2486-2497.
10. Chobanian AV, Bakris GL, Black HR, et al, for the National Heart, Lung, and Blood Institute Joint National Committee on Prevention, Detection, Evaluation, and Treatment of High Blood Pressure, National High Blood Pressure Education Program Coordinating Committee: The seventh report of the Joint National Committee on Prevention, Detection, Evaluation, and Treatment of High Blood Pressure, the JNC 7 report. *JAMA* 2003; 289:2560-2572.
11. Wilson PW, D'Angostino RB, Levy D, et al: Prediction of coronary heart disease using risk factor categories. *Circulation* 1998;97:1837-1847.
12. Becker L, Larsen MP, Eisenberg MS: Incidence of cardiac arrest during self-transport for chest pain. *Ann Emerg Med* 1996;28:612-616.
13. Brown AL, Mann NC, Daya M, et al: Demographic, belief, and situational factors influencing the decision to utilize emergency medical services among chest pain patients. Rapid Early Action for Coronary Treatment (REACT) study. *Circulation* 2000;102: 173-178.
14. Canto JG, Zalenski RJ, Ornato JP, et al: Use of emergency medical services in acute myocardial infarction and subsequent quality of care: observations from the National Registry of Myocardial Infarction 2. *Circulation* 2002;106:3018-3023.
15. Hutchings CB, Mann NC, et al: Patients with chest pain calling 911 or self-transporting to reach definitive care: which mode is quicker? *Am Heart J* 2004;147:35-41.
16. Roe MT, Messenger JC, et al: Treatments, trends, and outcomes of acute myocardial infarction and percutaneous coronary intervention. *J Am Coll Cardiol* 2010;56:254-263.
17. Faxon D, Lenfant C: Timing is everything: motivating patients to call 911 at onset of acute myocardial infarction. *Circulation* 2001;104:1210-1211.
18. Goff DC, Feldman HA, McGovern PG, et al, for the Rapid Early Action for Coronary Treatment (REACT) study group: Prehospital delay in patients hospitalized with heart attack symptoms in the United States: the REACT trial. *Am Heart J* 1999;138: 1046-1057.
19. Goldberg RJ, Steg PG, Sadiq I, et al: Extent of, and factors associated with, delay to hospital presentation in patients with acute coronary disease (the GRACE registry). *Am J Cardiol* 2002;89:791-796.
20. Canto JG, Shlipak MG, Rogers WJ, et al: Prevalence, clinical characteristics, and mortality among patients with myocardial infarction presenting without chest pain. *JAMA* 2000; 283:3223-3229.
21. Rathore SS, Weinfurt KP, Gersh BJ, et al: Treatment of patients with myocardial infarction who present with a paced rhythm. *Ann Intern Med* 2001;134:644-651.
22. Hallstrom AP, Ornato JP, Weisfeldt M, et al: Public-access defibrillation and survival after out-of-hospital cardiac arrest. *N Engl J Med* 2004;351:637-646.
23. Weisfeldt ML, Sitlani CM, Ornato JP, et al: Survival after application of automatic external defibrillators before arrival of the emergency medical system: evaluation in the resuscitation outcomes consortium population of 21 million. *J Am Coll Cardiol* 2010;55;1713-1720.
24. Perberdy MA, Callaway CW, Neumar RW, et al: Part 9: post-cardiac arrest care: 2010 American Heart Association Guidelines for Cardiopulmonary Resuscitation and Emergency Cardiac Care. *Circulation* 2010;122:S768-S786.
25. Field JM, Hazinski MF, Sayre MR, et al: Part 1: executive summary: 2010 American Heart Association Guidelines for Cardiopulmonary Resuscitation and Emergency Cardiac Care. *Circulation* 2010;122:S640-S656.
26. Bernard SA, Gray TW, Buist MD, et al: Treatment of comatose survivors of out of hospital cardiac arrest with induced hypothermia. *N Engl J Med* 2002;346:557-563.
27. HACA Study Group: Mild therapeutic hypothermia to improve the neurologic outcome after cardiac arrest. *N Engl J Med* 2002;346:549-556.
28. Jacobs AK, Antman EM, Faxon DP, et al: Development of systems of care for ST-elevation myocardial infarction patients: executive summary. *Circulation* 2007;116:217-230.
29. Krumholz HM, Bradley EH, Nallamothu BK, et al: A campaign to improve the timeliness of primary percutaneous coronary intervention: Door-to-Balloon: An Alliance for Quality. *J Am Coll Cardiol Cardiovasc Interv* 2008;1:97-103.
30. Kushner FG, Hand M, Smith SC Jr, et al: 2009 Focused Updates: ACC/AHA Guideline for the Management of Patients With ST-Elevation Myocardial Infarction (updating the 2004 Guideline and 2007 Focused Update) and ACC/AHA/SCAI Guidelines on Percutaneous Coronary Intervention (updating the 2005 Guideline and 2007 Focused Update). *J Am Coll Cardiol* 2009;54:2205-2241.
31. Dieker H, et al: Pre-hospital triage for primary angioplasty: direct referral to the intervention center versus interhospital transport. *J Am Coll Cardiol* 2010;3:705-711.
32. Fibrinolytic Therapy Trialists' (FTT) Collaborative Group: Indications for fibrinolytic therapy in suspected acute myocardial infarction: collaborative overviews of early mortality and major morbidity results from all randomised trials of more than 1000 patients. *Lancet* 1994;343:311-322.
33. Boersma E, Maas AC, Deckers JW, et al: Early thrombolytic treatment in acute myocardial infarction: reappraisal of the golden hour. *Lancet* 1996;348:771-775.
34. Danchin N, Blanchard D, Steg PG, et al: Impact of prehospital thrombolysis for acute myocardial infarction on 1-year outcome: results from the French Nationwide USIC 2000 Registry. *Circulation* 2004;110:1909-1915.
35. Sorensen JT, Terkelsen CJ, Norgaard BL, et al: Urban and rural implementation of prehospital diagnosis and direct referral for primary percutaneous coronary intervention in patients with acute ST-elevation myocardial infarction. *Eur Heart J* 2011;32:430-436.
36. Andersen HR, Nielsen TT, Rasmussen K, et al: A comparison of coronary angioplasty with fibrinolytic therapy in acute myocardial infarction. *N Engl J Med* 2003;349:733-742.
37. Dalby M, Brouzamondo A, Lechat P, et al: Transfer for primary angioplasty versus immediate thrombolysis in acute myocardial infarction: a meta-analysis. *Circulation* 2003;108:1809-1814.
38. Wijeysundera HC, Vijayaghavan R, Nallamothu BK, et al: Rescue angioplasty or repeat fibrinolysis after failed fibrinolytic therapy for ST-segment myocardial infarction: a meta-analysis of randomized trials. *J Am Coll Cardiol* 2007;49:422-430.
39. Borgia F, Goodman SG, Halvorsen S, et al: Early routine percutaneous coronary intervention after fibrinolysis vs. standard therapy in ST-segment elevation myocardial infarction: a meta-analysis. *Eur Heart J* 2010;31:2156-2169.
40. National Heart Attack Alert Program Coordinating Committee, 60 Minutes to Treatment Working Group: Emergency department: rapid identification and treatment of patients with acute myocardial infarction. *Ann Emerg Med* 1994;23:311-329.
41. Cannon CP: Time to treatment: a crucial factor in thrombolysis and primary angioplasty. *J Thromb Thrombolysis* 1996;3:249-255.
42. Brodie BR, et al: When is door-to-balloon time critical? *J Am Coll Cardiol* 2010;56:407-413.
43. Mauri F, Gasparini M, Barbonaglia L, et al: Prognostic significance of the extent of myocardial injury in acute myocardial infarction treated by streptokinase (the GISSI trial). *Am J Cardiol* 1989;63:1291-1295.
44. Kumar S, et al: Prognostic impact of Q waves on presentation and ST resolution in patients with ST-elevation myocardial infarction treated with primary percutaneous coronary intervention. *Am J Cardiol* 2009;104:780-785.
45. Wagner GS, et al: AHA/ACCF/HRS recommendations for the standardization and interpretation of the electrocardiogram. Part VI: acute ischemia/infarction. A scientific statement from the American Heart Association Electrocardiography and Arrhythmias Committee, Council on Clinical Cardiology; the American College of Cardiology Foundation; and the Heart Rhythm Society Endorsed by the International Society for Computerized Electrocardiology. *J Am Coll Cardiol* 2009;53:1003-1011.
46. Sgarbossa EB, Pinski SL, Barbagelata A, et al: Electrocardiographic diagnosis of evolving acute myocardial infarction in the presence of left bundle-branch block. GUSTO-1 (Global Utilization of Streptokinase and Tissue Plasminogen Activator for Occluded Coronary Arteries) investigators. *N Engl J Med* 1996;334:481-487.
47. de Winter RJ, Verouden NJ, Wellens HJ, et al: A new ECG sign of paroxysmal LAD occlusion. *N Engl J Med* 2008;359:2071.
48. Jong GP, Ma T, Chou P, et al: Reciprocal changes in 12-lead electrocardiography can predict left main coronary artery lesion in patients with acute myocardial infarction. *Int Heart J* 2006;47:13-20.
49. Wang K, Asinger RW, Marriott HJL: ST-segment elevation in conditions other than acute myocardial infarction. *N Engl J Med* 2003;349:2128-2135.
50. Fillmore SJ, Shapiro M, Killip T: Arterial oxygen tension in acute myocardial infarction: serial analysis of clinical state and blood gas changes. *Am Heart J* 1970;79:620-629.
51. ISIS-4 (Fourth International Study of Infarct Survival) collaborative group: ISIS-4: a randomized factorial trial assessing early oral captopril, oral mononitrate, and intravenous magnesium sulphate in 58,050 patients with suspected acute myocardial infarction. *Lancet* 1995;345:669-685.
52. Come PC, Pitt B: Nitroglycerin-induced severe hypotension and bradycardia in patients with acute myocardial infarction. *Circulation* 1976;54:624-628.
53. Cheitlin MD, Hutter AM, Brindis RG, et al: ACC/AHA expert consensus document on the use of sildenafil (Viagra) in patients with cardiovascular disease. American College of Cardiology/American Heart Association. *J Am Coll Cardiol* 1999;33:273-282.
54. Gislason GH, et al: Risk of death or reinfarction associated with the use of selective cyclooxygenase-2 inhibitors and nonselective nonsteroidal anti-inflammatory drugs after acute myocardial infarction. *Circulation* 2006;113:2906-2913.
55. ISIS-2 (Second International Study of Infarct Survival) collaborative group: Randomised trial of intravenous streptokinase, oral aspirin, both, or neither among 17,187 cases of suspected acute myocardial infarction: ISIS-2. *Lancet* 1988;2:349-360.
56. Roux S, Christeller S, Ludin E: Effects of aspirin on coronary reocculsion and recurrent ischemia after thrombolysis: a meta-analysis. *J Am Coll Cardiol* 1992;19:671-677.
57. Antithrombotic Trialists' Collaboration. Collaborative metaanalysis of randomised trials of antiplatelet therapy for prevention of death, myocardial infarction, and stroke in high-risk patients. *BMJ* 2002;324:71-86.
58. Mehta SR, et al: Dose comparisons of clopidogrel and aspirin in acute coronary syndromes. *N Engl J Med* 2010;363:930-942.
59. CAPRIE steering committee: A randomised, blinded trial of clopidogrel versus aspirin in patients at risk of ischaemic events (CAPRIE). *Lancet* 1996;348:1329-1339.
60. Chen ZM, Pan JC, Chen YP, et al: Addition of clopidogrel to aspirin in 45,852 patients with acute myocardial infarction: randomised placebo-controlled trial. *Lancet* 2005;366: 1607-1621.
61. Sabatine MS, Cannon CP, Gibson CM, et al: Addition of clopidogrel to aspirin and fibrinolytic therapy for myocardial infarction with ST-segment elevation. *N Engl J Med* 2005;352: 1179-1189.
62. Dangas G, et al: Role of clopidogrel loading dose in patients with ST elevation myocardial infarction undergoing primary angioplasty: results from the HORIZONS-AMI trial. *J Am Coll Cardiol* 2009;54:1438.
63. Peters RJ, Mehta SR, Fox KA, et al, for the Clopidogrel in Unstable angina to prevent Recurrent Events (CURE) trial investigators: Effects of aspirin dose when used alone or in combination with clopidogrel in patients with acute coronary syndromes: observations from the Clopidogrel in Unstable angina to prevent Recurrent Events (CURE) study. *Circulation* 2003;108:1682-1687.

64. Wiviott SD, et al: Prasugrel versus clopidogrel in patients with acute coronary syndromes. N. Engl J Med 2007;357:2001-2015.

65. Montalescot G, et al: Prasugrel compared with clopidogrel in patients undergoing percutaneous coronary intervention for ST-elevation myocardial infarction (TRITON-TIMI 38). Lancet 2009;373:723-731.

66. Wallentin L, et al, for the PLATO Investigators: Tricagrelor versus clopidogrel in patients with acute coronary syndromes. N Engl J Med 2009;361:1045-1057.

67. Topol EJ, for the GUSTO V investigators: Reperfusion therapy for acute myocardial infarction with fibrinolytic therapy or combination reduced fibrinolytic therapy and platelet glycoprotein IIb/IIIa inhibition: the GUSTO V randomised trial. Lancet 2001; 357:1905-1914.

68. Assessment of the Safety and Efficacy of a New Thrombolytic Regimen (ASSENT)-3 investigators: Efficacy and safety of tenecteplase in combination with enoxaparin, abciximab, or unfractionated heparin: the ASSENT-3 randomized trial in acute myocardial infarction. Lancet 2001;358:605-613.

69. Gurm H, et al: A comparison of abciximab and small molecule glycoprotein IIb/IIIa inhibitors in patients undergoing primary percutaneous coronary intervention: a meta-analysis of contemporary randomized controlled trials. Circ Cardiovasc Intervent 2009; 2:230-236.

70. De Luca G, et al: Benefits from small molecule administration as compared with abciximab among patients with ST-segment elevation myocardial infarction treated with primary angioplasty: a meta-analysis. J Am Coll Cardiol 2009;53:1668-1173.

71. Ellis SG, et al: Facilitated PCI in patients with ST-elevation myocardial infarction. N Engl J Med 2008;358:2205-2217.

72. Stone GW, et al: Bivalirudin during primary PCI in acute myocardial infarction. N Engl J Med 2008;358:2218-2230.

73. Mehilli J, et al: Abciximab in patients with acute ST-segment elevation myocardial infarction undergoing primary percutaneous coronary intervention after clopidogrel loading: a randomized double-blind trial. Circulation 2009;119:1933-1940.

74. Valgimigli M, et al: Comparison of angioplasty with infusion of tirofiban or abciximab and with implantation of sirolimus-eluting or uncoated stents for acute myocardial infaction: the MULTISTRATEGY randomized trial. JAMA 2008;299:1788-1799.

75. Van't Hof AW, et al: Prehospital initiation of tirofiban in patients with ST-elevation myocardial infarction undergoing primary angioplasty (ON-TIME 2): a multicentre, double-blind, randomized controlled trial. Lancet 2009;372:537-546.

76. Deibele AJ III, et al: Intracoronary eptifibatide bolus administration during percutaneous coronary stenting for acute coronary syndromes with evaluation of platelet glycoprotein IIb,IIIa receptor occupancy and platelet function: the ICE trial. Circulation 2010; 121:784-791.

77. Gu YL, et al: Intracoronary versus intravenous abciximab in ST-segment elevation myocardial infarction: rationale and design of the CICERO trial in patients undergoing primary percutaneous coronary intervention with thrombus aspiration. Trials 2009;10:90.

78. Collins R, Peto R, Baigent C, et al: Aspirin, heparin, and fibrinolytic therapy in suspected acute myocardial infarction. N Engl J Med 1997;336:847-860.

79. Wallentin L, Goldstein P, Armstrong PW, et al: Efficacy and safety of tenecteplase in combination with the low-molecular-weight heparin enoxabarin or unfractionated heparin in the prehospital setting: the Assessment of the Safety and Efficacy of a New Thrombolytic Regiment (ASSENT)-3 PLUS randomized trial in acute myocardial infarction. Circulation 2003;108:135-142.

80. Antman EM, Morrow DA, McCabe CH, et al, for the ExTRACT-TIMI 25 investigators: Enoxaparin versus unfractionated heparin with fibrinolysis for ST-elevated myocardial infarction. N Engl J Med 2006;354:1477-1488.

81. Antman EM, Morrow DA, McCabe CH, et al: Enoxaparin versus unfractionated heparin as antithrombin therapy in patients receiving fibrinolysis for ST-elevation myocardial infarction. Design and rationale for the Enoxaparin and Thrombolysis Reperfusion for Acute Myocardial Infarction Treatment-Thrombolysis in Myocardial Infarction study 25 (ExTRACT-TIMI 25). Am Heart J 2005;149:217-226.

82. Sabatine MS, Morrow DA, Montalescot G, et al: Angiographic and clinical outcomes in patients receiving low-molecular-weight heparin versus unfractionated heparin in ST-elevation myocardial infarction treated with fibrinolytics in the CLARITY-TIMI 28 trial. Circulation 2005;112:3846-3854.

83. Ferguson JJ, et al: Enoxaparin vs unfractionated heparin in high-risk patients with non ST segment elevation acute coronary syndromes managed with an intended early invasive strategy: primary results of the SYNERGY randomized trial. JAMA 2004;292:45-54.

84. Montalescot G, Zeymer U, Silvain J, et al: Intravenous enoxaparin or unfractionated heparin in primary percutaneous coronary intervention for ST-elevation myocardial infarction: the international randomised open-label ATOLL trial. Lancet 2011;378: 693-703.

85. Montalescot G, Ellis SG, de Belder MA, et al: Enoxaparin in primary and facilitated percutaneous coronary intervention. A formal prospective nonrandomized substudy of the FINESSE trial. JACC Interv 2010;3:203-212.

86. Goodman SG, et al: Acute ST-segment elevation myocardial infarction: American College of Chest Physicians Evidence-Based Clinical Practice Guidelines (8th edition). Chest 2008;133:708S.

87. Yusuf S, et al: Effects of fondaparinux on mortality and reinfarction in patients with acute ST-segment elevation myocardial infarction: the OASIS-6 randomized trial. JAMA 2006;295:1519-1530.

88. The MIAMI trial research group: Metoprolol in acute myocardial infarction: patient population. Am J Cardiol 1985;56:10G-14G.

89. First International Study of Infarct Survival Collaborative Group: Randomised trial of intravenous atenolol among 16 027 cases of suspected acute myocardial infarction: ISIS-1. Lancet 1986;2:57-66.

90. Roberts R, Rogers WJ, Mueller HS, et al: Immediate versus deferred beta-blockade following thrombolytic therapy in patients with acute myocardial infarction: results of the Thrombolysis in Myocardial Infarction (TIMI) II-B study. Circulation 1991;83:422-437.

91. Pfisterer M, Cox JL, Granger CB, et al: Atenolol use and clinical outcomes after thrombolysis for acute myocardial infarction: the GUSTO-I experience. Global Utilization of Streptokinase and TPA (alteplase) for Occluded Coronary Arteries. J Am Coll Cardiol 1998;32:634-640.

92. Chen ZM, Pan HC, Chen YP, et al: Early intravenous then oral metoprolol in 45,852 patients with acute myocardial infarction: randomised placebo-controlled trial. Lancet 2005;366:1622-1632.

93. De Luca G, Suryapranata J, Ottervanger JP, et al: Time delay to treatment and mortality in primary angioplasty for acute myocardial infarction: every minute of delay counts. Circulation 2004;109:1223-1225.

94. Ito H, Okamura A, Iwakura K, et al: Myocardial perfusion patterns related to thrombolysis in myocardial infarction perfusion grades after coronary angioplasty in patients with acute anterior wall myocardial infarction. Circulation 1996;93:1993-1999.

95. Morrison LJ, Verbeek PR, McDonald AC, et al: Mortality and prehospital thrombolysis for acute myocardial infarction: a meta-analysis. JAMA 2000;283:2686-2692.

96. Zeymer U, Tebbe U, Essen R, et al, for the ALKK-Study group: Influence of time to treatment on early infarct-related artery patency after different thrombolytic regimens. Am Heart J 1999;137:34-48.

97. Bonnefoy E, Lapostolle F, Leizorovicz A, et al, for the Comparison of Angioplasty and Prehospital Thrombolysis in Acute Myocardial Infarction Study Group: Primary angioplasty versus prehospital fibrinolysis in acute myocardial infarction: a randomised study. Lancet 2002;360:825-829.

98. Widimsky P, Budesinsky T, Vorac D, et al: Long distance transport for primary angioplasty vs. immediate thrombolysis in acute myocardial infarction: final results of the randomized national multicentre trial-PRAGUE-2. Eur Heart J 2003;24:94-104.

99. Steg PG, Bonnefoy E, Chabaud S, et al: Impact of time to treatment on mortality after inhospital fibrinolysis or primary angioplasty: data from the CAPTIM randomized clinical trial. Circulation 2003;108:2851-2856.

100. Lee KL, Woodlief LH, Topol EJ, et al, for the GUSTO-I investigators: Predictors of 30-day mortality in the era of reperfusion for acute myocardial infarction: results from an international trial of 41,021 patients. Circulation 1995;91:1659-1668.

101. Morrow DA, Antman EM, Charlesworth A, et al: TIMI risk score for ST-elevation myocardial infarction: a convenient, bedside, clinical score for risk assessment at presentation: an intravenous tPA for treatment of infarcting myocardium early II trial substudy. Circulation 2000;102:2031-2037.

102. Pieper KS, et al: Validity of a risk-prediction tool for hospital mortality: the Global Registry of Acute Coronary Events. Am Heart J 2009;157:1097-1105.

103. Stone GW, Grines CL, Browne KF, et al: Influence of acute myocardial infarction location on in-hospital and late outcome after primary percutaneous transluminal coronary angioplasty versus tissue plasminogen activator therapy. Am J Cardiol 1996;78:19-25.

104. Van't Hof AW, Henriques J, Ottervanger J-P, et al: No mortality benefit of primary angioplasty over thrombolytic therapy in patients with nonanterior myocardial infarction at long-term follow-up: results of the Zwolle trial [abstract]. J Am Coll Cardiol 2003;41:369A.

105. Wu AH, Parsons L, Every NR, et al, for the Second National Registry of Myocardial Infarction: Hospital outcomes in patients presenting with congestive heart failure complicating acute myocardial infarction: a report from the Second National Registry of Myocardial Infarction (NRMI-2). J Am Coll Cardiol 2002;40:1389-1394.

106. Hochman JS, Sleeper LA, Webb JG, et al, for the Should We Emergently Revascularize Occluded Coronaries for Cardiogenic Shock (SHOCK) investigators: Early revascularization in acute myocardial infarction complicated by cardiogenic shock. N Engl J Med 1999;341:625-634.

107. Kent DM, Schmid CH, Lau J, et al: Is primary angioplasty for some as good as primary angioplasty for all? J Gen Intern Med 2002;17:887-894.

108. Magid DJ, Calonge BN, Rumsfeld JS, et al, for the National Registry of Myocardial Infarction 2 and 3 investigators: Relation between hospital primary angioplasty volume and mortality for patients with acute MI treated with primary angioplasty vs. thrombolytic therapy. JAMA 2000;284:3131-3138.

109. Keeley EC, Boura JA, Grines CL: Primary angioplasty versus intravenous thrombolytic therapy for acute myocardial infarction: a quantitative review of 23 randomised trials. Lancet 2003;361:13-20.

110. Henriques JP, Haasdijk AP, Zijlstra F, for the Zwolle Myocardial Infarction Study Group: Outcome of primary angioplasty for acute myocardial infarction during routine duty hours versus during off-hours. J Am Coll Cardiol 2003;41:2138-2142.

111. Canto JG, Every NR, Magid DJ, et al, for the National Registry of Myocardial Infarction 2 Investigators: The volume of primary angioplasty procedures and survival after acute myocardial infarction. N Engl J Med 2000;342:1573-1580.

112. Ross JS, et al: Hospital volume and 30-day mortality for three common medical conditions. N Engl J Med 2010;362:1110-1118.

113. Nallamothu BK, Antman EM, Bates ER: Primary percutaneous coronary intervention versus fibrinolytic therapy in acute myocardial infarction: does the choice of fibrinolytic agent impact on the importance of time-to-treatment? Am J Cardiol 2004;94:772-774.

114. Andersen HR, Nielsen TT, Vesterlund T, et al: Danish multicenter randomized study on fibrinolytic therapy versus acute coronary angioplasty in acute myocardial infarction: rationale and design of the DANish trial in Acute Myocardial Infarction-2 (DANAMI-2). Am Heart J 2003;146:234-241.

115. Time-to-reperfusion in patients undergoing interhospital transfer for primary percutaneous coronary intervention in the U.S.: an analysis of 2005 and 2006 data from the National Cardiovascular Data Registry. J Am Coll Cardiol 2008;51:2442-2443.

116. Simoons ML, Maggioni AP, Knatterud G, et al: Individual risk assessment for intracranial haemorrhage during thrombolytic therapy. Lancet 1993;342:1523-1528.

117. Brass LM, Lichtman JH, Wang Y, et al: Intracranial hemorrhage associated with thrombolytic therapy for elderly patients with acute myocardial infarction: results from the Cooperative Cardiovascular Project. Stroke 2000;31:1802-1811.

118. The InTIME-II investigators: Intravenous NPA for the Treatment of Infarcting Myocardium Early: InTIME-II, a double-blind comparison of single-bolus lanoteplase vs. accelerated alteplase for the treatment of patients with acute myocardial infarction. Eur Heart J 2000;21:2005-2013.

119. Gruppo Italiano per lo Studio della Streptochinasi nell'Infarto Miocardico (GISSI): Effectiveness of intravenous thrombolytic treatment in acute myocardial infarction. *Lancet* 1986;1:397-402.
120. Wilcox RG, von der Lippe G, Olsson CG, et al: Trial of tissue plasminogen activator for mortality reduction in acute myocardial infarction. Anglo-Scandinavian Study of Early Thrombolysis (ASSET). *Lancet* 1988;2:525-530.
121. AIMS trial study group: Long-term effects of intravenous anistreplase in acute myocardial infarction: final report of the AIMS study. *Lancet* 1990;335:427-431.
122. Bates ER: Revisiting reperfusion therapy in inferior myocardial infarction. *J Am Coll Cardiol* 1997;30:334-342.
123. White HD: Thrombolytic therapy in the elderly. *Lancet* 2000;356:2028-2030.
124. Mahaffey KW, Granger CB, Sloan MA, et al: Neurosurgical evacuation of intracranial hemorrhage after thrombolytic therapy for acute myocardial infarction: experience from the GUSTO-I trial. Global Utilization of Streptokinase and tissue-plasminogen activator (tPA) for Occluded Coronary Arteries. *Am Heart J* 1999;138:493-499.
125. The GUSTO investigators: An international randomized trial comparing four thrombolytic strategies for acute myocardial infarction. *N Engl J Med* 1993;329:673-682.
126. The Global Use of Strategies to Open Occluded Coronary Arteries (GUSTO III) investigators: A comparison of reteplase with alteplase for acute myocardial infarction. *N Engl J Med* 1997;337:1118-1123.
127. Assessment of the Safety and Efficacy of a New Thrombolytic Investigators: Single-bolus tenecteplase compared with front-loaded alteplase in acute myocardial infarction: the ASSENT-2 double-blind randomised trial. *Lancet* 1999;354:716-722.
128. Bashore TM, et al: ACC/SCAI clinical expert consensus document on cardiac catheterization laboratory standards: a report of the ACC Task Force on Clinical Expert Consensus Documents endorsed by the AHA and the Diagnostic and Interventional Catheterization Committee of the Council on Clinical Cardiology of the AHA. *J Am Coll Cardiol* 2001;37:2170-2214.
129. Rogers WJ, Dean LS, Moore PB, et al, for the Alabama Registry of Myocardial Ischemia Investigators: Comparison of primary angioplasty versus thrombolytic therapy for acute myocardial infarction. *Am J Cardiol* 1994;74:111-118.
130. Every NR, Parsons LS, Hlatky M, et al, for the Myocardial Infarction Triage and Intervention Investigators: A comparison of thrombolytic therapy with primary coronary angioplasty for acute myocardial infarction. *N Engl J Med* 1996;335:1253-1260.
131. Tiefenbrunn AJ, Chandra NC, French WJ, et al: Clinical experience with primary percutaneous transluminal coronary angioplasty compared with alteplase (recombinant tissue type plasminogen activator) in patients with acute myocardial infarction: a report from the Second National Registry of Myocardial Infarction (NRMI-2). *J Am Coll Cardiol* 1998;31:1240-1245.
132. Wilson SH, Bell MR, Rihal CS, et al: Infarct artery reocclusion after primary angioplasty, stent placement, and thrombolytic therapy for acute myocardial infarction. *Am Heart J* 2001;141:704-710.
133. Zhu MM, Feit A, Chadow H, et al: Primary stent implantation compared with primary balloon angioplasty for acute myocardial infarction: a meta-analysis of randomized clinical trials. *Am J Cardiol* 2001;88:297-301.
134. Nordmann AJ, Hengstler P, Harr T, et al: Clinical outcomes of primary stenting versus balloon angioplasty in patients with myocardial infarction: a meta-analysis of randomized controlled trials. *Am J Med* 2004;116:253-262.
135. Stone GW, Ellis SG, Cox DA, et al: One-year clinical results with the slow-rease, polymer-based, paclitaxel-eluting TAXUS stent: the TAXUS-IV trial. *Circulation* 2004;109: 1942-1947.
136. Stone GW, Lansky AJ, Pocock SJ, et al: Paclitaxel-eluting stents versus bare-metal stents in acute myocardial infarction. *N Engl J Med* 2009;360:1946-1959.
137. Pan XH, Chen YX, Xiang MX, et al: A meta-analysis of randomized trials on clinical outcomes of paclitaxel-eluting stents versus bare-metal stents in ST-segment elevation myocardial infarction patients. *J Zhejiang Univ Sci B* 2010;11:754-761.
138. Hao PP, Chen YG, Wang XL, et al: Efficacy and safety of drug-eluting stents in patients with acute ST-segment-elevation myocardial infarction: a meta-analysis of randomized controlled trials. *Tex Heart Inst J* 2010;37:516-524.
139. Suh HS, Song HJ, Choi JE, et al: Drug-eluting stents versus bare metal stents in acute myocardial infarction: a systematic review and meta-analysis. *Int J Technol Assess Health Care* 2011;27:11-23.
140. Svilaas T, et al: Thrombus aspiration during primary percutaneous coronary intervention. *N Engl J Med* 2009;360:1283-1297.
141. Vlaar PJ, et al: Cardiac death and reinfarction after 1 year in the Thrombus Aspiration during Percutaneous Coronary Intervention in Acute Myocardial Infarction Study (TAPAS): a 1 year follow-up study. *Lancet* 2008;371:1915-1920.
142. Bavry AA, et al: Role of adjunctive thrombectomy and embolic protection devices in acute myocardial infarction: a comprehensive meta-analysis of randomized trials. *Eur Heart J* 2008;29:2989-3001.
143. Burzotta F, et al: Clinical impact of thrombectomy in acute ST-elevation myocardial infarction: an individual patient-data pooled analysis of 11 trials. *Eur Heart J* 2009;30: 2193-2203.
144. Gershlick AH, Stephens-Lloyd A, et al: Rescue angioplasty after failed thrombolytic therapy for acute myocardial infarction. *N Engl J Med* 2005;353:2758-2768.
145. ASSENT-4 PCI Investigators: Primary versus tenecteplase-facilitated percutaneous coronary intervention in patients with ST-segment elevation acute myocardial infarction (ASSENT-4 PCI): randomized trial. *Lancet* 2006;367:569-578.
146. Ellis SG, Armstrong P, et al: Facilitated percutaneous coronary intervention versus primary percutaneous coronary intervention: design and rationale of the Facilitated Intervention with Enhanced Reperfusion Speed to Stop Events (FINESSE) trial. *Am Heart J* 2004;147:E16.
147. Fernandez-Aviles F, Alonso JJ, et al: Routine invasive strategy within 24 hours of thrombolysis versus ischaemia-guided conservative approach for acute myocardial infarction with ST-segment elevation (GRACIA-1): a randomized controlled trial. *Lancet* 2004;364: 1045-1053.
148. Di Mario C, Dudek D, et al: Immediate angioplasty versus standard therapy with rescue angioplasty after thrombolysis in the Combined Abciximab Reteplase Stent Study in Acute Myocardial Infarction (CARESS-AMI): an open, prospective random mixed multicentre trial. *Lancet* 2008;371:559-568.
149. Cantor WJ, Figtchett D, et al: Routine early angioplasty after fibrinolysis for acute myocardial infarction. *N Engl J Med* 2009;360:2705-2718.
150. Bohmer E, Hoffman P, et al: Efficacy and safety of immediate angioplasty versus ischemia guided management after thrombolysis in acute myocardial infarction in areas with very long transfer distances. Results of the NORDISTEMI (Norwegian Study on District Treatment of ST-Elevation Myocardial Infarction). *J Am Coll Cardiol* 2009;55:102-110.
151. Wijeysundera HC, You JJ, et al: An early invasive strategy versus ischemia-guided management after fibrinolytic therapy for ST-segment elevation myocardial infarction: a meta-analysis of contemporary randomized controlled trials. *Am Heart J* 2008; 156(3):564-572.
152. Hochman JS, et al: Coronary intervention for persistent occlusion after myocardial infarction. *N Engl J Med* 2006;355:2395-2407.
153. Grzybowski M, Clements E, Parsons L, et al: Mortality benefit of immediate revascularization of acute ST-segment elevation myocardial infarction in patients with contraindications to thrombolytic therapy: a propensity analysis. *JAMA* 2003;290:1891-1898.
154. Wharton TP, McNamera NS, Fedele FA, et al: Primary angioplasty for the treatment of acute myocardial infarction: experience at two community hospitals without cardiac surgery. *J Am Coll Cardiol* 1999;33:1257-1265.
155. Aversano T, Aversano LT, Passamani E, et al, for the Atlantic Cardiovascular Patient Outcomes Research Team (C-PORT): Thrombolytic therapy vs. primary percutaneous coronary intervention for myocardial infarction in patients presenting to hospitals without on-site cardiac surgery: a randomized controlled trial. *JAMA* 2002;287:1943-1951.
156. Chae CU, Hennekens CH: Beta blockers. In Hennekens CH (ed): *Clinical Trials in Cardiovascular Disease: A Companion to Braunwald's Heart Disease.* Philadelphia, WB Saunders, 1999, pp 79-94.
157. Latini R, Maggioni AP, Flather M, et al: ACE inhibitor use in patients with myocardial infarction: summary evidence from clinical trials. *Circulation* 1995;92:3132-3127.
158. ACE Inhibitor Myocardial Infarction Collaborative Group: Indications for ACE inhibitors in the early treatment of acute myocardial infarction: systematic overview of individual data from 100,000 patients in randomized trials. *Circulation* 1998;97:2202-2212.
159. Flather MD, Yusuf S, Kober L, et al, for the ACE-Inhibitor Myocardial Infarction Collaborative Group: Long-term ACE inhibitor therapy in patients with heart failure or left-ventricular dysfunction: a systematic overview of data from individual patients. *Lancet* 2000;355:1575-1581.
160. Granger CB, McMurray JJ, Yusuf S, et al, for the CHARM investigators and committees: Effects of candesartan in patients with chronic heart failure and reduced left-ventricular systolic function intolerant to angiotensin-converting-enzyme inhibitors: the CHARM-Alternative trial. *Lancet* 2003;362:772-776.
161. Pfeffer MA, McMurray JJ, Velazquez EJ, et al: Valsartan, captopril or both in myocardial infarction complicated by heart failure, left ventricular dysfunction, or both. *N Engl J Med* 2003;349:1893-1906.
162. Pitt B, Zannad F, Remme WJ, et al, for the Randomized Aldactone Evaluation Study Investigators: The effect of spironolactone on morbidity and mortality in patients with severe heart failure. *N Engl J Med* 1999;341:709-717.
163. Pitt B, Remme W, Zannad F, et al, for the Eplerenone Post-Acute Myocardial Infarction Heart Failure Efficacy and Survival study investigators: Eplerenone, a selective aldosterone blocker, in patients with left ventricular dysfunction after myocardial infarction. *N Engl J Med* 2003;348:1309-1321.
164. Moghissi ES, Korythkowski MT, DiNardo M, et al: American Association of Clinical Endocrinologists and American Diabetes Association consensus statement on inpatient glycemic control. *Diabetes Care* 2009;32:1119-1131.
165. Finfer S, Chittock DR, Su SY, et al: Intensive versus conventional glucose control in critically ill patients. *N Engl J Med* 2009;360:1283-1297.
166. Weiner RS, Weiner DC, Larson RJ. Benefits and risks of tight gluconse control in critically ill adults: a meta-analysis. *JAMA* 2008;300:933-944.
167. Deedwania P, Kosiborod M, Barrett E, et al: Hyperglycemia and acute coronary syndrome: a scientific statement from the American Heart Association Diabetes Committee of the Council on Nutrition, Physical Activity, and Metabolism. *Anesthesiology* 2008;109:14-24.
168. Marfella R, Di Filippo C, Portoghese M, et al: Tight glycemic control reduces heart inflammation and remodeling during acute myocardial infarction in hyperglycemic patients. *J Am Coll Cardiol* 2009;53:1425-1436.
169. The Danish Study Group on Verapamil in Myocardial Infarction: Effect of verapamil on mortality and major events after acute myocardial infarction: the Danish Verapamil Infarction Trial II (DAVIT II). *Am J Cardiol* 1990;66:779-785.
170. Boden WE, van Gilst WH, Scheldewaert RG, et al: Diltiazem in acute myocardial infarction treated with thrombolytic agents: a randomized placebo-controlled trial. Incomplete Infarction Trial of European Research Collaborators Evaluating Prognosis post-Thrombolysis (INTERCEPT). *Lancet* 2000;355:1751-1756.
171. Furberg CD, Psaty BM, Meyer JV: Nifedipine: dose-related increase in mortality in patients with coronary heart disease. *Circulation* 1995;92:1326-1331.
172. Menon V, Slater JN, White HD, et al: Acute myocardial infarction complicated by systemic hypoperfusion without hypotension: report of the SHOCK trial registry. *Am J Med* 2000;108:374-380.
173. Hochman JS, Sleeper LA, White HD, et al, for the Should We Emergently Revascularize Occluded Coronaries for Cardiogenic Shock (SHOCK) investigators: One-year survival following early revascularization for cardiogenic shock. *JAMA* 2001;285:190-192.
174. Killip T, Kimball JT: Treatment of myocardial infarction in a coronary care unit: a two-year experience with 250 patients. *Am J Cardiol* 1967;20:457-464.
175. Bates ER, Topol EJ: Limitations of reperfusion therapy for acute myocardial infarction complicated by congestive heart failure and cardiogenic shock. *J Am Coll Cardiol* 1991;18:1077-1084.
176. The Acute Infarction Ramipril Efficacy (AIRE) study investigators: Effect of ramipril on mortality and morbidity of survivors of acute myocardial infarction with clinical evidence of heart failure. *Lancet* 2001;357:1385-1390.

177. Dargie HJ: Effect of carvedilol on outcome after myocardial infarction in patients with left-ventricular dysfunction: the CAPRICORN randomised trial. *Lancet* 2001;357: 1385-1390.
178. Hochman JS, Jaber W, Bates ER, et al: Angioplasty versus thrombolytics for patients presenting with congestive heart failure: GUSTO IIb substudy findings. *J Am Coll Cardiol* 1998;31:856-854.
179. Urban P, Stauffer JC, Bleed D, et al: A randomized evaluation of early revascularization to treat shock complicating acute myocardial infarction. The (Swiss) Multicenter Trial of Angioplasty for Shock-(S)MASH. *Eur Heart J* 1999;20:1030-1038.
180. Dzavik V, Sleeper LA, Cocke TP, et al, for the SHOCK investigators: Early revascularization is associated with improved survival in elderly patients with acute myocardial infarction complicated by cardiogenic shock: a report from the SHOCK trial registry. *Eur Heart L* 2003;24:828-837.
181. Dauerman HL, Goldberg RJ, Malinski M, et al: Outcomes and early revascularization for patients greater than or equal to 65 years of age with cardiogenic shock. *Am J Cardiol* 2001;87:844-848.
182. Antoniucci D, Valenti R, Migliorini A, et al: Comparison of impact of emergency percutaneous revascularization on outcome of patients >75 to those <75 years of age with acute myocardial infarction complicated by cardiogenic shock. *Am J Cardiol* 2003;91:1458-1460.
183. Ohman EM, Nannas J, Stomel RJ, et al: Thrombolysis and counterpulsation to improve survival in myocardial infarction complicated by hypotension and suspected cardiogenic shock or heart failure: results of the TACTICS trial. *J Thromb Thrombolysis* 2005;19:33-39.
184. Berger PB, Ryan TJ: Inferior myocardial infarction: high-risk subgroups. *Circulation* 1990;81:401-411.
185. Zehender M, Kasper W, Kauder E, et al: High right ventricular infarction as an independent predictor of prognosis after acute inferior myocardial infarction. *N Engl J Med* 1993;328:981-988.
186. Jacobs AK, Leopold JA, Bates E, et al: Cardiogenic shock caused by right ventricular infarction: a report from the SHOCK registry. *J Am Coll Cardiol* 2003;41:1273-1279.
187. Andersen HR, Falk E, Nielsen D: Right ventricular infarction: frequency, size, and topography in coronary heart disease: a prospective study comprising 107 consecutive autopsies from a coronary care unit. *J Am Coll Cardiol* 1987;10:1223-1232.
188. Lee FA: Hemodynamics of the right ventricle in normal and disease states. *Cardiol Clin* 1992;10:59-67.
189. Cross CE: Right ventricular pressure and coronary flow. *Am J Physiol* 1962;202:12-16.
190. Goldstein JA, Vlahakes GJ, Verrier ED, et al: The role of right ventricular systolic dysfunction and elevated intrapericardial pressure in the genesis of low output in experimental right ventricular infarction. *Circulation* 1982;65:513-522.
191. Ferguson JJ, Diver DJ, Boldt M, et al: Significance of nitroglycerin-induced hypotension with inferior wall acute myocardial infarction. *Am J Cardiol* 1989;64:311-314.
192. Goldstein JA, Tweddell JS, Barzilai B, et al: Importance of left ventricular function and systolic ventricular interaction to right ventricular performance during acute right heart ischemia. *J Am Coll Cardiol* 1992;19704-711.
193. Goldstein JA, Barzilai B, Rosamond TL, et al: Determinants of hemodynamic compromise with severe right ventricular infarction. *Circulation* 1990;82:359-368.
194. Dell'Italia LJ, Starling MR, O'Rourke RA: Physical examination for exclusion of hemodynamically important right ventricular infarction. *Ann Intern Med* 1983;99:608-611.
195. Dell'Italia LJ, Starling MR, Crawford MH, et al: Right ventricular infarction: identification by hemodynamic measurements before and after volume loading and correlation with noninvasive techniques. *J Am Coll Cardiol* 1984;4:931-939.
196. Robalino BD, Whitlow PL, Underwood DA, et al: Electrocardiographic manifestations of right ventricular infarction. *Am Heart J* 1989;118:138-144.
197. Braat SH, Brugada P, de Zwaan C, et al: Value of electrocardiogram in diagnosing right ventricular involvement in patients with an acute inferior wall myocardial infarction. *Br Heart J* 1983;49:368-372.
198. Manno BV, Bemis CE, Carver J, et al: Right ventricular infarction complicated by right to left shunt. *J Am Coll Cardiol* 1983;1:554-557.
199. Dell'Italia LJ, Starling MR, Blumhardt R, et al: Comparative effects of volume loading, dobutamine, and nitroprusside in patients with predominant right ventricular infarction. *Circulation* 1985;72:1327-1335.
200. Braat SH, de Zwaan C, Brugada P, et al: Right ventricular involvement with acute inferior wall myocardial infarction identifies high risk of developing atrioventricular nodal conduction disturbances. *Am Heart J* 1984;107:1183-1187.
201. Love JC, Haffajee CI, Gore JM, et al: Reversibility of hypotension and shock by atrial or atrioventricular sequential pacing in patients with right ventricular infarction. *Am Heart J* 1984;108-5-13.
202. Lamas GA, Mitchell GF, Flaker GC, et al, for the Survival and Ventricular Enlargement Investigators: Clinical significance of mitral regurgitation after acute myocardial infarction. *Circulation* 1997;96:827-833.
203. Byrne JG, Aranki SF, Cohn LH: Repair versus replacement of mitral valve for treating severe ischemic mitral regurgitation. *Coron Artery Dis* 2000;11:31-33.
204. Tepe NA, Edmunds LH: Operation for acute postinfarction mitral insufficiency and cardiogenic shock. *J Thorac Cardiovasc Surg* 1985;89:525-530.
205. Thompson CR, Buller CE, Sleeper LA, et al: Cardiogenic shock due to acute severe mitral regurgitation complicating acute myocardial infarction: a report from the SHOCK trial registry. SHould we emergently revascularize Occluded Coronaries cardiogenic shocK? *J Am Coll Cardiol* 2000;36:1104-1109.
206. Crenshaw BS, Granger CB, Birnbaum Y, et al, for the GUSTO (Global Utilization of Streptokinase and TPA for Occluded Coronary Arteries) trial investigators: Risk factors, angiographic patterns, and outcomes in patients with ventricular septal defect complicating acute myocardial infarction. *Circulation* 2000;27-32.
207. Menon V, Webb JG, Hillis LD, et al: Outcome and profile of ventricular septal rupture with cardiogenic shock after myocardial infarction: A report from the SHOCK trial registry. Should we emergently revascularize Occluded Coronaries in cardiogenic shocK? *J Am Coll Cardiol* 2000;36:1110-1116.
208. Thiele J, Kaulfersch C, Daehnert I, et al: Immediate primary transcatheter closure of postinfarction ventricular septal defects. *Eur Heart J* 2009;30:81-88.
209. Becker RC, Gore JM, Lambrew C, et al: A composite view of cardiac rupture in the United States National Registry of Myocardial Infarction. *J Am Coll Cardiol* 1996;27:1321-1326.
210. Honan MB, Harrell FE, Reime KA, et al: Cardiac rupture, mortality and timing of thrombolytic therapy: a meta-analysis. *J Am Coll Cardiol* 1990;16:359-367.
211. McMullan MH, Maples MD, Kilgor TL, et al: Surgical experience with left ventricular free wall rupture. *Ann Thorac Surg* 2001;71:1894-1898.
212. Slater J, Brown RJ, Antonelli TA, et al: Cardiogenic shock due to cardiac free-wall rupture or tamponade after acute myocardial infarction: a report from the SHOCK trial registry. Should we emergently revascularize Occluded Coronaries in cardiogenic shocK? *J Am Coll Cardiol* 2000;36:1117-1122.
213. Ohara K: Current surgical strategy for post-infarction left ventricular aneurysm: from linear aneurysmectomy to Dor's operation. *Ann Thorac Cardiovasc Surg* 2000;6: 289-294.
214. Vaitkus PT, Barnathan ES: Embolic potential, prevention and management of mural thrombus complicating anterior myocardial infarction: a meta-analysis. *J Am Coll Cardiol* 1993;22:1004-1009.
215. Seyfarth M, Sibbing D, Bauer I, et al: A randomized clinical trial to evaluate the safety and efficacy of a percutaneous left ventricular assist device versus intra-aortic balloon pumping for treatment of cardiogenic shock caused by myocardial infarction. *J Am Coll Cardiol* 2008;52:1584-1588.
216. Cheng JM, den Uil CA, Hoeks SE, et al: Percutaneous left ventricular assist devices vs. intra-aortic balloon pump counterpulsation for treatment of cardiogenic shock: a meta-analysis of controlled trials. *Eur Heart J* 2009;30:2102-2108.
217. Lopez-Sendon J, et al: Factors related to heart rupture in acute coronary syndromes in the Global Registry of Acute Coronary Events. *Eur Heart J* 2010;31:1449-1456.
218. Gregoratos G, Abrams J, Epstein AE, et al: ACC/AHA/NASPE 2002 guideline update for implantation of cardiac pacemakers and antiarrhythmia devices: summary article. *J Am Coll Cardiol* 2002;40:1703-1719.
219. Pedersen OD, Bagger J, Kober L, et al, for the TRAndolapril Cardiac Evaluation (TRACE) study group: The occurrence and prognostic significance of atrial fibrillation/flutter following acute myocardial infarction. *Eur Heart J* 1999;20:748-754.
220. Pizzetti F, Turazza FM, Franzoni MG, et al: Incidence and prognostic significance of atrial fibrillation in acute myocardial infarction: the GISSI-3 data. *Heart* 2001;86:527-532.
221. Behar S, Zahavi Z, Goldbourt U, et al, for the SPRINT study group: Long-term prognosis of patients with paroxysmal atrial fibrillation complicating acute myocardial infarction. *Eur Heart J* 1992;13:45-50.
222. Dahl DF, Ewy GA, Warner ED, et al: Myocardial necrosis from direct current countershock: effect of paddle electrode size and time interval between discharges. *Circulation* 1974;50:956-961.
223. Campbell RW, Murray A, Julian DG: Ventricular arrhythmias in first 12 hours of acute myocardial infarction: natural history study. *Br Heart J* 1981;46:351-357.
224. Ornato JP, Peberdy MA, Tadler SC, et al: Factors associated with the occurrence of cardiac arrest during hospitalization for acute myocardial infarction in the second National Registry of Myocardial Infarction in the U.S. *Resuscitation* 2001;48:117-123.
225. Antman EM, Berlin JA: Declining incidence of ventricular fibrillation in myocardial infarction: implications for the prophylactic use of lidocaine. *Circulation* 1992;86: 764-773.
226. Thompson CA, Yarzebski J, Goldberg RJ, et al: Changes over time in the incidence and case-fatality rates of primary ventricular fibrillation complicating acute myocardial infarction: perspectives from the Worcester Heart Attack Study. *Am Heart J* 2000; 139:1014-1021.
227. Behar S, Goldbourt U, Reicher-Reiss J, et al, for the Principal Investigators of the SPRINT study: Prognosis of acute myocardial infarction complicated by primary ventricular fibrillation. *Am J Cardiol* 1990;66:1208-1211.
228. MacMahon S, Collins R, Peto R, et al: Effects of prophylactic lidocaine in suspected acute myocardial infarction: An overview of results from the randomized, controlled trials. *JAMA* 1988;260:1910-1916.
229. Alexander JH, Granger CB, Sadowski Z, et al, for the GUSTO-I and GUSTO-IIb investigators: Prophylactic lidocaine use in acute myocardial infarction: incidence and outcome from two international trials. *Am Heart J* 1999;137:799-805.
230. Hjalmarson A, Herlitz J, Holmbeg S, et al: The Göteborg metoprolol trial: effects on mortality and morbidity in acute myocardial infarction. *Circulation* 1983;67:126-132.
231. The American Heart Association in collaboration with the International Liaison Committee on Resuscitation: Guidelines 2000 for cardiopulmonary resuscitation and emergency cardiovascular care: part 6: advanced cardiovascular life support: secton 5: pharmacology I: agents for arrhythmia. *Circulation* 2000;102:I112-I1128.
232. The Antiarrhythmics versus Implantable Defibrillators (AVID) investigators: A comparison of antiarrhythmic-drug therapy with implantable defibrillators in patients resuscitated from near-fatal ventricular arrhythmias. *N Engl J Med* 1997;337:1576-1583.
233. Siebels J, Kuck KH: Implantable cardioverter defibrillator compared with antiarrhythmic drug treatment in cardiac arrest survivors (the Cardiac Arrest Study Hamburg). *Am Heart J* 1994;127:1139-1144.
234. Connolly SJ, Gent M, Roberts RS, et al: Canadian Implantable Defibrillator Study (CIDS): a randomized trial of the implantable cardioverter defibrillator against amiodarone. *Circulation* 2000;101:1297-1302.
235. Moss AJ, Hall WJ, Cannom DS, et al, for the Multicenter Automatic Defibrillator Implantation Trial investigators: Improved survival with an implanted defibrillator in patients with coronary disease at high risk for ventricular arrhythmia. *N Engl J Med* 1996; 335:1933-1940.
236. Buxton AE, Lee KL, Fisher JD, et al, for the Multicenter Unsustained Tachycardia Trial investigators: A randomized study of the prevention of sudden death in patients with coronary artery disease. *N Engl J Med* 1999;341:1882-1890.
237. Moss AJ, Zareba W, Hall WJ, et al, for the Multicenter Automatic Defibrillator Implantation Trial II investigators: Prophylactic implantation of a defibrillator in patients with myocardial infarction and reduced ejection fraction. *N Engl J Med* 2002;346:877-883.

238. Zipes DP, Camm AJ, Borggrefe M, et al: ACC/AHA/ESC 2006 guidelines for management of patients with ventricular arrhythmias and the prevention of sudden cardiac death—executive summary. *J Am Coll Cardiol* 2006;48:1064-1108.
239. Ohman EM, Califf RM, Topol EJ, et al, for the TAMI study group: Consequences of reocclusion after successful reperfusion therapy in acute myocardial infarction. *Circulation* 1990;82:781-791.
240. Gibson CM, Karha J, Murphy SA, et al, for the TIMI study group: Early and long-term clinical outcomes associated with reinfarction following fibrinolytic administration in the thrombolysis In Myocardial Infarction trials. *J Am Coll Cardiol* 2003;42:7-16.
241. Tofler GH, Muller JE, Stone PH, et al: Pericarditis in acute myocardial infarction: characterization and clinical significance. *Am Heart J* 1989;117:86-92.
242. Wall TC, Califf RM, Harrelson-Woodlief L, et al, for the TAMI study group: Usefulness of a pericardial friction rub after thrombolytic therapy during acute myocardial infarction in predicting amount of myocardial damage. *Am J Cardiol* 1990;66:1418-1421.
243. Shahar A, Hod H, Barabash GM, et al: Disappearance of a syndrome: Dressler's syndrome in the era of thrombolysis. *Cardiology* 1994;85:255-258.
244. Berman J, Haffajee CI, Alpert JS: Therapy of symptomatic pericarditis after myocardial infarction: Retrospective and prospective studies of aspirin, indomethacin, prednisone, and spontaneous resolution. *Am Heart J* 1981;101:750-753.
245. Adler Y, Finkelstein Y, Guindo J, et al: Colchicine treatment for recurrent pericarditis: a decade of experience. *Circulation* 1998;97:2183-2185.
246. Bulkley BH, Roberts WC: Steroid therapy during acute myocardial infarction: a cause of delayed healing and of ventricular aneurysm. *Am J Med* 1974;56:244-250.
247. Figuras J, et al: Hospital outcome of moderate to severe pericardial effusion complicating ST-elevation acute myocardial infarction. *Circulation* 2010;122:1902-1909.
248. Tanne D, Gottleib S, Hod H, et al, for the Secondary Prevention Reinfarction Israeli Nifedipine Trial (SPRINT) and Israeli Thrombolytic Survey Groups: Incidence and mortality from early stroke associated with acute myocardial infarction in the prethrombolytic and thrombolytic eras. *J Am Coll Cardiol* 1997;30:1484-1490.
249. Mahaffey KW, Granger CB, Sloan MA, et al: Risk factors for inhospital nonhemorrhagic stroke in patients with acute myocardial infarction treated with thrombolysis: results from GUSTO-I. *Circulation* 1998;97:757-764.
250. Gore JM, Granger CB, Simoons ML, et al: Stroke after thrombolysis: mortality and functional outcomes in the GUSTO-I trial. Global Use of Strategies to Open Occluded Coronary Arteries. *Circulation* 1995;92:2811-2818.
251. Mooe T, Eriksson P, Stegmayr B: Ischemic stroke after acute myocardial infarction: a population-based study. *Stroke* 1997;28:762-767.
252. Sloan MA, Price TR, Terrin ML, et al: Ischemic cerebral infarction after rt-PA and heparin therapy for acute myocardial infarction: the TIMI-II pilot and randomized clinical trial combined experience. *Stroke* 1997;28:1107-1114.
253. Ringleb PA, Bhatt DL, Hirsch AT, et al, for the Clopidogrel Versus Aspirin in Patients at Risk of Ischemic Events investigators: Benefit of clopidogrel over aspirin is amplified in patients with a history of ischemic events. *Stroke* 2004;35:528-532.
254. Antman EM, et al: ACC/AHA guidelines for the management of patients with ST-elevation myocardial infarction: executive summary. *Circulation* 2004;110:588-636.
255. Turpie AG, Chin BS, Lip GY. Venous thromboembolism: pathophysiology, clinical features, and prevention. *Br Med J* 2002;325:887-90.
256. Dolovich LR, Ginsberg JS, Douketis JD, et al: A meta-analysis comparing low-molecular-weight heparins with unfractionated heparin in the treatment of venous thromboembolism: examining some unanswered questions regarding location of treatment, product type, and dosing frequency. *Arch Intern Med* 2000;160:181-188.
257. Ng TM, Tsai F, Khatri N, et al: Venous thromboembolism in hospitalized patients with heart failure: incidence, prognosis, and prevention. *Circ Heart Fail* 2010;3:165-173.
258. Rao SV, O'Grady K, Pieper KS, et al: Impact of bleeding severity on clinical outcomes among patients with acute coronary syndromes. *Am J Cardiol* 2005;96:1200-1206.
259. Wang TY, Xiao L, Alexander KP, et al: Antiplatelet therapy use after discharge among acute myocardial infarction patients with in-hospital bleeding. *Circulation* 2008;118: 2139-2145.
260. Rao SV, Ou FS, Wang TY, et al: Trends in the prevalence and outcomes of radial and femoral approaches to percutaneous coronary intervention: a report from the National Cardiovascular Data Registry. *JACC Cardiovasc Interv* 2008;1:379-386.
261. Marso SP, Amin AP, House JA, et al: Association between use of bleeding avoidance strategies and risk of periprocedural bleeding among patients undergoing percutaneous coronary intervention. *JAMA* 2010;303:2156-2164.
262. Koch CG, Li L, Sessler DI, et al: Duration of red-cell storage and complications after cardiac surgery. *N Engl J Med* 2008;358:1229-1239.
263. Rao SV, Jollis JG, Harrington RA, et al: Relationship of blood transfusion and clinical outcomes in patients with acute coronary syndromes. *JAMA* 2004;292:1555-1562.
264. Aroson D, Dann EJ, Bonstein L, et al: Impact of red blood cell transfusion on clinical outcomes in patients with acute myocardial infarction. *Am J Cardiol* 2008;102: 115-119.
265. Boden WE: Is it time to reassess the optimal timing of coronary artery bypass graft surgery following acute myocardial infarction? *Am J Cardiol* 2002;90:35-38.
266. Gersh BJ, Chesebro JH, Braunwald E, et al: Coronary artery bypass graft surgery after thrombolytic therapy in the Thrombolysis in Myocardial Infarction Trial, Phase II (TIMI II). *J Am Coll Cardiol* 1995;25:395-402.
267. Thielmann M, Neuhäuser M, Marr A, et al: Predictors and outcomes of coronary artery bypass grafting ST elevation myocardial infarction. *Ann Thorac Surg* 2007;84:17-24.
268. Parikh SV, de Lemos JA, Jessen ME, et al: Timing of in-hospital coronary artery bypass graft surgery for non-ST-segment elevation myocardial infarction patients results from the National Cardiovascular Data Registry ACTION Registry-GWTG (Acute Coronary Treatment and Intervention Outcomes Network Registry-Get With The Guidelines). *JACC Cardiovasc Interv* 2010;3:419-427.
269. Hillis LD, Smith PK, et al: 2011 ACCF/AHA guideline for coronary artery bypass graft surgery: executive summary. *Circulation* 2011;124:2610-2642.
270. Gibbons RJ, Balady GJ, Bricker JT, et al: ACC/AHA 2002 guideline update for exercise testing. Available at www.acc.org/clinical/guidelines/exercise/exercise_clean.pdf.
271. Gibson RS, Bishop HL, Stamm RB, et al: Value of early two dimensional echocardiography in patients with acute myocardial infarction. *Am J Cardiol* 1982;49:1110-1119.
272. Nishimura RA, Tajik AJ, Shub C, et al: Role of two-dimensional echocardiography in the prediction of in-hospital complications after acute myocardial infarction. *J Am Coll Cardiol* 1984;4:1080-1087.
273. Brown KA, Heller GV, Landin RS, et al: Early dipyridamole (99m)Tc-sestamibi single photon emission computed tomographic imaging 2 to 4 days after acute myocardial infarction predicts in-hospital and postdischarge cardiac events: comparison with submaximal exercise imaging. *Circulation* 1999;100:2060-2066.
274. Klocke FJ, et al: ACC/AHA/ASNC guidelines for the clinical use of cardiac radionuclide imaging: executive summary. *J Am Coll Cardiol* 2003;42:1318-1333.
275. The Multicenter Postinfarction Research Group: Risk stratification and survival after myocardial infarction. *N Engl J Med* 1983;309:331-336.
276. White HD, Norris RM, Brown MA, et al: Left ventricular end-systolic volume as the major determinant of survival after recovery from myocardial infarction. *Circulation* 1987;76:44-51.
277. Rahimtoola SH: The hibernating myocardium. *Am Heart J* 1989;117:211-221.
278. Braunwald E, Kloner RA: The stunned myocardium: prolonged, postischemic ventricular dysfunction. *Circulation* 1982;66:1146-1149.
279. Allman KC, Shaw LJ, Hachamovitch R, et al: Myocardial viability testing and impact of revascularization on prognosis in patients with coronary artery disease and left ventricular dysfunction: a meta-analysis. *J Am Coll Cardiol* 2002;39:1151-1158.
280. Bax JJ, Wijns W, Cornel H+JH, et al: Accuracy of currently available techniques for prediction of functional recovery after revascularization in patients with left ventricular dysfunction due to chronic coronary artery disease: comparison of pooled data. *J Am Coll Cardiol* 1997;30:1451-1460.
281. Beek Am, Kuhl HP, Bondarenko O, et al: Delayed contrast-enhanced magnetic resonance imaging for the prediction of regional functional improvement after acute myocardial infarction. *J Am Coll Cardiol* 2003;42:895-901.
282. Giannatsis E, et al: Cardiac magnetic resonance imaging study for quantification of infarct size comparing directly serial versus single time-point measurements of cardia troponin T. *J Am Coll Cardiol* 2008;51:307-314.
283. Topol EJ, Califf RM, George BS, et al: A randomized trial of immediate versus delayed elective angioplasty after intravenous tissue plasminogen activator in acute myocardial infarction. *N Engl J med* 1987;317:581-588.
284. Simoons ML, Arnold AE, Betriu A, et al: Thrombolysis with tissue plasminogen activator in acute myocardial infarction: no additional benefit from immediate percutaneous coronary angioplasty. *Lancet* 1988;1:197-203.
285. Should We Intervene Following Thrombolysis (SWIFT) trial study group: SWIFT trial of delayed elective intervention vs. conservative treatment after thrombolysis with anistreplase in acute myocardial infarction. *Br med J* 1991;302:555-560.
286. Barbash GI, Roth A, Hod H, et al: Randomized controlled trial of late in-hospital angiography and angioplasty versus conservative management after treatment with recombinant tissue-type plasminogen activator in acute myocardial infarction. *Am J Cardiol* 1990;66:538-545.
287. Rogers WJ, Baim DS, Gore JM, et al: Comparison of immediate invasive, delayed invasive, and conservative strategies after tissue-type plasminogen activator: results of the Thrombolysis in Myocardial Infarction (TIMI) Phase II-A trial. *Circulation* 1990;81: 1457-1476.
288. Jaski BE, et al: Outcome of urgent percutaneous transluminal coronary angioplasty in acute myocardial infarction: comparison of single-vessel versus multivessel coronary artery disease. *Am Heart J* 1992;124:1427-1433.
289. Muller DW, et al: Multivessel coronary artery disease: a key predictor of short-term prognosis after reperfusion therapy for acute myocardial infarction. Thrombolysis and Angioplasty in Myocardial Infarction (TAMI) study group. *Am Heart J* 1991;121:1042-1049.
290. Wilson SH, Bell MR: Infarct artery reocclusion after primary angioplasty, stent placement, and thrombolytic therapy for acute myocardial infarction. *Am Heart J* 2001;141: 704-710.
291. Erne P, et al: Effects of percutaneous coronary interventions in silent ischemia after myocardial infarction: the SWISSI II randomized controlled trial. *JAMA* 2007;297: 1985-1991.
292. Madsen JK, et al: Danish multicenter randomized study of invasive versus conservative treatment in patients with inducible ischemia after thrombolysis in acute myocardial infarction (DANAMI). DANish trial in Acute Myocardial Infarction. *Circulation* 1997;96: 748-755.
293. Newby LK, et al: Time-based risk assessment after myocardial infarction. Implications for timing of discharge and applications to medical decision-making. *Eur Heart J* 2003;24:182-189.
294. Goldenberg J, Gillespie J, Moss AJ, et al: Long-term benefit of primary prevention with an implantable cardioverter-defibrillator: an extended 8-year follow-up study of the Multicenter Automatic Defibrillator Implantation Trial II. *Circulation* 2010;122:1265-1271.
295. Bardy GH, Lee KL, Mark DB, et al: Amiodarone or an implantable cardioverter-defibrillator for congestive heart failure. *N Engl J Med* 2005;352:225-237.
296. Epstein AE, Dimarco JP, Ellenbogen KA, et al: ACC/AHA/HRS 2008 guidelines for evidence-based therapy of cardiac rhythm abnormalities: a report of the American College of Cardiology Task Force on Practice Guidelines. *J Am Coll Cardiol* 2008;51:e1-e62.
297. Hohnloser SH, Kuck KH, Dorian P, et al: Prophylactic use of an implantable cardioverter-defibrillator after acute myocardial infarction. *N Engl J Med* 2004;351:2481-2488.
298. Hohnloser SH, Franck P, Klingenheben T, et al: Open infarct artery, late potentials, and other prognostic factors in patients after acute myocardial infarction in the thrombolytic era: a prospective trial. *Circulation* 1994;90:1747-1756.
299. La Rovere MT, Bigger JT, Marcus FI, et al, for the ATRAMI (Autonomic Tone and Reflexes After Myocardial Infarction) investigators: Baroreflex sensitivity and heart-rate variability in prediction of total cardiac mortality after myocardial infarction. *Lancet* 1998;351:478-484.
300. Farrell TG, Paul V, Cripps TR, et al: Baroreflex sensitivity and electrophysiological correlates in patients after acute myocardial infarction. *Circulation* 1991;83:945-952.

301. Gold MR, Bloomfield DM, Anderson KP, et al: A comparison of T-wave alternans, signal averaged electrocardiography and programmed ventricular stimulation for arrhythmia risk stratification. *J Am Coll Cardiol* 2000;36:2247-2253.

302. Smith SC Jr, Benjamin EJ, Bonow RO, et al: AHA/ACCF secondary prevention and risk reduction therapy for patients with coronary and other atherosclerotic vascular disease: 2011 update. *Circulation* 2011;124:2458-2473.

303. Heart Protection Study Collaborative Group: MRC/BHF Heart Protection Study of cholesterol lowering with simvastatin in 20,536 high-risk individuals: a randomized placebo-controlled trial. *Lancet* 2002;360:7-22.

304. Myerburg RJ, Kessler KM, Castellanos A: Sudden cardiac death: epidemiology, transient risk, and intervention assessment. *Ann Intern Med* 1993;119:1187-1197.

305. Barry J, Mead K, Nabel EG, et al: Effect of smoking on the activity of ischemic heart disease. *JAMA* 1989;261:398-402.

306. Burling TA, Singleton EG, Bigelow GE, et al: Smoking following myocardial infarction: a critical review of the literature. *Health Psychol* 1984;3:83-96.

307. Glover ED, Glover PN, Payne TJ: Treating nicotine dependence. *Am J Med Sci* 2003;326:183-186.

308. Cannon CP, Braunwald E, McCabe CH, et al: Comparison of intensive and moderate lipid lowering with statins after acute coronary syndromes. *N Engl J Med* 2004;350:1562-1564.

309. Baigent C, Keech A, Kearney PM, et al: Efficacy and safety of cholesterol-lowering treatment: prospective meta-analysis of data from 90,056 participants in 14 randomised trials of statins. *Lancet* 2005;366:1267-1278.

310. Rubins HB, Robins SJ, Collins D, et al, for the Veterans Affairs High-Density Lipoprotein Cholesterol Intervention Trial study group: Gemfibrozil for the secondary prevention of coronary heart disease in men with low levels of high-density lipoprotein cholesterol. *N Engl J med* 1999;341:410-418.

311. Sacks FM, Pfeffer MA, Moye LA, et al, for the Cholesterol and Recurrent Events Trial investigators: The effect of pravastatin on coronary events after myocardial infarction in patients with average cholesterol levels. *N Engl J Med* 1996;335:1001-1009.

312. Aronow HD, Novaro GM, Lauer MS, et al: In-hospital initiation of lipid-lowering therapy after coronary intervention as a predictor of long-term utilization: a propensity analysis. *Arch Intern Med* 2003;163:2576-2582.

313. JNC 7: Seventh report of the Joint National Committee on the Prevention, Detection, Evaluation, and Treatment of High Blood Pressure (JNC 7): resetting the hypertension sails. *Hypertension* 2003;41:1178-1179.

314. Malmberg K, Ryden L, Efendic S, et al: Randomized trial of insulin-glucose infusion followed by subcutaneous insulin treatment in diabetic patients with acute myocardial infarction (DIGAMI study): Effects on mortality at 1 year. *J Am Coll Cardiol* 1995; 26:57-65.

315. The SOLVD investigators: Effect of enalapril on mortality and the development of heart failure in asymptomatic patients with reduced left ventricular ejection fractions. *N Engl J med* 1992;327:685-691.

316. Nesto RW, Bell D, Bonow RO, et al: Thiazolidinedione use, fluid retention, and congestive heart failure: a consensus statement from the American Heart Association and American Diabetes Association. *Circulation* 2003;108:2941-2948.

317. MacDonald TM, Wei L: Effect of ibuprofen on cardioprotective effect of aspirin. *Lancet* 2003;361:573-574.

318. Kurth T, Glynn RJ, Walder AM, et al: Inhibition of clinical benefits of aspirin on first myocardial infarction by nonsteroidal anti-inflammatory drugs. *Circulation* 2003;108: 1191-1195.

319. CAPRIE Steering Committee: A randomised, blinded trial of clopidogrel versus aspirin in patients at risk of ischaemic events (CAPRIE). *Lancet* 1996;348:1329-1339.

320. Gheorghiade M, Colucci WS, Swedberg K: Beta-blockers in chronic heart failure. *Circulation* 2003;107:1570-1575.

321. Sacks FM, Pfeffer MA, Moye LA, et al, for the Cholesterol and Recurrent Events Trial investigators: The effect of pravastatin on coronary events after myocardial infarction in patients with average cholesterol levels. *N Engl J Med* 1996;335:1001-1009.

322. The Long-Term Intervention with Pravastatin in Ischaemic Disease (LIPID) study group: Prevention of cardiovascular events and death with pravastatin in patients with coronary heat disease and a broad range of initial cholesterol levels. *N Engl J Med* 1998;339:1349-1357.

323. Cannon CP, Steinberg BA, Murphy SA, et al: Meta-analysis of cardiovascular outcomes trials comparing intensive versus moderate statin therapy. *J Am Coll Cardiol* 2006;48: 438-485.

324. Latini R, Maggioni AP, Flather M, et al: ACE inhibitor use in patients with myocardial infarction: summary evidence from clinical trials. *Circulation* 1995;92:3132-3137.

325. Pfeffer MA, Braunwald E, Moye LA, et al, for the SAVE investigators: Effect of captopril on mortality and morbidity in patients with left ventricular dysfunction after myocardial infarction: results of the survival and ventricular enlargement trial. *N Engl J med* 1992;342:821-828.

326. The Acute Infarction Ramipril Efficacy (AIRE) study investigators: Effect ramipril on mortality and morbidity of survivors of acute myocardial infarction with clinical evidence of heart failure. *Lancet* 1993;342:821-828.

327. Kober L, Torp-Pedersen C, Carlsen JE, et al, for the Trandolapril Cardiac Evaluation (TRACE) study group: A clinical trial of the angiotensin-converting enzyme inhibitor trandolapril in patients with left ventricular dysfunction after myocardial infarction. *N Engl J Med* 1995;333:1670-1676.

328. Yusuf S, Sleight P, Pogue J, et al, for the Heart Outcomes Prevention Evaluation study investigators: Effects of an angiotensin-converting-enzyme inhibitor, ramipril, on cardiovascular events in high-risk patients. *N Engl J med* 2000;342:145-153.

329. Fox KM, for the EURopean trial On reduction of cardiac events with Perinodopril in stable coronary Artery disease investigators: Efficacy of perindopril in reduction of cardiovascular events among patients with stable coronary artery disease: randomised, double-blind, placebo-controlled, multicentre trial (the EUROPA study). *Lancet* 2003;362: 782-788.

330. Pfeffer MA, McMurray JJ, Velazquez EJ, et al, for the Valsartan in Acute Myocardial Infarction trial investigators: Valsartan, captopril, or both in myocardial infarction complicated by heart failure, left ventricular dysfunction, or both. *N Engl J Med* 2003;349:1893-1906.

331. Granger CB, McMurray JJ, Yusuf S, et al, for the CHARM investigators and committees: Effects of candesartan in patients with chronic heart failure and reduced left-ventricular systolic function intolerant to angiotensin-converting –enzyme inhibitors: the CHARM-Alternative trial. *Lancet* 2003;362:772-776.

332. Brouwer MA, van den Bergh PJ, Aengevaeren WR, et al: Aspirin plus coumarin versus aspirin alone in the prevention of reocclusion after fibrinolysis for acute myocardial infarction: results of the Antithrombotics in the Prevention of Reocclusion In Coronary Thrombolysis (APRICOT)-2 trial. *Circulation* 2002;106:659-665.

333. Hurlen M, Abdelnoor M, Smith P, et al: Warfarin, aspirin, or both after myocardial infarction. *N Engl J Med* 2002;347:969-974.

334. Stenestrand U, Lindback J, Wallentin L: Anticoagulation therapy in atrial fibrillation in combination with acute myocardial infarction influences long-term outcome: a prospective cohort study from the Register of Information and Knowledge About Swedish Heart Intensive Care Admissions (RIKS-HIA). *Circulation* 2005;112:3225-3231.

335. Kushner FG, Antman EM: Oral anticoagulation for atrial fibrillation after ST-elevation myocardial infarction: new evidence to guide clinical practice. *Circulation* 2005;112: 3212-3214.

336. Hulley S, Grady D, Bush T, et al, for the Heart and Estrogen/progestin Replacement Study (HERS) research group: Randomized trial of estrogen plus progestin for secondary prevention of coronary heart disease in postmenopausal women. *JAMA* 1998;280: 605-613.

337. Grady D, Herrington D, Bittner V, et al, for the HERS research group: Cardiovascular disease outcomes during 6.8 years of hormone therapy: Heart and Estrogen/progestin Replacement Study follow-up (HERS II). *JAMA* 2002;288:49-57.

338. Rossouw JE, Anderson GL, Prentice RL, et al, for the Writing Group for the Women's Health Initiative investigators: Risks and benefits of estrogen plus progestin in healthy postmenopausal women: principal results from the Women's Health Initiative randomized controlled trial. *JAMA* 2002;288:321-323.

339. Pollock ML, Franklin BA, Balady GJ, et al: AHA science advisory: resistance exercise in individuals with and without cardiovascular disease: benefits, rationale, safety, and prescription: an advisory from the Committee on Exercise, Rehabilitation, and Prevention, Council on Clinical Cardiology, American Heart Association. Position paper endorsed by the American College of Sports Medicine. *Circulation* 2000;101:828-833.

340. Balady GJ, Ades PA, Comoss P, et al: Core components of cardiac rehabilitation/secondary prevention programs: a statement for healthcare professionals from the Americal Heart Association and the American Association of Cardiovascular and Pulmonary Rehabilitation Writing Group. *Circulation* 2000;102:1069-1073.

341. ENRICHD investigators: Enhancing Recovery in Coronary Heart Disease (ENRICHD) study intervention: rationale and design. *Psychosom Med* 2001;63:747-755.

342. Swenson JR, O'Connor CM, Barton D, et al, for the Sertraline Antidepressant Heart Attack Randomized Trial (SADHART) group: Influence of depression and effect of treatment with sertraline on quality of life after hospitalization for acute coronary syndrome. *Am J Cardiol* 2003;92:1271-1276.

CHAPTER 11

Advances in Coronary Revascularization

Suzanne J. Baron, Stephanie Mick, Prem S. Shekar, and Laura Mauri

OVERVIEW, 214

ADVANCES IN CORONARY STENTING, 214

Pre-Stent Era, 214
Bare-Metal Stents, 214
Drug-Eluting Stents, 215

ADVANCES IN REVASCULARIZATION IN SPECIFIC
CONDITIONS, 222

Saphenous Vein Graft Interventions, 222
Chronic Total Occlusion Intervention, 222
Bifurcation Lesion Treatment, 223

ADVANCES IN CATHETERIZATION TECHNIQUES, 223

Transradial Access, 223
Mechanical Support for High-Risk Percutaneous Coronary
    Intervention, 224
Intravascular Assessment of Lesion Severity, 224

ADVANCES IN SURGICAL CORONARY
REVASCULARIZATION, 225

Minimally Invasive Surgical Coronary Revascularization, 225
Non–Left Internal Mammary Arterial Conduits in Surgical
    Revascularization, 230
Hybrid Coronary Revascularization, 232
Future Directions, 233

REFERENCES, 234

Overview

The field of coronary revascularization was revolutionized more than 50 years ago, when the first successful coronary artery bypass surgery was performed, followed shortly thereafter by the first percutaneous procedure to dilate and open coronary arteries. Advances in operative techniques and biomedical engineering over the past decades have greatly expanded the indications and possibilities for coronary revascularization, so much so that in the United States alone, more than 800,000 revascularization procedures are performed each year. This chapter focuses on the recent advances in coronary revascularization in the catheterization laboratory and in the operating room.

Advances in Coronary Stenting

Pre-Stent Era

The concept of coronary angioplasty was first introduced in 1964, when Dotter and Judkins used serially larger sized, rigid dilators over a guidewire to enlarge the lumen of a stenotic blood vessel.[1] Unfortunately, the size and inflexibility of the dilators limited the ability of clinicians to deliver this therapy to small stenotic coronary arteries. Over the subsequent 15 years, a method designed specifically for coronary arteries was developed that utilized a small inflatable balloon to treat isolated lesions within atherosclerotic vessels; this was called *balloon angioplasty.*[2] Throughout the 1980s and 1990s, the techniques and equipment related to balloon angioplasty were further refined and included the development of a moveable guidewire system,[3] guidewires with tip designs of variable stiffness to aid in crossing complex lesions, and a collection of progressively smaller caliber guide catheters that could still provide necessary support during percutaneous interventions. These fundamental advances in balloon angioplasty allowed revascularization procedures to be performed percutaneously in a growing number of patients with coronary artery disease.

Despite these advances, the initial procedural success rate with balloon angioplasty was far from perfect, ranging between 60% and 80%.[4] Early studies demonstrated that balloon inflation within the coronary vessel often led to the embolization of plaque and thrombus with resulting poor flow in the distal vessel.[5,6] The risk of thrombotic complications was reduced with the use of systemic anticoagulation during balloon angioplasty.[7] However, other issues with balloon angioplasty surfaced. Studies demonstrated that balloon inflation in a stenotic vessel segment could result in vessel recoil, which could lead to abrupt closure early after the procedure. In addition, development of intimal hyperplasia with eventual restenosis of the vessel over the subsequent 6 months was common.[8-10] To address immediate elastic recoil and late restenosis that occurred commonly after balloon angioplasty, the concept of coronary stenting was born.

Bare-Metal Stents

The first stent was placed in a human coronary artery in 1987.[11] Over the following years, the design of the stent was refined to allow for delivery in more tortuous, stenotic, and distal vessels.[12-14] The benefits of stenting over balloon angioplasty were demonstrated in several studies. In the Belgium-Netherland Stent (BENESTENT) and Stent Restenosis Study (STRESS) randomized controlled trials (RCTs) in the early 1990s, intervention with the Palmaz-Schatz stent demonstrated lower rates of restenosis and cardiac events—including death, myocardial infarction (MI), stroke, or need for repeat angioplasty or coronary artery bypass grafting (CABG)—at 6 to 8 months when compared with balloon angioplasty (relative risk [RR], 0.68; 95% confidence interval [CI], 0.5 to 0.92; $P = .02$),[15,16] a benefit that persisted in long-term follow-up.[17]

Since the initial success of the Palmaz-Schatz stent, the physical design of stents has evolved to optimize their performance. Initial bare-metal stents were composed of stainless steel; however cobalt-chromium and cobalt-platinum alloys have allowed the engineering of stents with good radial strength but thinner and more flexible struts. The geometric configuration of stents has also undergone serial modifications. The Palmaz-Schatz stent was composed of rows of metallic slots, which would expand into diamond shapes with stent deployment ("slotted tube" formation). In an attempt to improve the flexibility of the stent, newer multicellular stents have been developed. These are generally categorized as either *open-cell* or *closed-cell* designs. Closed-cell stents have uniform patterns of cell shapes along the stent, which generally provide more constant vessel wall coverage but slightly less flexibility. Open-cell stents are more commonly used today and have patterns of varying cell sizes and shapes throughout the stent, thereby allowing for greater flexibility in the stent when maneuvering through a tortuous vessel.

Despite advances in stent deliverability, the risk of restenosis following bare-metal stent placement has remained fairly constant over time, with rates of restenosis as high as 20% to 40% on repeat angiography and a clinical need for repeat target lesion revascularization procedures in 14% to 17% of patients.[18] Although the placement of a stent prevents vessel recoil after angioplasty and stenting has lower overall rates of restenosis than balloon angioplasty, the presence of a stent is associated with a greater amount of later development of neointimal hyperplasia than angioplasty alone.[19] Diabetes mellitus, long lesion length, and small vessel diameter have all been identified as risk factors for higher rates of restenosis.[20]

Several pharmacologic and procedural interventions were investigated to prevent in-stent restenosis. Brachytherapy (intracoronary radiation) was shown to be effective in treating in-stent restenosis[21-24] but does not prevent it.[25] Oral drugs—including cilostazol, rosiglitazone, everolimus, tranilast, and rapamycin—have also been evaluated for the prevention of restenosis after baremetal stent placement,[26-30] but in general, the reduction in restenosis rates with oral or intravenous agents has been modest at best. With the lack of both effective and convenient methods to prevent and treat restenosis with bare-metal stent placement, the stage was set for the introduction of the drug-eluting stent.

Drug-Eluting Stents

DEVELOPMENT OF DRUG-ELUTING STENTS

To address the problem of high restenosis rates associated with bare-metal stents, researchers developed an intraarterial, localized, pharmacologic means to combat neointimal hyperplasia—the drug-eluting stent (DES). A successful DES would need to have three components: the drug, a delivery system for the pharmacologic agent (i.e., the polymer), and the stent platform itself. An ideal drug would need to target the proliferative response to vessel injury effectively without causing systemic side effects. An ideal drug delivery system would be able to store the drug effectively and release it in a measured time frame to provide the maximum effect on inhibition of restenosis, which would need to be accomplished without significant degradation or loss of function of either the drug or the drug vehicle. Lastly, the new stent platform would need to incorporate all the lessons learned from research with baremetal stents: the importance of thinner struts, flexibility and conformability to the vessel wall, and optimization of the stent design for consistent drug elution to all areas of the atherosclerotic vessel.

DES development was not immediately successful. Trials investigating stents that used a new antiproliferative agent, actinomycin D, on the Tetra-D stent (Guidant, Santa Clara, CA)[31]—or that used a tried-and-true paclitaxel derivative, taxane, but mounted into a novel polymer on the Quanam stent (Boston Scientific)[32]—demonstrated higher rates of restenosis and greater rates of major adverse cardiac events at 1 year with these new technologies. Local drug toxicity or adverse reactions to the polymer used were possible sources of these disappointing results.[33]

DRUG-ELUTING STENTS CURRENTLY AVAILABLE IN THE UNITED STATES

Sirolimus-Eluting Stents

Using the lessons learned from failed DESs, investigators eventually developed the sirolimus-eluting stent, Cypher (Cordis Corporation, Warren, NJ), in the late 1990s, and this technology has revolutionized interventional cardiology. Sirolimus was initially approved as an immunosuppressive agent for the prevention of organ transplant rejection; however, it was discovered that the drug also inhibits smooth muscle cell proliferation and migration, thus making it a good agent to inhibit neointimal hyperplasia.[34-36] Sirolimus was loaded into a polymer coat—a 2:1 combination of the polymers polyethylene-co-vinyl acetate and poly-n-butyl methacrylate, respectively—which acted to release the drug slowly over the following month; this polymer was subsequently placed onto a stainless steel, closed-cell metal stent, hence forming the Cypher stent.

In 1999, the first sirolimus-eluting stents were placed in 45 patients in Brazil.[37] Follow-up studies of this pilot population demonstrated significant suppression of restenosis at 1 year with the

sirolimus-eluting stent when compared with a bare-metal stent.[38] Given the promising results of these pilot studies, two randomized, controlled trials (RCTs), the Randomised Study with the Sirolimus-Coated BX Velocity Balloon-Expandable Stent (RAVEL) and the Sirolimus-Eluting Stent in de Novo Native Coronary Lesions (SIRUIS) trials, were conducted to evaluate further the sirolimus-eluting stent. In the RAVEL trial, 238 subjects with simple, discrete coronary stenoses were randomized to receive either the sirolimus-eluting stent or an analogous bare-metal stent. At 6 months, rates of angiographically detected in-stent restenosis were significantly lower with the sirolimus-eluting stent (26.6% vs. 0%; $P < .001$).[39] In the SIRIUS study, 1058 patients with more complex coronary artery disease (small vessels, long lesions) were randomized to receive either the sirolimus-eluting stent or the bare-metal stent. Again, rates of in-stent restenosis were significantly lower (35.4% vs. 3.2%; $P < .001$) with the sirolimus-eluting stent at 8 months, which translated to significantly lower rates of target lesion revascularization at 1 year and at 5 years.[40,41] The positive results of these two trials led to U.S. Food and Drug Administration (FDA) approval of the sirolimus-eluting stent in 2003. Subsequent studies of this stent in specific populations—including patients with diabetes, ST-elevation MI (STEMI), and complex disease—have all demonstrated the superiority of the sirolimus-eluting stent over bare-metal stents in reducing angiographic restenosis at 6 to 12 months and in reducing rates of repeat target revascularization for up to 5 years (Table 11-1).[42-56]

Paclitaxel-Eluting Stents

The Taxus paclitaxel-eluting stent (Boston Scientific, Natick, MA) was approved soon after the sirolimus-eluting stent. Paclitaxel is most commonly used as an antineoplastic agent because it has been shown to interfere with cell mitosis at high doses, thereby leading to cell death. At lower doses, paclitaxel can arrest the cell cycle without leading to cell death, and it can inhibit smooth muscle cell proliferation.[57,58] The Taxus stent releases paclitaxel from a stainless steel metal stent via the polymer poly styrene-b-isobutylene-b-styrene.

The first paclitaxel-eluting stent, Taxus-Express, was evaluated in the pilot Treatment of de novo Coronary Artery Disease Using a Single Paclitaxel-Eluting Stent (TAXUS) study, in which 61 patients with simple coronary lesions were randomized to receive either the paclitaxel-eluting stent or a bare-metal stent. The study demonstrated significantly lower rates of angiographic in-stent restenosis with the paclitaxel-eluting stent (10.4% vs. 0%; $P < .001$) and significantly lower rates of target lesion revascularization at 1 year (10% vs. 0%; $P < .05$).[59] The encouraging results of the first TAXUS study paved the way for several other trials—including TAXUS II, IV, V, and VI—larger RCTs that evaluated the use of paclitaxel-eluting stents in simple coronary lesions, complex lesions, and in the treatment of STEMI (Table 11-2).[50,60-68] In all these trials, paclitaxel was consistently associated with lower rates of angiographic restenosis and lower rates of target lesion revascularization for up to 5 years after stent placement.

Researchers subsequently refined the paclitaxel-eluting stent by changing the stent design to a hybrid of closed- and open-cell geometry, the result of which produced a more flexible stent (Taxus-Liberte, Boston Scientific) with thinner struts and more homogeneous drug delivery to the vascular wall.[69] The TAXUS Assessment of Treatment with Lisinopril and Survival (ATLAS) trial (polymer-based, paclitaxel-eluting TAXUS Liberte stent in de novo lesions) confirmed the preserved effectiveness of this stent modification.[69] Furthermore, in long coronary lesions (26 to 34 mm) in particular, the Taxus-Liberte stent was found to be associated with significantly lower rates of MI (1.4% vs. 6.5%; $P = .002$) when compared with the Taxus-Express stent,[70] presumably because of lower rates of side-branch occlusion by stent struts. Most recently, a platinum-based stent system for the Taxus drug and polymer was approved for use in the United States (discussed below).[71]

Several trials have compared paclitaxel-eluting stents with sirolimus-eluting stents. In general, the paclitaxel stent has been found to be associated with higher rates of angiographic restenosis

TABLE 11-1   Trials Involving Sirolimus-Eluting Stents

					SES vs. BMS (%)			
TRIAL	EXPERIMENTAL GROUP (N)	CONTROL GROUP (N)	CLINICAL POPULATION	ANGIOGRAPHIC/ CLINICAL FOLLOW-UP PERIOD (MO)	ANGIOGRAPHIC BINARY IN-STENT RESTENOSIS	DEATH	MI	TLR
RAVEL[39]	SES (120)	BMS (118)	Elective single lesions	6/12	0.0 vs. 26.6*	1.7 vs. 1.7	3.3 vs. 4.2	0.0 vs. 23.7*
SIRIUS[40,41]	SES (533)	BMS (525)	Complex disease	8/9 60	3.2 vs. 35.4* NA	0.9 vs. 0.6 8.4 vs. 8.4	2.8 vs. 3.2 6.2 vs. 6.5	4.1 vs. 16.6* 9.4 vs. 24.2*
SCANDSTENT[56]	SES (163)	BMS (159)	Complex disease	6/7	2.0 vs. 30.6*	0.6 vs. 0.6	1.2 vs. 3.1	2.5 vs. 29.3*
TYPHOON[54]	SES (355)	BMS (357)	STEMI	8/12	3.5 vs. 20.3*	2.3 vs. 2.2	1.1 vs. 1.4	5.6 vs. 13.4*
SESAMI[50,51]	SES (160)	BMS (160)	STEMI	12 36	9.3 vs. 21.3* NA	1.8 vs. 4.3 3.2 vs. 5.0	1.8 vs. 1.8 2.5 vs. 2.5	4.3 vs. 11.2* 7.0 vs. 13.5*
PASEO[49]	SES (90)	BMS (90)	STEMI	12 48	NA NA	3.3 vs. 6.7 7.8 vs. 12.2	4.4 vs. 6.7 8.9 vs. 13.3	3.3 vs. 14.4 * 5.6 vs. 21.1*
STRATEGY[52,53]	SES (87)	BMS (88)	STEMI	8 60	7.5 vs. 28.0* NA	8.0 vs. 9.1 18.0 vs. 16.0	6.9 vs. 9.1 22.0 vs. 25.0	5.7 vs. 20.5* 10.3 vs. 26.1*
Diaz de la Llera et al[46]	SES (60)	BMS (60)	STEMI	12	NA	5.0 vs. 3.6	NA	0.0 vs. 5.7*
DESSERT[44]	SES (75)	BMS (75)	Diabetes	8/12	3.6 vs. 38.8*	4.4 vs. 2.9	16.2 vs. 20.0	5.9 vs. 30.0*
SCORPIUS[45]	SES (98)	BMS (102)	Diabetes	8/12	8.8 vs. 42.1*	5.3 vs. 4.1	4.3 vs. 5.2	5.3 vs. 21.1*
DIABETES[42,43]	SES (80)	BMS (80)	Diabetes	9/24 48	3.9 vs. 31.7* NA	2.6 vs. 3.8 4.1 vs. 6.5	3.8 vs. 8.8 4.1 vs. 10.4	7.7 vs. 35.0* 8.1 vs. 37.7*

*P < .05.

BMS, bare-metal stent; MI, myocardial infarction; NA, not available; SES, sirolimus-eluting stent; STEMI, ST-elevation myocardial infarction; TLR, target lesion revascularization.

TABLE 11-2   Trials Involving Paclitaxel-Eluting Stents

					PES vs. BMS (%)			
TRIAL	EXPERIMENTAL GROUP (N)	CONTROL GROUP (N)	CLINICAL POPULATION	ANGIOGRAPHIC/ CLINICAL FOLLOW-UP PERIOD (MO)	ANGIOGRAPHIC BINARY IN-STENT RESTENOSIS	DEATH	MI	TLR
TAXUS-I[59]	PES (31)	BMS (30)	Elective simple lesions	6/12	0.0 vs. 10.4*	0.0 vs. 0.0	0.0 vs. 0.0	0.0 vs. 10.0*
TAXUS-II[60,61]	PES Slow Release (131)	BMS (136)	Elective simple lesions	6/12 60	2.3 vs. 17.9 * NA	0.0 vs. 1.5 2.4 vs. 1.5	2.4 vs. 5.3 4.7 vs. 7.1	4.7 vs. 12.9* 10.3 vs. 18.4*
	PES Moderate Release (135)	BMS (134)	Elective simple lesions	6/12 60	4.7 vs. 20.2 * NA	0.0 vs. 0.0 5.3 vs. 7.1	3.8 vs. 5.4 5.3 vs. 7.1	3.8 vs. 16.0* 4.5 vs. 18.4*
TAXUS-IV[62,63]	PES (662)	BMS (652)	Elective single lesions	9/9 60	5.5 vs. 24.4* NA	2.4 vs. 2.2 10.0 vs. 11.2	3.5 vs. 3.7 7.2 vs. 7.4	3.0 vs. 11.3* 9.1 vs. 20.5*
TAXUS-V[64]	PES (577)	BMS (579)	Complex lesions	9/9	13.7 vs. 31.9*	0.5 vs. 0.9	5.4 vs. 4.6	8.6 vs. 15.7*
TAXUS-VI[65,66]	PES (219)	BMS (227)	Complex lesions	9/9 60	9.1 vs. 32.9* NA	0.0 vs. 0.9 2.8 vs. 3.2	8.2 vs. 6.2 11.2 vs. 8.2	6.8 vs. 18.9* 14.6 vs. 21.4
PASEO[49]	PES (90)	BMS (90)	STEMI	12	NA	4.4 vs. 6.7	3.3 vs. 6.7	4.4 vs. 14.4*
HORIZONS-AMI[67]	PES (2257)	BMS (749)	STEMI	13/12	8.2 vs. 21.0*	3.5 vs. 3.5	3.6 vs. 4.4	4.3 vs. 7.2*
PASSION[68]	PES (310)	BMS (309)	STEMI	12	NA	4.6 vs. 6.5	1.7 vs. 2.0	5.3 vs. 7.8

*P < .05.

BMS, bare-metal stent; MI, myocardial infarction; NA, not available; PES, paclitaxel-eluting stent; STEMI, ST-elevation myocardial infarction; TLR, target lesion revascularization.

with higher rates of total lesion revascularization. In the Sirolimus-Eluting Stent Compared with Paclitaxel-Eluting Stent in Coronary Revascularization (SIRTAX) trial, 1011 patients requiring coronary stent placement were randomized to receive either the paclitaxel-eluting stent or a sirolimus-eluting stent.[72] At 8 months, the paclitaxel-eluting stent was associated with significantly higher levels of binary in-stent restenosis (7.5% vs. 3.2%; P < .05), which translated to higher rates of target lesion revascularization at 1 year (8.3% vs. 4.8%; P < .05), although the differences in target lesion revascularization had disappeared at 5 year follow-up (5.9% vs. 4.5%; P = not significant).[73] Comparisons of the two stents in specific populations—such as in patients with diabetes, STEMI, and in small vessels and long lesions—have also demonstrated that the paclitaxel stent is associated with slightly higher rates of angiographic in-stent restenosis and resulting increased rates of target lesion revascularization.[74-79] This finding may be exaggerated, however, by the performance of routine angiographic follow-up[80] because other studies without angiographic follow-up have demonstrated no significant difference in target lesion revascularization or in major adverse cardiac events between the two stents.[81,82]

Zotarolimus-Eluting Stents and Everolimus-Eluting Stents

The zotarolimus- and everolimus-eluting stents were approved by the FDA in 2008. Both use a cobalt-chromium stent, a durable polymer, and antiproliferative drugs that are analogues of sirolimus. The cobalt-chromium stent platform allowed for thinner stent struts and improved stent deliverability; hence, it was thought that these changes would allow for even lower rates of restenosis with the use of these two stents.

The zotarolimus-eluting stent has been shown to be superior to bare-metal stents in preventing in-stent restenosis, although it may not be superior to other drug-eluting stents on the market. The ENDEAVOR-II study randomized 1197 patients to receive either the zotarolimus-eluting stent or a bare-metal stent. Patients treated with the zotarolimus-eluting stent had significantly lower rates of angiographic restenosis at 9 months (33.5% vs. 9.4%; $P < .001$) and lower rates of target lesion revascularization (11.8% vs. 4.6%; $P < .001$).[83]

When compared with the sirolimus-eluting stent, the zotarolimus-eluting stent has been associated with higher rates of target lesion revascularization.[84] Compared with the paclitaxel-eluting stent, a slightly higher restenosis rate was also seen with the zotarolimus-eluting stent in studies with follow-up angiography.[85,86] Although significantly higher rates of in-stent late lumen loss were seen with the zotarolimus-eluting stent, this did not translate into a significant difference in the occurrence of target lesion revascularization (Table 11-3).[87]

The everolimus-eluting stent (Xience V, Abbott Vascular, Abbott Park, IL; Promus, Boston Scientific) was first evaluated in the SPIRIT FIRST trial, which was a study of 56 patients and compared the everolimus-eluting stent with the standard control of a bare-metal stent. The everolimus-eluting stent was found to have significantly lower rates of target lesion revascularization at 6 months and as far out as 5 years.[83,84] This small study paved the way for larger trials to be conducted in which the everolimus-eluting stent could be compared with other DESs (Table 11-4). Several randomized trials have compared the everolimus-eluting stent with the paclitaxel-eluting stent,[85,86,88,89] the largest of which was the SPIRIT-IV trial of more than 3600 patients. At 12 months, the everolimus-eluting stent was associated with significantly lower rates of target lesion revascularization (2.5% vs. 4.6%; $P = .001$) and lower rates of MI (1.9% vs. 3.1%; $P = .02$).[90] These results were essentially replicated in the smaller Second-Generation Everolimus-Eluting and Paclitaxel-Eluting Stents in Real-Life Practice (COMPARE) study, which also

TABLE 11-3 Trials Involving Zotarolimus-Eluting Stents

TRIAL	EXPERIMENTAL GROUP (N)	CONTROL GROUP(S) (N)	ANGIOGRAPHIC/ CLINICAL FOLLOW-UP PERIOD (MO)	ANGIOGRAPHIC BINARY IN-STENT RESTENOSIS	ZES vs. Control (%) DEATH	MI	TLR
ENDEAVOR I[291]	E-ZES (100)	N/A	12/12	5.4	0.0	1.0	2.0
ENDEAVOR II[292]	E-ZES (598)	BMS (599)	9/9	9.4 vs. 33.5*	1.2 vs. 0.5	2.7 vs. 3.9	4.6 vs. 11.8*
ENDEAVOR III[293]	E-ZES (323)	SES (113)	8/9	9.2 vs. 2.1*	0.6 vs. 0.0	0.6 vs. 3.5*	6.3 vs. 3.5
SORT OUT III[294]	E-ZES (1162)	SES (1170)	9	NA	2.0 vs. 2.0	1.4 vs. 0.5*	4.0 vs. 1.0*
			18	NA	4.4 vs. 2.7*	2.1 vs. 0.9*	6.1 vs. 1.7*
ENDEAVOR IV[87]	E-ZES (773)	PES (775)	8/12	13.3 vs. 6.7	1.1 vs. 1.1	1.6 vs. 2.7	4.5 vs. 3.2
ZEST[295]	E-ZES (880)	PES (880)	12	NA	0.7 vs. 1.1	5.3 vs.7.0	4.9 vs. 7.5
		SES (880)		NA	0.7 vs. 0.8	5.3 vs. 6.3	4.9 vs. 1.4*
RESOLUTE[152]	R-ZES (139)	NA	9/12	1.0%	2.2%	5.8%	0.7%
RESOLUTE US[296]	R-ZES (1376)	NA	8/12	9.2%	1.3%	1.4%	2.8%

*$P < .05$.

BMS, bare-metal stent; E-ZES, Endeavor zotarolimus-eluting stent; MI, myocardial infarction; NA, not available; PES, paclitaxel-eluting stent; SES, sirolimus-eluting stent; TLR, target lesion revascularization; R-ZES, Resolute zotarolimus-eluting stent.

TABLE 11-4 Trials Involving Everolimus-Eluting Stents

TRIAL	EXPERIMENTAL GROUP (N)	CONTROL GROUP (N)	ANGIOGRAPHIC/ CLINICAL FOLLOW-UP PERIOD (MO)	ANGIOGRAPHIC BINARY IN-STENT RESTENOSIS	EES vs. Control (%) DEATH	MI	TLR
SPIRIT FIRST[83,84]	EES (27)	BMS (29)	6/6	0.0 vs. 25.9*	0.0 vs 0.0	3.8 vs. 0.0	3.8 vs. 21.4
			60	NA	0.0 vs. 7.4	8.3 vs. 0.0	8.3 vs. 28.0
SPIRIT II[85,88]	EES (223)	PES (77)	6/6	1.3 vs. 3.5	0.0 vs. 1.3	0.9 vs. 3.9	2.7 vs. 6.5
			36	NA	0.5 vs. 4.3	3.6 vs. 7.2	4.6 vs. 10.1
SPIRIT III[86]	EES (669)	PES (333)	8/12	2.3 vs. 5.7	1.2 vs. 1.2	2.8 vs. 4.1	3.4 vs. 5.6
SPIRIT IV[90]	EES (2458)	PES (1229)	12	NA	1.0 vs. 1.3	1.9 vs. 3.1*	2.5 vs. 4.6*
COMPARE[89]	EES (897)	PES (903)	12	NA	2.0 vs. 1.6	2.8 vs. 5.3*	2.0 vs. 5.3*

*$P < .05$.

BMS, bare-metal stent; EES, everolimus-eluting stent; MI, myocardial infarction; NA, not available; PES, paclitaxel-eluting stent; TLR, target lesion revascularization.

showed lower rates of MI, stent thrombosis, and target lesion revascularization with the everolimus-eluting stent when compared with the paclitaxel-eluting stent.[89]

EFFICACY AND SAFETY OF DRUG-ELUTING STENTS

Efficacy of Drug-Eluting Stents

As described above, multiple studies have confirmed that DESs are extremely effective in reducing restenosis compared with bare-metal stents. Several meta-analyses have confirmed these findings,[91-93] the largest of which involved more than 18,000 patients and demonstrated that target lesion revascularization rates over 4 years are reduced by 70% with sirolimus-eluting stents and by 58% with paclitaxel-eluting stents when compared with bare-metal stents.[91] Furthermore, population-based studies and registries have shown a similar reduction in restenosis in patients who receive DESs for off-label indications (complex lesions, unstable clinical status), such as when the stents are used as initially studied for FDA approval.[94-96] Across stent types, some modest variation in efficacy exists, particularly in patients with higher restenosis risk—such as patients with diabetes or those with small vessels or long lesions—but in general, it is accepted that DESs are beneficial in reducing restenosis rates when compared with bare-metal stents.

Safety of Drug-Eluting Stents

Following approval in 2003, DESs were almost universally adopted for percutaneous coronary intervention (PCI); PCI was therefore concurrently applied to more complex lesion and patient cohorts.[97] It was in this environment that several reports surfaced in 2006 and 2007 suggesting that DESs may be associated with acute thrombotic occlusion a year or more after placement of the stent. The single-center Basel Stent Kosten Effectivitäts Trial–Late Thrombotic Events (BASKET-LATE) retrospectively analyzed the outcomes of 746 patients, who were randomized to receive either bare-metal stents or sirolimus-eluting stents for the treatment of both stable and unstable coronary artery disease. Excluding the first 6 months after treatment, when subjects with sirolimus-eluting stents had lower rates of repeat revascularization, death, and MI, the sirolimus-eluting stent was associated with a higher rate of death and MI between 7 and 18 months after stent placement.[98] Although the authors proposed that this finding was due to an increased rate of stent thrombosis with DESs, interestingly enough, no significant difference was found in the rates of stent thrombosis between the two groups. Subsequent examination of this trial revealed that the conclusion that DESs lead to increased mortality may have not been entirely accurate because of several factors, including small sample size with the resultant underpowering of the study to detect infrequent events, such as stent thrombosis, and the premature cessation of dual antiplatelet therapy at 6 months in all patients, which has since been shown to be a significant risk factor for stent thrombosis in patients with DESs.[99-102] More recently, the prospective, randomized 2300 patient BASKET Prospective Validation Examination (BASKET-PROVE) trial, which was designed specifically to address the safety concerns raised in the BASKET-LATE trial, demonstrated no significant difference in the rates of death, MI, or stent thrombosis among patients who received sirolimus-eluting stents, everolimus-eluting stents, or bare-metal stents.[103] Although a few other nonrandomized studies or meta-analyses have suggested that DESs may be associated with higher rates of mortality,[104-106] subsequent reanalyses using pooled patient-level data have demonstrated no significant differences in mortality between bare-metal stents and DESs.[107,108] Furthermore, several subsequent large meta-analyses and registry studies evaluating more than 200,000 patients have been reassuring in showing no apparent increased risk of death or MI with DESs at either short- or long-term follow-up.[91-94,96,109-113]

Despite these reassuring reports regarding the safety of DESs, the question of late stent thrombosis risk has remained. Although rare, stent thrombosis is associated with significant morbidity and mortality.[114] Although no randomized studies have demonstrated a significant difference in the overall rate of stent thrombosis between bare-metal stents and DESs, these studies have been limited in size.[91,92,107,109,111,115] On the other hand, analyses from several large registries and a number of meta-analyses have shown a higher risk of very late stent thrombosis with DES placement, although these findings should be considered critically, as residual confounding has been difficult to exclude.[92,109,111,116]

Investigation into the cause of stent thrombosis has implicated several different factors that likely contribute to the development of this serious complication. Patient factors—such as unstable coronary artery disease, diabetes, renal failure, and prior brachytherapy—and lesion characteristics that include small vessel diameter, high degrees of calcification, long lesions, or complex lesions may predispose a patient to developing stent thrombosis.[100,117-119] Characteristics of the DES itself may also predispose a patient to developing stent thrombosis. Although the purpose of a drug-coated stent is to interfere with neointimal hyperplasia and hence decrease restenosis, the side effect is that the endothelialization process is delayed, thereby increasing the exposure of thrombogenic molecules in the blood to the stent struts.[120-123] Furthermore, the polymer in which the drug is loaded in a DES can lead to hypersensitivity reactions and vascular inflammation, both of which can promote thrombotic events.[124-126] Procedural technique—such as if the stent is suboptimally expanded or undersized or if stent apposition is incomplete—has also been shown to be related to stent thrombosis.[127,128]

Premature cessation of dual antiplatelet therapy, particularly within the first month of stent placement, is one of the most potent factors associated with increased risk of stent thrombosis,[99-102] although the data as to what constitutes "premature cessation" are conflicting. The optimal duration of antiplatelet therapy after coronary stent placement therefore remains unknown. Although initial randomized trials of sirolimus-eluting stents used 3 months of dual antiplatelet therapy, observational studies suggest that at least 6 months,[102,129,130] or even 12 months, of dual antiplatelet therapy after DES placement has been associated with lower rates of stent thrombosis and improved mortality.[113,131,132] That said, the prolonged use of dual antiplatelet therapy is associated with an increased risk of bleeding. Although small RCTs have been performed to determine clinically significant differences in stent thrombosis or other cardiovascular events with varying durations of dual antiplatelet therapy, these studies have been underpowered.[133] But several large, randomized trials powered to provide more clarity on the duration of therapy after DES placement are enrolling patients[134] or have completed enrollment.[135] The current national and international society guidelines on dual antiplatelet therapy duration and use are summarized in Table 11-5.

WHEN TO USE DRUG-ELUTING STENTS

Although the benefits of the use of DESs are clear, such stents have generally been more expensive, and the precise risk of stent thrombosis has been uncertain.[136] Furthermore, the use of DESs does also obligate patients to a longer duration of dual antiplatelet therapy, even if the precise duration remains a topic of ongoing study. As a result of these differences in risk, cost, and benefit, it is reasonable to consider how stents can be optimally used in individual patients and in patient populations. Certain lesion characteristics and patient characteristics confer a higher risk for restenosis, and it is in the patient with a higher risk of restenosis that a DES may carry the most benefit. A model derived from a 10,000-subject, real-world registry suggested that patients younger than 60 years, those with prior PCI, an intervention being performed either on the left main artery or a saphenous vein graft (SVG), and a stent diameter of less than 2.5 mm or a lesion length greater than 40 mm were at an increased risk for restenosis after stent placement.[137] Similar results were demonstrated in the analysis of another larger registry, in which researchers reported that target vessel revascularization rates were no different between DESs and bare-metal stents in nondiabetic patients with short, noncomplex coronary lesions

TABLE 11-5	National and International Guidelines on Dual Antiplatelet Therapy After Stent Placement			
RECOMMENDATION		**SOCIETY**	**CLASS OF RECOMMENDATION**	**LEVEL OF EVIDENCE**
Aspirin				
After PCI, aspirin should be continued indefinitely.		ACCF/AHA/SCAI	I	A
After PCI, 81 mg aspirin is reasonable in preference to higher doses.		ACCF/AHA/SCAI	IIa	B
After elective PCI or PCI for NSTE-ACS or STEMI, a bolus of 150-300 mg aspirin should be given, followed by 75-100 mg/day.		ESC	I	A, B, C
After ACS, 75-162 mg aspirin should be continued indefinitely.		CCS	I	A
P2Y$_{12}$ Inhibitors				
After BMS or DES placement for ACS, P2Y$_{12}$ inhibitors—either clopidogrel, prasugrel, or ticragrelor—should be given for 12 months minimum.		ACCF/AHA/SCAI	I	B
After DES placement for a non-ACS indication, clopidogrel should be given for at least 12 months.		ACCF/AHA/SCAI	I	B
After BMS placement for a non-ACS indication, clopidogrel should be given for at least 1 month, ideally up to 12 months.		ACCF/AHA/SCAI	I	B
If bleeding risk is high and outweighs expected benefit of longer duration of P2Y$_{12}$ therapy, discontinuation of P2Y$_{12}$ therapy before 12 months is reasonable.		ACCF/AHA/SCAI	IIa	C
More than 12 months of P2Y$_{12}$ therapy may be considered in patients with DES placement.		ACCF/AHA/SCAI	IIb	C
After PCI for NSTE-ACS or STEMI, clopidogrel maintenance dosing for 9-12 months should be given.		ESC	I	B, C
After PCI for NSTE-ACS or STEMI, alternative P2Y$_{12}$ therapies (prasugrel or ticagrelor) can be given.		ESC	I, IIa	B
After PCI with BMS for ACS and elective PCI, clopidogrel should be continued for at least 1 month, up to 12 months in the absence of an excessive risk of bleeding.		CCS	I	B
After PCI with DES for ACS and elective PCI, clopidogrel should be continued for 12 months and can be considered for longer durations if the risk for stent thrombosis is high and risk of bleeding is low.		CCS	I, IIb	A, C
After PCI for ACS, prasugrel may be considered in patients with an increased risk of thrombosis.		CCS	IIa	B

Data from references 297, 298, 299and .
ACCF, American College of Cardiology Foundation; ACS, acute coronary syndrome; AHA, American Heart Association; BMS, bare-metal stent; CCS, Canadian Cardiovascular Society; DES, drug-eluting stent; ESC, European Society of Cardiology; NSTE, non–ST-segment elevation; PCI, percutaneous coronary intervention; SCAI, Society for Cardiac Angiography and Interventions; STEMI, ST-segment elevation myocardial infarction.

(<20 mm long) in vessels greater than 3 mm in diameter (5.3% vs. 5.9%; $P = .61$).[138] Studies consistently show that patients with small vessels, longer stents, and diabetes; treatment of multiple lesions; or treatment for restenosis itself are at the highest risk of restenosis with bare-metal stents. Therefore, models to predict the absolute risk reduction in restenosis associated with DES placement have been developed to identify patients who are most likely to benefit from DES placement.[139]

Before choosing a drug-eluting versus a bare-metal stent, consideration of obligate antiplatelet therapy is also important. Certain patients are at an increased risk for stopping dual antiplatelet therapy, such as those with preexisting anemia or upcoming surgeries,[101] which can lead to an even greater risk of stent thrombosis. Therefore, for each patient and clinical situation, the risk of restenosis must be balanced against the necessity of a prolonged period of dual antiplatelet therapy. If the risk of restenosis for a patient is low, and the risk of stent thrombosis, including the risk of premature cessation of dual antiplatelet therapy, plus the risk of bleeding with dual antiplatelet therapy is high, a bare-metal stent might be the more appropriate choice. Conversely, if the risk of restenosis for a patient is high and the risk of stent thrombosis plus the risk of bleeding with dual antiplatelet therapy is low, then a DES should be used.

NEW DRUG-ELUTING STENTS AVAILABLE OUTSIDE THE UNITED STATES OR UNDERGOING INVESTIGATION

Although many advances have been made in DES technology over the past 10 years, there continues to be room for improvement.

Research has focused on alterations involving the stent platform itself, the types of drugs to be delivered, and the polymer used to control the release of the drug. Many stents currently available outside the United States still require further clinical evaluation before U.S. approval because of the requirement of substantial evidence of safety beyond 1 year before new stents are introduced in the U.S. market.

Products Involving Changes to the Stent Platform

Traditional Stent Platforms

Because platinum in combination with chromium is a stronger alloy than stainless steel or cobalt-chromium, a stent with thinner struts can be designed.[140,141] Two DESs are available in Europe that use the platinum-chromium platform: the Promus Element stent (everolimus-eluting) and the Taxus Element stent (paclitaxel-eluting). A small, 100-subject, single-arm study evaluating the Promus Element stent demonstrated appropriate rates of late lumen loss (0.17 ± 0.25 mm) at 9 months.[142] Results of the larger Prospective, Randomized, Multicenter Trial to Assess an Everolimus-Eluting Coronary Stent System (Promus Element) for the Treatment of up to Two de Novo Coronary Artery Lesions (PLATINUM) trial, which randomized patients to either the Promus Element stent or an everolimus-eluting stent with a cobalt-chromium platform are pending. The Taxus Element stent is also being evaluated in the ongoing Prospective Evaluation in a Randomized Trial of the Safety and Efficacy of the Use of the TAXUS Element Paclitaxel-Eluting Coronary Stent System (PERSEUS) trial, and substudies of this trial have yielded favorable results for the Taxus Element stent in comparison to bare-metal stents and the earlier version of the Taxus Express stent in terms of in-stent late lumen loss.[71,143] Given these results, approval by the FDA for both the Taxus Element and the Promus Element stent is expected by 2013.

BIODEGRADABLE STENTS

Theoretical benefits of a biodegradable stent are similar to the benefits of a stent with a biodegradable polymer; with the eventual absence of a foreign material in the vessel wall, there is less possibility for residual inflammation there, leading to a lower theoretical incidence of in-stent thrombosis. Furthermore, with fully biodegradable stents, the issues surrounding the difficulty of performing later procedures across jailed side branches might be avoided.

Although biodegradable stents have theoretical benefits, their design poses several practical challenges. Current biodegradable stents under investigation are composed of either polymers or metal alloys. Biodegradable polymers have been studied in other medical implants, such as sutures and orthopedic devices, but stents composed entirely of polymer require thicker stent struts to maintain radial strength comparable with metallic stents; this may result in less flexibility in manipulating these stents into smaller vessels. Furthermore, biodegradable materials are usually not radiopaque and will still require metallic stent markers to be visualized

adequately. Lastly, although biodegradable, the deployment of the stent and the presence of the polymer, even if temporary, may still lead to neointimal hyperplasia and hence require drug suppression to achieve results comparable to DESs.

Several biodegradable stents are under investigation, but the most clinical data are currently available for the bioresorbable vascular scaffold (BVS) everolimus stent. This fully biodegradable stent utilizes the polymer poly-L-lactic acid combined with a coating of poly-D,L-lactic acid to release the drug everolimus to suppress neointimal hyperplasia. Clinical studies of this stent have shown that, although the acute gain in lumen diameter of these stents is slightly lower than conventional DESs, the combination of polymer and drug has good suppression of late neointimal hyperplasia.[144,145]

Products Involving Changes to Drug Coatings

The chemical structures and presumed mechanism of action of drugs currently used are shown in Figure 11-1. Several new derivatives of sirolimus have been applied to stent technology—including myolimus, biolimus, and novolimus—which, similar to sirolimus, inhibit mammalian target of rapamycin (mTOR). Besides sirolimus derivatives and antiproliferative agents, other novel agents have been applied to coronary stents that are currently available only

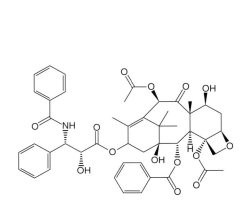

Paclitaxel
(stabilizes microtubules in centrosome and arrests cell cycle progression from G_0 to G_1 phase)

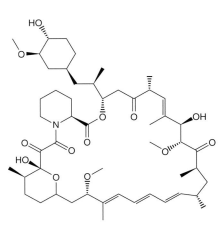

Sirolimus
(inhibits mTOR and arrests cell cycle progression from G_1 to S phase)

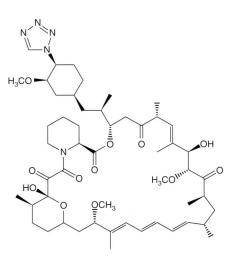

Everolimus
(inhibits mTOR and arrests cell cycle progression from G_1 to S phase)

Zotarolimus
(inhibits mTOR and arrests cell cycle progression from G_1 to S phase)

FIGURE 11-1   Molecular structure of compounds used in drug-eluting stents. mTOR, mammalian target of rapamycin.

in Europe. One example is CD34 antibodies, which have been shown to bind to endothelial progenitor cells circulating in the blood, and these can be used to coat the surface of a stent.[122,146] Titanium–nitride oxide is another coating that has been associated with reduced neointimal hyperplasia compared with stainless steel stents and is currently under investigation.[147]

Products Involving Changes to the Polymer Structure

Prior studies have demonstrated that the polymer drug delivery system may lead to prolonged inflammation in the arterial wall with delayed vessel wall healing; it therefore increases the risk of stent thrombosis.[148,149] In an attempt to minimize this histopathologic response, investigation has concentrated on modifying the polymer used to release the drug. These efforts have ranged from alterations to prior durable polymers to the development of biodegradable polymers that break down over time to stents free of polymers altogether.

STENTS WITH DURABLE POLYMERS

All the FDA-approved DESs currently available utilize durable polymers. Although these polymers have been successful in modulating sustained drug delivery during vascular healing, changes to durable polymers are being designed for existing stents to improve their clinical results. One such example is the Endeavor Resolute stent (Medtronic, Inc., Minneapolis, MN), which is similar to the Endeavor zotarolimus-eluting stent in that it uses a cobalt-chromium stent platform and zotarolimus as an antiproliferative agent. However, the polymer used to release the drug is novel and consists of three different polymers, which together allow for a delayed release of the drug compared with the Endeavor stent.[150,151] The result of this change in polymer has been greater efficacy, as measured by reduced mean late loss in clinical studies,[152] and similar clinical restenosis rates to current stents in randomized trials.[153] The Randomized Comparison of a Zotarolimus-Eluting Stent with an Everolimus-Eluting Stent for Percutaneous Coronary Intervention (RESOLUTE) All-Comers Trial randomized 2300 patients to receive either the Endeavor Resolute stent or the everolimus-eluting stent and found that the two stents had similar rates of major adverse cardiac events (8.2% vs. 8.3%; P for noninferiority < .001).[154]

STENTS WITH BIODEGRADABLE POLYMERS

There may be a benefit to biodegradable polymers that can release a drug over a defined period and be subsequently degraded, thereby limiting the duration of exposure of the vessel wall to the polymer. Several stents using biodegradable polymers are under investigation or are approved outside the United States, and they can be categorized by the drugs they release.

BIOLIMUS A9–BASED STENTS. There are two currently available stents—the Biomatrix stent (Biosensors International, Singapore) and the Nobori stent (Terumo Europe, Leuven, Belgium)—that use biolimus, an analogue of sirolimus. The two stents use the same biodegradable poly-lactic acid (PLA) polymer and the same stainless steel stent platform. The Nobori stent has demonstrated similar rates of angiographic restenosis when compared with the sirolimus-eluting stent,[155] and significantly lower rates of late lumen loss were noted when compared with the paclitaxel-eluting stent[156] in two small trials. In the randomized Limus Eluted from a Durable Versus Erodable Stent Coating (LEADERS) trial of more than 1700 patients, the Biomatrix stent showed lower angiographic restenosis and similar rates of major cardiac adverse events compared with the sirolimus-eluting stent.[157]

MYOLIMUS-BASED STENTS. Myolimus is another analogue of sirolimus that has been investigated as a component of a cobalt-chromium stent coated with a biodegradable PLA polymer. Small, single-arm studies have demonstrated good angiographic results with use of this stent.[158,159]

PACLITAXEL-BASED STENTS. Two stents with biodegradable polymers that use paclitaxel are currently being investigated, the Jactax stent (Boston Scientific) and the Infinnium stent (Sahajanand Medical Technologies, Gujarat, India). Although both stents are loaded with paclitaxel on a stainless steel platform, the

biodegradable polymer differs slightly between the two stents. Initial studies have demonstrated similar low rates of angiographic restenosis with the Jactax stent compared with a group of historic controls receiving the Taxus-Liberte stent.[69,160] The Infinnium stent has been tested in more than 200 subjects in the randomized, controlled Percutaneous Intervention (PAINT) trial, which compared the Infinnium stent and Supralimus stent (Sahajanand Medical Technologies; see below) to a bare-metal stent and demonstrated lower rates of target vessel revascularization at 9 months and less late lumen loss with the Infinnium stent.[161]

EVEROLIMUS-BASED STENTS. The SYNERGY stent (Boston Scientific) is composed of everolimus loaded onto a biodegradable poly-lactic-co-lactic acid (PLGA) polymer on a platinum-chromium platform. The efficacy and safety of this stent compared with a similar stent (everolimus-eluting stent on a platinum-chromium platform with a durable polymer) was demonstrated in the multicenter Evaluation of Cinacalcet Hydrochloride Therapy to Lower Cardiovascular Events (EVOLVE) trial.[162]

SIROLIMUS-BASED STENTS. Each of the three sirolimus-eluting stents with biodegradable polymers currently under investigation uses a different biodegradable polymer. The Excel stent (JW Medical System, Weihai, China) uses a polylactic acid polymer on a stainless steel platform to deliver sirolimus, and recent analyses from registry data involving more than 2000 subjects have demonstrated low rates of major adverse cardiac events (3.1%) over 18 months of follow-up.[163] The Supralimus stent also uses a stainless steel platform; the stent is then coated with a combination of biodegradable polymers loaded with sirolimus. In the small, randomized PAINT trial described above, the Supralimus stent was associated with significantly lower angiographic late lumen loss and lower target vessel revascularization than the bare-metal stent.[161] The Nevo stent (Cordis Corporation) is the third sirolimus-eluting stent with a biodegradable polymer being studied. Unlike the Excel stent and the Supralimus stent, the Nevo stent uses a polylactic-co-glycolic acid polymer loaded into microscopic reservoirs on a cobalt-chromium stent. By using reservoirs of drug-loaded polymer, as opposed to surface coating the stent platform, the exposure of vessel wall to polymer is theoretically decreased. Investigation of the Nevo stent in a 394-patient study demonstrated significantly lower levels of late lumen loss (0.13 vs. 0.36 mm; $P <$ .0001) compared with the Taxus Liberte stent.[164]

POLYMER-FREE STENTS

Removing the polymer as a drug delivery system altogether is another solution to the inflammation caused by the presence of a polymer; however, this is a challenge because the controlled release of the drug without a polymer delivery system is difficult to achieve. Direct-coating, microabrasion, and a microporous coating of the surface of the stents are all methods of drug delivery without polymers that have been investigated. Although initial pilot studies and observational studies have been promising, further RCTs are needed to evaluate the true safety and efficacy of this new technology.

Drug-Coated Balloons

Drug-coated balloons are designed to dilate the stenotic coronary artery while introducing medication to suppress neointimal hyperplasia. With a drug-eluting balloon, both the polymer and stent platform are absent; this completely eliminates the need for any foreign object within the vessel wall that might predispose to thrombus formation, and it could ease reintervention in jailed side branches or restenotic vessels. Furthermore, the absence of a stent would in theory lessen the need for a prolonged course of dual antiplatelet therapy, making it an attractive alternative for patients predisposed to bleeding. That said, the most immediate limitations of this technology are elastic recoil of the vessel and identification of effective carrier molecules for antiproliferative agents.

Most drug-coated balloons currently available in Europe or under investigation use paclitaxel as the antiproliferative agent of choice and have mostly been evaluated for treatment of in-stent restenosis and peripheral arterial stenosis, particularly in anatomic locations where stents are generally avoided because of mechanical stresses, such as the superficial femoral artery. In the Paclitaxel-Coated Balloon Catheter for In-Stent Restenosis (PAC-COCATH ISR) I study, 52 subjects with in-stent restenosis were randomized to treatment either with standard balloon angioplasty or angioplasty with a drug-coated balloon. The drug-coated balloon was associated with significantly lower rates of major adverse cardiac events at 1 year (4% vs. 31%; $P = .01$),[165] a finding that remained at the 2-year follow-up.[166] The drug-coated balloon also performed well compared with restenting using a paclitaxel-eluting stent in a study of 131 patients with in-stent restenosis, with a trend toward lower rates of target lesion revascularization.[167] Although these findings are promising, larger trials with longer term follow-up have yet to be conducted.

Although drug-coated balloons have showed promise in the treatment of in-stent restenosis, studies of drug-coated balloons in de novo coronary lesions have produced mixed results. The drug-coated balloon in combination with a bare-metal stent demonstrated better angiographic results compared with a bare-metal stent alone,[168] but it failed to exhibit superiority over the DES. In the Paclitaxel-Eluting PTCA-Balloon Catheter in Coronary Artery Disease (PEPCAD) III study, 637 patients were randomized to treatment with either a sirolimus-eluting stent or a combination of a bare-metal stent and drug-coated balloon. Not only was in-stent restenosis significantly higher in the drug-coated balloon arm (10% vs. 2.9%; $P < .01$), the rates of MI, stent thrombosis, and total lesion revascularization were also significantly higher at 9 months.[169] Similarly, the 57-subject Paclitaxel-Coated Balloon Versus Drug-Eluting Stent during PCI of Small Coronary Vessels (PICCO-LETO) study demonstrated significantly higher rates of in-stent restenosis (32.1% vs. 10.3%; $P = .043$) and showed an insignificant but highly suggestive trend toward more adverse cardiac events in patients receiving a combination of the drug-coated balloon and bare-metal stent compared with those receiving a paclitaxel-eluting stent (35.7% vs. 13.8%; $P = .54$).[170]

Advances in Revascularization in Specific Conditions

Saphenous Vein Graft Interventions

SVGs are commonly used during coronary artery bypass surgery in the treatment of multivessel coronary artery disease.[171] Unfortunately, such grafts are subject to accelerated atherosclerotic processes and recurrent ischemia as a result of graft degeneration; hence, they are often the target of PCI. In a recent analysis of all PCIs performed in a 5-year period from the National Cardiovascular Data Registry, SVG interventions accounted for 5.7% of all procedures.[172] Because this procedure is becoming more and more common, researchers have begun to study the optimal approach to this type of stenotic lesion.

Several small, randomized trials have compared DESs with bare-metal stents for SVG interventions. The Reduction of Restenosis in Saphenous Vein Grafts with Cypher Sirolimus-Eluting Stent (RRISC) study evaluated 75 patients, randomized to receive either a bare-metal stent or sirolimus-eluting stent for treatment of an SVG stenosis. Although in-stent restenosis was reduced at 6 months with use of the sirolimus-eluting stent,[173] long-term follow-up revealed higher rates of mortality (29% vs. 0%; $P < .001$) with the sirolimus-eluting stent at a median follow-up of 32 months and an absence of any benefit with regard to long-term target vessel revascularization rates (34% vs. 38%; $P = .74$).[174] These results were surprising given the multitude of retrospective data that have suggested DESs are safe and efficacious in SVG interventions.[175-179] A randomized study of 610 patients, the recent publication of which compared drug-eluting with bare-metal stents for SVG interventions and showed a reduction in the composite of death, MI, and target lesion revascularization associated with DESs at 1 year, with a similar rate of stent thrombosis (1%) in both treatment arms.[180] Taken together,

these results suggest that DESs should be the stent of choice for SVG interventions.

Because SVGs often harbor a sizable amount of atherosclerotic debris secondary to the large nature of the vessel itself, it follows that interventions for a lesion within an SVG carry a high risk of distal embolization and resulting myocardial damage. Early studies failed to show a benefit of glycoprotein (GP) IIb/IIIa inhibitors in preventing embolic events during SVG interventions,[181,182] so recent research has turned to the development of embolic protection devices for use during such interventions.

Three types of embolic protection devices are currently available. *Distal occlusion devices* consist of a balloon mounted on a wire that is passed beyond the lesion and inflated to occlude flow during lesion treatment, such that any embolic debris is trapped and can be aspirated prior to reperfusion of the coronary bed. The Saphenous Vein Graft Angioplasty Free of Emboli Randomized (SAFER) trial followed 801 patients who underwent SVG interventions either with a conventional guidewire or with the GuardWire distal occlusion device (Medtronic). At 30-day follow-up, a significant reduction was observed in major adverse cardiac event rates in patients treated with the GuardWire distal occlusion device (9.6% vs. 16.5%; $P = .004$).[183]

Distal embolic filter devices capture embolized debris while allowing perfusion of the target vessel. Several randomized trials have compared distal embolic filter devices (FilterWire EF, EZ [Boston Scientific], Interceptor PLUS [Medtronic]), and all have demonstrated noninferiority to the distal occlusion device in regard to major adverse cardiac events within 30 days of SVG interventions.[184-186]

Despite good results with distal embolic protection devices, embolization may still occur. *Proximally placed occlusion devices* have been developed to overcome some of the limitations of distally placed devices. Proximal devices consist of a guide catheter with a balloon placed proximal to the stenosis through which balloons, wires, and stents may be delivered, while antegrade flow is occluded. Embolic debris is aspirated after the intervention is complete, and antegrade flow is restored. This type of device may offer greater protection to a lesion that is so distal within an SVG that the distal device cannot be placed, or to a lesion that is located in a graft with a Y anastomosis, in which both limbs cannot be protected with a single distal device, or when a lesion is so narrow that it must be predilated before it can be crossed with a larger device. The Proximal Protection During Saphenous Vein Graft Intervention Using the Proxis Embolic Protection System (PROXIMAL) trial compared the Proxis proximal occlusion device (St. Jude Medical, St. Paul, MN) with both a distal occlusion and distal embolic device and found that the proximal occlusion device was noninferior to the distal embolic protection devices in the prevention of 30-day major adverse cardiac events.[187] Currently, embolic protection with either distal or proximal devices has become the standard of care when treating an SVG lesion.

Chronic Total Occlusion Intervention

Chronic total occlusions (CTOs) are a common angiographic finding, accounting for 15% to 30% of patients who undergo cardiac catheterization.[188] Nevertheless, clinical decision making regarding medications for revascularization, procedural technique in treating these lesions, or even whether a CTO should be opened may be challenging issues.

Observational studies have suggested that successful revascularization of a CTO is associated with reduced long-term mortality rates[189-192] and improvement in left ventricular (LV) function.[193,194] Because no randomized trials have been conducted, it is not clear whether these benefits are related to revascularization per se or that less complex cases are more likely to undergo successful procedures. Certain characteristics of CTO have been associated with a lower likelihood of success, including ostial or bifurcation lesions, lesions in difficult locations, an occlusive segment, significant calcification, or long lesions.[195] Furthermore, patients with no clinical symptoms or evidence of nonviable myocardium at the site of the CTO may not derive much benefit from revascularization of such an occlusion. Thus, numerous determinants need to be considered when deciding whether to attempt revascularization of a CTO.

Overall, the acute procedure success rate for CTO is 50% to 60%, and improvements in technology and technique have improved the feasibility of CTO treatment. The primary technical challenge during PCI of a total occlusion is the crossing of the occlusion with a wire. Several new wires have been specifically designed for crossing chronic occlusions, characterized by variable tip stiffness and increased hydrophilic characteristics. In addition, microcatheters with low profiles and hydrophilic coatings have been developed to aid in crossing the lesion. When crossing is not feasible from an antegrade approach, retrograde crossing of the lesion via collaterals is an alternative approach. After successful crossing of the lesion with the wire and recanalization, DES placement is preferred over bare-metal stents to reduce the restenosis rate of these complex, long lesions. The Primary Stenting of Totally Occluded Native Coronary Arteries (PRISON) II study randomized 200 patients with CTOs to receive either a sirolimus-eluting stent or a bare-metal stent and found that the sirolimus-eluting stent significantly reduced the rates of binary in-stent restenosis at 6 months (7% vs. 36%; $P < .001$),[196] which translated into significantly lower rates of target lesion revascularization at 3 years (7% vs. 27%;;$P < .001$).[197] These findings of lower rates of target lesion revascularization with DES placement in CTOs have been consistently replicated in other RCTs, observational studies, and meta-analyses.[191,198-201]

Bifurcation Lesion Treatment

Coronary bifurcation lesions are also relatively common and account for 15% to 20% of PCIs.[202] Although revascularization for bifurcation disease has historically been associated with lower acute success rates and higher restenosis and thrombosis rates than nonbifurcation lesions, the use of DESs and specific procedural techniques have improved success rates significantly.[203] First, several strategies are possible regarding where to place the stent or stents. One option is stenting the main branch of the diseased bifurcation but stenting the side branch only if significant stenosis remains in the side branch as determined by angiography, intravascular ultrasound, or fractional flow reserve measurements; this is called the *provisional approach*. Alternatively, a planned *two-stent approach* can be taken in which both the main vessel and the side branch are stented using a variety of catheterization techniques. Various techniques are possible for the two-stent approach, depending on the anatomic geometry of the bifurcation (e.g., *T-stenting, culotte, crush, kissing,* or *stenting*; Figure 11-2). Although certain anatomic characteristics may require a two-stent approach, such as larger diseased side branches or a large area of at-risk myocardium, several small randomized trials have demonstrated no benefit to routinely treating both branches with stents.[202,204-206] Furthermore, a recent meta-analysis involving 1553 patients suggested that a provisional strategy may be associated with a lower risk of MI (RR, 0.53; 95% CI, 0.37 to 0.78; $P = .001$).[207]

Whether a provisional strategy or two-stent approach is planned, neither approach is ideally suited to all types of bifurcations; lesion coverage therefore may be problematic. Several dedicated bifurcation stents (i.e., a single stent that will cover both the main vessel and the side branch) are being designed to maintain access to provide coverage for the entire lesion.[208-214] Although first-in-human studies and registries evaluating these new devices are promising, further studies are needed to determine whether they will improve angiographic and clinical outcomes in patients with coronary bifurcation lesions.

Advances in Catheterization Techniques

Transradial Access

Although transradial access during cardiac catheterization was initially described in the late 1940s,[215] lack of appropriate

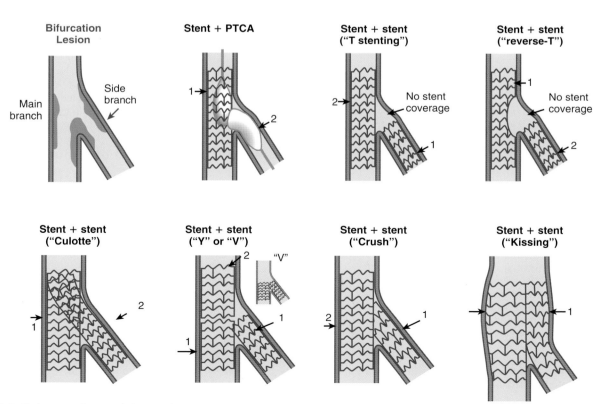

FIGURE 11-2 Techniques of treating bifurcation lesions. PTCA, percutaneous transluminal coronary angioplasty.

equipment hindered the technique from becoming widely used until recently. Recently, guide catheters specifically designed for a radial approach, hydrophilic sheaths, and lower profile stents that have allowed PCI to be performed via smaller catheters (5 or 6 Fr) have facilitated radial artery access and PCI. Furthermore, studies suggesting that the transradial approach may reduce bleeding and vascular complications have led to the radial artery becoming the access site of choice at many catheterization laboratories around the world.

When evaluating the success of transradial access, it is necessary to compare both procedural and clinical outcomes with the more commonly used transfemoral approach. Among operators with much experience in radial access, no significant difference was found in procedural success rates between the radial and femoral approach,[216] and as operator volume of transradial cases increases, rates of access failure and overall procedure time decrease significantly.[217] The largest randomized study to date to evaluate access techniques during PCI is the recently published Radial Versus Femoral Access for Coronary Intervention (RIVAL) trial, which randomized 3507 subjects undergoing PCI to either radial or femoral access. Researchers found that radial access was associated with a significantly lower rate of vascular access complications, and no difference was noted in a composite outcome of death, MI, stroke, or bleeding.[218] Although some large observational studies have shown reduced mortality associated with prevention of bleeding,[231,234,235] this benefit was not manifested in the RIVAL trial except within the subgroup of patients presenting with acute MI.[218]

Mechanical Support for High-Risk Percutaneous Coronary Intervention

Mechanical support devices during PCI are commonly used in two clinical scenarios: during intervention on complex coronary lesions, such as left main coronary artery interventions or multivessel interventions on a patient with compromised LV function, and in the setting of acute MI complicated by cardiogenic shock. The goal of a mechanical support device is to prevent or treat hemodynamic instability by unloading the left ventricle (LV) and decreasing myocardial oxygen consumption. Whereas the intra-aortic balloon pump (IABP) is the most commonly used mechanical support device, two new mechanical support devices, the TandemHeart (CardiacAssist, Inc, Pittsburgh, PA) and the Impella LP2.5 device (Texas Heart Institute, Houston, TX), are now frequently used.

Use of the IABP in patients with MI complicated by cardiogenic shock was first described in 1968.[219] Since then, several retrospective studies have suggested that IABP use in this class of patients is associated with significant reduction in mortality, particularly in patients treated with thrombolytics.[220-222] These data have resulted in a class I indication for IABP insertion in cardiogenic shock patients awaiting revascularization in the absence of improvement with pharmacologic therapies.[223]

The results for prophylactic IABP use during high-risk complex percutaneous interventions have been slightly less clear. Although initial observational studies supported the use of prophylactic IABPs,[224-226] a recent RCT has called this conclusion into question. The Balloon Pump Assisted Coronary Intervention Study (BCIS) 1 trial randomized 301 patients with depressed LV function and complex and extensive coronary disease to receive either an elective IABP prior to catheterization or to receive an IABP only if needed during the procedure. No significant difference was reported in major adverse cardiac events at discharge between the two groups (15.2% vs. 16%; $P = .85$). Furthermore, the Counterpulsation Reduces Infarct Size Pre-PCI for Acute MI (CRISP-AMI) study found that routine use of IABPs in patients who come to medical attention with anterior STEMIs did not result in a significant difference in mean infarct size as measured by cardiac magnetic resonance imaging (MRI; 42.1% with IABPs vs. 37.5%; $P = .07$).[227]

In contrast to the IABP, which acts to reduce afterload and improve diastolic coronary perfusion through counterpulsation, the TandemHeart (Cardiac Assist, Pittsburgh, PA) and the Impella LP2.5 (Abiomed, Danvers, MA) devices both act as percutaneous LV assist devices. Using the femoral vein and a transseptal puncture, the TandemHeart device is inserted into the left atrium, where it acts to aspirate oxygenated blood from the left atrium into an external, continuous-flow blood pump that subsequently delivers the blood back to the arterial system via the femoral arterial system. It is contraindicated in patients with ventricular septal defects because of the risk of hypoxemia from shunting; those with severe aortic regurgitation because of poor subendocardial perfusion; and those with severe peripheral disease because of the large-bore sheaths needed for device use. In small studies, the TandemHeart device was shown to be more effective than the IABP in improving cardiac index and other hemodynamic measures, such as pulmonary capillary wedge pressure or mean arterial pressure; however, no significant differences were observed in 30-day mortality.[228,229] Furthermore, one study reported significantly increased rates of complications, such as limb ischemia and bleeding, in patients who received the TandemHeart device.[228]

The Impella LP2.5 is an axial-flow pump that is placed across the aortic valve into the LV via the femoral artery and subsequently acts to draw blood from the LV and pump the blood into the ascending aorta, thereby reducing the work of the LV. Although required access is smaller than for the TandemHeart catheter, the output from the device is also less. The Impella LP2.5 device is contraindicated in patients with severe peripheral disease—again, because large-bore sheaths are needed to place the device—and in those with moderate to severe aortic stenosis or insufficiency; thrombus within the LV, which risks thrombus being propelled into the branch aortic vessels; and any significant aortic disease, such as aneurysm or dissection. The Efficacy Study of LV Assist Device to Treat Patients with Cardiogenic Shock (ISAR-SHOCK) trial studied 26 patients with MI complicated by cardiogenic shock and found that the Impella LP2.5 device resulted in a higher degree of increase in the cardiac index when compared with the IABP (0.49 L/min/m^2 vs. 0.11 L/min/m^2; $P = .02$), although no differences in mortality or ejection fraction at 30 days were found between the two groups.[230] Similarly, the Impella LP 2.5 device has been shown to be safe for use during elective high-risk PCI in a cohort of 20 patients.[231] The Prospective, Multi-Center, Randomized Controlled Trial of the IMPELLA RECOVER LP 2.5 System Versus the Intra-Aortic Balloon Pump (IABP) in Patients Undergoing Non Emergent High Risk PCI (PROTECT II), which had planned to randomize 654 patients to either IABP or Impella device for elective high-risk PCI, was recently halted when interim analyses determined that the study would not reach its prespecified endpoints.

Intravascular Assessment of Lesion Severity

Angiographic assessment of the severity of a coronary lesion plays a major role in the decision regarding whether to intervene in a lesion, particularly in the setting of stable angina. Coronary angiography can lead to both overestimation and underestimation of a coronary artery's true diameter.[232] Furthermore, in the presence of multiple coronary lesions, it can also be difficult to know which lesion, or lesions, are primarily responsible for ischemic symptoms.[233] Finally, angiography alone cannot demonstrate the physiologic significant of a stenosis. Hence, interventional cardiologists have turned to other techniques, including intravascular ultrasound and fractional flow reserve measurements, with which to assess lesion severity.

Intravascular ultrasound (IVUS) catheters use ultrasound waves to visualize the components of an arterial wall—the *intima, media,* and *adventitia*—and the vessel lumen, which can subsequently be measured along different points of the vessel to evaluate for any luminal stenosis. Because IVUS cannot provide a physiologic measurement of ischemia, it is used less for assessment of intermediate coronary lesions and more for guidance during planned interventions, such as guiding stent implantation and balloon angioplasty[234,235] or in diagnosing the causes of in-stent restenosis or stent thrombosis.[236] Another form of intravascular imaging is optical coherence tomography (OCT), which was approved for use in the United States in 2010. OCT provides greater axial resolution than IVUS and hence may be helpful for more refined imaging of stent struts and their interaction with plaque and vessel borders.[237]

Many lesions on angiography fall within an intermediate range, where their correlation with ischemia may be unclear. Fractional flow reserve (FFR) can provide a measurement of the hemodynamic significance of an angiographic lesion that appears intermediate. The FFR represents the ratio of flow in a stenotic lesion to the theoretical flow in the same vessel if there were no stenosis, and it is measured as a ratio of simultaneous mean pressures during intravenous adenosine infusion compared distal to the lesion and the aorta. FFR values of less than 0.75 to 0.8 have been associated with coronary ischemia.[238-240] In the Fractional Flow Reserve Versus Angiography in Multivessel Evaluation (FAME) trial, 1005 patients with multivessel coronary disease were randomized to receive PCI guided by angiography alone or by the combination of FFR measurements and angiography. In the FFR-guided arm, PCI was reserved for lesions with FFR below 0.80. At 1-year follow-up, patients receiving FFR-guided interventions had a significantly lower rate of the primary endpoint—a combination of death, MI, and repeat revascularization[241]—a finding confirmed at the 2-year follow-up.[242] With these rather definitive results, it follows that FFR should gain wider use in the assessment of lesion severity and for a more targeted approach to the treatment of multivessel coronary artery disease.

Advances in Surgical Coronary Revascularization

Many recent advances in surgical coronary revascularization have come in the form of newer, less invasive approaches, including off-pump CABG and smaller access surgeries. At the same time, additional information has been found in the area of arterial conduits as alternatives to the saphenous vein for bypass grafting. Finally, the use of hybrid revascularization procedures that combine the approaches of interventional cardiology and cardiac surgery has begun to be investigated. This section will describe the advancements in both knowledge and technique that have been made in these areas.

Minimally Invasive Surgical Coronary Revascularization

Many advances in surgical coronary revascularization in the past decade have come in the form of modifications to conventional CABG and fall under the broad rubric of minimally invasive coronary revascularization. When used in the context of cardiac surgery, the term *minimally invasive* carries more possible meanings than in other surgical specialties. In contrast to other surgical disciplines, in which the degree of invasiveness of a procedure is primarily defined by the size of access incisions, in cardiac surgery at least two levels of "invasion" can be altered. The trauma of physical access can be changed by the use of smaller incisions or incisions that involve less (or no) sternal splitting. Alternatively, the physiologic invasiveness can be altered by performing procedures off-pump, that is, without the use of cardiopulmonary bypass (CPB) and cardioplegic arrest. This at least theoretically modifies the degree of physiologic perturbation produced in performing the intervention.

The face of surgical coronary revascularization has been changed by innovations in both of these areas, and continued change is expected, as technological advances carry on in coming times. This section of the chapter describes the continuum of minimally invasive surgical (MIS) options and the recent data associated with each approach.

OFF-PUMP CORONARY ARTERY BYPASS GRAFTING

Surgical coronary revascularization was in fact originally described without the use of CPB in the 1960s,[243,245] but its use in surgical coronary revascularization took hold and became the standard of care. The use of CPB with myocardial protection provided a motionless, bloodless surgical field and created more optimal conditions for the construction of hand-sewn coronary anastomoses. Thus for decades the gold standard surgical approach to coronary revascularization was bypass grafting under cardioplegic arrest and CPB (on-pump coronary artery bypass [ONCAB]) via median sternotomy.[243]

During ONCAB, the aorta and venous components, typically the superior and inferior vena cava or right atrium, are cannulated for connection to an extracorporeal pump. Venous blood is drained into the heart-lung machine via polyvinyl chloride (PVC) tubing and is pumped through an oxygenator and into the systemic arterial tree. The ascending aorta is clamped, and the heart is arrested with cardioplegic solution. The pump maintains perfusion to the body while the heart is arrested (Figure 11-3).[246]

Because the coronary artery bypass procedure takes place on the surface of the heart and does not involve opening the heart, no theoretical reason demands that this surgery must take place on an arrested heart. The development of stabilizers that fix the portion of the epicardium where the anastomosis is being created and specialized retractors made in the late 1990s changed the landscape of this procedure and made coronary artery revascularization without extracorporeal support (off-pump coronary bypass surgery [OPCAB]) technically feasible.[243] OPCAB can be performed using a variety of surgical access approaches, ranging from traditional full median sternotomy to a robotic, totally endoscopic approach. The full range of incisions and approaches will be described below.

In its simplest incarnation, a full median sternotomy is used for the access to perform OPCAB. During the bypass procedure, the heart is maintained in its usual state of beating and providing systemic perfusion. Specialized retractors and stabilizing devices are used to expose the coronary arteries, which are individually occluded while conventional hand-sewn anastomoses are created (Figure 11-4).

In an OPCAB, the positioning of the heart carries with it the hazards of partial occlusion of venous inflow, as the angles of the heart relative to the vena cavae are altered to expose the lateral and inferior walls of the heart. The anesthesia team plays an active and critical role in maintaining hemodynamic stability during these maneuvers.[243] Access to and stabilization of the coronary arteries in this environment are the critical factors that determine the degree of difficulty of the procedure and perhaps decide the technical outcome (i.e., the patency of the anastomoses).[246]

As mentioned above, performing coronary bypass surgery without CPB represents an attempt to make the procedure less physiologically invasive—that is, to make it less physiologically disruptive. The use of CPB and cardioplegic arrest has a wide range of effects and is associated with many potential complications, although the great majority of patients tolerate its use without clinically apparent adverse effects.[247] The use of CPB is associated with derangements in the inflammatory and coagulation cascades; generation and delivery of microemboli; variations in regional organ perfusion, hemodilution, and hypothermia; and perturbations of acid-base homeostasis. These derangements result, at least in part, from the exposure of the patient's full blood volume to the nonendothelial surfaces of the pump and components within the surgical field. With exposure to the foreign surfaces of the pump, an intense systemic inflammatory reaction can follow, which may result in neurologic, renal, or pulmonary dysfunction.[247]

The deleterious effects of CPB have been extensively investigated over the past three decades, but limited evidence still suggests that OPCAB can offer significant advantages with respect to the already low morbidity and mortality associated with ONCAB.[248] The first sizable series of OPCAB was reported by Buffolo in 1989[248];

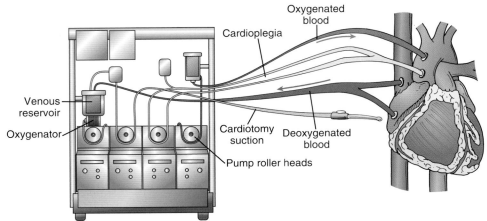

FIGURE 11-3 During cardiopulmonary bypass, the aorta and venous supply, here the superior and inferior venae cavae, are cannulated for connection to an extracorporeal pump. Venous blood, as well as blood from the field captured by the cardiotomy suction, is drained into the venous reservoir of the heart-lung machine via polyvinylchloride tubing, passed through an oxygenator, and pumped into the systemic arterial tree. The ascending aorta is clamped, and the heart is arrested with cardioplegic solution administered by the perfusionist using the pump. The pump maintains perfusion to the body while the heart is arrested.

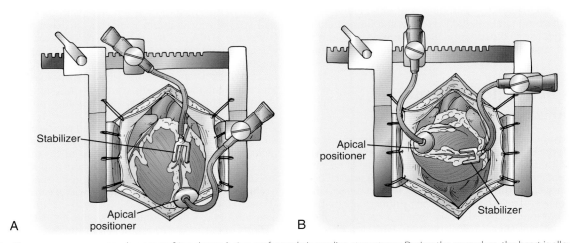

FIGURE 11-4 On-pump coronary artery bypass grafting shown being performed via median sternotomy. During the procedure, the heart is allowed to beat and continue in its usual state of function. An apical positioning device is used to position the heart for optimal exposure of the target vessel, and a stabilizing device is used to stabilize this target coronary artery. **A,** Typical positioning is shown for creation of a left anterior descending artery bypass. **B,** Positioning for obtuse marginal bypass.

since then, many studies comparing OPCAB with ONCAB have been conducted, with both prospective and retrospective designs, and multiple meta-analyses have been performed to try to address the superiority of one technique over the other.

In the early 2000s, several RCTs documented the safety and efficacy of OPCAB.[247] These trials were relatively small and did not show a mortality benefit to the technique, although many of the trials did demonstrate lower blood transfusion rates, decreased mechanical ventilator times, and shorter lengths of stay in the hospital and intensive care unit (ICU).[247] That said, these benefits were not without some cost. The early RCTs suggested no difference in early or long-term graft patency in comparing ONCAB and OPCAB, but questions regarding the completeness of revascularization in OPCAB have been raised.[247] A recent meta-analysis was performed, considering all of the RCT data before 2007, and the authors concluded that the data showed that use of OPCAB reduced the risk of postoperative atrial fibrillation but provided no significant benefit in measures such as death, MI, stroke, and renewed coronary revascularization.[249]

Since that meta-analysis, the largest RCT to be conducted on this question is the Veterans Affairs Randomized On/Off Bypass (ROOBY) trial. In this trial, 2203 patients scheduled for urgent or elective CABG were assigned to either OPCAB or ONCAB with follow-up for death or complications at 30 days and 1 year.[250] At 30 days, no significant differences were found between OPCAB and ONCAB for death (1.6% vs. 1.2% for OPCAB vs. ONCAB, respectively; $P = .47$) or for the composite of death, repeat revascularization, or MI (7.0% vs. 5.6%, respectively; $P = .19$). Similarly, no differences were found for other clinically important outcomes such as stroke, cardiac arrest, renal failure requiring dialysis, need for reintervention, and need for new mechanical support. At 1 year, all-cause death was not significantly different between groups (4.1% vs. 2.9% for OPCAB vs. ONCAB, respectively; $P = .15$); however, death from cardiac causes was significantly increased for OPCAB versus ONCAB at 1 year (2.7% vs. 1.3%; $P = .01$). Furthermore, a significant increase was observed in the 1-year primary composite outcome of death, repeat revascularization, or MI for the OPCAB group (9.9% vs. 7.4%; $P = .04$). Neuropsychologic outcomes were similar between groups at 1-year follow-up, but graft patency was reduced in the OPCAB group, although assessment of patency was incomplete; only one subgroup was available for imaging assessment during the study.

The ROOBY trial is not without limitations. In particular, a higher than usual conversion rate (12.4% in ROOBY vs. 8% in meta-analyses)[251] from OPCAB to ONCAB was noted in the trial, and this issue has been raised as a cause for concern regarding the level of experience of the practitioners involved,[252] with 55% of OPCABs performed by residents in the ROOBY trial. This high crossover rate may also have contributed to the rates of death and complications in the OPCAB arm of the ROOBY trial, because crossovers are (properly) analyzed by intention to treat in the OPCAB group—that is, they were analyzed in the group to which they were randomized, even though they did not receive OPCAB and instead underwent ONCAB by unplanned conversion. Furthermore, conversion to ONCAB surgery has been shown to increase the risk of death and serious complications for patients who were initially slated to undergo OPCAB.[251] Another important consideration when interpreting the ROOBY trial in the context of the totality of available evidence relates to the fact that this trial included only male patients and excluded high-risk patients. With observational data suggesting that OPCAB may be particularly beneficial for women, the elderly, and those with severe coexisting illnesses,[253] the ROOBY trial may have excluded the patients for whom the most benefit may have been expected.

The role of OPCAB in coronary revascularization remains a controversial and an as yet unanswered important question in cardiac surgery, and our understanding of this procedure's place in cardiac revascularization will undoubtedly continue to evolve over time. New trials are needed to more fully delineate the benefits of on- and off-pump coronary revascularization.

SMALL-ACCESS CORONARY REVASCULARIZATION

The remainder of this section describes surgical revascularization procedures using access incisions other than conventional median sternotomy, with or without the use of CPB (Table 11-6). The degree of revascularization possible with each intervention, whether single or multiple vessel, is discussed, as is some of the clinical literature available on the outcomes associated with these approaches.

Minimally Invasive Direct Coronary Artery Bypass

The term *minimally invasive direct coronary bypass* (MIDCAB), also referred to as *single-vessel small thoracotomy direct-vision bypass grafting* (SVST), is a procedure in which a limited, anterior, medially placed thoracotomy incision is used for both direct-vision left internal mammary artery (LIMA) harvest and for creation of an anastomosis of the LIMA to a coronary artery.[254] The procedure is performed off-pump and requires the use of a stabilizer, either placed directly through the operative incision or placed via a separate endoscopic port incision. To allow for takedown of the internal mammary artery (IMA) through this incision, a specialized chest wall retractor is needed, as is rib disarticulation or removal of cartilage (Figure 11-5). Furthermore, because of the difficulty of gaining access to the lateral and posterior surfaces of the beating heart during this procedure, coronary revascularization using MIDCAB is limited to the bypass of the left anterior descending artery (LAD) or its diagonal branches on the anterior surface of the heart.

The MIDCAB procedure was reintroduced in the mid-1990s, having originally been described in 1965 by Kolessov. The procedure was rapidly adopted at many U.S. and European centers after its reintroduction, and many early series demonstrated decreased lengths of stay compared with conventional CABG, decreased utilization of resources, earlier return to full activity, reduced transfusion requirement, and excellent graft patency.[255] When compared with a single-vessel OPCAB, data are more limited; however, small studies have suggested that durations of mechanical ventilation and total hospital stay were decreased with use of MIDCAB.[256] For instance, in one recent European report, Holzhey and colleagues reported their experience with 1347 MIDCABs.[257] This Leipzig group reported a 1.7% rate of conversion to sternotomy, 0.8% postoperative mortality rate, and 0.4% perioperative stroke rate. Routine postoperative angiograms showed 95.6% early graft patency, with a

TABLE 11-6 Small-Access Surgical Coronary Revascularization

PROCEDURE	DESCRIPTION	VESSELS BYPASSED	PUMP USE	NUMBER IN LITERATURE
LAST, MIDCAB, SVST	A limited anterior, medially placed thoracotomy incision is used for both direct-vision IMA harvest and creation of an anastomosis of the IMA to coronary artery in an off-pump fashion.	Single-vessel (LIMA-LAD or LIMA-diagonal) more often than multivessel (bilateral) procedures	Off pump	~5000[300]
Endo-ACAB; PACAB; robot-assisted, thoracoscopic, or video-assisted MIDCAB	The IMA is harvested thoracoscopically or robotically via small-access port incisions with direct-vision anastomosis creation through a minithoracotomy with minimal rib spreading.	Single-vessel (LIMA-LAD or LIMA-diagonal) more often than multivessel (bilateral) procedures	Off pump more often than on pump	~1000[301,302]
ALT-CAB, MVST	A larger left thoracotomy incision is used to harvest the LIMA and RIMA under direct vision with greater access to the heart, allowing all territories to be bypassed under direct vision through a single incision.	All territories	Off pump more often than on pump	<1000[262,303]
MICS CABG	A more laterally placed thoracotomy than a traditional MIDCAB uses a specialized pivoting retractor for IMA takedown through the thoracotomy with two port-site incisions for epicardial stabilizer and apical positioner. Multivessel OPCAB is performed through small incisions.	All territories	Off pump	~500[261]
AH-TECAB, BH-TECAB, TECAB	The IMA is harvested robotically with intracorporeal robotic anastomosis creation.	Anterior territories more often than multivessel procedures	On pump more often than off pump	<500[272,301]

AH, arrested heart; ALT-CAB, anterolateral thoracotomy coronary artery bypass; BH, beating heart; Endo-ACAB, endoscopic atraumatic coronary artery bypass; IMA, internal mammary artery; LAST, left anterior small thoracotomy direct-vision bypass grafting; LAD, left anterior descending artery; LIMA, left internal mammary artery; MICS CABG, minimally invasive coronary artery bypass grafting; MIDCAB, minimally invasive direct coronary bypass; MVST, multivessel small thoracotomy direct-vision bypass grafting; OPCAB, off-pump coronary artery bypass; PACAB, port access coronary artery bypass; RIMA, right internal mammary artery; SVST, single-vessel small thoracotomy direct-vision bypass grafting; TECAB, totally endoscopic coronary artery bypass.

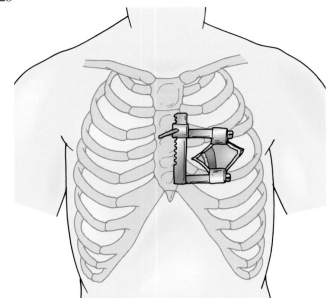

FIGURE 11-5 Small thoracotomy coronary artery bypass grafting. A limited anterior, medially placed thoracotomy incision is used for both direct-vision left internal mammary artery (LIMA) harvest and creation of an anastomosis of the LIMA to an anterior or anterolateral coronary artery. Because of the difficulty in gaining access to the lateral and posterior surfaces of the beating heart during this procedure, coronary revascularization is limited to the bypass of the left anterior descending artery or its diagonal branches on the anterior surface of the heart. To allow for takedown of the internal mammary artery through this incision, rib disarticulation or removal of cartilage is required along with a specialized chest-wall retractor.

short-term target vessel reintervention rate of 4.1%. Angiograms (n = 350) obtained at the 6-month interval demonstrated a 94.3% graft patency. MIDCAB procedures have also been used successfully for reoperations,[258] with some evidence of decreased operative mortality rates in these high-risk patients with this approach to coronary revascularization.

The main downside of the MIDCAB procedure is that the extensive chest wall retraction involved in LIMA harvest can result in challenging early postoperative pain control.[254] Even with a smaller incision, the difficulties with postoperative pain have contributed to the decrease in popularity of this procedure after its original introduction. Nevertheless, several centers skilled in this approach continue to perform it in large numbers and report excellent results.

Thoracoscopic Minimally Invasive Direct Coronary Bypass

In an effort to avoid the degree of chest retraction typically involved in the standard MIDCAB procedure, other approaches to LIMA takedown have been developed. In the video-assisted MIDCAB approach, the LIMA is harvested thoracoscopically via small access-port incisions. The LIMA-LAD anastomosis is created through a minithoracotomy with minimal rib spreading. It should be noted that thoracoscopic LIMA takedown requires chest cavity insufflation, and the patient's ability to tolerate diminished ventilation intraoperatively should be assessed preoperatively.[254]

The largest series of thoracoscopic MIDCAB was reported by Vassiliades and colleagues in 2007, who termed this approach *endoscopic atraumatic coronary artery bypass* (endo-ACAB). This group reported a 3.6% conversion rate to sternotomy or thoracotomy, a 1% postoperative mortality rate (compared with the STS National Database–predicted 30-day mortality rate of 2.7%), and a 0.3% stroke rate. Furthermore, these authors reported a 95% to 98.5% LIMA-LAD anastomosis patency rate with a mean follow-up of 18 months. The mean length of stay in the ICU was 11.2 ± 9.9 hours, and the mean hospital stay was 2.4 ± 1.3 days.[259]

Likely owing to the advanced thoracoscopic skills necessary for the LIMA takedown in this approach, with an estimated 25- to 50-case learning curve required for mastery of the technique, the thoracoscopic MIDCAB has not achieved widespread adoption at this time. Robot-assisted MIDCAB represents an alternative to thoracoscopic MIDCAB and will be discussed in conjunction with other robotic revascularization techniques below.

Multivessel Minimally Invasive Procedures

As described above, MIDCABs are generally restricted to the performance of a single LIMA-LAD or LIMA diagonal bypass. The benefits of this method can be expanded to patients with multivessel disease by combining MIDCAB with PCI for lesions on the posterior and lateral surfaces of the heart in a hybrid approach (discussed below). However, this hybrid method can be used only when such lesions are amenable to PCI, which has led some to create other minimally invasive alternatives for patients with multivessel disease.

The use of bilateral MIDCABs involving bilateral anterior (medially placed) minithoracotomies in conjunction with bilateral direct-vision IMA harvest and radial artery conduits has been reported[260] but has not been evaluated in large studies. The use of bilateral thoracoscopic IMA harvesting followed by right anterior thoracotomy for the bypass of right coronary artery and LAD territories has also been described. It should be noted, however, that in using this technique, bilateral thoracotomies were required to reach posterolateral vessels, and it is not possible for the posterior interventricular branch to be bypassed.[261]

Techniques involving a single thoracotomy for multivessel disease have also been reported. One procedure, termed the *anterolateral thoracotomy–coronary artery bypass* (ALT-CAB), uses a larger left thoracotomy. With this incision, both the LIMA and RIMA can be harvested under direct vision, and all territories of the heart can be bypassed. In addition, central cannulation is possible because of the greater exposure afforded by the larger incision. The procedure has not achieved widespread adoption but has been used in selected centers with acceptable results. In a series of 255 patients undergoing this procedure, complete revascularization was achieved in all patients, and there were no conversions to CPB. The mortality and stroke rate in this series was 1.2% and 0.8%, respectively, and 65.1% of patients were discharged within 48 hours of ALT-CAB.[262]

The newest minimally invasive option for multivessel disease was introduced in 2005 and is called *minimally invasive coronary artery bypass grafting* (MICS CABG)[261] or *multivessel small thoracotomy* (MVST).[263] This approach uses a more laterally placed thoracotomy than a traditional MIDCAB. A specialized pivoting retractor allows for LIMA takedown through the thoracotomy, and two port-site incisions allow for the use of an epicardial stabilizer and an apical positioner (Figure 11-6). Using the combination of the position of the access incision, the epicardial stabilizer, and the apical positioner, all territories of the heart can be bypassed with this technique. The procedure is performed off-pump and does not require the use of thoracoscopic or robotic equipment; it essentially amounts to a multivessel OPCAB performed through small incisions.

A dual-center series of 450 patients over 3.5 years was recently reported for this procedure with encouraging results. The authors reported a 1.3% mortality rate and a 0.4% stroke rate. Complete revascularization was reported in 95% of patients undergoing this technique. No angiographic evidence with respect to graft patency was reported; however, at 19-month mean follow-up, only 3% of patients required PCI. A 3.8% conversion to sternotomy was reported, and conversion to on-pump procedure (via peripheral cannulation) was reported in 7.6%. It is interesting to note that the report included the entire experience of the institutions with the procedure, including their initial experiences. The authors suggest that this implies that this procedure may be implemented and developed without a significant learning curve.

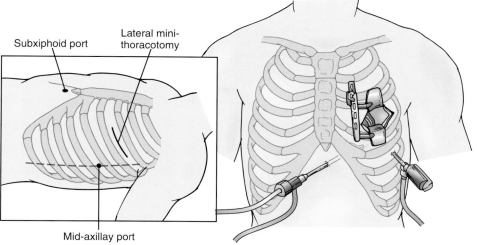

FIGURE 11-6 The minimally invasive coronary artery bypass grafting approach uses a more laterally placed thoracotomy than a traditional minimally invasive direct coronary artery bypass. A specialized pivoting retractor can be used that allows for left internal mammary artery takedown through the thoracotomy (not shown), and two port incisions allow an epicardial stabilizer and an apical positioner. Between the position of the access incision, the epicardial stabilizer, and the apical positioner, all territories of the heart can be bypassed using this technique.

Proponents of this procedure assert that it has a greater availability for all cardiothoracic surgeons because the procedure does not require the costly infrastructure and disposable materials associated with robotic or thoracoscopic procedures.[263] Additional data are needed to evaluate this novel procedure more fully, but it appears to have potential as a more widely adoptable, minimally invasive surgical option for patients with multivessel disease.

Robotically Assisted Revascularization

Robotic surgical systems are telemanipulators in which a surgeon controls microinstruments remotely from a console. The most widely used system is the da Vinci S (Intuitive Surgical, Mountain View, CA). The system conveys high-definition three-dimensional imaging to the surgeon at the console, and sensors register the surgeon's finger and wrist movements, which are translated (tremor free) into the motion of the microinstruments in the field.

The da Vinci robot was approved for cardiac surgery in 2002, and at present about 1700 robotic cardiac operations have been performed in the United States; the majority of these procedures take place in a small number of centers. The number of procedures is increasing by about 25% per year (~400 cases) but currently represents a tiny fraction of the total number of cardiac surgical interventions performed annually.[264]

The use of robotics in minimally invasive cardiac surgery was intended to overcome some of the limitations of thoracoscopy. For instance, thoracoscopic instruments offer only four degrees of freedom, a level inadequate for the delicacy required in cardiac surgery. The long-shafted instruments are subject to a fulcrum effect, and shear forces may be exerted at port sites, contributing to postoperative pain from intercostal nerve trauma. In addition, the surgical field images in thoracic surgical systems are presently two dimensional, and this loss of depth perception can impair surgical performance in delicate situations.[265]

Surgical robotic systems can be used in a number of ways in coronary revascularization. The procedures run the spectrum from robotic MIDCAB (robotic IMA harvest with hand-sewn anastomosis via anterior thoracotomy or sternotomy) to totally intrathoracic revascularization (IMA takedown and bypass creation) performed solely through small port-site incisions, with or without the use of CPB.

The earliest use of robotic technology in coronary revascularization, in the late 1990s to early 2000s, recapitulated the role of thoracoscopy in the thoracoscopically assisted MIDCAB described above. Namely, robotically assisted IMA harvest was performed and then followed by a single, hand-sewn anterior anastomosis via a small thoracotomy in an off-pump fashion. When compared with a single-vessel OPCAB, robotically assisted MIDCAB has been associated with a shorter hospital stay and quicker return to work.[266] As with thoracoscopically assisted MIDCABs, robotically assisted MIDCABs have also been described as key components of hybrid revascularizations (described below).

More recently, robotically assisted bilateral IMA (BIMA) harvest, combined with either a small thoracotomy or transabdominal approach for the creation of anastomoses, has been described for treatment of multivessel disease with good results. For instance, in Subramanian's series of 30 patients (mean number of grafts, 2.6), 97% of patients who underwent robotically assisted multivessel revascularization were extubated on the operating room table, and 77% were discharged in 48 hours. There were no deaths in this series, with only two patients requiring readmission and only one conversion to sternotomy.[267] The largest single-institution series of robotically assisted multivessel coronary revascularization comes from Srivastava and colleagues. In their series of 150 patients undergoing bilateral robotically assisted IMA harvest and small thoracotomy for hand-sewn anastomoses, the planned degree of arterial revascularization was completed in 148 patients. The mean number of arterial grafts per patient was 2.6 ± 0.8. The authors found that all coronary arteries could be reached as in situ BIMA or composite grafts with saphenous veins, and they had 0% mortality, stroke, MI, and wound infection rates. The mean postoperative length of stay was 3.6 ± 2.9 days in this series.[268]

In contrast to other minimally invasive approaches, the *totally endoscopic coronary bypass* (TECAB) does not involve the use of incisions larger than port sites (Figure 11-7). Both on-pump and off-pump TECABs have been described. First described in 1998, proponents of TECAB cite minimal surgical trauma and rapid recovery as the major advantages to this procedure. Scarring is reduced compared with minithoracotomy approaches, and no rib spreading is involved, which results in minimal intercostal nerve trauma and less postoperative pain. Series from the early 2000s showed short hospital stays, very early return of patients to full activities following TECAB, and very rare deep thoracic wound infections, owing to the minimal exposure of the operative field to the ambient environment.[269] It has been suggested that the obese may benefit more from TECAB with respect to wound complications, as the operative exposure is no different in obese versus nonobese patients using this approach.[269]

The majority of TECABs are on-pump single-vessel procedures (LIMA-LAD). These procedures involve robotic LIMA harvest through two instrument ports under conditions of double-lumen

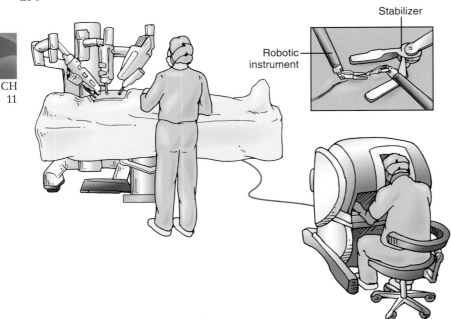

Stabilizer

Robotic
instrument

FIGURE 11-7 Totally endoscopic coronary artery bypass grafting. From the robotic console, the surgeon controls microinstruments placed through ports sites at the surgical field. The system conveys high-definition three-dimensional imaging to the surgeon at the console, and sensors register the surgeon's finger and wrist movements. These are translated into the motion of the microinstruments in the field. The position of the target vessel is stabilized with a stabilizer.

endotracheal intubation and single-lung ventilation. This is followed by systemic heparinization and peripheral arterial and venous cannulation for CPB. The arterial cannulation system involves an endoaortic balloon, which is positioned in the ascending aorta using transesophageal guidance; once deployed, it occludes the aorta and delivers antegrade cardioplegia. After cardiac arrest has been instigated and the patient is on CPB, the coronary arteriotomy and LIMA-LAD anastomosis is performed.[266]

Multiple trials have examined TECAB safety and efficacy. In a 2006 trial by Argeniazo et al, 98 patients who required LAD revascularization were enrolled in 12 centers, and 85 of these patients underwent TECAB. In these patients, the CPB time was 117 ± 44 minutes, cross-clamp time was 71 (± 26) minutes, and length of hospital stay was 5.1 ± 3.4 days. There was a 6% conversion rate to open techniques and one perioperative MI but 0% stroke and mortality rates. At 3 months, angiography in 75 patients revealed significant anastomotic stenosis or reocclusion in 7.1% of patients with a 91% overall freedom from reintervention or angiographic failure.

The largest multicenter series of robotically assisted coronary revascularization consisted of 228 patients undergoing TECAB (n = 117) or robotically assisted MIDCAB (n = 111) at five European institutions.[270] The overall mortality rate was 2.1%, although the conversion rate to nonrobotic procedures was 28%, but this decreased with time. Overall, procedural efficacy—defined by angiographic patency or lack of ischemic signs on stress electrocardiology—was 97% with a 5% incidence of major adverse cardiac events within 6 months. For both approaches, the rate of target vessel reintervention was slightly higher than that reported for open procedures in the Society of Thoracic Surgeons (STS) database, but graft patency rates and major adverse cardiac event rates were comparable to those reported in the database.[270]

The first off-pump, beating-heart TECAB (BH-TECAB) was described in 2001. Although case reports of even multivessel BH-TECAB[271] and small series of single-vessel BH-TECABs have been reported, by and large, CPB remains a prerequisite for TECAB, owing to the difficult target stabilization and totally endoscopic setup.[271] In the current era, BH-TECAB is in need of further procedural enhancement; however, as refinements in anastomotic devices,[266] endoscopic stabilization methods, and target vessel identification systems occur, both TECAB and BH-TECAB may become more widely used.[265]

Non—Left Internal Mammary Arterial Conduits in Surgical Revascularization

In addition to OPCAB and novel MIS techniques of myocardial revascularization, work has been ongoing to determine the role of non-SVG conduits in CABG (Table 11-7). The radial artery (RA), right internal mammary artery (RIMA), and gastroepiploic artery (GEA) have all been investigated.

BACKGROUND AND INTRODUCTION

For patients undergoing surgical revascularization, a clear advantage in clinical outcomes is seen when the LIMA is used to bypass the LAD. The LIMA-LAD graft has been shown to positively affect survival and has demonstrated 5-year patency rates between 92% and 95% and 10-year patency rates between 95% and 98%.[272] That said, for additional grafts in surgical coronary revascularization, the evidence has been less clear. The greater saphenous vein (GSV) is often used, but it is prone to intimal hyperplasia and graft atherosclerosis, causing late graft occlusion. SVG failure rates at 1 year range between 7% and 30%, and 40% to 50% of SVGs will fail or become atherosclerotic by 15 years.[272]

The superiority of the LIMA over SVG has prompted inquiry into the use of other arterial grafts, such as the RIMA, RA, and GEA. The use of the inferior epigastric artery (IEA) as an alternative arterial graft was reported and examined in the 1990s, but it is no longer widely used; its patency was not found to be superior to SVGs, and it was associated with abdominal wall hematomas and infections.[273] Because the RIMA, RA, and GEA are histologically, physiologically, and anatomically unique arteries, their behavior as conduits must be examined separately. The remainder of this section will outline the latest information on these arterial conduits in coronary revascularization.

RIGHT INTERNAL MAMMARY ARTERY FOR USE IN BILATERAL MAMMARY ARTERY GRAFTING

Like the LIMA, the RIMA has features of both elastic and muscular arteries, and this somatic artery is thus referred to as a *transitional artery*.[274,275] The media is thin, with fewer vascular smooth muscle cells than other arteries, and it shows a diminished proliferative response to mitogens such as platelet-derived growth factor and mechanical stretch. The nonfenestrated internal elastic lamina of

TABLE 11-7 Conduits for Surgical Revascularization: Advantages, Disadvantages, and Patency Rates

CONDUIT	ADVANTAGES	DISADVANTAGES	PATENCY RATES[278,279,283,285,304-307]	COMMENTS
SVG	Readily available	Prone to late graft occlusion	1 year: 78%-90% 10 years: 57%-61%	
LIMA	Readily available Resistant to atherosclerosis Well-established positive survival benefit to LIMA-LAD anastomosis		1 year: 95%-99% 10 years: 95%-99%	
RIMA (when used in association with LIMA, BIMA)	Readily available Resistant to atherosclerosis Not prone to spasm Graftable to any territory if used as free graft Survival benefit to BIMA grafting in retrospective studies	Longer harvest time Increased transfusion requirement Increased rate of sternal wound infection with BIMA grafting	1 year: 95%-99% 10 years: ~81%*	In situ grafting to PLV or PDA not possible because of short length May render future aortic surgery hazardous when used as in situ graft for left-sided targets Questionable benefit to RIMA grafting to right-sided targets with <70% occlusion
RA	Lower transfusion requirement with harvest compared to BIMA harvest Good surgical handling characteristics	Not always available† Proclivity to spasm requires vasodilator use postoperatively Risk of postoperative sensory/motor dysfunction	1 year: 70%-90% 5 years: 89%-98% 10 years: not available	Subject to flow competition; not recommended for use to bypass arteries with stenoses <75%
GEA	Able to be grafted to almost any territory in situ Available in reoperative surgical revascularization	Necessity of laparotomy for harvest Prone to flow competition	1 year: 92%-96% 10 years: ~62%	Use is contraindicated in certain patients (mesenteric ischemia, post gastric resection) Not recommended for LAD bypass
IEA	Available in reoperative surgical revascularization	Associated with abdominal wall hematomas, infection	Not significantly different from SVG patency rates	Not in common use

*Varies by target (e.g., LAD, 95%; OM, 90%; RCA or PDA, 83%).[304]
†Use is contraindicated in cases of forearm ischemia or arterial dissection from cannulation.
BIMA, bilateral internal mammary artery; GEA, gastroepiploic artery; IEA, inferior epigastric artery; LAD, left anterior descending artery; LIMA, left internal mammary artery; OM, obtuse marginal artery; PLV, posterior left ventricular artery; PDA, posterior descending artery; RA, radial artery; RCA, right coronary artery; RIMA, right internal mammary artery; SVG, saphenous vein graft.

the IMA may inhibit cellular migration, perhaps preventing the initiation of intimal hyperplasia and the initiation of atherosclerosis. Also, the endothelium of the IMA may have a greater predilection to vasodilation, as evidenced by its significantly higher basal production of vasodilators, such as prostacyclin and nitric oxide; its vasodilation in the presence of nitroglycerin; and its lack of vasoconstriction in response to norepinephrine.[276] Hence, these histopathologic characteristics of IMAs give them a unique resistance to atherosclerosis and a reduced proclivity to spasm.

Advantages to using the RIMA as a bypass graft include its reduced proclivity to spasm in comparison to the RA, the fact that it is nearly always available for use in grafting and is, at least theoretically, graftable to any territory as a composite free graft. That said, this grafting option does not come without disadvantages. The short length of the RIMA disallows grafting to the posterolateral or posterior descending artery in an in situ fashion. Furthermore, its thin wall is not suitable for aortic anastomosis, but it can be anastomosed to the LIMA, which is an accepted technique.[273,277] The downsides of the RIMA/LIMA combination include a longer harvest time, increased transfusion requirement, and a higher rate of sternal wound infection. In addition, if the RIMA is used as an in situ graft for left-sided grafts, and hence requires crossing the aorta in the midline, any future aortic surgery could be extremely hazardous, as the RIMA would be in danger of being damaged in this future procedure.[273]

With regard to sternal wound problems, recent studies have called into question the traditional wisdom that BIMA grafting is associated with a greater risk of such problems in diabetic patients. DePaulis and colleagues compared two groups of 450 patients undergoing single IMA (SIMA) or BIMA (n = 150) grafting and found that diabetes was not a significant risk factor for sternal wound issues. Instead, the pedicled harvesting technique was the

most significant risk factor, with a 4:1 odds ratio (OR) of sternal wound problems with this technique. In fact, these authors found a significantly higher rate of sternal problems in the pedicled SIMA group when compared with the skeletonized BIMA group (1.1% vs. 3.3%).

With regard to specific coronary targets, IMA grafts in general have shown increased patency to all coronary artery targets; however, IMA grafting to the right coronary artery (RCA) in particular bears further discussion. Sabik and colleagues evaluated the angiographic results of 2121 IMA (mostly LIMA) grafts and 8733 SVGs. They found that unadjusted 1-, 5-, and 10-year patency rates were 93%, 88%, and 90% for IMAs and 78%, 65%, and 57% for SVGs, respectively. At 10 years, IMAs were more likely than SVGs to be patent to the LAD in 99.1% of cases, to diagonal branches in 98.3%, to the circumflex artery in 98.3%, to the posterior descending artery in 98.5%, and to the RCA in 82.5%. For RCAs, SVG patency was equivalent to or better than internal thoracic artery patency early after surgery. However, by 10 years, the IMA demonstrated superior patency compared with SVGs to RCAs with 70% stenosis or greater. These findings led the authors to conclude that IMA grafts demonstrate better patency than SVGs in general, except in the case of RCA stenosis of less than 70%, in which case an SVG may be a better choice than the RIMA.[278]

With regard to the patency of the RIMA specifically, recent data from the investigators from the Radial Artery Patency and Clinical Outcomes (RAPCO) trial—a 10-year prospective, randomized, single-center trial aiming to evaluate the long-term patencies and clinical outcomes of the RA, RIMA, and SVG—has called the superiority of RIMA grafts into question. At 5-year angiographic follow-up, these investigators found no significant difference in patency among the RA, RIMA, and SVG.[279] However, other multiple retrospective studies have found that BIMA grafting is associated with a significant survival benefit. That said, these studies included a population of low-risk patients with a long life expectancy; hence, the results of these studies may not be applicable to the general population.[277,280] In one such recent study, a retrospective review of 4584 consecutive, isolated CABG operations was conducted that found improved long-term survival at 30 years in BIMA-grafted versus LIMA-only–grafted patients in nearly all of their propensity-matched groups, except those with the greatest propensity for single IMA grafting, in which late survival was not significantly different.[280] Although propensity matching was used in an effort to decrease selection bias, BIMA patients in this study were younger and less likely to have diabetes, renal dysfunction, vascular disease, congestive heart failure, and LV dysfunction. This has led surgeons to question whether such studies really do make a powerful argument for BIMA grafting, or whether the results are just a side effect of statistical confounding. Perhaps in part these concerns account for the reason that less than 4% of all coronary operations in the United States are currently done with bilateral IMAs.[274,280]

RADIAL ARTERY GRAFTS

The radial artery is a 20-cm-long somatic artery with a fenestrated internal elastic lamina, a thicker wall than the IMA, and a higher density of muscle cells in its medial layer. It has the same sensitivity to vasoconstrictive agents as the IMA, but its greater muscle mass generates a higher contractile force, and so it has a well-known propensity to spasm.[276]

The RA was first used as a conduit in the early 1970s by Carpentier and colleagues, who dealt with intraoperative spasm by using mechanical dilation. When 32% of the grafts were found to be occluded at 2 years, the RA was abandoned as an arterial conduit, only to be revived later, when some of these grafts were found to be fully patent 15 years later by angiogram.[273] The RA demonstrates good handling and is associated with lower transfusion rates and harvest times than, for instance, bilateral IMA harvesting; but the tendency to spasm requires the use of vasodilators in the postoperative period, and this can be difficult in the setting of postoperative hypotension. Additionally, the RA is not always available for use; it is contraindicated in cases of forearm ischemia, atherosclerosis, or dissection from cannulation, and it is associated with a 3% to 15% risk of postoperative sensory or motor dysfunction in the hand. It has also been shown to be subject to flow competition; hence, the RA is not recommended for use to bypass mildly (<75%) native coronary arteries.[273]

Although there was initial enthusiasm regarding the long-term patency of the RA in comparison to the SVG, more recent analyses have cast doubt on this matter. A recent meta-analysis of the RCTs did not show an advantage to the use of the RA, and the lack of superiority was attributed to a high incidence of severely impaired flow, possibly as a result of vasoreactivity.[281,282] As discussed above, investigators from the RAPCO trial recently reported their 5-year angiographic results of graft patencies and found no significant difference in patency between arterial and venous conduits.[279] An additional report from Fukui and colleagues[283] also found that there was only a 69.5% patency rate at 1 year with RA conduits, which was significantly worse than the RIMA (92%) and SVG (82.6%) patency. These results have led researchers to conclude that IMAs may be the most reliable conduit when multiple arterial conduits are used for grafting to the left coronary system.[278,283] Hence, there are still many questions regarding the superiority of the RA over the SVG in CABG, and further research is needed.

GASTROEPIPLOIC ARTERY GRAFTS

The GEA is a muscular artery with a thin intimal layer and a fenestrated internal elastic lamella. The medial layer has a thickness similar to the IMA but is less developed than the RA. In comparison with the IMA, the GEA's media is capable of generating a greater contractile force and is more prone to spasm than the IMA.[276,284]

The GEA, generally the right GEA, is more widely used in Japan than in Western countries as an arterial conduit. Its use was first described in 1987, with early descriptions mainly being its use as a free graft. However, when used in this way, its early patency was not favorable, and it is now used mainly as an in situ graft.[284] The GEA is desirable for its ability to be grafted to any territory as an in situ graft, although it is mainly used to graft the RCA,[284] and also for its availability in reoperative CABGs. The disadvantages of the GEA include the fact that its harvest requires laparotomy, and this can result in delayed postoperative oral intake. Furthermore, the GEA is more spasmodic than the IMA and more prone to flow competition given its 10- to 15-mm lower pressure than the IMA; hence, it may not be of appropriate size for grafting in some patients.[284] Its use is contraindicated in patients with previous gastric resection, prior endovascular instrumentation, or mesenteric vascular insufficiency.

A recent analysis of the available evidence on the patency of the GEA concluded that the right GEA as used for bypass of the RCA has a long-term patency similar to that of the saphenous vein: 80% to 90% patency at 5 years and approximately 62% at 10 years.[285] Of note, GEA grafts to the LAD perform much more poorly, with a midterm patency of about 59%.[284] Therefore it is not recommended as a conduit to the LAD.[285]

Hybrid Coronary Revascularization

INTRODUCTION AND DEFINITION

Hybrid coronary revascularization combines surgical and catheter-based therapies for the treatment of coronary artery disease. Usually, a LIMA graft to the LAD is placed in concert with PCI of non-LAD targets. Generally, the LIMA-LAD graft is performed with one of the minimally invasive techniques described in the earlier sections of this chapter, such as MIDCAB or TECAB. The hybrid concept can be extended to the treatment of combined coronary and valve diseases, such as a minimally invasive valve surgical procedure combined with PCI to coronary lesions with the intention, for example, of converting a high-risk valve/CABG into a lower risk, minimally invasive valve procedure, but these applications are not discussed here.

RATIONALE AND BACKGROUND

The hybrid approach attempts to bring together the "best of both worlds"—those of cardiac surgery and interventional cardiology—by combining the most effective treatment strategies from the two disciplines for the treatment of multivessel coronary artery disease.

It has been shown that the LIMA-LAD graft is the most effective and durable option for anterior wall revascularization, primarily related to its resistance to thrombosis and atherosclerosis. The LAD supplies the largest area of myocardium of any of the coronary arteries, including the anterior wall and septum, and the LIMA-LAD graft is known to improve survival, with 5-year patency rates between 92% and 95% and 10-year patency rates between 95% and 98%.[272] PCI with DESs offers equal if not better revascularization durability compared with vein and RA grafts. SVG failure rates at 1 year range between 7% and 30%, and 40% to 50% of SVGs will fail or become atherosclerotic by 15 years.[272] Furthermore, recent data (discussed above) regarding the use of arterial conduits other than the LIMA in CABG have cast doubt on improving patency rates by the use of these conduits.[279,285]

With these factors in mind, and in the context of the developing MIS procedures, interest in the potential advantages of hybrid approaches grew; beginning in the late 1990s, this growth has continued over the first decade of the new century. In 1996 Angelini and colleagues[286a] reported the first series of six patients treated with a MIDCAB LIMA-LAD and PTCA or PTCA and stent; since that time, a small number of centers have gained experience in this approach.

TECHNICAL AND TIMING ISSUES OF HYBRID INTERVENTIONS

Hybrid procedures generally involve a MIDCAB or TECAB surgical procedure for creation of the LIMA-LAD anastomosis along with catheter-based PCI interventions. The timing of the surgical procedure in relation to the PCI has been a subject of some discussion.

By their nature, all hybrid procedures are staged, and only the duration of the staging period and the order in which the procedures are performed can be varied. *Two-staged* hybrid procedures are those in which PCI and CABG are performed in separate operative locations, and the two procedures may be separated by hours, days, or weeks. *One-stop* procedures are performed in one setting, and the procedures are separated by minutes.[286] In a two-stage hybrid procedure, either the surgical or percutaneous intervention can be performed first. In a one-stop procedure, the surgical intervention is generally performed first.

The advantages and disadvantages of each approach are discussed below. Each approach has its theoretical relative merits and drawbacks, but at present, no data are available to support any of the approaches above the other. Indeed, clinicians must weigh the relative merits of each strategy in the context of their particular practice setting and then decide which approach is best for the individual patient.

Percutaneous Intervention Before Surgical Intervention

Performing the percutaneous revascularization before surgical revascularization is associated with several potential advantages. First, the revascularization of the non-LAD targets provides collateral circulation and decreases the risk of ischemia if LAD occlusion is used in a beating-heart surgical approach. Second, it allows the interventionalist the opportunity for aggressive multivessel revascularization, all the while knowing that if a complication occurs, or PCI is not successful, a conventional CABG can and will be performed at a later time. Third, the approach allows for a hybrid procedure in the setting of an acute infarct, when the target vessel is not the LAD; the acute lesion can be treated at that time, and the LAD can be revascularized later.

Unfortunately, this approach is associated with a number of disadvantages. It necessitates performing PCI in a setting in which no protection is afforded by a LIMA-LAD graft. Also, unless a third procedure (completion angiogram) is performed after the surgical procedure, there is no opportunity for midterm angiographic imaging of the LIMA-LAD graft. Most importantly, the risk of stent thrombosis and need for antiplatelet agents following PCI necessitates either performing the MIS revascularization on clopidogrel, which has been associated with a slightly increased risk of bleeding during cardiac surgery,[254] or maintaining in-hospital patients on a GP IIb/IIIa inhibitor until their surgical intervention.[254,286]

Surgical Intervention Before Percutaneous Intervention

Performing PCI after LIMA-LAD grafting makes it possible to avoid antiplatelet-related bleeding complications during the surgical procedure. Antiplatelet therapy can be started after surgery and may be continued long term in keeping with current recommendations following stent implantation. In addition, the PCIs can be performed with the protection afforded by the surgical revascularization, allowing interventionalists to more safely approach left main lesions.[254] A final benefit to this approach is that it allows for the LIMA-LAD anastomosis to be angiographically evaluated at the time of PCI. However, if there is a complication or failure of the PCI, a second, higher risk operation must be performed. This should be a rare occurrence, as the incidence of emergent CABG following PCI is less than 1%.[254] Given all of the above, most cardiologists and surgeons who perform two-staged hybrid procedures have adopted this strategy.

At present, the optimal duration of time between the two interventions is unclear; however, it seems reasonable to delay PCI until the inflammatory milieu that exists immediately after surgery resolves. This usually takes 3 to 5 days, but patients may need 7 to 10 days of mental and physical recovery following surgery. Ideally, PCI would be performed at the index hospitalization, so that the patient would be discharged fully revascularized; but economic issues can make this problematic, if long postsurgical recovery periods are required.[254]

Simultaneous Procedures

Although PCI and CABG can be performed in two separate procedures, these cases involve two teams, logistical challenges, increased costs, and possible hospitalization between the procedures. Additionally, many patients would simply prefer not to undergo two separate interventions.[286] In centers with hybrid operating rooms, where both percutaneous and surgical procedures can be performed, a one-stop procedure of simultaneous PCI and CABG can be performed.

With this approach, there is superb monitoring throughout the procedure under general anesthesia. Furthermore, any complications encountered can be resolved in one setting, and a completion angiogram can be done to evaluate the LIMA-LAD graft. Complete revascularization is ensured before patients leave the operating suite, and they experience the emotional and psychologic benefit of a complete "fix" in one anesthetic setting.[254] Potential drawbacks include the need for specialized hybrid facilities, increased operative times and cost, and inadequate hospital reimbursement. Concerns about performing PCI in the inflammatory milieu created by the surgical bypass have been raised, and additionally, bleeding risk remains a concern, as full antiplatelet therapy is required, and incomplete (or no) heparin reversal is needed following the combined procedure. At this point, the data regarding the effect of clopidogrel on bleeding in patients undergoing hybrid procedure are mixed, with some reporting increased bleeding and others reporting no such increase.[287-289] Furthermore, the effects of protamine reversal on stent patency are unknown.

CURRENT STATE OF HYBRID REVASCULARIZATION AND RECENT INFORMATION

At the time of this publication, experience with this hybrid revascularization is limited. No prospective randomized trials on hybrid revascularization have been published, and only case series with fewer than 500 patients total undergoing hybrid procedures, generally combining either MIDCAB or TECAB with PCI, have been reported in the literature, with the largest series a single-institution study of 70 patients followed over a 7-year period.[272,290]

The minimal amount of data available on the subject shows low mortality (0% to 2%) and low morbidity rates overall (average of 4.7% in-hospital morbidity across all studies), with shorter hospital and ICU stays than would be expected with conventional CABG.[286] Immediate LIMA-LAD patency rates range from 92% to 100%.[286] With respect to restenosis rates, the data are mixed: earlier series using bare-metal stents or angioplasty without stenting revealed 6 month stent restenosis rates ranging from 2.3% to 23%, with an average of 11% across all the literature.[286] However, in more recent series, in which DESs were used in procedures combining MIDCAB and PCI, 97% patency rates at 1 year were reported.[289]

Given the limited data available to evaluate hybrid revascularization, as well as the evolving nature of both the MIS approaches and percutaneous therapy, generalized statements regarding outcomes with hybrid revascularization are difficult to make at this time. Additional studies will be needed to fully evaluate this approach as time goes on.

Future Directions

The landscape has changed considerably since the inception of surgical coronary artery revascularization, and it continues to change as technological advances in the fields of cardiac surgery and cardiology occur. Research and development are needed in many areas of surgical revascularization, and new trials are needed to more fully delineate the benefits of on- and off-pump coronary revascularization, particularly with respect to the groups of patients who benefit from the off-pump approach. Robotic revascularization is still in its infancy, and better techniques and technologies need to be developed to serve patients who desire a minimally invasive approach. Hybrid revascularization is also still in its infancy, and rich opportunities are available going forward in developing this approach, both with respect to the "hard" technologies of procedural techniques involved and to the "soft" technologies of interdisciplinary cooperation between interventional cardiology and cardiac surgery teams. As these areas are developed, further outcomes data are needed to evaluate the efficacy and economic viability of the hybrid approach. With respect to the various arterial conduits possible for use in surgical revascularization, the cardiac surgical world awaits with interest the 10-year data from the RAPCO trial to better delineate the ultimate fate of the place of the radial artery graft in surgical revascularization.

REFERENCES

1. Dotter CT, Judkins MP. Transluminal treatment of arteriosclerotic obstruction. Description of a new technic and a preliminary report of its application. *Circulation* 1964;30:654-670.
2. Gruntzig AR, Senning A, Siegenthaler WE. Nonoperative dilatation of coronary-artery stenosis: percutaneous transluminal coronary angioplasty. *N Engl J Med* 1979;301(2):61-68.
3. Simpson JB, et al. A new catheter system for coronary angioplasty. *Am J Cardiol* 1982;49(5):1216-1222.
4. Detre K, et al. Percutaneous transluminal coronary angioplasty in 1985-1986 and 1977-1981. The National Heart, Lung, and Blood Institute Registry. *N Engl J Med* 1988;318(5):265-270.
5. Saber RS, et al. Coronary embolization after balloon angioplasty or thrombolytic therapy: an autopsy study of 32 cases. *J Am Coll Cardiol* 1993;22(5):1283-1288.
6. Piana RN, et al. Incidence and treatment of 'no-reflow' after percutaneous coronary intervention. *Circulation* 1994;89(6):2514-2518.
7. Ragosta M, et al. Effectiveness of heparin in preventing thrombin generation and thrombin activity in patients undergoing coronary intervention. *Am Heart J* 1999;137(2):250-257.
8. Holmes DR Jr, et al. Angiographic changes produced by percutaneous transluminal coronary angioplasty. *Am J Cardiol* 1983;51(5):676-683.
9. Black AJ, et al. Tear or dissection after coronary angioplasty. Morphologic correlates of an ischemic complication. *Circulation* 1989;79(5):1035-1042.
10. Ferguson JJ, et al. The relation of clinical outcome to dissection and thrombus formation during coronary angioplasty. Heparin Registry Investigators. *J Invasive Cardiol* 1995;7(1):2-10.
11. Sigwart U, Puel J, Mirkovitch V, Joffre F, Kappenberger L. Intravascular stents to prevent occlusion and restenosis after transluminal angioplasty. *N Engl J Med* 1987;316(12):701-706.
12. Palmaz JC, Sibbitt RR, Reuter SR, Tio FO, Rice WJ. Expandable intraluminal graft: a preliminary study. Work in progress. *Radiology* 1985;156(1):73-77.
13. Schatz RA. A view of vascular stents. *Circulation* 1989;79(2):445-457.
14. Schatz RA, Baim DS, Leon M, et al. Clinical experience with the Palmaz-Schatz coronary stent: initial results of a multicenter study. *Circulation* 1991;83(1):148-161.
15. Serruys PW, de Jaegere P, Kiemeneij F, et al. A comparison of balloon-expandable stent implantation with balloon angioplasty in patients with coronary artery disease. Benestent Study Group. *N Engl J Med* 1994;331(8):489-495.
16. Fischman DL, Leon MB, Baim DS, et al. A randomized comparison of coronary-stent placement and balloon angioplasty in the treatment of coronary artery disease. Stent Restenosis Study Investigators. *N Engl J Med* 1994;331(8):496-501.
17. Kimura T, Abe K, Shizuta S, et al. Long-term clinical and angiographic follow-up after coronary stent placement in native coronary arteries. *Circulation* 2002;105(25):2986-2991.
18. Cutlip DE, Chhabra AG, Baim DS, et al. Beyond restenosis: five-year clinical outcomes from second-generation coronary stent trials. *Circulation* 2004;110(10):1226-1230.
19. Gordon PC, Gibson CM, Cohen DJ, et al. Mechanisms of restenosis and redilation within coronary stents: quantitative angiographic assessment. *J Am Coll Cardiol* 1993;21(5):1166-1174.
20. Ho KK, Rodriguez O, Chauhan MS, Kuntz RE. Predictors of angiographic restenosis after stenting: pooled analysis of 1197 patients with protocol-mandated angiographic follow-up from five randomized stent trials. *Circulation* 1998;98(Suppl 1):362-368.
21. Teirstein PS, Massullo V, Jani S, et al. Catheter-based radiotherapy to inhibit restenosis after coronary stenting. *N Engl J Med* 1997;336(24):1697-1703.
22. Leon MB, Tiersteín PS, Moses JW, et al. Localized intracoronary gamma-radiation therapy to inhibit the recurrence of restenosis after stenting. *N Engl J Med* 2001;344(4):250-256.
23. Waksman R, White RL, Chan RC, et al. Intracoronary gamma-radiation therapy after angioplasty inhibits recurrence in patients with in-stent restenosis. *Circulation* 2000;101(18):2165-2171.
24. Popma J. Late clinical and angiographic outcomes after use of 90Sr/90Y beta radiation for the treatment of in-stent restenosis: results from the 90Sr Treatment of Angiographic Restenosis (START) Trial. *J Am Coll Cardiol* 2000;36:311-312.
25. Leon MB, Teirstein PS, Moses JW, et al. Declining long-term efficacy of vascular brachytherapy for in-stent restenosis: 5-year follow-up from the Gamma-1 randomized trial. *Am J Cardiol* 2004;94:144E.
26. Choi D, Kim SK, Choi SH, et al. Preventative effects of rosiglitazone on restenosis after coronary stent implantation in patients with type 2 diabetes. *Diabetes Care* 2004;27(11):2654-2660.
27. Guarda E, Marchant E, Fajuri A, et al. Oral rapamycin to prevent human coronary stent restenosis: a pilot study. *Am Heart J* 2004;148(2):e9.
28. Farb A, John M, Acampado E, et al. Oral everolimus inhibits in-stent neointimal growth. *Circulation* 2002;106(18):2379-2384.
29. Douglas JS Jr, Holmes DR Jr, Kereiakes DJ, et al. Coronary stent restenosis in patients treated with cilostazol. *Circulation* 2005;112(18):2826-2832.
30. Holmes DR Jr, Savage M, LaBlanche JM, et al. Results of Prevention of REStenosis with Tranilast and its Outcomes (PRESTO) trial. *Circulation* 2002;106(10):1243-1250.
31. Serruys PW, Ormiston JA, Sianos G, et al. Actinomycin-eluting stent for coronary revascularization: a randomized feasibility and safety study: the ACTION trial. *J Am Coll Cardiol* 2004;44(7):1363-1367.
32. Grube E, Lansky A, Hauptmann KE, et al. High-dose 7-hexanoyltaxol-eluting stent with polymer sleeves for coronary revascularization: one-year results from the SCORE randomized trial. *J Am Coll Cardiol* 2004;44(7):1368-1372.
33. Virmani R, Liistro F, Stankovic G, et al. Mechanism of late in-stent restenosis after implantation of a paclitaxel derivate–eluting polymer stent system in humans. *Circulation* 2002;106(21):2649-2651.
34. Marx SO, Jayaraman T, Go LO, Marks AR. Rapamycin-FKBP inhibits cell cycle regulators of proliferation in vascular smooth muscle cells. *Circ Res* 1995;76(3):412-417.
35. Poon M, Marx SO, Gallo R, et al. Rapamycin inhibits vascular smooth muscle cell migration. *J Clin Invest* 1996;98(10):2277-2283.
36. Marx SO, Marks AR. Bench to bedside: the development of rapamycin and its application to stent restenosis. *Circulation* 2001;104(8):852-855.
37. Sousa JE, Costa MA, Abizaid A, et al. Lack of neointimal proliferation after implantation of sirolimus-coated stents in human coronary arteries: a quantitative coronary angiography and three-dimensional intravascular ultrasound study. *Circulation* 2001;103(2):192-195.
38. Sousa JE, Costa MA, Abizaid AC, et al. Sustained suppression of neointimal proliferation by sirolimus-eluting: one-year angiographic and intravascular ultrasound follow-up. *Circulation* 2001;104(17):2007-2011.
39. Morice MC, Serruys PW, Sousa JE, et al. A randomized comparison of a sirolimus-eluting stent with a standard stent for coronary revascularization. *N Engl J Med* 2002;346(23):1773-1780.
40. Moses JW, Leon MB, Popma JJ, et al. Sirolimus-eluting stents versus standard stents in patients with stenosis in a native coronary artery. *N Engl J Med* 2003;349(14):1315-1323.
41. Weisz G, Leon MB, Holmes DR Jr, et al. Five-year follow-up after sirolimus-eluting stent implantation results of the SIRIUS (Sirolimus-Eluting Stent in De-Novo Native Coronary Lesions) Trial. *J Am Coll Cardiol* 2009;53(17):1488-1497.
42. Sabaté M, Jiménez-Quevedo P, Angiolillo DJ, et al. Randomized comparison of sirolimus-eluting stent versus standard stent for percutaneous coronary revascularization in diabetic patients: the diabetes and sirolimus-eluting stent (DIABETES) trial. *Circulation* 2005;112(14):2175-2183.
43. Jiménez-Quevedo P, Sabaté M, Angiolillo DJ, et al. Long-term clinical benefit of sirolimus-eluting stent implantation in diabetic patients with de novo coronary stenoses: long-term results of the DIABETES trial. *Eur Heart J* 2007;28(16):1946-1952.
44. Maresta A, Varani E, Balducelli M, et al. Comparison of effectiveness and safety of sirolimus-eluting stents versus bare-metal stents in patients with diabetes mellitus (from the Italian Multicenter Randomized DESSERT Study). *Am J Cardiol* 2008;101(11):1560-1566.
45. Baumgart D, Klauss V, Baer F, et al. SCORPIUS Study Investigators. One-year results of the SCORPIUS study: a German multicenter investigation on the effectiveness of sirolimus-eluting stents in diabetic patients. *J Am Coll Cardiol* 2007;50(17):1627-1634.
46. Diaz de la Llera LS, Ballesteros S, Nevado J, et al. Sirolimus-eluting stents compared with standard stents in the treatment of patients with primary angioplasty. *Am Heart J* 2007;154(1):164, e1-e6.
47. van der Hoeven BL, Liem SS, Jukema JW, et al. Sirolimus-eluting stents versus bare-metal stents in patients with ST-segment elevation myocardial infarction: 9-month angiographic and intravascular ultrasound results and 12-month clinical outcome results from the MISSION! Intervention Study. *J Am Coll Cardiol* 2008;51(6):618-626.
48. Atary JZ, van der Hoeven BL, Liem SS, et al. Three-year outcome of sirolimus-eluting versus bare-metal stents for the treatment of ST-segment elevation myocardial infarction (from the MISSION! Intervention Study). *Am J Cardiol* 2010;106(1):4-12.
49. Di Lorenzo E, Sauro R, Varricchio A, et al. Benefits of drug-eluting stents as compared to bare metal stent in ST-segment elevation myocardial infarction: four year results of the PaclitAxel or Sirolimus-Eluting stent vs bare metal stent in primary angiOplasty (PASEO) randomized trial. *Am Heart J* 2009;158(4):e43-e50.
50. Menichelli M, Parma A, Pucci E, et al. Randomized trial of Sirolimus-Eluting Stent Versus Bare-Metal Stent in Acute Myocardial Infarction (SESAMI). *J Am Coll Cardiol* 2007;49(19):1924-1930.
51. Violini R, Musto C, De Felice F, et al. Maintenance of long-term clinical benefit with sirolimus-eluting stents in patients with ST-segment elevation myocardial infarction 3-year results of the SESAMI (sirolimus-eluting stent versus bare-metal stent in acute myocardial infarction) trial. *J Am Coll Cardiol* 2010;55(8):810-814.
52. Tebaldi M, Arcozzi C, Campo G, et al. STRATEGY Investigators. The 5-year clinical outcomes after a randomized comparison of sirolimus-eluting versus bare-metal stent implantation in patients with ST-segment elevation myocardial infarction. *J Am Coll Cardiol* 2009;54(20):1900-1901.
53. Valgimigli M, Percoco G, Malagutti P, et al. STRATEGY Investivators. Tirofiban and sirolimus-eluting stent vs abciximab and bare-metal stent for acute myocardial infarction: a randomized trial. *JAMA* 2005;293(17):2109-2117.

54. Spaulding C, Henry P, Teiger E, et al. Sirolimus-eluting versus uncoated stents in acute myocardial infarction. *N Engl J Med* 2006;355(11):1093-1104.
55. Kelbaek H, Thuesen L, Helqvist S, et al. SCANDSTENT Investigators. The Stenting Coronary Arteries in Non-stress/benestent Disease (SCANDSTENT) trial. *J Am Coll Cardiol* 2006;47(2):449-455.
56. Kelbaek H, Kløvgaard L, Helqvist S, et al. Long-term outcome in patients treated with sirolimus-eluting stents in complex coronary artery lesions: 3-year results of the SCANDSTENT (Stenting Coronary Arteries in Non-Stress/Benestent Disease) trial. *J Am Coll Cardiol* 2008;51(21):2011-2016.
57. Axel DI, Kunert W, Göggelmann C, et al. Paclitaxel inhibits arterial smooth muscle cell proliferation and migration in vitro and in vivo using local drug delivery. *Circulation* 1997;96(2):636-645.
58. Giannakakou P, Robey R, Fojo T, Blagosklonny MV. Low concentrations of paclitaxel induce cell type–dependent p53, p21 and G1/G2 arrest instead of mitotic arrest: molecular determinants of paclitaxel-induced cytotoxicity. *Oncogene* 2001;20(29): 3806-3813.
59. Grube E, Silber S, Hauptmann KE, et al. TAXUS I: six- and twelve-month results from a randomized, double-blind trial on a slow-release paclitaxel-eluting stent for de novo coronary lesions. *Circulation* 2003;107(1):38-42.
60. Colombo A, Drzewiecki J, Banning A, et al. Randomized study to assess the effectiveness of slow- and moderate-release polymer-based paclitaxel-eluting stents for coronary artery lesions. *Circulation* 2003;108(7):788-794.
61. Silber S, Colombo A, Banning AP, et al. Final 5-year results of the TAXUS II trial: a randomized study to assess the effectiveness of slow- and moderate-release polymer-based paclitaxel-eluting stents for de novo coronary artery lesions. *Circulation* 2009;120(15): 1498-1504.
62. Stone GW, Ellis SG, Cox DA, et al. TAXUS-IV Investigators. A polymer-based, paclitaxel-eluting stent in patients with coronary artery disease. *N Engl J Med* 2004;350(3): 221-231.
63. Ellis SG, Stone GW, Cox DA, et al. TAXUS IV Investigators. Long-term safety and efficacy with paclitaxel-eluting stents: 5-year final results of the TAXUS IV clinical trial (TAXUS IV-SR: Treatment of De Novo Coronary Disease Using a Single Paclitaxel-Eluting Stent). *JACC Cardiovasc Interv* 2009;2(12):1248-1259.
64. Stone GW, Ellis SG, Cannon L, et al. Comparison of a polymer-based paclitaxel-eluting stent with a bare metal stent in patients with complex coronary artery disease: a randomized controlled trial. *JAMA* 2005;294(10):1215-1223.
65. Dawkins KD, Grube E, Guagliumi G, et al. Clinical efficacy of polymer-based paclitaxel-eluting stents in the treatment of complex, long coronary artery lesions from a multicenter, randomized trial: support for the use of drug-eluting stents in contemporary clinical practice. *Circulation* 2005;112(21):3306-3313.
66. Grube E, Dawkins K, Guagliumi G, et al. TAXUS VI final 5-year results: a multicentre, randomised trial comparing polymer-based moderate-release paclitaxel-eluting stent with a bare metal stent for treatment of long, complex coronary artery lesions. *EuroIntervention* 2009;4(5):572-577.
67. Stone GW, Lansky AJ, Pocock SJ, et al. Paclitaxel-eluting stents versus bare-metal stents in acute myocardial infarction. *N Engl J Med* 2009;360(19):1946-1959.
68. Laarman GJ, Suttorp MJ, Dirksen MT, et al. Paclitaxel-eluting versus uncoated stents in primary percutaneous coronary intervention. *N Engl J Med* 2006;355(11):1105-1113.
69. Turco MA, Ormiston JA, Popma JJ, et al. Polymer-based, paclitaxel-eluting TAXUS Liberte stent in de novo lesions: the pivotal TAXUS ATLAS trial. *J Am Coll Cardiol* 2007;49(16): 1676-1683.
70. Turco MA, Ormiston JA, Popma JJ, et al. Reduced risk of restenosis in small vessels and reduced risk of myocardial infarction in long lesions with the new thin-strut TAXUS Liberté stent: 1-year results from the TAXUS ATLAS program. *JACC Cardiovasc Interv* 2008;1(6):699-709.
71. Kereiakes DJ, Cannon LA, Feldman RL, et al. Clinical and angiographic outcomes after treatment of de novo coronary stenoses with a novel platinum chromium thin-strut stent: primary results of the PERSEUS (Prospective Evaluation in a Randomized Trial of the Safety and Efficacy of the Use of the TAXUS Element Paclitaxel-Eluting Coronary Stent System) trial. *J Am Coll Cardiol* 2010;56(4):264-271.
72. Windecker S, Remondino A, Eberli FR, et al. Sirolimus-eluting and paclitaxel-eluting stents for coronary revascularization. *N Engl J Med* 2005;353(7):653-662.
73. Raber L. SIRTAX-LATE: five-year clinical and angiographic follow-up from a prospective randomized trial of sirolimus-eluting and paclitaxel-eluting stents. *Transcatheter Cardiovascular Therapeutics* San Francisco, CA, 2009.
74. Lee SW, Park SW, Kim YH, et al. A randomized comparison of sirolimus- versus paclitaxel-eluting stent implantation in patients with diabetes mellitus 2-year clinical outcomes of the DES-DIABETES trial. *J Am Coll Cardiol* 2009;53(9):812-813.
75. Lee SW, Park SW, Kim YH, et al. A randomized comparison of sirolimus- versus Paclitaxel-eluting stent implantation in patients with diabetes mellitus. *J Am Coll Cardiol* 2008;52(9): 727-733.
76. Kim YH, Park SW, Lee SW, et al. Sirolimus-eluting stent versus paclitaxel-eluting stent for patients with long coronary artery disease. *Circulation* 2006;114(20):2148-2153.
77. Mehilli J, Dibra A, Kastrati A, et al. Randomized trial of paclitaxel- and sirolimus-eluting stents in small coronary vessels. *Eur Heart J* 2006;27(3):260-266.
78. Lee JH, Kim HS, Lee SW, et al. Prospective randomized comparison of sirolimus- versus paclitaxel-eluting stents for the treatment of acute ST-elevation myocardial infarction: pROSIT trial. *Catheter Cardiovasc Interv* 2008;72(1):25-32.
79. Dibra A, Kastrati A, Mehilli J, et al. ISA-DIABETES Study Investigators. Paclitaxel-eluting or sirolimus-eluting stents to prevent restenosis in diabetic patients. *N Engl J Med* 2005;353(7):663-670.
80. Pinto DS, Stone GW, Ellis SG, et al. TAXUS-IV Investigators. Impact of routine angiographic follow-up on the clinical benefits of paclitaxel-eluting stents: results from the TAXUS-IV trial. *J Am Coll Cardiol* 2006;48(1):32-36.
81. Morice MC, Colombo A, Meier B, et al. REALITY Trial Investigators. Sirolimus- vs paclitaxel-eluting stents in de novo coronary artery lesions: the REALITY trial: a randomized controlled trial. *JAMA* 2006;295(8):895-904.
82. Galloe AM, Thuesen L, Kelbaek H, et al. Comparison of paclitaxel- and sirolimus-eluting stents in everyday clinical practice: the SORT OUT II randomized trial. *JAMA* 2008; 299(4):409-416.
83. Serruys PW, Ong AT, Piek JJ, et al. A randomized comparison of a durable polymer Everolimus-eluting stent with a bare metal coronary stent: The SPIRIT first trial. *EuroIntervention* 2005;1(1):58-65.
84. Wiemer M, Serruys PW, Miquel-Hebert K, et al. Five-year long-term clinical follow-up of the XIENCE V everolimus eluting coronary stent system in the treatment of patients with de novo coronary artery lesions: the SPIRIT FIRST trial. *Catheter Cardiovasc Interv* 2010;75(7):997-1003.
85. Garg S, Serruys P, Onuma Y, et al; SPIRIT II Investigators. 3-year clinical follow-up of the XIENCE V everolimus-eluting coronary stent system in the treatment of patients with de novo coronary artery lesions: the SPIRIT II trial (Clinical Evaluation of the Xience V Everolimus Eluting Coronary Stent System in the Treatment of Patients with de novo Native Coronary Artery Lesions). *JACC Cardiovasc Interv* 2009;2(12):1190-1198.
86. Stone GW, Midei M, Newman W, et al; SPIRIT III Investigators. Comparison of an everolimus-eluting stent and a paclitaxel-eluting stent in patients with coronary artery disease: a randomized trial. *JAMA* 2008;299(16):1903-1913.
87. Leon MB, Mauri L, Popma JJ, et al. ENDEAVOR IV Investigators. A randomized comparison of the ENDEAVOR zotarolimus-eluting stent versus the TAXUS paclitaxel-eluting stent in de novo native coronary lesions 12-month outcomes from the ENDEAVOR IV trial. *J Am Coll Cardiol* 2010;55(6):543-554.
88. Serruys PW, Ruygrok P, Neuzner J, et al. A randomised comparison of an everolimus-eluting coronary stent with a paclitaxel-eluting coronary stent:the SPIRIT II trial. *EuroIntervention* 2006;2(3):286-294.
89. Kedhi E, Joesoef KS, McFadden E, et al. Second-generation everolimus-eluting and paclitaxel-eluting stents in real-life practice (COMPARE): a randomised trial. *Lancet* 2010;375(9710):201-209.
90. Stone GW, Rizvi A, Newman W, et al; SPIRIT IV Investigators. Everolimus-eluting versus paclitaxel-eluting stents in coronary artery disease. *N Engl J Med* 2010;362(18): 1663-1674.
91. Stettler C, Wandel S, Allemann S, et al. Outcomes associated with drug-eluting and bare-metal stents: a collaborative network meta-analysis. *Lancet* 2007;370(9591):937-948.
92. Stone GW, Moses JW, Ellis SG, et al. Safety and efficacy of sirolimus- and paclitaxel-eluting coronary stents. *N Engl J Med* 2007;356(10):998-1008.
93. Kastrati A, Dibra A, Spaulding C, et al. Meta-analysis of randomized trials on drug-eluting stents vs. bare-metal stents in patients with acute myocardial infarction. *Eur Heart J* 2007;28(22):2706-2713.
94. Kirtane AJ, Gupta A, Iyengar S, et al. Safety and efficacy of drug-eluting and bare metal stents: comprehensive meta-analysis of randomized trials and observational studies. *Circulation* 2009;119(25):3198-3206.
95. Lemos PA, Serruys PW, van Domburg RT, et al. Unrestricted utilization of sirolimus-eluting stents compared with conventional bare stent implantation in the "real world": the Rapamycin-Eluting Stent Evaluated At Rotterdam Cardiology Hospital (RESEARCH) registry. *Circulation* 2004;109(2):190-195.
96. Douglas PS, Brennan JM, Anstrom KJ, et al. Clinical effectiveness of coronary stents in elderly persons: results from 262,700 Medicare patients in the American College of Cardiology-National Cardiovascular Data Registry. *J Am Coll Cardiol* 2009;53(18): 1629-1641.
97. Jeremias A, Kirtane A. Balancing efficacy and safety of drug-eluting stents in patients undergoing percutaneous coronary intervention. *Ann Intern Med* 2008;148(3): 234-238.
98. Pfisterer M, Brunner-La Rocca HP, Buser PT, et al. Late clinical events after clopidogrel discontinuation may limit the benefit of drug-eluting stents: an observational study of drug-eluting versus bare-metal stents. *J Am Coll Cardiol* 2006;48(12):2584-2591.
99. Iakovou I, Schmidt T, Bonizzoni E, et al. Incidence, predictors, and outcome of thrombosis after successful implantation of drug-eluting stents. *JAMA* 2005;293(17):2126-2130.
100. van Werkum JW, Heestermans AA, Somer AC, et al. Predictors of coronary stent thrombosis: the Dutch Stent Thrombosis Registry. *J Am Coll Cardiol* 2009;53(16): 1399-1409.
101. Spertus JA, Kettelkamp R, Vance C, et al. Prevalence, predictors, and outcomes of premature discontinuation of thienopyridine therapy after drug-eluting stent placement: results from the PREMIER registry. *Circulation* 2006;113(24):2803-2809.
102. Airoldi F, Colombo A, Morici N, et al. Incidence and predictors of drug-eluting stent thrombosis during and after discontinuation of thienopyridine treatment. *Circulation* 2007;116(7):745-754.
103. Kaiser C, Galatius S, Erne P, et al; BASKET-PROVE Study Group. Drug-eluting versus bare-metal stents in large coronary arteries. *N Engl J Med* 2010;363(24):2310-2319.
104. Nordmann AJ, Briel M, Bucher HC. Mortality in randomized controlled trials comparing drug-eluting vs. bare metal stents in coronary artery disease: a meta-analysis. *Eur Heart J* 2006;27(23):2784-2814.
105. Camenzind E, Steg PG, Wijns W. Stent thrombosis late after implantation of first-generation drug-eluting stents: a cause for concern. *Circulation* 2007;115(11):1440-1455; discussion 1455.
106. Lagerqvist B, James SK, Stenestrand U, et al; SCAAR Study Group. Long-term outcomes with drug-eluting stents versus bare-metal stents in Sweden. *N Engl J Med* 2007;356(10): 1009-1019.
107. Spaulding C, Daemen J, Boersma E, Cutlip DE, et al. A pooled analysis of data comparing sirolimus-eluting stents with bare-metal stents. *N Engl J Med* 2007;356(10): 989-997.
108. James SK, Wallentin L, Lagerqvist B. The SCAAR-scare in perspective. *EuroIntervention* 2009;5(4):501-504.
109. Kastrati A, Mehilli J, Pache J, et al. Analysis of 14 trials comparing sirolimus-eluting stents with bare-metal stents. *N Engl J Med* 2007;356(10):1030-1039.
110. De Luca G, Stone GW, Suryapranata H, et al. Efficacy and safety of drug-eluting stents in ST-segment elevation myocardial infarction: a meta-analysis of randomized trials. *Int J Cardiol* 2009;133(2):213-222.

111. Roukoz H, Bavry AA, Sarkees ML, et al. Comprehensive meta-analysis on drug-eluting stents versus bare-metal stents during extended follow-up. *Am J Med* 2009;122(6):581, e1-e10.
112. James SK, Stenestrand U, Lindbäck J, et al; SCAAR Study Group. Long-term safety and efficacy of drug-eluting versus bare-metal stents in Sweden. *N Engl J Med* 2009;360(19):1933-1945.
113. Brar SS, Kim J, Brar SK, et al. Long-term outcomes by clopidogrel duration and stent type in a diabetic population with de novo coronary artery lesions. *J Am Coll Cardiol* 2008;51(23):2220-2227.
114. Serruys PW, Daemen J. Are drug-eluting stents associated with a higher rate of late thrombosis than bare metal stents? Late stent thrombosis: a nuisance in both bare metal and drug-eluting stents. *Circulation* 2007;115(11):1433-1439; discussion 1439.
115. Mauri L, Hsieh WH, Massaro JM, et al. Stent thrombosis in randomized clinical trials of drug-eluting stents. *N Engl J Med* 2007;356(10):1020-1029.
116. Bavry AA, Kumbhani DJ, Helton TJ, et al. Late thrombosis of drug-eluting stents: a meta-analysis of randomized clinical trials. *Am J Med* 2006;119(12):1056-1061.
117. Daemen J, Wenaweser P, Tsuchida K, et al. Early and late coronary stent thrombosis of sirolimus-eluting and paclitaxel-eluting stents in routine clinical practice: data from a large two-institutional cohort study. *Lancet* 2007;369(9562):667-678.
118. Wenaweser P, Daemen J, Zwahlen M, et al. Incidence and correlates of drug-eluting stent thrombosis in routine clinical practice: 4-year results from a large 2-institutional cohort study. *J Am Coll Cardiol* 2008;52(14):1134-1140.
119. Lasala JM, Cox DA, Dobies, D, et al; ARRIVE 1 and ARRIVE 2 Participating Physicians. Drug-eluting stent thrombosis in routine clinical practice: two-year outcomes and predictors from the TAXUS ARRIVE registries. *Circ Cardiovasc Interv* 2009; 2(4):285-293.
120. Joner M, Finn AV, Farb A, et al. Pathology of drug-eluting stents in humans: delayed healing and late thrombotic risk. *J Am Coll Cardiol* 2006;48(1):193-202.
121. Farb A, Burke AP, Kolodgie FD, Virmani R. Pathological mechanisms of fatal late coronary stent thrombosis in humans. *Circulation* 2003;108(14):1701-1706.
122. Finn AV, Joner M, Nakazawa G, et al. Pathological correlates of late drug-eluting stent thrombosis: strut coverage as a marker of endothelialization. *Circulation* 2007;115(18): 2435-2441.
123. Ong AT, McFadden EP, Regar E, et al. Late angiographic stent thrombosis (LAST) events with drug-eluting stents. *J Am Coll Cardiol* 2005;45(12):2088-2092.
124. Virmani R, Guagliumi G, Farb A, et al. Localized hypersensitivity and late coronary thrombosis secondary to a sirolimus-eluting stent: should we be cautious? *Circulation* 2004;109(6):701-705.
125. Nebeker JR, Virmani R, Bennett CL, et al. Hypersensitivity cases associated with drug-eluting coronary stents: a review of available cases from the Research on Adverse Drug Events and Reports (RADAR) project. *J Am Coll Cardiol* 2006;47(1):175-181.
126. Nakazawa G, Ladich E, Finn AV, Virmani R. Pathophysiology of vascular healing and stent mediated arterial injury. *EuroIntervention* 2008;(4 Suppl C):C7-C10.
127. Fujii K, Carlier SG, Mintz GS, et al. Stent underexpansion and residual reference segment stenosis are related to stent thrombosis after sirolimus-eluting stent implantation: an intravascular ultrasound study. *J Am Coll Cardiol* 2005;45(7):995-998.
128. Alfonso F, Suárez A, Pérez-Vizcayno MJ, et al. Intravascular ultrasound findings during episodes of drug-eluting stent thrombosis. *J Am Coll Cardiol* 2007;50(21):2095-2097.
129. Schulz S, Schuster T, Mehilli J, et al. Stent thrombosis after drug-eluting stent implantation: incidence, timing, and relation to discontinuation of clopidogrel therapy over a 4-year period. *Eur Heart J* 2009;30(22):2714-2721.
130. Kimura T, Morimoto T, Nakagawa Y, et al; j-Cypher Registry Investigators. Antiplatelet therapy and stent thrombosis after sirolimus-eluting stent implantation. *Circulation* 2009;119(7):987-995.
131. Eisenstein EL, Anstrom KJ, Kong DF, et al. Clopidogrel use and long-term clinical outcomes after drug-eluting stent implantation. *JAMA* 2007;297(2):159-168.
132. Tanzilli G, Greco C, Pelliccia F, et al. Effectiveness of two-year clopidogrel + aspirin in abolishing the risk of very late thrombosis after drug-eluting stent implantation (from the TYCOON [two-year ClOpidOgrel need] study). *Am J Cardiol* 2009;104(10): 1357-1361.
133. Park SJ, Park DW, Kim YH, et al. Duration of dual antiplatelet therapy after implantation of drug-eluting stents. *N Engl J Med* 2010;362(15):1374-1382.
134. Byrne RA, Schulz S, Mehilli J, et al. Rationale and design of a randomized, double-blind, placebo-controlled trial of 6 versus 12 months clopidogrel therapy after implantation of a drug-eluting stent: The Intracoronary Stenting and Antithrombotic Regimen: Safety And EFficacy of 6 Months Dual Antiplatelet Therapy After Drug-Eluting Stenting (ISAR-SAFE) study. *Am Heart J* 2009;157(4):620-624, e2.
135. Mauri L. Updates from ongoing DAPT studies: United States: DAPT randomized trial. *Transcatheter Cardiovascular Therapeutics*. San Francisco, CA, 2009.
136. Garg P, Cohen DJ, Gaziano T, Mauri L. Balancing the risks of restenosis and stent thrombosis in bare-metal versus drug-eluting stents: results of a decision analytic model. *J Am Coll Cardiol* 2008;51(19):1844-1853.
137. Stolker JM, Kennedy KF, Lindsey JB, et al; EVENT Investigators. Predicting restenosis of drug-eluting stents placed in real-world clinical practice: derivation and validation of a risk model from the EVENT registry. *Circ Cardiovasc Interv* 2010;3(4):327-334.
138. Tu JV, Bowen J, Chiu M, et al. Effectiveness and safety of drug-eluting stents in Ontario. *N Engl J Med* 2007;357(14):1393-1402.
139. Yeh RW, Normand SL, Wolf RE, et al. Predicting the restenosis benefit of drug-eluting versus bare metal stents in percutaneous coronary intervention. *Circulation* 2011;124(14): 1557-1564.
140. Kastrati A, Mehilli J, Dirschinger J, et al. Intracoronary stenting and angiographic results: strut thickness effect on restenosis outcome (ISAR-STEREO) trial. *Circulation* 2001;103(23): 2816-2821.
141. Pache J, Kastrati A, Mehilli J, et al. Intracoronary stenting and angiographic results: strut thickness effect on restenosis outcome (ISAR-STEREO-2) trial. *J Am Coll Cardiol* 2003;41(8):1283-1288.
142. Meredith I. PROMUS Element: First report of the QCA and IVUS study results. *Transcatheter Cardiovascular Therapeutics,* Washington, DC, 2010.
143. Cannon LA, Kereiakes DJ, Mann T, et al. A prospective evaluation of the safety and efficacy of TAXUS Element paclitaxel-eluting coronary stent implantation for the treatment of de novo coronary artery lesions in small vessels: the PERSEUS Small Vessel trial. *EuroIntervention* 2011;6(8):920-927, 921-922.
144. Ormiston JA, Serruys PW, Regar E, et al. A bioabsorbable everolimus-eluting coronary stent system for patients with single de-novo coronary artery lesions (ABSORB): a prospective open-label trial. *Lancet* 2008;371(9616):899-907.
145. Serruys PW, Ormiston JA, Onuma Y, et al. A bioabsorbable everolimus-eluting coronary stent system (ABSORB): 2-year outcomes and results from multiple imaging methods. *Lancet* 2009;373(9667):897-910.
146. Fujiyama S, Amano K, Uehira K, et al. Bone marrow monocyte lineage cells adhere on injured endothelium in a monocyte chemoattractant protein-1-dependent manner and accelerate reendothelialization as endothelial progenitor cells. *Circ Res* 2003; 93(10):980-989.
147. Windecker S, Mayer I, De Pasquale G, et al; Working Group on Novel Surface Coating of Biomedical Devices (SCOL). Stent coating with titanium-nitride-oxide for reduction of neointimal hyperplasia. *Circulation* 2001;104(8):928-933.
148. Finn AV, Kolodgie FD, Harnek J, et al. Differential response of delayed healing and persistent inflammation at sites of overlapping sirolimus- or paclitaxel-eluting stents. *Circulation* 2005;112(2):270-278.
149. Finn AV, Nakazawa G, Joner M, et al. Vascular responses to drug eluting stents: importance of delayed healing. *Arterioscler Thromb Vasc Biol* 2007;27(7):1500-1510.
150. Meredith IT, Worthley S, Whitbourn R, et al. The next-generation Endeavor Resolute stent: 4-month clinical and angiographic results from the Endeavor Resolute first-in-man trial. *EuroIntervention* 2007;3(1):50-53.
151. Udipi K, Melder RJ, Chen M, et al. The next generation Endeavor Resolute Stent: role of the BioLinx *Polymer System. EuroIntervention* 2007;3(1):137-139.
152. Meredith IT, Worthley S, Whitbourn R, et al; RESOLUTE Investigators. Clinical and angiographic results with the next-generation resolute stent system: a prospective, multicenter, first-in-human trial. *JACC Cardiovasc Interv* 2009;2(10):977-985.
153. Meredith IT, Worthley SG, Whitbourn R, et al. Long-term clinical outcomes with the next-generation Resolute Stent System: a report of the two-year follow-up from the RESOLUTE clinical trial. *EuroIntervention* 2010;5(6):692-697.
154. Serruys PW, Silber S, Garg S, et al. Comparison of zotarolimus-eluting and everolimus-eluting coronary stents. *N Engl J Med* 2010;363(2):136-146.
155. Ostojic M, Sagic D, Beleslin B, et al. First clinical comparison of Nobori-Biolimus A9 eluting stents with Cypher-Sirolimus eluting stents: Nobori Core nine months angiographic and one year clinical outcomes. *EuroIntervention* 2008;3(5):574-579.
156. Chevalier B, Silber S, Park SJ, et al; NOBORI 1 Clinical Investigators. Randomized comparison of the Nobori Biolimus A9-eluting coronary stent with the Taxus Liberte paclitaxel-eluting coronary stent in patients with stenosis in native coronary arteries: the NOBORI 1 trial—Phase 2. *Circ Cardiovasc Interv* 2009;2(3):188-195.
157. Garg S, Sarno G, Serruys PW, et al. The twelve-month outcomes of a biolimus eluting stent with a biodegradable polymer compared with a sirolimus eluting stent with a durable polymer. *EuroIntervention* 2010;6(2):233-239.
158. Rutsch W. Multi-center first-in-man study with the lowest known limus dose on the Elixir Medical myolimus-eluting coronary stent system with a durable polymer: nine-month clinical and six-month angiographic and IVUS follow-up. EuroPCR, Barcelona, Spain, 2009.
159. Schofer J. Multicentre, first-in-man study on the Elixir Myolimus-eluting coronary stent system with bioabsorbable polymer: 12-month clinical and angiographic/IVUS results. EuroPCR, Paris, 2010.
160. Grube E, Schofer J, Hauptmann KE, et al. A novel paclitaxel-eluting stent with an ultrathin abluminal biodegradable polymer 9-month outcomes with the JACTAX HD stent. *JACC Cardiovasc Interv* 2010;3(4):431-438.
161. Lemos PA, et al. Randomized evaluation of two drug-eluting stents with identical metallic platform and biodegradable polymer but different agents (paclitaxel or sirolimus) compared against bare stents: 1-year results of the PAINT trial. *Catheter Cardiovasc Interv* 2009;74(5):665-773.
162. Dawkins K. The element stent technology. *EuroPCR*, Paris, 2010.
163. Han Y, Jing Q, Xu B, et al; CREATE Investigators. Safety and efficacy of biodegradable polymer-coated sirolimus-eluting stents in "real-world" practice: 18-month clinical and 9-month angiographic outcomes. *JACC Cardiovasc Interv* 2009;2(4):303-309.
164. Ormiston JA, Abizaid A, Spertus J, et al; NEVO ResElution-I Investigators. Six-month results of the NEVO Res-Elution I (NEVO RES-I) trial: a randomized, multicenter comparison of the NEVO sirolimus-eluting coronary stent with the TAXUS Liberte paclitaxel-eluting stent in de novo native coronary artery lesions. *Circ Cardiovasc Interv* 2010; 3(6):556-564.
165. Scheller B, Hehrlein C, Bocksch W, et al. Treatment of coronary in-stent restenosis with a paclitaxel-coated balloon catheter. *N Engl J Med* 2006;355(20):2113-2124.
166. Scheller B, Hehrlein C, Bocksch W, et al. Two year follow-up after treatment of coronary in-stent restenosis with a paclitaxel-coated balloon catheter. *Clin Res Cardiol* 2008; 97(10):773-781.
167. Unverdorben M, Vellbracht C, Cremers B, et al. Paclitaxel-coated balloon catheter versus paclitaxel-coated stent for the treatment of coronary in-stent restenosis. *Circulation* 2009;119(23):2986-2994.
168. Herdeg C, Göhring-Frischholz K, Haase KK, et al. Catheter-based delivery of fluid paclitaxel for prevention of restenosis in native coronary artery lesions after stent implantation. *Circ Cardiovasc Interv* 2009;2(4):294-301.
169. Hamm C. Paclitaxel-eluting PTCA balloon in combination with the Coroflex Blue stent vs. the sirolimus-coated Cypher stent in the treatment of advanced coronary artery disease. American Heart Association Scientific Sessions, Orlando, FL, 2009.
170. Cortese B, Micheli A, Picchi A, et al. Paclitaxel-coated balloon versus drug-eluting stent during PCI of small coronary vessels, a prospective randomised clinical trial. The PICCOLETO study. *Heart* 2010;96(16):1291-1296.
171. Lee MS, Park SJ, Kandzari DE, et al. Saphenous vein graft intervention. *JACC Cardiovasc Interv* 2011;4(8):831-843.

172. Brilakis ES, Saeed B, Banerjee S. Drug-eluting stents in saphenous vein graft interventions: a systematic review. *EuroIntervention* 2010;5(6):722-730.
173. Vermeersch P, Agostoni P, Verheye S, et al. Randomized double-blind comparison of sirolimus-eluting stent versus bare-metal stent implantation in diseased saphenous vein grafts: six-month angiographic, intravascular ultrasound, and clinical follow-up of the RRISC Trial. *J Am Coll Cardiol* 2006;48(12):2423-2431.
174. Vermeersch P, Agostoni P, Verheye S, et al. Increased late mortality after sirolimus-eluting stents versus bare-metal stents in diseased saphenous vein grafts: results from the randomized DELAYED RRISC Trial. *J Am Coll Cardiol* 2007;50(3):261-267.
175. Ge L, Iakovou I, Sangiorgi GM, et al. Treatment of saphenous vein graft lesions with drug-eluting stents: immediate and midterm outcome. *J Am Coll Cardiol* 2005;45(7):989-994.
176. Lee MS, Shah AP, Aragon J, et al. Drug-eluting stenting is superior to bare metal stenting in saphenous vein grafts. *Catheter Cardiovasc Interv* 2005;66(4):507-511.
177. Hoffmann R, Pohl T, Köster R, et al. Implantation of paclitaxel-eluting stents in saphenous vein grafts: clinical and angiographic follow-up results from a multicentre study. *Heart* 2007;93(3):331-334.
178. Applegate RJ, Sacrinty M, Kutcher M, et al. Late outcomes of drug-eluting versus bare metal stents in saphenous vein grafts: propensity score analysis. *Catheter Cardiovasc Interv* 2008;72(1):7-12.
179. Brodie BR, Wilson H, Stuckey T, et al. Outcomes with drug-eluting versus bare-metal stents in saphenous vein graft intervention results from the STENT (strategic transcatheter evaluation of new therapies) group. *JACC Cardiovasc Interv* 2009;2(11):1105-1112.
180. Mehilli J, Pache J, Abdel-Wahab M, et al; ISAR-CABG Investigators. Drug-eluting versus bare-metal stents in saphenous vein graft lesions (ISAR-CABG): a randomised controlled superiority trial. *Lancet* 2011;378(9796):1071-1078.
181. Mak KH, Challapalli R, Eisenberg MJ, et al. Effect of platelet glycoprotein IIb/IIIa receptor inhibition on distal embolization during percutaneous revascularization of aortocoronary saphenous vein grafts. EPIC Investigators. Evaluation of IIb/IIIa platelet receptor antagonist 7E3 in Preventing Ischemic Complications. *Am J Cardiol* 1997;80(8):985-988.
182. Roffi M, Mukherjee D, Chew DP, et al. Lack of benefit from intravenous platelet glycoprotein IIb/IIIa receptor inhibition as adjunctive treatment for percutaneous interventions of aortocoronary bypass grafts: a pooled analysis of five randomized clinical trials. *Circulation* 2002;106(24):3063-3067.
183. Baim DS, Wahr D, George B, et al; SAFER Trial Investigators. Randomized trial of a distal embolic protection device during percutaneous intervention of saphenous vein aorto-coronary bypass grafts. *Circulation* 2002;105(11):1285-1290.
184. Kereiakes DJ, Turco MA, Breall J, et al; AMERthyst Study Investigators. A novel filter-based distal embolic protection device for percutaneous intervention of saphenous vein graft lesions: results of the AMEthyst randomized controlled trial. *JACC Cardiovasc Interv* 2008;1(3):248-257.
185. Halkin A, Masud AZ, Rogers C, et al. Six-month outcomes after percutaneous intervention for lesions in aortocoronary saphenous vein grafts using distal protection devices: results from the FIRE trial. *Am Heart J* 2006;151(4):915, e1-e7.
186. Stone GW, Rogers C, Hermiller, J, et al; FilterWire EX Randomized Evaluation Investigators. Randomized comparison of distal protection with a filter-based catheter and a balloon occlusion and aspiration system during percutaneous intervention of diseased saphenous vein aorto-coronary bypass grafts. *Circulation* 2003;108(5):548-553.
187. Mauri L, Cox D, Hermiller J, et al. The PROXIMAL trial: proximal protection during saphenous vein graft intervention using the Proxis Embolic Protection System: a randomized, prospective, multicenter clinical trial. *J Am Coll Cardiol* 2007;50(15):1442-1449.
188. Stone GW, Reifart NJ, Moussa I, et al. Percutaneous recanalization of chronically occluded coronary arteries: a consensus document: part II. *Circulation* 2005;112(16):2530-2537.
189. Olivari Z, Rubartelli P, Piscione F, et al; TOAST-GISE Investigators. Immediate results and one-year clinical outcome after percutaneous coronary interventions in chronic total occlusions: data from a multicenter, prospective, observational study (TOAST-GISE). *J Am Coll Cardiol* 2003;41(10):1672-1678.
190. Suero JA, Marso SP, Jones PG, et al. Procedural outcomes and long-term survival among patients undergoing percutaneous coronary intervention of a chronic total occlusion in native coronary arteries: a 20-year experience. *J Am Coll Cardiol* 2001;38(2):409-414.
191. Hoye A, van Domburg RT, Sonnenschein K, Surrys PW. Percutaneous coronary intervention for chronic total occlusions: the Thoraxcenter experience 1992-2002. *Eur Heart J* 2005;26(24):2630-2636.
192. Valenti R, Migliorini A, Signorini U, et al. Impact of complete revascularization with percutaneous coronary intervention on survival in patients with at least one chronic total occlusion. *Eur Heart J* 2008;29(19):2336-2342.
193. Chung CM, Nakamura S, Tanaka K, et al. Effect of recanalization of chronic total occlusions on global and regional left ventricular function in patients with or without previous myocardial infarction. *Catheter Cardiovasc Interv* 2003;60(3):368-374.
194. Cheng AS, Selvanayagam JB, Jerosch-Herold M, et al. Percutaneous treatment of chronic total coronary occlusions improves regional hyperemic myocardial blood flow and contractility: insights from quantitative cardiovascular magnetic resonance imaging. *JACC Cardiovasc Interv* 2008;1(1):44-53.
195. Jayasinghe R, Paul V, Rajendran S. A universal classification system for chronic total occlusions. *J Invasive Cardiol* 2008;20(6):302-304.
196. Suttorp MJ, Laarman GJ, Rahel BM, et al. Primary Stenting of Totally Occluded Native Coronary Arteries II (PRISON II): a randomized comparison of bare metal stent implantation with sirolimus-eluting stent implantation for the treatment of total coronary occlusions. *Circulation* 2006;114(9):921-928.
197. Rahel BM, Laarman GJ, Kelder JC, et al. Three-year clinical outcome after primary stenting of totally occluded native coronary arteries: a randomized comparison of bare-metal stent implantation with sirolimus-eluting stent implantation for the treatment of total coronary occlusions (Primary Stenting of Totally Occluded Native Coronary Arteries [PRISON] II study). *Am Heart J* 2009;157(1):149-155.
198. Rubartelli P, Petronio AS, Guiducci V, et al. Gruppo Italiano di Studio sullo Stent nelle Occlusioni Coronariche II GISE Ingestigators. Comparison of sirolimus-eluting and bare metal stent for treatment of patients with total coronary occlusions: results of the GISSOC II-GISE multicentre randomized trial. *Eur Heart J* 2010;31(16):2014-2020.
199. Werner GS, Krack A, Schwarz G, et al. Prevention of lesion recurrence in chronic total coronary occlusions by paclitaxel-eluting stents. *J Am Coll Cardiol* 2004;44(12): 2301-2306.
200. Nakamura S, Muthusamy TS, Bae JH, et al. Impact of sirolimus-eluting stent on the outcome of patients with chronic total occlusions. *Am J Cardiol* 2005;95(2):161-166.
201. Colmenarez HJ, Escaned J, Fernández C, et al. Efficacy and safety of drug-eluting stents in chronic total coronary occlusion recanalization: a systematic review and meta-analysis. *J Am Coll Cardiol* 2010;55(17):1854-1866.
202. Steigen TK, Maeng M, Wiseth R, et al; Nordic PCI Study Group. Randomized study on simple versus complex stenting of coronary artery bifurcation lesions: the Nordic bifurcation study. *Circulation* 2006;114(18):1955-1961.
203. Tsuchida K, Colombo A, Lefèvre T, et al. The clinical outcome of percutaneous treatment of bifurcation lesions in multivessel coronary artery disease with the sirolimus-eluting stent: insights from the Arterial Revascularization Therapies Study part II (ARTS II). *Eur Heart J* 2007;28(4):433-442.
204. Colombo A, Moses JW, Morice MC, et al. Randomized study to evaluate sirolimus-eluting stents implanted at coronary bifurcation lesions. *Circulation* 2004;109(10):1244-1249.
205. Pan M, de Lezo JS, Medina A, et al. Rapamycin-eluting stents for the treatment of bifurcated coronary lesions: a randomized comparison of a simple versus complex strategy. *Am Heart J* 2004;148(5):857-864.
206. Ferenc M, Gick M, Kienzle RP, et al. Randomized trial on routine vs. provisional T-stenting in the treatment of de novo coronary bifurcation lesions. *Eur Heart J* 2008;29(23): 2859-2867.
207. Zhang F, Dong L, Ge J. Simple versus complex stenting strategy for coronary artery bifurcation lesions in the drug-eluting stent era: a meta-analysis of randomised trials. *Heart* 2009;95(20):1676-1681.
208. Solar RJ. The Y Med sidekick stent delivery system for the treatment of coronary bifurcation and ostial lesions. *Cardiovascular Revascularization Therapies,* Washington, DC, 2007.
209. Lefèvre T, Ormiston J, Guagliumi G, et al. The Frontier stent registry: safety and feasibility of a novel dedicated stent for the treatment of bifurcation coronary artery lesions. *J Am Coll Cardiol* 2005;46(4):592-598.
210. Lefevre, T. Invatec twin rail bifurcation stent. Transcatheter Cardiovascular Therapeutics. Washington, DC, 2005.
211. Ormiston J, Webster M. El-Jack S, et al. The AST petal dedicated bifurcation stent: first-in-human experience. *Catheter Cardiovasc Interv* 2007;70(3):335-340.
212. Kaplan AV, Ramcharitar S, Louvard Y, et al. Tryton I, First-In-Man (FIM) Study: acute and 30 day outcome. A preliminary report. *EuroIntervention* 2007;3(1):54-59.
213. Costa RA. Preliminary results of the novel TMI (TriReme Medical Inc) Antares side branch adaptive system (Antares SAS Stent) for the treatment of de novo coronary bifurcation lesions - SCAI-ACCi2 Interventional E-Abstract 2900-123. *J Am Coll Cardiol* 2008;51:B51.
214. Doi H, Maehara A, Mintz GS, et al. Serial intravascular ultrasound analysis of bifurcation lesions treated using the novel self-expanding sideguard side branch stent. *Am J Cardiol* 2009;104(9):1216-1221.
215. Radner S. Thoracal aortography by catheterization from the radial artery; preliminary report of a new technique. *Acta Radiol* 1948;29(2):178-180.
216. Jolly SS, Amlani S, Hamon M, et al. Radial versus femoral access for coronary angiography or intervention and the impact on major bleeding and ischemic events: a systematic review and meta-analysis of randomized trials. *Am Heart J* 2009;157(1):132-140.
217. Spaulding C, Lefèvre T, Funck F, et al. Left radial approach for coronary angiography: results of a prospective study. *Cathet Cardiovasc Diagn* 1996;39(4):365-370.
218. Jolly SS, Yusuf S, Cairns J, et al; RIVAL trial group. Radial versus femoral access for coronary angiography and intervention in patients with acute coronary syndromes (RIVAL): a randomised, parallel group, multicentre trial. *Lancet* 2011;377(9775):1409-1420.
219. Kantrowitz A, Tjonneland S, Freed PS, et al. Initial clinical experience with intraaortic balloon pumping in cardiogenic shock. *JAMA* 1968;203(2):113-118.
220. Kovack PJ, Rasak MA, Bates ER, et al. Thrombolysis plus aortic counterpulsation: improved survival in patients who present to community hospitals with cardiogenic shock. *J Am Coll Cardiol* 1997;29(7):1454-1458.
221. Barron HV, Every NR, Parsons LS, et al; Investigators in the National Registry of Myocardial Infarction 2. The use of intra-aortic balloon counterpulsation in patients with cardiogenic shock complicating acute myocardial infarction: data from the National Registry of Myocardial Infarction 2. *Am Heart J* 2001;141(6):933-939.
222. Sjauw KD, Engström AE, Vis MM, et al. A systematic review and meta-analysis of intra-aortic balloon pump therapy in ST-elevation myocardial infarction: should we change the guidelines? *Eur Heart J* 2009;30(4):459-468.
223. Antman EM, Anbe DT, Armstrong PW, et al; American College of Cardiology; American Heart Association Task Force on Practice Guidelines; Canadian Cardiovascular Society. ACC/AHA guidelines for the management of patients with ST-elevation myocardial infarction: a report of the American College of Cardiology/American Heart Association Task Force on Practice Guidelines (Committee to Revise the 1999 Guidelines for the Management of Patients with Acute Myocardial Infarction). *Circulation* 2004;110(9): e82-e292.
224. Brodie BR, Stuckey TD, Hansen C, Muncy D. Intra-aortic balloon counterpulsation before primary percutaneous transluminal coronary angioplasty reduces catheterization laboratory events in high-risk patients with acute myocardial infarction. *Am J Cardiol* 1999;84(1):18-23.
225. Briguori C, Sarais C, Pagnotta P, et al. Elective versus provisional intra-aortic balloon pumping in high-risk percutaneous transluminal coronary angioplasty. *Am Heart J* 2003;145(4):700-707.
226. Mishra S, Chu WW, Torguson R, et al. Role of prophylactic intra-aortic balloon pump in high-risk patients undergoing percutaneous coronary intervention. *Am J Cardiol* 2006;98(5):608-612.
227. Patel MR, Smalling RW, Thiele H, et al. Intra-aortic balloon counterpulsation and infarct size in patients with acute anterior myocardial infarction without shock: the CRISP AMI randomized trial. *JAMA* 2011;306(12):1329-1337.

228. Thiele H, Sick P, Boudriot E, et al. Randomized comparison of intra-aortic balloon support with a percutaneous left ventricular assist device in patients with revascularized acute myocardial infarction complicated by cardiogenic shock. *Eur Heart J* 2005;26(13): 1276-1283.
229. Burkhoff D, Cohen H, Brunckhorst C, O'Neill WW; TandemHeart Investigators. A randomized multicenter clinical study to evaluate the safety and efficacy of the TandemHeart percutaneous ventricular assist device versus conventional therapy with intraaortic balloon pumping for treatment of cardiogenic shock. *Am Heart J* 2006;152(3):469, e1-e8.
230. Seyfarth M, Sibbing D, Bauer I, et al. A randomized clinical trial to evaluate the safety and efficacy of a percutaneous left ventricular assist device versus intra-aortic balloon pumping for treatment of cardiogenic shock caused by myocardial infarction. *J Am Coll Cardiol* 2008;52(19):1584-1588.
231. Dixon SR, Henriques JP, Mauri L, et al. A prospective feasibility trial investigating the use of the Impella 2.5 system in patients undergoing high-risk percutaneous coronary intervention (The PROTECT I Trial): initial U.S. experience. *JACC Cardiovasc Interv* 2009;2(2):91-96.
232. Topol EJ, Nissen SE. Our preoccupation with coronary luminology: the dissociation between clinical and angiographic findings in ischemic heart disease. *Circulation* 1995;92(8):2333-2342.
233. Fischer JJ, Samady H, McPherson JA, et al. Comparison between visual assessment and quantitative angiography versus fractional flow reserve for native coronary narrowings of moderate severity. *Am J Cardiol* 2002;90(3):210-215.
234. Stone GW, Hodgson JM, St Goar FB, et al. Improved procedural results of coronary angioplasty with intravascular ultrasound-guided balloon sizing: the CLOUT Pilot Trial. Clinical Outcomes With Ultrasound Trial (CLOUT) Investigators. *Circulation* 1997;95(8): 2044-2052.
235. de Jaegere P, Mudra H, Figulla H, et al. Intravascular ultrasound-guided optimized stent deployment. Immediate and 6 months clinical and angiographic results from the Multicenter Ultrasound Stenting in Coronaries Study (MUSIC Study). *Eur Heart J* 1998;19(8):1214-1223.
236. Castagna MT, Mintz GS, Leiboff BO, et al. The contribution of "mechanical" problems to in-stent restenosis: an intravascular ultrasonographic analysis of 1090 consecutive in-stent restenosis lesions. *Am Heart J* 2001;142(6):970-974.
237. Jang IK, Tearney GJ, MacNeill B, et al. In vivo characterization of coronary atherosclerotic plaque by use of optical coherence tomography. *Circulation* 2005;111(12):1551-1555.
238. Pijls NH, Van Gelder B, Van der Voort P, et al. Fractional flow reserve: a useful index to evaluate the influence of an epicardial coronary stenosis on myocardial blood flow. *Circulation* 1995;92(11):3183-3193.
239. Pijls NH, De Bruyne B, Peels K, et al. Measurement of fractional flow reserve to assess the functional severity of coronary-artery stenoses. *N Engl J Med* 1996;334(26):1703-1708.
240. De Bruyne B, Pijls NH, Bartunek J, et al. Fractional flow reserve in patients with prior myocardial infarction. *Circulation* 2001;104(2):157-162.
241. Tonino PA, De Bruyne B, Pijls NH, et al. Fractional flow reserve versus angiography for guiding percutaneous coronary intervention. *N Engl J Med* 2009;360(3):213-224.
242. Pijls NH, Fearon WF, Tonino PA, et al; FAME Study Investigators. Fractional flow reserve versus angiography for guiding percutaneous coronary intervention in patients with multivessel coronary artery disease: 2-year follow-up of the FAME (Fractional Flow Reserve Versus Angiography for Multivessel Evaluation) study. *J Am Coll Cardiol* 2010;56(3):177-184.
243. Hoff SJ. Off-pump coronary artery bypass: techniques, pitfalls, and results. *Semin Thorac Cardiovasc Surg* 2009;21(3):213-223.
244. Reference deleted in proofs.
245. Nwaejike N, Mansha M, Bonde P, Campalani G. Myocardial revascularization by off pump coronary bypass surgery (OPCABG): a ten year review. *Ulster Med J* 2008;77(2):106-109.
246. MacGillivray TE, Vlahakes GJ. Patency and the pump—the risks and benefits of off-pump CABG. *N Engl J Med* 2004;350(1):3-4.
247. Halkos ME, Puskas JD. Off-pump versus on-pump coronary artery bypass grafting. *Surg Clin North Am* 2009;89(4):913-922, ix.
248. Sedrakyan A, Wu AW, Parashar A, et al. Off-pump surgery is associated with reduced occurrence of stroke and other morbidity as compared with traditional coronary artery bypass grafting: a meta-analysis of systematically reviewed trials. *Stroke* 2006; 37(11):2759-2769.
249. Møller CH, Penninga L, Wetterslev J, et al. Clinical outcomes in randomized trials of off- vs. on-pump coronary artery bypass surgery: systematic review with meta-analyses and trial sequential analyses. *Eur Heart J* 2008;29(21):2601-2616.
250. Shroyer AL, Grover FL, Hattler B, et al; Veterans Affairs Randomized On/Off Bypass (ROOBY) Study Group. On-pump versus off-pump coronary-artery bypass surgery. *N Engl J Med* 2009;361(19):1827-1837.
251. Cheng DC, Martin J, Novick RJ. OPCAB surgery versus on-pump surgery: the beat goes on. *Innovations (Phila)* 2010;5(2):67-69.
252. Puskas JD, Mack MJ, Smith CR. On-pump versus off-pump CABG. *N Engl J Med* 2010;362(9):851; author reply 853-854.
253. Peterson ED. Innovation and comparative-effectiveness research in cardiac surgery. *N Engl J Med* 2009;361(19):1897-1899.
254. DeRose JJ. Current state of integrated "hybrid" coronary revascularization. *Semin Thorac Cardiovasc Surg* 2009;21(3):229-236.
255. Sellke FW, Chu LM, Cohn WE. Current state of surgical myocardial revascularization. *Circ J* 2010;74(6):1031-1037.
256. Karpuzoglu OE, Ozay B, Sener T, et al. Comparison of minimally invasive direct coronary artery bypass and off-pump coronary artery bypass in single-vessel disease. *Heart Surg Forum* 2009;12(1):E39-E43.
257. Holzhey DM, Jacobs S, Mochalski M, et al. Seven-year follow-up after minimally invasive direct coronary artery bypass: experience with more than 1300 patients. *Ann Thorac Surg* 2007;83(1):108-114.
258. Jacobs S, Holzhey D, Walther T, et al. Redo minimally invasive direct coronary artery bypass grafting. *Ann Thorac Surg* 2005;80(4):1336-1339.
259. Vassiliades TA Jr, Reddy VS, Puskas JD, Guyton RA. Long-term results of the endoscopic atraumatic coronary artery bypass. *Ann Thorac Surg* 2007;83(3):979-984; discussion 984-985.
260. Weerasinghe A, Bahrami T. Bilateral MIDCAB for triple vessel coronary disease. *Interact Cardiovasc Thorac Surg* 2005;4(6):523-525.
261. McGinn JT Jr, Usman S, Lapierre H, et al. Minimally invasive coronary artery bypass grafting: dual-center experience in 450 consecutive patients. *Circulation* 2009;120(11 Suppl):S78-S84.
262. Guida MC, Pecora G, Bacalao A, et al. Multivessel revascularization on the beating heart by anterolateral left thoracotomy. *Ann Thorac Surg* 2006;81(6):2142-2146.
263. Lapierre H, Chan V, Ruel M. Off-pump coronary surgery through mini-incisions: is it reasonable? *Curr Opin Cardiol* 2006;21(6):578-583.
264. Robicsek F. Robotic cardiac surgery: time told! *J Thorac Cardiovasc Surg* 2008;135(2): 243-246.
265. Modi P, Rodriguez E, Chitwood WR Jr. Robot-assisted cardiac surgery. *Interact Cardiovasc Thorac Surg* 2009;9(3):500-505.
266. Martens TP, Argenziano M, Oz MC. New technology for surgical coronary revascularization. *Circulation* 2006;114(6):606-614.
267. Subramanian VA, Patel NU, Patel NC, Loulmet DF. Robotic assisted multivessel minimally invasive direct coronary artery bypass with port-access stabilization and cardiac positioning: paving the way for outpatient coronary surgery? *Ann Thorac Surg* 2005;79(5):1590-1596; discussion 1590-1596.
268. Srivastava S, Gadasalli S, Agusala M, et al. Use of bilateral internal thoracic arteries in CABG through lateral thoracotomy with robotic assistance in 150 patients. *Ann Thorac Surg* 2006;81(3):800-806; discussion 806.
269. Katz MR, Bonatti JO. Totally endoscopic coronary artery bypass grafting on the arrested heart. *Heart Surg Forum* 2007;10(4):E338-E343.
270. de Cannière D, Wimmer-Greinecker G, Cichon R, et al. Feasibility, safety, and efficacy of totally endoscopic coronary artery bypass grafting: multicenter European experience. *J Thorac Cardiovasc Surg* 2007;134(3):710-716.
271. Ak K, Wimmer-Greinecker G, Dzemali O, et al. Totally endoscopic sequential arterial coronary artery bypass grafting on the beating heart. *Can J Cardiol* 2007; 23(5):391-392.
272. Popma JJ, Nathan S, Hagberg RC, Khabbaz KR. Hybrid myocardial revascularization: an integrated approach to coronary revascularization. *Catheter Cardiovasc Interv* 2010;75(Suppl 1):S28-S34.
273. Kobayashi J. Radial artery as a graft for coronary artery bypass grafting. *Circ J* 2009;73(7):1178-1183.
274. Kurlansky P. Thirty-year experience with bilateral internal thoracic artery grafting: where have we been and where are we going? *World J Surg* 2010;34(4):646-651.
275. Jorapur V, Cano-Gomez A, Conde CA. Should saphenous vein grafts be the conduits of last resort for coronary artery bypass surgery? *Cardiol Rev* 2009;17(5):235-242.
276. Cohn LH. *Cardiac Surgery in the Adult*, 3rd ed. New York, 2008. McGraw–Hill, p 1704.
277. Damgaard S, Steinbruchel DA, Kjaergard HK. An update on internal mammary artery grafting for coronary artery disease. *Curr Opin Cardiol* 2005;20(6):521-524.
278. Sabik JF 3rd, Lytle BW, Blackstone EH, et al. Comparison of saphenous vein and internal thoracic artery graft patency by coronary system. *Ann Thorac Surg* 2005;79(2):544-551; discussion 544-551.
279. Hayward PA, Gordon IR, Hare DL, et al. Comparable patencies of the radial artery and right internal thoracic artery or saphenous vein beyond 5 years: results from the Radial Artery Patency and Clinical Outcomes trial. *J Thorac Cardiovasc Surg* 2010;139(1):60-65; discussion 65-67.
280. Kurlansky PA, Traad EA, Dorman MJ, et al. Thirty-year follow-up defines survival benefit for second internal mammary artery in propensity-matched groups. *Ann Thorac Surg* 2010;90(1):101-108.
281. Benedetto U, Angeloni E, Refice S, Sinatra R. Radial artery versus saphenous vein graft patency: meta-analysis of randomized controlled trials. *J Thorac Cardiovasc Surg* 2010;139(1):229-231.
282. Slaughter MS. The ideal conduit for surgical revascularization: the quest for the holy grail continues. *Circulation* 2010;122(9):857-858.
283. Fukui T, Tabata M, Manabe S, et al. Graft selection and one-year patency rates in patients undergoing coronary artery bypass grafting. *Ann Thorac Surg* 2010;89(6): 1901-1905.
284. Sasaki H. The right gastroepiploic artery in coronary artery bypass grafting. *J Card Surg* 2008;23(4):398-407.
285. Malvindi PG, Jacob K, Kallikourdis A, Vitale N. What is the patency of the gastroepiploic artery when used for coronary artery bypass grafting? *Interact Cardiovasc Thorac Surg* 2007;6(3):397-402.
286. Byrne JG, Leacche M, Vaughan DE, Zhao DX. Hybrid cardiovascular procedures. *JACC Cardiovasc Interv* 2008;1(5):459-468.
286a. Angelini GD, Wilde P, Salerno TA, et al. Integrated left small thoracotomy and angioplasty for multivessel coronary artery revascularisation. *Lancet* 1996;347(9003):757-758.
287. Byrne JG, Leacche M, Unic D, et al. Staged initial percutaneous coronary intervention followed by valve surgery ("hybrid approach") for patients with complex coronary and valve disease. *J Am Coll Cardiol* 2005;45(1):14-18.
288. Bonatti J, Schachner T, Bonaros N, et al. Simultaneous hybrid coronary revascularization using totally endoscopic left internal mammary artery bypass grafting and placement of rapamycin eluting stents in the same interventional session. The COMBINATION pilot study. *Cardiology* 2008;110(2):92-95.
289. Kon ZN, Brown EN, Tran R, et al. Simultaneous hybrid coronary revascularization reduces postoperative morbidity compared with results from conventional off-pump coronary artery bypass. *J Thorac Cardiovasc Surg* 2008;135(2):367-375.
290. Gilard M, Bezon E, Cornily JC, et al. Same-day combined percutaneous coronary intervention and coronary artery surgery. *Cardiology* 2007;108(4):363-367.
291. Meredith IT, Ormiston J, Whitbourn R, et al. First-in-human study of the Endeavor ABT-578-eluting phosphorylcholine-encapsulated stent system in de novo native coronary artery lesions: Endeavor I Trial. *EuroIntervention* 2005;1(2):157-164.

292. Fajadet J, Wijns W, Laarman GJ, et al; ENDEAVOR II Investigators. Randomized, double-blind, multicenter study of the Endeavor zotarolimus-eluting phosphorylcholine-encapsulated stent for treatment of native coronary artery lesions: clinical and angiographic results of the ENDEAVOR II trial. *Circulation* 2006;114(8):798-806.

293. Kandzari DE, Leon MB, Popma JJ, et al; ENDEAVOR III Investigators. Comparison of zotarolimus-eluting and sirolimus-eluting stents in patients with native coronary artery disease: a randomized controlled trial. *J Am Coll Cardiol* 2006;48(12):2440-2447.

294. Rasmussen K, Maeng M, Kaltoft A, et al; SORT OUT III study group. Efficacy and safety of zotarolimus-eluting and sirolimus-eluting coronary stents in routine clinical care (SORT OUT III): a randomised controlled superiority trial. *Lancet* 2010;375(9720):1090-1099.

295. Park DW, Kim YH, Yun SC, et al. Comparison of zotarolimus-eluting stents with sirolimus- and paclitaxel-eluting stents for coronary revascularization: the ZEST (comparison of the efficacy and safety of zotarolimus-eluting stent with sirolimus-eluting and paclitaxel-eluting stent for coronary lesions) randomized trial. *J Am Coll Cardiol* 2010;56(15):1187-1195.

296. Yeung AC, Leon MB, Jain A, et al; RESOLUTE US Investigators. Clinical evaluation of the Resolute zotarolimus-eluting coronary stent system in the treatment of de novo lesions in native coronary arteries: the RESOLUTE US clinical trial. *J Am Coll Cardiol* 2011;57(17):1778-1783.

297. Levine GN, Bates ER, Blankenship JC, et al. 2011 ACCF/AHA/SCAI Guideline for Percutaneous Coronary Intervention: a report of the American College of Cardiology Foundation/American Heart Association Task Force on Practice Guidelines and the Society for Cardiovascular Angiography and Interventions. *Circulation* 2011;124(23):e574-651.

298. Wijns W, Kolh P, Canchin N, et al; Task Force on Myocardial Revascularization of the European Society of Cardiology (ESC) and the European Association for the Cardio-Thoracic Surgery (EACTS); European Association for Percutaneous Cardiovascular Interventions (EAPCI). Guidelines on myocardial revascularization. *Eur Heart J* 2010;31(20):2501-2555.

299. Bell AD, Roussin A, Cartier R, et al; Canadian Cardiovascular Society. The use of antiplatelet therapy in the outpatient setting: Canadian Cardiovascular Society guidelines. *Can J Cardiol* 2011;27(Suppl A):S1-S59.

300. Kettering K. Minimally invasive direct coronary artery bypass grafting: a meta-analysis. *J Cardiovasc Surg (Torino)* 2008;49(6):793-800.

301. Narasimhan S, Srinivas VS, DeRose JJ Jr. Hybrid coronary revascularization: a review. *Cardiol Rev* 2011;19(3):101-107.

302. Friedrich GJ, Bonatti J. Hybrid coronary artery revascularization: review and update 2007. *Heart Surg Forum* 2007;10(4):E292-E296.

303. Mishra YK, Collison SP, Malhotra R, et al. Ten-year experience with single-vessel and multivessel reoperative off-pump coronary artery bypass grafting. *J Thorac Cardiovasc Surg* 2008;135(3):527-532.

304. Tatoulis J, Buxton BF, Fuller JA. Patencies of 2127 arterial to coronary conduits over 15 years. *Ann Thorac Surg* 2004;77(1):93-101.

305. Albertini A, Lochegnies A, El Khoury G, et al. Use of the right gastroepiploic artery as a coronary artery bypass graft in 307 patients. *Cardiovasc Surg* 1998;6(4):419-423.

306. Goldman S, Sethi GK, Holman W, et al. Radial artery grafts vs saphenous vein grafts in coronary artery bypass surgery: a randomized trial. *JAMA* 2011;305(2):167-174.

307. Collins P, Webb CM, Chong CF, Moat NE; Radial Artery Versus Saphenous Vein Patency (RSVP) Trial Investigators. Radial artery versus saphenous vein patency randomized trial: five-year angiographic follow-up. *Circulation* 2008;117(22):2859-2864.

CH
11

ADVANCES IN CORONARY REVASCULARIZATION

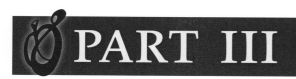

PART III

HEART FAILURE

CHAPTER **12**

Pharmacologic Management of Heart Failure in the Ambulatory Setting

Michael M. Givertz and Jay N. Cohn

PATHOPHYSIOLOGY AND STAGING SYSTEM: TARGETS OF THERAPY, 241

Diuretics and Sodium Restriction, 242
Renin-Angiotensin System Inhibitors, 245
β-Blockers, 250
Aldosterone Antagonists, 253
Hydralazine and Isosorbide Dinitrate, 255

Digoxin, 256
Calcium Channel Blockers, 257
Positive Inotropic Agents, 257
Antithrombotic Therapy, 258
Antiarrhythmic Therapy, 258
Special Considerations, 259

FUTURE DIRECTIONS IN PHARMACOLOGIC THERAPY, 263

Pharmacotherapy, 263
Comorbidities, 264

REFERENCES, 264

Heart failure is a growing public health problem.[1] Over the past 2 decades, considerable advancement has occurred in the understanding of the basic pathophysiologic mechanisms that underlie the clinical syndrome of heart failure (HF), the progressive nature of left ventricular (LV) remodeling, and the associated high mortality rates. Furthermore, randomized, controlled trials (RCTs) have demonstrated that medications such as angiotensin-converting enzyme (ACE) inhibitors, angiotensin receptor blockers (ARBs), β-blockers, and aldosterone antagonists reduce mortality rates and improve functional status. Nonetheless, the morbidity associated with HF remains high, and many patients are not optimally treated.[2] These observations have stimulated the formulation of specific guidelines for the management of patients with chronic HF.[3,4] A major emphasis in the coming years will include not only a continued search for more effective therapies, but also a significant educational effort to assist health care providers in the increased utilization of existing therapies.

This chapter reviews current pharmacologic treatment strategies for ambulatory patients with chronic HF. In each section, the most pertinent information regarding pathophysiologic mechanisms is presented, along with data from important clinical trials that provide the scientific rationale for the treatment recommendations. For areas in which there is strong agreement on medical management, evidence-based recommendations from the American College of Cardiology/American Heart Association (ACC/AHA) and the Heart Failure Society of America (HFSA) are provided.[3,4] For areas in which there are few data on mechanisms and treatment, the consensus opinion among HF specialists and empiric recommendations are discussed. In addition, each section includes practical recommendations that can be used in everyday clinical practice. A more detailed discussion of the drugs used in the treatment of HF can be found in Chapter 28 of the ninth edition of *Braunwald's Heart Disease.*

Pathophysiology and Staging System: Targets of Therapy

The basic pathophysiology of HF—including short-term adaptive mechanisms; chronic ventricular and vascular remodeling; and neurohormonal, paracrine, and autocrine adjustments—is extensively discussed in Braunwald's Chapter 25 and in other reviews.[5,6] Three important pathophysiologic concepts have had a substantial impact on the overall treatment strategy. The first concept recognizes the systemic nature of the clinical syndrome of HF. Although the primary problem is related to an abnormality in the myocardium, many of the presenting signs and symptoms are related to dysfunction of end organs, including the lungs, liver, kidneys, and skeletal muscle. The fact that HF is a systemic process makes it unlikely that any single therapy will offer a complete treatment response. A second important concept involves the interactions among myocardial dysfunction, activation of neurohormonal systems, and disease progression (Figure 12-1). This model emphasizes the fact that although HF is related to a primary abnormality in myocardial function, either genetic or acquired, further impairments in myocardial function and progressive hypertrophy, dilation, or both can occur in the absence of additional direct injury to the heart. This model can also help to explain the absence of signs and symptoms of HF in some patients who have significant ventricular dysfunction, and it provides the rationale for therapy with renin-angiotensin system inhibitors and β-blockers in patients with asymptomatic LV dysfunction. Finally, this model emphasizes the observation that treatments that do not have an intrinsic action on the primary myocardial abnormality can still have substantial benefits in HF. Thus, ACE inhibitors reduce vasoconstrictor tone and angiotensin-mediated toxicity in the heart, vasculature, and kidneys and are associated with marked improvement in symptoms and survival. In contrast, drugs that have been shown to activate neurohormonal pathways,

CH
12

such as oral positive inotropes, have a neutral or adverse effect on long-term survival.

A third concept that has evolved from randomized clinical trials is that all therapeutic interventions must be critically examined with respect to two different but equally important endpoints: 1) an improvement in symptoms or quality of life and 2) an improvement in survival. Although it is preferable that all interventions have a concordant effect on these endpoints, this is not always the case (Table 12-1). For example, diuretics are very effective in reducing signs and symptoms of HF, but their effects on survival are unknown. In contrast, β-blockers reduce hospitalizations and prolong survival, but their effects on exercise tolerance and quality of life are less evident. The distinction between the two endpoints is also reflected in prioritization of treatment for different patient subgroups. For example, patients with asymptomatic LV dysfunction do not require therapy that will reduce symptoms, but they benefit from treatment that slows disease progression and

prolongs life. In contrast, a patient with advanced HF is benefited by any treatment that relieves symptoms at the end of life.

In 2001, the writing committee of the ACC/AHA guidelines proposed a new approach to the classification of HF that emphasized both the development and progression of the disease. Stage A and B patients are at high risk for developing HF; this includes patients without structural heart disease (stage A) and those with structural heart disease but without signs or symptoms of HF (stage B). Stage C and D patients have structural heart disease with prior or current symptoms of HF (stage C) or refractory HF requiring specialized interventions (stage D; Figure 12-2). This staging system recognizes that 1) established risk factors and structural prerequisites exist for the development of HF; 2) therapies used before LV dysfunction or symptoms develop can reduce morbidity and mortality rates; 3) patients are expected to progress from one stage to the next unless slowed by treatment; and 4) all patients benefit from risk factor management that includes blood pressure control, lipid management, exercise, and smoking cessation. This chapter focuses primarily on stage C patients with reduced ejection fraction, for whom there is a large base of evidence available to guide therapy (Table 12-2). In contrast, a more limited discussion of empiric recommendations for patients with HF and preserved ejection fraction is presented.

Diuretics and Sodium Restriction

PATHOPHYSIOLOGIC MECHANISMS

A common abnormality in patients with HF is an expanded extracellular volume that manifests as pulmonary congestion, peripheral edema, ascites, elevated jugular venous pressure, and symptoms such as ankle swelling, dyspnea on exertion, and abdominal bloating. These abnormalities are related in part to avid sodium retention by the kidney caused by a complex interaction

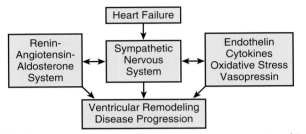

FIGURE 12-1 Proposed sequence of events in the progression of heart failure. After an initial injury, various secondary mediators such as norepinephrine, angiotensin, and mechanical stress act on the myocardium to cause ventricular remodeling. Additional biologic mediators—including endothelin, proinflammatory cytokines, and reactive oxygen species—are upregulated in heart failure and contribute to disease progression.

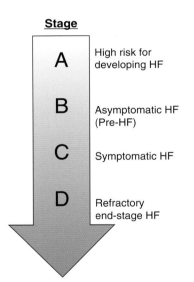

FIGURE 12-2 The American College of Cardiology/American Heart Association classification system for heart failure. CAD, coronary artery disease; HF, heart failure; LV, left ventricular; MI, myocardial infarction.

TABLE 12-1	Drugs in Heart Failure: Divergent Effects on Therapeutic Goals		
DRUG	**MORTALITY RATE**	**EXERCISE TOLERANCE**	**QUALITY OF LIFE**
ACE inhibitor	↓ 20%	Mild improvement	Mild improvement
β-Blocker	↓ 35%	Mild or no improvement	Mild or no improvement
Aldosterone antagonist	↓ 30%	Mild or no improvement	Mild improvement
Digoxin	No effect	Mild improvement	Unknown
Diuretic	Unknown	Moderate improvement	Moderate improvement

ACE, angiotensin-converting enzyme.

TABLE 12-2	Stage-Based Pharmacologic Therapy of Heart Failure	
STAGE	**DRUG**	**SELECTED INDICATIONS**
A	ACE inhibitor or ARB	Vascular disease, diabetes, hypertension
B	ACE inhibitor or ARB	Recent or remote MI, asymptomatic LVD, hypertensive LVH
	β-Blocker	Recent or remote MI, asymptomatic LVD
C	ACE inhibitor or ARB	All patients unless contraindicated
	β-Blocker	All patients unless contraindicated
	Diuretics	Fluid retention
	Aldosterone antagonist	Symptomatic LVD, post-MI heart failure, and LVD
	Hydralazine and nitrates	Symptomatic heart failure, African-American race
	ARB (on top of ACE inhibitor)	Symptomatic heart failure
	Digoxin	Symptomatic heart failure, atrial fibrillation
D	ACE inhibitor or ARB	All patients unless contraindicated or not tolerated
	β-Blocker	Stable NYHA class IV
	Diuretics	Fluid retention
	Digoxin	Atrial fibrillation with rapid ventricular response
	Positive inotropes	Bridge to transplantation or end of life

ACE, angiotensin-converting enzyme; ARB, angiotensin receptor blocker; LVD, left ventricular dysfunction; LVH, left ventricular hypertrophy; MI, myocardial infarction; NYHA, New York Heart Association.

TABLE 12-3	High-Sodium Foods	
FOOD	**PORTION**	**SODIUM (MG)**
American cheese	1 oz	406
Tuna, canned	3 oz	288
Ham	3 oz	1114
Hot dog	1	639
Spaghetti, canned	8 oz	1124
Bread, white	1 slice	114
Corn chips	2 oz	462
Chicken noodle soup	1 cup	1107
Beans, canned	1 cup	326
Soy sauce	1 tbsp	1029
Italian dressing	1 tbsp	116
Big Mac	1	1010
Whopper with cheese	1	1450

TABLE 12-4	Diuretic Therapy in Heart Failure	
GENERIC NAME	**USUAL ORAL DOSE**	**DURATION OF ACTION**
Loop Diuretics		
Furosemide	40-160 mg/day	6-8 hours
Bumetanide	0.5-4 mg/day	4-6 hours
Torsemide	10-40 mg/day	2-4 hours
Ethacrynic acid	50-150 mg/day	6-8 hours
Thiazide and Thiazide-Like Diuretics		
Chlorothiazide	500-1000 mg/day	6-12 hours
Hydrochlorothiazide	25-100 mg/day	>12 hours
Metolazone	2.5-10 mg/day	24-48 hours
Chlorthalidone	100 mg/day	24 hours
Indapamide	1.25-5 mg/day	24 hours
Potassium-Sparing Diuretics		
Spironolactone	25-100 mg/day	3 days after starting
Triamterene	100-200 mg/day	8-16 hours
Amiloride	5-10 mg/day	24 hours

among decreased cardiac output and renal perfusion, redistribution of intrarenal blood flow to the sodium-conserving medulla, systemic and local neurohormonal activation, and increased renal sympathetic nerve activity.[7] Diuretics are a cornerstone in the pharmacologic management of patients with signs and symptoms related to an expanded extracellular volume. Although restriction of dietary sodium intake is universally recommended for patients with HF who are treated with diuretics, this recommendation is inadequately implemented in many clinical settings. The failure to correctly implement a sodium-restricted diet diminishes the effectiveness of diuretics, increases the dosage requirement, and aggravates potassium loss.

SODIUM RESTRICTION

Few contemporary studies have specifically assessed the effect of dietary sodium intake in HF. Cody and colleagues[8] studied 10 patients with severe HF who were monitored in a clinical research center after all vasodilator and diuretic therapy was discontinued in conjunction with a diet containing very low sodium (~200 mg/day) or moderate sodium intake (~2000 mg/day). The very low sodium diet was associated with a significant reduction in weight, mean pulmonary artery pressure, and mean pulmonary capillary wedge pressure. In contrast, a high-salt diet in patients with mild HF has been shown to increase LV volumes, suppress renin and aldosterone concentrations, and reduce daily sodium excretion.[9] Thus, even in patients without signs or symptoms of congestion, the ability to excrete a sodium load is reduced. Other studies in patients with hypertensive heart disease[10] and HF with preserved ejection fraction[11] suggest that sodium restriction may reduce natriuretic peptides, attenuate ventricular remodeling, and improve clinical status.

The recommended level of sodium restriction depends on the history and severity of edema formation. In patients with asymptomatic LV dysfunction, judicious sodium restriction to no more than 3500 mg/day is probably reasonable. Patients with mild HF typically require restriction to less than 2500 mg/day, but those with moderate to severe HF should reduce intake to less than 2000 mg/day. Important principles include substituting herbs and other spices for table salt, avoiding common foods that contain large amounts of sodium (Table 12-3), reading food labels carefully, and cooking with fresh meats and vegetables. Keys to compliance are patient and family education by nurse specialists, referral to nutritionists, and use of patient-oriented texts and websites such as www.hfsa.org.[12]

DIURETICS

Mechanisms of Action

Diuretics inhibit sodium reabsorption in the kidney and lead to increased urinary sodium and water excretion.[13,14] Several diuretics are available (Table 12-4), usually classified according to site of action in the kidney. Thiazide diuretics inhibit the sodium-chloride symporter in the distal convoluted tubule, where approximately 30% to 35% of the filtered load of sodium is reabsorbed. However, as cardiac function and renal perfusion

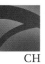

decrease, proximal tubular sodium reabsorption increases from approximately 65% to 80% to 90% of the filtered load, making thiazide diuretics less effective. Therefore, for most patients with HF and edema, a loop diuretic is the preferred initial agent; it will inhibit the sodium-potassium-chloride symporter in the thick ascending limb of the loop of Henle and lead to a marked increase in the fractional excretion of sodium. In addition, loop diuretics inhibit solute concentration in the medullary interstitium and thereby decrease the driving force for water reabsorption in the collecting duct. Because both loop diuretics and thiazides also cause potassium excretion, adjunctive therapy with potassium-sparing diuretics that act in the distal tubule and collecting duct may be required to maintain normokalemia. (For a detailed discussion of the pharmacology of diuretics, see Braunwald, Chapter 28).

Adverse Effects

Despite the wide acceptance of diuretics, they have a number of long-term adverse effects that include electrolyte depletion, neurohormonal activation, hypotension, and renal insufficiency. Chronic diuretic therapy can result in hypokalemia, hyponatremia, hypocalcemia, hypomagnesemia, and metabolic alkalosis. Hypokalemia and hypomagnesemia are of particular concern because they can precipitate arrhythmias in patients with HF. In addition to electrolyte depletion, diuretics may cause an increase in uric acid levels and contribute to the development or exacerbation of gout.[15] An adverse effect of diuretics that may be particularly important in patients with HF is activation of neurohormonal pathways.[16] The mechanisms by which diuretics stimulate renin and norepinephrine release have not been completely defined, but there are three important pathophysiologic consequences. First, renin secretion will result in increased secretion of aldosterone, which will promote sodium retention. Second, increased vasoconstriction secondary to increased levels of angiotensin II and norepinephrine may have a positive feedback effect, in which the increased impedance to ventricular emptying results in progressive ventricular dysfunction. Third, norepinephrine, angiotensin II, and aldosterone exert direct toxic effects on the myocardium that result in ventricular remodeling and proarrhythmia. Finally, neurohormonal activation is a strong predictor of increased mortality rate.[17] Therefore, it is possible that diuretic-associated neurohormonal stimulation could be associated with an adverse effect on long-term survival.[18]

The association of diuretic therapy with neurohormonal activation has an important influence on the optimal use of diuretics for patients with HF. As discussed, it is useful to reinforce dietary sodium restriction in patients who appear to require large doses of diuretics. Second, it is important to emphasize that many of the adverse effects of neurohormonal stimulation by diuretics can be blocked by the concomitant administration of an ACE inhibitor (or ARB) and β-blocker. With combination therapy, the beneficial effect of diuretics may be obtained but the increase in angiotensin II and aldosterone is blocked, and the effects of norepinephrine are inhibited. It is also important to understand the effects of secondary processes that can cause overall sodium balance to return to neutral despite continued diuretic administration. The response to a diuretic-induced reduction of extracellular volume is a further reduction in sodium and chloride excretion through stimulation of proximal tubular reabsorption, increased renal sympathetic nerve activity, and increased aldosterone.[19] In addition, long-term diuretic treatment induces a number of changes in the collecting duct and distal tubule, including increases in mitochondrial volume, adenosine triphosphatase activity, and cellular hypertrophy, that increase distal tubular reabsorption.[20]

The pharmacokinetics and pharmacodynamic effects of diuretics may be abnormal in patients with HF.[13] In patients with bowel wall edema and splanchnic hypoperfusion, the absorption of orally administered drugs can be reduced, thereby delaying the time to appearance and peak concentration of the diuretic in the urine. Unless the glomerular filtration rate (GFR) is less than 30 mL/min, the pharmacokinetics of intravenous (IV) formulations are largely normal in HF, which explains the effectiveness of the IV route in patients with acute decompensated HF (see Chapter 14). Furthermore, the pharmacodynamic response is attenuated in HF so that the rate of sodium excretion is reduced at any given renal tubular diuretic concentration. Thus, the "ceiling" dose, or dose above which further sodium excretion is minimal, is typically double in patients with HF compared with normal subjects. For this reason, prescribing a larger dose of diuretic is commonly more effective than increasing the frequency of administration.

Practical Considerations

Short-term studies have shown that diuretics reduce signs and symptoms of congestion and decrease cardiac filling pressures within hours to days of initiation, and intermediate-term studies demonstrate the beneficial effects of diuretics on exercise tolerance and quality of life. The effects of diuretics on morbidity and mortality in HF have not been tested. According to ACC/AHA guidelines, diuretics should be prescribed to all patients with current or prior symptoms of HF who have evidence of fluid retention and combined with an ACE inhibitor and β-blocker to maintain clinical stability.[4] Furthermore, inappropriately low doses of diuretics will result in fluid retention, which can attenuate the response to ACE inhibitors and increase the risk of β-blockade. The first step is to identify patients with fluid retention based on symptoms (shortness of breath, orthopnea, paroxysmal nocturnal dyspnea), signs (rales, elevated jugular venous pressure, peripheral edema), and other clinical characteristics such as weight gain, frequent outpatient visits, or recurrent hospitalizations. Noninvasive tools that may be helpful in recognizing hypervolemia include chest radiographs, natriuretic peptide levels, and echocardiography, although the sensitivity and specificity of these tests are limited.[21] Newer devices such as implantable hemodynamic and intrathoracic impedance monitors[22,23] and noninvasive Valsalva response recorders[24] have also been developed for use in HF. Direct assessment of blood volume using a radiolabeled albumin technique is available at specialized centers.[25] If the clinical evaluation is equivocal, a right heart catheterization to measure intracardiac filling pressures should be considered.

For patients with HF, the most commonly prescribed loop diuretic is furosemide, which is usually started at a low dose (20 to 40 mg once daily) and increased until urine output increases and weight loss occurs. The dose or frequency of diuretics may be titrated while monitoring several endpoints. Because one of the primary goals of therapy is symptom relief, the dose of diuretics may be reduced to maintenance levels once a satisfactory reduction is seen in dyspnea, orthopnea, and edema. In addition, careful attention to normalizing the jugular venous pressure and eliminating congestive hepatomegaly are keys to achieving euvolemia, especially in patients with advanced HF. The development of symptomatic hypotension or azotemia often necessitates holding diuretic therapy, but diuretics can often be resumed at a lower dose after adjustment of other HF medications, such as ACE inhibitors and β-blockers. Once fluid retention has resolved, a maintenance dose of diuretics is recommended to prevent recurrent volume overload. Selected patients with mild HF or asymptomatic LV dysfunction may not require maintenance diuretics if the patient is able to reduce dietary sodium intake, although a strategy of diuretic withdrawal has not been tested in randomized clinical trials. In a short-term study, diuretic withdrawal resulted in subclinical increases in volume status and markers of tubular dysfunction.[26] However, others have demonstrated stable clinical status with improved renal function and neurohormonal markers after 3 months of diuretic interruption.[27]

Some patients have refractory signs and symptoms of HF and are labeled *diuretic resistant*. However, these patients may be nonadherent with their medication regimens or ineffective in limiting sodium and fluid intake, and they require reinforcement of education. In patients with biventricular or right HF, significant bowel wall edema may limit oral absorption, so that IV formulations (furosemide or chlorothiazide) or loop diuretics with increased oral bioavailability (torsemide) may be effective in initiating a diuresis. In patients with low cardiac output, the problem is inadequate sodium delivery to the tubular lumen because of reduced renal perfusion and impaired tubular secretion of diuretics. Most patients will respond to doubling the dose rather than giving the same dose twice daily.

In other patients the combination of a loop diuretic with a thiazide diuretic or metolazone, which facilitates the action of the loop diuretic, may be particularly effective.[28] The mechanisms of diuretic synergism are not fully defined but are likely related to the fact that diuretics inhibit transport in different segments of the nephron. In addition, adding a thiazide diuretic may inhibit compensatory distal tubular adaptations and result in a sustained diuresis that would be much greater than simply increasing the dose of the loop diuretic. The addition of metolazone may also be used for transient episodes of fluid accumulation. This strategy maintains a constant dose of the loop diuretic, minimizes errors associated with frequent dosage changes, and reduces the long-term exposure to high-dose diuretics. However, close monitoring is required because this "booster pill" strategy can rapidly lead to overdiuresis with hypotension, hypokalemia, hyponatremia, and worsening renal function.

During long-term treatment, and particularly during changes in diuretic regimens, it is important to monitor levels of potassium, given the marked kaliuretic effects of diuretic drugs. Renal function as assessed by serum blood urea nitrogen (BUN) and creatinine levels should be monitored because they may be sensitive to changes in blood volume and/or vasoconstrictor hormones. Excessive volume depletion should be avoided because it may result in hypotension and renal dysfunction. In patients with coexistent HF and chronic kidney disease, the so-called *cardiorenal syndrome*,[29,30] potential nephrotoxic agents should be used with extreme caution. Nonsteroidal antiinflammatory drugs (NSAIDs), including cyclooxygenase-2 inhibitors, should be avoided; these agents can inhibit the natriuretic effects of diuretics and impair renal function, thereby exacerbating fluid retention. Other agents—such as thiazolidinediones[31] and pregabalin,[32] which cause edema—are relatively contraindicated in HF.

Patients should weigh themselves on a daily basis; if they do not own a scale, one should be provided for them. This process engages patients in their medical care, alerts them to the effect of dietary indiscretions, and facilitates fine-tuning of medications. For selected patients, electronic scales that transmit daily information on weight, vital signs, and symptoms may help to maintain accuracy and compliance. In the case of a rapid weight gain of 2 to 3 pounds, a temporary increase in diuretic dosage or the addition of metolazone or a thiazide diuretic for 1 to 3 days is often sufficient to return the patient to "dry" weight. In patients with advanced HF, it is important to remember that dry weight may decrease over time with loss of skeletal muscle mass and adipose tissue as a result of cardiac cachexia.[33] The use of IV diuretics and other fluid management strategies in hospitalized patients with acute decompensated HF is discussed in detail in Chapter 14.

Renin-Angiotensin System Inhibitors

PATHOPHYSIOLOGIC MECHANISMS

Nearly 35 years ago, an important advance in the treatment of HF was the recognition that pump function was critically dependent on the outflow resistance, against which the ventricle must empty.[34] Acute hemodynamic studies established that vasodilator drugs that relax peripheral arterioles shift the ventricular function curve upward and to the left, resulting in an increase in cardiac output without a large change in blood pressure. Moreover, drugs that increase venous capacitance redistribute blood volume from the central to peripheral reservoirs and therefore decrease the signs and symptoms of elevated cardiac filling pressures. Unlike hydralazine, which acts predominantly on the arterioles and leads to a reduction in impedance, or nitrates, which act on arterial compliance and venous tone, ACE inhibitors and ARBs have a balanced effect on arterioles, arteries, and veins.

The traditional view of ACE inhibitors was that their primary mechanism of action in HF was a reduction in angiotensin II–mediated vasoconstriction. In addition, the reduction of angiotensin II was noted to decrease the release of aldosterone from the adrenal gland and norepinephrine in the synaptic cleft.[35] However, subsequent studies have shown that the actions of ACE inhibitors are considerably more complex than a simple effect on circulating levels of angiotensin II (Figure 12-3). Because kininase is identical to converting enzyme, ACE inhibitors also reduce the metabolism of bradykinin, which can stimulate the release of nitric oxide and other endothelium-dependent vasodilators, including prostaglandins. More importantly, by inhibiting tissue renin-angiotensin systems in blood vessels, the kidney, and the heart, ACE inhibitors play a critical role in attenuating vascular and myocardial remodeling, reducing inflammation and the risk of thrombosis, and delaying the progression of renal disease. All these actions have an important impact on mediating the clinical efficacy of ACE inhibitors in HF.

Several nonenzymatic pathways independent of ACE exist for the conversion of angiotensin I to angiotensin II and may contribute to persistent availability of both circulating and tissue angiotensin despite treatment with ACE inhibitors (see Figure 12-3).[35] This *escape phenomenon* may be due in part to non-ACE pathways of angiotensin I metabolism (e.g., myocardial chymase); this has provided the rationale for the development of ARBs, which bind competitively to, and dissociate slowly from, angiotensin II type 1 receptors.[36] Circulating angiotensin II levels increase during therapy as a result of loss of negative feedback. Many ARBs are available, but only two are currently approved by the U.S. Food and

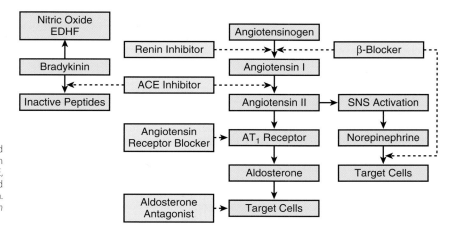

FIGURE 12-3 Pharmacologic agents (*yellow boxes*) used to manipulate the renin-angiotensin-aldosterone system (*blue boxes*). *Dashed lines* signify inhibitory pathways. ACE, angiotensin-converting enzyme; EDHF, endothelium-derived hyperpolarizing factor; SNS, sympathetic nervous system. (*Modified from Givertz MM. Manipulation of the renin-angiotensin system. Circulation 2001;104:e14-e18.*)

TABLE 12-5	ACE Inhibitor, Angiotensin Receptor Blocker, and β-Blocker Therapy in Heart Failure with Reduced Ejection Fraction	
GENERIC NAME	**INITIAL DAILY DOSE**	**MAXIMUM DOSE**
ACE Inhibitors		
Captopril	6.25 mg tid	50 mg tid
Enalapril	2.5 mg bid	10-20 mg bid
Fosinopril	5-10 mg qd	40 mg qd
Lisinopril	2.5-5 mg qd	20-40 mg qd
Quinapril	5 mg bid	20 mg bid
Ramipril	1.25-2.5 mg qd	10 mg qd
Trandolapril	1 mg qd	4 mg qd
Angiotensin Receptor Blockers		
Candesartan	4-8 mg qd	32 mg qd
Losartan	12.5-25 mg qd	100 mg qd
Valsartan	40 mg bid	160 mg bid
β-Blockers		
Bisoprolol	1.25 mg qd	10 mg qd
Carvedilol	3.125 mg bid	25 mg bid
Metoprolol succinate	12.5-25 mg qd	200 mg qd

Modified from Hunt SA, Abraham WT, Chin MH, et al. 2009 Focused update incorporated into the ACC/AHA 2005 Guidelines for the Diagnosis and Management of Heart Failure in Adults: a report of the American College of Cardiology Foundation/American Heart Association Task Force on Practice Guidelines: developed in collaboration with the International Society for Heart and Lung Transplantation. *Circulation* 2009;119:e391-e479.

Drug Administration (FDA) for the treatment of HF (Table 12-5). Valsartan is approved for the treatment of patients with New York Heart Association (NYHA) functional class II through IV heart failure and is indicated to reduce cardiovascular mortality in clinically stable patients with LV failure or dysfunction following myocardial infarction (MI). Candesartan is indicated to reduce cardiovascular mortality and hospitalizations in patients with NYHA functional class II through IV heart failure and reduced ejection fraction.

CLINICAL EFFICACY

Angiotensin-Converting Enzyme Inhibitors

Numerous prospective, placebo-controlled studies have demonstrated the beneficial effects of ACE inhibitors on exercise tolerance, salt and water balance, clinical signs and symptoms, neurohormonal stimulation, quality of life, and survival in patients with chronic HF (Table 12-6). The concordance of findings in these multicenter trials provides a strong scientific basis for the use of ACE inhibitors in the management of HF. Several multicenter trials deserve comment.

COOPERATIVE NORTH SCANDINAVIAN ENALAPRIL SURVIVAL STUDY (CONSENSUS)

CONSENSUS randomized 253 hospitalized patients with NYHA functional class IV symptoms to either enalapril or placebo in addition to treatment with digoxin, diuretics, and non-ACE vasodilators.[37] Based on an interim analysis, enalapril was associated with a highly significant survival benefit compared with placebo (52% vs. 36%), although no difference was reported in the combined risk of death or hospitalization for HF. The CONSENSUS trial was prematurely terminated, because it was deemed unethical to continue a trial in which half of the participants were randomized to placebo.

VASODILATOR HEART FAILURE TRIAL (V-HeFT) II

V-HeFT I was the first placebo-controlled trial to demonstrate that vasodilators could prolong survival in patients with HF.[38] V-HeFT II was designed to compare treatment with hydralazine–isosorbide dinitrate, the superior drug combination in V-HeFT I, to enalapril

in patients with mild to moderate HF as a result of ischemic or nonischemic cardiomyopathy.[39] The enalapril group had a lower 2-year mortality rate compared with those patients randomized to hydralazine–isosorbide dinitrate (18% vs. 25%; mortality reduction, 28%; $P = .016$). Interestingly, exercise time and LV function improved to a greater degree in the patients randomized to hydralazine–isosorbide dinitrate.

STUDIES OF LEFT VENTRICULAR DYSFUNCTION (SOLVD)

SOVLD was a prospective, double-blind placebo-controlled trial in patients with an ejection fraction of 35% or less.[40] The SOLVD Treatment trial randomized 2569 patients with NYHA functional class II or III heart failure, treated with digitalis and diuretics, to enalapril or placebo. After a mean follow-up of 41 months, significantly more deaths were reported in the placebo group compared with the enalapril group (510 vs. 452; mortality reduction, 16%; $P = .0036$). Furthermore, enalapril was associated with a 30% reduction in hospitalizations for HF.

The SOLVD Prevention trial[41] was run concurrently with the treatment trial and utilized the same experimental design except for the restriction to patients with minimal to no symptoms of HF who were on no treatment for overt HF. After an average follow-up of 37 months, 334 deaths were reported in the placebo group compared with 313 in the enalapril group. This 8% mortality reduction approached but did not achieve statistical significance ($P = .30$). More impressive were the highly significant reductions in the first hospitalization for HF (36%) and in the onset of HF requiring pharmacologic therapy (37%).

ASSESSMENT OF TREATMENT WITH LISINOPRIL AND SURVIVAL (ATLAS)

Despite controlled trials demonstrating the benefits of high-dose ACE inhibitor therapy (e.g., captopril 50 to 100 mg three times daily, enalapril 10 to 20 mg twice daily), much lower doses are used in clinical practice because of concerns regarding patient tolerance. The ATLAS study randomized 3164 patients with NYHA functional class II to IV heart failure and an ejection fraction of 30% or less to low-dose (2.5 to 5 mg/day) or high-dose (32.5 to 35 mg/day) lisinopril.[42] After a median follow-up of 46 months, high-dose lisinopril was modestly superior in decreasing the combined risk of death or hospitalization (12% reduction; $P = .0002$), but it had no significant effect on all-cause mortality. Although dizziness and renal insufficiency were more common in the high-dose group, the rate of drug withdrawal because of adverse effects (18%) was similar in the two groups.

Angiotensin Receptor Blockers

In early clinical studies in patients with chronic HF as a result of LV systolic dysfunction, angiotensin receptor blockade produced beneficial hemodynamic effects and was generally well tolerated.[43] The Evaluation of Losartan in the Elderly (ELITE) I study randomly assigned 722 patients aged 65 years or older with NYHA functional class II to IV heart failure and an ejection fraction of 40% or less to receive losartan or captopril for 48 weeks.[44] Although no difference was found between the drugs with regard to the primary safety endpoint (i.e., treatment effect on renal function), losartan unexpectedly decreased mortality rate by 46%. With a similar design as ELITE I, but powered to detect a difference in all-cause mortality, ELITE II randomized 3152 patients with mild to moderate HF to losartan (target dose 50 mg once daily) or captopril (target dose 50 mg three times daily) and demonstrated a nonsignificant 13% reduction in mortality rate in favor of captopril.[45] Trends were also seen in favor of ACE inhibitor therapy for the secondary endpoint of sudden cardiac death and the combined endpoint of death and hospitalization. Fewer patients randomized to losartan discontinued therapy because of side effects (9% vs. 15%; $P < .001$). The inferiority of losartan in ELITE II was likely due to underdosing; although losartan is not approved for the treatment of HF, the recommended daily dose in this setting is 100 mg.

There is theoretical reason to suggest that combined therapy with an ARB and an ACE inhibitor would be more clinically effective than therapy with either alone; this thesis has been tested in

TABLE 12-6   Randomized, Controlled Trials of Angiotensin-Converting Enzyme Inhibitors and Angiotensin Receptor Blockers

TRIAL	N	AGENT	ENTRY CRITERIA	FOLLOW-UP PERIOD	PRIMARY ENDPOINT	FINDINGS*
Heart Failure Trials						
CONSENSUS[37]	253	Enalapril vs. placebo	NYHA IV	188 days	Death	Placebo 52% Enalapril 36% (40% ↓)
V-HeFT II[39]	804	Hydralazine/ isosorbide dinitrate vs. enalapril	CTR >0.55 LVID >2.7 cm/m² LVEF <45% VO₂ <25 mL/kg/min	2.5 years	Death	Hyd/ISDN 25% Enalapril 18% (28% ↓)
SOLVD Treatment[40]	2569	Enalapril vs. placebo	LVEF ≤35% NYHA II-III	41 months	Death	Placebo 40% Enalapril 35% (16% ↓)
SOLVD Prevention[41]	4228	Enalapril vs. placebo	LVEF ≤35% No or minimal symptoms	37 months	Death	Placebo 16% Enalapril 15% (8% ↓, P = .30)
ATLAS[42]	3164	High-dose vs. low-dose lisinopril	LVEF ≤30% NYHA II-IV	39 to 58 months	Death	Low-dose 45% High-dose 43% (8% ↓, P = .13)
ELITE-II[45,71]	3152	Losartan vs. captopril	Age ≥60 years LVEF ≤40% NYHA II-IV	1.5 years	Death	Losartan 18% Captopril 16% (13% ↓, P = .16)
Val-HeFT[47]	5010	Valsartan vs. placebo	LVEF <40% LVID >2.9 cm/m² NYHA II-IV	23 months	Death Death and complications	Placebo 19% Valsartan 20% (P = .80) Placebo 32% Valsartan 29% (13% ↓)
CHARM-Added[48]	2548	Candesartan vs. placebo	LVEF ≤40% NYHA II-IV Treatment with ACE inhibitors	41 months	CV death or HF hospitalization	Placebo 42% Candesartan 38% (15% ↓)
CHARM-Alternative[49]	2028	Candesartan vs. placebo	LVEF ≤40% NYHA II-IV Intolerance to ACE inhibitors	34 months	CV death or HF hospitalization	Placebo 40% Candesartan 33% (23% ↓)
Postinfarction Trials						
SAVE[276]	2231	Captopril vs. placebo	LVEF ≤40% 3-16 days after MI	42 months	Death	Placebo 25% Captopril 20% (19% ↓)
CONSENSUS II[53]	6090	Enalapril IV/PO vs. placebo	24 hours after MI	6 months	Death	Placebo 10% Enalapril 11% (10% ↑, P = .26)
AIRE[277]	2006	Ramipril vs. placebo	HF 3-10 days after MI	15 months	Death	Placebo 23% Ramipril 17% (27% ↓)
GISSI-3[278]	19,394	Lisinopril vs. placebo	24 hours after MI	6 weeks	Death	Placebo 7.1% Lisinopril 6.3% (12% ↓)
SMILE[54]	1556	Zofenopril vs. placebo	24 hours after MI	6 weeks	Death or severe heart failure	Placebo 10.6% Zofenopril 7.1% (34% ↓)
TRACE[279]	1749	Trandolapril vs. placebo	LVEF ≤35% 3 days after MI	4 years	Death	Placebo 42% Trandolapril 35% (22% ↓)
ISIS-4[280]	58,050	Captopril vs. placebo	24 hours after MI	5 weeks	Death	Placebo 7.7% Captopril 7.2% (7% ↓)
VALIANT[55]	14,808	Valsartan vs. valsartan plus captopril vs. captopril	0.5-10 days after MI HF, LVEF ≤35%, or both	25 months	Death	Valsartan 20% Valsartan plus captopril 19% Captopril 20%

↓, reduction; ↑, increase.
*P < .05 unless noted.
ACE, angiotensin-converting enzyme; AIRE, Acute Infarction Ramipril Efficacy; ATLAS, Assessment of Treatment with Lisinopril and Survival; CHARM, Candesartan in Heart Failure: Assessment of Reduction in Mortality and Morbidity; CONSENSUS, Cooperative North Scandinavian Enalapril Survival Study; CTR, cardiothoracic ratio; CV, cardiovascular; GISSI-3, Grupo Italiano per lo Studio della Sopravivenza nell'infarto Miocardico; HF, heart failure; Hyd, hydralazine; ISDN, isosorbide dinitrate; ISIS-4, Fourth International Study of Infarct Survival; LVEF, left ventricular ejection fraction; LVID, left ventricular internal diameter at diastole; MI, myocardial infarction; NYHA, New York Heart Association functional class; SAVE, Survival and Ventricular Enlargement; SMILE, Survival of Myocardial Infarction Long-term Evaluation; SOLVD, Studies of Left Ventricular Dysfunction; TRACE, Trandolapril Cardiac Evaluation; Val-HeFT; Valsartan in Heart Failure Trial; VALIANT, Valsartan in Acute Myocardial Infarction; V-HeFT, Vasodilator Heart Failure Trial.

several clinical trials. In a small pilot study, the addition of losartan to maximally tolerated doses of ACE inhibitors was associated with a lower NYHA class and higher peak oxygen consumption.[46] The Valsartan in Heart Failure Trial (Val-HeFT) randomized 5010 patients with NYHA functional class II to IV heart failure to receive valsartan (target dose 160 mg twice daily) or placebo in addition to usual therapy that included ACE inhibitors in 93% and β-blockers in 36%.[47] Valsartan significantly reduced the combined endpoint of mortality and morbidity by 13% ($P = .009$), including a 28% reduction in HF hospitalization, but it had no effect on all-cause mortality. Despite post hoc analysis raising concern about adverse outcomes in patients receiving an ACE inhibitor, ARB, and β-blocker—so-called *triple therapy*—similar efficacy and safety results were reported from the Candesartan in Heart Failure: Assessment of Reduction in Mortality and Morbidity (CHARM)-Added study.[48] In CHARM-Added, 2548 patients with mild to moderate HF and reduced ejection fraction who were being treated with ACE inhibitors were randomized to receive candesartan (target dose 32 mg once daily) or placebo. During a median follow-up of 41 months, candesartan reduced the combined endpoint of cardiovascular death or HF hospitalizations by 15% ($P = .01$). Importantly, candesartan reduced this risk in patients treated with β-blockers in addition to an ACE inhibitor and was as effective among patients taking a recommended dose of ACE inhibitor as in those taking lower doses; however, the risk of worsening renal function and hyperkalemia were higher with add-on therapy.

For patients who are intolerant to ACE inhibition, angiotensin receptor blockade has proven effective as an alternative therapy. In the CHARM-Alternative study, 2028 patients with symptomatic LV dysfunction who were not receiving ACE inhibitors because of cough (72%), hypotension (13%), or renal dysfunction (12%) were randomized to receive candesartan (target dose 32 mg once daily) or placebo.[49] During a median follow-up period of 34 months, candesartan reduced the risk of cardiovascular death or HF hospitalization by 23% ($P = .004$). In addition, a trend was seen toward a decrease in all-cause mortality with candesartan (hazard ratio [HR], 0.87; 95% CI, 0.74 to 1.03; $P = .11$). A subgroup of 366 patients in the Val-HeFT study who were not taking ACE inhibitors at baseline also experienced a significant reduction in morbidity and mortality with angiotensin receptor blockade.[47]

In addition to targeting patients with HF, several large trials have studied the effects of ACE inhibitors and ARBs on mortality in patients following acute MI (see Table 12-6).[50] These trials focused on a patient population that is not comparable to patients with chronic HF and reduced ejection fraction that were enrolled in the V-HeFT, CONSENSUS, SOLVD, and CHARM trials. In addition, background drug therapy and study drug dosing differed significantly from the chronic HF trials. Nevertheless, the results of the postinfarction trials have several important implications when considering treatment for patients with LV systolic dysfunction and/or HF.

First, the majority of these trials demonstrated that treatment with an ACE inhibitor initiated early after MI had a small but significant benefit in reducing short-term mortality. This finding is significant because most of the patients enrolled in the postinfarction trials did not have HF. Furthermore, the Heart Outcomes Prevention Evaluation (HOPE) study demonstrated a reduction in mortality from the ACE inhibitor ramipril in patients with atherosclerosis in the absence of HF,[51] and the European Trial on Reduction of Cardiac Events with Perindopril in Stable Coronary Artery Disease (EUROPA) confirmed the vasculoprotective effect of ACE inhibitors in even lower risk patients.[52]

A second and more compelling issue is that early intervention with an ACE inhibitor can prevent or delay the onset of HF. In the Survival and Ventricular Enlargement (SAVE) trial, captopril was associated with a 37% reduction in the development of HF and a 22% reduction in hospitalizations for HF. CONSENSUS II demonstrated that enalapril reduced the need to change therapy for HF by 10%,[53] and the Survival of Myocardial Infarction Long-term Evaluation (SMILE) study demonstrated that early use of zofenopril reduced the likelihood of developing severe HF within

6 weeks of MI.[54] These data are consistent with the results of the SOLVD Prevention trial, which demonstrated a 20% reduction in hospitalizations for HF and a 29% reduction in the development of HF. In the HOPE study, ramipril reduced the risk of developing HF by 23%; and in EUROPA, perindopril reduced HF hospitalizations by 39%. These cumulative data suggest that ACE inhibitors have a significant clinical benefit even in relatively low-risk patients.

Third, results from the Valsartan in Acute Myocardial Infarction (VALIANT) trial[55] suggest that although ACE inhibitors and ARBs are equally effective at reducing morbidity and mortality in patients with acute MI and HF, LV systolic dysfunction, or both, combined therapy offers no advantages over ACE inhibition or angiotensin receptor blockade alone and increases the rate of adverse events.[55] These findings appear to be at odds with results from the Val-HeFT and CHARM studies demonstrating further cardiovascular risk reduction (RR) with the addition of angiotensin receptor blockade to background ACE inhibition; however, differences in patient population, drug regimens, and patterns of cardiovascular risk between patients with stable HF and those with acute MI likely explain these divergent results.[55]

PRACTICAL CONSIDERATIONS

Angiotensin-Converting Enzyme Inhibitors

Despite the overwhelming database from clinical trials and the adoption of consensus guidelines, the application—including utilization and dosing—of ACE inhibitors to the broad population of patients with HF remains suboptimal. Several factors are responsible for this. First, the use of ACE inhibitors appears to vary among different specialties, as evidenced by the fact that cardiologists are more likely to prescribe ACE inhibitors than are primary care physicians.[56] Second, it is a common perception that ACE inhibitors are associated with a high frequency of adverse effects when used at higher doses and/or in the elderly. However, the early experience from CONSENSUS and SOLVD in a large population of ambulatory patients suggests that the incidence of these complications is acceptably low given the potential benefit, and ATLAS demonstrated no increased risk of drug withdrawal with high-dose therapy.[42] Finally, management and avoidance of ACE inhibitor–related complications can be facilitated by knowledge of certain predisposing factors and by institution of precautionary measures. Other patient-related factors associated with physician underutilization of ACE inhibitors include older age, renal dysfunction, and preserved ejection fraction.[57]

The most important adverse effect to monitor for during the initiation of ACE inhibitors is hypotension (Table 12-7), although

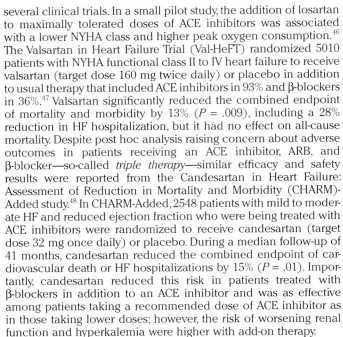

TABLE 12-7	Adverse Effects of Renin-Angiotensin-Aldosterone System Inhibitors		
ADVERSE EFFECT	ACE INHIBITOR	ANGIOTENSIN RECEPTOR BLOCKER	ALDOSTERONE ANTAGONIST
Hypotension	++	++	+
Renal insufficiency	++	++	+/−
Hyperkalemia	+	+	++
Cough	+	−	−
Angioedema	++	+	−
Skin rash	+	+/−	−
Neutropenia	+	+	+/−
Gynecomastia	−	−	+*
Impotence	−	−	+*

*Not seen with eplerenone, a selective mineralocorticoid receptor antagonist, with a hundredfold to a thousandfold lower affinity for androgen, glucocorticoid, and progesterone receptors than spironolactone.
ACE, angiotensin-converting enzyme.

the decrease in blood pressure is usually minor and the patient is often asymptomatic. Patients who are at highest risk for symptomatic hypotension are those who are volume depleted, receiving high doses of diuretics or concomitant vasodilator therapy, or older than 75 years. Patients with increased activation of the renin-angiotensin-aldosterone system, manifest by increased levels of plasma renin activity, are those who have angiotensin-mediated vasoconstriction and who are also at risk for hypotension.[58] Because measurements of plasma renin activity are not readily available, clinicians can take advantage of the relatively tight inverse correlation between plasma renin activity and serum sodium.[59] Patients with low serum sodium (<130 mmol/L) are more likely to develop hypotension during the initiation of therapy. Useful strategies in these patients include temporary withholding of diuretics, liberalizing of salt intake, and the use of a test dose of a short-acting ACE inhibitor (e.g., captopril 6.25 mg) followed by gradual uptitration over several weeks. If symptomatic hypotension occurs with the first dose, it may not recur with subsequent dosing.

Although mild renal insufficiency may concern clinicians, several misconceptions persist regarding the effects of ACE inhibitors on renal function. Many patients with HF actually have an improvement in renal function with the initiation of ACE inhibitors, which is likely mediated by an increase in cardiac output and renal perfusion. In addition, the incidence and magnitude of renal insufficiency in controlled trials are low, and only a small percentage of patients (<0.5%) are withdrawn from therapy. The mechanisms contributing to renal dysfunction are complex and are accentuated by concomitant drug therapy and hemodynamic abnormalities. Patients at risk for worsening renal function share many of the same features as those at risk for hypotension. In general, patients should be reassessed approximately 1 week after initiating an ACE inhibitor to monitor renal function and blood pressure. If there is an increase in serum creatinine of 0.5 mg/dL or more, the volume status and diuretic dose should be reassessed. In the majority of cases, renal function will return to baseline once volume status returns to normal or if the diuretic dose is decreased. It is also advisable to check for concomitant medications, such as NSAIDs, or medical conditions such as renal artery stenosis, which can aggravate renal function. Despite these concerns, ACE inhibitors may slow the progression of renal disease in HF patients with hypertensive and/or diabetic nephropathy.[60]

Hyperkalemia can occur in patients receiving ACE inhibitors because of the reduction in angiotensin II–mediated aldosterone secretion. Elevated potassium levels are more common in patients with diabetes or chronic kidney disease, especially if they are receiving potassium supplements or potassium-sparing diuretics, or if they are using salt substitutes that contain potassium chloride or iodide. Therefore, the dosage of potassium chloride and potassium levels should be monitored approximately 1 week after initiating ACE inhibitors, and potassium-sparing diuretics should be used with caution.

The other side effects of ACE inhibitors—such as dysgeusia, skin rash, and cough—are commonly self-limited or reversible with discontinuation of the drug. Clinicians must be particularly cautious about stopping ACE inhibitors because of cough, which has been reported in 5% to 15% of patients in clinical studies. ACE inhibitor–related cough is typically nonproductive, arises during the first few months of therapy, and disappears within 7 to 10 days of drug withdrawal; however, cough is a common manifestation of HF and may respond to an increased dose of diuretics, ACE inhibitors, or both. If the cough is intolerable, a smaller dose or temporary discontinuation can be tried. In the past, many patients would tolerate a mild cough in exchange for the important improvements in survival and quality of life; however, most patients can be easily switched to an ARB with expected clinical benefits.[49]

Angioedema is a rare but potentially life-threatening complication of ACE inhibitor therapy that can occur weeks to months following drug initiation. The causal mechanism is believed to be an accumulation of bradykinin or one of its metabolites. An ACE inhibitor should not be prescribed to any patient with a history of angioedema. Furthermore, if a patient develops angioedema while taking an ACE inhibitor, the drug should be stopped immediately.

Doses of ACE inhibitors should be titrated upward over several weeks until target doses—that is, doses that have been shown to reduce morbidity and mortality in clinical trials—are achieved (see Table 12-5). The issue of the optimal dose has been controversial because it is a common impression that many patients are being treated with substantially lower doses.[61] Although results from the ATLAS study[42] argue in favor of trying to achieve high-dose ACE inhibitor therapy to reduce the risk of hospitalization, lower doses showed similar effects on symptoms and mortality. For patients who cannot tolerate high-dose ACE inhibitors, low or intermediate doses should be continued while β-blockers are initiated. Once a maximally tolerated dose of ACE inhibitor has been achieved, patients can generally be maintained on this dose long-term despite changes in other HF medications. However, 20% to 25% of patients with advanced HF will develop a circulatory or renal limitation to ACE inhibitor therapy.[62] These patients tend to be older with longer duration of HF, lower blood pressure, and baseline renal dysfunction. ACE inhibitor intolerance is a marker of poor prognosis.

Another controversial issue is whether the beneficial effects of ACE inhibitors are class or drug specific. Captopril, enalapril, lisinopril, quinapril, and fosinopril are currently indicated for the treatment of symptomatic HF. Captopril, ramipril, and trandolapril are indicated for post-MI patients, and enalapril is the only ACE inhibitor indicated for the prevention of HF in asymptomatic patients. Although data are insufficient to prove that the benefits demonstrated in clinical trials are applicable to all ACE inhibitors or only to the specific drug studied, meta-analyses suggest an equivalent survival benefit for several different ACE inhibitors,[63] with consistent effects in a broad range of patients.[64] Although some differences in structure, pharmacokinetics, and pharmacodynamics are apparent, it is not known whether these differences have a significant impact on clinical outcomes. Furthermore, cost has become a dominant issue for many patients and providers.

Some evidence suggests that aspirin may attenuate the clinical benefits of ACE inhibitors by inhibiting bradykinin-mediated prostaglandin synthesis. In small pilot studies, aspirin inhibited the improvement in exercise duration and peak oxygen consumption and attenuated the hemodynamic effects of ACE inhibitors in patients with chronic HF.[65] Additional data from thromboembolic prevention studies also suggests that aspirin may have an adverse effect on the risk of HF hospitalizations.[66,67] In a post hoc analysis of SOLVD, the survival benefit of enalapril was not seen in patients receiving antiplatelet therapy at baseline.[68] However, a systematic overview of more than 22,000 patients from six large clinical trials found no difference in the benefits of ACE inhibitors on major clinical outcomes in patients taking or not taking aspirin (RR, 20% and 29%, respectively; interaction $P = .07$).[69] The attenuation of ACE inhibitor benefit appears less evident with clopidogrel. Although current guidelines recommend aspirin use for primary and secondary prevention of MI in patients with ischemic HF, there is no proven role for aspirin in patients with nonischemic cardiomyopathy.[66]

Angiotensin Receptor Blockers

Based on the clinical trials data and the ACC/AHA guidelines,[4] there are several indications for angiotensin receptor blockers (ARBs) in patients with HF and reduced ejection fraction. First, these agents may be used as alternative therapy in patients who are intolerant of ACE inhibitors, primarily due to persistent cough. Although ARBs were initially believed to be a safe alternative in patients with ACE inhibitor–induced angioedema, case reports suggest that life-threatening events may recur with the use of these agents,[70] and extreme caution is advised when substituting one for the other. Second, although ACE inhibitors remain the initial agents of choice for inhibition of the renin-angiotensin system, ARBs are a reasonable alternative and may be better tolerated in older patients,[71] although more recent data suggest that these agents are just as likely to produce hypotension, worsening renal function, and hyperkalemia as are ACE inhibitors (see Table 12-7). Finally, based on data from Val-HeFT and CHARM-Added, the addition of an ARB should be considered to reduce HF hospitalizations in patients who remain symptomatic despite ACE inhibitor and β-blocker therapy. Nevertheless, enthusiasm for combining an ACE inhibitor and ARB is somewhat diminished relative to the alternative of combining an ACE inhibitor or ARB with an aldosterone antagonist (see below). Until further information is available, the combined use of all three inhibitors of the renin-angiotensin system is not recommended[3,4] because of the high risk of hyperkalemia.[72]

Like ACE inhibitors, ARBs should be started at low doses (see Table 12-5) and titrated upward until target doses are achieved (e.g., candesartan 32 mg once daily, losartan 50 to 100 mg once daily, valsartan 160 mg twice daily). No large studies have compared efficacy and safety of high- versus low-dose angiotensin receptor blockade. The risks of hypotension, azotemia, and hyperkalemia are similar to those seen with ACE inhibitor monotherapy, and guidelines regarding clinical and laboratory follow-up discussed above should be followed. Greater caution is warranted when ARBs are added on top of ACE inhibitors as demonstrated by the higher rates of adverse events requiring drug withdrawal in the combined therapy group in the VALIANT study.[55]

β-Blockers

PATHOPHYSIOLOGIC RATIONALE

β-Blockers were traditionally contraindicated in patients with HF because of concerns that their negative inotropic actions could result in clinically important deterioration. It is now well established that chronic overactivity of the sympathetic nervous system plays an important role in the pathophysiology of HF (*Braunwald*, Chapter 25).[73] Adverse effects of circulating catecholamines and increased cardiac adrenergic drive include 1) myocardial hypertrophy, fibrosis, and apoptosis leading to ventricular remodeling and impaired contractile function; 2) β-receptor *downregulation*, a complex sequence of biochemical and molecular events that result in a decreased number of surface β-receptors and uncoupling of the β-receptor complex; 3) atrial and ventricular arrhythmias; 4) myocardial ischemia; 5) impaired renal sodium excretion; and 6) peripheral vasoconstriction. Regardless of the mechanism, it is clear that β-blockers slow or reverse ventricular remodeling, and in doing so, they reduce morbidity and mortality in patients with HF.

PHARMACOLOGY

Three classes of β-blockers are available for clinical use (see Chapter 7). *First-generation* agents, such as propranolol and timolol, are nonselective β-blockers with an equal affinity for β_1- and β_2-receptors. *Second-generation* β-blockers, such as metoprolol and bisoprolol, selectively inhibit β_1-receptors. *Third-generation* agents, such as carvedilol and bucindolol, were developed to include other pharmacologic properties in addition to β-blockade, in particular vasodilation. Carvedilol is a nonselective β_1-/β_2-blocker with potent α_1-blocking properties. In vitro studies also suggest that carvedilol exerts antioxidant effects,[74] although the clinical relevance of these findings remains unknown. Bucindolol is also a nonselective β-blocker with weak vasodilator properties, probably mediated via α_1-receptor blockade.[73] Nebivolol is a β_1-blocker with vasodilating properties related to increased bioavailability of nitric oxide.[75]

CLINICAL EFFICACY

In 1975, investigators at the University of Göteberg in Sweden first reported the beneficial effects of β-blockers when added to digoxin and diuretics in patients with dilated cardiomyopathy.[76] In the 1980s and early 1990s, several small clinical trials showed that

β-blockers, when administered carefully, can result in improved ventricular structure and function, hemodynamics, and β-receptor density.[77] Subsequent studies also demonstrated benefits of β-blockade on exercise tolerance and symptoms in patients with mild to moderate HF.[78] Finally, RCTs involving more than 20,000 patients with reduced ejection fraction treated with ACE inhibitors and diuretics (Table 12-8) demonstrated conclusively that β-blockers reduce hospitalizations and prolong survival in patients with chronic HF. As with ACE inhibitors, subgroup and meta-analyses show that β-blockers are equally effective in patients with ischemic and nonischemic HF and in a broad range of patients that includes women, those with diabetes, African Americans, and the elderly.[64,79,80] However, a recent study suggested that U.S. patients enrolled in β-blocker studies may have experienced a lower magnitude of survival benefit compared with patients from outside the United States,[81] and several multicenter trials deserve comment.

Cardiac Insufficiency Bisoprolol Studies (CIBIS) I and II

CIBIS I randomized 641 patients with ischemic or nonischemic cardiomyopathy and moderate to severe HF to either bisoprolol (up to 5 mg daily) or placebo.[82] After an average follow-up of 23 months, total mortality was slightly but not significantly reduced in the bisoprolol group (17% vs. 21%; $P = .22$). Subgroup analysis demonstrated that the mortality benefit was confined to patients with nonischemic cardiomyopathy. CIBIS II randomized 2647 patients with NYHA functional class III to IV heart failure and an ejection fraction of 35% or less to bisoprolol (up to 10 mg daily) or placebo for a mean of 1.3 years.[83] The study was stopped 18 months early because bisoprolol was associated with a 34% reduction in all-cause mortality. Bisoprolol also reduced sudden death by 44% and hospitalizations by 20%. Unlike CIBIS I, the treatment effects in CIBIS II were independent of the cause of HF. Notably, more than 90% of the patients enrolled in CIBIS II were in NYHA class III, and the annualized placebo mortality rate was only 13%, leading the investigators to warn against extrapolating the results to patents with severe HF.

U.S. Carvedilol Heart Failure Trials

The U.S. carvedilol HF trials program enrolled 1094 patients with NYHA functional class II to IV heart failure and an ejection fraction of 35% or less, on ACE inhibitors and diuretics, into one of four trials based on the distance walked in 6 minutes. The Prospective Randomized Evaluation of Carvedilol on Symptoms and Exercise (PRECISE) randomized 278 patients with moderate to severe HF to carvedilol or placebo for 6 to 8 months.[84] Carvedilol had no effect on the primary endpoint of exercise tolerance, but it reduced the combined endpoint of death or cardiovascular hospitalizations by 37%. The Multicenter Oral Carvedilol in Heart Failure Assessment (MOCHA) study randomized 345 patients with moderate to severe HF to one of three doses of carvedilol (12.5, 25, or 50 mg daily) or placebo.[85] As in PRECISE, treatment with carvedilol had no effect on exercise tolerance, but it reduced cardiovascular hospitalizations by 45% and all-cause mortality by 73%. The Mild Carvedilol Heart Failure study randomized 366 patients to carvedilol (50 to 100 mg daily) or placebo for up to 12 months.[86] Carvedilol reduced the risk of clinical progression—defined as death, HF hospitalization, or an increase in medications—by 48% and all-cause mortality by 77%. In the severe HF study, carvedilol had no effect on the primary endpoint, quality of life, but it improved global assessment by physicians and patients and increased ejection fraction.[87]

The U.S. Carvedilol Heart Failure Trials Program was stopped prematurely by the data safety monitoring board after a median follow-up of only 6.5 months because of a significant mortality benefit of carvedilol compared with placebo (RR, 65%; $P < .0001$).[88] Although the survival data were not considered conclusive because of the short follow-up period and small number of deaths (a total of 53), the combined results of the U.S. program led the FDA to approve carvedilol in 1997 for the treatment of patients with mild to moderate HF.

TABLE 12-8 Randomized, Controlled Trials of β-Blockers

TRIAL	N	AGENT	ENTRY CRITERIA	FOLLOW-UP PERIOD	PRIMARY ENDPOINT	FINDINGS*
CIBIS I[82]	641	Bisoprolol vs. placebo	LVEF <40% NYHA III-IV	23 months	Death	Placebo 21% Bisoprolol 17% (20% ↓, P = .22)
U.S. Carvedilol Heart Failure Trials[38,281]	1094	Carvedilol vs. placebo	LVEF ≤35% NYHA II-IV	6 months	Death	Placebo 7.8% Carvedilol 3.2% (65% ↓)
CIBIS II[83]	2647	Bisoprolol vs. placebo	LVEF ≤35% NYHA III-IV	16 months	Death	Placebo 17% Bisoprolol 12% (34% ↓)
MERIT-HF[89]	3991	Metoprolol CR/XL vs. placebo	LVEF ≤40% NYHA II-IV	12 months	Death	Placebo 11% Metoprolol 7% (34% ↓)
BEST[92,282]	2708	Bucindolol vs. placebo	LVEF <35% NYHA III-IV	2 years	Death	Placebo 33% Bucindolol 30% (10% ↓, P = .10)
COPERNICUS[95]	2289	Carvedilol vs. placebo	LVEF <25% NYHA IIIB-IV	10 months	Death	Placebo 17% Carvedilol 11% (35% ↓)
CAPRICORN[283]	1959	Carvedilol vs. placebo	LVEF ≤40% 3-21 days after MI	1.3 years	Death or CV hospitalization	Placebo 37% Carvedilol 35% (8% ↓, P = .30)
COMET[97]	3029	Carvedilol vs. metoprolol tartrate	LVEF ≤35% NYHA II-IV CV admission within 2 years	58 months	Death	Metoprolol 40% Carvedilol 34% (17% ↓)
SENIORS[98]	2128	Nebivolol vs. placebo	Age ≥70 years LVEF ≤35% or HF admission within 1 year	21 months	Death or CV admission	Placebo 35% Nebivolol 31% (14% ↓)

↓, reduction.
*P <.05 unless noted.
BEST, β-blocker Evaluation and Survival Trial; CAPRICORN, Carvedilol Post-Infarct Survival Control in Left Ventricular Dysfunction; CIBIS, Cardiac Insufficiency Bisoprolol Study; COMET, Carvedilol and Metoprolol European Trial; COPERNICUS, Carvedilol Prospective Randomized Cumulative Survival; CV, cardiovascular; HF, heart failure; LVEF, left ventricular ejection fraction; MERIT-HF, Metoprolol CR/XL Randomized Intervention Trial in Congestive Heart Failure; MI, myocardial infarction; NYHA, New York Heart Association functional class; SENIORS, Study of the Effects of Nebivolol Intervention on Outcomes and Rehospitalization in Seniors with Heart Failure.

Metoprolol CR/XL Randomised Intervention Trial in Congestive Heart Failure (MERIT-HF)

MERIT-HF enrolled 3991 patients with predominantly mild to moderate HF and an ejection fraction of 40% or less into a randomized placebo-controlled study of sustained-release metoprolol succinate (up to 200 mg daily).[89] After a mean follow-up of 1 year, an independent safety committee recommended early termination of the study because of a 34% lower risk of death in the metoprolol CR/XL group. In addition, metoprolol CR/XL reduced sudden deaths (by 41%), deaths as a result of worsening HF (by 49%), and total hospitalizations, and it improved NYHA functional class and quality of life.[90] A post hoc analysis of MERIT-HF and pooled data from other RCTs demonstrated that these benefits extend to women, including those with clinically stable severe HF.[91]

β-Blocker Evaluation and Survival Trial (BEST)

BEST randomized 2708 patients with moderate to severe HF to placebo or bucindolol and demonstrated a nonsignificant 10% reduction in total mortality (P = .10).[92] Preliminary subgroup analyses suggested that patients with NYHA functional class IV symptoms and African Americans tended to have worse outcomes on bucindolol therapy. An α-adrenergic receptor polymorphism that attenuates the norepinephrine-lowering effects of bucindolol may explain the differential racial effect.[93,94] The lower mortality benefit seen in BEST, when compared with MERIT-HF or CIBIS II, may be related to the population studied, the unique pharmacologic profile of bucindolol, or both. Bucindolol is not approved for clinical use in the United States.

Carvedilol Prospective Randomized Cumulative Survival Trial (COPERNICUS)

COPERNICUS was designed to test the efficacy of β-blockers in patients with severe HF.[95] This trial randomized 2289 patients with symptoms of HF at rest or on minimal exertion who were clinically euvolemic and had an ejection fraction of less than 25% to carvedilol or placebo. Patients could be enrolled during HF hospitalization but were excluded from participation if they required intensive care or were receiving IV vasoactive therapy. The trial was stopped early (mean follow-up, 10 months) by the data and safety monitoring board based on the finding of a 35% decrease in the risk of death with carvedilol. In addition, carvedilol decreased the combined risk of death or HF hospitalization by 31%.[96] The favorable effects of carvedilol were seen in all subgroups, including the highest-risk patients with recent or recurrent cardiac decompensation or ejection fraction less than 20%.

Carvedilol and Metoprolol European Trial (COMET)

Given the proven benefits of carvedilol and sustained-release metoprolol succinate relative to placebo, European investigators sought to compare the effects of carvedilol and metoprolol on clinical outcomes in HF. COMET randomized 3029 patients with NYHA functional class II to IV heart failure and an ejection fraction below 35% to receive carvedilol (target dose 25 mg twice daily) or immediate release metoprolol tartrate (target dose 50 mg twice daily).[97] After a mean follow-up of 58 months, all-cause mortality rate was 34% for carvedilol and 40% for metoprolol (HR, 0.83; 95% CI, 0.74 to 0.93; P = .0017), with the mortality benefit becoming apparent at about 6 months. Mean maintenance doses of carvedilol and metoprolol were 42 and 85 mg, respectively, with carvedilol exerting slightly greater blood pressure– and heart rate–lowering effects. The pattern of adverse events usually associated with β-blockade, including bradycardia and hypotension, was similar in the two groups.

Carvedilol Post-Infarct Survival Control in Left Ventricular Dysfunction (CAPRICORN)

The beneficial effects of β-blockers on survival following acute MI were first demonstrated in low-risk patients prior to the introduction of ACE inhibitors and thrombolysis. To determine the contemporary role of β-blocker therapy in higher-risk patients, CAPRICORN randomly assigned 1959 patients with an ejection fraction of 40% or less within 3 to 21 days following acute MI to receive carvedilol or placebo. Although no difference was noted in the primary combined endpoint of death or cardiovascular hospitalization, all-cause mortality was significantly reduced by carvedilol (HR, 0.77; 95% CI, 0.60 to 0.98; P = .03).

Study of the Effects of Nebivolol Intervention on Outcomes and Rehospitalization in Seniors with Heart Failure (SENIORS)

The pivotal β-blocker studies that preceded SENIORS enrolled patients with chronic HF, reduced ejection fraction, and an average age of 63 years. Accordingly, the SENIORS study was designed to test the effect of nebivolol, a β_1-selective blocker with vasodilating properties, on morbidity and mortality in elderly HF patients regardless of ejection fraction.[98] A total of 2128 patients aged 70 years or older with a history of HF, defined as a hospital admission within the previous year or ejection fraction less than or equal to 35%, were randomly assigned to receive nebivolol (target dose 10 mg once daily) or placebo for a mean of 21 months. The primary composite outcome of all-cause mortality or cardiovascular hospitalization occurred in 31.1% of the nebivolol group and 35.3% of the placebo group (HR, 0.86; 95% CI, 0.74 to 0.99; P = .039). In prespecified subgroup analyses, there was no evidence that age or ejection fraction modified the beneficial effects of nebivolol. At present, nebivolol is approved only for the treatment of hypertension.

PRACTICAL CONSIDERATIONS

Based on the results of controlled clinical trials, it is recommended that all stable patients with current or prior symptoms of HF and reduced ejection fraction be treated with a β-blocker unless contraindicated or not tolerated. Treatment with a β-blocker should be initiated as soon as LV dysfunction is diagnosed and should not be delayed until the patient's treatment with other drugs has failed (e.g., ACE inhibitors and diuretics). Patients with minimally symptomatic or asymptomatic LV dysfunction should also receive β-blockers to attenuate ventricular remodeling, slow disease progression, and reduce the risk of sudden death. Whether β-blockers are safe and effective in patients with refractory HF (stage D) remains unknown, although data from COPERNICUS suggest that the risk of clinical deterioration may be overstated.[96] In addition, the Initiation Management Predischarge: Process for Assessment of Carvedilol Therapy in Heart Failure (IMPACT-HF) trial demonstrated that initiation of β-blocker therapy prior to hospital discharge in stabilized patients is safe, that it does not increase length of stay, and that it enhances the long-term use of β-blockers.[99] The geographic variability in β-blocker treatment response recently described by O'Connor and colleagues[81] deserves additional study but may reflect population, genetic, cultural, or social differences.

When beginning therapy with β-blockers, patients should be stable on background therapy consisting of ACE inhibitors (or ARBs) and diuretics, although they do not need to be taking high doses of ACE inhibitors. Fluid retention should be minimal or absent, and patients should not be hospitalized in an intensive care unit and should not have recently received positive inotropic

therapy for acute decompensated HF. Volume depletion should also be corrected prior to initiating therapy. β-Blockers are relatively contraindicated in patients with moderate to severe asthma or chronic obstructive pulmonary disease (COPD) and in patients with severe bradycardia or conduction system disease that is not treated with a pacemaker. β-Blockers should be used with caution in patients with asymptomatic hypotension (e.g., systolic blood pressure <90 mm Hg). Although there is a theoretical concern that β-blockers may mask signs of hypoglycemia in the setting of diabetes, diabetic patients were not excluded from clinical trials and benefited equally compared to nondiabetic patients. Furthermore, carvedilol has been shown to have favorable metabolic effects and may delay the progression to microalbuminuria in patients with type 2 diabetes and hypertension.[100]

β-Blockers should be initiated at very low doses (e.g., bisoprolol 1.25 mg once daily, carvedilol 3.125 mg twice daily, metoprolol succinate 12.5 to 25 mg once daily), and they should be titrated slowly over several weeks as tolerated (see Table 12-5). During the titration phase, patients should be monitored closely for the development of adverse drug effects, including hypotension, worsening HF, or bradycardia. Family members should also be educated about potential side effects and how to monitor for drug intolerance. Hypotension is the most common side effect associated with β-blockers, especially with agents with concomitant α_1-blockade (e.g., carvedilol) and in the setting of volume depletion. Typically, patients describe mild lightheadedness, dizziness, or blurred vision that resolves after a few doses, but syncope may also occur. Strategies for managing hypotensive symptoms include taking β-blockers with food to slow absorption, staggering or reducing the doses of other vasodilators (e.g., ACE inhibitors or ARBs), or reducing diuretic therapy. If symptoms persist, the dose of β-blocker should be decreased, but abrupt withdrawal should be avoided.

Because the failing heart is dependent on adrenergic support, clinical HF status may worsen during the initiation of β-blocker therapy.[101] Although fluid retention and fatigue are less common than symptoms associated with hypotension, they are more likely to lead to β-blocker withdrawal.[88] Fluid retention, which may manifest as pulmonary and systemic venous congestion, can usually be managed with an increase in oral diuretics, whereas fatigue may require a decrease in the β-blocker dose. The management of acute decompensated HF in the setting of β-blocker initiation is discussed in Chapter 14. Another cause for hypotension or fatigue in patients recently started on β-blockers is bradycardia or heart block. Initial management includes assessing for laboratory or electrocardiographic (ECG) evidence of digoxin toxicity and lowering the dose of β-blocker. If other medications with negative chronotropic effects are contributing, such as amiodarone or antidepressants, they should either be stopped or permanent pacing should be considered. The role of permanent pacing to allow for β-blockade, especially in mildly symptomatic or asymptomatic patients, has not been studied.

Given the possibility of adverse effects occurring during initiation of β-blockers, uptitration should not occur until the patient is stable on the current dose. Overall, 10% to 15% of patients will not tolerate long-term therapy with β-blockers, although this rate may be higher in patients with more advanced disease[87] and in the elderly.[98] The optimal dosing of β-blockers in patients with HF is not known. In the MOCHA trial, in which patients were randomized to three different doses of carvedilol, trends were seen toward a dose-dependent increase in ejection fraction and decrease in mortality rates.[85] However, even patients randomized to low-dose carvedilol received significant clinical benefits. Similar clinical efficacy of high-dose versus low-dose metoprolol succinate was seen in MERIT-HF.[102] Therefore, although an attempt should be made to titrate β-blockers to the target doses used in controlled clinical trials (see Table 12-5), low-dose β-blocker therapy is preferred to no therapy. Patients should be advised that the clinical benefits of β-blockers may not become apparent for weeks to months, that they may feel worse before they feel better, and that the primary goals of therapy are to slow disease progression and prolong survival.

CHOICE OF β-BLOCKER

Three β-blockers have been shown to prolong survival and are approved by the FDA for the treatment of HF: *bisoprolol, sustained-release metoprolol succinate,* and *carvedilol.* Nebivolol prolonged the time to death or hospitalization and had a favorable safety profile in elderly HF subjects,[98] but it is only indicated for the treatment of hypertension. No controlled data are available on the use of atenolol or propranolol in HF. Although some remodeling[103] and survival data[97] suggest that carvedilol is superior to metoprolol, these studies were flawed by the use of immediate-release metoprolol at a lower β1-blocking dose. No studies have directly compared sustained-release metoprolol succinate and carvedilol at target doses, but review of the COPERNICUS and MERIT-HF studies suggests a similar reduction in all-cause mortality and sudden death. Once-daily β1-blocker therapy with metoprolol succinate or bisoprolol may be preferred in patients with reactive airway disease or in those for whom adherence or cost is an issue. Carvedilol may be more effective at lowering blood pressure in hypertensive patients and improving insulin sensitivity in diabetics,[100] and it has also been shown to be safe and effective in stable patients with severe HF.[95]

Aldosterone Antagonists

PATHOPHYSIOLOGY

In addition to systemic vasoconstriction and intravascular volume expansion, renal release of angiotensin in HF results in increased levels of aldosterone. Other stimuli of aldosterone release in HF include arginine vasopressin, endothelin, and catecholamines. Aldosterone is known to play an important role in the pathophysiology of HF by promoting sodium retention, sympathetic activation, and baroreceptor dysfunction and by causing myocardial and vascular fibrosis.[104] Although ACE inhibitors decrease aldosterone levels acutely, long-term inhibition of the renin-angiotensin system is associated with unsustained aldosterone suppression, referred to as *aldosterone escape.*[105]

Spironolactone and eplerenone competitively inhibit aldosterone-sensitive sodium channels in the cortical collecting tubule of the kidney and cause sodium and free water excretion and potassium retention. Similar to the antiremodeling effects of ACE inhibitors and ARBs, aldosterone antagonists inhibit mineralocorticoid receptors in the heart, kidney, and vasculature, which mediate pleiotropic effects that lead to ventricular and vascular remodeling and renal dysfunction.[106] Numerous studies in animals and humans have demonstrated salutary effects of aldosterone

receptor blockade on vasomotor reactivity, baroreceptor responsiveness, and norepinephrine uptake. In addition, myocardial injury can be attenuated by inhibiting the development of coronary inflammatory lesions. These experimental data provide an explanation for reduction in both HF and sudden death demonstrated in clinical trials of aldosterone antagonists (Table 12-9).

CLINICAL EFFICACY

In the past, spironolactone was used infrequently as a potassium-sparing diuretic in patients with advanced HF, refractory edema, and hypokalemia. With the recognition of aldosterone escape in HF and pilot studies demonstrating the safety of adding spironolactone to an ACE inhibitor,[107] a large mortality study of aldosterone antagonism was carried out. The Randomized Aldactone Evaluation Study (RALES) randomly assigned 1663 patients with severe HF and an ejection fraction of 35% or less to treatment with spironolactone (25 mg daily) or placebo.[108] The trial was stopped early after a mean follow-up of 24 months because of a 30% reduction in all-cause mortality by spironolactone. In addition, spironolactone improved symptoms and reduced the need for hospitalization as a result of HF. The striking results of RALES led to a rapid change in the prescribing patterns of health care providers and also to a heightened awareness of the risk of hyperkalemia (see below).[109]

Eplerenone is a selective mineralocorticoid receptor antagonist with a hundredfold to thousandfold lower affinity for androgen, glucocorticoid, and progesterone receptors than spironolactone. Pilot studies suggested that aldosterone receptor blockade exerted favorable effects on ventricular remodeling following MI. The Eplerenone Post-Acute Myocardial Infarction Heart Failure Efficacy and Survival Study (EPHESUS) was designed to test the hypothesis that treatment with eplerenone would reduce morbidity and mortality in patients with acute MI complicated by LV dysfunction and HF. EPHESUS randomly assigned 6632 patients within 3 to 14 days of acute MI with LV ejection fraction (LVEF) of 40% or less and HF as documented by the presence of pulmonary congestion or S3 gallop to receive eplerenone (target dose 50 mg once daily) or placebo. Patients with diabetes and LV dysfunction were not required to have clinical evidence of HF. During a mean follow-up of 16 months, eplerenone reduced the risk of death from any cause by 15% ($P = .008$) and reduced the combined endpoint of cardiovascular death or hospitalization by 13% ($P = .002$).[110] Eplerenone also reduced the risk of sudden cardiac death by 21%.

The results of EPHESUS and RALES demonstrated the benefits of aldosterone antagonists in HF patients with reduced ejection fraction after MI and with NYHA functional class III to IV symptoms, respectively. The aim of the Eplerenone in Mild Patients Hospitalization and Survival Study in Heart Failure (EMPHASIS-HF)

TABLE 12-9		Randomized, Controlled Trials of Aldosterone Antagonists				
TRIAL	**N**	**AGENT**	**ENTRY CRITERIA**	**FOLLOW-UP PERIOD**	**PRIMARY ENDPOINT**	**FINDINGS***
RALES	1663	Spironolactone vs. placebo	LVEF ≤35% NYHA III-IV	24 months	Death	Placebo 46% Spironolactone 35% (31% ↓)
EPHESUS	6632	Eplerenone vs. placebo	3-14 days post-MI LVEF ≤40% HF signs	16 months	Death	Placebo 16.7% Eplerenone 14.4% (15% ↓)
EMPHASIS-HF	2737	Eplerenone vs. placebo	Age >55 years LVEF ≤35% NYHA II Cardiac hospitalization within 6 months or elevated BNP or NT-proBNP	21 months	CV death or HF hospitalization	Placebo 25.9% Eplerenone 18.3% (37% ↓)

*$P < .05$.

BNP, B-type natriuretic peptide; CV, cardiovascular; EMPHASIS-HF, Eplerenone in Mild Patients Hospitalization and Survival Study in Heart Failure; EPHESUS, Eplerenone Post-Acute Myocardial Infarction Heart Failure Efficacy and Survival Study; HF, heart failure; LVEF, left ventricular ejection fraction; NT-proBNP, N-terminal pro-BNP; NYHA, New York Heart Association functional class; RALES, Randomized Aldactone Evaluation Study.

was to investigate the effects of eplerenone on clinical outcomes in patients with systolic HF and mild symptoms (i.e., NYHA functional class II). In this randomized, double-blind trial, 2737 patients with mild HF and LVEF of 35% or less were randomly assigned to receive eplerenone (up to 50 mg daily) or placebo in addition to standard therapy.[111] Additional inclusion criteria included a QRS duration greater than 130 ms for patients with an ejection fraction between 31% and 35%, a cardiovascular hospitalization within 6 months, and an elevated natriuretic peptide level. The executive committee stopped the trial prematurely after a median follow-up period of 21 months, when it was found that eplerenone reduced the primary composite endpoint of cardiovascular death or HF hospitalization by 37% ($P < .001$) and all-cause mortality by 24% ($P = .008$).

In an open-label study, spironolactone improved peak oxygen consumption, diastolic function, and symptoms in older women with at least one HF hospitalization and an ejection fraction of 50% or greater.[112] A multicenter RCT of Aldosterone Antagonist Therapy in Adults with Preserved Ejection Fraction Congestive Heart Failure (TOPCAT) is currently testing the effects of spironolactone on morbidity and mortality in patients with HF and preserved ejection fraction.

PRACTICAL CONSIDERATIONS

Based on the totality of the evidence from clinical trials, adjunctive therapy with aldosterone antagonists should be considered in all patients with symptomatic HF and reduced ejection fraction and in patients who have had an acute MI with LV dysfunction and HF. The major risk associated with aldosterone blockade is hyperkalemia, which in some cases may be exacerbated by worsening renal function. Although the incidence of serious hyperkalemia was minimal in the RALES trial (1% placebo, 2% spironolactone; $P = .42$), it is important to note that patients were not enrolled if serum creatinine exceeded 2.5 mg/dL, and the mean creatinine level at baseline was only 1.2 mg/dL. Similarly, patients were excluded from EMPHASIS-HF if their serum potassium level exceeded 5.0 mmol/L, or if the estimated GFR was less than 30 mL/min/1.73 m². In both studies, potassium supplements were discontinued, and electrolytes and renal function were monitored closely.

Following publication of RALES, the rates of spironolactone prescriptions, hospitalization for hyperkalemia, and associated mortality increased significantly.[109] Use of aldosterone antagonists in a broader patient population—the elderly, those with chronic kidney disease, and HF patients with preserved ejection fraction[113]—and less rigorous monitoring of serum potassium levels[114] were initially thought to explain these higher complication rates. However, a more recent community-based study suggests improved safety with aldosterone antagonists in HF,[115] possibly related to increased frequency of laboratory monitoring. In addition, although the rate of moderate hyperkalemia (serum potassium >5.5 mmol/L) was higher with eplerenone in EMPHASIS-HF (11.8% vs. 7.2% placebo; $P < .001$), the rate of severe hyperkalemia (serum potassium >6.0 mmol/L) was not different (2.5% vs. 1.9% placebo; $P = .29$), and placebo-treated patients had more hypokalemia.[111]

Antiandrogenic effects, which may also limit the use of spironolactone, include painful gynecomastia, impotence, and menstrual irregularities (see Table 12-7). These hormonal effects are generally not seen with the selective mineralocorticoid receptor antagonist eplerenone.

Spironolactone should be initiated at a dose of 12.5 mg once daily, and eplerenone should be initiated at a dose of 25 mg/day. Potassium supplementation should be decreased or discontinued, and follow-up laboratory tests should be checked within 1 week and then monthly for up to 3 months. Patients should be counseled on avoiding certain foods—such as bananas, avocados, and broccoli—and salt substitutes (Nu-Salt) that may contain high quantities of potassium. In addition, medications that can worsen renal function, such as NSAIDs, should be avoided. Any change in

cardiac medications that may affect renal function or volume status, such as ACE inhibitor titration or use of combination diuretics, requires reassessment of serum electrolytes and renal function. Depending on the severity of hyperkalemia, treatment may include permanent discontinuation of the aldosterone antagonist, temporary discontinuation of other renin-angiotensin system inhibitors and potassium supplements, and use of exchange resins. Hyperkalemia associated with cardiac dysrhythmias and/or hemodynamic instability should be treated according to the AHA Guidelines for Cardiopulmonary Resuscitation with IV sodium bicarbonate, calcium chloride, and glucose plus insulin.[116]

OPTIONS FOR PATIENTS WHO REMAIN SYMPTOMATIC DESPITE STANDARD THERAPY

Patients who have persistent signs and symptoms of HF despite intensive treatment with diuretics, ACE inhibitors or ARBs, β-blockers, and aldosterone antagonists present a difficult challenge for physicians treating patients with HF. Several pharmacologic, device, and surgical options are currently available and may require consultation with an HF specialist to optimize therapy for the individual patient. For patients with symptomatic HF, digoxin should be considered as adjunctive therapy to reduce morbidity and mortality related to progressive LV failure. The combination of hydralazine and isosorbide dinitrate is recommended to improve outcomes for African American patients with moderate to severe HF and reduced ejection fraction. For patients with advanced or refractory HF, several options can be considered individually or in combination (Table 12-10). Some patients will require combination diuretics, loop and thiazide, or multiple vasoactive agents, usually a combination of ACE inhibitors, ARBs, and/or hydralazine and isosorbide dinitrate. A small number of selected patients may be candidates for mechanical circulatory support and/or cardiac transplantation (see Chapter 15).

Cardiac resynchronization therapy improves contractile performance acutely in patients with dilated cardiomyopathy and intraventricular conduction delay, and it reduces morbidity and mortality in chronic HF (see Chapter 13). Also, high-risk coronary artery bypass grafting (CABG) and surgical mitral valvuloplasty (see Chapters 11 and 46, respectively) may reduce wall stress and may cause reverse ventricular remodeling in patients with ischemic or nonischemic cardiomyopathy. However, these procedures have not been shown to prolong survival compared with medical therapy alone,[117,118] and they are limited to specialized centers. Finally, continuous infusions of positive inotropic agents may be used as palliative care to bridge patients to end of life, or they may be used in selected patients as a bridge to cardiac transplant. The discussion below will focus on adjunctive pharmacologic therapy.

TABLE 12-10	Therapeutic Options for Patients with Advanced or Refractory Heart Failure	
APPROVED	**INVESTIGATIONAL**	
Combination diuretics	Novel vasodilators	
Additional vasodilators	Phosphodiesterase type 5 inhibitors	
Cardiac resynchronization therapy*	Erythropoiesis-stimulating agents	
Positive inotropic agents	Enhanced external counterpulsation	
Mechanical circulatory support	Implantable hemodynamic monitor	
Cardiac transplantation	Surgical or percutaneous mitral valvuloplasty	

*Also indicated for patients with mild heart failure symptoms, reduced ejection fraction, and prolonged QRS duration based on results of the Multicenter Automatic Defibrillator Implantation Trial with Cardiac Resynchronization Therapy (MADIT-CRT),[284] Resynchronization Reverses Remodeling in Systolic Left Ventricular Dysfunction (REVERSE),[285] and Resynchronization-Defibrillation for Ambulatory Heart Failure Trial (RAFT)[286] trials (see Chapter 13).

Hydralazine and Isosorbide Dinitrate

The combination of hydralazine and isosorbide dinitrate was shown in V-HeFT I to be an efficacious combination in terms of an improvement in survival compared to placebo.[38] Moreover, in V-HeFT II, this combination tended to increase exercise capacity and ejection fraction more than enalapril.[39] The experience from these two large trials clearly demonstrated the utility and benefits of this drug combination. Furthermore, retrospective analysis of the V-HeFT studies suggested particular efficacy in African Americans.[119] To test whether this combination provides additional benefit in this specialized population, the African American Heart Failure Trial (A-HeFT) randomized 1050 self-identified African Americans with NYHA functional class III to IV heart failure and dilated ventricles to receive a fixed dose of isosorbide dinitrate plus hydralazine (target daily doses of 120 mg and 225, respectively) or placebo in addition to standard therapy.[120] The vast majority were on an ACE inhibitor or ARB (86%) and β-blocker (74%). The study was stopped early because of a significantly higher mortality rate in the placebo group than in the group given isosorbide dinitrate plus hydralazine (10.2% vs. 6.2%; $P = .02$). Combination therapy also reduced the rate of HF hospitalizations by 33%, and it improved quality of life.

Although originally thought to be effective as vasodilators, emerging evidence suggests that the benefits of hydralazine and isosorbide dinitrate are related more to their biologic effects.[121] For example, nitrates may attenuate myocardial and vascular remodeling by increasing the bioavailability of nitric oxide,[122] and hydralazine has been shown to prevent nitrate tolerance through antioxidant activity.[123] Hydralazine attenuates nitrate tolerance through inhibition of NADH/NADPH oxidases and through direct scavenging of reactive oxygen species. By favorably altering the nitroso-redox balance in HF[122] the combination of nitrates and hydralazine may prevent myocardial hypertrophy, fibrosis, and apoptosis and may improve vascular compliance (Figure 12-4). Hydralazine has also been shown to have potent antiatherogenic effects.[124] Although these mechanisms have not been explored directly in RCTs, preliminary data from the A-HeFT study demonstrate clinical benefits independent of baseline blood pressure as well as reverse ventricular remodeling. It is also not known whether these mechanisms of benefit are of greater importance for African Americans than for other racial or ethnic groups. Preliminary studies demonstrate impaired flow-mediated vasodilation in blacks with hypertension compared with whites with hypertension, but these studies are limited by small numbers and potential confounders.[125] Others have shown a more generalized abnormality in endothelium-dependent vasodilation in HF,[126] which could be favorably affected by nitric oxide–enhancing therapy. Additional studies to understand the genetic and environmental determinants of the effect of hydralazine and nitrates on disease progression in HF are in progress.

PRACTICAL CONSIDERATIONS

A number of factors have limited the widespread application of hydralazine–isosorbide dinitrate to patients with HF. First, in V-HeFT II, the ACE inhibitor enalapril resulted in a significant improvement in survival compared with hydralazine–isosorbide dinitrate. Second, the combination of hydralazine and isosorbide dinitrate is considerably more cumbersome for patient adherence, because the target doses used in the V-HeFT studies were 160 mg of isosorbide dinitrate (40 mg four times daily) and 300 mg of hydralazine (75 mg four times daily). Although a fixed combination pill that can be taken three times daily is available, adherence and cost remain problematic for patients already taking several HF medications. Third, this combination has a number of side effects, including headaches and flushing associated with nitrate preparations and gastrointestinal symptoms from hydralazine. In the V-HeFT trials, 18% to 38% of patients discontinued one or both of the medications because of side effects. In A-HeFT, adverse effects of hydralazine–isosorbide dinitrate included headache (50%), dizziness (32%), and nausea (10%), with 1 in 5 patients discontinuing the fixed-dose combination.

In clinical practice, the combination of hydralazine and isosorbide dinitrate may be particularly useful in patients who have persistent symptoms of HF but are unable to tolerate renin-angiotensin system inhibitors. However, no studies have specifically targeted this patient population, and hydralazine and nitrates

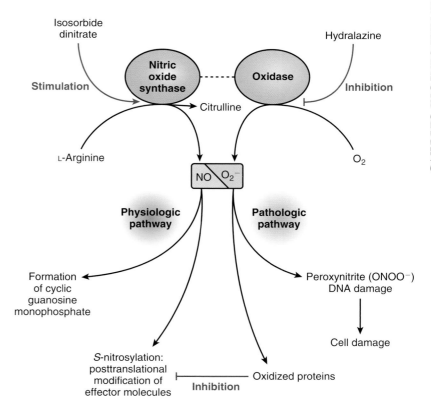

FIGURE 12-4 Consequences of disrupting the balance between nitric oxide and superoxide production in the cardiovascular system of patients with heart failure. The interaction between nitric oxide (*NO*) and superoxide (O_2^-) plays fundamental roles in cell and organ failure at key sites throughout the cardiovascular system. In patients with heart failure, the production of O_2^- is increased, and the level or location of NO is disrupted; this interrupts effector signaling and causes cellular dysfunction as a result of vasoconstriction and cardiac contractility or, if prolonged, it causes cell damage or cell death. Isosorbide dinitrate, a drug that stimulates the NO pathway, and hydralazine, an antioxidant that inhibits O_2^- synthesis, may restore nitroso-redox balance, converting pathologic pathways to physiologic pathways in the heart and blood vessels. (*Modified from Hare JM. Nitroso-redox balance in the cardiovascular system.* N Engl J Med *2004;351:2112-2114.*)

should not be substituted for ACE inhibitors or ARBs. Many physicians use nitrates in their patients with HF, especially those with underlying ischemic heart disease.[127] Based on both mechanistic and trial data, it would be prudent to administer nitrates in combination with hydralazine to African-American patients with HF and reduced ejection fraction. Furthermore, updated HFSA guidelines recommend the addition of a combination of hydralazine and isosorbide dinitrate for non–African-American patients with reduced ejection fraction who remain symptomatic despite optimized standard therapy.[3]

The most important recommendation regarding this regimen is to initiate therapy with low doses followed by gradual dose titration over several weeks. Initial doses greater than 10 mg of isosorbide dinitrate and 25 mg of hydralazine may produce headaches, but gradual uptitration is usually well tolerated. Prophylactic acetaminophen can reduce the problems associated with nitrate-induced headache, whereas NSAIDs should be avoided. Several long-acting nitrate preparations are now available, but the clinical experience with these formulations in patients with HF is limited.

Digoxin

PHARMACOLOGIC AND CLINICAL EFFECTS

The mechanisms of action and the pharmacology of digoxin are discussed in Chapter 28 of *Braunwald's Heart Disease* and in other reviews.[128] Through its inhibition of sodium-potassium adenosine triphosphatase, digoxin affects cellular processes in the heart (increased cardiac contractility), vagal afferents (decreased sympathetic outflow), and kidney (decreased renin secretion) that contribute to its cardiovascular effects. Although digoxin has been commonly used in the management of HF, considerable controversy has surrounded the precise documentation of its clinical efficacy. Early studies were conflicting, and interpretation was difficult because of small sample sizes and dependence on less precise clinical measures. Data from larger and more conclusive RCTs[129-133] have provided the scientific data to recommend the use of digoxin to improve symptoms and decrease hospitalizations for HF in patients with reduced ejection fraction and current or prior symptoms of HF.[3,4]

Many of the early trials that evaluated the efficacy of digoxin used a crossover design and sample sizes considered small compared with more recent multicenter trials. Subsequent trials used a parallel design in which digoxin was compared to placebo and other inotropic and/or vasodilator agents that included xamoterol, captopril, milrinone, and ibopamine. The German and Austrian Xamoterol Study Group randomized 433 patients to either placebo, digoxin, or xamoterol, a mixed β-agonist with some β-blocker activity.[129] Digoxin and xamoterol decreased symptoms of HF compared with placebo. The Captopril-Digoxin Multicenter Research Group randomized 300 patients to either placebo, digoxin, or captopril.[130] At 6 months, digoxin increased ejection fraction and reduced hospitalizations for HF, and captopril improved exercise duration and NYHA functional class. In other trials comparing digoxin with oral inotropic therapy, digoxin decreased neurohormonal activation and markedly decreased the frequency of clinical decompensation.[131,132] Two trials examined the effect of withdrawal of digoxin in HF patients who were treated with a diuretic only[134] or a diuretic and an ACE inhibitor.[135] In both trials, the withdrawal of digoxin resulted in a decrease in exercise tolerance, worsening HF symptoms, and lower ejection fraction.

Although these studies demonstrated the beneficial effects of digoxin on clinical endpoints, virtually all of these trials were unable to assess an effect on survival because of inadequate sample size. In addition, retrospective data in patients following acute MI suggested that digoxin increased mortality rate.[136] The effect of digoxin on mortality in patients with chronic HF was assessed in the Digitalis Investigation Group (DIG) trial. In the DIG trial, 6800 patients with mild to moderate HF and an ejection fraction of 45% or less were randomized to digoxin or placebo in addition to diuretics and ACE inhibitors. After a mean follow-up of 37 months, there were 1181 deaths in the digoxin group and 1194 deaths in the placebo group (RR, 0.99; $P = .80$). Digoxin reduced the risk of death or hospitalization as a result of worsening HF, but it tended to increase the risk of death from other causes.

The cumulative data from controlled trials suggests that digoxin is associated with important clinical improvements without adverse effects on survival. Furthermore, these benefits have been seen in a wide range of patients, regardless of the etiology of HF, the underlying rhythm, or concomitant medical therapy. The results of the DIG trial led the FDA to approve digoxin for the treatment of HF in 1997. According to the updated ACC/AHA guidelines, the goals of digoxin therapy should be to alleviate symptoms and improve clinical status in patients with HF who are being treated with diuretics, an ACE inhibitor or ARB, and a β-blocker.[4] Digoxin may also be added to the initial regimen in patients with severe symptoms who have not responded to standard treatment, but it is not indicated as a primary therapy to stabilize patients with acute decompensated HF (see Chapter 14). Digoxin has not been shown to be effective in patients with HF and preserved ejection fraction, and it may have adverse effects in patients with acute coronary syndromes. Furthermore, no data support the use of digoxin in patients with asymptomatic LV dysfunction.

PRACTICAL CONSIDERATIONS

Previous practice typically involved the use of full digitalizing doses to more rapidly achieve therapeutic levels. However, this is no longer recommended, and patients should simply be started on maintenance doses that range from 0.0625 to 0.25 mg/day. Steady-state levels will be reached in approximately 1 week. Because drug elimination is primarily via the kidneys, digoxin doses must be adjusted in patients with acute or chronic kidney disease. A number of drug interactions can significantly influence the efficacy and toxicity of digoxin.[128] Drugs known to increase digoxin levels include verapamil, spironolactone, and amiodarone. It is common practice to empirically reduce digoxin doses when initiating therapy with these drugs, with close follow-up of digoxin levels. In addition, lower doses are recommended in elderly patients with HF[137] and in those with low lean body mass.

Little evidence supports the routine use of serum digoxin concentrations to guide dose selection. However, it is reasonable to check the digoxin level in follow-up to identify patients who are receiving subtherapeutic doses, which in some cases is secondary to nonadherence. Digoxin levels are also very important in the evaluation of toxicity, for example, in patients who develop nausea, anorexia, arrhythmias, atrioventricular block, or confusion. Digoxin toxicity is usually associated with serum levels of more than 2.0 ng/mL, but it can occur with lower serum levels in the setting of hypokalemia or hypomagnesemia. Retrospective analyses from the DIG trial also suggest that serum digoxin concentrations in the high-normal range (e.g., 1.2 to 2.0 ng/mL) are associated with an increased risk of death in both men and women.[138,139] Taken together, these data suggest that the efficacy and safety of digoxin can be optimized by using doses that achieve a serum level in the range of 0.5 to 0.9 ng/mL. Of note, this recommendation has not yet been incorporated into reference ranges provided by most clinical laboratories.

For many years, digoxin has been used to control the ventricular response rate in atrial fibrillation. In many situations, however, digoxin may not provide adequate rate control, especially during exercise, in patients with high sympathetic tone and in the elderly. In patients with HF and atrial fibrillation already receiving a β-blocker, digoxin may be used as adjunctive therapy to control ventricular rate. Alternatively, amiodarone may be safely used for both ventricular rate control and restoration and maintenance of sinus rhythm.[140] In patients with symptomatic atrial fibrillation who do not respond to, or are intolerant of, antiarrhythmic therapy, options include atrioventricular junction ablation with back-up pacing or pulmonary vein isolation using radiofrequency or surgical ablation.[141,142] For more complete discussions of the pharmacologic and nonpharmacologic management of atrial fibrillation, see Chapters 20 and 21, and Chapter 40 in Braunwald.

Calcium Channel Blockers

Calcium channel blocking agents were initially considered useful in patients with HF because these drugs have potent vasodilator actions and may reduce ischemia in patients with LV dysfunction as a result of coronary artery disease.[143] Hemodynamic studies demonstrated that acute administration of calcium channel blockers reduced systemic vascular resistance and increased cardiac output. However, the acute hemodynamic effects of nifedipine, verapamil, and diltiazem have not been uniform, and short- and long-term treatment with these agents has been associated with serious adverse events and excess mortality, possibly related to negative inotropic effects or neurohormonal stimulation.

Second-generation calcium channel blockers with greater selectivity for vascular actions have also been evaluated in HF. Amlodipine, a long-acting dihydropyridine with potent vasodilator effects, is approved for the treatment of hypertension and angina. In the Prospective Randomized Amlodipine Survival Evaluation (PRAISE) study, 1153 patients with severe HF and an ejection fraction of less than 30% were randomized to amlodipine (up to 10 mg daily) or placebo for 6 to 33 months.[144] Amlodipine had no effect on the primary combined endpoint of death or major cardiovascular hospitalization but tended to reduce all-cause mortality (RR, 16%; $P = .07$), particularly in nonischemic cardiomyopathy. However, PRAISE II demonstrated no beneficial effects of amlodipine on neurohormonal stimulation or survival in this population.[145] Similar negative findings were seen in the V-HeFT III study, in which long-term therapy with felodipine had no beneficial effects on exercise tolerance, hospitalizations, or survival and was associated with a higher incidence of peripheral edema.[146] Finally, data from the Antihypertensive and Lipid-Lowering Treatment to Prevent Heart Attack Trial (ALLHAT) suggests that the antihypertensive benefits of amlodipine may be offset by an increased risk of developing HF.[147]

Based on these cumulative data, it is recommended that most calcium channel blockers should be avoided in patients with HF. The primary benefit may be mainly from control of hypertension or reduction of ischemia, although alternative agents such as nitrates or treatments such as revascularization are preferred. Of the available calcium channel blockers, only the vasoselective agents have not been shown to adversely affect survival in patients with HF and reduced ejection fraction. Calcium channel blockers may have a role in controlling heart rate or improving symptoms in patients with HF and preserved ejection fraction (see below).

Positive Inotropic Agents

ORAL POSITIVE INOTROPES

The search for safe and effective inotropic agents for patients with HF has been based on the observation that the clinical syndrome of HF results from a primary defect in myocardial contractility and that many patients have symptoms that are refractory to standard therapy. During the 1980s and early 1990s, an extraordinary effort was made to develop an orally administered inotropic agent.[148] The majority of studies focused on phosphodiesterase (PDE) inhibitors, which produce a marked hemodynamic benefit when administered acutely to patients with acute decompensated HF. However, enthusiasm for this class of drugs decreased significantly when multicenter trials failed to detect a significant improvement in symptoms and exercise tolerance,[149] and when the Prospective Randomized Milrinone Survival Evaluation (PROMISE) trial demonstrated increased mortality rates in patients treated with milrinone.[150] Other oral inotropes with PDE inhibitor effects have also

been associated with excess mortality in HF, including vesnarinone[151] and enoximone.[152]

INTRAVENOUS POSITIVE INOTROPES

An additional treatment that can be considered in patients with refractory HF is IV dobutamine or milrinone.[153] Dobutamine augments cardiac contractility primarily via stimulation of β-adrenergic receptors and is a modest vasodilator, whereas milrinone exerts potent inotropic and direct vasodilator effects via PDE type 3 inhibition in the myocardium and vasculature, respectively (see Chapter 14 for discussion of pharmacology and short-term use of positive inotropic therapy in acute decompensated HF). A small number of patients with end-stage HF cannot be weaned from acute inotropic therapy. Evidence of failure to wean includes the development of symptomatic hypotension, recurrent congestion, and/or worsening renal function. In practice, more than one attempt should be made to wean inotropes, and weaning should not be undertaken until the patient has achieved clinical stability. In addition, ACE inhibitors and β-blockers may need to be held to increase blood pressure and renal perfusion. Invasive monitoring and "optimization" of hemodynamics is generally not required, nor is it recommended,[154] except for the purpose of insurance approval for home infusion. For selected patients deemed to be inotrope dependent, chronic IV therapy may be used as a bridge to transplant or end of life.

Bridge to Transplantation

Because of the limited donor supply, the majority of patients who receive heart transplants require pharmacologic or mechanical circulatory support as a bridge to transplant (see Chapter 15). Options for inotrope-dependent patients include in-hospital or continuous home IV therapy. Criteria for discharge home include hemodynamic stability on a low-dose of a single agent, improved functional status, and family and nursing support. Implantable cardioverter-defibrillators (ICDs) are recommended to prevent sudden death. Home dobutamine and milrinone have been used successfully to bridge patients to transplant with improved functional capacity and renal function,[155] although readmissions and complications are common. In one study, 59% of patients required readmission: two thirds of readmissions resulted from worsening HF, and one third were due to infection or occlusion of the indwelling catheter.[156] Patients on home inotropes should be advised against driving.

Bridge to End of Life

For patients with refractory HF who are not transplant candidates, chronic inotropic therapy may be used to palliate symptoms at the end of life. This practice has become more common as cardiologists care for older patients who have exhausted their medical and surgical options. Also, the use of β-blockers and ICDs in the elderly has decreased the risk of sudden death in favor of progressive pump failure. Hershberger and colleagues[153] reported a 10-year experience with home inotropic infusions in nontransplant patients with end-stage HF. Although patients were ambulatory and pain-free at the time of discharge, the median survival was only 3 months, and one third died in the hospital. In practice, inotropic therapy in end-stage HF requires consultation with a palliative care service, collaboration with home hospice providers to facilitate coadministration of narcotics and anxiolytics, and a discussion with the patient and family about advanced directives and turning off ICDs.[157]

Positive inotropic agents have also been administered intermittently at home or in an infusion clinic.[158] Although initial uncontrolled studies suggested improvement in symptoms and decreased hospitalizations, some small randomized studies demonstrated either no benefit or excess mortality.[159] The primary mechanism responsible for increased mortality associated with chronic inotropic infusions is believed to be an increase in intracellular cyclic adenosine monophosphate (cAMP), which exerts a direct toxic effect on the myocardium and leads to further contractile dysfunction and proarrhythmia.[160] Hypersensitivity myocarditis with dobutamine may also contribute to hemodynamic deterioration.[161] Because of the lack of data demonstrating efficacy and the concerns about toxicity, the use of intermittent inotropic infusions is not recommended for the treatment of advanced HF.[4]

Antithrombotic Therapy

In the absence of specific contraindications, many clinicians have recommended anticoagulation for patients with dilated cardiomyopathy for prophylaxis against thromboembolism and stroke. This recommendation is based on older data that showed the presence of ventricular thrombi in up to 75% of cases of dilated cardiomyopathy[162] and on observations of a high incidence of embolic events in this patient population.[163,164] In addition, retrospective analyses have suggested that the incidence of embolic events[165] and all-cause mortality[166] is reduced in HF patients treated with anticoagulants. The mechanisms underlying the increased risk of thromboembolism in patients with HF include stasis of blood in the cardiac chambers and systemic venous circulation and hypercoagulability. Additionally, patients with HF are at increased risk for the development of atrial fibrillation,[167] which predisposes to cardiac thrombi formation.

Recommendations for the routine use of anticoagulants in patients with HF have been reconsidered in view of data from multicenter trials. In V-HeFT II, only 46 embolic events were reported in 804 patients followed for an average of 2.5 years.[168] Furthermore, V-HeFT II demonstrated an *increased* thromboembolic rate in patients who received anticoagulation compared with those who did not (4.9 vs. 2.1 per 100 patient-years; $P = .01$). In SOLVD, the annual incidence of thromboembolic events was only 2.4% in women and 1.8% in men. Furthermore, the use of anticoagulants as directed by individual physicians was not associated with a reduced incidence of thromboembolism.[169] Unfortunately, RCTs of anticoagulation in HF have been inconclusive because of small sample sizes[67] or premature cessation as a result of lack of enrollment.[170]

The Warfarin and Antiplatelet Therapy in Chronic Heart Failure (WATCH) trial was designed to determine the optimal antithrombotic agent for HF patients with reduced ejection fraction in normal sinus rhythm.[170] Between 1999 and 2002, the WATCH trial randomly assigned 1587 patients, rather than the planned 4500, with NYHA functional class II to IV heart failure and an LVEF of 35% or less to receive open-label warfarin (target international normalized ratio [INR] 2.5 to 3.0) or double-blind treatment with aspirin (162 mg once daily) or clopidogrel (75 mg once daily). During a mean follow-up of 19 months, the risk of the primary composite endpoint of all-cause mortality, nonfatal MI, and nonfatal stroke did not differ among the three groups. Compared with antiplatelet therapy, warfarin was associated with fewer nonfatal strokes and HF hospitalizations but more bleeding events. The investigators concluded that the data do not support the primary hypotheses that warfarin is superior to aspirin and that clopidogrel is superior to aspirin. The Warfarin Versus Aspirin in Reduced Cardiac Ejection Fraction (WARCEF) study was designed to compare warfarin (target INR of 2.0 to 3.5) and aspirin (325 mg/day) in patients with HF and reduced ejection fraction. In 2305 patients followed for up to 6 years, there was no difference in the rates of the composite endpoint (ischemic stroke, intercerebral hemorrhage, or death from any cause) between the two groups.[171] Although warfarin was associated with a reduction in ischemic stroke, this benefit was offset by an increased rate of major hemorrhage.

Because the risk of thromboembolism and the benefits of anticoagulants may not be as great as once considered, recommendations for anticoagulation for patients with HF should be made on an individual basis. Consensus indications for anticoagulation include atrial fibrillation (paroxysmal or persistent) and a history of venous or systemic thromboembolism,[3,4] but consideration of anticoagulation should also be given to patients with intracavitary thrombi or spontaneous contrast demonstrated by echocardiography, or with specific diagnoses associated with a higher thromboembolic risk, such as cardiac amyloid, LV noncompaction, and peripartum cardiomyopathy. Patients with a recent large anterior MI or recent MI with LV thrombus should be treated with warfarin for at least 3 months. Younger patients with genetic cardiomyopathies and a family history of thromboembolism should also be considered for anticoagulation. In patients with contraindications to warfarin, an alternate regimen is to use a single daily dose of aspirin, but no controlled data support this recommendation. In addition, as discussed above, aspirin may attenuate the benefits of ACE inhibition in HF and is not recommended in patients with nonischemic cardiomyopathy. The role of newer antiplatelet (prasugrel) and anticoagulant (dabigatran, apixaban, rivaroxaban) agents in reducing the risk of thromboembolism in HF has not been established.

Antiarrhythmic Therapy

The indications for, and the efficacy of, antiarrhythmic agents in the management of HF have been subjects of great controversy.[172] The original rationale for considering these agents as adjunctive therapy was based on the observation that as many as 30% to 50% of all deaths in patients with HF can be classified as sudden. Frequent ventricular premature contractions and nonsustained ventricular tachycardia on Holter recordings are almost universal in patients with HF and are frequent sources of concern in hospitalized patients who are on telemetry monitoring. These arrhythmias are likely related to a number of factors including fibrosis, wall stress, LV dilation, electrolyte imbalances, high levels of circulating catecholamines, and proarrhythmic effects of drugs such as digoxin and positive inotropes. All of these factors suggest that antiarrhythmic therapy and suppression of high-risk arrhythmias might be beneficial in this patient population. However, the understanding that sudden death in HF may be due to ischemia or bradyarrhythmias[173] and increased recognition of adverse events associated with antiarrhythmic therapy, including proarrhythmia and worsening HF[174] and excess mortality demonstrated in controlled trials,[175] has led to the recommendation to avoid the use of class I antiarrhythmic drugs.

Subsequent studies have focused on the role of class III agents—amiodarone, d-sotalol, and dofetilide—in HF. Amiodarone may substantially reduce the frequency and complexity of asymptomatic ventricular arrhythmias, and initial studies suggested that amiodarone may have a beneficial impact on morbidity and mortality in patients with HF.[176] The Congestive Heart Failure–Survival Trial of Antiarrhythmic Therapy (CHF-STAT) was a prospective, double-blind study in which 674 patients with HF, an ejection fraction of 40% or less, and asymptomatic ventricular ectopy were randomized to amiodarone or placebo for a median of 45 months.[177] As expected, amiodarone decreased ventricular ectopy compared with placebo. However, in contrast to a smaller, unblinded study, CHF-STAT demonstrated no beneficial effect of amiodarone on mortality. The Sudden Cardiac Death in Heart Failure Trial (SCD-HeFT) also demonstrated no effect of amiodarone on survival in more than 2500 patients with ischemic and nonischemic cardiomyopathy.[178]

Although amiodarone has no role in the treatment of HF per se, it may be useful in the management of symptomatic ventricular or atrial arrhythmias that complicate HF. In particular, amiodarone may be administered acutely to control ventricular response in HF patients with atrial fibrillation, and it may restore and maintain sinus rhythm when used long term.[179] Amiodarone may also be used to suppress symptomatic ventricular tachycardia, especially in patients who are receiving frequent ICD shocks. In the Optimal Pharmacological Therapy in Cardioverter Defibrillator Patients (OPTIC) study,[180] the combination of amiodarone plus β-blocker was effective in preventing ICD shocks in patients with reduced ejection fraction and a history of spontaneous or inducible ventricular tachycardia or fibrillation. However, the rate of drug discontinuation at 1 year was 18% for amiodarone and 5% for β-blocker alone. Monitoring for adverse reactions—including hepatic, pulmonary, and thyroid toxicity—and knowledge of drug interactions, such as increased digoxin levels and elevated INR, are critical to the safe use of amiodarone. In contrast to type I agents, amiodarone appears to be associated with a very low risk of proarrhythmia in patients with LV dysfunction.[181]

Other class III antiarrhythmic agents that have been tested in HF include dofetilide, dronedarone, and the potassium channel blocker d-sotalol. In the Survival With Oral d-sotalol (SWORD) trial, 3121 patients with ischemic cardiomyopathy were randomized to treatment with d-sotalol (200 mg twice daily) or placebo.[182] The trial was stopped early because of excess mortality in the d-sotalol group that appeared to be primarily arrhythmic. The Danish Investigations of Arrhythmia and Mortality on Dofetilide (DIAMOND) study group demonstrated no effect of dofetilide on mortality in 1518 patients with symptomatic LV dysfunction.[183] Like amiodarone, dofetilide was effective in converting atrial fibrillation to sinus rhythm; however, it was associated with a 3.3% incidence of torsades de pointes. Dronedarone is a noniodinated benzofuran derivative of amiodarone with similar electrophysiologic properties but without iodine-related side effects.[184] In a large trial of patients with atrial fibrillation, dronedarone reduced the incidence of cardiovascular hospitalization or death.[185] However, in a study of patients with acute decompensated HF, dronedarone was associated with increased early mortality as a result of worsening HF,[186] and in high-risk patients with permanent atrial fibrillation, dronedarone increased the rates of HF, stroke, and cardiovascular death.[187] These data have led to a black box warning against the use of dronedarone in patients with NYHA class IV heart failure or class II or III heart failure with a recent decompensation. The role of ICDs for primary and secondary prevention of sudden death in HF is discussed in Chapter 22.

Special Considerations

The majority of ambulatory patients with HF and reduced ejection fraction can be treated with medications according to the recommendations presented in this chapter. However, several subgroups of patients merit special consideration, because other pharmacologic therapy may provide important clinical benefits.

HEART FAILURE PATIENTS WITH PRESERVED EJECTION FRACTION

As many as one half of patients who come to medical attention with HF have a normal or near normal LVEF.[188] Although HF with preserved ejection fraction is relatively uncommon in young or middle-aged patients, the prevalence can exceed 50% in older patients, especially elderly women with hypertension.[189] In addition to hypertensive heart disease, other causes of HF with preserved ejection fraction include restrictive, hypertrophic, and infiltrative cardiomyopathies and constrictive pericarditis. Diastolic dysfunction is believed to be the primary mechanism responsible for this clinical syndrome,[190] but other pathophysiologic factors that may contribute to disease progression include arterial stiffness, sodium avidity, and renal dysfunction.[191] Although some data suggest that long-term survival is similar among patients with reduced versus preserved ejection fraction,[192] most studies show that HF with normal ejection fraction is associated with a lower risk of death (Table 12-11).[193]

Although large randomized trials have confirmed survival and other benefits of ACE inhibitors and β-blockers in patients with HF and reduced ejection fraction, trials in patients with preserved ejection fraction have been limited (Table 12-12). As a result, therapy is based primarily on the results of clinical investigations in small groups of patients and on pathophysiologic concepts.[194] Principles of therapy include blood pressure and heart rate control, reduction in cardiac filling pressures, and prevention of myocardial ischemia (Table 12-13). In HF as a result of hypertension, blood pressure control is important to prevent progression of LV hypertrophy and possibly to promote its regression. In addition, effective antihypertensive therapy may improve diastolic filling properties, relieve the load on the left atrium, and help preserve sinus rhythm.

Calcium channel blockers may reduce symptoms of HF with preserved ejection fraction not only by lowering blood pressure but also by improving ventricular relaxation.[195] Renin-angiotensin system inhibitors (e.g., ACE inhibitors and ARBs) may also improve ventricular relaxation, slow or reverse myocardial fibrosis, and prevent atrial fibrillation.[196] However, no evidence suggests that calcium channel blockers and renin-angiotensin system inhibitors improve survival or reduce HF hospitalization in patients with HF and preserved ejection fraction.[197]

Clinical Efficacy

The Perindopril in Elderly People with Chronic Heart Failure (PEP-CHF) study randomized 850 patients aged 70 years or older with preserved systolic function and diastolic dysfunction by echocardiography to receive perindopril (4 mg daily) or placebo.[198] The study population was predominantly nonischemic and hypertensive and had relatively normal renal function. An interval analysis at 1 year demonstrated a trend for reduced mortality and a significant reduction in HF hospitalization, along with improved functional capacity. However, no significant benefit was found in terms of death or unplanned HF hospitalization at 3 years (HR, 0.92; 95% CI, 0.70 to 1.21; $P = .55$). The discrepancy between outcomes noted at 1 year and at the end of follow-up has been attributed to limited power related to the high rate of crossover to open-label ACE inhibitor use after the first year and a relatively low overall event rate.

The effect of ARBs on morbidity and mortality has been tested in two large, multicenter clinical trials: CHARM-Preserved and the Irbesartan in Heart Failure with Preserved Systolic Function (I-PRESERVE) study. In CHARM-Preserved, 3023 patients with

TABLE 12-11	Mortality in Heart Failure with Reduced vs. Preserved Ejection Fraction					
STUDY	N	FOLLOW-UP	MORTALITY RATE WITH REDUCED EF (%)	MORTALITY RATE WITH PRESERVED EF (%)	RR OF DEATH WITH PRESERVED EF
Cohn et al[287]	623	2.3 years	19 (per year)	8 (per year)	0.42
Ghali et al[288]	78	2 years	46	26	0.56
McDermott et al[289]	192	27 months	35	35	0.97
Vasan et al[290]	73	5 years	64	32	0.50
McAlister et al[291]	566	3 years	38	34	NA
Philbin et al[292]	1291	6 months	18	15	0.69
Masoudi et al[293]	413	6 months	21	13	0.49

EF, ejection fraction; NA, not available; RR, relative risk.

TABLE 12-12 Randomized, Controlled Trials of Renin-Angiotensin System Inhibitors in Heart Failure with Preserved Ejection Fraction

TRIAL	N	AGENT	ENTRY CRITERIA	FOLLOW-UP PERIOD	PRIMARY ENDPOINT(S)	FINDINGS
PEP-CHF[198]	1000	Perindopril vs. placebo	Age ≥70 years LVEF ≥40%	26 months	Death or HF hospitalization	Placebo 25.1% Perindopril 23.6% (8% ↓; P = .55)
CHARM-Preserved[199]	3023	Candesartan vs. placebo	LVEF >40% NYHA II-IV Cardiac hospitalization	37 months	CV death or HF hospitalization	Placebo 24% Candesartan 22% (11% ↓; P = .12)
I-PRESERVE[200]	4128	Irbesartan vs. placebo	Age ≥60 years LVEF ≥45%	50 months	Death or CV hospitalization	Placebo 37% Irbesartan 36% (5% ↓; P = .35)
TOPCAT[112]	~3500	Spironolactone vs. placebo	Age ≥50 years LVEF ≥45% HF hospitalization within 12 months or elevated BNP or NT-proBNP	NA	Aborted cardiac arrest CV death or HF hospitalization	NA

BNP, B-type natriuretic peptide; CHARM, Candesartan in Heart Failure: Assessment of Reduction in Mortality and Morbidity; CV, cardiovascular; HF, heart failure; I-PRESERVE, Irbesartan in Heart Failure with Preserved Systolic Function; LVEF, left ventricular ejection fraction; NA, not available; NT-proBNP, N-terminal pro-BNP; NYHA, New York Heart Association functional class; PEP-CHF, Perindopril for Elderly Patients with Chronic Heart Failure; TOPCAT, Trial of Aldosterone Antagonist Therapy in Adults With Preserved Ejection Fraction Congestive Heart Failure.

TABLE 12-13 ACC/AHA Recommendations for Management of Heart Failure with Preserved Ejection Fraction

CLASS	RECOMMENDATION	LEVEL OF EVIDENCE
I	Control systolic and diastolic hypertension	A
	Control ventricular rate in atrial fibrillation	C
	Diuretics to control pulmonary congestion and peripheral edema	C
IIa	Coronary revascularization if ischemia is having an adverse effect on cardiac function in patients with CAD	C
IIb	Restore and maintain sinus rhythm to improve symptoms in patients with atrial fibrillation	C
	β-Blockers, ACE inhibitors, ARBs, or calcium antagonists to minimize symptoms in patients with controlled hypertension	C
	Digoxin to minimize symptoms of heart failure	C

ACC, American College of Cardiology; AHA, American Heart Association; ACE, angiotensin-converting enzyme; ARB, angiotensin receptor blocker; CAD, coronary artery disease.
Modified from Hunt SA, Abraham WT, Chin MH, et al. 2009 focused update incorporated into the ACC/AHA 2005 Guidelines for the Diagnosis and Management of Heart Failure in Adults: a report of the American College of Cardiology Foundation/American Heart Association Task Force on Practice Guidelines: developed in collaboration with the International Society for Heart and Lung Transplantation. *Circulation* 2009;119:e391-e479.

NYHA functional class II through IV heart failure and an ejection fraction greater than 40% were randomized to receive candesartan (target dose 32 mg once daily) or placebo and were followed for a median of 37 months.[199] Candesartan had no significant effect on the primary combined endpoint of cardiovascular death or HF hospitalization (HR 0.89; 95% CI, 0.77 to 1.03; P = .12), but it reduced the number of patients admitted once or multiple times for HF, and it decreased the risk of diabetes. Although nearly 70% of patients reached the target dose of candesartan by 6 months, the modest reduction in HF events was counterbalanced by an increased risk of serious adverse events, including hypotension, renal insufficiency, and hyperkalemia. I-PRESERVE randomly assigned 4128 older patients with symptoms of HF and an ejection fraction of at least 45% to receive irbesartan (target dose 300 mg daily) or placebo.[200] At a mean follow-up of 50 months, there was no difference between irbesartan and placebo in the composite of all-cause mortality or cardiovascular hospitalization, and there was no effect of irbesartan on hospitalization for worsening HF. During the study, 16% of patients in the irbesartan group and 14% of placebo-treated patients discontinued the study drug because of an adverse event (P = .07). The rates of serious adverse events because of hypotension, renal dysfunction, and hyperkalemia were not significantly different between the groups.

The effect of spironolactone on morbidity and mortality in patients with HF and preserved ejection fraction is currently being tested in the National Institutes of Health (NIH)-funded TOPCAT trial.[112]

Practical Considerations

Patients with LV hypertrophy are prone to subendocardial ischemia, even in the absence of ischemic heart disease. Ischemia increases myocardial diastolic stiffness and exacerbates diastolic dysfunction. Because most coronary flow occurs in diastole, tachycardia with reduced diastolic filling time compromises subendocardial perfusion. Therefore, heart rate control is central to preventing or treating ischemia associated with HF and preserved ejection fraction. β-Blockers and some calcium channel blockers (verapamil) are useful negative chronotropic agents. In patients with ischemic heart disease, percutaneous or surgical revascularization may be indicated to treat ischemia.

Pulmonary venous congestion associated with diastolic dysfunction usually responds rapidly to preload reduction with diuretics and/or nitrates. However, because of increased myocardial stiffness, a small decrease in LV volume can cause a marked decrease in left atrial filling pressure, stroke volume, and cardiac output. Therefore, it is important to avoid excessive preload reduction, which can cause symptomatic hypotension, especially in the elderly. Diuretic therapy should be initiated with a small dose of a loop diuretic (e.g., furosemide 20 mg, bumetanide 0.5 mg). If effective diuresis is not achieved, the dose should be increased, or a second diuretic agent, such as metolazone (2.5 to 5 mg), may be cautiously added.

Because of increased LV diastolic stiffness, some patients with HF and preserved ejection fraction have reduced passive ventricular filling in early and mid diastole and depend on an active atrial contribution to late ventricular filling. Thus a strong rationale has been set forth for maintaining sinus rhythm to achieve adequate stroke volume and cardiac output. However, trials that have tested rate versus rhythm control strategies in atrial fibrillation have failed to demonstrate benefits of rhythm control and show higher rates of hospitalization and adverse drug effects.[201] Unfortunately, these trials have included few patients with HF. Although data from ongoing clinical trials are awaited, β-blockers, calcium channel blockers, or digoxin may be used alone or in combination to control the ventricular response. If rate control is ineffective, options include chemical or electrical cardioversion, catheter ablation of atrial fibrillation (i.e., pulmonary vein isolation), or ablation of the atrioventricular junction with pacemaker implantation.[202] All patients with persistent or paroxysmal atrial fibrillation should be anticoagulated with warfarin unless contraindicated. For patients with nonvalvular atrial fibrillation, twice-daily administration of dabigatran, a new oral direct thrombin inhibitor, is now available and does not require anticoagulation monitoring.[203]

In general, positive inotropic agents should not be used in patients with HF and preserved ejection fraction, as such drugs may affect myocardial energetics adversely, induce ischemia, and promote tachyarrhythmias. In the DIG ancillary study, the administration of digoxin to patients with HF and an ejection fraction greater than 45% tended to reduce the combined endpoint of death or hospitalization from worsening HF (risk ratio, 0.82; 95% CI, 0.63 to 1.07) but had no effect on all-cause mortality.[133]

PATIENTS WITH ISCHEMIC HEART DISEASE

Ischemic heart disease can complicate the management of HF in several ways. Symptoms of angina pectoris and myocardial ischemia are often difficult to distinguish from the exertional dyspnea and fatigue associated with HF. However, patients who have myocardial ischemia frequently require additional antiischemic therapy to maximize clinical status (Table 12-14). Therefore, in addition to standard treatment with renin-angiotensin system inhibitors, β-blockers, and diuretics, such patients may improve

TABLE 12-14	Heart Failure Society of America Recommendations for Treatment of Heart Failure in the Setting of Ischemic Heart Disease	
RECOMMENDATION		**STRENGTH OF EVIDENCE**
Antiplatelet therapy to reduce vascular events in patients with HF and CAD		A (for aspirin) B (for clopidogrel)
ACE inhibitors in all patients with either reduced or preserved LVEF after an MI		A
β-blockers for the management of all patients with reduced LVEF or post MI		B
Early initiation (< 48 hr) of ACE inhibitor and β-blocker therapy in hemodynamically-stable post-MI patients with reduced LVEF or HF		A
Nitrates should be considered in patients with HF when additional medication is needed for relief of angina		B
Calcium channel blockers may be considered in patients with HF who have angina despite optimal use of β-blockers and nitrates. For patients with reduced LVEF, amlodipine and felodipine are preferred agents; diltiazem and verapamil should be avoided.		C
Coronary revascularization for patients with HF and suitable coronary anatomy for relief of refractory angina or ACS		B
Coronary revascularization should be considered in patients with HF and suitable coronary anatomy who have myocardial viability in areas of significant obstructive coronary disease or inducible ischemia.		C

ACE, angiotensin-converting enzyme; ACS, acute coronary syndrome; CAD, coronary artery disease; HF, heart failure; LVEF, left ventricular ejection fraction; MI, myocardial infarction.
Modified from Lindenfeld J, Albert NM, Boehmer JP, et al; Heart Failure Society of America. Executive Summary. HFSA 2010 Comprehensive Heart Failure Practice Guideline. *J Card Fail* 2010;16:475-539.

further with the addition of nitrates. As discussed above, a long-acting dihydropyridine calcium channel blocker such as amlodipine can be used as a second- or third-line agent to treat angina. Ranolazine—an inhibitor of the slow, inactivating sodium current (I_{Na})—has also been approved for the treatment of chronic angina.[204] Although the safety and efficacy of ranolazine have not been tested in HF, there is theoretical reason to believe that late I_{Na} inhibition could improve myocardial efficiency and lead to functional benefits,[205] although this remains unproven. In addition to I_{Na} inhibition, ranolazine inhibits the rapid inward rectifying current (I_{Kr}), thereby prolonging the ventricular action potential. Whereas ranolazine prolongs the QT interval in a dose-dependent fashion, an increased risk for proarrhythmia or sudden death has not been observed in acute coronary syndrome trials. In the Metabolic Efficiency With Ranolazine for Less Ischemia in Non–ST-Elevation Acute Coronary Syndrome Thrombolysis in Myocardial Infarction (MERLIN-TIMI) 36 trial, ranolazine actually *decreased* the incidence of ventricular and supraventricular tachycardia.[206]

Another oral agent that has shown clinical benefit in patients with refractory angina is allopurinol, a xanthine oxidase inhibitor that reduces systemic and vascular oxidative stress in animal models of cardiovascular disease.[207] In a proof-of-concept study, Noman and colleagues[208] enrolled 65 patients with coronary artery disease and chronic angina in a double-blind, randomized, placebo-controlled crossover study of high-dose allopurinol (600 mg daily) for 6 weeks. Compared with placebo, allopurinol increased total exercise time and the time to chest pain and ST-segment depression. Further mechanistic data from these investigators has shown that high-dose allopurinol improves endothelium-dependent vasodilation and abolishes vascular oxidative stress in patients with angina.[209] Given that oxidative stress has been implicated in the pathophysiology of ventricular remodeling, there is reason to believe that xanthine oxidase inhibition may have clinical benefits in chronic HF. This hypothesis is currently being tested in the NIH-sponsored Xanthine Oxidase Inhibition for Hyperuricemic Heart Failure Patients (EXACT-HF) study.

Other patients with ischemic heart disease may have periodic decompensations triggered by episodes of myocardial ischemia. In addition to antiischemic pharmacotherapy, these patients may benefit from coronary revascularization, with either coronary artery bypass graft (CABG) surgery or percutaneous coronary intervention (PCI). An important therapeutic consideration in these patients is the presence of hibernating myocardium.[210] Many patients will demonstrate marked improvement in LV function following bypass surgery, and assessment of myocardial viability has long been thought to be an important tool in predicting which patients will have a favorable response.[211] However, recent data from the Surgical Treatment for Ischemic Heart Failure (STICH) trial suggest limited benefit of surgical revascularization on top of medical therapy in patients with coronary artery disease and reduced ejection fraction.[117] In addition, the presence of myocardial viability in STICH did not identify patients with a differential survival benefit from bypass surgery compared with medical therapy alone.[212] For further discussion of the surgical treatment of ischemic heart disease see Chapter 31 in *Braunwald's Heart Disease* and other recent reviews.[213,214]

For patients with ischemia not amenable to direct revascularization, enhanced external counterpulsation (EECP) may reduce angina and improve quality of life. Acutely, the device reduces loading conditions in systole and increases coronary blood flow in diastole. However, the mechanisms responsible for a therapeutic response and the impact on long-term morbidity and mortality remain unknown.[215] Based on favorable data in ischemic heart disease, Feldman and colleagues[216] randomized 187 patients with mild to moderate HF to EECP and protocol-defined medical therapy or medical therapy alone. After 6 months of single-blind treatment, 35% of patients in the EECP group had increased their exercise time by at least 60 seconds (vs. 25% of control; $P = .016$). EECP also improved NYHA class and quality of life but had no effect on peak oxygen consumption. Further research is needed to define the impact of EECP in the treatment of HF and the mechanisms of benefit. Transmyocardial laser revascularization (TMLR) has also been used to treat refractory angina in patients with coronary artery disease not amenable to percutaneous or surgical revascularization.[217] However, a large placebo effect has been posited, and the only blinded study showed no benefit compared with medical therapy.[218] The safety and efficacy of TMLR in patients with ischemic HF remains undefined. For selected patients with end-stage ischemic cardiomyopathy, heart transplantation or destination LV assist device placement may be preferred (see Chapter 15).

PATIENTS WITH VALVULAR HEART DISEASE

Patients with significant regurgitant valvular heart disease represent another difficult patient subgroup. Many patients with significant LV dilation will have functional mitral regurgitation as a result of annular dilatation. Other patients will have concomitant pathology of the mitral apparatus because of a prior history of rheumatic heart disease, myxomatous degeneration, or ischemic heart disease and papillary muscle dysfunction. Frequently, the use of vasodilator and diuretic therapy will adequately reduce the regurgitant volume and result in hemodynamic and symptomatic improvement that may be long lasting.[219] In other patients in whom abnormalities of the mitral valve or subvalvular apparatus make a primary contribution to symptoms and LV dysfunction, valve repair or replacement may have important therapeutic benefit. However, no reliable method exists to consistently distinguish those who will benefit from mitral valve surgery from those who will experience a progressive decline in ventricular function afterward.

Mitral valvuloplasty has also been performed safely on patients with dilated cardiomyopathy and severe mitral regurgitation as a result of annular dilatation. Although initial surgical results were encouraging,[220] the long-term benefits of mitral valve repair compared with medical therapy in this subset of patients remain unproven.[118] Novel devices for percutaneous mitral valve repair are also under development for treatment of primary[221] and secondary[222] mitral regurgitation. A discussion of the management of aortic stenosis in patients with HF and/or low ejection fraction is beyond the scope of this chapter (see Chapters 45 through 47 and Chapter 66 in Braunwald for this discussion).

PATIENTS WITH DIABETES

In the HF population, several concerns exist regarding pharmacologic managment of diabetes, which is present in 25% to 35% of patients. The thiazolidinedione (TZD) class of oral hypoglycemic agents gained widespread popularity for the treatment of insulin resistance because of several advantageous ancillary effects on lipid metabolism, vascular endothelial function, and inflammatory cytokines.[223] However, these agents have been associated with an increase in fluid retention and exacerbation of HF symptoms. In general, TZDs produce a 6% to 7% increase in circulating intravascular volume and a 2- to 4-kg weight gain. In a study of diabetic patients with HF, initiation of TZDs was associated with a 17% increase in fluid retention as defined by a 10-lb involuntary weight gain.[224] Risk factors included older age, hypertension, and ischemic heart disease. TZD-induced fluid retention is dose related and is exacerbated by concomitant insulin use. Peripheral edema, rather than central, predominates and usually resolves upon drug withdrawal. These agents are contraindicated in patients with established NYHA functional class III or IV heart failure and are not recommended for use in patients with mild HF.[225] Furthermore, the use of rosiglitazone is restricted to patients with diabetes that cannot be controlled by other medications because of concerns about cardiovascular safety, in particular an increased risk of MI.[226]

Metformin is another popular oral insulin sensitizer. According to current labeling, however, metformin is contraindicated in patients with HF, in particular in those with unstable or acute HF that requires pharmacologic therapy because of the risk of lactic acidosis. Although the overall incidence of life-threatening lactic acidosis is low, the FDA assigned a black box warning in response to postmarketing reports of increased risk among patients with chronic hypoperfusion and hypoxia and in the very elderly.[227] Despite cautionary alerts, a review of prescribing patterns among Medicare beneficiaries hospitalized with HF reported that nearly one fourth of patients were discharged on either a TZD or metformin.[228] Further data are needed to examine the risk/benefit ratio of metformin in patients with mild to moderate HF or asymptomatic LV dysfunction.

GENDER, RACE, AND ETHNIC CONSIDERATIONS

With few exceptions, women, African Americans, and other racial minorities have been underrepresented in RCTs of new treatments for HF. However, most subgroup and meta-analyses have shown consistent benefits of standard therapy across a broad range of patient populations.[64] ACE inhibitors, ARBs, β-blockers, and aldosterone antagonists have all been shown to be equally effective in men and women with symptomatic LV dysfunction, whereas data on digoxin have been conflicting. In a post hoc subgroup analysis of the DIG trial, Rathore and colleagues[229] found that women who were randomized to digoxin had higher mortality rates compared with women who received placebo (33% vs. 29%), an effect that was not seen in men. Additional analyses, however, suggested that this sex/treatment interaction may have been the result of higher serum digoxin concentrations in women.[138] Other treatment recommendations specific to women with HF include avoiding ACE inhibitors, ARBs, and warfarin during pregnancy and exercising caution in the use of cardiotoxic chemotherapy (e.g., trastuzumab) in the treatment of breast cancer. For men with stable HF and erectile dysfunction, intermittent use of PDE type 5 inhibitors (sildenafil, vardenafil) is safe and effective.[230]

Compared to whites, African Americans appear to develop HF at an earlier age and have more rapid progression of symptoms.[231] The increased awareness of these differences in HF epidemiology has led to a greater emphasis by HF specialists in defining the most effective therapy in African Americans. Although retrospective analyses suggest that African Americans with hypertension or HF experience less efficacy with ACE inhibitors, a meta-analysis demonstrated similar mortality reduction in blacks and nonblacks with HF.[64] The data from RCTs of β-blockers is less clear, but carvedilol shows equal efficacy in black and nonblack patients,[80] whereas bucindolol tended to increase morbidity and mortality in African Americans,[92] possibly because of an adrenergic receptor polymorphism.[94] Excluding results from the BEST trial, Shekelle and colleagues[64] analyzed race-stratified data on β-blockers from the COPERNICUS, MERIT-HF, and U.S. carvedilol studies and found that the relative risk on the effect of mortality for black patients was 0.67 (95% CI, 0.38 to 1.16). As discussed above, the combination of hydralazine and isosorbide dinitrate reduces morbidity and mortality in self-identified African Americans with symptomatic LV systolic dysfunction, and it is now recommended as part of standard therapy in addition to ACE inhibitors and β-blockers.[121]

Like African Americans, Hispanics and other ethnic minorities have received little attention in HF trials. In the absence of data showing lack of efficacy or excess toxicity, renin-angiotensin-aldosterone system inhibitors, β-blockers, and other pharmacologic agents used to treat HF should be prescribed according to indications outlined in this chapter and to national guidelines.[3,4]

PATIENTS WITH MYOCARDITIS

The underlying causes, pathophysiology, clinical manifestations, and diagnostic evaluation of myocarditis are discussed in detail in Chapter 70 of *Braunwald's Heart Disease* and other reviews.[232,233] In brief, myocarditis is a rare disease whose pathophysiologic mechanism is not well understood and for which there is no diagnostic gold standard or proven therapy. Primary myocarditis is believed to be the result of viral and postviral immunologic effects on the heart,[234] and most therapies have been aimed at modulating the immune response. For patients with secondary myocarditis, inflammation of the myocardium from a known agent or disease process—such as *Aspergillus* or tuberculosis—frequently resolves with treatment of the causative agent.

Most patients with myocarditis have a history of an acute viral illness, although there is usually a delay between the initial viral symptoms and the onset of symptoms of heart muscle disease. This delay is probably dependent on the viral etiology and host response. Adults with fulminant myocarditis display the least delay and present with the most severe HF.[235] Rarely, patients may present with an embolic phenomenon, including MI or stroke, or sudden death. Although acute and convalescent viral titers may be of some value in determining the most likely cause of myocarditis, these tests only suggest an association and do not establish the diagnosis. Furthermore, noninvasive nuclear imaging studies with gallium or antimyosin antibody have relatively high false-negative rates and are too nonspecific to be of diagnostic use.[236] The diagnosis of myocarditis can be established by endomyocardial biopsy and requires evidence of myocyte damage associated with an inflammatory cell infiltrate not typical of damage as a result of ischemic heart disease. Because of sampling error, the false-negative rate of endomyocardial biopsy to diagnose myocarditis may be as high as 30% when up to five specimens are obtained.[237]

Currently, there are no clinically available antiviral agents for treating the enteroviruses that cause most cases of primary myocarditis: coxsackie B and A, echovirus, and adenovirus. In addition, immunization to prevent myocarditis is impossible because of the large number of potential causative agents. Because most cases of myocarditis are believed to be immune-mediated, immunosuppressive agents have received the most attention in the search for effective therapy; however, the results of controlled trials have generally been disappointing.[238,239]

The rate and degree of improvement in ventricular performance that has been observed in uncontrolled trials of immunosuppressive therapy has raised the possibility that many patients with myocarditis recover spontaneously. The Myocarditis Treatment Trial was a prospective, randomized, NIH-supported study that sought to determine the effect of immunosuppressive therapy on LV function in patients with myocarditis.[238] More than 2200 patients with HF of less than 2 years' duration and an ejection fraction less than 45% underwent endomyocardial biopsy. Two hundred patients (~10%) had biopsy-proven myocarditis; of these, only 111 were randomized to receive conventional therapy alone or combined with prednisone and either cyclosporine or azathioprine. After 28 weeks of therapy, the mean LVEF increased from 25% to 34% in the group as a whole but did not differ significantly between the groups. In addition, no difference in survival was noted, and overall 1- and 4-year mortality rates were 20% and 56%, respectively. Another immunomodulatory therapy that has been proposed for the treatment of myocarditis based on preclinical and uncontrolled clinical studies is IV immune globulin (IVIG).[240] However, an RCT of IVIG (2 g/kg) in 62 patients with new-onset HF and an ejection fraction of 40% or less failed to show a benefit over placebo. The mean ejection fraction increased dramatically in the group as a whole, from 25% to 42%, and prognosis was excellent, with a 2-year event-free survival of 88%.[239]

Frustaci and colleagues[241] reviewed outcomes in patients with acute myocarditis who were treated with prednisone and azathioprine after not responding to conventional medical therapy. Of 41 patients, 21 (51%) responded favorably to immunosuppressive therapy with improvement in ejection fraction (26% to 47% at 1 year; *P* < .001) and healing of myocarditis on follow-up biopsy. Nonresponders showed no change in cardiac function and myocyte degeneration. Viral genomes by polymerase chain reaction analysis were found in biopsy specimens of 17 nonresponders (85%) compared with 3 responders (14%, *P* < .001). Cardiac

autoantibodies were present in 19 responders (90%) and in none of the nonresponders (*P* < .001). Based on these data, Frustaci and colleagues randomly assigned 85 patients with viral genome–negative myocarditis and HF of at least 6 months' duration who were unresponsive to conventional medical therapy to receive prednisone and azathioprine or placebo. After 6 months of double-blind therapy, patients in the immunosuppression group had reverse LV remodeling with increase in ejection fraction (27% to 47%; *P* < .001) and decrease in volumes, whereas placebo-treated patients had worsening LV function (28% to 21%; *P* < .001).[242] Immunosuppressive therapy also resulted in improvement in NYHA class and in disappearance of myocardial inflammation with replacement fibrosis.

Given the clear lack of proven therapy, many referral centers have become less aggressive in performing endomyocardial biopsy to diagnose myocarditis. In addition, available data show no difference in survival between patients with myocarditis and those with idiopathic dilated cardiomyopathy.[243] However, in the subgroup of patients who come to medical attention with severe hemodynamic compromise, endomyocardial biopsy to confirm a diagnosis of fulminant myocarditis versus giant cell or hypersensitivity myocarditis can have important prognostic and therapeutic implications. Adults with fulminant lymphocytic myocarditis respond poorly to immunosuppressive therapy but may benefit from aggressive hemodynamic support, including mechanical circulatory support as a bridge to recovery.[244] Percutaneous ventricular assist and extracorporeal membrane oxygenation have also been used successfully as temporary support for patients with combined cardiogenic and respiratory failure.[245,246] By contrast, patients with giant cell myocarditis have a poor prognosis and should be urgently evaluated for mechanical assist and heart transplantation.[247] Although uncontrolled data suggest a role for immunosuppressive therapy with cyclosporine and steroids in giant cell myocarditis, posttransplant recurrences and death have been reported.[248] It is hoped that a better understanding of disease mechanisms will lead to improved diagnostic and therapeutic strategies for myocarditis.[249]

Future Directions in Pharmacologic Therapy

Pharmacotherapy

Future directions for HF parmacotherapy include novel vasodilators, sinus node inhibition, modulation of myocardial and vascular oxidant stress, and treatment of comorbidities such as anemia and pulmonary hypertension (see Table 12-10). Plasma levels of arginine vasopressin are elevated in patients with HF, which may contribute to hyponatremia and disease progression through stimulation of V_{1a} and V_2 receptors and cause vasoconstriction and free-water retention, respectively.[250] Short-term administration of vasopressin receptor antagonists in patients with acute decompensated HF improves symptoms and hemodynamics, increases urine output, and corrects hyponatremia without adversely effecting renal function.[251-253] However, long-term vasopressin receptor blockade had no effect on long-term mortality or recurrent hospitalizations in patients with HF.[254] Like vasopressin, renin may contribute to maladaptive volume regulation and systemic vasoconstriction in patients with HF through an increase in angiotensin II. Renin is released by the juxtaglomerular cells in the kidney in response to renal hypoperfusion, decreased sodium delivery, and sympathetic activation.[35] Although β-blockers inhibit renin release by the kidney, patients with HF on target doses of β-blockade have elevated circulating levels of renin. Aliskiren is a direct renin inhibitor that reduces plasma renin activity and angiotensin levels, and it is approved for the treatment of hypertension.[255] In a pilot study, aliskiren significantly reduced plasma natriuretic peptide and urinary aldosterone levels on top of ACE inhibitors in patients with symptomatic HF and reduced ejection fraction.[256] The Aliskiren

Trial to Mediate Outcome Prevention in Heart Failure (ATMO-SPHERE) is evaluating the efficacy and safety of aliskiren alone and in combination with enalapril compared with enalapril alone in more than 7000 patients with NYHA class II to IV heart failure. However, recent concerns have been raised about the risks of hypotension, renal dysfunction, and hyperkalemia with concomitant use of aliskiren and an ACE inhibitor in patients with cardiovascular disease. The Aliskiren Trial in Type 2 Diabetes Using Cardio-Renal Disease Endpoints (ALTITUDE) was stopped prematurely by the data monitoring committee due to futility and safety concerns, which included cardiorenal risks as well as an excess of strokes.[256a] Whether the preliminary results of ALTITUDE should alter the conduct of ATMOSPHERE, given the differences in patient populations and study design, remains controversial.

Another novel neurohormonal approach to managing patients with chronic HF is potentiation of the natriuretic peptide (NP) system. Although synthetic natriuretic peptides such as nesiritide (see Chapter 14) cause modest diuresis and natriuresis, improve hemodynamics, and inhibit neurohormonal activation acutely, they may be limited by hypotension and have unproven long-term effects on ventricular remodeling and disease progression. Cenderitide is a novel chimeric NP that consists of the human C-type natriuretic peptide and the C-terminus of *Dendroaspis* NP. Cenderitide activates guanylyl cyclase (GC) A and B receptors, with higher activity at GC-B, so as to be less hypotensive than nesiritide. Preliminary data in human HF suggests that cenderitide activates cyclic guanosine monophosphate (cGMP), unloads the heart, and preserves renal function at a nonhypotensive dose.[257] Phase II studies are currently underway to assess the safety, tolerability, and efficacy of cenderitide in HF.

Ivabradine is a selective inhibitor of the sinus node that reduces heart rate and may prove useful in HF patients with incomplete β-blockade. In a large RCT of patients with coronary artery disease and reduced ejection fraction, ivabradine reduced heart rate by 6 beats/min at 12 months (corrected for placebo).[258] Although ivabradine did not affect the primary composite endpoint of cardiovascular death or hospital admission for acute MI or HF in the overall cohort, there appeared to a benefit of ivabradine on secondary endpoints in patients with a heart rate of 70 beats/min or greater. The Systolic Heart Failure Treatment with the I_f Inhibitor Ivabradine Trial (SHIFT) randomly assigned 6558 patients with symptomatic HF and an ejection fraction of 35% or less, who were in sinus rhythm with a heart rate of 70 beats/min or greater, to receive ivabradine (target dose 7.5 mg twice daily) or placebo.[259] After a median follow-up of 23 months, 793 patients (24%) in the ivabradine group and 937 patients (29%) in the placebo group reached a primary endpoint of cardiovascular death or HF hospitalization (HR, 0.82; 95% CI, 0.75 to 0.90; $P < .0001$). Symptomatic bradycardia (5% vs. 1%) and visual side effects (3% vs. 1%) were more common in the ivabradine group. Additional data from SHIFT demonstrated a relationship between the reduction in heart rate and improvement in quality of life with ivabradine.[260] Despite these encouraging data, only 23% of the patients in SHIFT were receiving a target dose of β-blocker, and less than half were receiving 50% or more of the targeted β-blocker dose.[261] Also, patients receiving 50% or more of the target β-blocker dose at baseline had no significant benefit from ivabradine for the primary endpoint. In an observational cohort study of 2211 HF patients, "suitability" for ivabradine—that is, ejection fraction of 35% or less, sinus rhythm, and a resting heart rate of 70 beats/min or greater—was found in less than 10% of patients at 12 months.[262]

Finally, inhibition of myocardial and vascular oxidant stress is emerging as a novel therapeutic target in cardiovascular disease.[207] Allopurinol is a xanthine oxidase inhibitor that improves vascular endothelial function and myocardial efficiency when administered at high doses to patients with HF. Although treatment with oxypurinol, the active metabolite of allopurinol, had no clinical benefit in unselected HF patients with reduced ejection fraction, the subgroup of patients with hyperuricemia appeared to improve.[263] The EXACT-HF study is currently testing the hypothesis that in patients with symptomatic HF as a result of LV systolic dysfunction and elevated serum uric acid levels (≥9.5 mg/dL), treatment with allopurinol (target dose 600 mg daily) for 24 weeks will improve clinical outcomes compared with placebo.[264]

Comorbidities

Recognition and treatment of comorbidities is also a major focus of ongoing investigation in HF. Anemia is common in HF and may be due to increased plasma volume or decreased red cell mass.[265] Contributing factors include malnutrition with iron deficiency, bone marrow suppression from activation of proinflammatory cytokines, and chronic kidney disease. Anemia may contribute to ventricular remodeling and disease progression by stimulating neurohormonal and cytokine activation, promoting LV hypertrophy, and exacerbating ischemia. Short-term studies of erythropoiesis-stimulating agents (ESAs) in HF have shown that correction of anemia improves exercise tolerance and quality of life.[266] The Reduction of Events with Darbepoietin Alfa in Heart Failure (RED-HF) trial is currently testing the effect of a long-acting ESA on morbidity and mortality in approximately 2600 patients with NYHA functional class II to IV heart failure, an ejection fraction of 40% or less, and anemia defined as a hemoglobin between 9.0 and 12.0 g/dL.[267]

Like anemia, secondary pulmonary hypertension is common in patients with advanced HF and is associated with exercise intolerance and adverse outcomes.[268] Dysregulation of pulmonary vascular tone and structural remodeling are due in part to pulmonary vascular endothelial dysfunction that results in impaired nitric oxide availability and decreased levels of cGMP.[269] PDE-5 inhibitors such as sildenafil cause pulmonary vasodilation by promoting an enhanced and sustained level of cGMP. In patients with pulmonary arterial hypertension, acute administration of sildenafil decreases pulmonary vascular resistance and increases cardiac index,[270] whereas chronic oral administration improves exercise capacity and functional class.[271] Lewis and colleagues[272] assessed resting and exercise hemodynamics before and after acute administration of 50 mg of oral sildenafil in patients with moderate HF. Sildenafil improved peak oxygen consumption and ventilatory efficiency and acted as a selective pulmonary vasodilator. In a follow-up study, these investigators demonstrated improved exercise capacity and quality of life after 12 weeks of PDE-5 inhibition,[273] and others have demonstrated that sustained improvements in exercise ventilation and aerobic efficiency in HF are related to improved flow-mediated vasodilation.[274] The long-term effects of sildenafil in patients with HF and preserved ejection fraction are currently being tested,[275] although intermittent use of PDE-5 inhibitors appears to be safe in HF patients with erectile dysfunction.[230] Use of PDE-5 inhibitors is contraindicated in patients receiving organic nitrates for treatment of ischemic heart disease or HF.

REFERENCES

1. Roger VL, Go AS, Lloyd-Jones DM, et al. Heart disease and stroke statistics—2011 update: a report from the American Heart Association. *Circulation* 2011;123:e18.
2. Adams KF Jr, Fonarow GC, Emerman CL, et al. Characteristics and outcomes of patients hospitalized for heart failure in the United States: rationale, design, and preliminary observations from the first 100,000 cases in the Acute Decompensated Heart Failure National Registry (ADHERE). *Am Heart J* 2005;149:209.
3. Lindenfeld J, Albert NM, Boehmer JP, et al. HFSA 2010 Comprehensive Heart Failure Practice Guideline. *J Card Fail* 2010;16:e1.
4. Hunt SA, Abraham WT, Chin MH, et al. 2009 focused update incorporated into the ACC/AHA 2005 Guidelines for the Diagnosis and Management of Heart Failure in Adults: a report of the American College of Cardiology Foundation/American Heart Association Task Force on Practice Guidelines: developed in collaboration with the International Society for Heart and Lung Transplantation. *Circulation* 2009;119:e391.
5. McMurray JJ, Pfeffer MA. Heart failure. *Lancet* 2005;365:1877.
6. Konstam MA, Kramer DG, Patel AR, et al. Left ventricular remodeling in heart failure: current concepts in clinical significance and assessment. *JACC Cardiovasc Imaging* 2011;4:98.
7. Schrier RW, Abraham WT. Hormones and hemodynamics in heart failure. *N Engl J Med* 1999;341:577.

8. Cody RJ, Covit AB, Schaer GL, et al. Sodium and water balance in chronic congestive heart failure. *J Clin Invest* 1986;77:1441.

9. Volpe M, Tritto C, DeLuca N, et al. Abnormalities of sodium handling and of cardiovascular adaptations during high salt diet in patients with mild heart failure. *Circulation* 1993;88:1620.

10. Swift PA, Markandu ND, Sagnella GA, et al. Modest salt reduction reduces blood pressure and urine protein excretion in black hypertensives: a randomized control trial. *Hypertension* 2005;46:308.

11. Colin RE, Castillo ML, Orea TA, et al. Effects of a nutritional intervention on body composition, clinical status, and quality of life in patients with heart failure. *Nutrition* 2004;20:890.

12. Neily JB, Toto KH, Gardner EB, et al. Potential contributing factors to noncompliance with dietary sodium restriction in patients with heart failure. *Am Heart J* 2002;143:29.

13. Brater DC. Diuretic therapy. *N Engl J Med* 1998;339:387.

14. Weber KT. Furosemide in the long-term management of heart failure: the good, the bad, and the uncertain. *J Am Coll Cardiol* 2004;44:1308.

15. McAdams Demarco MA, Maynard JW, Baer AN, et al. Diuretic use, increased serum urate levels and risk of incident gout in a population-based study of adults with hypertension: The Atherosclerosis Risk in the Communities cohort study. *Arthritis Rheum* 2012;44:121.

16. Francis GS, Siegel RM, Goldsmith SR, et al. Acute vasoconstrictor response to intravenous furosemide in patients with chronic congestive heart failure. Activation of the neurohumoral axis. *Ann Intern Med* 1985;103:1.

17. Swedberg K, Eneroth P, Kjekshus J, et al. Effects of enalapril and neuroendocrine activation on prognosis in severe congestive heart failure (follow-up of the CONSENSUS trial). CONSENSUS Trial Study Group. *Am J Cardiol* 1990;66:40D.

18. Testani JM, Cappola TP, Brensinger CM, et al. Interaction between loop diuretic-associated mortality and blood urea nitrogen concentration in chronic heart failure. *J Am Coll Cardiol* 2011;58:375.

19. Ellison DH. The physiologic basis of diuretic synergism: its role in treating diuretic resistance. *Ann Intern Med* 1991;114:886.

20. Ellison DH, Velazquez H, Wright FS. Adaptation of the distal convoluted tubule of the rat. Structural and functional effects of dietary salt intake and chronic diuretic infusion. *J Clin Invest* 1989;83:113.

21. Sanders GP, Mendes LA, Colucci WS, et al. Noninvasive methods for detecting elevated left-sided cardiac filling pressure. *J Card Fail* 2000;6:157.

22. Abraham WT, Adamson PB, Bourge RC, et al. Wireless pulmonary artery haemodynamic monitoring in chronic heart failure: a randomised controlled trial. *Lancet* 2011;377:658.

23. Yu CM, Wang L, Chau E, et al. Intrathoracic impedance monitoring in patients with heart failure: correlation with fluid status and feasibility of early warning preceding hospitalization. *Circulation* 2005;112:841.

24. Sharma GV, Woods PA, Lindsey N, et al. Noninvasive monitoring of left ventricular end-diastolic pressure reduces rehospitalization rates in patients hospitalized for heart failure: a randomized controlled trial. *J Card Fail* 2011;17:718.

25. Androne AS, Hryniewicz K, Hudaihed A, et al. Relation of unrecognized hypervolemia in chronic heart failure to clinical status, hemodynamics, and patient outcomes. *Am J Cardiol* 2004;93:1254.

26. Damman K, Ng Kam Chuen MJ, MacFadyen RJ, et al. Volume status and diuretic therapy in systolic heart failure and the detection of early abnormalities in renal and tubular function. *J Am Coll Cardiol* 2011;57:2233.

27. Galve E, Mallol A, Catalan R, et al. Clinical and neurohumoral consequences of diuretic withdrawal in patients with chronic, stabilized heart failure and systolic dysfunction. *Eur J Heart Fail* 2005;7:892.

28. Jentzer JC, DeWald TA, Hernandez AF. Combination of loop diuretics with thiazide-type diuretics in heart failure. *J Am Coll Cardiol* 2010;56:1527.

29. Shah RV, Givertz MM. Managing acute renal failure in patients with acute decompensated heart failure: the cardiorenal syndrome. *Curr Heart Fail Rep* 2009;6:176.

30. Ronco C, Haapio M, House AA, et al. Cardiorenal syndrome. *J Am Coll Cardiol* 2008;52:1527.

31. Nesto RW, Bell D, Bonow RO, et al. Thiazolidinedione use, fluid retention, and congestive heart failure: a consensus statement from the American Heart Association and American Diabetes Association. October 7, 2003. *Circulation* 2003;108:2941.

32. Murphy N, Mockler M, Ryder M, et al. Decompensation of chronic heart failure associated with pregabalin in patients with neuropathic pain. *J Card Fail* 2007;13:227.

33. Anker SD, Negassa A, Coats AJ, et al. Prognostic importance of weight loss in chronic heart failure and the effect of treatment with angiotensin-converting-enzyme inhibitors: an observational study. *Lancet* 2003;361:1077.

34. Cohn JN, Franciosa JA. Vasodilator therapy of cardiac failure: (first of two parts). *N Engl J Med* 1977;297:27.

35. Givertz MM. Manipulation of the renin-angiotensin system. *Circulation* 2001;104:e14.

36. Burnier M, Brunner HR. Angiotensin II receptor antagonists. *Lancet* 2000;355:637.

37. The CONSENSUS Trial Study Group. Effects of enalapril on mortality in severe congestive heart failure. Results of the Cooperative North Scandinavian Enalapril Survival Study (CONSENSUS). *N Engl J Med* 1987;316:1429.

38. Cohn JN, Archibald DG, Ziesche S, et al. Effect of vasodilator therapy on mortality in chronic congestive heart failure. Results of a Veterans Administration Cooperative Study. *N Engl J Med* 1986;314:1547.

39. Cohn JN, Johnson G, Ziesche S, et al. A comparison of enalapril with hydralazine-isosorbide dinitrate in the treatment of chronic congestive heart failure. *N Engl J Med* 1991;325:303.

40. The SOLVD Investigators. Effect of enalapril on survival in patients with reduced left ventricular ejection fractions and congestive heart failure. *N Engl J Med* 1991;325:293.

41. The SOLVD Investigators. Effect of enalapril on mortality and the development of heart failure in asymptomatic patients with reduced left ventricular ejection fractions. *N Engl J Med* 1992;327:685.

42. Packer M, Poole-Wilson PA, Armstrong PW, et al. Comparative effects of low and high doses of the angiotensin-converting enzyme inhibitor, lisinopril, on morbidity and mortality in chronic heart failure. *Circulation* 2000;100:2312.

43. Crozier I, Ikram H, Awan N, et al. Losartan in heart failure. Hemodynamic effects and tolerability. Losartan Hemodynamic Study Group. *Circulation* 1995;91:691.

44. Pitt B, Segal R, Martinez FA, et al. Randomised trial of losartan versus captopril in patients over 65 with heart failure (Evaluation of Losartan in the Elderly Study, ELITE). *Lancet* 1997;349:747.

45. Pitt B, Poole-Wilson PA, Segal R, et al. Effect of losartan compared with captopril on mortality in patients with symptomatic heart failure: randomised trial—the Losartan Heart Failure Survival Study ELITE II. *Lancet* 2000;355:1582.

46. Hamroff G, Katz SD, Mancini D, et al. Addition of angiotensin II receptor blockade to maximal angiotensin-converting-enzyme inhibition improves exercise capacity in patients with severe congestive heart failure. *Circulation* 1999;99:990.

47. Cohn JN, Tognoni G. A randomized trial of the angiotensin-receptor blocker valsartan in chronic heart failure. *N Engl J Med* 2001;345:1667.

48. McMurray JJ, Ostergren J, Swedberg K, et al. Effects of candesartan in patients with chronic heart failure and reduced left-ventricular systolic function taking angiotensin-converting-enzyme inhibitors: the CHARM-Added trial. *Lancet* 2003;362:767.

49. Granger CB, McMurray JJ, Yusuf S, et al. Effects of candesartan in patients with chronic heart failure and reduced left-ventricular systolic function intolerant to angiotensin-converting-enzyme inhibitors: the CHARM-Alternative trial. *Lancet* 2003;362:772.

50. Pfeffer MA. ACE inhibitors in acute myocardial infarction: patient selection and timing. *Circulation* 1998;97:2192.

51. The Heart Outcomes Prevention Evaluation Study Investigators. Effects of an angiotensin-converting-enzyme inhibitor, ramipril, on cardiovascular events in high-risk patients. *N Engl J Med* 2000;342:145.

52. Fox KM, EURopean trial On reduction of cardiac events with Perindopril in stable coronary Artery disease Investigators. Efficacy of perindopril in reduction of cardiovascular events among patients with stable coronary artery disease: randomised, double-blind, placebo-controlled, multicentre trial (the EUROPA study). *Lancet* 2003;362:782.

53. Swedberg K, Held P, Kjekshus J, et al. Effects of the early administration of enalapril on mortality in patients with acute myocardial infarction. Results of the Cooperative New Scandinavian Enalapril Survival Study II (CONSENSUS II). *N Engl J Med* 1992;327:678.

54. Ambrosioni E, Borghi C, Magnani B. The effect of the angiotensin-converting-enzyme inhibitor zofenopril on mortality and morbidity after anterior myocardial infarction. The Survival of Myocardial Infarction Long-Term Evaluation (SMILE) Study Investigators. *N Engl J Med* 1995;332:80.

55. Pfeffer MA, McMurray JJ, Velazquez EJ, et al. Valsartan, captopril, or both in myocardial infarction complicated by heart failure, left ventricular dysfunction, or both. *N Engl J Med* 2003;349:1893.

56. Bello D, Shah NB, Edep ME, et al. Self-reported differences between cardiologists and heart failure specialists in the management of chronic heart failure. *Am Heart J* 1999;138:100.

57. Philbin EF, Andreaou C, Rocco TA, et al. Patterns of angiotensin-converting enzyme inhibitor use in congestive heart failure in two community hospitals. *Am J Cardiol* 1996;77:832.

58. Cody RJ, Laragh JH. Use of captopril to estimate renin-angiotensin-aldosterone activity in the pathophysiology of chronic heart failure. *Am Heart J* 1982;104:1184.

59. Packer M, Medina N, Yushak M. Relation between serum sodium concentration and the hemodynamic and clinical responses to converting enzyme inhibition with captopril in severe heart failure. *J Am Coll Cardiol* 1984;3:1035.

60. Barnett AH, Bain SC, Bouter P, et al. Angiotensin-receptor blockade versus converting-enzyme inhibition in type 2 diabetes and nephropathy. *N Engl J Med* 2004;351:1952.

61. Packer M. Do angiotensin-converting enzyme inhibitors prolong life in patients with heart failure treated in clinical practice? *J Am Coll Cardiol* 1996;28:1323.

62. Kittleson M, Hurwitz S, Shah MR, et al. Development of circulatory-renal limitations to angiotensin-converting enzyme inhibitors identifies patients with severe heart failure and early mortality. *J Am Coll Cardiol* 2003;41:2029.

63. Garg R, Yusuf S. Overview of randomized trials of angiotensin-converting enzyme inhibitors on mortality and morbidity in patients with heart failure. Collaborative Group on ACE Inhibitor Trials. *JAMA* 1995;273:1450.

64. Shekelle PG, Rich MW, Morton SC, et al. Efficacy of angiotensin-converting enzyme inhibitors and beta-blockers in the management of left ventricular systolic dysfunction according to race, gender, and diabetic status: a meta-analysis of major clinical trials. *J Am Coll Cardiol* 2003;41:1529.

65. Guazzi M, Marenzi G, Alimento M, et al. Improvement of alveolar-capillary membrane diffusing capacity with enalapril in chronic heart failure and counteracting effect of aspirin. *Circulation* 1997;95:1930.

66. Massie BM, Krol WF, Ammon SE, et al. The Warfarin and Antiplatelet Therapy in Heart Failure trial (WATCH): rationale, design, and baseline patient characteristics. *J Card Fail* 2004;10:101.

67. Cleland JG, Findlay I, Jafri S, et al. The Warfarin/Aspirin Study in Heart failure (WASH): a randomized trial comparing antithrombotic strategies for patients with heart failure. *Am Heart J* 2004;148:157.

68. Al Khadra AS, Salem DN, Rand WM, et al. Antiplatelet agents and survival: a cohort analysis from the Studies of Left Ventricular Dysfunction (SOLVD) trial. *J Am Coll Cardiol* 1998;31:419.

69. Teo KK, Yusuf S, Pfeffer M, et al. Effects of long-term treatment with angiotensin-converting-enzyme inhibitors in the presence or absence of aspirin: a systematic review. *Lancet* 2002;360:1037.

70. van Rijnsoever EW, Kwee-Zuiderwijk WJ, Feenstra J. Angioneurotic edema attributed to the use of losartan. *Arch Intern Med* 1998;158:2063.

71. Pitt B, Poole-Wilson PA, Segal R, et al. Effect of losartan compared with captopril on mortality in patients with symptomatic heart failure: randomised trial–the Losartan Heart Failure Survival Study ELITE II. *Lancet* 2000;355:1582.

72. Desai AS. Hyperkalemia in patients with heart failure: incidence, prevalence, and management. *Curr Heart Fail Rep* 2009;6:272.

73. Bristow MR. Beta-adrenergic receptor blockade in chronic heart failure. *Circulation* 2000;101:558.

74. Lopez BL, Christopher TA, Yue TL, et al. Carvedilol, a new beta-adrenoreceptor blocker antihypertensive drug, protects against free-radical-induced endothelial dysfunction. *Pharmacology* 1995;51:165.

75. Mason RP, Kalinowski L, Jacob RF, et al. Nebivolol reduces nitroxidative stress and restores nitric oxide bioavailability in endothelium of black Americans. *Circulation* 2005;112:3795.

76. Waagstein F, Hjalmarson A, Varnauskas E, et al. Effect of chronic beta-adrenergic receptor blockade in congestive cardiomyopathy. *Br Heart J* 1975;37:1022.

77. Heilbrunn SM, Shah P, Bristow MR, et al. Increased β-receptor density and improved hemodynamic response to catecholamine stimulation during long-term metoprolol therapy in heart failure from dilated cardiomyopathy. *Circulation* 1989;79:483.

78. Foody JM, Farrell MH, Krumholz HM. beta-Blocker therapy in heart failure: scientific review. *JAMA* 2002;287:883.

79. Ghali JK, Pina IL, Gottlieb SS, et al. Metoprolol CR/XL in female patients with heart failure: analysis of the experience in Metoprolol Extended-Release Randomized Intervention Trial in Heart Failure (MERIT-HF). *Circulation* 2002;105:1585.

80. Yancy CW, Fowler MB, Colucci WS, et al. Race and the response to adrenergic blockade with carvedilol in patients with chronic heart failure. *N Engl J Med* 2001;344:1358.

81. O'Connor CM, Fiuzat M, Swedberg K, et al. Influence of global region on outcomes in heart failure beta-blocker trials. *J Am Coll Cardiol* 2011;58:915.

82. CIBIS Investigators and Committees. A randomized trial of beta-blockade in heart failure. The Cardiac Insufficiency Bisoprolol Study (CIBIS). *Circulation* 1994;90:1765.

83. CIBIS II Investigators and Committees. The Cardiac Insufficiency Bisoprolol Study II (CIBIS-II): a randomised trial. *Lancet* 1999;353:9.

84. Packer M, Colucci WS, Sackner-Bernstein JD, et al. Double-blind, placebo-controlled study of the effects of carvedilol in patients with moderate to severe heart failure. The PRECISE Trial. Prospective Randomized Evaluation of Carvedilol on Symptoms and Exercise. *Circulation* 1996;94:2793.

85. Bristow MR, Gilbert EM, Abraham WT, et al. Carvedilol produces dose-related improvements in left ventricular function and survival in subjects with chronic heart failure. *Circulation* 1996;94:2807.

86. Colucci WS, Packer M, Bristow MR, et al. Carvedilol inhibits clinical progression in patients with mild symptoms of heart failure. US Carvedilol Heart Failure Study Group. *Circulation* 1996;94:2800.

87. Cohn JN, Fowler MB, Bristow MR, et al. Safety and efficacy of carvedilol in severe heart failure. The U.S. Carvedilol Heart Failure Study Group. *J Card Fail* 1997;3:173.

88. Packer M, Bristow MR, Cohn JN, et al. The effect of carvedilol on morbidity and mortality in patients with chronic heart failure. U.S. Carvedilol Heart Failure Study Group. *N Engl J Med* 1996;334:1349.

89. MERIT-HF Study Group. Effect of metoprolol CR/XL in chronic heart failure: Metoprolol CR/XL Randomised Intervention Trial in Congestive Heart Failure (MERIT-HF). *Lancet* 1999;353:2001.

90. Hjalmarson A, Goldstein S, Fagerberg B, et al. Effects of controlled-release metoprolol on total mortality, hospitalizations, and well-being in patients with heart failure: the Metoprolol CR/XL Randomized Intervention Trial in congestive heart failure (MERIT-HF). MERIT-HF Study Group. *JAMA* 2000;283:1295.

91. Ghali JK, Pina IL, Gottlieb SS, et al. Metoprolol CR/XL in female patients with heart failure: analysis of the experience in Metoprolol Extended-Release Randomized Intervention Trial in Heart Failure (MERIT-HF). *Circulation* 2002;105:1585.

92. The Beta-Blocker Evaluation of Survival Trial Investigators. A trial of the beta-blocker bucindolol in patients with advanced chronic heart failure. *N Engl J Med* 2001;344:1659.

93. Liggett SB, Mialet-Perez J, Thaneemit-Chen S, et al. A polymorphism within a conserved beta(1)-adrenergic receptor motif alters cardiac function and beta-blocker response in human heart failure. *Proc Natl Acad Sci U S A* 2006;103:11288.

94. Bristow MR, Murphy GA, Krause-Steinrauf H, et al. An alpha2C-adrenergic receptor polymorphism alters the norepinephrine-lowering effects and therapeutic response of the beta-blocker bucindolol in chronic heart failure. *Circ Heart Fail* 2010;3:21.

95. Packer M, Coats AJ, Fowler MB, et al. Effect of carvedilol on survival in severe chronic heart failure. *N Engl J Med* 2001;344:1651.

96. Packer M, Fowler MB, Roecker EB, et al. Effect of carvedilol on the morbidity of patients with severe chronic heart failure: results of the carvedilol prospective randomized cumulative survival (COPERNICUS) study. *Circulation* 2002;106:2194.

97. Poole-Wilson PA, Swedberg K, Cleland JG, et al. Comparison of carvedilol and metoprolol on clinical outcomes in patients with chronic heart failure in the Carvedilol Or Metoprolol European Trial (COMET): randomised controlled trial. *Lancet* 2003;362:7.

98. Flather MD, Shibata MC, Coats AJ, et al. Randomized trial to determine the effect of nebivolol on mortality and cardiovascular hospital admission in elderly patients with heart failure (SENIORS). *Eur Heart J* 2005;26:215.

99. Gattis WA, O'Connor CM, Gallup DS, et al. Predischarge initiation of carvedilol in patients hospitalized for decompensated heart failure: results of the Initiation Management Predischarge: Process for Assessment of Carvedilol Therapy in Heart Failure (IMPACT-HF) trial. *J Am Coll Cardiol* 2004;43:1534.

100. Bakris GL, Fonseca V, Katholi RE, et al. Metabolic effects of carvedilol vs metoprolol in patients with type 2 diabetes mellitus and hypertension: a randomized controlled trial. *JAMA* 2004;292:2227.

101. Hall SA, Cigarroa CG, Marcoux L, et al. Time course of improvement in left ventricular function, mass and geometry in patients with congestive heart failure treated with beta-adrenergic blockade. *J Am Coll Cardiol* 1995;25:1154.

102. Wikstrand J, Hjalmarson A, Waagstein F, et al. Dose of metoprolol CR/XL and clinical outcomes in patients with heart failure: analysis of the experience in metoprolol CR/XL randomized intervention trial in chronic heart failure (MERIT-HF). *J Am Coll Cardiol* 2002;40:491.

103. Metra M, Giubbini R, Nodari S, et al. Differential effects of beta-blockers in patients with heart failure: A prospective, randomized, double-blind comparison of the long-term effects of metoprolol versus carvedilol. *Circulation* 2000;102:546.

104. Weber KT. Aldosterone in congestive heart failure. *N Engl J Med* 2001;345:1689.

105. McKelvie RS, Yusuf S, Pericak D, et al. Comparison of candesartan, enalapril, and their combination in congestive heart failure: randomized evaluation of strategies for left ventricular dysfunction (RESOLVD) pilot study. The RESOLVD Pilot Study Investigators. *Circulation* 1999;100:1056.

106. Butler J, Ezekowitz J, Collins SP, et al. Update on aldosterone antagonists use in heart failure with reduced left ventricular ejection fraction: Heart Failure Society of America Guidelines Committee. *J Card Fail* 2012;18:265.

107. The RALES Investigators. Effectiveness of spironolactone added to an angiotensin-converting enzyme inhibitor and a loop diuretic for severe chronic congestive heart failure (the Randomized Aldactone Evaluation Study [RALES]). *Am J Cardiol* 1996;78:902.

108. Pitt B, Zannad F, Remme WJ, et al. The effect of spironolactone on morbidity and mortality in patients with severe heart failure. Randomized Aldactone Evaluation Study Investigators. *N Engl J Med* 1999;341:709.

109. Juurlink DN, Mamdani MM, Lee DS, et al. Rates of hyperkalemia after publication of the Randomized Aldactone Evaluation Study. *N Engl J Med* 2004;351:543.

110. Pitt B, Remme W, Zannad F, et al. Eplerenone, a selective aldosterone blocker, in patients with left ventricular dysfunction after myocardial infarction. *N Engl J Med* 2003;348:1309.

111. Zannad F, McMurray JJ, Krum H, et al. Eplerenone in patients with systolic heart failure and mild symptoms. *N Engl J Med* 2011;364:11.

112. Desai AS, Lewis EF, Solomon SD, et al. Rationale and design of the treatment of preserved cardiac function heart failure with an aldosterone antagonist trial: a randomized, controlled study of spironolactone in patients with symptomatic hear failure and preserved ejection fraction. *Am Heart J* 2011;162:966.

113. Bozkurt B, Agoston I, Knowlton AA. Complications of inappropriate use of spironolactone in heart failure: when an old medicine spirals out of new guidelines. *J Am Coll Cardiol* 2003;41:211.

114. Shah KB, Rao K, Sawyer R, et al. The adequacy of laboratory monitoring in patients treated with spironolactone for congestive heart failure. *J Am Coll Cardiol* 2005;46:845.

115. Wei L, Struthers AD, Fahey T, et al. Spironolactone use and renal toxicity: population based longitudinal analysis. *Br Med J* 2010;340:c1768.

116. Vanden Hoek TL, Morrison LJ, Shuster M, et al. Part 12: cardiac arrest in special situations: 2010 American Heart Association Guidelines for Cardiopulmonary Resuscitation and Emergency Cardiovascular Care. *Circulation* 2010;122:S829.

117. Velazquez EJ, Lee KL, Deja MA, et al. Coronary-artery bypass surgery in patients with left ventricular dysfunction. *N Engl J Med* 2011;364:1607.

118. Wu AH, Aaronson KD, Bolling SF, et al. Impact of mitral valve annuloplasty on mortality risk in patients with mitral regurgitation and left ventricular systolic dysfunction. *J Am Coll Cardiol* 2005;45:381.

119. Carson P, Ziesche S, Johnson G, et al. Racial differences in response to therapy for heart failure: analysis of the vasodilator-heart failure trials. Vasodilator-Heart Failure Trial Study Group. *J Card Fail* 1999;5:178.

120. Taylor AL, Ziesche S, Yancy C, et al. Combination of isosorbide dinitrate and hydralazine in blacks with heart failure. *N Engl J Med* 2004;351:2049.

121. Cole RT, Kalogeropoulos AP, Georgiopoulou VV, et al. Hydralazine and isosorbide dinitrate in heart failure: historical perspective, mechanisms, and future directions. *Circulation* 2011;123:2414.

122. Hare JM. Nitroso-redox balance in the cardiovascular system. *N Engl J Med* 2004;351:2112.

123. Daiber A, Oelze M, Coldewey M, et al. Hydralazine is a powerful inhibitor of peroxynitrite formation as a possible explanation for its beneficial effects on prognosis in patients with congestive heart failure. *Biochem Biophys Res Commun* 2005;338:1865.

124. Bouguerne B, Belkheiri N, Bedos-Belval F, et al. Antiatherogenic effect of bisvanillyl-hydralazone, a new hydralazine derivative with antioxidant, carbonyl scavenger, and antiapoptotic properties. *Antioxid Redox Signal* 2011;14:2093.

125. Kahn DF, Duffy SJ, Tomasian D, et al. Effects of black race on forearm resistance vessel function. *Hypertension* 2002;40:195.

126. Katz SD, Hryniewicz K, Hriljac I, et al. Vascular endothelial dysfunction and mortality risk in patients with chronic heart failure. *Circulation* 2005;111:310.

127. Bitar F, Akhter MW, Khan S, et al. Survey of the use of organic nitrates for the treatment of chronic congestive heart failure in the United States. *Am J Cardiol* 2004;94:1465.

128. Gheorghiade M, Adams KF, Jr., Colucci WS. Digoxin in the management of cardiovascular disorders. *Circulation* 2004;109:2959.

129. The German and Austrian Xamoterol Study Group. Double-blind placebo-controlled comparison of digoxin and xamoterol in chronic heart failure. *Lancet* 1988;1:489.

130. The Captopril-Digoxin Multicenter Research Group. Comparative effects of therapy with captopril and digoxin in patients with mild to moderate heart failure. *JAMA* 1988;259:539.

131. DiBianco R, Shabetai R, Kostuk W, et al. A comparison of oral milrinone, digoxin, and their combination in the treatment of patients with chronic heart failure. *N Engl J Med* 1989;320:677.

132. van Veldhuisen DJ, Man in 't Veld AJ, Dunselman PH, et al. Double-blind placebo-controlled study of ibopamine and digoxin in patients with mild to moderate heart failure: results of the Dutch Ibopamine Multicenter Trial (DIMT). *J Am Coll Cardiol* 1993;22:1564.

133. The Digitalis Investigation Group. The effect of digoxin on mortality and morbidity in patients with heart failure. *N Engl J Med* 1997;336:525.

134. Uretsky BF, Young JB, Shahidi FE, et al. Randomized study assessing the effect of digoxin withdrawal in patients with mild to moderate chronic congestive heart failure: results of the PROVED trial. PROVED Investigative Group. *J Am Coll Cardiol* 1993;22:955.

135. Packer M, Gheorghiade M, Young JB, et al. Withdrawal of digoxin from patients with chronic heart failure treated with angiotensin-converting-enzyme inhibitors. RADIANCE Study. *N Engl J Med* 1993;329:1.

136. Moss AJ, Davis HT, Conard DL, et al. Digitalis-associated cardiac mortality after myocardial infarction. *Circulation* 1981;64:1150.

137. Rich MW. Drug therapy of heart failure in the elderly. *Am J Geriatr Cardiol* 2003;12:235.

138. Rathore SS, Curtis JP, Wang Y, et al. Association of serum digoxin concentration and outcomes in patients with heart failure. *JAMA* 2003;289:871.

139. Adams KF, Jr., Patterson JH, Gattis WA, et al. Relationship of serum digoxin concentration to mortality and morbidity in women in the digitalis investigation group trial: a retrospective analysis. *J Am Coll Cardiol* 2005;46:497.

140. Weinfeld MS, Drazner MH, Stevenson WG, et al. Early outcome of initiating amiodarone for atrial fibrillation in advanced heart failure. *J Heart Lung Transplant* 2000;19:638.

141. Deedwania PC, Lardizabal JA. Atrial fibrillation in heart failure: a comprehensive review. *Am J Med* 2010;123:198.

142. Lubitz SA, Benjamin EJ, Ellinor PT. Atrial fibrillation in congestive heart failure. *Heart Fail Clin* 2010;6:187.

143. de Vries RJ, van Veldhuisen DJ, Dunselman PH. Efficacy and safety of calcium channel blockers in heart failure: focus on recent trials with second-generation dihydropyridines. *Am Heart J* 2000;139:185.

144. Packer M, O'Connor CM, Ghali JK, et al. Effect of amlodipine on morbidity and mortality in severe chronic heart failure. Prospective Randomized Amlodipine Survival Evaluation Study Group. *N Engl J Med* 1996;335:1107.

145. Wijeysundera HC, Hansen MS, Stanton E, et al. Neurohormones and oxidative stress in nonischemic cardiomyopathy: relationship to survival and the effect of treatment with amlodipine. *Am Heart J* 2003;146:291.

146. Cohn JN, Ziesche S, Smith R, et al. Effect of the calcium antagonist felodipine as supplementary vasodilator therapy in patients with chronic heart failure treated with enalapril: V-HeFT III. Vasodilator-Heart Failure Trial (V-HeFT) Study Group. *Circulation* 1997;96:856.

147. ALLHAT Officers and Coordinators for the ALLHAT Collaborative Research Group. Major outcomes in high-risk hypertensive patients randomized to angiotensin-converting enzyme inhibitor or calcium channel blocker vs diuretic: The Antihypertensive and Lipid-Lowering Treatment to Prevent Heart Attack Trial (ALLHAT). *JAMA* 2002;288:2981.

148. Colucci WS, Wright RF, Braunwald E. New positive inotropic agents in the treatment of congestive heart failure. Mechanisms of action and recent clinical developments. *N Engl J Med* 1986;314:349.

149. Massie B, Bourassa M, DiBianco R, et al. Long-term oral administration of amrinone for congestive heart failure: lack of efficacy in a multicenter controlled trial. *Circulation* 1985;71:963.

150. Packer M, Carver JR, Rodeheffer RJ, et al. Effect of oral milrinone on mortality in severe chronic heart failure. The PROMISE Study Research Group. *N Engl J Med* 1991;325:1468.

151. Cohn JN, Goldstein SO, Greenberg BH, et al. A dose-dependent increase in mortality with vesnarinone among patients with severe heart failure. Vesnarinone Trial Investigators. *N Engl J Med* 1998;339:1810.

152. Uretsky BF, Jessup M, Konstam MA, et al. Multicenter trial of oral enoximone in patients with moderate to moderately severe congestive heart failure. Lack of benefit compared with placebo. Enoximone Multicenter Trial Group. *Circulation* 1990;82:774.

153. Hershberger RE, Nauman D, Walker TL, et al. Care processes and clinical outcomes of continuous outpatient support with inotropes (COSI) in patients with refractory end-stage heart failure. *J Card Fail* 2003;9:180.

154. The ESCAPE Investigators and ESCAPE Study Coordinators. Evaluation study of congestive heart failure and pulmonary artery catheterization effectiveness: the ESCAPE trial. *JAMA* 2005;294:1625.

155. Upadya S, Lee FA, Saldarriaga C, et al. Home continuous positive inotropic infusion as a bridge to cardiac transplantation in patients with end-stage heart failure. *J Heart Lung Transplant* 2004;23:466.

156. Lang CC, Hankins S, Hauff H, et al. Morbidity and mortality of UNOS status 1B cardiac transplant candidates at home. *J Heart Lung Transplant* 2003;22:419.

157. Lewis EF. End of life care in advanced heart failure. *Curr Treat Options Cardiovasc Med* 2011;13:79.

158. Lopez-Candales AL, Carron C, Schwartz J. Need for hospice and palliative care services in patients with end-stage heart failure treated with intermittent infusion of inotropes. *Clin Cardiol* 2004;27:23.

159. Ewy GA. Inotropic infusions for chronic congestive heart failure: medical miracles or misguided medicinals? *J Am Coll Cardiol* 1999;33:572.

160. Abraham WT, Adams KF, Fonarow GC, et al. In-hospital mortality in patients with acute decompensated heart failure requiring intravenous vasoactive medications: an analysis from the Acute Decompensated Heart Failure National Registry (ADHERE). *J Am Coll Cardiol* 2005;46:57.

161. Takkenberg JJ, Czer LS, Fishbein MC, et al. Eosinophilic myocarditis in patients awaiting heart transplantation. *Crit Care Med* 2004;32:714.

162. Roberts WC, Siegel RJ, McManus BM. Idiopathic dilated cardiomyopathy: analysis of 152 necropsy patients. *Am J Cardiol* 1987;60:1340.

163. Fuster V, Gersh BJ, Giuliani ER, et al. The natural history of idiopathic dilated cardiomyopathy. *Am J Cardiol* 1981;47:525.

164. Stratton JR, Nemanich JW, Johannessen KA, et al. Fate of left ventricular thrombi in patients with remote myocardial infarction or idiopathic cardiomyopathy. *Circulation* 1988;78:1388.

165. Loh E, Sutton MS, Wun CC, et al. Ventricular dysfunction and the risk of stroke after myocardial infarction. *N Engl J Med* 1997;336:251.

166. Al Khadra AS, Salem DN, Rand WM, et al. Warfarin anticoagulation and survival: a cohort analysis from the Studies of Left Ventricular Dysfunction. *J Am Coll Cardiol* 1998;31:749.

167. Parkash R, Maisel WH, Toca FM, et al. Atrial fibrillation in heart failure: high mortality risk even if ventricular function is preserved. *Am Heart J* 2005;150:701.

168. Dunkman WB, Johnson GR, Carson PE, et al. Incidence of thromboembolic events in congestive heart failure. The V-HeFT VA Cooperative Studies Group. *Circulation* 1993;87:VI94.

169. Dries DL, Rosenberg YD, Waclawiw MA, et al. Ejection fraction and risk of thromboembolic events in patients with systolic dysfunction and sinus rhythm: evidence for gender differences in the studies of left ventricular dysfunction trials. *J Am Coll Cardiol* 1997;29:1074.

170. Massie BM, Collins JF, Ammon SE, et al. Randomized trial of warfarin, aspirin, and clopidogrel in patients with chronic heart failure: the Warfarin and Antiplatelet Therapy in Chronic Heart Failure (WATCH) trial. *Circulation* 2009;119:1616.

171. Homma S, Thompson JL, Pullicino PM, et al. Warfarin and aspirin in patients with heart failure and sinus rhythm. *N Engl J Med* 2012 May 2;366:1859.

172. Ellison KE, Stevenson WG, Sweeney MO, et al. Management of arrhythmias in heart failure. *Congest Heart Fail* 2003;9:91.

173. Luu M, Stevenson WG, Stevenson LW, et al. Diverse mechanisms of unexpected cardiac arrest in advanced heart failure. *Circulation* 1989;80:1675.

174. Gottlieb SS, Kukin ML, Medina N, et al. Comparative hemodynamic effects of procainamide, tocainide, and encainide in severe chronic heart failure. *Circulation* 1990;81:860.

175. Echt DS, Liebson PR, Mitchell LB, et al. Mortality and morbidity in patients receiving encainide, flecainide, or placebo. The Cardiac Arrhythmia Suppression Trial. *N Engl J Med* 1991;324:781.

176. Doval HC, Nul DR, Grancelli HO, et al. Randomised trial of low-dose amiodarone in severe congestive heart failure. Grupo de Estudio de la Sobrevida en la Insuficiencia Cardiaca en Argentina (GESICA). *Lancet* 1994;344:493.

177. Singh SN, Fletcher RD, Fisher SG, et al. Amiodarone in patients with congestive heart failure and asymptomatic ventricular arrhythmia. Survival Trial of Antiarrhythmic Therapy in Congestive Heart Failure. *N Engl J Med* 1995;333:77.

178. Bardy GH, Lee KL, Mark DB, et al. Amiodarone or an implantable cardioverter-defibrillator for congestive heart failure. *N Engl J Med* 2005;352:225.

179. Deedwania PC, Singh BN, Ellenbogen K, et al. Spontaneous conversion and maintenance of sinus rhythm by amiodarone in patients with heart failure and atrial fibrillation: observations from the veterans affairs congestive heart failure survival trial of antiarrhythmic therapy (CHF-STAT). The Department of Veterans Affairs CHF-STAT Investigators. *Circulation* 1998;98:2574.

180. Connolly SJ, Dorian P, Roberts RS, et al. Comparison of beta-blockers, amiodarone plus beta-blockers, or sotalol for prevention of shocks from implantable cardioverter defibrillators: the OPTIC Study: a randomized trial. *JAMA* 2006;295:165.

181. Hohnloser SH, Klingenheben T, Singh BN. Amiodarone-associated proarrhythmic effects. A review with special reference to torsade de pointes tachycardia. *Ann Intern Med* 1994;121:529.

182. Waldo AL, Camm AJ, deRuyter H, et al. Effect of d-sotalol on mortality in patients with left ventricular dysfunction after recent and remote myocardial infarction. The SWORD Investigators. *Lancet* 1996;348:7.

183. Torp-Pedersen C, Moller M, Bloch-Thomsen PE, et al. Dofetilide in patients with congestive heart failure and left ventricular dysfunction. Danish Investigations of Arrhythmia and Mortality on Dofetilide Study Group. *N Engl J Med* 1999;341:857.

184. Patel C, Yan GX, Kowey PR. Dronedarone. *Circulation* 2009;120:636.

185. Hohnloser SH, Crijns HJ, van Eickels M, et al. Effect of dronedarone on cardiovascular events in atrial fibrillation. *N Engl J Med* 2009;360:668.

186. Kober L, Torp-Pedersen C, McMurray JJ, et al. Increased mortality after dronedarone therapy for severe heart failure. *N Engl J Med* 2008;358:2678.

187. Connolly SJ, Camm AJ, Halperin JL, et al. Dronedarone in high-risk permanent atrial fibrillation. *N Engl J Med* 2011;365:2268.

188. Zile MR, Brutsaert DL. New concepts in diastolic dysfunction and diastolic heart failure: Part I: diagnosis, prognosis, and measurements of diastolic function. *Circulation* 2002;105:1387.

189. Lindenfeld J, Fiske KS, Stevens BR, et al. Age, but not sex, influences the measurement of ejection fraction in elderly patients hospitalized for heart failure. *J Card Fail* 2003;9:100.

190. Zile MR, Baicu CF, Gaasch WH. Diastolic heart failure: abnormalities in active relaxation and passive stiffness of the left ventricle. *N Engl J Med* 2004;350:1953.

191. Packer M. Can brain natriuretic peptide be used to guide the management of patients with heart failure and a preserved ejection fraction? The wrong way to identify new treatments for a nonexistent disease. *Circ Heart Fail* 2011;4:538.

192. Senni M, Redfield MM. Heart failure with preserved systolic function. A different natural history? *J Am Coll Cardiol* 2001;38:1277.

193. Yancy CW, Lopatin M, Stevenson LW, et al. Clinical presentation, management, and in-hospital outcomes of patients admitted with acute decompensated heart failure with perserved systolic function: a report from the Acute Decompensated Heart Failure National Registry (ADHERE) database. *J Am Coll Cardiol* 2006;47:76.

194. Zile MR, Brutsaert DL. New concepts in diastolic dysfunction and diastolic heart failure: Part II: causal mechanisms and treatment. *Circulation* 2002;105:1503.

195. Bonow RO, Dilsizian V, Rosing DR, et al. Verapamil-induced improvement in left ventricular diastolic filling and increased exercise tolerance in patients with hypertrophic cardiomyopathy: short- and long-term effects. *Circulation* 1985;72:853.

196. Maggioni AP, Latini R, Carson PE, et al. Valsartan reduces the incidence of atrial fibrillation in patients with heart failure: results from the Valsartan Heart Failure Trial (Val-HeFT). *Am Heart J* 2005;149:548.

197. Shah RV, Desai AS, Givertz MM. The effect of renin-angiotensin system inhibitors on mortality and heart failure hospitalization in patients with heart failure and preserved ejection fraction: a systematic review and meta-analysis. *J Card Fail* 2010;16:260.

198. Cleland JG, Tendera M, Adamus J, et al. The perindopril in elderly people with chronic heart failure (PEP-CHF) study. *Eur Heart J* 2006;27:2338.

199. Yusuf S, Pfeffer MA, Swedberg K, et al. Effects of candesartan in patients with chronic heart failure and preserved left-ventricular ejection fraction: the CHARM-Preserved Trial. *Lancet* 2003;362:777.

200. Massie BM, Carson PE, McMurray JJ, et al. Irbesartan in patients with heart failure and preserved ejection fraction. *N Engl J Med* 2008;359:2456.

201. Wyse DG, Waldo AL, DiMarco JP, et al. A comparison of rate control and rhythm control in patients with atrial fibrillation. *N Engl J Med* 2002;347:1825.

202. Stevenson WG, Stevenson LW. Atrial fibrillation and heart failure: five more years. *N Engl J Med* 2004;351:2437.

203. Connolly SJ, Ezekowitz MD, Yusuf S, et al. Dabigatran versus warfarin in patients with atrial fibrillation. *N Engl J Med* 2009;361:1139.

204. Chaitman BR, Pepine CJ, Parker JO, et al. Effects of ranolazine with atenolol, amlodipine, or diltiazem on exercise tolerance and angina frequency in patients with severe chronic angina: a randomized controlled trial. *JAMA* 2004;291:309.

205. Morrow DA, Givertz MM. Modulation of myocardial energetics: emerging evidence for a therapeutic target in cardiovascular disease. *Circulation* 2005;112:3218.

206. Scirica BM, Morrow DA, Hod H, et al. Effect of ranolazine, an antianginal agent with novel electrophysiological properties, on the incidence of arrhythmias in patients with non ST-segment elevation acute coronary syndrome: results from the Metabolic Efficiency With Ranolazine for Less Ischemia in Non ST-Elevation Acute Coronary Syndrome

Implantable Devices for the Management of Heart Failure

Jaimie Manlucu and William T. Abraham

IMPLANTABLE CARDIOVERTER-DEFIBRILLATORS IN THE MANAGEMENT OF HEART FAILURE, 270

MADIT II, 271
DEFINITE, 271
SCD-HeFT, 271

IMPLANTABLE CARDIOVERTER-DEFIBRILLATORS EARLY AFTER MYOCARDIAL INFARCTION, 272

DINAMIT, 272
IRIS, 272

INDICATIONS FOR PROPHYLACTIC CARDIOVERTER-DEFIBRILLATOR IMPLANTATION IN HEART FAILURE PATIENTS, 272

PRACTICAL CONSIDERATIONS IN IMPLANTABLE CARDIOVERTER-DEFIBRILLATOR THERAPY, 272

CONDUCTION ABNORMALITIES IN HEART FAILURE, 273

LANDMARK CARDIAC RESYNCHRONIZATION THERAPY CLINICAL TRIALS, 273

MUSTIC, 273
MIRACLE, 273
MIRACLE ICD, 274
CONTAK CD, 274
COMPANION, 274
CARE-HF, 275

CARDIAC RESYNCHRONIZATION THERAPY IN MILD HEART FAILURE, 275

REVERSE, 275
MADIT-CRT, 275
RAFT, 275

CARDIAC RESYNCHRONIZATION THERAPY, 276

Cardiac Resynchronization Therapy in Long-Term Right Ventricular Pacing, 276
Cardiac Resynchronization Therapy in Atrial Fibrillation, 276
Indications for Cardiac Resynchronization Therapy in Heart Failure Patients, 276
Future Directions of Cardiac Resynchronization Therapy, 276

MONITORING HEART FAILURE THROUGH IMPLANTABLE DEVICES, 276

FUTURE DIRECTIONS IN IMPLANTABLE DEVICES FOR THE MANAGEMENT OF HEART FAILURE, 278

SUMMARY, 278

REFERENCES, 279

After decades focused on pharmacologic management, the year 2001 ushered in a new era of implantable device therapies for the management of heart failure (HF) with the U.S. Food and Drug Administration (FDA) approval of the first cardiac resynchronization therapy (CRT) device. Soon thereafter, randomized controlled trials (RCTs) were published that supported the routine use of implantable cardioverter-defibrillators (ICDs) and combined CRT-ICD devices in the management of HF. Although ICDs had already been indicated for the management of resuscitated cardiac arrest, ventricular fibrillation, and hemodynamically destabilizing ventricular tachycardia in HF patients, these newer studies demonstrated mortality reduction with the prophylactic use of an ICD, substantially enlarging the population of patients eligible for an ICD. By 2005, the strength of evidence supporting the use of an ICD or CRT with or without a defibrillator in the management of HF was sufficiently strong to recommend use of these therapies in all eligible patients.[1] Despite the overwhelming evidence in support of device therapy for heart failure, ICDs and CRT remain underutilized.[2]

In addition to the therapeutic benefits of CRT and ICDs, implantable devices that monitor HF clinical status and/or hemodynamics have been developed and continue to be under investigation. One such device has been approved by the FDA. By using measurement of intrathoracic impedance, an available CRT-ICD device can track intrathoracic fluid volume changes. Another investigational approach to managing HF is through the use of implantable hemodynamic monitoring systems. These systems enable the day-to-day management of cardiac filling pressures and other physiologic parameters not otherwise available to the clinician. Initial reports suggest a substantial opportunity to reduce HF morbidity rates (e.g., HF hospitalizations), with the use of these devices. This chapter reviews the use of ICDs and CRT for the management of HF, previews the promise of implantable HF monitoring devices, and mentions other investigational device therapies for HF.

Implantable Cardioverter-Defibrillators in the Management of Heart Failure

ICDs were initially applied to survivors of sudden cardiac death (SCD) to treat second episodes of ventricular tachycardia or ventricular fibrillation (see Chapter 22 for a complete discussion of ICD use in secondary prevention of SCD). Patients with left ventricular dysfunction, either from ischemic or nonischemic etiologies, are at increased risk for SCD,[3,4] the leading cause of mortality in patients with HF, which occurs at a rate six to nine times that seen in the general population. The Metoprolol CR/XL Randomized Intervention Trial in Heart Failure (MERIT-HF) showed that patients with New York Heart Association (NYHA) functional class II or III symptoms die most frequently as a result of SCD.[5] This study estimated the proportion of total mortality attributable to SCD at 64% and 59% for NYHA class II and III patients, respectively. In contrast, the major cause of death in class IV patients in MERIT-HF was progressive or end-stage HF. Thus, all but the sickest HF patients are more likely to die suddenly rather than from worsening HF.

With this background, a series of studies published between 1996 and 2005 expanded the use of ICDs as prophylactic therapy in at-risk subjects (see Table 22-2).[6-11] These studies have focused on patients with coronary artery disease, usually after myocardial infarction (MI), and more recently on those with left ventricular (LV) systolic dysfunction of any cause. In the HF/LV dysfunction population, the Multicenter Automatic Defibrillator Implantation Trial (MADIT) was the first primary prevention study to show the benefit of prophylactic ICD implantation.[6] High-risk patients (n = 196) with prior MI, an LV ejection fraction (LVEF) of 35% or less, and nonsustained ventricular tachycardia at a rate of 3 to 30 beats higher than 120 beats/min underwent electrophysiologic testing and were randomized to an ICD versus conventional antiarrhythmic therapy, primarily amiodarone. Compared with conventional therapy, the ICD arm demonstrated an impressive reduction in all-cause mortality at 2 years (15.8% vs. 38.6%; P = .009). However, significantly more patients in the ICD group were receiving treatment with a β-blocker, which confounded the results of the trial.

MADIT was followed by a number of other encouraging studies of LV systolic dysfunction patients, such as the Coronary Artery Bypass Graft (CABG)-Patch trial and the Multicenter Unsustained Tachycardia Trial (MUSTT).[7,8] However, the landmark trials establishing a role for ICDs as primary prevention of mortality in HF patients are MADIT II and the National Institutes of Health (NIH)–sponsored Sudden Cardiac Death–Heart Failure Trial (SCD-HeFT).[9,11] Although underpowered to demonstrate a significant difference for its primary endpoint, the Prophylactic Defibrillator Implantation in Patients with Nonischemic Dilated Cardiomyopathy (DEFINITE) trial also contributed substantially to the burden of proof supporting prophylactic intervention with an ICD in the management of HF.[10]

MADIT II

MADIT II was a prospectively designed RCT powered to assess the survival benefit of ICDs in a population of post-MI patients with reduced ejection fraction (<30%). Importantly, this trial included no arrhythmic markers, such as nonsustained or inducible ventricular tachycardia, for inclusion. A total of 1232 patients were randomly assigned in a 3:2 ratio to receive an ICD (742 patients) or conventional medical therapy (490 patients). During an average follow-up of 20 months, the all-cause mortality rates were 19.8% in the conventional therapy arm and 14.2% in the ICD group (31% relative risk reduction [RR]; $P = .016$; Figure 13-1). The effect of ICD therapy on survival was similar in subgroup analyses stratified according to age, gender, ejection fraction, NYHA class, and the QRS interval. Moreover, β-blocker use was 72% in these patients and was well balanced between the ICD and conventional therapy groups.

Of note, the majority of patients enrolled in MADIT II fell into NYHA class II or III. NYHA class IV patients were excluded, and the NYHA class I cohort was relatively small. The average LVEF was 23%, and these findings suggest that HF patients with mild to moderate symptoms and a moderate to severe reduction in LVEF may benefit the most from a prophylactic ICD. Moreover, in contrast to MADIT I, in which the survival benefit of ICD therapy was seen early after randomization, the survival benefit observed in MADIT II began approximately 9 months after the device was implanted. The authors suggested that this difference might be due to a lower risk population being enrolled in MADIT II, the absence of arrhythmia as risk stratification for entry, or the use of more aggressive medical treatment. Regardless of the explanation, this observation may be important when considering the timing of device placement in eligible patients.

DEFINITE

Whereas MADIT II enrolled exclusively post-MI patients with an ischemic cause of LV systolic dysfunction and HF, the DEFINITE trial was the first randomized trial of primary prevention therapy with an ICD in nonischemic cardiomyopathy patients.[10] Such patients also exhibit high rates of SCD, but consensus had not been reached regarding the management of SCD risk in such patients. This was due, in part, to limitations in objective risk assessment, in

that no invasive or noninvasive testing procedure had been shown to accurately determine which nonischemic HF patient is likely to die suddenly. Also clouding the picture were older observations that suggested prophylactic administration of an antiarrhythmic agent such as amiodarone might prolong survival in nonischemic cardiomyopathy patients.[12]

The DEFINITE trial was a prospective evaluation of 458 patients with nonischemic cardiomyopathy. Entry criteria included an ejection fraction of 35% or less, a history of symptomatic HF, and the presence of ambient arrhythmias defined as episodes of nonsustained ventricular tachycardia or at least 10 premature ventricular contractions in 24 hours on continuous ambulatory electrocardiographic (ECG) monitoring. Patients (n = 458) were equally randomized to each arm of the study to receive either an ICD and standard medical therapy or standard medical therapy alone. Compliance with medical therapy was excellent and included an angiotensin-converting enzyme inhibitor (ACEI) in 86% of the cohort and a β-blocker in 85%. The patients were followed for a mean of 29 ± 14 months with a primary endpoint of all-cause mortality.

There were 68 deaths reported in the DEFINITE trial: 28 in the ICD group and 40 in the standard therapy group. The implantation of an ICD yielded a nonsignificant 35% reduction in death from any cause (hazard ratio [HR], 0.65; 95% confidence interval [CI], 0.40 to 1.06; $P = .08$) and significantly reduced the risk of sudden death by a remarkable 80% (HR, 0.20; 95% CI, 0.06 to 0.71; $P = .006$). In the subgroup of NYHA class III patients, all-cause mortality was significantly decreased in the ICD arm (HR, 0.37; 95% CI, 0.15 to 0.90; $P = .02$). Although this study was underpowered and did not reach statistical significance with respect to the primary endpoint of all-cause mortality for the entire randomized cohort, the results demonstrated a strong trend toward a survival advantage for patients receiving an ICD. It is worth mentioning that the all-cause mortality reduction seen in DEFINITE was 35%—a value strikingly similar to the 31% relative risk reduction observed in the ischemic population studied in MADIT II. The statistical power of DEFINITE was affected by a low rate of SCD in both groups, which may be related to aggressive use of ACEI and β-blockade in this trial.

SCD-HeFT

The results of the SCD-HeFT trial were published in 2005 and have had a substantial impact on current practice and reimbursement guidelines for ICDs.[11] This landmark RCT enrolled 2521 patients

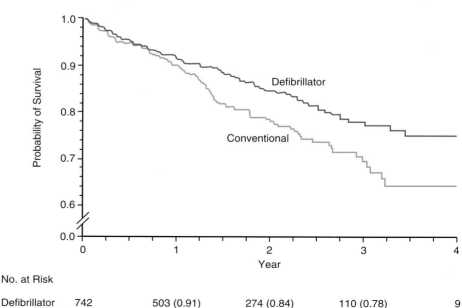

FIGURE 13-1 Kaplan-Meier estimates of survival in patients randomized to an implantable cardioverter-defibrillator compared with conventional medical therapy in the Multicenter Automatic Defibrillator Implantation II trial ($P = .007$ by log-rank test).

No. at Risk					
Defibrillator	742	503 (0.91)	274 (0.84)	110 (0.78)	9
Conventional	490	329 (0.90)	170 (0.78)	65 (0.69)	3

from 148 mostly U.S. centers between 1997 and 2001. Patients with NYHA class II (70%) or III (30%) HF and reduced LVEF (≤35% or less, mean ~25%) of either ischemic or nonischemic etiology were eligible for the study. SCD-HeFT was a three-arm trial, comparing treatment with an ICD with amiodarone and placebo. Thus, SCD-HeFT addressed at least two important issues in HF management: 1) whether empirical amiodarone therapy saves lives in well-treated NYHA class II and III heart failure patients with no arrhythmic indication for the drug and 2) whether a prophylactic ICD saves lives in such patients with HF from either an ischemic or nonischemic cause.

In SCD-HeFT, patients received standard HF therapy, if tolerated, which included an ACEI or angiotensin receptor blocker in 85%, β-blocker in 69%, and aldosterone antagonists in 19% (compatible with guideline recommendations at the time the study was conducted). The median follow-up was 45.5 months. Importantly, the cohort was equally divided between ischemic and nonischemic causes of HF, allowing an important subgroup analysis of these cohorts to be done. Mortality rates in the ICD, amiodarone, and placebo groups were 17.1%, 24%, and 22.3% at 3 years and 28.9%, 34.1%, and 35.9% at 5 years, respectively. The ICD was associated with a statistically significant 23% reduction in all-cause mortality compared with placebo (HR, 0.77; 97.5% CI, 0.62 to 0.96; $P = .007$). Outcomes on amiodarone were not significantly different from placebo across all subgroups (HR, 1.06; 97.5% CI, 0.86 to 1.30). Similar degrees of benefit were noted in patients with ischemic (21% mortality rate reduction) and nonischemic HF (27% mortality rate reduction), thus confirming the findings of MADIT II and DEFINITE, respectively. The SCD-HeFT trial provides the most robust evidence to date to support the prophylactic use of ICDs in patients with mild to moderate HF and reduced ejection fraction from virtually any cause.

Implantable Cardioverter-Defibrillators Early After Myocardial Infarction

Although many of the trials discussed above included patients with ischemic cardiomyopathy, the majority of those patients were months to years removed from their acute infarcts. The relative risk of SCD of those recovering from an acute ischemic event may be different from those with chronic infarct–related scar. In a subgroup analysis of patients enrolled in the Valsartan in Acute Myocardial Infarction Trial (VALIANT),[13] the risk of sudden death was highest within the first 30 days after MI. In those who had an event (occurring a median of 180 days following their infarct), 19% had either sudden death or an aborted cardiac arrest within the first 30 days. Although these findings suggested that an ICD in the early postinfarct period would significantly reduce mortality, the results of prospective randomized trials have proved otherwise. The role of an ICD in the initial weeks following MI has been defined by the landmark Defibrillator in Acute Myocardial Infarction Trial (DINAMIT)[14] and later confirmed by the Immediate Risk Stratification Improves Survival (IRIS) trial.[15]

DINAMIT

DINAMIT was the first trial to evaluate the role of prophylactic ICD implantation in the acute infarct period. The study randomized 674 patients who were within 6 to 40 days of MI, had an LVEF of 35% or less, and had impaired cardiac autonomic function, defined as either depressed heart rate variability or an elevated average 24-hour heart rate on Holter monitoring, to prophylactic ICD implant versus no ICD. Patients with sustained ventricular tachycardia more than 48 hours after MI, those with NYHA class IV heart failure, and those who were revascularized were excluded. After a mean follow-up of 30 months, no difference was observed in all-cause mortality between the two groups (HR for death in the ICD group, 1.08; 95% CI, 0.76 to 1.55; $P = .66$). The prespecified secondary endpoint, arrhythmic death, was more common in the control arm, whereas nonarrhythmic death was more common in the ICD arm. The results of this study provide the primary rationale for current guidelines that recommend deferring ICD implantation for at least 40 days following MI.

IRIS

The lack of benefit of an ICD in the immediate postinfarct period was confirmed by the large, multicenter IRIS trial, which randomized patients who were within 5 to 31 days of MI to an ICD or best medical therapy alone. Patients with an LVEF of 40% or less and a heart rate of 90 beats/min or greater on the first available ECG and/or those with a nonsustained ventricular tachycardia 150 beats/min or greater were included in the study. A total of 898 patients were followed for a mean of 37 months. Overall, no mortality reduction was observed in the ICD group relative to control (HR, 1.04; 95% CI, 0.81 to 1.35; $P = .78$). Similar to the DINAMIT findings, although SCDs decreased in the ICD group compared with the control group (HR, 0.55; 95% CI, 0.31 to 1.00; $P = .049$), this decrease was paralleled by an increase in non-SCD mortality in the ICD group (HR, 1.92; 95% CI, 1.29 to 2.84; $P = .001$).

Indications for Prophylactic Cardioverter-Defibrillator Implantation in Heart Failure Patients

Based on these trials, the indication for an ICD was extended to NYHA class II and III heart failure patients with a reduced ejection fraction (see Chapter 22). The 2009 ACC/AHA guidelines for HF promote class I indications for the use of an ICD as primary prevention of all-cause mortality in well-treated NYHA class II and III patients with either ischemic or nonischemic cardiomyopathy and an LVEF of 35% or less. Those with ischemic cardiomyopathy, NYHA class I functional status, and an ejection fraction less than 30% are also assigned a class I indication.[16] ICD implantation in those with a recent MI must be deferred until 40 days have passed from the date of acute MI. For those who have been surgically or percutaneously revascularized, the Centers for Medicare and Medicaid Services require waiting 3 months prior to ICD implant. In addition, the ACC/AHA guidelines qualify that ICD candidates should have a reasonable expectation of survival with a good functional status for more than 1 year.

Practical Considerations in Implantable Cardioverter-Defibrillator Therapy

Before ICD implantation, patients should have a thorough understanding of the risks and benefits of device therapy, as well as the need for routine follow-up and defibrillation threshold testing and the morbidity associated with appropriate and inappropriate ICD shocks. Patients should understand that ICDs have been shown to prolong survival, but they will not improve HF symptoms, nor will they slow disease progression. It should also be explained to the patient and family that the defibrillator function of an implantable device can be turned off as part of end-of-life care. Questions regarding exercise, driving, cellular telephones, and airport security, among others, should be anticipated and addressed in advance. The management of complications after ICD implantation is discussed in Chapter 22. Monitoring for bleeding or infection is paramount during the early postimplant period, although seeding of the device from a distant infectious source may occur at any time. For patients who develop new or recurrent ventricular arrhythmias that cause frequent ICD shocks, therapeutic options include antiarrhythmic drugs such as amiodarone or mexiletine, catheter ablation of ventricular tachycardia, or, in selected cases, consideration of mechanical circulatory support or heart transplant. In patients with ischemic heart disease, the occurrence of polymorphic ventricular tachycardia that leads to ICD shocks should warrant reassessment for ischemia. Patients who develop significant anxiety related to ICD shocks may benefit from anxiolytic therapy and/or referral to a therapist or support group. Finally, it is important to remember that ICDs may aggravate HF and result in increased HF hospitalizations. This may result from mechanical dyssynchrony induced by right ventricular pacing.[17]

Conduction Abnormalities in Heart Failure

A number of conduction abnormalities are seen in the setting of chronic HF. Approximately one third of patients with HF and reduced ejection fraction have a QRS duration greater than 120 ms, most commonly seen as a left bundle branch block (LBBB).[18,19] Such conduction delays produce suboptimal ventricular filling, a reduction in LV contractility, extended mitral regurgitation, and paradoxical septal wall motion.[20-23] These mechanical manifestations of ventricular conduction abnormalities have been referred to as *ventricular dyssynchrony*, especially because the septum and LV free wall no longer contract in a normal near-simultaneous fashion. This situation reduces the ability of the failing heart to eject blood and has been associated with increased mortality in HF patients.[24,25]

In the mid-1990s, the application of pacing therapies to overcome ventricular dyssynchrony began to be explored. In particular, atrial-synchronized biventricular pacing—now known as *cardiac resynchronization therapy* (CRT)—emerged as the most promising approach for the treatment of ventricular dyssynchrony. A series of studies confirmed the benefits of CRT in NYHA functional class III and IV heart failure patients with ventricular dyssynchrony and led to a strong contemporary recommendation for the use of this therapy.[16]

The first application of atrial-synchronized biventricular pacing was performed by Cazeau and colleagues,[26] who used four-chamber pacing in a 54-year-old man with NYHA class IV heart failure and significant atrial-ventricular and ventricular conduction disturbances. Standard transvenous pacing leads were placed in the right atrium and right ventricle. The left atrium was paced by a lead placed in the coronary sinus, whereas the LV was paced by an epicardial lead located on the LV free wall. After 6 weeks of pacing, the patient's clinical status improved markedly, with a weight loss of 17 kg and a disappearance of peripheral edema. His functional class improved remarkably to NYHA class II. Such favorable anecdotal experiences led to the inception of small studies to evaluate the acute effects of biventricular pacing on systemic hemodynamics. These studies provided additional proof of concept that CRT might reverse the deleterious consequences of ventricular dyssynchrony.[22,27] Several studies soon followed to further evaluate the acute and longer-term effects of CRT in HF.[28-36] The results were equally encouraging, with patients showing consistent, sustained improvement in exercise tolerance, quality of life (QOL), NYHA functional class, and cardiac output. With the advent of a transvenous, rather than an epicardial, approach for pacing the LV, larger-scale observational and randomized controlled trials of CRT were made possible.

Landmark Cardiac Resynchronization Therapy Clinical Trials

Substantial evidence supports the beneficial effects of CRT for the treatment of HF. Approximately 4000 patients have been evaluated in randomized single- or double-blind controlled trials, including large-scale morbidity and mortality studies. The most important of these trials are the Multisite Stimulation in Cardiomyopathy (MUSTIC) studies,[37,38] the Multicenter InSync Randomized Clinical Evaluation (MIRACLE) trial,[39,40] MIRACLE ICD,[41] the Safety and Effectiveness of Cardiac Resynchronization Therapy with

Defibrillation (CONTAK CD) trial,[42] the Cardiac Resynchronization in Heart Failure (CARE-HF) trial,[43,44] and the Comparison of Medical Therapy, Pacing, and Defibrillation in Heart Failure (COMPANION) trial.[45,46]

MUSTIC

The MUSTIC trials were designed to evaluate the safety and efficacy of cardiac resynchronization in patients with advanced HF, ventricular dyssynchrony, and either normal sinus rhythm[36] or atrial fibrillation.[37] They represent the first randomized single-blind trials of CRT for HF. The first study involved 58 randomized patients with NYHA class III heart failure, normal sinus rhythm, and a QRS duration of at least 150 ms. All patients were implanted with a CRT device, and after a run-in period, patients were randomized in a single-blind fashion to either active pacing or no pacing. After 12 weeks, patients were crossed over and remained in the alternate study assignment for 12 weeks. After completing this second 12-week period, the device was programmed to the patient's preferred mode of therapy.

The second MUSTIC study involved fewer patients (only 37 completers) with atrial fibrillation and a slow ventricular rate, either spontaneously or from radiofrequency ablation. A VVIR biventricular pacemaker and leads for each ventricle were implanted, and the same randomization procedure just described was applied; however, biventricular VVIR pacing versus single-site right ventricular VVIR pacing, rather than no pacing, was compared in this group of patients with atrial fibrillation. The primary endpoints for MUSTIC were exercise tolerance assessed by measurement of peak oxygen consumption (VO_2) or the 6-minute walk test and QOL determined using the Minnesota Living with Heart Failure questionnaire. Secondary endpoints included rehospitalizations and/or drug therapy modifications for worsening HF. Results from the normal sinus rhythm arm of MUSTIC provided strong evidence of benefit. The mean distance walked in 6 minutes was 23% greater with CRT than during the inactive pacing phase ($P < .001$). Significant improvement was also seen in quality of life and NYHA functional class, with fewer hospitalizations during active resynchronization therapy. The atrial fibrillation cohort evaluated in MUSTIC demonstrated similar improvements, although the magnitude of benefit was slightly less.

MIRACLE

MIRACLE was the first prospective, randomized, double-blind, parallel-controlled clinical trial designed to evaluate the merits of CRT and to further elucidate potential mechanisms of action of CRT.[38,39] Primary endpoints were NYHA class, QOL score (using the Minnesota Living with Heart Failure questionnaire), and 6-minute walk distance. Secondary endpoints included assessments of a composite clinical response, cardiopulmonary exercise performance, neurohormone and cytokine levels, QRS duration, cardiac structure and function (as determined by echocardiography), and a variety of measures of worsening HF and combined morbidity and mortality.

The MIRACLE trial was conducted between 1998 and 2000. Patients (n = 453) with moderate to severe symptoms of HF associated with an LVEF of 35% or less and a QRS duration of at least 130 ms were randomized (double-blind) to cardiac resynchronization (n = 228) or to a control group (n = 225) for 6 months while conventional therapy for HF was maintained.[37] Compared with the control group, patients randomized to CRT demonstrated a significant improvement in QOL score (−18.0 vs. −9.0 points; $P = .001$), 6-minute walk distance (+39 vs. +10 meters; $P = .005$), NYHA class (−1.0 vs. 0.0 class; $P < .001$), treadmill exercise time (+81 vs. +19 seconds; $P = .001$), peak VO_2 (+1.1 vs. 0.1 mL/kg/min; $P < .01$), and LVEF (+4.6% vs. −0.2%; $P < .001$) (Figure 13-2).

Patients randomized to CRT demonstrated a highly significant improvement in a composite clinical HF response endpoint compared with control subjects, suggesting an overall improvement in

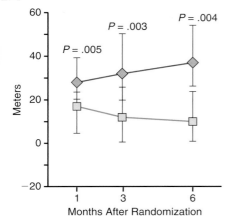
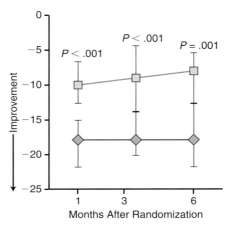

FIGURE 13-2 Effect of cardiac resynchronization therapy on 6-minute hall-walk distance (*left*) and quality of life (QOL) score (*right*) in the Multicenter InSync Randomized Clinical Evaluation trial. Shown are median changes and their respective 95% confidence intervals at 1, 3, and 6 months after randomization in the control (*squares*) and cardiac resynchronization groups (*diamonds*). A reduction in QOL score denotes improvement. *P* values denote significant between-group differences. For each variable, data are shown for patients who had values at all three time points.

HF clinical status. In addition, when compared with the control group, fewer patients in the CRT group required hospitalization (8% vs. 15%) or intravenous medications (7% and 15%) for the treatment of worsening HF (both $P < .05$). In the resynchronization group, the 50% reduction in hospitalization was accompanied by a significant reduction in length of stay, resulting in a 77% decrease in total days hospitalized over 6 months compared with the control group. The major limitation of the therapy was caused by unsuccessful implantation of the device in 8% of patients. The results of this trial led to the FDA approval of the InSync system (Medtronic, Inc., Minneapolis, MN) in August 2001, the first approved CRT system in the United States, allowing the introduction of CRT into clinical practice.

The MIRACLE trial also provided persuasive evidence supporting the occurrence of reverse LV remodeling with chronic CRT. In the MIRACLE trial, serial Doppler echocardiograms were obtained at baseline and at 3 months and 6 months in a subset of 323 patients.[44] CRT for 6 months was associated with reduced end-diastolic and end-systolic volumes (both $P < .001$), reduced LV mass ($P < .01$), increased ejection fraction ($P < .001$), reduced mitral regurgitation ($P < .001$), and improved myocardial performance index ($P < .001$) compared with controls. These effects are similar to those seen with β-blockade in HF, but in the MIRACLE trial, they were seen in patients already receiving β-blocker therapy.

MIRACLE ICD

The MIRACLE ICD study was designed to be almost identical to the MIRACLE trial. MIRACLE ICD was a prospective, multicenter, randomized, double-blind, parallel-controlled clinical trial intended to assess the safety and efficacy of a combined CRT-ICD system in patients with dilated cardiomyopathy (LVEF ≤35%, LV end diastolic dimension ≤55 mm), NYHA class III or IV heart failure, ventricular dyssynchrony (QRS ≥130 ms), and an indication for an ICD. Primary and secondary efficacy measures were essentially the same as those evaluated in the MIRACLE trial but also included measures of ICD function, including the efficacy of antitachycardia therapy with biventricular pacing.

Of 369 randomized patients who received devices, 182 were controls (ICD active, CRT inactive), and 187 were in the resynchronization group (ICD active, CRT active). At 6 months, patients assigned to active CRT had a greater improvement in median QOL score (−17.5 vs. −11.0; $P = .02$) and functional class (−1 vs. 0; $P = .007$) than controls but were no different than controls in the change in distance walked in 6 minutes (55 vs. 53 m; $P = .36$).[40] Peak oxygen consumption increased by 1.1 mL/kg/min in the resynchronization group, versus 0.1 mL/kg/min in controls ($P = .04$), and treadmill exercise duration increased by 56 seconds in the CRT group and decreased by 11 seconds in controls ($P = .0006$). The magnitude of improvement was comparable with that

seen in the MIRACLE trial, suggesting that HF patients with an ICD indication benefit as much from CRT as those patients without an indication for an ICD. The combined CRT-ICD device used in this study was approved in June 2002 by the FDA for use in NYHA class III and IV heart failure patients with reduced ejection fraction, ventricular dyssynchrony, and an ICD indication.

CONTAK CD

The CONTAK CD trial enrolled 581 symptomatic HF patients with ventricular dyssynchrony and malignant ventricular tachyarrhythmias, all of whom were candidates for an ICD.[41] Following unsuccessful implant attempts and withdrawals, 490 patients were available for analysis. The study did not meet its primary endpoint of a reduction in disease progression, defined by a composite endpoint of HF hospitalization, all-cause mortality, and ventricular arrhythmia requiring defibrillator therapies, although the trends were in a direction favoring improved outcomes with CRT. However, the CONTAK CD trial did show statistically significant improvements in peak oxygen uptake and quality of life in the resynchronization group compared with control subjects, although quality of life was improved only in NYHA class III and IV patients without right bundle branch block (RBBB). LV dimensions were also reduced, and LVEF increased, as seen in other trials of CRT. Importantly, the improvement seen in peak oxygen consumption with cardiac resynchronization was again comparable with that observed in the MIRACLE trial. Improvements in NYHA functional class were not observed in this study.

COMPANION

Begun in early 2000, COMPANION was a multicenter, prospective, randomized, controlled clinical trial designed to compare drug therapy alone with drug therapy in combination with cardiac resynchronization in patients with dilated cardiomyopathy, an intraventricular conduction defect (IVCD), NYHA class III or IV heart failure, and no indication for a device.[45,46] COMPANION randomized 1520 patients into one of three treatment groups in a 1:2:2 allocation. Group 1 (308 patients) received optimal medical care only, group II (617 patients) received optimal medical care and the Guidant (Indianapolis, IN) CONTAK TR (biventricular pulse generator), and group III (595 patients) received optimal medical care and the CONTAK CD (combined HF/bradycardia/tachycardia device). The primary endpoint of the COMPANION trial was a composite of all-cause mortality and all-cause hospitalization, measured as time to first event, beginning from time of randomization. Secondary endpoints included all-cause mortality and a variety of measures of cardiovascular morbidity.

When compared with optimal medical therapy alone, the combined endpoint of mortality or HF hospitalization was reduced by

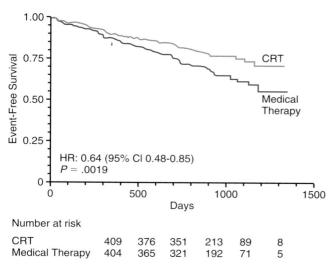

HR: 0.64 (95% CI 0.48-0.85)
P = .0019

Number at risk

CRT	409	376	351	213	89	8
Medical Therapy	404	365	321	192	71	5

FIGURE 13-3 Kaplan-Meier estimates of survival in patients randomized to cardiac resynchronization therapy (*CRT*) compared with conventional medical therapy in the CARE-HF trial. CI, confidence interval; HR, hazard ratio.

35% for patients receiving CRT and by 40% for patients receiving CRT-ICD (both $P < .001$). For the mortality endpoint alone, CRT patients had a 24% risk reduction ($P = .060$) and CRT-ICD patients had a 36% risk reduction ($P < .003$) compared with optimal medical therapy. COMPANION confirmed the results of earlier resynchronization therapy trials in improving symptoms, exercise tolerance, and quality of life for HF patients with ventricular dyssynchrony. In addition, COMPANION showed, for the first time, the impact of CRT-ICD in reducing all-cause mortality.

CARE-HF

The Cardiac Resynchronization–Heart Failure (CARE-HF) trial was designed to evaluate the effects of resynchronization therapy without an ICD on morbidity and mortality rates in patients with NYHA class III or IV heart failure and ventricular dyssynchrony.[42,43] Patients (n = 813) with an LVEF of 35% or less and ventricular dyssynchrony—defined as a QRS duration of 150 ms or greater, a QRS duration between 120 and 150 ms, with echocardiographic evidence of dyssynchrony—were enrolled in this randomized, unblinded, controlled trial and were followed up for an average of 29 months.[41] Optimal medical therapy alone was assigned to 404 patients, and 409 patients were randomized to optimal medical therapy plus resynchronization therapy. The risk of death from any cause or unplanned hospitalization for a major cardiac event, the primary endpoint analyzed as time to first event, was significantly reduced by 37% in the treatment group compared with control subjects (HR, 0.63; 95% CI, 0.51 to 0.77; $P < .001$). In the CRT group, 82 patients (20%) died during follow-up compared with 120 patients (30%) in the medical group, yielding a significant 36% reduction in all-cause mortality with resynchronization therapy (HR, 0.64; 95% CI, 0.48 to 0.85; $P < .002$; Figure 13-3). Resynchronization therapy also significantly reduced the risk of unplanned hospitalization for a major cardiac event by 39%, all-cause mortality plus HF hospitalization by 46%, and HF hospitalization by 52%.

Cardiac Resynchronization Therapy in Mild Heart Failure

Recent evidence from randomized clinical trials suggests that the beneficial effects of CRT on reverse remodeling, HF events, and mortality rate also extend to patients with ventricular dyssynchrony, reduced ejection fraction, and mild HF symptoms. Although these

patients were included in the MIRACLE ICD II and CONTAK-CD trials, they represented a relatively small proportion of the study populations. The main randomized trials that examined the effects of resynchronization therapy in mild HF are the Resynchronization Reverses Remodeling in Systolic Left Ventricular Dysfunction (REVERSE) study,[47] the Multicenter Automatic Defibrillator Implantation Trial with Cardiac Resynchronization Therapy (MADIT-CRT),[48] and the Resynchronization-Defibrillation for Ambulatory Heart Failure Trial (RAFT).[49]

REVERSE

Published in 2008,[47] the REVERSE trial was the first large, randomized clinical study to include patients with both NYHA class I and class II heart failure. The study randomized and followed 610 patients in sinus rhythm with an LVEF of 40% or less, a QRS duration of 120 ms or more, NYHA class I or II heart failure, and an LV end-diastolic diameter of at least 55 mm. All patients were implanted with a CRT device with or without ICD and were randomized in a 2:1 fashion to CRT-on or CRT-off. The primary endpoint was the HF clinical composite response; patients were considered worsened if they were hospitalized for HF, crossed over to the other study arm because of HF, had a deterioration in NYHA class, or died. The prespecified secondary endpoint was LV end-systolic volume index (LVESVI) as measured by echocardiography. Approximately 50% of patients had an ischemic cardiomyopathy, and more than 80% were in NYHA functional class II. Although the composite primary endpoint did not meet statistical significance at 1 year, a significant improvement was reported in LVESVI in the CRT-on arm (-18.4 ± 29.5 mL/m^2 vs. -1.3 ± 23.4 mL/m^2; $P < .0001$). Time to first HF hospitalization was also delayed with CRT-on (HR, 0.47; $P = .03$).

MADIT-CRT

MADIT-CRT was the largest trial of CRT in mild HF patients.[48] Over a 4.5-year period, 1820 patients with ischemic or nonischemic cardiomyopathy were enrolled. Inclusion criteria for the study were similar to the REVERSE trial in that patients were required to have dyssynchronous LV systolic dysfunction and NYHA class I or II heart failure, but with a slightly lower ejection fraction cutoff ($\leq 30\%$) and a slightly longer QRS duration (≥ 130 ms). Patients were randomized to receive an ICD with or without an LV lead (ICD vs. CRT-ICD). Neither patients nor treating physicians were blinded to the randomization assignment. The primary endpoint was all-cause mortality or occurrence of the first HF event, defined as a hospital admission for HF or outpatient treatment of HF requiring intravenous diuretic. The secondary endpoint was a change in LVESV. Over an average follow-up of 2.4 years, the primary endpoint occurred in 17.2% of the CRT-ICD group and in 25.3% of the ICD-only group (HR in CRT-ICD group 0.66; $P = .001$). The benefit of CRT-ICD was driven primarily by a 41% reduction in HF events, found primarily in those with QRS durations greater than 150 ms. Resynchronization therapy was also associated with a significant improvement in LV volumes and ejection fraction. No difference was observed between those with ischemic and nonischemic cardiomyopathy, and no difference was noted in the overall risk of death between those with CRT-ICD vs ICD only.

RAFT

The efficacy of CRT in mild to moderate HF was validated by the RAFT trial.[49] Patients (n = 1798) with an LVEF of 30% or less, an intrinsic QRS duration of 120 ms or more (or ≥ 200 ms paced QRS), and NYHA class II or III symptoms were randomized to CRT-ICD or ICD alone. More than 80% of the study population had NYHA class II heart failure, and two thirds of the patients had underlying ischemic heart disease. The primary outcome was death from any cause or HF hospitalization. Over a mean follow-up period of 40 months, the primary outcome occurred in 33.2% of the ICD-CRT group and in 40.3% of the group who received ICD alone (HR, 0.75; 95% CI, 0.69 to 0.87; $P < .001$). Resynchronization therapy was associated with decreased all-cause mortality (21% vs. 26%; $P = .003$) and fewer HF hospitalizations than ICD alone. However, at 30 days after implantation, the adverse event rate was higher in the CRT-ICD group (13% vs. 7%), with a higher incidence of hemothorax/pneumothorax, pocket hematomas and infections, lead dislodgements, and coronary sinus dissections.

RAFT was the first study to demonstrate that CRT offered a survival benefit beyond that provided by ICD therapy alone. In this population of patients with mild to moderate HF, the addition of resynchronization therapy to an ICD and optimal medical therapy reduced the absolute risk of death by 6% over 5 years compared with ICD and medications alone. Subgroup analyses also suggested that this benefit was more likely to occur in those with QRS durations of 150 ms or more and less likely in the presence of atrial fibrillation or RBBB.

Cardiac Resynchronization Therapy

Cardiac Resynchronization Therapy in Long-Term Right Ventricle Pacing

The potential detrimental effect of long-term RV pacing on LV function is a well-known phenomenon.[50] Regardless of the duration of the native QRS complex, evidence suggests that patients with LV dysfunction and a standard indication for pacing may benefit from resynchronization therapy. The Homburg Biventricular Pacing Evaluation (HOBIPACE) trial was a randomized crossover study in which 30 patients with LV systolic dysfunction (LV end-diastolic diameter ≥60 mm and LVEF ≤40%) were implanted with CRT systems.[51] Subjects received 3 months each of RV pacing and CRT. Compared with baseline and RV pacing, CRT was associated with reverse remodeling and lower N-terminal prohormone of brain natriuretic peptide (NT-proBNP) levels and also with improvements in LVEF, oxygen consumption, and HF symptoms. Similar results were seen in a small study of 60 patients with LV dysfunction and long-term RV pacing. In these patients, the addition of an LV pacing lead resulted in a significant improvement in NYHA functional class and LVEF.[52] According to the ACC/AHA guidelines, CRT is reasonable for patients with an LVEF of 35% or less and NYHA class III or ambulatory class IV symptoms who are receiving optimal medical therapy and who have frequent dependence on ventricular pacing (class IIa recommendation, level of evidence C).[16]

Cardiac Resynchronization Therapy in Atrial Fibrillation

Atrial fibrillation (AF) is a common comorbidity in patients who are candidates for resynchronization therapy. Subgroup analyses of some studies suggest that HF patients with AF may derive less benefit from CRT pacing than those in sinus rhythm.[41,49] One of the contributing factors may be inadequate ventricular rate control, resulting in fusion or pseudofusion and ultimately suboptimal levels of effective biventricular pacing. Some evidence suggests that AV node ablation as an adjunct to CRT in this population is superior to drug therapy alone. In a series of 673 patients with AF receiving CRT therapy for conventional indications (LVEF ≤35%, NYHA class ≥II, and a QRS duration ≥120 ms), only those who underwent AV node ablation demonstrated an improvement in LV function and functional capacity.[53] A recent study also suggests that among patients with AF and HF who receive CRT, AV node ablation not only improves NYHA class but may also provide a survival benefit over those treated medically with rate-control drugs alone.[54]

Indications for Cardiac Resynchronization Therapy in Heart Failure Patients

The 2009 ACC/AHA HF guidelines propose a class I indication for CRT in patients with an LVEF of 35% or less, a QRS duration of 120 ms or less, normal sinus rhythm, and NYHA functional class III or ambulatory class IV symptoms despite recommended optimal medical therapy.[16] In light of the growing evidence in favor of resynchronization therapy in mild HF, the most recent European Society of Cardiology (ESC) guidelines have broadened their CRT indications to incorporate the NYHA class II population.[55] The Heart Failure Society of America (HFSA) has also recently updated their guidelines to reflect these changes in data and clinical practice. At present, CRT is not recommended for patients with unstable or refractory HF.

Future Directions of Cardiac Resynchronization Therapy

Several issues related to CRT in HF are unresolved. Despite the widespread use of CRT, further advances in device and lead technology are needed. In up to 10% of patients, percutaneous LV lead placement cannot be performed because of failure of cardiac vein cannulation. Additionally, implant procedures may be complicated by coronary sinus dissection, and late lead malfunction or dislodgment may occur. Select patients are referred for surgical epicardial LV lead placement,[56] but outcomes are not well described. Newer lead systems and minimally invasive surgical procedures are now available, but randomized studies will be needed to determine the safety and efficacy of these new techniques.

Despite significant advancements in device technology and implant tools, up to a third of patients do not respond to resynchronization therapy. Although our understanding of this phenomenon remains incomplete, certain patient characteristics—such as scar burden, scar location relative to LV pacing site, ischemic cardiomyopathy, and RBBB—have been identified as poor prognosticators for CRT response. Alternatively, those with nonischemic cardiomyopathy and a QRS duration of at least 150 ms tend to experience significant clinical improvement and reverse remodeling.[57,58] More investigations are needed to further characterize the specific variables that will facilitate the differentiation between those who are optimal candidates for resynchronization and those unlikely to benefit.

Monitoring Heart Failure Through Implantable Devices

Either as stand-alone devices or combined with CRT and ICD devices, implantable monitoring technologies are rapidly being applied to the management of HF. Implantable devices can provide a wealth of physiologic information about the clinical status of HF patients, and the use of this information may improve HF outcomes. For example, many implantable CRT and ICD devices can provide information on atrial heart rate and rhythm, ventricular heart rate and rhythm, patient activity level, and heart rate variability (HRV), and an increasing number of FDA-approved implantable CRT-ICD devices can also track changes in intrathoracic impedance. By monitoring trends in such parameters, it may be possible to predict episodes of worsening HF.

HF patients are encouraged to remain active and to engage in regular submaximal aerobic exercise, such as walking, cycling, or swimming. The activity trend recorded by many implantable devices provides an objective record of the number of hours per day that patients are physically active. Thus, the activity report can serve as a useful teaching and reinforcement tool for both the patient and family about the importance and level of activity.

Because exercise intolerance is a hallmark of worsening HF, a decrease in measured patient activity level may provide one clue to disease progression or decompensation. This measurement may be viewed as complementary to the patient history and, perhaps, as more objective. The predictive value of objectively measured changes in patient activity level is currently under investigation, and anecdotal reports suggest that a reduction in measured patient activity level precedes overt HF decompensation.

Adamson and associates[59] evaluated the usefulness of monitoring changes in HRV as a marker of HF clinical status. HRV reflects the balance between sympathetic and parasympathetic nervous system activity in the heart, with a decrease in HRV serving as a sign of increased sympathetic and decreased parasympathetic tone.[60] This analysis showed that HRV diminished in the days to weeks leading up to a hospitalization for worsening HF, thereby suggesting that decreases in HRV can predict HF decompensation.[59] The notion that changes in continuously monitored HRV may be predictive of worsening HF is attractive, because it fits well with our understanding of the mechanisms leading to worsening HF or HF disease progression—specifically, activation of the sympathetic nervous system.

The ability of implantable devices to monitor fluid status was initially based on monitoring changes in intrathoracic impedance. Electrical impedance can be determined between the generator and the ICD lead residing within the right ventricle. Essentially, electrical impedance is measured across the lung, from the tip of the lead to the generator (Figure 13-4). Because water conducts electricity better than air, increasing lung water is associated with a decrease in electrical impedance. Using this technique, electrical impedance is assessed multiple times throughout the day and then plotted on a graph. The fluid volume thresholds can be adjusted by the clinician based on patient symptoms and can be reviewed to determine volume status. Clinical evaluation of intrathoracic impedance changes has shown its ability to predict hospitalizations for decompensated HF 10 to 14 days in advance of the event.[61] One such device has been approved by the FDA and is commercially available. Using measurements of intrathoracic impedance, this CRT-ICD device can reliably track intrathoracic fluid volume changes.[62] However, a recent study showed that an intrathoracic impedance-derived fluid index had low sensitivity and low positive predictive value for predicting HF hospitalizations in the early postimplant period.[63] In another study of 335 patients with ICDs or CRT-ICD devices, use of an implantable diagnostic tool to measure intrathoracic impedance with an audible patient alert did not improve outcome and actually increased HF hospitalizations and outpatient visits.[64]

A new generation of even more sophisticated implantable hemodynamic monitoring devices is under investigation. These systems enable the day-to-day management of ventricular filling pressures and other invasive physiologic parameters not otherwise available to the clinician. Early reports suggest a substantial opportunity to reduce HF morbidity rates (e.g., episodes of worsening HF requiring hospitalization) with the use of these devices. Each device varies in its platform, mechanism, and site of implant. Many of them are capable of securely transmitting hemodynamic information directly to the clinician, facilitating quick and easy therapeutic responses to clinical fluctuations. One of these implantable hemodynamic monitoring systems has undergone extensive evaluation in clinical trials. The platform of the Chronicle system (Medtronic) is similar to a single-lead permanent pacemaker system, consisting of a programmable generator placed in the pectoral area and a passive fixation transvenous electrode in the RV outflow tract. This device has been shown to be safe and effective to provide an accurate estimate of LV filling pressure and to predict HF events, such as an emergency room visit or hospitalization for worsening HF.[65-67] However, in the Chronicle Offers Management to Patients with Advanced Signs and Symptoms of Heart Failure (COMPASS-HF) study, an RCT of 274 patients, implantable hemodynamic monitor–guided care did not significantly reduce total HF-related events compared with optimal medical management.[67] In a prespecified subgroup analysis of patients with HF and preserved ejection fraction enrolled in COMPASS-HF, the addition of implantable hemodynamic monitor–guided care also did not lower HF event rates.[68] Based on these negative data, the FDA did not approve the Chronicle device for HF management.

A wireless sensor, without batteries or leads, has also been investigated as a tool for remote HF management (Figure 13-5, A). This implantable pressure monitor (CardioMEMS, Atlanta, GA) is seated into a distal branch of the descending pulmonary artery branch via a right heart catheter and is capable of continuous monitoring of pulmonary artery pressures and heart rate. A study in which 550 NYHA class III patients were implanted with this device and randomly assigned to an open (hemodynamic data available to the treating clinician) versus closed arm demonstrated a 30% reduction in HF hospitalizations with hemodynamic-guided therapy over a 6-month follow-up period (31% vs. 44%; HR, 0.70; 95% CI, 0.60 to 0.84).[69] Despite these positive findings, the FDA has not yet approved the CardioMEMS device for HF management.

Other systems empower patients to self-manage LV filling pressure in the same way that patients with diabetes self-manage glucose levels through the use of a glucometer. The potential for these devices to revolutionize the management of HF is substantial but remains under investigation. One such device, the LAPTOP (St. Jude Medical, St. Paul, MN), is designed to take continuous direct measurements of left atrial pressure; it consists of an abdominal generator attached to a sensor positioned in the interatrial septum (Figure 13-5, B). LAPTOP measurements reportedly correlate well with invasive measures of pulmonary capillary wedge pressure. Results of an observational study, in which patients used this technology to help manage their own therapy, showed a significant reduction in HF events.[70] The Left Atrial Pressure Monitoring to Optimize Heart Failure Therapy (LAPTOP-HF) study is currently enrolling NYHA class III heart failure patients to test the safety and efficacy of this device.[71]

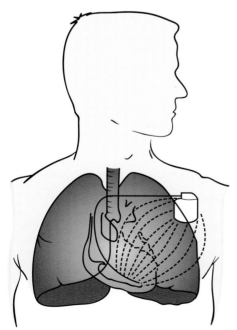

FIGURE 13-4 Diagram depicting the concept underlying intrathoracic impedance monitoring in heart failure. An electrical current is passed from the tip of the right ventricular lead to the "can," or generator. The impedance to the flow of electricity through the lung can be measured. Increased lung water is associated with a decrease in impedance, whereas a decrease in lung water is seen as an increase in intrathoracic impedance.

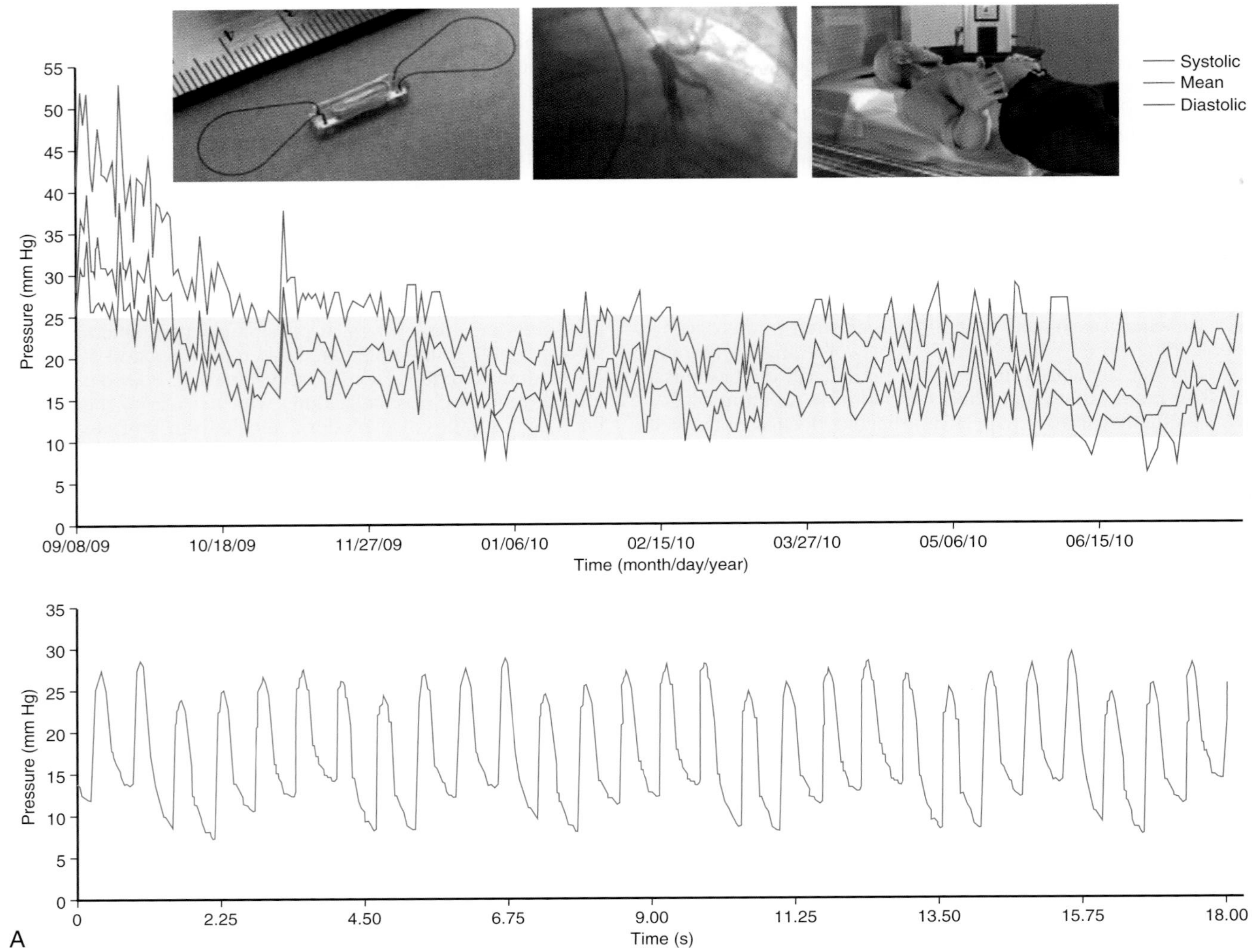

CH
13

FIGURE 13-5   Novel implantable hemodynamic monitors. **A,** CardioMEMS sensor (*top left*) is implanted through a catheter into a distal branch of the descending pulmonary artery (*top middle*). This platform enables the patient to take home measurements of pulmonary pressures (*top right*) and transmit them to clinicians for evaluation. Data can be transmitted in the form of general trends (*middle*) or individual pressure measurements (*bottom*). (**A** *Modified with permission from Abraham WT, Adamson PB, Bourge RC, et al. Wireless pulmonary artery haemodynamic monitoring in chronic heart failure: a randomised controlled trial.* Lancet *2011;377[9766]:658-666.*)

Future Directions in Implantable Devices for the Management of Heart Failure

A variety of other implantable devices are under evaluation for the management of HF. In many ways, we are now in a "device era" for the management of this disease. One promising approach is cardiac contractility modulation (CCM).[72] This implantable device delivers an intermittent electrical impulse to the heart during the absolute refractory period of the ventricle. Although the mechanism of action of this investigational therapy is incompletely understood, it may be thought of as a form of electrical conditioning of the heart, whereby electrically mediated changes in myocyte calcium handling improve contractility. This improvement in contractility occurs in association with a reduction in myocardial oxygen consumption, suggesting improved efficiency of the heart.[72] This favorable relationship between myocardial contractility and work has been associated with improved outcomes for other HF therapies, such as CRT. CCM has also been shown to contribute to LV reverse remodeling and improvement in ejection fraction.[73] Although a large-scale randomized trial examining the effect of CCM on moderate to severe HF patients with a narrow QRS and ejection fraction less than 35% was unable

to show an improvement in ventilatory anaerobic threshold over best medical therapy,[74] a subsequent subgroup analysis suggested that perhaps the benefit may be limited to those with NYHA class III symptoms and an ejection fraction greater than 25%.[75] Other implantable HF devices, including vagal nerve and spinal cord stimulators,[76] are in preclinical and early clinical evaluations.

Summary

Cardiac resynchronization therapy offers a new therapeutic approach for treating patients with ventricular dyssynchrony and moderate to severe HF. Substantial experience suggests that it is safe and effective; patients have shown significant improvement in clinical symptoms and multiple measures of functional status, exercise capacity, and outcomes. The beneficial effects of CRT on ventricular structure and function have also been demonstrated in multiple clinical studies. Prophylactic implantation of an ICD is also now of proven benefit in HF patients, at least in those with NYHA class II and III disease. Implantable monitoring technologies promise to improve our ability to avoid episodes of HF decompensation and may improve the natural history of the disease. Other investigational devices may add incremental benefit to the treatment of HF.

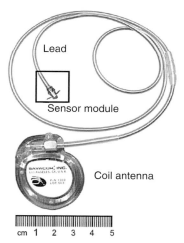

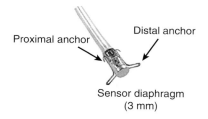

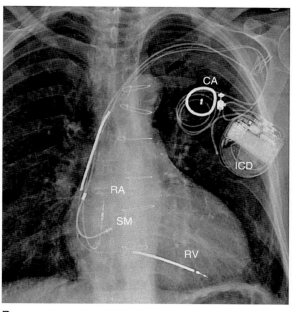

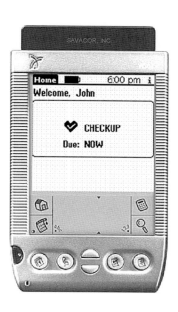

B

FIGURE 13-5, cont'd **B,** Illustration of the LAPTOP (St. Jude Medical) system, including the sensor lead that is implanted percutaneously into the interatrial septum and the coil antenna implanted in a prepectoral subcutaneous pocket. Below (*left*) is a chest radiograph of a patient with the LAPTOP system and a dual-chamber implantable cardioverter-defibrillator system alongside the patient advisor module (*right*) that patients can use to communicate with the sensor lead. (*B* *Modified with permission from Ritzema J, Troughton R, Melton I, et al. Physician-directed patient self-management of left atrial pressure in advanced chronic heart failure.* Circulation *2010;121[9]:1086-1095.*)

REFERENCES

1. Hunt SA, Abraham WT, Chin MH, et al. ACC/AHA 2005 guideline update for the diagnosis and management of chronic heart failure in the adult: a report of the American College of Cardiology/American Heart Association Task Force on Practice Guidelines (Writing Committee to Update the 2001 Guidelines for the Evaluation and Management of Heart Failure), developed in collaboration with the American College of Chest Physicians and the International Society for Heart and Lung Transplantation, endorsed by the Heart Rhythm Society. *Circulation* 2005;112(12):e154-e235.
2. Sims DB, Garcia LI, Mignatti A, et al. Utilization of defibrillators and resynchronization therapy at the time of evaluation at a heart failure and cardiac transplantation center. *Pacing Clin Electrophysiol* 2010;33(8):988-993.
3. Uretsky BF, Sheahan RG. Primary prevention of sudden cardiac death in heart failure: will the solution be shocking? *J Am Coll Cardiol* 1997;30(7):1589-1597.
4. Stevenson WG, Stevenson LW, Middlekauff HR, Saxon LA. Sudden death prevention in patients with advanced ventricular dysfunction. *Circulation* 1993;88(6):2953-2961.
5. Effect of metoprolol CR/XL in chronic heart failure: Metoprolol CR/XL Randomised Intervention Trial in Congestive Heart Failure (MERIT-HF). *Lancet* Jun 12 1999;353(9169):2001-2007.
6. Moss AJ, Hall WJ, Cannom DS, et al. Improved survival with an implanted defibrillator in patients with coronary disease at high risk for ventricular arrhythmia. Multicenter Automatic Defibrillator Implantation Trial Investigators. *N Engl J Med* 1996;335(26):1933-1940.
7. Bigger JT Jr. Prophylactic use of implanted cardiac defibrillators in patients at high risk for ventricular arrhythmias after coronary-artery bypass graft surgery. Coronary Artery Bypass Graft (CABG) Patch Trial Investigators. *N Engl J Med* 1997;337(22):1569-1575.
8. Buxton AE, Lee KL, Fisher JD, et al. A randomized study of the prevention of sudden death in patients with coronary artery disease. Multicenter Unsustained Tachycardia Trial Investigators. *N Engl J Med* 1999;341(25):1882-1890.
9. Moss AJ, Zareba W, Hall WJ, et al. Prophylactic implantation of a defibrillator in patients with myocardial infarction and reduced ejection fraction. *N Engl J Med* 2002;346(12):877-883.
10. Kadish A, Dyer A, Daubert JP, et al. Prophylactic defibrillator implantation in patients with nonischemic dilated cardiomyopathy. *N Engl J Med* 2004;350(21):2151-2158.
11. Bardy GH, Lee KL, Mark DB, et al. Amiodarone or an implantable cardioverter-defibrillator for congestive heart failure. *N Engl J Med* 2005;352(3):225-237.
12. Doval HC, Nul DR, Grancelli HO, et al. Randomised trial of low-dose amiodarone in severe congestive heart failure. Grupo de Estudio de la Sobrevida en la Insuficiencia Cardiaca en Argentina (GESICA). *Lancet* 1994;344(8921):493-498.
13. Solomon SD, Zelenkofske S, McMurray JJ, et al. Sudden death in patients with myocardial infarction and left ventricular dysfunction, heart failure, or both. *N Engl J Med* 2005;352(25):2581-2588.
14. Hohnloser SH, Kuck KH, Dorian P, et al. Prophylactic use of an implantable cardioverter-defibrillator after acute myocardial infarction. *N Engl J Med* 2004;351(24):2481-2488.
15. Steinbeck G, Andresen D, Seidl K, et al. Defibrillator implantation early after myocardial infarction. *N Engl J Med* 2009;361(15):1427-1436.

16. Hunt SA, Abraham WT, Chin MH, et al. 2009 focused update incorporated into the ACC/AHA 2005 guidelines for the diagnosis and management of heart failure in adults: a report of the American College of Cardiology Foundation/American Heart Association Task Force on Practice Guidelines, developed in collaboration with the International Society for Heart and Lung Transplantation. *Circulation* 2009;119(14):e391-e479.

17. Sweeney MO, Hellkamp AS, Ellenbogen KA, et al. Adverse effect of ventricular pacing on heart failure and atrial fibrillation among patients with normal baseline QRS duration in a clinical trial of pacemaker therapy for sinus node dysfunction. *Circulation* 2003;107(23):2932-2937.

18. Farwell D, Patel NR, Hall A, Ralph S, Sulke AN. How many people with heart failure are appropriate for biventricular resynchronization? *Eur Heart J* 2000;21(15):1246-1250.

19. Aaronson KD, Schwartz JS, Chen TM, et al. Development and prospective validation of a clinical index to predict survival in ambulatory patients referred for cardiac transplant evaluation. *Circulation* 1997;95(12):2660-2667.

20. Xiao HB, Brecker SJ, Gibson DG. Effects of abnormal activation on the time course of the left ventricular pressure pulse in dilated cardiomyopathy. *Br Heart J* 1992;68(4):403-407.

21. Littmann L, Symanski JD. Hemodynamic implications of left bundle branch block. *J Electrocardiol* 2000;33(Suppl):115-121.

22. Saxon LA, Kerwin WF, Cahalan MK, et al. Acute effects of intraoperative multisite ventricular pacing on left ventricular function and activation/contraction sequence in patients with depressed ventricular function. *J Cardiovascular Electrophysiol* 1998;9(1):13-21.

23. Kerwin WF, Botvinick EH, O'Connell JW, et al. Ventricular contraction abnormalities in dilated cardiomyopathy: effect of biventricular pacing to correct interventricular dyssynchrony. *J Am Coll Cardiol* 2000;35(5):1221-1227.

24. Xiao HB, Roy C, Fujimoto S, Gibson DG. Natural history of abnormal conduction and its relation to prognosis in patients with dilated cardiomyopathy. *Int J Cardiol* 1996;53(2):163-170.

25. Shamim W, Francis DP, Yousufuddin M, et al. Intraventricular conduction delay: a prognostic marker in chronic heart failure. *Int J Cardiol* 1999;70(2):171-178.

26. Cazeau S, Ritter P, Bakdach S, et al. Four chamber pacing in dilated cardiomyopathy. *Pacing Clin Electrophysiol* 1994;17(11 Pt 2):1974-1979.

27. Foster AH, Gold MR, McLaughlin JS. Acute hemodynamic effects of atrio-biventricular pacing in humans. *Ann Thorac Surg* 1995;59(2):294-300.

28. Cazeau S, Ritter P, Lazarus A, et al. Multisite pacing for end-stage heart failure: early experience. *Pacing Clin Electrophysiol* 1996;19(11 Pt 2):1748-1757.

29. Blanc JJ, Etienne Y, Gilard M, et al. Evaluation of different ventricular pacing sites in patients with severe heart failure: results of an acute hemodynamic study. *Circulation* 1997;96(10):3273-3277.

30. Leclercq C, Cazeau S, Le Breton H, et al. Acute hemodynamic effects of biventricular DDD pacing in patients with end-stage heart failure. *J Am Coll Cardiol* 1998;32(7):1825-1831.

31. Kass DA, Chen CH, Curry C, et al. Improved left ventricular mechanics from acute VDD pacing in patients with dilated cardiomyopathy and ventricular conduction delay. *Circulation* 1999;99(12):1567-1573.

32. Gras D, Mabo P, Tang T, et al. Multisite pacing as a supplemental treatment of congestive heart failure: preliminary results of the Medtronic Inc. InSync Study. *Pacing Clin Electrophysiol* 1998;21(11 Pt 2):2249-2255.

33. Auricchio A, Stellbrink C, Sack S, et al. The Pacing Therapies for Congestive Heart Failure (PATH-CHF) study: rationale, design, and endpoints of a prospective randomized multicenter study. *Am J Cardiol* 1999;83(5B):130D-135D.

34. Auricchio A, Klein H, Spinelli J. Pacing for heart failure: selection of patients, techniques and benefits. *Eur J Heart Fail* 1999;1(3):275-279.

35. Gras D, Leclercq C, Tang AS, et al. Cardiac resynchronization therapy in advanced heart failure the multicenter InSync clinical study. *Eur J Heart Fail* 2002;4(3):311-320.

36. Cazeau S, Leclercq C, Lavergne T, et al. Effects of multisite biventricular pacing in patients with heart failure and intraventricular conduction delay. *N Engl J Med* 2001;344(12):873-880.

37. Leclercq C, Walker S, Linde C, et al. Comparative effects of permanent biventricular and right-univentricular pacing in heart failure patients with chronic atrial fibrillation. *Eur Heart J* 2002;23(22):1780-1787.

38. Abraham WT. Rationale and design of a randomized clinical trial to assess the safety and efficacy of cardiac resynchronization therapy in patients with advanced heart failure: the Multicenter InSync Randomized Clinical Evaluation (MIRACLE). *J Card Fail* 2000;6(4):369-380.

39. Abraham WT, Fisher WG, Smith AL, et al. Cardiac resynchronization in chronic heart failure. *N Engl J Med* 2002;346(24):1845-1853.

40. Young JB, Abraham WT, Smith AL, et al. Combined cardiac resynchronization and implantable cardioversion defibrillation in advanced chronic heart failure: the MIRACLE ICD Trial. *JAMA* 2003;289(20):2685-2694.

41. Higgins SL, Hummel JD, Niazi IK, et al. Cardiac resynchronization therapy for the treatment of heart failure in patients with intraventricular conduction delay and malignant ventricular tachyarrhythmias. *J Am Coll Cardiol* 2003;42(8):1454-1459.

42. Cleland JG, Daubert JC, Erdmann E, et al. The CARE-HF study (CArdiac REsynchronisation in Heart Failure study): rationale, design and end-points. *Eur J Heart Fail* 2001;3(4):481-489.

43. Cleland JG, Daubert JC, Erdmann E, et al. The effect of cardiac resynchronization on morbidity and mortality in heart failure. *N Engl J Med* 2005;352(15):1539-1549.

44. Bristow MR, Feldman AM, Saxon LA. Heart failure management using implantable devices for ventricular resynchronization: Comparison of Medical Therapy, Pacing, and Defibrillation in Chronic Heart Failure (COMPANION) trial. COMPANION Steering Committee and COMPANION Clinical Investigators. *J Card Fail* 2000;6(3):276-285.

45. Bristow MR, Saxon LA, Boehmer J, et al. Cardiac-resynchronization therapy with or without an implantable defibrillator in advanced chronic heart failure. *N Engl J Med* 2004;350(21):2140-2150.

46. St John Sutton MG, Plappert T, Abraham WT, et al. Effect of cardiac resynchronization therapy on left ventricular size and function in chronic heart failure. *Circulation* 2003;107(15):1985-1990.

47. Linde C, Abraham WT, Gold MR, et al. Randomized trial of cardiac resynchronization in mildly symptomatic heart failure patients and in asymptomatic patients with left ventricular dysfunction and previous heart failure symptoms. *J Am Coll Cardiol* 2008;52(23):1834-1843.

48. Moss AJ, Hall WJ, Cannom DS, et al. Cardiac-resynchronization therapy for the prevention of heart-failure events. *N Engl J Med* 2009;361(14):1329-1338.

49. Tang AS, Wells GA, Talajic M, et al. Cardiac-resynchronization therapy for mild-to-moderate heart failure. *N Engl J Med* 2010;363(25):2385-2395.

50. Tantengco MV, Thomas RL, Karpawich PP. Left ventricular dysfunction after long-term right ventricular apical pacing in the young. *J Am Coll Cardiol* 2001;37(8):2093-2100.

51. Kindermann M, Hennen B, Jung J, et al. Biventricular versus conventional right ventricular stimulation for patients with standard pacing indication and left ventricular dysfunction: the Homburg Biventricular Pacing Evaluation (HOBIPACE). *J Am Coll Cardiol* 2006;47(10):1927-1937.

52. Baker CM, Christopher TJ, Smith PF, et al. Addition of a left ventricular lead to conventional pacing systems in patients with congestive heart failure: feasibility, safety, and early results in 60 consecutive patients. *Pacing Clin Electrophysiol* 2002;25(8):1166-1171.

53. Gasparini M, Auricchio A, Regoli F, et al. Four-year efficacy of cardiac resynchronization therapy on exercise tolerance and disease progression: the importance of performing atrioventricular junction ablation in patients with atrial fibrillation. *J Am Coll Cardiol* 2006;48(4):734-743.

54. Dong K, Shen WK, Powell BD, et al. Atrioventricular nodal ablation predicts survival benefit in patients with atrial fibrillation receiving cardiac resynchronization therapy. *Heart Rhythm* 2010;7(9):1240-1245.

55. Dickstein K, Vardas PE, Auricchio A, et al. 2010 Focused Update of ESC guidelines on device therapy in heart failure: an update of the 2008 ESC guidelines for the diagnosis and treatment of acute and chronic heart failure and the 2007 ESC guidelines for cardiac and resynchronization therapy. Developed with the special contribution of the Heart Failure Association and the European Heart Rhythm Association. *Eur Heart J* 2010;31(21):2677-2687.

56. Shah RV, Lewis EF, Givertz MM. Epicardial left ventricular lead placement for cardiac resynchronization therapy following failed coronary sinus approach. *Congest Heart Fail* 2006;12(6):312-316.

57. Yu CM, Wing-Hong Fung J, Zhang Q, Sanderson JE. Understanding nonresponders of cardiac resynchronization therapy: current and future perspectives. *J Cardiovascular Electrophysiol* 2005;16(10):1117-1124.

58. Shanks M, Delgado V, Ng AC, et al. Clinical and echocardiographic predictors of nonresponse to cardiac resynchronization therapy. *Am Heart J* 2011;161(3):552-557.

59. Adamson PB, Smith AL, Abraham WT, et al. Continuous autonomic assessment in patients with symptomatic heart failure: prognostic value of heart rate variability measured by an implanted cardiac resynchronization device. *Circulation* 2004;110(16):2389-2394.

60. Nolan J, Batin PD, Andrews R, et al. Prospective study of heart rate variability and mortality in chronic heart failure: results of the United Kingdom heart failure evaluation and assessment of risk trial (UK-heart). *Circulation* 1998;98(15):1510-1516.

61. Yu CM, Wang L, Chau E, et al. Intrathoracic impedance monitoring in patients with heart failure: correlation with fluid status and feasibility of early warning preceding hospitalization. *Circulation* 2005;112(6):841-848.

62. Abraham WT, Compton S, Haas G, et al. Intrathoracic impedance vs daily weight monitoring for predicting worsening heart failure events: results of the Fluid Accumulation Status Trial (FAST). *Congest Heart Fail* 2011;17(2):51-55.

63. Conraads VM, Tavazzi L, Santini M, et al. Sensitivity and positive predictive value of implantable intrathoracic impedance monitoring as a predictor of heart failure hospitalizations: the SENSE-HF trial. *Eur Heart J* 2011;32(18):2266-2273.

64. van Veldhuisen DJ, Braunschweig F, Conraads V, et al. Intrathoracic impedance monitoring, audible patient alerts, and outcome in patients with heart failure. *Circulation* 2011;124(16):1719-1726.

65. Magalski A, Adamson P, Gadler F, et al. Continuous ambulatory right heart pressure measurements with an implantable hemodynamic monitor: a multicenter, 12-month follow-up study of patients with chronic heart failure. *J Card Fail* 2002;8(2):63-70.

66. Adamson PB, Magalski A, Braunschweig F, et al. Ongoing right ventricular hemodynamics in heart failure: clinical value of measurements derived from an implantable monitoring system. *J Am Coll Cardiol* 2003;41(4):565-571.

67. Bourge RC, Abraham WT, Adamson PB, et al. Randomized controlled trial of an implantable continuous hemodynamic monitor in patients with advanced heart failure: the COMPASS-HF study. *J Am Coll Cardiol* 2008;51(11):1073-1079.

68. Zile MR, Bourge RC, Bennett TD, et al. Application of implantable hemodynamic monitoring in the management of patients with diastolic heart failure: a subgroup analysis of the COMPASS-HF trial. *J Card Fail* 2008;14(10):816-823.

69. Abraham WT, Adamson PB, Bourge RC, et al. Wireless pulmonary artery haemodynamic monitoring in chronic heart failure: a randomised controlled trial. *Lancet* 2011;377(9766):658-666.

70. Ritzema J, Troughton R, Melton I, et al. Physician-directed patient self-management of left atrial pressure in advanced chronic heart failure. *Circulation* 2010;121(9):1086-1095.

71. Left Atrial Pressure Monitoring to Optimize Heart Failure Therapy (LAPTOP-HF). NCT 01121107. www.ClinicalTrials.gov, January 2012.

72. Pappone C, Augello G, Rosanio S, et al. First human chronic experience with cardiac contractility modulation by nonexcitatory electrical currents for treating systolic heart failure: mid-term safety and efficacy results from a multicenter study. *J Cardiovascular Electrophysiol* 2004;15(4):418-427.

73. Yu CM, Chan JY, Zhang Q, et al. Impact of cardiac contractility modulation on left ventricular global and regional function and remodeling. *JACC Cardiovasc Imaging* 2009;2(12):1341-1349.

74. Kadish A, Nademanee K, Volosin K, et al. A randomized controlled trial evaluating the safety and efficacy of cardiac contractility modulation in advanced heart failure. *Am Heart J* Feb 2011;161(2):329-337 e321-322.

75. Abraham WT, Nademanee K, Volosin K, et al. Subgroup analysis of a randomized controlled trial evaluating the safety and efficacy of cardiac contractility modulation in advanced heart failure. *J Card Fail* 2011;17(9):710-717.

76. Cornelussen RN, Splett V, Klepfer RN, et al. Electrical modalities beyond pacing for the treatment of heart failure. *Heart Fail Rev* 2011;16(3):315-325.

CHAPTER 14 Strategies for Management of Acute Decompensated Heart Failure

Michael M. Givertz and Wilson S. Colucci

TERMINOLOGY, 281

EPIDEMIOLOGY, 281

PATHOPHYSIOLOGY, 282

Heart Failure with Reduced Versus Preserved Ejection Fraction, 282
Acute Compensatory Mechanisms, 283
Myocardial Injury, 284
Common Precipitating Factors of Heart Failure, 284

GENERAL MANAGEMENT, 285

Initial Patient Evaluation, 285
Risk Stratification, 285
Clinical Assessment of Intracardiac Filling Pressures, 285
Clinical Assessment of Systemic Perfusion, 287
Laboratory Assessment, 287
Noninvasive Versus Invasive Management, 288
Hemodynamic Profiles, 289
Hemodynamic Goals of Therapy, 290

FLUID MANAGEMENT, 290

Parenteral Diuretic Therapy, 290
Ultrafiltration, 291

VASOACTIVE THERAPY, 292

Nitroglycerin, 292
Nesiritide, 292
Nitroprusside, 293
Dobutamine, 293
Milrinone, 294
Dopamine, 295
Epinephrine and Norepinephrine, 296
Digoxin, 296

ADJUSTMENT OF ORAL MEDICATIONS, 296

Renin-Angiotensin-Aldosterone System Inhibitors, 296
Nitrates and Hydralazine, 297
β-Blockers, 297
Oral Diuretics, 297

OTHER MANAGEMENT ISSUES, 297

Sodium and Fluid Restriction, 297
Oxygen Supplementation, 297
Ventricular Arrhythmias, 298
Anticoagulation, 298
Comorbidities, 298
Discharge Planning and Immediate Postdischarge Care, 298

SPECIAL CONSIDERATIONS, 299

Mechanical Circulatory Support, 299
Acute Pulmonary Edema, 299
Heart Failure with Preserved Ejection Fraction, 301

UNFULFILLED PROMISES AND FUTURE DIRECTIONS, 301

REFERENCES, 303

Heart failure (HF) is a common reason for hospital admissions, especially in older adults.[1] Most patients hospitalized for HF have previously been diagnosed with HF but have subsequently developed progressive clinical and hemodynamic decompensation that leads to admission. All patients admitted to the hospital with HF should undergo a rapid clinical evaluation for risk stratification and to determine the degree of elevation in cardiac filling pressures and the adequacy of systemic perfusion. In addition, effective management should include a careful search for correctable or reversible factors. In selected cases, hemodynamic monitoring with a pulmonary artery catheter (PAC) may be indicated for the purpose of initiating and titrating positive inotropic, vasodilator, and diuretic therapy. Clinical and hemodynamic goals of therapy should be set, and specific pharmacologic agents must be chosen to meet these goals. In cases of refractory HF, evaluation for ventricular assist device (VAD) implantation or cardiac transplantation should be performed in select candidates. For those with end-stage HF who are not VAD or transplant candidates, strategies that focus on symptom management and end-of-life care are appropriate.

Terminology

Acute decompensated heart failure has been defined as HF with a relatively rapid onset of signs and symptoms, resulting in hospitalization or unplanned office or emergency department visits. A more recent term, *acute heart failure syndromes*, is defined more broadly as new onset or gradual or rapidly worsening HF that requires urgent therapy.[2] Most of these episodes result from worsening or decompensation of chronic HF. *Stage D heart failure*, as defined by the American College of Cardiology/American Heart Association (ACC/AHA) guidelines,[3] designates patients with refractory HF who might be eligible for specialized advanced treatment strategies (e.g., mechanical circulatory support [MCS], continuous inotropic infusions) or end-of-life care (Figure 14-1).[4] Approximately 20% of hospitalizations are due to new-onset HF, also termed *acute heart failure*, which may be caused by an acute coronary syndrome, uncontrolled hypertension, or acute valvular dysfunction. *Acute pulmonary edema* is a clinical term used to describe patients who are seen with rapid worsening of symptoms associated with physical and radiologic findings of pulmonary congestion as a result of acute elevation of the pulmonary capillary wedge pressure.

Epidemiology

It is estimated that 5,700,000 adults (2.4%) aged 20 years or older in the United States are being treated for HF, and 620,000 new cases are diagnosed each year.[5] The prevalence of HF increases dramatically with age, occurring in 1% to 2% of people aged 40 to 59 years and in up to 12% of individuals older than 80 years.[6] The annual rates per 1000 population of new HF events for white men are 15.2 for those aged 65 to 74 years, 31.7 for those aged 75 to 84 years, and 65.2 for those 85 years and older.[5] Between 1979 and 2006, the number of HF discharges rose from 390,000 to 1,100,000—an increase of 182% (Figure 14-2).[6] Approximately 80% of all HF admissions occur in patients older than 65 years; as a result, HF is the leading discharge diagnosis among Medicare beneficiaries, with an average length of stay of 5.3 days.[1] Hospitalizations are common after an HF diagnosis in the community, with 83% hospitalized once and 43% hospitalized at least four times.[7]

Over the past decade, large registries have defined the demographics and concomitant diseases associated with acute decompensated HF (Table 14-1). Approximately half of patients are women, and nearly 75% have a history of HF. Hypertension and coronary artery disease are present in more than 50% of patients, and 30% or more of hospitalized HF patients come to medical attention with diabetes, atrial fibrillation, and renal dysfunction.

Admission to the hospital with HF is associated with poor short- and long-term outcomes.[8] The Acute Decompensated Heart Failure National Registry (ADHERE) tracked outcomes of over 107,000 HF hospitalizations and found an in-hospital mortality rate of 4.0%.[9] In the EuroHeart Survey of more than 11,000 admissions, 6.9% of patients died during an HF hospitalization.[8] In community-based studies, crude mortality rates following an HF hospitalization range from 8% to 14% at 30 days and increase to 26% to 37% at 1 year.[10] For survivors, readmission with HF is common, ranging from 20% to 25% at 60 days and increasing to nearly 50% at 6 months.[11,12] With each subsequent admission, the risk of dying

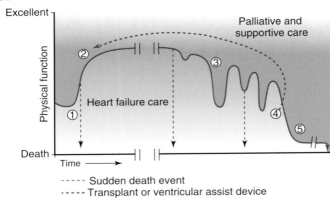

FIGURE 14-1 Time course of symptomatic heart failure. Patient comes to medical attention with symptoms of heart failure (*1*) and treatment is initiated. Stable functional status (*2*) is maintained for a variable length of time on optimal medical therapy but subsequently declines (*3*) with intermittent decompensation that responds to hospital-based therapy or ends in sudden death (*black dashed lines*). Patient subsequently develops refractory heart failure (*4*) that requires consideration of ventricular assist device, cardiac transplant (*blue dashed line*), or end-of-life care (*5*). (*From Goodlin SJ. Palliative care in congestive heart failure. J Am Coll Cardiol 2009;54:386.*)

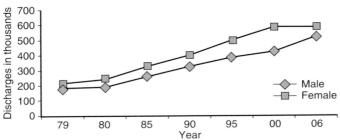

FIGURE 14-2 Hospital discharges for heart failure by sex in the United States between 1979 and 2006. Among men (*diamonds*), the number of discharges increased from 180,000 per year in 1979 to 520,000 per year in 2006. Among women (*squares*), the number of discharges increased from 210,000 per year in 1970 to 580,000 per year in 2006. (*From Lloyd-Jones D, Adams RJ, Brown TM, et al. Heart disease and stroke statistics—2010 update: a report from the American Heart Association. Circulation 2010;121:e46.*)

TABLE 14-1	Demographics and Comorbidities of Acute Decompensated Heart Failure		
	ADHERE[9] (N = 107,920)	EHFS[8,41] (N = 11,327)	OPTIMIZE-HF[256] (N = 48,612)
Mean age (yr)	75	71	73
Women (%)	52	47	52
Prior heart failure (%)	75	65	88
LVEF <40% (%)	59	35	52
CAD (%)	57	68	46
Hypertension (%)	72	53	71
Diabetes (%)	44	27	42
Atrial fibrillation (%)	31	43	31
Renal dysfunction (%)	30	17	20

ADHERE, Acute Decompensated Heart Failure National Registry; EHFS, Euro Heart Failure Survey; OPTIMIZE-HF, Organized Program to Initiate Lifesaving Treatment in Hospitalized Patients with Heart Failure; LVEF, left ventricular ejection fraction; CAD, coronary artery disease.

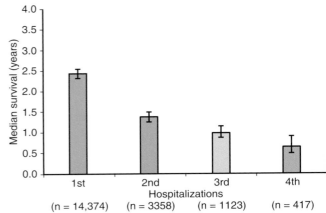

FIGURE 14-3 Repeat hospitalizations predict mortality in heart failure. Median survival (50% mortality rate) and 95% confidence limits in patients with heart failure after each heart failure hospitalization. (*From Setoguchi S, Stevenson LW, Schneeweiss S. Repeated hospitalizations predict mortality in the community population with heart failure.* Am Heart J *2007;154:260.*)

increases. In a Canadian cohort of more than 14,000 patients, median survival after the first, second, third, and fourth HF hospitalization was 2.4, 1.4, 1.0, and 0.6 years, respectively (Figure 14-3).[13]

As a result of direct medical costs, disability, and loss of employment, HF has an enormous economic impact on the U.S. health care system. In 2003, $3.6 billion ($5,456 per discharge) was spent on Medicare beneficiaries for the in-hospital management of HF.[14] Between 2000 and 2007, the mean costs to Medicare per patient for HF care in the last 6 months of life increased 26%—from $28,766 to $36,216—with chronic kidney and lung disease being independent predictors of higher costs.[15] In 2010, the total estimated direct and indirect cost of HF in the United States was $39.2 billion.[6] Notably, high-volume HF centers demonstrate improved quality of care and outcomes, but at higher costs, compared with low-volume hospitals.[16]

Pathophysiology

Heart Failure with Reduced Versus Preserved Ejection Fraction

In patients with reduced systolic function (i.e., ejection fraction <40%), HF reflects an abnormality of contractile function, in which the end-systolic pressure/volume relationship is shifted downward. End-systolic volume, end-diastolic volume, and end-diastolic pressure are increased, and elevated end-diastolic filling pressures are transmitted to the pulmonary venous circulation, resulting in signs and symptoms of pulmonary congestion. In some patients, elevated right-sided filling pressures cause systemic venous and hepatic congestion, leading to symptoms of abdominal discomfort. Contractile dysfunction may result from both direct and indirect insults to the myocardium, including loss of myocytes following myocardial infarction (MI); chronic volume or pressure overload; exposure to toxins, such as alcohol or doxorubicin; or a primary myocardial process, such as idiopathic dilated cardiomyopathy. Decreased contractility results in a fall in stroke volume, leading to symptoms of decreased cardiac output.

Up to 50% of patients admitted to the hospital with HF have normal or near normal left ventricular (LV) systolic function (see Table 14-1) and are presumed to have an abnormality in diastolic function.[17] The end-diastolic pressure/volume relationship may be shifted upward, reflecting impaired ventricular filling. Pulmonary vascular and systemic venous congestion results from an increase in left and right ventricular end-diastolic pressures, respectively. Diastolic dysfunction may be due to impaired early relaxation, increased chamber stiffness, or both of these,[18] and it is frequently associated with hypertension and abnormal vascular compliance.[19] Maladaptive volume regulation may also contribute to HF with preserved ejection fraction, and evidence suggests that in elderly hypertensive patients, volume expansion, renal dysfunction, and anemia play important roles in disease progression.[20] Common underlying causes of HF with preserved ejection fraction include ischemia and LV hypertrophy; restrictive, infiltrative, and hypertrophic cardiomyopathies are encountered less frequently.[21]

In an effort to promote standardization in practice, specific diagnostic criteria for heart failure with preserved ejection fraction, initially referred to as *diastolic heart failure*, were proposed.[22] However, it is important to remember that HF with reduced ejection fraction and HF with preserved ejection fraction are not mutually exclusive. Although use of older terms, such as *systolic* and *diastolic HF*, underscored a predominant pathophysiologic mechanism operating in the individual patient, many if not most patients with HF have abnormalities of both systole and diastole. In patients with ischemic cardiomyopathy, for example, HF with reduced ejection fraction is caused by both chronic loss of myocardium secondary to infarction and the acute loss of contractility as a result of ischemia; diastolic dysfunction is due to reduced compliance caused by chronic replacement fibrosis and the acute reduction in distensibility by ischemia.

From a mechanistic standpoint, studies using implantable hemodynamic monitors have shown that elevated diastolic pressures play a pivotal role in the underlying pathophysiology of acute decompensation in patients with either reduced or preserved ejection fraction.[23] Furthermore, for the purposes of in-hospital management, similar principles are often applied to patients regardless of ejection fraction. Although most of the approved diagnostic tools and treatment strategies have been validated in patients with reduced ejection fraction, recent acute HF trials have aimed to enroll a more heterogeneous population.[24] In the ADHERE national registry, in-hospital mortality rate was lower in patients with preserved ejection fraction (2.8% vs. 3.9%), although intensive care unit (ICU) stay and total length of stay were similar.[25] In the Organized Program to Initiate Lifesaving Treatment in Hospitalized Patients with Heart Failure (OPTIMIZE-HF), patients with an ejection fraction of 40% or higher also had similar lengths of stay and lower in-hospital mortality rates (2.9% vs. 3.9%), with no difference in death or rehospitalization rates at 60 to 90 days.[26] More complete discussions of HF with preserved ejection fraction may be found in Chapter 12 and elsewhere.[27]

Acute Compensatory Mechanisms

In the presence of a primary abnormality in contractile function, the heart depends on a number of compensatory mechanisms to maintain adequate cardiac output and vital organ perfusion (see *Braunwald*, Chapter 25). Acutely, ventricular performance may be maintained within normal limits by an increase in preload: the higher the preload, the greater the force of ventricular contraction and the greater the stroke volume. However, the Frank-Starling mechanism is advantageous only if the relationship between preload and contractility is positive. Although this may hold true in the setting of acute ischemia with normal chamber dimensions, in chronic systolic HF associated with LV dilation, the ventricular function curve may be flat at higher diastolic volumes (Figure 14-4, *A*). Increased filling may result in little augmentation in cardiac output, and further elevation in end-diastolic pressures may result in increased wall stress, decreased subendocardial perfusion, and worsening mitral regurgitation. Hemodynamic studies in patients with acute decompensated HF have shown that maximal stroke volumes can be achieved by lowering pulmonary capillary wedge pressure (PCWP) into the normal range with parenteral vasodilator (Figure 14-4, *B*) and diuretic therapy.[28] This improvement in ventricular function may be due in large part to a reduction in secondary mitral or tricuspid regurgitation or both, which often complicates dilated ischemic or nonischemic cardiomyopathy

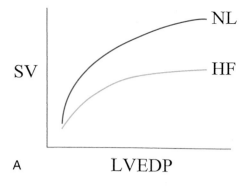

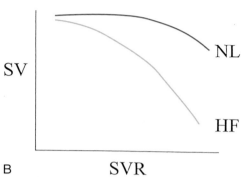

FIGURE 14-4 Preload and afterload effects on cardiac output/stroke volume in patients with normal (*NL*) and decreased (*HF*) left ventricular systolic function. **A**, Ventricular function curve in patients with HF may be flat at higher filling pressures. Thus, further increases in left ventricular end-diastolic pressure (*LVEDP*) may result in no change in stroke volume (*SV*). **B**, Alternatively, a reduction in systemic vascular resistance (*SVR*) by vasodilator therapy may result in a significant increase in SV.

but may also reflect improved myocardial oxygen supply and demand.

In addition to the beat-to-beat alterations in contractile function determined by the Frank-Starling mechanism, short-term stabilization of cardiac output or blood pressure may be achieved by activation of the renin-angiotensin-aldosterone system (RAAS) and sympathetic nervous system. Decreased perfusion pressure sensed by carotid sinus and aortic arch receptors results in increased sympathetic and decreased parasympathetic nervous system activity. Consequences of an increase in circulating catecholamines during cardiac decompensation include increased heart rate and contractility to augment cardiac output, systemic vasoconstriction to increase preload and maintain systolic blood pressure, and redistribution of blood flow away from the skin and splanchnic beds to the heart and central nervous system. Activation of the RAAS acts in concert with increased sympathetic activity to maintain arterial pressure. Elevated levels of circulating angiotensin II result in systemic vasoconstriction and intravascular volume expansion, and the latter leads to increased aldosterone secretion by the adrenal cortex and sodium and water retention by the kidney. Elevated circulating levels of arginine vasopressin[29] and endothelin[30] may also contribute to volume expansion and vasoconstriction in acute decompensated HF. In response to an increase in intracardiac pressure and volume, atrial and B-type natriuretic peptides are secreted from cardiac chambers and act as counterregulatory hormones by causing vasodilation, diuresis, natriuresis, and aldosterone and endothelin antagonism.

Myocardial Injury

Circulating levels of cardiac troponin are increased in the serum of patients with advanced HF[31] and may increase further during episodes of acute decompensation in the absence of ischemia.[32] Furthermore, elevated cardiac troponins predict adverse short-term outcomes, including worsening HF and in-hospital mortality, independent of ischemia (Figure 14-5).[33] Even patients with negative troponin levels on admission may develop positive levels during admission, and troponin conversion predicts worse outcomes at 60 days that are not significantly different from the risk of positive troponin at baseline.[34] These clinical observations raise the possibility that acute HF syndromes are associated with an accelerated loss of cardiac myocytes, which in turn contributes to ventricular remodeling and disease progression.[32] Underlying mechanisms of myocyte loss include necrosis and apoptosis. In addition to ischemia, several apoptotic stimuli are active in the setting of acute decompensation, including oxidative stress, mechanical strain, and neurohormones (e.g., norepinephrine and angiotensin).

Common Precipitating Factors of Heart Failure

Patients with HF may be asymptomatic or mildly symptomatic, either because the cardiac impairment is mild or because compensatory mechanisms help to balance or normalize cardiac function. Symptoms of HF that necessitate hospital admission may develop when one or more precipitating factors increases cardiac workload and disrupts the balance in favor of decompensation (Box 14-1). Specific factors may be identified in 50% to 90% of admissions and are often correctable.[35,36] In a report from the Randomized Evaluation of Strategies for Left Ventricular Dysfunction (RESOLVED) pilot study, the most commonly identified causes of HF exacerbation included excessive salt intake in 22%, other noncardiac disorders in 20%, arrhythmias in 13%, and upper respiratory tract infections in 11%.[36] In the OPTIMIZE-HF registry, one or more precipitating factors was identified in 61% of patients, with pneumonia (15%), ischemia (15%), and arrhythmia (14%) being the most common.[35]

In a study of 435 patients admitted nonelectively to an urban hospital with the diagnosis of HF, acute chest pain and noncompliance with medications or diet were the precipitating factors in 33% and 21%, respectively.[37] The rate of nonadherence with HF medications is particularly high among the elderly,[38] although it has improved modestly over time.[39] Despite a higher risk profile, nonadherent patients have been shown to have a lower in-hospital mortality rate and shorter length of stay,[40] suggesting that it may be easier to achieve clinical stability by reinstituting sodium and/or fluid restriction and resuming medical therapy. Failure to take prescribed HF medications and adhere to dietary restrictions may result in progressive fluid retention and worsening congestion; however, inadequate therapy is not always the result of patient nonadherence. Physician underutilization of RAAS inhibitors and β-blockers in patients with HF is well documented.[41] Likewise, digoxin may be withdrawn because of concerns about toxicity,[42] or the diuretic dose may be decreased in the face of worsening renal function,[43] thereby precipitating HF hospitalization.

Cardiac arrhythmias are common in patients with HF and often precipitate or exacerbate episodes of moderate to severe decompensation.[44] Atrial fibrillation with rapid ventricular response results in elevated atrial pressures and may further reduce cardiac output in a patient with limited baseline systolic reserve.[45,46] In patients with ischemic heart disease, tachycardia may induce or intensify ischemia and result in worsening systolic or diastolic function or both by increasing myocardial oxygen demands. In addition, a regular, narrow complex tachycardia may occasionally be misinterpreted as sinus in origin, when in fact atrial flutter or atrioventricular nodal reentry tachycardia is present. In some cases, atrial arrhythmias may be the primary cause of a tachycardia-mediated cardiomyopathy, which is potentially reversible with effective antiarrhythmic therapy or radiofrequency ablation.[47] New onset of atrial arrhythmias warrants assessment of thyroid function, particularly in the elderly.

Although less common than atrial arrhythmias, sustained or paroxysmal nonsustained ventricular tachycardia often associated with implantable cardioverter-defibrillator (ICD) therapies may precipitate admission to the hospital in a patient with impaired LV function.[48] In patients with HF and either reduced or preserved ejection fraction, symptomatic bradyarrhythmias may be due to intrinsic sinus or atrioventricular nodal dysfunction, adverse drug effects, or electrolyte abnormalities (e.g., hyperkalemia). Early recognition and aggressive management of cardiac arrhythmias may be critical to achieving the goal of recompensation; however, it should be remembered that in addition to precipitating HF, arrhythmias may be caused by HF, or they may result from proarrhythmic effects of drugs used in the management of HF. Although not an arrhythmia per se, ventricular dyssynchrony induced by right ventricular (RV) pacing is associated with an increased risk of HF hospitalization and atrial fibrillation and warrants consideration of biventricular pacing.[49]

Myocardial ischemia or infarction should be considered as a possible precipitant, not only in patients with known ischemic heart disease presenting with HF, but also in patients with other forms of heart disease. For example, patients with previous HF secondary to hypertension or valvular heart disease may be well compensated until they develop unstable angina or an acute

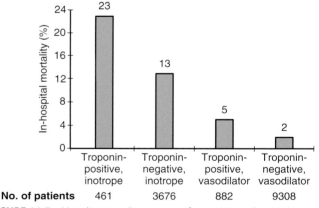

No. of patients   461   3676   882   9308

FIGURE 14-5 Mortality according to type of treatment and troponin status. In-hospital mortality in patients with acute decompensated heart failure enrolled in the ADHERE registry stratified by baseline troponin status and in-hospital treatment with an intravenous inotrope or vasodilator. (From Peacock WF 4th, De Marco T, Fonarow GC, et al. Cardiac troponin and outcome in acute heart failure. N Engl J Med 2008;358:2117.)

> ### Box 14-1 Potentially Reversible Factors Contributing to Acute Decompensation in Patients with Heart Failure
>
> Myocardial ischemia
> Uncontrolled hypertension
> Tachyarrhythmias or bradyarrhythmias
> Nonadherence with medications and/or salt and fluid restriction
> Heavy alcohol consumption
> Periodic hypoxia (e.g., as a result of sleep apnea, COPD)
> Anemia
> Recent viral illness
> Noncardiac medication causing fluid retention (e.g., NSAIDs, pregabalin)
> Acute kidney injury or worsening renal function with diuretic refractoriness
> Hyperthyroidism

COPD, chronic obstructive pulmonary disease; NSAIDs, nonsteroidal antiinflammatory drugs.

coronary syndrome. Diabetic patients with silent ischemia or infarction may also come to medical attention with insidious HF.[50] Infection is another common precipitating cause of HF. In one study, 11% of patients with an exacerbation of HF had pneumonia.[36] Common viral infections, including influenza A and respiratory syncytial virus (RSV),[51] may also cause acute-on-chronic impairment of ventricular function and precipitate an admission with acute decompensated HF. It is not known whether direct viral infection of the myocardium, myocardial inflammation, or myocardial dysfunction secondary to circulating or local cytokines plays a significant role in such patients. Guidelines recommend that all patients with current or prior symptoms of HF receive yearly influenza vaccinations,[3] which have been shown to be safe and effective in reducing the risk of hospitalization for pneumonia and death,[52,53] especially in older patients.

Comorbid conditions common in patients with HF that may exacerbate symptoms leading to hospitalization include uncontrolled hypertension and anemia. In addition, the development of acute kidney injury or worsening renal function with or without diuretic refractoriness (see Cardiorenal Syndrome below) may further impair the ability of patients with HF to excrete sodium or free water and thus may exacerbate fluid retention.[54,55] Other potentially correctable factors contributing to acute decompensation in HF include excessive alcohol consumption[56,57] and medications that either depress myocardial function (β-blockers, amiodarone) or cause salt and water retention (nonsteroidal antiinflammatory drugs, thiazolidinediones, pregabalin).[58-60] It is essential to search for these and other less common precipitating causes, such as hyperthyroidism or pulmonary embolism, in patients admitted to the hospital with HF because failure to recognize such conditions may lead to refractory or recurrent HF.

General Management

Initial Patient Evaluation

Regardless of the etiology or underlying precipitant, patients admitted to the hospital for the treatment of HF have the potential for hemodynamic deterioration, including the development of cardiogenic shock. Therefore, a rapid bedside evaluation of circulatory status and cardiac rhythm and assessment for ischemia should be performed even before the medical records or diagnostic studies are reviewed. In addition to ruling out an acute coronary syndrome that may require urgent revascularization or thrombolysis, evidence for marked elevation of intracardiac filling pressures and/or inadequacy of systemic perfusion should be sought. In selected cases, positive inotropic or vasopressor therapy may need to be initiated prior to obtaining additional diagnostic data or invasive hemodynamic measurements. However, in the majority of patients who are clinically more stable, a complete review of the medical history and a detailed physical exam may provide important information regarding the underlying cause and acute precipitants of HF as well as appropriate targets of therapy.

Risk Stratification

Clinical information obtained at the time of an HF admission may help to predict outcomes during the hospitalization and after discharge. Chin and Goldman[61] first sought to determine the risk of a major complication or death in 435 patients admitted to an urban university hospital with worsening HF. Two thirds of the patients had a previous history of HF. Compared with those with new onset HF, these patients were older and had more comorbidities, lower LV ejection fraction (LVEF), and lower initial blood pressure. In a multivariate analysis, independent predictors of in-hospital death or major complications noted at the time of admission were a systolic blood pressure less than 90 mm Hg, respiratory rate greater than 30 breaths/min, serum sodium less than or equal to 135 mEq/L, and ischemic electrocardiographic changes not known to be old.

TABLE 14-2 Risk Stratification for in-Hospital Mortality in the ADHERE Registry

BUN ≥43 MG/DL	SBP <115 MM HG	CREATININE ≥2.75 MG/DL	MORTALITY RATE (%)
−	−	−	2.3
+	−	−	5.7
−	+	−	5.7
+	+	−	13.2
+	+	+	19.8

ADHERE, Acute Decompensated Heart Failure National Registry; BUN, blood urea nitrogen; SBP, systolic blood pressure; −, absent; +, present.
Modified from Fonarow GC, Adams KF Jr, Abraham WT, et al. Risk stratification for in-hospital mortality in acutely decompensated heart failure: classification and regression tree analysis. *JAMA* 2005;293:572.

Using data from the ADHERE registry, Fonarow and colleagues[9] sought to develop a practical bedside tool for risk stratification of patients with acute decompensated HF. Derivation and validation cohorts of more than 65,000 patient records were subjected to classification and regression tree (CART) analysis to identify predictors of in-hospital mortality. Based on this empirical analysis, the single best predictor for mortality was an elevated admission level of blood urea nitrogen (BUN) of 43 mg/dL or higher; followed by systolic blood pressure less than 115 mm Hg; and serum creatinine of 2.75 mg/dL or higher. A simple risk tree identified patient groups with mortality rates ranging from 2.3% to 19.8% (Table 14-2). Similarly, the OPTIMIZE-HF investigators developed a risk-prediction nomogram based on data derived from 48,612 HF admissions. Multivariable predictors of mortality included age, heart rate, systolic blood pressure, sodium, creatinine, HF as a primary cause of hospitalization, and presence or absence of LV systolic dysfunction (Table 14-3, Figure 14-6).[62] Additional clinical and laboratory predictors of adverse outcomes obtained at the time of hospital admission include presence of congestion,[63] reduced LVEF,[25] ischemic etiology,[64,65] anemia,[66,67] elevated natriuretic peptide levels,[68,69] and positive cardiac troponins.[31,33]

Clinical Assessment of Intracardiac Filling Pressures

Most hospitalizations for acute decompensated HF occur because of congestion rather than low cardiac output.[8,70] Although congestion is often readily apparent in patients with de novo or acute HF, marked elevation in filling pressures may be underappreciated in patients with chronic HF.[71] In one study of nonedematous HF patients, unrecognized hypervolemia was present in 65% and predicted reduced survival.[72] Recent studies using implantable hemodynamic monitors demonstrate that cardiac filling pressures gradually rise over the days and weeks preceding an HF admission, with signs and symptoms lagging behind or not appreciated at all.[73] Increased capacity for pulmonary lymphatic drainage resulting from chronic pulmonary congestion may lead to clinical situations in which PCWPs exceeding 30 to 35 mm Hg are tolerated. Conversely, a history of dyspnea on exertion is common in patients with HF and lacks the specificity to detect elevated cardiac filling pressures. Alternative mechanisms of dyspnea include decreased pulmonary function, increased ventilatory drive, and respiratory muscle fatigue.[74] Not surprisingly, investigators have been unable to demonstrate a close correlation between symptoms or exercise tolerance and measures of resting LV performance in patients with HF. However, dyspnea on minimal exertion or at rest, including orthopnea and paroxysmal nocturnal dyspnea, are more specific historic clues to increased left-sided filling pressures in patients with known LV failure. In patients with biventricular HF, abdominal discomfort, early satiety, nausea, vomiting, and anorexia

TABLE 14-3	Nomogram for Predicting Risk of in-Hospital Mortality		
PARAMETER	SCORE	PARAMETER	SCORE
Age (yr)		110	10
20	0	120	8
25	2	130	6
30	3	140	4
35	5	150	2
40	6	160	0
45	8	**Sodium (mEq/L)**	
50	9	110	13
55	11	115	11
60	13	120	9
65	14	125	7
70	16	130	4
75	17	135	2
80	19	140	0
85	20	145	2
90	22	150	4
95	24	160	8
Heart Rate (beats/min)		165	10
65	0	170	12
70	1	**Serum Creatinine (mg/dL)**	
75	1	0	0
80	2	0.5	2
85	3	1	5
90	4	1.5	7
95	4	2	10
100	5	2.5	12
105	6	3	15
110	6	3.5	17
SBP (mm Hg)		**Primary Cause of Admission**	
50	22	Heart failure	0
60	20	Other	3
70	18	**Left Ventricular Systolic Dysfunction**	
80	16	No	0
90	14	Yes	1
100	12		

From Abraham WT, Fonarow GC, Albert NM, et al. Predictors of in-hospital mortality in patients hospitalized for heart failure: insights from the Organized Program to Initiate Lifesaving Treatment in Hospitalized Patients with Heart Failure (OTPIMIZE-HF). *J Am Coll Cardiol* 2008;52:347.

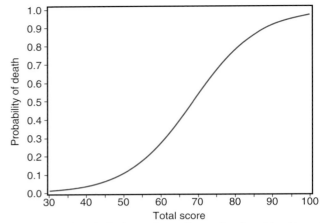

FIGURE 14-6 The risk of in-hospital mortality as a function of the risk prediction nomogram score shown in Table 14-3. *(From Abraham WT, Fonarow GC, Albert NM, et al. Predictors of in-hospital mortality in patients hospitalized for heart failure: Insights from the Organized Program to Initiate Lifesaving Treatment in Hospitalized Patients with Heart Failure [OPTIMIZE-HF]. J Am Coll Cardiol 2008;52:347.)*

specific clinical situations, such as with right ventricular infarction or pulmonary embolism, jugular venous distension may occur without signs of left-sided congestion. Recent data also suggest that mismatch between right- and left-heart pressures may be present in up to one third of acute HF patients.[77] Significant interobserver variability regarding the extent of jugular venous elevation further limits its usefulness at the bedside.[78] Both ascites and peripheral edema are less sensitive signs of volume overload than jugular venous distension, particularly in young adults, and may be preceded by the development of tender hepatomegaly. A third heart sound may suggest the presence of previously undiagnosed cardiomyopathy and carries prognostic value,[79] but it is neither sensitive nor specific for acute decompensated HF. Increased intensity of the pulmonic component of the second heart sound in association with a holosystolic murmur suggests pulmonary hypertension as a result of chronic HF and associated mitral regurgitation, tricuspid regurgitation, or both.

Rarely, experienced examiners may use the bedside Valsalva maneuver with sphygmomanometric determination of arterial blood pressure response to help clarify the LV filling pressure.[71] However, arrhythmias and limited patient effort because of dyspnea or discomfort may interfere with this exam. An automated device that quantifies the blood pressure response to the Valsalva maneuver,[80] as well as contrast-enhanced and tissue Doppler echocardiographic techniques,[81] have been developed for the noninvasive determination of left ventricular filling pressures. In addition, intrathoracic impedance monitoring,[82] plasma volume analysis,[72] and lung ultrasound[83] are newer methods to assess fluid status in HF patients; however, these techniques may lack accuracy in a heterogeneous population of patients with acute decompensated HF,[84,85] and prospective data demonstrating the utility of these tools in patient management are lacking.

Like the physical exam, routine chest radiography has been shown to be an insensitive clinical tool for demonstrating the presence of worsening HF. In an initial report, 68% of patients with advanced HF and PCWP of 25 mm Hg or more had minimal or no evidence of pulmonary congestion on admission chest radiograph.[86] In the ADHERE registry, 15,937 of 85,376 patients (19%) had no signs of congestion on emergency department chest radiography, and these patients were more likely to be given a non-HF diagnosis.[87] When present, however, interstitial or alveolar edema suggests markedly elevated filling pressures. Bilateral or unilateral pleural effusions are common in acute decompensated HF[88] and may not necessarily respond to diuresis. In these instances, ultrasound-guided thoracentesis[89] or chest tube thoracostomy may be necessary to relieve respiratory distress and improve arterial oxygenation.

suggest increased right-sided cardiac filling pressures. In addition, changes in baseline symptoms in an individual patient may suggest a clinically important worsening of HF.

Rales are a relatively specific but insensitive sign of pulmonary vascular congestion. In a series of patients with chronic HF and reduced ejection fraction, rales were present in only 60% of patients with an elevated PCWP.[75] However, rales were also detected in 16% of patients with normal PCWP and may be due to coexistent pulmonary or pleural disease. In both the ADHERE and OPTIMIZE-HF registries, rales were present in approximately two thirds of patients with acute decompensated HF.[25,26] Signs of increased right-sided filling pressures—including jugular venous distension, ascites, and peripheral edema—are generally reliable indicators of increased left-sided filling pressures.[76] However, in

Clinical Assessment of Systemic Perfusion

Fatigue and weakness, which are commonly reported in patients with HF, may be due to reduced cardiac output and poor perfusion of skeletal muscles. In addition, abnormal endothelium-dependent vasodilation respiratory muscle fatigue and altered skeletal muscle structure and function may contribute to exercise intolerance in HF.[90] However, fatigue is a nonspecific symptom that may be caused by many noncardiopulmonary diseases (anemia, chronic kidney disease, hypothyroidism, depression), disordered sleep (from sleep apnea, restless legs), drugs (β-blockers, sedatives), or electrolyte abnormalities. If a patient is admitted to the hospital with acute decompensated HF, mental obtundation or anuria is highly suggestive of critically reduced perfusion. A more subtle history of altered mentation, such as lack of concentration or memory, may be obtained from a family member. In severe low-output states, the patient may appear anxious or diaphoretic or may exhibit signs of air hunger. Patients with advanced HF may be cachectic from a low-output state and may have a catabolic/anabolic imbalance,[91] whereas those with more recent onset HF will be well nourished. Other physical signs of acute hypoperfusion include cool extremities, digital or circumoral cyanosis, and marked hypotension with a rapid, thready pulse. *Pulsus alternans* signifies advanced myocardial disease and tends to be present during tachycardia.

When measuring blood pressure noninvasively, it is important to deflate the cuff slowly and listen closely to define the systolic blood pressure and pulse pressure, especially in patients with atrial fibrillation. Prior studies have shown that when the pulse pressure is less than 25% of the systolic blood pressure, the likelihood is high that the cardiac index is below 2.2 L/min/m^2 in such a patient.[76] Thus, in someone with severe HF, a blood pressure of 100/90 mm Hg may be more worrisome than a blood pressure of 80/50 mm Hg. However, data from the Evaluation Study of Congestive Heart Failure and Pulmonary Artery Catheterization Effectiveness (ESCAPE) demonstrated a weak relationship between estimated and measured cardiac index.[92]

Laboratory Assessment

Routine chemistry and hematology studies obtained on admission may be helpful in the initial assessment of patients with acute decompensated HF and may assist in formulating a therapeutic plan. Dilutional hyponatremia may result from a combination of sodium restriction, aggressive diuresis, and an impaired ability to excrete free water.[93] Increased circulating levels of renin and vasopressin are also important mediators of hyponatremia in HF.[29] Although angiotensin-converting enzyme (ACE) inhibitors alone or in combination with loop diuretics may acutely correct hyponatremia in severely ill patients with HF, overactivity of the RAAS may predispose these same patients to the development of hypotension, worsening renal function, and hyperkalemia upon initiation of, or rechallenge with, an ACE inhibitor. Use of nonsteroidal antiinflammatory agents should be avoided in hyponatremic patients, as they may aggravate hemodynamic abnormalities and cause worsening renal function.[58]

Prolonged, high-dose diuretics may predispose patients to hypokalemia and hypomagnesemia,[94] both of which are associated with an increased risk of ventricular arrhythmias. Hyperkalemia may result from marked reductions in glomerular filtration rate (GFR) and inadequate delivery of sodium to the distal renal tubule. Excess total body potassium may be exacerbated by the use of RAAS inhibitors, potassium-sparing diuretics, or potassium supplements.[95] The risk of hyperkalemic arrhythmias appears to be highest during potassium replacement, when intracellular potassium concentrations are still low; and hyperkalemia is a common cause of iatrogenic morbidity, and even mortality, during an HF hospitalization. Other laboratory abnormalities that may complicate management of acute decompensated HF include increased liver enzymes, hyperbilirubinemia, and elevated international normalized ratio. If right-sided HF is long-standing, cardiac cirrhosis

Box 14-2 Potential Consequences of Worsening Renal Function During a Heart Failure Admission

Hospital discharge is delayed.
Diuretic doses are decreased, often despite persistent congestion.
ACE inhibitors, ARBs, and aldosterone receptor antagonists are discontinued.
Noncardiac medications (e.g., antibiotics) are dose-adjusted.
Positive inotropic agents are initiated to increase renal perfusion.
A pulmonary artery catheter is placed to assess hemodynamics.
A urinary catheter is placed to record urine output.
Renal ultrasound is ordered to rule out postobstructive uropathy.

ACE, angiotensin-converting enzyme; ARB, angiotensin receptor blocker.

may result in hypoalbuminemia and an exacerbation of extravascular fluid accumulation as well as inappropriate vasodilation.[96] Low serum prealbumin levels and elevated C-reactive protein levels are proinflammatory markers associated with cachexia in patients with end-stage HF.

In patients with chronic HF, BUN, and serum creatinine levels are elevated secondary to reductions in renal blood flow and glomerular filtration rate (GFR). Decreased renal perfusion can precipitate bouts of acute tubular necrosis and lead to reduced renal mass. Other factors contributing to the presentation of combined cardiac and renal dysfunction, or *cardiorenal syndrome*,[97] include an altered balance of vasoconstrictor and vasodilating hormones and comorbidities such as diabetes, hypertension, and peripheral arterial disease. In patients with advanced HF, several commonly used classes of drugs, including inhibitors of the RAAS and diuretics, may exacerbate renal impairment. During an HF hospitalization, between 15% and 30% of patients will develop worsening renal function, defined variably as an increase in serum creatinine by 0.3 mg/dL or more or reduction in estimated GFR by 25% or more.[98] The mechanisms underlying worsening renal function remain unknown but are thought to include diuretic-induced reductions in GFR, neurohormonal activation, and a fall in systolic blood pressure.[99] From a clinical standpoint, worsening renal function may be transient or persistent[100] and often results in interruption of diuretic therapy and discontinuation of other disease-modifying agents such as ACE inhibitors and aldosterone receptor antagonists (Box 14-2). Most studies show that worsening renal function is an independent predictor of increased length of stay and excess mortality both in the hospital and after discharge,[54] although emerging data suggest that baseline renal dysfunction primarily impacts outcomes.[98]

B-TYPE NATRIURETIC PEPTIDE

B-type natriuretic peptide (BNP) is synthesized and secreted by the cardiac ventricles in response to an increase in wall stress or filling pressure. N-terminal pro-BNP (NT-proBNP) is an inactive fragment that results from cleavage of BNP from its prohormone. Both BNP and NT-proBNP can be used to help diagnose and risk stratify patients with acute decompensated HF according to risk.[68,69,101] In patients with chronic HF and reduced ejection fraction, BNP levels are elevated in relation to disease severity and provide strong independent prognostic information. Plasma natriuretic peptide levels are also elevated in patients with HF and preserved ejection fraction, correlate with wall stress,[102] and can predict morbidity and mortality.[103,104] In the acute setting, low or normal BNP (<100 pg/mL) or NT-proBNP (<500 pg/mL) levels have a reasonably high negative predictive value for excluding HF as the cause of dyspnea. According to current practice guidelines, BNP or NT-proBNP levels should be measured in patients being evaluated for dyspnea in which the contribution of HF is not known, but these must be interpreted in the context of all available clinical data.[3,105]

In one study of patients presenting to the emergency room with shortness of breath, patients with HF and preserved ejection fraction had lower BNP levels compared with those with HF and reduced ejection fraction (median, 413 pg/mL vs. 812 pg/mL, respectively; Figure 14-7).[106] However, BNP added only modest discriminatory value in differentiating these two groups. In patients with advanced HF, BNP levels correlate only modestly with LV filling pressures,[107] and the diagnostic accuracy of BNP for predicting an elevated PCWP is limited by a high false-negative rate. BNP levels decrease in parallel with a reduction in filling pressures during acute diuretic and vasoactive therapy.[108] Change in BNP (Figure 14-8, *A*) and predischarge BNP (Figure 14-8, *B*), as well as in NT-proBNP, are independent predictors of subsequent events.[68,109] In practice, however, natriuretic peptide levels can vary substantially among individuals with the same degree of HF (see Table 14-4). For example, natriuretic peptide levels are higher in women, increase with age and renal dysfunction, and decrease

with obesity.[110] Currently, no proven role has been established for natriuretic peptide–guided therapy in the inpatient or outpatient setting,[111] although a BNP level obtained at the time of presentation to the emergency room may decrease resource utilization.[112] Novel biomarkers that include ST2, galectin-3, and neutrophil gelatinase-associated lipocalin are currently under development for use in the diagnosis and treatment of acute decompensated HF.[113]

Noninvasive Versus Invasive Management

Although practice patterns differ greatly, the majority of patients with acute decompensated HF can be managed safely and effectively on a cardiac telemetry unit without invasive monitoring. Admission to an intensive care unit should be reserved for patients with 1) hemodynamic instability that requires titration of vasoactive therapy, placement of a PAC, or mechanical circulatory support; 2) unstable cardiac rhythms that require cardioversion, defibrillation, or temporary pacing; 3) acute respiratory failure that requires noninvasive or mechanical ventilation; or 4) severe renal impairment that requires electrolyte management and urgent consideration of dialysis. For all patients, clinical goals of therapy should be set (Table 14-5), including the relief of congestion-related symptoms, such as orthopnea and

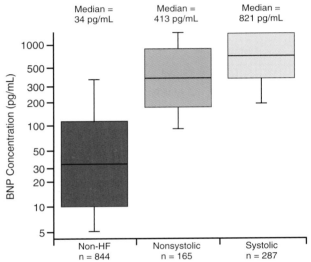

FIGURE 14-7 Box and whisker plots showing median B-type natriuretic peptide (*BNP*) levels in patients who came to the emergency department with dyspnea that was not the result of heart failure (*non-HF*) compared with patients with a final adjudicated diagnosis of preserved ejection fraction (nonsystolic) versus reduced ejection fraction heart failure. (*From Maisel AS, McCord J, Nowak RM, et al. Bedside B-type natriuretic peptide in the emergency diagnosis of heart failure with reduced or preserved ejection fraction: results from the Breathing Not Properly Study. J Am Coll Cardiol 2003;41;2010.)*

TABLE 14-4	Biologic and Clinical Variability of B-Type Natriuretic Peptide Levels	
INCREASED LEVELS	**DECREASED LEVELS**
Older age	Overweight and obesity
Female sex	Heart failure with preserved ejection fraction
Acute or chronic kidney disease	
Non–heart failure conditions	Pharmacologic therapy
Myocardial infarction	Angiotensin receptor blockers
Pulmonary embolism	β-Blockers
Cor pulmonale	Spironolactone
	Device therapy
	Cardiac resynchronization therapy
	Ventricular assist device

A

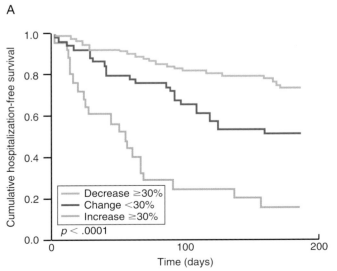

B

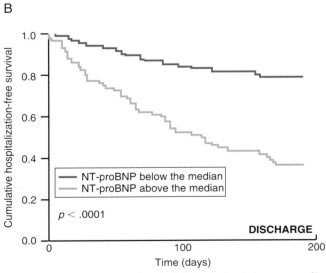

FIGURE 14-8 Hospitalization-free survival. **A,** Patterns of response of N-terminal pro–B-type natriuretic peptide (*NT-proBNP*) during in-hospital treatment of heart failure: decreased by ≥30%, changed by <30%, or increased by ≥30% of baseline. **B,** NT-proBNP level at discharge (median, 4137 pg/mL). (*From Bettencourt P, Azevedo A, Pimenta J, et al. N-terminal pro–brain natriuretic peptide predicts outcome after hospital discharge in heart failure patients. Circulation 2004;110:2168.)*

TABLE 14-5 General Goals in the Treatment of Acute Decompensated Heart Failure

GOAL	CLINICAL ENDPOINT	HEMODYNAMIC ENDPOINT
Decrease left-sided filling pressure	Absence of orthopnea, dyspnea on minimal exertion	PCWP ≤16 mm Hg
Decrease right-sided filling pressure	Absence of gastrointestinal symptoms Resolution of edema or hepatomegaly JVP <8 cm H₂O	RAP ≤8 mm Hg
Decrease peripheral resistance	Warm extremities	SVR 1000-1200 dynes/sec/cm⁻⁵
Maintain adequate perfusion pressure	SBP ≥80 mm Hg Stable (or improved) renal function	SBP ≥80 mm Hg
Increase cardiac output	Proportional pulse pressure >25%	CI ≥2.2 L/min/m²
Restore normal oxygenation	Oxygen saturation on room air >90%	NA

CI, cardiac index; JVP, jugular venous pressure; NA, not applicable; PCWP, pulmonary capillary wedge pressure; RAP, right atrial pressure; SBP, systolic blood pressure; SVR, systemic vascular resistance

abdominal fullness, and improvement in symptoms of low cardiac output (fatigue, anorexia) if present. Physical findings of volume overload—including jugular venous distension, lower extremity edema, hepatomegaly, and ascites—should also be targets of therapy. Despite optimal care, not all patients will be free of congestion at the time of discharge, including patients in whom diuresis is limited by worsening renal function, hypotension, or both. If possible, the patient should be discharged with a systolic blood pressure above 80 mm Hg and warm extremities.

The insertion of a PAC for the purpose of hemodynamic monitoring may be helpful in selected patients but is not recommended for the routine management of acute decompensated HF.[105] As described above, a reasonable noninvasive assessment of volume status and adequacy of perfusion may be obtained by history and physical exam. If severely elevated filling pressures or critically reduced perfusion are evident, placement of a PAC should not take precedence over initiation of appropriate therapy, such as parenteral diuretics, positive inotropic drugs, or vasopressor agents. In selected cases, hemodynamic measurements will be helpful in the choice and titration of parenteral agents to optimize loading conditions and improve clinical status rapidly. However, routine clinical use of the PAC for HF management has not proven effective in observational or controlled clinical studies.

In an observational study of critically ill patients with a variety of conditions—including acute respiratory failure, multisystem organ failure, and HF—right-heart catheterization was associated with an increased 30-day mortality and increased utilization of resources.[114] However, this study was methodologically flawed; control for the collection, interpretation, and use of hemodynamic data was lacking, and post hoc matching was used. In the subgroup of patients with HF, the relative hazard of death was 1.02 (P = .94).

The ESCAPE trial sought to determine whether PAC use is safe and whether it improves clinical outcomes in patients hospitalized with severe HF.[115] In this study, 433 patients were randomized to receive therapy guided by clinical assessment and PAC or by clinical assessment alone. The target of therapy in both groups was resolution of congestion, with additional hemodynamic targets (right atrial pressure 8 mm Hg, PCWP 15 mm Hg) set for the invasive group. Therapy in both groups led to substantial reduction in signs and symptoms of congestion, but no difference in morbidity or mortality was observed in the two groups (Table 14-6). In a meta-analysis of randomized clinical trials in critically ill patients that included data from ESCAPE, use of the PAC had no effect on hospital length of stay or mortality.[116]

Despite these negative findings, there may be selected indications for invasive hemodynamic monitoring during treatment of acute decompensated HF, especially in patients who are refractory to initial therapy or in those whose volume status is uncertain.[3,105] These include evidence of severe hypoperfusion; marked congestion at rest, associated with acute ischemia, infarction, or renal failure; fluid retention refractory to high-dose or

TABLE 14-6 Impact of Pulmonary Artery Catheter vs. Clinical Assessment During Heart Failure Hospitalization: The ESCAPE Study[115]

VARIABLE	PAC GROUP	CLIN GROUP	P VALUE
Days alive out of hospital (mean)	133	135	.99
Mortality at 180 days (%)	20.0	17.4	.95
Hospitalizations per patient (median)	2.0	2.0	NA
Δ Global symptom score	25 ± 25	24 ± 24	.45
Weight loss (kg)	4.0 ± 5.4	3.4 ± 4.2	.32
Δ Creatinine (mg/dL)	0.0 ± 0.4	0.1 ± 0.1	.02
Line infection (%)	1.9	0	.03

ESCAPE, Evaluation Study of Congestive Heart Failure and Pulmonary Artery Catheterization Effectiveness; PAC, pulmonary artery catheter; CLIN, clinical assessment.
Modified from Nohria A, Mielniczuk LM, Stevenson LW. Evaluation and monitoring of patients with acute heart failure syndromes. *Am J Cardiol* 2005;96:32G.

combination diuretics; hypoxemia with coexistent cardiac and pulmonary disease; and shock of unclear etiology. In addition, hemodynamic assessment is routine in considering patients for cardiac transplantation; and the degree and reversibility of pulmonary hypertension[117] are important predictors of posttransplant outcomes.[118] Similarly, invasive hemodynamic measurements are helpful in the evaluation of patients for VAD implantation, either as a bridge to cardiac transplant or as permanent therapy, and in their perioperative management (see Chapter 15). In patients with end-stage HF being considered for home inotropic support,[119] documentation of an adequate hemodynamic response to the inotropic agent is recommended. The benefits of PAC use may be more evident at centers experienced with hemodynamic monitoring for advanced HF.[120]

Hemodynamic Profiles

Initial *clinical assessment* of cardiac filling pressures and systemic perfusion can be used to categorize patients into broad *hemodynamic profiles* that help guide medical management and provide prognostic information.[63] If the patient is found to be *clinically well-compensated* despite presenting with shortness of breath at rest, an evaluation for intermittent ischemia or paroxysmal arrhythmias is indicated. In addition, noncardiac causes of dyspnea, both pulmonary and extrapulmonary, as well as psychologic causes such as anxiety should be considered.

The most common hemodynamic profile encountered in patients with acute decompensated HF is pulmonary and/or systemic venous *congestion with normal perfusion*. In these patients, symptoms will generally respond to diuresis using an intravenous (IV) loop diuretic or the combination of a loop and thiazide diuretic. If the patient does not respond to initial attempts at diuresis, vasodilator therapy—either oral or IV—may require titration, as elevated filling pressures can be exacerbated by systemic and pulmonary vasoconstriction in addition to volume expansion. If the patient is already taking an ACE inhibitor or angiotensin receptor blocker (ARB), the dose should be titrated after an effective diuresis has been achieved, while monitoring closely for orthostatic hypotension and worsening renal function. In selected patients, a combination of vasodilators may be used, such as isosorbide dinitrate, hydralazine, or an ARB in addition to an ACE inhibitor. Large pleural effusions or ascites that do not respond to diuresis may require thoracentesis or paracentesis, respectively. Symptomatic goals of diuretic therapy include resolution of orthopnea and dyspnea at rest or on minimal exertion. Although symptoms of congestion often improve significantly within the first 12 to 24 hours of therapy, several additional days of hospitalization are often necessary to achieve optimal volume status.[105] For patients in whom a PAC has been placed, hemodynamic goals are discussed below.

Hypoperfusion without pulmonary venous congestion, manifested by progressive fatigue and anorexia and often accompanied by azotemia, may precipitate hospitalization in patients with severe HF. Use of positive inotropic agents is often necessary when perfusion is critically limited, although open-label and controlled studies, as well as registry data,[121] suggest that short-term exposure to an inotrope is associated with an increased risk of adverse events, including death. Use of parenteral vasodilators may be considered, if systemic vasoconstriction is suspected, but these are usually poorly tolerated if filling pressures are not also elevated. They can precipitate hypotension[12] and lead to worsening renal function[122] in the setting of low or normal cardiac filling pressures. In addition, further reflex neurohormonal activation can lead to clinically significant arrhythmias. In patients with underlying ischemic heart disease, decreased coronary artery perfusion pressure and reflex tachycardia may aggravate ischemia. Finally, some patients may develop significant hypoperfusion secondary to overdiuresis. In this situation, the judicious use of IV fluids may be considered, but patients should be observed closely to avoid the onset of congestive symptoms.

For patients who come to medical attention with a combination of *pulmonary and/or systemic venous congestion and inadequate systemic perfusion*, simultaneous reduction in filling pressures and optimization of systemic vascular resistance (SVR; see Figure 14-4, *B*) can generally be accomplished with IV vasodilator therapy, with intermittent or continuous infusion diuretics, over 1 to 3 days. Once clinical goals are achieved, conversion to an oral regimen that maintains stability of clinical and laboratory parameters may require an additional 24 to 48 hours of treatment.

Hemodynamic Goals of Therapy

When a PAC has been placed to guide treatment, the ideal goal of parenteral therapy in the management of acute decompensated HF is to achieve an effective cardiac output at relatively normal filling pressures. For patients with severe hemodynamic compromise, a reduction in filling pressures and SVR is often associated with a 30% to 50% increase in forward stroke volume. Although the optimal hemodynamics for a given patient cannot be predicted with certainty, specific goals of hemodynamically guided therapy should be set (see Table 14-5). A PCWP less than or equal to 16 mm Hg is appropriate for most patients with chronic HF, whereas a slightly higher filling pressure may be necessary to maintain cardiac output in the setting of acute MI (i.e., decreased LV compliance without significant dilation). A right atrial pressure less than or equal to 8 mm Hg is optimal in most settings, as long as the PCWP is not reduced excessively. With exceptions such as RV infarction and pulmonary embolism associated with hypotension, a higher right atrial pressure may be required. Maintaining

a cardiac index greater than or equal to 2.2 L/min/m² is often necessary to avoid cerebral, renal, or hepatic hypoperfusion. However, lower cardiac indices may cause relatively little organ dysfunction, if the low-output state has developed gradually. SVR is optimal in the range of 1000 to 1200 dynes/sec/cm⁻⁵. Although cardiac output may be increased further with additional lowering of the SVR, in the range of 800 to 900 dynes/sec/cm⁻⁵, a reflex increase in sympathetic tone may result in unwanted tachycardia, orthostatic hypotension, and renal dysfunction. Finally, the above goals should be aimed for while maintaining a systolic blood pressure of 80 mm Hg or greater and a mean arterial pressure of 60 mm Hg or greater.

It should be remembered that thermodilution measurements may overestimate the cardiac output in patients with low-output states, possibly because of a loss of the cold indicator across the myocardium. Thermodilution measurements may also be unreliable in the setting of significant tricuspid regurgitation or marked respiratory variation, although one study showed a good correlation between thermodilution and Fick outputs in patients with chronic HF and moderate to severe tricuspid regurgitation.[123] Alternatively, mixed venous oxygen saturations may be used to calculate cardiac output using the Fick equation with oxygen consumption measured by a metabolic rate meter. Given that oxygen consumption may be influenced markedly by infection, other stresses, or sedation and that it has been shown to vary greatly among adults at the time of cardiac catheterization, the use of "assumed" Fick outputs are not recommended. An alternative is to follow changes in the mixed venous oxygen saturation to estimate cardiac output trends.[124] For patients who require hemodynamic monitoring, but with a contraindication to PAC placement (e.g., poor venous access), several minimally invasive devices that measure cardiac output are now available,[125] although most have been used to manage postoperative cardiac surgical patients, and none has been shown to improve outcomes in acute decompensated HF.

In choosing an initial parenteral agent, particular attention should be paid to the SVR (see the following discussion on specific agents). Patients with an elevated SVR will generally tolerate initiation of a vasodilator, such as nitroglycerin or nesiritide, without hypotension and will achieve significant hemodynamic benefit. On the other hand, patients with a low SVR, such as that secondary to concomitant sepsis or anesthesia, often will not tolerate further vasodilation without developing symptomatic hypotension. Dobutamine, which provides inotropic support in addition to mild vasodilation, is the preferred initial agent in this situation. An alternative choice would be dopamine at lower doses (3 to 5 μg/kg/min). Higher doses may increase filling pressures and elevate the SVR by stimulating α-adrenergic receptors. In patients with an SVR in the normal range, both vasodilators and positive inotropes are often effective and may be used in combination. An alternative to the combination of a vasodilator and inotrope is the phosphodiesterase (PDE) inhibitor milrinone, which exerts both direct inotropic and vasodilator effects in patients with acute decompensated HF. The incidence of hypotension is higher with milrinone as a result of greater peripheral vasodilation.

Fluid Management

Parenteral Diuretic Therapy

The initiation of an effective diuresis is integral to the management of elevated cardiac filling pressures associated with acute decompensated HF. For patients admitted to the hospital, this can best be accomplished with parenteral diuretics, as the IV route will more reliably deliver high drug concentrations to the renal tubular lumen.[126] Furosemide is the most widely used loop diuretic, although bumetanide and torsemide are also available for patients with documented intolerance or unresponsiveness to furosemide. Furosemide can be given intravenously in doses ranging from 20 to 240 mg or higher depending on the patient's diuretic history and as frequently as every 4 to 6 hours. If patients are already receiving loop diuretics, the initial IV dose should equal or exceed the chronic oral dose (ACC/AHA class I recommendation, level of evidence C).[3] Addition of a thiazide-type diuretic, such as metolazone (2.5 to 10 mg orally) or chlorothiazide (250 to 500 mg IV), often potentiates the diuresis. A continuous infusion of loop diuretic (e.g., furosemide 5 to 40 mg/h) may be used to treat refractory fluid retention, but the benefit of this approach as an initial diuretic strategy remains unproven.[127]

A Cochrane review of eight trials in 254 patients found that urine output was significantly greater with a continuous infusion, although the difference was modest (mean difference, 271 mL/day), and less tinnitus and hearing loss occurred with continuous infusion.[128] The Diuretic Optimization Strategies in Acute Heart Failure (DOSE-AHF) study used a 2 × 2 factorial design and randomly assigned 308 patients within 24 hours of HF admission to receive high-dose versus low-dose and continuous versus bolus IV diuretics. No differences were observed in symptom relief (Figure 14-9,A), renal function, net fluid loss, or death and rehospitalization

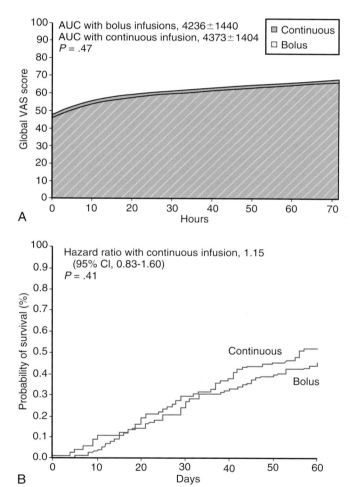

FIGURE 14-9 Bolus versus continuous infusion diuretic strategy: the Diuretic Optimization Strategies in Acute Heart Failure study. **A,** Patients' global assessment of symptoms was measured by visual analogue scale (*VAS*) and quantified as the area under the curve (*AUC*) from baseline to 72 hours. There was no significant difference between the two treatment groups in the primary efficacy endpoint (*P* = .47). **B,** Likewise, Kaplan-Meier curves for death, rehospitalization, or emergency department visit during the 60-day follow-up period show no difference between the continuous infusion and bolus groups (67 and 63 events, respectively; hazard ratio with continuous infusion, 1.15; 95% confidence interval [*CI*], 0.83 to 1.60; *P* = .41). *(From Felker GM, Lee KL, Bull DA, et al. Diuretic strategies in patients with acute decompensated heart failure. N Engl J Med 2011;364:797.)*

at 60 days (Figure 14-9, *B*) among patients receiving bolus versus continuous-infusion diuretics.[129] Although the higher dose strategy was associated with greater diuresis and more favorable outcomes in some secondary measures, including weight loss and relief from dyspnea, it was also associated with transient worsening renal function. Although not demonstrated in DOSE-AHF, transient worsening renal function during treatment of acute decompensated HF may actually be associated with improved outcomes, when it is related to aggressive diuresis.[130]

With regard to timing of the initiation of IV diuretics, the ACC/AHA guidelines strongly recommend that treatment begin in the emergency department or outpatient clinic, as early intervention may be associated with better outcomes. In an analysis from the ADHERE registry, delay in initiation of IV diuretics was associated with less symptom relief at discharge and a modest increased risk of in-hospital mortality, independent of other prognostic variables.[131] The addition of hypertonic saline to IV furosemide may result in more rapid achievement of dry weight, but this novel strategy remains to be tested in a multicenter study.[132]

For patients with hypokalemia that requires significant potassium supplementation, a potassium-sparing diuretic, such as spironolactone or triamterene, may be used; however, serum potassium levels should be followed closely to avoid the development of hyperkalemia, which can be precipitated by worsening renal function. Aldosterone receptor antagonists are additionally beneficial in the management of fluid retention associated with cirrhosis,[133] and chronic therapy with spironolactone or eplerenone reduces morbidity and mortality in patients with New York Hospital Association (NYHA) class II to IV heart failure[134,135] or LV dysfunction complicating acute MI (see Chapter 12).[136] For patients with marked fluid overload unresponsive to diuretics, or for those who develop worsening renal function that requires discontinuation of diuretics, ultrafiltration or hemodialysis may be considered if there is coexistent renal failure; this will be discussed later in this chapter.

In the setting of acute pulmonary edema, the rapid clearance of congestion by parenteral diuretics is mediated by natriuresis and diuresis, decreased intravascular volume, and systemic vasodilation. In patients with acute decompensated HF, the goals of diuretic therapy include the elimination of edema and orthopnea (see Table 14-5). Reduction in atrial and ventricular diastolic pressures reduces wall stress and ventricular volumes and may improve subendocardial perfusion and reduce valvular regurgitation, respectively. Frequent reevaluation of clinical status and renal function, as well as hemodynamics if available, is necessary to guide frequency and duration of therapy. Mild worsening of renal function may be tolerated in order to achieve hemodynamic compensation, and diuretic-induced hemoconcentration may be a marker for improved outcomes in this group of patients.[130] On the other hand, persistent worsening renal function may identify high-risk patients who require closer follow-up after discharge.[100] Fluid and sodium restriction and cautious replacement of potassium and magnesium are important adjunctive measures that should not be overlooked. Once treatment goals are achieved, the patient should be converted to an oral diuretic regimen that maintains stable weight and renal function. Adverse effects of aggressive diuresis also include electrolyte abnormalities and associated arrhythmias, metabolic alkalosis, muscle cramps, and ototoxicity.[137]

Ultrafiltration

Ultrafiltration removes excess plasma volume without causing a significant change in electrolytes. In patients with chronic HF and diuretic resistance, ultrafiltration may improve symptoms, neurohormones, and hemodynamics without hypotension.[138] Reductions in peripheral and pulmonary edema and a subsequent increase in diuretic efficacy have been reported. Recent pilot studies in acute decompensated HF suggest that early ultrafiltration is associated with greater fluid removal and symptom relief than medical therapy alone[139] and may decrease length of stay and readmission rates.[140] The Ultrafiltration versus Intravenous Diuretics for Patients Hospitalized for Acute Decompensated Congestive Heart Failure (UNLOAD) trial randomized 200 patients within 24 hours of hospitalization for HF to ultrafiltration or IV diuretics. At 48 hours, weight loss (5.0 vs. 3.1 kg; $P = .001$) and net fluid loss (4.6 vs. 3.3 L; $P = .001$) were greater in the ultrafiltration group. At 90 days, ultrafiltration had reduced the risk of rehospitalization for HF compared with IV diuretics ($P = .037$), but no differences were found between the two groups in symptoms, quality of life, 6-minute walk test, BNP levels, renal function, or hospital length of stay. It has been hypothesized that greater sodium removal during ultrafiltration (hypotonic plasma water) compared with furosemide (hypotonic urine) explains a sustained improvement.[141] The Heart Failure Society of America (HFSA) guidelines acknowledge the apparent effectiveness of ultrafiltration but raise concerns about safety, cost, need for venous access, and nursing support.[105] The ACC/AHA guidelines suggest consultation with a renal specialist before opting for any mechanical strategy to effect volume removal.[3]

The effects of ultrafiltration on renal function and outcomes in patients with acute decompensated HF and cardiorenal syndrome are currently being tested in the multicenter randomized Cardiorenal Rescue Study in Acute Decompensated Heart Failure (CARRESS) trial sponsored by the National Institutes of Health (NIH).[142] In this study, 200 patients with worsening renal function at the time of admission or during the first 7 days of inpatient therapy, defined as an increase in serum creatinine by at least 0.3 mg/dL, are being randomized to stepped pharmacologic care versus ultrafiltration. The change in serum creatinine *and* weight together as a "bivariate" endpoint will be assessed at 96 hours after enrollment.

Vasoactive Therapy

Nitroglycerin

When administered intravenously, nitroglycerin has an immediate onset of action and a plasma half-life of 1 to 4 minutes. It is cleared by the vascular endothelium, hydrolyzed in the blood, and metabolized in the liver. At lower infusion rates, its main cardiovascular effect is venodilation with a resultant fall in ventricular volumes and filling pressures (Table 14-7). At higher infusion rates, nitroglycerin also causes arterial dilation that results in decreases in both pulmonary and systemic vascular resistance.[12,143] Nitroglycerin may be of particular use in patients refractory to diuretic therapy and in those who continue to manifest elevated filling pressures, have disproportionate right-sided failure or unstable ischemia, or are intolerant to nitroprusside.

Intravenous nitroglycerin is usually started at a low infusion rate of 20 to 30 μg/min and increased by 10 to 20 μg/min every 5 to 10 minutes, until the desired response is observed or a dose of 400 μg/min is reached. If a PAC is present, cardiac filling pressures and SVR are used to guide titration, although careful noninvasive monitoring of blood pressure may be adequate in the absence of severely reduced perfusion. As with other vasodilators, use of

nitroglycerin may be limited by hypotension, requiring cessation of the drug, infusion of IV fluids, or leg elevation. In addition, vasodilation may be associated with headache, flushing, and diaphoresis. Patients with significant right-sided HF may be resistant to the acute administration of nitroglycerin but will often respond following diuresis. Pharmacologic tolerance to nitroglycerin because of free radical generation may also develop,[144] and preventive strategies include avoidance of excessive dosing, limiting fluid retention, and the use of intermittent dosing. In relatively small clinical trials, IV nitrates were shown to improve dyspnea during the first hours of administration.[12] Cotter and colleagues randomly assigned 110 patients with severe pulmonary edema to receive repeated high-dose IV boluses of nitroglycerin after low-dose IV furosemide versus low-dose IV nitroglycerin plus high-dose furosemide.[145] In this open-label study, the use of high-dose IV nitroglycerin and low-dose diuretics was associated with reduced need for mechanical ventilation (17% vs. 40%; $P = .004$) and reduced risk of MI (17% vs. 37%; $P = .05$).

Nesiritide

As discussed above, natriuretic peptide levels 1) are elevated in patients with HF, 2) correlate with severity of illness, and 3) provide prognostic information. The physiologic effects of BNP include vasodilation, diuresis, natriuresis, and antagonism of the RAAS and endothelin system.[146] Based on these favorable actions, recombinant human BNP (nesiritide) was developed for the treatment of HF. In early clinical studies in patients with mild to moderate HF, nesiritide was shown to exert potent vasodilatory (see Table 14-7)[147] and modest natriuretic effects,[148] and it improved dyspnea and fatigue when compared with placebo.[149] To compare the efficacy and safety of nesiritide with another vasodilator, the Vasodilation in the Management of Acute CHF (VMAC) study randomized 489 patients with acute decompensated HF to receive IV nitroglycerin or nesiritide in addition to standard therapy.[12] At 24 hours, the reduction in PCWP was greater with nesiritide than with nitroglycerin (−8.2 vs. −6.3 mm Hg; $P = .04$) with no evidence of tachyphylaxis, although a similar improvement in dyspnea was seen in both groups. The duration of symptomatic hypotension, which occurred in approximately 5% of patients in both groups, was greater with nesiritide; headache and abdominal pain were more common with nitroglycerin.

In 2001, the U.S. Food and Drug Administration (FDA) approved nesiritide for the treatment of patients with acute decompensated HF and dyspnea at rest or with minimal activity. Although clinical use grew rapidly, meta-analyses soon raised concerns about the effects of nesiritide on renal function and survival,[122,150] and rapid deadoption followed.[151] An independent panel of experts recommended that a large clinical trial be performed to test the effectiveness and safety of nesiritide.[152] Accordingly, the Acute Study of Clinical Effectiveness of Nesiritide in Decompensated Heart Failure (ASCEND-HF) trial randomly assigned 7141 patients with acute HF to receive either nesiritide or placebo for 1 to 7 days in addition to standard therapy.[153] Patients treated with nesiritide reported greater relief from dyspnea at 6 and 24 hours but experienced no improvement in the rates of worsening renal function, HF readmission, or death from any cause at 30 days (Figure 14-10). Hypotension was more common with nesiritide (27% vs. 15%; $P < .001$).

Despite these negative results, nesiritide is still occasionally used in patients who remain symptomatic despite IV diuretic therapy. The recommended starting dose of nesiritide is a 2 μg/kg IV bolus followed by a continuous infusion of 0.01 μg/kg/min. Although the dose may be increased by 0.005 μg/kg/min to a maximum of 0.03 μg/kg/min to achieve the desired clinical or hemodynamic effects (see Table 14-7), higher doses are associated with increased rates of hypotension[12] and worsening renal function.[122] Thus, nesiritide is not recommended for use in patients with a systolic blood pressure below 90 mm Hg or in those suspected of having low cardiac filling pressures. If uncertainty exists regarding volume status, an initial infusion rate of 0.005 μg/kg/min without a bolus

TABLE 14-7	Hemodynamic Effects of Parenteral Vasodilators		
	PCWP	SVR	CO
Nitroglycerin	↓↓	↔↓	↑↔↓
Nesiritide	↓↓	↓	↑
Nitroprusside	↓↓	↓↓	↑↑
Milrinone	↓↓	↓↓	↑↑

CO, cardiac output; PCWP, pulmonary capillary wedge pressure; SVR, systemic vascular resistance.

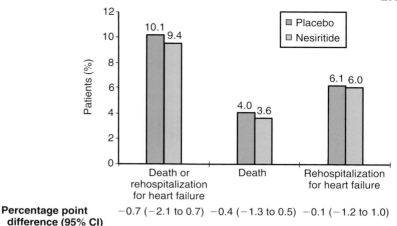

FIGURE 14-10 Primary clinical endpoints in the Acute Study of Clinical Effectiveness of Nesiritide in Decompensated Heart Failure. Rehospitalization for heart failure or death from any cause at 30 days occurred in 321 patients (9.4%) in the nesiritide group vs. 345 patients (10.1%) in the placebo group (P = .31; hazard ratio, 0.93; 95% confidence interval, 0.8-1.8). The individual components are also shown and do not differ significantly between the groups. CI, confidence interval. (*From O'Connor CM, Starling RC, Hernandez AF, et al. Effect of nesiritide in patients with acute decompensated heart failure. N Engl J Med 2011;365:32.*)

is recommended. If symptomatic hypotension occurs, the infusion rate should be immediately decreased or discontinued. In patients with cardiorenal syndrome, no evidence suggests that nesiritide improves renal function or enhances diuresis[154]; however, the potential renoprotective and nonhypotensive effects of very low dose nesiritide (0.005 μg/kg/min)[155] are being compared with low-dose dopamine (2 μg/kg/min) and placebo in a randomized controlled trial of acute decompensated HF.[156]

In patients with secondary pulmonary hypertension who are awaiting cardiac transplant, continuous nesiritide infusion for days to weeks has been used alone or in combination with a positive inotrope (e.g., dobutamine) to lower pulmonary artery pressures and pulmonary vascular resistance.[157] It is recommended that nesiritide be discontinued several hours prior to induction of cardiac anesthesia to avoid the development of catecholamine-refractory vasoplegia following cardiopulmonary bypass.[158] Serial outpatient nesiritide infusions have shown no proven benefit over intensive disease management in patients with advanced or refractory HF.[159]

Nitroprusside

For patients with acute decompensated HF characterized by low cardiac output, high filling pressures, and elevated SVR, nitroprusside can be used either alone or in combination with an inotropic agent to rapidly improve hemodynamics.[160] The drug's potent vasodilator effect is mediated by the local production of nitric oxide.[161] The onset of action is rapid, from 1 to 2 minutes, making it an ideal agent for use in urgent situations that require rapid dose titration and a predictable hemodynamic effect. Nitroprusside is a balanced arterial and venous dilator, and it reduces both filling pressures and systemic and pulmonary vascular resistance (see Table 14-7). Stroke volume and cardiac output increase, and pulmonary artery pressure, PCWP, and right atrial pressure decrease (Figure 14-11). In patients with chronic HF, heart rate is generally unchanged or may fall as a result of reflex sympathetic withdrawal.[143] Nitroprusside infusion may be started at a rate of 10 to 20 μg/min and increased by 20 μg/min every 5 to 15 minutes, until the hemodynamic goals are achieved, while maintaining a systolic blood pressure of 80 mm Hg or higher. Doses of 300 μg/min or higher are seldom required and increase the risk of toxicity. Cardiac output and SVR should be measured frequently during titration.

Nitroprusside is a potent vasodilator, and its use may be limited by hypotension. In patients with ischemic heart disease, decreases in coronary perfusion pressure accompanied by reflex tachycardia may worsen myocardial ischemia. In patients with acute decompensated HF, hemodynamic deterioration may occur immediately following the withdrawal of nitroprusside because

of a transient increase in systemic vascular tone (Figure 14-12).[162] Hemodynamic rebound may be avoided by initiating oral vasodilator therapy prior to nitroprusside withdrawal. Other adverse effects of nitroprusside are due to the accumulation of its metabolites, cyanide and thiocyanate.[163] Cyanide toxicity, which is most likely to occur in patients with hepatic dysfunction or following prolonged infusions, results in lactic acidosis and methemoglobinemia and may manifest as nausea, restlessness, and dysphoria. If cyanide toxicity is suspected, the infusion should be stopped, and serum levels should be checked. Thiocyanate toxicity may occur gradually in patients with renal insufficiency and is manifested by nausea, confusion, weakness, tremor or seizures, and rarely, coma. If mild, cessation of the infusion is usually sufficient to resolve symptoms; however, in severe cases, hemodialysis may be necessary.

Dobutamine

Dobutamine is a direct-acting synthetic sympathomimetic amine that stimulates β_1-, β_2-, and α-adrenergic receptors in the myocardium and vasculature.[164] Its primary cardiovascular effect is to increase cardiac output by increasing myocardial contractility (Table 14-8). Although dobutamine does not stimulate dopaminergic receptors in the kidney, renal blood flow often increases in proportion to the increase in cardiac output. In contrast to other β-adrenergic agonists (i.e., isoproterenol), the positive inotropic effect of dobutamine is associated with less increase in heart rate. The drug causes modest decreases in LV filling pressure and SVR (see Figure 14-11) because of a combination of direct vascular effects and the withdrawal of sympathetic tone. Dobutamine also directly improves LV relaxation via stimulation of myocardial β-adrenergic receptors.[165]

Dobutamine may be a useful agent for the initial management of patients with acute decompensated HF characterized by a low cardiac output and end-organ dysfunction. It can be initiated at a dose of 2 μg/kg/min and titrated upward by 1 to 2 μg/kg/min, until clinical or hemodynamic goals are achieved or until a dose-limiting event occurs, such as unacceptable tachycardia or an arrhythmia. Doses of 3 to 5 μg/kg/min are often adequate for good clinical response. Maximum effects are usually achieved at a dose of 15 μg/kg/min, although higher infusion rates may occasionally be used. The inotropic response to dobutamine may be attenuated as a result of desensitization of the β-adrenergic receptor pathway.[166] If the maximally tolerated infusion rate of dobutamine does not result in a sufficient increase in cardiac index or improved end-organ perfusion, a second positive inotropic agent such as milrinone may be added.[167] In patients with elevated cardiac filling pressures and/or SVR, the coadministration of a vasodilator may be required. In patients who remain hypotensive on dobutamine,

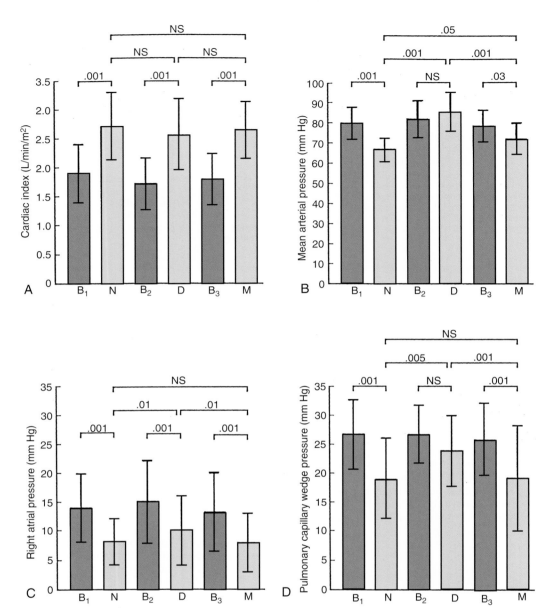

FIGURE 14-11 Comparative effects of nitroprusside (*N*), dobutamine (*D*), and milrinone (*M*) on cardiac index, mean arterial pressure, right atrial pressure, and pulmonary capillary wedge pressure (PCWP) in patients with severe heart failure (B_1, B_2, and B_3 = baseline measurements). **A,** The three agents were administered in doses that caused comparable increases in cardiac index. **B,** Under these conditions, nitroprusside and milrinone significantly reduced arterial pressure, but dobutamine had no effect. **C,** All three agents reduced right atrial pressure, although the effect of dobutamine was slightly less pronounced. **D,** Both nitroprusside and milrinone significantly reduced PCWP, an effect that was more pronounced than the effect of dobutamine. NS, not significant. *(Modified from Monrad ES, Baim DS, Smith HS, et al. Milrinone, dobutamine, and nitroprusside: comparative effects on hemodynamics and myocardial energetics in patients with severe congestive heart failure. Circulation 1986;73:III168.)*

high-dose dopamine may be added, while considering mechanical circulatory support and cardiac transplantation (see Chapter 15) if indicated.

Dobutamine may increase heart rate, thereby limiting the dose that can be infused; however, in some patients with very depressed cardiac output, the improvement in hemodynamic function may cause a withdrawal of sympathetic tone such that heart rate actually decreases. Hypotension is uncommon but can occur in patients who are hypovolemic. Arrhythmias, including supraventricular and ventricular tachycardia, may also limit the dose. Likewise, myocardial ischemia secondary to increased myocardial oxygen consumption may occur. Some patients with severe HF may show pharmacologic tolerance to dobutamine, or tolerance may develop after several days of a continuous infusion. In patients awaiting cardiac transplant, chronic dobutamine

therapy may cause hypersensitivity myocarditis[168] and lead to hemodynamic deterioration. In these situations, the addition or substitution of a PDE inhibitor may be necessary.

Milrinone

In myocardium and vascular smooth muscle, inhibition of the membrane-bound enzyme PDE results in an increase in intracellular cyclic adenosine monophosphate. Milrinone is a selective inhibitor of the type III isoform of PDE. In the myocardium, milrinone exerts both positive inotropic and lusitropic effects,[169] and it is a potent vasodilator in the systemic and pulmonary circulation (see Figure 14-11).[170] In patients with acute decompensated HF, milrinone increases cardiac output because of an increase in stroke volume (see Table 14-8). Balanced arterial and venous

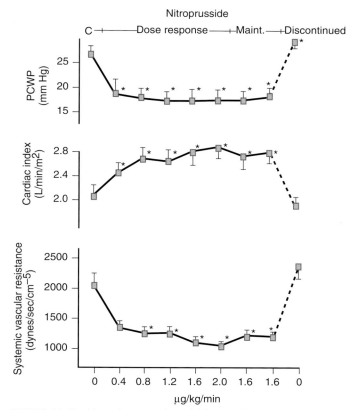

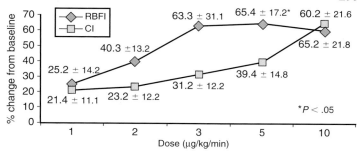

FIGURE 14-13 Renal vasodilatory action of dopamine in heart failure. Thirteen patients with moderate to severe heart failure as a result of left ventricular systolic dysfunction who were undergoing diagnostic cardiac catheterization were instrumented for assessment of renal and systemic blood flow during intravenous dopamine infusion. Shown are the percent changes from baseline in renal blood flow index (*RBFI*) and cardiac index (*CI*) at increasing doses of dopamine. The percentage increases in RBFI appeared to be greater than those for CI, reaching statistical significance at 5 μg/kg/min. In addition, renal vascular resistance significantly decreased at doses of 2 μg/kg/min through 10 μg/kg/min. (*Modified from Elkayam U, Ng TMH, Hatamizadeh P, et al. Renal vasodilatory action of dopamine in patients with heart failure.* Circulation *2008;117:200.*)

FIGURE 14-12 Hemodynamic rebound following discontinuation of nitroprusside in patients with moderate to severe heart failure. Graphs show changes in pulmonary capillary wedge pressure (*PCWP; top*), cardiac index (*middle*), and systemic vascular resistance (*bottom*) during dose response, maintenance, and discontinuation of nitroprusside infusion. Thirty minutes following discontinuation, PCWP and systemic vascular resistance increased significantly above, and cardiac index decreased significantly below, control values. (*Modified from Leier CV, Bambach D, Thompson MJ, et al. Central and regional hemodynamic effects of intravenous isosorbide dinitrate, nitroglycerin, and nitroprusside in patients with congestive heart failure.* Am J Cardiol *1981;48:1115.*)

TABLE 14-8	Hemodynamic Effects of Positive Inotropic Agents			
	+dP/dt	**PCWP**	**SVR**	**CO**
Dobutamine	↑↑	↓	↓	↑
Dopamine (low dose)	↔	↔	↓	↔↑
Dopamine (high dose)	↑↑	↑	↑↑	↑↔↓
Milrinone	↑	↓↓	↓↓	↑

CO, cardiac output; +dP/dt, maximum rate of rise of left ventricular systolic pressure; PCWP, pulmonary capillary wedge pressure; SVR, systemic vascular resistance.

dilation causes decreases in right atrial, pulmonary artery, pulmonary capillary wedge, and mean arterial pressures (see Table 14-7). For a comparable increase in cardiac output, milrinone decreases SVR and LV filling pressure to a greater extent than dobutamine. Conversely, for a comparable decrease in arterial blood pressure, milrinone increases cardiac output to a greater extent than nitroprusside.[171]

Milrinone may be useful for the treatment of refractory HF characterized by low cardiac output, high filling pressures, and elevated or normal SVR. It may also be used as a bridge to cardiac transplant[172] or end of life,[119] especially in patients who develop tolerance to dobutamine, or to test pulmonary vasoreactivity in patients with secondary pulmonary hypertension being evaluated

for cardiac transplant or mechanical circulatory support.[170] The positive inotropic effects of milrinone are additive to those of digoxin and may be synergistic with those of dobutamine.[173]

In patients with acute decompensated HF, milrinone is usually administered as a 25 to 50 μg/kg IV bolus over 10 minutes followed by a constant infusion at 0.25 to 0.75 μg/kg/min, although an infusion may be initiated without a bolus, and lower doses (e.g., 0.10 μg/kg/min) may be used. Although the pharmacologic half-life of milrinone is less than 1 hour in patients with HF, it is prolonged in the setting of renal dysfunction, and physiologic effects of discontinuation may not be fully apparent for more than 12 hours. Thus for patients undergoing cardiac surgery, it is recommended that milrinone be discontinued several hours before induction of anesthesia to avoid the development of vasoplegia. The major dose-limiting effects of milrinone are tachycardia and atrial or ventricular arrhythmias.[11] In addition, relatively volume-depleted patients may not tolerate the vasodilator effects of this agent and will experience hypotension that requires drug discontinuation. Other adverse effects of milrinone include liver function test abnormalities, fever, and nausea.

The occurrence of adverse events with short-term therapy and the observed association with increased in-hospital[121] and post-discharge mortality[174] has led clinicians to question the wisdom of using positive inotropes routinely in the management of acute decompensated HF. In a large study of patients admitted with an exacerbation of systolic HF, a 48-hour infusion of milrinone did not reduce the subsequent need for hospitalization and was associated with an increased risk of arrhythmias and sustained hypotension compared with placebo.[11] However, this study was criticized for enrolling patients who did not require inotropic therapy. With the evolution of VAD technology, long-term milrinone support is being replaced by continuous flow VADs as a bridge to transplant (see Chapter 15).

Dopamine

Dopamine is the immediate biosynthetic precursor of epinephrine and norepinephrine and has both cardiac and vascular sites of action, depending in part on the dose used.[175] At low doses (1 to 3 μg/kg/min), dopamine directly activates dopaminergic receptors in the kidney, causing vasodilation (Figure 14-13).[176] A small increase in cardiac output and a decrease in SVR may also be observed (see Table 14-8). The resultant increase in renal blood flow leads to increased urine output and sodium excretion. At moderate doses (3 to 8 μg/kg/min), dopamine is a weak partial agonist at myocardial β₁-receptors and exerts positive chrono-tropic and inotropic effects. In addition, increased release of norepinephrine from nerve terminals in the vasculature may result in stimulation of α-adrenergic receptors and may have a mild vasoconstrictor effect. At moderate to high doses (5 to 20 μg/kg/min), peripheral α-adrenergic stimulation becomes apparent, resulting in vasoconstriction and increases in mean arterial pressure and SVR. As dopaminergic vasodilator effects in the kidney are overshadowed, renal blood flow decreases, and urine output may decline.

In patients with acute decompensated HF, dopamine is occa-sionally used at low infusion rates to improve renal function by increasing renal blood flow (see Figure 14-13). Increased water and sodium excretion results in a decrease in cardiac filling pressures; however, the safety and efficacy of *low dose*, or *renal dose*, dopamine in this setting have not been proven. Giamouzis and colleagues randomized 60 patients with acute decompen-sated HF to either high-dose furosemide (20 mg/h) or low-dose furosemide (5 mg/h) plus low-dose dopamine (5 μg/kg/min) for 8 hours.[177] No differences were observed in urine output (272 vs. 278 mL; *P* = .97) or dyspnea scores between the two groups during the 8 hours of protocol treatment, and no differences were found in hospital length of stay or 60-day death and rehospi-talization rates. However, worsening renal function, defined as an increase in serum creatinine of more than 0.3 mg/dL from baseline to 24 hours, was more frequent in the high-dose furose-mide group (30% vs. 7%; *P* = .042). The NIH-sponsored Renal Opti-mization Strategies Evaluation in Acute Heart Failure (ROSE-AHF) trial is currently studying the safety and efficacy of adjuvant renal protective therapies with low-dose dopamine and low-dose nesirit-ide with added optimal diuretic dosing in 360 patients with acute decompensated HF and moderate to severe chronic kidney disease.[156]

To achieve clinical or hemodynamic goals, low-dose dopamine may be combined with other inotropic or vasodilator therapies.[167] In patients with significant hypotension or frank cardiogenic shock, higher doses of dopamine are used to increase SVR. When it is necessary to use vasoconstrictor doses of dopamine in the setting of myocardial failure, it is often useful to add dobutamine to augment the level of positive inotropic support beyond that provided by dopamine alone. If used alone at vasoconstrictor doses in patients with advanced HF, dopamine may increase both left- and right-heart filling pressures.[175] To counteract increased afterload and peripheral venoconstriction, high-dose dopamine may be combined with a vasodilator such as nitroglycerin.

As with dobutamine, the inotropic response to dopamine may be attenuated in patients with advanced HF[178] as a result of β-receptor downregulation and depletion of myocardial catechol-amine stores.[179] Although generally well tolerated at low doses, higher infusion rates of dopamine may result in sinus tachycardia and supraventricular or ventricular arrhythmias. Other adverse effects of dopamine include digital gangrene in patients with peripheral artery disease, tissue necrosis at sites of infiltration, and nausea at high doses.

Epinephrine and Norepinephrine

Epinephrine stimulates β₁- and β₂-adrenergic receptors in the myocardium, thereby causing marked positive chronotropic and inotropic responses. It also has potent agonist effects at vascular α-adrenergic receptors, causing increased arterial and venous constriction. Because of this latter effect, epinephrine, like high-dose dopamine, plays little role in the management of acute decompensated HF, except when complicated by severe hypoten-sion. Epinephrine may be useful for the treatment of low cardiac output, with or without bradycardia, immediately following car-diopulmonary bypass or cardiac transplantation.[180] Continuous infusions may be started at a low dose of 0.5 to 1 μg/min, and titrated upward to 10 μg/min as needed. The use of epinephrine may be limited by tachycardia, arrhythmias, ischemia as a result

of increased myocardial oxygen consumption, and oliguria from renal vasoconstriction.

The myocardial and peripheral vascular effects of norepineph-rine are similar to those of epinephrine, except that norepineph-rine causes little stimulation of vascular β₂-adrenergic receptors and therefore causes more intense vasoconstriction. Norepineph-rine may be used to provide temporary circulatory support in the setting of severe hypotension, such as following cardiac surgery or with cardiogenic shock complicating acute MI. Norepinephrine is infused at doses of 2 to 10 μg/min. As with epinephrine, the use of norepinephrine may be limited by arrhythmias, myocardial ischemia, and renal impairment.

Digoxin

Although digoxin can be given intravenously, it is seldom used as a positive inotropic agent in the management of acute decompen-sated HF, although it may occasionally be useful to control heart rate in a patient with HF complicated by atrial fibrillation or atrial flutter with rapid ventricular response. In this setting, digoxin is given as a 0.5 to 1 mg IV load in divided doses over 12 to 24 hours. If the patient is markedly symptomatic with hemodynamic com-promise, prompt synchronized electrical cardioversion should be performed. Less commonly, IV amiodarone or ibutilide may be tried for urgent chemical cardioversion, while the patient is sup-ported with an inotrope, a vasodilator, or both. As there is a signifi-cant risk of proarrhythmia (*torsades de pointes*) with ibutilide administration, patients should be monitored closely on telemetry. Given the lack of safe positive inotropic agents for short-term use, some have called for studies to assess the clinical, hemodynamic, and neurohormonal effects of digoxin in patients with acute HF syndromes and normal sinus rhythm, followed by a large outcomes study.[181]

Adjustment of Oral Medications

Renin-Angiotensin-Aldosterone System Inhibitors

For patients without symptomatic hypotension or evidence of hypoperfusion, ACE inhibitors can often be initiated or increased empirically; however, in patients with hyponatremia or a resting systolic blood pressure below 90 mm Hg, marked hypotension may develop with the initial dose of an ACE inhibitor. In such patients, therapy should be initiated with low-dose captopril (e.g., 6.25 mg). For patients who have been stabilized on an IV vasodila-tor, such as nesiritide or nitroprusside, ACE inhibitors should be titrated upward gradually as the IV vasodilator is weaned. With captopril, the dose can be increased every 6 to 8 hours, until the desired level of vasodilation is achieved, while avoiding orthostatic vital signs. For patients whose medication compliance has been suboptimal, switching over to a once-daily ACE inhibitor (e.g., lisinopril or ramipril) at the time of discharge may be helpful; however, not all patients tolerate ACE inhibition. Data suggest that approximately 25% of patients with advanced HF previously treated with an ACE inhibitor develop a circulatory or renal limitation—such as symptomatic hypotension, worsening renal function, or hyperkalemia—to continued use. ACE inhibitor intolerance identi-fies patients with severe HF and poor prognosis.[182]

An ARB may be substituted for an ACE inhibitor in patients who develop a persistent and troublesome cough that is not due to HF or concomitant pulmonary disease (see Chapter 12). Updated ACC/AHA guidelines also suggest that although ACE inhibitors remain the first choice for inhibition of the RAAS in HF, ARBs are a reasonable alternative.[3] Furthermore, addition of an ARB may be considered in persistently symptomatic patients with reduced ejection fraction already treated with an ACE inhibitor,[183] although ARBs are as likely to produce hypotension, worsening renal function, and hyperkalemia as are ACE inhibitors. Limited data are available on the efficacy and safety of adding an ARB to therapy with both an ACE inhibitor and aldosterone antagonist. Given the growing use of aldosterone antagonists to reduce morbidity and mortality in patients with symptomatic LV dysfunction[134,135] and HF after MI,[136] increasing awareness of the risk of worsening renal function and hyperkalemia is critical in patient management, as discussed above. However, as stated in the ACC/AHA guidelines, "until further information is available, the routine combined use of all three inhibitors of the renin-angiotensin-aldosterone system cannot be recommended."

Nitrates and Hydralazine

The addition of isosorbide dinitrate to captopril frequently reduces SVR and ventricular filling pressures more effectively than does captopril alone. In some patients who cannot tolerate captopril, isosorbide dinitrate may be used alone as an effective vasodilator.[184] Isosorbide dinitrate is typically initiated at a dose of 10 mg three times daily and may be increased up to a total daily dose of 180 to 240 mg. The development of nitrate tolerance may be minimized by use of a nitrate-free interval of 10 to 12 hours.[144] As with ACE inhibitors, compliance may be enhanced by switching to a once-daily formulation (e.g., isosorbide mononitrate) before discharge.

For patients who are difficult to wean off IV agents, or in those who do not tolerate ACE inhibitors or whose clinical or hemodynamic status cannot be adequately optimized, hydralazine may be of value, often in combination with oral nitrates. The African-American Heart Failure Trial (A-HeFT) showed that adjunctive therapy with hydralazine and isosorbide dinitrate improves survival in blacks with advanced HF.[185] The usual starting dose of hydralazine is 10 to 25 mg, and the maximum dose is 75 to 100 mg three or four times daily. Side effects are common, and in A-HeFT, these included headache (48%), dizziness (29%), and nausea (10%). Hydralazine may also precipitate ischemic events in patients with HF as a result of ischemic cardiomyopathy.[186]

β-Blockers

As discussed in Chapter 12, and as recommended in the ACC/AHA guidelines,[3] all patients with HF and reduced ejection fraction should be treated with a β-blocker, unless a contraindication (e.g., moderate to severe reactive airway disease) or documented intolerance to treatment is evident. Although no studies demonstrate the long-term benefits of β-blockade in patients with HF and preserved ejection fraction, most patients with this clinical syndrome have another indication for antiadrenergic therapy, such as ischemic heart disease or hypertension. In the management of acute decompensated HF, a frequent question that arises at the time of hospital admission is what to do with background β-blocker therapy. At present, only empiric recommendations can be made based on the severity of presentation. If the patient is on a stable dose of β-blocker and comes to medical attention with mild HF exacerbation, the outpatient dose of β-blocker should be continued. If the acute decompensation is moderate in severity and/or precipitated by recent β-blocker titration, the dose should be decreased by at least 50%. If the patient comes in with severe HF with hemodynamic instability that is not due to tachyarrhythmias or uncontrolled hypertension, the β-blocker should be withheld until clinical and hemodynamic stabilization has been achieved.

If treatment with a β-adrenergic agonist such as dobutamine is being considered, it is important to remember that chronic β-blocker therapy, especially with carvedilol, may attenuate the hemodynamic response[187] and should therefore be discontinued. For patients with atrial or ventricular arrhythmias complicating severe decompensated HF, the hemodynamic effects of milrinone do not appear to be compromised by concomitant β-blocker therapy.[187] For stable patients with new-onset HF who have not yet received a β-blocker, cautious initiation prior to discharge appears safe, does not increase length of stay, and improves the

use of long-term β-blockade.[188] Optimizing oral medications, including ACE inhibitors and β-blockers, prior to discharge has become a key performance measure for hospitals and individual practitioners. Failure to use β-blockers in particular is independently associated with an increased risk of death or rehospitalization within 60 to 90 days.[189]

Oral Diuretics

Once fluid balance has been restored, the selection of an oral diuretic dose is empiric, and further adjustment is usually required both in the hospital and after discharge. It should be noted that most patients have a different salt and fluid intake at home than in the hospital. As a first approximation, the dose of IV diuretic that was effective may be given as an oral dose twice daily. Daily weights should be recorded along with fluid intake and output. Renal function and electrolytes should be monitored closely until discharge, and predischarge education regarding home weight monitoring and flexible diuretic dosing reduces the likelihood of an HF readmission.[190] In most cases, clinical and laboratory stability for 24 hours after discontinuation of IV diuretic therapy is sufficient to assess the likelihood that the patient will continue to improve on an oral regimen.[105] No data are available to compare the effect of different loop diuretics (e.g., furosemide vs. torsemide) on clinical outcomes following an HF hospitalization. The choice is often empiric and based on recent patient use or documented intolerance, such as a sulfa allergy that prevents the use of furosemide.

Other Management Issues
Sodium and Fluid Restriction

The majority of patients with advanced HF should be put on a sodium-restricted diet (2 g/day) while in the hospital, except in rare cases in which oral nutrition is of overriding importance. In addition, education regarding the sodium content of common foods may be enhanced during an admission with the intent to improve outcomes after discharge.[191] Patients with intense neurohormonal activation, as indicated by a low serum sodium, may have marked thirst. Diuresis may intensify thirst initially, but this usually improves over 1 to 2 weeks, as a lower volume status is maintained, and the thirst mechanism "resets" itself. Restricting fluid intake to 2 L/day is usually adequate for most hospitalized patients. In cases of severe or symptomatic hyponatremia, fluid should be restricted to 1 to 1.5 L/day, and administration of oral salt or normal saline and diuretics may be necessary. Although vasopressin receptor antagonists are also available to treat symptomatic hyponatremia associated with acute decompensated HF,[29,192] these agents have limiting side effects (dry mouth, thirst), do not improve long-term outcomes,[193] and are not approved for ambulatory HF management.

Oxygen Supplementation

In the absence of acute respiratory failure, concomitant pulmonary or pulmonary vascular disease, or significant right-to-left shunting, patients with chronic HF rarely exhibit arterial desaturation. In such patients, supplemental oxygen does not improve systemic oxygen delivery and has the drawbacks of causing airway irritation and limiting movement. The use of nasal oxygen is often empiric and may provide subjective benefit, perhaps through suppression of central dyspnea. In some patients, oxygen may decrease elevated pulmonary vascular resistance and improve right-heart function, although 100% oxygen has been shown to depress cardiac output and increase PCWP in patients with moderate to severe HF.[194] Mechanistic data also show that hyperoxemia can cause coronary vasoconstriction in patients with ischemic heart disease.[195] Nevertheless, supplemental oxygen is recommended in patients with acute MI complicated by HF and may be of benefit alone or in combination with continuous positive airway pressure (CPAP) in patients with central or obstructive sleep apnea, respectively.[196]

Ventricular Arrhythmias

Premature ventricular contractions and nonsustained ventricular tachycardia may occur in up to 80% of patients hospitalized with HF. Their appearance correlates with the severity of HF and all-cause mortality,[197] but no evidence shows that suppression with antiarrhythmic agents improves prognosis. Ventricular arrhythmias that compromise perfusion or cause symptoms should be treated. Suppression with agents such as lidocaine is rarely necessary and is often complicated by toxicity. Amiodarone is the antiarrhythmic of choice in patients with acute decompensated HF and can be given as an IV or oral load,[198] while monitoring closely for toxicity related to acute negative inotropic effects or, rarely, acute pulmonary toxicity.[199] Less efficacious alternatives include oral mexilitene or dofetilide, and dronedarone is contraindicated in HF. A search for reversible factors such as ischemia, electrolyte disturbances or drug-induced QT prolongation is also indicated. Drug-refractory ventricular tachycardia as a result of myocardial scarring may be amenable to radiofrequency, alcohol, or surgical ablation (see Chapter 23).[200] For patients with unstable ventricular arrhythmias that complicate cardiogenic shock, intraaortic balloon counterpulsation or percutaneous VADs may be necessary to improve coronary perfusion and reduce ventricular afterload.[201] Patients with chronic ischemic or nonischemic cardiomyopathy with a reasonable likelihood of 1 year survival should be considered for placement of an ICD based on primary prevention studies[202,203] and revised Centers for Medicare and Medicaid Services guidelines (see Chapter 22 and the Appendix).

Anticoagulation

Although patients with a low ejection fraction and a dilated ventricle are at increased risk of thromboembolism, no prospective data support the routine use of anticoagulation in chronic HF. Anticoagulation is indicated for patients with additional risk factors such as atrial fibrillation (paroxysmal or persistent), history of an embolic event, or echocardiographic evidence of intracavitary thrombus. Consideration should also be given to anticoagulating HF patients with spontaneous echocontrast, apical akinesis or aneurysm, or underlying disorders that may be associated with increased thromboembolic risk—amyloidosis, left ventricle noncompaction, or familial dilated cardiomyopathy with a history of thromboembolism in first-degree relatives—as well as patients with acute HF as a result of peripartum cardiomyopathy or fulminant myocarditis.[3] During hospitalization, such patients can be treated with IV unfractionated heparin, which can be discontinued for invasive procedures. Screening for venous thromboembolism is indicated when patients come to medical attention with unilateral or asymmetric bilateral lower extremity edema, pleuritic chest pain, increased shortness of breath, and/or presyncope. An unexplained elevation in pulmonary vascular resistance and RV failure should also raise the possible diagnosis of chronic thromboembolic pulmonary hypertension.[204] Hospitalized patients should be prophylaxed against venous thromboembolism with low-dose unfractionated heparin, low-molecular-weight heparin, or fondaparinux unless contraindicated.[3,105] For patients with a contraindication to anticoagulation, intermittent pneumatic compression devices or graded compression stockings may be used.

Comorbidities

A hospitalization for acute decompensated HF is an ideal time to assess for, and optimize treatment of, comorbidities such as diabetes, anemia, and sleep apnea (see Chapter 12). The long-term cardiovascular benefits of tight glycemic control with insulin have been well documented.[205] For patients treated with oral agents, it is important to recognize that thiazolidinediones, which have important ancillary effects on lipid metabolism and endothelial function,[206] may increase fluid retention and exacerbate HF, and this effect is exacerbated by concomitant administration of insulin. In addition, metformin, another popular insulin sensitizer, is associated with a low risk of life-threatening lactic acidosis and is contraindicated in patients with unstable or acute HF who are at risk of hypoperfusion, worsening renal function, and hypoxemia. Anemia is also common in patients with advanced HF and is associated with increased morbidity and mortality.[67,207] Pilot studies suggest that correction of anemia with erythropoiesis-stimulating agents (ESAs) and iron improves symptoms and functional status and may reduce readmission rates in HF.[208] However, large clinical trials of ESAs in patients with anemia, diabetes, and chronic kidney disease have raised concerns about increased cardiovascular risk, including stroke.[209] Definitive data on the balance of risks and benefits of anemia treatment in HF awaits completion of randomized controlled trials.

Discharge Planning and Immediate Postdischarge Care

Following treatment for acute decompensated HF, readmission rates are high, reaching 25% at 60 days and up to 50% at 6 months.[11,12] Patients at high risk for hospital readmission can be predicted based on a number of predischarge clinical and laboratory parameters, including use of positive inotropes or nonuse of ACE inhibitors, persistent congestion, worsening renal function, and elevated natriuetic peptide levels (Table 14-9). Following discharge, the ability to maintain freedom from congestion identifies a population with good survival despite a history of severe HF.[210] Although objective criteria for determining the optimal timing of discharge have not been established, empiric guidelines have been proposed (Box 14-3). Ideally, all patients should achieve near-optimal volume status and should transition successfully to oral diuretics. As discussed above, use of ACE inhibitors and β-blockers, or documentation of intolerance, is indicated for

TABLE 14-9	Predictors of Heart Failure Readmission Assessed Prior to Discharge
FACTOR	**PREDICTOR**
Clinical	
Functional capacity	Reduced submaximal exercise capacity during admission[257]
Congestion	Clinical or hemodynamic evidence of congestion at discharge[258] or soon after[211]
Arrhythmias	New atrial or ventricular arrhythmias during admission[259]
Dyssynchrony	Prolonged QRS duration (≥120 ms)[260]
Parenteral therapy	Use of positive inotropes during admission[174] or at discharge[119]
Oral therapy	Nonuse of ACE inhibitors or β-blockers at discharge[189]
Laboratory	
Natriuretic peptides	Increase in natriuretic peptide levels during admission or elevated levels at discharge[68]
Renal function	Worsening renal function during admission[261] or elevated serum creatinine at discharge[98]
Serum sodium	Persistent hyponatremia during admission[262]
Troponin	Conversion from negative to positive troponin during admission[34]

ACE, angiotensin-converting enzyme.
Modified from Gheorghiade M, Pang PS. Acute heart failure syndromes. *J Am Coll Cardiol* 2009;53:557.

Box 14-3 Discharge Criteria

Recommended for All Heart Failure Patients

Exacerbating factors addressed
Near optimal volume status achieved
Transition from intravenous to oral diuretics successfully completed
Patient and family education provided
Left ventricular ejection fraction documented
Smoking cessation counseling initiated
Optimal pharmacologic therapy (ACE inhibitor/ARB and β-blocker) achieved or intolerance documented*
Follow-up visit scheduled within 7 to 10 days

Should be Considered for Patients with Advanced or Refractory Heart Failure

No intravenous vasoactive agent given and oral medication regimen stable for 24 hours
Ambulation before discharge to assess functional capacity after therapy
Plans for postdischarge management in place (e.g., with VNA or via telephone follow-up)
Referral for disease management (if available)

*For patients with reduced left ventricular ejection fraction.
ACE, angiotensin-converting enzyme; ARB, angiotensin receptor blocker; VNA, visiting nurse association.
Modified from Lindenfeld J, Albert NM, Boehmer JP, et al. HFSA 2010 Comprehensive Heart Failure Practice Guideline. *J Card Fail* 2010;16:e1.

patients with HF and reduced ejection fraction and serves as a national quality measure. Patient and family education, along with written discharge instructions, should address activity level, sodium and fluid restriction, medications, weight monitoring, and follow-up appointments. Importantly, patients and their caregivers need to know what to do and who to contact if symptoms worsen. Failure to provide predischarge education is strongly associated with an increased risk of HF readmission.[190]

For patients with advanced HF or those at high risk for readmission, including the elderly, referral to a disease-management program can be an important adjunct to maintaining clinical stability and preventing early readmission.[211] In addition, effective multidisciplinary programs may improve HF outcomes, such as survival and quality of life, without increasing health care costs.[212] The first follow-up visit should take place within 1 to 2 weeks of discharge. Visiting nurses with expertise in HF care can assist in disease management for patients with transportation or travel limitations.[213]

Special Considerations

Mechanical Circulatory Support

For patients with severe hemodynamic compromise who do not respond to positive inotropic or vasopressor agents, urgent consideration should be given to support with an intraaortic balloon pump (IABP) or percutaneous VAD. In the setting of cardiogenic shock complicating acute MI, intraaortic balloon counterpulsation is commonly used to reduce ischemia by improving diastolic coronary blood flow and improve hemodynamics by reducing myocardial afterload, while awaiting more definitive treatment, such as percutaneous or surgical revascularization or repair of a mechanical complication (papillary muscle rupture, ventricular septal defect). In addition, balloon counterpulsation may support a patient awaiting spontaneous recovery of stunned myocardium as a result of ischemia, acute myocarditis, or stress cardiomyopathy.[214] Absolute contraindications to IABP include aortic insufficiency and aortic dissection. Significant peripheral arterial disease involving the abdominal aorta or iliofemoral arteries is also a contraindication. For further discussion of the use of balloon counterpulsation in the setting of acute MI that includes insertion technique, monitoring, and complications, see Chapter 10 and the Appendix.

Percutaneous VADs are also available for temporary hemodynamic support of patients with cardiogenic shock.[215] These continuous-flow devices typically withdraw blood from the left atrium using a transseptal cannula or from the left ventricle using a catheter placed retrograde across the aortic valve, and they eject blood into the femoral artery or ascending aorta, respectively. Percutaneous VADs can generate up to 5 L/min of blood flow, and they rapidly reverse end-organ dysfunction associated with severe, refractory cardiogenic shock. Although open-label studies to compare percutaneous VADs with balloon counterpulsation have demonstrated superior hemodynamic benefit, they have failed to show any difference in short-term morbidity or mortality.[216,217] Major risks associated with these devices include bleeding, stroke, infection, and vascular complications.

In patients with end-stage HF, worsening hemodynamics, and end-organ dysfunction, IABP or percutaneous VADs have also been used successively as a bridge to surgical VAD placement, a so-called *bridge to bridge*, or to cardiac transplantation.[218] In this setting, systemic perfusion may be maintained, and end-organ function preserved, while awaiting a donor heart. However, given the increase in waiting list times in many regions, IABP and percutaneous VAD are not feasible methods of providing prolonged support lasting weeks to months, and they preclude pretransplant rehabilitation. Surgically placed durable VADs offer the best alternative for extended circulatory support, allowing for physical and nutritional rehabilitation and reversal of renal and hepatic dysfunction prior to transplant[219] or, rarely, prior to myocardial recovery.[220] VADs are also increasingly being implanted for permanent, so-called destination therapy in selected patients who are ineligible for cardiac transplant because of age or comorbidites.[221]

General indications and surgical techniques for placement of an LV assist device (LVAD), biventricular assist device (BIVAD), or total artificial heart (TAH) and perioperative care of VAD patients are discussed in Chapter 15 and in the Appendix. Decisions regarding the use of MCS should be made in consultation with an advanced heart disease cardiologist and a VAD/transplant surgeon, and such decisions require evaluation and management by a multidisciplinary team.[222]

Acute Pulmonary Edema

The principles described above have been developed primarily to treat acute decompensation of chronic HF. Similar principles apply to acute pulmonary edema, sometimes referred to as *acute HF*, with some special considerations. Unlike the approach to an exacerbation of chronic HF, the primary goal of therapy for acute pulmonary edema is temporary stabilization of the patient until definitive mechanical intervention or spontaneous recovery can occur. The design of an effective oral regimen for outpatient stabilization is not a major goal.

HF in the setting of acute MI can develop and progress rapidly, and the patient may suffer from intense precordial pain. Unless cardiogenic shock is present, arterial pressure is usually elevated as a result of adrenergically mediated vasoconstriction, and it may be suspected incorrectly that the pulmonary edema is due to hypertensive heart disease. However, hypertensive crises are now uncommon,[223] and fundoscopic examination will usually indicate whether hypertensive heart disease is actually present. In addition, echocardiography may be useful in defining the pathogenesis of acute pulmonary edema. In most patients with hypertensive pulmonary edema and normal LV function, the edema is due to an exacerbation of diastolic dysfunction, rather than to transient systolic dysfunction, myocardial ischemia, or severe mitral regurgitation (Figure 14-14).[224] The Studying the Treatment of Acute Hypertension (STAT) registry is a U.S., multicenter, observational survey of the management practices and outcomes for patients with acute severe hypertension who receive parenteral antihypertensive therapy.[225] A recent STAT report on a subset of patients with acute hypertensive HF, defined as pulmonary edema on a chest radiograph or elevated natriuretic peptide level, demonstrated that

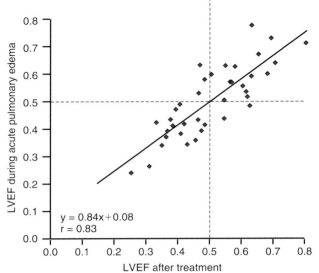

$y = 0.84x + 0.08$
$r = 0.83$

FIGURE 14-14 Relationship between left ventricular ejection fraction (*LVEF*) during acute pulmonary edema and 1 to 3 days after treatment in 38 patients (14 men and 24 women, aged 67 ± 13 years). *Dotted lines* indicate normal values for LVEF. (*Modified from Gandhi SK, Powers JC, Nomeir AM, et al. The pathogenesis of acute pulmonary edema associated with hypertension.* N Engl J Med *2001;344:17.*)

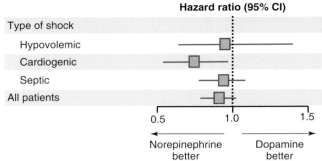

FIGURE 14-15 Norepinephrine versus dopamine for the treatment of shock: the Sepsis Occurrence in Acutely Ill Patients II trial. Shown is a forest plot for predefined subgroup analysis according to type of shock. A total of 1044 patients were in septic shock, 280 were in cardiogenic shock, and 263 were in hypovolemic shock. CI, confidence interval. (*Modified from De Backer D, Biston P, Devriendt J, et al. Comparison of dopamine and norepinephrine in the treatment of shock.* N Engl J Med *2010;362:779.*)

hypertensive HF patients had worse renal function and lower ejection fraction and were more likely to require ICU admission and noninvasive positive-pressure ventilation compared with non-HF patients with hypertensive urgency.[226] Readmission rate at 90 days was also higher (46% vs. 35%; *P* = .001). As demonstrated with acute decompensated HF (see Table 14-9), factors at discharge associated with readmission included higher serum BUN and creatinine levels and elevated BNP.

Diagnosis of cardiogenic shock complicating acute MI is occasionally delayed when blood pressure is maintained by sinus tachycardia. IV positive inotropic support should not be postponed because of concern about increasing myocardial oxygen demand, which is also raised by increased ventricular filling pressures. Dobutamine can be initiated while a PAC is being placed to monitor loading conditions and response to therapy. In contrast to the hemodynamic goals in the chronically dilated heart, low systemic blood pressure and reduced cardiac output may be less well tolerated in patients with previously normal hemodynamics, and higher filling pressures may be required to maximize cardiac output. In the setting of marked hypotension, dopamine or norepinephrine should be initiated to support a systolic blood pressure above 80 mm Hg. In a recent randomized study of patients requiring vasopressor therapy for the treatment of shock,[227] the rate of death at 28 days was significantly higher among patients with cardiogenic shock who were treated with dopamine compared with those who were treated with norepinephrine (*P* = .03; Figure 14-15).

Sublingual followed by IV nitroglycerin can be used to decrease ischemia and associated symptoms and may also provide arterial vasodilation when the SVR is high. If symptoms are not immediately relieved with nitroglycerin, morphine sulfate given intravenously may be effective by causing mild venodilation and preload reduction. However, some data suggest an association between morphine use and adverse outcomes in acute decompensated HF that include mechanical ventilation, ICU admission, and increased mortality.[228] Nitroprusside has the potential to cause a "coronary steal" in the setting of acute ischemia and should be avoided except in patients with severe hypertension. As total body volume status is usually normal, diuretics are infrequently needed during acute infarction except as initial therapy for pulmonary edema.

IABP or percutaneous VAD should be considered if cardiac output is markedly reduced, filling pressures are severely elevated, or ongoing ischemia is evident. Evaluation for definitive intervention, such as revascularization, should not be delayed by prolonged attempts to stabilize a patient on pharmacologic therapy. In a landmark trial of cardiogenic shock complicating acute MI, overall mortality at 30 days did not differ between patients randomized to emergency revascularization or initial medical stabilization, although 6 month mortality was lower in the revascularization group (50% vs. 63%; *P* = .027).[229]

Patients with acute HF secondary to new mitral or aortic valve regurgitation (e.g., from acute bacterial endocarditis) are exquisitely sensitive to afterload reduction. Arterial vasodilation with IV nitroprusside, followed by oral vasodilators, often improves forward flow markedly[230] and allows for elective consideration of valve replacement. Nitroprusside has also been used successfully to stabilize critically ill patients with severe aortic stenosis and LV dysfunction (Figure 14-16) awaiting definitive aortic valve replacement[231] or percutaneous balloon valvuloplasty as a bridge to aortic valve surgery.[232]

The use of noninvasive positive-pressure ventilation (NIPPV) in the emergency department or ICU has been advocated to relieve dyspnea and improve outcomes in patients with acute cardiogenic pulmonary edema. Although early studies raised concerns about precipitating an MI, subsequent randomized studies and a meta-analysis suggested that noninvasive ventilation reduced the need for intubation and reduced mortality.[233] The Three Interventions in Cardiogenic Pulmonary Oedema (3CPO) trial randomly assigned 1060 patients to oxygen therapy, CPAP (5 to 15 cm H_2O), or NIPPV (inspiratory pressure, 8 to 20 cm H_2O; expiratory pressure, 4 to 10 cm H_2O).[234] At 7 days, no significant difference in mortality rate was found between patients receiving oxygen therapy (9.8%) and those undergoing noninvasive ventilation (9.5%; *P* = .87; Figure 14-17), and no difference was seen in the combined endpoint of death or intubation. However, noninvasive ventilation induced a more rapid improvement in dyspnea, heart rate, hypercapnia, and acidosis. Based on these data, the HFSA guidelines recommend considering the use of NIPPV for severely dyspneic patients with clinical evidence of pulmonary edema.[105]

The evaluation and management of patients with acute myocarditis is discussed in Chapter 12. Lieberman and colleagues[235] classified myocarditis as *fulminant, acute (nonfulminant), chronic active,* or *chronic persistent* on the basis of clinicopathologic criteria. Patients with fulminant myocarditis display the least delay between initial viral symptoms and the onset of HF and are initially seen with severe hemodynamic compromise. However, they are more likely to recover LV function and have an excellent long-term prognosis.[236] When this distinct clinical entity is suspected and confirmed by endomyocardial biopsy, aggressive hemodynamic support that includes the use of positive inotropic agents and mechanical circulatory assist is warranted to bridge patients to recovery. One exception is giant cell myocarditis, in which patients are unlikely to recover even with adjuvant immunosuppressive therapy, and such patients should be considered for urgent cardiac transplant.[237,238]

Heart Failure with Preserved Ejection Fraction

The pathophysiology of HF with preserved ejection fraction is discussed above, in Chapter 12, and in other reviews.[21,27,239] Common precipitants of acute decompensation include ischemia, hypertension, and volume overload, all of which should be treated aggressively. Although cardiac output may be reduced, IV positive inotropic agents are seldom necessary to maintain vital organ perfusion and may exacerbate tachycardia or arrhythmias. Low-dose dopamine therapy (2 to 3 μg/kg/min) may help with diuresis in some cases. Systemic hypertension is a common target of therapy, and vasodilators, often used in combination, can be adjusted without the need for hemodynamic monitoring. ACE inhibitors, ARBs, and calcium channel blockers can lower blood pressure and improve ventricular compliance. Oral, topical, or IV nitrates may be used to reduce ventricular filling pressures and improve exertional tolerance and also to treat myocardial ischemia. In some patients, however, postural hypotension may limit the use of nitrates or other vasodilators.

In addition to the management of blood pressure and fluid status, heart rate control is central to preventing or treating ischemia associated with HF with preserved ejection fraction. Also, β-blockers and calcium channel blockers are useful negative chronotropic agents. For patients who come to medical attention with new-onset atrial arrhythmias, restoration of sinus rhythm is important for achieving adequate cardiac output. While awaiting therapeutic anticoagulation, β-blockers, calcium channel blockers, or digoxin may be used to control the ventricular response. For patients with a contraindication to chronic anticoagulation, a transesophageal echocardiogram should be performed prior to cardioversion to assess for intracardiac thrombus.[180] Electrical or chemical cardioversion should also be considered for patients with chronic HF and atrial fibrillation in whom adequate rate control cannot be achieved. Alternatively, ablation of the atrioventricular junction with back-up ventricular pacing may be considered. In this scenario, if LVEF is even mildly reduced (40% to 50%), consideration should be given to placement of a cardiac resynchronization therapy pacemaker to prevent further LV dysfunction and recurrent HF from RV apical pacing.[240]

Unfulfilled Promises and Future Directions

The last approved vasoactive agent for the treatment of acute decompensated HF was nesiritide in 2001. As discussed above, initial enthusiasm was tempered by concerns for renal injury[122]

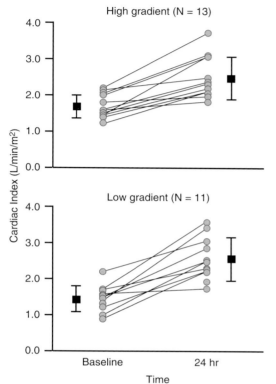

FIGURE 14-16 Change in cardiac index 24 hours after the start of nitroprusside infusion in subgroups of patients with left ventricular dysfunction and severe aortic stenosis according to the mean aortic valve pressure gradient at baseline (≤30 mm Hg [low gradient] vs. >30 mm Hg [high gradient]; *P* = 0.20). *(Modified from Khot UN, Novaro GM, Popovic ZB, et al. Nitroprusside in critically ill patients with left ventricular dysfunction and aortic stenosis. N Engl J Med 2003;348:1756.)*

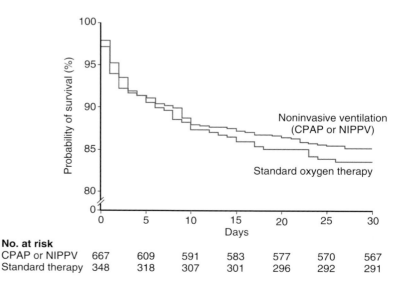

FIGURE 14-17 Role of noninvasive ventilation in patients with acute cardiogenic pulmonary edema. Kaplan-Meier survival curves show the comparison between noninvasive ventilation (with continuous positive airway pressure [*CPAP*] or noninvasive positive pressure ventilation [*NIPPV*]) and standard oxygen therapy. No significant difference was reported in the primary endpoint of 7-day mortality between patients receiving noninvasive ventilation (9.5%) and those receiving oxygen (9.8%; odds ratio, 0.97; 95% confidence interval, 0.63 to 1.48; *P* = .87). *(Modified from Gray A, Goodacre S, Newby DE, et al. Noninvasive ventilation in acute cardiogenic pulmonary edema. N Engl J Med 2008;359:142.)*

No. at risk							
CPAP or NIPPV	667	609	591	583	577	570	567
Standard therapy	348	318	307	301	296	292	291

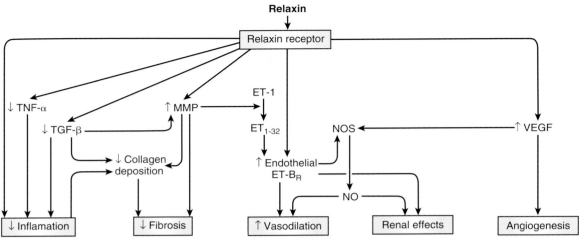

FIGURE 14-18 Biology of relaxin and potential beneficial effects in heart failure. Human data indicate that relaxin reverses systemic and renal vasoconstriction and increases vascular compliance, leading to normalization of central and regional hemodynamics. Experimental data suggest that relaxin also has antiinflammatory and antifibrotic effects that may attenuate ventricular remodeling. ET, endothelin; MMP, matrix metalloproteinase; NO, nitric oxide; NOS, nitric oxide synthase; TGF, transforming growth factor; TNF, tumor necrosis factor; VEGF, vascular endothelial growth factor. *(Modified from Teichman SL, Unemori E, Teerlink JR, et al. Relaxin: review of biology and potential role in treating heart failure.* Curr Heart Fail Rep *2010;7:75.)*

and mortality,[150] and the ASCEND-HF study recently demonstrated, in about 7000 patients, no benefit compared with placebo in 30-day morbidity or mortality.[153] Given the potential toxicity of positive inotropic agents[121,174] and the increased recognition of the cardiorenal syndrome contributing to adverse outcomes, recent clinical investigations have focused on the development of alternative vasodilators, renal-sparing agents, and safer inotropes.[241]

Plasma levels of arginine vasopressin are elevated in patients with HF and correlate with poor outcomes.[29] Adverse effects of vasopressin are mediated by V_{1a} receptors in the vasculature and myocardium, causing vasoconstriction and positive inotropy respectively, and V_2 receptors in the kidney cause water retention. Vasopressin receptor antagonists are a new class of agents that were developed to improve hemodynamics, attenuate disease progression, and improve survival in HF.[29,242] However, based on neutral outcomes data, these agents have been approved only for the treatment of hyponatremia. In patients with advanced HF, conivaptan, a combined V_{1a}/V_2 receptor antagonist, reduced PCWP and right atrial pressure and caused a dose-dependent increase in urine output.[243] Tolvaptan, an oral selective V_2 receptor antagonist, increased urine volume and decreased body weight compared with placebo in patients with acute decompensated HF,[244] and it increased serum sodium concentrations in patients with hyponatremia.[245]

The Efficacy of Vasopressin Antagonism in Heart Failure Outcome Study with Tolvaptan (EVEREST)[193] randomly assigned 4133 patients with worsening HF within 48 hours of admission to receive oral tolvaptan (30 mg once daily) or placebo in addition to standard therapy. During a median follow-up of 10 months, no difference in mortality (tolvaptan, 25.9%; placebo, 26.3%; *P* = .68) or in the combined endpoint of cardiovascular death or HF hospitalization was found between the two groups. Although tolvaptan significantly improved edema at 7 days, drug discontinuation because of increased thirst and dry mouth occurred more frequently. In phase II pilot studies in acute decompensated HF, conivaptan was no different than placebo for multiple clinical outcomes, and like tolvaptan, it is approved only for the treatment of euvolemic or hypervolemic hyponatremia.

Relaxin is a naturally occurring human peptide initially identified as a reproductive hormone. Produced by the corpus luteum of the ovary and the placenta, relaxin exerts systemic vasodilatory effects through stimulation of endothelin type B receptors on vascular endothelial cells.[246] Additional beneficial effects in HF suggested by emerging understanding of the biology of relaxin include sodium and water excretion, reduced inflammation, and

cardioprotection (Figure 14-18). Teerlink and colleagues[247] performed a multicenter, randomized, placebo-controlled dose-finding study of relaxin (10 to 250 μg/kg/day) in 234 patients with acute HF and mild to moderate renal dysfunction. Compared with placebo, relaxin improved dyspnea and tended to reduce short-term morbidity and mortality, although hypotension and worsening renal function were observed at higher doses. The Efficacy and Safety of Relaxin for the Treatment of Acute Heart Failure (RELAX-AHF) study aims to randomize 1160 patients with acute decompensated HF and systolic blood pressure above 125 mm Hg to receive a 48-hour infusion of relaxin 30 μg/kg/day or placebo. The primary outcome measure is relief of dyspnea for up to 5 days.

A limitation of most positive inotropic agents, such as dobutamine and milrinone, is that they act by increasing intracellular calcium in the myocyte and therefore may cause tachycardia and arrhythmias. Levosimendan is a pyridazinone-dinitrile derivative, which enhances calcium sensitivity of myofilaments via calcium-dependent binding to troponin C.[250] Other pharmacologic actions include mild PDE inhibition and activation of potassium channels. In patients with moderate to severe HF as a result of ischemic or nonischemic cardiomyopathy, a 6-hour infusion of levosimendan caused rapid, dose-dependent increases in stroke volume and cardiac index and resulted in decreases in PCWP and right atrial pressure with only a modest increase in heart rate.[249] Levosimendan was well tolerated and appeared to improve symptoms without proarrhythmia. However, additional phase II data[250] suggested that hypotension and arrhythmias might limit the use of levosimendan in patients with acute decompensated HF, and a randomized, controlled, double-blind study showed no difference between levosimendan and dobutamine in all-cause mortality at 180 days (26% vs. 28%, respectively; hazard ratio, 0.91; 95% confidence interval, 0.74 to 1.13; *P* = .40).[251] Levosimendan is not approved for use in the United States.

Clinically available inotropes, including levosimendan, increase cardiac contractility indirectly through signaling cascades. Omecantiv mecarbil is a small molecule that selectively activates cardiac myosin by increasing the transition rate of myosin into the strongly actin-bound force-generating state.[252] In animal models of HF, omecantiv mecarbil induced sustained increases in cardiac function by increasing the duration of LV ejection without changing the rate of contraction (LV dP/dt).[253] Furthermore, this positive inotropic effect occurred without an increase in myocardial oxygen consumption or desensitization, as seen with dobutamine. Small proof-of-concept studies in normal humans[254] and in patients with systolic HF[255] provide additional support for the development of omecantiv mecarbil for the treatment of acute decompensated HF, with dose-dependent increases in stroke volume and ejection fraction. However, early clinical studies have also raised concerns about dose-limiting hypotension and ischemia. A larger study (n = 600) is currently underway to assess the risk/benefit ratio of this agent in acute HF.

REFERENCES

1. Ko DT, Tu JV, Masoudi FA, et al. Quality of care and outcomes of older patients with heart failure hospitalized in the United States and Canada. *Arch Intern Med* 2005;165:2486.
2. Gheorghiade M, Pang PS. Acute heart failure syndromes. *J Am Coll Cardiol* 2009;53:557.
3. Hunt SA, Abraham WT, Chin MH, et al. 2009 focused update incorporated into the ACC/AHA 2005 Guidelines for the Diagnosis and Management of Heart Failure in Adults: a report of the American College of Cardiology Foundation/American Heart Association Task Force on Practice Guidelines: developed in collaboration with the International Society for Heart and Lung Transplantation. *Circulation* 2009;119:e391-e479.
4. Goodlin SJ. Palliative care in congestive heart failure. *J Am Coll Cardiol* 2009;54:386.
5. Roger VL, Go AS, Lloyd-Jones DM, et al. Heart disease and stroke statistics—2011 update: a report from the American Heart Association. *Circulation* 2011;123:e18-e209.
6. Lloyd-Jones D, Adams RJ, Brown TM, et al. Heart disease and stroke statistics—2010 update: a report from the American Heart Association. *Circulation* 2010;121:e46-e215.
7. Dunlay SM, Redfield MM, Weston SA, et al. Hospitalizations after heart failure diagnosis: a community perspective. *J Am Coll Cardiol* 2009;54:1695.
8. Cleland JG, Swedberg K, Follath F, et al. The EuroHeart Failure survey programme—a survey on the quality of care among patients with heart failure in Europe. Part 1: patient characteristics and diagnosis. *Eur Heart J* 2003;24:442.
9. Fonarow GC, Adams KF Jr, Abraham WT, et al. Risk stratification for in-hospital mortality in acutely decompensated heart failure: classification and regression tree analysis. *JAMA* 2005;293:572.
10. Jong P, Gong Y, Liu PP, et al. Care and outcomes of patients newly hospitalized for heart failure in the community treated by cardiologists compared with other specialists. *Circulation* 2003;108:184.
11. Cuffe MS, Califf RM, Adams KF Jr, et al. Short-term intravenous milrinone for acute exacerbation of chronic heart failure: a randomized controlled trial. *JAMA* 2002;287:1541.
12. Publication Committee for the VMAC Investigators. Intravenous nesiritide vs nitroglycerin for treatment of decompensated congestive heart failure: a randomized controlled trial. *JAMA* 2002;287:1531.
13. Setoguchi S, Stevenson LW, Schneeweiss S. Repeated hospitalizations predict mortality in the community population with heart failure. *Am Heart J* 2007;154:260.
14. Centers for Medicare & Medicaid Services. *2003 data compendium*. Available at http://www.cms.gov/research-statistics-data-and-systems/statistics-trends-and-reports/datacompendium/19_2003datacompendium.html.
15. Unroe KT, Greiner MA, Hernandez AF, et al. Resource use in the last 6 months of life among medicare beneficiaries with heart failure, 2000-2007. *Arch Intern Med* 2011;171:196.
16. Joynt KE, Orav EJ, Jha AK. The association between hospital volume and processes, outcomes, and costs of care for congestive heart failure. *Ann Intern Med* 2011;154:94.
17. Baicu CF, Zile MR, Aurigemma GP, et al. Left ventricular systolic performance, function, and contractility in patients with diastolic heart failure. *Circulation* 2005;111:2306.
18. Zile MR, Baicu CF, Gaasch WH. Diastolic heart failure—abnormalities in active relaxation and passive stiffness of the left ventricle. *N Engl J Med* 2004;350:1953.
19. Kawaguchi M, Hay I, Fetics B, et al. Combined ventricular systolic and arterial stiffening in patients with heart failure and preserved ejection fraction: implications for systolic and diastolic reserve limitations. *Circulation* 2003;107:714.
20. Klapholz M, Maurer M, Lowe AM, et al. Hospitalization for heart failure in the presence of a normal left ventricular ejection fraction: results of the New York Heart Failure Registry. *J Am Coll Cardiol* 2004;43:1432.
21. Zile MR, Brutsaert DL. New concepts in diastolic dysfunction and diastolic heart failure: Part II: causal mechanisms and treatment. *Circulation* 2002;105:1503.
22. Vasan RS, Levy D. Defining diastolic heart failure: a call for standardized diagnostic criteria. *Circulation* 2000;101:2118.
23. Zile MR, Bennett TD, St John SM, et al. Transition from chronic compensated to acute decompensated heart failure: pathophysiological insights obtained from continuous monitoring of intracardiac pressures. *Circulation* 2008;118:1433.
24. Felker GM, Pang PS, Adams KF, et al. Clinical trials of pharmacological therapies in acute heart failure syndromes: lessons learned and directions forward. *Circ Heart Fail* 2010;3:314.
25. Yancy CW, Lopatin M, Stevenson LW, et al. Clinical presentation, management, and in-hospital outcomes of patients admitted with acute decompensated heart failure with preserved systolic function: a report from the Acute Decompensated Heart Failure National Registry (ADHERE) database. *J Am Coll Cardiol* 2006;47:76.
26. Fonarow GC, Stough WG, Abraham WT, et al. Characteristics, treatments, and outcomes of patients with preserved systolic function hospitalized for heart failure: a report from the OPTIMIZE-HF Registry. *J Am Coll Cardiol* 2007;50:768.
27. Redfield MM. Heart failure with normal ejection fraction. In Libby P, Bonow RO, Mann D, Zipes DP, editors: *Braunwald's heart disease: a textbook of cardiovascular medicine*, 8th edition. Philadelphia, 2008, Saunders Elsevier, pp 641-664.
28. Stevenson LW, Tillisch JH. Maintenance of cardiac output with normal filling pressures in patients with dilated heart failure. *Circulation* 1986;74:1303.
29. Goldsmith SR, Gheorghiade M. Vasopressin antagonism in heart failure. *J Am Coll Cardiol* 2005;46:1785.
30. Ooi H, Colucci WS, Givertz MM. Endothelin mediates increased pulmonary vascular tone in patients with heart failure: demonstration by direct intrapulmonary infusion of sitaxsentan. *Circulation* 2002;106:1618.
31. Horwich TB, Patel J, MacLellan WR, et al. Cardiac troponin I is associated with impaired hemodynamics, progressive left ventricular dysfunction, and increased mortality rates in advanced heart failure. *Circulation* 2003;108:833.
32. Kociol RD, Pang PS, Gheorghiade M, et al. Troponin elevation in heart failure prevalence, mechanisms, and clinical implications. *J Am Coll Cardiol* 2010;56:1071.
33. Peacock WF, De Marco T, Fonarow GC, et al. Cardiac troponin and outcome in acute heart failure. *N Engl J Med* 2008;358:2117.
34. O'Connor CM, Fiuzat M, Lombardi C, et al. Impact of serial troponin release on outcomes in patients with acute heart failure: analysis from the PROTECT pilot study. *Circ Heart Fail* 2011;4:724.
35. Fonarow GC, Abraham WT, Albert NM, et al. Factors identified as precipitating hospital admissions for heart failure and clinical outcomes: findings from OPTIMIZE-HF. *Arch Intern Med* 2008;168:847.
36. Tsuyuki RT, McKelvie RS, Arnold JM, et al. Acute precipitants of congestive heart failure exacerbations. *Arch Intern Med* 2001;161:2337.
37. Chin MH, Goldman L. Factors contributing to the hospitalization of patients with congestive heart failure. *Am J Public Health* 1997;87:643.
38. Cline CM, Bjorck-Linne AK, Israelsson BY, et al. Non-compliance and knowledge of prescribed medication in elderly patients with heart failure. *Eur J Heart Fail* 1999;1:145.
39. Setoguchi S, Choudhry NK, Levin R, et al. Temporal trends in adherence to cardiovascular medications in elderly patients after hospitalization for heart failure. *Clin Pharmacol Ther* 2010;88:548.
40. Ambardekar AV, Fonarow GC, Hernandez AF, et al. Characteristics and in-hospital outcomes for nonadherent patients with heart failure: findings from Get With The Guidelines-Heart Failure (GWTG-HF). *Am Heart J* 2009;158:644.
41. Lenzen MJ, Boersma E, Reimer WJ, et al. Under-utilization of evidence-based drug treatment in patients with heart failure is only partially explained by dissimilarity to patients enrolled in landmark trials: a report from the Euro Heart Survey on Heart Failure. *Eur Heart J* 2005;26:2706.
42. Rathore SS, Curtis JP, Wang Y, et al. Association of serum digoxin concentration and outcomes in patients with heart failure. *JAMA* 2003;289:871.
43. Felker GM, O'Connor CM, Braunwald E. Loop diuretics in acute decompensated heart failure: Necessary? Evil? A necessary evil? *Circ Heart Fail* 2009;2:56.
44. Ebinger MW, Krishnan S, Schuger CD. Mechanisms of ventricular arrhythmias in heart failure. *Curr Heart Fail Rep* 2005;2:111.
45. Efremidis M, Pappas L, Sideris A, et al. Management of atrial fibrillation in patients with heart failure. *J Card Fail* 2008;14:232.
46. DiMarco JP. Atrial fibrillation and acute decompensated heart failure. *Circ Heart Fail* 2009;2:72.
47. Gopinathannair R, Sullivan R, Olshansky B. Tachycardia-mediated cardiomyopathy: recognition and management. *Curr Heart Fail Rep* 2009;6:257.
48. Stevenson WG, Wilber DJ, Natale A, et al. Irrigated radiofrequency catheter ablation guided by electroanatomic mapping for recurrent ventricular tachycardia after myocardial infarction: the multicenter thermocool ventricular tachycardia ablation trial. *Circulation* 2008;118:2773.
49. Sweeney MO, Hellkamp AS, Ellenbogen KA, et al. Adverse effect of ventricular pacing on heart failure and atrial fibrillation among patients with normal baseline QRS duration in a clinical trial of pacemaker therapy for sinus node dysfunction. *Circulation* 2003;107:2932.
50. Nguyen MT, Cosson E, Valensi P, et al. Transthoracic echocardiographic abnormalities in asymptomatic diabetic patients: association with microalbuminuria and silent coronary disease. *Diabetes Metab* 2011;37:343.
51. Falsey AR, Hennessey PA, Formica MA, et al. Respiratory syncytial virus infection in elderly and high-risk adults. *N Engl J Med* 2005;352:1749.
52. Nichol KL, Nordin JD, Nelson DB, et al. Effectiveness of influenza vaccine in the community-dwelling elderly. *N Engl J Med* 2007;357:1373.
53. Wu J, Xu F, Lu L, et al. Safety and effectiveness of a 2009 H1N1 vaccine in Beijing. *N Engl J Med* 2010;363:2416.
54. Forman DE, Butler J, Wang Y, et al. Incidence, predictors at admission, and impact of worsening renal function among patients hospitalized with heart failure. *J Am Coll Cardiol* 2004;43:61.
55. Shah RV, Givertz MM. Managing acute renal failure in patients with acute decompensated heart failure: the cardiorenal syndrome. *Curr Heart Fail Rep* 2009;6:176.
56. Piano MR. Alcohol and heart failure. *J Card Fail* 2002;8:239.
57. Lucas DL, Brown RA, Wassef M, et al. Alcohol and the cardiovascular system: research challenges and opportunities. *J Am Coll Cardiol* 2005;45:1916.
58. Page J, Henry D. Consumption of NSAIDs and the development of congestive heart failure in elderly patients: an underrecognized public health problem. *Arch Intern Med* 2000;160:777.
59. Tang WH, Francis GS, Hoogwerf BJ, et al. Fluid retention after initiation of thiazolidinedione therapy in diabetic patients with established chronic heart failure. *J Am Coll Cardiol* 2003;41:1394.
60. Page RL, Cantu M, Lindenfeld J, et al. Possible heart failure exacerbation associated with pregabalin: case discussion and literature review. *J Cardiovasc Med (Hagerstown)* 2008;9:922.
61. Chin MH, Goldman L. Correlates of major complications or death in patients admitted to the hospital with congestive heart failure. *Arch Intern Med* 1996;156:1814.
62. Abraham WT, Fonarow GC, Albert NM, et al. Predictors of in-hospital mortality in patients hospitalized for heart failure: insights from the Organized Program to Initiate Lifesaving Treatment in Hospitalized Patients with Heart Failure (OPTIMIZE-HF). *J Am Coll Cardiol* 2008;52:347.
63. Nohria A, Tsang SW, Fang JC, et al. Clinical assessment identifies hemodynamic profiles that predict outcomes in patients admitted with heart failure. *J Am Coll Cardiol* 2003;41:1797.
64. Felker GM, Benza RL, Chandler AB, et al. Heart failure etiology and response to milrinone in decompensated heart failure: results from the OPTIME-CHF study. *J Am Coll Cardiol* 2003;41:997.
65. Flaherty JD, Bax JJ, De Luca L, et al. Acute heart failure syndromes in patients with coronary artery disease: early assessment and treatment. *J Am Coll Cardiol* 2009;53:254.

66. Felker GM, Leimberger JD, Califf RM, et al. Risk stratification after hospitalization for decompensated heart failure. *J Card Fail* 2004;10:460.

67. Tarantini L, Oliva F, Cantoni S, et al. Prevalence and prognostic role of anaemia in patients with acute heart failure and preserved or depressed ventricular function. *Intern Emerg Med* May 5, 2011. Epub ahead of print.

68. Bettencourt P, Azevedo A, Pimenta J, et al. N-terminal-pro-brain natriuretic peptide predicts outcome after hospital discharge in heart failure patients. *Circulation* 2004;110:2168.

69. Januzzi JL, van Kimmenade R, Lainchbury J, et al. NT-proBNP testing for diagnosis and short-term prognosis in acute destabilized heart failure: an international pooled analysis of 1256 patients. The International Collaborative of NT-proBNP Study. *Eur Heart J* 2006;27:330.

70. Adams KF, Jr., Fonarow GC, Emerman CL, et al. Characteristics and outcomes of patients hospitalized for heart failure in the United States: rationale, design, and preliminary observations from the first 100,000 cases in the Acute Decompensated Heart Failure National Registry (ADHERE). *Am Heart J* 2005;149:209.

71. Sanders GP, Mendes LA, Colucci WS, et al. Noninvasive methods for detecting elevated left-sided cardiac filling pressure. *J Card Fail* 2000;6:157.

72. Androne AS, Hryniewicz K, Hudaihed A, et al. Relation of unrecognized hypervolemia in chronic heart failure to clinical status, hemodynamics, and patient outcomes. *Am J Cardiol* 2004;93:1254.

73. Bourge RC, Abraham WT, Adamson PB, et al. Randomized controlled trial of an implantable continuous hemodynamic monitor in patients with advanced heart failure: the COMPASS-HF study. *J Am Coll Cardiol* 2008;51:1073.

74. Wang CS, FitzGerald JM, Schulzer M, et al. Does this dyspneic patient in the emergency department have congestive heart failure? *JAMA* 2005;294:1944.

75. Chakko S, Woska D, Martinez H, et al. Clinical, radiographic, and hemodynamic correlations in chronic congestive heart failure: conflicting results may lead to inappropriate care. *Am J Med* 1991;90:353.

76. Stevenson LW, Perloff JK. The limited reliability of physical signs for estimating hemodynamics in chronic heart failure. *JAMA* 1989;261:884.

77. Campbell P, Drazner MH, Kato M, et al. Mismatch of right- and left-sided filling pressures in chronic heart failure. *J Card Fail* 2011;17:561.

78. McGee SR. Physical examination of venous pressure: a critical review. *Am Heart J* 1998;136:10.

79. Drazner MH, Rame JE, Stevenson LW, et al. Prognostic importance of elevated jugular venous pressure and a third heart sound in patients with heart failure. *N Engl J Med* 2001;345:574.

80. Givertz MM, Slawsky MT, Moraes DL, et al. Noninvasive determination of pulmonary artery wedge pressure in patients with chronic heart failure. *Am J Cardiol* 2001;87:1213.

81. Prasad A, Hastings JL, Shibata S, et al. Characterization of static and dynamic left ventricular diastolic function in patients with heart failure with a preserved ejection fraction. *Circ Heart Fail* 2010;3:617.

82. Yu CM, Wang L, Chau E, et al. Intrathoracic impedance monitoring in patients with heart failure: correlation with fluid status and feasibility of early warning preceding hospitalization. *Circulation* 2005;112:841.

83. Volpicelli G, Caramello V, Cardinale L, et al. Bedside ultrasound of the lung for the monitoring of acute decompensated heart failure. *Am J Emerg Med* 2008;26:585.

84. Mullens W, Borowski AG, Curtin RJ, et al. Tissue Doppler imaging in the estimation of intracardiac filling pressure in decompensated patients with advanced systolic heart failure. *Circulation* 2009;119:62.

85. Kamath SA, Drazner MH, Tasissa G, et al. Correlation of impedance cardiography with invasive hemodynamic measurements in patients with advanced heart failure: the Bio-Impedance CardioGraphy (BIG) substudy of the Evaluation Study of Congestive Heart Failure and Pulmonary Artery Catheterization Effectiveness (ESCAPE) Trial. *Am Heart J* 2009;158:217.

86. Mahdyoon H, Klein R, Eyler W, et al. Radiographic pulmonary congestion in end-stage congestive heart failure. *Am J Cardiol* 1989;63:625.

87. Collins SP, Lindsell CJ, Storrow AB, et al. Prevalence of negative chest radiography results in the emergency department patient with decompensated heart failure. *Ann Emerg Med* 2006;47:13.

88. Kataoka H. Pericardial and pleural effusions in decompensated chronic heart failure. *Am Heart J* 2000;139:918.

89. Kataoka H, Takada S. The role of thoracic ultrasonography for evaluation of patients with decompensated chronic heart failure. *J Am Coll Cardiol* 2000;35:1638.

90. Pina IL, Apstein CS, Balady GJ, et al. Exercise and heart failure: a statement from the American Heart Association committee on exercise, rehabilitation, and prevention. *Circulation* 2003;107:1210.

91. Anker SD, Negassa A, Coats AJ, et al. Prognostic importance of weight loss in chronic heart failure and the effect of treatment with angiotensin-converting-enzyme inhibitors: an observational study. *Lancet* 2003;361:1077.

92. Drazner MH, Hellkamp AS, Leier CV, et al. Value of clinician assessment of hemodynamics in advanced heart failure: the ESCAPE trial. *Circ Heart Fail* 2008;1:170.

93. Ghali JK, Tam SW. The critical link of hypervolemia and hyponatremia in heart failure and the potential role of arginine vasopressin antagonists. *J Card Fail* 2010;16:419.

94. Milionis HJ, Alexandrides GE, Liberopoulos EN, et al. Hypomagnesemia and concurrent acid–base and electrolyte abnormalities in patients with congestive heart failure. *Eur J Heart Fail* 2002;4:167.

95. Juurlink DN, Mamdani MM, Lee DS, et al. Rates of hyperkalemia after publication of the Randomized Aldactone Evaluation Study. *N Engl J Med* 2004;351:543.

96. Gelow JM, Desai AS, Hochberg CP, et al. Clinical predictors of hepatic fibrosis in chronic advanced heart failure. *Circ Heart Fail* 2010;3:59.

97. Ronco C, Haapio M, House AA, et al. Cardiorenal syndrome. *J Am Coll Cardiol* 2008;52:1527.

98. Nohria A, Hasselblad V, Stebbins A, et al. Cardiorenal interactions: insights from the ESCAPE trial. *J Am Coll Cardiol* 2008;51:1268.

99. Voors AA, Davison BA, Felker GM, et al. Early drop in systolic blood pressure and worsening renal function in acute heart failure: renal results of Pre-RELAX-AHF. *Eur J Heart Fail* 2011;13:961.

100. Aronson D, Burger AJ. The relationship between transient and persistent worsening renal function and mortality in patients with acute decompensated heart failure. *J Card Fail* 2010;16:541.

101. Maisel AS, Krishnaswamy P, Nowak RM, et al. Rapid measurement of B-type natriuretic peptide in the emergency diagnosis of heart failure. *N Engl J Med* 2002;347:161.

102. Iwanaga Y, Nishi I, Furuichi S, et al. B-type natriuretic peptide strongly reflects diastolic wall stress in patients with chronic heart failure: comparison between systolic and diastolic heart failure. *J Am Coll Cardiol* 2006;47:742.

103. Grewal J, McKelvie RS, Persson H, et al. Usefulness of N-terminal pro-brain natriuretic peptide and brain natriuretic peptide to predict cardiovascular outcomes in patients with heart failure and preserved left ventricular ejection fraction. *Am J Cardiol* 2008;102:733.

104. Komajda M, Carson PE, Hetzel S, et al. Factors associated with outcome in heart failure with preserved ejection fraction: findings from the Irbesartan in Heart Failure with Preserved Ejection Fraction Study (I-PRESERVE). *Circ Heart Fail* 2011;4:27.

105. Lindenfeld J, Albert NM, Boehmer JP, et al. HFSA 2010 Comprehensive Heart Failure Practice Guideline. *J Card Fail* 2010;16:e1.

106. Maisel AS, McCord J, Nowak RM, et al. Bedside B-type natriuretic peptide in the emergency diagnosis of heart failure with reduced or preserved ejection fraction. Results from the Breathing Not Properly Multinational Study. *J Am Coll Cardiol* 2003;41:2010.

107. Parsonage WA, Galbraith AJ, Koerbin GL, et al. Value of B-type natriuretic peptide for identifying significantly elevated pulmonary artery wedge pressure in patients treated for established chronic heart failure secondary to ischemic or idiopathic dilated cardiomyopathy. *Am J Cardiol* 2005;95:883.

108. Cioffi G, Tarantini L, Stefenelli C, et al. Changes in plasma N-terminal proBNP levels and ventricular filling pressures during intensive unloading therapy in elderly with decompensated congestive heart failure and preserved left ventricular systolic function. *J Card Fail* 2006;12:608.

109. Waldo SW, Beede J, Isakson S, et al. Pro–B-type natriuretic peptide levels in acute decompensated heart failure. *J Am Coll Cardiol* 2008;51:1874.

110. Wang TJ, Larson MG, Levy D, et al. Impact of obesity on plasma natriuretic peptide levels. *Circulation* 2004;109:594.

111. Pfisterer M, Buser P, Rickli H, et al. BNP-guided vs symptom-guided heart failure therapy: the Trial of Intensified vs Standard Medical Therapy in Elderly Patients With Congestive Heart Failure (TIME-CHF) randomized trial. *JAMA* 2009;301:383.

112. Mueller C, Scholer A, Laule-Kilian K, et al. Use of B-type natriuretic peptide in the evaluation and management of acute dyspnea. *N Engl J Med* 2004;350:647.

113. Yanavitski M, Givertz MM. Novel biomarkers in acute heart failure. *Curr Heart Fail Rep* 2011;8:206.

114. Connors AF Jr, Speroff T, Dawson NV, et al. The effectiveness of right heart catheterization in the initial care of critically ill patients. SUPPORT Investigators. *JAMA* 1996;276:889.

115. The ESCAPE Investigators and ESCAPE Study Coordinators. Evaluation study of congestive heart failure and pulmonary artery catheterization effectiveness: the ESCAPE trial. *JAMA* 2005;294:1625.

116. Shah MR, Hasselblad V, Stevenson LW, et al. Impact of the pulmonary artery catheter in critically ill patients: meta-analysis of randomized clinical trials. *JAMA* 2005;294:1664.

117. Cappola TP, Felker GM, Kao WH, et al. Pulmonary hypertension and risk of death in cardiomyopathy: patients with myocarditis are at higher risk. *Circulation* 2002;105:1663.

118. Moraes DL, Colucci WS, Givertz MM. Secondary pulmonary hypertension in chronic heart failure: the role of the endothelium in pathophysiology and management. *Circulation* 2000;102:1718.

119. Hershberger RE, Nauman D, Walker TL, et al. Care processes and clinical outcomes of continuous outpatient support with inotropes (COSI) in patients with refractory endstage heart failure. *J Card Fail* 2003;9:180.

120. Nohria A, Mielniczuk LM, Stevenson LW. Evaluation and monitoring of patients with acute heart failure syndromes. *Am J Cardiol* 2005;96:32G.

121. Abraham WT, Adams KF, Fonarow GC, et al. In-hospital mortality in patients with acute decompensated heart failure requiring intravenous vasoactive medications: an analysis from the Acute Decompensated Heart Failure National Registry (ADHERE). *J Am Coll Cardiol* 2005;46:57.

122. Sackner-Bernstein JD, Skopicki HA, Aaronson KD. Risk of worsening renal function with nesiritide in patients with acutely decompensated heart failure. *Circulation* 2005;111:1487.

123. Hamilton MA, Stevenson LW, Woo M, et al. Effect of tricuspid regurgitation on the reliability of the thermodilution cardiac output technique in congestive heart failure. *Am J Cardiol* 1989;64:945.

124. Nunez S, Maisel A. Comparison between mixed venous oxygen saturation and thermodilution cardiac output in monitoring patients with severe heart failure treated with milrinone and dobutamine. *Am Heart J* 1998;135:383.

125. Alhashemi JA, Cecconi M, della RG, et al. Minimally invasive monitoring of cardiac output in the cardiac surgery intensive care unit. *Curr Heart Fail Rep* 2010;7:116.

126. Kramer BK, Schweda F, Riegger GA. Diuretic treatment and diuretic resistance in heart failure. *Am J Med* 1999;106:90.

127. Dormans TP, van Meyel JJ, Gerlag PG, et al. Diuretic efficacy of high dose furosemide in severe heart failure: bolus injection versus continuous infusion. *J Am Coll Cardiol* 1996;28:376.

128. Salvador DR, Rey NR, Ramos GC, et al. Continuous infusion versus bolus injection of loop diuretics in congestive heart failure. *Cochrane Database Syst Rev* 2005;CD003178.

129. Felker GM, Lee KL, Bull DA, et al. Diuretic strategies in patients with acute decompensated heart failure. *N Engl J Med* 2011;364:797.

130. Testani JM, Chen J, McCauley BD, et al. Potential effects of aggressive decongestion during the treatment of decompensated heart failure on renal function and survival. *Circulation* 2010;122:265.

131. Maisel AS, Peacock WF, McMullin N, et al. Timing of immunoreactive B-type natriuretic peptide levels and treatment delay in acute decompensated heart failure: an ADHERE

(Acute Decompensated Heart Failure National Registry) analysis. *J Am Coll Cardiol* 2008;52:534.

132. Paterna S, Di Pasquale P, Parrinello G, et al. Changes in brain natriuretic peptide levels and bioelectrical impedance measurements after treatment with high-dose furosemide and hypertonic saline solution versus high-dose furosemide alone in refractory congestive heart failure: a double-blind study. *J Am Coll Cardiol* 2005;45:1997.

133. Santos J, Planas R, Pardo A, et al. Spironolactone alone or in combination with furosemide in the treatment of moderate ascites in nonazotemic cirrhosis. A randomized comparative study of efficacy and safety. *J Hepatol* 2003;39:187.

134. Pitt B, Zannad F, Remme WJ, et al. The effect of spironolactone on morbidity and mortality in patients with severe heart failure. Randomized Aldactone Evaluation Study Investigators. *N Engl J Med* 1999;341:709.

135. Zannad F, McMurray JJ, Krum H, et al. Eplerenone in patients with systolic heart failure and mild symptoms. *N Engl J Med* 2011;364:11.

136. Pitt B, Remme W, Zannad F, et al. Eplerenone, a selective aldosterone blocker, in patients with left ventricular dysfunction after myocardial infarction. *N Engl J Med* 2003;348:1309.

137. Cody RJ. Diuretic Therapy. In Poole-Wilson P, Colucci WS, Massie BM, Chatterjee K, Coats AJ, editors: *Heart failure*. New York, 1997, Churchill Livingstone, pp 635-648.

138. Marenzi G, Lauri G, Grazi M, et al. Circulatory response to fluid overload removal by extracorporeal ultrafiltration in refractory congestive heart failure. *J Am Coll Cardiol* 2001;38:963.

139. Bart BA, Boyle A, Bank AJ, et al. Ultrafiltration versus usual care for hospitalized patients with heart failure: the Relief for Acutely Fluid-Overloaded Patients with Decompensated Congestive Heart Failure (RAPID-CHF) trial. *J Am Coll Cardiol* 2005;46:2043.

140. Costanzo MR, Saltzberg M, O'Sullivan J, et al. Early ultrafiltration in patients with decompensated heart failure and diuretic resistance. *J Am Coll Cardiol* 2005;46:2047.

141. Bart BA. Treatment of congestion in congestive heart failure: ultrafiltration is the only rational initial treatment of volume overload in decompensated heart failure. *Circ Heart Fail* 2009;2:499.

142. Accessed online August 19, 2011 at www.hfnetwork.org/hf-trials/carress-trial.

143. Leier CV, Bambach D, Thompson MJ, et al. Central and regional hemodynamic effects of intravenous isosorbide dinatrate, nitroglycerin, and nitroprusside in patients with congestive heart failure. *Am J Cardiol* 1981;48:1115.

144. Gori T, Parker JD. Nitrate tolerance: a unifying hypothesis. *Circulation* 2002;106:2510.

145. Cotter G, Metzkor E, Kaluski E, et al. Randomised trial of high-dose isosorbide dinitrate plus low-dose furosemide versus high-dose furosemide plus low-dose isosorbide dinitrate in severe pulmonary oedema. *Lancet* 1998;351:389.

146. Silver MA, Maisel A, Yancy CW, et al. BNP Consensus Panel 2004: A clinical approach for the diagnostic, prognostic, screening, treatment monitoring, and therapeutic roles of natriuretic peptides in cardiovascular diseases. *Congest Heart Fail* 2004;10:1.

147. Mills RM, LeJemtel TH, Horton DP, et al. Sustained hemodynamic effects of an infusion of nesiritide (human B-type natriuretic peptide) in heart failure: a randomized, double-blind, placebo-controlled clinical trial. Natrecor Study Group. *J Am Coll Cardiol* 1999;34:155.

148. Marcus LS, Hart D, Packer M, et al. Hemodynamic and renal excretory effects of human brain natriuretic peptide infusion in patients with congestive heart failure. A double-blind, placebo-controlled, randomized crossover trial. *Circulation* 1996;94:3184.

149. Colucci WS, Elkayam U, Horton DP, et al. Intravenous nesiritide, a natriuretic peptide, in the treatment of decompensated congestive heart failure. Nesiritide Study Group. *N Engl J Med* 2000;343:246.

150. Sackner-Bernstein JD, Kowalski M, Fox M, et al. Short-term risk of death after treatment with nesiritide for decompensated heart failure: a pooled analysis of randomized controlled trials. *JAMA* 2005;293:1900.

151. Hauptman PJ, Schnitzler MA, Swindle J, et al. Use of nesiritide before and after publications suggesting drug-related risks in patients with acute decompensated heart failure. *JAMA* 2006;296:1877.

152. Topol EJ. The lost decade of nesiritide. *N Engl J Med* 2011;365:81.

153. O'Connor CM, Starling RC, Hernandez AF, et al. Effect of nesiritide in patients with acute decompensated heart failure. *N Engl J Med* 2011;365:32.

154. Wang DJ, Dowling TC, Meadows D, et al. Nesiritide does not improve renal function in patients with chronic heart failure and worsening serum creatinine. *Circulation* 2004;110:1620.

155. Chen HH, Sundt TM, Cook DJ, et al. Low-dose nesiritide and the preservation of renal function in patients with renal dysfunction undergoing cardiopulmonary-bypass surgery: a double-blind placebo-controlled pilot study. *Circulation* 2007;116:I134-I138.

156. Accessed online August 11, 2011 at www.hfnetwork.org/hf-trials/rose-trial.

157. Michaels AD, Chatterjee K, De Marco T. Effects of intravenous nesiritide on pulmonary vascular hemodynamics in pulmonary hypertension. *J Card Fail* 2005;11:425.

158. Leyh RG, Kofidis T, Struber M, et al. Methylene blue: the drug of choice for catecholamine-refractory vasoplegia after cardiopulmonary bypass? *J Thorac Cardiovasc Surg* 2003;125:1426.

159. Yancy CW, Krum H, Massie BM, et al. Safety and efficacy of outpatient nesiritide in patients with advanced heart failure: results of the Second Follow-Up Serial Infusions of Nesiritide (FUSION II) trial. *Circ Heart Fail* 2008;1:9.

160. Miller RR, Awan NA, Joye JA, et al. Combined dopamine and nitroprusside therapy in congestive heart failure: greater augmentation of cardiac performance by addition of inotropic stimulation to afterload reduction. *Circulation* 1977;55:881.

161. Dixon LJ, Morgan DR, Hughes SM, et al. Functional consequences of endothelial nitric oxide synthase uncoupling in congestive cardiac failure. *Circulation* 2003;107:1725.

162. Packer M, Meller J, Medina N, et al. Rebound hemodynamic events after the abrupt withdrawal of nitroprusside in patients with severe chronic heart failure. *N Engl J Med* 1979;301:1193.

163. Friederich JA, Butterworth JF. Sodium nitroprusside: twenty years and counting. *Anesth Analg* 1995;81:152.

164. Ruffolo RR, Jr. The pharmacology of dobutamine. *Am J Med Sci* 1987;294:244.

165. Parker JD, Landzberg JS, Bittl JA, et al. Effects of beta-adrenergic stimulation with dobutamine on isovolumic relaxation in the normal and failing human left ventricle. *Circulation* 1991;84:1040.

166. Hare JM, Givertz MM, Creager MA, et al. Increased sensitivity to nitric oxide synthase inhibition in patients with heart failure: potentiation of beta-adrenergic inotropic responsiveness. *Circulation* 1998;97:161.

167. Uretsky BF, Hua J. Combined intravenous pharmacotherapy in the treatment of patients with decompensated heart failure. *Am Heart J* 1991;121:1679.

168. Takkenberg JJ, Czer LS, Fishbein MC, et al. Eosinophilic myocarditis in patients awaiting heart transplantation. *Crit Care Med* 2004;32:714.

169. DiBianco R. Acute positive inotropic intervention: the phosphodiesterase inhibitors. *Am Heart J* 1991;121:1871.

170. Givertz MM, Hare JM, Loh E, et al. Effect of bolus milrinone on hemodynamic variables and pulmonary vascular resistance in patients with severe left ventricular dysfunction: a rapid test for reversibility of pulmonary hypertension. *J Am Coll Cardiol* 1996;28:1775.

171. Colucci WS, Wright RF, Jaski BE, et al. Milrinone and dobutamine in severe heart failure: differing hemodynamic effects and individual patient responsiveness. *Circulation* 1986;73:III-175-III-183.

172. Lang CC, Hankins S, Hauff H, et al. Morbidity and mortality of UNOS status 1B cardiac transplant candidates at home. *J Heart Lung Transplant* 2003;22:419.

173. Colucci WS, Denniss AR, Leatherman GF, et al. Intracoronary infusion of dobutamine to patients with and without severe congestive heart failure: dose–response relationships, correlation with circulating catecholamines, and effect of phosphodiesterase inhibition. *J Clin Invest* 1988;81:1103.

174. Elkayam U, Tasissa G, Binanay C, et al. Use and impact of inotropes and vasodilator therapy in hospitalized patients with severe heart failure. *Am Heart J* 2007;153:98.

175. Givertz MM, Fang JC. Approach to the patient with hypotension and hemodynamic instability. In Irwin RS, Rippe JM, editors: *Intensive care medicine*, ed 6. Philadelphia, 2008, Lippincott, Williams & Wilkins, pp 327-336.

176. Elkayam U, Ng TM, Hatamizadeh P, et al. Renal vasodilatory action of dopamine in patients with heart failure: magnitude of effect and site of action. *Circulation* 2008;117:200.

177. Giamouzis G, Butler J, Starling RC, et al. Impact of dopamine infusion on renal function in hospitalized heart failure patients: results of the Dopamine in Acute Decompensated Heart Failure (DAD-HF) Trial. *J Card Fail* 2010;16:922.

178. Ungar A, Fumagalli S, Marini M, et al. Renal, but not systemic, hemodynamic effects of dopamine are influenced by the severity of congestive heart failure. *Crit Care Med* 2004;32:1125.

179. Port JD, Gilbert EM, Larrabee P, et al. Neurotransmitter depletion compromises the ability of indirect-acting amines to provide inotropic support in the failing human heart. *Circulation* 1990;81:929.

180. McKinlay KH, Schinderle DB, Swaminathan M, et al. Predictors of inotrope use during separation from cardiopulmonary bypass. *J Cardiothorac Vasc Anesth* 2004;18:404.

181. Gheorghiade M, Braunwald E. Reconsidering the role for digoxin in the management of acute heart failure syndromes. *JAMA* 2009;302:2146.

182. Kittleson M, Hurwitz S, Shah MR, et al. Development of circulatory-renal limitations to angiotensin-converting enzyme inhibitors identifies patients with severe heart failure and early mortality. *J Am Coll Cardiol* 2003;41:2029.

183. McMurray JJ, Ostergren J, Swedberg K, et al. Effects of candesartan in patients with chronic heart failure and reduced left-ventricular systolic function taking angiotensin-converting-enzyme inhibitors: the CHARM-Added trial. *Lancet* 2003;362:767.

184. Metra M, Teerlink JR, Voors AA, et al. Vasodilators in the treatment of acute heart failure: what we know, what we don't. *Heart Fail Rev* 2009;14:299.

185. Taylor AL, Ziesche S, Yancy C, et al. Combination of isosorbide dinitrate and hydralazine in blacks with heart failure. *N Engl J Med* 2004;351:2049.

186. Packer M, Meller J, Medina N, et al. Provocation of myocardial ischemic events during initiation of vasodilator therapy for severe chronic heart failure: clinical and hemodynamic evaluation of 52 consecutive patients with ischemic cardiomyopathy. *Am J Cardiol* 1981;48:939.

187. Metra M, Nodari S, D'Aloia A, et al. Beta-blocker therapy influences the hemodynamic response to inotropic agents in patients with heart failure: a randomized comparison of dobutamine and enoximone before and after chronic treatment with metoprolol or carvedilol. *J Am Coll Cardiol* 2002;40:1248.

188. Gattis WA, O'Connor CM, Gallup DS, et al. Predischarge initiation of carvedilol in patients hospitalized for decompensated heart failure. Results of the Initiation Management Predischarge: Process for Assessment of Carvedilol Therapy in Heart Failure (IMPACT-HF) trial. *J Am Coll Cardiol* 2004;43:1534.

189. O'Connor CM, Abraham WT, Albert NM, et al. Predictors of mortality after discharge in patients hospitalized with heart failure: an analysis from the Organized Program to Initiate Lifesaving Treatment in Hospitalized Patients with Heart Failure (OPTIMIZE-HF). *Am Heart J* 2008;156:662.

190. Koelling TM, Johnson ML, Cody RJ, et al. Discharge education improves clinical outcomes in patients with chronic heart failure. *Circulation* 2005;111:179.

191. Koelling TM, Johnson ML, Cody RJ, et al. Discharge education improves clinical outcomes in patients with chronic heart failure. *Circulation* 2005;111:179.

192. Goldsmith SR. Treatment options for hyponatremia in heart failure. *Heart Fail Rev* 2009;14:65.

193. Konstam MA, Gheorghiade M, Burnett JC Jr, et al. Effects of oral tolvaptan in patients hospitalized for worsening heart failure: the EVEREST Outcome Trial. *JAMA* 2007;297:1319.

194. Haque WA, Boehmer J, Clemson BS, et al. Hemodynamic effects of supplemental oxygen administration in congestive heart failure. *J Am Coll Cardiol* 1996;27:353.

195. Moradkhan R, Sinoway LI. Revisiting the role of oxygen therapy in cardiac patients. *J Am Coll Cardiol* 2010;56:1013.

196. Kasai T, Bradley TD. Obstructive sleep apnea and heart failure: pathophysiologic and therapeutic implications. *J Am Coll Cardiol* 2011;57:119.

197. Benza RL, Tallaj JA, Felker GM, et al. The impact of arrhythmias in acute heart failure. *J Card Fail* 2004;10:279.

198. Weinfeld MS, Drazner MH, Stevenson WG, et al. Early outcome of initiating amiodarone for atrial fibrillation in advanced heart failure. *J Heart Lung Transplant* 2000;19:638.
199. Vassallo P, Trohman RG. Prescribing amiodarone: an evidence-based review of clinical indications. *JAMA* 2007;298:1312.
200. Raymond JM, Sacher F, Winslow R, et al. Catheter ablation for scar-related ventricular tachycardias. *Curr Probl Cardiol* 2009;34:225.
201. Saidi A, Akoum N, Bader F. Management of unstable arrhythmias in cardiogenic shock. *Curr Treat Options Cardiovasc Med* 2011;13:354.
202. Bardy GH, Lee KL, Mark DB, et al. Amiodarone or an implantable cardioverter-defibrillator for congestive heart failure. *N Engl J Med* 2005;352:225.
203. Moss AJ, Zareba W, Hall WJ, et al. Prophylactic implantation of a defibrillator in patients with myocardial infarction and reduced ejection fraction. *N Engl J Med* 2002;346:877.
204. Piazza G, Goldhaber SZ. Chronic thromboembolic pulmonary hypertension. *N Engl J Med* 2011;364:351.
205. Nathan DM, Cleary PA, Backlund JY, et al. Intensive diabetes treatment and cardiovascular disease in patients with type 1 diabetes. *N Engl J Med* 2005;353:2643.
206. Inzucchi SE. Oral antihyperglycemic therapy for type 2 diabetes: scientific review. *JAMA* 2002;287:360.
207. Horwich TB, Fonarow GC, Hamilton MA, et al. Anemia is associated with worse symptoms, greater impairment in functional capacity and a significant increase in mortality in patients with advanced heart failure. *J Am Coll Cardiol* 2002;39:1780.
208. Felker GM, Adams KF Jr, Gattis WA, et al. Anemia as a risk factor and therapeutic target in heart failure. *J Am Coll Cardiol* 2004;44:959.
209. Pfeffer MA, Burdmann EA, Chen CY, et al. A trial of darbepoetin alfa in type 2 diabetes and chronic kidney disease. *N Engl J Med* 2009;361:2019.
210. Lucas C, Johnson W, Hamilton MA, et al. Freedom from congestion predicts good survival despite previous class IV symptoms of heart failure. *Am Heart J* 2000;140:840.
211. Phillips CO, Wright SM, Kern DE, et al. Comprehensive discharge planning with postdischarge support for older patients with congestive heart failure: a meta-analysis. *JAMA* 2004;291:1358.
212. McAlister FA, Stewart S, Ferrua S, et al. Multidisciplinary strategies for the management of heart failure patients at high risk for admission: a systematic review of randomized trials. *J Am Coll Cardiol* 2004;44:810.
213. Kwok T, Lee J, Woo J, et al. A randomized controlled trial of a community nurse-supported hospital discharge programme in older patients with chronic heart failure. *J Clin Nurs* 2008;17:109.
214. Akashi YJ, Goldstein DS, Barbaro G, et al. Takotsubo cardiomyopathy: a new form of acute, reversible heart failure. *Circulation* 2008;118:2754.
215. Kar B, Gregoric ID, Basra SS, et al. The percutaneous ventricular assist device in severe refractory cardiogenic shock. *J Am Coll Cardiol* 2011;57:688.
216. Burkhoff D, Cohen H, Brunckhorst C, et al. A randomized multicenter clinical study to evaluate the safety and efficacy of the TandemHeart percutaneous ventricular assist device versus conventional therapy with intraaortic balloon pumping for treatment of cardiogenic shock. *Am Heart J* 2006;152:469.
217. Seyfarth M, Sibbing D, Bauer I, et al. A randomized clinical trial to evaluate the safety and efficacy of a percutaneous left ventricular assist device versus intra-aortic balloon pumping for treatment of cardiogenic shock caused by myocardial infarction. *J Am Coll Cardiol* 2008;52:1584.
218. Sanchez L, I, Almenar BL, Martinez-Dolz L, et al. Effect of circulatory assistance on premature death and long-term prognosis. *Transplant Proc* 2008;40:3025.
219. Wilson SR, Givertz MM, Stewart GC, et al. Ventricular assist devices the challenges of outpatient management. *J Am Coll Cardiol* 2009;54:1647.
220. Burkhoff D, Klotz S, Mancini DM. LVAD-induced reverse remodeling: basic and clinical implications for myocardial recovery. *J Card Fail* 2006;12:227.
221. Kirklin JK, Naftel DC, Kormos RL, et al. Third INTERMACS Annual Report: the evolution of destination therapy in the United States. *J Heart Lung Transplant* 2011;30:115.
222. Wilson SR, Mudge GH Jr, Stewart GC, et al. Evaluation for a ventricular assist device: selecting the appropriate candidate. *Circulation* 2009;119:2225.
223. Deshmukh A, Kumar G, Kumar N, et al. Effect of Joint National Committee VII Report on Hospitalizations for Hypertensive Emergencies in the United States. *Am J Cardiol* 2011;108:1277.
224. Gandhi SK, Powers JC, Nomeir AM, et al. The pathogenesis of acute pulmonary edema associated with hypertension. *N Engl J Med* 2001;344:17.
225. Katz JN, Gore JM, Amin A, et al. Practice patterns, outcomes, and end-organ dysfunction for patients with acute severe hypertension: the Studying the Treatment of Acute hyper-Tension (STAT) registry. *Am Heart J* 2009;158:599.
226. Peacock F, Amin A, Granger CB, et al. Hypertensive heart failure: patient characteristics, treatment, and outcomes. *Am J Emerg Med* 2011;29:855.
227. De Backer D, Biston P, Devriendt J, et al. Comparison of dopamine and norepinephrine in the treatment of shock. *N Engl J Med* 2010;362:779.
228. Peacock WF, Hollander JE, Diercks DB, et al. Morphine and outcomes in acute decompensated heart failure: an ADHERE analysis. *Emerg Med J* 2008;25:205.
229. Hochman JS, Sleeper LA, Webb JG, et al. Early revascularization in acute myocardial infarction complicated by cardiogenic shock. SHOCK Investigators. Should We Emergently Revascularize Occluded Coronaries for Cardiogenic Shock. *N Engl J Med* 1999;341:625.
230. Capomolla S, Pozzoli M, Opasich C, et al. Dobutamine and nitroprusside infusion in patients with severe congestive heart failure: hemodynamic improvement by discordant effects on mitral regurgitation, left atrial function, and ventricular function. *Am Heart J* 1997;134:1089.
231. Khot UN, Novaro GM, Popovic ZB, et al. Nitroprusside in critically ill patients with left ventricular dysfunction and aortic stenosis. *N Engl J Med* 2003;348:1756.
232. Ben Dor I, Pichard AD, Satler LF, et al. Complications and outcome of balloon aortic valvuloplasty in high-risk or inoperable patients. *JACC Cardiovasc Interv* 2010;3:1150.
233. Masip J, Roque M, Sanchez B, et al. Noninvasive ventilation in acute cardiogenic pulmonary edema: systematic review and meta-analysis. *JAMA* 2005;294:3124.
234. Gray A, Goodacre S, Newby DE, et al. Noninvasive ventilation in acute cardiogenic pulmonary edema. *N Engl J Med* 2008;359:142.
235. Lieberman EB, Hutchins GM, Herskowitz A, et al. Clinicopathologic description of myocarditis. *J Am Coll Cardiol* 1991;18:1617.
236. McCarthy RE III, Boehmer JP, Hruban RH, et al. Long-term outcome of fulminant myocarditis as compared with acute (nonfulminant) myocarditis. *N Engl J Med* 2000;342:690.
237. Cooper LT Jr, Berry GJ, Shabetai R. Idiopathic giant-cell myocarditis—natural history and treatment. Multicenter Giant Cell Myocarditis Study Group Investigators. *N Engl J Med* 1997;336:1860.
238. Cooper LT Jr, Hare JM, Tazelaar HD, et al. Usefulness of immunosuppression for giant cell myocarditis. *Am J Cardiol* 2008;102:1535.
239. Zile MR, Brutsaert DL. New concepts in diastolic dysfunction and diastolic heart failure: Part I: diagnosis, prognosis, and measurements of diastolic function. *Circulation* 2002;105:1387.
240. Brignole M, Botto G, Mont L, et al. Cardiac resynchronization therapy in patients undergoing atrioventricular junction ablation for permanent atrial fibrillation: a randomized trial. *Eur Heart J* 2011;32:2420.
241. Campia U, Nodari S, Gheorghiade M. Acute heart failure with low cardiac output: can we develop a short-term inotropic agent that does not increase adverse events? *Curr Heart Fail Rep* 2010;7:100.
242. Lee CR, Watkins ML, Patterson JH, et al. Vasopressin: a new target for the treatment of heart failure. *Am Heart J* 2003;146:9.
243. Udelson JE, Smith WB, Hendrix GH, et al. Acute hemodynamic effects of conivaptan, a dual V(1A) and V(2) vasopressin receptor antagonist, in patients with advanced heart failure. *Circulation* 2001;104:2417.
244. Gheorghiade M, Niazi I, Ouyang J, et al. Vasopressin V2-receptor blockade with tolvaptan in patients with chronic heart failure: results from a double-blind, randomized trial. *Circulation* 2003;107:2690.
245. Schrier RW, Gross P, Gheorghiade M, et al. Tolvaptan, a selective oral vasopressin V2-receptor antagonist, for hyponatremia. *N Engl J Med* 2006;355:2099.
246. Teichman SL, Unemori E, Teerlink JR, et al. Relaxin: review of biology and potential role in treating heart failure. *Curr Heart Fail Rep* 2010;7:75.
247. Teerlink JR, Metra M, Felker GM, et al. Relaxin for the treatment of patients with acute heart failure (Pre-RELAX-AHF): a multicentre, randomised, placebo-controlled, parallel-group, dose-finding phase IIb study. *Lancet* 2009;373:1429.
248. Haikala H, Nissinen E, Etemadzadeh E, et al. Troponin C-mediated calcium sensitization induced by levosimendan does not impair relaxation. *J Cardiovasc Pharmacol* 1995; 25:794.
249. Slawsky MT, Colucci WS, Gottlieb SS, et al. Acute hemodynamic and clinical effects of levosimendan in patients with severe heart failure. *Circulation* 2000;102:2222.
250. Kivikko M, Lehtonen L, Colucci WS. Sustained hemodynamic effects of intravenous levosimendan. *Circulation* 2003;107:81.
251. Mebazaa A, Nieminen MS, Packer M, et al. Levosimendan vs dobutamine for patients with acute decompensated heart failure: the SURVIVE Randomized Trial. *JAMA* 2007; 297:1883.
252. Malik FI, Hartman JJ, Elias KA, et al. Cardiac myosin activation: a potential therapeutic approach for systolic heart failure. *Science* 2011;331:1439.
253. Teerlink JR, Clarke CP, Saikali KG, et al. Dose-dependent augmentation of cardiac systolic function with the selective cardiac myosin activator, omecamtiv mecarbil: a first-in-man study. *Lancet* 2011;378:667.
254. Shen YT, Malik FI, Zhao X, et al. Improvement of cardiac function by a cardiac myosin activator in conscious dogs with systolic heart failure. *Circ Heart Fail* 2010;3:522.
255. Cleland JG, Teerlink JR, Senior R, et al. The effects of the cardiac myosin activator, omecamtiv mecarbil, on cardiac function in systolic heart failure: a double-blind, placebo-controlled, crossover, dose-ranging phase 2 trial. *Lancet* 2011;378:676.
256. Fonarow GC, Abraham WT, Albert NM, et al. Influence of a performance-improvement initiative on quality of care for patients hospitalized with heart failure: results of the Organized Program to Initiate Lifesaving Treatment in Hospitalized Patients With Heart Failure (OPTIMIZE-HF). *Arch Intern Med* 2007;167:1493.
257. Alahdab MT, Mansour IN, Napan S, et al. Six-minute walk test predicts long-term all-cause mortality and heart failure rehospitalization in African-American patients hospitalized with acute decompensated heart failure. *J Card Fail* 2009;15:130.
258. Sharma GV, Woods PA, Lindsey N, et al. Noninvasive monitoring of left ventricular end-diastolic pressure reduces rehospitalization rates in patients hospitalized for heart failure: a randomized controlled trial. *J Card Fail* 2011;17:718.
259. Aziz EF, Kukin M, Javed F, et al. Right ventricular dysfunction is a strong predictor of developing atrial fibrillation in acutely decompensated heart failure patients. ACAP-HF data analysis. *J Card Fail* 2010;16:827.
260. Wang NC, Maggioni AP, Konstam MA, et al. Clinical implications of QRS duration in patients hospitalized with worsening heart failure and reduced left ventricular ejection fraction. *JAMA* 2008;299:2656.
261. Metra M, Nodari S, Parrinello G, et al. Worsening renal function in patients hospitalised for acute heart failure: clinical implications and prognostic significance. *Eur J Heart Fail* 2008;10:188.
262. Gheorghiade M, Rossi JS, Cotts W, et al. Characterization and prognostic value of persistent hyponatremia in patients with severe heart failure in the ESCAPE Trial. *Arch Intern Med* 2007;167:1998.

CHAPTER **15**

Cardiac Transplantation and Circulatory Support Devices

Jeffrey Teuteberg, Michael A. Mathier, and Michael A. Shullo

OVERVIEW, 307

PATIENT SELECTION FOR ADVANCED HEART FAILURE
THERAPIES, 307

CARDIAC TRANSPLANTATION, 307

Patient Selection, 307
Pretransplantation Patient Management, 309
Cardiac Transplantation Surgical Technique, 309

Management of the Patient After Cardiac Transplantation, 309
Prevention and Treatment of Posttransplant
    Complications, 310
Future Directions, 314

MECHANICAL CIRCULATORY SUPPORT, 314

Benefits of Mechanical Circulatory Support, 314
Configuration of Mechanical Circulatory Support, 314

Indications for Mechanical Circulatory Support, 315
Timing of Support, 315
Considerations Prior to Long-Term Mechanical Circulatory
    Support, 317

REFERENCES, 319

Overview

Despite treatment with new drug regimens and high-risk cardiac surgery, many patients with heart failure (HF) progress to advanced stages characterized by marked symptomatic limitation and profound hemodynamic compromise. Cardiac transplantation is the first-line therapy for select patients with end-stage HF. In the United States, 135 transplant centers perform approximately 2000 procedures annually. Unfortunately, the limited supply of donor hearts has restricted the growth of cardiac transplantation and has led to the search for alternative strategies, such as mechanical circulatory support (MCS). The recent explosion in MCS technology offers the promise of a universally available therapy to decrease morbidity and mortality rates in all patients with end-stage HF. Taken together, cardiac transplantation and MCS are often referred to as *advanced HF therapies*, and their availability is generally limited to advanced HF centers.

Patient Selection for Advanced Heart Failure Therapies

Although important differences exist in patient selection for cardiac transplantation and MCS, a number of considerations are shared. An algorithm for patient selection for advanced HF therapies is shown in Figure 15-1. Selection issues specific to each modality are addressed in their respective sections of this chapter.

Cardiac Transplantation

Human cardiac transplantation was first performed in 1967. Over more than 4 decades, cardiac transplantation has evolved into the gold standard therapy for many patients with end-stage HF. This evolution has been made possible by significant advances in every aspect of cardiac transplantation: recipient and donor selection and management, organ preservation, surgical technique, immunosuppression, and management of acute and chronic posttransplantation complications. More than 3000 cardiac transplantations are performed worldwide each year, and the 1-, 5-, and 10-year survival rates after cardiac transplantation are approximately 88%, 75%, and 56%, respectively.[1] Long-term survival (more than 15 years) is not uncommon, with a graft half-life in the modern era of transplant of 12.9 years, largely as a result of more limited and targeted immunosuppression. The total number of cardiac transplantations performed annually has not changed substantially in the past 20 years, mostly owing to limited donor availability.[2]

During this same period, dramatic advances have been made in the medical and nontransplant surgical therapy of patients with advanced HF. Comprehensive pharmacotherapy has significantly delayed the progression of HF to its advanced stages. Biventricular

pacemakers and implantable cardioverter-defibrillator devices (ICDs) have contributed importantly to reductions in the rates of HF morbidity and mortality. In addition, surgical advances have allowed the benefits of coronary revascularization and valvular repair to be extended to patients with poor ventricular function. Nevertheless, cardiac transplantation remains the best option for many patients with advanced HF.

Patient Selection

Although cardiac transplantation offers excellent patient outcomes, it has several important limitations. Among these are inadequate donor availability, significant perioperative risk, and substantial posttransplantation morbidity and mortality. Consequently, optimizing patient selection for the procedure is critical. The overriding principle is to select patients whose cardiac dysfunction substantially impairs their lifestyle and threatens their life span, but who do not have sufficient extracardiac comorbidities to importantly compromise posttransplant outcome.[3] Individual transplant programs establish their own inclusion and exclusion criteria; a representative list of criteria is shown in Box 15-1.

Cardiac transplantation is most commonly performed for chronic severe left ventricular (LV) systolic dysfunction, although it is occasionally used in patients with other advanced cardiac pathology such as coronary artery disease, hypertrophic cardiomyopathy, restrictive cardiomyopathy, and others. A standard array of cardiac tests is generally performed to thoroughly assess each patient's cardiac status. The goals of cardiac testing are to determine that 1) the cardiac disease limits functional status or anticipated survival to a degree sufficient to warrant consideration of transplantation; 2) no acceptable alternative therapies, medical or surgical, are available for the cardiac disease; 3) irreversible pulmonary hypertension is not present; and 4) appropriate therapy is chosen to bridge the patient to transplantation.

ASSESSMENT OF CARDIAC DISEASE SEVERITY

The assessment of the severity of cardiac disease is based on anatomic, functional, and hemodynamic data. The functional assessment includes a determination of New York Heart Association (NYHA) class, as well as more objective measures of exercise capacity, such as peak oxygen consumption (VO_2) or 6-minute walk distance. Peak VO_2 is measured by breath-to-breath respiratory gas analysis during either bicycle ergometry or graded treadmill exercise. In a seminal study, peak VO_2 was found to predict death in patients with advanced HF.[4] Based on this study, a peak VO_2 of 14 mL/kg/min or less is commonly used as a threshold for listing the patient for cardiac transplantation. Studies have suggested that in patients with advanced HF who are treated with β-adrenergic antagonists, this threshold may be too high, and a

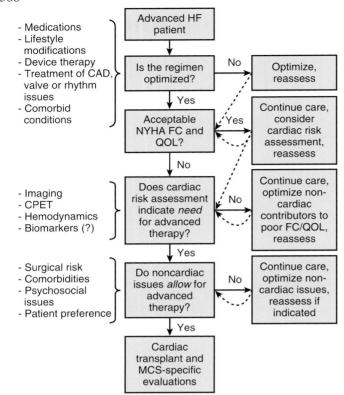

- Medications
- Lifestyle modifications
- Device therapy
- Treatment of CAD, valve or rhythm issues
- Comorbid conditions

- Imaging
- CPET
- Hemodynamics
- Biomarkers (?)

- Surgical risk
- Comorbidities
- Psychosocial issues
- Patient preference

FIGURE 15-1 Approach to the patient with advanced heart failure (*HF*). CAD, coronary artery disease; CPET, cardiopulmonary exercise testing; FC, functional class; MCS, mechanical circulatory support; NYHA, New York Heart Association; QOL, quality of life.

Box 15-1 Selection Criteria for Cardiac Transplantation

Candidates
1. Advanced heart failure with refractory New York Hospital Association class III and IV symptoms and markedly shortened life expectancy
2. Advanced coronary artery disease with refractory angina
3. Malignant ventricular arrhythmias unresponsive to standard therapies

Exclusion Criteria
1. Advanced age
2. Irreversible pulmonary hypertension
3. Chronic noncardiac illness that compromises survival and functional recovery
4. Severe peripheral vascular disease
5. Morbid obesity
6. Active or recent malignancy
7. Active infection (excluding chronic drive line infections of mechanical circulatory support devices)
8. Human immunodeficiency virus seroconversion
9. Drug, tobacco, or alcohol abuse within the previous 6 months
10. Psychiatric or psychosocial instability

lower peak VO$_2$ may be more appropriate for transplant listing.[5] Other parameters obtained during these studies—including minute ventilation/carbon dioxide (VE/CO$_2$) slope, a measure of ventilatory efficiency—have been shown to predict outcome, and these measures may be useful in the evaluation of a patient's candidacy for cardiac transplantation.[6]

The 6-minute walk distance has been shown to correlate well with peak VO$_2$, suggesting that this simpler measure of functional capacity can be used in place of the more cumbersome oxygen-consumption study.[7] A number of readily available clinical and laboratory parameters—such as hyponatremia, azotemia, anemia,

and cachexia—along with intolerance of neurohormonal antagonists or dependence on inotropic support identify patients with a poor prognosis.[8] Calculation of a risk score based on clinical variables has been advocated by some as a more refined predictor of outcome in patients with advanced HF.[9,10]

ASSESSMENT OF THE PULMONARY VASCULATURE

An important determinant of candidacy for cardiac transplantation is the status of the pulmonary circulation. Patients with long-standing left-sided HF frequently develop pulmonary hypertension, which may or may not reverse with acute or chronic vasodilator therapy. Agents commonly used to assess pulmonary vasoreactivity acutely include sodium nitroprusside, prostaglandin E1 (PGE1), milrinone, and inhaled nitric oxide. Patients with reversible pulmonary hypertension have posttransplant survival rates similar to those with normal pulmonary pressures prior to transplant. Patients with irreversible pulmonary hypertension (pulmonary vascular resistance persistently >2.5 U) have a significantly worse posttransplant survival, largely due to failure of the donor right ventricle (RV).[11] For these patients, alternative strategies may be considered, such as MCS as a bridge to a decision on transplant candidacy, combined heart-lung transplantation, or heterotopic heart transplantation with retention of the native heart to take advantage of its "trained" RV.[12]

OTHER CARDIAC TRANSPLANTATION CANDIDACY ISSUES

Age

Many adult cardiac transplant programs establish an upper age cutoff of 65 years for transplant candidacy. Data from the International Society for Heart and Lung Transplantation (ISHLT) Registry have suggested that survival after cardiac transplantation declines with increasing recipient age after 50 years of age; this effect is most striking above 70 years of age.[1,2] Among the possible explanations for this association is the apparent increased risk of post-transplantation malignancy in older versus younger patients. Despite this, several reports of acceptable outcomes in an older patient population have emerged.[13,14]

Comorbidities

Many cardiac transplantation programs list significant, irreversible, noncardiac organ dysfunction as an exclusion criterion. Examples include intrinsic kidney disease with a creatinine clearance of 40 mL/min or less, intrinsic lung disease with spirometric values less than 50% of predicted, and biopsy-proven liver cirrhosis. However, a number of successful multiorgan transplantations have been reported, most commonly combined heart-kidney, heart-lung, and heart-liver transplants.[15,16] Moreover, some of these abnormalities may reverse with MCS. Similarly, significant noncardiac comorbidities, such as diabetes with end-organ dysfunction, may exclude patients from cardiac transplantation, although reports of acceptable outcomes in these populations do exist.[17] Other relative contraindications to transplant include conditions that are likely to worsen with corticosteroid therapy, such as obesity and osteoporosis.

Immunologic Sensitization

Although rarely an exclusion for cardiac transplantation by itself, immunologic sensitization of potential transplant recipients—that is, the presence of anti–human leukocyte antigen (HLA) donor-specific antibodies—can pose a significant challenge. All potential recipients undergo immunologic assessment, usually via a complement-dependent cytotoxicity assay or panel-reactive antibodies (PRA). If elevated (>10%), further evaluation of antibody specificity is warranted using a more sensitive solid-phase assay, such as flow cytometry.[18] Highly sensitized candidates commonly have a history of multiple pregnancies, prior transfusions, or prior placement of an MCS device; they require careful donor

TABLE 15-1	United Network of Organ Sharing Heart Allocation System
STATUS	**DEFINITION**
1A	Patient admitted to the listing center with: 1. Mechanical ventilation 2. Intraaortic balloon pump 3. Extracorporeal membrane oxygenator 4. All VADs receive 30 days of the highest status at some time after implantation or in the setting of device complication 5. Single high-dose or multiple low-dose inotrope infusion with pulmonary artery catheter monitoring
1B	Patient on low-dose single inotrope or on uncomplicated mechanical VAD for more than 30 days
2	Patient not meeting 1A or 1B criteria
7	Patient listed but temporarily unsuitable for cardiac transplantation

VAD, ventricular assist device.

selection and perioperative immunologic management, which will be described here.

Listing for Cardiac Transplantation

The United Network of Organ Sharing (UNOS) was created in 1986 by the United States Congress to oversee the allocation of organs on a nationwide basis to recipients who have been registered by transplant programs on regional waiting lists. Local Organ Procurement Organizations (OPOs) are nonprofit agencies responsible for evaluating the suitability of potential donor organs and for coordinating organ recovery, preservation, and transport to the transplant center. Organs are allocated according to ABO blood typing, size matching, duration on the waiting list, and severity of disease. In 1999, UNOS updated the criteria by which disease severity affects patient priority on the waiting list. Table 15-1 summarizes the current UNOS status criteria.

Improved success rates with cardiac transplantation have inevitably led to efforts to expand the procedure to previously excluded patient populations. One controversial strategy that has been used by some centers is the creation of a second or alternate list for those candidates deemed to be at higher risk.[19,20] Organs accepted for patients on this list are those judged to be marginal, such as organs from older donors or from donors with single-vessel coronary disease, and are therefore not acceptable for most candidates who meet standard listing criteria, although some have argued that using suboptimal donor organs for higher risk candidates will lead to worse outcomes.

Pretransplantation Patient Management

Patients deemed to be acceptable candidates for cardiac transplantation require careful management as they await the procedure. Standard pharmacologic and device therapies for HF, as well as appropriate lifestyle modifications, are recommended for all patients. Patients with intractable signs and symptoms related to low cardiac output and end-organ hypoperfusion (kidney or liver dysfunction or poor nutritional status) may require continuous inotropic therapy or MCS, both of which affect the priority status of the patient in the UNOS system. Patients managed with continuous intravenous (IV) inotropic therapy or MCS require careful surveillance for, and aggressive therapy of, infection. Similarly, patients with evidence of pulmonary hypertension require careful follow-up of their pulmonary pressures. Chronic LV unloading with MCS may prevent worsening of pulmonary hypertension, and it may even reverse previously refractory pulmonary hypertension and allow for successful transplantation.[21]

Patients found to be highly immunologically sensitized may benefit from immunomodulatory therapy before undergoing cardiac transplantation. Numerous protocols have been described

in the literature, including those that use immunoglobulin, rituximab, and plasmapheresis.[22,23] The goal of these protocols is to reduce the patient's burden of preformed antibodies to commonly encountered antigens, both to increase the possibility of finding a donor with a negative prospective crossmatch, thus shortening the waiting time, and to decrease the chance of rejection of the transplanted heart.

Cardiac Transplantation Surgical Technique

The surgical technique for cardiac transplantation has remained fairly constant for the last two decades. One significant modification of the original operation has been the adoption of a bicaval anastomotic technique in place of the standard biatrial anastomosis. With both techniques, the donor left atrium is anastomosed to a retained cuff of recipient left atrium with the pulmonary veins left intact. In the bicaval technique, the donor and recipient vena cavae are anastomosed after complete excision of the recipient right atrium. Studies indicate that the bicaval technique results in improved atrial function and decreased incidence of atrial arrhythmias.[24,25] A further modification, termed *total orthotopic cardiac transplantation,* combines a bicaval anastomosis with pulmonary vein anastomoses. This technique has not as yet been shown to offer significant benefit over biatrial or bicaval techniques.[26]

Advances have also been made in the area of organ preservation after harvest.[27] This may have contributed to the observation that outcomes with longer donor ischemic times are not markedly worse compared with those with shorter ischemic times.[28] Further technological development, including beating-heart donor transport, may improve outcomes further. In addition, immediate postoperative management has improved with the judicious use of inotropic agents, acute pulmonary vasodilators, and even temporary mechanical cardiac support for instances of transient allograft dysfunction related to ischemia, elevated pulmonary pressures, or both.[29-31]

Management of the Patient After Cardiac Transplantation

The management of the patient after cardiac transplantation involves three main strategies: 1) optimization of immunosuppressive therapy, 2) prevention of allograft rejection and complications resulting from the transplant or the immunosuppressive agents, and 3) treatment of allograft rejection and associated complications when they arise. The relative impact of these various conditions on mortality rates varies over time after cardiac transplantation.[2]

Rejection is an important cause of morbidity and mortality after cardiac transplantation. Rejection after transplantation is due to an alloimmune response involving naïve and memory lymphocytes. Specifically, after foreign antigen recognition and appropriate presentation, the immune response is activated, targeting the allograft. The response may be humoral (antibody), cell mediated (T cell), or a combination of both. Current immunosuppression focuses on multiple pharmacologic targets in this cascade.[32]

Despite intensive investigation of potential noninvasive indicators of rejection, transvenous endomyocardial biopsy remains the diagnostic tool of choice; current ISHLT criteria for grading acute rejection are shown in Table 15-2.[33] Of note, however, a recently published multicenter study suggested that peripheral blood gene expression profiling of circulating leukocytes may be able to identify low-risk patients for whom it is safe to defer endomyocardial biopsy.[34] The risk of acute cellular rejection is highest in the first year after cardiac transplantation and declines significantly thereafter. This observation underlies the strategy of more intensive immunosuppression and surveillance for rejection early after transplantation, with a gradual decrease in both over time (Table 15-3). The incidence of infection correlates with the degree of immunosuppression and is higher in the months following transplantation, and it declines thereafter. Accordingly, prophylaxis against opportunistic infections is generally indicated early after transplantation, when the level of immunosuppression is highest.[35,36]

After cardiac transplantation, other conditions assume greater importance over time in determining patient outcome. Hypertension, diabetes, and dyslipidemia are quite common, occurring in 76%, 27%, and 74% of patients within the first year after cardiac transplantation, respectively.[2] The high incidence of these conditions reflects the fact that they are frequent comorbidities in patients who require transplantation and that immunosuppressive therapy can cause or exacerbate these conditions. Aggressive therapy of each is recommended, although data indicating that this improves outcomes in patients following cardiac transplantation are limited.[37] Among the important sequelae that may be prevented or delayed with such therapy are cardiac allograft vasculopathy (CAV) and renal insufficiency. Late mortality after cardiac transplantation is predominantly related to CAV, renal failure, and malignancy.[2]

The risk of rejection is at its maximum during the initial period of exposure to the allograft, and consequently the level of immunosuppression is maintained at its highest level during the first 6 months posttransplant. For long-term survival, limiting the complications of immunosuppression is of primary importance and leads to a critical additional management goal: to limit rejection with the lowest level of immunosuppression possible.

PREVENTION AND TREATMENT OF CARDIAC REJECTION

The primary management goal of immunosuppressive therapy is to limit episodes of acute rejection and minimize long-term drug-related morbidity. Strategies to achieve these goals may vary from center to center, but several underlying fundamental approaches are commonly used, based on the timing of medication and its mechanism of action or its origin. Immunosuppressants can be classified in one of three ways: by use as 1) induction therapy,

2) maintenance therapy, or 3) therapy of rejection. Some medications can be used for dual purposes. Induction therapy is generally administered immediately prior to transplant, intraoperatively, or in the immediate postoperative period in an effort to minimize the immune response immediately after transplantation. Maintenance therapy is taken indefinitely from the time of transplant to minimize the long-term risk of rejection. Medications used for treatment of rejection are generally used as a short course of therapy to reverse the ongoing immunologic attack on the allograft.

Classification of immunosuppressive therapy by mechanism of action and origin reveals several distinct classes of medications: monoclonal antibodies, polyclonal antibodies, calcineurin inhibitors, antimetabolites, proliferation signal inhibitors, and corticosteroids (Tables 15-4 and 15-5).[18,32,38]

Postoperative immunosuppression can vary greatly from program to program; however, the combination of tacrolimus, mycophenolate mofetil (MMF) or mycophenolic acid, and prednisone continue to be the most commonly prescribed immunosuppressive choices after heart transplantation. Several centers have published data describing rapid steroid weaning after transplantation with similar rejection rates compared with more traditional extended corticosteroid use.[39,40] Also, with the use of newer induction agents, it is possible to safely minimize or completely avoid maintenance corticosteroid use.[41] The use of induction immunosuppression has gradually increased over the last 15 years with 54% of centers worldwide using induction therapy. The majority of these patients receive an interleukin-2 receptor (IL2R) antagonist, and slightly fewer receive polyclonal antilymphocytic antibodies.[2]

DRUG INTERACTIONS

Drug interactions are a common concern with immunosuppressants.[18] Prescription and over-the-counter medications, supplements, and nutraceuticals can have both pharmacodynamic and pharmacokinetic effects on many immunosuppressive agents (Box 15-2) Frequently, interactions can occur with tacrolimus, cyclosporine, sirolimus, and everolimus, which are all metabolized by the cytochrome P450 3A4 isoenzyme. Numerous drugs that inhibit or induce this system are known to increase (diltiazem, allopurinol, amiodarone) or decrease (nafcillin, phenobarbitol, phenytoin) immunosuppressant exposure. Some drug interactions with immunosuppressants are significant enough to cause major morbidity,[42] therefore careful consideration is required before initiation of additional drug therapy in this patient population.

Prevention and Treatment of Posttransplant Complications

The major complications that occur following cardiac transplantation include infection, hypertension, diabetes, dyslipidemia, osteoporosis, CAV, renal insufficiency, and malignancy. The top three

TABLE 15-2	International Society for Heart and Lung Transplantation Standardized Cardiac Biopsy Grading: Acute Cellular Rejection*
Grade 0 R	No rejection
Grade 1 R, mild	Interstitial and/or perivascular infiltrate with up to one focus of myocyte damage
Grade 2 R	Two or more foci of infiltrate with moderate associated myocyte damage
Grade 3 R	Diffuse infiltrate with multifocal myocyte damage ± edema ± hemorrhage ± vasculitis

*The presence or absence of acute antibody-mediated rejection (AMR) may be recorded as AMR 0 or AMR 1, as required.

TABLE 15-3	Frequency of Follow-up Evaluations After Cardiac Transplantation				
	DISCHARGE TO WEEK 4	MONTH 1 TO MONTH 3	MONTH 4 TO YEAR 1	YEAR 1 TO YEAR 5	AFTER YEAR 5
Office visit	1 week	2 week	1-2 months	3-6 months	6 months to 1 year
Bloodwork	1 week	2 week	1-2 months	3 months	3 months
Right heart catheterization and biopsy	1 week	2 week	1-2 months	3 months to 1 year	As needed
Echocardiogram	As needed	At month 3	3 months	6 months to 1 year	As needed
Dopamine stress echocardiogram	—	—	At year 1	1 year	1 year
Coronary angiogram	—	—	At year 1	2 year	As needed

Blood work includes serum chemistries, complete blood count, liver function testing, serum levels of calcineurin inhibitor and sirolimus, lipid profile, glycosylated hemoglobin, uric acid, and, less frequently, thyroid studies.
From Mathier MA, McNamara DM. Management of the patient after heart transplant. *Curr Treat Options Cardiovasc Med* 2004;6:459-469.

TABLE 15-4 Polyclonal and Monoclonal Antibodies Used as Immunosuppressants in Heart Transplantation

DRUG	DESCRIPTION	MECHANISM	USE*	TOXICITY AND COMMENTS
Basiliximab	Chimeric monoclonal antibody against CD25	Binds to and blocks the IL-2 receptor on activated T cells, depleting them and inhibiting IL-2–induced T-cell activation	Induction	Hypersensitivity reactions (uncommon); 2 doses required; no monitoring required
Alemtuzumab	Humanized monoclonal antibody against CD52	Binds to CD52 on all B and T cells, most monocytes, macrophages, and natural killer cells, causing cell lysis and prolonged depletion	Induction/ACR	Mild cytokine release syndrome, neutropenia, anemia, idiosyncratic pancytopenia, autoimmune thrombocytopenia, thyroid disease
Antithymocyte globulin	Polyclonal IgG from horses or rabbits immunized with human thymocytes	Blocks T-cell membrane proteins, causing altered function, lysis, and prolonged T-cell depletion	Induction/ACR	Cytokine release syndrome (fever, chills, hypotension), thrombocytopenia, leukopenia, serum sickness
Rituximab	Chimeric monoclonal antibody against CD20	Binds to CD20 on B cells and mediates B-cell lysis	AMR	Infusion reactions, hypersensitivity reactions (uncommon)

*Most common clinical indications.
ACR, acute cellular rejection treatment; AMR, antibody-mediated rejection treatment; Ig, immunoglobulin; IL, interleukin.
Modified from Halloran PF. Immunosuppressive drugs for kidney transplantation. *N Engl J Med* 2004;351:2715-2729.

TABLE 15-5 Common Maintenance Immunosuppressants Used in Heart Transplantation

DRUG	CLASS	MECHANISM	MONITORING†	TOXICITY AND COMMENTS
Cyclosporine	CI	Binds to cyclophilin; complex inhibits calcineurin phosphatase and T-cell activation	2-hour postdose blood level or trough: initially 200-375 ng/mL, decreasing to 150-250 ng/mL ≥6 months from transplant*	Nephrotoxicity, hemolytic-uremic syndrome, hypertension, neurotoxicity, gum hyperplasia, skin changes, hirsutism, posttransplantation diabetes mellitus, hyperlipidemia
Tacrolimus	CI	Binds to FKBP12; complex inhibits calcineurin phosphatase and T-cell activation	Trough: Initially 10-15 ng/mL, decreasing to 5-10 ng/mL ≥6 months from transplant	Effects similar to those of cyclosporine but with a lower incidence of hypertension, hyperlipidemia, skin changes, hirsutism, and gum hyperplasia and a higher incidence of posttransplantation diabetes mellitus and neurotoxicity
Sirolimus	PSI	Binds to FKBP12; complex inhibits target of rapamycin and interleukin-2–driven T-cell proliferation	Trough: 4-12 ng/mL when used with a CI	Hyperlipidemia, increased toxicity of calcineurin inhibitors, thrombo-cytopenia, delayed wound healing, delayed graft function, mouth ulcers, pneumonitis, interstitial lung disease; lipid monitoring required; recipients whose risk of rejection is low to moderate can stop cyclosporine treatment 2 to 4 mo after transplantation
Everolimus	PSI	Derivative of sirolimus	Trough: 3-8 ng/mL when used with a CI	Similar to sirolimus
Mycophenolate mofetil or myco-phenolic acid	AM	Inhibits synthesis of guanosine monophosphate nucleotides; blocks purine synthesis, preventing proliferation of T and B cells	Routine monitoring of MPA levels; cannot be recommended at this time	Gastrointestinal symptoms (mainly diarrhea), colitis, neutropenia, mild anemia; absorption reduced by cyclosporine
Azathioprine	AM	Converts 6-mercaptopurine to tissue inhibitor of metalloproteinase, which is converted to thioguanine nucleotides that interfere with DNA synthesis; prevents proliferation of T and B cells	No routine blood level monitoring available; blood count monitoring required	Leukopenia, bone marrow suppression, macrocytosis, liver toxicity (uncommon)
Prednisone	Steroid	Block cytokine activation, interfere with cell migration, recognition, and cytotoxic effector mechanisms	No routine blood level monitoring available	Glucose intolerance, osteopenia, skeletal myopathy, hypertension, hyperlipidemia, weight gain, and cataracts

*Abbott TDX assay.
†Depending on programmatic protocol.
AM, antimetabolite; CI, calcineurin inhibitor; PSI, proliferation signal inhibitor
Modified from Halloran PF. Immunosuppresive drugs for kidney transplantation. *N Engl J Med* 2004;351:2715-2729; and Costanzo MR, Dipchand A, Starling R, et al. The International Society of Heart and Lung Transplantation Guidelines for the care of heart transplant receipients. *J Heart Lung Transplant* 2010;29(8):914-956.

Box 15-2 Common Drugs that Interfere with Cyclosporine, Tacrolimus, Sirolimus, or Everolimus

Decrease Immunosuppression Levels

Antimicrobials
Caspofungin
Nafcillin
Rifabutin
Rifampin
Rifapentine

Antiepileptics
Carbamazepine
Fosphenytoin
Phenytoin
Phenobarbital

Antiretroviral Therapy
Efavirenz
Etravirine
Nevirapine

Others
Antacids containing magnesium, calcium, or aluminum (tacrolimus only)
Deferasirox
Modafinil
St. John's wort
Thalidomide
Ticlopidine
Troglitazone

Increase Immunosuppression Levels

Antimicrobials
Clarithromycin
Erythromycin
Metronidazole
Tinidazole
Quinupristin/dalfopristin

Antifungals
Clotrimazole
Itraconazole

Ketoconazole
Fluconazole
Posaconazole
Voriconazole

Antiretroviral Therapy
Protease inhibitors (general)
Amprenavir
Atazanavir
Darunavir
Fosamprenavir
Indinavir
Nelfinavir
Ritonavir
Saquinavir
Tipranavir

Cardiovascular
Amiodarone
Diltiazem
Verapamil
Nutraceuticals
Bitter orange
Grapefruit juice
Pomegranate

Others
Rilonacept
Theophylline
Cimetidine
Fluvoxamine
Glipizide
Glyburide
Imatinib
Nefazodone

Modified from Costanzo MR, Dipchand A, Starling R, et al. The International Society of Heart and Lung Transplantation Guidelines for the care of heart transplant receipients. *J Heart Lung Transplant* 2010;29(8):914-956.

causes of mortality in patients who survive more than 5 years after transplant are malignancy, CAV, and graft failure.[2] Changes in immunosuppression, alternative drug therapy, and lifestyle modification are techniques employed to minimize posttransplant morbidity and mortality.

INFECTIONS

Infections after transplantation occur in three distinct phases, with different risks associated with each. The *early phase* (<1 month) includes donor/recipient derived infections and nosocomial infections. The *intermediate phase* (1 to 6 months) includes infections by a number of viruses and bacteria—most notably herpesviruses, cytomegalovirus (CMV), *Pneumocystis carinii* pneumonia, *Listeria, Toxoplasma gondii, Nocardia,* and oropharyngeal *Candida.* The late phase (>6 months) includes more traditional infections: urinary tract infections, community-acquired pneumonia, late CMV, *Aspergillus, Nocardia,* and polyomavirus.[35] The major focus of infection prophylaxis is in the early and intermediate phases.

The risk of viral opportunistic infection is related to the intensity and type of immunosuppression and the viral status of both the donor and the recipient. A recipient without prior CMV exposure who receives a heart from a CMV-positive donor has a 50% to 75% risk of developing CMV disease; a recipient with prior CMV exposure has a 10% to 15% chance, regardless of donor status.[43] Patients at high risk for CMV disease generally receive oral ganciclovir (1000 mg PO three times daily) or valganciclovir (900 mg/day PO) with adjustment for renal function for 3 to 6 months *or* IV

ganciclovir (5 to 10 mg/kg/day) for 1 to 3 months; some centers add CMV immune globulin. Patients at lower risk may use these regimens or preemptive therapy, monitoring with nucleic acid testing or CMV antigenemia assays and treating when patients test positive.[18]

CMV disease is notorious for nonspecific symptoms and findings: the clinical presentation can range from a mild influenza-like illness to life-threatening pneumonitis or enteritis; therefore a high index of suspicion for CMV is required when evaluating constitutional, respiratory, or gastrointestinal (GI) complaints.

Pneumocystis carinii pneumonia is infrequently seen with current prophylactic strategies. The risk of this disease is greatest during the period of highest corticosteroid dosing, prompting the use of prophylactic trimethoprim-sulfamethoxazole (single-strength 80/400 mg tablet PO every day or double strength on alternate days) for the first 6 to 12 months, with less frequent dosing or discontinuation thereafter. This agent also appears to be effective against a variety of other pathogens, including *Toxoplasma gondii, Listeria,* and urinary tract pathogens.[44] Atovaquone or dapsone may be acceptable alternatives in patients with sulfa allergy or in those who develop renal insufficiency or hyperkalemia on trimethoprim-sulfamethoxazole, and nystatin liquid or mycostatin troches are usually effective in preventing oropharyngeal candidiasis. Although these pathogens represent the most common targets for antibiotic prophylaxis in patients following cardiac transplantation, many other opportunistic and nonopportunistic infections can occur, and a high index of suspicion for opportunistic infections is required. A full discussion of the therapy of established infections is beyond the scope of this chapter.[45]

HYPERTENSION

Hypertension occurs frequently in cardiac transplant recipients; the incidence in long-term follow-up has been reported to be more than 70% at 1 year and as much as 95% at 5 years. Hypertension after cardiac transplantation may have several etiologies, including preexisting essential hypertension, chronic use of calcineurin inhibitors, chronic kidney disease, and alterations in function of the renin-angiotensin-aldosterone system.[46]

Most standard antihypertensive agents are safe and are likely to be effective in patients following cardiac transplantation. A randomized comparison of diltiazem and lisinopril in hypertensive transplant patients found both agents to be safe, but neither consistently provided adequate blood pressure control when used as monotherapy.[47] Diltiazem may have the ancillary benefits of raising calcineurin levels and, in one study, of slowing the development of CAV.[48] In practice, multidrug regimens for the control of hypertension are common and often include adrenergic antagonists such as α-blockers or clonidine. A thorough understanding of potential drug interactions is mandatory.

DIABETES

Cardiac transplantation in patients with diabetes at the time of surgery appears to offer a similar outcome to transplant in patients without diabetes.[49] In the first year after cardiac transplantation, however, preexisting diabetes frequently becomes much more difficult to treat. In addition, many patients will develop diabetes for the first time during this period, primarily as a result of corticosteroid and calcineurin therapy.[50] This is why many innovative immunosuppression strategies have been used to either minimize steroid exposure or use no steroids after transplantation.[38,51]

Either oral agents or insulin may be effective in the treatment of transplant-related diabetes.[52] Metformin is generally avoided because of concerns over renal dysfunction. Referral to a diabetes management specialist or program can help to optimize glycemic control and address modifiable factors such as obesity. Consensus guidelines for the management of diabetes in transplant recipients have been published.[53]

DYSLIPIDEMIA

Dyslipidemia develops in 50% of patients at 1 year and in more than 80% at 5 years and appears to be more severe in patients treated with cyclosporin A as compared with tacrolimus; fewer patients treated with tacrolimus require lipid-lowering therapy.[54,55] A small, randomized trial in patients with posttransplant dyslipidemia compared simvastatin, gemfibrozil, and cholestyramine and demonstrated superior total and LDL cholesterol–lowering effects for simvastatin, whereas gemfibrozil improved triglyceride levels.[56] A larger, longer-term randomized trial of simvastatin started early after heart transplantation versus dietary therapy alone revealed significant reduction in mortality, rates of CAV, and severe rejection without significant adverse effects in the simvastatin group.[57] This and other studies suggest that statins may have beneficial immunomodulatory effects independent of their effects on lipids. A head-to-head nonrandomized comparison of simvastatin and pravastatin suggested greater safety and efficacy of pravastatin.[58] Atorvastatin also appears to be safe and effective in the treatment of dyslipidemia in the transplant patient.[59] Accordingly, pravastatin and atorvastatin are the generally preferred agents. The risk of myositis and rhabdomyolysis is increased with statin use in patients following cardiac transplantation, necessitating use of lower doses and less aggressive lipid targets along with heightened clinical surveillance for such complications when using higher doses or combinations of agents.

CARDIAC ALLOGRAFT VASCULOPATHY

CAV is now the most common cause of late allograft dysfunction in patients following cardiac transplantation.[2] Risk factors for the development of CAV include the frequency and severity of cellular rejection,[60] smoking, dyslipidemia, diabetes, antecedent coronary artery disease in either the recipient or donor, and older age of either the recipient or donor.[61] Studies indicate a potential role of systemic inflammation and infectious agents in the development of CAV,[62] which is associated with both worse functional status[63] and worse survival,[64,65] with late manifestations that include refractory HF and sudden cardiac death. During transplantation, the innervation to the heart is disrupted, and the transplanted heart becomes reinnervated only infrequently, and only partially; because of this, most patients do not develop angina, so a regular screening strategy is necessary. Intravascular ultrasound is the most sensitive diagnostic test for the detection of CAV, but it is infrequently used because of cost considerations and center inexperience. Thus coronary angiography, radionuclide perfusion imaging, and dobutamine stress echocardiography are the screening tests of choice (see Table 15-3). CAV may be a diffuse, concentric, and often distal process not amenable to percutaneous or surgical revascularization. On occasion, however, it may manifest as discrete, proximal stenoses treatable by standard revascularization techniques.[66]

Medical therapy of CAV generally includes the use of a statin to aggressively lower cholesterol and changes in maintenance immunosuppression. In addition to their beneficial effects on serum lipid levels, statins preserve coronary endothelial function and modulate the elaboration of proinflammatory cytokines in the transplanted heart.[67] Long-term follow-up data also suggest that statins improve survival in heart transplant recipients.[68] When combined with CsA, corticosteroids, and statins, everolimus decreased the incidence of CAV within the first year after cardiac transplantation compared with azathioprine added to the same combination.[69] In patients with established CAV, substituting sirolimus for azathioprine or MMF, in combination with corticosteroids and a calcineurin inhibitor, may attenuate disease progression.[70] Coronary angioplasty[64,65] and stenting[66,71] have both been used with acceptable results in the treatment of CAV. In addition, standard, off-pump,[72] and minimally invasive coronary artery bypass grafting (CABG)[73] have been successfully performed in highly select patients who have undergone cardiac transplantation. Retransplantation for CAV appears to have greater success than when it is used for acute graft failure or acute cellular rejection.[74] Although the rate of early mortality following retransplantation for CAV is comparable with that of initial transplantation, long-term survival is worse.[75]

RENAL INSUFFICIENCY

The risk of renal insufficiency is related to patient age, baseline renal function, and the development of hypertension.[76,77] The incidence of end-stage renal disease after cardiac transplantation is 6.3% in patients who survive 10 years, and survival in those who experience renal failure is significantly worse than in those with preserved renal function.[2] It is generally accepted that calcineurin inhibitor use increases the risk of renal insufficiency. The conversion of patients from a calcineurin inhibitor–based immunosuppressive regimen to one based on MMF and sirolimus or everolimus appears to be safe and effective and is associated with an improvement in renal function.[78,79] Hemodialysis, peritoneal dialysis, and renal transplantation have all been reported to be acceptable therapies for end-stage renal disease in cardiac transplant patients.[80]

MALIGNANCY

The final major cause of morbidity and mortality in patients after cardiac transplantation is malignancy, which is the leading cause of death in patients who survive more than 5 years after transplantation.[81,82] Additionally, according to the heart transplant registry data, 14% of 5-year and 30% of 10-year survivors after transplant have had some form of malignancy.[2] Recipients of organ transplants have a greater risk of developing most cancers,[83,84] and heart transplant recipients in particular seem to have a significantly higher risk of developing lymphomas (Epstein-Barr virus–associated posttransplant lymphoproliferative disease [PTLD]) and skin cancers.[85,86] One large study of patients after heart transplantation found an overall incidence of PTLD of 6% and an incidence among long-term survivors of 15%.[87] In general, the risk of malignancy appears to correlate with the intensity and duration of immunosuppression. Patients exposed to lytic induction therapy and those who receive lytic therapy for treatment of severe rejection are at particularly high risk.[83,84] Although younger recipients of cardiac transplants may be at higher risk for PTLD,[86] patients who are older at the time of transplantation appear to be at significantly increased risk for non-PTLD cancers.[88] PTLD often responds to a decrease in the intensity of immunosuppression, with or without concomitant antineoplastic therapy. Disease progression can often be monitored with serial positron emission tomography (PET) or computed tomography (CT) scanning. An anti-CD20 monoclonal antibody, rituximab, has been reported to be of benefit in select cases.[89]

Skin cancers that develop in transplant recipients, particularly squamous or basal cell carcinomas, generally respond well to local excision. Additional treatment may include oral retinoids or topical chemotherapy agents[90]; however, recurrence is common regardless of therapy. Because of this high rate of recurrence, many programs may choose to alter maintainance immunosuppression in an effort to decrease risk. Specifically, calcineurin-free therapy, utilizing either sirolimus or everolimus in addition to a low-dose MMF product has been used in stable, low-risk patients. The majority of these data are from the renal and liver transplant populations, but the results are impressive, with up to a threefold reduction in risk of solid organ and skin cancer. These benefits can occur as early as 2 years after calcineurin discontinuation.[81,82,84] Alterations in long-standing maintenance immunosuppression carry inherent risks of rejection, therefore close immunologic and histologic surveillance is necessary.

Future Directions

The last several decades have seen significant improvements in the management of patients before and after cardiac transplantation. One challenge for the future will be to extend the life expectancy of patients following transplantation. This will depend on our ability to prevent and treat the long-term complications of transplantation, including many of the long-term consequences of immunosuppression. Toward this end, extensive investigation is underway into possible strategies for minimization of maintenance immunosuppression. If successful, such strategies would likely yield an optimal posttransplant outcome. Ongoing investigation in the fields of xenotransplantation and regenerative medicine may offer the possibility of an unlimited supply of donor organs and allow for expansion of transplantation to increasing numbers of patients.

Mechanical Circulatory Support

Since it was first introduced into clinical use nearly 50 years ago, MCS has grown from being able to provide only partial support for short periods to select patient populations to providing permanent support of the entire circulation for many years in most patients with chronic systolic HF. The past decade has also seen a substantial change in device technology with bulky, less durable pulsatile devices giving way to substantially smaller and more durable continuous-flow pumps.

Benefits of Mechanical Circulatory Support

HEMODYNAMIC

As the LV fails, there is a concomitant increase in intracardiac filling pressures and eventually a decrease in cardiac output. The primary focus of MCS is to restore perfusion while decompressing the failing ventricle.[91] Restoration of cardiac output provides end-organ perfusion and eventually allows for improvement in exercise capacity. The chronic reduction of LV filling pressures decreases the severity of mitral regurgitation and reduces pulmonary arterial hypertension, which in turn can improve RV function. Relief of the HF state with MCS also leads to a reduction in neurohormonal activation, which may alleviate the cardiorenal syndrome and may even allow for myocardial recovery.[92]

BIOLOGIC

The hemodynamic benefits of MCS are also accompanied by concomitant improvements in the myriad of negative cellular and extracellular effects of chronic HF. Isolated myocytes after MCS have shown improved contractile function and greater responsiveness to β-adrenergic stimulation.[93-96] MCS has also been shown to alter myocyte gene and protein expression and to reduce the degree of fibrosis and collagen content within the cardiac extracellular matrix.[97,98]

Configuration of Mechanical Circulatory Support

Devices are categorized by several general categories: the duration of support, the ventricles supported, and the mechanism of pump flow. The duration of support can be temporary, such as post cardiotomy or in acute shock or for stabilization prior to the implantation of a more permanent device. In the United States, two major indications are approved for MCS, as a bridge to transplant (BTT) or as long-term support in the transplant ineligible, known as *destination therapy* (DT). Devices allow for support of the RV alone (RV assist device, or RVAD) or the LV alone (LVAD) or for biventricular (BiVAD) support, or in the case of the total artificial heart (TAH), the device can be implanted in place of the native heart. Although most pumps are implanted within the thoracic and/or abdominal cavity with only a percutaneous drive line to provide for pump power and monitoring, some are extracorporeal or paracorporeal in location, with the pump outside of the body and transcutaneous cannulae that allow for inflow and outflow of blood.

PULSATILE FLOW

Most prior generations of MCS were pulsatile pumps, which sequentially filled and emptied a volume displacement chamber, thus generating pulsatile flow. These pumps typically filled passively or with only a modest ability to augment their filling and were operated in a mode that was asynchronous to the native hearts. With less preload, the pumps filled less quickly; with more preload, the pump filled more quickly, thus maintaining decompression of the LV. But there are many disadvantages to pulsatile pumps: the need for a volume displacement chamber necessitated a larger pump size, maintenance of unidirectional flow required the use of valves, and the resultant mechanical wear led to shorter pump life, often less than 18 months.

CONTINUOUS FLOW

Continuous-flow pumps move blood with a rotating impeller, which results in a continuous, active unloading of the LV and provides forward flow with limited pulsatility. The degree of LV unloading is dependent upon the set speed of the device. Speeds are typically set to maintain a constant unloading of the LV such that the aortic valve infrequently opens. Continuous-flow pumps are categorized as either *axial* or *centrifugal* pumps. The impeller in an axial-flow pump spins in the same axis as the blood flow; in contrast, centrifugal pumps accelerate the blood perpendicularly to the axis of inflow. The only moving part is the impeller, which is

HeartMate II LVAD   HeartMate XVE LVAD

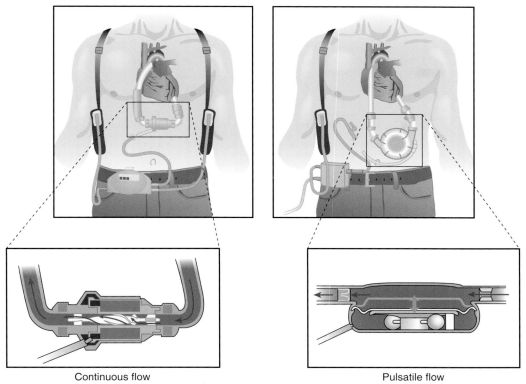

Continuous flow   Pulsatile flow

FIGURE 15-2   Representative HeartMate (Thoratec Corporation) pulsatile and continuous-flow left ventricular assist devices (*LVAD*). *(From Wilson SR, Givertz MM, Stewart GC, Mudge GH Jr. Ventricular assist devices: the challenges of outpatient management.* J Am Coll Cardiol *2009;54:1647-1659.)*

supported by mechanical bearings, or it can be magnetically or hydrodynamically suspended to result in minimal wear. Eliminating the volume-displacement chamber has allowed for dramatic reductions in the pump size; substantially longer pump life, owing to reductions in mechanical wear; and generally superior adverse-event profiles that have resulted in substantial improvements in quality of life and functional capacity for patients.[99] Given these benefits, continuous-flow pumps are now the dominant pump technology. Representative pulsatile- and continuous-flow pumps are shown in Figure 15-2.

CANNULATION

Most MCS is implanted in parallel with the native left or right ventricle. For LV support, an inflow cannula is placed into the LV apex, and outflow is through a cannula anastomosed to the ascending aorta just above the aortic valve. For temporary percutaneous systems, the pump can receive inflow transseptally from the left atrium, or from the LV itself, with a pump positioned across the aortic valve. When supporting the RV, inflow is typically from the right atrium, which provides more reliable flow than RV apical cannulation. Temporary devices may access venous blood from the cavae or femoral veins. The outflow cannula of the RVAD is anatomosed to the main pulmonary artery just distal to the pulmonic valve.

Indications for Mechanical Circulatory Support

Mechanical support can be used for several days or for long-term support over many years. Although a variety of short-term devices are placed to allow for revascularization or recovery, this chapter will focus primarily on the devices meant for more durable long-term support. The primary indication for MCS had been as a bridge to transplant (BTT), but a growing proportion of patients

who are not transplant eligible receive MCS in lieu of transplant (DT).[100-102]

UNIVENTRICULAR VERSUS BIVENTRICULAR SUPPORT

Although either or both ventricles may be supported, an LVAD alone is the preferred modality for those who require long-term support, because the current generation of small, continuous-flow devices are designed for LV support alone. On the other hand, long-term biventricular support can only be accomplished with two separate paracorporeal devices (BiVAD), one for each ventricle, or with a TAH.[103] Although the BiVAD and TAH are reasonable options for those who need such support, the degree of anticoagulation, side-effect profile, and patient-device interface are inferior to continuous flow LVAD support.

The adequacy of native RV function becomes the critical factor in choosing between LV versus biventricular support. When an LVAD is implanted in the setting of RV failure, the filling of the LV, and hence the LVAD, will be insufficient and the LVAD will not function properly.[104] Therefore for patients with concomitant severe RV dysfunction, biventricular support may be necessary. Determining the adequacy of RV function can be difficult (see below); despite efforts to predict and mitigate it, the rate of RV failure requiring an RVAD after an LVAD is approximately 7%.[105-110]

Timing of Support

Emergent mechanical support is usually reserved for those who come to medical attention because of an acute insult: an extensive myocardial infarction, postcardiotomy shock, or fulminant myocarditis. For such patients, the focus is on hemodynamic stabilization, because a comprehensive assessment of the patient prior to MCS is not feasible. Furthermore, the consideration of long-term goals

CH
15

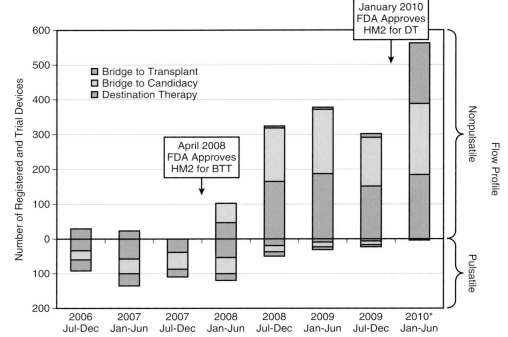

FIGURE 15-3 Evolution of device type and strategy over time. BTT, bridge to transplant; DT, destination therapy; FDA, Food and Drug Administration; HM2, Heart-Mate II (Thoratec Corporation). *(From Stewart GC, Stephenson LW. Keeping left ventricular assist device acceleration on track.* Circulation *2011;123:1559-1568.)*

(BTT or DT) is not the immediate consideration, but often patients with an acute presentation may have some degree of recovery of ventricular function that allows eventual weaning of the device. Given this, many such patients are supported with temporary devices to allow for the possibility of ventricular recovery. However, if the ventricle does not recover sufficiently, MCS allows for end-organ recovery and provides time to determine whether the patient is suitable for long-term support.[111] Despite reasonable outcomes for those who are supported emergently, such patients have higher rates of both morbidity and mortality.[112]

Given the worse outcomes in those who are implanted emergently, centers prefer to implant MCS electively. Even with chronic inotropy for those awaiting heart transplant, there can be repeated hospitalizations, progressive end-organ dysfunction, and an increased risk of adverse events.[113] Thus the appropriate timing for referral for assessment and implantation of MCS is critical.

When approaching patients who do not require emergent support, the timing of MCS becomes paramount. A few patients may have an identifiable and treatable cause of their decompensation, such as ischemia or dysrhythmia, and they should be given time to respond to medical therapy. However, the issue of timing of MCS is most germane to those with chronic, progressive systolic dysfunction. For those who are eligible or are already listed for transplantation, the risks and benefits of earlier implantation of MCS must be balanced against continuing aggressive medical support in hopes of obtaining a suitable organ.[114] The major reason to wait for transplantation would be to avoid the potential morbidity and mortality of the surgery for, and life with, MCS. Some patients may have surgical or anatomic considerations that may make MCS relatively contraindicated.[115] The risk to delaying MCS include a higher risk of transplant in the setting of acute or prolonged decompensation, the need for emergent mechanical support, and progression of HF, which leads to transplant or MCS ineligibility or death. The benefit to earlier MCS is that patients who are less ill at the time of implant have superior outcomes. Once patients recover from the MCS implant, the HF state resolves, and they can undergo physical rehabilitation; hence, the transplant can be performed in the setting of clinical stability. The expected wait time for organs also weighs heavily in the decision regarding the timing of MCS.

The wait time may be affected by patient size, blood type, where they live, and the types and strengths of the patient's preformed antibodies. Of the patients currently implanted with noninvestigational devices in the United States, only half are actively listed at the time of MCS (Figure 15-3). Many patients have relative contraindications to listing for transplant, but a period of mechanical support may allow the patient to become a transplant candidate; this is colloquially referred to as a *bridge to decision*. Such contraindications may be medical problems that MCS will alleviate, such as pulmonary hypertension or renal dysfunction, or MCS may allow time for an issue to be adequately addressed, such as substance abuse or obesity, or treated, such as localized prostate or bladder cancer.

The relatively poor long-term outcome with the prior generation of pulsatile devices dampened enthusiasm for earlier implantation. The 6- and 12-month survival rates after pulsatile devices were roughly 75% and 60%, respectively; however, with modern continuous-flow devices, survival at 6 and 12 months is 95% and 90%, respectively.[116] Not only has survival improved with the current generation of devices, but the adverse event profiles have improved, and the pumps are much smaller and more suitable for a much broader population of patients.[116,117] Much of the early morality after MCS has been attributed to patient selection, which has led to the search for risk factors and risk scores to allow for improved patient selection.

Many of the available risk models were developed from single-center experiences with small numbers of patients, based mostly on pulsatile devices, or they are from a prior era of MCS management and thus may not be applicable to the devices available today.[118-120] Despite these limitations, many of these risk scores continue to be used clinically. The most common of these is the Lietz-Miller risk score, also known as the *Destination Therapy Risk Score (DTRS)*; however, recent data show that the DTRS is not predictive of post-MCS outcomes for continuous-flow MCS when implanted as BTT and is only modestly predictive for DT.[121-122] The Seattle Heart Failure Model (SHFM) comprises risk factors from multiple clinical trials of HF but included very few patients with end-stage HF.[123] However, those patients with lower SHFM scores prior to implantation have better outcomes after MCS.[124] In general,

TABLE 15-6 Intermacs Profiles

PROFILE	DESCRIPTIONS	TIME FRAME FOR INTERVENTION
1: Critical cardiogenic shock	Patients with life-threatening hypertension despite rapidly escalating inotropic support; critical organ hypoperfusion, often confirmed by worsening acidosis and/or lacate levels ("crash and burn")	Definitive intervention needed within hours
2: Progressive decline	Patient with declining function despite inotropic support; may be manifested by worsening renal function, nutritional depletion, inability to restore volume balance ("strong on inotropes"); also describes declining status in patients unable to tolerate inotropic therapy	Definitive intervention needed within a few days
3: Stable but inotrope dependent	Patient with stable blood pressure, organ function, nutrition, and symptoms on continuous intravenous inotropic support (or a temporary circulatory support device, or both), but demonstrating repeated failure to wean from support because of recurrent symptomatic hypotension or renal dysfunction ("dependent stability")	Definitive intervention elective over a period of weeks to a few months
4: Resting symptoms	Patient can be stabilized close to normal volume status but experiences daily symptoms of congestion at rest or during ADLs. Doses of diuretics generally fluctuate at very high levels. More intensive management and surveillance strategies should be considered, which may, in some cases, reveal poor compliance that would compromise outcome with any therapy (some patients may move between profiles 4 and 5)	Definitive intervention elective over a period of weeks to a few months
5: Exertion intolerant	Comfortable at rest and with ADLs but unable to engage in any other activity, staying predominantly within the house; patients are comfortable at rest without congestive symptoms but may have underlying, refractory, elevated volume status, often with renal dysfunction; with marginal underlying nutritional status and organ function, patient may be more at risk than at profile 4 and may require definitive intervention	Variable urgency, depends on maintenance of nutrition, organ function, and activity level
6: Exertion limited	Patient without evidence of fluid overload, comfortable at rest and with ADLs and minor activities outside the home, but fatigues after the first few minutes of any meaningful activity; attention to cardiac limitation requires careful measurement of peak oxygen consumption, in some cases with hemodynamic monitoring to confirm severity of cardiac impairment ("walking wounded")	Variable urgency, depends on maintenance of nutrition, organ function, and activity level
7: Advanced New York Heart Association class II	A placeholder for more precise specification in the future; includes patients who are without current or recent episodes of unstable fluid balance, living comfortably with meaningful activity limited to mild physical exertion	Transplantation or circulatory support may not be currently indicated

ADLs, activities of daily living.
From Stevenson LW, Pagani FD, Young JB, et al. INTERMACS profiles of advanced heart failure: the current picture. *J Heart Lung Transplant* 2009;28:535-541.

the high-risk features found in those studies—such as RV failure, respiratory failure, renal and hepatic dysfunction, and infection—are typically markers of a higher degree of illness at the time of implantation.

The Interagency Registry for Mechanically Assisted Circulatory Support (INTERMACS) is a registry of approved durable devices in the United States. Patients entered into INTERMACS are assigned one of seven profiles according to the their level of illness, ranging from 7 (NYHA class IIIb) to 1 (patients in acute shock), as seen in Table 15-6.[125] Outcomes stratified by INTERMACS profiles demonstrate that those with lower profiles—that is, sicker patients—have worse outcomes than those with higher INTERMACS profiles, as shown in Figure 15-4.[126] Patients who have advanced HF but are not yet inotrope dependent, INTERMACS profiles 4 through 7, have been shown to have significantly greater survival at 18 months (96% vs. 73%, $P < .01$) than those who are inotrope dependent.[127]

Considerations Prior to Long-Term Mechanical Circulatory Support

CARDIAC CONSIDERATIONS

Right Ventricular Function

Adequate RV function is critical for a patient being considered for an LVAD. RV dysfunction results in inadequate filling of the left heart and thus the LVAD, and it is associated with high rates of morbidity and mortality. Furthermore, most durable MCS approved as bridge and destination therapy only support the LV. Although BiVADs and the artificial heart can be used as a BTT, they are associated with worse survival, are less suitable for long-term support, and are not approved as DT. RV dysfunction can result from the underlying myopathy, may be exacerbated by left-sided

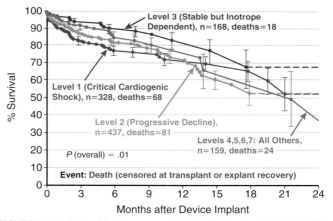

FIGURE 15-4 Survival by Interagency Registry for Mechanically Assisted Circulatory Support (INTERMACS) profile. *(From Kirklin JK, Naftel DC, Kormos RL, et al. Second INTERMACS annual report: more than 1,000 primary left ventricular assist device implants.* J Heart Lung Transplant *2010;29:1-10.)*

failure, or may arise from other factors such as lung disease, pulmonary hypertension, pulmonary vascular disease, or from complications during surgery. Continuous-flow pumps can even induce RV dysfunction by shifting the intraventricular septum to the left.

Echocardiography alone is often inadequate to determine the degree of RV dysfunction.[128] A full assessment of the RV requires pulmonary arterial catheterization. A high right atrial pressure in conjunction with low pulmonary arterial pressures is often indicative of severe RV failure.[129] Numerous risk-prediction models are available for RV failure, but they are limited by being small, single-center experiences with mostly pulsatile pumps.[108,109,130] A single, large study of continuous-flow devices found that the multivariate predictors of RV failure were preoperative ventilator support (odds ratio [OR], 5.5), a central venous pressure to pulmonary capillary wedge pressure ratio greater than 0.63 (OR, 2.3), and a blood urea nitrogen (BUN) level above 39 (OR, 2.1).[131]

Valvular Disease

Aortic insufficiency can adversely affect LVAD performance by creating a "blind loop" of flow from the LV, through the LVAD, into the aortic root, then back to the LV. Patients with more than mild aortic insufficiency should have the valve surgically repaired, replaced, or oversewn at the time of LVAD placement. Mechanical aortic valves can become thrombosed in the setting of an LVAD because of decreased transvalvular flow; such valves should be replaced with a tissue valve or should be oversewn.[132] Mitral stenosis can affect inflow of blood into the LVAD, and this must be addressed at the time of implantation.

Arrhythmias

Most supraventricular arrhythmias are well tolerated with an LVAD. However, persistent ventricular tachycardia or ventricular fibrillation is not well tolerated in the setting of an LVAD because these rhythms lead to RV dysfunction. Patients with VT storm often require biventricular support.

Other Cardiac Abnormalities

A comprehensive survey should also investigate for the presence of atrial or ventricular septal defects that need to be repaired. Complex congenital heart disease may necessitate unusual pump orientations or may preclude the use of MCS altogether. Lastly, mural thrombus must be identified and removed at the time of implantation to avoid systemic embolization or thrombus being drawn into the pump.

NONCARDIAC CONSIDERATIONS

Other chronic medical conditions, many of which are exacerbated by advanced HF, should be optimized prior to implantation of long-term MCS. Patients must be assessed for signs of infection, and if found, should be treated aggressively prior to implantation. Active infection at the time of implantation can be catastrophic, as septicemia can result in device infection, which may be chronically suppressed, but rarely cured, with antibiotic therapy. If the pump or the pocket in which it sits becomes infected, the only recourse is urgent transplant, if indicated, because device exchanges in these situations often result in recurrent infection.[133] Renal dysfunction at the time of presentation is common, and it stems from a variety of causes: poor renal perfusion, high central venous pressures, preexisting renal dysfunction, high doses of diuretics, and the adverse neurohormonal milieu of HF. If the patient has decompensated hemodynamics, the use of inotropes, intraaortic balloon pump, or even temporary mechanical support may allow for renal recovery. Improvement of renal function is often seen with restoration of cardiac output and resolution of the HF state after MCS, but it is not the rule, especially when patients are implanted in the setting of significant renal dysfunction.[134,135] Renal failure requiring dialysis after MCS remains a highly morbid event, likely reflecting the patient's level of illness at surgery and an additional, persistent nidus of infection as a result of vascular access.[136]

Intrinsic pulmonary disease also has a number of implications for long-term MCS. Advanced lung disease impacts mortality and morbidity from the implantation surgery itself, and it also affects the patient's ability to rehabilitate postoperatively and can continue to affect long-term functional status. Hypoxic pulmonary vasoconstriction from intrinsic lung disease may also exacerbate preexisting pulmonary hypertension. Severe chronic pulmonary disease with an FEV_1 of less than 1 L should raise concerns about a patient's suitability for MCS.[132] Intubation and mechanical

ventilation prior to implantation is also a strong predictor of poor outcomes.[106] Hepatic dysfunction is occasionally a result of shock from acute decompensation, but chronic occult hepatic dysfunction is not uncommon with chronic HF, especially in the setting of poor RV function with persistently high right atrial pressures or in those with a Fontan circulation.[132] These patients may have significant hepatic dysfunction without substantial baseline abnormalities of aspartate aminotransferase (AST), alanine transaminase (ALT), or total bilirubin. The threshold should be low to screen such patients with ultrasonography, or even with CT scanning, to assess hepatic architecture for signs of cirrhosis. If cirrhosis is evident, early involvement of hepatologists is essential, and transjugular biopsy of the liver is often performed. Patients with marginal hepatic function frequently have massive transfusion requirements during implantation, which can place them at risk for allosensitization. Careful management of antiplatelet and anticoagulant therapy around the time of VAD implantation may be critical to minimizing the risk of perioperative bleeding. Extensive carotid or peripheral arterial disease may increase the risk of extracardiac vascular events following MCS and must be evaluated appropriately with noninvasive preoperative testing.[132] In patients who present acutely, nutrition is not often a pressing issue, but nutritional impairment in patients with chronic HF can be quite profound, and low BMI is a risk factor for poor outcomes.[137] Poor nutrition impacts T-cell function and is another risk factor for infection and poor wound healing postoperatively. For patients at nutritional risk, supplemental feeding may be of some use but should not delay implantation when MCS is indicated. For carefully selected obese patients, mechanical support can be performed reasonably safely but with an increased risk of infectious complications.[138,139] Such patients are often supported in the hope that they will be able to lose a sufficient amount of weight to become eligible for cardiac transplantation; however, such a strategy is rarely successful.[139]

SURGICAL CONSIDERATIONS

Whenever patients are being considered for MCS, the surgical team should be involved, not only to help assess a patient's suitability for support but to allow them time to properly survey the patient for additional factors that may impact outcomes. The number of prior sternotomies will impact the ease of surgical approach, the operative time, the risk of postoperative bleeding, and perhaps even the overall candidacy for MCS. The presence and degree of aortic insufficiency, the presence of mechanical valves, the number and location of prior bypass grafts, the presence of intraventricular thrombus, and the details of congenital abnormalities and subsequent surgical corrections should be determined and communicated to the surgical team. The details of past surgical ventricular reconstruction should be sought, as these surgeries usually involve the LV apex, the site of inflow cannulation for all long-term LVADs, and may present significant technical challenges. Body size is also an important variable that the surgeon may need to assess when considering the specific LVAD.

OTHER CONSIDERATIONS

Aside from the many and varied medical and surgical considerations are emotional, physical, and social considerations. The acute nature of many patients' illness often precludes a detailed assessment of such issues, but for nonemergent situations, addressing these issues prior to implantation is ideal. Physical limitations may impact the patient's ability to care for the device; for example, the manual dexterity needed to change batteries and the ability hear alarms are a critical part of such a review. Adequate cognitive ability is needed to understand the importance of the device and its components, and the ability to troubleshoot problems and to recognize when to ask for assistance are also important. The emotional stability to adapt to the device, its implications, potential limitations, and adverse events is also important to maximize

TABLE 15-7 Adverse Event Rates with Pulsatile-Flow vs. Continuous-Flow Left Ventricular Assist Devices

ADVERSE EVENT	PULSATILE FLOW (n = 59)	CONTINUOUS FLOW (n = 133)	P VALUE FOR INTERACTION
Ischemic stroke	0.10	0.06	.38
Hemorrhagic stroke	0.12	0.07	.33
LVAD-related infection	0.90	0.48	.01
Sepsis	1.11	0.39	<.001
Bleeding requiring transfusion	2.45	1.66	.06
Bleeding requiring surgery	0.29	0.23	.57
Right heart failure managed with inotropes	0.46	0.14	<.001
Right heart failure managed with RVAD	0.07	0.02	.12
LVAD thrombosis	0.00	0.02	—
Pump replacement	0.51	0.06	<.001

All values are number of events per patient-year.
LVAD, left ventricular assist device; RVAD, right ventricular assist device.
Modified from Slaughter MS, Rogers JG, Milano CA, et al. Advanced heart failure treated with continuous-flow left ventricular assist device. *N Engl J Med* 2009;361:2241-2251.

long-term outcomes and quality of life. Lastly, patients must have an adequate social support network; although having an implanted VAD does not typically require around-the-clock supervision, a background of reliable support must be established for assistance in an emergency, for long-term emotional support, and to help with the drive line dressing changes and device care.

Adverse Events

With modern continuous-flow devices, the rates of adverse events are generally lower than with pulsatile-flow devices (Table 15-7). Although a discussion of all of the potential adverse events is beyond the scope of this text, several of the most common are worth addressing. Adverse events are either found early, as a result of the surgical procedure, or late, as a consequence of the device itself. Bleeding is among the most common early adverse events as a result of the median sternotomy required to place most devices. Multivariate predictors of perioperative bleeding include dialysis, lower INTERMACS profiles, concomitant surgery at the time of MCS, prior CABG, and older age. Bleeding also occurs in the chronic phase of MCS. Continuous-flow devices require anticoagulation with warfarin to an international normalized ratio (INR) between 1.5 and 2.5, depending on the device type. Antiplatelet therapy is also typically used for most patients, although there is no accepted standard dosing regimen. In addition to the bleeding risk associated with chronic anticoagulation, continuous-flow devices also appear to have a unique risk of bleeding from an acquired von Willebrand disease. The rotation of the impeller causes the unfolding of large multimers of von Willebrand factor (vWF), which eventually leads to their enzymatic breakdown.[140] Bleeding usually occurs from GI ateriovenous malformation, which may be more likely to form in the setting of the minimal or reduced pulsatility of continuous-flow devices. Rates of GI bleeding with continuous-flow devices range from 9% to 22% in various series, about a third of which are attributable to bleeding from ateriovenous malformations.[141] The bleeding itself may place patients at additional risk during support, but the need for transfusions leads to an increased chance for HLA sensitization, which may make it more difficult to find a suitable donor organ.[142]

The most common adverse events during long-term mechanical support are infection, particularly in the drive line; thromboembolism; and stroke. The devices in use today require a percutaneous drive line, through which power is delivered to the pump and from which pump performance may be assessed. Meticulous care is needed to keep the drive line free of infection, but despite intensive education about proper care, the rate of drive line infections is 7% to 18% in BTT populations and up to 32% in DT populations.[101,116,126] Once established, infections can be difficult to fully eradicate; patients may need prolonged courses of IV or oral antibiotics along with surgical debridement, more urgent transplantation, or even pump replacement.[143] Even with therapeutic anticoagulation, the risk of thromboembolism and stroke is still present. With the use of continuous-flow pumps, the rate of ischemic stroke is 4% to 7%, with similar rates of hemorrhagic stroke.[101,116,126] De novo thrombus formation or the drawing of thrombus into the pump are the most common causes of device malfunction, but these have an incidence of less than 5% in most BTT trials; however, use as DT may be associated with a higher incidence because of the longer duration of support. The development of aortic insufficiency is a recently noted complication of long-term support with continuous-flow devices.[144] In setting of little to no aortic valve opening, the valve leaflets may become partially fused and may fail to coapt properly, leading to aortic insufficiency. Inadequate control of blood pressure during MCS therapy may also be a contributing factor, but the precise etiology and risk factors are not known at this time. If the aortic insufficiency becomes severe, the patient may require aortic valve repair or replacement.

REFERENCES

1. OPTN/SRTR Annual Report 2010. Available at http://www.srtr.org/annual_reports/2010/. Accessed September 2011.
2. Stehlik J, Edwards LB, Kucheryavaya AY, et al. Registry of the International Society for Heart and Lung Transplantation: twenty-seventh official adult heart transplant report—2010. *J Heart Lung Transplant* 2010;29:1089-1101.
3. Cimato TR, Jessup M. Recipient selection in cardiac transplantation: contraindications and risk factors for mortality. *J Heart Lung Transplant* 2002;21:1161-1173.
4. Mancini D, Eisen H, Kussmaul W, et al. Value of peak exercise oxygen consumption for optimal timing of cardiac transplantation in ambulatory patients with heart failure. *Circulation* 1991;82:778-786.
5. Pohwani AL, Murali S, Mathier MA, et al. Impact of beta-blocker therapy on functional capacity criteria for heart transplant listing. *J Heart Lung Transplant* 2003;22:78-86.
6. Gitt AK, Wasserman K, Kilkowski C, et al. Exercise anaerobic threshold and ventilatory efficiency identify heart failure patients for high risk of early death. *Circulation* 2002;106:3079-3084.
7. Cahalin LP, Mathier MA, Semigran MJ, et al. The six-minute walk test predicts peak oxygen uptake and survival in patients with advanced heart failure. *Chest* 1996;110:325-332.
8. Rose EA, Gelijns AC, Moskowitz AJ, et al. Long-term mechanical left ventricular assistance for end-stage heart failure. *N Engl J Med* 2001;345:1435-1443.
9. Aaronson KD, Schwartz JS, Chen TM, et al. Development and prospective validation of a clinical index to predict survival in ambulatory patients referred for cardiac transplant evaluation. *Circulation* 1997;95:2660-2667.
10. Levy WC, Mozaffarian D, Linker DT, et al. The Seattle Heart Failure Model: prediction of survival in heart failure. *Circulation* 2006;113:1424-1433.
11. Costard-Jackle A, Fowler MB. Influence of preoperative pulmonary artery pressure on mortality after heart transplantation: testing of potential reversibility of pulmonary hypertension with nitroprusside is useful in defining a high risk group. *J Am Coll Cardiol* 1992;19:48-54.
12. Kadner A, Chen RH, Adams DH. Heterotopic heart transplantation: experimental development and clinical experience. *Eur J Cardiothorac Surg* 2000;17:474-481.

13. Baran DA, Galin ID, Courtney MC, et al. Cardiac transplantation in the older recipient: Excellent long-term survival based on pretransplant screening. *Transplant Proc* 2003;35: 2465-2467.
14. Blanche C, Blanche DA, Kearney B, et al. Heart transplantation in patients seventy years of age and older: a comparative analysis of outcome. *J Thorac Cardiovasc Surg* 2001;121:532-541.
15. Murali S, Tokarczyk T, Ristich J, et al. Short-term survival with combined heart-kidney or combined heart-liver transplantation with allografts from a single donor. *J Heart Lung Transplant* 2001;20:168.
16. Blanche C, Kamlot A, Blanche DA, et al. Combined heart-kidney transplantation with single-donor allografts. *J Thorac Cardiovasc Surg* 2001;122:495-500.
17. Morgan JA, John R, Weinberg AD, et al. Heart transplantation in diabetic recipients: a decade review of 161 patients at Columbia Presbyterian. *J Thorac Cardiovasc Surg* 2004;127:1486-1492.
18. Costanzo et al. The International Society of Heart and Lung Transplantation Guidelines for the care of heart transplant recipients. *J Heart Lung Transplant* 2010;29:914-956.
19. Laks H, Marelli D, Fonarow GC, et al, UCLA Heart Tranplant Group. Use of two recipient lists for adults requiring heart transplantation. *J Thorac Cardiovasc Surg* 2003;125:49-59.
20. Chen JM, Russo MJ, Hammond KM, et al. Alternate waiting list strategies for heart transplantation maximize donor organ utilization. *Ann Thorac Surg* 2005;80:224-228.
21. Martin J, Siegenthaler MP, Friesewinkel O, et al. Implantable left ventricular assist device for treatment of pulmonary hypertension in candidates for orthotopic heart transplantation: a preliminary study. *Eur J Cardiothorac Surg* 2004;25:971-977.
22. Pisani BA, Mullen GM, Malinowska K, et al. Plasmapheresis with intravenous immunoglobulin G is effective in patients with elevated panel reactive antibody prior to cardiac transplantation. *J Heart Lung Transplant* 1999;18:701-706.
23. John R, Lietz K, Burke E, et al. Intravenous immunoglobulin reduces anti-HLA alloreactivity and shortens waiting time to cardiac transplantation in highly sensitized left ventricular assist device recipients. *Circulation* 1999;100(19 Suppl):II229-II235.
24. Beniaminovitz A, Savoia MT, Oz M, et al. Improved atrial function in bicaval versus standard orthotopic techniques in cardiac transplantation. *Am J Cardiol* 1997;80: 1631-1635.
25. Brandt M, Harringer W, Hirt SW, et al. Influence of bicaval anastomoses on late occurrence of atrial arrhythmia after heart transplantation. *Ann Thorac Surg* 1997;64:70-72.
26. Morgan JA, Edwards NM. Orthotopic cardiac transplantation: comparison of outcome using biatrial, bicaval, and total techniques. *J Card Surg* 2005;20:102-106.
27. Faggian G, Forni A, Mazzucco A. Donor organ preservation in high-risk cardiac transplantation. *Transplant Proc* 2004;36:617-619.
28. Morgan JA, John R, Weinberg AD, et al. Prolonged donor ischemic time does not adversely affect long-term survival in adult patients undergoing cardiac transplantation. *J Thorac Cardiovasc Surg* 2003;126:1624-1633.
29. Stobierska-Dzierzek B, Awad H, Michler RE. The evolving management of acute right-sided heart failure in cardiac transplant recipients. *J Am Coll Cardiol* 2001;38:923-931.
30. Ardehali A, Hughes K, Sadeghi A, et al. Inhaled nitric oxide for pulmonary hypertension after heart transplantation. *Transplantation* 2001;72:638-641.
31. Kavarana MN, Sinha P, Naka Y, et al. Mechanical support for the failing cardiac allograft: A single-center experience. *J Heart Lung Transplant* 2003;22:542-547.
32. Halloran PF. Immunosuppressive drugs for kidney transplantation. *N Engl J Med* 2004;351:2715-2729.
33. Stewart S, Winters GL, Fishbein MC, et al. Revision of the 1990 working formulation for the standardization of nomenclature in the diagnosis of heart rejection. *J Heart Lung Transplant* 2005;24:1710-1720.
34. Pham MX, Teuteberg JT, Kfoury AG, et al. Gene-expression profiling for rejection surveillance after cardiac transplantation. *N Engl J Med* 2010;362:1890-1900.
35. Fishman JA. Infection in solid-organ transplant recipients. *New Engl J Med* 2007; 357:2601-2614.
36. Brann WM, Bennett LE, Keck BM, et al. Morbidity, functional status, and immunosuppressive therapy after heart transplantation: an analysis of the Joint International Society for Heart and Lung Transplantation/United Network for Organ Sharing Thoracic Registry. *J Heart Lung Transplant* 1998;17:374-382.
37. Kobashigawa JA, Katznelson S, Laks H, et al. Effect of pravastatin on outcomes after cardiac transplantation. *N Engl J Med* 1995;333:621-627.
38. Teuteberg JJ, Shullo M. Aggressive steroid weaning after cardiac transplantation is possible without the additional risk of significant rejection. *Clin Transplant* 2008;22: 730-737.
39. Baran DA, Zucker, MJ, Arroyo LH, et al. Randomized trial of tacrolimus monotherapy: Tacrolimus In Combination, Tacrolimus Alone Compared (the TICTAC Trial). *J Heart Lung Transplant* 2007;26:992-997.
40. Teuteberg JJ, Shullo MA, Zomak R, et al. Aggressive steroid weaning after cardiac transplantation is possible without the additional risk of significant rejection. *Clin Transplant* 2008;22:730-737.
41. Teuteberg JJ, Shullo MA, Zomak R, et al. Alemtuzumab induction prior to cardiac transplantation with lower intensity maintenance immunosuppression: one-year outcomes. *Am J Transplantation* 2010;10:382-388.
42. Schonder K, Shullo MA, Okusanya O. Tacrolimus and lopinavir/ritonavir interaction in liver transplantation. *Ann Pharmacother* 2003;37:1793-1796.
43. Rubin RH. Prevention and treatment of cytomegalovirus disease in heart transplant patients. *J Heart Lung Transplant* 2000;19:731-735.
44. Keay S. Cardiac transplantation: Pre-transplant infectious diseases evaluation and post-transplant prophylaxis. *Curr Infect Dis Rep* 2002;4:285-292.
45. Haddad F, Deuse T, Pham M, et al. Changing trends in infectious disease in heart transplantation. *J Heart Lung Transplant* 2010;29:306-315.
46. Eisen HJ. Hypertension in heart transplant recipients: more than just cyclosporine. *J Am Coll Cardiol* 2003;41:433-434.
47. Brozena SC, Johnson MR, Ventura H, et al. Effectiveness and safety of diltiazem or lisinopril in treatment of hypertension after heart transplantation. *J Am Coll Cardiol* 1996;27:1707-1712.
48. Schroeder JS, Gao SZ, Alderman EL, et al. A preliminary study of diltiazem in the prevention of coronary artery disease in heart-transplant recipients. *N Engl J Med* 1993; 328:164-170.
49. Lang CC, Beniaminovitz A, Edwards N, et al. Morbidity and mortality in diabetic patients following cardiac transplantation. *J Heart Lung Transplant* 2003;22:244-249.
50. Vincenti F, Jensik SC, Filo RS, et al. A long-term comparison of tacrolimus (FK506) and cyclosporine in kidney transplantation: evidence for improved allograft survival at five years. *Transplantation* 2002;73:775-778.
51. Teuteberg JJ, Shullo MA. Alemtuzumab induction prior to cardiac transplantation with lower intensity maintenance immunosuppression: one-year outcomes. *Am J Transplant* 2010;10:382-388.
52. Marchetti P. New-onset diabetes after transplantation. *J Heart Lung Transplant* 2004;23:S194-S201.
53. Davidson J, Wilkinson A, Dantal J, et al. New-onset diabetes after transplantation: 2003 International Consensus Guidelines. *Transplantation* 2003;75:SS3-SS24.
54. Taylor DO, Barr ML, Radovancevic B, et al. A randomized, multicenter comparison of tacrolimus and cyclosporine immunosuppressive regimens in cardiac transplantation: decreased hyperlipidemia and hypertension with tacrolimus. *J Heart Lung Transplant* 1999;18:336-345.
55. Fatemeh A, Jackson CH, Parameshwar J, et al. Risk factors for the development and progression of dyslipidemia after heart transplantation. *Transplantation* 2003;73: 1258-1264.
56. Pflugfelder PW, Huff M, Oskalns R, et al. Cholesterol-lowering therapy after heart transplantation: a 12-month randomized trial. *J Heart Lung Transplant* 1995;14:613-622.
57. Wenke K, Meiser B, Thiery J, et al. Simvastatin initiated early after heart transplantation. *Circulation* 2003;107:93-97.
58. Keogh A, Macdonald P, Kaan A, et al. Efficacy and safety of pravastatin vs. simvastatin after cardiac transplantation. *J Heart Lung Transplant* 2000;19:529-537.
59. Bonet LA, Martinez-Dolz L, Vives MA, et al. Lipid-lowering effect of atorvastatin in heart transplantation. *Transplantation Proc* 2002;34:179-181.
60. Jimenez J, Kapadia SR, Yamani MH, et al. Cellular rejection and rate of progression of transplant vasculopathy: a 3-year serial intravascular ultrasound study. *J Heart Lung Transplant* 2001;20:393-398.
61. Valantine H. Cardiac allograft vasculopathy after heart transplantation: risk factors and management. *J Heart Lung Transplant* 2004;23:S187-S193.
62. Subramanian AK, Quinn TC, Kickler TS, et al. Correlation of *Chlamydia pneumoniae* infection and severity of accelerated graft arteriosclerosis after cardiac transplantation. *Transplantation* 2002;73:761-764.
63. Schwaiblmair M, von Scheidt W, Uberfuhr P, et al. Lung function and cardiopulmonary exercise performance after heart transplantation: influence of cardiac allograft vasculopathy. *Chest* 1999;116:332-339.
64. Aranda JM, Pauly DF, Kerensky RA, et al. Percutaneous coronary intervention versus medical therapy for coronary allograft vasculopathy. *J Heart Lung Transplant* 2002;21: 860-866.
65. Schnetzler B, Drobinski G, Dorent R, et al. The role of percutaneous transluminal coronary angioplasty in heart transplant recipients. *J Heart Lung Transplant* 2000;19: 557-565.
66. Lee MS, Tarantini G, Xhaxho J, et al. Sirolimus- versus paclitaxel-eluting stents for the treatment of cardiac allograft vasculopathy. *J Am Coll Cardiol Int* 2010;3:378-382.
67. Weis M, Pehlivanli S, Meiser BM, et al. Simvastatin treatment is associated with improvement in coronary endothelial function and decreased cytokine activation in patients after heart transplantation. *J Am Coll Cardiol* 2001;38:814-818.
68. Kobashigawa JA, Moriguchi JD, Laks H, et al. Ten-year follow-up of a randomized trial of pravastatin in heart transplant patients. *J Heart Lung Transplant* 2005;24:1736-1740.
69. Eisen HJ, Tuzcu EM, Dorent R, et al. Everolimus for the prevention of allograft rejection and vasculopathy in cardiac-transplant recipients. *N Engl J Med* 2003;349:847-858.
70. Mancini D, Pinney S, Burkhoff D, et al. Use of rapamycin slows progression of cardiac transplantation vasculopathy. *Circulation* 2003;108:48-53.
71. Doshi AA, Rogers J, Kern MJ, et al. Effectiveness of percutaneous coronary intervention in cardiac allograft vasculopathy. *Am J Cardiol* 2004;93:90-92.
72. Ono M, Michler RE. Beating heart coronary artery bypass surgery after orthotopic heart transplantation. *J Card Surg* 2003;18:545-549.
73. Aleksic I, Piotrowski JA, Kamler M, et al. Minimally invasive direct coronary artery bypass in a cardiac transplant recipient with allograft vasculpathy. *Ann Thorac Surg* 2004;77:1433-1434.
74. Radovancevic B, McGiffin DC, Kobashigawa JA, et al. Reptransplantation in 7,290 primary transplant patients: a 10-year multi-institutional study. *J Heart Lung Transplant* 2003;22: 862-868.
75. Topkara VK, Dang NC, John R, et al. A decade experience of cardiac retransplantation in adult recipients. *J Heart Lung Transplant* 2005;24:1745-1750.
76. Sehgal V, Radhakrishnan J, Appel GB, et al. Progressive renal insufficiency following cardiac transplantation: cyclosporine, lipids and hypertension. *Am J Kidney Dis* 1995;26: 193-201.
77. Vossler MR, Ni H, Toy W, et al. Pre-operative renal function predicts development of chronic renal insufficiency after orthotopic heart transplantation. *J Heart Lung Transplant* 2002;21:874-881.
78. Groetzner J, Meiser B, Landwehr P, et al. Mycophenolate mofetil and sirolimus as calcineurin inhibitor–free immunosuppression for late cardiac-transplant recipients with chronic renal failure. *Transplantation* 2004;77:568-574.
79. Engelen MA, Almer S et al. Prospective study of everolimus with calcineurin inhibitor-free immunosuppression in maintenance heart transplant patients: results at 2 years *Transplantation* 2011;91:1159-1165.
80. Frimat L, Villemot JP, Cormier L, et al. Treatment of end-stage renal failure after heart transplantation. *Nephrol Dial Transplant* 1998;13:2905-2908.
81. Gutierrez-Dalmau A, Campistol JM. Immunosuppressive therapy and malignancy in organ transplant recipients: a systematic review. *Drugs* 2007;67(8):1167-1198.
82. Domhan S, Zeier M, Abdollahi A. Immunosuppressive therapy and posttransplant malignancy. *Nephrol Dial Transplant* 2009;24:1097-1103.

83. Kiberd BA, Rose C, Gill JS. Cancer mortality in kidney transplantation. *Am J Transplantation* 2009;9:1868-1875.

84. Vajdic CM, van Leeuwen MT. Cancer incidence and risk factors after solid organ transplantation. *Int J Cancer* 2009;125:1747-1754.

85. Jemec GBE, Holm EA. Nonmelanoma skin cancer in organ transplant patients. *Transplantation* 2003;75:253-257.

86. Fortina AB, Caforio AL, Piaserico S, et al. Skin cancer in heart transplant recipients: frequency and risk factor analysis. *J Heart Lung Transplant* 2000;19:249-255.

87. Gao SZ, Chaparro SV, Perlroth M, et al. Post-transplantation lymphoproliferative disease in heart and heart-lung transplant recipients: 30-year experience at Stanford University. *J Heart Lung Transplant* 2003;22:505-514.

88. Demers P, Moffatt S, Oyer PE, et al. Long-term results of heart transplantation in patients older than 60 years. *J Thorac Cardiovasc Surg* 2003;126:224-231.

89. DiNardo CD, Tsai DE. Treatment advances in posttransplant lymphoproliferative disease. *Curr Opin Hematol* 2010;17:368-374.

90. Chen K, Craig JC, Shumack S. Oral retinoids for the prevention of skin cancers in solid organ transplant recipients: a systematic review of randomized controlled trials. *Br J Dermatol* 2005;152:518-523.

91. Dandel M, Weng Y, Siniawski H, et al. Prediction of cardiac stability after weaning from left ventricular assist devices in patients with idiopathic dilated cardiomyopathy. *Circulation* 2008;118:S94-S105.

92. Birks EJ, Tansley PD, Hardy J, et al. Left ventricular assist device and drug therapy for the reversal of heart failure. *N Engl J Med* 2006;355:1873-1884.

93. Latif N, Yacoub MH, George R, Barton PJ, Birks EJ. Changes in sarcomeric and non-sarcomeric cytoskeletal proteins and focal adhesion molecules during clinical myocardial recovery after left ventricular assist device support. *J Heart Lung Transplant* 2007; 26:230-235.

94. Rodrigue-Way A, Burkhoff D, Geesaman BJ, et al. Sarcomeric genes involved in reverse remodeling of the heart during left ventricular assist device support. *J Heart Lung Transplant* 2005;24:73-80.

95. Bruggink AH, van Oosterhout MF, de Jonge N, et al. Reverse remodeling of the myocardial extracellular matrix after prolonged left ventricular assist device support follows a biphasic pattern. *J Heart Lung Transplant* 2006;25:1091-1098.

96. Ogletree-Hughes ML, Stull LB, Sweet WE, et al. Mechanical unloading restores beta-adrenergic responsiveness and reverses receptor downregulation in the failing human heart. *Circulation* 2001;104:881-886.

97. Bruckner BA, Stetson SJ, Perez-Verdia A, et al. Regression of fibrosis and hypertrophy in failing myocardium following mechanical circulatory support. *J Heart Lung Transplant* 2001;20:457-464.

98. Beltrami AP, Urbanek K, Kajstura J, et al. Evidence that human cardiac myocytes divide after myocardial infarction. *N Engl J Med* 2001;344:1750-1757.

99. Allen JG, Weiss ES, Schaffer JM, et al. Quality of life and functional status in patients surviving 12 months after left ventricular assist device implantation. *J Heart Lung Transplant* 2010;29:278-285.

100. Rose EA, Gelijns AC, Moskowitz AJ, et al. Long-term mechanical left ventricular assistance for end-stage heart failure. *N Engl J Med* 2001;345:1435-1443.

101. Slaughter MS, Rogers JG, Milano CA, et al. HeartMate II Investigators. Advanced heart failure treated with continuous-flow left ventricular assist device. *N Engl J Med* 2009;361:2241-2251.

102. Stevenson LW, Rose EA. Left ventricular assist devices: bridges to transplantation, recovery, and destination for whom? *Circulation* 2003;108:3059-3063.

103. Morris RJ. Total artificial heart: concepts and clinical use. *Semin Thorac Cardiovasc Surg* 2008;20:247-254.

104. Fukamachi K, McCarthy PM, Smedira NG, et al. Preoperative risk factors for right ventricular failure after implantable left ventricular assist device insertion. *Ann Thorac Surg* 1999;68:2181-2184.

105. Bhama JK, Kormos RL, Toyoda Y, et al. Clinical experience using the Levitronix CentriMag system for temporary right ventricular mechanical circulatory support. *J Heart Lung Transplant* 2009;28:971-976.

106. Ochiai Y, McCarthy PM, Smedira NG, et al. Predictors of severe right ventricular failure after implantable left ventricular assist device insertion: analysis of 245 patients. *Circulation* 2002;106:I198-I202.

107. Kavarana MN, Pessin-Minsley MS, Urtecho J, et al. Right ventricular dysfunction and organ failure in left ventricular assist device recipients: a continuing problem. *Ann Thorac Surg* 2002;73:745-750.

108. Tsukui H, Teuteberg JJ, Murali S, et al. Biventricular assist device utilization for patients with morbid congestive heart failure: a justifiable strategy. *Circulation* 2005;112:165-I72.

109. Fitzpatrick JR 3rd, Frederick JR, Hiesinger W, et al. Early planned institution of biventricular mechanical circulatory support results in improved outcomes compared with delayed conversion of a left ventricular assist device to a biventricular assist device. *J Thorac Cardiovasc Surg* 2009;137:971-977.

110. Zahr F, Ootaki Y, Starling RC, et al. Preoperative risk factors for mortality after biventricular assist device implantation. *J Card Fail* 2008;14:844-849.

111. Okuda M. A multidisciplinary overview of cardiogenic shock. *Shock* 2006;25:557-570.

112. Kirklin JK, Naftel DC, Stevenson LW, et al. INTERMACS database for durable devices for circulatory support: first annual report. *J Heart Lung Transplant* 2008;27:1065-1072.

113. Rogers JG, Butler J, Lansman SL, et al. Chronic mechanical circulatory support for inotrope-dependent heart failure patients who are not transplant candidates: results of the INTrEPID Trial. *J Am Coll Cardiol* 2007;50:741-747.

114. Taylor DO, Edwards LB, Aurora P, et al. Registry of the International Society for Heart and Lung Transplantation: twenty-fifth official adult heart transplant report—2008. *J Heart Lung Transplant* 2008;27:943-956.

115. Wilson SR, Mudge GH, Stewart GC, Givertz MM. Evaluating for ventricular assist device: selecting the appropriate candidate. *Circulation* 2009;119:2225-2232.

116. Strueber M, O'Driscoll G, Jansz P, et al. Multicenter evaluation of an intrapericardial left ventricular assist system. *J Am Coll Cardiol* 2011;57:1375-1382.

117. Starling RA, Naka Y, Boyle AJ, et al. Results of the post-US Food and Drug Administration-approval study with a continuous flow left ventricular assist device as a bridge to transplantation: A prospective study using INTERMACS. *J Am Coll Cardiol* 2011;57:1890-1898.

118. Levy WC, Mozaffarian D, Linker DT, Farrar DJ, Miller LW. Can the Seattle heart failure model be used to risk-stratify heart failure patients for potential left ventricular assist device therapy? *J Heart Lung Transplant* 2009;28:231-236.

119. Deng MC, Loebe M, El-Banayosy A, et al. Mechanical circulatory support for advanced heart failure: effect of patient selection on outcome. *Circulation* 2001;103:231-237.

120. Oz MC, Goldstein DJ, Pepino P, et al. Screening scale predicts patients successfully receiving long-term implantable left ventricular assist devices. *Circulation* 1995;92:II169-II73.

121. Lietz K, Long JW, Kfoury AG, et al. Outcomes of left ventricular assist device implantation as destination therapy in the post-REMATCH era: implications for patient selection. *Circulation* 2007;116:497-505.

122. Teuteberg JJ, Ewald G, Adamson R, et al. Application of the destination therapy risk score to HeartMateII clinical trial data. *J Heart Lung Transplant* 2011;30:S31.

123. Levy WC, Mozaffarian D, Linker DT, et al. The Seattle Heart Failure Model: prediction of survival in heart failure. *Circulation* 2006;113:1424-1433.

124. Ketchum ES, Moorman AJ, Fishbein DP, et al. Predictive value of the Seattle Heart Failure Model in patients undergoing left ventricular assist device placement. *J Heart Lung Transplant* 2010;29:1021-1025.

125. Stevenson LW, Pagani FD, Young JB, et al. INTERMACS profiles of advanced heart failure: the current picture. *J Heart Lung Transplant* 2009;28:535-541.

126. Pagani FD, Miller LW, Russell SD, et al. Extended mechanical circulatory support with a continuous-flow rotary left ventricular assist device. *J Am Coll Cardiol* 2009;54:312-321.

127. Boyle AJ, Teuteberg JJ, Ascheim DD, et al. LVADs for less acutely ill patients: Do current data justify the strategy? *ASAIO* 2008;54:A22.

128. Mandarino WA, Winowich S, Gorcsan J, 3rd, et al. Right ventricular performance and left ventricular assist device filling. *Ann Thorac Surg* 1997;63:1044-1049.

129. Matthews JC, Koelling TM, Pagani FD, Aaronson KD. The right ventricular failure risk score a pre-operative tool for assessing the risk of right ventricular failure in left ventricular assist device candidates. *J Am Coll Cardiol* 2008;51:2163-7212.

130. Wilson SR, Mudge GH Jr, Stewart GC, Givertz MM. Evaluation for a ventricular assist device: selecting the appropriate candidate. *Circulation* 2009;119:2225-2232.

131. Kormos RL, Teuteberg JJ, Pagani FD, et al. Right ventricular function in patients with the HeartMateII continuous-flow left ventricular assist device: Incidence, risk factors, and effect on outcomes. *J Thoracic Cardiovasc Surg* 2010;139:1316-1324.

132. Holman WL, Kormos RL, Naftel DC. Predictors of death and transplant in patients with a mechanical circulatory support device: a multi-institutional study. *J Heart Lung Transplant* 2009;28:44-50.

133. Schulman AR, Martens TP, Russo MJ, et al. Effect of left ventricular assist device infection on post-transplant outcomes. *J Heart Lung Transplant* 2009;28:237-242.

134. Sandner SE, Zimpfer D, Zrunek P, et al. Renal function and outcome after continuous flow left ventricular assist device implantation. *Ann Thorac Surg* 2009;87:1072-1078.

135. Butler J, Geisberg C, Howser R, et al. Relationship between renal function and left ventricular assist device use. *Ann Thorac Surg* 2006;81:1745-1751.

136. Topkara VK, Dang NC, Barili F, et al. Predictors and outcomes of continuous veno-venous hemodialysis use after implantation of a left ventricular assist device. *J Heart Lung Transplant* 2006;25:404-408.

137. Mano A, Fujita K, Uenomachi K, et al. Body mass index is a useful predictor of prognosis after left ventricular assist system implantation. *J Heart Lung Transplant* 2009;28:428-433.

138. Butler J, Howser R, Portner PM, Pierson RN III. Body mass index and outcomes after left ventricular assist device placement. *Ann Thorac Surg* 2005;79:66-73.

139. Zahr F, Genovese E, Mathier M, et al. Obese patients and mechanical circulatory support: weight loss, adverse events, and outcomes. *Ann Thorac Surg* 2011;92:1420-1427.

140. Klovaite J, Gustafsson F, Mortensen SA, et al. Severely impaired vonWillebrand factor–dependent platelet aggregation in patients with a continuous flow left ventricular assist device (HeartMateII). *J Am Coll Cardiol* 2009;53:2162-2167.

141. Demirozu ZT, Radovancevic R, Hochman LF, et al. Ateriovenous malformations and gastrointestinal bleeding in patients with the HeartMateII left ventricular assist device. *J Heart Lung Transplant* 2011;30:849-853.

142. Mehra MR, Uber PA, Uber WE, Scott RL, Park MH. Allosensitization in heart transplantation: implications and management strategies. *Curr Opin Cardiol* 2003;18:153-158.

143. Holman WL, Park SJ, Long JW, et al. Infection in permanent circulatory support: experience from the REMATCH trial. *J Heart Lung Transplant* 2004;23:1359-1365.

144. Pak SW, Uriel N, Takayama H, et al. Prevalence of de novo aortic insufficiency during long-term support with left ventricular assist devices. *J Heart Lung Transplant* 2010;29:1172-1176.

CHAPTER 16

Regenerative Therapy for Heart Failure

Annarosa Leri, Jan Kajstura, and Piero Anversa

CIRCULATING PROGENITOR CELLS AND MYOCARDIAL REGENERATION, 322

HEMATOPOIETIC STEM CELL TRANSDIFFERENTIATION, 323

BONE MARROW CELLS AND CLINICAL STUDIES, 324

ENDOGENOUS CARDIAC PROGENITORS, 326

AGE, CARDIAC DISEASE, AND HUMAN CARDIAC STEM CELL FUNCTION, 327

REFERENCES, 331

This chapter discusses the fundamental observations that have profoundly changed our view of the adult human heart, resulting in the experimental use of stem/progenitor cells as a potential form of therapy for the failing heart. For nearly a century, the general view was that the heart is a terminally differentiated postmitotic organ in which the number of cardiomyocytes is established at birth, and these cells persist throughout the lifespan of the organ and organism.[1] From birth to adulthood and senescence, the increase in myocardial mass was assumed to be dictated by a parallel increase in volume of cardiomyocytes; the changes in cell size were considered equivalent to the changes in ventricular weight. Myocyte enlargement was regarded as the exclusive mechanism available to the heart to increase its muscle compartment. In the absence of coronary artery disease and other pathologic conditions, the number of cardiomyocytes was thought to remain constant throughout life.[1,2] Cardiac hypertrophy and its regression were conditioned, respectively, by cellular enlargement and atrophy; the 250- to 300-g human heart was presumed to contain the same number of myocytes present in the markedly hypertrophied heart, weighing 1000 g or more. Myocytes may quadruple their volume, and they modulate their age and mechanical behavior by turnover of their cytoplasmic proteins and mitochondrial organelles. Myocytes may live and function up to 90 years or longer, coinciding with an individual's lifespan. This notion of *cardiac biology* has dictated basic and clinical research in the last century.

A series of studies in humans appeared in the late 1990s and early 2000s documenting that cardiac hypertrophy is characterized by a chronic loss of myocytes mediated by cell apoptosis and necrosis, together with an increase in volume and number of parenchymal cells. Myocyte formation, hypertrophy, and death occur in humans with systemic hypertension or aortic stenosis and after acute and chronic myocardial infarction (MI) or idiopathic dilated cardiomyopathy.[3,4] Similar observations have been made experimentally, strengthening the notion that myocyte growth in its two aspects, *hypertrophy* and *proliferation*, and myocyte death in its two forms, *apoptosis* and *necrosis* (Figure 16-1,*A*), are important determinants of cardiac mass and function. The plasticity of the myocardium cannot be restricted to cellular hypertrophy but must include myocyte death and regeneration. These three interrelated variables determine the balance between pathologic overloads and the adaptive capacity of the human heart, structurally and functionally. Collectively, these results have offered a more biologically valid interpretation of the growth reserve of the heart and its myocyte population. Activation of the components of the cell cycle machinery, *karyokinesis* and *cytokinesis*, have been detected in cardiomyocytes, imposing a reinterpretation of the growth mechanisms of the adult heart. At all ages, the heart contains a pool of replicating myocytes that express the cell cycle proteins CDC6, Ki67, MCM5, phospho-H3, or aurora B kinase (Figure 16-1, *B*). But whether dividing myocytes are transit-amplifying cells generated by commitment of endogenous or exogenous stem cells, or whether they constitute a pool of cells that retains the ability to reenter the cell cycle and divide, remains unclear. The possibility has also been raised that myocytes possess a certain degree of developmental plasticity and are able to dedifferentiate, acquire a

proliferative state, multiply, and form functionally competent cells.[5] These findings challenge stem cell differentiation as the predominant source of myocytes, pointing to alternative mechanisms of myocyte renewal in the adult heart. However, these studies fell short in providing evidence in favor of the formation of cardiomyocytes independently from stem cell commitment.[6] Therefore, stem cell–based therapy is, at present, the most promising option for the potential reconstitution of damaged myocardium.

Circulating Progenitor Cells and Myocardial Regeneration

The documentation that stem/progenitor cells are present within the myocardium raised the question as to whether these primitive cells reside in the heart or derive from distant organs such as the bone marrow. The first evidence supporting the notion that the heart is a stem cell–regulated organ was provided by the identification of male cells in female hearts transplanted in male recipients.[7] In these cases of sex-mismatched cardiac transplants, the female heart in a male host had a significant number of Y chromosome–positive myocytes and coronary vessels. Although discrepancies exist among groups in terms of the magnitude of chimerism, these results documented that male cells colonize the female heart and differentiate into cardiovascular structures (Figure 16-1,*C*). A comparison has also been made between the degree of chimerism of cardiomyocytes and coronary vessels in cardiac allografts and in hearts of patients who received allogeneic bone marrow transplants.[8] In the latter case, only 2% to 5% chimeric myocytes were detected, but 14% to 16% chimeric myocytes and endothelial cells were observed in the transplanted heart. Host cells may migrate from the residual atrial stumps to the donor heart or may reach the myocardium through the circulation.

In the presence of tissue injury, the bone marrow may sense distant signals that favor the translocation of bone marrow cells (BMCs) to the site of damage, promoting organ repair. The physiologic relevance of circulating stem/progenitor cells to hematopoiesis is well known. Migration represents a fundamental step in the determination of hematopoietic stem cell (HSC) fate through the relocation of daughter HSCs to distinct marrow niches. A similar phenomenon may be involved in the contribution of circulating HSCs and BMCs to the regeneration of injured nonhematopoietic organs (Figure 16-2).

Migration, homing, and proliferation of endothelial progenitor cells (EPCs) in ischemic regions of the heart and the hind limb lead to de novo formation of vascular structures.[9,10] In addition, circulating EPCs participate, together with resident vascular progenitors, in the reendothelialization of the damaged vessel wall.[11] EPCs are a subset of bone marrow mononuclear cells, which give rise to functionally competent endothelial cells and result in neovascularization of ischemic parenchyma. The bone marrow mononuclear cells, which express the CD34 antigen, share some of the properties of EPCs. However, CD34-positive cells exhibit superior efficacy in the preservation of myocardial integrity and function after infarction than unselected circulating mononuclear cells.[12]

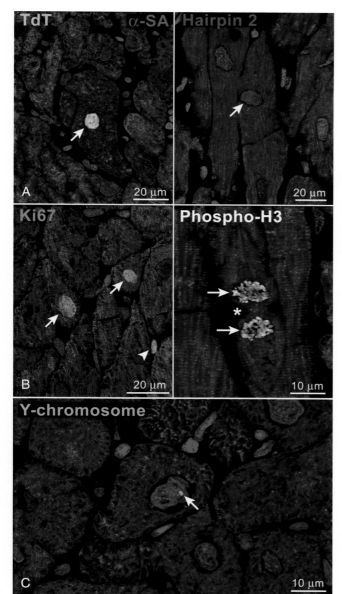

FIGURE 16-1 Myocyte death and regeneration. **A,** TdT (*left, arrow*) and hairpin 2 (*right, arrow*) labeling of human myocyte nuclei undergoing apoptosis and necrosis, respectively. **B,** Replicating (*left*) and dividing (*right*) myocyte nuclei are positive for the cell cycle protein Ki67 (*arrows*) and phospho-H3 (*arrows*), respectively; the *asterisk* indicates the site of myocyte cytokinesis. The myocyte cytoplasm is illustrated by α-sarcomeric actin staining (α-SA, *red*). **C,** A newly formed male cardiomyocyte within a transplanted donor female heart is identified by the localization of the Y chromosome (*light blue dot; arrow*).

telomere attrition. Telomeric shortening in patient-derived EPCs conditions their reduced migratory response to vascular endothelial growth factor (VEGF) and stromal-derived factor-1 (SDF-1), suggesting that age-associated telomere erosion contributes to impaired EPC function. Collectively, these observations indicate that cardiovascular risk factors profoundly affect the therapeutic benefit of EPCs.[13]

Hematopoietic Stem Cell Transdifferentiation

In the past decade, major discoveries have been made concerning the biology of adult HSCs. They can differentiate into cell lineages distinct from the organ in which they reside and into cells derived from a different germ layer.[14] These properties were considered to be restricted to embryonic stem cells, and because of their dramatic biologic and clinical implications, they triggered a vigorous debate in the scientific community. The controversy reached unexpected levels of intensity when HSCs were shown to be able to migrate to sites of injury, repairing damage in various organs and in the heart in particular. The heart has always been viewed as a nonpermissive organ for exogenous and endogenous tissue regeneration. Studies presenting positive results[14] were confronted by negative reports,[15] which challenged stem cell plasticity and the emerging new paradigm of organ and organism homeostasis and repair. However, molecular and genetic tools have been used to obtain unequivocal evidence of HSC transdifferentiation; HSCs acquire the cardiomyocyte and vascular lineages, promoting the structural and functional recovery of the damaged heart.[16]

HSCs express the receptor tyrosine kinase c-kit, and when injected in the border zone of a MI or mobilized systemically into the circulation with cytokines, HSCs lead experimentally to the repair of the necrotic tissue and the formation of functionally competent myocardium.[16,17] These observations were confirmed in multiple laboratories[18-21] and argue in favor of the differentiation of bone marrow–derived cells into the myogenic and vascular cell phenotypes as the mechanism of cardiac repair (Figure 16-3, *A*). The formed cardiac cells in female infarcted hearts carry the fluorescent tag and the Y chromosome of the injected enhanced green fluorescent protein (EGFP)-positive male HSCs (Figure 16-3, *B*).

In addition, BMC transdifferentiation was shown by the delivery to the infarcted heart of c-kit–positive HSCs carrying a reporter gene under the control of a myocyte-specific promoter (Figure 16-3, *C*). These findings, and the paucity of effective new drugs for the treatment of heart failure, have prompted cardiologists to the rapid implementation of bone marrow–derived cells in the management of the infarcted human heart.[22,23] However, a mixed population of BMCs, rather than a highly purified stem cell pool, has commonly been used for the restoration of the injured myocardium. Thus far, c-kit–positive HSCs have not been used in clinical trials.

If c-kit–positive HSCs attain the properties of cardiac stem cells (CSCs) when they home to the myocardium and give rise to cardiomyocytes and coronary vessels, the concept of transdifferentiation has to be accepted. And understanding whether CSCs and HSCs are separate stem cell categories becomes extremely important. Hypothetically, stem cells that reside in the heart should be more effective in making new myocardium than stem/progenitor cells from other organs, including the bone marrow. CSCs are programmed to generate heart structures and, upon activation, can rapidly form parenchymal cells and coronary vessels, possibly rescuing the failing heart. Conversely, HSCs have to acquire a different phenotype, which necessitates chromatin remodeling and reprogramming of genes before they transdifferentiate and create functionally competent myocardium. To date, the HSC appears to be the most versatile stem cell in crossing lineage boundaries and the most prone to break the law of tissue fidelity.

In addition to HSCs, the bone marrow contains a population of mesenchymal stromal cells (MSCs). The high degree of plasticity

An increased number of circulating EPCs and CD34-positive cells have been reported during the early phases of MI, although these cells have partly lost their functional integrity.[11] Patients with type 1 and type 2 diabetes have a reduced pool of EPCs, a decrease proportional to the severity of the diabetic vasculopathy. The functional impairment of EPCs is conditioned by dysregulation of nitric oxide synthase, enhanced production of reactive oxygen species, and activation of proinflammatory protein kinases. Other cardiovascular risk factors—including hypercholesterolemia, hypertension, and smoking—are coupled with dysfunctional EPCs. In addition, chronologic age in healthy individuals and in patients with coronary artery disease is associated with decreased number and function of circulating EPCs.[11] Aging is accompanied by shortening of telomeres in leukocytes and other bone marrow–derived cells, and coronary artery disease and heart failure further enhance

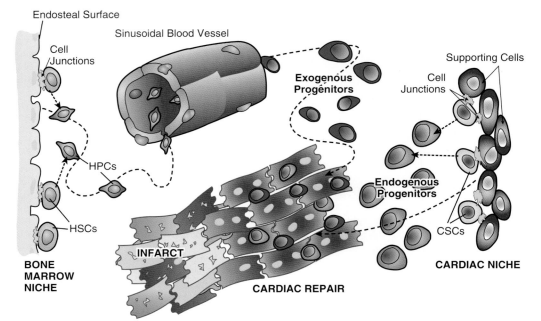

FIGURE 16-2 Myocardial repair by exogenous and endogenous progenitor cells. Hematopoietic stem cells (*HSCs*) and hematopoietic progenitor cells (*HPCs*) may reach the damaged myocardium through the circulation. In addition, cardiac stem cells (*CSCs*), stored in niches, and committed progenitors may translocate to the injured area to promote myocyte regeneration.

of MSCs supports their phenotypic flexibility and the ability to switch from one cell type to another.[24] Because MSCs are multipotent and can be easily expanded in culture, there has been significant interest in their potential for tissue regeneration. MSCs appear to possess a capacity for cardiac repair that exceeds their ability to differentiate into cardiomyocytes.[25] Recently, it has been shown that bone marrow–derived MSCs injected in a large animal model of MI promote cardiac repair by activating resident c-kit–positive CSCs and by enhancing the proliferation of host transit amplifying myocytes.[25] The interaction between recipient CSCs and delivered MSCs may reflect the cell-to-cell communication, which is operative within stem cell niches.

Bone Marrow Cells and Clinical Studies

Shortly after the experimental evidence that HSCs induce myocardial regeneration after infarction,[17] pilot clinical studies documented that intracoronary infusion of BMCs is feasible and may improve functional recovery in patients with acute myocardial infarction (AMI).[26] The Transplant of Progenitor Cells and Regeneration Enhancement in Acute Myocardial Infarction (TOPCARE-AMI) trial was the first randomized study to investigate the outcome of this approach in 59 patients with successfully reperfused AMI.[27] At 5 years, the results of the trial demonstrated the long-term safety of intracoronary BMC administration and suggested that this form of cell therapy has a beneficial effect on left ventricular (LV) function.[28] Magnetic resonance imaging (MRI) analysis of 31 patients confirmed a significant 11% increase in LV ejection fraction (LVEF) and a reduction in functional infarct size. LV end-systolic volume (LVESV) remained stable, but LV end-diastolic volume (LVEDV) enlarged.[13]

The first double-blind, placebo-controlled, randomized multicenter Reinfusion of Enriched Progenitor Cells and Infarct Remodeling in Acute Myocardial Infarction (REPAIR-AMI) study was then designed.[29] Following successful reperfusion of AMI, patients underwent bone marrow aspiration, and a heterogeneous population of mononuclear cells containing a small fraction of stem/progenitor cells was obtained by Ficoll gradient. These cells were infused intracoronarily within the segment containing the stent. With respect to controls, LVEF increased by 2.8% points at 12 months. In patients with baseline LVEF less than the median, cell

therapy was associated with a 6.6% points improvement in LVEF, which was coupled with abrogation of LVESV expansion and attenuation in LVEDV enlargement.[30] The incidence of the prespecified combined clinical endpoints of death, reinfarction, and coronary revascularization was significantly lower in the BMC-treated patients than in placebo controls, and these positive effects persisted at 2 years.[31]

Concurrently, a similar study, the Autologous Stem Cell Transplantation in Acute Myocardial Infarction (ASTAMI) trial, was conducted in patients with anterior-wall AMI.[32] At 6-month and 3-year follow-up, the 7.6% points increase in LVEF was similar in control and stem cell–treated groups. End-diastolic volume, infarct size, and global LV systolic function measured by echocardiography and MRI did not differ in control and stem cell–treated patients. A small improvement in exercise time was observed in treated patients 3 years after cell infusion.[33] The difference between the REPAIR-AMI and ASTAMI trial has been attributed to the protocols used for the isolation and storage of BMCs. Compared with BMCs used in the REPAIR-AMI, those used in the ASTAMI trial had a decreased migratory capacity in vitro and a reduced vasculogenic potential in vivo.[34]

Isolation procedures, sorting protocols, and preservation media have a major impact on the bioactivity of progenitor cells. The importance of these variables became apparent when the functional properties of BMCs were found to parallel the degree of contractile improvement of patients enrolled in the REPAIR-AMI trial. The level of contamination of the final BMC product with red blood cells (RBCs) correlated with the reduced recovery of LVEF.[35] The presence of RBCs was associated with lower BMC viability, decreased colony formation and invasion ability in vitro, and impaired capacity to form new capillaries in vivo. These factors conditioned the therapeutic efficacy of BMCs, diminishing the extent of LVEF improvement.

The conflicting results of the REPAIR-AMI and ASTAMI trials are just one example of the controversy in the field. The substantial disparity among studies was investigated by designing meta-analyses that involved subgroups of trials, in which one or more unifying parameters were identified: route of delivery, type of cardiac disease, age and gender of the patients, and presence of comorbidities. Intracoronary injection of BMCs in patients with AMI was found to be safe and effective, with an average 3.79%

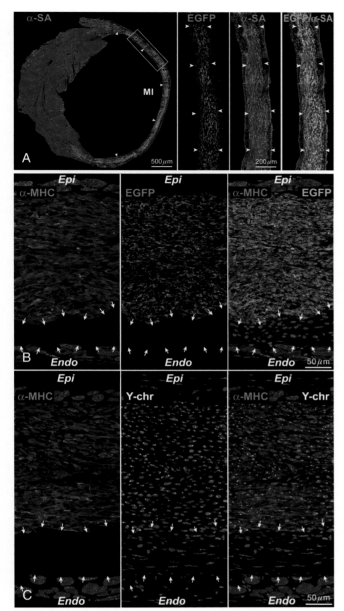

FIGURE 16-3 Hematopoietic stem cell (HSC) transdifferentiation. **A,** The c-kit–positive HSCs obtained from a mouse, in which enhanced green fluorescent protein (EGFP) is under the control of the α-MHC promoter, were injected in the border zone of an infarcted heart. The area included in the large transverse section is shown at higher magnification in the adjacent panels. Newly formed EGFP-positive (*green*) α-sarcomeric–positive (*red*) myocytes partly replaced the necrotic myocardium. Epi, epicardium; Endo, endocardium. **B,** The c-kit-positive HSCs obtained from a mouse, in which EGFP is under the control of the ubiquitous β-actin promoter, were injected in the border zone of an infarcted heart. A large portion of the transmural infarct (*left*) is replaced by myocytes positive for α-myosin heavy chain (α-MHC, *red*); the new myocytes are positive for EGFP (*center, green*). **C,** Male c-kit–positive HSCs were injected in the border zone of an infarcted heart. A large portion of the transmural infarct (*left*) is replaced by myocytes positive for α-myosin heavy chain (α-MHC, *red*); the new myocytes carry the Y chromosome (*center, white dots in nuclei*). In these three examples, the regenerated myocytes derive from HSC differentiation.

points increase in ejection fraction with respect to baseline.[36] However, the persistence of the beneficial effects of intracoronary injection of BMCs over time remained controversial. The Bone Marrow Transfer to Enhance ST-Elevation Infarct Regeneration (BOOST) trial showed that BMC therapy did not improve LVEF at 5-year follow-up,[37] whereas the Treatment of Hyponatremia Based

on Lixivaptan in New York Hospital Association (NYHA) Class III/ IV Cardiac Patient Evaluation (BALANCE) study demonstrated a long-term benefit of autologous cell administration.[38] Patients enrolled in the BOOST trial had ST-segment elevation myocardial infarction (STEMI) and relatively preserved systolic function. A single intracoronary infusion of BMCs led to a significant (6% points) improvement in LVEF at 6 months, which declined to 2.8% points at 18 months.[37] After 5 years, major adverse cardiac events occurred with similar frequency in cell-treated and untreated patients. With respect to baseline, LVEF by MRI decreased 3.3% points in controls and by 2.5% points in BMC-treated patients. When the subgroup of patients with infarct transmurality higher than the median was evaluated independently, the initial benefit of BMC administration persisted throughout the 61-month study period.

In the BALANCE trial, cells infused directly into the infarct-related artery led to a significant improvement of contractility in the border zone of the infarct and to reduction of arrhythmogenic events at 12 and 60 months. Compared with controls, mortality rate was significantly reduced in BMC-treated patients.[38] Because of the conflicting results of the BOOST and BALANCE trials, meta-analyses have been conducted to address specifically the question concerning the durability of BMC therapy. The evaluation of randomized controlled trials with 1 year or more of follow-up documented a significant 4.37% points increase of LVEF in BMC-treated patients with respect to controls.[23] This functional improvement was accompanied by reductions in LVEDV, LVEDS, and infarct size. By meta-regression analyses, BMC therapy was found to be more successful in older and diabetic patients and less effective in males.[36]

BMCs have been administered more frequently via the intracoronary route; however, intramyocardial BMC transplantation was introduced during cardiac artery bypass graft (CABG) surgery in about 20 trials. In six cases, the homogeneity among studies in patients affected by chronic ischemic cardiomyopathy was considered sufficient for a meaningful comparison.[39] With respect to controls, in which CABG was not combined with cell infusion, BMC delivery resulted in a 5.4% points increase in LVEF and a small decrease in LVEDV. Despite the relative homogeneity of these six clinical trials, a relevant source of inconsistency has been found in the type and dose of delivered cells. In three clinical trials, CD133-positive or CD34-positive BMCs were used; these cell pools are highly enriched for stem/progenitor cells of hematopoietic and endothelial lineages.

Patients affected by dilated cardiomyopathy have been enrolled in a few pilot studies. The prospective, open-label Transplantation of Progenitor Cells and Recovery of Left Ventricular Function in Patients with Nonischemic Dilatative Cardiomyopathy (TOPCARE-DCM) trial involved 33 patients with LVEF lower than 40% and left ventricular end-diastolic dimension (LVEDD) greater than 60 mm.[40] With respect to baseline, a measurable improvement of regional wall motion was detected at 3 months and persisted at 12 months, when an absolute 3.2% points increase in LVEF was accompanied by a reduction in serum levels of N-terminal prohormone brain natriuretic peptide (NT-proBNP). No significant changes were seen in LVEDV and LVESV.

Similar results were obtained in a recent open-label randomized study that involved 55 patients with dilated cardiomyopathy and severe ventricular dysfunction (LVEF <30%). Patients received CD34-positive cells by intracoronary infusion. This intervention resulted at 3 months in a 5% points increase in LVEF above control value, which persisted at 12 months.[41] Cell therapy did not decrease LVEDV; however, untreated patients showed expansion in cavitary volume over time. Cell administration improved exercise capacity and significantly reduced the serum levels of NT-proBNP. The combined cardiac mortality/heart transplantation rate was significantly lower in the BMC-treated group, and the excellent safety profile of these two pilot trials supports the rationale for larger, multicenter studies.

Patients with refractory angina have been enrolled in a double-blind, randomized, placebo-controlled dose-escalating study.[42]

After 5 days of treatment with granulocyte colony-stimulating factor (G-CSF), CD34-positive cells were immunosorted and injected intramyocardially. Efficacy parameters that included angina frequency, nitroglycerine usage, exercise time, and Canadian Cardiovascular Society class showed trends that favored CD34-positive cell-treated patients versus controls. A larger phase IIb study is currently ongoing.

Allogeneic and autologous MSCs have been used in small clinical trials, with encouraging results.[43,44] A safety study based on the intravenous delivery of allogeneic MSCs was conducted in 53 reperfused AMI patients. Global symptom score in all patients and ejection fraction in the subset of subjects with anterior AMI were significantly better in MSC-treated versus placebo controls. Based on a large amount of preclinical data obtained in porcine models of ischemic cardiomyopathy, a phase I pilot study was conducted in eight patients who received intramyocardial injection of autologous mononuclear or mesenchymal BMCs in the LV scar and border zone.[44] This safe therapeutic strategy produced functional recovery of the scarred myocardium and reverse remodeling of the LV. At 1 year, MRI analysis demonstrated a significant decrease in LVEDV and infarct size, and a trend toward decreased LVESV was observed. Improved regional function of the infarct zone strongly correlated with reduction of LVEDV and LVESV.

The mechanisms involved in the positive impact of BMC therapy on patients remains to be identified. The impossibility to permanently label the cells to be delivered and the difficulty to obtain cardiac biopsies to assess parameters consistent with myocardial regeneration leaves uncertain our understanding of the cellular processes mediating partial myocardial recovery. Measurements of coronary flow suggest that vasculogenesis may be operative, but the contribution of de novo myocyte formation is uncertain. Reductions in infarct scar size speak in favor of myocardial regeneration, although unequivocal data have not been obtained as yet.[22,23] The recent identification of CSCs has shifted the attention to endogenous cell mechanisms as a novel target of cell therapy for the failing heart.

Endogenous Cardiac Progenitors

The most logical and potentially powerful cell to be employed for cardiac repair is a primitive cell that resides in the adult heart. The appreciation that the heart is a dynamic organ that constantly renews its cell populations has generated great enthusiasm in the scientific and clinical communities.[45,46] Understanding the mechanisms of cardiac homeostasis would offer the extraordinary opportunity to potentiate this naturally occurring process and promote myocardial regeneration following injury. Two phase I clinical trials (NCT00474461 [SCIPIO] and NCT00893360 [CADUCEUS]; www.ClinicalTrials.gov) currently are in progress.[47,48] Two distinct populations of autologous cardiac-derived cells are being delivered to patients with subacute and chronic ischemic cardiomyopathy: c-kit–positive CSCs[49,50] and progenitors making cardiospheres in vitro.[51] The Stem Cell Infusion in Patients with Ischemic Cardiomyopathy (SCIPIO) trial involves the delivery of autologous c-kit–positive, lineage-negative CSCs for the treatment of severe chronic heart failure of ischemic origin.[47] Patients with an EF less than 40% at 4 months after CABG were enrolled in the treatment and control groups. Treated patients received a single intracoronary infusion of 1 million autologous CSCs. The primary endpoint was short-term safety of treatment, and the secondary endpoint was efficacy. Importantly, no CSC-related adverse effects were reported. In 14 CSC-treated patients who were analyzed, EF increased from 30% to 38% at 4 months after infusion. In contrast, seven control patients during the corresponding time interval did not show any change in this functional parameter. The beneficial effects of CSCs were even more pronounced at 1 year. In seven treated patients, in whom cardiac MRI could be done, infarct size decreased 24% and 30% at 4 and 12 months, respectively.

Before infusion in patients enrolled in SCIPIO, c-kit–positive CSCs were extensively characterized by immunolabeling and confocal microscopy and fluorescence-activated cell sorter analysis. In each of the 20 treated patients, the fraction of c-kit–positive cells varied from 75% to 98%. The markers of cellular proliferative potential, telomere length, and telomerase activity documented that, after passaging in culture, CSCs retained a significant growth reserve. The characterization of the telomere-telomerase axis should be introduced as standard quality control assay for the evaluation of the functional properties of cells to be administered to patients.

The prospective, randomized CardioSphere-Derived Autologous Stem Cells to Reverse Ventricular Dysfunction (CADUCEUS) trial included patients with subacute MI and an EF of 25% to 45%. Autologous cells grown from endomyocardial biopsy specimens were infused into the infarct-related artery 1.5 to 3 months after infarction. The primary endpoint consisted of the proportion of patients at 6 months who died from arrhythmic events or had MI after cell infusion, new cardiac tumor, or a major adverse cardiac event (MACE). In addition, preliminary data concerning the efficacy of the treatment were collected by MRI at 6 months.

At baseline, mean EF was 39% and the scar occupied 24% of the left ventricular mass. At 6 months, no patients had died, developed cardiac tumors, or had an MACE in either group. However, four patients in the cell-treated group had serious adverse events compared with one control subject. Cell therapy resulted in a reduction in scar mass, an increase in viable heart mass, and enhanced regional contractility and regional systolic wall thickening. End-diastolic volume, end-systolic volume, and EF did not differ between treated and untreated groups. The initial results of SCIPIO and CADECEUS trials are highly encouraging and warrant further, larger phase 2 studies.

The isolation of cells from self-renewing organs and their culture in serum-free media and nonadhesive substrates may lead to the formation of spherical clusters of cells known as *floating spheres*. This suspension culture method is employed for large-scale expansion of stem/progenitor cells as an alternative technique to single-cell deposition and clone generation. This protocol, however, does not result in the formation of a homogenous population of identical cells; this peculiar form of anchorage-independent growth has been used for the expansion of cardiospheres from endomyocardial biopsies.[51] Cardiospheres contain a core of c-kit–positive primitive cells, several layers of differentiating cells that express myocyte proteins and connexin 43, and an outer sheet composed of cells positive for CD105, a classic epitope of MSCs.[24] Biologically, cardiospheres can be regarded as a simplified in vitro system of cardiac differentiation (Figure 16-4).

Clinically, cardiosphere-derived cells (CDCs) may represent the ideal combination of primitive and early committed cells for the treatment of cardiac diseases. But whether the utilization of cells already committed to the myocyte, endothelial cell, and smooth muscle cell lineages is preferable to the use of a pure population of undifferentiated human CSCs (hCSCs) is currently unknown. Clonal cells have a larger growth reserve but may need more time to acquire the differentiated state. Conversely, the committed cells may have a reduced capacity to proliferate but may attain more rapidly the adult phenotype. However, the clinical implementation of a partially defined heterogeneous cell preparation may result in a vaster array of unpredictable, undesired effects than a uniform population of identical cells with well-established biologic characteristics. Analogous to pharmacologic therapy, the combination of different drugs in the same pill is associated with ease of administration but may not allow flexibility in dosing and personalized therapy.

Cardiospheres may recapitulate the microenvironment of the stem cell niche. Mesenchymal-like and committed cells of the external layer may act as supporting cells for the internally distributed c-kit–positive CSCs. It has been suggested that direct implantation of niche-like cardiospheres in the damaged myocardium may be associated with a homing advantage with respect to monolayer-cultured CDCs.[52] The presence of supporting cells may transiently protect the adjacent primitive cells, enhancing

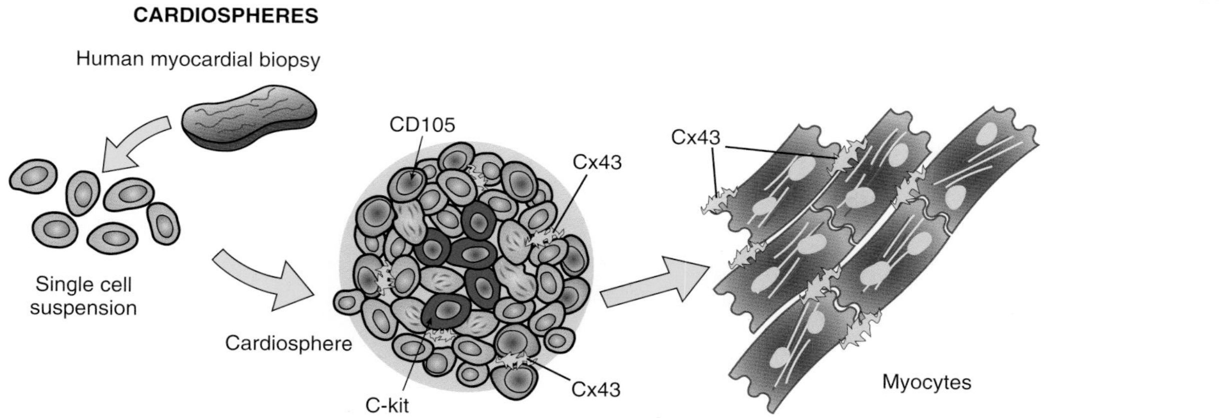

CARDIOSPHERES

FIGURE 16-4 Schematic of a cardiosphere. Cardiac tissue is dissociated into a single cell suspension, and the cells are plated. With time, they form three-dimensional structures composed of differentiated cells on the surface and primitive dividing cells in the core. Cx43, connexin 43.

their survival in the hostile environment of the damaged myocardium. However, direct contact between the delivered and recipient cardiac cells is required for actual engraftment in the host tissue and acquisition of the cardiogenic fate. Donor stem cells have to integrate structurally within the surrounding myocardium by forming junctional and adhesion complexes with adjacent myocytes and fibroblasts.[53] In the absence of engraftment, adoptively transferred cells die by apoptosis.[16] The formation of these chimeric temporary niches creates the microenvironment necessary for the engrafted cells to adopt the cardiac destiny and form de novo myocardium.

Importantly, successful cell-based therapy has to achieve two fundamental objectives: 1) reconstitution of the lost muscle mass by replacement of the necrotic and scarred tissue with functionally competent cardiomyocytes and vascular structures and 2) repopulation of depleted, empty, or dysfunctional hCSC niches. The persistence of malfunctioning niches will sustain the inevitable progression of the cardiac disease and attenuate the beneficial effects of cell administration. Restoration of cardiac niches can only be obtained by delivery of a population of highly primitive hCSCs; this process may ensure long-term benefit in terms of cardiac cell renewal and repair following injury.

The c-kit–positive CSC was the first stem cell identified in the adult heart.[48] C-kit, a receptor tyrosine kinase, was originally thought to be located exclusively on the membrane of a class of murine HSCs with long-term repopulating ability in irradiated recipients. C-kit identifies a population of resident CSCs that are self-renewing, clonogenic, and multipotent in vitro and that replace necrotic tissue with functional myocardium in vivo, thereby improving ventricular performance.[49,50,54,55] Quantitative data have shown that there is one CSC for about every 30,000 cardiac cells. Similarly, the frequency of c-kit–positive pluripotent HSCs in the bone marrow has been estimated to be about one every 10,000 to 100,000 cells.[56]

C-kit–positive hCSCs are present throughout the ventricular myocardium, although they are preferentially distributed to the atria and apex,[53] and hCSCs do not express hematopoietic and endothelial cell epitopes, which strongly suggests that they do not originate from the bone marrow but rather constitute a compartment of resident undifferentiated cells. Stem cell niches have been discovered in the cardiac microenvironment[49,57]; they consist of discrete ellipsoidal structures located in the myocardial interstitium, where hCSCs are clustered together and connected to adjacent myocytes and fibroblasts by adherens and gap junctions (Figure 16-5, A). Myocytes and fibroblasts operate as supporting cells within the cardiac niches,[49,57] providing the necessary permissive milieu for the long-term residence, survival, and growth of hCSCs (Figure 16-5, B and C). The identification of cardiac niches, and the documentation that hCSCs have

phenotypic characteristics distinct from HSCs, offers further evidence in support of the notion that the heart is a self-renewing organ regulated by a stem cell compartment.

Also, hCSCs divide both symmetrically and asymmetrically. By asymmetric division, hCSCs create new stem cells and cells destined to acquire specialized function[49,57]; hCSCs commit to the myocyte, smooth muscle cell, and endothelial cell lineages. The delivery of hCSCs to the infarcted mouse heart generates a chimeric organ in which human and rodent cardiomyocytes and coronary vessels are integrated structurally and functionally, documenting the critical role that hCSCs have in organ homeostasis and repair (Figure 16-6, A and B).

The identification of a pool of resident hCSCs in the adult human heart is apparently at variance with the small foci of myocardial regeneration (Figure 16-6, C) present following MI[58] or chronic aortic stenosis.[59] This limitation has been interpreted as unequivocal documentation of the inability of the adult heart to undergo spontaneous tissue repair.[1,2] A possible explanation of this apparent paradox has been obtained in animal models of the human disease. Stem cells are present throughout the infarcted myocardium, but in spite of the postulated resistance of these cells to death stimuli, they follow the same pathway of cardiomyocytes and die by apoptosis and necrosis. The fate of hCSCs is comparable to that of the surrounding cells, and myocyte formation by hCSCs is predominantly restricted to the viable portion of the infarcted heart.[60]

It might come as a surprise, but a similar phenomenon occurs in other solid and nonsolid organs that include the skin, liver, intestine, bone marrow, and kidney. In all cases, occlusion of a supplying artery leads to scar formation that mimics cardiac pathology.[61-65] In the presence of polyarteritis nodosa and vasculitis, microinfarcts develop in the intestine and skin, and resident stem cells do not repair the damaged organs.[61] Similarly, infarcts of the bone marrow are frequently seen with sickle cell anemia.[65] Thus, the stem cell compartment appears to be properly equipped to modulate growth during postnatal development and to regulate homeostasis in adulthood. However, the stem cell pool does not respond effectively to ischemic injury or, late in life, to aging and senescence of the organ and organism.[45,46,66] These constraints may be overcome by intramyocardial delivery of stem cells expanded in vitro or by local stimulation of resident stem cells by growth factors.

Age, Cardiac Disease, and Human Cardiac Stem Cell Function

In analogy with other stem cells, the life cycle of hCSCs is regulated by telomerase activity and telomere length.[49] Telomeric

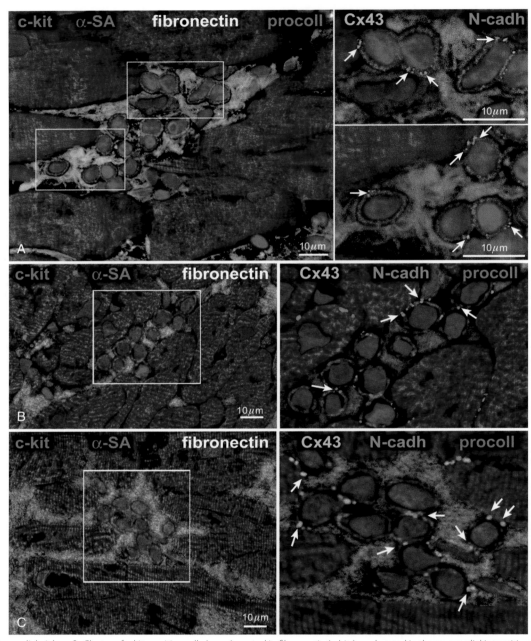

FIGURE 16-5 Myocardial niches. **A,** Cluster of c-kit–positive cells (*green*), nested in fibronectin (*white*), are located in the myocardial interstitium. The areas included in the rectangles are shown at higher magnification in the adjacent panels. Connexin 43 (*Cx43; yellow arrows*) and N-cadherin (*N-cadh; bright blue, bottom arrows*) are detected between c-kit–positive cells and myocytes (α-SA, *red*) and fibroblasts (procollagen [*procoll*]; *magenta*). **B** and **C,** Two additional examples of cardiac niches.

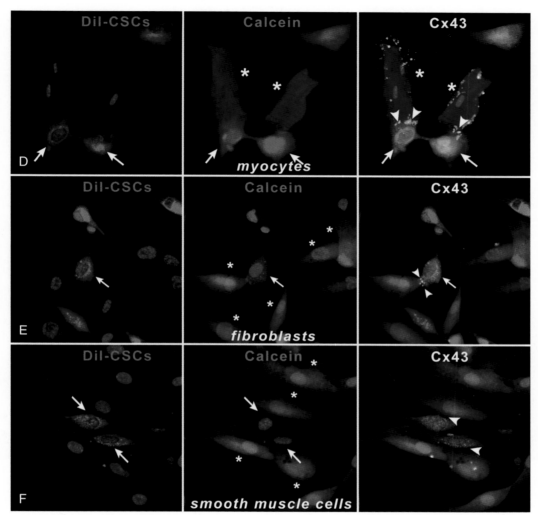

FIGURE 16-5, cont'd   D to **F,** Dye transfer assay. **D,** DiI-labeled (*left; red, arrows*) and calcein-labeled (*center; green, arrows*) human CSCs were cocultured with unlabeled adult rat cardiomyocytes that acquired green fluorescence (*center; green, asterisks*). Cx43 was detected between coupled CSCs and myocytes (*right; arrowheads*). **E,** DiI-labeled human CSCs (*left; red, arrow*) were cocultured with calcein-labeled human fibroblasts (*center; green, asterisks*). Green fluorescence of calcein was detected in CSCs (*center; arrow*) together with red fluorescence of DiI (*right; red-green, arrow*). Cx43 (*white*) was expressed between CSCs and fibroblasts (*right; arrowheads*). **F,** DiI-labeled human CSCs (*left; red, arrows*) were cocultured with calcein-labeled human SMCs (*center; green, asterisks*). Green fluorescence of calcein was not detected in CSCs (*center; arrows*). Cx43 (*white*) was not expressed between CSCs and SMCs (*right; arrowheads*). DiI, 1,1′-Dioctadecyl-3,3,3′,3′-tetramethylindocarbocyanine iodide.

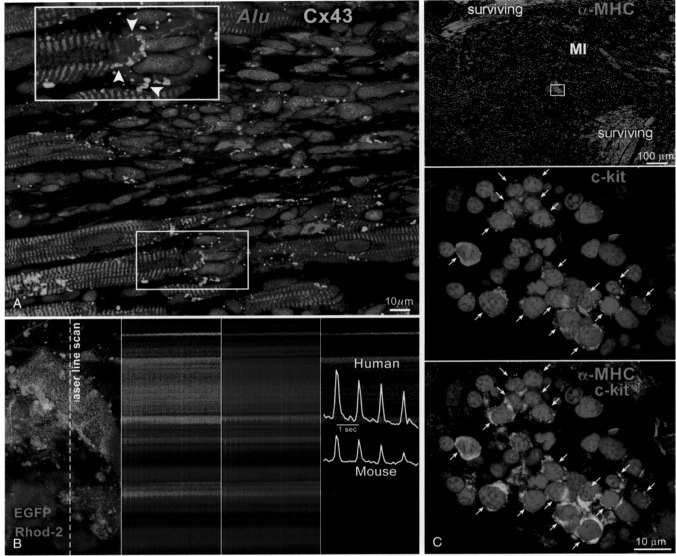

FIGURE 16-6 Structural and functional integration of newly formed cardiomyocytes. **A,** Myocardial regeneration 3 weeks after coronary artery ligation and injection of human cardiac stem cells (CSCs). Connexin 43 (*Cx43, yellow*) is present between human myocytes (α-SA, *red;* Alu, *green*) and spared rat myocytes (α-SA, *red;* Alu-negative). See inset for higher magnification. **B,** Calcium transient in enhanced green fluorescent protein (EGFP)-positive human myocytes and EGFP-negative mouse myocytes recorded by two-photon microscopy and laser line-scan imaging (calcium indicator Rhod-2, *red*). Note the synchronicity in calcium transient between human (EGFP-positive) and mouse (EGFP-negative) cardiomyocytes. **C,** Area of regenerating myocardium within an acute infarct in a human heart. The area included in the rectangle is shown at higher magnification in the lower panels. A cluster of c-kit–positive CSCs (*green, arrows*) at times expressing cardiac myosin (α-MHC, *red*) is visible.

shortening occurs in aging hCSCs, and those with critically shortened or dysfunctional telomeres undergo replicative senescence and apoptosis. Loss of telomere integrity is a critical variable of the decline of stem cell growth in the failing human heart.[46,58,59,66] The number of hCSCs increases with age, but the fraction of functionally competent cells decreases.[46] The accumulation of old, dysfunctional hCSCs conditions myocardial aging; hCSCs carrying short telomeres generate a progeny that rapidly attains the senescent phenotype.[46] The compartment of old cardiomyocytes progressively increases, defining the aging myopathy.[46,66-68] A pool of hCSCs with intact telomeres, 8 to 12 kbp, is present in the female and male heart at 90 to 104 years of age[46]; this cell category is expected to generate a young myocyte progeny within the senescent heart.

Myocyte regeneration in the physiologically aging heart takes place at previously unexpected levels. In the female heart, myocyte replacement occurs at a rate of 10%, 14%, and 40% per year at 20, 60, and 100 years of age, respectively. Corresponding values in the male heart are 7%, 12%, and 32% per year, documenting that myocyte turnover involves a large and progressively increasing number of parenchymal cells with aging.[46] These growth processes are potentiated in pathologic states.[45,58,59] From a clinical perspective, the recognition that a subset of telomerase-competent hCSCs with long telomeres persists at all ages and in the presence of cardiac diseases raises the possibility that autologous cell-based therapy may be feasible in patients with chronic heart failure. Recently, a methodology has been developed to isolate from endomyocardial biopsies of very sick patients this compartment of functionally competent hCSCs to be expanded in vitro prior to their intracoronary or intramyocardial delivery.[69] Although this approach remains to be used clinically, it generates a therapeutically relevant quantity of cells in the absence of invasive surgical techniques. This strategy is in the process of being implemented in forthcoming clinical trials.

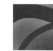

REFERENCES

1. Parmacek MS, Epstein JA. Cardiomyocyte renewal. *N Engl J Med* 2009;361:86-88.
2. Musunuru K, Domian IJ, Chien KR. Stem cell models of cardiac development and disease. *Annu Rev Cell Dev Biol* 2010;26:667-687.
3. Anversa P, Kajstura J. Ventricular myocytes are not terminally differentiated in the adult mammalian heart. *Circ Res* 1998;83:1-14.
4. Leri A, Kajstura J, Anversa P. Cardiac stem cells and mechanisms of myocardial regeneration. *Physiol Rev* 2005;85:1373-1416.
5. Bersell K, Arab S, Haring B, et al. Neuregulin1/ErbB4 signaling induces cardiomyocyte proliferation and repair of heart injury. *Cell* 2009;138:257-270.
6. Bailey B, Izarra A, Alvarez R, et al. Cardiac stem cell genetic engineering using the alphaMHC promoter. *Regen Med* 2009;4:823-833.
7. Quaini F, Urbanek K, Beltrami AP, et al. Chimerism of the transplanted heart. *N Engl J Med* 2002;346:5-15.
8. Thiele J, Varus E, Wickenhauser C, et al. Mixed chimerism of cardiomyocytes and vessels after allogeneic bone marrow and stem-cell transplantation in comparison with cardiac allografts. *Transplantation* 2004;77:1902-1905.
9. Urbich C, Heeschen C, Aicher A, et al. Cathepsin L is required for endothelial progenitor cell-induced neovascularization. *Nat Med* 2005;11:206-213.
10. Hamada H, Kim MK, Iwakura A, et al. Estrogen receptors alpha and beta mediate contribution of bone marrow–derived endothelial progenitor cells to functional recovery after myocardial infarction. *Circulation* 2006;114:2261-2270.
11. Dimmeler S, Leri A. Aging and disease as modifiers of efficacy of cell therapy. *Circ Res* 2008;102:1319-1330.
12. Kawamoto A, Iwasaki H, Kusano K, et al. CD34-positive cells exhibit increased potency and safety for therapeutic neovascularization after myocardial infarction compared with total mononuclear cells. *Circulation* 2006;114:2163-2169.
13. Britten MB, Abolmaali ND, Assmus B, et al. Infarct remodeling after intracoronary progenitor cell treatment in patients with acute myocardial infarction (TOPCARE-AMI): mechanistic insights from serial contrast-enhanced magnetic resonance imaging. *Circulation* 2003;108:2212-2218.
14. Anversa P, Leri A, Kajstura J. Cardiac regeneration. *J Am Coll Cardiol* 2006;47:1769-1776.
15. Murry CE, Reinecke H, Pabon LM. Regeneration gaps: observations on stem cells and cardiac repair. *J Am Coll Cardiol* 2006;47:1777-1785.
16. Rota M, Kajstura J, Hosoda T, et al. Bone marrow cells adopt the cardiomyogenic fate in vivo. *Proc Natl Acad Sci USA* 2007;104:17783-17788.
17. Orlic D, Kajstura J, Chimenti S, et al. Bone marrow cells regenerate infarcted myocardium. *Nature* 2001;410:701-705.
18. Yoon YS, Wecker A, Heyd L, et al. Clonally expanded novel multipotent stem cells from human bone marrow regenerate myocardium after myocardial infarction. *J Clin Invest* 2005;115:326-338.
19. Murasawa S, Kawamoto A, Horii M, et al. Niche-dependent translineage commitment of endothelial progenitor cells, not cell fusion in general, into myocardial lineage cells. *Arterioscler Thromb Vasc Biol* 2005;25:1388-1394.
20. Koyanagi M, Brandes RP, Haendeler J, et al. Cell-to-cell connection of endothelial progenitor cells with cardiac myocytes by nanotubes: a novel mechanism for cell fate changes? *Circ Res* 2005;96:1039-1041.
21. Kubo H, Jaleel N, Kumarapeli A, et al. Increased cardiac myocyte progenitors in failing human hearts. *Circulation* 2008;118:649-657.
22. Abdel-Latif A, Bolli R, Tleyjeh IM, et al. Adult bone marrow-derived cells for cardiac repair: a systematic review and meta-analysis. *Arch Intern Med* 2007;167:989-997.
23. Zhang C, Sun A, Zhang S, et al. Efficacy and safety of intracoronary autologous bone marrow–derived cell transplantation in patients with acute myocardial infarction: insights from randomized controlled trials with 12 or more months follow-up. *Clin Cardiol* 2010;33:353-360.
24. Bianchi G, Muraglia A, Daga A, et al. Microenvironment and stem properties of bone marrow-derived mesenchymal cells. *Wound Repair Regen* 2001;9:460-466.
25. Hatzistergos KE, Quevedo H, Oskouei BN, et al. Bone marrow mesenchymal stem cells stimulate cardiac stem cell proliferation and differentiation. *Circ Res* 2010;107:913-922.
26. Strauer BE, Brehm M, Zeus T, et al. Repair of infarcted myocardium by autologous intracoronary mononuclear bone marrow cell transplantation in humans. *Circulation* 2002;106:1913-1918.
27. Assmus B, Schächinger V, Teupe C, et al. Transplantation of Progenitor Cells and Regeneration Enhancement in Acute Myocardial Infarction (TOPCARE-AMI). *Circulation* 2002;106:3009-3017.
28. Leistner DM, Fischer-Rasokat U, Honold J, et al. Transplantation of progenitor cells and regeneration enhancement in acute myocardial infarction (TOPCARE-AMI): final 5-year results suggest long-term safety and efficacy. *Clin Res Cardiol* 2011;100(10):925-934.
29. Assmus B, Honold J, Schächinger V, et al. Transcoronary transplantation of progenitor cells after myocardial infarction. *N Engl J Med* 2006;355:1222-1232.
30. Dill T, Schächinger V, Rolf A, et al. Intracoronary administration of bone marrow-derived progenitor cells improves left ventricular function in patients at risk for adverse remodeling after acute ST-segment elevation myocardial infarction: results of the Reinfusion of Enriched Progenitor cells And Infarct Remodeling in Acute Myocardial Infarction study (REPAIR-AMI) cardiac magnetic resonance imaging substudy. *Am Heart J* 2009;157:541-547.
31. Assmus B, Rolf A, Erbs S, et al. Clinical outcome 2 years after intracoronary administration of bone marrow–derived progenitor cells in acute myocardial infarction. *Circ Heart Fail* 2010;3:89-96.
32. Lunde K, Solheim S, Aakhus S, et al. Intracoronary injection of mononuclear bone marrow cells in acute myocardial infarction. *N Engl J Med* 2006;355:1199-1209.
33. Beitnes JO, Hopp E, Lunde K, et al. Long-term results after intracoronary injection of autologous mononuclear bone marrow cells in acute myocardial infarction: the ASTAMI randomised, controlled study. *Heart* 2009;95:1983-1989.
34. Seeger FH, Tonn T, Krzossok N, et al. Cell isolation procedures matter: a comparison of different isolation protocols of bone marrow mononuclear cells used for cell therapy in patients with acute myocardial infarction. *Eur Heart J* 2007;28:766-772.
35. Assmus B, Tonn T, Seeger FH, et al. Red blood cell contamination of the final cell product impairs the efficacy of autologous bone marrow mononuclear cell therapy. *J Am Coll Cardiol* 2010;55:1385-1394.
36. Bai Y, Sun T, Ye P. Age, gender and diabetic status are associated with effects of bone marrow cell therapy on recovery of left ventricular function after acute myocardial infarction: a systematic review and meta-analysis. *Ageing Res Rev* 2010;9:418-423.
37. Meyer GP, Wollert KC, Lotz J, et al. Intracoronary bone marrow cell transfer after myocardial infarction: eighteen months' follow-up data from the randomized, controlled BOOST (BOne marrOw transfer to enhance ST-elevation infarct regeneration) trial. *Circulation* 2006;113:1287-1294.
38. Yousef M, Schannwell CM, Köstering M, et al. The BALANCE Study: clinical benefit and long-term outcome after intracoronary autologous bone marrow cell transplantation in patients with acute myocardial infarction. *J Am Coll Cardiol* 2009;53:2262-2269.
39. Donndorf P, Kundt G, Kaminski A, et al. Intramyocardial bone marrow stem cell transplantation during coronary artery bypass surgery: a meta-analysis. *J Thorac Cardiovasc Surg* 2011;142(4):911-920.
40. Fischer-Rasokat U, Assmus B, Seeger FH, et al. A pilot trial to assess potential effects of selective intracoronary bone marrow–derived progenitor cell infusion in patients with nonischemic dilated cardiomyopathy: final 1-year results of the transplantation of progenitor cells and functional regeneration enhancement pilot trial in patients with nonischemic dilated cardiomyopathy. *Circ Heart Fail* 2009;2:417-423.
41. Vrtovec B, Poglajen G, Sever M, et al. Effects of intracoronary stem cell transplantation in patients with dilated cardiomyopathy. *J Card Fail* 2011;17:272-281.
42. Losordo DW, Schatz RA, White CJ, et al. Intramyocardial transplantation of autologous CD34+ stem cells for intractable angina: a phase I/IIa double-blind, randomized controlled trial. *Circulation* 2007;115:3165-3172.
43. Hare JM, Traverse JH, Henry TD, et al. A randomized, double-blind, placebo-controlled, dose-escalation study of intravenous adult human mesenchymal stem cells (prochymal) after acute myocardial infarction. *J Am Coll Cardiol* 2009;54:2277-2286.
44. Williams AR, Trachtenberg B, Velazquez DL, et al. Intramyocardial stem cell injection in patients with ischemic cardiomyopathy: functional recovery and reverse remodeling. *Circ Res* 2011;108:792-796.
45. Kajstura J, Urbanek K, Perl S, et al. Cardiomyogenesis in the adult human heart. *Circ Res* 2010;107:305-315.
46. Kajstura J, Gurusamy N, Ogórek B, et al. Myocyte turnover in the aging human heart. *Circ Res* 2010;107:1374-1386.
47. Bolli R, Chugh AR, D'Amario D, et al. Cardiac stem cells in patients with ischaemic cardiomyopathy (SCIPIO): initial results of a randomised phase 1 trial. *Lancet* 2001;378:1847-1857.
48. Makkar RR, Smith RR, Cheng K, et al. Intracoronary cardiosphere-derived cells for heart regeneration after myocardial infarction (CADUCEUS): a prospective, randomised phase 1 trial. *Lancet* 2012;379:895-904.
49. Bearzi C, Rota M, Hosoda T, et al. Human cardiac stem cells. *Proc Natl Acad Sci USA* 2007;104:14068-14073.
50. Hosoda T, D'Amario D, Cabral-Da-Silva MC, et al. Clonality of mouse and human cardiomyogenesis in vivo. *Proc Natl Acad Sci USA* 2009;106:17169-17174.
51. Smith RR, Barile L, Cho HC, et al. Regenerative potential of cardiosphere-derived cells expanded from percutaneous endomyocardial biopsy specimens. *Circulation* 2007;115:896-908.
52. Li TS, Cheng K, Lee ST, et al. Cardiospheres recapitulate a niche-like microenvironment rich in stemness and cell-matrix interactions, rationalizing their enhanced functional potency for myocardial repair. *Stem Cells* 2010;28:2088-2098.
53. Urbanek K, Cesselli D, Rota M, et al. Stem cell niches in the adult mouse heart. *Proc Natl Acad Sci USA* 2006;103:9226-9231.
54. Hosoda T, Zheng H, Cabral-Da-Silva M, et al. Human cardiac stem cell differentiation is regulated by a mircrine mechanism. *Circulation* 2011;123:1287-1296.
55. D'Amario D, Cabral-Da-Silva M, Zheng H, et al. The IGF-1 receptor identifies a pool of human cardiac stem cells with superior therapeutic potential for myocardial regeneration. *Circ Res* 2011;108:1467-1481.
56. Orlic D, Fischer R, Nishikawa S, et al. Purification and characterization of heterogeneous pluripotent hematopoietic stem cell populations expressing high levels of c-kit receptor. *Blood* 1993;82:762-770.
57. Bearzi C, Leri A, Lo Monaco F, et al. Identification of a coronary vascular progenitor cell in the human heart. *Proc Natl Acad Sci USA* 2009;106:15885-15890.
58. Urbanek K, Torella D, Sheikh F, et al. Myocardial regeneration by activation of multipotent cardiac stem cells in ischemic heart failure. *Proc Natl Acad Sci USA* 2005;102:8692-8697.
59. Urbanek K, Quaini F, Tasca G, et al. Intense myocyte formation from cardiac stem cells in human cardiac hypertrophy. *Proc Natl Acad Sci USA* 2003;100:10440-10445.
60. Beltrami AP, Urbanek K, Kajstura J, et al. Evidence that human cardiac myocytes divide after myocardial infarction. *N Engl J Med* 2001;344:1750-1757.
61. Lopez LR, Schocket AL, Stanford RE, et al. Gastrointestinal involvement in leukocytoclastic vasculitis and polyarteritis nodosa. *J Rheumatol* 1980;7:677-684.
62. Saegusa M, Takano Y, Okudaira M. Human hepatic infarction: histopathological and postmortem angiological studies. *Liver* 1993;13:239-245.
63. Watanabe K, Abe H, Mishima T, et al. Polyangitis overlap syndrome: a fatal case combined with adult Henoch-Schönlein purpura and polyarteritis nodosa. *Pathol Int* 2003;53:569-573.
64. Leong FT, Freeman LJ. Acute renal infarction. *J R Soc Med* 2005;98:121-122.
65. Dang NC, Johnson C, Eslami-Farsani M, et al. Bone marrow embolism in sickle cell disease: a review. *Am J Hematol* 2005;79:61-67.
66. Chimenti C, Kajstura J, Torella D, et al. Senescence and death of primitive cells and myocytes lead to premature cardiac aging and heart failure. *Circ Res* 2003;93:604-613.
67. Gonzalez A, Rota M, Nurzynska D, et al. Activation of cardiac progenitor cells reverses the failing heart senescent phenotype and prolongs lifespan. *Circ Res* 2008;102:597-606.
68. Bergmann O, Bhardwaj RD, Bernard S, et al. Evidence for cardiomyocyte renewal in humans. *Science* 2009;324:98-102.
69. D'Amario D, Fiorini C, Campbell PM, et al. Functionally competent cardiac stem cells can be isolated from endomyocardial biopsies of patients with advanced cardiomyopathies. *Circ Res* 2011;108:857-861.

CHAPTER **17** # Hypertrophic, Restrictive, and Infiltrative Cardiomyopathies

Neal K. Lakdawala and G. William Dec Jr.

HYPERTROPHIC CARDIOMYOPATHY, 332

MANAGEMENT OF LEFT VENTRICULAR OUTFLOW TRACT OBSTRUCTION, 332

Therapies for Nonobstructive Hypertrophic
    Cardiomyopathy, 335
Prevention of Sudden Cardiac Death in Hypertrophic
    Cardiomyopathy, 335

Management of Atrial Fibrillation in Hypertrophic
    Cardiomyopathy, 335
Screening at-Risk Family Members for Hypertrophic
    Cardiomyopathy, 336

RESTRICTIVE AND INFILTRATIVE CARDIOMYOPATHIES, 336

Idiopathic Restrictive Cardiomyopathy, 336
Cardiac Amyloidosis, 336

Cardiac Sarcoidosis, 337
Cardiac Hemochromatosis, 338
Storage Diseases of the Myocardium, 339
Endomyocardial Disorders, 339

REFERENCES, 340

Hypertrophic, restrictive, and infiltrative cardiomyopathies are a diverse group of heart muscle diseases that can culminate in the development of heart failure (HF) with associated risks of sudden death and thromboembolism. Much progress has been made elucidating the molecular pathways involved in these disorders, and the reader is directed to Chapters 68 and 69 of the ninth edition of *Braunwald's Heart Disease* for details of natural history and pathophysiology. A contemporary approach to diagnosis and management is presented in this chapter.

Hypertrophic Cardiomyopathy

Hypertrophic cardiomyopathy (HCM) is the most common inherited cardiomyopathy, with an estimated prevalence of 0.2%.[1] It is defined as left ventricular hypertrophy (LVH) that develops in the absence of excess hemodynamic load (hypertension) or other systemic conditions known to cause increased ventricular wall thickness.[2] Mutations in sarcomere genes cause HCM and are transmitted in an autosomal-dominant fashion.[1] Carriers of pathogenic sarcomere mutations typically do not develop LVH until later in life (*age-dependent penetrance*), and clinical expression may vary dramatically, even within the same family. The general therapeutic considerations for individuals with HCM are symptom management, prevention of sudden death, prevention of thromboembolism, and screening of at-risk family members. The principal pathophysiologic mechanisms of symptoms in HCM are LV outflow tract obstruction with or without mitral regurgitation, diastolic dysfunction, and in a subset, atrial fibrillation.[3]

Management of Left Ventricular Outflow Tract Obstruction

Left ventricular outflow tract obstruction (LVOTO) is caused by Venturi and drag forces, which cause systolic anterior motion (SAM) of the mitral valve and obstruction to the flow through the outflow tract.[4] Mitral regurgitation caused by malapposition of mitral leaflets often accompanies LVOTO. Up to 70% of HCM patients have clinically significant LVOTO (≥30 mm Hg) at rest and/or with provocation by exercise, Valsalva maneuver, or pharmaceuticals.[4] Lifestyle adjustment and medical therapy are usually sufficient to control symptoms related to LVOTO, but about 5% to 10% of patients require nonpharmacologic intervention with either surgical myectomy or alcohol septal ablation (ASA). Patients are advised to avoid medications and situations that worsen obstruction via reduced preload or afterload or increased contractility. Commonly prescribed drugs that worsen LVOTO include vasodilators such as angiotensin-converting enzyme (ACE) inhibitors, diuretics, and digoxin. Culprit recreational activities include alcohol consumption and activities associated with vasodilation and/or dehydration, such as sauna use.

Standard medical therapies for LVOTO are β-blockers and non-dihydropyridine calcium channel blockers, such as verapamil and diltiazem, either alone or in combination.[3] Doses of these medications are escalated until symptoms are relieved or limiting side effects develop. Patients who remain symptomatic may derive benefit from the addition of disopyramide, and β-blockers have been shown to reduce the severity of LVOTO and improve angina. Verapamil, and to a lesser extent diltiazem, may also improve symptoms and exercise tolerance, but the vasodilating properties of verapamil may actually contribute to worsening LVOTO in some patients.

Disopyramide, a class I antiarrhythmic drug, reduces LVOTO through its negative inotropic properties. In a multicenter retrospective study of 118 patients with obstructive HCM treated with controlled-release disopyramide (200 to 300 mg twice daily), 66% had a clinical response and avoided surgical myectomy, pacing, or ASA. Clinical responders had a drop in LV outflow tract gradient (from 75 ± 33 to 40 ± 32 mm Hg; $P < .001$), whereas clinical nonresponders had a more modest hemodynamic benefit (from 75 ± 35 to 63 ± 31 mm Hg).[5] The annual risk of sudden death while taking disopyramide was 0.8%, which was not increased compared with a matched HCM cohort not taking disopyramide.[5] Because disopyramide can increase the QT interval, in-hospital initiation of this medication is advised to allow for continuous electrocardiographic (ECG) monitoring. If the baseline QTc is prolonged, or if the QTc increases by 25%, disopyramide should not be used, nor should it be trialed at a lower dose. Verapamil, diltiazem, or a β-blocker should be prescribed with disopyramide because it can accelerate atrioventricular (AV) nodal conduction. Anticholinergic side effects of disopyramide—such as constipation, dry mouth, and urinary retention—can limit its use, especially in elderly patients. In a multicenter HCM study, 7% of patients discontinued disopyramide because of these side effects.[5]

Patients with significant LVOTO, either resting or provoked, and moderate-to-severe effort intolerance that is refractory to medical therapy should be considered for surgical myectomy.[3] The current surgical approach involves resection of a rectangular section of septal muscle (trough) from the base to midventricle, resulting in increased LV outflow tract area and decreased SAM (Figure 17-1). Typically less than 10 g of muscle tissue is excised, but this should include the area of mitral-septal contact to relieve LVOTO.[6] Unlike the rectangular muscle trough described by Morrow and colleagues,[6a] some surgeons advocate extending the myectomy trough toward the apex, where the trough is wider than at the base of the heart.[6] It has become standard practice to perform intraoperative transesophageal echocardiography (TEE) with all myectomies. In a retrospective series, the use of intraoperative TEE has been shown to alter surgical intervention in 9% to 20% of cases, often through the detection of residual obstruction that requires further myectomy.[7]

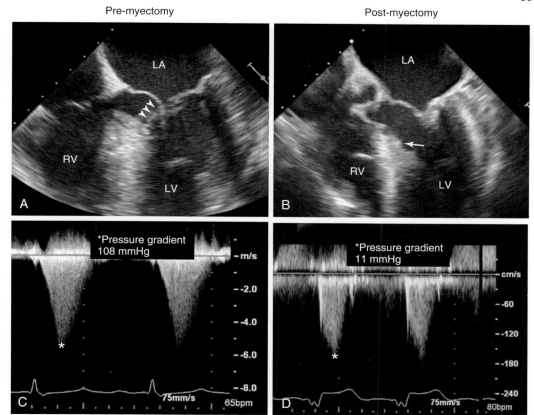

Pre-myectomy

Post-myectomy

FIGURE 17-1 Myectomy effectively abolishes left ventricular (*LV*) outflow tract obstruction. Intraoperative transesophageal images reveal characteristic findings before and after myectomy. Premyectomy systolic anterior motion of the mitral valve (*arrowheads*) and postmyectomy trough (*arrow*) are shown in **A** and **B,** respectively. The corresponding spectral Doppler images in **C** and **D** demonstrate resolution of significant obstruction. LA, left atrium; RV, right ventricle.

Mitral regurgitation associated with LVOTO is caused by SAM and incomplete coaptation of anterior and posterior mitral leaflets. This results in posteriorly directed regurgitation, which corresponds in severity to the magnitude of the outflow tract obstruction. Septal myectomy alone—that is, *without* mitral valve surgery—will effectively resolve mitral regurgitation secondary to LVOTO (Figure 17-2).[8] In contrast, about 10% of HCM patients with mitral regurgitation have structural disease of the mitral apparatus, such as mitral valve prolapse, which results in centrally or anteriorly directed regurgitation. These patients often require mitral valve repair or replacement. Anomalies of the submitral apparatus, including abnormal papillary muscle insertion or orientation, are present in 10% to 20% of patients and may require operative intervention, such as extended myectomy and/or papillary muscle reorientation.[9] Nevertheless, valve *replacement* is infrequently required to correct anomalies of the mitral apparatus.

Contemporary myectomy at highly experienced referral centers typically results in elimination of LVOTO and improvement in symptoms for the vast majority of patients (Table 17-1).[10-12] Severe effort intolerance after myectomy is uncommon (<20%) and is associated with advanced age and female gender, not residual LVOTO.[10] Perioperative death is also uncommon (<2%) in the modern era. The postoperative risk of AV block requiring permanent pacing is 5% to 10%. Because most patients will develop left bundle branch block (LBBB) after myectomy, the risk of complete AV block is much higher in patients with preoperative *right* bundle branch block (RBBB). Late survival after myectomy is good and is similar to age-matched individuals without HCM.[12] Risk factors for cardiovascular events late after myectomy are increased age, concomitant coronary artery disease, female gender, preoperative atrial fibrillation, and atrial enlargement.[10]

ASA is a less invasive approach to septal reduction, and it can effectively relieve LVOTO in selected patients (Table 17-2). ASA involves selective delivery of concentrated ethanol (1 to 3 mL) into a septal perforator artery, causing infarction and thinning of the obstructing myocardium. Coronary anatomy is not always

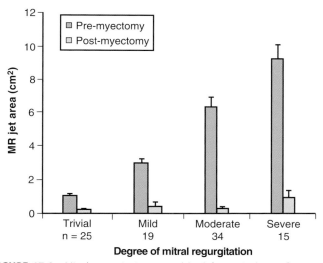

FIGURE 17-2 Mitral regurgitation caused by left ventricular outflow tract obstruction (LVOTO) is relieved by myectomy. Regardless of severity, mitral regurgitation (*MR*) associated with LVOTO is relieved by myectomy and does not require mitral valve repair or replacement. Systolic anterior motion of the mitral leaflets can cause incomplete coaptation of the anterior and posterior leaflets and lead to posteriorly directed regurgitation. (*Data from Yu EH, Omran AS, Wigle ED, et al. Mitral regurgitation in hypertrophic obstructive cardiomyopathy: relationship to obstruction and relief with myectomy. J Am Coll Cardiol 2000;36[7]:2219-2225.*)

suitable to allow ASA,[13] and inappropriate ASA where coronary anatomy is not favorable may be ineffective or may even cause inadvertent infarction of the right ventricle or papillary muscles— with disastrous outcomes. The use of periprocedural contrast echocardiography has been shown to affect 15% to 20% of ASA cases by leading to procedural termination (6%) or target vessel

TABLE 17-1   Outcomes with Surgical Myectomy in Selected Contemporary Series

REFERENCE	N	AGE (YR)	LVOTO (mm Hg, Mean ± SD) BEFORE	AFTER	OPERATIVE MORTALITY (%)	Survival (%) 1 YR	3 YR	5 YR	REOPERATION (%)	PPM (%)
11	323	50 ± 14	68 ± 43	17 ± 11	0	99	98	96	3	7.9
10	338*	47 ± 14	66 ± 32	†	1.5	98	95	83	NR	6
12	289	45 ± 19	67 ± 41	3 ± 8	0.8	98	NR	96	NR	NR

Unless otherwise noted, outcomes are for patients undergoing myectomy alone.
LVOTO, left ventricular outflow tract obstruction; NR, not reported; PPM, postoperative requirement for permanent pacemaker placement; SD, standard deviation.
*249 underwent myectomy alone, 89 as part of a combined surgical procedure.
†98% had no postoperative gradient.

TABLE 17-2   Outcomes with Alcohol Septal Ablation in Selected Contemporary Series

REFERENCE	N	AGE (YR)	ETHANOL (ML)	LVOTO (mm Hg) BEFORE	AFTER	PROCEDURAL MORTALITY (%)	IN-HOSPITAL VF/VT (%)	1-YEAR SURVIVAL (%)	PPM (%)
16	138	64 ± 21	1.8 ± 0.5	80 ± 50	10 ± 19	1.4	0.7	93.5	20
88	91	54 ± 15	3.5 ± 1.5	92 ± 25	8 ± 17	2.2	4.4	NA	4
89	329*	58 ± 15	0.8 ± 0.4	72 ± 43	16 ± 22	0.6	NA	NR	NR
90	629	54 ± 15	2.6 ± 1.0	77 ± 31	26 ± 27	1.0	NA	97	8.2
18	279	59 ± 14	2.2 ± 0.8	58†[34,89]	12†[8,24]	0.3	2.8	97	20

Values are mean ± standard deviation unless otherwise noted.
LVOTO, left ventricular outflow tract obstruction; NR, not reported; PPM, postprocedural requirement for permanent pacemaker placement; VF, ventricular fibrillation; VT, ventricular tachycardia.
*Cohort underwent contemporary therapy of lower dose ethanol injection.
†Median and interquartile range.

change (11%).[14] Septal thickness should be at least 15 mm to prevent iatrogenic ventricular septal rupture. Patients with midcavitary obstruction do not benefit from ASA.

Similar to myectomy, ASA results in substantial reductions in LVOTO (see Table 17-2) and in symptoms for most patients. In a meta-analysis of 42 studies with 2959 patients undergoing ASA, the resting and provoked gradients were reduced from 65 to 16 mm Hg and from 125 to 32 mm Hg, respectively.[15] Although LVOTO improves immediately after ASA, the maximum benefit usually does not develop until adequate thinning of the infarcted segment has occurred, typically after several weeks. When performed at experienced centers, less than 20% of patients are left with significant LVOTO after ASA.[16] Predictors of long-term procedural failure are operator inexperience, immediate postprocedural LVOTO of 25 mm Hg or higher, and low post-ASA peak creatine kinase.[13,17] The reduction in LVOTO translates into improved symptoms, as most patients are New York Hospital Association (NYHA) class I or II after ASA.[15,16] In a multicenter Scandinavian series, the percentage of patients who experienced severe effort intolerance (NYHA class III to IV) was reduced from 94% before ASA to 21% at 1 year follow-up.[18] Persistent symptoms after ASA may reflect persistent LVOTO but are more likely to result from concomitant cardiopulmonary comorbidities.[18] Approximately 2% of patients who undergo ASA will die within 30 days, and 2% to 4% will be resuscitated because of ventricular tachyarrhythmias. Patients who die during or immediately after ASA are often critically ill before the procedure.[16] AV block that requires permanent pacing complicates 10% to 20% of ASA procedures. In addition, RBBB commonly develops afterward; accordingly, patients with preexisting LBBB more commonly require a pacemaker. Coronary artery dissection, pericardial tamponade, and iatrogenic ventricular septal rupture are rare complications of ASA that complicate less than 2% of cases. Late complications of ASA are relatively infrequent, although the associated risk of ventricular arrhythmias and sudden death is debated.[19]

It remains controversial whether myectomy or ASA should be considered the preferred treatment modality for patients with LVOTO and medically refractory symptoms.[20,21] It is unlikely that any controlled, prospective study will compare the efficacy and safety of surgical myectomy to ASA. As such, comparisons are based on retrospective analyses that are subject to considerable selection bias. Meta-analyses have compared ASA to myectomy and found no significant difference in postintervention NYHA functional class or mortality.[22] The American Heart Association/American College of Cardiology (AHA/ACC) consensus document on HCM recommends surgical myectomy as the preferred therapy for patients with medically refractory obstructive HCM. Nevertheless, ASA far outnumbers myectomy, and institutional practice varies considerably. Ultimately, patient preference is often the major factor driving this decision, and providers should appropriately inform patients of the relative merits of each procedure.[20,21] Nevertheless, certain patient-specific factors do constitute either absolute or relative indications for myectomy over ASA or vice versa. Patients with a need for concomitant surgery, such as coronary artery bypass grafting (CABG) or mitral valve repair, should undergo myectomy. Surgical myectomy is also preferred for individuals with coronary anatomy unsuitable to ASA, severe hypertrophy (interventricular septum [IVS] >30 mm), papillary muscle anomalies, or unusual patterns of hypertrophy. Likewise, most experts agree that young patients are better served with surgical myectomy. Alternatively, patients with medical comorbidities associated with high cardiac surgical risk should undergo ASA.

Ventricular pacing showed initial promise for reducing LVOTO in small studies. In the Multicenter Pacing Therapy (M-PATHY) study, 44 medically refractory patients with a resting outflow tract gradient of 50 mm Hg or higher underwent implantation of a dual-chamber pacer.[23] In this randomized, double-blind crossover study, pacing did not improve exercise capacity or symptoms. The severity of obstruction was improved after 3 months of pacing (76 ± 32 vs. 48 ± 32 mm Hg; $P < .001$), but gradient reduction did not correlate with symptom improvement or exercise capacity. Accordingly, implantation of a pacemaker is not recommended as a routine treatment of symptomatic outflow tract obstruction.[24] However, if patients have a pacemaker for another indication (e.g., heart block), a trial of pacing can be considered for refractory symptoms. In this setting, it is advised that AV delay be sufficient to allow AV synchrony while maximizing the amount of ventricular pacing.

Therapies for Nonobstructive Hypertrophic Cardiomyopathy

Patients with nonobstructive HCM may experience significant effort intolerance related to diastolic dysfunction and/or microvascular ischemia. Few therapies have been systematically studied in nonobstructive HCM; however, nondihydropyridine calcium channel blockers (verapamil and diltiazem) and β-blockers are empiric first-line therapies. In nonobstructive HCM, diuretics are used as required without excess risk of hemodynamic compromise; this stands in contrast to the situation of LVOTO, in which obstruction can be acutely worsened by decreased preload.[3] In a small, double-blind crossover study of 16 patients with mild symptoms and predominantly nonobstructive HCM, neither nadolol nor verapamil improved exercise capacity or oxygen consumption compared with placebo. However, a trend was seen toward improved symptoms with drug therapy.[25]

Abnormal myocardial energy utilization is an important feature of HCM that is present early in disease pathogenesis and represents a new therapeutic target.[26] One drug that improves myocardial oxygen utilization and has been shown to improve ejection fraction and quality of life in HF[27] is perhexiline, which was studied in a double-blind, placebo-controlled trial of 46 patients with nonobstructive HCM; it significantly improved NYHA functional classification, symptoms, and exercise capacity.[28] These changes were associated with improved myocardial energetics (as assessed by ^{31}P magnetic resonance [MR] spectroscopy) and diastolic function (as assessed by radionuclide angiography). Although these results are promising, perhexiline is not approved for use by the U.S. Food and Drug Administration (FDA) because of concerns about hepatotoxicity.

Approximately 5% of patients will develop end-stage HCM, characterized by reduced LV ejection fraction with or without dilated remodeling.[29] Survival is substantially reduced in end-stage HCM, and although medical therapy has not been studied in this population, conventional therapies for HF with reduced ejection fraction are advised[2,30]—β-blockers, ACE inhibitors, and aldosterone antagonists—as is withdrawal of verapamil, diltiazem, and disopyramide. Consensus guidelines do not yet address the appropriateness of cardiac resynchronization therapy in end-stage HCM.

Cardiac transplantation is an option for patients with refractory HF or intractable arrhythmias. Registry data have shown that transplanted patients have favorable long-term survival but wait longer for transplantation than non-HCM patients.[31] Patients with HCM were not included in the pivotal trials of left ventricular assist devices (LVADs) for advanced HF. The feasibility of LVAD therapy has been shown in a small series of patients with end-stage HCM.[32]

Prevention of Sudden Cardiac Death in Hypertrophic Cardiomyopathy

The leading cause of sudden cardiac death (SCD) in young people is HCM. Ventricular tachyarrhythmias underlie these events and are unpredictable. Nevertheless, SCD affects only a minority of patients with HCM, and in patients diagnosed as adults, overall survival is similar to age-matched individuals without HCM.[33] Patients at risk can be identified through comprehensive evaluation for established risk factors of SCD, which include 1) unexplained syncope, 2) family history of SCD, 3) failure to augment systolic blood pressure of 20 mm Hg or more with exercise, 4) nonsustained ventricular tachycardia (VT), and 5) maximal wall thickness of 30 mm or more.[33] Of these, unexplained syncope and family history of sudden death carry the greatest prognostic value. Multiple risk

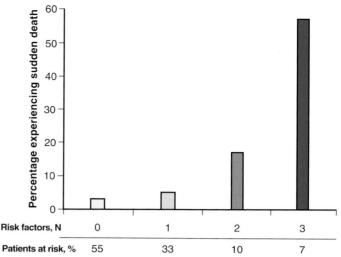

FIGURE 17-3 Risk factors for sudden death in hypertrophic cardiomyopathy increase cumulative risk in an additive fashion. Risk of sudden cardiac death increased with the number of risk factors, whereas the proportion of patients with multiple risk factors was low. Risk factors include abnormal blood pressure response to exercise, nonsustained ventricular tachycardia, syncope, massive hypertrophy (>30 mm), and family history of sudden cardiac death. *(Modified from Elliot PM, Poloniecki J, Dickie S, et al. Sudden death in hypertrophic cardiomyopathy: identification of high-risk patients. J Am Coll Cardiol 2000;36[7]:2212-2218.)*

factors identify patients at highest risk (Figure 17-3).[34] The prognostic implications are unresolved for several emerging risk factors, including end-stage remodeling,[29] extensive delayed enhancement on cardiac magnetic resonance imaging (MRI),[35] genotype,[36] possibly LVOTO,[37] and paced ventricular electrogram fractionation.[38] Programmed ventricular stimulation (electrophysiology [EP] testing) is not predictive and is therefore not recommended for risk stratification.[33] No controlled studies of SCD prevention strategies in HCM have been done, but all patients should be advised to avoid activities perceived to increase the risk of SCD, including competitive sports and high-intensity athletic training.[2] Routine physical fitness, however, is not prohibited. Placement of an implantable cardioverter-defibrillator (ICD) is advised for all patients with a history of resuscitated SCD or sustained VT. ICD therapy is an option for primary prevention of SCD in patients judged to be at high risk based on the presence of one or more established risk factors.[24] Medical therapy is largely unproven for prevention of SCD in HCM. Consensus guidelines recommend amiodarone in patients at high risk of SCD who are not candidates for an ICD.[39] Combined epicardial and endocardial mapping and ablation has also been used in selected HCM patients to treat refractory monomorphic VT.[40]

Management of Atrial Fibrillation in Hypertrophic Cardiomyopathy

Atrial fibrillation (AF) is a common arrhythmia in patients with HCM, with an overall prevalence of about 20%. In some patients, the development of AF may significantly worsen symptoms through loss of AV synchrony and/or increased ventricular rate. A strategy of heart-rate control versus rhythm management has not been specifically tested in HCM, but in selected patients, restoration of sinus rhythm can be beneficial.[3] Both amiodarone and disopyramide have been studied in HCM and have an acceptable safety profile in these patients.[41] Because disopyramide can increase AV nodal conduction and accelerate ventricular response to AF, it should be used in conjunction with verapamil, diltiazem, or a β-blocker. The role of nonpharmacologic therapy for AF, such as a surgical Maze procedure or radiofrequency ablation (RFA), is not well established in HCM.

Based on large cohort studies, patients with HCM have an annual risk of stroke and arterial embolic events of approximately 1%. AF further increases the risk of these events by as much as 18-fold.[42] Conventional strategies of assessing risk for stroke and assigning antithrombotic therapy for AF, such as the CHADS$_2$ score, were not developed for patients with HCM.[41,43] Consensus guideline recommendations call for anticoagulation of patients with HCM and either persistent or permanent AF. Anticoagulation for paroxysmal AF should be considered for patients otherwise at increased risk for thromboembolism.[41]

Screening at-Risk Family Members for Hypertrophic Cardiomyopathy

All first-degree family members of patients with HCM should be screened for LVH with transthoracic echocardiography and 12-lead ECG. The presence of mild hypertrophy (IVS ≥13 mm or Z score ≥2 in children) is sufficient to make a diagnosis of overt HCM. In addition, findings on ECG may be nonspecific, particularly increased QRS voltage, but these can serve as supportive or confirmatory findings.[43a] Because disease may not develop until later in life, screening should be performed on a longitudinal basis, beginning in childhood and concentrated during adolescence and young adulthood, when development of the overt phenotype is most common.[44] Genetic testing is recommended because it can simplify family evaluations by definitively identifying risk, and it can restrict clinical evaluations except where truly needed.[44] A pathogenic sarcomere mutation can be identified in about 50% of patients with HCM. Complete sequencing of a panel of sarcomere genes should be performed on the proband because pathogenic mutations are typically "private" or unique to a family. If present in the index family member (proband), relatives can be tested for the presence of the same mutation; those who are carriers will require clinical follow-up. The clinical management of asymptomatic mutation carriers who have not (yet) developed LVH is undefined. Abnormal myocardial function can be demonstrated in preclinical mutation carriers, including abnormal diastolic function, increased myocardial fibrosis, and abnormal energetics.[45] Nevertheless, medical therapy is not currently indicated in this population, and proscription from competitive athletics is not mandated.[46]

Restrictive and Infiltrative Cardiomyopathies

Restrictive cardiomyopathies (RCMs) are a less commonly encountered type of heart muscle disease and are generally divided into those that affect the myocardium—such as primary RCM, amyloidosis, sarcoidosis, and hemochromatosis—and those that affect the endocardium, such as endomyocardial fibrosis (Box 17-1).[47,48] RCM must be differentiated from constrictive pericarditis, so computed tomography (CT), MRI, and invasive hemodynamics are quite useful for differentiating the two conditions.[48]

Idiopathic Restrictive Cardiomyopathy

The pathogenesis of idiopathic RCM is unknown, and a familial form, although extremely rare, does exist. Endomyocardial biopsy is useful in excluding secondary causes of infiltrative or restrictive disease, but findings may be nondiagnostic because of sampling error and/or end-stage fibrosis. Medical management consists of diuretics to control diastolic HF symptoms, management of supraventricular arrhythmias, and pacemaker insertion if high-grade AV block develops. Cardiac transplantation is often necessary in patients who progress to NYHA class IV symptoms of HF. Multivariate analysis has identified male sex, marked left atrial enlargement, age greater than 70 years, and higher NYHA functional class as

Box 17-1 Etiology of Restrictive Cardiomyopathies

Myocardial Diseases
Noninfiltrative
Idiopathic restrictive
Scleroderma
Pseudoxanthoma elasticum
Diabetic cardiomyopathy
Mitochondrial cardiomyopathy

Infiltrative
Amyloidosis*
Sarcoidosis*
Gaucher disease*
Hunter/Hurler disease*

Storage Diseases
Hemochromatosis*
Fabry disease*
Danon disease
PRKAG2 mutations†
Glycogen storage diseases*

Endocardial Diseases
Endomyocardial fibrosis
Hypereosinophilic syndrome*
Carcinoid heart disease*
Metastatic tumors
Radiation injury
Drug toxicities (anthracycline, serotonin, ergotamine, busulfan)

*Disease-specific therapy available.
†*PRKAG2* encodes the gamma subunit of adenosine monophosphate–activated protein kinase.
Modified from Kushwaha S, Fallon JT, Fuster V. Restrictive cardiomyopathy. *N Engl J Med* 1997;336[4]:267-276.

predictors of poor survival in adults.[48] However, end-stage liver disease may result from long-standing right HF and may preclude cardiac transplantation. This highlights the importance of early identification of patients who would benefit from cardiac transplantation prior to the development of cardiac cirrhosis. In one retrospective study, hepatic fibrosis was more common in end-stage HF if concomitant renal failure, tricuspid regurgitation, and/or abnormal liver function tests were evident.[49]

Cardiac Amyloidosis

Primary amyloidosis (AL) accounts for 85% of cases of cardiac amyloidosis and is associated with the deposition of monoclonal κ- or λ-immunoglobulin light chains. A familial autosomal form of amyloidosis occurs through deposition of mutated transthyretin-related (ATTR$_m$) protein.[50,51] Senile cardiac amyloidosis (SCA) results from deposition of either atrial natriuretic peptide or wild-type transthyretin-related (ATTR$_{wt}$) protein.[51] Most patients who come to medical attention do so with right-sided HF signs and symptoms. Orthostatic hypotension and syncope are also common. SCA is usually asymptomatic, although HF is the most common presentation when symptoms do exist.

It is essential to obtain a tissue diagnosis and determine amyloid type prior to initiating therapy. Although endomyocardial biopsy is the most sensitive technique, less invasive tissue biopsies—including abdominal fat pad aspiration or rectal biopsy—are often initially performed. Serum protein electrophoresis will demonstrate an M component in only 50% of cases of AL amyloid. The presence of serum or urine monoclonal paraproteins is highly suggestive of AL amyloid but does not definitely establish the diagnosis. Immunofixation electrophoresis of serum or urine is more sensitive and is thus the preferred method for detecting abnormal light chains. Familial amyloidosis is generally confirmed through genetic testing. MRI findings are highly suggestive of cardiac amyloidosis, and the technique may be used for initial screening of family members.[52]

Therapy should focus on two aspects: 1) general supportive measures of cardiac-related symptoms and 2) specific treatment to reduce further amyloid deposition.[50,51] Management and prognosis differ by type of amyloidosis, but diuretics are the mainstay of HF therapy; high doses or intravenous administration may be required, if ascites is marked or hypoalbuminemia is present as a result of concomitant nephrotic syndrome. Recurrent pleural effusions may necessitate repeated thoracentesis or occasional pleurodesis. ACE inhibitors and angiotensin receptor antagonists are poorly tolerated, even at low doses, because of orthostatic hypotension.[50,51] Data are lacking on the effectiveness of β-blockade on survival in amyloidosis, but these agents may not be tolerated because of heart rate slowing in the face of a fixed stroke volume. Calcium channel antagonists are contraindicated because of their negative inotropic effects. Amyloid fibrils directly bind digoxin and may increase susceptibility to digoxin toxicity. Renal-dose dopamine (1 to 3 μg/kg) may be a useful adjunct in the treatment of anasarca,[51] and amiodarone is useful for maintaining sinus rhythm among patients who have worsening of symptoms during bouts of AF.

Anticoagulation is indicated in patients with paroxysmal or permanent AF because the risk of intracardiac thrombus is high.[50,53] It should be recognized, however, that amyloidosis may be associated with vascular infiltration and coagulopathy and may thus pose a theoretical increased risk of hemorrhage. The role of anticoagulation among patients in sinus rhythm is uncertain. Atrial contractile failure and diastolic dysfunction, even in the presence of sinus rhythm, are associated with an increased risk of atrial thrombus formation. Anticoagulation is often recommended when a small transmitral A wave (<20 cm/s) is seen on ECG.[53] TEE may reveal left atrial appendage thrombus or left atrial appendage spontaneous echo contrast.[53] Dual-chamber pacemaker insertion is indicated for high-grade AV block or for symptomatic bradycardic rhythms, whereas ICDs have not been shown to prolong survival; death is usually the result of electromechanical dissociation or progressive HF.[54]

Definitive treatment for AL amyloid is aimed at eliminating abnormal protein production. Standard treatment for cardiac amyloid patients has generally involved a combination of melphalan and prednisone, although complete remission is uncommon. Survival is best among patients who demonstrate a substantial reduction in circulating free light chains.[55] A regimen of "continuous" oral melphalan may have slight benefit over "pulsed" melphalan and prednisone regimens among patients with severe cardiac disease; nonetheless, median survival still falls below 6 months.[50] Low-dose oral melphalan-prednisone regimens have largely been replaced by melphalan-dexamethasone protocols for cardiac AL patients. Short courses of oral melphalan (0.25 mg/kg daily on days 1 through 4 every 28 days) combined with dexamethasone (40 mg/day in a similar protocol) has resulted in overall response rates of 67%, and complete remissions have been reported for up to 3 years.[56] However, the vast majority of these patients did not have advanced cardiac involvement. A variety of new chemotherapeutic regimens are being evaluated that include thalidomide, lenalidomide, rituximab, and bortezomib either alone or in combination.[57] Unfortunately, significant cardiac involvement is a contraindication for several of these new agents.

Heart transplantation is rarely performed because of substantial amyloid deposition in other organs. Small initial case series demonstrated that AL amyloid recurred in the donor heart and resulted in unacceptable short-term survival rates.[58] More recently, sequential heart transplantation followed by autologous stem cell transplantation has been undertaken in a small number of highly selected patients at referral centers.[59,60] Ideal candidates include younger patients with HF symptoms but preserved renal, gastrointestinal (GI), and autonomic function. Standard immunosuppressive therapy has been utilized following transplantation. Myeloablative high-dose melphalan therapy followed by autologous stem cell infusion typically occurs 6 to 12 months after successful heart transplantation. Median survival has been reported at 75.5 months with over 70% of patients surviving 5 years following transplantation.[59]

Patients with ATTR$_m$ typically have less severe cardiac involvement, and liver transplantation is curative in most patients.[51] Heart transplantation in ATTR$_m$ amyloid is rarely required but has been reported to be successful. Clinical trials are ongoing to assess novel therapies that stabilize ATTR$_m$ and prevent further amyloid deposition.[61]

Cardiac Sarcoidosis

Clinical manifestations of cardiac sarcoidosis depend on the location and extent of granulomatous inflammation. The heart is involved in approximately 25% of cases of generalized sarcoidosis.[62] Myocardial involvement is uncommon when cardiac symptoms are absent. Symptoms result from either infiltration of the conduction system, the myocardium, or both. Patients may be seen with arrhythmias or heart block with normal ventricular function, or they may be seen with HF resulting from either a dilated or restrictive cardiomyopathy.[48,62] Sudden death is an uncommon, but feared, initial presentation.

Initial cardiac evaluation should include a detailed history, physical examination, ECG, and echocardiography. Among patients in whom the suspicion of cardiac sarcoidosis is low and initial evaluation proves normal, periodic clinical and ECG follow-up is recommended.

When initial evaluation suggests cardiac sarcoidosis, many clinicians will proceed directly to endomyocardial biopsy.[62,63] Although the biopsy is the gold standard for confirming myocardial sarcoidosis, sensitivity is poor—10% to 50% depending on clinical presentation and number of samples—and it is not always capable of differentiating cardiac sarcoidosis from giant cell myocarditis, which has a substantially worse prognosis.[63] Current ACC/American Heart Association (AHA) guidelines indicate biopsy as a 2B recommendation that should be considered for patients with HF of longer than 3 months' duration associated with a dilated cardiomyopathy (DCM) and either new ventricular arrhythmias or second- or third-degree heart block.[64,65] Many clinicians have abandoned biopsy as a confirmatory technique and instead rely on noninvasive imaging modalities to evaluate cardiac involvement.

Echocardiography may demonstrate normal ventricular function, abnormal diastolic function, global or regional LV systolic dysfunction, RCM, aneurysm formation, or pericardial effusion. Myocardial perfusion imaging using either thallium-201 or technetium-99 scintigraphy typically reveals reversible or fixed defects that correspond to abnormalities of the coronary microvasculature and/or the presence of scar or granulomatous formation. Although not specific, these may indicate potential responsiveness to corticosteroid treatment.[62] Positron emission tomography (PET) using ^{18}F fluorodeoxyglucose (FDG) has recently proven useful for diagnosing cardiac sarcoidosis.[66] PET imaging has the advantage of being able to acquire perfusion images that may permit better assessment of disease activity in addition to visualization of the extent of fibrogranulomatous replacement of the myocardium. Cardiac MRI has become the noninvasive procedure of choice for evaluating patients with suspected sarcoidosis.[62,67] MRI may show segmental wall motion abnormalities or regions of focal wall thickening or thinning. The pattern of late gadolinium enhancement (LGE) may represent a combination of fibrous and granulomatous replacement in addition to ongoing inflammation. Recent studies have documented a relationship between extent of LGE and clinical disease severity. MRI evidence of myocardial involvement predicts a 9-fold higher rate of adverse events (17% per year vs. 2%) and an 11.5-fold higher risk of cardiac death (11.5% vs. 1%).[68]

FDG-PET and cardiac MRI are also useful for monitoring therapeutic responsiveness.[69] If neither imaging modality is available, technetium 99m scintigraphy can be used. The optimal time for follow-up imaging after initiation of treatment is not known, but 2 to 3 months is generally recommended.[62,69]

Ambulatory 24-hour ECG monitoring of cardiac sarcoid patients to assess extent of ventricular arrhythmias is recommended.[62] EP testing is usually reserved for patients with syncope or wide complex tachycardia.[48,62] Although reproducibility is low, some clinicians still advocate EP testing for risk stratification.[62] Patients with spontaneous or inducible ventricular arrhythmias are at higher risk for future life-threatening events despite treatment with β-blockers. For patients who have documented high-grade ventricular arrhythmias, ICD placement should be considered regardless of EP testing results.[48,62]

TREATMENT

Prospective randomized trials to evaluate therapy for cardiac sarcoidosis are lacking. Conservative treatment of asymptomatic patients appears warranted and should include yearly clinical evaluation, ECG, and echocardiography. Cardiac pacing should be considered for patients with second-degree AV block, even if asymptomatic. Whether these patients would also benefit from prophylactic ICD insertion is uncertain, although many clinicians advocate this approach to try to lower the risk of SCD.[62]

Corticosteroid therapy is the mainstay of treatment for sarcoidosis.[48,62] Although most data have been obtained from small retrospective case series, improvement or even complete resolution of abnormal findings on MRI, PET, echocardiography, and myocardial perfusion studies have been reported during steroid treatment.[62,66,68,69] Among patients with RCM, no deterioration in ejection fraction has been reported during treatment.[70] Among patients with ejection fractions between 30% and 50%, treatment often results in significantly improved ventricular function. Treatment is seldom successful when LV ejection fraction is below 30%.[70] Prednisone is typically initiated at 30 to 60 mg daily and rapidly tapered over 3 to 6 months to 5 to 15 mg daily. Treatment is typically continued for 6 to 12 months, although some investigators recommend lifelong low-dose treatment to prevent relapses.[70] Patients should be monitored closely for relapse after discontinuation of corticosteroids, and follow-up imaging studies at 3, 6, and 12 months and then yearly have been advocated.[70] Other immunosuppressive agents—including infliximab, methotrexate, azathioprine, cyclophosphamide, and thalidomide—have been used in combination with steroids in the treatment of generalized sarcoidosis; however, the responsiveness of cardiac disease to some newer agents is uncertain. Although 5- and 10-year survival rates are significantly higher in DCM patients treated with immunosuppression, it is unknown whether this approach can improve survival in RCM patients. For patients with persistent systolic dysfunction, standard pharmacologic therapy with ACE inhibitors, angiotensin receptor antagonists, diuretics, and β-blockers is recommended.

Ventricular arrhythmias in cardiac sarcoidosis respond poorly to antiarrhythmic therapy. ICD therapy is indicated for the secondary prevention of survivors of sudden death or for patients with refractory ventricular arrhythmias who remain at risk for sudden death.[24] The role of prophylactic ICD therapy among patients with ejection fractions above 35% has not been studied, but ICD placement may be considered among patients with significant late gadolinium enhancement because their risk of sudden death is high.[68] Catheter ablation may occasionally reduce or eliminate VT in patients with recurrent ventricular arrhythmias,[71] but recurrence of the same or different VT is common.

Surgery is occasionally necessary to correct progressive mitral regurgitation or for ventricular aneurysm resection for refractory ventricular arrhythmias.[48] Cardiac transplantation is a therapeutic option for end-stage cardiomyopathy or refractory arrhythmias, and survival rates following transplantation exceed those for other forms of cardiomyopathy.[72] Although recurrent sarcoidosis in the allograft can occur, it is highly responsive to enhanced immunosuppression and does not affect long-term prognosis, which exceeds 80% at 5 years.[72]

Cardiac Hemochromatosis

Iron overload cardiomyopathy may present as systolic or diastolic cardiac dysfunction.[73,74] Excessive iron accumulation usually occurs either by increased GI iron absorption (hemochromatosis) or excessive administration of exogenous iron by dietary sources or transfusions. Early iron-overload cardiomyopathy is characterized by restrictive disease, which progresses to end-stage DCM if untreated.[73,74]

The clinical presentation in systemic hemochromatosis may include hepatomegaly, abnormal liver function tests, and arthritis. Right-sided HF findings predominate. ECG abnormalities occur in 25% to 65% of patients with cardiac hemochromatosis and may include nonspecific repolarization abnormalities, low QRS voltage, conduction delays, AF, and AV block.[73,75] Unlike most infiltrative cardiomyopathies, LV wall thickening on ECG is seldom observed. Systolic function remains normal until late in the disease process. Conventional ECG measures of diastolic function are insensitive for detecting early myocardial iron overload. Cardiac MRI can quantitatively assess myocardial iron content because the paramagnetic effects of iron shorten T2 and T2* relaxation times. Patients with ventricular dysfunction demonstrate myocardial T2* duration less than 20 ms.[76] T2* duration is highly predictive in a step-wise manner for the subsequent development of HF, which is rarely observed when T2* is more than 10 ms but exceeds 50% when T2* is less than 8 ms.[76]

The diagnostic approach to a patient with RCM should include transthoracic ECG, serum iron studies, and cardiac MRI with T2* imaging. If T2* is confirmed to be normal (>20 ms), iron overload is unlikely, and further evaluation is unnecessary unless the patient remains at continued risk for iron overload.[74]

TREATMENT

The optimal treatment of asymptomatic patients identified by genetic screening remains uncertain. Phlebotomy therapy may minimize cardiac injury, and strain rate imaging has been suggested as a sensitive tool for early detection of contractile dysfunction in this population at risk, but this approach remains unproven.

Primary therapy for primary or secondary hemochromatosis should promote whole-body iron removal.[74] Patients should eliminate consumption of iron-rich foods, such as red meat; minimize alcohol intake, which increases iron absorption; and avoid multivitamin tablets containing iron and vitamin C. Phlebotomy is the gold standard for treating hereditary hematochromatosis and causes iatrogenic anemia by removing 200 to 250 mg of iron per session. Early in the disease, phlebotomy can be performed up to twice a week to lower ferritin to below 20 ng/mL.[74] The frequency of maintenance phlebotomy is determined by follow-up serum iron and ferritin levels with a goal of keeping the serum ferritin concentration below 50 ng/mL. Phlebotomy, when initiated early, can result in normal life span among patients with mild restrictive disease and can also improve LV function among those with advanced disease.[73-75]

Iron chelation therapy is the mainstay of treatment for RCM patients; it decreases excess myocardial iron by binding it and excreting the compound in urine and bile. The primary parenteral iron chelator, deferoxamine, or oral iron chelators, such as deferiprone or deferasirox, are clinically useful. Deferoxamine has a very high affinity for binding to the trivalent ferric iron that accumulates in the myocardial tissue. Long-term subcutaneous deferoxamine has been shown to improve survival and decrease cardiac complications in transfusion-dependent iron-overloaded patients with restrictive or dilated cardiomyopathies.[73] High intravenous doses can rapidly lower iron levels in advanced disease, improve T2* values, increase LV ejection fraction, and reduce LV volume and mass.[77] The need for frequent intravenous administration and the high maintenance cost contribute to poor compliance. Oral deferiprone is more effective than deferoxamine in removing myocardial iron, and combination therapy with deferoxamine and deferiprone has been shown to be more effective in improving LV function than either agent alone.[78,79] Newer chelating agents—deferitrin, desferrithiocin, and hydroxybenzyl ethylenediamine-diacetic acid—are undergoing clinical investigation.[78]

Heart transplantation should be considered for patients who progress from a restrictive to a dilated phase with advanced HF symptoms. Combined heart and liver transplantation may sometimes be required because of advanced cardiac and hepatic disease. Actuarial 10-year survival rates for isolated heart transplantation approximate 50%.[80] Rarely, pacemaker therapy is required to treat symptomatic bradyarrhythmias or conduction system disease.

Storage Diseases of the Myocardium

FABRY DISEASE

Fabry disease is an X-linked autosomal-recessive disorder that results from deficiency of the lysosomal enzyme, α-galactosidase A, which degrades neutral glycosphingolipids.[47] Intracellular accumulation of ceramide trihexoside occurs in myocardium; full expression occurs in males, and incomplete expression occurs in females. Cardiac involvement frequently mimics morphologic and clinical features of hypertrophic cardiomyopathy, including very thick ventricular walls. Approximately 1% of cases initially diagnosed as HCM are, in fact, due to Fabry disease.[47] Cardiac MRI typically shows focal inferolateral midwall LGE that spares the subendocardium.[47] The ECG typically shows LVH, and preexcitation may also be present. The disease is diagnosed by detection of low α-galactosidase levels in plasma, the identification of a pathogenic mutation in *GLA*, or the presence of lamellar inclusion bodies on myocardial biopsy specimens. Recombinant enzyme replacement therapy has been shown to improve symptoms, reduce LV wall thickness, and improve regional myocardial function, but its effects on long-term survival have not been adequately determined.[47] A randomized, controlled trial of replacement therapy with recombinant human α-galactosidase A demonstrated substantial clearance of microvascular globotriaosyl ceramide in posttreatment endomyocardial biopsies.[81] Capillary endothelial cells remain free of accumulation for up to 5 years, suggesting that long-term treatment may halt the progression of vascular pathology.[81,82]

CARDIOMYOPATHY ASSOCIATED WITH MUTATIONS IN *LAMP2* (DANON DISEASE), *PRKAG2*, OR MITOCHONDRIAL GENES

Danon disease is a rare, semidominant X-linked disorder that results from primary deficiency of lysosome-associated membrane protein 2 (*LAMP2*).[47,83] Cardiac symptoms typically begin during adolescence with progressive HF that results in death or cardiac transplantation in the third decade. Patients may develop lethal ventricular tachyarrhythmias that cannot be terminated by ICD therapies.[84] Echocardiographic characteristics include massive LVH (wall thickness of 20 to 60 mm) and a prominent increase in right ventricular wall thickness (≥10 mm). Similar to Fabry's disease, preexcitation on surface ECG is often seen, but genetic testing for *LAMP2* gene mutations is the definitive diagnostic test. At present, no specific treatment is available for Danon disease; however, a low threshold to refer for cardiac transplantation is advised, given the precipitous decline experienced by many patients.

Mutations in genes that encode adenosine monophosphate–activated protein kinase (*PRKAG2*) may also be seen with marked LVH and preexcitation, for which no specific therapy is currently available.[47] The prognosis cardiomyopathy associated with *PRKAG2* mutations is better than what is seen with Danon disease.

Mutations in mitochondrial genes cause multisystem disorders that can include cardiomyopathy with conduction disease and arrhythmia.[65] Cardiac remodeling is typically hypertrophic but may progress to dilation and systolic dysfunction. Diagnosis may

be suspected if inheritance is matrilinear or if associated features include hearing loss, epilepsy, diabetes, and/or skeletal myopathy. Genetic testing can allow definitive diagnosis, and suggestive features may be present by histopathologic examination. Standard HF therapies are recommended, and there may be a role for agents that improve myocardial energetics, including creatine, carnitine, and coenzyme Q10.[85]

Endomyocardial Disorders

ENDOMYOCARDIAL FIBROSIS

Endomyocardial fibrosis (EMF) is a myocardial disorder typically seen in equatorial countries, and it accounts for approximately 20% of all HF cases and 15% of cardiac deaths in equatorial Africa. The heart size is normal or small with prominent obliterative fibrosis that restricts inflow of the right and/or left ventricles. EMF is biventricular in approximately 50% of patients, purely involves the left ventricle in 40%, and involves only the right ventricle in the remaining 10%. Fibrosis also involves the papillary muscles and chordae tendineae, distorting AV valvular anatomy and producing regurgitation. EMF is a disease of the young and occurs in children, adolescents, and young adults. ECG features include myocardial calcification, intracavity thrombi, thickening of the anterior right ventricular wall, and small pericardial effusions.[48] Right and/or left ventricular apical cavity obliteration by thrombus or fibrous tissue is common, as is severe biatrial enlargement and varying degrees of mitral and tricuspid regurgitation. EMF may be visualized as a linear band of calcification *within* the myocardium, thereby differentiating it from constrictive pericardial disease. Endomyocardial biopsy is not clinically indicated and, in fact, it is contraindicated with LV disease, as it may be complicated by systemic emboli. Sudden death and syncopal episodes appear to be more common in EMF compared with other etiologies of RCM.[48]

Medical management of EMF consists of sodium and fluid restriction and diuretics.[48] As most patients come to medical attention with end-stage disease, annual mortality rates often approach 25% despite medical therapy.[86] The development of AF is a poor prognostic indicator. Diuretic refractoriness develops with progressive right-sided failure and ascites. Surgical treatment involves resection of the fibrous endocardium and, often, replacement of the mitral and tricuspid valves. Operative mortality rates have historically ranged from 10% to 30%, but more recent series have found lower perioperative mortality rates.[48,87] Patients with NYHA functional class III or IV symptoms derive the most benefit from surgical treatment that produces sustained hemodynamic improvement with reduction in filling pressures and increased cardiac output. Surgically treated patients have 5-year survival rates of 60% to 70%, but fibrosis may occasionally recur.

LÖFFLER HYPEREOSINOPHILIC SYNDROME

Hypereosinophilic EMF, also known as *Löffler syndrome*, is observed in temperate zones. Restrictive disease occurs in more than 75% of patients, and an eosinophilic count exceeding 1500 mm[3] for at least 6 months is typically observed. Hypereosinophilia may be secondary to leukemia, parasitic infections, drug allergies, granulomatous disease, hypersensitivity, or neoplastic disorders. Both right and left ventricles are involved, with endocardial thickening of the inflow regions and the ventricular apices.[48] Varying degrees of eosinophilic myocarditis may be observed within the myocardium and thrombosis, and inflammation of small intramural coronary arteries is common. Clinical presentations typically include fever, cough, rash, weight loss, HF, and systemic emboli. AF, apical thrombus formation, and varying degrees of AV valve regurgitation are often present.

Medical therapy typically consists of corticosteroids in combination with cytotoxic drugs, particularly hydroxyurea, and interferon therapy has been reported as being useful for patients with refractory symptoms.[48] Pharmacologic therapy with diuretics, ACE inhibitors or angiotensin receptor blockers, and anticoagulants are also appropriate. In addition, surgical resection of the fibrotic endocardial material and valve replacement or repair may offer significant symptomatic improvement, once the fibrotic stage of the disease has become evident.

REFERENCES

1. Wang L, Seidman JG, Seidman CE. Narrative review: harnessing molecular genetics for the diagnosis and management of hypertrophic cardiomyopathy. *Ann Intern Med* 2010;152(8):513-520, W181.
2. Gersh BJ, Maron BJ, Bonow RO, et al. 2011 ACCF/AHA guideline for the diagnosis and treatment of hypertrophic cardiomyopathy: executive summary: a report of the American College of Cardiology Foundation/American Heart Association Task Force on Practice Guidelines. *Circulation* 2011;124(24):2761-2796.
3. Fifer MA, Vlahakes GJ. Management of symptoms in hypertrophic cardiomyopathy. *Circulation* 2008;117(3):429-439.
4. Ommen SR, Shah PM, Tajik AJ. Left ventricular outflow tract obstruction in hypertrophic cardiomyopathy: past, present and future. *Heart* 2008;94(10):1276-1281.
5. Sherrid MV, Barac I, McKenna WJ, et al. Multicenter study of the efficacy and safety of disopyramide in obstructive hypertrophic cardiomyopathy. *J Am Coll Cardiol* 2005;45(8): 1251-1258.
6. Dearani JA, Ommen SR, Gersh BJ, et al. Surgery Insight: septal myectomy for obstructive hypertrophic cardiomyopathy—the Mayo Clinic experience. *Nat Clin Pract Cardiovasc Med* 2007;4(9):503-512.

6a. Morrow AG, Reitz BA, Epstein SE, et al. Operative treatment in hypertrophic subaortic stenosis. Techniques, and the results of pre and postoperative assessments in 83 patients. *Circulation* 1975;52:88-102.

7. Ommen SR, Park SH, Click RL, et al. Impact of intraoperative transesophageal echocardiography in the surgical management of hypertrophic cardiomyopathy. *Am J Cardiol* 2002;90(9):1022-1024.
8. Yu EHC, Omran AS, Wigle ED, et al. Mitral regurgitation in hypertrophic obstructive cardiomyopathy: relationship to obstruction and relief with myectomy. *J Am Coll Cardiol* 2000;36(7):2219-2225.
9. Kwon DH, Smedira NG, Thamilarasan M, et al. Characteristics and surgical outcomes of symptomatic patients with hypertrophic cardiomyopathy with abnormal papillary muscle morphology undergoing papillary muscle reorientation. *J Thorac Cardiovasc Surg* 2010;140(2):317-324.
10. Woo A, Williams WG, Choi R, et al. Clinical and echocardiographic determinants of long-term survival after surgical myectomy in obstructive hypertrophic cardiomyopathy. *Circulation* 2005;111(16):2033-2041.
11. Smedira NG, Lytle BW, Lever HM, et al. Current effectiveness and risks of isolated septal myectomy for hypertrophic obstructive cardiomyopathy. *Ann Thorac Surg* 2008;85(1):127-133.
12. Ommen SR, Maron BJ, Olivotto I, et al. Long-term effects of surgical septal myectomy on survival in patients with obstructive hypertrophic cardiomyopathy. *J Am Coll Cardiol* 2005;46(3):470-476.
13. Fifer MA, Sigwart U. Hypertrophic obstructive cardiomyopathy: alcohol septal ablation. *Eur Heart J* 2011;32(9):1059-1064.
14. Faber L, Seggewiss H, Welge D, et al. Echo-guided percutaneous septal ablation for symptomatic hypertrophic obstructive cardiomyopathy: 7 years of experience. *Eur J Echocardiogr* 2004;5(5):347-355.
15. Alam M, Dokainish H, Lakkis N. Alcohol septal ablation for hypertrophic obstructive cardiomyopathy: a systematic review of published studies. *J Interv Cardiol* 2006;19(4): 319-327.
16. Sorajja P, Valeti U, Nishimura RA, et al. Outcome of alcohol septal ablation for obstructive hypertrophic cardiomyopathy. *Circulation* 2008;118(2):131-139.
17. van der Lee C, Scholzel B, ten Berg JM, et al. Usefulness of clinical, echocardiographic, and procedural characteristics to predict outcome after percutaneous transluminal septal myocardial ablation. *Am J Cardiol* 2008;101(9):1315-1320.
18. Jensen MK, Almaas VM, Jacobsson L, et al. Long-term outcome of percutaneous transluminal septal myocardial ablation in hypertrophic obstructive cardiomyopathy. *Circ Cardiovasc Interv* 2011;4.
19. Nishimura RA, Ommen SR. Septal reduction therapy for obstructive hypertrophic cardiomyopathy and sudden death: what statistics cannot tell you. *Circ Cardiovasc Interv* 2010;3(2):91-93.
20. Fifer MA. Most fully informed patients choose septal ablation over septal myectomy. *Circulation* 2007;116(2):207-216.
21. Maron BJ. Surgical myectomy remains the primary treatment option for severely symptomatic patients with obstructive hypertrophic cardiomyopathy. *Circulation* 2007;116(2):196-206.
22. Agarwal S, Tuzcu EM, Desai MY, et al. Updated meta-analysis of septal alcohol ablation versus myectomy for hypertrophic cardiomyopathy. *J Am Coll Cardiol* 2010;55(8): 823-834.
23. Maron BJ, Nishimura RA, McKenna WJ, et al. Assessment of permanent dual-chamber pacing as a treatment for drug-refractory symptomatic patients with obstructive hypertrophic cardiomyopathy: a randomized, double-blind, crossover study (M-PATHY). *Circulation* 1999;99(22):2927-2933.
24. Epstein AE, DiMarco JP, Ellenbogen KA, et al. ACC/AHA/HRS 2008 Guidelines for Device-Based Therapy of Cardiac Rhythm Abnormalities: a report of the American College of Cardiology/American Heart Association Task Force on Practice Guidelines (Writing Committee to Revise the ACC/AHA/NASPE 2002 Guideline Update for Implantation of Cardiac Pacemakers and Antiarrhythmia Devices): developed in collaboration with the American Association for Thoracic Surgery and Society of Thoracic Surgeons. *Circulation* 2008;117(21):e350-e408.
25. Gilligan DM, Chan WL, Joshi J, et al. A double-blind, placebo-controlled crossover trial of nadolol and verapamil in mild and moderately symptomatic hypertrophic cardiomyopathy. *J Am Coll Cardiol* 1993;21(7):1672-1679.
26. Horowitz JD, Chirkov YY. Perhexiline and hypertrophic cardiomyopathy: a new horizon for metabolic modulation. *Circulation* 2010;122(16):1547-1549.
27. Lee L, Campbell R, Scheuermann-Freestone M, et al. Metabolic modulation with perhexiline in chronic heart failure: a randomized, controlled trial of short-term use of a novel treatment. *Circulation* 2005;112(21):3280-3288.
28. Abozguia K, Elliott P, McKenna W, et al. Metabolic modulator perhexiline corrects energy deficiency and improves exercise capacity in symptomatic hypertrophic cardiomyopathy. *Circulation* 2010;122(16):1562-1569.
29. Harris KM, Spirito P, Maron MS, et al. Prevalence, clinical profile, and significance of left ventricular remodeling in the end-stage phase of hypertrophic cardiomyopathy. *Circulation* 2006;114(3):216-225.
30. Jessup M, Abraham WT, Casey DE, et al. 2009 Focused Update: ACCF/AHA Guidelines for the Diagnosis and Management of Heart Failure in Adults: a report of the American College of Cardiology Foundation/American Heart Association Task Force on Practice Guidelines: developed in collaboration with the International Society for Heart and Lung Transplantation. *Circulation* 2009;119(14):1977-2016.
31. Maron MS, Kalsmith BM, Udelson JE, et al. Survival after cardiac transplantation in patients with hypertrophic cardiomyopathy/clinical perspective. *Circ Heart Fail* 2010;3(5):574-579.
32. Topilsky Y, Pereira NL, Shah DK, et al. LVAD Therapy in patients with restrictive and hypertrophic cardiomyopathy. *Circ Heart Fail* 2011;4(3):266-275.
33. Maron BJ. Contemporary insights and strategies for risk stratification and prevention of sudden death in hypertrophic cardiomyopathy. *Circulation* 2010;121(3):445-456.
34. Elliott PM, Poloniecki J, Dickie S, et al. Sudden death in hypertrophic cardiomyopathy: identification of high-risk patients. *J Am Coll Cardiol* 2000;36(7):2212-2218.
35. Rubinshtein R, Glockner JF, Ommen SR, et al. Characteristics and clinical significance of late gadolinium enhancement by contrast-enhanced magnetic resonance imaging in patients with hypertrophic cardiomyopathy. *Circ Heart Fail* 2010;3(1):51-58.
36. Olivotto I, Girolami F, Ackerman MJ, et al. Myofilament protein gene mutation screening and outcome of patients with hypertrophic cardiomyopathy. *Mayo Clin Proc* 2008;83(6): 630-638.
37. Maron MS, Olivotto I, Betocchi S, et al. Effect of left ventricular outflow tract obstruction on clinical outcome in hypertrophic cardiomyopathy. *N Engl J Med* 2003;348(4):295-303.
38. Saumarez RC, Pytkowski M, Sterlinski M, et al. Paced ventricular electrogram fractionation predicts sudden cardiac death in hypertrophic cardiomyopathy. *Eur Heart J* 2008;29(13): 1653-1661.
39. Zipes DP, Camm AJ, Borggrefe M, et al. ACC/AHA/ESC 2006 Guidelines for Management of Patients with Ventricular Arrhythmias and the Prevention of Sudden Cardiac Death: a report of the American College of Cardiology/American Heart Association Task Force and the European Society of Cardiology Committee for Practice Guidelines (Writing Committee to Develop Guidelines for Management of Patients with Ventricular Arrhythmias and the Prevention of Sudden Cardiac Death), Developed in Collaboration with the European Heart Rhythm Association and the Heart Rhythm Society. *Circulation* 2006;114(10):e385-e484.
40. Dukkipati SR, d'Avila A, Soejima K, et al. Long-term outcomes of combined epicardial and endocardial ablation of monomorphic ventricular tachycardia related to hypertrophic cardiomyopathy/clinical perspective. *Circ Arrhythm Electrophysiol* 2011;4(2): 185-194.
41. Fuster V, Ryden LE, Cannom DS, et al. 2011 ACCF/AHA/HRS Focused Updates incorporated into the ACC/AHA/ESC 2006 Guidelines for the Management of Patients with Atrial Fibrillation: a report of the American College of Cardiology Foundation/American Heart Association Task Force on Practice Guidelines. *Circulation* 2011;123(10):e269-e367.
42. Olivotto I, Cecchi F, Casey SA, et al. Impact of atrial fibrillation on the clinical course of hypertrophic cardiomyopathy. *Circulation* 2001;104(21):2517-2524.
43. Camm AJ, Kirchhof P, Lip GY, et al.; European Heart Rhythm Association; European Association for the Cardio-Thoracic Surgery. Guidelines for the management of atrial fibrillation: the Task Force for the Management of Atrial Fibrillation of the European Society of Cardiology (ESC). *Eur Heart J* 2010;31(19):2369-2429.

43a. Lakdawala NK, Thune JJ, Maron BJ, et al. Electrocardiographic features of sarcomere mutation carriers with and without clinically overt hypertrophic cardiomyopathy. *Am J Cardiol* 2011;108:1606-1613.

44. Hershberger RE, Lindenfeld J, Mestroni L, et al. Genetic evaluation of cardiomyopathy: a Heart Failure Society of America practice guideline. *J Card Fail* 2009;15(2):83-97.
45. Ho CY. Genetics and clinical destiny: improving care in hypertrophic cardiomyopathy. *Circulation* 2010;122(23):2430-2440; discussion 2440.
46. Maron BJ, Ackerman MJ, Nishimura RA, et al. Task Force 4: HCM and other cardiomyopathies, mitral valve prolapse, myocarditis, and Marfan syndrome. *J Am Coll Cardiol* 2005;45(8):1340-1345.
47. Seward JB, Casaclang-Verzosa G. Infiltrative cardiovascular diseases: cardiomyopathies that look alike. *J Am Coll Cardiol* 2009;55(17):1769-1779.
48. Perreira N, Dec GW. Restrictive and infiltrative cardiomyopathies. In Crawford MH, DiMarco JP, editors: *Cardiology*, 3rd ed. 2009, New York, Mosby, p 1113-1124.
49. Gelow JM, Desai AS, Hochberg CP, et al. Clinical predictors of hepatic fibrosis in chronic advanced heart failure. *Circ Heart Fail* 2010;3(1):59-64.
50. Selvanayagam JB, Hawkins PN, Paul B, et al. Evaluation and management of the cardiac amyloidosis. *J Am Coll Cardiol* 2007;50(22):2101-2110.
51. Falk RH. Diagnosis and management of the cardiac amyloidoses. *Circulation* 2005;112(13): 2047-2060.
52. Syed IS, Glockner JF, Feng D, et al. Role of cardiac magnetic resonance imaging in the detection of cardiac amyloidosis. *JACC Cardiovasc Imaging* 2010;3(2):155-164.
53. Feng D, Syed IS, Martinez M, et al. Intracardiac thrombosis and anticoagulation therapy in cardiac amyloidosis. *Circulation* 2009;119(18):2490-2497.
54. Kristen AV, Dengler TJ, Hegenbart U, et al. Prophylactic implantation of cardioverter-defibrillator in patients with severe cardiac amyloidosis and high risk for sudden cardiac death. *Heart Rhythm* 2008;5(2):235-240.

55. Palladini G, Lavatelli F, Russo P, et al. Circulating amyloidogenic free light chains and serum N-terminal natriuretic peptide type B decrease simultaneously in association with improvement of survival in AL. *Blood* 2006;107(10):3854-3858.

56. Jaccard A, Moreau P, Leblond V, et al. High-dose melphalan versus melphalan plus dexamethasone for AL amyloidosis. *N Engl J Med* 2007;357(11):1083-1093.

57. Wechalekar AD, Goodman HJ, Lachmann HJ, et al. Safety and efficacy of risk-adapted cyclophosphamide, thalidomide, and dexamethasone in systemic AL amyloidosis. *Blood* 2007;109(2):457-464.

58. Kpodonu J, Massad MG, Caines A, et al. Outcome of heart transplantation in patients with amyloid cardiomyopathy. *J Heart Lung Transplant* 2005;24(11):1763-1765.

59. Dey BR, Chung SS, Spitzer TR, et al. Cardiac transplantation followed by dose-intensive melphalan and autologous stem-cell transplantation for light chain amyloidosis and heart failure. *Transplantation* 2010;90(8):905-911.

60. Lacy MQ, Dispenzieri A, Hayman SR, et al. Autologous stem cell transplant after heart transplant for light chain (Al) amyloid cardiomyopathy. *J Heart Lung Transplant* 2008;27(8):823-829.

61. Safety and Efficacy Study of Fx-1006A in Patients with Familial Amyloidosis: NCT00409175. Accessed at http://www.clinicaltrials.gov.

62. Kim JS, Judson MA, Donnino R, et al. Cardiac sarcoidosis. *Am Heart J* 2009;157(1):9-21.

63. Magnani JW, Dec GW. Myocarditis: current trends in diagnosis and treatment. *Circulation* 2006;113(6):876-890.

64. Cooper LT, Baughman KL, Feldman AM, et al. The role of endomyocardial biopsy in the management of cardiovascular disease: a scientific statement from the American Heart Association, the American College of Cardiology, and the European Society of Cardiology. *Circulation* 2007;116(19):2216-2233.

65. Lakdawala NK, Givertz MM. Dilated cardiomyopathy with conduction disease and arrhythmia. *Circulation* 2010;122(5):527-534.

66. Ishimaru S, Tsujino I, Takei T, et al. Focal uptake on 18F-fluoro-2-deoxyglucose positron emission tomography images indicates cardiac involvement of sarcoidosis. *Eur Heart J* 2005;26(15):1538-1543.

67. Smedema JP, Snoep G, van Kroonenburgh MP, et al. Evaluation of the accuracy of gadolinium-enhanced cardiovascular magnetic resonance in the diagnosis of cardiac sarcoidosis. *J Am Coll Cardiol* 2005;45(10):1683-1690.

68. Patel MR, Cawley PJ, Heitner JF, et al. Detection of myocardial damage in patients with sarcoidosis. *Circulation* 2009;120(20):1969-1977.

69. Tadamura E, Yamamuro M, Kubo S, et al. Multimodality imaging of cardiac sarcoidosis before and after steroid therapy. *Circulation* 2006;113(20):e771-e773.

70. Chiu CZ, Nakatani S, Zhang G, et al. Prevention of left ventricular remodeling by long-term corticosteroid therapy in patients with cardiac sarcoidosis. *Am J Cardiol* 2005;95(1):143-146.

71. Jefic D, Joel B, Good E, et al. Role of radiofrequency catheter ablation of ventricular tachycardia in cardiac sarcoidosis: report from a multicenter registry. *Heart Rhythm* 2009;6(2):189-195.

72. Zaidi AR, Zaidi A, Vaitkus PT. Outcome of heart transplantation in patients with sarcoid cardiomyopathy. *J Heart Lung Transplant* 2007;26(7):714-717.

73. Murphy CJ, Oudit GY. Iron-overload cardiomyopathy: pathophysiology, diagnosis, and treatment. *J Card Fail* 2010;16(11):888-900.

74. Gujja P, Rosing DR, Tripodi DJ, et al. Iron overload cardiomyopathy: better understanding of an increasing disorder. *J Am Coll Cardiol* 2010;56(13):1001-1012.

75. Qaseem A, Aronson M, Fitterman N, et al. Screening for hereditary hemochromatosis: a clinical practice guideline from the American College of Physicians. *Ann Intern Med* 2005;143(7):517-521.

76. Kirk P, Roughton M, Porter JB, et al. Cardiac T2* magnetic resonance for prediction of cardiac complications in thalassemia major. *Circulation* 2009;120(20):1961-1968.

77. Anderson LJ, Westwood MA, Holden S, et al. Myocardial iron clearance during reversal of siderotic cardiomyopathy with intravenous desferrioxamine: a prospective study using T2* cardiovascular magnetic resonance. *Br J Haematol* 2004;127(3):348-355.

78. Tanner MA, Galanello R, Dessi C, et al. A randomized, placebo-controlled, double-blind trial of the effect of combined therapy with deferoxamine and deferiprone on myocardial iron in thalassemia major using cardiovascular magnetic resonance. *Circulation* 2007;115(14):1876-1884.

79. Tanner MA, Galanello R, Dessi C, et al. Combined chelation therapy in thalassemia major for the treatment of severe myocardial siderosis with left ventricular dysfunction. *J Cardiovasc Magn Reson* 2008;10:12.

80. Caines AE, Kpodonu J, Massad MG, et al. Cardiac transplantation in patients with iron overload cardiomyopathy. *J Heart Lung Transplant* 2005;24(4):486-488.

81. Thurberg BL, Fallon JT, Mitchell R, et al. Cardiac microvascular pathology in Fabry disease: evaluation of endomyocardial biopsies before and after enzyme replacement therapy. *Circulation* 2009;119(19):2561-2567.

82. Mehta A, Beck M, Elliott P, et al. Enzyme replacement therapy with agalsidase alfa in patients with Fabry's disease: an analysis of registry data. *Lancet* 2009;374(9706):1986-1996.

83. Yang Z, McMahon CJ, Smith LR, et al. Danon disease as an underrecognized cause of hypertrophic cardiomyopathy in children. *Circulation* 2005;112(11):1612-1617.

84. Maron BJ, Roberts WC, Arad M, et al. Clinical outcome and phenotypic expression in LAMP2 cardiomyopathy. *JAMA* 2009;301(12):1253-1259.

85. Partington SL, Givertz MM, Gupta S, et al. Cardiac magnetic resonance aids in the diagnosis of mitochondrial cardiomyopathy. *Circulation* 2011;123(6):e227-e229.

86. Mocumbi AO, Ferreira MB, Sidi D, et al. A population study of endomyocardial fibrosis in a rural area of Mozambique. *N Engl J Med* 2008;359(1):43-49.

87. Schneider U, Jenni R, Turina J, et al. Long-term follow up of patients with endomyocardial fibrosis: effects of surgery. *Heart* 1998;79(4):362-367.

88. ten Cate FJ, Soliman OII, Michels M, et al. Long-term outcome of alcohol septal ablation in patients with obstructive hypertrophic cardiomyopathy: clinical perspective. *Circ Heart Fail* 2010;3(3):362-369.

89. Kuhn H, Lawrenz T, Lieder F, et al. Survival after transcoronary ablation of septal hypertrophy in hypertrophic obstructive cardiomyopathy (TASH): a 10 year experience. *Clin Res Cardiol* 2008;97(4):234-243.

90. Fernandes VL, Nielsen C, Nagueh SF, et al. Follow-up of alcohol septal ablation for symptomatic hypertrophic obstructive cardiomyopathy: the Baylor and Medical University of South Carolina experience 1996 to 2007. *JACC Cardiovasc Interv* 2008;1(5):561-570.

CH
17

HYPERTROPHIC, RESTRICTIVE, AND INFILTRATIVE CARDIOMYOPATHIES

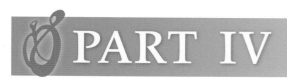

PART IV

ARRHYTHMIAS AND CONDUCTION DISTURBANCES

CHAPTER **18**

Clinical Pharmacology of Antiarrhythmic Drugs

Klaus Romero and Raymond L. Woosley

CLASSIFICATION OF ANTIARRHYTHMIC DRUGS, 344

DRUGS, 344

Lidocaine, 344
Mexiletine, 347
Procainamide, 348
Disopyramide, 349

Quinidine, 350
Propafenone, 351
Flecainide, 352
Sotalol, 352
Amiodarone, 353
Ibutilide, 355
Dofetilide, 356

Adenosine, 357
Dronedarone, 358

APPENDIX, 359

REFERENCES, 360

Antiarrhythmic drugs were developed with the expectation that they would extend and improve life for many patients with cardiovascular (CV) disease and those with a history of life-threatening arrhythmias. The usefulness of such drugs, however, has been limited by their ineffectiveness and/or toxicity. In mortality trials, benefit has not been clearly demonstrated, and worsened mortality has been observed with several drugs. A thorough clinical evaluation must therefore be conducted when deciding the mode of treatment or when deciding whether to treat at all.

The use of antiarrhythmic drugs has been dramatically altered by the findings of the Cardiac Arrhythmia Suppression Trial (CAST).[1] This landmark study was designed to test the hypothesis that suppression of asymptomatic ventricular arrhythmias in patients with recent myocardial infarction (MI) would reduce mortality rate from cardiac arrest and arrhythmic sudden death. Prior to the CAST study, antiarrhythmic drugs were prescribed for these patients to suppress asymptomatic arrhythmias, a therapy aimed at reducing mortality. Based on the results of a feasibility and planning trial, the Cardiac Arrhythmia Pilot Study (CAPS), the CAST study evaluated encainide, flecainide, and moricizine. These drugs were chosen because they appeared to reasonably suppress symptomatic ventricular arrhythmias. In April 1989, the CAST study was interrupted by the Data Safety and Monitoring Committee, and encainide and flecainide were removed because they had been found to increase mortality rates twofold to threefold. The CAST II study continued to evaluate the remaining drug, moricizine; however, CAST II was also terminated prematurely, in August 1991, when it became apparent that moricizine was producing a similar trend toward harm and that there was no reasonable chance a beneficial effect on mortality could be detected.[2] These results shocked the medical community but have influenced thinking in this and many other areas of medicine. Hine and colleagues[3] reported a meta-analysis of CAST and similar studies with sodium channel–blocking antiarrhythmic drugs and found overall support for the conclusion of the CAST study, which has also led to recommendations by the Food and Drug Administration (FDA) for more restrictive labeling for all sodium channel–blocking antiarrhythmic drugs. In 1991, these drugs were given class labeling with indications for the treatment of documented ventricular arrhythmias that, in the judgment of the prescribing physician, are life threatening. Exceptions among sodium channel–blocking drugs are quinidine, propafenone, and flecainide, which have an additional indication for supraventricular arrhythmias.

With the loss of confidence in sodium channel blockers, attention turned to drugs that prolong cardiac refractoriness, such as amiodarone. Although these drugs are effective in controlling symptomatic arrhythmias, their effects on mortality rate have been unclear but seem neutral, except for an increase in noncardiac mortality in heart failure (HF) class III patients.[4,5] Dofetilide, ibutilide, dronedarone, and the d-isomer of sotalol all prolong the action potential duration (APD) and were developed in the hope that they would have the efficacy of amiodarone but with a more favorable adverse event profile. However, the first of these drugs to be evaluated in a mortality trial, d-sotalol, was found to increase mortality rate after MI.[6,7] Development of d-sotalol was halted, but the other two have been marketed with restrictions placed on their indications and clinical use. Clearly, antiarrhythmic drugs are some of the most complex drugs in clinical use today, and they require care in their selection and use.

Another development in the treatment of serious ventricular arrhythmias has been the automated internal cardioverter-defibrillator (ICD). The Antiarrhythmics Versus Implantable Defibrillators (AVID) trial found that devices are associated with a greater improvement in mortality rates.[8,9] More recent evidence shows that ICDs reduce the rate of cardiac mortality and sudden death presumed to be ventricular tachyarrhythmic in case of sudden death in patients with HF, but ICDs have no effect on HF mortality.[5]

In any case, patients with devices may continue to require treatment with antiarrhythmics, and interactions, both desirable and undesirable, between drugs and devices have been documented. In general, drugs that block sodium channels can increase pacing and defibrillation thresholds, and drugs that prolong refractoriness, such as potassium-blocking drugs, lower the defibrillation threshold.[10-12]

Classification of Antiarrhythmic Drugs

Antiarrhythmic drugs are often classified according to their electrophysiologic effects.[13] The scheme most often used was originally proposed by Vaughan Williams, who suggested it should be viewed as a class of drug actions that should be antiarrhythmic, not a classification of drugs. This is a subtle but important distinction that is made for the following reasons:

- Most antiarrhythmic drugs have multiple actions; hence their pharmacology is more complex than indicated by a simple drug-classification scheme.
- The actions of a given drug differ in the various kinds of cardiac tissues.
- Many antiarrhythmic agents have pharmacologically active metabolites, whose activity may be quite different in magnitude and in a class other than that of the parent compound.
- The relative amounts of these metabolites produced are genetically determined for several of these drugs, and they often vary extensively within the population.

Drugs having class I action possess "local anesthetic" or "membrane stabilizing" activity. Their predominant action is to block the fast, inward sodium channel. This produces a decrease in the maximum depolarization rate (V_{max}) of the action potential (phase 0) and slows intracardiac conduction. These agents have been further subclassified as belonging to either class IA, IB, or IC on the basis of their relative effects on specific aspects of intracardiac conduction and refractoriness.[14,15] Drugs having class IA action include quinidine, procainamide, and disopyramide. These agents also produce measurable increases in ventricular refractoriness and prolongation of the QT interval. Lidocaine, mexiletine, and tocainide have actions belonging to class IB. Their potency for blocking sodium channels is only moderate, and in isolated tissues, they shorten the APD and refractoriness. At usual dosages, they generally exert little effect on PR, QRS, or QT intervals. Drugs with class IC actions are the more potent agents, flecainide and propafenone. Because these are potent sodium channel inhibitors, slowing conduction velocity but having little effect on repolarization, they increase the PR and QRS intervals at usual dosages. For these drugs, a prolonged QRS may be mistakenly interpreted as QT prolongation, but in fact these drugs with the exception of flecainide, cause little change in cardiac repolarization.

Class II action refers to β-adrenergic antagonism, possessed by agents such as propranolol, timolol, and metoprolol. Although these drugs are effective for treatment of supraventricular arrhythmias and tachyarrhythmias secondary to excessive sympathetic activity, they are not very effective in the treatment of severe arrhythmias, such as recurrent ventricular tachycardia (VT). With several proposed mechanisms of action, they are the only antiarrhythmic drugs found to be clearly effective in preventing sudden cardiac death in patients with prior MI.

Drugs whose predominant effect is to prolong the duration of the cardiac action potential and refractoriness have *class III action:* amiodarone, dronedarone, sotalol, bretylium, ibutilide, dofetilide, and N-acetylprocainamide (NAPA), the major metabolite of procainamide. It should be noted, however, that these drugs have mechanisms that overlap with other classes. *Class IV action* is calcium channel antagonism; antiarrhythmic drugs with this action include verapamil, bepridil, diltiazem, and nifedipine.

Because of the many limitations of the Vaughan Williams classification of antiarrhythmic drug mechanisms, another approach has been proposed,[16] termed the *Sicilian gambit*. This classification system is based on the differential effects of antiarrhythmic drugs on 1) channels, 2) receptors, and 3) transmembrane pumps. The grouping is based primarily on the predominant action of drugs but also considers the other ancillary actions that may be clinically relevant. As shown in Figure 18-1, because of the sequence of drugs listed, the symbols for these primary actions are generally aligned diagonally. For example, in this system quinidine is a sodium channel antagonist with potassium channel– and α-blocking activity. This provides a more complete

and accurate description of the pharmacologic actions of the drugs than simply designating it as "class Ia." When combined with an understanding of the electrophysiologic role of these actions, predictions about the effects likely to occur in vivo can be made more easily. In the case of quinidine, the three main actions produce conduction slowing, along with increased APD, and refractoriness, as well as vasodilation.

The Sicilian gambit also creates a framework in which newly discovered actions of drugs can be readily added. It emphasizes the multiple actions of drugs and the subtle differences and similarities that exist, and it is more complete. At present, the general understanding of the pharmacology of these drugs has progressed to the point that oversimplification can be misleading. The increased detail of this system reflects the current state of knowledge at a level necessary for optimal use of these drugs.

Because of the low level of efficacy of any one agent by itself, the treatment of acute or chronic ventricular arrhythmias frequently necessitates the use of multiple drugs, sequentially or in combination. For example, the astute clinician may produce increased sodium channel blockade and, hopefully, increase drug efficacy by using combinations of drugs with different kinetics of interaction with the sodium channel. Basic to these considerations is an understanding of the regulation of sodium channel function. Hodgkin and Huxley[17] proposed that sodium channels exist in three distinct states: *open, closed,* and *inactivated.* According to the modulated receptor theory of cardiac sodium channel regulation proposed by Hille and by Hondeghem and Katzung,[18,19] sodium channels in each of these states have differing affinities for drugs that block these channels.

This theory also provides a potential explanation for the phenomenon of "frequency dependence," or "use dependence," the increase in conduction block observed at an increasing rate of stimulation in response to sodium channel–blocking antiarrhythmic agents. Because an increase in the rate of stimulation increases the number of sodium channels in the open and inactivated states, antiarrhythmic agents that have greater affinity for activated (open) or inactivated channels, as opposed to rested channels, would have a greater opportunity to bind to the receptor and reduce conduction; therefore greater block will occur during tachycardia, leaving less drug action at normal heart rates. Also, antiarrhythmic drugs have different affinities for the different states of the sodium channel, and this is manifested as different rates for onset or recovery from block. Drugs that slowly associate with the receptor will cause block to accumulate over the first few cardiac cycles. Drugs that associate more rapidly, such as lidocaine, produce little additional block after the first beat in a train of stimuli. Likewise, drugs dissociate from the sodium channel at different rates, leading to differences in rates of recovery from block. The rate of onset of block of sodium channels has been proposed as a means to subclassify antiarrhythmic drugs.[20] This is the electrophysiologic correlate of the subclassification of sodium channel blockers proposed by Harrison that was based on differences in clinical effects of the drugs.[15]

This chapter reviews the clinical pharmacology and applications of the currently available antiarrhythmic drugs, excluding digoxin, β-receptor antagonists, and calcium channel blockers, which are addressed in other chapters. The drugs appear in the same order as listed in Figure 18-1, an updated revision of the Sicilian gambit classification.

Drugs

Lidocaine

CLINICAL APPLICATIONS

Introduced as a local anesthetic, lidocaine was first used as an antiarrhythmic agent in the 1950s for the treatment of arrhythmias arising during cardiac catheterization.[21] Although lidocaine was historically used as a first-line antiarrhythmic agent for ventricular arrhythmias, this drug is now rarely recommended. It is

ANTIARRHYTHMIC DRUG ACTIONS

Vaughn-Williams Class	DRUG	ECG Changes	Ca++	Na+	K+	α	β	ACh	Ado	Pro-Arrhy	Extra Cardiac	LV FX	Heart Rate
A	Quinidine			M	M	L		M		H	M		
	Procainamide	A		M	M					M	H		
	Disopyramide (Norpace)			M	M			M		L	M	↓↓	
B	Lidocaine (Xylocaine)	B		L						L	M		
	Mexiletine (Mexitil)			L						L	M		
C	Propafenone (Rythmol)	C		H			M			M	L	↓↓	↓
	Flecainide (Tambocor)			H						H	L	↓↓	
II	β-Adrenergic antagonists							H			L	L	↓	↓↓
III	Dronedarone (Multaq)		L	L	H	M	M	M		L	H	↓	↓
	Amiodarone (Cordarone)		L	L	H	M	M	M		L	H	↓	↓
	Sotalol (Betapace)				H		H			H	L	↓	↓
	Ibutilide (Corvert)			△	H					H	L		
	Dofetilide (Tikosyn)				H					H	L		
IV	Verapamil (Calan, Isoptin)		M							L	L	↓↓	↓
	Diltiazem (Cardizem)		M							L	L	↓	↓
Misc	Adenosine (Adenocard)								△	L	L		↓

Antagonist relative potency
L = Low
M = Moderate
H = High

△ = Agonist
● = ECG Changes related to Ca++ channel block
● = ECG Changes related to Na+ channel block
● = ECG Changes related to K+ channel block

FIGURE 18-1 A modification of the Sicilian gambit drug classification system that includes designation by the Vaughan-Williams system. The sodium channel blockers are subdivided into groups A, B, and C based on their relative potency. The electrocardiographic tracings indicate the changes caused by usual dosages of the drug: PR interval (*red*), QRS interval (*yellow*), and QT interval (*blue*). The target ion channels for antiarrhythmic drugs (calcium, sodium, and potassium) are listed in columns with the relative potency for each agent indicated as the letters *H*, *M*, and *L* for "high," "medium," and "low." Listed next, and using the same convention for relative potency, are additional targets: α-adrenergic (*α*), β-adrenergic (*β*), cholinergic (*ACh*), and adenosinergic (*Ado*) receptors. Clinical effects are listed next: proarrhythmic (*ProArrhy*), extracardiac adverse effects (*Extra Card*), inotropic (left ventricular function, *LV FX*), and chronotropic (*Heart Rate*). The direction of the *arrows* indicates the direction of effects; the number of arrows indicates the magnitude. ECG, electrocardiogram.

considered a second choice behind amiodarone for the treatment of immediately life-threatening or symptomatic ventricular arrhythmias since publication of the ECC/AHA 2005 guidelines for cardiopulmonary resuscitation.[22,23] Because extensive first-pass metabolism makes it unsatisfactory for oral use, congeners such as mexiletine were developed that would possess similar sodium channel–blocking actions and be active when taken orally.

Although lidocaine can be used for the acute suppression of ventricular arrhythmias, it has been shown to be ineffective for prophylaxis of arrhythmias in patients after MI.[22,23] Because of lidocaine's complex pharmacokinetics, a monitored environment is desirable to permit evaluation of patient response and detection of toxicity.

Lidocaine has little effect on atrial tissue in vitro,[24,25] consistent with the clinical observation that it has no value in treating supraventricular tachyarrhythmias. Although lidocaine has been used to decrease the ventricular response during atrial fibrillation (AF) in patients whose atrioventricular (AV) conduction follows an accessory pathway, this is not an FDA-approved indication.[26] In addition, some researchers have reported accelerated conduction[27-30] and lack of efficacy in an unselected sample of AF patients.[31]

MECHANISM OF ACTION

In concentrations similar to those attained during clinical use, lidocaine reduces V_{max} and produces shortening or no change in APD and the effective refractory period of normal Purkinje fibers. This contrasts with quinidine and procainamide, which

additionally block potassium channels and produce lengthening of APD.[32,33] At usual concentrations, lidocaine has little effect on the electrophysiology of the normal conduction system, but in patients with abnormalities in this system, it has produced variable effects. Some studies have failed to detect significant changes in conduction,[34] whereas others have found slowing of ventricular rate or potentiation of infranodal block in patients with conduction-system defects.[35] Variability in dosage and pharmacokinetics may explain some of these discrepancies.

CLINICAL PHARMACOLOGY

Orally administered lidocaine is well absorbed, but it has poor bioavailability, because it undergoes extensive first-pass hepatic metabolism. Lidocaine clearance is well approximated by measurement of liver blood flow.[36,37] The two desethyl metabolites, which are excreted by the kidneys, have less antiarrhythmic potency than the parent drug and may contribute to the production of central nervous system side effects that occur with lidocaine.[38,39] Following intravenous (IV) administration, lidocaine's biphasic disposition is well represented by a two-compartment pharmacokinetic model.[40] Because antiarrhythmic activity is correlated with lidocaine's concentration in the central compartment, and the half-life of distribution out of this compartment is rapid (~8 minutes), regimens that use a series of multiple loading doses and a maintenance infusion are able to achieve and then maintain a therapeutic concentration in plasma and myocardial tissue.

Regardless of the initial regimen used, during prolonged constant infusion, the lidocaine concentration eventually reaches a steady state dependent only on drug-infusion rate and lidocaine clearance. The time required to reach steady-state conditions is approximately 8 to 10 hours in normal individuals and up to 20 to 24 hours in some patients with HF or liver disease. This is longer than often anticipated because of the failure to recognize the relatively long elimination half-life: 1.5 to 2 hours in normal subjects and longer in patients with HF or hepatic disease.

DOSAGE AND ADMINISTRATION

Lidocaine's primary use is for acute and rapid suppression of highly symptomatic and life-threatening ventricular arrhythmias. Single IV boluses will achieve only transient therapeutic effects because the drug is rapidly distributed out of the plasma and myocardium; therefore, multiple loading doses should be used to rapidly achieve and sustain therapeutic plasma levels of lidocaine. Based on pharmacokinetic models validated in clinical studies, several regimens have been designed to maintain a relatively constant therapeutic level. For a stable patient, a total loading dose of lidocaine should be approximately 3 to 4 mg/kg body weight administered over 20 to 30 minutes. After injection of an initial dose of 1 mg/kg over 2 minutes, a series of three loading boluses can be administered slowly (approximately 50 mg each over 2 minutes) 8 to 10 minutes apart, while the patient is continuously observed for the development of side effects. Loading should be stopped if the transient, usually mild, central nervous system side effects persist, or if serious unwanted effects occur.

Another effective and well-tolerated loading regimen was suggested by Wyman and associates.[41] For a 75-kg person, an initial bolus of 75 mg is recommended, followed by 50 mg every 5 minutes, repeated three times to a total dose of 225 mg. This regimen usually achieves and maintains plasma concentrations within usual therapeutic guidelines (1.5 to 5 μg/mL). A priming dose of 75 mg followed by a loading infusion of 150 mg over 18 minutes has also been used successfully.[42] At the time of initiation of the loading regimen, a maintenance infusion should be started, designed to replace ongoing losses resulting from drug elimination. This may be calculated as the product of the desired plasma concentration (~3 μg/mL) and the expected clearance (see below). This calculation usually yields a dosage in the range of 20 to 60 μg/kg/min.

Even in normal individuals, wide variability occurs in peak plasma concentration; consequently, variability is seen in the calculated size of the central compartment for lidocaine. Therefore during loading, the patient's electrocardiogram (ECG), blood pressure, and mental status should be monitored, and the process should be stopped at the first sign of lidocaine excess. When symptomatic arrhythmias persist in the presence of documented adequate dosage, defined by side effects or plasma concentration in excess of 5 to 7 μg/mL, another agent should be used.

If the maintenance infusion has reached steady state, but the concentration is below the level needed to prevent recurrence, and the arrhythmia reappears while side effects are absent, the appropriate actions are to 1) obtain a plasma sample for measurement of lidocaine concentration for future reference, 2) administer a small bolus of lidocaine (25 to 50 mg over 2 minutes), and 3) increase the maintenance infusion rate proportionally. The plasma concentration can be used to estimate clearance for calculation of the final maintenance infusion with the following formulas:

$$\text{Maintenance dose} = \text{Clearance} \times \text{Plasma concentration}$$

$$\text{Clearance} = \text{Infusion rate/Steady state plasma concentration}$$

In effect, *maintenance dose* equals clearance multiplied by the desired plasma concentration, and *clearance* equals infusion rate divided by the plasma concentration measured at steady state. Little therapeutic effect is evident at lidocaine plasma concentrations below 1.5 μg/mL, whereas the risk of toxicity increases above 5 μg/mL. In some patients, however, concentrations in the range of 5 to 9 μg/mL may be required for arrhythmia suppression, which can safely be achieved with cautious drug administration.[43]

Once steady state conditions have been achieved, simply terminating a lidocaine infusion will result in a gradual decline in plasma levels over the subsequent 8 to 10 hours as elimination occurs. Not only is there no reason to taper lidocaine infusions, but also it may be dangerous if oral antiarrhythmic therapy is initiated too early, because unpredictable additive effects may occur between lidocaine and newly started oral therapy. If a patient has reached steady state equilibrium, it is possible to estimate when the plasma lidocaine concentration will fall below the usual therapeutic levels. The plasma lidocaine concentration should be determined when the infusion is terminated, and the number of half-lives needed for that level to reach approximately 1.5 μg/mL can be estimated. The half-life of lidocaine for an individual patient can be estimated from the following equation, where V_D is the final volume of distribution:

$$T_{1/2} = \frac{\text{Plasma concentration} \times V_D \times 0.693}{\text{Infusion rate}}$$

The measured plasma concentration and the infusion rate are known components of the equation. V_D is usually 1.1 L/kg, but it may be reduced by 50% or more in patients with HF.

MODIFICATION OF DOSAGE IN DISEASE STATES

Initial loading regimens require no adjustment in patients with renal or liver disease[40]; however, maintenance infusions must be decreased in liver disease and HF to compensate for decreased clearance. Because clearance alone is altered in liver disease with little change in the volume of distribution, the half-life of elimination is prolonged greatly, to as much as 5 hours, and steady state conditions may not be achieved until 20 to 25 hours after the institution of an IV infusion. Despite the fact that lidocaine metabolites are excreted by the kidneys, renal disease has not been reported to exert any significant effect on lidocaine dosing regimens, and dose adjustment may only be required in patients with severe renal insufficiency who are not receiving hemodialysis.[44] With mechanical ventilation, cardiac output and hepatic blood flow are often decreased, so a decrease in lidocaine dosage may be required.[45] Patients with congestive heart failure (CHF) achieve lidocaine levels that are almost double those in normal individuals administered the same dose.[40] Because the central volume of distribution is generally halved in HF, loading doses should be reduced by 50%. Because clearance is also approximately halved, maintenance doses should be reduced proportionally from an infusion rate of 30 μg/kg/min for the typical patient to about half that. The time required to achieve steady state conditions following the initiation of a maintenance infusion is still 8 to 10 hours in many patients with HF because of concomitant changes in V_D and clearance, resulting in a half-life similar to that seen in patients without HF.[40]

In summary, general recommendations for initial lidocaine dosage selection should be adjusted for each patient based on clinical presentation and response and the results of plasma-level monitoring. Some patients with CHF may experience toxicity when given an infusion even as low as 0.5 mg/mL, so blood level monitoring is essential for proper dosage adjustment. In post-MI patients who receive lidocaine infusions for more than 24 hours, plasma lidocaine levels can increase, and the elimination phase half-life can increase up to 50%.[46] This increase could be due in part to changes that occur in the protein binding of lidocaine during the first few days of therapy. Assays for plasma lidocaine measure the sum of both protein-bound and free lidocaine as total lidocaine and thus do not give a true picture of the amount of free drug available. An increase in plasma lidocaine occurring at this time often reflects an elevation in plasma levels of α-1–acid glycoprotein (AAG), to which it binds,[47] which does not always indicate an increase in free, active drug. In this case, the lidocaine dosage should not be reduced to compensate for the higher total plasma concentration as long as the patient displays no adverse effects. Subsequent decreases in AAG concentrations will result in an apparent decrease in plasma lidocaine, which may reflect a drop in only the fraction bound to AAG.

ADVERSE REACTIONS

Central nervous system symptoms are the most frequent side effects of lidocaine administration. A rapid bolus can induce tinnitus or seizures. With more gradual attainment of excessive levels, drowsiness, dysarthria, confusion, hallucinations, and dysesthesia may occur. Excessive lidocaine can also cause coma, which should be a consideration in patients after cardiac arrest.[48] Lidocaine can depress cardiac function, which decreases its clearance and produces an even greater increase in lidocaine concentrations. Advanced degrees of sinus node dysfunction have been reported in isolated instances.[49-51] In patients with known conduction abnormalities below the AV node, lidocaine should be administered cautiously, if at all, unless a temporary pacemaker is readily available.

DRUG INTERACTIONS

An additive or synergistic depression of myocardial function or conduction may occur when using lidocaine combined with other antiarrhythmic agents,[52] especially during conversion from lidocaine to another antiarrhythmic agent. Lidocaine is metabolized in the liver into two active compounds, monoethylglycinexylidide (MEGX) and glycinexylidide (GX). The major metabolic pathway, sequential N-deethylation to MEGX and GX, is primarily mediated by CYP1A2 with a minor role for CYP3A4.[53-56] A pharmacokinetic drug interaction between propranolol and lidocaine has been described experimentally and in humans in which β-adrenergic blockade caused decreases in cardiac output and liver blood flow with a resultant decreased lidocaine clearance.[57] Lidocaine is considered a high hepatic extraction ratio drug, and cimetidine has been reported to reduce splanchnic, and hence hepatic, blood flow (see the Appendix at the end of this chapter); however, it appears that cimetidine has a greater effect on intrinsic hepatic metabolism of drugs as a result of CYP1A2 and CYP3A4 inhibition. Thus the effect of cimetidine on systemic clearance is less than the effect on oral clearance for a high extraction ratio drug such as lidocaine.[58] Because lidocaine is administered parenterally, the magnitude of decrease in lidocaine clearance caused by cimetidine (12% to 25%) is unlikely to be of clinical significance.[58] Nevertheless, patients who receive lidocaine should be monitored for the possibility of lidocaine toxicity, and both loading and maintenance dosages may require downward adjustment if cimetidine is added.

Mexiletine

CLINICAL APPLICATIONS

Mexiletine is indicated for the treatment of documented ventricular arrhythmias, such as sustained ventricular tachycardia, that, in the judgment of the physician, are life-threatening. Initiation of therapy should be in the hospital with ECG monitoring. It also has been used successfully in the treatment of pain associated with diabetic neuropathy.[59] Success rates vary between 6% and 60%, and more than half of the studies suggest limited efficacy (less than 20%).[60,61] Mexiletine does not prolong the QT interval, it can therefore be useful for patients with a history of drug-induced torsades de pointes (TdP) or long QT syndrome when quinidine, sotalol, procainamide, or disopyramide are contraindicated. Although the rate of response to mexiletine is low when used alone, it has been combined successfully with quinidine,[60] propranolol,[62] or procainamide for ventricular arrhythmias.[63] This mode of therapy takes advantage of the additive, and perhaps synergistic, antiarrhythmic response produced by the combination of these agents. Lower than usual dosages of both agents can be used, so that dosage-related adverse effects are reduced concomitantly. Mexiletine exerts minimal effects on both hemodynamics and myocardial contractility, even in patients with severe CHF.[64]

MECHANISM OF ACTION

Mexiletine is an orally active lidocaine congener with class IB sodium channel–blocking activity and structural similarity to tocainide. It was originally developed as an anorexiant and anticonvulsant agent, and its antiarrhythmic properties were only later recognized. Mexiletine blocks fast sodium channels, decreasing V_{max} and shortening the repolarization phase of ventricular myocardium.[65]

CLINICAL PHARMACOLOGY

Mexiletine's systemic bioavailability approximates 90%,[66] with a large volume of distribution (5.5 to 9.5 L/kg) reflecting extensive tissue uptake. Approximately 1% of total body content of mexiletine is in the plasma compartment, with roughly 70% of this bound to serum proteins. Mexiletine has little first-pass metabolism but is eliminated primarily by hepatic metabolism, with only 10% to 15% being excreted unchanged in the urine. Its half-life of elimination is between 8 and 20 hours (9 and 12 hours for healthy subjects), with the time needed to reach steady state ranging between 1 and 3 days.[65] Mexiletine undergoes extensive hepatic metabolism by CYP2D6[67-69]; consequently, clearance is extremely variable (discussed later in this chapter).[70]

DOSAGE AND ADMINISTRATION

Mexiletine therapy should be initiated at a low dose and increased at 2- to 3-day intervals, until efficacy or intolerable side effects develop, such as tremor or other central nervous system symptoms. With normal renal function, the recommended initial oral mexiletine dosage is 200 mg every 8 hours.[71] As with most drugs that have extensive liver metabolism, clearance will be widely variable within the general population. This is especially true for mexiletine, because CYP2D6, which is responsible for its metabolism, is absent in 7% to 9% of the white population. Also, it is necessary to consider dosage adjustment to compensate for the action of agents (discussed below) that induce or inhibit hepatic mexiletine metabolism.

MODIFICATION OF DOSAGE IN DISEASE STATES

Patients with renal failure who also are genetically deficient in hepatic CYP2D6 are likely to have extremely slow elimination for mexiletine.[72] For this reason, all patients with renal failure should be given low initial doses. Elimination half-life and clearance may be prolonged by overt CHF[73] and hepatic failure,[74] and dosage reduction is required.

ADVERSE REACTIONS

The most frequently reported adverse events with mexiletine are gastrointestinal or neurologic in nature and include tremor, visual blurring, dizziness, dysphoria, nausea, dyspepsia, and, less frequently, dysphagia.[75] Thrombocytopenia has been reported to occur infrequently with mexiletine therapy,[76,77] and a positive antinuclear antibody test rarely occurs. Severe bradycardia and abnormal prolongation of sinus node recovery time have been reported in patients with the sick sinus syndrome,[78] and at high concentrations, worsening of heart block has been reported.[79] Oral mexiletine appears to have a reduced risk of causing worsened CHF compared with IV administration, which is not available in the United States.[80-82]

DRUG INTERACTIONS

Mexiletine's hepatic metabolism can be increased by phenobarbital, phenytoin (Dilantin), or rifampicin, which reduce the half-life of mexiletine, possibly changing an effective dose to an ineffective one.[65,83,84] Conversely, if treatment with an inducing agent is stopped, a previously effective dose may become toxic.

In one study, mexiletine decreased the clearance and increased plasma concentrations of theophylline.[85] Quinidine inhibits the CYP2D6 enzyme primarily responsible for mexiletine's metabolic clearance, and plasma concentration of mexiletine may increase in those individuals who express the enzyme—91% to 93% of whites.

Procainamide

CLINICAL APPLICATIONS

Procainamide is indicated for the treatment of documented ventricular arrhythmias, such as sustained ventricular tachycardia, that, in the judgment of the physician, are life-threatening. Initiation of therapy should be in the hospital with ECG monitoring. Procainamide has been found to be useful in the acute management of patients with reentrant supraventricular tachycardia, AF, and the flutter associated with Wolff-Parkinson-White syndrome.[87]

Procainamide has also been used intravenously to suppress ventricular arrhythmias that occur immediately following MI or to convert sustained VT. One randomized study found procainimide (10 mg/kg) to be superior to lidocaine (1.5 mg/kg) for termination of hemodynamically stable VT.[88] However, because it takes approximately 20 minutes to administer a loading dose of procainamide safely, its use is limited to situations when adequate time is available. An advantage over lidocaine is the potential for conversion to oral therapy using the same agent.

The active metabolite of procainamide, N-acetylprocainamide (acecainide [NAPA]), produces class III antiarrhythmic activity in some patients, although not always in those who respond to procainamide.[89] This is most likely due to the very different electrophysiologic actions of procainamide and NAPA.[90] NAPA was investigated as an antiarrhythmic drug and was shown to be effective in the treatment of some types of ventricular arrhythmias, but its use was limited by a narrow therapeutic index, and development was therefore halted.[89]

MECHANISM OF ACTION

As with other agents that demonstrate class I activity, procainamide slows conduction and decreases automaticity and excitability of atrial and ventricular myocardium and Purkinje fibers.[91] Because of its effect on potassium channels, it also prolongs APD and refractoriness. Compared with quinidine, procainamide has very little vagolytic activity and does not prolong the QT interval to as great an extent.[92] NAPA has predominantly class III antiarrhythmic activity; it prolongs APD and refractoriness in both atrial and ventricular myocardium and prolongs the QT interval.[93,94] It has little or no effect on V_{max}, in either Purkinje fibers or ventricular cells, and it does not alter His-Purkinje conduction velocity because of its very low potency as a sodium channel antagonist.

CLINICAL PHARMACOLOGY

Procainamide is rapidly absorbed and 100% orally bioavailable. About 15% of procainamide is bound to serum proteins, and its short elimination half-life of 2 to 4 hours in patients with normal renal function necessitates dosing every 3 to 6 hours. Dosing every 6, 8, or 12 hours is possible with sustained-release preparations. The varied formulations and their very different dosing requirements often create confusion and can lead to dangerous mistakes in dosing.

Slightly more than half of the general population are phenotypic rapid acetylators of procainamide and quickly convert it to NAPA,

a metabolite with very pure class III antiarrhythmic action.[95] As would be expected, however, the response to one agent does not predict response to the other. When each is given as the sole agent, the plasma concentration that is usually effective is 4 to 8 μg/mL for procainamide and 7 to 15 μg/mL for NAPA.[95] During oral procainamide therapy, both agents are present in variable amounts, and there is no way to readily determine the contribution of NAPA to arrhythmia suppression under these conditions. Consequently, the utility of measuring plasma levels of procainamide during chronic therapy is limited because of this variable hepatic conversion to NAPA; however, monitoring plasma concentrations for determination of compliance or prevention of toxicity is both feasible and recommended (see below).

DOSAGE AND ADMINISTRATION

Procainamide is available for either IV or oral use. For patients with normal renal and cardiac function, the initial recommended oral maintenance dose is 50 mg/kg/day. Frequent administration is required for oral procainamide, which is inconvenient and makes compliance difficult. Sustained-release forms of procainamide are available that permit dosing every 6, 8, or 12 hours, depending upon the formulation. During long-term therapy, levels of NAPA may accumulate to effective or toxic levels in some individuals, resulting in achievement of maximum pharmacologic effect long after procainamide has reached steady state.[90,95] Therefore, the elimination half-life of 2 to 4 hours for procainamide may be misleading as a predictor of time to occurrence of stable pharmacologic action. Thus dosage should be initiated at conservative levels, and the patient should be carefully monitored until both procainamide and its metabolite have reached a steady state. Because the electrophysiologic effects of procainamide and NAPA are quite different, monitoring patients receiving procainamide should at some point include measurement of plasma concentrations of both agents to determine their relative concentrations. Patients who are rapid acetylators or who have impaired renal function usually have plasma concentrations of NAPA that are higher than procainamide at steady state. These individuals should be monitored for excessive accumulation of NAPA during dose titration to maintain plasma levels of NAPA below 20 μg/mL. The practice of using the sum of the plasma concentration of procainamide and NAPA is without basis and is not recommended.

When administered IV, procainamide can be given as a constant 25-minute loading infusion of 275 μg/min/kg or by a series of doses (100 mg delivered over 3 minutes) given every 5 minutes, up to a total dose of 1 g.[96,97] If the loading infusion is well tolerated, with no hypotension and less than 25% QRS or QT widening, a maintenance IV infusion of 20 to 60 μg/kg/min can then be given. Larger and more rapid loading infusions of 1 g over 15 to 20 minutes have been given in the electrophysiology laboratory to prevent induction of VT by programmed ventricular stimulation. A second loading infusion of 0.5 to 1 g has been given in some instances when an initial loading infusion was well tolerated but ineffective, but these large dosages are accompanied by a higher incidence of hypotension and conduction disturbance and often result in attainment of unacceptably high plasma concentration.

MODIFICATION OF DOSAGE IN DISEASE STATES

With renal dysfunction or a low cardiac output, both procainamide and NAPA in the usual doses may accumulate to potentially toxic levels, and the dose should be reduced.[98] Increased plasma levels of procainamide and/or NAPA may occur with CHF because of decreased urinary excretion and hydrolysis of procainamide.[99] However, two studies of procainamide pharmacokinetics following a single IV bolus revealed no difference in volume of distribution, clearance, elimination half-life, unbound drug fraction, and peak procainamide concentrations between patients with CHF and normal individuals.[100,101] Although IV procainamide does depress myocardial contractility and also lowers blood pressure, worsening of HF is uncommon during oral therapy, when the usual dosages and plasma concentrations are maintained.

ADVERSE REACTIONS

Side effects associated with long-term procainamide therapy limit its usefulness. Up to 40% of patients discontinue therapy in the first 6 months because of adverse reactions. The potential exists for arrhythmia aggravation, including the development of TdP with procainamide or, more often, due to NAPA.[102] Therefore, as with all agents that possess class IA activity, procainamide should not be used in patients with long QT syndrome, a history of TdP, or hypokalemia.[103,104] To reduce the occurrence of proarrhythmia, potassium levels should be maintained above 4 mEq/L when taking procainamide. Heart block and sinus node dysfunction can occur in patients with preexisting conduction system abnormalities.[105,106]

Between 15% and 20% of patients who receive long-term oral procainamide therapy develop a lupuslike syndrome that is often difficult to recognize but regresses with discontinuation of treatment. If necessary, corticosteroid treatment may be used to treat unresolved symptoms after drug withdrawal.[107] The syndrome usually begins insidiously as mild arthralgia but progresses to frank arthritis, fever, malar erythematous rash, and pleural and/or pericardial effusions, with serum antibodies against nucleoprotein (histone) appearing as antinuclear antibodies with a smooth or diffuse pattern. These symptoms abate if procainamide is discontinued and generally resolve at a rate proportional to their duration.[108,109] Approximately 80% of patients who receive prolonged therapy with the drug demonstrate an increased titer of antinuclear antibodies, early evidence of lupus, usually within 1 to 12 months of therapy initiation,[110] but only 15% to 20% develop symptoms of the lupus syndrome.[111] Therefore, it is unnecessary to discontinue therapy solely because of the positive antinuclear antibody titer. Slow acetylation status may indicate a higher risk for lupus symptoms or an increased rate of development of antinuclear antibodies, especially in patients with renal impairment.[112,113] The patient should be fully informed of the symptoms, which should be reported, so therapy can be discontinued at the earliest signs or symptoms of the syndrome. Continuing procainamide after the development of the early symptoms of the lupus syndrome is dangerous because of the possibility of pleural effusion and potentially lethal pericardial tamponade.[114]

Procainamide therapy has also been associated with the development of agranulocytosis.[115-120] Although more research is needed, it has been suggested that the sustained-release form of the drug may be especially capable of inducing this toxicity.[121-125] The manufacturer recommends that a white blood count be obtained every week for the first 3 months and periodically thereafter.[107]

DRUG INTERACTIONS

Unlike quinidine, procainamide does not cause an increase in digoxin levels.[126] Its clearance is reduced between 30% and 50% by cimetidine, which blocks the renal tubular secretion of procainamide.[126-129] A similar competition has been found between procainamide and its predominant metabolite, NAPA.[130] Ranitidine affects procainamide pharmacokinetics by reducing both its renal clearance and its absorption, the former by 14% to 23% and the latter by 10% to 24%, depending on the dose.[131]

Disopyramide

CLINICAL APPLICATIONS

Disopyramide is effective against a broad range of supraventricular and ventricular arrhythmias, but it is only approved by the FDA for treatment of documented ventricular arrhythmias, such as sustained ventricular tachycardia, that, in the judgment of the physician, are life-threatening.[132] Initiation of therapy should be in the hospital with ECG monitoring. Its antiarrhythmic profile is similar to that of quinidine and procainamide; although newer than these, disopyramide is still one of the older antiarrhythmic agents, having been in use in the United States since 1977. Its negative inotropic and anticholinergic actions occur frequently and limit its usefulness.

MECHANISMS OF ACTION

Disopyramide's class IA antiarrhythmic effects are predominantly those associated with sodium and potassium channel blockade. Its effects are similar to those of quinidine and procainamide on automaticity, conduction, and refractoriness in atrial and ventricular tissue.[133,134]

CLINICAL PHARMACOLOGY

Disopyramide's oral bioavailability is 80% to 90%.[135] Its half-life of elimination, usually 6 to 8 hours, is lengthened to as long as 15 hours in cardiac patients.[136] About half of the compound is eliminated by the kidneys unchanged, and the remainder is eliminated as an active metabolite resulting from hepatic N-dealkylation.[137] Protein binding of disopyramide is complex, with between 20% and 50% of disopyramide being bound to plasma proteins. For most drugs, the percentage bound to plasma protein is a constant over the usual range of therapeutic concentrations. The saturation of disopyramide-binding sites on plasma proteins at usual doses means increases in levels of free drug in plasma are disproportionate compared with the magnitude of dosage increment.[138]

DOSAGE AND ADMINISTRATION

Loading doses are not recommended with disopyramide. The usual effective dosage for disopyramide is 100 to 200 mg three to four times daily, up to a maximum dose of 800 mg/day. Dosages up to 1600 mg/day have been required for some refractory arrhythmias. Therapy should be very carefully titrated, beginning with low doses and allowing ample time for achievement of steady state equilibrium.

Although rapid fluctuations in plasma concentration are undesirable, they are difficult to avoid because of disopyramide's saturable protein binding. The controlled-release form of disopyramide may be useful in reducing adverse effects by decreasing fluctuations in the concentration of free disopyramide in plasma.[139] Because of saturable protein binding,[140] the generally accepted therapeutic range for total disopyramide in plasma of 2 to 5 µg/mL should not be relied on with confidence. Although monitoring the plasma concentrations of free disopyramide has been recommended,[141] the range of concentrations associated with arrhythmia suppression has not been clearly delineated and overlaps with that associated with adverse effects.

MODIFICATION OF DOSAGE IN DISEASE STATES

Patient response to disopyramide should be monitored especially closely after acute MI, when both the absorption and elimination of disopyramide are decreased.[142] In fact, in view of disopyramide's negative inotropic actions and changes in levels of binding proteins in plasma following MI, other antiarrhythmic agents should be considered first.

Disopyramide is contraindicated in patients with uncompensated HF because it can worsen such failure.[143] The initial dosage of disopyramide should be reduced to 50 to 100 mg every 12 hours in patients with renal insufficiency[144] or decreased hepatic function.[145]

ADVERSE REACTIONS

The predominant side effects of disopyramide include new or worsened CHF and symptoms resulting from dose-related anticholinergic actions, including urinary retention, constipation, dry mouth, and esophageal reflux. Because of this anticholinergic action, patients with obstructive uropathy or glaucoma should not take this agent.[146] For some patients, the anticholinergic side effects can be prevented or alleviated by concomitant use of cholinesterase inhibitors such as physostigmine and neostigmine without reduction in antiarrhythmic efficacy.[147,148] As with all agents that prolong repolarization, disopyramide should not be used in patients with long QT syndrome, hypokalemia, or a history of TdP[149,150] because of the potential for arrhythmia aggravation. Direct actions of disopyramide on the sinus node can lead to excessive bradycardia in patients with sinus node dysfunction,[151,152] which may contribute to development of TdP in patients with hypokalemia.[153]

DRUG INTERACTIONS

Disopyramide does not increase digoxin levels,[154] and the effects of warfarin are not potentiated by disopyramide.[155] Phenytoin, rifampicin, and phenobarbital induce CYP3A4, thus enhancing hepatic metabolism of disopyramide, which leads to an increase in its elimination and to the potential loss of antiarrhythmic effect.[156,157] Significant depression of myocardial contractility may result from the combined administration of disopyramide with β-adrenergic or calcium channel antagonists; this combination should be avoided in patients with impairment of ventricular function.[158]

Quinidine

CLINICAL APPLICATIONS

Quinidine is an old drug that, in the past, has been used successfully for a variety of supraventricular and ventricular arrhythmias, including conversion of AF or atrial flutter,[159-161] supraventricular tachycardia,[162] VT, and ventricular fibrillation.[163,164] On the other hand, a grouped analysis of six small placebo-controlled trials in patients with AF showed a statistically significant increase in mortality rate for the patients treated with quinidine, and another meta-analysis also showed a threefold increased mortality rate with quinidine.[165] Because of the similar negative effects on mortality seen in CAST and CAST II, quinidine's risk/benefit ratio must be carefully considered in each patient. The FDA recommends it only in refractory patients for conversion of symptomatic AF or flutter, prevention of recurrences of AF, and the treatment of documented ventricular arrhythmias, such as sustained ventricular tachycardia, that, in the judgment of the physician, are life-threatening.

MECHANISM OF ACTION

Quinidine has multiple actions, but the action thought by many to be primarily responsible for its efficacy is block of the rapid inward sodium channel. This results in a decrease in V_{max} of the action potential upstroke and slowed conduction that is more marked in the His-Purkinje system than in the atria. Quinidine's effects on sodium channels are greatest at increased heart rate and less negative membrane potential—that is, they are pH, rate, and voltage dependent. Dose-related changes in the ECG are manifested as increases in PR, QRS, and QTc intervals, which reflect quinidine's multiple actions.[166]

CLINICAL PHARMACOLOGY

Quinidine's effective dosage varies among individuals because of several factors. Although quinidine sulfate is usually administered every 6 hours, wide interindividual differences are seen in its elimination half-life, which varies from 3 to 19 hours.[167] Plasma protein binding also varies widely, ranging from 50% to 95%.[167] Oral bioavailability is approximately 70%, and clearance after oral administration ranges from 200 to 400 mL/min. Quinidine is inactivated or eliminated by both hepatic metabolism (50% to 90%) and renal elimination (10% to 30%). Several potentially active metabolites are formed in amounts that vary among individuals,[168] but for most, their clinical role has not been determined. One of quinidine's metabolites, 3-hydroxyquinidine, has been shown to possess antiarrhythmic activity when given to humans.[168] Experimental data indicate some contribution by metabolites of quinidine to its antiarrhythmic action.[169-171]

DOSAGE AND ADMINISTRATION

Quinidine therapy (as the sulfate) is usually initiated with an oral dosage of 200 mg every 6 hours, and the dosage is titrated every 3 or more days. Elderly patients often require lower dosages of quinidine because of both reduced clearance and volume of distribution.

Quinidine is available commercially in at least two different forms: quinidine sulfate and quinidine gluconate. Because the quinidine content varies between these at 83% and 62%, respectively, the need for dose adjustment should be considered if one form is substituted for another. The usually effective dosage of quinidine sulfate ranges from 800 to 2400 mg/day, with the maximum recommended single dose being 600 mg. Because the half-life varies from 3 to 19 hours, a delay of 4 days between dosage increases is recommended to prevent unexpected drug accumulation. The range of therapeutic plasma concentrations measured using assays that differentiate quinidine from its metabolites is 0.7 to 5.5 µg/mL.[172,173] Rapid escalation in quinidine dosage has been used to convert AF, but this therapy is no longer recommended because of unnecessary toxicity.

IV therapy with quinidine is usually avoided if alternatives are feasible. Vasodilation and hypotension result from quinidine-induced α-adrenergic blockade. If quinidine is administered intravenously as quinidine gluconate, the patient should be carefully monitored, and the infusion rate should be no more rapid than 16 mg/min. The infusion should be discontinued if hypotension is observed, or if the QRS is prolonged by more than 30%.

MODIFICATION OF DOSAGE IN DISEASE STATES

No adjustment in initial dosage is usually needed for patients with renal or hepatic disease,[174,175] although because of decreased protein binding in patients with hepatic failure, lower than usual total plasma concentration can produce toxicity.[176] Slower dose titration is advisable to permit attainment of steady state and complete accumulation of active metabolites; however, because the usual range of effective dosages is wide, dosage for these patients is not markedly different. Patients with rapid quinidine elimination may require higher dosages, up to 600 mg every 6 hours. This is often due to induction of hepatic metabolism caused by other drugs.

Patients with congenital long QT syndrome, hypokalemia, or a history of TdP should not be given quinidine because of their increased risk for this form of proarrhythmic event.[177] For patients with CHF, more serious problems associated with use of quinidine are proarrhythmia and digitalis toxicity, either with digitoxin or digoxin. Prudent use of quinidine in individuals taking digitalis requires 1) that titration begin at a reduced dosage; 2) that dosage of any cardiac glycoside being administered concomitantly be reduced; and 3) that plasma electrolyte levels, especially potassium, be maintained above 4 mEq/L.

Although quinidine does possess some direct negative inotropic effects, these are usually counteracted by its vasodilatory effect; therefore, oral quinidine is well tolerated hemodynamically when given at dosages that produce usual plasma concentrations, even in patients with reduced ventricular function.[178] In a study of more than 650 patients, 35% of whom had CHF, quinidine therapy resulted in no induction or worsening of CHF.[179] On the other hand, a significant problem for patients with CHF who receive quinidine therapy is proarrhythmia, with quinidine-induced TdP being potentiated in the setting of bradycardia and low serum levels of magnesium or potassium.[180,181]

ADVERSE REACTIONS

Marked prolongation of the QT interval has been seen in some patients receiving low or usual dosages of quinidine, and the risk of TdP is markedly increased. This arrhythmia may be responsible for all cases of quinidine-induced death and quinidine-induced syncope, which occur in as many as 5% to 10% of patients within the first days of quinidine treatment.[182] TdP usually occurs in patients with low concentrations of quinidine, hypokalemia, hypomagnesemia, poor ventricular function, and bradycardia, and females have an increased susceptibility.[182,183] In a study by Drici and colleagues, dihydrotestosterone reduced the sensitivity to the effects of quinidine on the QT interval in animals.[184] Additional studies showed women to be more sensitive to the effects of quinidine on the QT interval,[185,186] providing evidence that sex hormones have direct effects on cardiac tissue that may be responsible for the differences in baseline QT interval[187] and incidence of TdP in men and women.[183,188]

The first steps for the treatment of patients who develop TdP are to stop medications known to prolong the QT interval[189] and to correct electrolyte imbalances. Observational studies support the use of magnesium sulfate (2 g IV bolus with 2 to 4 g repeated once, if necessary) to treat TdP.[190] The efficacy of magnesium is supported by the findings of a prospective controlled trial of two 5-g doses of magnesium that showed it reduced the incidence of TdP and improved the efficacy of ibutilide in 476 patients with AF or flutter.[191] One case series showed that isoproterenol or ventricular pacing can be effective in terminating TdP associated with bradycardia and drug-induced QT prolongation.[192] It is essential to clinically distinguish TdP from polymorphic VT in the setting of a normal QT interval, because in this setting, magnesium is likely to be ineffective. Because quinidine acts via α-adrenergic blockade to induce vasodilation, hypotension may occur, especially in patients concomitantly receiving nitrates or other vasodilators.[193] Other adverse effects include a high incidence of diarrhea and vomiting, tinnitus at high plasma levels, thrombocytopenia, and conduction block in patients with existing conduction-system disease.[179,194,195] In patients treated with quinidine for atrial flutter without prior AV nodal blockade by digitalis, there have been reports of sudden increases in AV conduction and rapid ventricular rates.[193] This is the result of a slight reduction of the flutter rate and enhanced AV nodal conduction because of the anticholinergic effects of quinidine. This allows one-to-one conduction through the AV node, often at 200 to 250 beats/min. This may be of particular concern for patients receiving other drugs that prolong conduction time through the AV node, such as β-adrenergic agonists.

DRUG INTERACTIONS

Quinidine metabolism is inhibited by cimetidine and induced by phenytoin, phenobarbital, and rifampicin, with the latter agents leading to reduced, often subtherapeutic quinidine concentrations.[195-197] Clinical digoxin toxicity has been described in 20% to 40% of patients receiving quinidine and digoxin concurrently.[196] The magnitude of this interaction is dependent on quinidine dosage, and in some patients, it may not appear until the dosage is increased to higher levels.[198,199] The rise in digoxin levels appears with the first dose of quinidine, therefore it is suggested that digoxin dosage be halved when quinidine therapy is initiated. A similar interaction has been reported for quinidine and digitoxin.

Although quinidine is a substrate of the hepatic cytochrome P450 (CYP) 3A4 isozyme, it is a potent inhibitor of CYP2D6.[200-203] Thus, it may interfere with the biotransformation and actions of pharmacologic agents dependent on this cytochrome for their metabolism, which include propafenone, mexiletine, flecainide, metoprolol, timolol, sparteine, and bufuralol.[204] Quinidine worsens neuromuscular blockade in patients with myasthenia gravis and may prolong the effects of succinylcholine.[205,206]

Propafenone

CLINICAL APPLICATIONS

Propafenone was developed in Germany, where it has been marketed since 1977. Propafenone is used primarily to treat atrial arrhythmias, paroxysmal supraventricular tachycardia, and ventricular arrhythmias in patients with no or minimal heart disease and preserved ventricular function.[207]

CLINICAL PHARMACOLOGY

Propafenone has a marked structural similarity to propranolol, and studies have shown that propafenone can accumulate during continued administration to levels capable of producing clinically significant β-adrenergic inhibition.[208]

Like mexiletine and flecainide, propafenone is eliminated by a metabolic pathway that has a polymorphic pattern of inheritance. Patients deficient in CYP2D6 activity have very slow elimination of propafenone and fail to form measurable quantities of the potentially active metabolite, 5-hydroxypropafenone.[209-211] The accumulation of high concentrations of propafenone leads to significant β-receptor antagonism at both low and high doses in poor metabolizers but only at high dosages in extensive metabolizers of propafenone.[212] Although metabolic phenotype does not seem to dramatically influence the antiarrhythmic response to propafenone in many patients, it clearly influences the degree of β-blockade that occurs during therapy.[209]

DOSAGE AND ADMINISTRATION

Effective dosages range from 300 to 900 mg/day in two to four divided doses. To prevent unexpected accumulation of pharmacologic action, propafenone dosage should not be changed more frequently than every 3 days; elimination of the parent drug is slow in poor metabolizers, and accumulation of the metabolites is slow in extensive metabolizers.

Patients with reduced ventricular function, especially those receiving propafenone, should be carefully monitored for deterioration in ventricular function, which may result from β-adrenergic receptor antagonism and/or the direct negative inotropic effect.[213]

MODIFICATION OF DOSAGE IN DISEASE STATES

A reduction of approximately 20% to 30% in the normal oral dosage for immediate-release tablets is recommended for patients with hepatic dysfunction; no reduction is recommended for patients with renal insufficiency. Severe liver dysfunction increases propafenone bioavailability to approximately 70% compared with 3% to 40% for normal hepatic function. Although specific guidelines are not available, the manufacturer recommends consideration of dosage reduction for the extended-release capsules (Rythmol SR) in patients with hepatic impairment.[214]

DRUG INTERACTIONS

It is very likely that drug interactions will occur between propafenone and other agents that utilize or inhibit CYP2D6 for their metabolism. Such an interaction has been documented already between propafenone and metoprolol and should be expected with timolol, many antidepressants, many neuroleptics, and perhaps other agents.[215] Quinidine, which inhibits this cytochrome, inhibits the formation of 5-hydroxypropafenone in extensive metabolizers; however, the clinical consequence of such inhibition is unknown and difficult to predict.[216] Greater β-blockade occurs after combining quinidine with propafenone therapy because of the resulting higher propafenone concentrations and its actions to block β receptors.[217]

Flecainide

CLINICAL APPLICATIONS

As a result of the CAST study, flecainide is not considered a first-line agent in patients with structural heart disease because of its propensity for fatal proarrhythmic effects.

Like propafenone, flecainide is used primarily to treat atrial arrhythmias, paroxysmal supraventricular tachycardia, and ventricular arrhythmias in patients with no or minimal heart disease and preserved ventricular function.

MECHANISM OF ACTION

Flecainide has sodium channel–blocking activity and is considered to have class IC actions. It has also been found to block the delayed rectifier potassium channel in feline ventricular myocytes, and this action may be clinically relevant.[218]

Flecainide slows intraventricular conduction velocity more than it prolongs effective refractory periods.[219] It prolongs A-H and H-V intervals and measurably increases PR and QRS intervals on the surface ECG at therapeutic doses. The QTc interval is slightly increased, primarily as a result of prolongation of the QRS, but its ability to block the delayed rectifier potassium channel may contribute to QT changes.[220]

CLINICAL PHARMACOLOGY

The systemic bioavailability of oral flecainide is 90% to 95%, and most of the flecainide is metabolized in the liver into compounds that are not pharmacologically active at the concentrations usually found in plasma.[221,222] Like many other antiarrhythmic agents, flecainide is metabolized by CYP2D6.[223] Because flecainide is also eliminated by the kidneys to a considerable extent, the enzyme deficiency has little effect on its pharmacokinetics; however, if those patients without the enzyme develop renal insufficiency, or when patients with renal failure are given a drug that blocks flecainide's metabolism, extremely high plasma concentrations are likely to occur.[224] Flecainide has a very slow elimination, with a half-life that ranges from 7 to 23 hours in normal individuals and tends to be even longer, from 14 to 26 hours, in patients with cardiac disease, even in the absence of HF.[221,225]

DOSAGE AND ADMINISTRATION

After an initial dose of 100 mg every 12 hours, maximum dosage of flecainide for ventricular arrhythmias is 150 mg every 12 hours in patients without cardiac or renal failure. The recommended dose for patients with supraventricular tachyarrhythmias is 50 or 100 mg every 12 hours as a starting dose. The range of therapeutic plasma concentrations of flecainide is reported to be between 200 and 1000 ng/mL. However, adverse effects may occur in some patients at concentrations within this range, although other patients may tolerate concentrations well above it.[226,227] To reduce the incidence of adverse effects, flecainide therapy should start with a low dose that is maintained until steady state has been reached (at least 4 days) and altered relative to clinical response.

MODIFICATION OF DOSAGE IN DISEASE STATES

With cardiac failure, the usual initial dose is 50 to 100 mg every 12 hours. Because 7% to 9% of white patients with renal failure will not have the CYP2D6 enzyme, and because flecainide is usually eliminated by both metabolism and renal excretion, all patients with renal failure should be given very low dosages, titrated very slowly and carefully.[228] Plasma concentration monitoring is essential in patients with renal disease or cardiac or hepatic dysfunction. Any significant reduction in ejection fraction should be expected to lengthen elimination half-life and hence the time needed to attain steady state equilibrium, and reductions in clearance may occur in renal or hepatic dysfunction that lead to higher plasma concentrations at steady state.

ADVERSE REACTIONS

Flecainide has the potential to induce proarrhythmic events, even when prescribed as recommended. This is especially true in patients with severe heart disease, and when flecainide is given in higher dosages.[229] Because of its negative inotropic effects at dosages necessary to suppress arrhythmias, flecainide produces a measurable decrease in left ventricular (LV) function in most patients.[230,231] Because of the increased mortality rate seen in the CAST study, flecainide is not considered a first-line agent because of its propensity for fatal proarrhythmic effects. Additionally, its negative inotropic actions restrict its use to patients with moderately well-preserved ventricular function.

Other side effects of flecainide include depression of sinus node activity in patients with preexisting sinus node dysfunction and prolongation of QRS and PR intervals on the surface ECG.[232] In addition, flecainide increases pacing thresholds by as much as 200% and should therefore be used with caution in patients dependent on pacemakers.[233] It also increases the threshold for electrical defibrillation, so patients with implanted devices should be evaluated carefully.[234]

DRUG INTERACTIONS

Cimetidine reduces flecainide clearance and prolongs its elimination half-life.[235] Studies in normal volunteers have shown an increase in the plasma concentrations of digoxin and propranolol when flecainide is coadministered.[236,237] Not unexpectedly, propranolol and flecainide have been found to have additive negative inotropic effects. An interaction with amiodarone has been described that results in elevation of plasma flecainide concentration and necessitates reduction of flecainide dosage.[238]

Sotalol

CLINICAL APPLICATIONS

Sotalol is a unique β-blocker that shows class II and III antiarrhythmic effects, but as a nonselective β-blocker, it lacks intrinsic sympathomimetic and membrane-stabilizing activity. Like amiodarone, sotalol prolongs the APD and increases refractoriness. Sotalol is used in the treatment of atrial arrhythmias or life-threatening ventricular arrhythmias, including sustained VT. However, it should not be used for minor arrhythmias, because it is known to be proarrhythmic with an increased risk for TdP. Although sotalol is effective for the maintenance of sinus rhythm in patients with AF,[239] amiodarone was shown to be superior for maintaining sinus rhythm in this population, as data from the Solatol Amiodarone Atrial Fibrillation Efficacy Trial (SAFE-T), the Clinical Trial of Atrial Fibrillation (CTAF), and the Atrial Fibrillation Follow-up Investigation of Rhythm Management (AFFIRM) indicate.[240-242]

Nonetheless, it has not yet been determined whether the survival rate is improved with sotalol use versus use of an implanted defibrillator alone. Sotalol was originally approved by the FDA under the brand name Betapace for the treatment of life-threatening ventricular arrhythmias in October 1992. The d-isomer of sotalol—with virtually no β-blocking activity, and considered to have only class III antiarrhythmic effects—was studied as an antiarrhythmic in high-risk patients after MI in the Survival With Oral d-Sotalol (SWORD) trial, but the study was terminated prematurely because of a higher mortality rate in the d-sotalol group compared with the placebo group. This finding was presumably due to increased arrhythmic deaths.[243] The present commercial product, Betapace AF, is intended for use in AF, with the caveat that sotalol is not effective for conversion of AF to sinus rhythm, but it may be used to prevent AF.[244] Although both commercial presentations contain sotalol, Betapace should not be substituted for Betapace AF because of significant differences in the labeling sections on indications, dosing, administration, and safety profile.[245,246] The injectable form of sotalol was approved by the FDA in July 2009.

Although sotalol can also be used to treat paroxysmal supraventricular tachycardia, the higher risk for proarrhythmia makes AV nodal blocking agents—such as adenosine, calcium channel blockers, and β-blockers—more desirable agents, with the exception of patients with preexcited atrial arrhythmias, in whom such AV blockers are contraindicated.[86]

MECHANISM OF ACTION

In addition to its β-blocking effects, sotalol markedly prolongs refractoriness in atrial and ventricular tissues, a class III antiarrhythmic action. These actions slow heart rate, decrease AV nodal conduction, and increase refractoriness of atrial, ventricular, AV nodal, and AV accessory pathways in both the anterograde and retrograde directions.[247] When given in dosages between 160 and 640 mg/day, increases of 40 to 100 ms are seen in the QT interval, and 10 to 40 ms increases are observed in the QTc.[248]

CLINICAL PHARMACOLOGY

Oral bioavailability of sotalol is greater than 90%, and peak concentrations are seen 2.5 to 4 hours after a dose. It is not bound to plasma proteins and is eliminated by the kidneys unchanged, with an elimination half-life of approximately 12 hours. Because of the relatively long half-life and the twice-daily dosing regimen, it is recommended that testing for efficacy be conducted near the end of the dosing interval at steady state. Age, per se, does not influence the pharmacokinetics of sotalol other than those effects that are due to the natural decline in renal function that occurs with age.

DOSAGE AND ADMINISTRATION

The recommended initial oral dose of sotalol is 80 mg every 12 hours. In patients with relatively normal renal function, steady state is reached in 2 to 3 days. If evaluation at this dosage indicates a lack of desired response without evidence of excessive effects on repolarization (QT >500 ms), the dosage may be increased to 160 mg twice daily and, if necessary, to 240 mg twice daily. Some patients with life-threatening arrhythmias have required dosages of 640 mg/day. Accelerated titration regimens have been used with close monitoring without any apparent increase in adverse events.[249]

It is recommended that before starting therapy or increasing the dose of sotalol, the QT interval, heart rate, and creatinine clearance (CLCR) be evaluated. IV sotalol is contraindicated if the baseline QT is greater than 450 ms, heart rate is less than 50 beats/min, or if CLCR is less than 40 mL/min. According to the FDA-approved label, corresponding doses are 80 mg PO equals 75 mg IV, 120 mg PO equals 112.5 mg IV, and 160 mg PO equals 150 mg IV.[245,246]

Two placebo-controlled trials that studied patients in sinus rhythm who had at least one documented prior episode of AF found sotalol to be safe and effective at doses ranging from 80 to 160 mg twice daily.[239,250] However, clinicians should be aware of the fact that QT monitoring is essential during treatment with sotalol; an absolute QT greater than 500 ms, or a QT prolongation greater than 60 ms regardless of absolute value, excessively increases the risk of TdP.

A randomized double-blind study found that a 5-minute IV infusion of sotalol 100 mg was more effective than a 5-minute infusion of 100 mg lidocaine in patients with spontaneous, hemodynamically stable, sustained monomorphic VT within a hospital setting.[251] Another study in 109 patients with a history of spontaneous and inducible sustained VT showed that the infusion of 1.5 mg/kg of sotalol over 5 minutes or less was effective.[252]

MODIFICATION OF DOSAGE IN DISEASE STATES

Because sotalol is mainly eliminated unchanged in the urine, the dosage must be adjusted for altered renal function. For patients with a CLCR greater than 60 mL/min, the usual dosing interval is every 12 hours. If the CLCR is between 30 and 60 mL/min, the recommended interval between doses is 24 hours. For patients with CLCR between 10 and 30 mL/min, the interval should be every 36 to 48 hours, or the usual dose may be halved and given every 24 hours. The dosage for patients with CLCR less than 10 mL/min should be individualized. Because of the increased risk of proarrhythmia and CHF, patients with reduced cardiac output should be given lower doses and should be monitored carefully.

ADVERSE REACTIONS

A major concern with sotalol treatment has been the occurrence of TdP. As of the fourth quarter of 2011, a total of 244 reports of TdP had been reported to the FDA's Adverse Events Reporting System (AERS). Clearly, hypokalemia, hypomagnesemia, and bradycardia are predisposing factors for the development of this arrhythmia during sotalol therapy, as they are with quinidine, disopyramide, and procainamide. It is more common in females, in patients with CHF, and in those with a history of sustained VT. The incidence of TdP should be minimized by careful screening and consideration of predisposing factors such as female gender, bradycardia, baseline prolongation of the QT interval, and electrolyte disturbances, especially hypokalemia; careful dose escalation, beginning at 160 mg/day; and limitation of the maximum QT interval prolongation to less than 500 ms. Sotalol should not be administered with other drugs that prolong the QT interval. A list of such drugs can be found at www.QTdrugs.org.

The incidence of new or worsened CHF is about 3%. This may be attenuated because of the increased inotropy produced by its action to prolong repolarization. Other side effects typical of β-blockers are to be expected, including bronchospasm in asthmatic patients, masking the signs and symptoms of hypoglycemia in diabetic patients, and catecholamine hypersensitivity withdrawal syndrome.

DRUG INTERACTIONS

Concomitant use of sotalol with agents that prolong repolarization has the potential to increase the likelihood of TdP. No pharmacokinetic interactions have been seen with sotalol and/or warfarin, digoxin, cholestyramine, or hydrochlorothiazide. Because of the β-blocking actions of sotalol, it is likely that there would be increased pharmacologic effect, if the drug were to be combined with amiodarone, calcium channel blockers, antihypertensive agents, clonidine, or antiarrhythmic agents.

Amiodarone

CLINICAL APPLICATIONS

Amiodarone has been reported to have efficacy in a wide range of arrhythmias. Numerous trials in the literature describe the efficacy of amiodarone in the conversion and slowing of AF, AV nodal reentrant tachycardia, and tachycardias associated with the Wolff-Parkinson-White syndrome.[244,253,254]

After the results of CAST, antiarrhythmic drugs were examined for their effects on mortality rate. The Veteran's Administration trial, Congestive Heart Failure Survival Trial of Antiarrhythmic Therapy

(CHF STAT),[255] examined the effects of amiodarone on total mortality in patients with a history of CHF, more than 10 premature ventricular contractions per hour on ambulatory monitoring, and an ejection fraction less than 40%. The study found no difference in the placebo and amiodarone arms. Two other major trials evaluated amiodarone in patients with recent MI. The Canadian Myocardial Infarction Amiodarone Trial (CAMIAT)[256] and the European Myocardial Infarction Amiodarone Trial (EMIAT)[257] were completed in the last decade. The results of these trials were mixed in that neither found amiodarone to reduce overall mortality, but the Canadian trial reported a reduced incidence of ventricular fibrillation or arrhythmic death among survivors of MI with ventricular ectopy. Importantly, no increase in mortality was noted, as has been seen with other antiarrhythmic drugs. Meta-analyses of the many trials with amiodarone[258-261] have generally confirmed a slight reduction in mortality rate in cardiac patients. The NIH-sponsored Antiarrhythmics Versus Implanted Devices (AVID)[262] trial found that the devices were superior to amiodarone in reducing mortality in patients who had been resuscitated from sudden death or in those who had sustained VT.

In 1993, an IV formulation of amiodarone became available in the United States. Three completed controlled trials demonstrated the value of amiodarone in patients with recurrent life-threatening VT or fibrillation, and a comparison of three dosages (125, 500, and 1000 mg/day) found that the recurrence of arrhythmia was lowest at the higher dosages.[263] Hypotension was the major side effect seen, but it occurred equally, about 26%, in all groups. The second study in a similar group of patients was a comparison of bretylium to two doses of amiodarone.[264] The arrhythmia event rate for the first 48 hours of therapy was equivalent for the high dose of amiodarone and bretylium, and both were more effective than the low dose of amiodarone. Hypotension was common in all groups but was significantly higher in the bretylium group. Amiodarone was approved for IV therapy of ventricular arrhythmia by the FDA in 1998. Although not yet approved in labeling, a study found IV amiodarone effective for prevention of postoperative AF.[265]

MECHANISM OF ACTION

Amiodarone is an iodinated benzofuran that has structural similarity to thyroxine and procainamide and was originally developed as an antianginal agent. It was incidentally noted to suppress a wide variety of ventricular and supraventricular arrhythmias. It has been assumed that this efficacy is caused by its prolongation of refractoriness and APD in myocardial tissue (Vaughan Williams class III antiarrhythmic activity), although amiodarone has been found to have many diverse pharmacologic actions. The actions responsible for its high degree of antiarrhythmic efficacy remain unidentified.

In intracellular recordings of rabbit cardiac myocytes, amiodarone prolongs APD and increases refractoriness of both atrial and ventricular myocardium and of Purkinje fibers and sinus and AV nodal tissues. Amiodarone decreases phase 3 depolarization of myocardial cells, blocks sodium channels that are in the inactivated state, slows phase 4 depolarization of the sinus node, and slows conduction through the AV node.[266,267] The electrophysiologic actions of the major metabolite of amiodarone, desethyl-amiodarone (DEA), differ from those of amiodarone, with the metabolite having greater effects on conduction because of its effects on sodium channels and therefore on conduction.[268] Intracoronary injection of amiodarone has shown little cardiac effect compared with DEA's ability to prolong cardiac refractoriness.[269]

Electrophysiologic changes in humans depend on the route of administration and the duration of therapy. Following acute IV amiodarone administration, prolongation of the AH interval and an increase in the refractory periods of the AV node and bypass tracts are seen, but this may be due to the presence of the solubilizing agent, polysorbate 80 (Tween 80), in the IV formulation. No acute changes occur in either sinus rate or atrial or ventricular refractoriness, whereas these are prolonged during chronic oral therapy. Chronic amiodarone therapy also prolongs the AH and HV intervals and the PR and QT intervals of the surface ECG. Conflicting reports on the time course of these changes are found, and it is not clear how they might relate to antiarrhythmic efficacy.

Changes in APD and refractoriness are seen in hypothyroidism similar to changes resulting from oral amiodarone therapy.[270] These changes can be prevented in animals by coadministration of thyroid hormone with amiodarone,[271] leading to the conclusion that amiodarone's antiarrhythmic efficacy is attributed to production of "cardiac hypothyroidism." This is supported by the observation that amiodarone's major metabolite causes noncompetitive inhibition of thyroid hormone binding to nuclear receptors.[272] On the other hand, amiodarone also causes noncompetitive blockade of α- and β-receptors,[273] muscarinic receptors,[274] and both calcium and sodium channel blockade, any combination of which may contribute to its antiarrhythmic efficacy.

CLINICAL PHARMACOLOGY

Amiodarone is a highly lipid-soluble compound with extremely variable and complex pharmacokinetics. It is slowly absorbed from the gastrointestinal tract, and bioavailability varies over a fourfold range.[275] Amiodarone is extensively metabolized to DEA by CYP3A4 and CYP2C8,[276,277] and little if any is excreted unchanged in the urine. Concentrations of DEA in plasma vary from 0.4 to 2.0 times that of amiodarone during long-term therapy.[278] This metabolite has antiarrhythmic potency equal to or greater than amiodarone in in vitro and in animal models.[279] Amiodarone is rapidly concentrated in some tissues, including myocardium, but it accumulates more slowly in others, such as adipose tissue. It redistributes out of myocardial tissue while still accumulating in adipose and other tissues.[278,280] Until all tissues are saturated, rapid redistribution out of the myocardium may be responsible for early recurrence of arrhythmias after discontinuation of therapy or rapid reduction of dosage. Because of drug accumulation in tissues, the volume of distribution for amiodarone is very large, 20 to 200 L/kg.[280] After IV administration, the measured half-life in plasma is from 4.8 to 68.2 hours,[281] with tissue uptake being the primary factor responsible for the decline in plasma concentration. As tissues become saturated, however, the decline in plasma levels is slow, reflecting mainly elimination and slow redistribution of the drug out of adipose and muscle tissues. This leads to slow and extremely variable elimination from plasma, with half-lives ranging from 13 to 103 days at steady state.[280] It is also possible that amiodarone inhibits its own elimination after chronic therapy, contributing to the differences between half-life early in therapy to that after prolonged therapy.

DOSAGE AND ADMINISTRATION

Without a loading-dose regimen, amiodarone requires several weeks to months before producing its antiarrhythmic action; however, large IV doses or oral loading doses can hasten the onset of therapeutic effects. From small prospective studies, loading doses have varied from 600 to 1400 mg/day for 2 to 21 days.[282] Recent large clinical trials have used a lower loading dose of 600 to 800 mg/day for 14 days.[283,284] Because of relatively rapid redistribution out of myocardial tissue, the dosage should be tapered over a period of several weeks. The usual maintenance dose varies from 200 to 600 mg/day, and because of the severe nature of adverse reactions, the lowest effective dose should be prescribed. Patients with supraventricular arrhythmias may respond to lower doses than those with ventricular arrhythmias, but there are many exceptions. Because of the variable pharmacokinetics and oral bioavailability, generalizations such as this may be unreliable. Some patients with extensive absorption (80% to 90% bioavailability) of even low doses may have the same drug exposure as a person with limited bioavailability given a high dose.

For IV administration, the manufacturer recommends a three-phase infusion over the first 24 hours: 150 mg over 10 minutes, followed by 360 mg over the next 6 hours, followed by 0.5 mg/min. The drug can be continued at this rate, but monitoring of plasma concentrations is recommended. An additional 150 mg can be infused over 10 minutes for patients who continue to have recurrent VT or fibrillation or those whose arrhythmia recurs during downward titration of the infusion. Concentrations of drug greater than 3 mg/mL should be infused through a central catheter to prevent phlebitis. Also, the surfactant properties of the drug alter the size of a drop of infusate, and pumps that count drops will give approximately 30% less drug than intended.

Amiodarone concentrations are usually between 1 and 2 µg/mL during effective oral therapy.[285,286] Similar concentrations of DEA accumulate during therapy, and although this is unproven, it is likely to contribute to antiarrhythmic efficacy. Because of extensive overlap between the range of concentrations required for arrhythmia suppression and those associated with toxicity, monitoring of plasma concentrations is of limited value. Levels of amiodarone above 3 to 4 µg/mL for prolonged periods of time are clearly associated with a higher incidence of adverse effects.[287]

MODIFICATION OF DOSAGE IN DISEASE STATES

Long-term oral therapy with amiodarone appears to be well tolerated hemodynamically in patients with CHF. In the Veteran's Administration trial discussed above, amiodarone failed to prolong life for CHF patients with arrhythmias but was associated with improved ventricular function as measured by radionuclide ejection fraction.[283]

ADVERSE REACTIONS

IV amiodarone at dosages greater than 5 mg/kg decreases cardiac contractility and peripheral vascular resistance and produces severe hypotension in some instances. Because oral administration at usual dosages improves myocardial contractility, some of this effect, like the electrophysiologic effects described earlier, may be due to the effects of polysorbate 80 or benzyl alcohol.

The safety of amiodarone is controversial. Early reports found it to be very well tolerated and described it as the "ideal" antiarrhythmic drug. Some studies continue to find that it is relatively safe and effective, even in the treatment of arrhythmias in children.[288] The early experience with amiodarone in the United States, with a very high incidence of intolerable and sometimes lethal reactions, may have been the result of high dosages required for control of life-threatening arrhythmias. Under less urgent conditions, lower dosages are given and are much better tolerated. Determination of the incidence of adverse reactions is difficult because of highly variable dosages and durations of treatment.[289,290]

The most serious adverse reaction is lethal interstitial pneumonitis,[291,292] which may be more frequent in patients with preexisting lung disease. Monitoring is essential, because the pneumonitis is reversible if detected early. A chest radiograph every 3 months may be useful, but serial pulmonary function tests are of little value for follow-up. Hyperthyroidism or hypothyroidism occurs in about 4% of patients treated long-term.[293] Accumulation of corneal microdeposits is almost uniform during long-term therapy and in many cases can progress to the point of interfering with vision.[294] Some white patients develop a slate gray or bluish discoloration of sun-exposed areas of the skin.[295] Many also report photosensitivity, which can sometimes be prevented or alleviated with sunscreens and garments, and 30% or more patients have abnormally elevated serum hepatic enzyme levels, and progression to jaundice and cirrhosis has been reported in some of these patients.[296,297] Serial laboratory tests to screen for amiodarone toxicity can be costly and generally are of limited value; however, it is wise to obtain a reliable assessment of baseline tests, including complete blood count, blood chemistry, tests of thyroid and pulmonary function, a slit-lamp examination, and measurement of blood levels of other drugs whenever possible due to frequent drug interactions.

DRUG INTERACTIONS

Amiodarone interferes with the clearance of many drugs. This may involve the formation of a metabolically inactive CYP Fe(II)–metabolite complex, which has been described in animals treated with amiodarone[298] and may explain the reduced metabolism and unexpected accumulation of warfarin,[299] quinidine, procainamide, disopyramide, mexiletine, and propafenone[300] and the resulting bleeding, heart block, or TdP.[301-303] It does not, however, explain interaction with drugs eliminated predominantly by the kidneys, such as digoxin.[304] Here the effect is mediated by inhibition of P-glycoprotein. The elimination of other drugs may be impaired by amiodarone, and the lowest effective dosage should be sought.

Ibutilide

CLINICAL APPLICATIONS

In 1995, ibutilide was given FDA approval for the rapid conversion of recent-onset AF or atrial flutter,[305] and testing in other arrhythmias and in patients with AF or atrial flutter of long duration (>90 days) was completed. Ibutilide should not be given to patients who have hypokalemia, hypomagnesemia, or QTc prolongation at baseline greater than 440 ms. In placebo-controlled studies summarized in the manufacturer's labeling, the placebo conversion rate for AF or atrial flutter was approximately 2%. Ibutilide terminated the arrhythmia in approximately 43% to 48% of patients treated with 1 mg followed by either 0.5 or 1 mg. Approximately 20% of patients responded to the first infusion, and approximately 25% of those who did not respond to the first infusion responded to the second infusion. Response usually occurred at 20 to 30 minutes but ranged from 5 to 88 minutes after infusion. The response in patients with AF and atrial flutter was not significantly different in the early trials performed. However, in patients with postoperative arrhythmias, a greater response was seen in patients with atrial flutter, with a conversion rate of 53% to 72% compared with 20% with placebo.[306] Ibutilide may have value in conversion of AF in patients with Wolff-Parkinson-White syndrome.[307,308]

MECHANISM OF ACTION

Ibutilide is a remarkably potent methanesulfonamide analogue of sotalol that prolongs cardiac APD and has class III action (i.e., it prolongs cardiac refractoriness and APD), and it appears that ibutilide has multiple mechanisms of action. The manufacturer's data indicate that the drug's class III action is due to an increase in inward sodium current, as observed in guinea pig ventricular myocytes at 10^{-7} mol/L concentrations. They observed that higher concentrations (10^{-5} mol/L) increase an outward potassium current to shorten APD.[309] Other investigators reported that, as has been seen with dofetilide, sotalol, and other methanesulfonamides, 10^{-8} mol/L concentrations of ibutilide block the rapid component of the delayed rectifier potassium current, I_{Kr}, in mouse and human cardiac cells.[310]

CLINICAL PHARMACOLOGY

Ibutilide is only available for IV administration. When given over 10 minutes, it distributes rapidly in a multiexponential fashion, and the relevant component has a half-life from 2 to 12 hours (mean, 6 hours). The plasma concentration and pharmacokinetics are highly variable, and dosing is recommended on the basis of weight. The drug is mainly eliminated by oxidative hepatic metabolism with sequential β-oxidation to eight metabolites, systemic clearance is rapid (approximately 29 mL/min/kg), and protein binding is about 40%. According to animal models, only one metabolite possesses class III antiarrhythmic effects similar to those of ibutilide; however, the plasma concentration of this metabolite is less than 10% of that of ibutilide.[305] Because formal drug interaction studies have not been performed, it is not possible to anticipate which enzymes are likely responsible for its biotransformation.

DOSAGE AND ADMINISTRATION

Ibutilide is administered undiluted or diluted in saline as an infusion over 10 minutes. The recommended dose for a patient heavier than 60 kg is 1 mg, and a dose of 0.01 mg/kg is recommended for a patient weighing less than 60 kg. For patients whose arrhythmias have not converted by 10 minutes after completion of the first dose, a second dose of equal magnitude can be administered. Because conversion of arrhythmias is usually associated with peak levels, slower infusion rates are not likely to be as effective.

Because of ibutilide's significant risk of TdP, it is essential that patients who receive this drug be treated in a monitored environment for at least 4 hours after administration. The FDA-approved labeling recommends that skilled personnel, facilities, and medication for defibrillation or resuscitation be readily available.[305] A retrospective analysis indicated that pretreatment with magnesium sulfate can reduce the estimated 3% to 4% incidence of TdP by approximately 20% to 30%.[311] A subsequent controlled trial found that two 5-g doses of magnesium sulfate reduced the incidence of TdP associated with ibutilide administration.

MODIFICATION OF DOSAGE IN DISEASE STATES

Specific studies with HF and renal or hepatic disease have not been conducted. Patients with severe LV dysfunction have a higher risk of developing ventricular arrhythmias, including TdP. Because the duration of drug effect is determined by distribution, it is very possible that patients with severe CHF will have decreased volumes of distribution and hence an exaggerated and prolonged duration of effect.

According to the manufacturer, it is unlikely that dosage adjustments are necessary in patients with impaired renal or hepatic function, based on the considerations that ibutilide is indicated for rapid IV therapy (duration of 30 minutes or less) and is dosed to a well-defined goal (termination of arrhythmia) and that drug distribution appears to be one of the primary mechanisms responsible for termination of the pharmacologic effect. Nonetheless, patients with abnormal hepatic function should be monitored for longer than the recommended 4-hour interval afterward.[305]

ADVERSE REACTIONS

The most serious adverse reaction to ibutilide is TdP; however, only 586 patients participated in trials before marketing, and patients with a QTC greater than 440 ms or potassium concentrations less than 4 mEq/L were excluded. Despite these precautions, the incidence of sustained polymorphic VT requiring cardioversion was 1.7%. Another 2.7% developed nonsustained polymorphic VT, 4.9% had nonsustained monomorphic VT, 1.5% had AV block, and 1.9% had bundle branch block. The risk of polymorphic VT in some studies was highest in patients who were female and in those who had evidence of reduced ventricular performance. The incidence of these adverse effects may well be higher in general clinical use, in which electrolyte disorders and concomitant therapies may be more common. As of the fourth quarter of 2011, a total of 114 reports of TdP were reported to be associated with ibutilide in the FDA's AERS database. Bradycardia and multiple episodes of sinus arrest have also been reported,[311,312] along with a single case of acute renal failure.[313]

DRUG INTERACTIONS

No specific drug interaction studies have been performed. Concomitant β-receptor or calcium channel antagonists do not apparently interact, although data are limited. The manufacturer's labeling warns against combining ibutilide with other drugs that prolong the QT interval (see www.QTdrugs.org).[305] During ibutilide's development, these drugs were discontinued for at least five half-lives prior to administration of ibutilide and were not allowed until at least 4 hours after administration.

Dofetilide

CLINICAL APPLICATIONS

Dofetilide was approved and marketed in 2000 for oral therapy of AF and atrial flutter. In controlled trials of approximately 1000 patients, about 30% of those with AF who were given a dosage of 500 μg twice daily converted to normal sinus rhythm compared with 6% in the control group treated with sotalol and 1% of patients given placebo. Prevention of recurrence was demonstrated with 62% to 71% remaining in sinus rhythm after 6 months compared with 59% for sotalol and 26% to 37% for placebo (S. Singh, personal communication). A large mortality trial, the Danish Investigators of Arrhythmia and Mortality on Dofetilide (DiAMOND) trial, examined the effects of dofetilide on mortality rate and AF in 1518 patients with reduced ejection fraction and symptoms of HF. A decrease in the incidence of hospitalization for HF was observed. Although dofetilide's antiarrhythmic efficacy was confirmed in the lower incidence of AF, a positive effect on mortality was not observed.[314] This is in stark contrast to the previously observed increases in mortality rate with sodium channel blockers (CAST and CAST-II) and with d-sotalol (SWORD). A caveat to this safety finding was the potentially important role of extensive screening and monitoring for potential harm. Even with these efforts, 3.3% of patients in this trial developed TdP. Because of the risk of TdP, the manufacturer requires physicians to receive special training before prescribing dofetilide, and the FDA has required that labeling include a boxed warning that therapy should be initiated in the hospital with continuous ECG monitoring for at least 3 days.

MECHANISM OF ACTION

Dofetilide is one of the most potent I_{KR} blockers ever synthesized. Perhaps an additional advantage is the twofold greater ability to prolong APD in atrial compared with ventricular tissue.[315] It does not appear to depress cardiac function at usual dosages even in patients with reduced ejection fraction.

CLINICAL PHARMACOLOGY

Dofetilide is well absorbed after oral administration and is partially metabolized by CYP3A4[316] to inactive metabolites, and it is excreted predominantly in urine. In most patients, the elimination half-life ranges from 8 to 10 hours but is prolonged, and clearance is reduced, in patients with renal failure. Dofetilide is susceptible to several drug interactions, because it is metabolized by CYP3A4 (see below). It is very likely that some of these interactions increase the risk of TdP.

DOSAGE AND ADMINISTRATION

The recommended dosage of dofetilide is 500 μg twice daily. Lower dosages are recommended for patients who develop excessive QT-interval prolongation on 500 μg twice daily. In the largest clinical trial, "excessive" was defined as greater than 550 ms or more than 20% longer than baseline.

MODIFICATION OF DOSAGE IN DISEASE STATES

Dosage should be reduced in patients with renal disease (250 μg twice daily for CLCR 60 to 40 mL/min and 250 μg four times a day for CLCR 40 to 20 mL/min). Data are not available for adjustment of dosage in patients with liver disease, and it is not clear whether the greater risk of TdP in women is influenced by a pharmacokinetic difference between the sexes.

ADVERSE DRUG REACTIONS

The major adverse effect of dofetilide is TdP, and the overall incidence during clinical development was 0.9%. In the DiAMOND trial, 3.3% of patients with a history of HF developed TdP.

DRUG INTERACTIONS

Concomitant administration of dofetilide with verapamil, ketoconazole, or cimetidine—but not ranitidine—results in increased plasma concentrations of dofetilide, especially in patients with reduced renal function.[317] Because it is known to be a substrate for CYP3A4, there may be other potential interactions with erythromycin, other macrolides, or antifungals. No interactions have been seen between dofetilide and digoxin or warfarin.

Adenosine

CLINICAL APPLICATIONS

Adenosine is very effective for the acute conversion of paroxysmal supraventricular tachycardia (PSVT) caused by reentry involving accessory bypass pathways. At a dose of 6 mg, 60% of patients respond, and an additional 32% respond when given a 12-mg dose. Because of the fleeting and relatively selective action of adenosine on the AV node, some have suggested that it be used as a diagnostic tool in patients with narrow and wide complex tachycardia.[318] However, when possible, it is preferable to make the correct diagnosis before giving any drugs because of their risk of adverse effects.

MECHANISM OF ACTION

Adenosine is a nucleoside formed in the body by serial dephosphorylation of adenosine triphosphate (ATP), from cyclic adenosine monophosphate or from hydrolysis of S-adenosylhomocysteine. It is formed both inside and outside the cell, and its actions are rapidly terminated by active transport into cells, followed by metabolism. The actions of adenosine are highly dependent on the rate and route of administration. A rapid IV injection into a central venous line is thought to activate carotid body chemoreceptors and usually produces an initial increase in blood pressure of 10 to 15 mm Hg, followed by a small and transient decrease. These reflexes are attenuated during surgery, and in this setting, adenosine decreases peripheral vascular resistance, increases cardiac output, and increases heart rate moderately. Bolus injections also produce biphasic effects on heart rate. Approximately 20 seconds after injection, sinus bradycardia occurs for 10 to 15 seconds, followed by sinus tachycardia thought to be due to chemoreceptor activation. Activation of the carotid chemoreceptors stimulates respiration and causes secondary activation of pulmonary stretch receptors. Adenosine has a direct effect of slowing AV nodal conduction, which can result in transient AV block. Although adenosine has no direct effect on the His-Purkinje system, it does attenuate the effects of catecholamine stimulation and, in patients with heart block, it can block acceleration of the ventricular escape rate by isoproterenol. Adenosine usually has no effect on anterograde or retrograde accessory pathway conduction. Pathways that demonstrate decremental conduction often respond to adenosine, probably because they are partially depolarized and can be hyperpolarized by adenosine. Slow injections into a peripheral line often produce no clinical benefit or changes in blood pressure or heart rate.

The development of synthetic agonists and antagonists of adenosine receptors has made possible the subclassification of A_1 and A_2 receptor subtypes. The A_1 receptors are present in myocardial cells and mediate the negative inotropic, dromotropic, and chronotropic actions of adenosine. The A_2 receptors are present in the endothelium and vascular smooth muscle cells and cause coronary vasodilation when activated.

The efficacy of adenosine in PSVT is most likely a result of actions in atrial myocardium and in the AV node, such as 1) hyperpolarization of sinoatrial (SA) node cells and slowing of firing rate, 2) shortening of the action potential duration of atrial cells, and 3) depression of conduction velocity in the AV node. These actions are due to activation of A_1 adenosine receptor subtypes, which leads to activation of cyclic adenosine monophosphate (cAMP)–independent, acetylcholine/adenosine-regulated potassium current, $I_{ACh,Ado}$.

CLINICAL PHARMACOLOGY

After IV injection, adenosine is rapidly transported into red blood cells and endothelial cells. Half-life of elimination has ranged from 1.5 to 10 seconds, and the drug is rapidly metabolized in the plasma and in cells to form inosine and AMP. Maximal pharmacologic effects are seen within 30 seconds after injection into a peripheral IV line but occur within 10 to 20 seconds when given into a central line.

DOSAGE AND ADMINISTRATION

Adenosine should be injected intravenously into a proximal tubing site and flushed quickly with 20 mL saline. For adults, the initial dose is 6 mg injected over 1 to 2 seconds. If the arrhythmia persists, a 12-mg dose can be injected 1 to 2 minutes later. This can be repeated, but doses larger than 12 mg are not recommended by the manufacturer. A dosage regimen based on body weight has been proposed, with an initial dose of 50 µg/kg incremented by 50 µg/kg until the PSVT is terminated, or side effects become intolerable.[319] Higher doses may be required for patients who have received caffeine or theophylline because of their antagonistic effects at A_1 receptors. Lower doses are recommended for patients receiving dipyridamole or carbamazepine.

MODIFICATION OF DOSAGE IN DISEASE STATES

Although the pharmacokinetics of adenosine are unlikely to be altered in patients with renal or hepatic disease, these patients often have electrolyte imbalances that could alter the clinical response. Although patients with CHF have not been reported to respond abnormally, heart transplant recipients appear to require one third to one fifth of the usual dose because of denervation hypersensitivity.[320]

ADVERSE REACTIONS

Adenosine is contraindicated in patients with sick sinus syndrome or second- or third-degree heart block, unless the patient has a functioning artificial pacemaker. Because of the rapid clearance of adenosine, side effects such as facial flushing, dyspnea, or chest pressure last less than 60 seconds. Although intrapulmonary administration of adenosine has precipitated bronchospasm in asthmatic patients, this has not been reported with IV administration. Other less frequent side effects include nausea, lightheadedness, headache, sweating, palpitations, hypotension, and blurred vision. IV theophylline, which has been recommended to reverse the effects of adenosine, should be prepared and ready for injection in high-risk patients.

DRUG INTERACTIONS

Several proven interactions can increase or decrease the activity of adenosine. Dipyridamole pretreatment increases the potency of adenosine, probably because it blocks cellular uptake of adenosine.[320] On the other hand, caffeine and theophylline antagonize the actions of adenosine,[318,321] and the manufacturer cautions that carbamazepine may potentiate the actions of adenosine.[322]

Dronedarone

CLINICAL APPLICATIONS

Dronedarone was approved by the FDA in July 2009 to reduce the risk of hospitalization for persistent or recurring AF and atrial flutter. Dronedarone is an antiarrhythmic agent developed with the aim of achieving an efficacy similar to that of amiodarone with an improved safety and tolerability profile. A comparison among dronedarone, amiodarone, and placebo in the trial to evaluate the Efficacy and Safety of Dronedarone versus Amiodarone for the Maintenance of Sinus Rhythm in Patients with Atrial Fibrillation (DIONYSOS) employed a primary composite efficacy endpoint of recurrence of AF that included unsuccessful electrical cardioversion, no spontaneous conversion, and no electrical cardioversion or premature study discontinuation and a main safety endpoint that aggregated the occurrence of events specific to the eyes, skin, and thyroid and hepatic, pulmonary, neurologic, and gastrointestinal systems, or premature study drug discontinuation following an adverse event. Results showed that the composite efficacy endpoint was met in 75.1% and 58.8% with dronedarone and amiodarone respectively at 12 months (hazard ratio [HR], 1.59; 95% confidence interval [CI], 1.28 to 1.98; $P < .0001$), driven mainly by AF recurrence with dronedarone compared with amiodarone (63.5% vs. 42.0%). AF recurrence after successful cardioversion was 36.5% and 24.3% with dronedarone and amiodarone, respectively. Premature drug discontinuation tended to be less frequent with dronedarone (10.4% vs 13.3%). The frequency of the main safety endpoint was 39.3% and 44.5% with dronedarone and amiodarone, respectively, at 12 months (HR, 0.80; 95% CI, 0.60 to 1.07; $P = .129$). These results were driven mainly by fewer thyroid, neurologic, skin, and ocular events in the dronedarone group.[323]

The dronedarone label contains a boxed warning that contraindicates its use in patients with New York Heart Association (NYHA) class IV heart failure or NYHA class II to III heart failure with a recent decompensation requiring hospitalization or referral to a specialized HF clinic.[324] This warning is due to results from the European Trial of Dronedarone in Moderate to Severe Congestive Heart Failure (ANDROMEDA), which led to the trial's premature discontinuation.[325] As opposed to previous dronedarone trials,[326,327] ANDROMEDA enrolled high-risk patients with symptomatic HF and severe LV systolic dysfunction. The twofold increase in mortality seen in ANDROMEDA was predominately owed to worsening HF.[325] Because of modifications in the chemical structure of dronedarone—that is, removal of the iodine moiety and addition of a methanesulfonyl group—dronedarone has lower lipophilicity, thus resulting in a shorter half-life of 13 to 19 hours, compared with 58 days for amiodarone, and lower tissue accumulation compared with amiodarone. These characteristics of the dronedarone molecule are postulated to account for the proposed improved safety profile seen with dronedarone; however, trials lasting longer than 12 months have not been conducted. Dronedarone is indicated to reduce the risk of CV hospitalization in patients with paroxysmal or persistent AF who are in sinus rhythm or will be cardioverted and who have had a recent episode of AF and have associated CV risk factors: age greater than 70 years, hypertension, diabetes, prior cerebrovascular accident, left atrial diameter of 50 mm or more, or LV ejection fraction less than 40%. (See Chapter 20 for a discussion of the PALLAS trial.)

MECHANISM OF ACTION

Dronedarone is a benzofuran analogue of amiodarone. The exact mechanism of action of dronedarone is yet unknown, but like amiodarone, dronedarone has complex electrophysical effects belonging to all four Vaughan Williams classes. As a drug with class III effects, dronedarone prolongs the cardiac action potential and refractory periods by inhibiting the potassium currents I_{Kr}, I_{K1}, I_{KACh}, and I_{sus}. It also inhibits sodium channels, which results in a decreased slope of the depolarization phase of the action potential, a class IB effect, and also inhibits the slow L-type calcium channels, a class IV effect. Additionally, dronedarone has shown antiadrenergic effects (class II). In healthy subjects, dronedarone was found to significantly prolong the R-R and QT interval in a dose-dependent manner.[328,329] The removal of the iodine moiety described above was also aimed at reducing the risk of thyroid function abnormalities known to occur with amiodarone therapy. Animal studies indicate dronedarone does not affect circulating plasma thyroid hormones.[330,331]

CLINICAL PHARMACOLOGY

Dronedarone is administered orally. Dronedarone and its metabolites are more than 98% bound to plasma proteins, mainly albumin, and this protein binding is not saturable. Dronedarone is extensively metabolized, mainly involving the CYP3A4 isoenzyme. The main active metabolite, desbutyl-dronedarone, is 0.1 to 0.3 times as potent as dronedarone. Approximately 30 other uncharacterized metabolites of dronedarone also exist. About 6% of radiolabeled dronedarone is excreted in urine, and 84% is excreted in feces, mainly as metabolites. The elimination half-life of dronedarone is 13 to 19 hours.[332]

Dronedarone possesses electrophysiologic properties of all four Vaughan Williams classes. Dronedarone was evaluated in healthy volunteers receiving repeated oral doses of up to 1600 mg once daily or 800 mg twice daily for 14 days and 1600 mg twice daily for 10 days. A dose-dependent increase in the PR interval of 5 ms occurred in the group that received 400 mg twice daily, and an increase of up to 50 ms occurred in the 1600 mg twice-daily group. A similar dose-related effect occurred in the QT interval with an increase of 10 ms in the 400 mg twice daily group and an increase of up to 25 ms in the 1600 mg twice daily group.[333]

INDIVIDUALIZATION OF DOSAGE

Two trials, European Trial in Atrial Fibrillation Patients Receiving Dronedarone for the Maintenance of Sinus Rhythm (EURIDIS) and the American-Australian-African Trial with Dronedarone in Atrial Fibrillation Patients for the Maintenance of Sinus Rhythm (ADONIS), were identical multicenter, double-blind, randomized trials to evaluate the efficacy of dronedarone (400 mg twice daily; $n = 828$) vs. placebo ($n = 409$) for the maintenance of sinus rhythm in AF or atrial flutter over a 12-month study period. The median time to first recurrence of arrhythmia was significantly longer in the dronedarone group compared with the placebo group (EURIDIS: 96 vs. 41 days, $P = .01$; ADONIS: 158 vs. 59 days, $P = .002$). In addition, the rates of recurrence of AF were significantly lower for the dronedarone group compared with placebo for both trials (EURIDIS: 67.1% vs. 77.5%, respectively; ADONIS: 61.1% vs. 72.8%, respectively).[334]

A Placebo-Controlled, Double-Blind, Parallel-Arm Trial to Assess the Efficacy of Dronedarone 400 mg bid for the Prevention of Cardiovascular Hospitalization or Death from any Cause in Patients with Atrial Fibrillation/Atrial Flutter (ATHENA) involved 4628 patients with AF or atrial flutter. The trial included patients with stable HF but excluded patients who were clinically decompensated. The primary endpoint was time to first hospitalization owing to cardiovascular (CV) events or death from any cause. CV hospitalization or death occurred in 917 patients (39.4%) in the placebo group and in 734 patients (31.9%) in the dronedarone group. There were 116 deaths (5%) in the dronedarone group and 139 deaths (6%) in the placebo group. Of these deaths, 63 (2.7%) were from CV causes—nonarrhythmic cardiac causes, cardiac arrhythmia, noncardiac vascular causes—in the dronedarone group, and 90 (3.9%) were from CV events in the placebo group, which was due to the difference in cardiac arrhythmia seen between the dronedarone and placebo groups (26 [1.1%] vs 48 [2.1%], respectively).[335]

MODIFICATION OF DOSAGE IN DISEASE STATES

Limited data are available, but according to the FDA-approved label, dosage adjustments are not needed in mild to moderate hepatic impairment. However, dronedarone is considered contraindicated in patients with severe liver impairment. Specific guidelines are not available for dosage adjustments in renal impairment.[324]

ADVERSE REACTIONS

An increase in serum creatinine concentration of 10% or more after 5 days of treatment initiation was seen in 51% of patients receiving dronedarone compared with 21% of those receiving placebo.[336]

CV effects of dronedarone are difficult to differentiate from extensions of its normal pharmacologic activity. In the ATHENA outcomes trial, bradycardia was reported in 3.5% of patients in the dronedarone group compared with 1.2% of patients taking placebo.[335] In combined data from EURIDIS and ADONIS, bradycardia was reported in 2.7% of patients in the dronedarone group compared with 2% in the placebo group ($P = .56$), and baseline heart rate was reduced in the dronedarone group by 6.8% ($P < .001$).[334]

According to the manufacturer, QT prolongation, defined as greater than 450 ms for males and greater than 470 ms for females, occurred in 28% of patients receiving dronedarone in clinical trials compared with 19% of those receiving placebo. One patient in the ATHENA trial developed TdP while receiving dronedarone. Combined data from EURIDIS and ADONIS show that when compared with placebo, dronedarone prolonged the QT_C interval by 9 ms ($P < .001$) with no significant effects on QRS duration. As of the fourth quarter of 2011, a total of 47 reports of TdP associated with dronedarone were filed in the FDA's registry of adverse events (AERS).

Dronedarone is associated with worsening HF and increased mortality rate in patients with NYHA class IV heart failure or NYHA class II to III heart failure with a recent decompensation requiring hospitalization or referral to a specialized HF clinic, and these conditions are considered absolute contraindications for dronedarone in FDA-approved labeling.[324,327]

Additional contraindications include use in pregnant or nursing women; the coadministration of strong CYP3A4 inhibitors such as ketoconazole, clarithromycin, or certain antiretrovirals such as nelfinavir or ritonavir; AV block of second or third degree; sick sinus syndrome, except when used in conjunction with pacing; a heart rate less than 50 beats/min; QT_C of 500 ms or more; and PR greater than 280 ms.[324]

The FDA-approved label also includes a warning on the potential for hepatotoxicity that includes life-threatening liver failure.[324] Several reports of hepatocellular liver injury and hepatic failure have been reported in patients treated with dronedarone. Two cases of acute hepatic failure requiring transplantation occurred in patients with previously normal hepatic serum enzymes. In both cases, the patients were female and approximately 70 years of age, and hepatic failure occurred within 6 months of therapy. In the first case, the patient presented with jaundice, coagulopathy, elevated hepatic enzymes, and hyperbilirubinemia, which then progressed to hepatic encephalopathy. In the second case, the patient presented with weakness, abdominal pain, coagulopathy, elevated hepatic enzymes, and hyperbilirubinemia. In both cases, alternative etiology for liver failure was not identified, and extensive hepatic necrosis was seen in the explanted liver. Although it is not known whether monitoring of hepatic serum enzymes will prevent the development of severe hepatic injury, clinicians are advised to consider obtaining periodic hepatic serum enzymes in patients treated with dronedarone, especially during the first 6 months of treatment. Dronedarone treatment should be discontinued immediately if hepatic injury is suspected, and serum liver enzymes and bilirubin concentrations should be obtained. Dronedarone should not be restarted in patients who experience hepatic injury during treatment without another explanation for the injury.[337]

DRUG INTERACTIONS

Dronedarone is both a substrate for and an inhibitor of CYP3A4, and it is a CYP2D6 inhibitor that can also inhibit P-glycoprotein transport.[332] Therefore caution is advised in the setting of other drugs metabolized by these hepatic CYP450 systems. There is an almost twofold increase in digoxin concentrations and a twofold to fourfold increase in simvastatin concentrations when these agents are used concomitantly with dronedarone. β-Blockers and calcium channel blockers (diltiazem and verapamil) also interact with dronedarone.[338,339] Because these CV drugs are frequently used in patients being treated for AF, clinicians are advised to be aware of these potential interactions and to closely monitor patients to adjust the doses to help prevent bradycardia or potential toxicity as appropriate.

Appendix

The elimination of a drug from the systemic circulation (central compartment) by liver, kidney, lung, and so on can be considered from the fundamental concepts of mass balance, the rate of drug entry, and the rate of drug exit. If steady state conditions are assumed—that is, the drug in the eliminating organ or gland is assumed to have reached distribution equilibrium—the elimination process becomes the only reason that explains any difference between arterial and venous concentrations of the drug. For the major eliminating organ (kidney) and gland (liver), this state will usually be achieved rapidly after IV administration because of high blood flow through these tissues. Where Q represents blood flow, and C_a is the arterial drug concentration, the rate of drug entry D_i into an organ or gland of elimination can be expressed as follows:

$$D_i = Q \times C_a$$

Thus, where Q still represents blood flow, and C_v is the venous drug concentration, the rate at which a drug flows out of the eliminating tissue (R_o) can be expressed as follows:

$$R_o = Q \times C_v$$

Considering the two equations above, the extraction rate (R_E, elimination of the drug by the eliminating tissue) can be expressed as follows:

$$R_E = Q \times C_a - C_v$$

An important parameter is the extraction ratio (E), which can have any value between 0 and 1 to indicate the fraction of drug extracted and can be expressed as follows:

$$E = \frac{C_a - C_v}{C_a}$$

Hepatic extraction can be influenced by modulating effects on the drug-metabolizing enzymes (e.g., CYP450 inhibition or induction). This has a strong impact on the hepatic clearance of drugs with low extraction ratios. Hepatic elimination may be decreased if two or more drugs administered concomitantly compete for the same enzyme, or if the enzyme's capacity becomes saturated, for example, as a result of the administration of high doses.

Such a dose-dependent metabolism during the first-pass effect has been reported for several drugs such as propranolol, metoprolol, lorcainide, and phenytoin. In the context of a drug-drug interaction, an increase of intrinsic clearance because of enzymatic induction will result in an increased extraction ratio as well as an increased bioavailability of the target compound. On the other hand, in the case of enzymatic inhibition, both extraction ratio and bioavailability will decrease.

REFERENCES

1. CAST investigators. Preliminary report: effect of encainide and flecainide on mortality in a randomized trial of arrhythmia suppression after myocardial infarction. *N Engl J Med* 1989;321(6):406-412.

2. Greene HL, Roden DM, Katz RJ, et al. The Cardiac Arrhythmia Suppression Trial: first CAST ... then CAST-II. *J Am Coll Cardiol* 1992;19(5):894-898.

3. Hine LK, Laird N, Hewitt P, Chalmers TC. Meta-analytic evidence against prophylactic use of lidocaine in acute myocardial infarction. *Arch Intern Med* 1989;149(12):2694-2698.

4. Kudenchuk PJ, Cobb LA, Copass MK, et al. Amiodarone for resuscitation after out-of-hospital cardiac arrest as a result of ventricular fibrillation. *N Engl J Med* 1999;341:871-878.

5. Packer DL, Prutkin JM, Hellkamp AS, et al. Impact of implantable cardioverter-defibrillator, amiodarone, and placebo on the mode of death in stable patients with heart failure: analysis from the Sudden Cardiac Death in Heart Failure trial. *Circulation* 2009;120(22):2170-2176.

6. Waldo AL, Camm AJ, deRuyter H, et al.; SWORD Investigators. Effect of d-sotalol on mortality in patients with left ventricular dysfunction after recent and remote myocardial infarction. Survival With ORal D-sotalol. *Lancet* 1996;348(9019):7-12.

7. Pratt CM, Camm AJ, Cooper W, et al. Mortality in the Survival With ORal D-sotalol (SWORD) trial: why did patients die? *Am J Cardiol* 1998;81(7):869-876.

8. The Antiarrhythmics versus Implantable Defibrillators (AVID) Investigators. A comparison of antiarrhythmic-drug therapy with implantable defibrillators in patients resuscitated from near-fatal ventricular arrhythmias. *N Engl J Med* 1997;337(22):1576-1583.

9. Sharma A, Epstein AE, Herre JM, et al. DAVID Investigators. A comparison of the AVID and DAVID trials of implantable defibrillators. *Am J Cardiol* 2005;95(12):1431-1435.

10. Krol RB, Saksena S, Prakash A. Interactions of antiarrhythmic drugs with implantable defibrillator therapy for atrial and ventricular tachyarrhythmias. *Curr Cardiol Rep* 1999;1(4):282-288.

11. Dorian P. Combination ICD and drug treatments: best options. *Resuscitation* 2000;45(3):S3-S6.

12. Singer I, Al-Khalidi HR, et al. Placebo-controlled, randomized clinical trial of azimilide for prevention of ventricular tachyarrhythmias in patients with an implantable cardioverter defibrillator. *Circulation* 2004;110:3646-3654.

13. Vaughan Williams EM. A classification of antiarrhythmic actions reassessed after a decade of new drugs. *J Clin Pharmacol* 1984;24(4):129-147.

14. Milne JR, Hellestrand KJ, Bexton RS, et al. Class 1 antiarrhythmic drugs: characteristic electrocardiographic differences when assessed by atrial and ventricular pacing. *Eur Heart J* 1984;5(2):99-107.

15. Harrison DC. Antiarrhythmic drug classification: new science and practical applications. *Am J Cardiol* 1985;56:185-187.

16. Task Force of the Working Group on Arrhythmias of the European Society of Cardiology. The Sicilian gambit: a new approach to the classification of antiarrhythmic drugs based on their actions on arrhythmogenic mechanisms. *Circulation* 1991;84(4):1831-1851.

17. Hodgkin AL, Huxley AF. A quantitative description of membrane current and its application to conduction and excitation in nerve. *J Physiol* 1952;117(4):500-544.

18. Hondeghem LM, Katzung BG. Antiarrhythmic agents: the modulated receptor mechanism of action of sodium and calcium channel blocking drugs. *Annu Rev Pharmacol Toxicol* 1984;24:387-423.

19. Hondeghem LM, Katzung BO. Time- and voltage-dependent interactions of antiarrhythmic drugs with cardiac sodium channels. *Biochim Biophys Acta* 1977;474:373-398.

20. Varro A, Elharrar V, Surawicz B. Frequency-dependent effects of several class I antiarrhythmic drugs on V_{max} of action potential upstroke in canine Purkinje fibers. *J Cardiovasc Pharmacol* 1985;7:482-492.

21. Gianelly R, von der Groeben JO, Spivack AP, et al. Effect of lidocaine on ventricular arrhythmias in patients with coronary heart disease. *N Engl J Med* 1967;277:1215-1219.

22. Kushner FG, Hand M, Smith SC Jr, et al. 2009 Focused updates: ACC/AHA guidelines for the management of patients with ST-elevation myocardial infarction (updating the 2004 guideline and 2007 focused update) and ACC/AHA/SCAI guidelines on percutaneous coronary intervention (updating the 2005 guideline and 2007 focused update): a report of the American College of Cardiology Foundation/American Heart Association Task Force on Practice Guidelines. *Circulation* 2009;120(22):2271-2306.

23. ECC Committee, Subcommittees and Task Forces of the American Heart Association. 2005 American Heart Association Guidelines for Cardiopulmonary Resuscitation and Emergency Cardiovascular Care. Advanced Cardiac Life Support Part 7.2: Management of Cardiac Arrest. *Circulation* 2005;112:IV-58-IV-66.

24. Mandel WJ, Bigger JT Jr. Electrophysiologic effects of lidocaine on isolated canine and rabbit atrial tissue. *J Pharmacol Exp Ther* 1971;178(1):81-93.

25. Aomine M. Electrophysiological effects of lidocaine on isolated guinea pig Purkinje fibers: comparison with its effects on papillary muscle. *Gen Pharmacol* 1989;20(1):99-104.

26. Xylocaine (lidocaine hydrochloride injection, USP) package insert. 2012, Wilmington, DE, AstraZeneca LP.

27. Sinatra ST, Jeresaty RM. Enhanced atrioventricular conduction atrial fibrillation after lidocaine administration. *JAMA* 1977;237(13):1356-1357.

28. Danahy DT, Aronow WS. Lidocaine-induced cardiac rate changes in atrial fibrillation and atrial flutter. *Am Heart J* 1978;95(4):474-482.

29. Endresen K, Amlie JP. Acute effects of lidocaine on repolarization and conduction in patients with coronary artery disease. *Clin Pharmacol Ther* 1989;45(4):387-395.

30. Marrouche NF, Reddy RK, Wittkowsky AK, Bardy GH. High-dose bolus lidocaine for chemical cardioversion of atrial fibrillation: a prospective, randomized, double-blind crossover trial. *Am Heart J* 2000;139(6):E8-E11.

31. Dangman KH, Hoffman BF. In vivo and in vitro antiarrhythmic and arrhythmogenic effects of N-acetyl procainamide. *J Pharmacol Exp Ther* 1981;217(3):851-862.

32. Roden DM, Reele SB, Higgins SB, et al. Antiarrhythmic efficacy, pharmacokinetics and safety of N-acetylprocainamide in human subjects: comparison with procainamide. *Am J Cardiol* 1980;46(3):463-468.

33. Thompson KA, Blair IA, Woosley RL, Roden DM. Comparative in vitro electrophysiology of quinidine, its major metabolites and dihydroquinidine. *J Pharmacol Exp Ther* 1987;241(1):84-90.

34. Kunkel F, Rowland M, Scheinman MM. The electrophysiologic effects of lidocaine in patients with intraventricular conduction defects. *Circulation* 1974;49(5):894-899.

35. Roos JC, Dunning AJ. Effects of lidocaine on impulse formation and conduction defects in man. *Am Heart J* 1975;89(6):686-699.

36. Stenson RE, Constantino RT, Harrison DC. Interrelationships of hepatic blood flow, cardiac output, and blood levels of lidocaine in man. *Circulation* 1971;43(2):205-211.

37. Zito RA, Reid PR. Lidocaine kinetics predicted by indocyanine green clearance. *N Engl J Med* 1978;298(21):1160-1163.

38. Blumer J, Strong JM, Atkinson AJ Jr. The convulsant potency of lidocaine and its N-dealkylated metabolites. *J Pharmacol Exp Ther* 1973;186(1):31-36.

39. Narang PK, Crouthamel WG, Carliner NH, Fisher ML. Lidocaine and its active metabolites. *Clin Pharmacol Ther* 1978;24:654-662.

40. Thomson PD, Melmon KL, Richardson JA, et al. Lidocaine pharmacokinetics in advanced heart failure, liver disease, and renal failure in humans. *Ann Intern Med* 1973;78(4):499-508.

41. Wyman MG, Slaughter RL, Farolino DA, et al. Multiple bolus technique for lidocaine administration in acute ischemic heart disease. II. Treatment of refractory ventricular arrhythmias and the pharmacokinetic significance of severe left ventricular failure. *J Am Coll Cardiol* 1983;2(4):764-769.

42. Stargel WW, Shand DG, Routledge PA, Barchowsky A, Wagner GS. Clinical comparison of rapid infusion and multiple injection methods for lidocaine loading. *Am Heart J* 1981;102(5):872-876.

43. Alderman EL, Kerber RE, Harrison DC. Evaluation of lidocaine resistance in man using intermittent large-dose infusion techniques. *Am J Cardiol* 1974;34(3):342-349.

44. De Martin S, Orlando R, Bertoli M, Pegoraro P, Palatini P. Differential effect of chronic renal failure on the pharmacokinetics of lidocaine in patients receiving and not receiving hemodialysis. *Clin Pharmacol Ther* 2006;80(6):597-606.

45. Richard C, Berdeaux A, Delion F, et al. Effect of mechanical ventilation on hepatic drug pharmacokinetics. *Chest* 1986;90(6):837-841.

46. LeLorier J, Grenon D, Latour Y, et al. Pharmacokinetics of lidocaine after prolonged intravenous infusions in uncomplicated myocardial infarction. *Ann Intern Med* 1977;87(6):700-706.

47. Routledge PA, Shand DG, Barchowsky A, Wagner G, Stargel WW. Relationship between alpha 1-acid glycoprotein and lidocaine disposition in myocardial infarction. *Clin Pharmacol Ther* 1981;30(2):154-157.

48. Reference deleted in proofs.

49. Dhingra RC, Deedwania PC, Cummings JM, et al. Electrophysiologic effects of lidocaine on sinus node and atrium in patients with and without sinoatrial dysfunction. *Circulation* 1978;57(3):448-454.

50. Ishii Y, Mitsuda H, Eno S, et al. Electrophysiological effects of lidocaine in sick sinus syndrome. *Jpn Heart J* 1980;21(1):27-34.

51. Keidar S, Grenadier E, Palant A. Sinoatrial arrest due to lidocaine injection in sick sinus syndrome during amiodarone administration. *Am Heart J* 1982;104(6):1384-1385.

52. Côte P, Harrison DC, Basile J, Schroeder JS. Hemodynamic interaction of procainamide and lidocaine after experimental myocardial infarction. *Am J Cardiol* 1973;32(7):937-942.

53. Olkkola KT, Isohanni MH, Hamunen K, et al. The effect of erythromycin and fluvoxamine on the pharmacokinetics of intravenous lidocaine. *Anesth Analg* 2005;100:1352-1356.

54. Orlando R, Piccoli P, De Martin S, et al. Cytochrome P450 1A2 is a major determinant of lidocaine metabolism in vivo: effects of liver function. *Clin Pharmacol Ther* 2004;75:80-88.

55. Wang JS, Backman JT, Wen X, et al. Fluvoxamine is a more potent inhibitor of lidocaine metabolism than ketoconazole and erythromycin in vitro. *Pharmacol Toxicol* 1999;85:201-205.

56. Wang JS, Backman JT, Taavitsainen P, et al. Involvement of CYP1A2 and CYP3A4 in lidocaine N-deethylation and 3-hydroxylation in humans. *Drug Metab Dispos* 2000;28:959-965.

57. Ochs HR, Carstens G, Greenblatt DJ. Reduction in lidocaine clearance during continuous infusion and by coadministration of propranolol. *N Engl J Med* 1980;303(7):373-377.

58. Powell JR, Donn KH. Histamine H2-antagonist drug interactions in perspective: mechanistic concepts and clinical implications. *Am J Med* 1984;77(Suppl 5B):57-84.

59. Stracke J, Meyer UE, Schumacher HE, et al. Mexiletine in the treatment of diabetic neuropathy. *Diabetes Care* 1992;15:1550-1555.

60. Duff HJ, Roden D, Primm RK, Oates JA, Woosley RL. Mexiletine in the treatment of resistant ventricular arrhythmias: enhancement of efficacy and reduction of dose-related side effects by combination with quinidine. *Circulation* 1983;67(5):1124-1128.

61. Mason JW; Electrophysiologic Study versus Electrocardiographic Monitoring Investigators. A comparison of seven antiarrhythmic drugs in patients with ventricular tachyarrhythmias. *N Engl J Med* 1993;329(7):452-458.

62. Kobayashi A, Yamazaki N, Kobayashi T, et al. Efficacy of combination therapy with mexiletine and a low dose of propranolol for premature ventricular arrhythmias. *Jpn Circ J* 1990;54(12):1486-1496.

63. Yeung-Lai-Wah JA, Murdock CJ, Boone J, Kerr CR. Propafenone-mexiletine combination for the treatment of sustained ventricular tachycardia. *J Am Coll Cardiol* 1992;20(3):547-551.

64. Morita H, Hirabayashi K, Nozaki S, et al. Chronic effect of oral mexiletine administration on left ventricular contractility in patients with congestive heart failure: a study based on mitral regurgitant flow velocity measured by continuous-wave Doppler echocardiography. *J Clin Pharmacol* 1995;35(5):478-483.

65. Woosley RL, Wang T, Stone W, et al. Pharmacology, electrophysiology, and pharmacokinetics of mexiletine. *Am Heart J* 1984;107(5 Pt 2):1058-1065.

66. Prescott LF, Clemens JA, Pottage A. Absorption, distribution, and elimination of mexiletine. *Postgrad Med J* 1977;53(Suppl 1):50-55.

67. Brown JE, Shand DG. Therapeutic drug monitoring of antiarrhythmic agents. *Clin Pharmacokinet* 1982;7(2):125-148.
68. Beckett AH, Chidomere EC. The distribution, metabolism and excretion of mexiletine in man. *Postgrad Med J* 1977;53(Suppl 1):60-68.
69. Otani M, Fukuda T, Naohara M, et al. Impact of CYP2D6*10 on mexiletine pharmacokinetics in healthy adult volunteers. *Eur J Clin Pharmacol* 2003;59(5-6):395-399.
70. Campbell NP, Kelly JG, Adgey AA, Shanks RG. The clinical pharmacology of mexiletine. *Br J Clin Pharmacol* 1978;6(2):103-108.
71. Moak JP, Smith RT, Garson A Jr. Mexilitine: an effective antiarrhythmic drug for treatment of ventricular arrhythmias in congenital heart disease. *J Am Coll Cardiol* 1987;10:824-828.
72. El Allaf D, Henrard L, Crochelet L, et al. Pharmacokinetics of mexiletine in renal insufficiency. *Br J Clin Pharmacol* 1982;14(3):431-435.
73. Leahey EB, Jr, Giardina E-GV, Bigger JT Jr. Effect of ventricular failure on steady state kinetics of mexiletine. *Clin Res* 1980;26:239A.
74. Pentikäinen PJ, Hietakorpi S, Halinen MO, Lampinen LM. Cirrhosis of the liver markedly impairs the elimination of mexiletine. *Eur J Clin Pharmacol* 1986;30(1):83-88.
75. Mexiletine package insert. North Wales, PA, Teva Pharmaceuticals.
76. Girmann G, Pees H, Scheurlen PG. Pseudothrombocytopenia and mexiletine. *Ann Intern Med* 1984;100(5):767.
77. Fasola GP, D'Osualdo F, de Pangher V, Barducci E. Thrombocytopenia and mexiletine. *Ann Intern Med* 1984;100(1):162.
78. Gambhir DS, Yadav BS, Gupta R, Bahl VK, Khalilullah M. Electrophysiological effects of mexiletine in patients of sinus node dysfunction and intraventricular conduction defects. *Indian Heart J* 1986;38(3):173-178.
79. Kolecki PF, Curry SC. Poisoning by sodium channel blocking agents. *Crit Care Clin* 1997;13(4):829-848.
80. Ravid S, Podrid PJ, Lampert S, Lown B. Congestive heart failure induced by six of the newer antiarrhythmic drugs. *J Am Coll Cardiol* 1989;14(5):1326-1330.
81. Ballas SL, Baughman KL, Griffith LS, Veltri EP. Mexiletine-associated left ventricular dysfunction: a case study. *Md Med J* 1991;40(6):519-520.
82. Gottlieb SS, Weinberg M. Cardiodepressant effects of mexiletine in patients with severe left ventricular dysfunction. *Eur Heart J* 1992;13(1):22-27.
83. Campbell RW. Mexiletine. *N Engl J Med* 1987;316(1):29-34.
84. Pentikäinen PJ, Koivula IH, Hiltunen HA. Effect of rifampicin treatment on the kinetics of mexiletine. *Eur J Clin Pharmacol* 1982;23(3):261-266.
85. Bigger JT Jr. The interaction of mexiletine with other cardiovascular drugs. *Am Heart J* 1984;107(5 Pt 2):1079-1085.
86. Neumar RW, Otto CW, Link MS, et al. Part 8: adult advanced cardiovascular life support—2010 American Heart Association Guidelines for Cardiopulmonary Resuscitation and Emergency Cardiovascular Care. *Circulation* 2010;122(18 Suppl 3):S729-S767.
87. Simonian SM, Lotfipour S, Wall C, Langdorf MI. Challenging the superiority of amiodarone for rate control in Wolff-Parkinson-White and atrial fibrillation. *Intern Emerg Med* 2010;5(5):421-426.
88. Gorgels AP, van den Dool A, Hofs A, et al. Comparison of procainamide and lidocaine in terminating sustained monomorphic ventricular tachycardia. *Am J Cardiol* 1996;78:43-46.
89. Roden DM, Reele SB, Higgins SB, et al. Antiarrhythmic efficacy, pharmacokinetics and safety of N-acetylprocainamide in human subjects: comparison with procainamide. *Am J Cardiol* 1980;46(3):463-468.
90. Funck-Brentano C, Light RT, Lineberry MD, et al. Pharmacokinetic and pharmacodynamic interaction of N-acetyl procainamide and procainamide in humans. *J Cardiovasc Pharmacol* 1989;14(3):364-373.
91. Dangman KH, Miura DS. Effects of therapeutic concentrations of procainamide on transmembrane action potentials of normal and infarct zone Purkinje fibers and ventricular muscle cells. *J Cardiovasc Pharmacol* 1989;13(6):846-852.
92. Zipes DP. Proarrhythmic effects of antiarrhythmic drugs. *Am J Cardiol* 1987;59(11):26E-31E.
93. Hondeghem LM, Snyders DJ. Class III antiarrhythmic agents have a lot of potential but a long way to go: reduced effectiveness and dangers of reverse use dependence. *Circulation* 1990;81(2):686-690.
94. Roden DM. Current status of class III antiarrhythmic drug therapy. *Am J Cardiol* 1993;72(6):44B-49B.
95. Roden DM, Reele SB, Higgins SB, et al. Antiarrhythmic efficacy, pharmacokinetics and safety of N-acetylprocainamide in human subjects: comparison with procainamide. *Am J Cardiol* 1980;46(3):463-468.
96. Giardina EG, Heissenbuttel RH, Bigger JT Jr. Intermittent intravenous procaine amide to treat ventricular arrhythmias: correlation of plasma concentration with effect on arrhythmia, electrocardiogram, and blood pressure. *Ann Intern Med* 1973;78(2):183-193.
97. Lima JJ, Goldfarb AL, Conti DR, et al. Safety and efficacy of procainamide infusions. *Am J Cardiol* 1979;43(1):98-105.
98. Karlsson E. Clinical pharmacokinetics of procainamide. *Clin Pharmacokinet* 1978;3(2):97-107.
99. du Souich P, Erill S. Metabolism of procainamide in patients with chronic heart failure, chronic respiratory failure and chronic renal failure. *Eur J Clin Pharmacol* 1978;14(1):21-27.
100. Kessler KM, Kayden DS, Estes DM, et al. Procainamide pharmacokinetics in patients with acute myocardial infarction or congestive heart failure. *J Am Coll Cardiol* 1986;7(5):1131-1139.
101. Tisdale JE, Rudis MI, Padhi ID, et al. Disposition of procainamide in patients with chronic congestive heart failure receiving medical therapy. *J Clin Pharmacol* 1996;36(1):35-41.
102. Chow MJ, Piergies AA, Bowsher DJ, et al. Torsade de pointes induced by N-acetylprocainamide. *J Am Coll Cardiol* 1984;4(3):621-624.
103. Stratmann HG, Walter KE, Kennedy HL. Torsade de pointes associated with elevated N-acetylprocainamide levels. *Am Heart J* 1985;109(2):375-377.
104. Piergies AA, Ruo TI, Jansyn EM, Belknap SM, Atkinson AJ Jr. Effect kinetics of N-acetylprocainamide-induced QT interval prolongation. *Clin Pharmacol Ther* 1987;42(1):107-112.
105. Pronestyl (procainamide HCL) package insert. 2012, New York, NY, Bristol-Myers Squibb.
106. Lertora JJ, King LW, Donkor KA. The inotropic actions of N-acetylprocainamide: blockade and reversal by propranolol. *Angiology* 1986;37(12 Pt 2):939-949.
107. Kim HG, Friedman HS. Procainamide-induced sinus node dysfunction in patients with chronic renal failure. *Chest* 1979;76(6):699-701.
108. Ladd AT. Procainamide-induced lupus erythematosus. *N Engl J Med* 1962;267:1357-1358.
109. Sanford HS, Michaelson AK, Halpern MM. Procainamide-induced lupus erythematosus syndrome. *Dis Chest* 1967;51(2):172-176.
110. Yung R, Chang S, Hemati N, Johnson K, Richardson B. Mechanisms of drug-induced lupus. IV. Comparison of procainamide and hydralazine with analogs in vitro and in vivo. *Arthritis Rheum* 1997;40(8):1436-1443.
111. Reidenberg MM, Drayer DE. Procainamide, N-acetylprocainamide, antinuclear antibody and systemic lupus erythematosus. *Angiology* 1986;37(12 Pt 2):968-971.
112. Clark DW. Genetically determined variability in acetylation and oxidation. Therapeutic implications. *Drugs* 1985;29(4):342-375.
113. Lessard E, Hamelin BA, Labbé L, et al. Involvement of CYP2D6 activity in the N-oxidation of procainamide in man. *Pharmacogenetics* 1999;9(6):683-696.
114. Ghose MK. Pericardial tamponade: a presenting manifestation of procainamide-induced lupus erythematosus. *Am J Med* 1975;58(4):581-585.
115. Rothman IK, Amorosi EL. Procainamide-induced agranulocytosis and thrombocytopenia. *Arch Intern Med* 1979;139(2):246-247.
116. Wang RI, Schuller G. Agranulocytosis following procainamide administration. *Am Heart J* 1969;78(2):282-284.
117. Konttinen YP, Tuominen L. Reversible procainamide-induced agranulocytosis twice in one patient. *Lancet* 1971;2(7730):925.
118. Riker J, Baker J, Swanson M. Bone marrow granulomas and neutropenia associated with procainamide: report of a case. *Arch Intern Med* 1978;138(11):1731-1732.
119. Crook JE, Woosley RL, Leftwich RB, Natelson EA. Agranulocytosis during combined procainamide and phenytoin therapy. *South Med J* 1979;72(12):1599-1601.
120. Nagesh KG, Poulose KP, Tseng TH, Schadchehr A. Procainamide-induced agranulocytosis: report of two cases and review. *J Kans Med Soc* 1980;81(1):18-24.
121. Berger BE, Hauser DJ. Agranulocytosis due to new sustained-release procainamide. *Am Heart J* 1983;105(6):1035-1036.
122. Meisner DJ, Carlson RJ, Gottlieb AJ. Thrombocytopenia following sustained-release procainamide. *Arch Intern Med* 1985;145(4):700-702.
123. Malters PB, Salem AG. Agranulocytosis secondary to extended-release procainamide: a case report and review of the literature. A case of agranulocytosis caused by procainamide in a patient who had undergone open-heart surgery. *S D J Med* 1987;40(2):7-10.
124. Freed JS, Reiner MA. Septic complications of procainamide-induced agranulocytosis: report of two cases. *Mt Sinai J Med* 1988;55(2):194-197.
125. Abe H, Suzuka H, Tasaki H, Kuroiwa A. Sustained-release procainamide-induced reversible granulocytopenia after myocardial infarction. *Jpn Heart J* 1995;36(4):483-487.
126. Leahey EB Jr, Reiffel JA, Giardina EG, Bigger JT Jr. The effect of quinidine and other oral antiarrhythmic drugs on serum digoxin: a prospective study. *Ann Intern Med* 1980;92(5):605-608.
127. Christian CD Jr, Meredith CG, Speeg KV Jr. Cimetidine inhibits renal procainamide clearance. *Clin Pharmacol Ther* 1984;36(2):221-227.
128. Higbee MD, Wood JS, Mead RA. Procainamide-cimetidine interaction: a potential toxic interaction in the elderly. *J Am Geriatr Soc* 1984;32(2):162-164.
129. Bauer LA, Black D, Gensler A. Procainamide–cimetidine drug interaction in elderly male patients. *J Am Geriatr Soc* 1990;38(4):467-469.
130. Somogyi A, McLean A, Heinzow B. Cimetidine–procainamide pharmacokinetic interaction in man: evidence of competition for tubular secretion of basic drugs. *Eur J Clin Pharmacol* 1983;25(3):339-345.
131. Somogyi A, Bochner F. Dose and concentration dependent effect of ranitidine on procainamide disposition and renal clearance in man. *Br J Clin Pharmacol* 1984;18(2):175-181.
132. Norpace (disopyramide) package insert. 2012, New York, NY, Pfizer US Pharmaceuticals.
133. Birkhead JS, Vaughan Williams EM. Dual effect of disopyramide on atrial and atrioventricular conduction and refractory periods. *Br Heart J* 1977;39(6):657-660.
134. Spurrell RA, Thorburn CW, Camm J, Sowton E, Deuchar DC. Effects of disopyramide on electrophysiological properties of specialized conduction system in man and on accessory atrioventricular pathway in Wolff-Parkinson-White syndrome. *Br Heart J* 1975;37(8):861-867.
135. Dubetz DK, Brown NN, Hooper WD, Eadie MJ, Tyrer JH. Disopyramide pharmacokinetics and bioavailability. *Br J Clin Pharmacol* 1978;6(3):279-281.
136. Rangno RE, Warnica W, Ogilvie RI, Kreeft J, Bridger E. Correlation of disopyramide pharmacokinetics with efficacy in ventricular tachyarrhythmia. *J Int Med Res* 1976;4(1 Suppl):54-58.
137. Hinderling PH, Garrett ER. Pharmacodynamics of the antiarrhythmic disopyramide in healthy humans: correlation of the kinetics of the drug and its effects. *J Pharmacokinet Biopharm* 1976;4(3):231-242.
138. Meffin PJ, Robert EW, Winkle RA, et al. Role of concentration-dependent plasma protein binding in disopyramide disposition. *J Pharmacokinet Biopharm* 1979;7(1):29-46.
139. Davies RF, Siddoway LA, Shaw L, et al. Immediate- versus controlled-release disopyramide: importance of saturable binding. *Clin Pharmacol Ther* 1993;54(1):16-22.
140. Pedersen LE, Bonde J, Graudal NA, et al. Quantitative and qualitative binding characteristics of disopyramide in serum from patients with decreased renal and hepatic function. *Br J Clin Pharmacol* 1987;23(1):41-46.
141. Edvardsson N, Olsson SB. Clinical value of plasma concentrations of antiarrhythmic drugs. *Eur Heart J* 1987;8(Suppl A):83-89.

142. Kumana CR, Rambihar VS, Tanser PH, et al. A placebo-controlled study to determine the efficacy of oral disopyramide phosphate for the prophylaxis of ventricular dysrhythmias after acute myocardial infarction. *Br J Clin Pharmacol* 1982;14(4):519-527.
143. Podrid PJ, Schoeneberger A, Lown B. Congestive heart failure caused by oral disopyramide. *N Engl J Med* 1980;302(11):614-617.
144. Johnston A, Henry JA, Warrington SJ, Hamer NA. Pharmacokinetics of oral disopyramide phosphate in patients with renal impairment. *Br J Clin Pharmacol* 1980;10(3):245-248.
145. Bonde J, Graudal NA, Pedersen LE, et al. Kinetics of disopyramide in decreased hepatic function. *Eur J Clin Pharmacol* 1986;31(1):73-77.
146. Woosley RL, Funck-Brentano C. Overview of the clinical pharmacology of antiarrhythmic drugs. *Am J Cardiol* 1988;61(2):61A-69A.
147. Frucht J, Freimann I, Merin S. Ocular side effects of disopyramide. *Br J Ophthalmol* 1984;68(12):890-891.
148. Brown JH, Wetzel GT, Dunlap J. Activation and blockade of cardiac muscarinic receptors by endogenous acetylcholine and cholinesterase inhibitors. *J Pharmacol Exp Ther* 1982;223(1):20-24.
149. Tzivoni D, Keren A, Stern S, Gottlieb S. Disopyramide-induced torsade de pointes. *Arch Intern Med* 1981;141(7):946-947.
150. Keren A, Tzivoni D, Gottlieb S, Benhorin J, Stern S. Atypical ventricular tachycardia (torsade de pointes) induced by amiodarone: arrhythmia previously induced by quinidine and disopyramide. *Chest* 1982;81(3):384-386.
151. Wilkinson PR, Desai J, Hollister J, et al. Electrophysiologic effects of disopyramide in patients with atrioventricular nodal dysfunction. *Circulation* 1982;66(6):1211-1216.
152. LaBarre A, Strauss HC, Scheinman MM, et al. Electrophysiologic effects of disopyramide phosphate on sinus node function in patients with sinus node dysfunction. *Circulation* 1979;59(2):226-235.
153. Hayashi Y, Ikeda U, Hashimoto T, et al. Torsades de pointes ventricular tachycardia induced by clarithromycin and disopyramide in the presence of hypokalemia. *Pacing Clin Electrophysiol* 1999;22(4 Pt 1):672-674.
154. Risler T, Burk M, Peters U, Grabensee B, Seipel L. On the interaction between digoxin and disopyramide. *Clin Pharmacol Ther* 1983;34(2):176-180.
155. Sylvén C, Anderson P. Evidence that disopyramide does not interact with warfarin. *Br Med J (Clin Res Ed)* 1983;286(6372):1181.
156. Echizen H, Tanizaki M, Tatsuno J, et al. Identification of CYP3A4 as the enzyme involved in the mono-N-dealkylation of disopyramide enantiomers in humans. *Drug Metab Dispos* 2000;28(8):937-944.
157. Kessler JM, Keys PW, Stafford RW. Disopyramide and phenytoin interaction. *Clin Pharm* 1982;1(3):263-264.
158. Cumming AD, Robertson C. Interaction between disopyramide and practolol. *Br Med J* 1979;2(6200):1264.
159. Naccarelli GV, Dorian P, Hohnloser SH, Coumel P; Flecainide Multicenter Atrial Fibrillation Study Group. Prospective comparison of flecainide versus quinidine for the treatment of paroxysmal atrial fibrillation/flutter. *Am J Cardiol* 1996;77(3):53A-59A.
160. Juul-Moller S, Edvardson N, Rehnqvist-Ahlberg N. Sotalol versus quinidine for the maintenance of sinus rhythm after direct cardioversion of atrial fibrillation. *Circulation* 1990;82:1932-1939.
161. Borgeat A, Goy JJ, Maendly R, et al. Flecainide versus quinidine for conversion of atrial fibrillation to sinus rhythm. *Am J Cardiol* 1986;58(6):496-498.
162. Makynen PJ, Kossinen PJ, Saaristo TE, Liisanantti RK. Comparison of encainide and quinidine for supraventricular tachyarrhythmias. *Am J Cardiol* 1988;62(Suppl):55L-59L.
163. Sheldon R, Duff H, Koshman ML. Antiarrhythmic activity of quinine in humans. *Circulation* 1995;92(10):2944-2950.
164. Mason JW; Electrophysiologic Study versus Electrocardiographic Monitoring Investigators. A comparison of seven antiarrhythmic drugs in patients with ventricular tachyarrhythmias. *N Engl J Med* 1993;329(7):452-458.
165. Morganroth J, Goin JE. Quinidine-related mortality in the short-to-medium-term treatment of ventricular arrhythmias: a meta-analysis. *Circulation* 1991;84(5):1977-1983.
166. Holford NH, Coates PE, Guentert TW, Riegelman S, Sheiner LB. The effect of quinidine and its metabolites on the electrocardiogram and systolic time intervals: concentration–effect relationships. *Br J Clin Pharmacol* 1981;11(2):187-195.
167. Sokolow M, Edgar AL. Blood quinidine concentrations as a guide in the treatment of cardiac arrhythmias. *Circulation* 1950;1:576-592.
168. Vozeh S, Oti-Amoako K, Uematsu T, Follath F. Antiarrhythmic activity of two quinidine metabolites in experimental reperfusion arrhythmia: relative potency and pharmacodynamic interaction with the parent drug. *J Pharmacol Exp Ther* 1987;243(1):297-301.
169. Vozeh S, Bindschedler M, Ha HR, et al. Pharmacodynamics of 3-hydroxyquinidine alone and in combination with quinidine in healthy persons. *Am J Cardiol* 1987;59(6):681-684.
170. Kavanagh KM, Wyse DG, Mitchell LB, et al. Contribution of quinidine metabolites to electrophysiologic responses in human subjects. *Clin Pharmacol Ther* 1989;46(3):352-358.
171. Thompson KA, Blair IA, Woosley RL, Roden DM. Comparative in vitro electrophysiology of quinidine, its major metabolites and dihydroquinidine. *J Pharmacol Exp Ther* 1987;241(1):84-90.
172. Drayer DE, Lorenzo B, Reidenberg MM. Liquid chromatography and fluorescence spectroscopy compared with a homogeneous enzyme immunoassay technique for determining quinidine in serum. *Clin Chem* 1981;27(2):308-310.
173. Lehmann CR, Boran KJ, Pierson WP, Melikian AP, Wright GJ. Quinidine assays: enzyme immunoassay versus high performance liquid chromatography. *Ther Drug Monit* 1986;8(3):336-339.
174. Drayer DE, Lowenthal DT, Restivo KM, et al. Steady-state serum levels of quinidine and active metabolites in cardiac patients with varying degrees of renal function. *Clin Pharmacol Ther* 1978;24(1):31-39.
175. Kessler KM, Humphries WC Jr, Black M, Spann JF. Quinidine pharmacokinetics in patients with cirrhosis or receiving propranolol. *Am Heart J* 1978;96(5):627-635.
176. Ochs HR, Greenblatt DJ, Woo E. Clinical pharmacokinetics of quinidine. *Clin Pharmacokinet* 1980;5(2):150-168.
177. Kay GN, Plumb VJ, Arciniegas JG, Henthorn RW, Waldo AL. Torsade de pointes: the long-short initiating sequence and other clinical features: observations in 32 patients. *J Am Coll Cardiol* 1983;2(5):806-817.
178. Gottlieb SS, Weinberg M. Hemodynamic and neurohormonal effects of quinidine in patients with severe left ventricular dysfunction secondary to coronary artery disease or idiopathic dilated cardiomyopathy. *Am J Cardiol* 1991;67(8):728-731.
179. Cohen IS, Jick H, Cohen SI. Adverse reactions to quinidine in hospitalized patients: findings based on data from the Boston Collaborative Drug Surveillance Program. *Prog Cardiovasc Dis* 1977;20(2):151-163.
180. Roden DM, Hoffman BF. Action potential prolongation and induction of abnormal automaticity by low quinidine concentrations in canine Purkinje fibers: relationship to potassium and cycle length. *Circ Res* 1985;56(6):857-867.
181. Dargie HJ, Cleland JG, Leckie BJ, et al. Relation of arrhythmias and electrolyte abnormalities to survival in patients with severe chronic heart failure. *Circulation* 1987;75(5 Pt 2):IV98-IV107.
182. Roden DM, Woosley RL, Primm RK. Incidence and clinical features of the quinidine-associated long QT syndrome: implications for patient care. *Am Heart J* 1986;111(6):1088-1093.
183. Makkar RR, Fromm BS, Steinman RT, Meissner MD, Lehmann MH. Female gender as a risk factor for torsades de pointes associated with cardiovascular drugs. *JAMA* 1993;270(21):2590-2597.
184. Drici MD, Burklow TR, Haridasse V, Glazer RI, Woosley RL. Sex hormones prolong the QT interval and downregulate potassium channel expression in the rabbit heart. *Circulation* 1996;94(6):1471-1474.
185. Benton RE, Sale M, Flockhart DA, Woosley RL. Greater quinidine-induced QTc interval prolongation in women. *Clin Pharmacol Ther* 2000;67(4):413-418.
186. El-Eraky H, Thomas SH. Effects of sex on the pharmacokinetic and pharmacodynamic properties of quinidine. *Br J Clin Pharmacol* 2003;56(2):198-204.
187. Bidoggia H, Maciel JP, Capalozza N, et al. Sex differences on the electrocardiographic pattern of cardiac repolarization: possible role of testosterone. *Am Heart J* 2000;140(4):678-683.
188. Ebert SN, Liu XK, Woosley RL. Female gender as a risk factor for drug-induced cardiac arrhythmias: evaluation of clinical and experimental evidence. *J Womens Health* 1998;7(5):547-557.
189. Woosley RL. QT drug lists by risk group. Arizona Center for Education and Research on Therapeutics. Available at http://www.azcert.org/medical-pros/drug-lists/drug-lists.cfm. Accessed May 2012.
190. Tzivoni D, Banai S, Schuger C, et al. Treatment of torsades de pointes with magnesium sulfate. *Circulation* 1988;77:392-397.
191. Patsilinakos S, Christou A, Kafkas N, et al. Effect of high doses of magnesium on converting ibutilide to a safe and more effective agent. *Am J Cardiol* 2010;106:673-676.
192. Keren A, Tzivoni D, Gavish D, et al. Etiology, warning signs and therapy of torsade de pointes: a study of 10 patients. *Circulation* 1981;64:1167-1174.
193. Schmid PG, Nelson LD, Mark AL, Heistad DD, Abboud FM. Inhibition of adrenergic vasoconstriction by quinidine. *J Pharmacol Exp Ther* 1974;188(1):124-134.
194. Quinidine gluconate injection package insert. Indianapolis, IN, Eli Lilly Co.
195. Nair MR, Duvernoy WF, Leichtman DA. Severe leukopenia and thrombocytopenia secondary to quinidine. *Clin Cardiol* 1981;4(5):247-257.
196. Polish LB, Branch RA, Fitzgerald GA. Digitoxin–quinidine interaction: potentiation during administration of cimetidine. *South Med J* 1981 May;74(5):633-634.
197. Data JL, Wilkinson GR, Nies AS. Interaction of quinidine with anticonvulsant drugs. *N Engl J Med* 1976;294(13):699-702.
198. Leahey EB Jr, Reiffel JA, Drusin RE, et al. Interaction between quinidine and digoxin. *JAMA* 1978;240(6):533-534.
199. Bussey HI. The influence of quinidine and other agents on digitalis glycosides. *Am Heart J* 1982;104(2 Pt 1):289-302.
200. Brinn R, Brøsen K, Gram LF, Haghfelt T, Otton SV. Sparteine oxidation is practically abolished in quinidine-treated patients. *Br J Clin Pharmacol* 1986;22(2):194-197.
201. Speirs CJ, Murray S, Boobis AR, Seddon CE, Davies DS. Quinidine and the identification of drugs whose elimination is impaired in subjects classified as poor metabolizers of debrisoquine. *Br J Clin Pharmacol* 1986;22(6):739-743.
202. Guengerich FP, Müller-Enoch D, Blair IA. Oxidation of quinidine by human liver cytochrome P-450. *Mol Pharmacol* 1986;30(3):287-295.
203. Mikus G, Ha HR, Vozeh S, et al. Pharmacokinetics and metabolism of quinidine in extensive and poor metabolisers of sparteine. *Eur J Clin Pharmacol* 1986;31(1):69-72.
204. Brøsen K, Gram LF, Haghfelt T, Bertilsson L. Extensive metabolizers of debrisoquine become poor metabolizers during quinidine treatment. *Pharmacol Toxicol* 1987;60(4):312-314.
205. Kornfeld P, Horowitz SH, Genkins G, Papatestas AE. Myasthenia gravis unmasked by antiarrhythmic agents. *Mt Sinai J Med* 1976;43(1):10-14.
206. Gogono AW. Anaesthesia for atrial defibrillation: effect of quinidine on muscular relaxation. *Lancet* 1963;2(7316):1039-1040.
207. Siddoway LA, Roden DM, Woosley RL. Clinical pharmacology of propafenone: pharmacokinetics, metabolism and concentration-response relations. *Am J Cardiol* 1984;54(9):9D-12D.
208. McLeod AA, Stiles GL, Shand DG. Demonstration of beta adrenoceptor blockade by propafenone hydrochloride: clinical pharmacologic, radioligand binding and adenylate cyclase activation studies. *J Pharmacol Exp Ther* 1984;228(2):461-466.
209. Siddoway LA, Thompson KA, McAllister CB, et al. Polymorphism of propafenone metabolism and disposition in man: clinical and pharmacokinetic consequences. *Circulation* 1987;75(4):785-791.
210. Cai WM, Chen B, Cai MH, Chen Y, Zhang YD. The influence of CYP2D6 activity on the kinetics of propafenone enantiomers in Chinese subjects. *Br J Clin Pharmacol* 1999;47(5):553-556.
211. Chen B, Cai WM. Influence of CYP2D6*10B genotype on pharmacokinetics of propafenone enantiomers in Chinese subjects. *Acta Pharmacol Sin* 2003;24(12):1277-1280.
212. Lee JT, Kroemer HK, Silberstein DJ, et al. The role of genetically determined polymorphic drug metabolism in the beta-blockade produced by propafenone. *N Engl J Med* 1990;322(25):1764-1768.

213. Baker BJ, Dinh H, Kroskey D, et al. Effect of propafenone on left ventricular ejection fraction. *Am J Cardiol* 1984;54(9):20D-22D.

214. Rythmol SR *(propafenone hydrochloride) package insert*. 2012, Philadephia, GlaxoSmithKline.

215. Wagner F, Kalusche D, Trenk D, Jähnchen E, Roskamm H. Drug interaction between propafenone and metoprolol. *Br J Clin Pharmacol* 1987;24(2):213-220.

216. Funck-Brentano C, Kroemer HK, Pavlou H, Woosley RL, Roden DM. Genetically-determined interaction between propafenone and low dose quinidine: role of active metabolites in modulating net drug effect. *Br J Clin Pharmacol* 1989;27(4):435-444.

217. Mörike KE, Roden DM. Quinidine-enhanced beta-blockade during treatment with propafenone in extensive metabolizer human subjects. *Clin Pharmacol Ther* 1994; 55(1):28-34.

218. Hondeghem LM, Katzung BG. Antiarrhythmic agents: the modulated receptor mechanism of action of sodium and calcium channel–blocking drugs. *Annu Rev Pharmacol Toxicol* 1984;24:387-423.

219. Hellestrand KJ, Bexton RS, Nathan AW, Spurrell RA, Camm AJ. Acute electrophysiological effects of flecainide acetate on cardiac conduction and refractoriness in man. *Br Heart J* 1982;48(2):140-148.

220. Paul AA, Witchel HJ, Hancox JC. Inhibition of the current of heterologously expressed HERG potassium channels by flecainide and comparison with quinidine, propafenone and lignocaine. *Br J Pharmacol* 2002;136(5):717-729.

221. Conard GJ, Ober RE. Metabolism of flecainide. *Am J Cardiol* 1984;53(5):41B-51B.

222. Roden DM, Woosley RL. Drug therapy: flecainide. *N Engl J Med* 1986;315(1):36-41.

223. Haefeli WE, Bargetzi MJ, Follath F, Meyer UA. Potent inhibition of cytochrome P450IID6 (debrisoquin 4-hydroxylase) by flecainide in vitro and in vivo. *J Cardiovasc Pharmacol* 1990;15(5):776-779.

224. Johnston A, Warrington S, Turner P. Flecainide pharmacokinetics in healthy volunteers: the influence of urinary pH. *Br J Clin Pharmacol* 1985;20(4):333-338.

225. Franciosa JA, Wilen M, Weeks CE, et al. Pharmacokinetics and hemodynamic effects of flecainide in patients with chronic low output heart failure (abstract). *J Am Coll Cardiol* 1983;1:669.

226. Winkelman BR, Leinberger H. Life-threatening flecainide toxicity: a pharmacodynamic approach. *Ann Intern Med* 1987;106:807-814.

227. Salerno DM, Granrud G, Sharkey P, et al. Pharmacodynamics and side effects of flecainide acetate. *Clin Pharmacol Ther* 1986;40(1):101-107.

228. Evers J, Eichelbaum M, Kroemer HK. Unpredictability of flecainide plasma concentrations in patients with renal failure: relationship to side effects and sudden death? *Ther Drug Monit* 1994;16(4):349-351.

229. Morganroth J. Risk factors for the development of proarrhythmic events. *Am J Cardiol* 1987;59(11):32E-37E.

230. Josephson MA, Ikeda N, Singh BN. Effects of flecainide on ventricular function: clinical and experimental correlations. *Am J Cardiol* 1984;53(5):95B-100B.

231. Falk RH. Flecainide-induced ventricular tachycardia and fibrillation in patients treated for atrial fibrillation. *Ann Intern Med* 1989;111(2):107-111.

232. Morganroth J, Horowitz LN. Flecainide: its proarrhythmic effect and expected changes on the surface electrocardiogram. *Am J Cardiol* 1984;53(5):89B-94B.

233. Hellestrand KJ, Nathan AW, Bexton RS, Camm AJ. Electrophysiologic effects of flecainide acetate on sinus node function, anomalous atrioventricular connections, and pacemaker thresholds. *Am J Cardiol* 1984;53(5):30B-38B.

234. Dopp AL, Miller JM, Tisdale JE. Effect of drugs on defibrillation capacity. *Drugs* 2008;68(5):607-630.

235. Tjandra-Maga TB, van Hecken A, van Melle P, Verbesselt R, de Schepper PJ. Altered pharmacokinetics of oral flecainide by cimetidine. *Br J Clin Pharmacol* 1986;22(1):108-110.

236. Weeks CE, Conard GJ, Kvam DC, et al. The effect of flecainide acetate, a new antiarrhythmic, on plasma digoxin levels. *J Clin Pharmacol* 1986;26(1):27-31.

237. Lewis GP, Holtzman JL. Interaction of flecainide with digoxin and propranolol. *Am J Cardiol* 1984;53(5):52B-57B.

238. Shea P, Lal R, Kim SS, Schechtman K, Ruffy R. Flecainide and amiodarone interaction. *J Am Coll Cardiol* 1986;7(5):1127-1130.

239. Benditt DG, Williams JH, Jin J, et al. Maintenance of sinus rhythm with oral d,l-sotalol therapy in patients with symptomatic atrial fibrillation and/or atrial flutter. *Am J Cardiol* 1999;84:270-277.

240. Roy D, Talajic M, Dorian P, et al. Amiodarone to prevent recurrence of atrial fibrillation. Canadian Trial of Atrial Fibrillation Investigators. *N Engl J Med* 2000;342:913-920.

241. Singh BN, Singh SN, Reda DJ, et al; Sotalol Amiodarone Atrial Fibrillation Efficacy Trial (SAFE-T) Investigators. Amiodarone versus sotalol for atrial fibrillation. *N Engl J Med* 2005;352(18):1861-1872.

242. The AFFIRM First Antiarrhythmic Drug Substudy Investigators. Maintenance of sinus rhythm in patients with atrial fibrillation. *J Am Coll Cardiol* 2003;42:20-29.

243. Waldo AL, Camm AJ, DeRuyter H; The SWORD Investigators. Effect of d-sotalol on mortality in patients with left ventricular dysfunction after recent and remote myocardial infarction: Survival With Oral D-sotalol. *Lancet* 1996;348:7-12.

244. Fuster V, Rydén LE, Cannom DS, et al. ACC/AHA/ESC 2006 Guidelines for the Management of Patients with Atrial Fibrillation: a report of the American College of Cardiology/American Heart Association Task Force on practice guidelines and the European Society of Cardiology Committee for Practice Guidelines (Writing Committee to Revise the 2001 Guidelines for the Management of Patients with Atrial Fibrillation) developed in collaboration with the European Heart Rhythm Association and the Heart Rhythm Society. *Europace* 2006;8(9):651-745.

245. Betapace (sotalol) package insert. 2012, Montville, NJ, Bayer Healthcare Pharmaceuticals.

246. Betapace AF *(sotalol hydrochloride) package insert*. 2003, Montville, NJ, Bayer Healthcare Pharmaceuticals.

247. Touboul P, Atallah G, Kirkorian G, Lamaud M, Moleur P. Clinical electrophysiology of intravenous sotalol, a beta-blocking drug with class III antiarrhythmic properties. *Am Heart J* 1984;107(5 Pt 1):888-895.

248. Wang T, Bergstrand RH, Thompson KA, et al. Concentration-dependent pharmacologic properties of sotalol. *Am J Cardiol* 1986;57(13):1160-1165.

249. Barbey JT, Sale ME, Woosley RL, et al. Pharmacokinetic, pharmacodynamic, and safety evaluation of an accelerated dose titration regimen of sotalol in healthy middle-aged subjects. *Clin Pharmacol Ther* 1999;66(1):91-99.

250. Wanless RS, Anderson K, Joy M, Joseph SP. Multicenter comparative study of the efficacy and safety of sotalol in the prophylactic treatment of patients with paroxysmal supraventricular tachyarrhythmias. *Am Heart J* 1997;133:441-446.

251. Ho DS, Zecchin RP, Richards DA, Uther JB, Ross DL. Double-blind trial of lignocaine versus sotalol for acute termination of spontaneous sustained ventricular tachycardia. *Lancet* 1994;344:18-23.

252. Ho DSW, Zecchin RP, Cooper MJ, et al. Rapid intravenous infusion of d-1 sotalol: time to onset of effects on ventricular refractoriness and safety. *Eur Heart J* 1995; 16:81-86.

253. Leak D, Eydt JN. Control of refractory cardiac arrhythmias with amiodarone. *Arch Intern Med* 1979;139(4):425-428.

254. Podrid PJ, Lown B. Amiodarone therapy in symptomatic, sustained refractory atrial and ventricular tachyarrhythmias. *Am Heart J* 1981;101(4):374-379.

255. Singh SN, Fletcher RD, Fisher S, et al. Veterans Affairs congestive heart failure antiarrhythmic trial. CHF STAT Investigators. *Am J Cardiol* 1993;72(16):99F-102F.

256. Crystal E, Kahn S, Roberts R, et al. Long-term amiodarone therapy and the risk of complications after cardiac surgery: results from the Canadian Amiodarone Myocardial Infarction Arrhythmia Trial (CAMIAT). *J Thorac Cardiovasc Surg* 2003;125(3):633-637.

257. Milliez P, Leenhardt A, Maisonblanche P, et al; EMIAT Investigators. Usefulness of ventricular repolarization dynamicity in predicting arrhythmic deaths in patients with ischemic cardiomyopathy (from the European Myocardial Infarct Amiodarone Trial). *Am J Cardiol* 2005;95(7):821-826.

258. Lafuente-Lafuente C, Mouly S, Longás-Tejero MA, Mahé I, Bergmann JF. Antiarrhythmic drugs for maintaining sinus rhythm after cardioversion of atrial fibrillation: a systematic review of randomized controlled trials. *Arch Intern Med* 2006;166(7):719-728.

259. Lafuente-Lafuente C, Mouly S, Longas-Tejero MA, Bergmann JF. Antiarrhythmics for maintaining sinus rhythm after cardioversion of atrial fibrillation. *Cochrane Database Syst Rev* 2007;(4):CD005049.

260. Piccini JP, Berger JS, O'Connor CM. Amiodarone for the prevention of sudden cardiac death: a meta-analysis of randomized controlled trials. *Eur Heart J* 2009;30(10):1245-1253.

261. Doyle JF, Ho KM. Benefits and risks of long-term amiodarone therapy for persistent atrial fibrillation: a meta-analysis. *Mayo Clin Proc* 2009;84(3):234-242.

262. The Antiarrhythmics versus Implantable Defibrillators (AVID) Investigators. A comparison of antiarrhythmic-drug therapy with implantable defibrillators in patients resuscitated from near-fatal ventricular arrhythmias. *N Engl J Med* 1997;337(22):1576-1583.

263. Scheinman MM, Levine JH, Cannom DS, et al; Intravenous Amiodarone Multicenter Investigators Group. Dose-ranging study of intravenous amiodarone in patients with life-threatening ventricular tachyarrhythmias. *Circulation* 1995;92(11):3264-3272.

264. Kowey PR, Levine JH, Herre JM, et al; Intravenous Amiodarone Multicenter Investigators Group. Randomized, double-blind comparison of intravenous amiodarone and bretylium in the treatment of patients with recurrent, hemodynamically destabilizing ventricular tachycardia or fibrillation. *Circulation* 1995;92(11):3255-3263.

265. Daoud EG, Strickberger SA, Man KC, et al. Preoperative amiodarone as prophylaxis against atrial fibrillation after heart surgery. *N Engl J Med* 1997;337(25):1785-1791.

266. Yabek SM, Kato R, Singh BN. Effects of amiodarone and its metabolite, desethylamiodarone, on the electrophysiologic properties of isolated cardiac muscle. *J Cardiovasc Pharmacol* 1986;8(1):197-207.

267. Ikeda N, Nademanee K, Kannan R, Singh BN. Electrophysiologic effects of amiodarone: experimental and clinical observation relative to serum and tissue drug concentrations. *Am Heart J* 1984;108(4 Pt 1):890-898.

268. Kato R, Venkatesh N, Kamiya K, et al. Electrophysiologic effects of desethylamiodarone, an active metabolite of amiodarone: comparison with amiodarone during chronic administration in rabbits. *Am Heart J* 1988;115(2):351-359.

269. Veltri EP, Reid PR, Platia EV, Griffith LS. Results of late programmed electrical stimulation and long-term electrophysiologic effects of amiodarone therapy in patients with refractory ventricular tachycardia. *Am J Cardiol* 1985;55(4):375-379.

270. Hohnloser SH, Klingenheben T, Singh BN. Amiodarone-associated proarrhythmic effects: a review with special reference to torsade de pointes tachycardia. *Ann Intern Med* 1994;121(7):529-535.

271. Kodama I, Kamiya K, Toyama J. Cellular electropharmacology of amiodarone. *Cardiovasc Res* 1997;35(1):13-29.

272. van Beeren HC, Bakker O, Wiersinga WM. Structure-function relationship of the inhibition of the 3,5,3'-triiodothyronine binding to the alpha1- and beta1-thyroid hormone receptor by amiodarone analogs. *Endocrinology* 1996;137(7):2807-2814.

273. Kowey PR, Marinchak RA, Rials SJ, Filart RA. Intravenous amiodarone. *J Am Coll Cardiol* 1997;29(6):1190-1198.

274. Cohen-Armon M, Schreiber G, Sokolovsky M. Interaction of the antiarrhythmic drug amiodarone with the muscarinic receptor in rat heart and brain. *Cardiovasc Pharmacol* 1984;6(6):1148-1155.

275. Pourbaix S, Berger Y, Desager JP, Pacco M, Harvengt C. Absolute bioavailability of amiodarone in normal subjects. *Clin Pharmacol Ther* 1985;37(2):118-123.

276. Libersa CC, Brique SA, Motte KB, et al. Dramatic inhibition of amiodarone metabolism induced by grapefruit juice. *Br J Clin Pharmacol* 2000;49(4):373-378.

277. Ohyama K, Nakajima M, Nakamura S, et al. A significant role of human cytochrome P450 2C8 in amiodarone N-deethylation: an approach to predict the contribution with relative activity factor. *Drug Metab Dispos* 2000;28(11):1303-1310.

278. Adams PC, Holt DW, Storey GC, et al. Amiodarone and its desethyl metabolite: tissue distribution and morphologic changes during long-term therapy. *Circulation* 1985; 72(5):1064-1075.

279. Nattel S, Davies M, Quantz M. The antiarrhythmic efficacy of amiodarone and desethylamiodarone, alone and in combination, in dogs with acute myocardial infarction. *Circulation* 1988;77(1):200-208.

280. Holt DW, Tucker GT, Jackson PR, McKenna WJ. Amiodarone pharmacokinetics. *Br J Clin Pract Suppl* 1986;44:109-114.

281. Plomp TA, van Rossum JM, Robles de Medina EO, van Lier T, Maes RA. Pharmacokinetics and body distribution of amiodarone in man. *Arzneimittelforschung* 1984;34(4):513-520.

282. Siddoway LA, McAllister CB, Wilkinson GR, Roden DM, Woosley RL. Amiodarone dosing: a proposal based on its pharmacokinetics. *Am Heart J* 1983;106(4 Pt 2):951-956.

283. Singh SN, Fletcher RD, Fisher SG, et al. Amiodarone in patients with congestive heart failure and asymptomatic ventricular arrhythmia. Survival Trial of Antiarrhythmic Therapy in Congestive Heart Failure. *N Engl J Med* 1995;333(2):77-82.

284. Cairns JA, Connolly SJ, Gent M, Roberts R. Post-myocardial infarction mortality in patients with ventricular premature depolarizations. Canadian Amiodarone Myocardial Infarction Arrhythmia Trial Pilot Study. *Circulation* 1991;84(2):550-557.

285. Escoubet B, Coumel P, Poirier JM, et al. Suppression of arrhythmias within hours after a single oral dose of amiodarone and relation to plasma and myocardial concentrations. *Am J Cardiol* 1985;55(6):696-702.

286. Mostow ND, Vrobel TR, Noon D, Rakita L. Rapid suppression of complex ventricular arrhythmias with high-dose oral amiodarone. *Circulation* 1986;73(6):1231-1238.

287. Greenberg ML, Lerman BB, Shipe JR, Kaiser DL, DiMarco JP. Relation between amiodarone and desethylamiodarone plasma concentrations and electrophysiologic effects, efficacy and toxicity. *J Am Coll Cardiol* 1987;9(5):1148-1155.

288. Figa FH, Gow RM, Hamilton RM, Freedom RM. Clinical efficacy and safety of intravenous Amiodarone in infants and children. *Am J Cardiol* 1994;74(6):573-577.

289. Singh BN. Amiodarone: the expanding antiarrhythmic role and how to follow a patient on chronic therapy. *Clin Cardiol* 1997;20(7):608-618.

290. Lafuente-Lafuente C, Alvarez JC, Leenhardt A, et al. Amiodarone concentrations in plasma and fat tissue during chronic treatment and related toxicity. *Br J Clin Pharmacol* 2009;67(5):511-519.

291. Martin WJ 2nd, Rosenow EC 3rd. Amiodarone pulmonary toxicity: recognition and pathogenesis (Part I). *Chest* 1988;93(5):1067-1075.

292. Martin WJ 2nd, Rosenow EC 3rd. Amiodarone pulmonary toxicity: recognition and pathogenesis (Part 2). *Chest* 1988;93(6):1242-1248.

293. Harjai KJ, Licata AA. Effects of amiodarone on thyroid function. *Ann Intern Med* 1997;126(1):63-73.

294. Pollak PT, Sharma AD, Carruthers SG. Correlation of amiodarone dosage, heart rate, QT interval and corneal microdeposits with serum amiodarone and desethylamiodarone concentrations. *Am J Cardiol* 1989;64(18):1138-1143.

295. Granstein RD, Sober AJ. Drug- and heavy metal–induced hyperpigmentation. *J Am Acad Dermatol* 1981;5(1):1-18.

296. Lewis JH, Ranard RC, Caruso A, et al. Amiodarone hepatotoxicity: prevalence and clinicopathologic correlations among 104 patients. *Hepatology* 1989;9(5):679-685.

297. Simon JB, Manley PN, Brien JF, Armstrong PW. Amiodarone hepatotoxicity simulating alcoholic liver disease. *N Engl J Med* 1984;311(3):167-172.

298. Larrey D, Tinel M, Letteron P, et al. Formation of an inactive cytochrome P-450Fe(II)-metabolite complex after administration of amiodarone in rats, mice and hamsters. *Biochem Pharmacol* 1986;35(13):2213-2220.

299. Almog S, Shafran N, Halkin H, et al. Mechanism of warfarin potentiation by amiodarone: dose- and concentration-dependent inhibition of warfarin elimination. *Eur J Clin Pharmacol* 1985;28(3):257-261.

300. Marcus FI. Drug interactions with amiodarone. *Am Heart J* 1983;106(4 Pt 2):924-930.

301. Ha HR, Bigler L, Wendt B, Maggiorini M, Follath F. Identification and quantitation of novel metabolites of amiodarone in plasma of treated patients. *Eur J Pharm Sci* 2005;24(4):271-279.

302. Ha HR, Bigler L, Binder M, et al. Metabolism of amiodarone (part I): identification of a new hydroxylated metabolite of amiodarone. *Drug Metab Dispos* 2001;29(2):152-158.

303. Yamreudeewong W, DeBisschop M, Martin LG, Lower DL. Potentially significant drug interactions of class III antiarrhythmic drugs. *Drug Saf* 2003;26(6):421-438.

304. Fenster PE, White NW Jr, Hanson CD. Pharmacokinetic evaluation of the digoxin-amiodarone interaction. *J Am Coll Cardiol* 1985;5(1):108-112.

305. Corvert (ibutilide) package insert. 2002, Kalamazoo, Pharmacia and Upjohn Company.

306. VanderLugt JT, Mattioni T, Denker S, et al. Efficacy and safety of ibutilide fumarate for the conversion of atrial arrhythmias after cardiac surgery. *Circulation* 1999;100(4):369-375.

307. Glatter KA, Dorostkar PC, Yang Y, et al. Electrophysiological effects of ibutilide in patients with accessory pathways. *Circulation* 2001;104(16):1933-1939.

308. Varriale P, Sedighi A, Mirzaietehrane M. Ibutilide for termination of atrial fibrillation in the Wolff-Parkinson-White syndrome. *Pacing Clin Electrophysiol* 1999;22(8):1267-1269.

309. Lee KS, Tsai TD, Lee EW. Membrane activity of class III antiarrhythmic compounds: a comparison between ibutilide, d-sotalol, E-4031, sematilide and dofetilide. *Eur J Pharmacol* 1993;234(1):43-53.

310. Yang T, Snyders DJ, Roden DM. Ibutilide, a methanesulfonanilide antiarrhythmic, is a potent blocker of the rapidly activating delayed rectifier K+ current (IKr) in AT-1 cells.

311. Amin NB, Borzak S, Housholder S, Tisdale JE. Sinus bradycardia and multiple episodes of sinus arrest following administration of ibutilide. *Heart* 1998;79(6):628-629.

312. Neumayr G, Gatterer H, Erne B. Ibutilide and sinus arrest. *Herz* 2007;32(4):342.

313. Franz M, Geppert A, Kain R, Hörl WH, Pohanka E. Acute renal failure after ibutilide. *Lancet* 1999;353(9151):467.

314. Pedersen OD, Bagger H, Keller N, et al. Efficacy of dofetilide in the treatment of atrial fibrillation-flutter in patients with reduced left ventricular function: a Danish investigations of arrhythmia and mortality on dofetilide (DiAMOND) substudy. *Circulation* 2001;104(3):292-296.

315. Sedgwick ML, Dalrymple I, Rae AP, Cobbe SM. Effects of the new class III antiarrhythmic drug dofetilide on the atrial and ventricular intracardiac monophasic action potential in patients with angina pectoris. *Eur Heart J* 1995;16(11):1641-1646.

316. Walker DK, Alabaster CT, Congrave GS, et al. Significance of metabolism in the disposition and action of the antidysrhythmic drug, dofetilide. In vitro studies and correlation with in vivo data. *Drug Metab Dispos* 1996;24(4):447-455.

317. Lenz TL, Hilleman DE. Dofetilide, a new class III antiarrhythmic agent. *Pharmacotherapy* 2000;20(7):776-786.

318. DiMarco JP, Sellers TD, Lerman BB, et al. Diagnostic and therapeutic use of adenosine in patients with supraventricular tachyarrhythmias. *J Am Coll Cardiol* 1985;6(2):417-425.

319. Lerman BB, Belardinelli L. Cardiac electrophysiology of adenosine: basic and clinical concepts. *Circulation* 1991;83(5):1499-1509.

320. Ellenbogen KA, Thames MD, DiMarco JP, Sheehan H, Lerman BB. Electrophysiological effects of adenosine in the transplanted human heart: evidence of supersensitivity. *Circulation* 1990;81(3):821-828.

321. Lerman BB, Wesley RC, Belardinelli L. Electrophysiologic effects of dipyridamole on atrioventricular nodal conduction and supraventricular tachycardia: role of endogenous adenosine. *Circulation* 1989;80(6):1536-1543.

322. Adenocard (adenosine) package insert. 2012, Deerfield, IL, Astellas Pharma US.

323. Le Heuzey JY, De Ferrari GM, Radzik D, et al. A short-term, randomized, double-blind, parallel-group study to evaluate the efficacy and safety of dronedarone versus amiodarone in patients with persistent atrial fibrillation: the DIONYSOS study. *J Cardiovasc Electrophysiol* 2010;21(6):597-605.

324. Multaq (dronedarone) package insert. Bridgewater, NJ, 2012, Sanofi-Aventis.

325. Køber L, Torp-Pedersen C, McMurray JJ, et al. Increased mortality after dronedarone therapy for severe heart failure. *N Engl J Med* 2008;358(6):2678-2687.

326. Singh BN, Connolly SJ, Crijns HJ, et al. Dronedarone for maintenance of sinus rhythm in atrial fibrillation or flutter. *N Engl J Med* 2007;357:987-999.

327. Hohnloser SH, Crijns H, van Eickels M, et al. Effect of dronedarone on cardiovascular events in atrial fibrillation. *N Engl J Med* 2009;360:668-678.

328. Wadhani N, Sarma J, Singh BN, et al. Dose-dependent effects of oral dronedarone on the circadian variation of RR and QT intervals in healthy subjects: implications for antiarrhythmic actions. *J Card Pharmacol Ther* 2006;11(3):184-190.

329. Wegener FT, Ehrlich JR, Hohnloser SH, et al. Dronedarone: an emerging agent with rhythm- and rate-controlling effects. *J Cardiovasc Electrophysiol* 2006;17(Suppl 2):S17-S20.

330. Van Beeren HC, Jong WC, Kaptein E, et al. Dronedarone acts as a selective inhibitor of 3,5,3′-triiodothyronine binding to thyroid hormone receptor-alpha: in vitro and in vivo evidence. *Endocrinology* 2003;144(2):552-558.

331. Han TS, Williams GR, Vanderpump MJ. Benzofuran derivatives and the thyroid. *Clin Endocrinol* 2009;70:2-13.

332. Patel C, Yan GX, Kowey PR. New drugs and technology: Dronedarone. *Circulation* 2009;120:636-644.

333. Touboul P, Brugada J, Capucci A, et al. Dronedarone for prevention of atrial fibrillation: a dose-ranging study. *Eur Heart J* 2003;24(16):1481-1487.

334. Singh BN, EURIDIS/ADONIS Study Investigators. Abstract 3699: Dronedarone is effective in maintaining sinus rhythm in atrial fibrillation patients in whom previous antiarrhythmic drug therapy has failed. *Circulation* 2006;114: II_790.

335. Page RL, Connolly SJ, Crijns HJ, et al; ATHENA Investigators. Rhythm- and rate-controlling effects of dronedarone in patients with atrial fibrillation (from the ATHENA Trial). *Am J Cardiol* 2011;107(7):1019-1022.

336. Tschuppert Y, Buclin T, Rothuizen LE, et al. Effect of dronedarone on renal function in healthy subjects. *Br J Clin Pharmacol* 2007;64(6):785-791.

337. FDA Drug Safety Communication. Severe liver injury associated with the use of dronedarone (marketed as Multaq). Accessed 2011 Jan 14 at www.fda.gov/Drugs/DrugSafety/ucm240011.htm.

338. Wolbrette D, Gonzalez M, Samii S, et al. Dronedarone for the treatment of atrial fibrillation and atrial flutter: approval and efficacy. *Vasc Health Risk Manag* 2010;6:517-523.

339. Dorian P. Clinical pharmacology of dronedarone: implications for the therapy of atrial fibrillation. *J Cardiovasc Pharmacol Ther* 2010;15(4 Suppl):15S-18S.

CHAPTER 19

Pharmacologic Management of Supraventricular Tachycardias

John P. DiMarco, J. Michael Mangrum, and John D. Ferguson

PHARMACOLOGY OF SUPRAVENTRICULAR
TACHYCARDIAS, 365

EVALUATION OF THERAPY, 365

PAROXYSMAL SUPRAVENTRICULAR
TACHYCARDIA, 366

MECHANISMS OF PAROXYSMAL SUPRAVENTRICULAR
TACHYCARDIA, 366

Management of Acute Episodes of Paroxysmal Supraventricular
Tachycardia, 367
Long-Term Therapy of Premature Supraventricular
Tachycardia, 369
Long-Term Pharmacologic Therapy, 369

ATRIAL FLUTTER, 369

Short-Term Management of Atrial Flutter, 370
Long-Term Management of Atrial Flutter, 370
Multifocal Atrial Tachycardia, 370
Inappropriate Sinus Tachycardia, 371

JUNCTIONAL ECTOPIC TACHYCARDIA, 371

REFERENCES, 371

Electrophysiologic study with catheter ablation is now the primary mode of therapy for most forms of recurrent supraventricular tachycardia. However, pharmacologic therapy for acute episodes and for the long-term management of patients for whom electrophysiologic studies and ablation are not available or appropriate is still an important clinical consideration. The proper use of drugs in these patients requires an understanding of multiple factors: the electrophysiologic mechanism responsible for the arrhythmia, the functional roles of the anatomic pathways involved, the pharmacology of the target tissues, and the properties of the drugs themselves.

Drugs may be used both as immediate therapy to terminate episodes of tachycardia or for long-term prophylactic therapy to maintain sinus rhythm long term. The most common supraventricular tachycardias (SVTs) involve reentry over a single circuit, and a very short duration of drug effect may be all that is necessary to break a single tachycardia episode. Prophylaxis of recurrent arrhythmias requires a different strategy than that for termination. In reentrant arrhythmias, complete and permanent conduction block in the circuits involved is achievable with drug therapy only rarely, and if the tissue is required for normal conduction, fixed block will not be desirable. Effective strategies may include facilitation of early termination via rate-related block in the atrioventricular (AV) node, drug-induced changes in conduction times, or production of block only in abnormal conduction pathways. Long-term suppression of automatic arrhythmias often requires approaches that eliminate or modify precipitating stimuli or that suppress or eliminate selectively the responsible anatomic focus. This chapter deals primarily with therapy for paroxysmal supraventricular tachycardia (PSVT) and atrial flutter.

Pharmacology of Supraventricular Tachycardias

Drug therapy of supraventricular arrhythmias is typically based on the concept of a "vulnerable target" at which drug treatment may be directed.[1] The sinus node and the AV node have calcium-mediated action potentials and are more sensitive to direct effects of calcium channel blockers (CCBs) and adenosine and indirect, autonomically mediated effects of adenosine, β-adrenergic blockers, or cardiac glycosides. The primary pacemaker current in the sinus node—the "funny current," or I_f—is a new target for arrhythmias originating in the sinus node.[2] Atrial muscle conduction is depressed by sodium channel blockers, and refractory periods are prolonged by potassium channel blockers. Enhanced or abnormal automaticity in atrial muscle may be due to many mechanisms; therefore drugs that block adenosine or β-adrenergic receptors, and calcium, sodium, and potassium channels may all be effective in selected cases. Most accessory pathways have electrophysiologic properties similar to those of atrial or ventricular muscle. Conduction and refractory periods of accessory pathways are most susceptible to sodium and potassium channel blockers, but some pathways sensitive to adenosine have been described. Although there are limitations to the Vaughan Williams classification of antiarrhythmic drugs,[3] it may still be useful as a general guide for the selection of drug therapy (Table 19-1).

Evaluation of Therapy

Several types of studies have been used to establish the effectiveness of drug therapy in patients with supraventricular arrhythmias. The most reliable studies are randomized trials that compare the study drug with either a placebo control or a second active agent. The range of doses studied during the course of drug evaluation should include both minimally and maximally effective doses. When two agents are compared, it is important that each drug be tested at a dose expected to produce a maximal or near-maximal response.

For acute termination of an episode of tachycardia, the efficacy of a drug is relatively easy to evaluate. Patients who come to medical attention with an appropriate arrhythmia are entered into the trial; both spontaneous and stimulation-induced episodes of arrhythmia may be included. After an observation period to establish stability of the tachycardia, the patient is administered one or more doses of the drug under study or the active or inactive control. Total response is determined by the proportion of episodes converted within a specified period. The maintenance of normal rhythm after conversion for some prespecified time can serve as a secondary endpoint.

The prevention of arrhythmia induction in an electrophysiologic study during drug therapy is rarely used as an endpoint in patients with supraventricular arrhythmias for several reasons. First, radio-frequency ablation (RFA) has become the primary therapy for many supraventricular arrhythmias owing to its high success and low complication rates. The administration of a drug that blocks conduction in the target tissue during the study might interfere with the primary goal of the procedure. Second, the role of autonomic nervous system influences on arrhythmia initiation and maintenance may be profound, and in many cases, changes in autonomic tone can override drug effects.

Most of the common forms of PSVT and many cases of atrial flutter are now treated with catheter ablation as a first option when that modality is available; therefore only limited contemporary data are available about long-term drug therapy for common varieties of PSVT and atrial flutter. When placebo-controlled studies have been performed, they typically have used endpoints such as the total number of episodes and the time to first recurrence.[4,5]

TABLE 19-1   Drug Actions in Supraventricular Arrhythmias

CLASS AND AGENTS	Electrocardiography				Electrophysiology		
	PR	QRS	QTC	JTC	AV	AP	AVN
Class Ia: Na⁺ channel blockers (quinidine, procainamide, disopyramide)	NC	(↑)	↑	↑	ERP ↑ COND ↓	ERP ↑ COND ↓	ERP NC COND NC
Class Ic: Na⁺ channel blockers (flecainide, propafenone, moricizine)	↑	↑↑	(↑)	NC	ERP ↑ COND ↓↓	ERP ↑ COND ↓↓	ERP ↑ COND ↓
Class II: β-Adrenergic blockers (many preparations)	↑	NC	NC	NC	ERP NC COND NC	ERP NC COND NC	ERP ↑ COND ↓
Class III: K⁺ channel blockers (amiodarone, sotalol, dofetilide)*	↑	NC	↑↑	↑↑	ERP (↑) COND ↑	ERP ↑ COND ↑	ERP ↑ COND ↓
Class IV: Ca²⁺ channel blockers (verapamil, diltiazem)	↑	NC	NC	NC	ERP NC COND NC	ERP NC COND NC	ERP ↑↑ COND ↓↓
Adenosine	↑	NC	NC	NC	ERP (A) ↓ ERP (V) NC COND NC	ERP ↓ COND ↑	ERP ↑↑ COND ↓↓
Digoxin	↑	NC	NC	NC	ERP (A) ↓ ERP (V) NC COND NC	ERP ↓/NC COND ↑/NC	ERP ↑ COND ↑

*Clinically available agents have other actions not related to K⁺ channel blockade.
↓, decreased; ↑, increased; ↑↑, marked increase; ↓↓, marked decrease; parentheses indicate slight effect.
A, atrium; AP, accessory pathway; AVN, atrioventricular node; COND, conduction velocity or capability; ERP, effective refractory period; JTc, corrected JT; NC, no change; QTc, corrected QT; V, ventricle.

Paroxysmal Supraventricular Tachycardia

PSVT is a common arrhythmia with a prevalence of about 2.5 per 1000 adults.[6-10] PSVT in the absence of structural heart disease can manifest at any age, but the first episode commonly occurs between age 12 and 30 years. In most patients, PSVT as a result of atrioventricular nodal reentrant tachycardia (AVNRT) or atrioventricular reentrant tachycardia (AVRT) is not causally associated with structural heart disease, although exceptions exist (e.g., Ebstein's anomaly, familial preexcitation with cardiomyopathy). Atrial tachycardias may occur either in structurally normal or abnormal hearts. In normal patients, the physical examination during PSVT is significant mainly for the rapid heart rate. Prominent jugular venous pulsations, the "frog's neck" finding, which are due to atrial contraction against closed AV valves, are characteristic of AVNRT. The patient's history, physical examination, and ECG constitute an appropriate initial evaluation. Further diagnostic studies are indicated only if signs or symptoms that suggest structural heart disease are present. In patients with incessant tachycardia, the clinician should remember that a tachycardia-induced cardiomyopathy may develop that is completely reversible if the tachycardia is eliminated.

Mechanisms of Paroxysmal Supraventricular Tachycardia

Figure 19-1 illustrates the common forms of PSVT.[6] The AV node sits in the triangle of Koch in the floor of the right atrium. Separate pathways, characterized by their conduction velocities as fast or slow, provide input into the AV node. If these pathways have different refractory periods, reentry using one pathway for anterograde conduction and one for retrograde conduction may occur. The P-wave position during AVNRT depends on the types of pathways used. In the most common form (slow pathway anterograde–fast pathway retrograde) the P wave is either not seen or is visible only in the terminal portion of the QRS (Figure 19-2). If two slow pathways or fast anterograde and slow retrograde pathways form the circuit, the R-P′ interval will either be short or long, respectively. Although uncommon, AV block is possible during AVNRT if the block occurs distal to the turnaround point, where the pathways join.

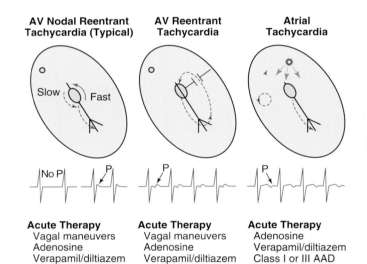

FIGURE 19-1   The common forms of paroxysmal supraventricular tachycardia (PSVT). AV, atrioventricular; AAD, antiarrhythmic drug. (*Modified from Ferguson JD, DiMarco JP. Contemporary management of supraventricular tachycardia. Circulation 2003;107:1096-1099.*)

In AVRT, an extranodal accessory pathway connects the atrium and ventricle. Accessory pathways may exhibit both anterograde and retrograde conduction, or they may show only antegrade (uncommon) or retrograde conduction. In the latter situation, the pathway is called a *concealed pathway*. When the pathway manifests anterograde conduction, ventricular preexcitation with a delta wave will be present on the surface ECG. A diagnosis of Wolff-Parkinson-White syndrome is made if the patient has PSVT. Accessory pathways usually manifest rapid AV conduction with no change in conduction velocity over a range of cycle lengths,

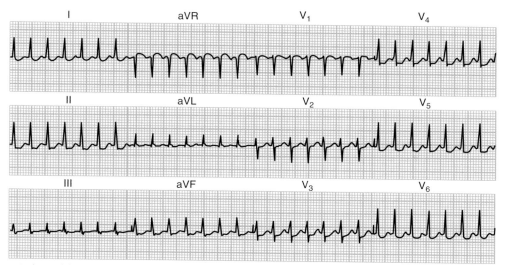

FIGURE 19-2 Atrioventricular nodal reentrant tachycardia. In this patient, the QRS duration is short, and retrograde activity is seen as small, sharp, negative deflection at the end of the QRS in leads II and III. Lead V1 is also a common site for this finding.

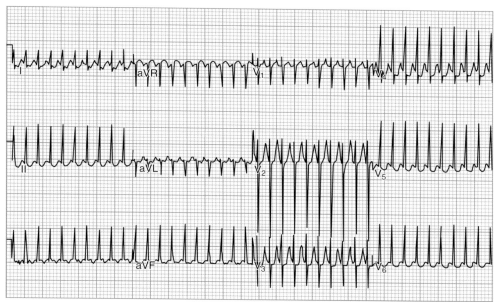

FIGURE 19-3 Orthodromic atrioventricular reentrant tachycardia in a patient with baseline preexcitation. Note that during tachycardia, the delta wave is absent, because the pathway is used for retrograde conduction. The retrograde P wave is seen in the early ST segment.

but a minority of pathways may manifest longer conduction times at all rates. The most common form of AV reentry, termed *orthodromic AVRT*, uses the accessory pathway as the retrograde limb and the AV node–His as the anterograde limb, resulting in a narrow QRS (Figure 19-3). Functional or fixed bundle branch block, a reversal of the circuit, termed *antidromic AVRT*, or the presence of two accessory pathways can lead to a wide QRS complex during PSVT owing to AV reentry. Accessory pathways can also conduct as passive bystanders during AVNRT or atrial tachycardias, but these patterns are less common. In AVRT the ventricle is an obligate part of the circuit; therefore AV block cannot occur.

Atrial tachycardia is the least common form of PSVT in normal individuals but may predominate in patients who have significant atrial scarring, especially those who have undergone earlier atrial surgery. Atrial tachycardias may be due to enhanced or triggered

automaticity or to reentry. Because the AV node and ventricle are not required participants in the arrhythmia, AV block commonly occurs if there is a short atrial cycle length. The P-R and apparent R-P′ intervals depend on the response of the AV conduction system to the atrial rate. P-wave morphology is determined by the site of origin in the atrium. If the site of origin is within or involves the sinus node region, the terms *sinus node reentrant* or *inappropriate sinus tachycardia* are often applied.

Management of Acute Episodes of Paroxysmal Supraventricular Tachycardia

PSVT rarely is so poorly tolerated that it requires immediate termination with electrical cardioversion. Most episodes can be managed with physiologic maneuvers or drugs. The most common

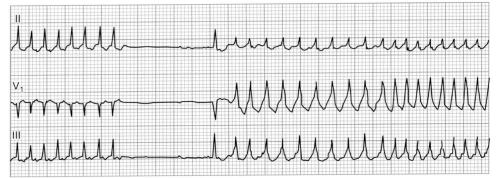

FIGURE 19-4 Adenosine-induced atrial fibrillation. This patient with Wolff-Parkinson-White syndrome came to medical attention with an orthodromic atrioventricular reentrant tachycardia. She received 6 mg adenosine intravenously just before the start of this rhythm strip. The tachycardia is terminated, but then preexcited atrial fibrillation is seen.

types of PSVT require intact one-to-one AV nodal conduction for continuation and are classified as AV nodal–dependent tachycardias. Because the refractory period of the AV node may be modified by vagal maneuvers and by many pharmacologic agents, and because prolongation of AV nodal refractoriness can lead to transient block, AV nodal conduction is the weak link targeted by most short-term therapies.

Many patients learn to terminate acute episodes of PSVT by using vagal maneuvers early during an episode. Valsalva is the most effective technique for adults, but carotid massage may also be effective.[5] Facial immersion is the most reliable method for infants. Vagal maneuvers are less effective once a sympathetic response to PSVT has become established; therefore patients should try them soon after onset.

Oral antiarrhythmic drug tablets are not reliably absorbed during rapid PSVT, but some patients may respond to self-administration of crushed medications. In one small study,[11] a combination of diltiazem (120 mg) plus propranolol (80 mg) was shown to be superior to both placebo and oral flecainide (approximately 3 mg/kg). Hypotension and bradycardia after termination are rare complications of this approach in otherwise healthy individuals.

Adenosine and the nondihydropyridine calcium antagonists, verapamil and diltiazem, are the intravenous (IV) drugs of choice for termination of PSVT.[6-10] Adenosine is an endogenous purine nucleoside that slows AV nodal conduction and results in transient AV nodal block when administered during an episode of PSVT.[12,13] Conduction in rapidly conducting accessory pathways is not affected by adenosine, but pathways with long refractory periods or slow conduction may exhibit block. Exogenous adenosine is cleared extremely rapidly from the circulation by cellular uptake and metabolism with an estimated half-life of less than 5 seconds. Adenosine effect is typically seen 15 to 30 seconds after rapid peripheral infusion as a first-pass phenomenon. Administration via a central line requires dose reduction. The effective dose range in adults is 2.5 to 25 mg. If no upper dosage limit is imposed, at least transient termination of AV node–dependent PSVT can be produced in essentially all patients. The recommended adult dosage is 6 mg followed if needed by a 12-mg dose. In pediatric patients, the dose range is 50 to 250 µg/kg using an upward dose titration. Because of the ultrashort duration of action, cumulative effects of sequential doses are not seen.

Minor side effects of transient dyspnea or chest pain are common with adenosine. Sinus arrest or bradycardia may occur but resolves quickly if appropriate upward dose titration is used. Atrial and ventricular premature beats are frequently seen with PSVT termination. A few patients with adenosine-induced polymorphic ventricular tachycardia (VT) and ventricular fibrillation have been reported.[13-16] The majority of these patients had long baseline QT intervals during tachycardia and had long pauses during adenosine-induced AV block that led to bradycardia-dependent polymorphic VT. Adenosine shortens the atrial

refractory period, and critically timed atrial ectopic beats may induce atrial fibrillation (Figure 19-4). This may be a dangerous situation if the patient has an accessory pathway capable of rapid anterograde conduction, because adenosine may further shorten the effective refractory period of the pathway. Because adenosine is cleared so rapidly, reinitiation of PSVT after initial termination may occur. Repeat administration of the same dose of adenosine or substitution of a CCB is likely to be effective.

Adenosine mediates its effects via a specific cell surface receptor, the A_1 receptor. In some countries, adenosine triphospate (ATP) is used in place of adenosine. Most, if not all, of the effects of ATP in PSVT are produced after it is metabolized to adenosine. Theophylline and other methylxanthines block the A_1 receptor. However, caffeine levels seen after moderate beverage ingestion do not usually interfere with the clinical efficacy of adenosine. Dipyridamole blocks adenosine elimination, thereby potentiating and prolonging its effects. Cardiac transplant recipients are also unusually sensitive to adenosine. If adenosine is chosen in these patients, much lower starting doses (approximately 1 mg) should be selected.

The AV node action potential is calcium channel dependent, and the nondihydropyridine CCBs, verapamil and diltiazem, are highly effective for terminating AV node–dependent PSVT.[7,17,18] The recommended initial dosage of verapamil is 5 mg intravenously over 2 minutes, followed in 5 to 10 minutes by a second 5- to 7.5-mg dose. The recommended initial dosage of diltiazem is 20 mg followed by a second dose of 25 to 35 mg if necessary. PSVT termination should occur within 5 minutes of the end of the infusion, and more than 90% of patients with AV node–dependent PSVT respond to these dosages.

As with adenosine, transient arrhythmias that include atrial and ventricular ectopy, atrial fibrillation, and bradycardia may be seen after PSVT termination with CCBs. Persistent hypotension may occur with CCBs, particularly if the PSVT does not terminate. CCBs are not recommended in infants and neonates with PSVT because of reports of cardiovascular collapse.[19] Extreme bradycardia after PSVT termination may rarely be seen if CCBs are given to a patient who has just received an IV β-adrenergic blocker.

Adenosine and verapamil have been shown to have similar efficacy in several randomized clinical trials.[6,17,18,20] The authors of a meta-analysis by the Cochrane Group covering eight trials that included 577 patients found no major differences between adenosine and CCBs.[20] Most PSVT patients can be acutely managed with either (Table 19-2). To minimize the potential for adverse effects, adenosine should be selected for patients with severe hypotension or heart failure, for infants and neonates, and for those at risk for severe bradycardia. Verapamil and diltiazem should be chosen for patients with poor venous access, for patients with bronchospasm, and for those receiving agents that interfere with adenosine action or metabolism. Patients with more than a single recurrent episode may do better if they are switched to a CCB rather than receiving repeated bolus injections of adenosine.

AV node–dependent PSVT can manifest with a wide QRS complex in patients with fixed or functional aberration or when an accessory pathway is used for anterograde conduction. However, most wide-complex tachycardias are due to mechanisms that may worsen after IV administration of adenosine and CCBs. Unless there is strong evidence that a wide QRS tachycardia is AV node dependent, test doses of adenosine, verapamil, or diltiazem should be discouraged.

Data are limited on the acute pharmacologic therapy of atrial tachycardias.[6,21] Automatic or triggered atrial tachycardias and those as a result of sinus node reentry are likely to terminate with adenosine, verapamil, diltiazem, or β-adrenergic blockers. Tachycardias caused by scar-related atrial reentry are more likely to manifest AV block with an unchanged atrial cycle length after administration of these agents.

Long-Term Therapy of Premature Supraventricular Tachycardia

Patients with well-tolerated episodes of PSVT that either always terminate spontaneously or can be broken quickly and reliably by the patient do not require long-term prophylactic therapy. Rarely, patients may medicate themselves only for acute episodes as mentioned earlier. For other PSVT patients, catheter ablation is preferred, but drug therapy may be appropriate for some patients (Figure 19-5). Current guidelines consider catheter ablation to be the treatment of choice for patients with more than minimal symptoms.[6,7] Previously asymptomatic patients with preexcitation on ECG may also benefit from ablation, if they have inducible PSVT at electrophysiologic study[22] or other clinical or electrophysiologic findings that suggest increased risk with conservative management. A suggested treatment algorithm is shown in Figure 19-5.

Long-Term Pharmacologic Therapy

For AV node–dependent PSVT, CCBs and β-adrenergic blockers will improve but rarely totally eliminate symptoms in 60% to 80% of patients.[6] Flecainide (50 to 100 mg twice daily) and propafenone (150 to 300 mg twice daily) have effects on both the AV node and the accessory pathways and will also reduce episode frequency.[23,24] These agents can be used safely if patients with ischemic heart disease and/or congestive heart failure are excluded from therapy.[25] Sotalol (80 to 320 mg daily in divided doses), dofetilide (125 to 500 μg twice daily), and amiodarone (100 to 200 mg daily) should be considered second-line agents.[6] Because sympathetic stimulation can antagonize the effects of many antiarrhythmic agents, concomitant therapy with a β-adrenergic blocker may improve clinical efficacy.

Pharmacologic treatment strategies for atrial tachycardias have not been well evaluated in controlled clinical trials. Depending on the mechanism responsible for the arrhythmia, β-adrenergic blockers, CCBs, and class I or class III antiarrhythmic drugs may reduce or eliminate symptoms. Scar-related atrial tachycardias, particularly those associated with earlier surgery for congenital heart disease, may be particularly difficult to control with ablation techniques or drug therapy. It is often necessary to use AV nodal blocking agents to control ventricular rates during ongoing tachycardia in these patients.

Atrial Flutter

Clinical investigations during the last 20 years in patients with atrial flutter have greatly expanded our understanding of this relatively common arrhythmia.[6,26] In atrial flutter, the ECG will show an organized atrial rhythm at a rate of approximately 300 ± 50 beats/min. Patients with atrial flutter share many clinical and electrophysiologic characteristics with patients with atrial fibrillation, and many patients will manifest both arrhythmias. In most cases, atrial flutter is due to reentry over a large, well-defined circuit within the atria. In typical atrial flutter, a counterclockwise circuit is present in the right atrium, with the cavotricuspid isthmus forming a critical portion that is susceptible to ablation. In classic or typical atrial flutter, this circuit produces an ECG pattern with negative flutter waves in the inferior leads and a positive atrial deflection in lead V_1. The same isthmus-dependent circuit can also be used in a clockwise fashion with reversal of these ECG findings. Because the atrial cycle length in atrial flutter is less than the refractory period of the AV node, 2:1 or greater block in the AV node is most commonly seen, but 1:1 conduction may be seen if adrenergic tone is high or if the flutter cycle length is relatively slow. Other ECG patterns in regular rhythms with rates consistent with atrial flutter may also be observed. Some atrial flutters, although still isthmus dependent, will involve circulation around the inferior vena cava from slow conduction across the *crista terminalis*, a pattern described as "lower-loop reentry."[6,26-28] If the reentry circuit does not involve the cavotricuspid isthmus, the patient is said to have *atypical flutter*, and a variety of ECG patterns may occur, some of which can mimic the patterns seen in typical atrial flutter. Atypical flutters can arise in either atria. Many are scar related, from either catheter ablation or surgical procedures (Figure 19-6). Focal tachycardias as a result of reconnection of pulmonary veins and mitral annular flutter circuits are common problems after atrial fibrillation ablation.[29,30]

TABLE 19-2	Short-Term Therapy for Paroxysmal Supraventricular Tachycardia	
ADENOSINE PREFERRED	**NEUTRAL**	**CALCIUM BLOCKER PREFERRED**
Neonates	Routine PSVT	Poor IV access
Hypotension	Central line*	Dipyridamole*
Uncertain diagnosis		Transplant*
Prior IV β-blocker		Theophylline

*Dose reduction for adenosine is required.
IV, intravenous; PSVT, paroxysmal supraventricular tachycardia.

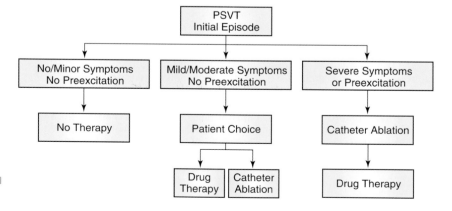

FIGURE 19-5 Algorithm for the management of paroxysmal supraventricular tachycardia (PSVT).

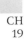

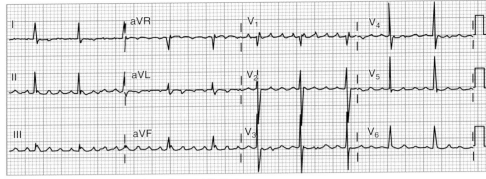

FIGURE 19-6 Left atrial tachycardia after a catheter ablation for atrial fibrillation.

Atrial flutter can be associated with a wide range of symptoms that are largely dependent on ventricular rate. Some patients may be asymptomatic despite a ventricular rate of 150 beats/min and 2:1 AV block. Patients with advanced forms of heart disease may not tolerate atrial flutter, even when ventricular rates can be controlled.

Short-Term Management of Atrial Flutter

Management of the patient who presents with atrial flutter may involve termination of the arrhythmia, control of ventricular rate, and prevention of thromboembolism. Although data that specifically relate to patients with atrial flutter are limited, guidelines for the prevention of embolic events in patients with atrial flutter are the same as those for patients with atrial fibrillation.

As with other arrhythmias, the immediate management strategy for patients with atrial flutter will depend on the clinical situation, the patient's symptoms, and the patient's hemodynamic status. Cardioversion with a direct current shock is highly effective in atrial flutter but is rarely required as an urgent intervention and does not protect against recurrence. Rapid atrial pacing is also quite effective. Stable rate control in atrial flutter is often difficult to achieve because concealed conduction in the AV node is not prominent at the atrial cycle lengths seen in atrial flutter. IV diltiazem and verapamil may slow the ventricular rate, but their effects are often transient, and hypotension may complicate therapy.[31-33] IV β-adrenergic blockers and amiodarone may also be used for rate control in critically ill patients. Selected patients with conduction-system disease may achieve stable ventricular rates during drug therapy for atrial flutter, but most patients will require termination of the arrhythmia.

Although several antiarrhythmic drugs have been reported to be effective for terminating atrial flutter, the response rates in clinical practice are often disappointing (see Chapter 18). Class III drugs have been the most successful, presumably because they slow conduction velocity and prevent wavelength shortening.[34] IV ibutilide (1 to 2 mg) is the agent that has been studied most thoroughly. In placebo-controlled trials, ibutilide has shown efficacy rates of 38% to 76%,[35,36] and it has been shown to be superior to both procainamide and sotalol for terminating atrial flutter.[6,35,36] The major problem with ibutilide is the risk of proarrhythmia; 1% to 2% of patients in clinical trials of ibutilide developed QT prolongation and sustained polymorphic ventricular tachycardia. Nonsustained ventricular tachycardia episodes after ibutilide occur with an incidence of 1.8% to 6.7%. Assessment of serum potassium levels and the QT interval are important steps to take before ibutilide administration. Pretreatment with IV magnesium before ibutilide infusion would be a reasonable precaution, but only limited data about the efficacy of this approach are available.[37,38] IV dofetilide is also quite effective for conversion of atrial flutter, but dofetilide is available now only in an oral formulation.[38,39] Oral administration of dofetilide is effective at converting atrial flutter but has a delayed onset of effect.[39,40] The class IC agents, propafenone and flecainide, have limited efficacy in atrial flutter, and should they slow the atrial cycle length, they may allow 1:1 AV conduction with a paradoxical increase in ventricular rate.[41]

Long-Term Management of Atrial Flutter

Atrial flutter is less commonly recurrent or persistent compared with atrial fibrillation. As a result, few studies are available that specifically focus on the long-term efficacy of drug therapy for atrial flutter. Long-term rate control may be an option in selected patients who have intrinsic conduction system disease. In most others, concealed conduction in the AV node is not prominent owing to the regularity of the atrial cycle length and, as a result, effective long-term rate control is usually very difficult to maintain. The approach to prophylactic drug therapy in atrial flutter is similar to that used in patients with atrial fibrillation (see Chapter 18). If class Ia, class Ic, or class III drugs are used, AV nodal blocking agents are usually also prescribed to protect against one-to-one conduction, should atrial flutter recur with a cycle length prolonged by the drug.

As discussed in Chapter 21, catheter ablation of isthmus-dependent atrial flutter is often the therapy of choice for many patients. In this procedure, a linear ablation line is drawn from the tricuspid valve isthmus to the inferior vena cava that is highly (>90%) successful in the short term. Although early recurrence rates were found to be high when this technique was first used, this was probably because of incomplete lesions that failed to produce complete bidirectional block in the cavotricuspid isthmus. Current techniques have reduced the incidence of recurrence of typical atrial flutter after the initial ablation procedure. However, many patients, particularly those who have associated structural heart disease, will remain at risk for developing atrial fibrillation despite a previously successful ablation for atrial flutter.[42,43]

Multifocal Atrial Tachycardia

Multifocal atrial tachycardia is characterized by three or more distinct P-wave morphologies at an irregular rate that ranges from 110 to 180 beats/min. It is usually associated with a severe underlying illness, often respiratory insufficiency or methylxanthine toxicity. Rate control is difficult, because there is little concealed conduction in the AV node, and the patient's background sympathetic tone is often high. β-Adrenergic blockers may slow the rate but are often contraindicated by bronchospasm. IV CCBs often produce hypotension. High-dose IV magnesium has been reported to facilitate conversion, but hypotension and nausea may complicate use.[44] Therapy therefore is best directed at the underlying disease process. AV junctional ablation and pacemaker insertion may be effective in selected patients.

Inappropriate Sinus Tachycardia

Inappropriate sinus tachycardia may be diagnosed when a persistent, nonparoxysmal tachycardia with a P-wave morphology identical to that seen in sinus rhythm is present during the waking hours.[45] Secondary systemic causes should be excluded. Typical symptoms include palpitations, dizziness, fatigue, dyspnea, and chest pain. Many patients alternate between periods of tachycardia and relative bradycardia. The latter makes drug therapy difficult. β-Blockers have traditionally been the agents selected initially for therapy, but some patients will respond to verapamil or diltiazem. Ivabradine, a highly selective I_f channel blocker currently available in some European countries, has been shown to be effective in a small number of patients with inappropriate sinus tachycardia.[46,47]

Junctional Ectopic Tachycardia

This rhythm occurs primarily in infants and children, and a congenital form and the more common postoperative form have been described.[48,49] The congenital form usually manifests with congestive heart failure in infancy. The postoperative form is seen after surgery to repair tetralogy of Fallot, transposition of the great vessels, and other forms of complex congenital heart disease. The mechanism for both arrhythmias is believed to be enhanced automaticity in the AV junction proximal to the region that gives rise to the His potential. Because of the incessant nature of the tachycardia and its resistance to cardioversion and most forms of drug therapy, mortality rates are high when the arrhythmia is seen in critically ill postoperative patients. Limited experience with sotalol, propafenone, flecainide, and amiodarone suggests that trials with these drugs are warranted. In addition, total body cooling may be helpful in postoperative patients. Rarely, catheter ablation with permanent pacing may be required for patients who fail to respond to drugs.

REFERENCES

1. Task Force of the Working Group on Arrhythmias of the European Society of Cardiology. The Sicilian gambit: a new approach to the classification of antiarrhythmic drugs based on their actions on arrhythmogenic mechanisms. *Circulation* 1991;84:1831-1851.
2. DiFrancesco D. Funny channel–based pacemaking. *Heart Rhythm* 2010;7:276-279.
3. Vaughan Williams EM. A classification of antiarrhythmic actions reassessed after a decade of new drugs. *J Clin Pharmacol* 1984;24:129-147.
4. Tendera M, Wnuk-Wojnar AM, Kulakowski P, et al. Efficacy and safety of dofetilide in the prevention of symptomatic episodes of paroxysmal supraventricular tachycardia: a 6-month double-blind comparison with propafenone and placebo. *Am Heart J* 2001;142:93-98.
5. Page RL, Connolly SJ, Wilkinson WE, et al. Antiarrhythmic effects of azimilide in paroxysmal supraventricular tachycardia: efficacy and dose-response. *Am Heart J* 2002;143:643-649.
6. Blomstrom-Lundqvist C, Scheinman MM, Aliot EM, et al. ACC/AHA/ESC guidelines for the management of patients with supraventricular arrhythmias. *Circulation* 2003;108:1871-1909.
7. Ferguson JD, DiMarco JP. Contemporary management of supraventricular tachycardia. *Circulation* 2003;107:1096-1099.
8. Orejarena LA, Vidaillet H Jr, DeStefano F, et al. Paroxysmal supraventricular tachycardia in the general population. *J Am Coll Cardiol* 1998;31:150-157.
9. Fox DJ, Tischenko A, Krahn AD, et al. Supraventricular tachycardia: diagnosis and management. *Mayo Clin Proc* 2008;83:1400-1411.
10. Delacretaz E. Supraventricular tachycardia. *N Engl J Med* 2006;354:1039-1051.
11. Alboni P, Tomasi C, Menozzi C, et al. Efficacy and safety of out-of-hospital self-administered single-dose oral drug treatment in the management of infrequent, well-tolerated paroxysmal supraventricular tachycardia. *J Am Coll Cardiol* 2001;37:548-553.
12. DiMarco JP. Adenosine and digoxin. In Zipes DP, Jalife J, editors: *Cardiac electrophysiology: from cell to bedside*, 4th ed. 2004, Philadelphia, WB Saunders, pp 693-694.
13. Wltzschig HK. Adenosine: an old drug newly discovered. *Anesthesiology* 2009;111:904-915.
14. Shah CP, Gupta AK, Thakur RK, et al. Adenosine-induced ventricular fibrillation. *Indian Heart J* 2001;53:208-210.
15. Strickberger SA, Man KC, Daoud EG, et al. Adenosine-induced atrial arrhythmia: a prospective analysis. *Ann Int Med* 1997;127:417-422.
16. Mallet ML. Proarrhythmic effects of adenosine: a review of the literature. *Emerg Med J* 2004;21:408-410.
17. Dougherty AH, Jackman WM, Naccarelli GV, et al.; IV Diltiazem Study Group. Acute conversion of paroxysmal tachycardia with intravenous diltiazem. *Am J Cardiol* 1992;70:587-592.
18. Singh BN. β-Blockers and calcium channel blockers as antiarrhythmic drugs. In Zipes DP, Jalife J, editors: *Cardiac electrophysiology from cell to bedside*, 4th ed. 2004, Philadelphia, WB Saunders, pp 918-931.
19. Lim SH, Anantharaman V, Teo WS. Slow-infusion of calcium channel blockers in the emergency management of supraventricular tachycardia. *Resuscitation* 2002;52:167-174.
20. Holdgate A, Foo A. Adenosine versus intravenous calcium channel antagonists for the treatment of supraventricular tachycardia in adults. *Cochrane Database System Rev* (4): CD005154, 2006.
21. Glatter KA, Cheng J, Dorostkar P, et al. Electrophysiologic effects of adenosine in patients with supraventricular tachycardia. *Circulation* 1999;99:1034-1040.
22. Pappone C, Santinelli V, Rosanio S, et al. Usefulness of invasive electrophysiologic testing to stratify risk of arrhythmic events in patients with Wolff-Parkinson-White pattern. *J Am Coll Cardiol* 2003;15:889-897.
23. Dorian P, Naccarelli GV, Coumel P, et al.; Flecainide Multicenter Investigators Group. A randomized comparison of flecainide versus verapamil in paroxysmal supraventricular tachycardia. *Am J Cardiol* 1996;77:89A-95A.
24. UK Propafenone PSVT Study Group. A randomized, placebo-controlled trial of propafenone in the prophylaxis of paroxysmal supraventricular tachycardia and paroxysmal atrial fibrillation. *Circulation* 1995;92:2550-2557.
25. Wehling M. Meta-analysis of flecainide safety in patients with supraventricular arrhythmias. *Arzneimittel-Forschung* 2002;52:507-514.
26. Saoudi N, Cosio F, Waldo A, et al. Classification of atrial flutter and regular atrial tachycardia according to electrophysiological mechanism and anatomic basis: a statement from the joint expert group from the Working Group of Arrhythmias of the European Society of Cardiology and the North American Society of Pacing and Electrophysiology. *J Cardiovasc Electrophys* 2001;12:852-866.
27. Yang Y, Cheng J, Bochoeyer A, et al. Atypical right atrial flutter patterns. *Circulation* 2001;103:3092-3098.
28. Cheng J, Cabeen WR Jr, Scheinman MM. Right atrial flutter due to lower loop reentry: mechanism and anatomic substrates. *Circulation* 1999;99:1700-1705.
29. Gerstenfeld EP, Dixit S, Bata R, et al. Surface electrocardiogram characteristics of atrial tachycardias occurring after pulmonary vein isolation. *Heart Rhythm* 2007;4:1136-1143.
30. Veenhuyzen GD, Knecht S, O'Neill MD, et al. Atrial tachycardias encountered during and after catheter ablation for atrial fibrillation. Part I: Classification, incidence and management. *PACE* 2009;32:393-398.
31. Ellenbogen KA, Dias VC, Plumb VJ, et al. A placebo-controlled trial of continuous intravenous diltiazem infusion for 24-hour rate control during atrial fibrillation and atrial flutter: a multicenter study. *J Am Coll Cardiol* 1991;18:891-897.
32. Goldenberg IF, Lewis WR, Dias VC, et al. Intravenous diltiazem for the treatment of patients with atrial fibrillation or flutter and moderate to severe congestive heart failure. *Am J Cardiol* 1994;74:884-889.
33. Phillips BG, Ghandi AJ, Sanoski CA, et al. Comparison of intraveous diltiazem and verapamil for the acute treatment of atrial fibrillation and flutter. *Pharmacotherapy* 1997;17:1238-1245.
34. Cosio FG, Delpon E. New antiarrhythmic drugs for atrial flutter and atrial fibrillation: a conceptual breakthrough at last? *Circulation* 2002;105:276-278.
35. Stambler BS, Wood MA, Ellenbogen KA, et al.; Ibutilide Repeat Dose Study Investigators. Efficacy and safety of repeated intravenous doses of ibutilide for rapid conversion of atrial flutter or fibrillation. *Circulation* 1996;94:1623-1631.
36. Ellenbogen KA, Stambler BS, Wood MA, et al. Efficacy of intravenous ibutilide for rapid termination of atrial fibrillation and atrial flutter: a dose-response study. *J Am Coll Cardiol* 1996;28:130-136.
37. Tercius AJ, Kluger J, Coleman CJ, White CM. Intravenous magnesium sulfate enhances the ability of intravenous ibutilide to successfully convert atrial fibrillation or flutter. *PACE* 2007;30:1331-1335.
38. Coleman CI, Sood N, Chawla D, et al. Intravenous magnesium sulfate enhances the ability of dofetilide to successfully cardiovert atrial fibrillation or flutter: results of the Dofetilide and Intravenous Magnesium Evaluation. *Europace* 2009;11:892-895.
39. Singh S, Zoble RG, Yellen L, et al. Efficacy and safety of oral dofetilide in converting to and maintaining sinus rhythm in patients with chronic atrial fibrillation or atrial flutter: the Symptomatic Atrial Fibrillation Investigative Research on Dofetilide (SAFIRE-D) study. *Circulation* 2000;102:2385-2390.
40. Banchs JE, Wolbrette DL, Samii SM, et al. Efficacy and safety of dofetilide in patients with atrial fibrillation and atrial flutter. *J Interv Card Electrophysiol* 2008;23:111-115.
41. Falk RH. Proarrhythmia in patients treated for atrial fibrillation or flutter. *Ann Int Med* 1992;117:141-150.
42. Gilligan DM, Zakaib JS, Fuller I, et al. Long-term outcome of patients after successful radiofrequency ablation for typical atrial flutter. *Pacing Clin Electrophysiol* 2003;26:53-58.
43. Calkins H, Canby R, Weiss R, et al. Results of catheter ablation of typical atrial flutter. *Am J Cardiol* 2004;94:437-442.
44. McCord JK, Borzak S, Davis T, Gheorghiade M. Usefulness of intravenous magnesium for multifocal atrial tachycardia in patients with chronic obstructive pulmonary disease. *Am J Cardiol* 1998;91:91-96.
45. Still AM, Raatikainen P, Ylitalo A, et al. Prevalence, characteristics and natural course of inappropriate sinus tachycardia. *Europace* 2005;7:104-112.
46. Zellerhoff S, Hinterseer M, Krull BF, et al. Ivabradine in patients with inappropriate sinus tachycardia. *Nuanyn-Schmied Arch Phamacol* 2010;382:433-436.
47. Cato L, Rebecchi M, Sette A, et al. Efficacy of ivabradine administration in patients affected by inappropriate sinus tachycardia. *Heart Rhythm* 2010;7:1318-1323.
48. Haas NA, Plumpton K, Justo R, et al. Postoperative junctional ectopic tachycardia (JET). *Zeitschr Kardiol* 2004;373-380.
49. Hoffman TM, Bush DM, Wernovsky G, et al. Postoperative junctional ectopic tachycardia in children: incidence, risk factors, and treatment. *Ann Thorac Surg* 2002;74:1607-1611.

CHAPTER 20

Atrial Fibrillation

Peter Zimetbaum and Rodney H. Falk

CLASSIFICATION, 372

DECISION FOR RHYTHM OR RATE CONTROL, 372

Rate Control, 373
Rhythm Control, 374

MAINTENANCE OF SINUS RHYTHM, 375

Pharmacologic Approaches, 375
Adjunctive Therapy for the Maintenance of Sinus Rhythm, 377

Nonpharmacologic Approaches to the Maintenance of Sinus Rhythm, 377
Pacing for the Maintenance of Sinus Rhythm, 378
Thromboembolic Prophylaxis, 378
Pericardioversion Anticoagulation, 379

ATRIAL FIBRILLATION FOLLOWING CARDIAC SURGERY, 379

CONCLUSIONS, 380

REFERENCES, 380

Atrial fibrillation (AF) is the most common arrhythmia in clinical practice, and in many ways it is the most complex to manage. Understanding of this disorder has increased immensely in the past decade, and new therapeutic options are developing at a rapid pace. AF is increasingly recognized as a heterogenous disease that cannot be managed with a "one size fits all" solution. Instead, the approach to the optimal treatment of a patient with AF requires the clinician to address the underlying heart disease and its interactions with potential therapies, the individual's estimated risk of thromboembolism associated with the arrhythmia, and the presence and severity of arrhythmia-related symptoms. The general physician and cardiologist treating AF should know when to refer the patient for an electrophysiologic intervention, and the cardiac electrophysiologist should know when to stay the course and when to offer one of several invasive approaches.

Classification

AF may be classified by the underlying disease,[1] the frequency and duration of its occurrence,[2] or a combination of both. *Paroxysmal AF* is defined as a self-terminating arrhythmia, usually lasting less than 48 hours and rarely lasting more than 7 days. *Persistent AF* is an arrhythmia that fails to spontaneously convert but will do so with intervention, usually cardioversion or drug therapy. *Permanent AF* is an arrhythmia that is resistant to conversion to sinus rhythm and is the loosest term of the three; its definition in many cases depends on the vigor with which the physician pursues sinus rhythm restoration. With the advent of ablation procedures for AF, a new term, *long-standing persistent AF*, has been introduced to describe patients with a history of continuous AF longer than 1 year in whom an ablation procedure is attempted. To these categories is added the term *new-onset AF* to represent the initial documented event, since the outcome of a first episode of arrhythmia is not known. These temporal categories are not static and may merge with one another over time, as new-onset or paroxysmal AF become persistent in a significant percentage of patients. The presence or absence of symptoms, their severity, and an assessment of whether they are related to inadequate ventricular rate control or loss of normal AV synchrony is a helpful adjunct to the classification of AF, but it should be recognized that thromboembolic risk is unrelated to the presence or absence of arrhythmia-related symptoms.

Decision for Rhythm or Rate Control

A series of randomized, controlled trials of rhythm control compared with rate control were published 10 years ago.[3-5] These studies were generally conducted in older patients with AF and clinical risk factors for thromboembolism. The study methods varied, and anticoagulation in the rhythm-control group was not mandated in most instances, although it was used in the majority of patients. In the largest of these trials, the Atrial Fibrillation Follow-up Investigation of Rhythm Management (AFFIRM) study,[6] the primary endpoint was death, and the uniform finding of all these studies was that neither strategy was superior to the other in terms of any of the primary endpoints. When a post hoc analysis was done as to outcomes *by rhythm*, regardless of assigned strategy, the presence of sinus rhythm in the AFFIRM trial favored survival; the presence of coronary disease, diabetes, and/or smoking were adverse factors in terms of mortality.[7] However, to maintain sinus rhythm, antiarrhythmic agents generally had to be used and were associated with a decreased likelihood of survival, which offset any potential benefit of sinus rhythm. Although this observation might be used to argue that an optimal strategy is sinus rhythm maintenance by nonpharmacologic means, the complexity of this retrospective analysis is such that it should only be thought of as a hypothesis-generating observation, not a well-supported conclusion. Indeed, a subsequent analysis of the Comparison of Rate Control and Rhythm Control in Patients with Recurrent Persistent Atrial Fibrillation (RACE) trial data performed by actual rhythm failed to demonstrate any benefit of sinus rhythm over AF,[8] although functional status was slightly better in the AFFIRM trial among patients in sinus rhythm regardless of assigned group.[9]

The trials of rate versus rhythm control are not the last word in this controversy because large groups of patients—including the young and very old, those with congestive heart failure (CHF), and those with highly symptomatic AF—were underrepresented.[10,11] The role of restoration of sinus rhythm in a group of patients with CHF and an ejection fraction of 35% or less was subsequently investigated in the Atrial Fibrillation and Congestive Heart Failure (AF-CHF) trial.[12] Amiodarone was the predominant drug used to maintain sinus rhythm, and there was no difference in outcome in patients randomized either to the rhythm or to the rate control groups. Despite all these apparently negative outcomes for a strategy of vigorous restoration and maintenance of sinus rhythm, it should be recognized that for many patients, the onset of persistent AF is associated with troublesome symptoms and a diminished overall quality of life despite adequate rate control.[13] Many such patients were likely excluded from clinical trials, and data do support restoration of sinus rhythm for improving quality of life.[14] Thus, when faced with a patient with recent-onset AF, the clinician should take a comprehensive history and have a low threshold for at least one attempt at sinus rhythm restoration to assess whether this leads to an improved sense of well-being. As a consequence, debate is ongoing regarding the relative merits of these two approaches in large numbers of AF patients. Regardless of the unanswered questions left by these trials, an important and consistent finding was that stroke risk was not reduced by the strategy of rhythm control when compared with that of rate control and anticoagulation. Although most of the patients in both groups received warfarin, it was stopped in the earlier trials more often in the group in whom sinus rhythm had apparently been restored; recurrent sustained or paroxysmal AF in this group was most likely responsible for thromboembolic events. Decisions regarding rhythm compared with rate control must therefore not be based on the desire to withdraw or withhold warfarin because recurrence is common and may be both asymptomatic and paroxysmal, rendering its detection on routine examination difficult. Although the decision to attempt to maintain sinus rhythm or choose rate control should be an individualized decision based on a careful assessment of clinical and echocardiographic features in each patient, younger patients with severe symptoms are generally preferred candidates for attempted rhythm control, whereas older patients with minimal symptoms may be equally if not better served by a rate-control strategy.

Rate Control

In patients with new-onset AF, the average ventricular response is 100 to 150 beats/min.[15] The irregular R-R intervals are associated with a marked variation in stroke volume,[16,17] and this possibly contributes to the uncomfortable sensation of AF with a poorly controlled heart rate. With stimuli that result either in vagal tone withdrawal or an increase in sympathetic tone—such as exertion, fever, hyperthyroidism, or blood loss—the ventricular rate in AF may increase markedly. Thus, a good question for the clinician to ask is whether the patient would have sinus tachycardia in sinus rhythm. If the answer is affirmative, the rapid ventricular response may reflect the presence of one of these conditions, which will need to be corrected before rate control can be achieved.

For some patients, particularly those with paroxysmal AF, a rapid ventricular response is associated with uncomfortable symptoms, most commonly of palpitations or dyspnea.[18] In persistent AF, a disproportionate rise in heart rate with exertion may lead to dyspnea or fatigue.

PHARMACOLOGIC RATE CONTROL IN ATRIAL FIBRILLATION: OPTIMAL VENTRICULAR RATE

Control of the ventricular rate in AF has a twofold aim: elimination of symptoms and improvement of cardiac efficiency. As heart rate increases in AF, stroke volume tends to decrease, but cardiac output is generally maintained over a relatively wide range, probably decreasing when mean heart rate exceeds 110 to 120 beats/min.[19] However, a higher resting heart rate probably is inefficient because it is associated with a higher myocardial oxygen demand. Thus, it is appropriate to attempt to reduce heart rate during AF.

The AFFIRM investigators empirically defined *adequate rate control* as an average heart rate of 80 beats/min or fewer at rest and either a maximum heart rate of 110 beats/min or fewer during a 6-minute walk or, during 24 hours of ambulatory monitoring, an average heart rate of 100 beats/min or less with no heart rate greater than 110% maximum predicted age-adjusted exercise heart rate.[20] Using this definition, β-blocking agents were the most effective initial drug for rate control, with 70% success if used either alone or with digoxin, compared with 54% for calcium channel antagonists and 54% with digoxin alone.[20]

These results, based on an older population with cardiac disease, document not only the apparent superiority of β-blockers but also that digoxin alone, although not effective in everyone, still has a role to play in heart-rate control in patients with AF. Furthermore, digoxin is synergistic both with calcium channel blockers and β-blockers and may decrease the required dosages of these agents and their associated side effects.[21]

It is important to recognize that tighter heart rate control based on the number of beats per minute does not necessarily translate into improved symptoms. Although calcium channel antagonists are less effective than β-blockade for heart rate control, trials of β-blockers in patients with sustained AF have failed to show an improved exercise tolerance. Moreover, if peak heart rate is excessively blunted, exercise tolerance may decrease.[22] A comparison of more stringent rate control that used criteria similar to the AFFIRM trial, with lenient rate control (resting heart rate <110 beats/min), showed no difference in outcome over a 3-year follow-up; this suggests that tight rate control may not be necessary in all patients.[23]

When considering agents for ventricular rate control in AF, therapies are often divided into β-blocking agents, calcium channel antagonists, and digoxin—as though each of these classes of agents was mutually exclusive (Table 20-1). Although monotherapy may be effective in a significant number of patients, the addition of digoxin and intermediate dose of a β-blocker or calcium channel blocker may produce excellent heart rate control, even when a high-dose single agent has failed. Evaluation of information from the AFFIRM trial shows that physicians frequently use a combination of agents for heart rate control and that combination

TABLE 20-1	**Pharmacologic Heart Rate Control in Atrial Fibrillation**		
DRUG	**CONTROL OF ACUTE EPISODE**	**CONTROL OF SUSTAINED AF**	**COMMENTS**
Calcium Channel Blockers			
Diltiazem	20 mg bolus followed, if necessary, by 25 mg given 15 min later; maintenance infusion of 5-15 mg/h	Oral controlled-release diltiazem 180-360 mg/day	Long-term rate control may be better with the addition of digoxin.
Verapamil	5-10 mg IV over 2-3 min repeated once 30 min later; maintenance infusion rate is not reliably documented	Slow-release verapamil 120-240 mg qd or bid	Use causes elevation in digoxin level; may have more negative inotropic effect than diltiazem.
β-Blockers*			
Esmolol	0.5 mg/kg IV, repeated if necessary; follow with infusion at 0.05 mg/kg/min, increasing as needed to 0.2 mg/kg/min	Not available in oral form	Hypotension may be troublesome but responds to drug discontinuation.
Metoprolol	5-mg IV bolus repeated twice q2min; no data on maintenance infusion	50-400 mg/day in divided doses	Metoprolol is useful if concomitant coronary disease present.
Propranolol	1-5 mg IV given over 10 min	30-360 mg in divided doses or as long-acting form qd	Noncardioselective; use with caution in patients with history of bronchospasm.
Digoxin	1.0-1.5 mg IV or PO over 24 h in increments of 0.25-0.5 mg	0.125-0.25 mg/day	Digoxin is renally excreted, with a slow onset of action IV and less effective control than other agents, although it may be synergistic with them. The least effective agent but may be acceptable monotherapy in sedentary patients.

*Several other oral β-blockers have similar efficacy for rate control.
AF, atrial fibrillation; IV, intravenous.

therapy seems to have a greater likelihood of tight rate control compared with monotherapy with any agent.[20] In a small but well-designed crossover trial, it was shown that the addition of digoxin to either diltiazem or to a β-blocker resulted in superior rate control than when any of these agents was used as monotherapy.[21] Furthermore, rate control could be achieved with a combination that included digoxin at a lower dose than the other agent and with a reduced prevalence of side effects. However, clinicians should recognize that the negative chronotropic effects of the combination may produce significant sinus bradycardia, should sinus rhythm return. If verapamil is chosen, the verapamil-digoxin interaction is likely to necessitate a lower dose of digoxin than would be required if it were used alone or with diltiazem.[24]

NONPHARMACOLOGIC APPROACH TO RATE CONTROL

Interruption of atrioventricular (AV) nodal function with catheter ablation and concomitant pacemaker implantation is a highly effective strategy for rate control. It is a relatively simple procedure that is associated with a significant and sustained improvement in quality of life.[25] Data suggest, however, that at least in the setting of impaired ventricular function, right ventricular (RV) pacing may aggravate heart failure in some patients.[26-28] This realization has tempered enthusiasm for this procedure, except in cases for which pharmacologic management and catheter ablation of the atrial arrhythmia prove impossible. An alternative to RV pacing is biventricular pacing, which preserves ventricular synchrony to a greater degree and thus may not have the adverse effects associated with RV pacing.[29,30]

Rhythm Control

The strategy of rhythm control involves the restoration and maintenance of sinus rhythm. AF may spontaneously revert to sinus rhythm or may persist indefinitely unless cardioversion is performed. Spontaneous return of sinus rhythm occurs most often within 48 hours of arrhythmia onset.[31] If this does not occur, sinus rhythm can be restored through the use of antiarrhythmic drugs or direct current (DC) electrical cardioversion. Before cardioversion, appropriate precautions must be taken to prevent thromboembolic events.

PHARMACOLOGIC CARDIOVERSION

Intravenous and oral drugs are available for pharmacologic cardioversion (Table 20-2). This approach is most successful when used within 24 to 48 hours of onset of AF,[32] and the use of pharmacologic agents for conversion should be followed by electrical therapy if this approach fails. The currently available intravenous (IV) agents in the United States are limited to procainamide and ibutilide (see Chapter 18). The success rate of these agents for the conversion of AF is poorer with procainamide than with ibutilide, and ibutilide is better for the conversion of atrial flutter than it is for AF.[33]

Electrocardiographic (ECG) monitoring should be used when administering these drugs because of the risk of torsades de pointes (TdP) with procainamide and ibutilide—as high as 3% to 5% with ibutilide[34]—and hypotension with procainamide.[33] Patients must be monitored for proarrhythmia for at least 2 hours following the termination of the infusion. It had been shown that the combination of the class 1C agent propafenone administered orally with IV ibutilide increases the likelihood of conversion to sinus rhythm and is well tolerated, but experience with this combination is limited to one publication.[35]

An alternative approach to IV therapy is the use of high-dose oral antiarrhythmic drugs for the conversion of AF to sinus rhythm. Quinidine in an initial dose of 200 mg, repeated at a dose of 200 mg every 2 hours for three separate doses, has a high success rate for conversion,[36] but it has fallen into disfavor because of a high incidence of side effects, including TdP.[37] High-dose oral therapy has been widely studied with high doses of type 1C medications (450 to 600 mg of propafenone[38] or 300 to 400 mg of flecainide).[39,40] These drugs should be avoided in patients with bundle branch block, structural heart disease, or ventricular pre-excitation because of a risk of proarrhythmia, including atrial flutter with 1:1 AV nodal conduction, hemodynamic collapse, and ventricular tachycardia.

TABLE 20-2	Recommended Doses of Drugs Proven Effective for Pharmacologic Cardioversion of Atrial Fibrillation			
DRUG	ROUTE OF ADMINISTRATION	DOSAGE*		POTENTIAL ADVERSE EFFECTS
Amiodarone	PO	Inpatient: 1.2-1.8 g qd in divided doses until 10 g total, then 200-400 mg/day maintenance or 30 mg/kg as a single dose		Hypotension, QT prolongation, torsades de pointes (rare), GI upset, constipation, phlebitis (IV)
	PO	Outpatient: 600-800 mg/day in divided doses until 10 g total, then 200-400 mg/day maintenance		
	IV/PO	5-7 mg/kg over 30-60 min, then 1.2-1.8 g/day continuous IV or in divided oral doses until 10 g total, then 200-400 mg/day maintenance		
Dofetilide	PO	Creatinine clearance (mL/min): >60 40-60 20-40 <20	Dose (μg bid): 500 250 125 Contraindicated	QT prolongation, torsades de pointes; adjust dose for renal function, body size, and age
Flecainide	PO/IV	PO: 200-300 mg† IV: 1.5-3.0 mg/kg over 10-20 min†		Hypotension, atrial flutter with high ventricular rate
Ibutilide	IV	1 mg over 10 min; repeat 1 mg when necessary		QT prolongation, torsades de pointes
Propafenone	PO/IV	600 mg 1.5-2.0 mg/kg over 10-20 min†		Hypotension, atrial flutter with high ventricular rate
Quinidine‡	PO	0.75-1.5 g in divided doses over 6-12 h, usually with a rate-slowing drug		QT prolongation, torsades de pointes, GI upset, hypotension

*Dosages given may differ from those recommended by the manufacturers.
†Insufficient data are available on which to base specific recommendations for the use of one loading regimen over another for patients with ischemic heart disease or impaired left ventricular function; these drugs should be used cautiously or not at all in such patients.
‡The use of quinidine loading to achieve pharmacologic conversion of atrial fibrillation is controversial, and safer methods are available with the alternative agents listed in the table.
AF, atrial fibrillation; BID, twice a day; GI, gastrointestinal; IV, intravenous.
Modified from ACC/AHA/ESC guidelines for the management of patients with atrial fibrillation. Circulation 2006;114:e257-e354.

The initial administration of these drugs should be in a monitored setting with the capability for defibrillation. If found to be successful without adverse effects, oral therapy can subsequently be self-administered by selected patients with a structurally normal heart, the so-called *pill-in-the-pocket* approach.[41] Oral amiodarone has been extensively studied for the conversion of AF and has been shown to be safe to load during AF in the outpatient setting; it is also associated with a rate of successful cardioversion of up to 80% after 24 hours in AF of 48 hours' duration or less,[42] although the rate is much lower for longer duration arrhythmia.[43]

ELECTRICAL CARDIOVERSION

Electrical cardioversion can restore sinus rhythm in AF more than 90% of the time.[44] *Successful cardioversion* is defined as the restoration of sinus rhythm, if even for only one beat, and it is inversely related to the duration of AF and the size of the left atrium. Biphasic defibrillator waveforms are more successful than monophasic waveforms,[45] and anteroposterior electrode positioning is somewhat more successful than anterolateral placement, although this is not a consistent finding.[46,47] Reversion to AF immediately after a single beat of sinus rhythm or within the subsequent 24 hours occurs frequently,[48] and these phenomena are called *immediate recurrence of AF* (IRAF) or *early recurrence of AF* (ERAF).[49] Early recurrences may be prevented by antiarrhythmic drugs such as ibutilide.[50,51]

If cardioversion fails at the maximum energy output of the device, a second shock at the same energy level a minute or so later may succeed, as transthoracic impedance falls with each shock. Alternatively, a change to another orientation will occasionally be successful. Application of pressure to the anterior electrode will also diminish the transthoracic impedance and improve success rates.[52] Finally, pretreatment with an intravenous or oral antiarrhythmic drug can facilitate cardioversion by

lowering defibrillation thresholds and reducing early recurrence of AF.[50,51]

Maintenance of Sinus Rhythm
Pharmacologic Approaches

Antiarrhythmic drugs are widely prescribed for the maintenance of sinus rhythm. In general, these agents have a similar efficacy, with a 50% rate of recurrence at 1 year compared with 20% to 25% maintenance of sinus rhythm in the absence of antiarrhythmic drugs. Amiodarone has consistently been shown to be more efficacious than other available antiarrhythmic drugs, with up to a 75% rate of AF suppression at 1 year.[53] If one agent fails to maintain sinus rhythm, a second agent may be successful, particularly one from another group of drugs.[54] It is unrealistic to expect complete suppression of AF with any of these agents. Instead, the goal should be a significant reduction in the frequency of AF compared with pretreatment patterns.

The major toxicities of antiarrhythmic drugs include both proarrhythmia and noncardiovascular adverse effects. The noncardiovascular toxicities differ by drug and range from benign changes in taste to life-threatening pulmonary or liver toxicity (Table 20-3). All antiarrhythmic drugs alter cardiac sodium and/or potassium channel function.[55] It is believed that these drugs prevent or terminate AF by prolonging the refractory period (potassium channel blockers) or slowing the conduction (sodium channel blockers) of atrial cells. Prolongation of the refractory period (prolongation of repolarization) results in QT prolongation, which may be excessive if dosing is too high, excretion is reduced, or the patient has either a genetic predisposition to a prolonged QT or a genetically prolonged drug metabolism.[56] Prolongation in conduction such as that produced by the class IC agents causes QRS prolongation, which is more marked at faster heart rates.[57] QT

TABLE 20-3 Antiarrhythmic Drugs, Dosages, and Toxicities

DRUG	DOSE (24 H)	CARDIAC TOXICITY	NONCARDIAC TOXICITY	RECOMMENDED MONITORING AND DRUG INTERACTIONS
Amiodarone	200-400 mg (initial load 600-1200 mg for 1-2 wk) with lower dosing for smaller and older patients	Bradycardia, TdP (rare)	Pulmonary toxicity, photosensitivity, hepatic toxicity, GI upset and neurologic toxicity (dose related), thyroid dysfunction, rise in INR with warfarin	LFTs: q6mo, PFTs at baseline and only with symptoms of potential toxicity; CXR yearly TFTs: baseline, 3 mo, then q6mo; potentiates warfarin, digoxin, dilantin, tricyclics
Dronedarone	400 mg bid	None; avoid in patients with congestive heart failure or permanent AF	Hepatic toxicity; impairs secretion of creatinine	Monitor for recurrent AF at least q3mo
Dofetilide	500-1000 μg	TdP	NS	In-hospital initiation for 72 h, creatinine clearance q3mo QT interval; levels increased by multiple drugs (e.g., verapamil)
Sotalol	160-320 mg	TdP, CHF, sinus bradycardia	Bronchospasm	QT interval
Flecainide	200-300 mg	Ventricular tachycardia, atrial flutter with 1:1 conduction	Dizziness	NS
Propafenone	450-900 mg	Ventricular tachycardia, atrial flutter with 1:1 conduction	Metallic taste	NS
Quinidine	600-1500 mg	TdP, enhanced AV nodal conduction	Thrombocytopenia, fever, nausea, diarrhea	QT interval; platelet count; will increase digoxin levels; can potentiate warfarin
Procainamide	1-4 g	TdP	Agranulocytosis, lupuslike syndrome	QT interval; NAPA increased by ethanol
Disopyramide	400-750 mg	TdP, CHF	Urinary retention, dry mouth; contraindicated in glaucoma	QT interval

AV, atrioventricular; CHF, congestive heart failure; CXR, chest x-ray; GI, gastrointestinal; INR, International Normalized Ratio; LFTs, liver function tests; NAPA, N-acetyl procainamide; NS, not significant/not stated; PFTs, pulmonary function tests; TdP, torsades de pointes; TFT, thyroid function tests.

prolongation may result in TdP[57,58] and antiarrhythmic drugs that block the delayed rectifier potassium channel (I_{kr} and/or I_{ks}) may cause TdP in up to 5% of patients.[57] Drug-related TdP is more likely to occur in association with slow heart rates, electrolyte abnormalities (hypokalemia or hypomagnesemia), female gender, prior unrecognized congenital long QT syndrome, and pauses associated with the conversion of AF to sinus rhythm.[59] The concomitant use of drugs that interfere with the hepatic metabolism of antiarrhythmic drugs may also result in QT prolongation,[60] and a reduced urinary clearance of renally excreted medications may result in toxicity.[61] In some instances, such as with sotalol or dofetilide, the risk of TdP is proportional to blood levels and is related to renal excretion[62]; with quinidine it may be idiosyncratic and not dose related. A metabolite of procainamide, N-acetyl procainamide, prolongs the QT interval, whereas the parent compound has little effect on repolarization. Slow acetylators produce less N-acetyl procainamide and have a lower risk of TdP. Rapid acetylators develop more N-acetyl procainamide and are more prone to TdP.[63]

Ventricular tachycardia may occur in patients taking antiarrhythmic drugs. This complication is well described in patients taking type 1C medications (flecainide and propafenone) who have had a prior myocardial infarction (MI) and have impaired ventricular function.[64] Atrial flutter with a slow atrial rate and one-to-one AV nodal conduction, producing a widened QRS duration with hemodynamic collapse, may also occur, particularly with class 1C drugs.[65] This latter complication can generally be avoided with the addition of AV node–blocking medications.

Bradyarrhythmias develop most often as a result of sinus node suppression or slowing of conduction through the AV node. Both of these complications are more frequently seen in elderly patients with underlying sick sinus syndrome.[66] Ambulatory monitoring and appropriate dose reduction or discontinuation can prevent serious consequences.[67]

CHOICE OF DRUG

The toxicity of antiarrhythmic drugs can be reduced by the selection of agents in the context of the patient's clinical history. In brief, the risk factors for adverse effects include myocardial scarring (most commonly as a result of earlier MI), left ventricular (LV) systolic dysfunction, and possibly LV hypertrophy. The presence of any of these clinical features should be evaluated before choosing an antiarrhythmic drug (Figure 20-1). For patients without structural heart disease, the choice of drugs is wider, but it is still important to evaluate noncardiac comorbidity.

INITIATION AND MONITORING OF ANTIARRHYTHMIC DRUGS

The toxicity of antiarrhythmic drugs can also be reduced with the appropriate choice of dosage and method of monitoring during the loading phase. For example, unexpected bradycardia can often be avoided by reducing the usual loading dose of amiodarone or by starting with a low dose of sotalol and increasing to therapeutic dose as tolerated. This strategy is particularly important in patients with suspected sinus node dysfunction.

Some controversy exists regarding the need for in-hospital initiation of antiarrhythmic drugs for the treatment of AF, the major concern being the precipitation of TdP. This proarrhythmic effect occurs in drugs that prolong repolarization, and it is almost never seen with flecainide and propafenone. In-hospital monitoring for 72 hours is incorporated into the drug labeling of dofetilide and is therefore mandatory for this drug, regardless of the presence or absence of structural heart disease.[68] Quinidine is rarely used nowadays because of its significant and idiosyncratic propensity for provoking TdP,[69] but it is an effective atrial antiarrhythmic agent. Experimental data suggest that the risk of TdP can be reduced by the concomitant use of verapamil. Two large trials of quinidine, for paroxysmal AF or for maintenance of sinus rhythm after an episode of persistent AF, demonstrated that when quinidine was combined with verapamil, it was as effective as sotalol, but with less TdP risk.[70,71] As previously noted, a pause associated with the conversion of AF to sinus rhythm may promote the development of TdP. Consequently, in patients with paroxysmal AF, it is advisable to initiate antiarrhythmic drugs with the potential for TdP while the patient is in sinus rhythm.

In contrast to QT-prolonging agents, in-hospital initiation of type 1C agents, which should only be used in patients with a structurally normal heart, and amiodarone, which may be used in any form of heart disease, is generally not required. There is considerable experience with the initiation of amiodarone in the outpatient setting during AF without significant toxicity.[43,67,72] QT prolongation is common with amiodarone, but it is not generally associated with a great risk of TdP (<1%), unless the corrected QT interval is significantly prolonged (>500 ms).[73]

Dronedarone has been approved for the treatment of AF and can be started in the outpatient setting. It is similar in chemical structure to amiodarone but lacks the iodine moiety, so thyroid dysfunction is less of a concern. However, it is less effective at maintaining sinus rhythm than amiodarone[74] and should not be used in patients with recently decompensated heart failure because of an increased risk of death.[75] A Placebo-Controlled, Double-Blind, Parallel-Arm Trial to Assess the Efficacy of Dronedarone 400 mg BID for the Prevention of Cardiovascular Hospitalization or Death from Any Cause in Patients with Atrial Fibrillation/ Atrial Flutter (ATHENA) was the first trial to demonstrate prospectively a decrease in cardiovascular hospitalizations in patients with AF,[76] although this has been shown with dronedarone in a retrospective analysis and is probably simply a function of maintenance of sinus rhythm.[77] In a post hoc analysis of the ATHENA trial, stroke incidence was also lower in patients treated with dronedarone.[78] The main side effect of dronedarone is diarrhea, and there may be a previously unrecognized risk of hepatic toxicity associated with

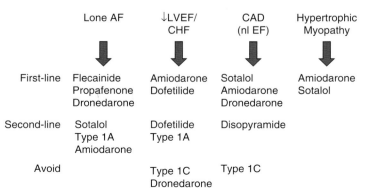

Antiarrhythmic Medications

	Lone AF	↓LVEF/ CHF	CAD (nl EF)	Hypertrophic Myopathy
First-line	Flecainide Propafenone Dronedarone	Amiodarone Dofetilide	Sotalol Amiodarone Dronedarone	Amiodarone Sotalol
Second-line	Sotalol Type 1A Amiodarone	Dofetilide Type 1A	Disopyramide	
Avoid		Type 1C Dronedarone	Type 1C	

FIGURE 20-1 Algorithm for the choice of antiarrhythmic drug based on the patient's clinical characteristics. AF, atrial fibrillation; CAD, coronary artery disease; CHF, congestive heart failure; EF, ejection fraction; LVEF, left ventricular ejection fraction.

this therapy. Data from the Permanent Afibrillation Outcome Study Using Dronedarone on Top of Standard Therapy (PALLAS) trial, which used dronedarone in patients with persistent AF, showed increased toxicity and was stopped. Specifically, there was an increase in stroke, cardiovascular hospitalization, and cardiovascular mortality rate in patients taking dronedarone. At present, it is recommended to only use dronedarone if frequent monitoring (at least every 3 months) fails to show AF recurrence.

The concern with type 1C agents is the conversion of AF to atrial flutter with 1 : 1 conduction to the ventricles and hemodynamic instability. It is therefore strongly recommended that AV node–blocking agents be used in conjunction with a type 1C agent.[79] Particular caution should be exercised for patients who are athletic because the development of atrial flutter during exercise may be associated with 1 : 1 conduction, even in the presence of digoxin or calcium channel blockers. Theoretically, the antisympathetic aspects of β-blockade should be more effective in such patients.

Amiodarone may be initiated in an outpatient setting during AF given the widespread safety data with this practice. If there is no CHF, and if the patient is in sinus rhythm, it may be possible to initiate other antiarrhythmic drugs, with the exception of dofetilide, in the ambulatory setting. To increase the safety of this approach, patients can be monitored with a continuous event recorder. The transmission of a single 30-second tracing daily permits monitoring for bradycardia, QT prolongation, and tachyarrhythmias. This protocol is continued for 10 days and has been shown to be quite effective.[67]

Despite safe initiation of an antiarrhythmic drug, the long-term possibility of proarrhythmic effects still exists. It is therefore important that both physicians and patients are aware of circumstances that may render previously tolerated medications dangerous. Examples of these situations include the initiation of diuretics or certain antibiotics in patients taking QT-prolonging drugs and the development of renal dysfunction in patients receiving renally excreted antiarrhythmic drugs such as sotalol.

Adjunctive Therapy for the Maintenance of Sinus Rhythm

Advances in the understanding of the electrical and mechanical remodeling of the atrium that occurs during AF have led to the evaluation of drugs that are not primarily antiarrhythmic in nature as an adjunct to maintaining sinus rhythm. The calcium channel–blocking agents may blunt electrical remodeling of the atrium, and several trials have evaluated their efficacy in the pericardioversion state. As single agents, diltiazem and verapamil do not appear to prevent recurrence of AF in humans.[80] However, when given for a few weeks before cardioversion and continued for a few weeks after cardioversion of AF in the setting of an antiarrhythmic agent, there appears to be a modest, synergistic benefit.[81] In large clinical trials of losartan versus atenolol for hypertension, AF was reduced in the group treated with losartan,[82] and several small trials seem to demonstrate a benefit of pericardioversion use of these agents,[83] although the results are more consistent with angiotensin receptor blockers (ARBs) than with calcium channel antagonists.[84] Inflammation is believed to play a role in recurrence of AF, although small trials of statins, which reduce C-reactive protein, have shown contradictory results.[85,86] The Gruppo Italiano per lo Studio Della Sopravvivenza nell'Infarto Miocardio–Atrial Fibrillation (GISSI-AF), the largest trial to date of valsartan compared with placebo, failed to demonstrate a reduction in recurrent episodes of AF in patients taking the ARB valsartan.[87] Thus, if the proposed effect is class specific rather than drug specific, it seems unlikely that ARBs have any role in preventing postcardioversion AF. Currently, no specific recommendations about the use of either calcium channel antagonists or angiotensin-converting enzyme (ACE) inhibitors as an adjunctive therapy can be made.

Nonpharmacologic Approaches to the Maintenance of Sinus Rhythm

The invasive approach to the management of AF is rapidly evolving. As noted above, certain antiarrhythmic agents may transform AF into atrial flutter. Advantage has been taken of this transformation, because atrial flutter may be cured by the application of a line of ablation from the tricuspid valve to the inferior vena cava. This *hybrid therapy*, defined as the conversion of AF to atrial flutter by an antiarrhythmic drug, most commonly flecainide or propafenone, with subsequent ablation of atrial flutter[88] is most commonly unplanned and is suitable for only a small minority of patients with AF in whom flutter fortuitously occurs.

Percutaneous left atrial ablation is now used widely for the attempted prevention of AF recurrence. Multiple permutations of this procedure exist, but all involve the electrical isolation of the pulmonary veins to prevent atrial premature beats from entering the left atrium and triggering the onset of AF.[89-91] Some clinicians choose to create additional linear lesions in the left atrium to impair the perpetuation of AF, should it become triggered by a nonpulmonary vein source or an incomplete pulmonary vein isolation (PVI). The optimal ablation procedure and the best choice of patient population for this procedure continue to evolve. Although relatively uncommon, the risks include pulmonary vein stenosis, pericardial tamponade, stroke, and atrial-esophageal fistula formation.[92]

This procedure is associated with a 60% to 70% rate of suppression of AF during a 12- to 24-month follow-up period.[93-96] Left atrial tachycardia, flutter, or recurrent AF is seen in the remaining patients, and these arrhythmias often require treatment that includes repeat ablation. Five years after AF ablation, the majority of patients have at least one recurrence of the arrhythmia, and the need for repeat procedures is common.[97]

Studies of arrhythmia surveillance after PVI have demonstrated significant rates of asymptomatic AF.[98] It is therefore commonly advised to continue anticoagulation in patients with clinical risk factors for stroke, irrespective of the perceived success of the PVI procedure.

The surgical correlate of the percutaneous PVI procedure is the Maze procedure. The modern Maze procedure is a series of ablations performed on the endocardial surface, most often in conjunction with a coronary artery bypass or valve operation.[99] The left atrial appendage (LAA) is generally oversewn as part of this procedure. Data on patients with preoperative AF undergoing the Maze procedure along with mitral valve surgery reported a 78% to 81% actuarial rate of sinus rhythm at 5 years compared with less than 10% in a group with mitral surgery but no Maze procedure.[100] The efficacy of this procedure has been reported to be substantially higher in patients with paroxysmal AF, and the overall efficacy will vary from center to center, as it is dependent on the experience of the surgeon and the selection of patients. The obliteration of the LAA as part of the Maze procedure carries the potential additional advantage of reducing stroke risk. Nevertheless, caution must be taken in discontinuing warfarin after this procedure, because no data confirm that the combined Maze and LAA obliteration completely abolish thromboembolic risk.

A minimally invasive variant of the Maze procedure involves the creation of lesions around the pulmonary veins through a thoracoscopic or minithoracotomy approach. The LAA can also be obliterated from the epicardial surface. This procedure is under investigation, and the long-term efficacy is awaited.

The early recurrence of AF after the surgical Maze procedure approaches 30%, but these early recurrences do not necessarily predict long-term failure of the primary procedure. To reduce short-term postoperative AF after the Maze procedure, amiodarone is often prescribed for 1 to 3 months after surgery. If AF redevelops after discontinuation of amiodarone, the procedure is recognized as unsuccessful.

Intravenous β-blockers and calcium channel blockers, such as diltiazem and verapamil, have been shown to be effective in controlling ventricular rate in postoperative patients.[150] Digoxin is generally not as effective as the calcium channel blockers or β-blockers because digoxin performs poorly in the setting of high sympathetic tone. However, digoxin may be a useful adjunctive drug for rate control, and it should certainly be considered in a patient with AF and impaired systolic ventricular function.

No trials in patients with postoperative arrhythmia have compared a strategy of restoration of sinus rhythm with anticoagulation and rate control to allow spontaneous resolution of the AF. If a patient deteriorates with the onset of AF and does not improve with rate control, electrical cardioversion should be attempted. However, the recurrent nature of postoperative AF often requires an antiarrhythmic agent to maintain sinus rhythm and prevent recurrence. Special considerations for antiarrhythmic agents in the postoperative patient include rapid shifts in electrolytes that pose a potential increased risk of TdP and depressed ventricular function that may increase other proarrhythmic effects. If LV dysfunction is present, amiodarone is considered the drug of choice if conversion to, and maintenance of, sinus rhythm is needed. In patients with normal ventricular function, ibutilide may be used to restore sinus rhythm, but it cannot be used for sinus rhythm maintenance. Sotalol may be a reasonable choice, given its β-blocking properties, although excessive bradycardia may occur with sotalol in the postoperative patient.

Conclusions

The management of AF has undergone considerable change in the past decade and will doubtlessly continue to evolve. Advances have been made in the field of anticoagulation with the release of the direct thrombin inhibitor dabigatran, which does not need constant monitoring,[133] and the development of oral factor Xa inhibitors.[151] Constant refinements are being made in ablation procedures, and new antiarrhythmic drugs are under development. It is possible that the adjunctive therapy of AF will be applied as prophylaxis in high-risk populations. With all these measures, the goal should be to reverse the increasing incidence and prevalence of this common arrhythmia and to make it easier to effectively treat patients in whom it still occurs.[152-154]

REFERENCES

1. Falk RH. Etiology and complications of atrial fibrillation: insights from pathology studies. *Am J Cardiol* 1998;82:10N-17N.
2. Gallagher MM, Camm J. Classification of atrial fibrillation. *Am J Cardiol* 1998; 82:18N-28N.
3. Van Gelder IC, Hagens VE, Bosker HA, et al. A comparison of rate control and rhythm control in patients with recurrent persistent atrial fibrillation. *N Engl J Med* 2003;347:1834-1840.
4. Carlsson J, Miketic S, Windeler J, et al. Randomized trial of rate-control versus rhythm-control in persistent atrial fibrillation: the Strategies of Treatment of Atrial Fibrillation (STAF) study. *J Am Coll Cardiol* 2003;41:1690-1696.
5. Hohnloser SH, Kuck KH. Randomized trial of rhythm or rate control in atrial fibrillation: the Pharmacological Intervention in Atrial Fibrillation Trial (PIAF). *Eur Heart J* 2001;22:801-802.
6. Wyse DG, Waldo AL, DiMarco JP, et al; Artial Fibrillation Follow-Up Investigation of Rhythm Management (AFFIRM) Investigators. A comparison of rate control and rhythm control in patients with atrial fibrillation. *N Engl J Med* 2002;347:1825-1833.
7. Corley SD, Epstein AE, DiMarco JP, et al. Relationships between sinus rhythm, treatment, and survival in the Atrial Fibrillation Follow-Up Investigation of Rhythm Management (AFFIRM) Study. *Circulation* 2004;109:1509-1513.
8. Rienstra M, Van Gelder IC, Hagens VE, et al. Mending the rhythm does not improve prognosis in patients with persistent atrial fibrillation: a subanalysis of the RACE study. *Eur Heart J* 2004;27:357-364.
9. Chung MK, Shemanski L, Sherman DG, et al. Functional status in rate- versus rhythm-control strategies for atrial fibrillation: results of the Atrial Fibrillation Follow-Up Investigation of Rhythm Management (AFFIRM) functional status substudy. *J Am Coll Cardiol* 2005;46:1891-1899.
10. Zimetbaum P. Is rate control or rhythm control preferable in patients with atrial fibrillation? An argument for maintenance of sinus rhythm in patients with atrial fibrillation. *Circulation* 2005;111:3150-3156; discussion 3156-3157.
11. Falk RH. Is rate control or rhythm control preferable in patients with atrial fibrillation? Rate control is preferable to rhythm control in the majority of patients with atrial fibrillation. *Circulation* 2005;111:3141-3150; discussion 3157.
12. Roy D, Talajic M, Nattel S, et al. Rhythm control versus rate control for atrial fibrillation and heart failure. *N Engl J Med* 2008;358:2667-2677.
13. Singh SN, Tang XC, Singh BN, et al. Quality of life and exercise performance in patients in sinus rhythm versus persistent atrial fibrillation: a Veterans Affairs Cooperative Studies Program Substudy. *J Am Coll Cardiol* 2006;48:721-730.
14. Falk RH. Atrial fibrillation or sinus rhythm? Controversy and contradiction in quality of life outcomes. *J Am Coll Cardiol* 2006;48:731-733.
15. Rawles JM, Metcalfe MJ, Jennings K. Time of occurrence, duration, and ventricular rate of paroxysmal atrial fibrillation: the effect of digoxin. *Br Heart J* 1990;63:225-227.
16. Gosselink ATM, Blanksma PK, Crijns H, et al. Left ventricular beat-to-beat performance in atrial fibrillation: contribution of Frank-Starling mechanism after short rather than long RR intervals. *J Am Coll Cardiol* 1995;26:1516-1521.
17. Hardman SMC, Noble MIM, Biggs T, Seed WA. Evidence for an influence of mechanical restitution on beat-to-beat variations in haemodynamics during chronic atrial fibrillation in patients. *Cardiovasc Res* 1998;38:82-90.
18. van den Berg MP, Hassink RJ, Tuinenburg AE, et al. Quality of life in patients with paroxysmal atrial fibrillation and its predictors: importance of the autonomic nervous system. *Eur Heart J* 2001;22:247-253.
19. Rawles JM. What is meant by a "controlled" ventricular rate in atrial fibrillation? *Br Heart J* 1990;63:157-161.
20. Olshansky B, Rosenfeld LE, Warner AL, et al. The Atrial Fibrillation Follow-up Investigation of Rhythm Management (AFFIRM) study: approaches to control rate in atrial fibrillation. *J Am Coll Cardiol* 2004;43:1201-1208.
21. Farshi R, Kistner D, Sarma JSM, Longmate JA, Singh BN. Ventricular rate control in chronic atrial fibrillation during daily activity and programmed exercise: a crossover open-label study of five drug regimens. *J Am Coll Cardiol* 1999;33:304-310.
22. Atwood JE, Sullivan M, Forbes S, et al. Effect of beta-adrenergic blockade on exercise performance in patients with chronic atrial fibrillation. *J Am Coll Cardiol* 1987;10:314-320.
23. Van Gelder IC, Groenveld HF, Crijns HJ, et al. Lenient versus strict rate control in patients with atrial fibrillation. *N Engl J Med* 2010;362:1363-1373.
24. Klein HO, Lang R, Weiss E, et al. The influence of verapamil on serum digoxin concentration. *Circulation* 1982;65:998-1003.
25. Wood MA, Brown-Mahoney C, Kay GN, Ellenbogen KA. Clinical outcomes after ablation and pacing therapy for atrial fibrillation: a meta-analysis. *Circulation* 2000;101:1138-1144.
26. Sweeney MO, Hellkamp AS, Ellenbogen KA, et al. Adverse effect of ventricular pacing on heart failure and atrial fibrillation among patients with normal baseline QRS duration in a clinical trial of pacemaker therapy for sinus node dysfunction. *Circulation* 2003;107:2932-2937.
27. Szili-Torok T, Kimman GP, Theuns D, et al. Deterioration of left ventricular function following atrio-ventricular node ablation and right ventricular apical pacing in patients with permanent atrial fibrillation. *Europace* 2002;4:61-65.
28. Poci D, Backman L, Karlsson T, Edvardsson N. New or aggravated heart failure during long-term right ventricular pacing after AV junctional catheter ablation. *Pacing Clin Electrophysiol* 2009;32:209-216.
29. Orlov MV, Gardin JM, Slawsky M, et al. Biventricular pacing improves cardiac function and prevents further left atrial remodeling in patients with symptomatic atrial fibrillation after atrioventricular node ablation. *Am Heart J* 2010;159:264-270.
30. Patel D, Natale A, Di Biase L, et al. Catheter ablation for atrial fibrillation: a promising therapy for congestive heart failure. *Expert Rev Cardiovasc Ther* 2009;7:779-787.
31. Azpitarte J, Alvarez M, Baun O, et al. Value of single oral loading dose of propafenone in converting recent-onset atrial fibrillation: results of a randomized, double-blind, controlled study. *Eur Heart J* 1997;18:1649-1654.
32. Tieleman RG, Van Gelder IC, Bosker HA, et al. Does flecainide regain its antiarrhythmic activity after electrical cardioversion of persistent atrial fibrillation? *Heart Rhythm* 2005;2:223-230.
33. Volgman AS, Carberry PA, Stambler B, et al. Conversion efficacy and safety of intravenous ibutilide compared with intravenous procainamide in patients with atrial flutter or fibrillation. *J Am Coll Cardiol* 1998;31:1414-1419.
34. Stambler BS, Wood MA, Ellenbogen KA, et al. Efficacy and safety of repeated intravenous doses of ibutilide for rapid conversion of atrial flutter or fibrillation. *Circulation* 1996;94:1613-1621.
35. Korantzopoulos P, Kolettis TM, Papathanasiou A, et al. Propafenone added to ibutilide increases conversion rates of persistent atrial fibrillation. *Heart* 2006;92:631-634.
36. Halinen MO, Huttunen M, Paakkinen S, Tarssanen L. Comparison of sotalol with digoxin-quinidine for conversion of acute atrial fibrillation to sinus rhythm (the Sotalol-Digoxin-Quinidine Trial). *Am J Cardiol* 1995;76:495-498.
37. Coplen SE, Antman EM, Berlin JA, Hewitt P, Chalmers TC. Efficacy and safety of quinidine therapy for maintenance of sinus rhythm after cardioversion: a meta-analysis of randomized control trials [published erratum, 1991;83(2):714]. *Circulation* 1990;82:1106-1116.
38. Boriani G, Biffi M, Capucci A, et al. Oral propafenone to convert recent-onset atrial fibrillation in patients with and without underlying heart disease: a randomized, controlled trial. *Ann Intern Med* 1997;126:621-625.
39. Crijns HJ, van Wijk LM, van Gilst WH, et al. Acute conversion of atrial fibrillation to sinus rhythm: clinical efficacy of flecainide acetate—comparison of two regimens. *Eur Heart J* 1988;9:634-638.
40. Khan IA. Oral loading single dose flecainide for pharmacological cardioversion of recent-onset atrial fibrillation. *Int J Cardiol* 2003;87:121-128.
41. Alboni P, Botto GL, Baldi N, et al. Outpatient treatment of recent-onset atrial fibrillation with the "pill-in-the-pocket" approach. *N Engl J Med* 2004;351:2384-2391.
42. Peuhkurinen K, Niemela M, Ylitalo A, et al. Effectiveness of amiodarone as a single oral dose for recent-onset atrial fibrillation. *Am J Cardiol* 2000;85:462-465.
43. Tieleman RG, Gosselink ATM, Crijns H, et al. Efficacy, safety, and determinants of conversion of atrial fibrillation and flutter with oral amiodarone. *Am J Cardiol* 1997;79:53-57.
44. Scholten M, Szili-Torok T, Klootwijk P, Jordaens L. Comparison of monophasic and biphasic shocks for transthoracic cardioversion of atrial fibrillation. *Heart* 2003;89:1032-1034.

45. Mittal S, Ayati S, Stein KM, et al. Transthoracic cardioversion of atrial fibrillation: comparison of rectilinear biphasic versus damped sine wave monophasic shocks. *Circulation* 2000;101:1282-1287.

46. Mathew TP, Moore A, McIntyre M, et al. Randomised comparison of electrode positions for cardioversion of atrial fibrillation. *Heart* 1999;81:576-579.

47. Chen CJ, Guo GB. External cardioversion in patients with persistent atrial fibrillation: a reappraisal of the effects of electrode pad position and transthoracic impedance on cardioversion success. *Jpn Heart J* 2003;44:921-932.

48. Siaplaouras S, Jung J, Buob A, Heisel A. Incidence and management of early recurrent atrial fibrillation (ERAF) after transthoracic electrical cardioversion. *Europace* 2004; 6:15-20.

49. Schwartzman D, Musley SK, Swerdlow C, Hoyt RH, Warman EN. Early recurrence of atrial fibrillation after ambulatory shock conversion. *J Am Coll Cardiol* 2002;40:93-99.

50. Sticherling C, Ozaydin M, Tada H, et al. Comparison of verapamil and ibutilide for the suppression of immediate recurrences of atrial fibrillation after transthoracic cardioversion. *J Cardiovasc Pharmacol Ther* 2002;7:155-160.

51. Oral H, Souza JJ, Michaud GF, et al. Facilitating transthoracic cardioversion of atrial fibrillation with ibutilide pretreatment. *N Engl J Med* 1999;340:1849-1854.

52. Cohen TJ, Ibrahim B, Denier D, Haji A, Quan WL. Active compression cardioversion for refractory atrial fibrillation. *Am J Cardiol* 1997;80:354 ff.

53. Roy D, Talajic M, Dorian P, et al. Amiodarone to prevent recurrence of atrial fibrillation. *N Engl J Med* 2000;342:913-920.

54. Crijns HJ, Van Gelder IC, Van Gilst WH, et al. Serial antiarrhythmic drug treatment to maintain sinus rhythm after electrical cardioversion for chronic atrial fibrillation or atrial flutter. *Am J Cardiol* 1991;68:335-341.

55. Roden M. Antiarrhythmic drugs: from mechanisms to clinical practice. *Heart* 2000;84: 339-346.

56. Roden DM. Pharmacogenetics and drug-induced arrhythmias. *Cardiovasc Res* 2001;50: 224-231.

57. Nattel S. The molecular and ionic specificity of antiarrhythmic drug actions. *J Cardiovasc Electrophysiol* 1999;10:272-282.

58. Falk RH. Proarrhythmia in patients treated for atrial fibrillation or flutter. *Ann Intern Med* 1992;117:141-150.

59. Roden DM. Taking the "idio" out of "idiosyncratic": predicting torsades de pointes. *Pacing Clin Electrophysiol* 1998;21:1029-1034.

60. Salata J, Jurkiewics N, Wallace A. Cardiac electrophysiologic actions of the histamine H1-receptor antagonists astemizole and terfenadine compared with chlorpheniramine and purilamine. *Circ Res* 1995;76:110-119.

61. Basta MN, Leitch JW, Fletcher PJ. Sotalol proarrhythmia: a report of five cases and an audit of the use of sotalol in a teaching hospital. *Aust N Z J Med* 1996;26:167-170.

62. Abel S, Nichols DJ, Brearley CJ, Eve MD. Effect of cimetidine and ranitidine on pharmacokinetics and pharmacodynamics of a single dose of dofetilide. *Br J Clin Pharmacol* 2000;49:64-71.

63. Stevenson WG, Weiss J. Torsades de pointes due to n-acetylprocainamide. *Pacing Clin Electrophysiol* 1985;8:528-531.

64. The Cardiac Arrhythmia Suppression Trial (CAST) Investigators. Preliminary report: effect of encainide and flecainide on mortality in a randomized trial of arrhythmia suppression after myocardial infarction. *N Engl J Med* 1989;321:406-412.

65. Crijns H, van Gelder IC, Lie KI. Supraventricular tachycardia mimicking ventricular tachycardia during flecainide treatment. *Am J Cardiol* 1988;62:1303-1306.

66. Maisel WH, Kuntz KM, Reimold SC, et al. Risk of initiating antiarrhythmic drug therapy for atrial fibrillation in patients admitted to a university hospital. *Ann Intern Med* 1997;127:281-284.

67. Hauser TH, Pinto DS, Josephson ME, Zimetbaum P. Safety and feasibility of a clinical pathway for the outpatient initiation of antiarrhythmic medications in patients with atrial fibrillation or atrial flutter. *Am J Cardiol* 2003;91:1437-1441.

68. Falk RH, DeCara JM. Dofetilide: a new pure class III antiarrhythmic agent. *Am Heart J* 2000;140:697-706.

69. Roden DM, Woosley RL, Primm RK. Incidence and clinical features of the quinidine-associated long QT syndrome: implications for patient care. *Am Heart J* 1986;111: 1088-1093.

70. Patten M, Maas R, Bauer P, et al. Suppression of paroxysmal atrial tachyarrhythmias—results of the SOPAT trial. *Eur Heart J* 2004;1395-1404.

71. Fetsch T, Bauer P, Engberding R, et al. Prevention of atrial fibrillation after cardioversion: results of the PAFAC trial. *Eur Heart J* 2004;25:1385-1394.

72. Kochiadakis GE, Igoumenidis NE, Parthenakis FI, Chlouverakis GI, Vardas PE. Amiodarone versus propafenone for conversion of chronic atrial fibrillation: results of a randomized, controlled study. *J Am Coll Cardiol* 1999;33:966-971.

73. Hohnloser SH, Klingenheben T, Singh BN. Amiodarone-associated proarrhythmic effects: a review with special reference to torsades de pointes tachycardia. *Ann Intern Med* 1994;121:529-535.

74. Piccini JP, Hasselblad V, Peterson ED, et al. Comparative efficacy of dronedarone and amiodarone for the maintenance of sinus rhythm in patients with atrial fibrillation. *J Am Coll Cardiol* 2009;54:1089-1095.

75. Køber L, Torp-Pedersen C, McMurray JJV, et al; Dronedarone Study Group. Increased mortality after dronedarone therapy for severe heart failure. *N Engl J Med* 2008;358: 2678-2687.

76. Hohnloser SH, Crijns HJ, van Eickels M, et al. Effect of dronedarone on cardiovascular events in atrial fibrillation. *N Engl J Med* 2009;360:668-678.

77. Falk RH, Camm AJ. Rethinking the reasons to treat atrial fibrillation? The role of dronedarone in reducing cardiovascular hospitalizations. *Eur Heart J* 2009;30:2438-2440.

78. Connolly SJ, Crijns HJ, Torp-Pedersen C, et al. Analysis of stroke in ATHENA: a placebo-controlled, double-blind, parallel-arm trial to assess the efficacy of dronedarone 400 mg BID for the prevention of cardiovascular hospitalization or death from any cause in patients with atrial fibrillation/atrial flutter. *Circulation* 2009;120:1174-1180.

79. Fuster V, Ryden LE, Asinger RW, et al. ACC/AHA/ESC Guidelines for the Management of Patients with Atrial Fibrillation: executive summary. A report of the American College of Cardiology/American Heart Association Task Force on Practice Guidelines and the European Society of Cardiology Committee for Practice Guidelines and Policy Conferences (Committee to Develop Guidelines for the Management of Patients with Atrial Fibrillation): developed in collaboration with the North American Society of Pacing and Electrophysiology. *J Am Coll Cardiol* 2001;38:1231-1266.

80. Van Noord T, Van Gelder IC, Tieleman RG, et al. VERDICT: the verapamil versus digoxin cardioversion trial—a randomized study on the role of calcium lowering for maintenance of sinus rhythm after cardioversion of persistent atrial fibrillation. *J Cardiovasc Electrophysiol* 2001;12:766-769.

81. De Simone A, De Pasquale M, De Matteis C, et al. Verapamil plus antiarrhythmic drugs reduce atrial fibrillation recurrences after an electrical cardioversion (VEPARAF Study). *Eur Heart J* 2003;24:1425-1429.

82. Wachtell K, Lehto M, Gerdts E, et al. Angiotensin II receptor blockade reduces new-onset atrial fibrillation and subsequent stroke compared to atenolol: the Losartan Intervention For End Point Reduction in Hypertension (LIFE) study. *J Am Coll Cardiol* 2005;45: 712-719.

83. Madrid AH, Bueno MG, Rebollo JM, et al. Use of irbesartan to maintain sinus rhythm in patients with long-lasting persistent atrial fibrillation: a prospective and randomized study. *Circulation* 2002;106:331-336.

84. Lindholm CJ, Fredholm O, Moller SJ, et al. Sinus rhythm maintenance following DC cardioversion of atrial fibrillation is not improved by temporary precardioversion treatment with oral verapamil. *Heart* 2004;90:534-538.

85. Ozaydin M, Varol E, Aslan SM, et al. Effect of atorvastatin on the recurrence rates of atrial fibrillation after electrical cardioversion. *Am J Cardiol* 2006;97:1490-1493.

86. Almroth H, Hoglund N, Boman K, et al. Atorvastatin and persistent atrial fibrillation following cardioversion: a randomized placebo-controlled multicentre study. *Eur Heart J* 2009;30:827-833.

87. Disertori M, Latini R, Barlera S, et al. Valsartan for prevention of recurrent atrial fibrillation. *N Engl J Med* 2009;360:1606-1617.

88. Huang DT, Monahan KM, Zimetbaum P, et al. Hybrid pharmacologic and ablative therapy: a novel and effective approach for the management of atrial fibrillation. *J Cardiovasc Electrophysiol* 1998;9:462-469.

89. Jais P, Sanders P, Hsu LF, Hocini M, Haissaguerre M. Catheter ablation for atrial fibrillation. *Heart* 2005;91:7-9.

90. Takahashi Y, Rotter M, Sanders P, et al. Left atrial linear ablation to modify the substrate of atrial fibrillation using a new nonfluoroscopic imaging system. *Pacing Clin Electrophysiol* 2005;28(Suppl 1):S90-S93.

91. Shah DC, Haissaguerre M, Jais P. Current perspectives on curative catheter ablation of atrial fibrillation. *Heart* 2002;87:6-8.

92. Pappone C, Oral H, Santinelli V, et al. Atrio-esophageal fistula as a complication of percutaneous transcatheter ablation of atrial fibrillation. *Circulation* 2004;109:2724-2726.

93. Hsieh MH, Tai CT, Lee SH, et al. Catheter ablation of atrial fibrillation versus atrioventricular junction ablation plus pacing therapy for elderly patients with medically refractory paroxysmal atrial fibrillation. *J Cardiovasc Electrophysiol* 2005;16:457-461.

94. Bourke JP, Dunuwille A, O'Donnell D, Jamieson S, Furniss SS. Pulmonary vein ablation for idiopathic atrial fibrillation: six month outcome of first procedure in 100 consecutive patients. *Heart* 2005;91:51-57.

95. Wazni OM, Marrouche NF, Martin DO, et al. Radiofrequency ablation vs antiarrhythmic drugs as first-line treatment of symptomatic atrial fibrillation: a randomized trial. *JAMA* 2005;293:2634-2640.

96. Hsieh MH, Tai CT, Tsai CF, et al. Clinical outcome of very late recurrence of atrial fibrillation after catheter ablation of paroxysmal atrial fibrillation. *J Cardiovasc Electrophysiol* 2003;14:598-601.

97. Weerasooriya R, Khairy P, Litalien J, et al. Catheter ablation for atrial fibrillation: are results maintained at 5 years of follow-up? *J Am Coll Cardiol* 2011;57:160-166.

98. Senatore G, Stabile G, Bertaglia E, et al. Role of transtelephonic electrocardiographic monitoring in detecting short-term arrhythmia recurrences after radiofrequency ablation in patients with atrial fibrillation. *J Am Coll Cardiol* 2005;45:873-876.

99. Nitta T. Surgery for atrial fibrillation. *Ann Thorac Cardiovasc Surg* 2005;11:154-158.

100. Bando K, Kobayashi J, Kosakai Y, et al. Impact of Cox maze procedure on outcome in patients with atrial fibrillation and mitral valve disease. *J Thorac Cardiovasc Surg* 2002;124:575-583.

101. Lamas GA, Lee KL, Sweeney MO, et al. Ventricular pacing or dual-chamber pacing for sinus-node dysfunction. *N Engl J Med* 2002;346:1854-1862.

102. Maisel WH, Epstein AE; American College of Chest Physicians. The role of cardiac pacing: American College of Chest Physicians Guidelines for the Prevention and Management of Postoperative Atrial Fibrillation after Cardiac Surgery. *Chest* 2005;128(2 Suppl):36S-38S.

103. Archbold RA, Schilling RJ. Atrial pacing for the prevention of atrial fibrillation after coronary artery bypass graft surgery: a review of the literature. *Heart* 2004;90:129-133.

104. Wolf PA, Abbott RD, Kannel WB. Atrial fibrillation: a major contributor to stroke in the elderly. The Framingham Study. *Arch Int Med* 1987;147:1561-1564.

105. Lin HJ, Wolf PA, Kellyhayes M, et al. Stroke severity in atrial fibrillation: the Framingham Study. *Stroke* 1996;27:1760-1764.

106. Lamassa M, Di Carlo AA, Pracucci G, et al. Characteristics, outcome, and care of stroke associated with atrial fibrillation in Europe: data from a multicenter multinational hospital-based registry (The European Community Stroke Project). *Stroke* 2001;32: 392-398.

107. The Boston Area Anticoagulation Trial for Atrial Fibrillation Investigators. The effect of low-dose warfarin on the risk of stroke in patients with nonrheumatic atrial fibrillation. *N Engl J Med* 1990;323:1505-1511.

108. The Stroke Prevention in Atrial Fibrillation Investigators. Stroke Prevention in Atrial Fibrillation Study: final results. *Circulation* 1991;84:527-539.

109. Ezekowitz MD, Bridgers SL, James KE, et al; Veterans Affairs Stroke Prevention in Nonrheumatic Atrial Fibrillation Investigators. Warfarin in the prevention of stroke associated with nonrheumatic atrial fibrillation. *N Engl J Med* 1992;327:1406-1412.

110. European Atrial Fibrillation Trial Study Group. Secondary prevention in non-rheumatic atrial fibrillation after transient ischaemic attack or minor stroke. *Lancet* 1993;342: 1255-1262.

111. McBride R, Chesebro JH, Wiebers DO, et al. Warfarin versus aspirin for prevention of thromboembolism in atrial fibrillation: Stroke Prevention in Atrial Fibrillation II Study. *Lancet* 1994;343:687-691.

112. Connolly SJ, Laupacis A, Gent M, et al. Canadian Atrial Fibrillation Anticoagulation (CAFA) Study. *J Am Coll Cardiol* 1991;18:349-355.

113. Blackshear JL, Baker VS, Rubino F, et al. Adjusted-dose warfarin versus low-intensity, fixed-dose warfarin plus aspirin for high-risk patients with atrial fibrillation: Stroke Prevention in Atrial Fibrillation III randomised clinical trial. *Lancet* 1996;348:633-638.

114. Gullov AL, Koefoed BG, Petersen P, et al. Fixed minidose warfarin and aspirin alone and in combination vs adjusted-dose warfarin for stroke prevention in atrial fibrillation: Second Copenhagen Atrial Fibrillation, Aspirin, and Anticoagulation Study. *Arch Int Med* 1998;158:1513-1521.

115. Albers GW. Atrial fibrillation and stroke: three new studies, three remaining questions. *Arch Int Med* 1994;154:1443-1448.

116. Go AS, Hylek EM, Phillips KA, et al. Implications of stroke risk criteria on the anticoagulation decision in nonvalvular atrial fibrillation: the anticoagulation and risk factors in atrial fibrillation (ATRIA) study. *Circulation* 2000;102:11-13.

117. Gage BF, Waterman AD, Shannon W, et al. Validation of clinical classification schemes for predicting stroke: results from the National Registry of Atrial Fibrillation. *JAMA* 2001;285:2864-2870.

118. Hart RG, Halperin JL, Pearce LA, et al. Lessons from the Stroke Prevention in Atrial Fibrillation trials. *Ann Intern Med* 2003;138:831-838.

119. Zabalgoitia M, Halperin JL, Pearce LA, et al. Transesophageal echocardiographic correlates of clinical risk of thromboembolism in nonvalvular atrial fibrillation. *J Am Coll Cardiol* 1998;31:1622-1626.

120. Labovitz AJ, Bransford TL. Evolving role of echocardiography in the management of atrial fibrillation. *Am Heart J* 2001;141:518-527.

121. Gage BF, van Walraven C, Pearce L, et al. Selecting patients with atrial fibrillation for anticoagulation: stroke risk stratification in patients taking aspirin. *Circulation* 2004;110:2287-2292.

122. van Walraven C, Hart RG, Singer DE, et al. Oral anticoagulants vs aspirin in nonvalvular atrial fibrillation: an individual patient meta-analysis. *JAMA* 2002;288:2441-2448.

123. Cleland JG, Kaye GC. Long term anticoagulation or antiplatelet treatment: only warfarin has been shown to reduce stroke risk in patients with atrial fibrillation. *Br Med J* 2001;323:233; discussion 235-236.

124. Connolly SJ, Pogue J, Hart RG, et al. Effect of clopidogrel added to aspirin in patients with atrial fibrillation. *N Engl J Med* 2009;360:2066-2078.

125. Palareti G, Leali N, Coccheri S, et al. Bleeding complications of oral anticoagulant treatment: an Inception-Cohort, Prospective Collaborative Study (Iscoat). *Lancet* 1996;348:423-428.

126. Gullov AL, Koefoed BG, Petersen P. Bleeding during warfarin and aspirin therapy in patients with atrial fibrillation: the AFASAK 2 Study. *Arch Int Med* 1999;159:1322-1328.

127. Torn M, van der Meer FJ, Rosendaal FR. Lowering the intensity of oral anticoagulant therapy: effects on the risk of hemorrhage and thromboembolism. *Arch Int Med* 2004;164:668-673.

128. Lip GY, Frison L, Halperin JL, Lane DA. Comparative validation of a novel risk score for predicting bleeding risk in anticoagulated patients with atrial fibrillation: the HAS-BLED (Hypertension, Abnormal Renal/Liver Function, Stroke, Bleeding History or Predisposition, Labile INR, Elderly, Drugs/Alcohol Concomitantly) score. *J Am Coll Cardiol* 2011;57:173-180.

129. Gage BF, Yan Y, Milligan PE, et al. Clinical classification schemes for predicting hemorrhage: results from the National Registry of Atrial Fibrillation (NRAF). *Am Heart J* 2006;151:713-719.

130. Johnston JA, Cluxton RJ Jr, Heaton PC, et al. Predictors of warfarin use among Ohio medicaid patients with new-onset nonvalvular atrial fibrillation. *Arch Int Med* 2003;163:1705-1710.

131. Guo GBF, Chang HW, Chen MC, Yang CH. Underutilization of anticoagulation therapy in chronic atrial fibrillation. *Jpn Heart J* 2001;42:55-65.

132. Cohen N, Almoznino-Sarafian D, Alon I, et al. Warfarin for stroke prevention still underused in atrial fibrillation: patterns of omission. *Stroke* 2000;31:1217-1222.

133. Connolly SJ, Ezekowitz MD, Yusuf S, et al. Dabigatran versus warfarin in patients with atrial fibrillation. *N Engl J Med* 2009;361:1139-1151.

134. Nagarakanti R, Ezekowitz MD, Oldgren J, et al. Dabigatran versus warfarin in patients with atrial fibrillation: an analysis of patients undergoing cardioversion. *Circulation* 2011;123:131-136.

135. Patel M, Mahaffey K, Garg J, et al. Rivaroxaban versus warfarin in nonvalvular atrial fibrillation. *N Engl J Med* 2011;365:883-891.

136. Granger CC, Alexander J, McMurray J, et al; ARISTOTLE Committee and Investigators. Apixaban versus warfarin in patients with atrial fibrillation. *N Engl J Med* 2011;365:981-992.

137. Khan IA. Atrial stunning: determinants and cellular mechanisms. *Am Heart J* 2003;145:787-794.

138. Pollak A, Falk RH. Aggravation of postcardioversion atrial dysfunction by sotalol. *J Am Coll Cardiol* 1995;25:665-671.

139. Klein AL, Murray RD, Grimm RA. Role of transesophageal echocardiography-guided cardioversion of patients with atrial fibrillation. *J Am Coll Cardiol* 2001;37:691-704.

140. Singer DE, Albers GW, Dalen JE, et al. Antithrombotic therapy in atrial fibrillation: the Seventh ACCP Conference on Antithrombotic and Thrombolytic Therapy. *Chest* 2004;126:429S-456S.

141. Jasper SE, Lieber EA, Murray RD, et al. Impact of cardioversion strategy on functional capacity in patients with atrial fibrillation: the Assessment of Cardioversion Using Transesophageal Echocardiography (ACUTE) study. *Am Heart J* 2005;149:309-315.

142. Klein AL, Murray RD, Becker ER, et al. Economic analysis of a transesophageal echocardiography-guided approach to cardioversion of patients with atrial fibrillation: the ACUTE economic data at eight weeks. *J Am Coll Cardiol* 2004;43:1217-1224.

143. Asher CR, Klein AL. The ACUTE trial: transesophageal echocardiography to guide electrical cardioversion in atrial fibrillation:—assessment of cardioversion using transesophageal echocardiography. *Cleve Clin J Med* 2002;69:713-718.

144. Bradley D, Creswell LL, Hogue CW Jr, et al. Pharmacologic prophylaxis: American College of Chest Physicians guidelines for the prevention and management of postoperative atrial fibrillation after cardiac surgery. *Chest* 2005;128:39S-47S.

145. Aasbo JD, Lawrence AT, Krishnan K, Kim MH, Trohman RG. Amiodarone prophylaxis reduces major cardiovascular morbidity and length of stay after cardiac surgery: a meta-analysis. *Ann Intern Med* 2005;143:327-336.

146. Daoud EG, Strickberger SA, Man KC, et al. Preoperative amiodarone as prophylaxis against atrial fibrillation after heart surgery. *N Engl J Med* 1997;337:1785-1791.

147. Song YB, On YK, Kim JH, et al. The effects of atorvastatin on the occurrence of postoperative atrial fibrillation after off-pump coronary artery bypass grafting surgery. *Am Heart J* 2008;156:373.e9-373.e16.

148. Patti G, Chello M, Candura D, et al. Randomized trial of atorvastatin for reduction of postoperative atrial fibrillation in patients undergoing cardiac surgery: results of the ARMYDA-3 (Atorvastatin for Reduction of MYocardial Dysrhythmia After cardiac surgery) study. *Circulation* 2006;114:1455-1461.

149. Epstein AE, Alexander JC, Gutterman, DD, Maisel W, Wharton JM; American College of Chest Physicians. Anticoagulation: American College of Chest Physicians guidelines for the prevention and management of postoperative atrial fibrillation after cardiac surgery. *Chest* 2005;128(2 Suppl):24S-27S.

150. Martinez EA, Epstein AE, Bass EB. Pharmacologic control of ventricular rate: American College of Chest Physicians guidelines for the prevention and management of postoperative atrial fibrillation after cardiac surgery. *Chest* 2005;128:56S-60S.

151. Schirmer SH, Baumhakel M, Neuberger HR, et al. Novel anticoagulants for stroke prevention in atrial fibrillation: current clinical evidence and future developments. *J Am Coll Cardiol* 2010;56:2067-2076.

152. Wattigney WA, Mensah GA, Croft JB. Increased atrial fibrillation mortality: United States, 1980-1998. *Am J Epidemiol* 2002;155:819-826.

153. De Caterina R, Connolly SJ, Pogue J, et al. Mortality predictors and effects of antithrombotic therapies in atrial fibrillation: insights from ACTIVE-W. *Eur Heart J* 2010;31:2133-2140.

154. Asbach S, Olschewski M, Faber TS, et al. Mortality in patients with atrial fibrillation has significantly decreased during the last three decades: 35 years of follow-up in 1627 pacemaker patients. *Europace* 2008;10:391-394.

CHAPTER 21

Nonpharmacologic Treatment of Tachyarrhythmias

David J. Callans and Elad Anter

CATHETER ABLATION FOR THE TREATMENT OF TACHYARRHYTHMIAS, 383

PRACTICAL CONSIDERATIONS, 383

CATHETER ABLATION BY SPECIFIC ARRHYTHMIA SYNDROME, 383

Catheter Ablation for Supraventricular Tachyarrhythmias, 383

ATRIAL FIBRILLATION, 386

ATRIOVENTRICULAR JUNCTION ABLATION FOR VENTRICULAR RATE CONTROL, 390

Catheter Ablation for Ventricular Tachyarrhythmias, 390

SUMMARY, 392

REFERENCES, 392

For many arrhythmia syndromes, catheter ablation has replaced pharmacologic therapy. Multicenter studies over the past 3 decades have demonstrated disappointing efficacy, frequent nuisance, and even life-threatening side effects of antiarrhythmic drug therapy, particularly in patients with structural heart disease.[1-3] Antiarrhythmic drugs are still used as part of a rhythm control strategy for atrial fibrillation (AF) and for the reduction of implantable cardioverter-defibrillator (ICD) shocks in patients with these devices. For most other syndromes, catheter ablation has become the first-line treatment in patients with significant symptoms (Box 21-1).

This chapter provides an arrhythmia-specific overview of the available techniques, current efficacy, procedural side effects, and future considerations of nonpharmacologic therapy. Although broadly speaking, this topic could well include a discussion of surgical ablation and pacing therapy, the predominant focus is on catheter ablation. Discussion of the use of implantable electrical devices for the management of sudden cardiac death (SCD) is found in Chapter 22.

Catheter Ablation for the Treatment of Tachyarrhythmias

The results of catheter ablation are syndrome specific. Although it can be curative for many paroxysmal supraventricular arrhythmias, catheter ablation is largely palliative for ventricular tachycardia (VT) in the setting of structural heart disease and is rapidly evolving as a method for treatment of AF (Table 21-1). Cost, efficacy, and patient preference are important considerations in determining the role of catheter ablation versus drug therapy in specific arrhythmia syndromes.

Practical Considerations

The general principle of ablation therapy, either surgical or catheter based, involves the selective destruction of a "vulnerable parameter" of the tachycardia circuit. Depending on the arrhythmia, this parameter can be identified electrophysiologically (e.g., bypass tract) or anatomically (e.g., slow pathway). Catheter positioning at this critical component is achieved based on electrical recording and fluoroscopic, echocardiographic, and/or magnetic resonance imaging (MRI) information, often in conjunction with three-dimensional (3D) electroanatomic mapping data. Ablation is performed by delivery of some form of energy to the tip of the catheter, resulting in focal destruction of the myocardium. Alternative energy sources—such as cryothermy, microwave, high-frequency ultrasound, and laser—are available for specific indications, but radiofrequency energy is the workhorse of catheter ablation at present because of its excellent efficacy and safety profiles. Radiofrequency energy damages tissue by resistive heating

in the myocardium directly in contact with the distal catheter electrode.[4] Irreversible tissue death occurs at temperatures in excess of 50° C.[5] Radiofrequency lesions are homogeneous and precise, with necrotic centers 5 to 6 mm in diameter and 2 to 3 mm deep, surrounded by a hemorrhagic periphery (Figure 21-1).[6] Two biophysical considerations fundamentally limit the size of radiofrequency lesions: first, heat transmission diminishes by distance from the energy source to the fourth power and, second, temperatures greater than 100° C at the catheter/myocardial surface interface lead to coagulum and gas bubble formation that prevents subsequent current delivery. Although this is a fundamental limitation, the development of new ablation catheters—such as irrigated-tip radiofrequency ablation (RFA) devices, which allow for the production of larger and deeper lesions—is helpful in selected applications, particularly for VT in the setting of healed myocardial infarction (MI).

Catheter Ablation by Specific Arrhythmia Syndrome

Catheter ablation therapy for most paroxysmal supraventricular arrhythmias is safe, cost effective, and virtually curative. The success rate of catheter ablation for AF is more variable and depends on its paroxysmal or persistent nature (see Table 21-1).

Catheter Ablation for Supraventricular Tachyarrhythmias

ACCESSORY PATHWAY–MEDIATED TACHYCARDIAS

Accessory pathways are microscopic muscular bundles that connect the atrium and ventricle, providing a "bypass" of the normal conduction system. Manifest pathways, those capable of antegrade conduction, are present in the Wolff-Parkinson-White (WPW) syndrome. Concealed pathways are not apparent on the surface electrocardiogram (ECG) but can still mediate reentry. Most symptomatic arrhythmias in patients with accessory bypass tracts are associated with a narrow QRS complex—that is, *orthodromic supraventricular tachycardia*, conducted antegrade through the atrioventricular (AV) node and retrograde through the bypass tract. Less frequently, *circus movement tachycardia* occurs in the reverse order: the bypass tract serves as the anterograde limb of the reentrant circuit. The QRS complex during this tachycardia is fully preexcited, resulting in a wide QRS, or *antidromic supraventricular tachycardia*. Importantly, in patients with AF, rapid antegrade conduction over the accessory pathway can lead to ventricular fibrillation (VF) and cardiac arrest (estimated annual risk, 0.05% to 0.5%).[7]

The target for ablation in accessory pathway–mediated reentry is the accessory pathway itself (Figure 21-2). The AV node is

Box 21-1 Indications for Catheter Ablation

First-Line Therapy in Symptomatic Patients
Accessory pathways
AV node reentry
Atrial flutter
Idiopathic VT

Potentially Helpful in Patients with Symptoms Despite Pharmacologic Therapy
Atrial tachycardia
Atrial fibrillation
VT in structural heart disease
Anatomic ablation of poorly tolerated VT
AV junction ablation for rate control of AF
Inappropriate sinus tachycardia

AF, atrial fibrillation; AV, atrioventricular; VT, ventricular tachycardia.

TABLE 21-1	Success Rates for Catheter Ablation at Referral Centers	
TACHYARRHYTHMIA	**SUCCESS (%)**
SVT	
Accessory pathway mediated	>90
Atrioventricular nodal reentry	>97
Atrial tachycardia	>80
Atrial flutter	>90
Paroxysmal atrial fibrillation	>75
Atrioventricular junction ablation	>97
VT	
Idiopathic VT	>85
VT in structural heart disease	>70

SVT, supraventricular tachycardia; VT, ventricular tachycardia.

another vulnerable site, but its ablation may ultimately necessitate pacemaker therapy if antegrade bypass tract conduction fails, a phenomenon that can occur in up to 20% of patients. Accessory pathways can occur at any location along the tricuspid and mitral annulus, except between the left and right fibrous trigones, where the left atrial myocardium is not in direct juxtaposition with the left ventricular (LV) myocardium, the region of the aortomitral continuity. The distribution of bypass tracts along the AV groove is not homogenous: 46% to 60% of bypass tracts are found within the left free wall space; 25% are within the posteroseptal space; 13% to 21% are within the right free wall space; and 2% are within the right superoparaseptal (formerly called the *anteroseptal*) space.[8] Right-sided pathways are ablated by a venous approach, typically at the atrial insertion of the pathway. Left-sided pathways are ablated either by a retrograde aortic approach or a transseptal approach to the left atrium.[9,10] A small percentage of posterior septal accessory pathways can be successfully ablated with a catheter positioned within the proximal coronary sinus, often within the middle cardiac vein or within a venous malformation.[11]

Ablation is a highly effective and curative therapy (>90%) for accessory pathway–mediated tachycardia. Acute success is usually persistent, and late recurrence of bypass tract conduction after ablation is rare (4%), typically observed during the first month after ablation. In a contemporary survey of 6065 patients undergoing ablation of an accessory pathway between 1997 and 2002, the long-term success rate was 98%, and a repeat procedure was necessary in 2.2% of cases.[12] Serious complications—cardiac tamponade, AV block, coronary artery injury, or stroke—occurred in 0.6% of patients, with one fatality (0.02%). The highly favorable risk/benefit ratio justifies the use of catheter ablation as first-line

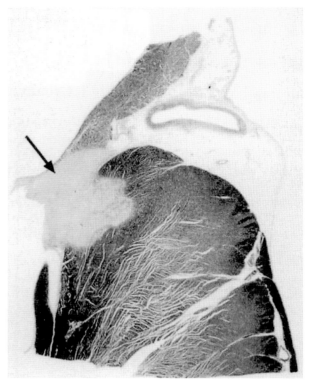

FIGURE 21-1 Histology of radiofrequency ablation lesion. The atrioventricular (AV) junction is seen (atrial wall is superior, coronary artery is seen in the AV groove) with an ablation lesion (*arrow*) at the annulus. Note the homogeneous nature of the lesion. *(From Morady F. Radio-frequency ablation as treatment for cardiac arrhythmias. N Engl J Med 1999; 340:535.)*

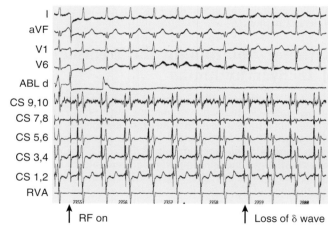

FIGURE 21-2 Surface electrocardiogram (leads I, aVF, V1, V6) and intracardiac electrograms during ablation of accessory pathway with antegrade conduction. Note the presence of preexcitation and short PR interval on the surface leads on the left side of the tracing (start of radiofrequency [RF] application). After seven QRS complexes, the PR interval increases, and preexcitation (delta wave) is lost. CS, coronary sinus catheter; ABL d, distal ablation catheter; RVA, right ventricular apical catheter.

therapy for any patient with accessory pathway–dependent tachycardia that requires treatment. This is particularly true for young patients who want to avoid long-term pharmacologic therapy.

Treatment of asymptomatic patients with incidentally detected accessory pathways is controversial. Most patients with asymptomatic preexcitation have a good prognosis; cardiac arrest is rarely the first manifestation of the disease. Prior studies have reported that approximately 20% of asymptomatic patients will demonstrate a rapid ventricular rate, but in AF, that is induced during electrophysiology (EP) testing. However, during clinical follow-up, few patients developed symptomatic arrhythmias, and none had cardiac arrest.[13] An EP study can be useful to risk stratify patients with asymptomatic preexcitation.[14] One study reported the follow-up of 212 patients with asymptomatic preexcitation, all of whom underwent a baseline EP study. After a mean follow-up of 38 months, 33 patients became symptomatic; 3 of these patients had VF, and 1 died. The most important factors in predicting outcome were the inducibility of AF during the study and the short bypass tract anterograde refractory period. Despite this study, the positive predictive value of invasive EP testing is considered to be too low to justify routine use in asymptomatic patients.[13] The decision to risk stratify patients and possibly ablate pathways in asymptomatic individuals with high-risk occupations—such as school bus drivers, pilots, and scuba divers—is made on the basis of individual clinical considerations.[13]

ATRIOVENTRICULAR NODE REENTRY

The most common mechanism of paroxysmal supraventricular tachycardia (PSVT) is atrioventricular node reentrant tachycardia (AVNRT). The slow pathway is the vulnerable parameter in AVNRT, and radiofrequency energy is applied at the posteroseptal right atrial sites near the ostium of the coronary sinus (Figure 21-3). In a survey of a pooled sample of 8230 patients with AVNRT who underwent ablation between 1997 and 2002, the long-term success rate for AVNRT elimination was 99%.[12] A repeat ablation procedure was necessary in 1.3% of patients, and high-grade AV block that required implantation of a pacemaker occurred in 0.4% of patients. These results confirm the highly favorable risk/benefit ratio of radiofrequency slow pathway ablation.

AVNRT is not a life-threatening arrhythmia, but many patients have bothersome symptoms of tachycardia. Because of a very favorable risk/benefit ratio, radiofrequency catheter ablation of AVNRT has become the treatment of choice for most symptomatic patients. Many patients elect to undergo catheter ablation as first-line therapy to avoid the need for antiarrhythmic drug therapy. A cost analysis study demonstrated that catheter ablation improved quality-adjusted survival and resulted in cost savings over pharmacologic therapy in symptomatic patients with AVNRT.[15]

ATRIAL TACHYCARDIA

Atrial tachycardias may be focal or *macroreentrant* (also known as *atrial flutter*). *Focal atrial tachycardia* is characterized by centrifugal spread of activation away from the site of origin and most commonly arises in the right atrium along the crista terminalis, near the tricuspid annulus, or near the coronary sinus ostium.[16,17] Approximately 5% of focal atrial tachycardias arise in the left atrium, commonly along the mitral annulus.[18] Experience gained during catheter ablation of AF revealed that focal tachycardias can also arise in the pulmonary veins,[19] the superior vena cava,[20] the vein of Marshall,[21] or other atrial sites. Targets for ablation of focal atrial tachycardias are identified by the site of earliest activation, or activation mapping, or by pacemapping. Because focal atrial tachycardias are relatively uncommon, literature that describes results of catheter ablation is limited. In seven studies that included a total of 112 patients with focal atrial tachycardia, the short-term success rate of RFA was approximately 90%, with 7% late recurrence and no major complications.[22-28] However, these success rates may overestimate the true efficacy of catheter ablation for focal atrial tachycardia, as these patients had uncomplicated diagnostic studies and reproducible atrial tachycardia amenable for mapping. Nonetheless, these studies did not use either a 3D mapping system or a cooled-tip ablation catheter, both of which are widely available today. With these advanced mapping tools, and with ablation catheters capable of creating larger lesions, clinical failures are more often related to the emergence of new foci rather than the inability to ablate a particular tachycardia.

Given the high probability of successful ablation and the low risk of serious complications, it is appropriate to consider the option of catheter ablation for any patient with a clinically significant atrial tachycardia that requires therapy. However, pharmacologic therapy is more appropriate if multiple atrial foci are present. In these patients, even if all the atrial tachycardia foci are mapped and ablated, new foci may emerge later. In older patients with multifocal atrial tachycardia who are highly symptomatic and drug

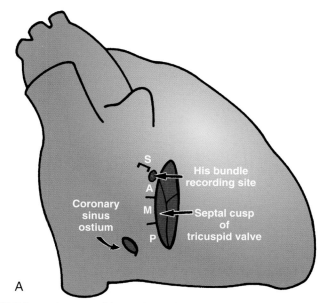
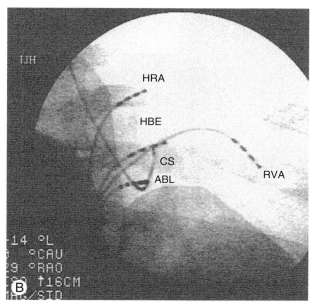

FIGURE 21-3 Anatomy of slow-pathway ablation. **A,** Schematic of the atrioventricular junction in the right atrium. The slow pathway is usually ablated just anterior to the coronary sinus ostium at the posterior septal isthmus. S, septum; A, anterior septal isthmus; M, midseptal isthmus; P, posterior septal isthmus. **B,** Right anterior oblique fluoroscopic view of the ablation catheter location. HRA, high right atrial catheter; HBE, His bundle catheter; CS, coronary sinus catheter; ABL, ablation catheter; RVA, right ventricular catheter. *(Modified from Jazayeri MR, Hempe SL, Sra JS, et al. Selective transcatheter ablation of the fast and slow pathways using radiofrequency energy in patients with atrioventricular nodal reentrant tachycardia.* Circulation *1992;85:1318-1328.)*

refractory, AV node ablation and pacemaker insertion may be more appropriate.

Inappropriate sinus tachycardia is a nonparoxysmal tachyarrhythmia characterized by a persistent increase in resting sinus rate unrelated to, or out of proportion with, the level of physical, emotional, pathologic, or pharmacologic stress. These patients also exhibit an exaggerated heart rate response to minimal exertion.[29] Sinus node modification targets the site of most rapid discharge, generally at the superior aspect of the crista terminalis. RFA is at best an only modestly effective technique for managing patients with inappropriate sinus tachycardia, and long-term success rate ranges between 23% and 83%.[30]

ATRIAL FLUTTER

Isthmus-Dependent Atrial Flutter

The most common type of atrial flutter is isthmus-dependent atrial flutter, in which the reentry circuit is confined to the right atrium, between the tricuspid annulus and the inferior vena cava, with the wavefront progressing either in a counterclockwise or clockwise direction across the cavotricuspid isthmus. This isthmus forms the vulnerable parameter of the circuit and is the target for ablation.[31] Strategies for ablation have evolved in terms of procedural endpoint, from termination of atrial flutter to durable bidirectional block (Figure 21-4), and technology that includes 4 mm to larger or irrigated RFA. In a randomized study that compared the 8-mm tip and irrigated-tip catheters, complete isthmus block was achieved in 99 of 100 patients, with equal efficacy between the two catheters.[32] Early recurrence is unusual, although not well studied, in contemporary series, and complications are virtually absent. In light of the high efficacy and safety of RFA for isthmus-dependent atrial flutter, catheter ablation is an appropriate therapeutic option for drug-refractory patients and for those who prefer curative therapy over pharmacologic therapy. An important disadvantage to an ablation strategy for atrial flutter is the high incidence of AF in intermediate-term follow-up.

Other Atrial Flutters

Atypical atrial flutters—that is, noncavotriscuspid isthmus-dependent flutters—are relatively uncommon and are usually related to atrial scarring (i.e., idiopathic or secondary to surgical incisions or incomplete ablation lines); it is increasingly seen after ablation of AF. The most frequent locations of right atrial ablation lines used to treat incisional flutters are between a lateral atriotomy scar and the inferior vena cava, superior vena cava, or tricuspid annulus.[33,34] Success rates ranging between 80% and 85% were reported in early studies that did not use 3D mapping systems. A more contemporary study incorporated electroanatomic mapping and demonstrated that macroreentrant right atrial tachycardias often use relatively narrow channels between scars.[35] Detailed voltage mapping has allowed identifications of these channels and elimination of the tachycardia with only a few applications of radiofrequency energy.[35] Left atrial flutters may be a proarrhythmic complication of heart surgery, such as mitral valve surgery or a Maze procedure,[36] or left atrial catheter ablation may be a proarrhythmic complication of AF.[37-39] Many of these left atrial flutters use the isthmus between the mitral annulus and the left inferior pulmonary vein; hence, this is usually the target of ablation. In a series of 78 patients who underwent RFA of left atrial arrhythmias that occurred after pulmonary vein isolation (PVI), catheter ablation was successful in 85% of patients. After a mean follow-up of 1 year, 77% of patients were free of atrial arrhythmias without antiarrhythmic medications.[40] Atrial arrhythmias that occur after RFA for AF are often persistent, difficult to suppress with rhythm control medications, and associated with rapid ventricular rates. Catheter ablation may therefore offer the best chance either to cure the arrhythmia or to render patients asymptomatic.

Atrial Fibrillation

A landmark study by Haissaguerre and colleagues in 1998 focused attention on the importance of the pulmonary veins in the

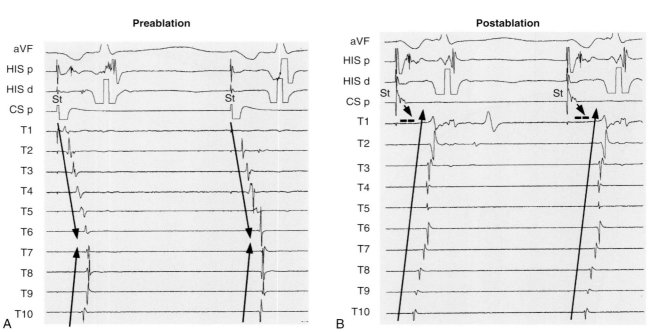

FIGURE 21-4 Activation sequence around the tricuspid annulus before and after cavotricuspid isthmus ablation for atrial flutter. A circular mapping catheter is placed on the atrial side of the tricuspid valve annulus. T10 is the proximal electrode, which sits at the superior annulus; T1 is the distal electrode, which sits at the inferolateral annulus. During pacing from the coronary sinus (*CS*) before ablation, activation spreads in two directions around the tricuspid valve (note the "Christmas tree" pattern of activation on the mapping catheter around the tricuspid valve annulus). After ablation, activation is blocked at the ablation line, which is just medial to T1 and spreads in a counterclockwise direction around the annulus (from T10 to T1). HIS p and HIS d, proximal and distal His catheter; CS p, proximal coronary sinus catheter.

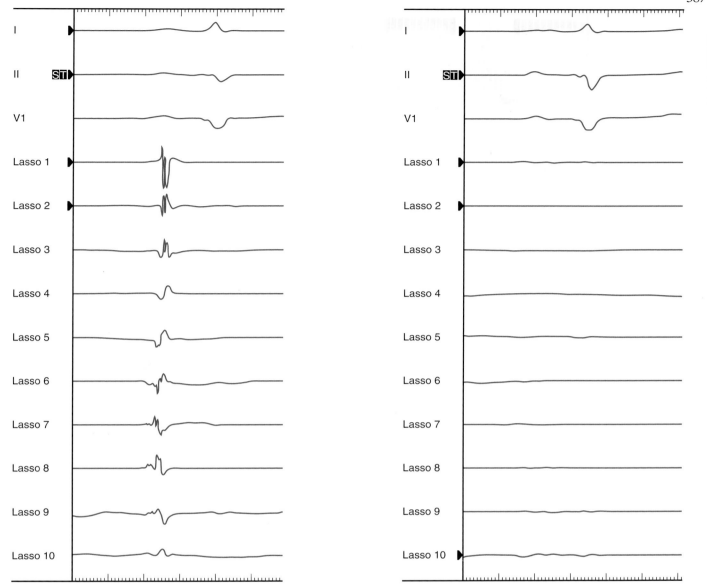

FIGURE 21-5 Endpoint of segmental ostial ablation. The ablation catheter is positioned at the ostium of the left superior pulmonary vein, and multiple bipolar electrograms recorded at the circumference of the vein ostium are shown before (*left*) and after (*right*) ostial applications of radiofrequency energy. Abl, ablation catheter.

generation of AF.[19] This began a period of rapid progress in the search for the optimal ablation strategy. *Trigger-based strategies* evolved from point-source ablation within individual veins to selective arrhythmogenic PVI (Figure 21-5)[41] to more proximal, four-vein antral isolation facilitated by 3D mapping systems (Figure 21-6).[42,43] This wider, circumferential ablation approach, originally developed to prevent pulmonary vein stenosis, has several potential advantages over segmental ostial isolation: 1) elimination of anchor points for "mother waves" or rotors near the pulmonary vein ostium; 2) ablation of other potential trigger sites, such as the vein of Marshall and the posterior left atrial wall; 3) atrial debulking, to provide less space for circulating wavelets; and 4) atrial denervation (i.e., vagal denervation by ablation lines).

Substrate-based strategies aim to prevent the atrium from sustaining fibrillation. Such strategies began as recapitulation of the surgical Maze[43] and evolved to additional ablation of complex, fractionated atrial electrograms (CAFÉ)[44] and developed to a stepwise ablation approach through to termination of AF.[45] Comparisons between the two general strategies have been contentious and have led to variable results, depending on intensity of ECG

monitoring, categorization of AF versus atrial tachycardia/flutter at recurrence, and the effect of repeat procedures and adjuvant antiarrhythmic drugs. In most contemporary studies, success rates of catheter ablation for paroxysmal AF are greater than 70%.[44-60] Although many different techniques are used to achieve these results, most investigators acknowledge the primacy of PVI in patients with paroxysmal AF.

Persistent AF, especially long-lasting (>1 year since last episode of sinus rhythm) persistent AF, has proven more challenging to address, and the discussion regarding adjuvant substrate-based ablation is still topical. As reviewed by Brooks and coworkers,[61] more extensive ablation appears to have an advantage in single-procedure efficacy, but efficacy is still fairly limited and variable, ranging from 21% to 74%. Alternative mechanisms perhaps are related to the significant structural and EP remodeling of the left atrium instilled by the long-standing arrhythmia. PVI alone is associated with a single-procedure, drug-free success rate ranging from 37% to 56% at 1 year.[43,62-64] Repeat procedures (mean, 1.3 per patient) increases the drug-free success rate to 59%. Efforts to improve outcomes for persistent AF have led to investigation of

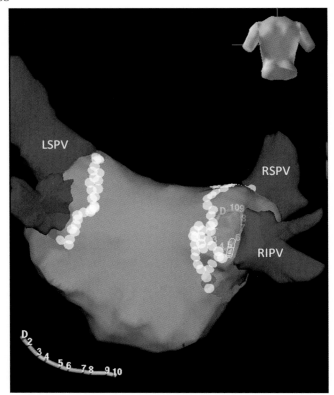

FIGURE 21-6 Registered three-dimensional surface reconstruction of the left atrium during circumferential antral pulmonary vein isolation of the right pulmonary veins. Contiguous radiofrequency lesions are deployed (*circles*) in the left atrium, proximal to the pulmonary vein ostia, creating a circumferential line around the veins. LSPV, left superior pulmonary vein; RSPV, right superior pulmonary vein; RIPV, right inferior pulmonary vein.

alternative and adjunctive targets, such as fractionated electrograms,[44,63] ganglionic plexi,[65] extensive modification of the posterior and inferior wall,[66] or ablation to the point of AF termination.[67] As we continue to understand more about the persistent fibrillatory process, it is hoped that the evolution of more specific ablation techniques will improve the efficacy and safety of ablation in this patient population.

Compared with drug therapy, the available evidence supports the superiority of catheter ablation in terms of efficacy in maintaining sinus rhythm. Studies that directly compared catheter ablation and antiarrhythmic drug therapy confirmed that sinus rhythm is better maintained following catheter ablation.[52,68-74] Moreover, in an intention-to-treat analysis, catheter ablation resulted in freedom of atrial arrhythmia in 79% of patients compared with only 32% in the antiarrhythmic drug group. These data were mostly driven by the larger number of patients with paroxysmal disease; however, favorable outcomes with ablation were also observed in the patients with persistent disease. In addition to being superior to drug therapy in maintaining sinus rhythm, catheter ablation resulted in better symptomatic relief and better exercise tolerance compared with drug treatment.[70]

Complications of catheter ablation procedures are usually directly related to the intervention. Mortality rate following catheter ablation of AF is 1 per 1000 procedures according to a recently published international survey.[75] Major complications occurred in 4.5% of procedures. The most frequently occurring complications included pericardial tamponade, pneumothorax, diaphragmatic paralysis, vascular complications (femoral pseudoaneurysm, arteriovenous fistula), atrioesophageal fistula, pulmonary vein stenosis, and transient and permanent embolic strokes (0.7%, and 0.3%, respectively).

With increasing success and concomitant use of catheter ablation for AF, a question of major importance is whether long-term maintenance of sinus rhythm after successful ablation eliminates the risk for stroke and thereby permits discontinuation of oral anticoagulation therapy. Unfortunately, only limited long-term outcome studies have been published.[57,76-80] In a single-center study by Tzou and colleagues[78] of 239 patients with both paroxysmal and persistent AF who underwent circumferential PVI and were free of AF at 1 year, the majority of patients (84%) remained free of AF after 5 years. Recurrence of AF occurred in 7% of patients per year, and the strongest predictors for recurrence were persistent AF and older age. Moreover, in the patients who underwent repeat ablation, the mechanism of late recurrence was overwhelmingly associated with pulmonary vein reconnection.[78]

The management of anticoagulation in patients who have undergone AF ablation has largely been left to the judgment of the treating physician. However, several practice patterns have emerged based on the apparent presence or absence of AF, duration of recurrent episodes, and the CHADS$_2$ stroke risk stratification (congestive heart failure, hypertension, age >75 years, diabetes mellitus, and prior stroke or transient ischemic attack).[81] In a multicenter study, Themistoclakis and colleagues[80] studied the largest multicenter experience to date to address this issue. In this study, 3355 patients were monitored for a mean of 2.3 years. In 2692 patients (80%), warfarin therapy was discontinued 3 to 6 months after ablation (347 patients had a CHADS$_2$ score ≥2). Although the decision to stop warfarin was made on an individual basis, as a general rule, these patients did not have any recurrence of atrial arrhythmias. The annual incidence of stroke in the group off warfarin was 0.03%. This compared with an annual incidence of stroke of 0.2% in those continuing warfarin. Although this study suggests a very low incidence of stroke following successful ablation, caution must be exercised when applying these data to patients typically seen in practice, who may have only limited symptoms and for whom freedom of atrial arrhythmias after ablation is not as rigorously monitored. Current guidelines advocate continuing anticoagulation therapy guided by CHADS$_2$ score, at least until these data are confirmed by large, prospective, randomized trials.[82]

Left atrial appendage (LAA) closure devices have emerged as novel nonpharmacologic approaches to reduce the risk of stroke in patients with AF. The first device tested in humans was the percutaneous LAA transcatheter occlusion (PLAATO; ev3 Endovascular, Inc., Plymouth, MN) system, a self-expanding, membrane-covered, spherical nitinol cage inserted into the LAA transseptally to occlude it in patients with contraindications to chronic warfarin therapy.[83] However, because of high complication rates, the device was withdrawn from the market. The Watchman device (Atritech, Inc., Plymouth, MN) is also composed of a self-expanding nitinol frame. It has fixation barbs and a permeable polyester fabric that covers the left atrial–facing surface of the device (Figure 21-7). In the Watchman Left Atrial Appendage System for Embolic Protection in Patients with AF (PROTECT-AF) study, the Watchman device was compared with conventional warfarin treatment in patients with AF and a CHADS$_2$ score of 1 or higher.[84] Patients were anticoagulated with warfarin in the postimplantation period and were switched to aspirin/clopidogrel for 6 months and then indefinite aspirin alone if transesophageal echocardiogram (TEE) at 45 days after implantation confirmed adequate LAA closure. The device was noninferior to warfarin in the primary efficacy outcome—stroke, systemic emboli, and cardiovascular or other death—with fewer hemorrhagic strokes, and 90% of patients were able to stop warfarin. However, 12.3% of patients had serious procedural complications, most often pericardial effusions, but these complications also included acute ischemic stroke as a result of air embolism or thromboembolism. In addition, 2.2% of attempted implantations resulted in the need for cardiac surgery because of device-related complications.

Importantly, all percutaneous techniques to date require transseptal puncture; deploy long, hollow sheaths in the left atrium (another source of thrombus); and deposit residual hardware

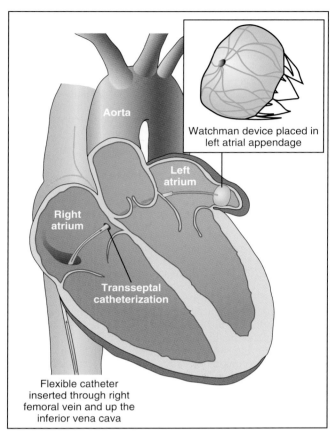

FIGURE 21-7 The Watchman device (Atritech, Inc.) is a self-expanding nitinol structure delivered percutaneously via a transseptal approach to the left atrial appendage. The device is positioned with the use of angiography and transesophageal echocardiography.

in the left atrium, necessitating postprocedural anticoagulation. These factors may all contribute to procedural implant complications. Also, because of the complexity and variability of LAA anatomy, current devices may not always be suitable for deployment, and optimal positioning of the device to ensure complete closure may be difficult. Moreover, although LAA occluding devices may have a role in thromboprophylaxis in patients at high stroke risk with contraindications to warfarin, they will not prevent embolism that originates outside the atrial appendage, and long-term efficacy is uncertain.

Surgical techniques for treatment of AF began in the early 1980s. The majority of these have only historic significance now, as they were unable to address major detrimental sequelae of AF, including vulnerability to systemic thromboembolism and hemodynamic compromise. The prototype surgical ablation procedure for AF was developed in the late 1980s by James Cox.[85-87] The Cox Maze procedure was an operation involving multiple incisions in both the left and right atria, designed to interrupt the macroreentrant circuits thought to be responsible for AF. The procedure appeared to be highly successful in preventing recurrent AF, although it was never subjected to modern ECG monitoring in follow-up; it appeared not to compromise atrial transport function and significantly reduced the risk of thromboembolism and stroke.[88] After two iterations to address late complications and technical difficulty, the Cox Maze III emerged and become the gold standard for the surgical treatment of AF. In a long-term study of patients who had the Cox Maze III procedure, 97% of patients at late follow-up were free of symptomatic AF.[89-92] Despite these excellent results, the Cox Maze procedure did not gain widespread acceptance because of its complexity and technical difficulty. In the most recent iteration of the procedure, the Cox Maze IV (Figure 21-8), bipolar RFA lesions had replaced the surgical incisions.[93] This iteration supported efforts to develop a limited set of lesions that can be performed less invasively through a small thoracotomy on a beating heart, without a need for cardiopulmonary bypass. However, the major shortcoming of this procedure is its inability

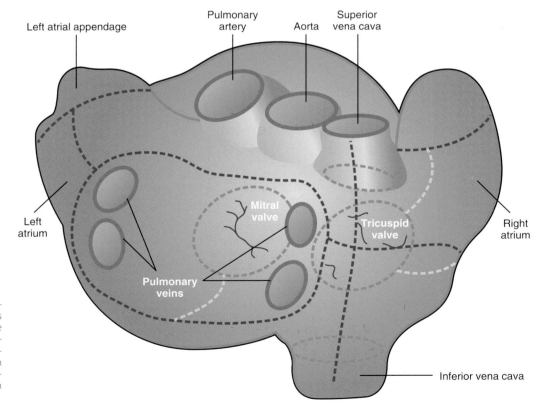

FIGURE 21-8 The Cox Maze IV procedure lesion set. Most of the incisions of the original Cox Maze III procedure have been replaced with bipolar radiofrequency ablation (*dashed lines*). Modification included independent isolation of the pulmonary veins with connecting lesion and no atrial septal incision (originally used for exposure).

to reliably create permanent transmural atrial lesions. Importantly, both incomplete and complete ablation lesions created during surgical ablation procedures can be proarrhythmic by promoting macroreentrant circuits.[94-96] In a study of 50 patients who underwent minimally invasive PVI and were followed up for at least 1 year, 20 patients (40%) developed recurrent atrial tachyarrhythmias. Thirteen of these patients underwent EP study. Pulmonary vein reconnection was the most common finding in patients with recurrent AF and occurred in 50% of all pulmonary veins examined despite achieving entrance and exit block in the operating room. Macroreentrant atrial flutter was the second most common arrhythmia.[97]

One of the major obstacles for adaptation of surgical AF ablation, either as a combined or stand-alone procedure, has been the lack of controlled studies and the absence of postprocedure rhythm monitoring in particular.[98,99] A recent prospective study of a minimally invasive surgical (MIS) approach for the treatment of paroxysmal AF used postprocedure long-term rhythm monitoring—24-hour Holter, 14-day event, or pacemaker interrogation—for a follow-up period of at least 1 year.[100] The procedure consisted of circumferential PVI, partial autonomic denervation, and selective excision of the LAA. No major adverse events were reported, and average hospital stay was 5.2 days. Freedom from any atrial tachyarrhythmia was 80.8% at 1 year, and antiarrhythmic drugs were stopped in 90% of patients. These results are in line with the reported outcomes of percutaneous ablation procedures for paroxysmal AF, although important differences in patient selection may well exist.

Excision/exclusion of the LAA is a critical component of the surgical approach for the treatment of AF. However, the efficacy of this approach in preventing stroke has only recently been critically examined. In a meta-analysis of five clinical trials studying 1400 patients who underwent LAA exclusion, no clear benefit was shown. One reason for this may be the inability to achieve acceptably high occlusion success rates (55% to 93%).[101] A study that examined success rates associated with different surgical techniques to exclude the LAA demonstrated that excision of the LAA was significantly more effective than exclusion of the LAA (73% versus 23%, respectively).[102]

The indications in the 2011 American College of Cardiology Foundation (ACCF)/American Heart Association (AHA)/Heart Rhythm Society (HRS) Focused Update on the Management of Patients with Atrial Fibrillation for catheter or surgical ablation for AF include reduction in AF-related symptoms and improved quality of life in patients who had not responded to medical therapy with at least one antiarrhythmic drug.[103]

Atrioventricular Junction Ablation for Ventricular Rate Control

Treatment of AF with either restoration of sinus rhythm or control of the ventricular rate can sometimes be difficult. Moreover, growing evidence suggests that uncontrolled ventricular rates during AF frequently cause tachycardia-related cardiomyopathy.[104-107] This is of special concern in the presence of preexisting structural heart disease because these patients are at high risk of complications from antiarrhythmic therapy and are less likely to tolerate the negative inotropic effects of AV node–blocking agents. Catheter ablation of the AV junction was the first routinely successful strategy to use radiofrequency energy, and the overall success rate for AV junction ablation is essentially 100% in recent reports,[108-112] although a recurrence of AV conduction occurs in about 3% to 5% of patients. Randomized comparisons of ablation versus medical therapy demonstrated better symptomatic control and improvement in LV function in patients with severe symptoms.[108-114] Despite this success, there are two important limitations in regard to AV junction ablation: the requisite pacemaker dependency and the potential risk to develop right ventricular (RV) pacing–related cardiomyopathy. A large body of evidence has recently emerged that

underscores the harmful effects of long-term RV pacing. LV dyssynchrony imposed by RV pacing can lead to LV remodeling with dilation and decreases in LV ejection fraction (LVEF).[115] In response, the Left Ventricular–Based Cardiac Stimulation Post–AV Nodal Ablation Evaluation (PAVE) study investigated the prophylactic implantation of biventricular pacemakers in patients undergoing AV junction ablation and showed that patients treated with a biventricular pacemaker performed modestly better on a 6-minute walk test and had preserved LVEF compared with patients with RV pacing only.[116]

Catheter Ablation for Ventricular Tachyarrhythmias

IDIOPATHIC VENTRICULAR TACHYCARDIA

Idiopathic ventricular tachycardias are VTs that occur in the absence of clinically apparent structural heart disease. The outflow tract is the most common origin of idiopathic VT, and approximately 70% to 80% of these arrhythmias originate from the RV outflow tract.[117-123] Other origins include the pulmonary artery, the LV outflow tract; the aortic sinuses of Valsalva, near the bundle of His; the coronary sinus and cardiac veins; the mitral and tricuspid valve annuli; and the epicardium.[124-135] These VTs can often be recognized by specific ECG characteristics.[119,125,136] The typical QRS morphology during outflow tract VT shows a left bundle branch block (LBBB) configuration with an inferior (right or left) axis. Idiopathic focal outflow tract VT is typically seen between 20 and 50 years of age and occurs more frequently in women. The two typical forms are *exercise-induced VT* and *repetitive monomorphic VT* occurring at rest. Repetitive salvos of nonsustained VT (NSVT) are frequent and comprise 60% to 92% of reported series, but sustained VT occasionally occurs. RV outflow tract VTs are usually mapped to the area just below the pulmonary valve on the septal aspect of the outflow tract.[137] In a case report series of RV outflow tract ablation, acute success rates typically exceeded 80%, and recurrence of arrhythmia was reported in up to 5% of cases.[128,137,138] Complications are rare, but perforation, tamponade, and death have been reported.[134]

One frequently seen reason for failed ablation of an RV outflow tract VT is incorrect mapping. VT with an LBBB configuration and inferior axis QRS morphology can also originate from the LV outflow tract, including the sinus of Valsalva, and the anterior epicardium. VT arising from the RV outflow tract typically shows an R/S transition zone in the precordial leads at V4, whereas an R/S transition at V1 or V2 indicates an LV origin.[128,139,140] VTs originating from extension of ventricular myocardium above the aortic annulus are ablated from within the sinuses of Valsalva. These VTs account for about 20% of all idiopathic outflow tract VTs. Activation mapping typically shows a two-component electrogram with the earliest deflection preceding the QRS complex by an average 39-ms ablation.[141,142] The majority are ablated from the left coronary cusp, followed in frequency by the right coronary cusp, the junction between the right and left coronary cusp, and rarely the noncoronary cusp.[143]

Although idiopathic outflow tract VTs have a benign course, potentially malignant forms of VT that resemble idiopathic VT may also arise from the outflow tract region, including VT in arrhythmogenic RV dysplasia/cardiomyopathy,[144-146] polymorphic catecholaminergic VT, Brugada syndrome,[117] and also idiopathic polymorphic VT (PMVT)/VF. All patients who come to medical attention with outflow tract VT require an evaluation for organic heart diseases or genetic syndromes associated with sudden death.

Intrafascicular verapamil-sensitive reentrant tachycardia typically presents as exercise-related VT in individuals between the ages of 15 and 40 years, and 60% to 80% of patients are male.[122,147-150] The QRS morphology has a right bundle branch block (RBBB) configuration with RS complexes in the midprecordial leads. The mechanism is reentry in or near portions of Purkinje fascicles of the left bundle, and often Purkinje fiber activation precedes local ventricular activation at the site of origin both in sinus rhythm and during VT.[147,150] The overall success rate of intrafascicular VT ablation is greater than 95%.[122,147-153] Although complications related to left-heart catheterization are expected, no serious complications were reported in these studies. Given its high efficacy and low risk, catheter ablation should be considered in patients with persistent symptoms despite the use of drug therapy (β-blockers or calcium channel antagonists) or in patients who prefer curative therapy over long-term drug therapy.

VENTRICULAR TACHYCARDIA IN PATIENTS WITH STRUCTURAL HEART DISEASE

Sustained monomorphic VT can complicate several forms of heart disease, including coronary heart disease, nonischemic dilated cardiomyopathy, hypertrophic cardiomyopathy, RV dysplasia/cardiomyopathy, and sarcoid heart disease. The most frequent and well-understood anatomic substrate for VT is healed MI, in which slow, discontinuous conduction in the surviving border zone of the infarct allows the establishment of stable reentrant circuits.[154] Sites of arrhythmia origin are recognized by low-amplitude, fractionated endocardial electrograms, an EP marker for the slow conduction necessary for reentry (Figure 21-9).[155] Similar endocardial electrogram abnormalities have been demonstrated in other forms of heart disease, however, the abnormal electrograms are typically localized to perivalvular areas and the epicardium.[156-160] Because the majority of VTs are hemodynamically unstable, and patients usually exhibit multiple VT morphologies as a result of separate reentry circuits (or shared areas of slow conduction with variable exits from the scar), activation and entrainment mapping, which require mapping during ongoing VT, have been increasingly supplemented by substrate-mapping approaches (Figure 21-10).[161]

Catheter ablation has proved effective in well-selected patients with VT in the setting of healed infarction. It results in improved arrhythmia control in two thirds of patients who have mappable scar-related VT, decreases episodes of VT-triggering ICD therapies, and can be lifesaving for patients with incessant VT.[162,163] In single-center studies that included 800 patients who underwent VT ablation since 2000, the clinical VT was abolished in 72% to 96% of patients, and all inducible VTs were ablated in 38% to 72% of patients.[162,164-181] Procedure-related mortality rate was 0.5%. For the 13 studies with mean follow-up of at least 1 year, 50% to 88% of patients were free of any VT. Contemporary large, multicenter series have reported postablation outcomes following combined entrainment and substrate-mapping approaches. The Multicentre Thermocool Ventricular Tachycardia Ablation Trial reported outcomes for 231 patients who underwent ablation with an open irrigation catheter.[182] This was a representative population of postinfarction VT patients who had had a median LVEF of 25% and a median of three VTs; only one third had mappable-only VTs. The targeted VT was successfully ablated in 81% of patients, and all VTs were ablated in almost 50% of patients. Although 51% of patients had a recurrent episode at 6 months, the frequency of episodes was markedly reduced in most patients. Similar acute and midterm successes were reported in the Euro-VT study in 63 patients with healed myocardial infarction VT.[183] The randomized controlled Substrate Mapping and Ablation in Sinus Rhythm to Halt Ventricular Tachycardia (SMASH-VT) multicenter trial examined the feasibility of using substrate-based ablation as a prophylactic strategy in 128 patients with ischemic cardiomyopathy who had received secondary prevention ICD.[184] During an average follow-up of 23 months, 33% of the control group, but only 12% of the ablation group, received appropriate ICD therapy for VT or VF, and a nonsignificant trend was observed toward better survival in the ablation group. However, at this time, prophylactic VT ablation in patients with ICDs is investigational, and further trials are needed to assess this approach.

Catheter ablation for sustained VT with healed MI is recommended for patients whose symptoms recur despite antiarrhythmic drug therapy and for those patients for whom antiarrhythmic drugs are not tolerated or not desired. Even in relatively ill populations, procedural mortality and morbidity rates are acceptable. Ablation usually reduces the frequency of VT episodes, although isolated recurrences remain a risk. Death from heart failure is a concern, but this appears to be related largely to the severity of underlying heart disease. Many opinion leaders believe that ablation should be considered relatively early, before multiple recurrences of VT and repeated courses of drug therapy.[185]

Patients with nonischemic dilated cardiomyopathy and VT may also benefit from RFA.[161,186] Approximately 80% of VTs in nonischemic patients are due to scar-related reentrant circuits, with the remainder caused by bundle branch reentry of focal origin.[186,187]

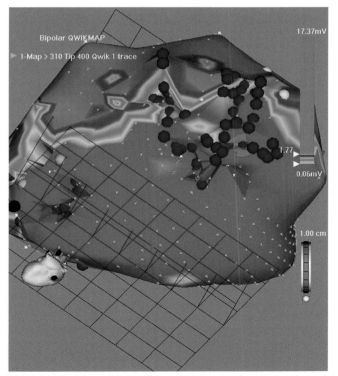

FIGURE 21-10 Linear ablation of scar-related ventricular tachycardia. Inferior view of left ventricle. Myocardial scar is displayed in *red* (low voltage). Normal myocardium is displayed in *purple* (normal voltage). Two lines of radiofrequency lesions (*red dots*) are seen at the base of the left ventricle, extending from deep within the scar across the border zone to normal myocardium.

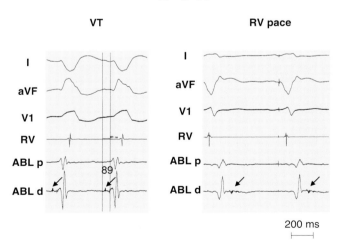

FIGURE 21-9 Electrogram (EGM) from an area of slow conduction in a ventricular tachycardia (*VT*) circuit. *Left,* Recording during VT. The ablation catheter (*ABL*) is in the left ventricle at the exit of the VT circuit. Note a low-voltage presystolic deflection 89 ms before the onset of the surface QRS and before the larger component of the EGM. *Right,* The same recording site during right ventricular (*RV*) pacing. The larger component of the EGM now precedes the low-voltage deflection, indicating slow conduction into scar during RV pacing. RV, right ventricle; ABL p, proximal ablation catheter; ABL d, distal ablation catheter.

Bundle branch reentrant VT uses the left and right bundle branches in a circuit that can be easily treated by ablation of the right bundle branch.

Catheter ablation for VT in the setting of nonischemic cardiomyopathy uses approaches similar to those described for scar-related VT. For patients with mappable VTs, ablation targets the critical isthmus of the reentrant circuit defined by activation and entrainment mapping techniques. For unmappable VTs, linear ablation lesions are guided by the VT QRS morphology, pacemapping in the border zone, and the local abnormal electrograms. Linear lesions usually connect the border zone with an anatomic barrier, such as valve annulus.[161] The success of endocardial ablation is lower than that observed for post-MI VT. Reentry circuits deep to the endocardium and in the epicardium appear to be the likely explanation, and combined endocardial and epicardial mapping approaches improve outcome. In a series of 22 patients, epicardial mapping and ablation were performed if endocardial ablation failed.[158] Scar-related reentry circuits were identified in the endocardium in 12 patients and in the epicardium in all 7 who underwent epicardial mapping after failed endocardial ablation. At least one VT was successfully ablated in 16 of 22 patients, and all VTs were abolished in 12 of 22 patients. During a mean follow-up of 1 year, VT recurred in 46% of patients, 1 patient died of heart failure, and cardiac transplantation was performed in 2 patients.

Although ablation of VT in this patient population can be more difficult when compared with that in the post-MI population, it usually results in improved arrhythmia control, and it can be life-saving for patients with incessant VT. Therefore, indications for catheter ablation in this group of patients are similar to the ones discussed for patients with healed infarction.[185]

Surgical ablation for the treatment of healed-infarction VTs has been largely replaced by catheter-based ablation approaches. However, surgical ablation should still be considered for patients with symptomatic VT refractory to percutaneous endocardial and epicardial ablations. In 2010, we reported our surgical ablation experience in patients with recurrent symptomatic VTs who had not responded to medical therapy or endocardial or epicardial ablations. All eight patients had nonischemic cardiomyopathy, and the underlying substrate frequently involved a midmyocardial or epicardial scar in proximity to a coronary vessel. Surgical cryoablation guided by preoperative EP study led to significant reduction in the VT burden with no significant perioperative complications.[188]

VENTRICULAR FIBRILLATION AND POLYMORPHIC VENTRICULAR TACHYCARDIA

Caused in part by the success of ablation for AF, the trigger hypothesis of arrhythmia initiation has been applied to the treatment of VF with ablative techniques. Selected patients with VF and PMVT owing to varied etiologies—such as Brugada syndrome, long QT syndrome,[117] postinfarction VT,[189] and idiopathic VF[121]—have achieved control of VF through mapping and ablation of the triggering premature ventricular beats that initiate the tachyarrhythmia. These premature beats most often originate from the Purkinje system but may also arise from the RV outflow tract.[117,121,189] The current literature is limited to case reports and case series; therefore ICD implantation remains the preferred therapy, whereas ablation can be considered in patients with frequent ICD shocks in the setting of uncontrolled arrhythmia.

Summary

Developments in nonpharmacologic therapy have eclipsed the results possible with antiarrhythmic drugs in many arrhythmia syndromes. Catheter ablation therapy is highly effective in a variety of supraventricular arrhythmias; extension of this success to the majority of patients with VT and VF, particularly in the setting of structural heart disease, awaits improvements in understanding of the arrhythmia substrate as well as technologic enhancements.

REFERENCES

1. The Cardiac Arrhythmia Suppression Trial (CAST) Investigators. Preliminary report: effect of encainide and flecainide on mortality in a randomized trial of arrhythmia suppression after myocardial infarction. N Engl J Med 1989;321(6):406-412.
2. Flaker GC, Blackshear JL, McBride R, et al. Stroke Prevention in Atrial Fibrillation Investigators. Antiarrhythmic drug therapy and cardiac mortality in atrial fibrillation. J Am Coll Cardiol 1992;20(3):527-532.
3. Steinberg JS, Sadaniantz A, Kron J, et al. Analysis of cause-specific mortality in the Atrial Fibrillation Follow-up Investigation of Rhythm Management (AFFIRM) study. Circulation 2004;109(16):1973-1980.
4. Borggrefe M, Hindricks G, Havercamp W, Breithardt G. Catheter ablation using radiofrequency energy. Clin Cardiol 1990;13(2):127-131.
5. Nath S, Lynch C 3rd, Whayne JG, Haines DE. Cellular electrophysiological effects of hyperthermia on isolated guinea pig papillary muscle: implications for catheter ablation. Circulation 1993;88(4 Pt 1):1826-1831.
6. Simmers TA, Wittkampf FH, Hauer RN, Robles de Medina EO. In vivo ventricular lesion growth in radiofrequency catheter ablation. Pacing Clin Electrophysiol 1994;17(3 Pt 2):523-531.
7. Hogenhuis W, Stevens SK, Wang P, et al. Cost-effectiveness of radiofrequency ablation compared with other strategies in Wolff-Parkinson-White syndrome. Circulation 1993;88(5 Pt 2):II437-II446.
8. Scheinman MM, Huang S. The 1998 NASPE Prospective Catheter Ablation Registry. Pacing Clin Electrophysiol 2000;23(6):1020-1028.
9. Swartz JF, Tracy CM, Fletcher RD. Radiofrequency endocardial catheter ablation of accessory atrioventricular pathway atrial insertion sites. Circulation 1993;87(2):487-499.
10. Deshpande SS, Bremner S, Sra JS, et al. Ablation of left free-wall accessory pathways using radiofrequency energy at the atrial insertion site: transseptal versus transaortic approach. J Cardiovasc Electrophysiol 1994;5(3):219-231.
11. Haissaguerre M, Gaita F, Fischer B, et al. Radiofrequency catheter ablation of left lateral accessory pathways via the coronary sinus. Circulation 1992;86(5):1464-1468.
12. Morady F. Catheter ablation of supraventricular arrhythmias: state of the art. J Cardiovasc Electrophysiol 2004;15(1):124-139.
13. Priori SG, Aliot E, Blomstrom-Lundqvist C, et al. Task Force on Sudden Cardiac Death of the European Society of Cardiology. Eur Heart J 2001;22(16):1374-1460.
14. Pappone C, Santinelli V, Rosanio S, et al. Usefulness of invasive electrophysiologic testing to stratify the risk of arrhythmic events in asymptomatic patients with Wolff-Parkinson-White pattern: results from a large prospective long-term follow-up study. J Am Coll Cardiol 2003;41(2):239-244.
15. Cheng CH, Sanders GD, Hlatky MA, et al. Cost-effectiveness of radiofrequency ablation for supraventricular tachycardia. Ann Intern Med 2000;133(11):864-876.
16. Poty H, Saoudi N, Haissaguerre M, et al. Radiofrequency catheter ablation of atrial tachycardias. Am Heart J 1996;131(3):481-489.
17. Kalman JM, Olgin JE, Karch MR, et al. "Cristal tachycardias": origin of right atrial tachycardias from the crista terminalis identified by intracardiac echocardiography. J Am Coll Cardiol 1998;31(2):451-459.
18. Kistler PM, Sanders P, Hussin A, et al. Focal atrial tachycardia arising from the mitral annulus: electrocardiographic and electrophysiologic characterization. J Am Coll Cardiol 2003;41(12):2212-2219.
19. Haissaguerre M, Jais P, Shah DC, et al. Spontaneous initiation of atrial fibrillation by ectopic beats originating in the pulmonary veins. N Engl J Med 1998;339(10):659-666.
20. Tsai CF, Tai CT, Hsieh MH, et al. Initiation of atrial fibrillation by ectopic beats originating from the superior vena cava: electrophysiological characteristics and results of radiofrequency ablation. Circulation 2000;102(1):67-74.
21. Hwang C, Wu TJ, Doshi RN, Peter CT, Chen PS. Vein of Marshall cannulation for the analysis of electrical activity in patients with focal atrial fibrillation. Circulation 2000;101(13):1503-1505.
22. Pappone C, Stabile G, De Simone A, et al. Role of catheter-induced mechanical trauma in localization of target sites of radiofrequency ablation in automatic atrial tachycardia. J Am Coll Cardiol 1996;27(5):1090-1097.
23. Walsh EP, Saul JP, Hulse JE, et al. Transcatheter ablation of ectopic atrial tachycardia in young patients using radiofrequency current. Circulation 1992;86(4):1138-1146.
24. Kay GN, Chong F, Epstein AE, Dailey SM, Plumb VJ. Radiofrequency ablation for treatment of primary atrial tachycardias. J Am Coll Cardiol 1993;21(4):901-909.
25. Tracy CM, Swartz JF, Fletcher RD, et al. Radiofrequency catheter ablation of ectopic atrial tachycardia using paced activation sequence mapping. J Am Coll Cardiol 1993;21(4):910-917.
26. Goldberger J, Kall J, Ehlert F, et al. Effectiveness of radiofrequency catheter ablation for treatment of atrial tachycardia. Am J Cardiol 1993;72(11):787-793.
27. Chen SA, Chiang CE, Yang CJ, et al. Sustained atrial tachycardia in adult patients: electrophysiological characteristics, pharmacological response, possible mechanisms, and effects of radiofrequency ablation. Circulation 1994;90(3):1262-1278.
28. Lesh MD, Van Hare GF, Epstein LM, et al. Radiofrequency catheter ablation of atrial arrhythmias: results and mechanisms. Circulation 1994;89(3):1074-1089.
29. Morillo CA, Klein GJ, Thakur RK, et al. Mechanism of 'inappropriate' sinus tachycardia: role of sympathovagal balance. Circulation 1994;90(2):873-877.
30. Shen WK, Low PA, Jahangir A, et al. Is sinus node modification appropriate for inappropriate sinus tachycardia with features of postural orthostatic tachycardia syndrome? Pacing Clin Electrophysiol 2001;24(2):217-230.
31. Feld GK, Fleck RP, Chen PS, et al. Radiofrequency catheter ablation for the treatment of human type 1 atrial flutter: identification of a critical zone in the reentrant circuit by endocardial mapping techniques. Circulation 1992;86(4):1233-1240.
32. Schreieck J, Zrenner B, Kumpmann J, et al. Prospective randomized comparison of closed cooled-tip versus 8-mm-tip catheters for radiofrequency ablation of typical atrial flutter. J Cardiovasc Electrophysiol 2002;13(10):980-985.

33. Kalman JM, VanHare GF, Olgin JE, et al. Ablation of 'incisional' reentrant atrial tachycardia complicating surgery for congenital heart disease: use of entrainment to define a critical isthmus of conduction. *Circulation* 1996;93(3):502-512.

34. Baker BM, Lindsay BD, Bromberg BI, et al. Catheter ablation of clinical intraatrial reentrant tachycardias resulting from previous atrial surgery: localizing and transecting the critical isthmus. *J Am Coll Cardiol* 1996;28(2):411-417.

35. Nakagawa H, Shah N, Matsudaira K, et al. Characterization of reentrant circuit in macro-reentrant right atrial tachycardia after surgical repair of congenital heart disease: isolated channels between scars allow "focal" ablation. *Circulation* 2001;103(5):699-709.

36. Jais P, Shah DC, Haissaguerre M, et al. Mapping and ablation of left atrial flutters. *Circulation* 2000;101(25):2928-2934.

37. Gerstenfeld EP, Callans DJ, Dixit S, et al. Mechanisms of organized left atrial tachycardias occurring after pulmonary vein isolation. *Circulation* 2004;110(11):1351-1357.

38. Oral H, Scharf C, Chugh A, et al. Catheter ablation for paroxysmal atrial fibrillation: segmental pulmonary vein ostial ablation versus left atrial ablation. *Circulation* 2003;108(19):2355-2360.

39. Chugh A, Oral H, Good E, et al. Catheter ablation of atypical atrial flutter and atrial tachycardia within the coronary sinus after left atrial ablation for atrial fibrillation. *J Am Coll Cardiol* 2005;46(1):83-91.

40. Chae S, Oral H, Good E, et al. Atrial tachycardia after circumferential pulmonary vein ablation of atrial fibrillation: mechanistic insights, results of catheter ablation, and risk factors for recurrence. *J Am Coll Cardiol* 2007;50(18):1781-1787.

41. Haissaguerre M, Shah DC, Jais P, et al. Electrophysiological breakthroughs from the left atrium to the pulmonary veins. *Circulation* 2000;102(20):2463-2465.

42. Pappone C, Rosanio S, Oreto G, et al. Circumferential radiofrequency ablation of pulmonary vein ostia: a new anatomic approach for curing atrial fibrillation. *Circulation* 2000;102(21):2619-2628.

43. Pappone C, Oreto G, Rosanio S, et al. Atrial electroanatomic remodeling after circumferential radiofrequency pulmonary vein ablation: efficacy of an anatomic approach in a large cohort of patients with atrial fibrillation. *Circulation* 2001;104(21):2539-2544.

44. Nademanee K, Schwab MC, Kosar EM, et al. Clinical outcomes of catheter substrate ablation for high-risk patients with atrial fibrillation. *J Am Coll Cardiol* 2008;51(8):843-849.

45. Jais P, Hocini M, Sanders P, et al. Long-term evaluation of atrial fibrillation ablation guided by noninducibility. *Heart Rhythm* 2006;3(2):140-145.

46. Arentz T, Weber R, Burkle G, et al. Small or large isolation areas around the pulmonary veins for the treatment of atrial fibrillation? Results from a prospective randomized study. *Circulation* 2007;115(24):3057-3063.

47. Hocini M, Jais P, Sanders P, et al. Techniques, evaluation, and consequences of linear block at the left atrial roof in paroxysmal atrial fibrillation: a prospective randomized study. *Circulation* 2005;112(24):3688-3696.

48. Verma A, Patel D, Famy T, et al. Efficacy of adjuvant anterior left atrial ablation during intracardiac echocardiography-guided pulmonary vein antrum isolation for atrial fibrillation. *J Cardiovasc Electrophysiol* 2007;18(2):151-156.

49. Fassini G, Riva S, Chiodelli R, et al. Left mitral isthmus ablation associated with PV isolation: long-term results of a prospective randomized study. *J Cardiovasc Electrophysiol* 2005;16(11):1150-1156.

50. Della Bella P, Fassini G, Cireddu M, et al. Image integration-guided catheter ablation of atrial fibrillation: a prospective randomized study. *J Cardiovasc Electrophysiol* 2009; 20(3):258-265.

51. Van Belle Y, Janse P, Theuns D, Szili-Torok T, Jordaens L. One year follow-up after cryoballoon isolation of the pulmonary veins in patients with paroxysmal atrial fibrillation. *Europace* 2008;10(11):1271-1276.

52. Jais P, Cauchemez B, Macle L, et al. Catheter ablation versus antiarrhythmic drugs for atrial fibrillation: the A4 study. *Circulation* 2008;118(24):2498-2505.

53. Fiala M, Chovancik J, Nevralova R, et al. Termination of long-lasting persistent versus short-lasting persistent and paroxysmal atrial fibrillation by ablation. *Pacing Clin Electrophysiol* 2008;31(8):985-997.

54. Yoshida K, Ulfarsson M, Tada H, et al. Complex electrograms within the coronary sinus: time- and frequency-domain characteristics, effects of antral pulmonary vein isolation, and relationship to clinical outcome in patients with paroxysmal and persistent atrial fibrillation. *J Cardiovasc Electrophysiol* 2008;19(10):1017-1023.

55. Wang XH, Liu X, Sun YM, et al. Pulmonary vein isolation combined with superior vena cava isolation for atrial fibrillation ablation: a prospective randomized study. *Europace* 2008;10(5):600-605.

56. Fiala M, Chovancik J, Nevralova R, et al. Pulmonary vein isolation using segmental versus electroanatomical circumferential ablation for paroxysmal atrial fibrillation: over 3-year results of a prospective randomized study. *J Interv Card Electrophysiol* 2008;22(1):13-21.

57. Dixit S, Gerstenfeld EP, Ratcliffe SJ, et al. Single procedure efficacy of isolating all versus arrhythmogenic pulmonary veins on long-term control of atrial fibrillation: a prospective randomized study. *Heart Rhythm* 2008;5(2):174-181.

58. Chang SL, Tai CT, Lin YJ, et al. The efficacy of inducibility and circumferential ablation with pulmonary vein isolation in patients with paroxysmal atrial fibrillation. *J Cardiovasc Electrophysiol* 2007;18(6):607-611.

59. Sheikh I, Krum D, Cooley R, et al. Pulmonary vein isolation and linear lesions in atrial fibrillation ablation. *J Interv Card Electrophysiol* 2006;17(2):103-109.

60. Oral H, Chugh A, Lemola K, et al. Noninducibility of atrial fibrillation as an end point of left atrial circumferential ablation for paroxysmal atrial fibrillation: a randomized study. *Circulation* 2004;110(18):2797-2801.

61. Brooks AG, Stiles MK, Laborderie J, et al. Outcomes of long-standing persistent atrial fibrillation ablation: a systematic review. *Heart Rhythm* 2010;7(6):835-846.

62. Oral H, Chugh A, Yoshida K, et al. A randomized assessment of the incremental role of ablation of complex fractionated atrial electrograms after antral pulmonary vein isolation for long-lasting persistent atrial fibrillation. *J Am Coll Cardiol* 2009;53(9):782-789.

63. Elayi CS, Verma A, Di Biase L, et al. Ablation for longstanding permanent atrial fibrillation: results from a randomized study comparing three different strategies. *Heart Rhythm* 2008;5(12):1658-1664.

64. Cheema A, Dong J, Dalal D, et al. Circumferential ablation with pulmonary vein isolation in permanent atrial fibrillation. *Am J Cardiol* 2007;99(10):1425-1428.

65. Pokushalov E, Romanov A, Shugayev P, et al. Selective ganglionated plexi ablation for paroxysmal atrial fibrillation. *Heart Rhythm* 2009;6(9):1257-1264.

66. Bhargava M, Di Biase L, Mohanty P, et al. Impact of type of atrial fibrillation and repeat catheter ablation on long-term freedom from atrial fibrillation: results from a multicenter study. *Heart Rhythm* 2009;6(10):1403-1412.

67. O'Neill MD, Wright M, Knecht S, et al. Long-term follow-up of persistent atrial fibrillation ablation using termination as a procedural endpoint. *Eur Heart J* 2009;30(9):1105-1112.

68. Wazni OM, Marrouche NF, Martin DO, et al. Radiofrequency ablation vs antiarrhythmic drugs as first-line treatment of symptomatic atrial fibrillation: a randomized trial. *JAMA* 2005;293(21):2634-2640.

69. Pappone C, Augello G, Sala S, et al. A randomized trial of circumferential pulmonary vein ablation versus antiarrhythmic drug therapy in paroxysmal atrial fibrillation: the APAF Study. *J Am Coll Cardiol* 2006;48(11):2340-2347.

70. Forleo GB, Mantica M, De Luca L, et al. Catheter ablation of atrial fibrillation in patients with diabetes mellitus type 2: results from a randomized study comparing pulmonary vein isolation versus antiarrhythmic drug therapy. *J Cardiovasc Electrophysiol* 2009;20(1):22-28.

71. Stabile G, Bertaglia E, Senatore G, et al. Catheter ablation treatment in patients with drug-refractory atrial fibrillation: a prospective, multi-centre, randomized, controlled study (Catheter Ablation For The Cure Of Atrial Fibrillation Study). *Eur Heart J* 2006;27(2):216-221.

72. Oral H, Pappone C, Chugh A, et al. Circumferential pulmonary-vein ablation for chronic atrial fibrillation. *N Engl J Med* 2006;354(9):934-941.

73. Krittayaphong R, Raungrattanaamporn O, Bhuripanyo K, et al. A randomized clinical trial of the efficacy of radiofrequency catheter ablation and amiodarone in the treatment of symptomatic atrial fibrillation. *J Med Assoc Thai* 2003;86(Suppl 1):S8-S16.

74. Wilber DJ, Pappone C, Neuzil P, et al. Comparison of antiarrhythmic drug therapy and radiofrequency catheter ablation in patients with paroxysmal atrial fibrillation: a randomized controlled trial. *JAMA* 2010;303(4):333-340.

75. Cappato R, Calkins H, Chen SA, et al. Updated worldwide survey on the methods, efficacy, and safety of catheter ablation for human atrial fibrillation. *Circ Arrhythm Electrophysiol* 2010;3(1):32-38.

76. Mainigi SK, Sauer WH, Cooper JM, et al. Incidence and predictors of very late recurrence of atrial fibrillation after ablation. *J Cardiovasc Electrophysiol* 2007;18(1):69-74.

77. Hsieh MH, Tai CT, Tsai CF, et al. Clinical outcome of very late recurrence of atrial fibrillation after catheter ablation of paroxysmal atrial fibrillation. *J Cardiovasc Electrophysiol* 2003;14(6):598-601.

78. Tzou WS, Marchlinski FE, Zado ES, et al. Long-term outcome after successful catheter ablation of atrial fibrillation. *Circ Arrhythm Electrophysiol* 2010;3(3):237-242.

79. Oral H, Chugh A, Ozaydin M, et al. Risk of thromboembolic events after percutaneous left atrial radiofrequency ablation of atrial fibrillation. *Circulation* 2006;114(8):759-765.

80. Themistoclakis S, Corrado A, Marchlinski FE, et al. The risk of thromboembolism and need for oral anticoagulation after successful atrial fibrillation ablation. *J Am Coll Cardiol* 2010;55(8):735-743.

81. Gage BF, Waterman AD, Shannon W, et al. Validation of clinical classification schemes for predicting stroke: results from the National Registry of Atrial Fibrillation. *JAMA* 2001;285(22):2864-2870.

82. Calkins H, Brugada J, Packer DL, et al. HRS/EHRA/ECAS Expert Consensus Statement on Catheter and Surgical Ablation of Atrial Fibrillation: Recommendations for Personnel, Policy, Procedures and Follow-Up: a report of the Heart Rhythm Society (HRS) Task Force on Catheter and Surgical Ablation of Atrial Fibrillation, developed in partnership with the European Heart Rhythm Association (EHRA) and the European Cardiac Arrhythmia Society (ECAS); in collaboration with the American College of Cardiology (ACC), American Heart Association (AHA), and the Society of Thoracic Surgeons (STS). Endorsed and approved by the governing bodies of the American College of Cardiology, the American Heart Association, the European Cardiac Arrhythmia Society, the European Heart Rhythm Association, the Society of Thoracic Surgeons, and the Heart Rhythm Society. *Europace* 2007;9(6):335-379.

83. Ostermayer SH, Reisman M, Kramer PH, et al. Percutaneous left atrial appendage transcatheter occlusion (PLAATO system) to prevent stroke in high-risk patients with non-rheumatic atrial fibrillation: results from the international multi-center feasibility trials. *J Am Coll Cardiol* 2005;46(1):9-14.

84. Holmes DR, Reddy VY, Turi ZG, et al. Percutaneous closure of the left atrial appendage versus warfarin therapy for prevention of stroke in patients with atrial fibrillation: a randomised non-inferiority trial. *Lancet* 2009;374(9689):534-542.

85. Cox JL. The surgical treatment of atrial fibrillation. IV. Surgical technique. *J Thorac Cardiovasc Surg* 1991;101(4):584-592.

86. Cox JL, Canavan TE, Schuessler RB, et al. The surgical treatment of atrial fibrillation. II. Intraoperative electrophysiologic mapping and description of the electrophysiologic basis of atrial flutter and atrial fibrillation. *J Thorac Cardiovasc Surg* 1991;101(3):406-426.

87. Cox JL, Schuessler RB, D'Agostino HJ Jr, et al. The surgical treatment of atrial fibrillation. III. Development of a definitive surgical procedure. *J Thorac Cardiovasc Surg* 1991; 101(4):569-583.

88. Cox JL, Ad N, Palazzo T. Impact of the maze procedure on the stroke rate in patients with atrial fibrillation. *J Thorac Cardiovasc Surg* 1999;118(5):833-840.

89. Prasad SM, Maniar HS, Camillo CJ, et al. The Cox maze III procedure for atrial fibrillation: long-term efficacy in patients undergoing lone versus concomitant procedures. *J Thorac Cardiovasc Surg* 2003;126(6):1822-1828.

90. McCarthy PM, Gillinov AM, Castle L, Chung M, Cosgrove D III. The Cox-Maze procedure: the Cleveland Clinic experience. *Semin Thorac Cardiovasc Surg* 2000;12(1):25-29.

91. Raanani E, Albage A, David TE, Yau TM, Armstrong S. The efficacy of the Cox/maze procedure combined with mitral valve surgery: a matched control study. *Eur J Cardiothorac Surg* 2001;19(4):438-442.

92. Schaff HV, Dearani JA, Daly RC, Orszulak TA, Danielson GK. Cox-Maze procedure for atrial fibrillation: Mayo Clinic experience. *Semin Thorac Cardiovasc Surg* 2000;12(1):30-37.

93. Gaynor SL, Diodato MD, Prasad SM, et al. A prospective, single-center clinical trial of a modified Cox maze procedure with bipolar radiofrequency ablation. *J Thorac Cardiovasc Surg* 2004;128(4):535-542.

94. McElderry HT, McGiffin DC, Plumb VJ, et al. Proarrhythmic aspects of atrial fibrillation surgery: mechanisms of postoperative macroreentrant tachycardias. *Circulation* 2008;117(2):155-162.

95. Akar JG, Al-Chekakie MO, Hai A, et al. Surface electrocardiographic patterns and electrophysiologic characteristics of atrial flutter following modified radiofrequency Maze procedures. *J Cardiovasc Electrophysiol* 2007;18(4):349-355.

96. Magnano AR, Argenziano M, Dizon JM, et al. Mechanisms of atrial tachyarrhythmias following surgical atrial fibrillation ablation. *J Cardiovasc Electrophysiol* 2006;17(4):366-373.

97. Kron J, Kasirajan V, Wood MA, et al. Management of recurrent atrial arrhythmias after minimally invasive surgical pulmonary vein isolation and ganglionic plexi ablation for atrial fibrillation. *Heart Rhythm* 2010;7(4):445-451.

98. Shemin RJ, Cox JL, Gillinov AM, Blackstone EH, Bridges CR. Guidelines for reporting data and outcomes for the surgical treatment of atrial fibrillation. *Ann Thorac Surg* 2007;83(3):1225-1230.

99. Pacifico A, Henry PD. Ablation for atrial fibrillation: are cures really achieved? *J Am Coll Cardiol* 2004;43(11):1940-1942.

100. Edgerton JR, Brinkman WT, Weaver T, et al. Pulmonary vein isolation and autonomic denervation for the management of paroxysmal atrial fibrillation by a minimally invasive surgical approach. *J Thorac Cardiovasc Surg* 2010;140(4):823-828.

101. Saltman AE, Gillinov AM. Surgical approaches for atrial fibrillation. *Cardiol Clin* 2009;27(1):179-188.

102. Kanderian AS, Gillinov AM, Pettersson GB, Blackstone E, Klein AL. Success of surgical left atrial appendage closure: assessment by transesophageal echocardiography. *J Am Coll Cardiol* 2008;52(11):924-929.

103. Wann LS, Curtis AB, January CT, et al. 2011 ACCF/AHA/HRS Focused Update on the Management of Patients with Atrial Fibrillation (Updating the 2006 Guideline): a report of the American College of Cardiology Foundation/American Heart Association Task Force on Practice Guidelines. *Circulation* 2011;123(1):104-123.

104. Grogan M, Smith HC, Gersh BJ, Wood DL. Left ventricular dysfunction due to atrial fibrillation in patients initially believed to have idiopathic dilated cardiomyopathy. *Am J Cardiol* 1992;69(19):1570-1573.

105. Zupan I, Rakovec P, Budihna N, Brecelj A, Kozelj M. Tachycardia induced cardiomyopathy in dogs; relation between chronic supraventricular and chronic ventricular tachycardia. *Int J Cardiol* 1996;56(1):75-81.

106. Wilson JR, Douglas P, Hickey WF, et al. Experimental congestive heart failure produced by rapid ventricular pacing in the dog: cardiac effects. *Circulation* 1987;75(4):857-867.

107. Zipes DP. Atrial fibrillation: a tachycardia-induced atrial cardiomyopathy. *Circulation* 1997;95(3):562-564.

108. Brignole M, Gianfranchi L, Menozzi C, et al. Assessment of atrioventricular junction ablation and DDDR mode-switching pacemaker versus pharmacological treatment in patients with severely symptomatic paroxysmal atrial fibrillation: a randomized controlled study. *Circulation* 1997;96(8):2617-2624.

109. Brignole M, Menozzi C, Gianfranchi L, et al. Assessment of atrioventricular junction ablation and VVIR pacemaker versus pharmacological treatment in patients with heart failure and chronic atrial fibrillation: a randomized, controlled study. *Circulation* 1998;98(10):953-960.

110. Fitzpatrick AP, Kourouyan HD, Siu A, et al. Quality of life and outcomes after radiofrequency His-bundle catheter ablation and permanent pacemaker implantation: impact of treatment in paroxysmal and established atrial fibrillation. *Am Heart J* 1996;131(3):499-507.

111. Buys EM, van Hemel NM, Kelder JC, et al. Exercise capacity after His bundle ablation and rate response ventricular pacing for drug refractory chronic atrial fibrillation. *Heart* 1997;77(3):238-241.

112. Rodriguez LM, Smeets JL, Xie B, et al. Improvement in left ventricular function by ablation of atrioventricular nodal conduction in selected patients with lone atrial fibrillation. *Am J Cardiol* 1993;72(15):1137-1141.

113. Brignole M, Gianfranchi L, Menozzi C, et al. Influence of atrioventricular junction radiofrequency ablation in patients with chronic atrial fibrillation and flutter on quality of life and cardiac performance. *Am J Cardiol* 1994;74(3):242-246.

114. Kay GN, Bubien RS, Epstein AE, Plumb VJ. Effect of catheter ablation of the atrioventricular junction on quality of life and exercise tolerance in paroxysmal atrial fibrillation. *Am J Cardiol* 1988;62(10 Pt 1):741-744.

115. O'Keefe JH Jr, Abuissa H, Jones PG, et al. Effect of chronic right ventricular apical pacing on left ventricular function. *Am J Cardiol* 2005;95(6):771-773.

116. Doshi RN, Daoud EG, Fellows C, et al. Left ventricular-based cardiac stimulation post AV nodal ablation evaluation (the PAVE study). *J Cardiovasc Electrophysiol* 2005;16(11):1160-1165.

117. Haissaguerre M, Extramiana F, Hocini M, et al. Mapping and ablation of ventricular fibrillation associated with long-QT and Brugada syndromes. *Circulation* 2003;108(8):925-928.

118. Bunch TJ, Day JD. Right meets left: a common mechanism underlying right and left ventricular outflow tract tachycardias. *J Cardiovasc Electrophysiol* 2006;17(10):1059-1061.

119. Callans DJ, Menz V, Schwartzman D, Gottlieb CD, Marchlinski FE. Repetitive monomorphic tachycardia from the left ventricular outflow tract: electrocardiographic patterns consistent with a left ventricular site of origin. *J Am Coll Cardiol* 1997;29(5):1023-1027.

120. Chinushi M, Aizawa Y, Takahashi K, Kitazawa H, Shibata A. Radiofrequency catheter ablation for idiopathic right ventricular tachycardia with special reference to morphological variation and long-term outcome. *Heart* 1997;78(3):255-261.

121. Haissaguerre M, Shoda M, Jais P, et al. Mapping and ablation of idiopathic ventricular fibrillation. *Circulation* 2002;106(8):962-967.

122. Kaseno K, Tada H, Ito S, et al. Ablation of idiopathic ventricular tachycardia in two separate regions of the outflow tract: prevalence and electrocardiographic characteristics. *Pacing Clin Electrophysiol* 2007;30(Suppl 1):S88-S93.

123. Miles WM. Idiopathic ventricular outflow tract tachycardia: where does it originate? *J Cardiovasc Electrophysiol* 2001;12(5):536-537.

124. Tada H, Tadokoro K, Miyaji K, et al. Idiopathic ventricular arrhythmias arising from the pulmonary artery: prevalence, characteristics, and topography of the arrhythmia origin. *Heart Rhythm* 2008;5(3):419-426.

125. Ouyang F, Fotuhi P, Ho SY, et al. Repetitive monomorphic ventricular tachycardia originating from the aortic sinus cusp: electrocardiographic characterization for guiding catheter ablation. *J Am Coll Cardiol* 2002;39(3):500-508.

126. Good E, Desjardins B, Jongnarangsin K, et al. Ventricular arrhythmias originating from a papillary muscle in patients without prior infarction: a comparison with fascicular arrhythmias. *Heart Rhythm* 2008;5(11):1530-1537.

127. Movsowitz C, Schwartzman D, Callans DJ, et al. Idiopathic right ventricular outflow tract tachycardia: narrowing the anatomic location for successful ablation. *Am Heart J* 1996;131(5):930-936.

128. Coggins DL, Lee RJ, Sweeney J, et al. Radiofrequency catheter ablation as a cure for idiopathic tachycardia of both left and right ventricular origin. *J Am Coll Cardiol* 1994;23(6):1333-1341.

129. Hachiya H, Aonuma K, Yamauchi Y, et al. Electrocardiographic characteristics of left ventricular outflow tract tachycardia. *Pacing Clin Electrophysiol* 2000;23(11 Pt 2):1930-1934.

130. Hirasawa Y, Miyauchi Y, Iwasaki YK, Kobayashi Y. Successful radiofrequency catheter ablation of epicardial left ventricular outflow tract tachycardia from the anterior interventricular coronary vein. *J Cardiovasc Electrophysiol* 2005;16(12):1378-1380.

131. Ito S, Tada H, Naito S, et al. Simultaneous mapping in the left sinus of Valsalva and coronary venous system predicts successful catheter ablation from the left sinus of Valsalva. *Pacing Clin Electrophysiol* 2005;28 Suppl 1:S150-154.

132. Kanagaratnam L, Tomassoni G, Schweikert R, et al. Ventricular tachycardias arising from the aortic sinus of Valsalva: an under-recognized variant of left outflow tract ventricular tachycardia. *J Am Coll Cardiol* 2001;37(5):1408-1414.

133. Sekiguchi Y, Aonuma K, Takahashi A, et al. Electrocardiographic and electrophysiologic characteristics of ventricular tachycardia originating within the pulmonary artery. *J Am Coll Cardiol* 2005;45(6):887-895.

134. Timmermans C, Rodriguez LM, Crijns HJ, Moorman AF, Wellens HJ. Idiopathic left bundle-branch block-shaped ventricular tachycardia may originate above the pulmonary valve. *Circulation* 2003;108(16):1960-1967.

135. Yamauchi Y, Aonuma K, Takahashi A, et al. Electrocardiographic characteristics of repetitive monomorphic right ventricular tachycardia originating near the His-bundle. *J Cardiovasc Electrophysiol* 2005;16(10):1041-1048.

136. Dixit S, Gerstenfeld EP, Callans DJ, Marchlinski FE. Electrocardiographic patterns of superior right ventricular outflow tract tachycardias: distinguishing septal and free-wall sites of origin. *J Cardiovasc Electrophysiol* 2003;14(1):1-7.

137. Movsowitz C, Schwartzman D, Callans DJ, et al. Idiopathic right ventricular outflow tract tachycardia: narrowing the anatomic location for successful ablation. *Am Heart J* 1996;131(5):930-936.

138. Klein LS, Shih HT, Hackett FK, Zipes DP, Miles WM. Radiofrequency catheter ablation of ventricular tachycardia in patients without structural heart disease. *Circulation* 1992;85(5):1666-1674.

139. Ito S, Tada H, Naito S, et al. Development and validation of an ECG algorithm for identifying the optimal ablation site for idiopathic ventricular outflow tract tachycardia. *J Cardiovasc Electrophysiol* 2003;14(12):1280-1286.

140. Wilber DJ, Baerman J, Olshansky B, Kall J, Kopp D. Adenosine-sensitive ventricular tachycardia: clinical characteristics and response to catheter ablation. *Circulation* 1993;87(1):126-134.

141. Yamada T, Yoshida N, Murakami Y, et al. Electrocardiographic characteristics of ventricular arrhythmias originating from the junction of the left and right coronary sinuses of Valsalva in the aorta: the activation pattern as a rationale for the electrocardiographic characteristics. *Heart Rhythm* 2008;5(2):184-192.

142. Bala R, Marchlinski FE. Electrocardiographic recognition and ablation of outflow tract ventricular tachycardia. *Heart Rhythm* 2007;4(3):366-370.

143. Kumagai K, Fukuda K, Wakayama Y, et al. Electrocardiographic characteristics of the variants of idiopathic left ventricular outflow tract ventricular tachyarrhythmias. *J Cardiovasc Electrophysiol* 2008;19(5):495-501.

144. Bakir I, Brugada P, Sarkozy A, Vandepitte C, Wellens F. A novel treatment strategy for therapy refractory ventricular arrhythmias in the setting of arrhythmogenic right ventricular dysplasia. *Europace* 2007;9(5):267-269.

145. Tada H, Hiratsuji T, Naito S, et al. Prevalence and characteristics of idiopathic outflow tract tachycardia with QRS alteration following catheter ablation requiring additional radiofrequency ablation at a different point in the outflow tract. *Pacing Clin Electrophysiol* 2004;27(9):1240-1249.

146. Boulos M, Lashevsky I, Gepstein L. Usefulness of electroanatomical mapping to differentiate between right ventricular outflow tract tachycardia and arrhythmogenic right ventricular dysplasia. *Am J Cardiol* 2005;95(8):935-940.

147. Nakagawa H, Beckman KJ, McClelland JH, et al. Radiofrequency catheter ablation of idiopathic left ventricular tachycardia guided by a Purkinje potential. *Circulation* 1993;88(6):2607-2617.

148. Chen M, Yang B, Zou J, et al. Non-contact mapping and linear ablation of the left posterior fascicle during sinus rhythm in the treatment of idiopathic left ventricular tachycardia. *Europace* 2005;7(2):138-144.

149. Lin D, Hsia HH, Gerstenfeld EP, et al. Idiopathic fascicular left ventricular tachycardia: linear ablation lesion strategy for noninducible or nonsustained tachycardia. *Heart Rhythm* 2005;2(9):934-939.

150. Tada H, Nogami A, Naito S, et al. Retrograde Purkinje potential activation during sinus rhythm following catheter ablation of idiopathic left ventricular tachycardia. *J Cardiovasc Electrophysiol* 1998;9(11):1218-1224.

151. Kaseno K, Tada H, Tanaka S, et al. Successful catheter ablation of left ventricular epicardial tachycardia originating from the great cardiac vein: a case report and review of the literature. *Circ J* 2007;71(12):1983-1988.

152. Wen MS, Yeh SJ, Wang CC, Lin FC, Wu D. Successful radiofrequency ablation of idiopathic left ventricular tachycardia at a site away from the tachycardia exit. *J Am Coll Cardiol* 1997;30(4):1024-1031.

153. Nogami A, Naito S, Tada H, et al. Demonstration of diastolic and presystolic Purkinje potentials as critical potentials in a macroreentry circuit of verapamil-sensitive idiopathic left ventricular tachycardia. *J Am Coll Cardiol* 2000;36(3):811-823.

154. de Bakker JM, van Capelle FJ, Janse MJ, et al. Reentry as a cause of ventricular tachycardia in patients with chronic ischemic heart disease: electrophysiologic and anatomic correlation. *Circulation* 1988;77(3):589-606.

155. Cassidy DM, Vassallo JA, Miller JM, et al. Endocardial catheter mapping during sinus rhythm: relation of underlying heart disease and ventricular arrhythmia. *Circulation* 1986;73:645-652.

156. Hsia HH, Marchlinski FE. Characterization of the electroanatomic substrate for monomorphic ventricular tachycardia in patients with nonischemic cardiomyopathy. *Pacing Clin Electrophysiol* 2002;25(7):1114-1127.

157. Hsia HH, Callans DJ, Marchlinski FE. Characterization of endocardial electrophysiological substrate in patients with nonischemic cardiomyopathy and monomorphic ventricular tachycardia. *Circulation* 2003;108(6):704-710.

158. Soejima K, Stevenson WG, Sapp JL, et al. Endocardial and epicardial radiofrequency ablation of ventricular tachycardia associated with dilated cardiomyopathy: the importance of low-voltage scars. *J Am Coll Cardiol* 2004;43(10):1834-1842.

159. Nazarian S, Bluemke DA, Lardo AC, et al. Magnetic resonance assessment of the substrate for inducible ventricular tachycardia in nonischemic cardiomyopathy. *Circulation* 2005;112(18):2821-2825.

160. Delacretaz E, Stevenson WG, Ellison KE, Maisel WH, Friedman PL. Mapping and radiofrequency catheter ablation of the three types of sustained monomorphic ventricular tachycardia in nonischemic heart disease. *J Cardiovasc Electrophysiol* 2000;11(1):11-17.

161. Marchlinski FE, Callans DJ, Gottlieb CD, Zado E. Linear ablation lesions for control of unmappable ventricular tachycardia in patients with ischemic and nonischemic cardiomyopathy. *Circulation* 2000;101(11):1288-1296.

162. Soejima K, Suzuki M, Maisel WH, et al. Catheter ablation in patients with multiple and unstable ventricular tachycardias after myocardial infarction: short ablation lines guided by reentry circuit isthmuses and sinus rhythm mapping. *Circulation* 2001;104(6):664-669.

163. Calkins H, Epstein A, Packer D, et al.; Cooled RF Multi Center Investigators Group. Catheter ablation of ventricular tachycardia in patients with structural heart disease using cooled radiofrequency energy: results of a prospective multicenter study. *J Am Coll Cardiol* 2000;35(7):1905-1914.

164. Dalal D, Jain R, Tandri H, et al. Long-term efficacy of catheter ablation of ventricular tachycardia in patients with arrhythmogenic right ventricular dysplasia/cardiomyopathy. *J Am Coll Cardiol* 2007;50(5):432-440.

165. Bogun F, Li YG, Groenefeld G, et al. Prevalence of a shared isthmus in postinfarction patients with pleiomorphic, hemodynamically tolerated ventricular tachycardias. *J Cardiovasc Electrophysiol* 2002;13(3):237-241.

166. Ventura R, Klemm HU, Rostock T, et al. Stable and unstable ventricular tachycardias in patients with previous myocardial infarction: a clinically oriented strategy for catheter ablation. *Cardiology* 2008;109(1):52-61.

167. Della Bella P, Riva S, Fassini G, et al. Incidence and significance of pleomorphism in patients with postmyocardial infarction ventricular tachycardia: acute and long-term outcome of radiofrequency catheter ablation. *Eur Heart J* 2004;25(13):1127-1138.

168. Callans DJ, Ren JF, Narula N, et al. Effects of linear, irrigated-tip radiofrequency ablation in porcine healed anterior infarction. *J Cardiovasc Electrophysiol* 2001;12(9):1037-1042.

169. Ciaccio EJ, Chow AW, Kaba RA, et al. Detection of the diastolic pathway, circuit morphology, and inducibility of human postinfarction ventricular tachycardia from mapping in sinus rhythm. *Heart Rhythm* 2008;5(7):981-991.

170. Arenal A, del Castillo S, Gonzalez-Torrecilla E, et al. Tachycardia-related channel in the scar tissue in patients with sustained monomorphic ventricular tachycardias: influence of the voltage scar definition. *Circulation* 2004;110(17):2568-2574.

171. Bogun F, Kim HM, Han J, et al. Comparison of mapping criteria for hemodynamically tolerated, postinfarction ventricular tachycardia. *Heart Rhythm* 2006;3(1):20-26.

172. Borger van der Burg AE, de Groot NM, van Erven L, et al. Long-term follow-up after radiofrequency catheter ablation of ventricular tachycardia: a successful approach? *J Cardiovasc Electrophysiol* 2002;13(5):417-423.

173. Strickberger SA, Knight BP, Michaud GF, Pelosi F, Morady F. Mapping and ablation of ventricular tachycardia guided by virtual electrograms using a noncontact, computerized mapping system. *J Am Coll Cardiol* 2000;35(2):414-421.

174. Segal OR, Chow AW, Markides V, et al. Long-term results after ablation of infarct-related ventricular tachycardia. *Heart Rhythm* 2005;2(5):474-482.

175. Reddy VY, Neuzil P, Taborsky M, Ruskin JN. Short-term results of substrate mapping and radiofrequency ablation of ischemic ventricular tachycardia using a saline-irrigated catheter. *J Am Coll Cardiol* 2003;41(12):2228-2236.

176. Kottkamp H, Wetzel U, Schirdewahn P, et al. Catheter ablation of ventricular tachycardia in remote myocardial infarction: substrate description guiding placement of individual linear lesions targeting noninducibility. *J Cardiovasc Electrophysiol* 2003;14(7):675-681.

177. Kautzner J, Cihak R, Peichl P, Vancura V, Bytesnik J. Catheter ablation of ventricular tachycardia following myocardial infarction using three-dimensional electroanatomical mapping. *Pacing Clin Electrophysiol* 2003;26(1 Pt 2):342-347.

178. Arenal A, Glez-Torrecilla E, Ortiz M, et al. Ablation of electrograms with an isolated, delayed component as treatment of unmappable monomorphic ventricular tachycardias in patients with structural heart disease. *J Am Coll Cardiol* 2003;41(1):81-92.

179. Klemm HU, Ventura R, Steven D, et al. Catheter ablation of multiple ventricular tachycardias after myocardial infarction guided by combined contact and noncontact mapping. *Circulation* 2007;115(21):2697-2704.

180. de Chillou C, Lacroix D, Klug D, et al. Isthmus characteristics of reentrant ventricular tachycardia after myocardial infarction. *Circulation* 2002;105(6):726-731.

181. Soejima K, Stevenson WG, Maisel WH, Sapp JL, Epstein LM. Electrically unexcitable scar mapping based on pacing threshold for identification of the reentry circuit isthmus: feasibility for guiding ventricular tachycardia ablation. *Circulation* 2002;106(13):1678-1683.

182. Stevenson WG, Wilber DJ, Natale A, et al. Irrigated radiofrequency catheter ablation guided by electroanatomic mapping for recurrent ventricular tachycardia after myocardial infarction: the multicenter thermocool ventricular tachycardia ablation trial. *Circulation* 2008;118(25):2773-2782.

183. Aliot EM, Stevenson WG, Almendral-Garrote JM, et al. EHRA/HRS Expert Consensus on Catheter Ablation of Ventricular Arrhythmias, developed in a partnership with the European Heart Rhythm Association (EHRA), a Registered Branch of the European Society of Cardiology (ESC), and the Heart Rhythm Society (HRS); in collaboration with the American College of Cardiology (ACC) and the American Heart Association (AHA). *Heart Rhythm* 2009;6(6):886-933.

184. Reddy VY, Reynolds MR, Neuzil P, et al. Prophylactic catheter ablation for the prevention of defibrillator therapy. *N Engl J Med* 2007;357(26):2657-2665.

185. Aliot EM, Stevenson WG, Almendral-Garrote JM, et al. EHRA/HRS Expert Consensus on Catheter Ablation of Ventricular Arrhythmias: developed in a partnership with the European Heart Rhythm Association (EHRA), a Registered Branch of the European Society of Cardiology (ESC), and the Heart Rhythm Society (HRS); in collaboration with the American College of Cardiology (ACC) and the American Heart Association (AHA). *Europace* 2009;11(6):771-817.

186. Soejima K, Stevenson W, Sapp J, et al. Endocardial and epicardial radiofrequency ablation of ventricular. *J Am Coll Cardiol* 2004;43(10):1834-1842.

187. Delacretaz E, Stevenson WG, Ellison KE, Maisel WH, Friedman PL. Mapping and radiofrequency catheter ablation of the three types of sustained monomorphic ventricular tachycardia in nonischemic heart disease. *J Cardiovasc Electrophysiol* 2000;11(1):11-17.

188. Anter E, Haqqani H, Callans DJ, Marchlinski F, Dixit S. Electrophysiologic and electroanatomic characterization of ventricular tachycardia to guide precise surgical ablation. *Heart Rhythm Soc* 2010;7(5S):S454.

189. Szumowski L, Sanders P, Walczak F, et al. Mapping and ablation of polymorphic ventricular tachycardia after myocardial infarction. *J Am Coll Cardiol* 2004;44(8):1700-1706.

CHAPTER 22

Role of Implantable Cardioverter-Defibrillators in Primary and Secondary Prevention of Sudden Cardiac Death

Mark A. Wood and Kenneth A. Ellenbogen

SUDDEN CARDIAC DEATH, 396

IMPLANTABLE CARDIOVERTER-DEFIBRILLATOR SYSTEMS AND TECHNOLOGY, 396

Implantable Cardioverter-Defibrillators for Secondary Prevention of Sudden Death, 396
Implantable Cardioverter-Defibrillators for Primary Prevention of Sudden Cardiac Death, 397

Risk Stratification for Sudden Cardiac Death, 398
Comorbidities and Implantable Cardioverter-Defibrillator Benefit, 400
Cardiac Resynchronization Implantable Cardioverter-Defibrillators, 401

Guidelines for Cardioverter-Defibrillator Implantation, 401
Special Patient Groups, 404
Clinical Issues, 405

REFERENCES, 406

Sudden Cardiac Death

Sudden cardiac death (SCD) remains a major health care problem despite the progressive decline in the incidence of coronary artery disease (CAD) over the past 50 years. Approximately 310,000 patients die each year from SCD, which accounts for half of all deaths in patients with CAD.[1] Approximately 80% of cases are associated with underlying CAD, 10% to 15% with nonischemic cardiomyopathies, and 5% with primary electrical diseases.[2] SCD is defined as sudden unexpected death from a cardiac cause within 1 hour after the onset of cardiac symptoms. Approximately 80% of cases occur at home, and 40% are unwitnessed.[3,4] The overall survival rate to hospital discharge for out-of-hospital cardiac arrest in North America is about 8% despite the presence of advanced emergency response systems.[4]

When the cardiac rhythm is assessed within 4 minutes of witnessed arrest, ventricular fibrillation (VF) is present in 95% of cases, and asystole is present in 5%.[5] As the time from collapse to rhythm assessment increases to 12 minutes, VF is present in only 71% of cases, and asystole is present in 29%. Resuscitation outcome is thus critically dependent on time from arrest. Because no antiarrhythmic agent has been shown to prevent SCD in a meaningful way, and because survival is greatest when defibrillation is performed in the first 4 minutes of arrest, the implantable cardioverter-defibrillator (ICD) is a powerful therapeutic agent for prevention of sudden death. However, ICDs are expensive and carry long-term consequences in many patients. Identification of patients who will benefit most from an ICD and those who will not remains an important ongoing clinical challenge.

Although a patient profile at very high risk for sudden death can be defined, the majority of patients who manifest SCD do not fit this profile.[6] Indeed, SCD is the first manifestation of heart disease in 50% of those who die suddenly. Thus, although patients previously diagnosed with CAD, heart failure, and left ventricular (LV) dysfunction have the highest annual risk of sudden death, in terms of absolute numbers, this patient group accounts for only a minority of all patients who will die from cardiac arrest (Figure 22-1).

Implantable Cardioverter-Defibrillator Systems and Technology

Current ICD generator size is as small as 35 cc, compared with 10 cc for a pacemaker. ICD leads may be transvenous, epicardial, or subcutaneous (Figure 22-2). Basic arrhythmia detection by the ICD requires a sensed heart rate greater than a programmable cut-off value for a prescribed duration or number of cardiac cycles. Additional analysis of tachycardia rate variation, electrogram morphology, and atrial/ventricular electrogram relationship may be applied to discriminate ventricular tachycardia (VT) from supraventricular tachycardia (SVT). Antiarrhythmic therapies include high-voltage shocks or antitachycardia pacing. All current ICDs provide bradycardia pacing. Patients with high defibrillation energy requirements may have a subcutaneous coil lead in place, and a completely subcutaneous ICD system is under development.[7] Epicardial leads are now primarily limited to cases in which implantation of transvenous leads for resynchronization therapy fail. For patients with temporary contraindications to ICD implantation or for those with a temporary risk for ventricular arrhythmias, a wearable defibrillator vest is available for use over weeks or months (see Figure 22-2). ICDs are considered to be cost effective, with estimated costs of $40,000 to $60,000 per life-year saved.[8]

Implantable Cardioverter-Defibrillators for Secondary Prevention of Sudden Death

The evidence that ICDs reduce mortality rates in those who have survived previous cardiac arrest derives from three randomized clinical trials (Table 22-1). A significant mortality benefit with an ICD was demonstrated in the Antiarrhythmic Drug Versus Defibrillator (AVID) trial, but nonsignificant trends toward reduced mortality rates with an ICD were noted in the Cardiac Arrest Survival in Hamburg (CASH) and the Canadian Implantable Defibrillator Study (CIDS) trials.[9-11] The latter two trials are believed to have been underpowered to detect a mortality benefit; however, both were found to have contributed more deaths in a meta-analysis of all three studies.[12] This was due in part to longer follow-up in CASH and CIDS compared with AVID.[12] This meta-analysis found a significant 25% relative reduction in mortality rate with an ICD compared with amiodarone therapy (hazard ratio [HR], 0.75; 95% confidence interval [CI], 0.64 to 0.87). The benefit was entirely due to a 50% relative reduction in sudden death (HR, 0.50; 95% CI, 0.34 to 0.62). The absolute reduction in all-cause mortality was 7% (95% CI, 5% to 10%). Fifteen patients needed to be treated with ICD to prevent one death.

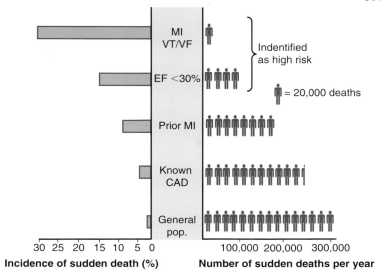

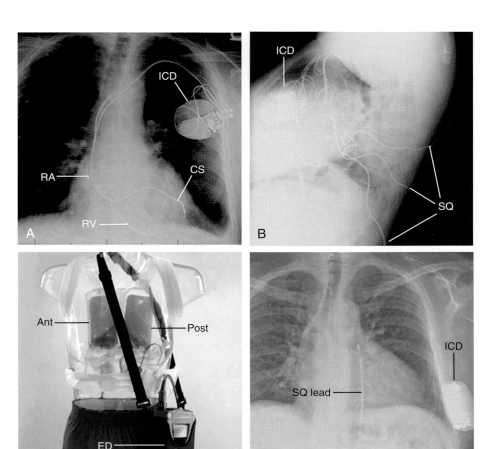

FIGURE 22-1 Incidence of sudden death in the United States as a percentage of the population (*left*) and by absolute numbers (*right*) according to risk profile. Those with prior sustained ventricular tachycardia (*VT*) or ventricular fibrillation (*VF*) and left ventricular ejection fraction (*EF*) <30% are at highest statistical risk (*left*). Although at low statistical risk, those with known coronary artery disease (*CAD*) or in the general population comprise the majority of sudden death fatalities because of their overwhelming numbers. (*Modified from Myerberg RJ, Interian A, Mitrani RM, et al. Frequency of sudden cardiac death and profiles at risk. Am J Cardiol 1997;80:10F-19F.*)

FIGURE 22-2 Implantable cardioverter-defibrillator (ICD) systems. **A,** Anteroposterior radiograph of a transvenous cardiac resynchronization ICD system with generator (*ICD*), right atrial lead (*RA*), right ventricular lead (*RV*), and coronary sinus lead (*CS*). **B,** Lateral radiograph of an ICD system with subcutaneous array lead (*SQ*). **C,** Wearable external defibrillator vest. The anterior (*Ant*) and posterior (*Post*) shocking patch electrodes are shown incorporated into a mesh vest. ED, external defibrillator unit. **D,** Anteroposterior radiograph of an entirely subcutaneous ICD system. The anteriorly placed parasternal subcutaneous defibrillation lead (*SQ lead*) is shown. (**B,** *Courtesy LifeVest, Inc.* **D,** *From Bardy GH, Smith WM, Hood MA, et al. An entirely subcutaneous implantable cardioverter-defibrillator. N Engl J Med 2010;363:36-44.*)

Implantable Cardioverter-Defibrillators for Primary Prevention of Sudden Cardiac Death

CLINICAL TRIALS

Based on success with ICD therapy for the secondary prevention of SCD, numerous trials have been performed for primary prevention in patients at high risk for fatal ventricular arrhythmias but who had not had an arrest (Table 22-2). These trials have a common feature in that the major inclusion criterion was reduced LV ejection fraction (LVEF), which was proven in epidemiologic studies to be a powerful predictor of total mortality rate and SCD. Patients with infarct-related cardiomyopathy initially were targeted by ICD trials because of the known risk of SCD in this patient population. These trials include patients with a reduced LVEF who received ICD late after myocardial infarction (MI).[13-15] All three of these studies found benefit with prophylactic ICD implantation, with HRs of 0.46 to 0.73 for total mortality. The evidence for benefit to primary prevention treatment is strongest for the cohort of patients with ischemic cardiomyopathy who received ICDs late

TABLE 22-1	Secondary Prevention Implantable Cardioverter-Defibrillator Trials								
TRIAL	PATIENTS (N)	FOLLOW-UP	PATIENT GROUP	TRIAL DESIGN	PRIMARY ENDPOINT	MORTALITY CONTROL*	MORTALITY ICD*	RR WITH ICD	NNT*
AVID[9]	1013	18 mo	Resuscitated from VF or sustained VT with syncope or sustained VT plus EF ≤40% and hemodynamic compromise	Randomized ICD vs. amiodarone	All-cause mortality	24%	15.8%	0.73 (P < .02)	4.6
CIDS[10]	659	3 y	Resuscitated VF or VT or unmonitored syncope	Randomized amiodarone vs. ICD	All-cause mortality	21%	14.7%	0.70 (P = .142)	11
CASH[11]	228	57 mo	Cardiac arrest secondary to VF or VT	Randomized to ICD vs. amiodarone vs. metoprolol	All-cause mortality	44%	36%	0.61 (P =.2)	5.6

*At 2 years.
AVID, Antiarrhythmic Drug Versus Defibrillator; CASH, Cardiac Arrest Survival in Hamburg; CIDS, Canadian Implantable Defibrillator Study; EF, ejection fraction; ICD, implantable cardioverter-defibrillator; NNT, number needed to treat to prevent one death; RR, relative risk; VF, ventricular fibrillation; VT, ventricular tachycardia.

after MI. Patients with reduced LVEF who received ICDs early (<40 days) after MI (Defibrillator in Acute Myocardial Infarction Trial [DINAMIT] and Insulin Resistance Intervention After Stroke [IRIS] Trial) or patients with a reduced LVEF who underwent surgical revascularization (coronary artery bypass graft [CABG][16-18]) did not show benefit in controlled trials. In these trials, reduced rates of sudden death were offset by higher non-sudden death rates in ICD patients. In two very small studies, patients with a reduced LVEF and nonischemic cardiomyopathy showed no benefit to prophylactic ICD (Cardiomyopathy Trial [CAT] and Amiodarone Versus Implantable Cardioverter-Defibrillator Trial [AMIOVIRT]).[19,20] The much larger Defibrillators in Non-Ischemic Cardiomyopathy Treatment Evaluation (DEFINITE) of nonischemic cardiomyopathy patients showed a strong trend toward improved total mortality rate in nonischemic cardiomyopathy patients (relative risk [RR], 0.65; 95% CI, 0.40 to 1.06; P = .08).[21] The largest primary prevention trial to enroll ischemic and nonischemic cardiomyopathy patients, the Sudden Cardiac Death-Heart Failure Trial (SCD-HeFT) of 2521 patients, showed benefit to ICD implantation for all patients combined and for ischemic and nonischemic subgroups (Figure 22-3).[22] Although no single trial has shown a statistically significant reduction in total mortality rate (as a primary endpoint) for nonischemic cardiomyopathy patients treated with primary prevention ICDs, these devices are considered to benefit this patient cohort based on the overall weight of the results from these multiple studies.

Risk Stratification for Sudden Cardiac Death

ICD therapy is expensive and is associated with long-term consequences. Ideal patient selection criteria would identify those at high risk for malignant arrhythmias *and* exclude those unlikely to benefit from ICDs because of low risk of SCD or competing nonarrhythmic death. All variables studied to date have limited positive predictive value for SCD. No other risk factor, other than reduced ejection fraction, is currently required for ICD implantation. The following risk stratification measures have received the greatest attention (Table 22-3).

EJECTION FRACTION

The risk for SCD and total mortality increases dramatically when ejection fraction (EF) falls below 40%. As EF falls lower, the relative risk for non-sudden cardiac death exceeds that for SCD; and whereas EF is highly predictive of total mortality, it has poor sensitivity for SCD, ranging from 22% to 72% in clinical trials.[23-25] In addition, patients with additional risk factors for SCD but an EF of 30% to 40% may have SCD rates higher than patients with lower

EFs alone. Two thirds of those who experience SCD have normal or near-normal EFs,[26] and no screening strategy has yet been devised to identify these patients for prophylactic management.[24]

ELECTROPHYSIOLOGIC STUDIES

Inducible sustained ventricular arrhythmias may identify patients with a twofold to 15-fold increased risk of SCD after MI.[24] In many studies, the absolute risk of SCD remains unacceptably high in noninducible patients as well.[13,23] The sensitivity and specificity of electrophysiologic testing for patients with nonischemic cardiomyopathies are quite low.

NONSUSTAINED VENTRICULAR ARRHYTHMIAS

Nonsustained ventricular arrhythmias are frequent in patients with reduced EF. This finding has limited specificity for predicting benefit from ICD therapy.[23] The duration of nonsustained ventricular arrhythmias has no influence on outcomes.[24]

SIGNAL-AVERAGED ELECTROCARDIOGRAM

The signal-averaged electrocardiogram (ECG) has limited positive predictive value, and time-dependent reversal of abnormal test results may occur after acute MI.[27] Results may also differ based on infarct location, on infarct-related vessel patency, and for patients with nonischemic cardiomyopathies.

T-WAVE ALTERNANS

Many studies have demonstrated a high negative predictive value for arrhythmic events but a low positive predictive value.[28] The test gives indeterminant results in up to one third of patients. Several recent studies suggest that as a single test, microvolt T-wave alternans does not have a role in stratifying patients for an ICD.[29,30]

AUTONOMIC FUNCTION

A vast array of heart rate variability measures has been investigated. Heart rate variability may better predict nonarrhythmic death than arrhythmic death.[27] Baroreflex sensitivity carries a relatively low positive predictive value for identifying patients at risk for VT after MI.[31]

LEFT VENTRICULAR SCAR BURDEN

The presence and extent of late myocardial enhancement on magnetic resonance imaging (MRI) has been correlated with the

ROLE OF IMPLANTABLE CARDIOVERTER-DEFIBRILLATORS IN PREVENTION OF SUDDEN CARDIAC DEATH

TABLE 22-2 Primary Prevention Implantable Cardioverter-Defibrillator Trials

TRIAL	PATIENTS (N)	FOLLOW-UP	PATIENT GROUP	TRIAL DESIGN	PRIMARY ENDPOINT	RR (95% CI) WITH ICD	NNT
MADIT[15]	1232	20 mo	NYHA class I-III, LVEF ≤30% post MI	Randomized ICD vs. no ICD	All-cause mortality	0.69 (0.51-0.93), P = .016; 0.74 after extended follow-up at 7.6 y	8 at 20 mo
AMIOVIRT[20]	103	2 y	Nonischemic cardiomyopathy and nonsustained VT	Randomized amiodarone vs. ICD	Total mortality	Stopped due to futility	
CAT[19]	104	5.5 y	Dilated cardiomyopathy and LVEF ≤30%	Randomized ICD vs. no ICD	All-cause mortality	No difference between groups	
DEFINITE[21]	458	29 mo	Nonischemic cardiomyopathy, LVEF <36%, history of heart failure and >10 PVCs/h or nonsustained VT	Randomized ICD vs. no ICD	All-cause mortality	0.65 (0.40-1.06), P = .08	24
SCD-HeFT[22]	2521	45.5 mo	NYHA class II-III and EF ≤35%, ischemic or nonischemic heart disease	Randomized ICD vs. amiodarone vs. placebo	All-cause mortality	0.77 (0.62-0.96), P = .007); absolute decrease in mortality of 7.2%	14
DINAMIT[16]	674	30 mo	6-40 days post MI with EF ≤35% and depressed heart rate variability or elevated resting heart rate	Randomized to ICD or no ICD <40 days after MI	All-cause mortality	1.08 (0.76-1.55), P = .66	
IRIS[17]	898	37 mo	5-31 days post MI with EF ≤40%, nonsustained VT, or heart rate >90 beats/min	Randomized to ICD vs. no ICD <31 days after MI	All-cause mortality	1.04 (0.81-1.35), P = .78	
MADIT[14]	196	27 mo	NYHA class I-II, prior MI, LVEF ≤35%, nonsustained VT and inducible VT not suppressed with procainamide	Randomized to ICD vs. best medical therapy (amiodarone in 74%)	All-cause mortality	0.46 (0.26-0.82), P = .009	2
MUSTT[13]	704	39 mo	Prior MI, LVEF ≤40%, and inducible sustained VT	Randomized medical therapy vs. EPS-guided therapy (58% received ICDs)	Cardiac arrest or arrhythmic death	0.73 (0.53-0.99), P < .004	2.5
CABG-Patch[18]	900	2.7 y	LVEF ≤35% with abnormal SAECG and elective CABG	Randomized epicardial ICD or no ICD	All-cause mortality	1.07 (0.81-1.42), P = .64	

AMIOVIRT, Amiodarone Versus Implantable Cardioverter-Defibrillator Trial; CABG, coronary artery bypass grafting; CAT, Cardiomyopathy Trial; CI, confidence interval; DEFINITE, Defibrillators in Non-Ischemic Cardiomyopathy Treatment Evaluation; DINAMIT, Defibrillator in Acute Myocardial Infarction Trial; EPS, electrophysiology study; ICD, implantable cardioverter-defibrillator; IRIS, Insulin Resistance After Stroke; LVEF, left ventricular ejection fraction; MADIT, Multicenter Automatic Defibrillator Implantation Trial; MI, myocardial infarction; MUSTT, Multicenter Unsustained Tachycardia Trial; NNT, number needed to treat to prevent one death; NYHA, New York Heart Association; PVC, premature ventricular contraction; RR, relative risk; SAECG, signal-averaged electrocardiogram; SCD-HeFT, Sudden Cardiac Death-Heart Failure Trial; VT, ventricular tachycardia.

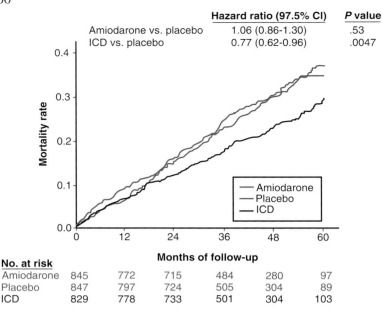

	Hazard ratio (97.5% CI)	P value
Amiodarone vs. placebo	1.06 (0.86-1.30)	.53
ICD vs. placebo	0.77 (0.62-0.96)	.0047

No. at risk

	0	12	24	36	48	60
Amiodarone	845	772	715	484	280	97
Placebo	847	797	724	505	304	89
ICD	829	778	733	501	304	103

FIGURE 22-3 Total survival curves for heart failure patients treated with amiodarone, placebo, or implantable cardioverter-defibrillator (ICD) for primary prevention of sudden death in the Sudden Cardiac Death-Heart Failure Trial (SCD-HeFT). CI, confidence interval. *(From Bardy GH, Lee KL, Mark DB, et al. Amiodarone or an implantable cardioverter-defibrillator for congestive heart failure. N Engl J Med 2005;352:225-237.)*

TABLE 22-3   Risk Stratification for Sudden Cardiac Death

VARIABLE	CRITICAL MEASURE	PPV	NPV	COMMENT	KEY REFERENCE(S)
LVEF	LVEF <30%-40%	10%	75%	For VT after MI	13,14,15
Electrophysiologic study	Inducible MMVT >15 to 30 sec duration or requiring DCC or sustained PMVT with 1 or 2 extra stimuli	11%	95%	CAD patients, value of EPS in nonischemic cardiomyopathy patients limited 1-year follow-up	13
Nonsustained ventricular tachycardia	10 PVCs/h	19%	94%	For VT post MI	13
Signal-averaged ECG	Filtered QRS >120 ms; RMS40 <20 uV or LAS40 >38 ms	17%	96%	From post-MI patients	27
T-Wave alternans	>1 min with V_{alt} ≥1.9 uV at heart rate <110 beats/min	9%	95%	CAD patients for ICD implant	30
Baroreflex slope	<3 ms/mm Hg	21%	95%	Post MI	31
Heart rate variability		22%	91%		
Ventricular scar burden	Late myocardial enhancement presence or extant	Hazard ratio, 5.2		Nonischemic cardiomyopathy	32

CAD, coronary artery disease; DCC, direct current cardioversion; ECG, electrocardiogram; EPS, electrophysiologic study; ICD, implantable cardioverter-defibrillator; LAS40, low-amplitude signal duration <40 uV; LVEF, left ventricular ejection fraction; MI, myocardial infarction; MMVT, monomorphic ventricular tachycardia; NPV, negative predictive value; PMVT, polymorphic ventricular tachycardia; PPV, positive predictive value; PVCs, premature ventricular contractions; RMS40, root mean square voltage terminal 40 ms; V_{alt}, alternans amplitude; VT, ventricular tachycardia.

---

risk for SCD and ventricular arrhythmias in patients with dilated cardiomyopathies.[32]

GENETIC TESTING

The occurrence of SCD in one parent confers an 80% increased risk of SCD, and SCD in both parents confers a ninefold risk of sudden death.[33] Common variants in sodium and potassium channel genes are associated with SCD.[34] In the future, genetic testing may play a role in risk stratification for sudden death.

Many factors—such as inducible VT, heart failure, QRS duration, and EF—predict SCD and demonstrate interactive effects. For example, a patient with heart failure, left bundle branch block (LBBB), and an LVEF of 35% may have a greater risk of SCD than a patient with no heart failure and a narrow QRS but EF less than 30%.[24] Nevertheless, no single measure has been accepted to refine inclusion criteria for primary prevention ICD implantation over LVEF alone. Some measures predict total mortality, but none adequately predicts arrhythmic death; therefore they have not been incorporated into routine clinical care. These risk factors may have the best utility when used for their negative predictive value. Theoretically, combinations of these measures may reduce ICD implantation by more than 50% by excluding patients with very low risk of SCD.[31] For example, the combination of a nonpositive T-wave alternans study and a negative electrophysiologic test was associated with a 1-year arrhythmic event rate of 2.3% in the Alternans Before Cardioverter Defibrillator (ABCD) trial.[30] A model to predict mode of death in heart failure patients based on common clinical variables has also been developed.[35] Those with the lowest scores had an incidence rate for SCD of 3.8 per 100 person-years versus 24.9 per 100 person-years for the highest score group. Defining a lower limit of acceptable risk at which to exclude patients from ICD implantation remains a scientific and ethical challenge.

Comorbidities and Implantable Cardioverter-Defibrillator Benefit

Patients with severe comorbid conditions were excluded from the landmark randomized ICD trials. Current implant guidelines do not specify any comorbid conditions as contraindications to ICD implantation, unless patient survival is expected to be less than 1 year. As a result, population-based ICD patient cohorts may differ greatly from those of controlled trials, with up to 80% of patients with ischemic heart disease, 60% with New York Heart Association class III or IV heart failure, 50% with renal disease, 8% with strokes, and 3% with cancer.[36,37] The most studied comorbid conditions that may influence benefit from the ICD are age, renal disease, and heart failure.

AGE

Age alone has not been considered a contraindication to ICD implantation, although 30% percent of patients receiving ICDs are 70 to 79 years old, and 12% are older than 80 years.[38] With advancing age, the annual risk of both SCD and total mortality increase, but total mortality increases at a greater rate.[39] Nevertheless, median survival for octogenarians receiving ICDs is 3.6 years (95% CI, 2.3 to 4.9), which appears acceptable from both clinical and cost-effective perspectives.[40] Older patients with an LVEF less than 20% or with severe renal disease derive greatly reduced ICD benefit, however.[41] As with all patients, recommendations for ICD implantation must be highly individualized for those at advanced ages.

KIDNEY DISEASE

Renal dysfunction is a powerful predictor of death in the ICD population. Retrospective studies have shown diminishing benefits and progressive renal dysfunction from ICDs. In the Multicenter Automatic Defibrillator Implantation Trial (MADIT) II, patients with estimated glomerular filtration rate (eGFR) less than 35 mL/min/1.74 m^2 derived no benefit from ICD implantation compared with medically treated patients.[42] Although patients who undergo dialysis (hemodialysis and peritoneal dialysis) have annual mortality rates up to 21%, with 26% of all deaths from sudden death, the benefits of primary prevention ICD therapy in these patients appears to be markedly less than for those without severe renal disease.[43,44] It is unclear whether any benefit is achieved because of the lack of randomized trials of ICD versus no ICD in dialysis patients. As secondary prevention, ICDs may reduce total mortality rate by 42% in highly selected dialysis patients.[43] A recent analysis of arrhythmic and nonarrhythmic death in more than 3000 patients with chronic kidney disease showed that the benefits of ICDs in patients with more advanced disease is limited by the preponderance of nonarrhythmic death.[45]

HEART FAILURE

Within the range of class II and III heart failure patients enrolled in clinical trials, those with lower LVEFs generally derived the greatest survival benefit from primary prevention ICDs.[46,47] A threshold value for an LVEF below which ICD implantation is futile has not yet been established, but class IV heart failure is a contraindication to ICD therapy (without cardiac resynchronization therapy [CRT]) unless anticipating cardiac transplantation ("bridge" to cardiac transplantation).

EFFECTS OF MULTIPLE COMORBID CONDITIONS

Multiple comorbid conditions have been assessed to identify patients at greatest risk for early death after ICD implantation. Risk factors for death in primary prevention ICD patients include age greater than 70 years, heart failure class II or greater, atrial fibrillation, QRS greater than 0.12 seconds, and blood urea nitrogen (BUN) level greater than 26 mg/dL.[48] Patients with no risk factors or those at very high risk of total mortality (serum creatinine ≥2.5 mg/dL) derived no benefit from primary prevention ICDs compared with medically treated patients (Figure 22-4).[48] These data indicate that some patient groups are either too well or too sick to benefit from ICDs. However, these findings have not been incorporated into formal guidelines. For patients at the extremes of comorbid risk, recommendations for ICD implantation must be highly individualized.

Cardiac Resynchronization Implantable Cardioverter-Defibrillators

Indications for CRT defibrillator implantation include the above indications associated with LVEF of 35% or less, class III or IV congestive heart failure despite optimal medical therapy, and QRS duration greater than 120 ms.[49] Patients with LBBB pattern, nonischemic cardiomyopathy, and QRS duration greater than 150 ms are most likely to respond. CRT improves heart failure symptoms in 70% of patients with prolonged (>120 ms) QRS durations.[49] In the Comparison of Medical Therapy, Pacing, and Defibrillation in Heart Failure (COMPANION) trial, implantation of a cardiac resynchronization defibrillator reduced all-cause mortality by 36% over optimal medical therapy alone (Table 22-4, Figure 22-5).[50] The subset of class IV heart failure patients in this trial showed a reduction in sudden death, but not total mortality, compared with patients treated with resynchronization pacemakers or medical therapy alone.[51] The MADIT with Cardiac Resynchronization Therapy trial (MADIT-CRT) demonstrated a reduced combined endpoint of death or heart failure hospitalization with CRT compared with non-CRT ICDs, but no benefit in mortality rate alone was demonstrated for the CRT device.[52] The Resynchronization/Defibrillation for Ambulatory Heart Failure Trial (RAFT) demonstrated improved survival and better heart failure hospitalization rates for patients receiving CRT ICDs compared with standard ICDs.[53] The MADIT-CRT trial demonstrated improved outcomes for patients with class I and II heart failure in the setting of LBBB, QRS duration greater than 130 ms, and LVEF less than 30%.[52]

Guidelines for Cardioverter-Defibrillator Implantation

The 2008 ACC/AHA/ESC guidelines for ICD implantation are listed in Box 22-1 and are summarized in Figure 22-6.[49]

CLASS I INDICATIONS

Class I indications for secondary prevention ICDs are SCD, hemodynamically unstable ventricular arrhythmias, or unexplained syncope with LV dysfunction and inducible ventricular arrhythmias not a result of reversible causes.

Class I indications for primary prevention ICDs in patients with ischemic cardiomyopathy are LVEF of 35% or less with class II or III heart failure more than 40 days after infarction or LVEF of 30% or less with class I heart failure more than 40 days after infarction. In addition, inducible sustained ventricular arrhythmias in a patient with nonsustained spontaneous ventricular tachycardia, LVEF less than 40%, and prior MI is a class I indication for ICD.

Class I indications for ICD implantation in patients with nonischemic cardiomyopathy are LVEF of 35% or less with class II or III heart failure. The presence of class I heart failure in these patients constitutes a class IIb indication. For reimbursement, nonischemic patients should demonstrate persistently low EF after 3 to 9 months of medical therapy.

CLASS II INDICATIONS

ICD implantation is considered reasonable (class II indication) for patients with nonischemic cardiomyopathy and unexplained syncope, primary electrical disease, familial heart disease, or cardiac sarcoidosis with disease-specific risk factors for SCD.

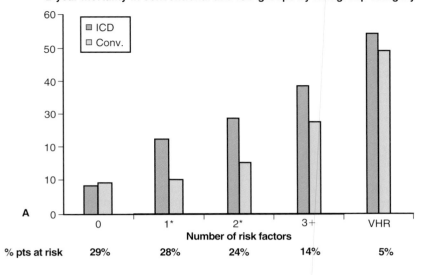

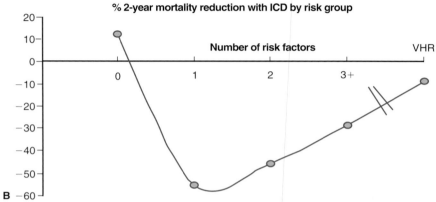

FIGURE 22-4   A, Two-year mortality rates for patients treated with implantable cardioverter-defibrillator (*ICD*) vs. conventional medical therapy alone (*Conv.*) by number of comorbidities in the Multicenter Automatic Defibrillator Implantation Trial II (MADIT II). The five clinical factors assessed were New York Hospital Association functional class higher than II, age older than 70 years, blood urea nitrogen level greater than 26 mg/dL, QRS duration longer than 120 ms, and atrial fibrillation. *$P < .05$ ICD vs. conventional therapy. **B,** Corresponding 2-year mortality risk reduction with ICD by number of risk factors. Note that at the extremes of risk-factor burden, the ICD has no effect on mortality rate; this suggests some patient groups are too well or too sick to benefit from ICD therapy. VHR, very high risk.

TABLE 22-4	Selected Cardiac Resynchronization Therapy Implantable Cardioverter-Defibrillator Trials			
TRIAL	**PATIENTS (N)**	**FOLLOW-UP**	**PATIENT GROUP AND TRIAL DESIGN**	**PRIMARY ENDPOINT**	**RESULTS**
COMPANION[50]	1520	12 mo	NYHA class III-IV CHF, QRS >120 ms, EF <35%	All-cause mortality or heart failure hospitalization	
			CRT-ICD vs. medical therapy alone		RR, 0.80; 95% CI, 0.68-0.95; *P* = .010
			CRT pacemaker vs. medical therapy		RR, 0.81; 95% CI, 0.69-0.96; *P* = .14
			Secondary endpoint total mortality		RR, 0.64; 95% CI, 0.48-0.86; *P* = .003
			CRT-ICD vs. medical therapy		
			CRT pacemaker vs. medical therapy		RR, 0.76; 95% CI, 0.58-1.01; *P* = .59; NNT = 5
MADIT-CRT[52]	1820	30 mo	NYHA class I-II and QRS ≥130 ms, ICD vs. CRT-ICD	All-cause mortality or heart failure event	For CRT-ICD: RR, 0.34; 95% CI, 0.52-0.84; *P* = .001
					Driven by HF events and no benefit of CRT vs. CRT-D on mortality alone
RAFT[53]	1798	40 mo	NYHA class II-III and QRS ≥120 ms, ICD vs. CRT-ICD	All-cause mortality	For CRT-ICD: RR, 0.75; 95% CI, 0.64-0.87; *P* < .001

CHF, congestive heart failure; CI, confidence interval; COMPANION, Comparison of Medical Therapy, Pacing, and Defibrillation in Heart Failure; CRT, cardiac resynchronization therapy; CRT-D, CRT-defibrillation; HF, heart failure; ICD, implantable cardioverter-defibrillator; MADIT-CRT, Multicenter Automatic Defibrillator Implantation Trial Cardiac Resynchronization Therapy; NNT, number needed to treat to prevent one death; NYHA, New York Heart Association; RAFT, Resynchronization/Defibrillation for Ambulatory Heart Failure Trial; RR, relative risk.

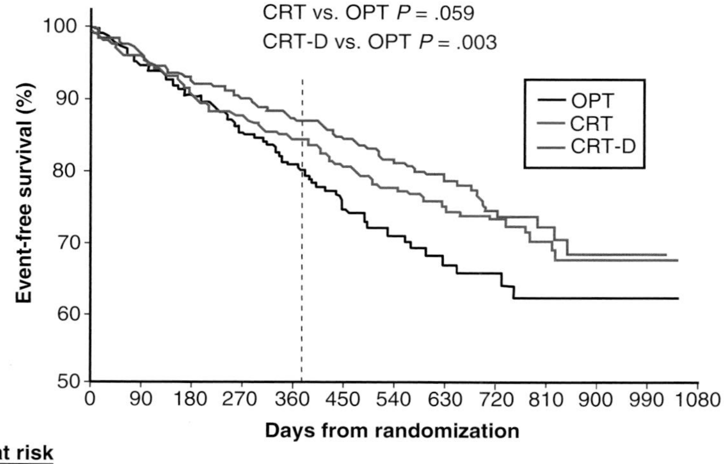

CRT vs. OPT *P* = .059
CRT-D vs. OPT *P* = .003

FIGURE 22-5 Total survival curves for heart failure patients treated with cardiac resynchronization implantable cardioverter-defibrillator (*CRT-D*), cardiac resychronization pacemaker without defibrillator (*CRT*), or optimal medical therapy alone (*OPT*) for primary prevention of sudden death in the Comparison of Medical Therapy, Pacing, and Defibrillation in Heart Failure (COMPANION) rial. The endpoint was determined at 12 months of follow-up (*dashed line*). (*From Bristow MR, Saxon LA, Boehmer J, et al. Cardiac-resynchronizaiton therapy with or without an implantable defibrillator in advanced heart failure. N Engl J Med 2004:350:2140-2150.*)

No. at risk

OPT	308	284	255	217	186	141	94	57	45	25	4	2
CRT	617	579	520	488	439	355	251	164	104	60	25	5
CRT-D	595	555	517	470	420	331	219	148	95	47	21	1

ROLE OF IMPLANTABLE CARDIOVERTER-DEFIBRILLATORS IN PREVENTION OF SUDDEN CARDIAC DEATH

CH 22

Box 22-1 ACC/AHA/ESC/HRS 2008 Indications for Cardioverter-Defibrillator Implantation

Class I

1. Patients who are survivors of cardiac arrest as a result of VF or hemodynamically unstable sustained VT after evaluation to define the cause of the event and to exclude any completely reversible causes (*level of evidence: A*).
2. Patients with structural heart disease and spontaneous sustained VT, whether hemodynamically stable or unstable (*level of evidence: B*).
3. Patients with syncope of undetermined origin with clinically relevant, hemodynamically significant sustained VT or VF induced at electrophysiologic study (*level of evidence: B*).
4. Patients with LVEF <35% as a result of prior MI who are at least 40 days after MI and are in NYHA functional class II or III (*level of evidence: A*).
5. Patients with nonischemic DCM who have an LVEF ≤35% and who are in NYHA functional class II or III (*level of evidence: B*).
6. Patients with LV dysfunction because of prior MI who are at least 40 days post MI, have an LVEF <30%, and are in NYHA functional class I (*level of evidence: A*).
7. Patients with nonsustained VT because of prior MI, LVEF <40%, and inducible VF or sustained VT at electrophysiologic study (*level of evidence: B*).

Class IIA

1. Patients with unexplained syncope, significant LV dysfunction, and nonischemic DCM (*level of evidence: C*).
2. Patients with sustained VT and normal or near-normal ventricular function (*level of evidence: C*).
3. Patients with HCM who have ≥1 major risk factor for SCD (*level of evidence: C*).
4. Patients with ARVD/C to prevent SCD in those who have ≥1 risk factors for SCD (*level of evidence: C*).
5. Patients with long QT syndrome who are experiencing syncope and/or VT while receiving β-blockers, to reduce SCD (*level of evidence: B*).
6. Nonhospitalized patients awaiting heart transplantation (*level of evidence: C*).
7. Patients with Brugada syndrome who have had syncope (*level of evidence: C*).
8. Patients with Brugada syndrome who have documented VT that has not resulted in cardiac arrest (*level of evidence: C*).

9. Patients with catecholaminergic polymorphic VT who have syncope and/or documented sustained VT while receiving β-blockers (*level of evidence: C*).
10. Patients with cardiac sarcoidosis, giant cell myocarditis, or Chagas disease (*level of evidence: C*).

Class IIB

1. Patients with nonischemic heart disease who have an LVEF of ≤35% and who are in NYHA functional class I (*level of evidence: C*).
2. Patients with long QT syndrome and risk factors for SCD (*level of evidence: B*).
3. Patients with syncope and advanced structural heart disease in whom thorough invasive and noninvasive investigations have failed to define a cause (*level of evidence: C*).
4. Patients with a familial cardiomyopathy associated with sudden death (*level of evidence: C*).
5. Patients with LV noncompaction (*level of evidence: C*).

Class III

1. ICD therapy is not indicated for patients who do not have a reasonable expectation of survival with an acceptable functional status for at least 1 year, even if they meet ICD implantation criteria specified in the class I, IIa, and IIb recommendations (*level of evidence: C*).
2. ICD therapy is not indicated for patients with incessant VT or VF (*level of evidence: C*).
3. ICD therapy is not indicated in patients with significant psychiatric illnesses that may be aggravated by device implantation or that may preclude systematic follow-up (*level of evidence: C*).
4. ICD therapy is not indicated for NYHA class IV patients with drug-refractory congestive heart failure who are not candidates for cardiac transplantation or CRT-D (*level of evidence: C*).
5. ICD therapy is not indicated for syncope of undetermined cause in a patient without inducible ventricular tachyarrhythmias and without structural heart disease (*level of evidence: C*).
6. ICD therapy is not indicated when VF or VT is amenable to surgical or catheter ablation, such as in atrial arrhythmias associated with the Wolff-Parkinson-White syndrome, RV or LV outflow tract VT, idiopathic VT, or fascicular VT in the absence of structural heart disease (*level of evidence: C*).

ICD therapy is not indicated for patients with VT as a result of a completely reversible disorder in the absence of structural heart disease, such as electrolyte imbalance, drug use, or trauma (level of evidence: B).
ACC, American College of Cardiology; AHA, American Heart Association; ARVD/C, arrhythmogenic right ventricular dysplasia/cardiomyopathy; CRT-D, cardiac resynchronization therapy/defibrillation; DCM, dilated cardiomyopathy; ESC, European Society of Cardiology; HCM, hypertrophic cardiomyopathy; HRS, Heart Rhythm Society; ICD, implantable cardioverter-defibrillator; LV, left ventricle; LVEF, left ventricular ejection fraction; MI, myocardial infarction; NYHA, New York Heart Association; SCD, sudden cardiac death; VF, ventricular fibrillation; VT, ventricular tachycardia.
From Zipes DP, Camm AJ, Borggrefe M, et al. ACC/AHA/ESC 2006 Guidelines for Management of Patients with Ventricular Arrhythmias and the Prevention of Sudden Cardiac Death: a report of the American College of Cardiology/American Heart Association Task Force and the European Society of Cardiology Committee for Practice Guidelines. *J Am Coll Cardiol* 2006;48, e247-e346; and Epstein AE, DiMarco JP, Ellenbogen KE, et al. ACC/AHA/HRS 2008 Guidelines for Device-Based Therapy of Cardiac Rhythm Abnormalities: executive summary. A report of the American College of Cardiology/American Heart Association Task Force on Practice Guidelines. *Heart Rhythm* 2008;5:934-955.

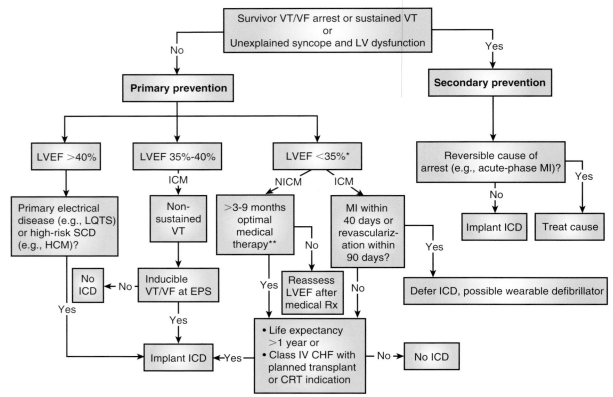

FIGURE 22-6 Flowchart summarizing indications for an implantable cardioverter-defibrillator (*ICD*). CHF, congestive heart failure; CRT, cardiac resynchronization therapy; EPS, electrophysiologic study; HCM, hypertrophic cardiomyopathy; ICM, ischemic cardiomyopathy; LQTS, long QT syndrome; LV, left ventricle; LVEF, left ventricular ejection fraction; MI, myocardial infarction; NICM, nonischemic cardiomyopathy; Rx, therapy; SCD, sudden cardiac death; VF, ventricular fibrillation; VT, ventricular tachycardia. *LVEF <35% with class II or III heart failure or <30% with class I heart failure. **Period of 3 to 9 months on medical therapy after new diagnosis of NICM not part of scientific guidelines but required for reimbursement in the United States with or without surgical or percutaneous procedures.

CLASS III INDICATIONS

ICD therapy is not recommended in patients who do not have a reasonable expectation of survival with an acceptable functional status for at least 1 year, even if class I or II implantation criteria are present. Patients with class IV or inotrope-dependent heart failure are not expected to benefit from ICD implantation except as a bridge to transplantation or combined with CRT.

Special Patient Groups

AFTER CORONARY ARTERY BYPASS GRAFT/REVASCULARIZATION

The CABG Patch Trial demonstrated no survival benefit to primary prevention ICD implantation at the time of CABG in patients with EFs less than 35% and abnormal signal-averaged ECG.[18] Guidelines for primary prevention ICD after percutaneous or surgical revascularization recommend waiting 3 months after the procedure.[49]

IMMEDIATELY AFTER MYOCARDIAL INFARCTION

Primary prevention ICD implantation within 40 days of acute infarction is associated with reduced rates of sudden death but offsetting increased rates of non-sudden death to confer no overall survival advantage.[16,17] The impact of the ICD therapy seems time dependent relative to acute MI. For example, in the MADIT II trial, the time from MI to enrollment was approximately 6.5 years.[15] Analyses of subgroups from ICD trials are consistent with an increased risk of ventricular tachyarrhythmias over time, potentially because of ventricular remodeling.

LONG QT SYNDROME

ICD implantation is recommended for patients who have syncope or ventricular arrhythmias during β-blocker therapy. Primary prevention ICDs may be considered for patients at high risk for sudden death, but at experienced centers, the majority of patients with long QT syndrome may be managed without ICD implantation.[54] The routine implantation of an ICD in all patients diagnosed with long QT syndrome is an overuse of these devices.

HYPERTROPHIC CARDIOMYOPATHY

Risk factors for sudden death include syncope, wall thickness greater than 3 cm, nonsustained ventricular tachycardia, abnormal blood pressure response to exercise, and family history of SCD.[55] The presence of any one risk factor is accepted as indication for ICD implantation, although randomized trials are lacking. In addition, some genotypes appear to be associated with higher risk of sudden death, although genetic testing has not proven useful for patient selection for ICDs because of the great variability in gene expression.

ARRHYTHMOGENIC RIGHT VENTRICULAR DYSPLASIA

ICD therapy is recommended by the American College of Cardiology Foundation (ACCF)/American Heart Association (AHA)/Heart Rhythm Society (HRS) guidelines as a class I indication for sustained VT with right ventricular dysplasia and a class II indication for primary prevention. No randomized clinical trials have been performed in this patient population, so these recommendations are based on observational data. A high incidence of appropriate

ICD shocks has been reported in this patient group with right ventricular dysplasia. The response to programmed electrical stimulation has not been identified as a risk factor; rather, the patients with syncope or LV involvement should be considered for a primary prevention device.[56]

BRUGADA SYNDROME

The indications for primary prevention ICDs in this population remain controversial. At this time, a spontaneously occurring type 1 ECG pattern or inducible type 1 pattern with a history of syncope is believed to warrant consideration for ICD implantation.[57,58]

CARDIOVERTER-DEFIBRILLATOR THERAPY

Indications for CRT combined with an implantable defibrillator are LVEF of 35% or less, class III or IV heart failure symptoms on optimal medical therapy, and QRS duration of 120 ms or more.[49] Combined resynchronization and defibrillator therapy is also approved for patients with class I or II heart failure symptoms in the setting of nonischemic cardiomyopathy, LVEF less than 30%, and LBBB QRS morphology longer than 150 ms.

Clinical Issues

FOLLOW-UP

The recommended ICD follow-up is every 3 to 6 months. At the follow-up visits, pacing and sensing thresholds are measured, lead integrity is assessed, battery status is determined, and data regarding detected arrhythmias and delivered therapies are retrieved[59] so the characteristics of events that trigger arrhythmia therapy can be examined. Patients receiving audible or vibratory alerts from their devices should undergo immediate interrogation.

One recent development is remote ICD monitoring. This technology allows the patient to send data to the monitoring physician regularly and automatically. A device therefore may be continually monitored, such as for an increase in pacing impedance heralding the onset of lead failure before an inappropriate shock is delivered. In the Lumos-T Safely Reduces Routine Office Device Follow-up Trial (TRUST), the remote monitoring group had less than a 2-day delay in the evaluation of arrhythmic events compared with a 36-day delay in patients undergoing in-office monitoring only.[60] More than 85% of 6- and 12-month visits were made with remote monitoring, reducing in-office monitoring by 45% without an increase in morbidity. At the present time, devices cannot be programmed remotely.

IMPLANTABLE CARDIOVERTER-DEFIBRILLATOR SHOCKS

Shocks occur with an annual incidence of 5% per year for primary prevention devices and 20% to 60% per year in patients with advanced heart failure or secondary prevention indications for implantation.[22,61,62] Isolated single ICD shocks should prompt ICD interrogation within 1 week of the event (Figure 22-7). Two or more ICD shocks within 24 hours warrant immediate evaluation, which includes history of medication changes, heart failure symptoms, activities preceding the shock, and physical examination.[63] Assessment of serum electrolyte level, drug levels, renal function, and myocardial ischemia should be considered, and patients taking amiodarone should have thyroid function tests performed every 4 to 6 months. Device interrogation confirms the appropriateness of the shock. In addition, occasional appropriate ICD therapies for ventricular arrhythmias are expected events, but they may require alterations of drug therapy or catheter ablation for suppression. Device reprogramming with antitachycardia pacing may terminate most ventricular arrhythmias without shocks. Guidelines for management of ICD shocks have been recently published,[63] and state-specific driving restrictions should be reviewed for each patient after appropriate ICD therapies.

Inappropriate shocks occur in more than 20% of ICD patients.[61] These shocks are most often because of SVT, especially atrial fibrillation and sinus tachycardia, and oversensing or lead failure. For patients who experience repeated inappropriate shocks, the

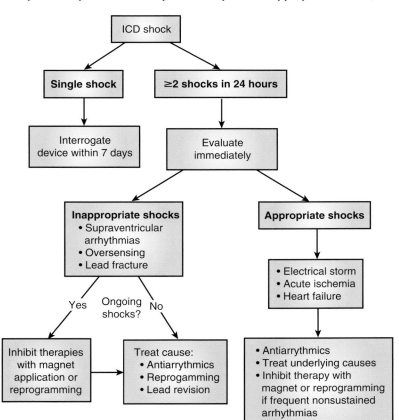

FIGURE 22-7 Management strategy for patients receiving implantable cardioverter-defibrillator (*ICD*) shocks.

tachycardia therapies can be disabled in most devices without interfering with pacemaker functions by application of a pacemaker magnet.

ELECTRICAL STORM

Electrical storm is defined as more than two or three appropriate ICD therapies within 24 hours.[64] Hundreds of shocks are sometimes delivered. Causes of electrical storm include heart failure, ischemia, metabolic disturbances, and drug proarrhythmia, although in many cases a specific etiology is not evident. Treatment includes β-blockade for patients with ischemic heart disease, amiodarone, and management of electrolyte disorders and heart failure. Intubation and sedation may also be necessary, and emergency catheter ablation may be attempted in medically refractory cases. The occurrence of electrical storm portends an increased mortality rate after the event. Patients who receive multiple shocks for any reason may experience a posttraumatic syndrome with anxiety and depression.

ELECTROMAGNETIC INTERFERENCE AND PERIOPERATIVE CARE

Electrosurgical cautery may trigger inappropriate therapy in ICD patients. Patients should have antitachycardia therapies disabled by programming prior to surgery, and the device should be fully interrogated and reprogrammed postoperatively. In emergency situations, a pacemaker magnet maintained over the device, taped on the skin, will inhibit antitachycardia therapy delivery but will not alter bradycardia pacing. Evaluation of the patient with an ICD undergoing a surgical procedure is described in detail in the joint guidelines from the HRS and the American Society of Anesthesiology.[65] After magnet application, the device should be interrogated. Although MRI has been reported to be safe with certain ICDs and specialized pulse sequences, it is generally considered contraindicated for patients with ICDs.[66] MRI of a patient with an ICD currently requires preprocedure preparation, monitoring during the procedure, and reinterrogation of the device after the procedure. Radiation therapy may damage the circuitry in unshielded ICDs and may cause late failure of the device. Nuclear radioisotope studies, radiographs and fluoroscopy, ultrasound, and computed tomography (CT) examinations have no effect on ICD function.

DRIVING

Commercial driving is prohibited in patients with ICDs, and personal driving is prohibited for 3 to 6 months in most states after syncope following ICD implantation.

REFERENCES

1. Lloyd-Jones D, Adams R, Brown T, et al. Heart disease and stroke statistics: 2010 update. *Circulation* 2010;e1-e170.
2. Zipes DP. Epidemiology and mechanisms of sudden cardiac death. *Can J Cardiol* 2005;21(Suppl A):37A-40A.
3. de Vreede Swagermakers JJ, Gorgels AP, Dubois-Arouw WI, et al. Out-of-hospital cardiac arrest in the 1990s: a population based study in the Maastricht area on incidence, characteristics and survival. *J Am Coll Cardiol* 1997;30:1500-1505.
4. Chugh SS, Jui J, Gunson K, et al. Current burden of sudden cardiac death: multiple source surveillance versus retrospective death certificate–based review in a large U.S. community. *J Am Coll Cardiol* 2004;44:1268-1275.
5. Hallstrom AP, Eisenberg MS, Bergner L. The persistence of ventricular fibrillation and its implications for evaluating EMS. *Emerg Health Serv Q* 1983;1:41-47.
6. Myerberg RJ, Interian A, Mitrani RM, et al. Frequency of sudden death and profiles of risk. *Am J Cardiol* 1997;80:10F-19F.
7. Bardy GH, Smith WM, Hood MA, et al. An entirely subcutaneous implantable cardioverter-defibrillator. *N Eng J Med* 2010;363:36-44.
8. Kupersmith J, Holmes-Rover N, Hogan A, Rovner D, Gardiner J. Cost-effectiveness analysis in heart disease, Part III. Ischemia, congestive heart failure, and arrhythmias. *Prog Cardiovasc Dis* 1995;37:307-346.
9. The Antiarrhythmics versus Implantable Defibrillators (AVID) Investigators. A comparison of antiarrhythmic-drug therapy with implantable defibrillators in patients resuscitated from near-fatal ventricular arrhythmias. *N Engl J Med* 1997;337:1576-1584.
10. Connolly SJ, Gent M, Roberts RS, et al. Canadian Implantable Defibrillator Study (CIDS): a randomized trial of the implantable cardioverter defibrillator against amiodarone. *Circulation* 2000;101:1297-1302.
11. Kuck CH, Cappato R, Siebels J, et al. Randomized comparison of antiarrhythmic drug therapy with implantable cardioverter defibrillators in patients resuscitated from cardiac arrest: the Cardiac Arrest Study Hamburg (CASH). *Circulation* 2000;102:748-754.
12. Lee DS, Green LD, Liu PP, et al. Effectiveness of implantable defibrillators for preventing arrhythmic events and death: a meta-analysis. *J Am Coll Cardiol* 2003;41:1573-1582.
13. Buxton AE, Lee KL, Fisher JD, et al; Multicenter Unsustained Tachycardia Trial Investigators. A randomized study of the prevention of sudden death in patients with coronary artery disease. *N Engl J Med* 1999;341:1882-1890.
14. Moss A, Hall WJ, Cannom DS, et al; Multicenter Automatic Defibrillator Implantation Trial Investigators. Improved survival with an implanted defibrillator in patients with coronary disease at high risk for ventricular arrhythmia. *N Engl J Med* 1996;335:1933-1940.
15. Moss A, Zareba W, Hall WJ, et al; Multicenter Automatic Defibrillator Implantation Trial II Investigators. Prophylactic implantation of a defibrillator in patients with myocardial infarction and reduced ejection fraction. *N Engl J Med* 2002;346:877-883.
16. Hohnloser SH, Kuck KH, Dorian P, et al; DINAMIT Investigators. Prophylactic use of an implantable cardioverter-defibrillator after acute myocardial infarction. *N Engl J Med* 2004;351:2481-2488.
17. Steinbeck G, Andersen D, Seidi K, et al. Defibrillator implantation early after myocardial infarction. *N Eng J Med* 2009;361:1427-1436.
18. Bigger JJ; Coronary Artery Bypass Graft (CABG) Patch Trial Investigators. Prophylactic use of implanted cardiac defibrillators in patients at high risk for ventricular arrhythmias after coronary-artery bypass graft surgery. *N Engl J Med* 1997;337:1569-1575.
19. Bansch D, Antz M, Boczor S, et al. Primary prevention of sudden cardiac death in idiopathic dilated cardiomyopathy: the Cardiomyopathy Trial (CAT). *Circulation* 2002;105:1453-1458.
20. Strickberger SA, Hummel JD, Bartlett TG, et al; the AMIOVIRT Investigators. Amiodarone versus implantable cardioverter-defibrillator: randomized trial in patients with nonischemic dilated cardiomyopathy and asymptomatic nonsustained ventricular tachycardia–AMIOVIRT. *J Am Coll Cardiol* 2003;41:1707-1712.
21. Kadish A, Dyer A, Daubert JP, et al; Defibrillators in Non-Ischemic Cardiomyopathy Treatment Evaluation (DEFINITE) Investigators. Prophylactic defibrillator implantation in patients with nonischemic dilated cardiomyopathy. *N Engl J Med* 2004;350:2151-2158.
22. Bardy GH, Lee KL, Mark DB, et al; Sudden Cardiac Death in Heart Failure Trial (SCD-HeFT) Investigators. Amiodarone or an implantable cardioverter-defibrillator for congestive heart failure. *N Engl J Med* 2005;352:225-237.
23. Buxton AE. Risk stratification for sudden death in patients with coronary artery disease. *Heart Rhythm* 2009;6:836-847.
24. Buxton AE, Lee KL, Hafley GE, et al. Limitations of ejection fraction for prediction of sudden death risk in patients with coronary artery disease. *J Am Coll Cardiol* 2007;50:1150-1157.
25. Buxton AE, Ellison KE, Lorvidhaya P, Ziv O. Left ventricular ejection fraction for sudden death risk stratification and guiding implantable cardioverter-defibrillator implantation. *J Cardiovasc Pharmacol* 2010;55:450-455.
26. Zipes DP, Wellens HJ. Sudden cardiac death. *Circulation* 1998;98:2334-2351.
27. Stein KM. Noninvasive risk stratification for sudden death: signal-averaged electrocardiography, nonsustained ventricular tachycardia, heart rate variability, baroreflex sensitivity, and QRS duration. *Prog Cardiovasc Dis* 2008;51:106-117.
28. Cutler MJ, Rosenbaum DS. Risk stratification for sudden cardiac death: Is there a clinical role for T wave alternans? *Heart Rhythm* 2009;6:S56-S61.
29. Gold MR, Ip JH, Constantini O, et al. Role of T-wave alternans in assessment of arrhythmia vulnerability among patients with heart failure and systolic dysfunction: primary results from the T-wave alternans sudden cardiac death in heart failure trial substudy. *Circulation* 2008;118:2022-2028.
30. Costantini O, Hohnloser SH, Kirk MM, et al. The ABCD (Alternans Before Cardioverter Defibrillator) Trial. *J Am Coll Cardiol* 2009;53:471-479.
31. La Rovere MT, Pinna DP, Hohnloser SH, et al. Baroreflex sensitivity and heart rate variability in the identification of patients at risk for life-threatening arrhythmias: implications for clinical trials. *Circulation* 2001;103:2072-2077.
32. Assomull RG, Preasad SK, Lyne J, et al. Cardiovascular magnetic resonance, fibrosis, and prognosis in dilated cardiomyopathy. *J Am Coll Cardiol* 2006;48:1977-1985.
33. Jouven X, Desnos M, Guerot C, et al. Predicting sudden death in the population: the Paris Prospective Study. *Circulation* 1999;99:1978-1983.
34. Noseworthy PA, Newton-Cheh C. Genetic determinants of sudden cardiac death. *Circulation* 2008;118:1854-1863.
35. Mozaffarian D, Anker SD, Anand I, et al. Prediction of mode of death in heart failure: the Seattle Heart Failure Model. *Circulation* 2007;116:392-398.
36. Lee DS, Tu JV, Austin PC, et al. Effect of cardiac and noncardiac conditions on survival after defibrillator implantation. *J Am Coll Cardiol* 2007;49:2408-2415.
37. Bruch C, Bruch C , Sindermann J, et al. Prevalence and prognostic impact of comorbidities in heart failure patients with implantable cardioverter-defibrillator. *EuroPace* 2007;9:681-686.
38. Epstein AE, Kay GN, Plumb VJ, et al. Implantable cardioverter-defibrillator prescription in the elderly. *Heart Rhythm* 2009;6:1136-1143.
39. Krahn AD, Connolly SJ, Roberts RS, et al. Diminishing proportional risk of sudden death with advancing age: implications for prevention of sudden death. *Am Heart J* 2004;147:837-840.
40. Heidenreich PA, Tsai V. Is anyone too old for an implantable cardioverter-defibrillator? *Circ Cardiovasc Qual Outcomes* 2009;2:6-8.
41. Ertel D, Phatak K, Makati K, et al. Predictors of early mortality in patients age 80 and older receiving implantable defibrillators. *PACE* 2010:33:1-7.
42. Goldenberg I, Moss AJ, McNitt S, et al. Relations among renal function, risk of sudden cardiac death and benefit of the implantable cardiac defibrillator in patients with ischemic left ventricular dysfunction. *Am J Cardiol* 2006;98:485-490.

43. Herzog CA, Li S, Weinhandl ED, et al. Survival of dialysis patients after cardiac arrest and the impact of implantable cardioverter defibrillators. *Kidney Int* 2005;68:818-825.

44. Sakhuja R, Keebler M, Lai T-S, et al. Meta-analysis of mortality in dialysis patients with an implantable cardioverter defibrillator. *Am J Cardiol* 2009;103:735-741.

45. Korantzopoulos P, Liu T, Li L, Goudevenos JA, Li G. Implantable cardioverter defibrillator therapy in chronic kidney disease: a meta-analysis. *Europace* 2009;11:1469-1475.

46. Salukhe TV, Briceno NI, Ferenczi EA, Sutton R, Francis DP. Is there benefit in implanting defibrillators in patients with severe heart failure? *Heart* 2010;96:599-603.

47. Moss AJ. Implantable cardioverter defibrillator therapy: the sickest patients benefit the most. *Circulation* 2000;101;1638-1640.

48. Goldenberg I, Vyas AK, Hall WJ, et al. Risk stratification for primary implantation of a cardioverter-defibrilator in patients with ischemic left ventricular dysfunction. *J Am Coll Cardiol* 2008;51:288-296.

49. Epstein AE, DiMarco JP, Ellenbogen KE, et al. ACC/AHA/HRS 2008 Guidelines for Device-based Therapy of Cardiac Rhythm Abnormalities: executive summary. A report of the American College of Cardiology/American Heart Association Task Force on Practice Guidelines (Writing Committee to Revise the ACC/AHA/NASPE 2002 Guideline Update for Implantation of Cardiac Pacemakers and Antiarrhythmia Devices). *Heart Rhythm* 2008;5:934-955.

50. Bristow MR, Saxon LA, Boehmer J, et al. Cardiac-resynchronization therapy with or without an implantable defibrillator in advanced heart failure. *N Eng J Med* 2004:350: 2140-2150.

51. Lindenfeld J, Feldman AM, Saxon L, et al. Effects of cardiac resynchronization therapy with or without a defibrillator on survival and hospitalizations in patients with New York Heart Association class IV heart failure. *Circulation* 2007;115:204-212.

52. Moss A, Hall WJ, Cannom DS, et al. Cardiac-resynchronization therapy for the prevention of heart-failure events. *N Engl J Med* 2009;361:1329-1338.

53. Tang ASL, Wells GA, Talajic M, et al. Cardiac resynchronization therapy for mild-moderate heart failure. *N Engl J Med* 2010; 363:2385-2395.

54. Horner JM, Kinoshita M, Webster TL, et al. Implantable cardioverter defibrillator therapy for congenital long QT syndrome: a single center experience. *Heart Rhythm* 2010:7: 1616-1622.

55. Maron BJ. Contemporary insights and strategies for risk stratification and prevention of sudden death in hypertrophic cardiomyopathy. *Circulation* 2010;121:445-456.

56. Corrado D, Calkins H, Link M, et al. Prophylactic implantable defibrillator in patients with arrhythmogenic right ventricular cardiomyopathy/dysplasia and no prior ventricular fibrillation or sustained ventricular tachycardia. *Circulation* 2010;122:1144-1152.

57. Kaufman ES. Mechanisms and clinical management of inherited channelopathies: long QT syndrome, Brugada syndrome, catecholaminergic polymorphic ventricular tachycardia, and short QT syndrome. *Heart Rhythm* 2009;6:S51-S55.

58. Probst V, Veltmann C, Eckardt L, et al. Long-term prognosis of patients diagnosed with Brugada syndrome: results from the FINGER Brugada Syndrome Registry. *Circulation* 2010;121:635-643.

59. Chugh SS, Wood MA. ICD follow-up and troubleshooting. In Ellenbogen K, Wood M, editors: *Cardiac pacing and ICDs*. 2008, Oxford, UK, Blackwell, pp. 463-497.

60. Varma N, Epstein AE, Irimpen A, et al. Efficacy and safety of automatic remote monitoring for implantable cardioverter-defibrillator follow-up: the Lumos-T Safely Reduces Routine Office Device Follow-Up (TRUST) trial. *Circulation* 2010;122:325-332.

61. Connolly SJ, Dorian P, Roberts RS, et al. Comparison of beta-blockers, amiodarone plus beta-blockers or sotalol for prevention of shocks from implantable cardioverter defibrillators: the OPTIC study—a randomized trial. *JAMA* 2006;295;165-171.

62. Desai AD, Burke MC, Hong TE, et al. Predictors of appropriate defibrillator therapy among patients with an implantable defibrillator that delivers resynchronization therapy. *J Cardiovasc Electrophysiol* 2006;17:486-490.

63. Braunschweig F, Boriani G, Bauer A, et al. Management of patients receiving implantable cardioverter defibrillator shocks. *Europace* 2010;12:1673-1690.

64. Huang DT, Traub D. Recurrent ventricular arrhythmia storms in the age of implantable cardioverter defibrillator therapy: a comprehensive review. *Prog Cardiovasc Dis* 2008;51: 229-236.

65. Zaidan JR, Atlee JL, Belott P, et al. Practice advisory for the perioperative management of patients with cardiac rhythm management devices: pacemakers and implantable cardioverter-defibrillators. *Anesthesiology* 2005;103:186-198.

66. Shinbane JS, Colleti PM, Shellock FG. MR in patients with pacemakers and ICDs: defining the issues. *J Cardiovasc Magn Reson* 2007;9:5-13.

ROLE OF IMPLANTABLE CARDIOVERTER-DEFIBRILLATORS IN PREVENTION OF SUDDEN CARDIAC DEATH

Treatment of Ventricular Tachycardia and Cardiac Arrest

Stephen Trzeciak, Andrea M. Russo, and Joseph E. Parrillo

VENTRICULAR TACHYCARDIA: ACUTE
MANAGEMENT, 408

Sustained Monomorphic Ventricular Tachycardia with a
 Pulse, 408
Polymorphic Ventricular Tachycardia, 413

MANAGEMENT OF CARDIAC ARREST, 414

Epidemiology and General Principles, 414
Cardiopulmonary Resuscitation and Advanced Cardiac Life
 Support, 414
Post–Cardiac Arrest Care, 417

REFERENCES, 418

Sudden cardiac death (SCD) represents a major public health problem in the United States and throughout the world, with a frequently cited estimate of more than 300,000 adult sudden deaths occurring annually in the United States, and an overall incidence of 0.1% to 0.2% per year, accounting for more than half of all cardiovascular deaths.[1,2] Contemporary evidence demonstrates that the risk of SCD has declined over the past 50 years, based on data from the Framingham Heart Study, coincident with the decline in deaths from coronary disease.[3] In Seattle, a decline in annual incidence of treated SCD occurred, and if this data were applied nationally, there would be 184,000 sudden deaths annually, in contrast to earlier estimates.[4] This is similar to 2008 data from the American Heart Association (AHA) Statistics Committee, which reports that approximately 166,200 out-of-hospital cardiac arrests occur annually in the United States.[5]

Myerburg and colleagues illustrated the relationship between the incidence and the total number of SCDs per year for the overall adult population in the United States and for higher risk subgroups (Figure 23-1).[2] With identification of more powerful risk factors, the incidence progressively increases, but this higher incidence is associated with a progressive decrease in the number of patients identified. Primary and secondary prevention implantable cardioverter-defibrillator (ICD) trials have focused on the higher risk subgroups that have either already demonstrated a sustained ventricular arrhythmia or have been identified to have underlying coronary disease with prior infarction or cardiomyopathy (see Chapter 22). However, most of the individuals in the general population who have had a cardiac arrest were not previously identified to be at risk based on traditional risk factors.

Epidemiologic studies show that most cardiac arrests occur outside the hospital, and initial recordings by emergency personnel reveal that ventricular tachyarrhythmias are the most common mechanisms leading to SCD. In an older study, ventricular fibrillation (VF) was the initial recorded rhythm in 75% of patients who had a cardiac arrest in Seattle, a city with an effective rapid response system.[6] More updated evidence reveals that the annual incidence of cardiac arrest with VF as the first identified rhythm has decreased significantly from 1980 to 2000.[7] Defining the initial rhythm at the time of the arrest may be difficult because of delay between the onset of the event and time of arrival of emergency personnel because ventricular tachycardia (VT) may rapidly degenerate to VF, and tachyarrhythmias may change to bradyarrhythmias, pulseless electrical activity, or asystole within a short period of time. Study of patients who were wearing ambulatory monitors at the time of death reveals that the most frequent cause of sudden death was related to ventricular tachyarrhythmias, observed in 84% of cases, most often VT degenerating into VF in 62% of cases.[8] Rapid defibrillation is the most effective therapy for resuscitation of these patients. Use of automated external defibrillators (AEDs) by trained lay responders or by Good Samaritans with little or no training in community-based programs can increase survival after SCD, with impressive results seen in studies examining use in airports, airplanes, and casinos.[9-11] Unfortunately,

similar results were not seen with home AEDs, where overall survival was not improved when compared with reliance on conventional resuscitation methods.[12] Most out-of-hospital cardiac arrests occur in the home, and this location presents a particular challenge for provision of timely care by emergency medical services.

Patients who have a cardiac arrest or sustained VT frequently have underlying structural heart disease, most frequently coronary artery disease (CAD); such structural disease accounts for approximately 62% to 80% of cases of SCD.[13,14] Other etiologies include left ventricular (LV) hypertrophy, cardiomyopathy (dilated, hypertrophic, and right ventricular [RV] cardiomyopathy/ dysplasia), valvular disease, myocarditis, and congenital heart disease. Ion channel defects, preexcitation syndromes, and proarrhythmic effects of antiarrhythmic drugs are less frequently seen etiologies. In addition, sudden cardiac arrest may rarely occur in patients without any identified structural defect. This is called *idiopathic VF*. Because the substrate abnormality is continually present, there must also be a trigger that initiates sustained ventricular arrhythmias. For example, common triggers include heart failure, transient ischemia, and electrolyte disturbances, such as hypokalemia.

Myerburg and colleagues described a model of SCD showing the interactions among structure, function, and electrogenesis of VT/VF (Figure 23-2).[15] Structural abnormalities such as myocardial infarction (MI), hypertrophy, myopathic ventricle, and primary structural electrical abnormalities interact with one or more functional perturbations that can lead to transient destabilization. The major categories of functional influences include transient ischemia and reperfusion, metabolic and hemodynamic abnormalities, neurochemical or neurophysiologic fluctuations, and toxins. This interaction between structural abnormalities and functional perturbations may convert chronic, benign, ambient arrhythmias such as premature ventricular contractions (PVCs) into triggering events for sustained VT/VF.[2,15]

Treatment of cardiac arrest and sustained VT has evolved over the years, and advancements in therapy have improved outcome. This chapter will focus on the pharmacologic treatment of acute episodes of monomorphic VT, drug use during cardiac arrest, and early management of cardiac arrest survivors.

Ventricular Tachycardia: Acute Management

Sustained Monomorphic Ventricular Tachycardia with a Pulse

Sustained monomorphic VT may occur with a variety of clinical features and symptoms. Most patients have underlying structural heart disease, including CAD and nonischemic cardiomyopathy in the setting of LV systolic dysfunction, and VT is most often related to scar-related reentry. Monomorphic VT may also occur in the

FIGURE 23-1 Relationship between the incidence and total number of sudden cardiac deaths annually in specific population subgroups. The incidence (percent per year) and the total number of events per year are illustrated for the overall adult population in the United States and for increasingly higher risk subgroups. With identification of increasingly powerful risk factors, the incidence increases progressively, but this is accompanied by a progressive reduction in the number of patients identified. The population affected by multicenter, randomized, primary and secondary prevention implantable cardioverter-defibrillator trials is also noted. AVID, Antiarrhythmic Drug Versus Defibrillator; CASH, Cardiac Arrest Survival in Hamburg; CIDS, Canadian Implantable Defibrillator Study; EF, ejection fraction; HF, heart failure; MADIT, Multicenter Automatic Defibrillator Implantation Trial; MI, myocardial infarction; MUSTT, Multicenter Unsustained Tachycardia Trial; SCD-HeFT, Sudden Cardiac Death-Heart Failure Trial. (Data from Myerburg RJ, Spooner PM. Opportunities for sudden death prevention: directions for new clinical and basic research. Cardiovasc Res 2001;50:177-185.)

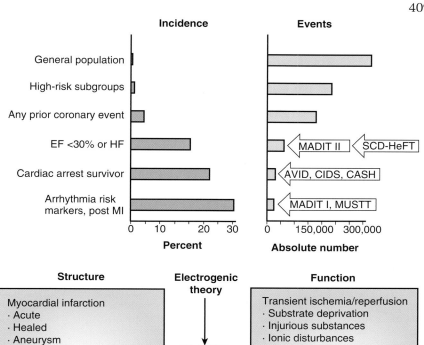

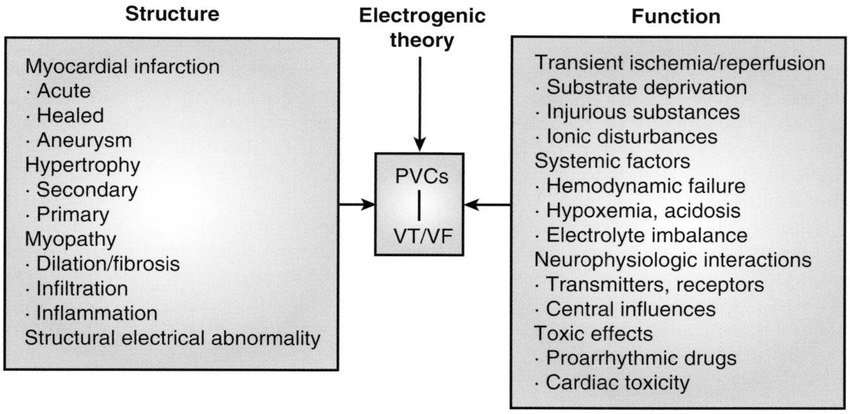

FIGURE 23-2 Interactions among structure, function, and electrogenesis of ventricular tachycardia (VT)/ventricular fibrillation (VF). Four common structural abnormalities are identified that may interact with functional perturbations to cause transient destabilization. This interaction may convert chronic, ambient, benign arrhythmias such as premature ventricular contractions (PVCs) into triggering events for VT/VF. (Modified from Myerburg RJ, Kessler KM, Bassett AL, Castellanos A. A biological approach to sudden cardiac death: structure, function and cause. Am J Cardiol 1989;63:1512-1516.)

setting of RV cardiomyopathy/dysplasia, again likely related to a reentrant mechanism. Automatic VT may also occur, although this is seen more often in a periinfarction setting. Bundle branch reentry VT, which is related to a macroreentrant circuit, should be treated the same as scar-related VT. Less frequently, special forms of VT or idiopathic VT may occur in the setting of a structurally normal heart. The latter may respond to adenosine, β-blocker, or calcium channel blocker therapy and are not discussed in this chapter. If these special forms of VT cannot be recognized with certainty, the arrhythmia should be treated similarly to VT related to scar and underlying structural heart disease.

A wide spectrum of clinical presentations and symptoms are associated with sustained monomorphic VT. Patients may present with pulseless VT or cardiac arrest or may come to medical attention with less severe symptoms—palpitations, lightheadedness, shortness of breath, or chest pain. Others may experience presyncope or brief loss of consciousness. Although loss of consciousness may occur during sustained monomorphic VT because of transient severe hypotension while upright, patients may awaken as blood pressure improves after assuming a supine position. Underlying cardiac disease and LV function, as well as the cycle length of the tachycardia, are important factors that influence clinical presentation.

The most rapid and effective way to terminate sustained VT is electrical cardioversion, but this requires use of anesthesia for appropriate sedation. Intravenous (IV) antiarrhythmic drugs can be used for the treatment of hemodynamically stable VT, and they may also help prevent recurrent ventricular arrhythmias. A retrospective study showed that 77% of patients who came to the emergency department with sustained VT were initially classified

as hemodynamically stable, and 33 (60%) of 55 patients had their VT terminated with first-line IV antiarrhythmic therapy.[16] If hemodynamic instability occurs during or after IV antiarrhythmic drug therapy without termination of VT, direct current cardioversion is the class I treatment recommendation per the American College of Cardiology (ACC)/AHA/European Society of Cardiology (ESC) Guidelines for the Treatment of Patients with Ventricular Arrhythmias.[17]

According to the current AHA Advanced Cardiovascular Life Support (ACLS) recommendations, IV amiodarone is the first-line therapy for sustained monomorphic VT.[18] Although other parenteral antiarrhythmic agents for life-threatening ventricular arrhythmias are discussed in this section for historic purposes, these drugs are selected for use either as single agents or in combination with amiodarone for treatment of recurrent, incessant VT. In particular, VT storm—recurrent, incessant, sustained monomorphic VT—may require the combination of multiple antiarrhythmic agents for continued suppression of recurrent arrhythmias until more definitive therapy, such as catheter ablation or surgical approaches for the treatment of arrhythmias, can be instituted.

LIDOCAINE

Lidocaine is a class Ib antiarrhythmic agent that has been used for many years for the treatment of ventricular arrhythmias associated with ischemia and acute MI. However, the efficacy of lidocaine in terminating sustained monomorphic VT is low—only 8% to 27%.[19-23] Because of poor efficacy, it is no longer recommended as first-line therapy for the treatment of monomorphic VT in the ACLS protocol. According to the 2000 version of the AHA Guidelines for Cardiopulmonary Resuscitation and Emergency Cardiac Care, if electrical cardioversion is not possible, desirable, or successful, IV procainamide, IV sotalol (not available in the United States), or IV amiodarone is preferred over IV lidocaine.[24] A randomized study that compared the efficacy of IV procainamide with lidocaine revealed that procainamide was superior to lidocaine in terminating spontaneously occurring monomorphic VT.[19]

Although the ACLS protocol no longer recommends lidocaine as an initial treatment option, the ACC/AHA/ESC Guidelines for the Treatment of Patients with Ventricular Arrhythmias state that IV lidocaine might be reasonable for the initial treatment of patients with stable, sustained monomorphic VT specifically associated with acute myocardial ischemia or infarction, with a class IIb recommendation (level of evidence C).[17] It is thought that lidocaine may be useful in suppressing automatic VT associated with acute MI. Although lidocaine was previously used routinely for prophylaxis against VF in the setting of acute MI, a meta-analysis suggested that this antiarrhythmic agent may actually increase overall mortality rate, and this practice has long since been abandoned.[25]

The recommended IV loading dose of lidocaine is 100 mg (or 1.0 to 1.5 mg/kg), administered slowly, for attempted termination of VT (Table 23-1); this is followed by a maintenance infusion at 1 to 4 mg/min. Dosage adjustments are required for patients with heart failure or hepatic disease. An advantage of this antiarrhythmic drug is that it can be infused rapidly with minimal hemodynamic effects at therapeutic levels. In addition, it is also less likely than other agents to cause bradycardia when maintained at therapeutic levels.

Although lidocaine is no longer recommended as initial therapy in the ACLS protocol, our group still finds this agent useful as adjunctive therapy in patients with recurrent, incessant, sustained VT, particularly following initiation of amiodarone, which may take several days to suppress ventricular arrhythmias. In addition, it can be useful in suppressing ambient frequent ventricular ectopy, which may promote spontaneous induction of sustained monomorphic VT in some situations, including periinfarction. In the setting of recurrent sustained VT, a second dose of 50 mg may be administered after the initial 100-mg bolus, which tends to be initially well tolerated in most patients; however, drug levels need to be closely monitored on a maintenance drip because central nervous system side effects often occur in patients with rising lidocaine levels, particularly in patients with abnormal hepatic function or low cardiac output.

PROCAINAMIDE

Procainamide is a class Ia antiarrhythmic agent that has been available for over 50 years and has demonstrated clinical utility for treatment of VT. It has been studied in the electrophysiology (EP)

laboratory for suppression of inducibility of VT by programmed ventricular stimulation, with an efficacy of 33% to 61%.[26-28] With respect to acute termination of sustained monomorphic VT, the efficacy of IV procainamide is 80% to 93%.[19,29] In contrast, one retrospective analysis reported a much lower efficacy, only 30%, for the termination of sustained, stable monomorphic VT, perhaps because of a lower infusion rate in this study, although it did appear to be more effective when used as the initial antiarrhythmic medication with termination in 57% of patients.[30] In a randomized study that compared the efficacy of IV procainamide with lidocaine, procainamide was superior to lidocaine in terminating spontaneously occurring monomorphic VT.[19] Although it is no longer listed as an early treatment option in the ACLS protocol, IV procainamide is reasonable for initial treatment of patients with stable sustained monomorphic VT, according to the ACC/AHA/ESC guidelines, as a class IIa recommendation (level of evidence B).[17] This is consistent with the 2010 International Consensus on Cardiopulmonary Resuscitation and Emergency Cardiovascular Care, which states that procainamide is recommended for patients with hemodynamically stable monomorphic VT and without concomitant severe congestive heart failure or acute MI.[31]

Procainamide is also administered with the aim to prevent recurrent VT in an acute setting. Even when VT recurs in patients taking this antiarrhythmic agent, it may be better tolerated because of its effects on prolongation of the VT cycle length. This increase in VT cycle length may help in pace termination of the arrhythmia, although less often it may actually stabilize the reentrant circuit and make it more difficult to terminate with pacing maneuvers.[32] The ability of the drug to terminate the arrhythmia does not necessarily correlate with the ability of the drug to prevent inducibility in the EP laboratory.[29]

Procainamide may be administered orally, intravenously, or intramuscularly, although the latter is rare. For the acute termination of VT, it is typically used intravenously. The recommended IV loading dose of procainamide is 10 to 15 mg/kg (see Table 23-1). The drug may be administered at a rate of 20 mg/min, not to exceed 50 mg/min, for a maximum dose of 1 to 1.5 g. Administration of procainamide may lead to hypotension; therefore blood pressure should be monitored at least every 5 minutes, and electrocardiographic (ECG) monitoring should be continuous. Slowing the rate of infusion may help prevent hypotension because the initial fall in blood pressure may be related to the vasodilatory effect; volume repletion may also be useful. When a maintenance drip is required, dosing should be individualized because the half-life for elimination is no longer present in patients with reduced renal function and/or low cardiac output. Drip rates typically range from 2 to 4 mg/min. In addition, N-acetylprocainamide (NAPA) is an active metabolite with class III antiarrhythmic effects, and further dosage adjustment may be needed in the setting of renal insufficiency because this metabolite is also renally excreted. Serum levels of procainamide and NAPA are available for clinical monitoring, and therapeutic procainamide levels are reported to be 3 to 10 μg/mL. Frequent ECGs should also be performed to monitor the QT interval because procainamide prolongs repolarization and can lead to proarrhythmia in the form of polymorphic VT with a long QT interval or to torsades de pointes (TdP).

Although this antiarrhythmic agent is no longer included in the ACLS protocol, our group still finds this drug useful for some patients who have frequent episodes of sustained monomorphic VT in the critical care setting. Because it may take days for amiodarone to suppress VT, procainamide significantly slows the VT rate and may be used initially as adjunctive therapy to help reduce the need for external cardioversions or internal ICD shocks. This slowing of the tachycardia rate may make the arrhythmia hemodynamically better tolerated and more amenable to pace termination, thereby reducing painful shock therapy. It is also occasionally used in the EP laboratory during VT catheter ablation procedures to help slow the VT rate and improve hemodynamic tolerance to allow entrainment mapping, although newer substrate-mapping techniques and electroanatomic mapping have reduced this

TABLE 23-1	Recommended Doses of IV Antiarrhythmic Agents for Termination of Hemodynamically Tolerated Sustained Monomorphic Ventricular Tachycardia	
DRUG	**LOADING DOSE**	**MAINTENANCE DRIP**
Lidocaine	1-1.5 mg/kg over 2-3 min; may repeat 0.5-0.75 mg/kg over 2-3 min in 5-10 min (max. total, 3 mg/kg)	1-4 mg/min
Procainamide	10-15 mg/kg, up to 1-1.5 g (typically 20 mg/min, not to exceed 50 mg/min)	2-4 mg/min
Sotalol	0.2-1.5 mg/kg over 30 min	0.008 mg/kg/min
Amiodarone	150 mg over 10 min (additional loading doses as needed, up to max. 2.2 g/24 h)	1 mg/min for 6 h, then 0.5 mg/min

IV, intravenous

need. In a closely monitored setting such as the EP laboratory, procainamide may be administered at a rate of up to 50 mg/min, with careful attention to blood pressure and QT interval changes.

SOTALOL

Although the IV formulation of sotalol is not currently marketed in the United States, efficacy in acute termination of hemodynamically tolerated VT has been shown. IV sotalol was superior to lidocaine for the acute termination of spontaneous sustained VT in a randomized double-blind study, with acute termination of VT occurring in 69% of patients versus 18%, respectively.[33] In fact, the 2000 version of the AHA Guidelines for Cardiopulmonary Resuscitation and Emergency Cardiac Care recommended IV sotalol over lidocaine for treatment of hemodynamically stable VT.[24]

The recommended dose of sotalol is 1.5 mg/kg or 100 mg intravenously (see Table 23-1). It is renally excreted and should be used with caution in patients with renal insufficiency. With its negative inotropic effects, it may precipitate congestive heart failure in patients with depressed LV systolic function.

AMIODARONE

Although already available for many years in other countries, IV amiodarone was approved by the FDA for use in the United States in 1995 for the acute suppression of hemodynamically unstable VT or VF refractory to therapy with conventional antiarrhythmic drugs. Amiodarone is a class III antiarrhythmic agent with class I, II, and IV antiarrhythmic properties. The IV form of amiodarone has initial sympatholytic and calcium channel–blocking effects,

with class I and III activity appearing later. Kowey and colleagues[34] reviewed the use of IV amiodarone, including efficacy of this agent for treatment of frequently recurrent destabilizing VT and VF, with suppression rates of 63% to 91% in uncontrolled trials. IV amiodarone reduced the frequency of recurrent VT/VF and terminated arrhythmias in severely ill patients. However, these studies were either retrospective reviews or uncontrolled studies with relatively small numbers of patients who might also have concomitantly received other antiarrhythmic agents.

Three prospective trials confirmed these findings, and one study demonstrated a dose-response relationship, with an efficacy at least comparable to bretylium, an antiarrhythmic agent no longer available in the United States (and therefore not discussed in this chapter).[35-37] In all three studies, enrollment criteria included at least two episodes of hemodynamically unstable VT or VF within 24 hours despite treatment with lidocaine, procainamide, and bretylium (except in the bretylium comparison study). Most of the patients enrolled in these trials had VT, and few initially presented with VF. Because placebo-controlled studies would not be ethical in this cohort, a dose ranging study design was used in two of the studies, and a placebo-controlled comparison with bretylium was used in the third study. In these studies, 40% to 43% of patients were event free at 24 hours after administration of 1000 mg. The time to first event showed significant differences among the three IV amiodarone dose groups ($P = .0247$), and the most significant contribution to that difference was the paired comparison between the 1000- and 125-mg dose groups (Figure 23-3).[37] The higher dose of amiodarone (1000 mg) and bretylium had similar efficacy rates (Figure 23-4).[35] However, there was a high crossover rate from bretylium to amiodarone as a result of hypotensive effects that

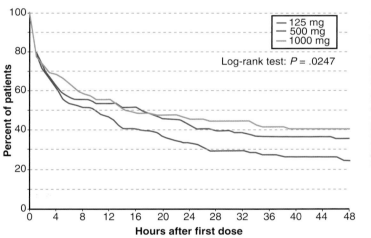

FIGURE 23-3 Comparison of three different doses of intravenous amiodarone in patients with life-threatening ventricular arrhythmias. The graph of the analysis of time to first event demonstrates significant differences among the dose groups ($P = .0247$). The most important contribution to that difference was the paired comparison between the 1000-mg and 125-mg dose groups ($P = .030$). *(Data from Scheinman MM, Levine JH, Cannom DS, et al.; Intravenous Amiodarone Multicenter Investigators Group. Dose-ranging study of intravenous amiodarone in patients with life-threatening ventricular tachyarrhythmias. Circulation 1995;92:3264-3272.)*

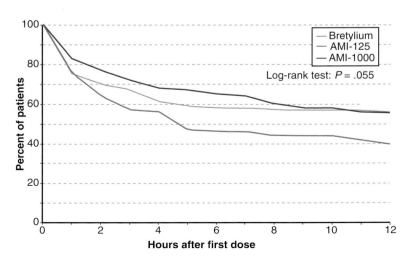

FIGURE 23-4 Comparison of two doses of intravenous amiodarone to bretylium in the treatment of recurrent ventricular tachycardia (VT) and ventricular fibrillation (VF). The graph shows the cumulative percentage of patients who remained VT/VF event free at each hour after initial dose administration for the first 12 hours only, when the majority of events occurred. There appears to be separation between the low-dose amiodarone curve and the bretylium and high-dose amiodarone curves. The differences among groups approached statistical significance ($P = .0545$). AMI, amiodarone. *(Data from Kowey PR, Levine JH, Herre JM, et al, for the Intravenous Amiodarone Multicenter Investigators Group. Randomized, double-blind comparison of intravenous amiodarone and bretylium in the treatment of patients with recurrent, hemodynamically destabilizing ventricular tachycardia or fibrillation. Circulation 1995;92:3255-3263.)*

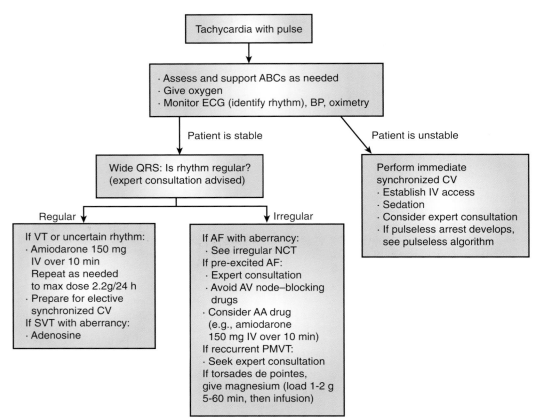

FIGURE 23-5 Algorithm for tachycardia with a pulse. AA, antiarrhythmic; AF, atrial fibrillation; AV, atrioventricular; BP, blood pressure; CV, cardioversion; ECG, electrocardiograph; IV, intravenous; NCT, narrow complex tachycardia; PMVT, polymorphic ventricular tachycardia; SVT, supraventricular tachycardia; VT, ventricular tachycardia. *(Modified from ACLS protocol: approach to stable tachycardia. In Field JM, editor:* Advanced cardiovascular life support provider manual. *Dallas, TX, 2006, American Heart Association, pp 97-100.)*

occurred more often with bretylium than with amiodarone. The specific presenting arrhythmia—hypotensive VT, VF, or incessant VT—or severity of LV dysfunction did not influence efficacy of amiodarone.[36]

Despite its incorporation into the ACLS guidelines (Figure 23-5), limited direct evidence supports the use of IV amiodarone for the rapid termination of hemodynamically stable, sustained monomorphic VT. Retrospective case reviews of relatively small numbers of patients revealed that IV amiodarone at a dosage of 150 to 300 mg was relatively ineffective for acute termination of hemodynamically well-tolerated monomorphic VT, with pharmacologic termination within 15 to 20 minutes in 15% to 29% of patients.[38,39] Efficacy with respect to acute termination of hemodynamically well-tolerated VT was slightly higher in one study, in which termination occurred within 31 minutes in 42% of patients.[40] In a more recent study to evaluate the aqueous formulation of amiodarone, acute termination of previous shock-resistant VT occurred in 78% of patients, with two thirds of these terminating after a single bolus of 150 mg.[22] Amiodarone was superior to lidocaine in the treatment of shock-resistant VT.[22]

Even if VT recurs after initial therapy with amiodarone, it may be slower and better tolerated. Amiodarone slows conduction, prolongs refractoriness, and prolongs the VT cycle length. Combination therapy with other class I antiarrhythmic agents may be useful in some patients with recurrent refractory VT. The combination of a class I antiarrhythmic agent with amiodarone often results in additional slowing of the VT rate, which further improves hemodynamic tolerance and occasionally results in suppression of inducibility.[41,42]

A large individual variation is seen in the time to respond to amiodarone during initiation of IV therapy; therefore close observation and dosage adjustments are suggested. Hypotension may be seen during initial rapid infusion and may improve by slowing

the rate of infusion. Transient negative inotropic effects may also be seen during the bolus infusion, which may be more pronounced in patients with severe LV dysfunction. These adverse effects may improve with a more prolonged period of loading. Despite initial loading, supplemental boluses may be needed in some patients who have early recurrence of VT. The recommended IV loading dose of amiodarone is 150 mg administered over 10 minutes, followed by infusion of 1 mg/min for 6 hours and then 0.5 mg/min. Additional loading doses can be repeated as needed to a maximum dose of 2.2 g in 24 hours (see Table 23-1).

A newer aqueous formulation of IV amiodarone has a significant advantage related to a low risk of drug-induced hypotension over the previous formulation.[43] Hypotension is the most frequent adverse effect of IV amiodarone, attributed to the vasoactive solvents in the standard formulation, specifically polysorbate 80 (Tween 80) and benzyl alcohol; these are used to keep amiodarone in solution because it is not water soluble. In previous controlled studies, hypotension occurred in 15% to 26% of patients receiving the original formulation of IV amiodarone, which contained polysorbate 80.[35-37] In a study to compare rapid administration of a new aqueous formulation of IV amiodarone with lidocaine, hypotension occurred in a similar percentage of patients who received amiodarone versus lidocaine (11% vs. 19%, respectively; *P* = not significant).[43] Aqueous amiodarone was concluded to be at least as safe as lidocaine in terms of causing hypotension during rapid administration.

In the clinical setting of recurrent, incessant, sustained VT, our group's experience has been that multiple amiodarone boluses may be required, administered over 2 g/day for the first 2 to 3 days. In this setting of VT storm, it may be necessary to leave the maintenance drip at 1 mg/min for 24 to 48 hours if tolerated, particularly if VT ablation therapy is not readily available. In the setting of very frequent VT, combination antiarrhythmic therapy may be required for the first few days. Combination therapy with amiodarone, lidocaine, and procainamide may be required to suppress or reduce incessant arrhythmias or to improve hemodynamic tolerance. If VT is not suppressible with drugs and VT ablation is not successful, cardiac transplantation may be considered if the patient is a candidate.

MAGNESIUM

IV magnesium has been used to treat drug-induced TdP and digoxin-induced ventricular arrhythmias. Its efficacy may be related to suppressing triggered activity, leading to more homogenous transmural ventricular repolarization. In contrast, magnesium appears to have no role in the treatment of sustained monomorphic VT. In normomagnesemic patients with CAD, magnesium is not effective for acute termination of induced hemodynamically stable sustained monomorphic VT caused by reentry.[44]

OVERDRIVE VENTRICULAR PACING

In addition to antiarrhythmic drugs, overdrive pacing is an effective way to terminate sustained monomorphic VT and potentially reduce or avoid the need for multiple cardioversions (Figure 23-6). This form of "painless" therapy is routinely delivered through ICDs in the form of *antitachycardia pacing,* although overdrive pacing can also be performed through a temporary transvenous pacing catheter inserted through the subclavian or femoral vein into the right ventricle. The ability to terminate the arrhythmia effectively depends on several factors, including the VT rate. Many antiarrhythmic agents may slow the VT rate, often making the tachycardia more amenable to pace termination. In the case of recurrent, incessant, sustained monomorphic VT (VT storm), intermittent pace termination may be a reasonable option until IV antiarrhythmic agents have had their full effects, or until a more definitive therapy, such as catheter ablation, can be instituted. Pace termination may sometimes result in acceleration of the tachycardia or degeneration of a hemodynamically well-tolerated monomorphic VT into polymorphic VT or VF; therefore, external cardioversion capabilities should be readily available.

According to the ACC/AHA/ESC Guidelines for the Treatment of Patients with Ventricular Arrhythmias, transvenous catheter pace termination can be useful in the treatment of patients with sustained monomorphic VT that is refractory to cardioversion or is frequently recurrent despite antiarrhythmic medication, with a class IIa recommendation (level of evidence C).[17]

CARDIOVERSION

For patients who have a pulse during sustained VT, synchronized cardioversion is recommended if IV amiodarone is ineffective in terminating VT.[18] The amount of energy that should be selected for initial attempts has been controversial, but it should be sufficient to result in prompt conversion in an attempt to avoid the need for multiple shocks and repeated failures. The latter could result in ischemia from prolonged VT and injury from multiple shocks. The energy requirement for termination of monomorphic VT is typically less than 100 J. The ACLS protocol recommends delivery of shocks starting with 100 J for sustained monomorphic VT with a pulse, followed by 200, 300, and then 360 J if initial shocks are unsuccessful.[18] Current defibrillators typically deliver energy in the form of biphasic shocks, which have efficacy superior to monophasic shocks. Appropriate sedation should be administered prior to cardioversion attempts.

EVALUATION TO EXCLUDE POTENTIALLY REVERSIBLE CAUSES OF VENTRICULAR TACHYCARDIA

Although sustained monomorphic VT suggests that a primary arrhythmic substrate is present in the setting of structural heart disease, evaluation to exclude reversible causes should be performed. Ischemia or acute infarction should be excluded by ECG, troponin testing, and imaging techniques. Cardiac catheterization or stress testing should be performed to determine whether the potential for ongoing ischemia exists and to exclude the need for revascularization. Electrolyte abnormalities or drug proarrhythmia should also be excluded. In the Antiarrhythmics Versus Implantable Defibrillator (AVID) trial, a secondary prevention ICD trial, patients with a potentially transient or correctable cause for their VT/VF (who were not eligible for randomization and were followed in a registry), remained at high risk for death. The mortality rate was no different, or was perhaps even worse, than that of the primary VT/VF population.[45] This suggests that factors such as electrolyte abnormalities or ischemia were not primary causes but perhaps were precipitants of arrhythmias in patients with underlying arrhythmogenic substrates.

Polymorphic Ventricular Tachycardia

Polymorphic VT associated with a normal QT interval is most often caused by acute ischemia or infarction and may rapidly degenerate into VF. When polymorphic VT is associated with a long QT interval, the syndrome is called *torsades de pointes* (Figure 23-7). TdP is associated with prolonged repolarization and is frequently pause dependent, with a late coupled PVC (long-short initiating interval). The tachycardia is often nonsustained and self-terminating, but it may recur frequently and may require preventive therapy and correction or removal of any precipitating factors, such as those outlined in Box 23-1.

The recommended treatment of polymorphic VT with a long QT interval is administration of IV magnesium at a dosage of 1 to 2 g

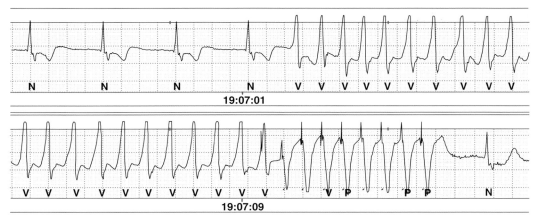

FIGURE 23-6 Antitachycardia pacing. Monomorphic ventricular tachycardia is effectively terminated with overdrive pacing.

CH
23

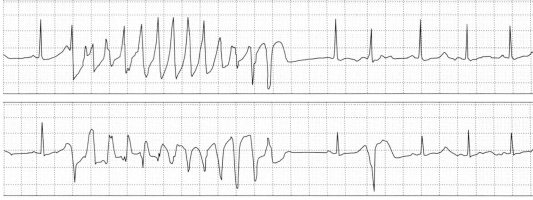

FIGURE 23-7 Torsades de pointes. Polymorphic ventricular tachycardia with a changing axis of the QRS complex ("twisting" around the baseline); a long QT interval.

> **Box 23-1 Frequently Implicated Causes of Torsades de Pointes**
>
> Antiarrhythmics
> - Class Ia (quinidine, disopyramide, procainamide)
> - Class III (sotalol, ibutilide, dofetilide, dronedarone)
>
> Antibiotics (erythromycin, azithromycin, ciprofloxacin, clarithromycin, levofloxacin, trimethoprim-sulfa)
> Antihistamines (terfenadine, astemizole)
> Antianginals (bepridil)
> Antimalarials (halofantrine, chloroquine)
> Antifungals (ketoconazole)
> Antilipemics (probucol)
> Tricyclic antidepressants (amitriptyline, imipramine, nortriptyline)
> Neuroleptics (haloperidol, chlorpromazine, risperidone, thioridazine)
> Narcotics (methadone)
> Stimulants (cocaine)
> Gastrointestinal stimulants (cisapride)
> Hypocholesterolemics (probucol)
> Electrolyte abnormalities
> - Hypokalemia
> - Hypomagnesemia
> Ion channel defects (congenital long QT syndrome)
> Bradycardia

over 5 to 60 minutes followed by an infusion according to the ACLS protocol (see Figure 23-5).[18] The efficacy of IV magnesium is supported by a case series in which all 12 patients responded to a single or repeated bolus of 2 g plus infusion (3 to 20 mg/min), until the QT interval was below 500 ms, without adverse effects.[46] Discontinuation of precipitating drugs, repletion of potassium, isoproterenol administration, or temporary pacing (if associated with bradycardia) may also be useful.

Management of Cardiac Arrest

Epidemiology and General Principles

When VT results in a loss of effective circulation (pulseless VT), a *cardiac arrest* has occurred. Approximately 350,000 persons in North America undergo resuscitation for sudden cardiac arrest each year. Approximately 25% of sudden cardiac arrest events are attributable to pulseless ventricular arrhythmias.[47] Cardiac arrest patients who come to medical attention with pulseless ventricular arrhythmias, including pulseless VT or ventricular fibrillation (VF), have a much higher chance of surviving cardiac arrest compared with those who are seen with other initial rhythms, such as asystole or pulseless electrical activity (PEA).[48] The better prognosis for pulseless ventricular arrythmias is largely related to two factors. First, pulseless ventricular arrhythmias are potentially treatable

with defibrillation (a "shockable" rhythm) to restore circulation, whereas the other initial rhythms are not. Second, pulseless ventricular arrhythmias are typically a manifestation of a cardiac etiology for the sudden cardiac arrest, whereas the other initial rhythms are more likely to be related to a noncardiac etiology and perhaps an underlying condition that is less amenable to treatment. Therefore, therapeutic interventions for cardiac arrest because of pulseless ventricular arrhythmias can be truly lifesaving, and the basic principles of treating this condition are an integral part of training for health care providers (HCPs).

A number of critical actions, a so-called *chain of survival*, must occur in response to a sudden cardiac arrest. The chain of survival paradigm (Figure 23-8) for the treatment of cardiac arrest has five elements: 1) immediate recognition of cardiac arrest and activation of the emergency response system, 2) effective cardiopulmonary resuscitation (CPR), 3) early defibrillation, 4) advanced cardiac life support, and 5) provision of post–cardiac arrest care (e.g., therapeutic hypothermia).[49] The remainder of this chapter is focused on the elements in this paradigm for treating cardiac arrest in adult patients.

Cardiopulmonary Resuscitation and Advanced Cardiac Life Support

For CPR to be effective, it must be applied without delay. Immediate recognition of cardiac arrest and activation of the emergency response system is therefore essential. With the onset of cardiac arrest, the patient becomes unresponsive. Although breathing ceases, agonal gasps may be observed in the early moments after cardiac arrest. Pulse checks—that is, palpation of large arteries for the presence or absence of a pulse—are often unreliable, even when performed by trained HCPs.[50] Because prolonged attempts to detect a pulse may result in a delay in initiating CPR, resuscitation should be started immediately if the patient is unconscious and not breathing or if agonal gasping occurs.[49]

CHEST COMPRESSIONS

Chest compressions provide circulation to the heart and brain until effective spontaneous circulation can be restored. Chest compressions generate cardiac output through an increase in intrathoracic pressure and direct compression of the heart. Compressions are applied to the patient's sternum with the patient in the supine position. The heel of one hand is placed over the lower half of the sternum and the heel of the other hand on top in an overlapping and parallel fashion. The recommended compression depth in adults is two inches, which typically requires considerable force. The recommended rate of compressions is 100 or more per minute. The current AHA teaching maxim is "push hard, push fast." This

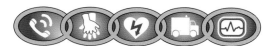

FIGURE 23-8 The chain of survival paradigm from the American Heart Association. The links in the chain represent the critical actions to optimize the chances of survival from cardiac arrest. From left to right, the links include 1) immediate recognition of cardiac arrest and activation of the emergency response system; 2) early and effective cardiopulmonary resuscitation; 3) defibrillation, if applicable; 4) advanced life support; and 5) post–cardiac arrest care, including therapeutic hypothermia if appropriate. *(From Travers AH, Rea TD, Bobrow BJ, et al. Part 4. CPR overview: 2010 American Heart Association guidelines for cardiopulmonary resuscitation and emergency cardiovascular care. Circulation 2010;122[18 Suppl 3]:S676-684.)*

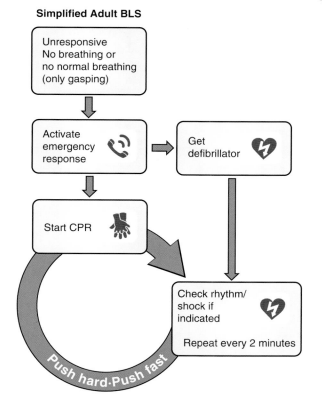

Simplified Adult BLS

FIGURE 23-9 American Heart Association simplified basic life support (*BLS*) algorithm. CPR, cardiopulmonary resuscitation. *(From Travers AH, Rea TD, Bobrow BJ, et al. Part 4. CPR overview: 2010 American Heart Association Guidelines for Cardiopulmonary Resuscitation and Emergency Cardiovascular Care. Circulation 2010;122[18 Suppl 3]:S676-S684.)*

simple instruction underscores the critical importance of vigorous chest compressions in achieving return of spontaneous circulation (ROSC).[51] In addition, it is important to allow the chest wall to recoil completely between compressions because incomplete recoil impairs the cardiac output that is generated. Due to fatigue, the quality of chest compressions typically decreases as the time providing compressions increases. Importantly, the person providing chest compressions may not perceive the fatigue or the decrease in the quality of compressions[52]; rotation of chest compressors every 2 minutes is therefore recommended. Although numerous automated mechanical devices are currently available for the provision of chest compressions, no long-term clinical outcome data support routine use of these products.

The quality of CPR is one of the most important determinants of outcome from cardiac arrest.[53] One of the most important goals related to CPR quality is minimization of interruptions in chest compressions. Historically, interruptions in chest compressions during CPR occurred frequently, and the "hands off" time comprised a substantial amount of the total resuscitation time.[53] Potential reasons for interruptions in compressions include pulse checks, rhythm analysis, switching compressors, procedures such as airway placement, and pauses before shocks are delivered ("preshock pause"). All these potential reasons for interruptions should be minimized as much as possible. Pauses for switching compressors or pulse checks by HCPs should take no longer than a few seconds.[51] Minimization of the preshock pause has been associated with higher rates of successful defibrillation and improved clinical outcome.[54]

DEFIBRILLATION

The other vital step in the resuscitation of patients with cardiac arrest as a result of pulseless ventricular arrhythmias is defibrillation. The length of the time interval from arrest to defibrillation is a critical determinant of outcome, with a sharp decrease in survival as the time to defibrillation increases.[55] Defibrillation should therefore be performed as soon as possible. With the advent of automatic external defibrillators AEDs and their dissemination into public places, both elements of effective CPR, chest compressions and defibrillation, can be performed by lay rescuers for victims of out-of-hospital cardiac arrest. The AHA algorithm for adult basic life support that incorporates these elements appears in Figure 23-9.

RESCUE BREATHING

The current AHA recommendations regarding ventilation during CPR are a function of the level of training of the rescuers.[51] For trained HCPs, the recommended ventilation strategy is a 30:2 compression/ventilation ratio—that is, a cycle of 30 chest compressions to 2 breaths—until an advanced airway is placed, and then continuous chest compressions with 1 breath every 6 to 8 seconds after the advanced airway is placed. An excessive number of ventilations ("overbagging" the patient) could be deleterious from a hemodynamic perspective, related to increased intrathoracic

pressure and decreased cardiac output with CPR, and should be avoided.

For untrained laypersons who are attempting to resuscitate a victim of out-of-hospital cardiac arrest, rescue breathing is no longer recommended. Rather, the recommended strategy is compression-only, or "hands only," CPR.[51] The rationale behind this recommendation is twofold: first, compression-only CPR can increase the number of effective chest compressions delivered to the patient because CPR does not need to be interrupted for rescue breaths; second, it does not require mouth-to-mouth contact, which may reduce the perceived barriers to CPR in the community and result in an increase in bystander CPR. The available data for out-of-hospital cardiac arrest shows that compression-only CPR is noninferior to CPR with rescue breaths; therefore it can be concluded that compression-only CPR is at least safe if not more efficacious.[56-58] For these reasons, compression-only CPR appears to be the preferred technique to teach to the general public.

ADVANCED CARDIAC LIFE SUPPORT

There are several additional, important considerations for the treatment of patients with cardiac arrest that are intended specifically for trained HCPs, specifically pharmacologic therapy. The AHA algorithm for ACLS appears in Figure 23-10.[59]

The primary goal of pharmacologic therapy is to assist the achievement and maintenance of spontaneous circulation. The mainstay of pharmacologic interventions is vasopressor agents. Epinephrine (1 mg) is recommended by IV or via the intraosseous (IO) route every 3 to 5 minutes during resuscitative efforts until spontaneous circulation is restored.[59] If IV/IO access cannot be established, epinephrine can be administered via an endotracheal tube at a higher dose (2 to 2.5 mg). If desired, vasopressin (40 mg IV/IO) could be substituted for the first or second dose of

416

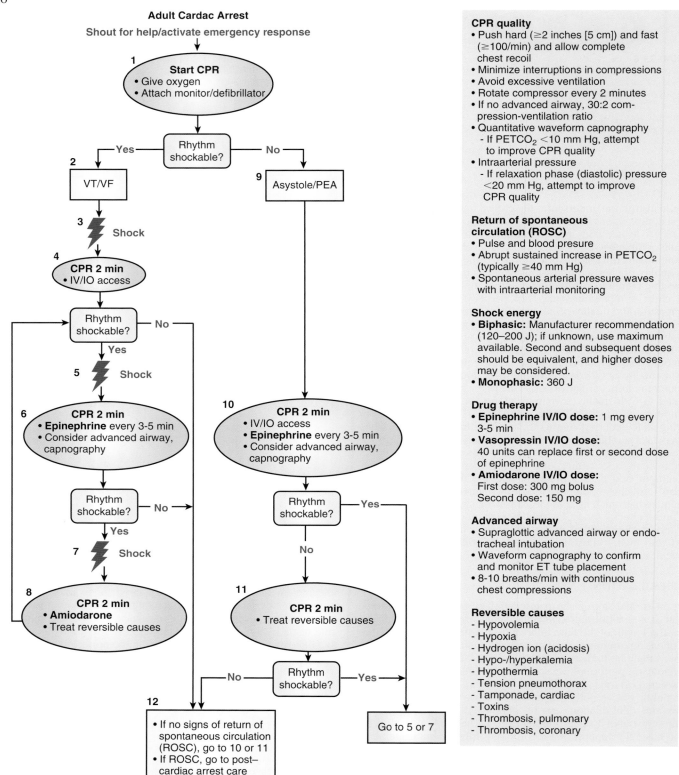

Adult Cardiac Arrest

Shout for help/activate emergency response

1 Start CPR
• Give oxygen
• Attach monitor/defibrillator

Rhythm shockable?

Yes → **2 VT/VF**

No → **9 Asystole/PEA**

3 ⚡ Shock

4 CPR 2 min
• IV/IO access

Rhythm shockable? — No

Yes

5 ⚡ Shock

6 CPR 2 min
• **Epinephrine** every 3-5 min
• Consider advanced airway, capnography

Rhythm shockable? — No

Yes

7 ⚡ Shock

8 CPR 2 min
• **Amiodarone**
• Treat reversible causes

10 CPR 2 min
• IV/IO access
• **Epinephrine** every 3-5 min
• Consider advanced airway, capnography

Rhythm shockable? — Yes

No

11 CPR 2 min
• Treat reversible causes

Rhythm shockable? — Yes → **Go to 5 or 7**

No

12
• If no signs of return of spontaneous circulation (ROSC), go to 10 or 11
• If ROSC, go to post–cardiac arrest care

CPR quality
• Push hard (≥2 inches [5 cm]) and fast (≥100/min) and allow complete chest recoil
• Minimize interruptions in compressions
• Avoid excessive ventilation
• Rotate compressor every 2 minutes
• If no advanced airway, 30:2 compression-ventilation ratio
• Quantitative waveform capnography
  - If $PETCO_2$ <10 mm Hg, attempt to improve CPR quality
• Intraarterial pressure
  - If relaxation phase (diastolic) pressure <20 mm Hg, attempt to improve CPR quality

Return of spontaneous circulation (ROSC)
• Pulse and blood presure
• Abrupt sustained increase in $PETCO_2$ (typically ≥40 mm Hg)
• Spontaneous arterial pressure waves with intraarterial monitoring

Shock energy
• **Biphasic:** Manufacturer recommendation (120–200 J); if unknown, use maximum available. Second and subsequent doses should be equivalent, and higher doses may be considered.
• **Monophasic:** 360 J

Drug therapy
• **Epinephrine IV/IO dose:** 1 mg every 3-5 min
• **Vasopressin IV/IO dose:** 40 units can replace first or second dose of epinephrine
• **Amiodarone IV/IO dose:** First dose: 300 mg bolus Second dose: 150 mg

Advanced airway
• Supraglottic advanced airway or endotracheal intubation
• Waveform capnography to confirm and monitor ET tube placement
• 8-10 breaths/min with continuous chest compressions

Reversible causes
- Hypovolemia
- Hypoxia
- Hydrogen ion (acidosis)
- Hypo-/hyperkalemia
- Hypothermia
- Tension pneumothorax
- Tamponade, cardiac
- Toxins
- Thrombosis, pulmonary
- Thrombosis, coronary

FIGURE 23-10 American Heart Association advanced cardiac life support algorithm. CPR, cardiopulmonary resuscitation; ET, endotracheal; IV, intravenous; IO, intraosseous; PEA, pulseless electrical activity; $PETCO_2$, end-tidal pressure of carbon dioxide; ROSC, return of spontaneous circulation. VF, ventricular fibrillation; VT, ventricular tachycardia. *(From Neumar RW, Otto CW, Link MS, et al. Part 8. Adult advanced cardiovascular life support: 2010 American Heart Association Guidelines for Cardiopulmonary Resuscitation and Emergency Cardiovascular Care. Circulation 2010;122[18 Suppl 3]:S729-S767.)*

epinephrine. Amiodarone is the preferred antiarrhythmic agent for resuscitation. In patients with VF/VT that does not respond to CPR, defibrillation, and vasopressor therapy, amiodarone is recommended (first dose: 300 mg IV/IO; second dose: 150 mg IV/IO).[59] It should be noted that the use of atropine for PEA/asystole was recently removed from the ACLS algorithm, and evidence is insufficient to recommend routine administration of sodium bicarbonate during resuscitation.

Another important consideration is the fact that some studies have shown that ACLS interventions did not improve clinical outcomes when compared with basic life support alone[60]; therefore, the impact of these therapies on outcome in the setting of cardiac arrest remains a matter of debate.

Post–Cardiac Arrest Care

Even if the heart is successfully restarted and a pulse is restored, cardiac arrest patients remain at high risk of death. Among out-of-hospital cardiac arrests, approximately 60% of patients who are successfully resuscitated do not survive to hospital discharge. Return of spontaneous circulation involves global ischemia/reperfusion (I/R) injury with potentially devastating neurologic consequences. The primary mode of death in these patients is the brain injury that typically follows a severe I/R insult, and it is now recognized that early therapeutic interventions initiated after ROSC can improve the trajectory of this condition. Specifically, clinical trials have shown that a mild therapeutic hypothermia strategy after ROSC can improve neurologic outcome and survival, providing the first meaningful evidence that anoxic brain injury is in fact a treatable disease. Accordingly, the post-ROSC phase of therapy is now considered to be a crucial link in the chain of survival paradigm for treating cardiac arrest (see Figure 23-8).[61] If a pulse is restored with CPR and defibrillation, post–cardiac arrest care should be started immediately.

GENERAL APPROACH

Patients resuscitated from cardiac arrest should be admitted to an intensive care unit (ICU) capable of providing comprehensive post–cardiac arrest care. These capabilities should include[62]:

- Critical care support to optimize cardiovascular indices and vital organ perfusion
- Therapeutic hypothermia to limit neurologic injury
- An evidence-based approach to neurologic prognostication to prevent inappropriately early determinations of poor neurologic prognosis
- An interventional cardiac catheterization laboratory for possible percutaneous coronary intervention before admission to the ICU if the cause of the cardiac arrest is thought to be acute MI

CRITICAL CARE SUPPORT

Approximately half of patients resuscitated from cardiac arrest will have major hemodynamic instability after ROSC, which should be anticipated.[63] Although no clinical trials haved tested whether targeting specific goals for hemodynamic indexes could improve outcome in post–cardiac arrest patients,[64] expert opinion advocates a general approach in which hemodynamics and organ perfusion are optimized.[61] Despite the fact that no interventional trials have been performed, it is prudent to be aggressive about raising the blood pressure in patients who remain markedly hypotensive after resuscitation because postresuscitation arterial hypotension has been associated with sharply higher mortality rates.[63]

Exposure to hyperoxia, the excessively high arterial partial pressure of oxygen, has been associated with poor clinical outcome among adult patients resuscitated from cardiac arrest and admitted to an ICU.[65] These data support the findings of numerous experimental studies in animal models in which hyperoxia exposure after ROSC worsened brain histopathologic changes and

neurologic function.[67-70] There appears to be a paradox regarding oxygen delivery to the injured brain; insufficient oxygen delivery can exacerbate cerebral anoxia, but excessive oxygen delivery can exacerbate oxygen free radical formation and subsequent reperfusion injury. Although no clinical trials of a rapidly titrated rexoygenation strategy after cardiac arrest have been performed, expert opinion advocates limiting unnecessary exposure to an excessively high fraction of inspired oxygen and maintaining an arterial oxygen saturation of 94% or more.[61]

THERAPEUTIC HYPOTHERMIA

Therapeutic hypothermia (TH), also called *mild therapeutic hypothermia,* is a treatment strategy that reduces the body temperature for neuroprotection in a patient resuscitated from cardiac arrest. The body temperature is typically reduced to 33° to 34° C for 12 to 24 hours. The brain sustains I/R injury after resuscitation from cardiac arrest, and although the severity of the initial ischemic injury (i.e., the no-flow time) has already occurred and cannot be mitigated, the severity of the reperfusion injury after restoration of blood flow can, in fact, be reduced. Neuronal cell death is not instantaneous after an I/R injury from cardiac arrest; in fact, in experimental models, it has been shown to take up to 72 hours after ROSC for histopathologic changes to manifest.[61] This indicates that a window of opportunity exists in which the brain injury is potentially treatable. In theory, therapeutic hypothermia can protect the brain by reducing at the cellular or subcellular level the cellular metabolic requirements, mitochondrial dysfunction, derangements of calcium ion homeostasis, oxygen free radical production, and apoptosis.

Two landmark clinical trials of TH were published in 2002, one randomized, controlled trial and one quasiexperimental trial.[71,72] These trials showed improved outcomes with TH for comatose survivors of witnessed out-of-hospital cardiac arrest with VF as the initial rhythm.

The AHA algorithm for post–cardiac arrest care appears in Figure 23-11.[62] If the patient lacks a meaningful response to verbal commands after ROSC, this indicates that brain injury may be present, and TH should be strongly considered. Clinicians should initiate TH as soon as possible after ROSC, and multiple potential methods are available for inducing TH: external cooling devices, intravascular cooling devices, or a combination of ice packs, conventional cooling blankets, and cold (4° C) IV saline. The advantage of using devices specifically intended for targeted temperature management is that the devices typically have computer modules that regulate the cooling rate based on a feedback loop that continuously monitors the patient's core body temperature. This approach may help the patient reach target temperature faster, and it may limit the risk of overshoot (temperature <89° C), which is not uncommon with ice packs and conventional cooling blankets.[73] The main disadvantage of the device-based approach compared with conventional cooling methods is cost. Regardless of what methods are used, effective achievement of target temperature may be aided by the use of a uniform physician order set for TH induction.[74] The current recommendation is to maintain TH for 12 to 24 hours.[62] Whether a longer duration of therapy might be beneficial is currently unknown.

Clinicians should be mindful of a number of potential complications associated with TH; these include coagulopathy, hypovolemia (cold diuresis), hyperglycemia, bradycardia, and the potential increased risk of secondary infection. However, these complications are often not severe when they do occur, and in terms of risk/benefit determinations, the risk of anoxic brain injury typically outweighs risks associated with complications.

NEUROLOGIC PROGNOSTICATION

Neurologic prognostication is challenging in the first few days after resuscitation from cardiac arrest.[75] Although some findings may suggest poor neurologic prognosis, few of these signs are

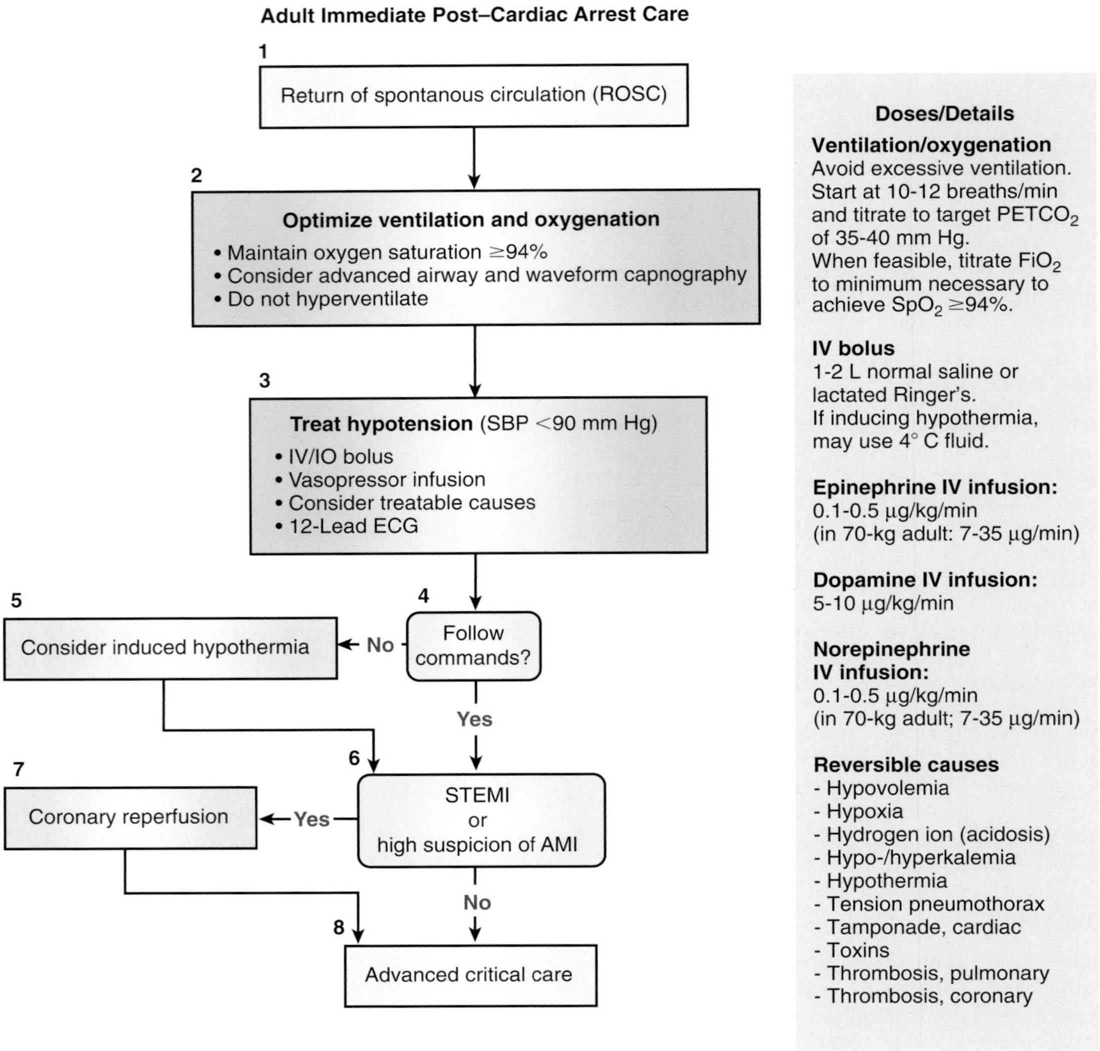

Adult Immediate Post–Cardiac Arrest Care

1 Return of spontanous circulation (ROSC)

2
Optimize ventilation and oxygenation
- Maintain oxygen saturation ≥94%
- Consider advanced airway and waveform capnography
- Do not hyperventilate

3
Treat hypotension (SBP <90 mm Hg)
- IV/IO bolus
- Vasopressor infusion
- Consider treatable causes
- 12-Lead ECG

5 Consider induced hypothermia ← No

4 Follow commands?

Yes

7 Coronary reperfusion ← Yes

6 STEMI or high suspicion of AMI

No

8 Advanced critical care

Doses/Details

Ventilation/oxygenation
Avoid excessive ventilation. Start at 10-12 breaths/min and titrate to target PETCO$_2$ of 35-40 mm Hg. When feasible, titrate FiO$_2$ to minimum necessary to achieve SpO$_2$ ≥94%.

IV bolus
1-2 L normal saline or lactated Ringer's. If inducing hypothermia, may use 4° C fluid.

Epinephrine IV infusion:
0.1-0.5 µg/kg/min (in 70-kg adult: 7-35 µg/min)

Dopamine IV infusion:
5-10 µg/kg/min

Norepinephrine IV infusion:
0.1-0.5 µg/kg/min (in 70-kg adult: 7-35 µg/min)

Reversible causes
- Hypovolemia
- Hypoxia
- Hydrogen ion (acidosis)
- Hypo-/hyperkalemia
- Hypothermia
- Tension pneumothorax
- Tamponade, cardiac
- Toxins
- Thrombosis, pulmonary
- Thrombosis, coronary

FIGURE 23-11 American Heart Association post–cardiac arrest care algorithm. AMI, acute myocardial infarction; ECG, electrocardiogram; FiO$_2$, forced inspiratory oxygen; IV, intravenous; IO, intraosseous; PETCO$_2$, end-tidal pressure of carbon dioxide; ROSC, return of spontaneous circulation; SBP, systolic blood pressure; SpO$_2$, oxygen saturation; STEMI, ST-segment–elevation myocardial infarction. *(From Peberdy MA, Callaway CW, Neumar RW, et al. Part 9. Post–cardiac arrest care: 2010 American Heart Association Guidelines for Cardiopulmonary Resuscitation and Emergency Cardiovascular Care. Circulation 2010;122[18 Suppl 3]:S768-786.)*

sufficiently reliable that treatment decisions such as withdrawal of support for poor prognosis can be made. The general approach should be to base such decisions on neurologic findings in which the false-positive rate (FPR)—that is, the rate of predicting a poor outcome that ultimately proves not to be poor—approaches zero. A plethora of data exist on hypoxic-ischemic encephalopathy after cardiac arrest, and few neurologic findings on physical exam have a sufficiently low FPR in the first 72 hours after cardiac arrest to justify making decisions on limitation of support based on them.[61,76] Neurologic prognostication in the first 24 hours after cardiac arrest is especially unreliable. Survivors of cardiac arrest who are initially comatose may have the potential for full recovery, especially if TH is used. In general, the recommended approach is to wait a minimum of 72 hours after ROSC before attempting neurologic prognostication.[76] However, it is important to recognize that the vast majority of data on neurologic prognostication of hypoxic-ischemic encephalopathy from cardiac arrest were generated before the efficacy of TH was realized; that is, before there was a known treatment for the brain injury. In the population of patients treated with TH, the optimal time course for neurologic prognostication may be significantly different—first, because the therapy can modulate the brain injury, and second, because low body temperature typically decreases the metabolism of sedative agents

used during TH induction. After TH, it often takes longer for the effects of sedation to wear off. Small contemporary studies have shown that good neurologic outcome can occur even with poor neurologic findings at 72 hours, suggesting that the optimal time interval to wait before attempting neurologic prognostication in the population treated with TH may be longer than that.[77] Our general approach is to withhold neurologic prognostication until 72 hours after ROSC in all patients. In the population treated with TH, we perform daily neurologic assessments beyond the 72-hour mark, and we withhold neurologic prognostication as long as the patient continues to improve. If there are no signs (even subtle signs) of neurologic improvement over 2 consecutive days, we usually deem neurologic prognostication to be reliable at that time.

REFERENCES

1. Myerburg RJ, Castellanos A. Cardiac arrest and sudden cardiac death. In Bonow RO, Mann DL, Zipes DP, et al (editors): *Braunwald's heart disease: a textbook of cardiovascular medicine*, 9th ed. 2012, Philadelphia, WB Saunders, pp 845-884.
2. Myerburg RJ, Kessler KM, Castellanos A. Sudden cardiac death: structure, function, and time-dependence of risk. *Circulation* 1992;85:I2-I10.
3. Fox CS, Evans JC, Larson MG, Kannel WB, Levy D. Temporal trends in coronary heart disease mortality and sudden cardiac death from 1950 to 1999: the Framingham Heart Study. *Circulation* 2004;110:522-527.

4. Cannom DS. Prevention of sudden cardiac death. *J Cardiovasc Electrophysiol* 2005;16: S21-S24.
5. Rosamond W, Flegal K, Furie K, et al.; American Heart Association Statistics Committee and Stroke Statistics Subcommittee. Heart disease and stroke statistics—2008 update: a report from the American Heart Association Statistics Committee and Stroke Statistics Subcommittee. *Circulation* 2008;117:e25-e146.
6. Weaver WD, Cobb LA, Hallstrom AP, et al. Considerations for improving survival from out-of-hospital cardiac arrest. *Ann Emerg Med* 1986;15:1181-1186.
7. Cobb LA, Fahrenbruch CE, Olsufka M, Copass MK. Changing incidence of out-of-hospital ventricular fibrillation, 1980-2000. *JAMA* 2002;288:3008-3013.
8. Bayés de Luna A, Coumel P, Leclercq JF. Ambulatory sudden cardiac death: mechanisms of production of fatal arrhythmia on the basis of data from 157 cases. *Am Heart J* 1989;117:151-159.
9. Page RL, Joglar JA, Kowal RC, et al. Use of automated external defibrillators by a U.S. airline. *N Engl J Med* 2000;343:1210-1216.
10. Valenzuela TD, Roe DJ, Nichol G, et al. Outcomes of rapid defibrillation by security officers after cardiac arrest in casinos. *N Engl J Med* 2000 26;343(17):1206-1209.
11. Caffrey SL, Willoughby PJ, Pepe PE, Becker LB. Public use of automated external defibrillators. *N Engl J Med* 2002;347(16):1242-1247.
12. Bardy GH, Lee KL, Mark DB, et al.; HAT Investigators. Home use of automated external defibrillators for sudden cardiac arrest. *N Engl J Med* 2008;358:1793-1804.
13. Myerburg RJ, Interian A Jr, Mitrani RM, Kessler KM, Castellanos A. Frequency of sudden cardiac death and profiles of risk. *Am J Cardiol* 1997;80:10F-19F.
14. Zheng ZJ, Croft JB, Giles WH, Mensah GA. Sudden cardiac death in the United States, 1989 to 1998. *Circulation* 2001;104:2158-2163.
15. Myerburg RJ, Kessler KM, Bassett AL, Castellanos A. A biological approach to sudden cardiac death: structure, function and cause. *Am J Cardiol* 1989;63:1512-1516.
16. Domanovits H, Paulis M, Nikfardjam M, et al. Sustained ventricular tachycardia in the emergency department. *Resuscitation* 1999;42:19-25.
17. Zipes DP, Camm AJ, Borggrefe M, et al. ACC/AHA/ESC 2006 Guidelines for Management of Patients with Ventricular Arrhythmias and the Prevention of Sudden Cardiac Death: a report of the American College of Cardiology/American Heart Association Task Force and the European Society of Cardiology Committee for Practice Guidelines (Writing Committee to Develop Guidelines for Management of Patients with Ventricular Arrhythmias and the Prevention of Sudden Cardiac Death). *J Am Coll Cardiol* 2006;48:e247-e346.
18. Approach to stable tachycardia. In Field JM (editor): *Advanced cardiovascular life support provider manual*. 2006, Dallas, TX, American Heart Association, pp. 97-100.
19. Gorgels AP, van den Dool A, Hofs A, et al. Comparison of procainamide and lidocaine in terminating sustained monomorphic ventricular tachycardia. *Am J Cardiol* 1996; 78:43-46.
20. Nasir N Jr, Taylor A, Doyle TK, Pacifico A. Evaluation of intravenous lidocaine for the termination of sustained monomorphic ventricular tachycardia in patients with coronary artery disease with or without healed myocardial infarction. *Am J Cardiol* 1994;74:1183-1186.
21. Armengol RE, Graff J, Baerman JM, Swiryn S. Lack of effectiveness of lidocaine for sustained, wide QRS complex tachycardia. *Ann Emerg Med* 1989;18:254-257.
22. Somberg JC, Bailin SJ, Haffajee CI, et al.; Amio-Aqueous Investigators. Intravenous lidocaine versus intravenous amiodarone (in a new aqueous formulation) for incessant ventricular tachycardia. *Am J Cardiol* 2002;90:853-859.
23. Marill KA, Greenberg GM, Kay D, Nelson BK. Analysis of the treatment of spontaneous sustained stable ventricular tachycardia. *Acad Emerg Med* 1997;4:1122-1128.
24. Guidelines 2000 for Cardiopulmonary Resuscitation and Emergency Cardiovascular Care. Part 6: advanced cardiovascular life support. Section 1: introduction to ACLS 2000—overview of recommended changes in ACLS from the Guidelines 2000 Conference. The American Heart Association in collaboration with the International Liaison Committee on Resuscitation. *Circulation* 2000;102:186-189.
25. Hine LK, Laird N, Hewitt P, Chalmers TC. Meta-analytic evidence against prophylactic use of lidocaine in acute myocardial infarction. *Arch Intern Med* 1989;149:2694-2698.
26. Wynn J, Torres V, Flowers D, et al. Antiarrhythmic drug efficacy at electrophysiology testing: predictive effectiveness of procainamide and flecainide. *Am Heart J* 1986;111: 632-638.
27. Waxman HL, Buxton AE, Sadowski LM, Josephson ME. The response to procainamide during electrophysiologic study for sustained ventricular tachyarrhythmias predicts the response to other medications. *Circulation* 1983;67:30-37.
28. Interian A Jr, Zaman L, Velez-Robinson E, et al. Paired comparisons of efficacy of intravenous and oral procainamide in patients with inducible sustained ventricular tachyarrhythmias. *J Am Coll Cardiol* 1991;17:1581-1586.
29. Callans DJ, Marchlinski FE. Dissociation of termination and prevention of inducibility of sustained ventricular tachycardia with infusion of procainamide: evidence for distinct mechanisms. *J Am Coll Cardiol* 1992;19:111-117.
30. Marill KA, deSouza IS, Nishijima DK, et al. Amiodarone or procainamide for the termination of sustained stable ventricular tachycardia: an historical multicenter comparison. *Acad Emerg Med* 2010;17:297-306.
31. Morrison LJ, Deakin CD, Morley PT, et al.; Advanced Life Support Chapter Collaborators. Part 8. Advanced life support: 2010 international consensus on cardiopulmonary resuscitation and emergency cardiovascular care science with treatment recommendations. *Circulation* 2010;122:S345-S421.
32. Roy D, Waxman HL, Buxton AE, et al. Termination of ventricular tachycardia: role of tachycardia cycle length. *Am J Cardiol* 1982;50:1346-1350.
33. Ho DS, Zecchin RP, Richards DA, Uther JB, Ross DL. Double-blind trial of lignocaine versus sotalol for acute termination of spontaneous sustained ventricular tachycardia. *Lancet* 1994;344(8914):18-23.
34. Kowey PR, Marinchak RA, Rials SJ, Filart RA. Intravenous amiodarone. *J Am Coll Cardiol* 1997;29:1190-1198.
35. Kowey PR, Levine JH, Herre JM, et al.; Intravenous Amiodarone Multicenter Investigators Group. Randomized, double-blind comparison of intravenous amiodarone and bretylium in the treatment of patients with recurrent, hemodynamically destabilizing ventricular tachycardia or fibrillation. *Circulation* 1995;92:3255-3263.
36. Levine JH, Massumi A, Scheinman MM, et al.; Intravenous Amiodarone Multicenter Trial Group. Intravenous amiodarone for recurrent sustained hypotensive ventricular tachyarrhythmias. *J Am Coll Cardiol* 1996;27(1):67-75.
37. Scheinman MM, Levine JH, Cannom DS, et al.; Intravenous Amiodarone Multicenter Investigators Group. Dose-ranging study of intravenous amiodarone in patients with life-threatening ventricular tachyarrhythmias. *Circulation* 1995;92:3264-3272.
38. Tomlinson DR, Cherian P, Betts TR, Bashir Y. Intravenous amiodarone for the pharmacological termination of haemodynamically-tolerated sustained ventricular tachycardia: is bolus dose amiodarone an appropriate first-line treatment? *Emerg Med J* 2008;25:15-18.
39. Marill KA, deSouza IS, Nishijima DK, et al. Amiodarone is poorly effective for the acute termination of ventricular tachycardia. *Ann Emerg Med* 2006;47:217-224.
40. Schützenberger W, Leisch F, Kerschner K, Harringer W, Herbinger W. Clinical efficacy of intravenous amiodarone in the short term treatment of recurrent sustained ventricular tachycardia and ventricular fibrillation. *Br Heart J* 1989;62:367-371.
41. Marchlinski FE, Buxton AE, Miller JM, et al. Amiodarone versus amiodarone and a type IA agent for treatment of patients with rapid ventricular tachycardia. *Circulation* 1986;74: 1037-1043.
42. Toivonen L, Kadish A, Morady F. A prospective comparison of class IA, B, and C antiarrhythmic agents in combination with amiodarone in patients with inducible, sustained ventricular tachycardia. *Circulation* 1991;84:101-108.
43. Somberg JC, Timar S, Bailin SJ, et al.; Amio-Aqueous Investigators. Lack of a hypotensive effect with rapid administration of a new aqueous formulation of intravenous amiodarone. *Am J Cardiol* 2004;93:576-581.
44. Farouque HM, Sanders P, Young GD. Intravenous magnesium sulfate for acute termination of sustained monomorphic ventricular tachycardia associated with coronary artery disease. *Am J Cardiol* 2000;86:1270-1272, A9.
45. Wyse DG, Friedman PL, Brodsky MA, et al.; AVID Investigators. Life-threatening ventricular arrhythmias due to transient or correctable causes: high risk for death in follow-up. *J Am Coll Cardiol* 2001;38:1718-1724.
46. Tzivoni D, Banai S, Schuger C, et al. Treatment of torsades de pointes with magnesium sulfate. *Circulation* 1988;77:392-397.
47. Nichol G, Thomas E, Callaway CW, et al. Regional variation in out-of-hospital cardiac arrest incidence and outcome. *JAMA* Sep 24 2008;300(12):1423-1431.
48. Nadkarni VM, Larkin GL, Peberdy MA, et al. First documented rhythm and clinical outcome from in-hospital cardiac arrest among children and adults. *JAMA* 2006;295(1):50-57.
49. Travers AH, Rea TD, Bobrow BJ, et al. Part 4. CPR overview: 2010 American Heart Association Guidelines for Cardiopulmonary Resuscitation and Emergency Cardiovascular Care. *Circulation* 2010;122(18 Suppl 3):S676-684.
50. Field JM, Hazinski MF, Sayre MR, et al. Part 1. Executive summary: 2010 American Heart Association Guidelines for Cardiopulmonary Resuscitation and Emergency Cardiovascular Care. *Circulation* 2010;122(18 Suppl 3):S640-S656.
51. Berg RA, Hemphill R, Abella BS, et al. Part 5. Adult basic life support: 2010 American Heart Association Guidelines for Cardiopulmonary Resuscitation and Emergency Cardiovascular Care. *Circulation* 2010;122(18 Suppl 3):S685-S705.
52. Manders S, Geijsel FE. Alternating providers during continuous chest compressions for cardiac arrest: every minute or every two minutes? *Resuscitation* 2009;80(9):1015-1018.
53. Abella BS, Alvarado JP, Myklebust H, et al. Quality of cardiopulmonary resuscitation during in-hospital cardiac arrest. *JAMA* 2005;293(3):305-310.
54. Edelson DP, Abella BS, Kramer-Johansen J, et al. Effects of compression depth and pre-shock pauses predict defibrillation failure during cardiac arrest. *Resuscitation* 2006; 71(2):137-145.
55. Kitamura T, Iwami T, Kawamura T, et al. Conventional and chest-compression–only cardiopulmonary resuscitation by bystanders for children who have out-of-hospital cardiac arrests: a prospective, nationwide, population-based cohort study. *Lancet* 2010; 375(9723):1347-1354.
56. Hupfl M, Selig HF, Nagele P. Chest-compression–only versus standard cardiopulmonary resuscitation: a meta-analysis. *Lancet* 2010;376:1552-1557.
57. Rea TD, Fahrenbruch C, Culley L, et al. CPR with chest compression alone or with rescue breathing. *N Engl J Med* 2010;363(5):423-433.
58. Svensson L, Bohm K, Castren M, et al. Compression-only CPR or standard CPR in out-of-hospital cardiac arrest. *N Engl J Med* 2010;363(5):434-442.
59. Neumar RW, Otto CW, Link MS, et al. Part 8: adult advanced cardiovascular life support: 2010 American Heart Association Guidelines for Cardiopulmonary Resuscitation and Emergency Cardiovascular Care. *Circulation* 2010;122(18 Suppl 3):S729-767.
60. Stiell IG, Wells GA, Field B, et al. Advanced cardiac life support in out-of-hospital cardiac arrest. *N Engl J Med.* 2004;351(7):647-656.
61. Neumar RW, Nolan JP, Adrie C, et al. Post-cardiac arrest syndrome: epidemiology, pathophysiology, treatment, and prognostication. A consensus statement from the International Liaison Committee on Resuscitation (American Heart Association, Australian and New Zealand Council on Resuscitation, European Resuscitation Council, Heart and Stroke Foundation of Canada, InterAmerican Heart Foundation, Resuscitation Council of Asia, and the Resuscitation Council of Southern Africa); the American Heart Association Emergency Cardiovascular Care Committee; the Council on Cardiovascular Surgery and Anesthesia; the Council on Cardiopulmonary, Perioperative, and Critical Care; the Council on Clinical Cardiology; and the Stroke Council. *Circulation* 2008;118(23):2452-2483.
62. Peberdy MA, Callaway CW, Neumar RW, et al. Part 9. Post–cardiac arrest care: 2010 American Heart Association Guidelines for Cardiopulmonary Resuscitation and Emergency Cardiovascular Care. *Circulation* 2010;122(18 Suppl 3):S768-786.
63. Trzeciak S, Jones AE, Kilgannon JH, et al. Significance of arterial hypotension after resuscitation from cardiac arrest. *Crit Care Med* 2009;37(11):2895-2903; quiz 2904.
64. Jones AE, Shapiro NI, Kilgannon JH, Trzeciak S. Goal-directed hemodynamic optimization in the post–cardiac arrest syndrome: a systematic review. *Resuscitation* 2008;77(1):26-29.
65. Kilgannon JH, Jones AE, Shapiro NI, et al. Association between arterial hyperoxia following resuscitation from cardiac arrest and in-hospital mortality. *JAMA* 2010;303(21): 2165-2171.
66. Danilov CA, Fiskum G. Hyperoxia promotes astrocyte cell death after oxygen and glucose deprivation. *Glia* 2008;56(7):801-808.

CH
23

67. Fiskum G, Danilov CA, Mehrabian Z, et al. Postischemic oxidative stress promotes mitochondrial metabolic failure in neurons and astrocytes. *Ann N Y Acad Sci* 2008; 1147:129-138.

68. Richards EM, Fiskum G, Rosenthal RE, Hopkins I, McKenna MC. Hyperoxic reperfusion after global ischemia decreases hippocampal energy metabolism. *Stroke* 2007;38(5): 1578-1584.

69. Richards EM, Rosenthal RE, Kristian T, Fiskum G. Postischemic hyperoxia reduces hippocampal pyruvate dehydrogenase activity. *Free Radic Biol Med* 2006;40(11):1960-1970.

70. Vereczki V, Martin E, Rosenthal RE, et al. Normoxic resuscitation after cardiac arrest protects against hippocampal oxidative stress, metabolic dysfunction, and neuronal death. *J Cereb Blood Flow Metab* 2006;26(6):821-835.

71. Hypothermia After Cardiac Arrest (HACA) study group. Mild therapeutic hypothermia to improve the neurologic outcome after cardiac arrest. *N Engl J Med* 2002;346(8):549-556.

72. Bernard SA, Gray TW, Buist MD, et al. Treatment of comatose survivors of out-of-hospital cardiac arrest with induced hypothermia. *N Engl J Med* 2002;346(8):557-563.

73. Merchant RM, Abella BS, Peberdy MA, et al. Therapeutic hypothermia after cardiac arrest: unintentional overcooling is common using ice packs and conventional cooling blankets. *Crit Care Med* 2006;34(12 Suppl):S490-S494.

74. Kilgannon JH, Roberts BW, Stauss M, et al. Use of a standardized order set for achieving target temperature in the implementation of therapeutic hypothermia after cardiac arrest: a feasibility study. *Acad Emerg Med* 2008;15(6):499-505.

75. Young GB. Clinical practice: neurologic prognosis after cardiac arrest. *N Engl J Med* 2009;361(6):605-611.

76. Wijdicks EF, Hijdra A, Young GB, Bassetti CL, Wiebe S. Practice parameter: prediction of outcome in comatose survivors after cardiopulmonary resuscitation (an evidence-based review): report of the Quality Standards Subcommittee of the American Academy of Neurology. *Neurology* 2006;67(2):203-210.

77. Al Thenayan E, Savard M, Sharpe M, Norton L, Young B. Predictors of poor neurologic outcome after induced mild hypothermia following cardiac arrest. *Neurology* 2008;71(19): 1535-1537.

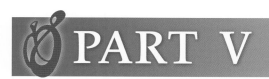

PART V

DYSLIPOPROTEINEMIAS AND ATHEROSCLEROSIS

CHAPTER **24** **Drugs for Elevated Low-Density Lipoprotein Cholesterol**

Neil J. Stone

EFFECTS ON LIPIDS AND LIPOPROTEINS, 421

PHARMACOKINETIC PROPERTIES, 422

Drug Interactions, 422
Efficacy, 423

MECHANISM OF BENEFIT OF STATINS, 424

Safety, 424

REFERENCES, 431

Inhibitors of 3-hydroxy-3-methylglutaryl coenzyme A (HMG-CoA) reductase, also known as *statins*, are competitive inhibitors of the rate-limiting step of hepatic cholesterol synthesis. This leads to a reduction in hepatocyte cholesterol concentration with subsequent upregulation of low-density lipoprotein (LDL) receptors that enhance clearance of LDL.[1] Statins lower both large and small LDL subclasses.[2] In addition to its effects on LDL, intermediate-density lipoprotein (IDL) and very-low-density lipoprotein (VLDL) are decreased by statin therapy.[3] Both fractions are decreased to similar percentages by statin therapy; thus statins are effective drugs for lowering both elevated LDL cholesterol (LDL-c) and triglyceride-rich lipoproteins. Statins are indicated in individuals with elevations of these lipoproteins because of genetics, as in familial hypercholesterolemia, familial defective apolipoprotein B (ApoB), familial combined hyperlipidemia, and type 3 hyperlipoproteinemia (remnant removal disease). They are also indicated in most adults with diabetes,[4] renal dysfunction,[5] and for the dyslipidemia found in renal and cardiac transplantation recipients.[6] The Adult Treatment Panel III (ATP III) recommends statins as the most effective class of drugs for lowering LDL-c to reduce the risk for coronary heart disease (CHD) in both primary and secondary prevention.[7]

A current controversy is whether statins are as effective in the primary prevention of cardiovascular disease (CVD) as they are in the secondary prevention of CVD, especially for women.[8-11] These meta-analyses must be analyzed carefully; inclusions and exclusions, as well as length of exposure to statin therapy, must be considered to put this controversy in perspective. Statins do not always lower risk in those at very high risk (>5% per year), as demonstrated by clinical trials of statins,[12] which fail to show significant benefit in patients on long-term hemodialysis with end-stage renal disease[13,14] and in those with chronic, symptomatic, systolic ischemic[15] heart failure or those with heart failure of any cause. These studies raise the issue as to whether mechanisms other than the prevention of plaque rupture in those with atherosclerotic vascular disease, for which the evidence for statin benefit appears strong, are operable and for which statin therapy is not an important solution (e.g., fatal arrhythmia, recurrent reperfusion injury, and/or progressive left ventricular dysfunction).[16] Preprocedural statin use to reduce the incidence of myocardial infarction (MI) after invasive procedures—such as angioplasty, coronary artery bypass grafting (CABG), or noncardiac surgery—has been

proposed.[17] Emerging data suggest that the administration of statin therapy, if the preventive data hold up, should precede percutaneous coronary angioplasty (PCI) by approximately 1 to 7 days, or it should occur approximately 4 weeks before noncardiac surgical procedures to result in a reduced incidence of postoperative MI. For noncardiac surgical trials, fluvastatin was used in more than 90% of studies and conferred benefit despite its less potent LDL-c lowering effects compared with other statins.[18] One speculation is that its longer half-life allows it to be withheld the first postoperative day without a diminution in its effects. Caution must be exercised, however, about attributing benefits of statin or any other therapy based on short-term trial results. Although short-term trials that used more sensitive atrial fibrillation (AF) detection methods suggest statin therapy can reduce the risk of AF, a recent meta-analysis that looked at longer term studies as well could not confirm this effect.[19]

Effects on Lipids and Lipoproteins

All members of the statin class reduce LDL-c levels in a dose-dependent fashion. This dose/response relationship is log linear, which means that although the initial dose lowers LDL-c from 25% to 45%, additional doublings of the statin dose result in only an additional 6% to 7% of LDL-c lowering.[20] Responsiveness to statins by individuals varies, and individuals who are hyporesponsive or hyperresponsive to one statin maintain that response with other statins.[21] In familial combined hyperlipidemia, use of a moderate dosage of a potent statin generates lowered cholesterol not only in LDL but also in triglyceride-rich remnant lipoproteins (TGRLs) in both the fasting and fed state.[22] This allows attainment of both LDL and non–high-density lipoprotein (HDL) goals.

The initially available statins—lovastatin, pravastatin, and simvastatin—were derived from fungal fermentation.[23] Subsequently, synthetic forms such as fluvastatin, atorvastatin, cerivastatin, and rosuvastatin have become available.[24] The newest available synthetic statin, pitavastatin, has a unique cyclopropyl group on its base structure that potently inhibits HMG-CoA reductase and inhibits synthesis of cholesterol in the liver.[25] It is not a substrate for 3A4 cytochrome P450, but the *Medical Letter* noted that pitavastatin's use is contraindicated with cyclosporine and ritonavir/lopinavir.[26] The concentration of pitavastatin can be raised 30% by adding rifampin, atazanavir, and gemfibrozil. No large-scale clinical trial data are currently available on outcome and safety data from such trials. Finally, cerivastatin, the most potent of all the statins introduced to date, was withdrawn from the market after it was found to have an unacceptable incidence of myositis and rhabdomyolysis.[27,28] The latter reaction was more likely when cerivastatin was combined with gemfibrozil.

A review of clinical trial data indicated that initial doses of statins should provide at least a 30% reduction in LDL-c.[24] Table 24-1 shows the dose of currently available statins that would provide this. Triglycerides are lowered with statins approximately proportional to the degree of LDL-c lowering.[29] This is a modest effect (15% to 30%) and is usually not adequate to normalize moderate elevations of triglycerides. Statin therapy does not result in removal of triglyceride-laden chylomicrons; thus statins should not be used when severe hypertriglyceridemia suggesting chylomicronemia is present. Statins affect HDL-c levels to a variable degree, and no relationship has been found between degree of LDL-c lowering and change in HDL-c.[30] Rosuvastatin, simvastatin, and pravastatin appear to raise HDL-c more than atorvastatin, for example. In the Pravastatin or Atorvastatin Evaluation and Infection Therapy–Thrombolysis in Myocardial Infarction (PROVE-IT–TIMI) 22 trial, standard LDL-c lowering with pravastatin in subjects with acute coronary syndrome (ACS) was associated with a greater percent increase in HDL-c than that seen with the intensive LDL-c lowering with atorvastatin. In PROVE-IT–TIMI 22, those individuals with the greatest LDL-c lowering had the greatest event reduction.[31] Statins in moderate doses do not lower lipoprotein A [Lp(a)], which can account for apparent reduced effectiveness of statin therapy in reducing LDL-c if the latter is determined by the Friedewald formula.[32] Statins lower markers of inflammation and oxidation, such as high-sensitivity C-reactive protein (hs-CRP), and they reduce lipoprotein-associated phospholipase A2 (Lp-PLA2).[33] Statins lower hs-CRP in primary and secondary prevention patients, a result seen in as little as 12 weeks.[34] For hs-CRP, the lowering is mainly independent of LDL-c lowering,[35] unlike that seen with Lp-PLA2, which is largely mediated by the statin-induced reduction in LDL-c. Lovastatin was effective among individuals with a ratio of total cholesterol to HDL-c that was lower than the median and an hs-CRP level higher than the median in a primary prevention trial.[36] In contrast, lovastatin was ineffective among subjects in this trial, with both a ratio of total cholesterol to HDL-c and an hs-CRP level that were lower than the median. Also, patients with ACS who have low hs-CRP levels after statin therapy have better clinical outcomes than those with higher hs-CRP levels, regardless of the resultant level of LDL-c.[37] The primary prevention study Justification for the use of Statins in Primary Prevention: An Intervention Trial Evaluating Rosuvastatin (JUPITER) used an hs-CRP of 2.0 mg/L or more as an entry criteria in men aged 50 years and older and women aged 60 years and older.[38] All the subjects had LDL-c below 130 mg/dL. Controversy is ongoing as to the merits of using hs-CRP to identify those who should receive statin therapy.[39]

Pharmacokinetic Properties

The available statins differ in terms of lipid solubility, half-life, and hepatic and renal clearance (see Table 24-2).[40,41] These properties can have clinical importance; for example, in patients with impaired renal function, atorvastatin and fluvastatin are important choices because of their limited renal clearance.

Drug Interactions

Table 24-3 shows various drug interactions for simvastatin; however, it should be recognized that safety is not a class effect because statins vary in their routes of excretion and in their metabolism by other drugs, especially those that affect the P450 system.[42] Knowledge of drug interactions is important in all patients, but it is critical in older patients, who are prone to acquire a long list of medications from multiple physicians. Fluvastatin is metabolized by P450 2C9, whereas lovastatin, simvastatin, and atorvastatin are metabolized by P450 3A4. Rosuvastatin is only weakly metabolized by 2C9, and pravastatin concentrations are not affected by the P450 system at all. Drugs such as erythromycin, clarithromycin, or ketoconazole—but not azithromycin or fluoconazole—affect statins metabolized by the P450 3A4 pathway, and this should influence the choice of a statin. Large amounts of grapefruit juice can inhibit intestinal P450 3A4 irreversibly, with effects that last up to 3 days, which may increase steady-state concentrations of statins with the potential to cause rhabdomyolysis.[43,44] Drug interactions with grapefruit juice are likely to be clinically significant for drugs with a narrow therapeutic index and/or in cases where the magnitude of the interaction is large.

A clinically useful tactic is to substitute pravastatin for a statin metabolized by the 3A4 system, if a prolonged course of therapy with a known inhibitor of the 3A4 system is needed, as may occur in the common example of sinusitis treated with a prolonged course of clarithromycin.

TABLE 24-1	Effective Clinical Doses for Statins	
STATIN	**DAILY DOSE (MG) TO LOWER LDL >30%**	**MAXIMAL DOSE (MG)**
Lovastatin	40	80
Pravastatin	40	80
Simvastatin	20	40
Fluvastatin XL	80	80
Atorvastatin	10	80
Rosuvastatin	5	40
Pitavastatin	2	4

TABLE 24-2	Statin Pharmacokinetics						
STATIN	**ATORVASTATIN**	**FLUVASTATIN/XL**	**LOVASTATIN**	**PITAVASTATIN**	**PRAVASTATIN**	**ROSUVASTATIN**	**SIMVASTATIN**
Origin	Synthetic	Synthetic	Fungal	Synthetic	Semisynthetic	Synthetic	Semisynthetic
Lipophilicity	Yes	Yes	Yes	No	No	No	Yes
Protein binding	>98%	>99%	>95%	>99%	50%	88%	95%
CYP	3A4	2C9	3A4	Minimal	None	2C9 minor	3A4
$T_{1/2}$	Long acting	Short acting	Short acting	Long acting	Short acting	Long acting	Short acting
Renal adjustments to statin dosage	None	If severe impairment, use with caution	If severe impairment, use doses >20 mg/day with caution	Maximum 2 mg/day	Monitor if impairment	No more than 10 mg/day if severe impairment	Monitor if severe impairment

Short acting, <5 hours; *long acting,* >10 hours. Of the long-acting statins, rosuvastatin has a longer action than atorvastatin, which acts longer than pitavastatin.
Modified from references 18, 19, 24and .

TABLE 24-3	Federal Drug Administration Ruling on Drug-Drug Interaction for Simvastatin as of June 2011

PREVIOUS SIMVASTATIN LABEL	CURRENT SIMVASTATIN LABEL
Avoid simvastatin with: • Itraconazole • Ketoconazole • Erythromycin • Clarithromycin • Telithromycin • HIV protease inhibitors • Nefazodone	Contraindicated with simvastatin: • Itraconazole • Ketoconazole • Posaconazole (new) • Erythromycin • Clarithromycin • Telithromycin • HIV protease inhibitors • Nefazodone • Gemfibrozil • Cyclosporine • Danazol
Do not exceed 10 mg/day simvastatin with: • Gemfibrozil • Cyclosporine • Danazol	Do not exceed 10 mg/day simvastatin with*: • Amiodarone • Verapamil • Diltiazem
Do not exceed 20 mg/day simvastatin with: • Amiodarone • Verapamil	Do not exceed 20 mg/day simvastatin with: • Amlodipine (new) • Ranolazine (new)
Do not exceed 40 mg/day simvastatin with: • Diltiazem	
Avoid large quantities of grapefruit juice (>1 quart/day)	Avoid large quantities of grapefruit juice (>1 quart/day)

*These drugs are contraindicated with Simcor, which is only available with 20 mg or 40 mg of simvastatin.
HIV, human immunodeficiency virus
From http://www.fda.gov/Drugs/DrugSafety/ucm256581.htm. Accessed June 26, 2011.

Certain populations need to be especially aware of drug-drug interactions when given statins. A detailed review of patients with CHD and human immunodeficiency virus (HIV) advised that, because protease inhibitors (PIs) inhibit the P450 3A4 cytochrome system, lovastatin and simvastatin are contraindicated to avoid elevated statin concentrations.[45] The authors instead recommended pravastatin and rosuvastatin for patients taking PIs. Of note, this expert review proposed that atorvastatin was an acceptable choice with PIs, in that it does not seem to be affected as greatly as lovastatin and simvastatin by inhibitors of the P450 3A4 system. They further suggested that clinicians who treat patients taking PIs who require statins be aware of the following limitations of such therapy:

- Pravastatin should not be prescribed with boosted darunavir.
- Ritonavir and ritonavir-boosted PI combinations cause the most significant increases in lipids.
- Fluvastatin data are limited.
- Efavirenz, not a PI, in contrast to effects seen with a PI, lowers levels of simvastatin, pravastatin, and atorvastatin.

Cardiac patients are another group for whom vigilance is required to avoid statin-drug interactions; these are detailed in Table 24-3. Both amiodarone and verapamil inhibit the P450 3A4 system; when either is started, it is important to consider whether a statin-drug interaction is likely. The U.S. Food and Drug Administration (FDA) has warned that the dose of simvastatin used should not exceed 10 mg/day with these drugs to avoid myopathy and its most serious consequence, rhabdomyolysis.[46] Safer statins include pravastatin, fluvastatin, or rosuvastatin. All statins may interact with cyclosporine and with other lipid-lowering drugs such as fibrates, nicotinic acid, warfarin, and digoxin.[47] Cyclosporine is used extensively in transplant recipients; it is highly lipid soluble, a significant portion is bound to lipoproteins, and it increases LDL-c and Lp(a) concentrations, although it affects fluvastatin less so.[48] Gemfibrozil

affects glucuronidation of statins and results in a higher concentration of statins and increased toxicity in turn, which results in an unacceptably high incidence of rhabdomyolysis when gemfibrozil was combined with a statin, especially cerivastatin.[49] Coadministered fenofibrate does not raise statin concentrations[50] and is therefore considered the fibrate of choice when fibrate and statin therapy are combined. Both fluvastatin and warfarin are metabolized by the P450 2C9 pathway. Because case reports have indicated changes in warfarin levels with other statins not metabolized this way, until more definitive data are available, patients on warfarin should have their international normalized ratio (INR) monitored closely after starting statin therapy[51] because statins may increase digoxin concentrations by inhibiting P-glycoprotein transport.[52]

Although there were early reports of myositis with statin and nicotinic acid combinations, this has not been reported in studies of an extended-release form of nicotinic acid.[53] This may relate to the higher incidence of hepatotoxicity with long-acting forms of nicotinic acid and the increased levels of statins that results from hepatic damage.

Efficacy

ANGIOGRAPHIC TRIALS

A decade of double-blind, randomized, controlled angiographic trials has demonstrated that treatment with statins could significantly decrease progression of atherosclerosis.[54] Thompson emphasized the importance of statins in lowering non-HDL and LDL cholesterol in these trials. The Post Coronary Artery Bypass Graft Trial (Post CABG) demonstrated the value of lower LDL-c attained with more intensive statin (lovastatin) therapy in subjects who had undergone CABG.[55] The higher dose lovastatin group attained an LDL-c of approximately 100 mg/dL compared with the reduction of LDL-c to only 132 to 136 mg/dL. The investigators found delayed atherosclerotic progression in the grafts at 4 to 5 years. An informative angiographic trial enrolled 341 subjects with stable coronary disease, relatively normal left ventricular function, and an LDL-c higher than 115 mg/dL who were referred for angioplasty.[56] Those assigned to the high-dose statin therapy (atorvastatin) had a significantly longer time to the first ischemic CHD event compared with those who were assigned to angioplasty and usual medical care.

Although the CHD event rate was 36% lower in the statin group, the *P* value obtained was not statistically significant because of the adjustment for multiple on-trial analyses. On closer inspection, the intensive statin therapy had its greatest effect in reducing revascularization procedures and hospitalizations for worsening angina. With the use of intravascular ultrasound, a multicenter study showed that intensive statin therapy (atorvastatin 80 mg/day) had a significantly greater effect on the primary endpoint, the percentage change in atheroma volume, than a moderate dose of a statin (pravastatin 40 mg/day).[57] Importantly, progression did not occur in those assigned to atorvastatin 80 mg/day, whereas it did in those assigned to pravastatin 40 mg/day. Of note, those assigned to atorvastatin 80 mg/day had significantly lower hs-CRP levels than those assigned to pravastatin 40 mg/day. O'Keefe and colleagues plotted out the results of major angiographic trials showing the increasing benefit of LDL-c lowering down to an LDL-c of less than 80 mg/day (Figure 24-1).[58]

Surface/transesophageal magnetic resonance imaging (MRI) has been used to monitor statin-induced atherosclerotic plaque (AP) reduction.[59] AP regression and reverse remodeling was detected accurately by MRI in just 6 months after statin therapy initiation and, not surprisingly, was associated with LDL-c reduction.

LARGE-SCALE CLINICAL TRIALS

Statins have proven effective in primary prevention and secondary prevention trials (Tables 24-4 and 24-5). As might be expected, the

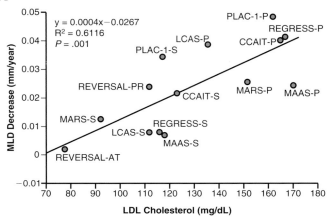

FIGURE 24-1 Atherosclerosis progression varies directly with low-density lipoprotein (*LDL*). This regression line indicates that atherosclerosis does not progress when LDL is 67 mg/dL or below. Data from randomized, placebo-controlled trials using statins to prevent atherosclerosis progression or coronary heart disease events in primary or secondary prevention were used for computation of the univariate regression lines correlating LDL with outcomes. Regression estimates, model R^2, and P values for LDL effect were obtained from the unweighted regression lines. AT, atorvastatin; CCAIT, Canadian Coronary Atherosclerosis Intervention Trial; LCAS, Lipoprotein and Coronary Atherosclerosis Study; MAAS, Multicentre Anti-Atheroma Study; MARS, Monitored Atherosclerosis Regression Study; MLD, mean luminal diameter; P, placebo; PLAC, Pravastatin Limitation of Atherosclerosis in the Coronary Arteries study; PR, pravastatin; REGRESS, Regression Growth Evaluation Statin Study; REVERSAL, Reversal of Atherosclerosis with Aggressive Lipid Lowering; S, statin. *(From O'Keefe JH, Cordain L, Harris WH, Moe RH, Vogel R. Optimal low-density lipoprotein is 50 to 70 mg/dL; lower is better and physiologically normal. J Am Coll Cardiol 2004;43:2142-2146.)*

absolute risk reduction is greater in the secondary prevention trials, resulting in a steeper LDL-c event reduction curve than that seen in primary prevention trials. The large Heart Protection Study (HPS) demonstrated significant benefit for total mortality rate and CHD events in subjects at high risk of a coronary event who were assigned to simvastatin 40 mg/day compared with placebo.[60] This substantial benefit occurred regardless of baseline LDL-c, and it was seen in all subgroups, including women and the elderly, and benefit increased with duration of therapy. Ischemic stroke incidence was also substantially reduced by statin therapy.[61] No significant increase in liver or muscle toxicity was reported, and statin therapy was not associated with an increase in cancer, respiratory disease, or suicide. The advantage of using large-scale trials to demonstrate negatives of statin therapy was seen in trials of the 80-mg dose of simvastatin. Whereas 40 mg of simvastatin appeared safe in the HPS, two clinical trials using an 80-mg dose of simvastatin showed an excess of myopathy incidence compared with placebo.[62,63]

The mechanism for this may be due to a polymorphism in one of the several hepatic membrane transporters. For example, a common single-nucleotide variation in the *SLCO1B1* gene that encodes organic anion transporter polypeptide (OATP) 1B1 decreases the transporting activity of OATP1B1 and results in elevated statin concentrations, especially of simvastatin acid. In the Study of the Effectiveness of Additional Reductions in Cholesterol (SEARCH), a genome association study, the risk for myopathy in those assigned to simvastatin was increased by a factor of 4.5 per copy of a common *SLCO1B1* variant found to be present in 15% of the population who developed myopathy during the trial.[64]

Numerous primary and secondary prevention trials of statin therapy led to the prospective meta-analysis of data from 90,056 subjects in 14 randomized trials of statins.[65] Known as the Cholesterol Treatment Trialists' (CTT) collaboration, the LDL-c reductions owing to statin therapy at 1 year ranged from 14 mg/dL to 69 mg/dL with a mean of 42 mg/dL. After 5 years, a highly significant

reduction in all-cause mortality was observed, as was a significant 19% reduction in coronary mortality (Figure 24-2). Nonsignificant rate reductions were also seen in noncoronary vascular mortality and nonvascular mortality. Statin therapy substantially reduced MI and CHD death and coronary revascularization by about 25%, and the rates for fatal or nonfatal stroke were reduced by 17% on average. The proportional reduction in major vascular events differed significantly ($P < .0001$) according to the absolute reduction in LDL-c achieved, but it remained similar throughout the range of LDL-c studied. These benefits were significant within the first year but were greater in subsequent years. Moreover, statin therapy was demonstrated to be safe with no increase in cancer risk. Taken as a whole, this large dataset suggested that the promise of prolonged statin treatment with substantial LDL-c reductions in those at risk over a wide range of LDL-c was clinically meaningful. A follow-up report from the CTT was a meta-analysis of data from 170,000 participants in 26 randomized trials that included trials with high-dose versus low-dose statin therapy; it indicated that further reduction in LDL-c can be shown to produce further reductions in cardiovascular (CV) outcomes such as MI, revascularization, and ischemic stroke.[66] Across all 26 trials, which included primary and secondary prevention, all-cause mortality was reduced by 10% per 1.0 mmol/L (38.8 mg/dL) LDL-c reduction. This was due primarily to effects on CHD, but with no significant effects on stroke. These data support the use of a maximally tolerated safe dose of a statin to lower LDL-c in those at increased CV risk.

Mechanism of Benefit of Statins

Although LDL lowering appears to be the major reason why statins produce CV benefit, some investigators hold that there are pleiotropic effects on endothelial dysfunction, inflammation, coagulation, and plaque regression that more fully explain how statins work (Box 24-1).[67] They argue that pleiotropic effects may explain the early benefit seen with statins in ACS[68] as contrasted with beneficial but delayed effects in nondrug trials of LDL-c lowering by partial ileal bypass.[69] Whether these effects are truly cholesterol-independent and mediated by their ability to block the synthesis of isoprenoid intermediates is actively debated.[70] Some argue that LDL-c reduction may serve as a marker for the pleiotropic effects seen with statins, which is supported by increasing benefit from statins at the higher dosage range.

Safety

As can be seen from the large-scale meta-analysis, in clinical trials, statins are very well tolerated. The two major side effects that clinicians encounter are those involving the liver and muscles.

LIVER

An ACC/AHA/National Heart, Lung and Blood Institute (NHLBI) clinical advisory on statins noted that statin-induced elevated hepatic transaminases generally are infrequent, with rates below 2%.[71] These elevations were dose dependent and were more likely at the highest dosages. The setting may be important as well; in the PROVE-IT–TIMI 22 trial, the percentage of participants with significant liver transaminase elevations, more than three times the upper limit of normal (ULN), was 3.3% in the atorvastatin group versus 1.1% in the pravastatin group.[31] In the setting of chronic, stable coronary disease, the Treat to New Targets (TNT) trial showed a low order of liver toxicity that did not differentiate between the low- and high-dose atorvastatin regimens used. Indeed, it has been questioned whether low-level transaminase elevation (more than twice the ULN) constitutes true hepatotoxicity.

Statin-associated hepatotoxicity has several characteristic features.[72] Elevations of liver transaminases usually are noted within the first 12 weeks of therapy. Unlike the situation with nicotinic acid hepatotoxicity, in which symptoms often herald liver damage, statin-associated elevations of liver transaminases are usually

TABLE 24-4   Cardiovascular Benefits of Statins in Placebo-Controlled Secondary Prevention Clinical Trials

STUDY	POPULATION	STATIN AND DOSE USED (N)	LDL-C REDUCTION	EFFICACY AGAINST CHD	EFFICACY AGAINST STROKE
HPS	Age 40-80 y with coronary disease, other occlusive disease, diabetes	Simvastatin 40 mg/day (10,269) vs. placebo (10,267)	37%	Significant reductions in total mortality, fatal and nonfatal MI, revascularization	Yes
PROSPER	Age 70-82 y with history of, or risk factors for, vascular disease	Pravastatin 40 mg/day (2891) vs. placebo (2913); mean follow-up, 3.2 y	3%	No reduction in total mortality, but significant reduction in fatal and nonfatal CHD	No, although a decrease in TIA (low rate of stroke in placebo group)
PROVE-IT–TIMI 22	4162 subjects with ACS; mean age, 58 y	Atorvastatin 80 mg (2099) vs. pravastatin 40 mg (2063); mean follow-up, 2.0 y	10% with pravastatin, 42% with atorvastatin	Greater reduction in combined endpoint with atorvastatin than with pravastatin	No
CARE	4159 subjects post MI; mean age, 59 y	Pravastatin 40 mg vs. placebo; mean follow-up, 5 y	28%	Significant reduction of primary endpoint	Yes
LIPID	9014 subjects aged 31-75 y with MI and ACS	Pravastatin 40 mg/day (4512) vs. placebo (4502); mean follow-up, 5 y	25%	Significant reduction of primary endpoint	Yes
TNT	10,001 subjects age 35-75 y with stable CHD	Atoravastatin 10 mg/day (5006) vs. 80 mg/day (4995); follow-up, 4.9 y	80 mg/day: 77 mg/dL 10 mg/day; 101 mg/dL Further reduction: 23% Further LDL-c reduction: 22%	Significant reduction in primary endpoint; significant improvement in fatal and nonfatal MI and major coronary events, but no improvement in mortality	Yes
IDEAL	8888 subjects < 80 y with prior MI	Simvastatin 20 mg/day (4449) vs. atorvastatin 80 mg/day (4439)	Simvastatin: 104 mg/dL Atorvastatin: 81 mg/dL (22%)	No significant lowering of primary combined endpoint of coronary death, confirmed nonfatal MI, or cardiac arrest with resuscitation; no significant decrease in any coronary event	No

ACS, acute coronary syndrome; CARE, Cholesterol and Recurrent Events; CHD, coronary heart disease; HPS, Heart Protection Study; IDEAL, Incremental Decrease in Clinical Endpoints Through Aggressive Lipid Lowering; LDL-c; low-density lipoprotein cholesterol; LIPID, Long-Term Intervention in Ischaemic Patients; MI, myocardial infarction; PROSPER, Prospective Study of Pravastatin in the Elderly at Risk; PROVE-IT–TIMI 22, Pravastatin or Atorvastatin Evaluation and Infection Therapy–Thrombolysis in Myocardial Infarction; TIA, transient ischemic attack; TNT, Treat to New Targets.

TABLE 24-5   Cardiovascular Benefits of Statins in Primary Prevention Clinical Trials (Statin vs. Placebo)

PRIMARY PREVENTION CLINICAL TRIALS	POPULATION	STATIN DOSAGE	LDL-C REDUCTION	EFFECTIVE AGAINST CHD	EFFECTIVE AGAINST STROKE
AFCAPS/TEXCAPS	5608 men aged 45-73 y and 997 women aged 55-73 y with lipid entry criteria (low HDL-c required)	Lovastatin 20 mg and 40 mg/day (3304) vs. placebo (3301)	25%	Yes	NR
WOSCOPS	High-risk men aged 45-64 y without prior MI, followed up for 4.9 y	Pravastatin 40 mg/day (3302) vs. placebo (3293)	26%	Yes	No
ASCOT-LLA	10,305 hypertensive patients aged 40-79 y with at least three other cardiovascular risk factors; followed up for 3.3 y before study was halted by the DSMB	Atorvastatin 10 mg/day (5168) vs. placebo (5137)	29%	Yes	Yes
ALLHAT-LLA	10,355 subjects aged ≥55 y who met lipid criteria, monitored for up to 8 y	Pravastatin 40 mg/day	16.7% (related to drop-ins in placebo group plus drop-outs in treatment groups)	No; 18% difference in LDL-c between groups because of high crossover and dropout rates	No
JUPITER	17,802 apparently healthy men and women with LDL-c <130 mg/dL and hs-CRP 2.0 or higher	Rosuvastatin 20 mg (8901) vs. placebo (8901)	50%	Yes	Yes
CARDS	2838 men and women with type 2 diabetes and ≥1 other risk factor[29]	Atorvastatin 10 mg/day	40%	Yes	Yes

AFCAPS/TEXCAPS, Air Force/Texas Coronary Atherosclerosis Prevention Study; ALLHAT-LLA, Antihypertensive and Lipid Lowering to Prevent Heart Attack Trial; ASCOT-LLA, Anglo-Scandinavian Cardiac Outcomes Trial Lipid Lowering Arm; CARDS, Collaborative Atorvastatin Diabetes Study; CHD, coronary heart disease; JUPITER, Justification for the Use of Statins in Prevention: An Intervention Trial Evaluating Rosuvastatin; LDL-c, low-density lipoprotein cholesterol; MI, myocardial infarction; NR, not reported; WOSCOPS, West of Scotland Coronary Prevention Study.

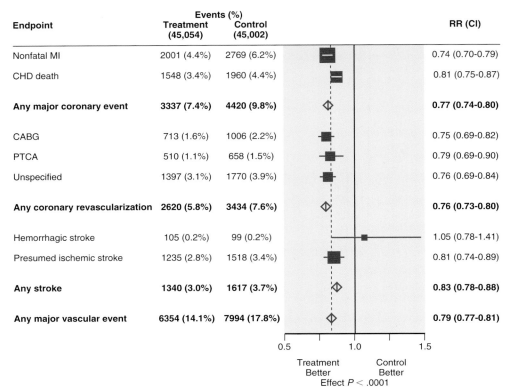

Endpoint	Events (%) Treatment (45,054)	Control (45,002)		RR (CI)
Nonfatal MI	2001 (4.4%)	2769 (6.2%)		0.74 (0.70-0.79)
CHD death	1548 (3.4%)	1960 (4.4%)		0.81 (0.75-0.87)
Any major coronary event	**3337 (7.4%)**	**4420 (9.8%)**		**0.77 (0.74-0.80)**
CABG	713 (1.6%)	1006 (2.2%)		0.75 (0.69-0.82)
PTCA	510 (1.1%)	658 (1.5%)		0.79 (0.69-0.90)
Unspecified	1397 (3.1%)	1770 (3.9%)		0.76 (0.69-0.84)
Any coronary revascularization	**2620 (5.8%)**	**3434 (7.6%)**		**0.76 (0.73-0.80)**
Hemorrhagic stroke	105 (0.2%)	99 (0.2%)		1.05 (0.78-1.41)
Presumed ischemic stroke	1235 (2.8%)	1518 (3.4%)		0.81 (0.74-0.89)
Any stroke	**1340 (3.0%)**	**1617 (3.7%)**		**0.83 (0.78-0.88)**
Any major vascular event	**6354 (14.1%)**	**7994 (17.8%)**		**0.79 (0.77-0.81)**

0.5   1.0   1.5

Treatment Better   Control Better

Effect $P < .0001$

FIGURE 24-2 Proportional effects on major vascular events per mmol/L low-density lipoprotein cholesterol (LDL-c) reduction. Broken vertical line indicates overall relative risk (*RR*) for any type of major vascular event. The Lescol Intervention Prevention Study (LIPS) only provided data on fatal strokes and does not contribute to the stroke analyses. Totals and subtotals are shown as *diamonds* (95% confidence interval [*CI*]); *squares* represent individual categories; and *horizontal lines* are 95% CIs, with the area of square proportional to the amount of statistical information in that category. RR values are weighted to represent reduction in rate per 1 mmol/L of LDL-c reduction achieved by treatment at 1 year after randomization. CABG, coronary artery bypass graft; CHD, coronary heart disease; PTCA, percutaneous transluminal coronary angioplasty. *(From Cholesterol Treatment Trialists' Collaborators. Efficacy and safety of cholesterol-lowering treatment: prospective meta-analysis of data from 90,056 participants in 14 randomised trials of statins. Lancet 2005;366:1267.)*

Box 24-1 Pleiotropic Effects of Statin Drugs

- Improve impaired endothelial vasodilation
- Produce antithrombotic effects
- Decrease vascular inflammation
- Decrease vascular smooth muscle proliferation
- Increase plaque stability

asymptomatic. Evidence of cholestasis with jaundice and hyperbilirubinemia is rare. Progression to liver failure shown to be specifically due to statins is also rare; indeed, despite the large number of subjects assigned to statins in large-scale clinical trials, statin-induced liver failure was not seen. When the statin dose is reduced, or when there is rechallenge with another statin, elevations of liver transaminases often do not occur. When statin therapy is stopped, liver transaminases return to normal. The National Lipid Association Statin Safety Assessment Task Force expressed its concern that the benefits of routine liver screening were so small, and the potential consequences of having needed statin treatment either temporarily or permanently withdrawn were so dire, that they urged the FDA to reconsider its current labeling.[73] In 2012, the FDA indicated that if pre-statin liver test results were normal, routine monitoring of liver enzyme levels was no longer needed because monitoring was not found to be effective in predicting cases of serious liver injury. Instead, monitoring of liver enzyme levels was to be done if clinically indicated.[73a]

Information may be gleaned from those patients with more than mildly elevated transaminases on statins. For example, a study of health maintenance organization (HMO) cases of severe hepatic transaminase elevation, defined as more than 10 times the ULN, indicated that in 14 of 17 cases in which hepatotoxicity was directly attributable to statin use, a drug interaction was apparent.[74]

The more difficult situation is when statins are considered for those with existing liver disease. A double-blind placebo-controlled trial of pravastatin 80 mg in those with well-compensated chronic liver disease—including nonalcoholic fatty liver, infection, or causes such as hepatitis B, hemochromatosis, autoimmune hepatitis, liver cirrhosis as a result of primary biliary cirrhosis, or cryptogenic cirrhosis—confirmed pravastatin's safe use with no significant increase in alanine transaminase (ALT) levels compared with controls. Furthermore, no difference was seen in event rates among liver disease groups despite the fact that some patients had elevations up to five times the ULN in baseline transaminase levels. These findings favor the safe use of pravastatin in patients with well-compensated chronic liver disease and hypercholesterolemia if clinically appropriate. A reasonable and useful approach was recently published in *Mayo Clinic Proceedings* (Figure 24-3).[75]

Cholestasis and active liver disease are listed as contraindications to statin use. Patients with acute liver disease, such as acute viral hepatitis or alcoholic hepatitis, should not take statins until they have recovered, and then they should be reassessed to see whether this therapy is appropriate.

Thus if the patient is at high risk of CVD, and a statin drug is indicated to lower LDL-c and thereby lower that risk, minor elevations of liver transaminase tests unrelated to adverse clinical consequences should not keep such therapy from proceeding. In the patient with known *stable* liver disease, such as fatty liver disease, who merits statin therapy, low doses of statins can be used initially, but screening should be more frequent. Statin therapy should be stopped if transaminase elevations exceed two times the upper limit of the starting levels, and the patient should then be carefully reassessed. Statins should not be prescribed or continued in those with acute decompensated liver problems. For these patients, statin use is contraindicated and could result in safety issues.

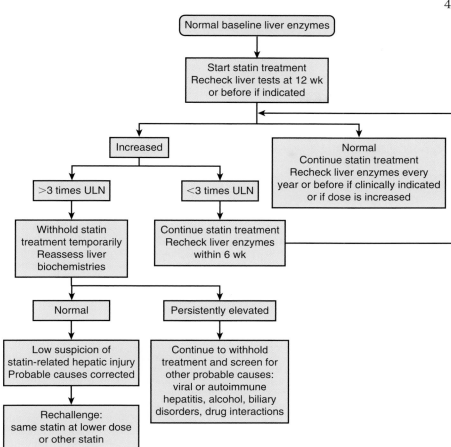

FIGURE 24-3 Algorithm for managing patients with abnormal liver transaminase measurements before and during statin management. ULN, upper limit of normal. *(From Calderon RM, Cubeddu LX, Goldberg RB, Schiff ER. Statins in the treatment of dyslipidemia in the presence of elevated liver aminotransferase levels: a therapeutic dilemma. Mayo Clin Proc 2010;85:349-356.)*

MUSCLE

Since statins were clinically introduced more than 20 years ago, the most serious reports of adverse drug effects to the FDA have been statin-related muscle problems, usually triggered by a drug-drug interaction.[76] Despite several quality reviews of the literature,[77-80] there are differences in definitions and solutions to this important clinical problem. Patients commonly come to medical attention with muscular symptoms that include persistent pain, soreness, cramps, and muscular weakness. Fortunately, the most feared complication, rhabdomyolysis, is rare. Rhabdomyolysis can have a variety of causes and can be thought of qualitatively as a syndrome of skeletal muscle breakdown with leakage of muscle contents, hence the elevated creatine kinase (CK) levels; it is frequently accompanied by myoglobinuria, and if sufficiently severe, by acute renal failure with potentially life-threatening metabolic consequences.[81]

The frequency and severity of muscular complaints can depend, at least in part, on the statin dosage. An observational study of almost 8000 patients in France who received high-dose statin therapy that included at least 40 mg of simvastatin, pravastatin, atorvastatin, or fluvastatin XL reported a questionnaire prevalence of 10.5%, occurring at a median time of onset of 1 month after starting statin therapy.[82] Despite the limitations of the study design, muscular pain prevented even moderate physical effort during daily activity in 38%, and 4% were confined to bed or were unable to work. Recognition of statin-related muscle effects is important, because most patients recover fully after stopping the statin and attending to the cause of the problem. In a systematic review of inpatient and outpatient data over 13 years in Wisconsin, to uncover cases of statin-associated myopathy, the mean (standard deviation) duration of statin therapy before symptom onset was 6.3 (9.8) months. Resolution of the muscle symptoms required

2.3 (3.0) months after discontinuation of the statin.[83] Of note, in those with statin-associated myopathy who recovered and were rechallenged with another statin, more than 40% of patients tolerated the new statin well and without symptoms.

Few patients who begin statin therapy require the determination of a baseline CK level. Some physicians may wish to obtain a pretreatment level of CK if they consider their patient at high risk for statin myopathy. Frequent monitoring of CK in *asymptomatic* patients does not appear to be useful. CK values do not uniformly predict underlying statin-associated skeletal muscle injury, and in fact, such values may be in the normal range in patients on statin therapy who come to medical attention with weakness as the primary complaint.[84,85] Patients are rarely seen with findings of persistent proximal muscle weakness and elevated CK levels, ongoing after 3 to 4 weeks of statin discontinuation, who have abnormal muscle biopsies that require immunosuppressive agents for improvement.[86] When patients on statins develop muscle symptoms, their total CK level should be measured and carefully evaluated for treatable causes of muscle weakness, such as hypothyroidism, polymyalgia rheumatica, and vitamin D deficiency.[87]

Although there is concern for statin-associated myopathy, the low risk of statins for causing a low-grade myopathy must be balanced against the substantial benefit in those who require these drugs to minimize adverse CV outcomes.[88] A reasonable approach is to look for predisposing conditions of myopathy, listed by the ACC/AHA/NHLBI panel, that include advanced age (these patients may not complain of pain, just weakness), relatively low body weight, female sex, multisystem disease, acute illnesses, and use of certain medications or of multiple medications.[67] Additional predisposing factors to consider are alcohol use, compromised liver or renal function, diabetes, and hypothyroidism (Box 24-2).[89]

One useful clinical maneuver for those with vague muscle complaints not clearly a result of the statin therapy is to provide a 2- to

Box 24-2 Suggestions for Statin Use

1. Understand who benefits from statin therapy; do a careful cardiovascular risk assessment and medication history before starting statin therapy.

2. If you use statins, lower LDL-c by at least 30% to 40%. For those who require statins for the secondary prevention of coronary heart disease, try to use maximally tolerated statin therapy before adding other lipid medications to lower LDL-c.

3. Do not consider safety or properties a class effect of statins. Statins differ in pharmacologic properties, which can be helpful in deciding which statin to use in an individual patient. Simvastatin 80 mg should not be started, and drug-drug interactions with simvastatin are noted in Table 24-3.

4. Consider that muscle and liver toxicity, although uncommon, can occur. Get a baseline liver panel, a urine analysis for protein, and a recent thyroid function test (such as TSH) before starting statin therapy. Carefully review the medication list for drug-drug statin interactions. Mild elevations of transaminases are often transient and nonserious. If AST is consistently greater than ALT, consider alcohol excess.

5. Do not measure CK routinely on follow-up blood tests, as it varies widely, especially in those who exercise regularly. Remember that statins can exacerbate exercise-induced skeletal muscle injury; but if the patient develops muscle symptoms such as weakness, discomfort, or cramps, stop the statin and perform a careful history. Helpful tests include total CK, 25-OH vitamin D, sedimentation rate, and TSH.

6. If a nonserious adverse reaction occurs with a patient on a statin, consider rechallenging with a lower dose after the patient is back to baseline, especially if that dose was well tolerated in the past. Gastrointestinal active drugs can be used to obtain the additional LDL-c lowering required, if higher-dose statins cannot be safely taken. It is useful to point out to patients that a diet high in fiber and low in saturated and trans fats and low in dietary cholesterol can lower LDL-c by 6% to 8%, which is roughly the lowering obtained by doubling the statin dose.

ALT, alanine transaminase; AST, aspartate aminotransferase; CK, creatine kinase; LDL-c, low-density lipoprotein cholesterol; TSH, thyroid-stimulating hormone. Modified from Stone NJ. In Grundy S, editor: *Atlas on atherosclerosis.* 2005, Philadelphia, Current Science.

3-week holiday off statins, with a view toward rechallenging with either the same or a lowered dose of the statin, to see whether the statin is truly causing the symptoms noted. An analysis of the TNT trial showed that discontinuing statins for a short time during the run-in phase did not result in an increased risk of CHD events.[90] For patients with familial muscle disorders or those presenting with new-onset weakness, it is important to recognize that symptoms can result from both an acquired and inherited muscle disorder. A suggested workup should include an inquiry into exogenous substances (alcohol, grapefruit juice, or drugs that increase statin concentrations), systemic causes (hypothyroidism, collagen vascular disease [polymyalgia rheumatica if older than 50 years] or vitamin D deficiency), and/or a primary muscular cause; therefore it is important to take a family history and consider muscle biopsy if appropriate before a consideration of whether and when to start statin therapy is undertaken. For the patient with persistent weakness despite stopping the statin, neurologic referral may be useful, and these patients may fare best when given bile acid sequestrants and niacin for control of their LDL-c. For those who experience myalgias with daily statins, short trials of multiple statins can be undertaken, if muscle pains or cramps, not weakness, are the statin-related complaints. Some physicians find that a once- or twice-weekly long-acting statin, such as rosuvastatin, can allow otherwise statin-intolerant patients to get to goal.[91,92]

Lovastatin, the first statin on the U.S. market, was not synthetic but was extracted from yeast rice. A partially purified extract of red yeast with multiple components, known as *Xuezhikang* (XZK), was given in a randomized trial to survivors of MI with mean LDL-c of about 129 mg/dL,[93] an LDL-c value similar to initial LDL-c levels in the Heart Protection Study. In this placebo-controlled trial, LDL-c was reduced by 20% in the XZK group and by 3% in the placebo group, and this was associated with a significant decrease in the frequency of major coronary events. Treatment with XZK produced a relative risk (45%) and absolute risk (4.7%) reduction in major coronary events compared with placebo. Those patients on XZK also had a highly significant decrease of approximately 30% to 32% in both CV (6.1% vs. 4.3%) and total mortality (7.7% vs. 5.2%) compared with those treated with placebo. Although only 50% to 60% of subjects were on β-blockers, the use of aspirin was at the 95% level. Because of a lack of standardized preparations, most physicians prefer to use statins tested in large-scale clinical trials first. Despite this intriguing preliminary outcome data of red yeast rice in China and short-term clinical trials in the United States,[94,95] showing tolerability and LDL-c lowering efficacy similar to pravastatin 20 mg/day, it would seem prudent not to recommend red yeast rice as an alternative to statins approved and regulated by the FDA until needed standardization is at hand.[96]

The JUPITER trial called attention to a slight but significant risk for diabetes. This was confirmed by a meta-analysis of 13 large statin trials of at least 1-year duration, excluding those on dialysis or posttransplant, which demonstrated that in 91,140 participants, statin use increased the risk for incident diabetes by 9%.[97] This risk, which is equivalent to one additional case of diabetes for every 255 people treated with a statin for 4 years, is generally outweighed by the statin-mediated reduction in clinical events. Not unexpectedly, this incidence was high in older patients and resulted in an extra case of diabetes over a 4-year period for every 255 patients treated. Thus, statins can be added to the list of treatments, such as niacin and hydrochlorothiazide (HCTZ), which improve CV outcomes but have a small but associated risk of diabetes. This makes a strong point for associated lifestyle counseling with the statin prescription.

Fibrates and nicotinic acid can lower LDL-c, but they are mainly used to treat atherogenic dyslipidemia. Fenofibrate can reduce LDL-c by at least 20% in patients with normal triglyceride levels.[98] In those with elevated triglyceride levels at baseline, LDL-c lowering is much less pronounced, and LDL-c may actually increase. In patients with diabetes, adding fenofibrate to simvastatin did not result in improved CV outcomes.[99] Nicotinic acid lowers LDL-c in a dose-related fashion, but there are concerns about adding it to statin therapy. The Atherothrombosis Intervention in Metabolic Syndrome with low HDL/High Triglycerides: Impact on Global Health Outcomes (AIM-HIGH) trial was stopped prematurely when it was determined that it did not improve outcomes to add high-dose extended-release niacin at 2000 mg/day to statin therapy in participants with established CHD who had reached LDL-c targets of 40 to 80 mg/day but still had low HDL-c (mean, approximately 35 mg/dL). Moreover, an increased risk of ischemic stroke was reported in the niacin group. Further analysis of these trials of combination therapy are required to fully understand their implications, but at present, it seems prudent to use maximally tolerated doses of statins in those with atherogenic dyslipidemia before adding drugs to improve triglycerides and/or HDL-c.[100]

For patients who require LDL-c lowering above and beyond what statins can provide—for example, those with familial hypercholesterolemia—or those whose intolerance of statin therapy, most often because of muscle symptoms, prevents them reaching goal levels for LDL-c, drugs that have a primary effect on the gastrointestinal (GI) tract are recommended with first preference to those that have an outcomes evidence base.

Three classes of drugs are available: *bile acid sequestrants*, resins such as cholestyramine and colestipol and a polymer such as colesevelam; less well-proven therapies, including *cholesterol absorption inhibitors*, such as ezetimibe; and *plant stanol esters*.

BILE ACID SEQUESTRANTS

Bile acid sequestrant (BAS) therapy lowers LDL-c by interfering with bile acid absorption in the ileum. Sequestrants promote fecal excretion of the bound bile acids and result in a compensatory increased LDL receptor synthesis to replenish hepatic cholesterol pools, thus producing enhanced LDL clearance. They are

TABLE 24-6 Bile Acid Sequestrants

BILE ACID SEQUESTRANT	INITIAL DOSAGE	MAINTENANCE DOSAGE	LDL-C REDUCTION	COMMENTS
Cholestyramine resin	8 g/day in divided doses	16-24 g/day as monotherapy; lower doses if used with statins	Varies from 8.7% to 28% depending on dosage of resin	Take other drugs 1 h before or 3 h after; psyllium augments action
Colestipol resin	10 g/day in divided doses	16-24 g/day as monotherapy; lower doses if used with statins	Similar to cholestyramine, varies with dosage of resin	Take other drugs 1 h before or 3 h after; psyllium augments action
Colesevelam	Two or three 625-mg tabs twice daily (7 tabs/day max.)	625 mg tid; can be administered as 7 tabs/day if needed; also available in a suspension equivalent to 6 tabs/day	19% (3.8 g/day)	Take with a large glass of water; lowers HbA1c in type 2 diabetics

HbA1c, hemoglobin A1c; LDL-c, low-density lipoprotein cholesterol.

TABLE 24-7 Clinical Efficacy of Bile Acid Sequestrants

TRIAL	POPULATION	DRUG	LDL-C REDUCTION	EFFICACY AGAINST CHD
LRC CPPT	3806 men, no CHD	Cholestyramine 16-24 g/day	20.3%	19% reduction in fatal and nonfatal MI noted at 7.4 years
STARS	26 men, CHD	Cholestyramine 16 g/day	35.7%	Improvement seen on angiography at 2 years
NHLBI type 2 trial	116 men and women, CHD	Cholestyramine 16 g/day average	26%	Yes, if narrowing was >50% at baseline at 5 years
CLAS	162 men, CHD	Colestipol 30 g/day + nicotinic acid 4.3 g/day	43%	Patients treated had significantly more regression noted on angiography at 2 years
FH-SCOR	72 men and women, familial hypercholesterolemia	Colestipol, nicotinic acid, and lovastatin*	39%	Angiographic change correlated with change in LDL-c at 2 years
FATS	120 men, CHD	Colestipol 30 g/day and either lovastatin 20 mg bid or nicotinic acid 4 g/day	46% (lovastatin), 36% (nicotinic acid)	Nicotinic acid group had higher HDL-c than lovastatin group; significant angiographic and clinical improvement seen at 2.5 years

*No dosages available.
BAS, bile acid sequestrant; CHD, coronary heart disease; CLAS, Cholesterol-Lowering Atherosclerosis Study; HDL-c, high-density lipoprotein cholesterol; LDL-c, low-density lipoprotein cholesterol; LRC PPT, Lipid Research Clinics Coronary Primary Prevention; MI, myocardial infarction, STARS, St. Thomas' Atherosclerosis Regression Study.

nonsystemic drugs for LDL-c lowering, either singly or in combination with statins (see Tables 24-6 and 24-7).

Effects on Lipids and Lipoproteins

For decades, the only BAS resins available were cholestyramine and colestipol. Before the introduction of statins, these were given in higher dosages than are used currently. They were difficult drugs to use at high dosages because of the limiting GI side effects. These resins bound other drugs avidly, especially thyroid replacement hormone, digoxin, and antibiotics. Colesevelam, a polymer gel, was introduced in tablet form.[101] It has the advantage of greater specificity for bile acids, and except for verapamil, it has markedly fewer drug interactions than the resins.[102] Combining colesevelam with a low dose of simvastatin (10 mg/day) resulted in a mean reduction in LDL-c of 42%, which exceeded the reduction usually seen with simvastatin 40 mg/day alone.[103] The effects of combination therapy on serum HDL-c and triglyceride levels were similar to those for simvastatin alone. BAS drugs lower LDL-c in a dose-related fashion, and such therapies are an essential part of a multidrug regimen in patients with markedly elevated LDL levels owing to familial hypercholesterolemia (FH), because their LDL-c–lowering effects are additive to those seen with statins. BAS drugs allow those who cannot tolerate a higher dose of statin to obtain further LDL-c lowering that is more substantial than that seen with doubling the statin dose. BAS drugs should not be given to those with triglycerides higher than 250 mg/dL because of an increased secretion of triglyceride-rich particles that can produce marked hypertriglyceridemia in some cases. HDL-c levels are increased to a mild degree with BAS drugs, but they do not lower Lp(a).

A new indication for colesevelam is in type 2 diabetes; colesevelam therapy added to metformin was found at week 26 not only to significantly lower LDL-c (15.9%), non HDL-c (10.3%), and

ApoB (7.9%) but also to reduce A1c level (mean reduction of 0.54%).[104] Although further studies are needed to clarify its role in the therapy of type 2 diabetes, colesevelam is an attractive option for patients with diabetes who are taking maximally tolerated statins and are still not at goal; however, it is not approved for use in type 1 diabetes.

Efficacy

In primary prevention, cholestyramine was used in the Lipid Research Clinics Primary Prevention Trial. It reduced rates of fatal and nonfatal MI, but the trial was not powered to reduce the total mortality rate.[105] In two small angiographic trials, the NHLBI Type II Intervention Study[106] and the STARS[107] trial, hypercholesterolemic men with CHD who were taking cholestyramine had reduced progression on serial angiograms. In the Familial Atherosclerosis Treatment Study (FATS), colestipol was added to either nicotinic acid or lovastatin and contributed to the decreased progression on angiography and to the event reduction seen in that trial when compared with a placebo group.[109]

Safety/Compliance Issues

BAS medications are not absorbed and should not be considered systemic drugs. Indeed, GI side effects, such as constipation and aggravation of hemorrhoidal bleeding, can be limiting. Resins, such as cholestyramine and colestipol, are available as powders that must be mixed with water or applesauce. Colestipol is also available in tablet form. Colesevelam is available in tablet form (average dose 6 tablets/day, 3 after lunch and 3 after supper) and in a suspension that only needs to be taken once daily. It is important that patients be told to always take these medications with a large glass of water and to dissolve any residue with additional water. All drugs in this class must be taken 90 minutes after or at least 3 to 4 hours before other drugs are taken (at least 4 hours before phenytoin, glyburide, levothyroxine, warfarin, and oral contraceptives). They may interfere with fat-soluble vitamin absorption, so they should be taken in the morning and not taken after lunch and dinner. These drugs require patient instruction to be sure that measures are taken to minimize constipation—for example, adding psyllium powder if tolerated—and to keep well hydrated during the day. Physicians should not start these drugs if triglycerides exceed 300 mg/dL, as resins especially can raise triglyceride levels. The package insert should be consulted, and caution is advised before starting these medications if the patient complains of significant swallowing or motility disorders.

EZETIMIBE AND CHOLESTEROL ABSORPTION INHIBITORS

Ezetimibe, a 2-azetidione, is a potent inhibitor of cholesterol absorption. Using a genetic approach, investigators identified Niemann–Pick C1-Like 1 (*NPC1L1*) as a critical mediator of cholesterol absorption and the direct target of this drug.[110] After absorption, ezetimibe is rapidly glucuronidated by the liver and recycled by the enterohepatic circulation to its target site in the brush border of the small intestine. It prevents the absorption of cholesterol from dietary and especially biliary sources, and it markedly reduces absorption of plant sterols.

Two cotransporters, ABCG5 and ABCG 8, are responsible for resecreting absorbed plant sterols back into the intestinal lumen. Defects of either of these leads to the rare inherited disease phytosterolemia, characterized by hyperabsorption and diminished biliary excretion of plant sterols. Because ezetimibe interferes with *NPC1L1*, reducing the intestinal uptake of cholesterol and plant sterols, it is a novel treatment for this rare disorder.[111]

Effect on Lipids/Lipoproteins

Ezetimibe is used at a single dosage of 10 mg/day. It lowers LDL-c approximately 20%, and its LDL-c–lowering effects are additive to those obtained with statins. Although it has been proposed as monotherapy in patients intolerant to statins, limited outcome data from clinical trials confirm that the combination of a lower dose of statin plus ezetimibe is as efficacious as a larger dose of statin. For statin-intolerant patients or those with FH, combination of ezetimibe and a BAS such as colestipol results in an additional 20% reduction in LDL-c than with either one alone.[112] For optimal efficacy, patients should be advised to avoid taking a BAS and ezetimibe at the same time.

Efficacy

Although patients with the homozygous form of FH are often resistant to statins, they appear to respond to ezetimibe,[113] thus ezetimibe becomes a fourth drug—alongside statins, BAS drugs, and nicotinic acid—to treat this type of FH. A clinical role for ezetimibe was suggested by the Study of Heart and Renal Protection (SHARP) trial, in which simvastatin 20 mg plus ezetimibe 10 mg was compared with placebo in a randomized, double-blind clinical trial of 9720 patients with chronic kidney disease that included more than 3000 patients on dialysis. The investigators reported a 17% reduction seen after 4.9 years in the prespecified outcome of first major atherosclerotic event—nonfatal MI or CHD death, nonhemorrhagic stroke, or any arterial revascularization—without significant excess adverse events. Importantly, no increased risk of cancer was seen. The authors noted that in contrast to earlier trials with statins that showed no benefit for those on hemodialysis, the significant difference in the SHARP trial could have been due both to the much smaller numbers of the prior trials and the much smaller proportion of vascular events noted in primary outcomes that were related to atherosclerotic vascular disease and hence amenable to therapy to lower LDL-c.[114] Data on efficacy and safety from a large-scale clinical trial of patients with ACS are eagerly awaited.[115]

Safety

For most patients, ezetimibe is remarkably well tolerated, and its safety profile is similar to that seen with placebo. In patients who previously had experienced myalgia with statin therapy, with or without elevated CK levels, myalgia has occurred with ezetimibe. Patients with a history of statin intolerance should be monitored for adverse muscle events during treatment with ezetimibe.[116] Elevations of liver transaminases and cases of hepatitis have been reported in patients treated with ezetimibe. Drug interactions include cyclosporine, so cyclosporine concentrations should be monitored; fibrates, which should not be added to fenofibrate if the patient has a history of gallstones; and bile acid resins, which can decrease concentrations of ezetimibe.

Patients who begin ezetimibe should have a liver panel at baseline. After 6 to 12 weeks, measurement of hepatic transaminases is recommended. This should be repeated if ezetimibe is combined with a statin. Whether taken alone or with a statin, ezetimibe is contraindicated for patients with active liver disease or unexplained persistent elevations of liver transaminases, and it should not be given to pregnant women or nursing mothers.

PLANT STANOL ESTERS

Plant sterols are ubiquitous in nature and have the familiar multiring nuclear structure of the sterol family. They differ from cholesterol—found in animals as a key component of cell membranes, vitamin D, and adrenal and gonadal steroids—only in the structure of their side chain. Saturated sterols, termed *stanols*, lack the five-numbered double bond in their B-ring.[117] Saturation of *sitosterol*, the most commonly occurring plant sterol, gives rise to *sitostanol;* saturation of *campesterol* gives rise to *campestanol.* Plant sterols and cholesterol are consumed approximately in equal amounts, but phytosterols occur in human plasma in a concentration that is normally less than 0.5% that of cholesterol. Plant stanols are even less well absorbed from the intestine and have a plasma level that is only one tenth as high (i.e., 0.05% that of cholesterol). The ATP III report suggested that addition of plant stanol or sterol esters and fiber could help patients reach LDL-c goals without having to resort to medications. Because there had been no rigorous comparison of plant stanols and sterols, ATP III recommended either one.[118] Data that became available subsequent to the ATP III report indicate a possible advantage to using plant stanol esters, rather than plant sterols, to lower LDL-c.[119] The efficacy of plant sterol esters for lowering LDL-c tends to diminish over time; in contrast, plant stanol esters maintain their LDL-c–lowering efficacy at about 10% from baseline. Also, plant stanols were found not to effect bile acid synthesis, unlike plant sterols. Finally, dietary plant stanol esters reduce statin-induced elevations of serum plant sterol levels, whereas serum plant sterol levels are not lowered when dietary plant sterol ester is fed.[120]

Effect on Lipids/Lipoproteins

An important practical observation is that the margarine-based stanol ester is as effective in a single dose as it is when taken in three divided doses.[121] The persistence of the single-dose effect suggests that stanols not only compete with cholesterol for micellar solubilization but also have an additional, longer-lasting effect on intestinal mucosal cells. There are practical limits to how much margarine an individual can ingest; maximal LDL-c lowering with plant stanols occurs with 2 g/day of plant stanol esters.[122] In a study of postmenopausal women, LDL-c levels were lowered 13%, which might allow low-risk patients to avoid drug therapy. Older patients appear to be more responsive than younger ones to the effects of plant stanol esters.[123]

Efficacy Against Coronary Heart Disease

There are no CHD endpoint studies available, and some researchers have raised concerns that elevated plant sterol concentrations could increase CHD risk. To determine whether plasma levels of plant sterols were associated with coronary atherosclerosis in humans, 2542 subjects, aged 30 to 67 years, who underwent electron-beam computed tomography had plasma levels of cholesterol and plant sterols measured.[124] Plasma levels of cholesterol, but not sitosterol or campesterol, were significantly higher in subjects with coronary calcium. In addition, in the same paper, investigators could not show that elevated plasma levels of plant sterols (sitosterol and campesterol) were associated with atherosclerosis in genetically modified mice.

Safety

A meta-analysis presented at a workshop on plant stanol esters indicated that levels of vitamins A and D are not affected by stanols or sterols.[125] Alpha carotene, lycopene, and vitamin E levels are carried on LDL particles and remain stable relative to LDL levels. Although β-carotene levels were observed to decline, the panel did not expect adverse health outcomes; indeed, adverse health outcomes have been reported from β-carotene supplementation. This panel concluded that present evidence is sufficient to promote use of plant sterols and stanols for lowering LDL-c levels in those at increased risk for CHD.[126] Some have suggested that sources of carotenoids be ingested at meals other than those in which plant sterol esters are eaten.

A final note: The safe use of the medications mentioned here requires a review of the individual patient's indications, potential liver or kidney issues that could affect drug concentrations and efficacy, and a review for potential drug-drug and food-drug interactions. A review of the manufacturer's Web site and physician prescribing information can be valuable and is highly recommended for safe use of these products.

REFERENCES

1. Goldstein JL, Brown MS. Molecular medicine: the cholesterol quartet. *Science* 2001; 292(5520):1310-1312.
2. Sacks FM, Campos H. Clinical review 163: cardiovascular endocrinology—low-density lipoprotein size and cardiovascular disease: a reappraisal. *J Clin Endocrinol Metab* 2003; 88(10):4525-4532.
3. Vega GL, Grundy SM. Effect of statins on metabolism of apo-B-containing lipoproteins in hypertriglyceridemic men. *Am J Cardiol* 1998;81(4A):36B-42B.
4. Snow V, Aronson MD, Hornbake ER, et al. Lipid control in the management of type 2 diabetes mellitus: a clinical practice guideline from the American College of Physicians. *Ann Int Med* 2004;140:644-649.
5. Tonelli M, Isles C, Craven T, et al. Effect of pravastatin on rate of kidney function loss in people with or at risk for coronary disease. *Circulation* 2005;112(2):171-178.
6. Davidson M. Considerations in the treatment of dyslipidemia associated with chronic kidney failure and renal transplantation. *Prev Cardiol* 2005;8(4):244-249.
7. Third Report of the National Cholesterol Education Program (NCEP) Expert Panel on Detection, Evaluation, and Treatment of High Blood Cholesterol in Adults. (Adult Treatment Panel III) final report. *Circulation* 2002;106(25):3143-3421.
8. Taylor F, Ward K, Moore TH, et al. Statins for the primary prevention of cardiovascular disease. *Cochrane Database Syst Rev* 2011 Jan 19;(1):CD004816.
9. Ray KK, Seshasai SR, Erqou S, et al. Statins and all-cause mortality in high-risk primary prevention: a meta-analysis of 11 randomized controlled trials involving 65,229 participants. *Arch Intern Med* 2010;170(12):1024-1031.
10. Thavendiranathan P, Bagai A, Brookhart MA, Choudhry NK. Primary prevention of cardiovascular diseases with statin therapy: a meta-analysis of randomized controlled trials. *Arch Intern Med* 2006;166(21):2307-2313.
11. Mora S, Glynn RJ, Hsia J, et al. Statins for the primary prevention of cardiovascular events in women with elevated high-sensitivity C-reactive protein or dyslipidemia: results from the Justification for the Use of Statins in Prevention: An Intervention Trial Evaluating Rosuvastatin (JUPITER) and meta-analysis of women from primary prevention trials. *Circulation* 2010;121(9):1069-1077.
12. Tavazzi L, Maggioni AP, Marchioli R, et al. Gissi-HF Investigators. Effect of rosuvastatin in patients with chronic heart failure (the GISSI-HF trial): a randomised, double-blind, placebo-controlled trial. *Lancet* 2008;372:1231-1239.
13. Wanner C, Krane V, Marz W, et al. German Diabetes and Dialysis Study Investigators. Atorvastatin in patients with type 2 diabetes mellitus undergoing hemodialysis. *N Engl J Med* 2005;353:238-248.
14. Fellstrom BC, Jardine AG, Schmieder RE, et al. AURORA Study Group. Rosuvastatin and cardiovascular events in patients undergoing hemodialysis. *N Engl J Med* 2009;360: 1395-1407.
15. Kjekshus J, Apetrei E, Barrios V, et al. CORONA Group. Rosuvastatin in older patients with systolic heart failure. *N Engl J Med* 2007;357(22):2248-2261.
16. Sniderman AD, Solhpour A, Alam A, et al. Cardiovascular death in dialysis patients: lessons we can learn from AURORA. *Clin J Am Soc Nephrol* 2010;5(2):335-340.
17. Winchester DE, Wen X, Xie L, Bavry AA. Evidence of pre-procedural statin therapy a meta-analysis of randomized trials. *J Am Coll Cardiol* 2010;56(14):1099-1109.
18. Dunkelgrun E, Boersma E, Schouten O, et al. Bisoprolol and fluvastatin for the reduction of perioperative cardiac mortality and myocardial infarction in intermediate-risk patients undergoing noncardiovascular surgery: a randomized controlled trial (DECREASE-IV). *Ann Surg* 2009;249: 921-992.
19. Rami K, Martin J, Emberson J, et al. Effect of statins on atrial fibrillation: collaborative meta-analysis of published and unpublished evidence from randomized controlled trials. *Br Med J* 2011;342:d1250.
20. Roberts WC. The rule of 5 and the rule of 7 in lipid-lowering by statin drugs. *Am J Cardiol* 1997;80(1):106-107.
21. Schaefer EJ, McNamara JR, Tayler T, et al. Comparisons of effects of statins (atorvastatin, fluvastatin, lovastatin, pravastatin, and simvastatin) on fasting and postprandial lipoproteins in patients with coronary heart disease versus control subjects. *Am J Cardiol* 2004;93(1):31-39.
22. Stein DT, Devaraj S, Balis D, Adams-Huet B, Jialal I. Effect of statin therapy on remnant lipoprotein cholesterol levels in patients with combined hyperlipidemia. *Arterioscler Thromb Vasc Biol* 2001;21(12):2026-2031.
23. Maron DJ, Fazio S, Linton MF. Current perspectives on statins. *Circulation* 2000; 101;207-213.
24. Grundy SM, Cleeman JI, Merz CN, et al. Implications of recent clinical trials for the National Cholesterol Education Program Adult Treatment Panel III Guidelines. *Circulation* 2004; 110:227-239.
25. Gotto AM Jr, Moon J. Pitavastatin for the treatment of primary hyperlipidemia and mixed dyslipidemia. *Expert Rev Cardiovasc Ther* 2010;8(8):1079-1090.
26. Pitavastatin (Livalo): the seventh statin. *Med Lett Drugs Ther* 2010;52:57-58.
27. Pasternak RC, Smith SC, Bairey-Merz CN, et al. ACC/AHA/NHLBI clinical advisory on the use and safety of statins. *J Am Coll Cardiol* 2002;40:567-572.
28. Garcia-Valdecasas-Campelo E, Gonzalez-Reimers E, Lopez-Lirola A, Rodriguez-Rodriguez E, Santolaria-Fernandez F. Acute rhabdomyolysis associated with cerivastatin therapy. *Arch Intern Med* 2001;161:893.
29. Stein EA, Lane M, Laskarzewski P. Comparison of statins in hypertriglyceridemia. *Am J Cardiol* 1998;81(4A):66B-69B.
30. Jones PH, Davidson MH, Stein EA, et al. Comparison of the efficacy and safety of rosuvastatin versus atorvastatin, simvastatin, and pravastatin across doses (STELLAR trial). *Am J Cardiol* 2003;92:152-160.
31. Cannon CP, Braunwald E, McCabe CH, et al. Pravastatin or Atorvastatin Evaluation and Infection Therapy–Thrombolysis in Myocardial Infarction 22 Investigators. Intensive versus moderate lipid lowering with statins after acute coronary syndromes. *N Engl J Med* 2004;350:1495-1504.
32. Scanu A. Lipoprotein(a), Friedewald formula, and NCEP guidelines. National Cholesterol Education Program. *Am J Cardiol* 2001;87(5):608-609, A9.
33. Albert MA, Glynn RJ, Wolfert RL, Ridker PM. The effect of statin therapy on lipoprotein associated phospholipase A2 levels. *Atherosclerosis* 2005;182;193-198.
34. Albert MA, Danielson E, Rifai N, Ridker PM. PRINCE Investigators. Effect of statin therapy on C-reactive protein levels: the pravastatin inflammation/CRP evaluation (PRINCE): a randomized trial and cohort study. *JAMA* 2001;286:64-70.
35. Peters SA, Palmer MK, Grobbee DE, et al. C-reactive protein lowering with rosuvastatin in the METEOR study. *J Intern Med* 2010;268(2):155-161.
36. Ridker PM, Rifai N, Clearfield M, et al. Air Force/Texas Coronary Atherosclerosis Prevention Study Investigators. Measurement of C-reactive protein for the targeting of statin therapy in the primary prevention of acute coronary events. *N Engl J Med* 2001;344(26): 1959-1965.
37. Ridker PM, Cannon CP, Morrow D, et al. Pravastatin or Atorvastatin Evaluation and Infection Therapy–Thrombolysis in Myocardial Infarction 22 (PROVE IT–TIMI 22) Investigators. C-reactive protein levels and outcomes after statin therapy. *N Engl J Med* 2005; 352(1):20-28.
38. Ridker PM, Danielson E, Fonseca FA, et al. JUPITER Study Group. Rosuvastatin to prevent vascular events in men and women with elevated C-reactive protein. *N Engl J Med* 2008;359(21):2195-2207.
39. Kaul S, Morrissey RP, Diamond GA. By Jove! What is a clinician to make of JUPITER? *Arch Intern Med* 2010;170(12):1073-1077.
40. Ballantyne CM, Corsini A, Davidson MH, et al. Risk for myopathy with statin therapy in high-risk patients. *Arch Intern Med* 2003;163(5):553-564.
41. Corsini A, Bellosta S, Davidson MH. Pharmacokinetic interactions between statins and fibrates. *Am J Cardiol* 2005;96(9A):44K-49K.
42. Stone NJ. Strategies for treating abnormal lipid profiles with drugs. In Grundy SM, editor: *Atlas of atherosclerosis, risk factors and treatment,* 4th ed. Philadelphia, 2005, Current Medicine, pp143-166.
43. Kane GC, Lipsky JJ. Drug–grapefruit juice interactions. *Mayo Clin Proc* 2000;75:933-942.
44. Hanley MJ, Cancalon P, Widmer WW, Greenblatt DJ. The effect of grapefruit juice on drug disposition. *Expert Opin Drug Metab Toxicol* 2011;7(3):267-286.
45. Malvestutto CD, Aberg JA. Coronary heart disease in people infected with HIV. *Cleve Clin J Med* 2010;77(8):547-556.
46. U.S. Food and Drug Administration. *FDA drug safety communication: new restrictions, contraindications, and dose limitations for zocor (simvastatin) to reduce the risk of muscle injury.* Available at http://www.fda.gov/drugs/drugsafety/ucm256581.htm. Accessed June 25, 2012.
47. McKenney JM. Efficacy and safety of rosuvastatin in treatment of dyslipidemia. *Am J Health Syst Pharm* 2005;62(10):1033-1047.
48. Holdaas H, Fellstrom B, Jardine AG, et al. Assessment of Lescol in Renal Transplantation (ALERT) Study Investigators. Effect of fluastatin on cardiac outcomes in renal transplant recipients: a multicentre, randomized, placebo controlled trial. *Lancet* 2003;361: 2024-2031.
49. Jones PH, Davidson MH. Reporting rate of rhabdomyolysis with fenofibrate + statin versus gemfibrozil + any statin. *Am J Cardiol* 2005;95:120-122.
50. Bergman AJ, Murphy G, Burke J, et al. Simvastatin does not have a clinically significant pharmacokinetic interaction with fenofibrate in humans. *J Clin Pharmacol* 2004;44: 1054-1062.

51. Andrus MR. Oral anticoagulant drug interactions with statins: case report of fluvastatin and review of the literature. *Pharmacotherapy* 2004;24(2):285-290.

52. Williams D, Feely J. Pharmacokinetic-pharmacodynamic drug interactions with HMG-CoA reductase inhibitors. *Clin Pharmacokinet* 2002;41(5):343-370.

53. Guyton JR, Capuzzi DM. Treatment of hyperlipidemia with combined niacin-statin regimens. *Am J Cardiol* 1998;82(12A):82U-84U.

54. Thompson GR. Angiographic evidence for the role of triglyceride-rich lipoproteins in progression of coronary artery disease. *Eur Heart J* 1998;(19 Suppl):H31-H36.

55. Knatterud GL, Rosenberg Y, Campeau L, et al.; Post CABG Investigators. Long-term effects on clinical outcomes of aggressive lowering of low-density lipoprotein cholesterol levels and low-dose anticoagulation in the post coronary artery bypass graft trial. *Circulation* 2000;102(2):157-165.

56. Pitt B, Waters D, Brown WV, et al. Aggressive lipid-lowering therapy compared with angioplasty in stable coronary artery disease. *N Engl J Med* 1999;341:70-76.

57. Nissen SE, Tuzcu EM, Schoenhagen P, et al. REVERSAL Investigators. Effect of intensive compared with moderate lipid-lowering therapy on progression of coronary atherosclerosis: a randomized controlled trial. *JAMA* 2004;291(9):1071-1080.

58. O'Keefe JH Jr, Cordain L, Harris WH, Moe RM, Vogel R. Optimal low-density lipoprotein is 50 to 70 mg/dL: lower is better and physiologically normal. *J Am Coll Cardiol* 2004;43(11):2142-2146.

59. Lima JA, Desai MY, Steen H, et al. Statin-induced cholesterol lowering and plaque regression after 6 months of magnetic resonance imaging–monitored therapy. *Circulation* 2004;110(16):2336-2341.

60. Heart Protection Study Collaborative Group. MRC/BHF Heart Protection Study of cholesterol-lowering with simvastatin in 20 536 high-risk individuals: a randomized placebo-controlled trial. *Lancet* 2002;360:7-22.

61. Collins R, Armitage J, Parish S, Sleight P, Peto R. Heart Protection Study Collaborative Group. Effects of cholesterol-lowering with simvastatin on stroke and other major vascular events in 20 536 people with cerebrovascular disease or other high-risk conditions. *Lancet* 2004;363(9411):757-767.

62. de Lemos JA, Blazing MA, Wiviott SD, et al. Early intensive vs a delayed conservative simvastatin strategy in patients with acute coronary syndromes: phase Z of the A to Z trial. *JAMA* 2004;292:1307-1316.

63. Armitage J, Bowman L, Wallendszus K, et al. Study of the Effectiveness of Additional Reductions in Cholesterol and Homocysteine (SEARCH) Collaborative Group. Intensive lowering of LDL cholesterol with 80 mg versus 20 mg simvastatin daily in 12,064 survivors of myocardial infarction: a double-blind randomised trial. *Lancet* 2010;376(9753):1658-1669.

64. SEARCH Collaborative Group. SLCO1B1 variants and statin-induced myopathy—a genome-wide study. *N Engl J Med* 2008;359(8):789-799.

65. Baigent C, Keech A, Kearney PM, et al. Cholesterol Treatment Trialists' (CTT) Collaborators. Efficacy and safety of cholesterol-lowering treatment: prospective meta-analysis of data from 90,056 participants in 14 randomised trials of statins. *Lancet* 2005;366(9493):1267-1278.

66. Baigent C, Blackwell L, Emberson J, et al. Cholesterol Treatment Trialists' (CTT) Collaboration. Efficacy and safety of more intensive lowering of LDL cholesterol: a meta-analysis of data from 170,000 participants in 26 randomised trials. *Lancet* 2010;376(9753):1670-1681.

67. Ray KK, Cannon CP. The potential relevance of the multiple lipid-independent (pleiotropic) effects of statins in the management of acute coronary syndromes. *J Am Coll Cardiol* 2005;46:1425-1433.

68. Schwartz GG, Olsson AG, Ezekowitz MD, et al. Effects of atorvastatin on early recurrent ischemic events in acute coronary syndromes: the MIRACL study. A randomized controlled trial. *JAMA* 2001;285:1711-1718.

69. Buchwald H, Campos CT, Varco RL, et al. Effective lipid modification and morbidity: five-year posttrial follow-up report from the POSCH. *Arch Intern Med* 1998;158:1253-1261.

70. Palinski W, Napoli C. Unraveling pleiotropic effects of statins on plaque rupture. *Arterioscler Thromb Vasc Biol* 2002;22:1745-1750.

71. Pasternak RC, Smith SC Jr, Bairey-Merz CN, et al. American College of Cardiology; American Heart Association; National Heart, Lung and Blood Institute. ACC/AHA/NHLBI clinical advisory on the use and safety of statins. *Circulation* 2002;106(8):1024-1028.

72. Russo M, Jacobson I. How to use statins with chronic liver disease. *Cleve Clinic J Med* 2004;71:58-62.

73. Report of the National Lipid Association's Statin Safety Task Force. *Am J Card* 2006;97 (Suppl 1):S89-S94.

73a. Available at http://www.fda.gov/ForConsumers/ConsumerUpdates/ucm293330.htm. Accessed May 28, 2012.

74. Charles EC, Olson KL, Sandhoff BG, McClure DL, Merenich JA. Evaluation of cases of severe statin-related transaminitis within a large health maintenance organization. *Am J Med* 2005;118(6):618-624.

75. Calderon RM, Cubeddu LX, Goldberg RB, Schiff ER. Statins in the treatment of dyslipidemia in the presence of elevated liver aminotransferase levels: a therapeutic dilemma. *Mayo Clin Proc* 2010;85:349-356.

76. Chang JT, Staffa JA, Parks M, Green L. Rhabdomyolysis with HMG-CoA reductase inhibitors and gemfibrozil combination therapy. *Pharmacoepidemiol Drug Saf* 2004;13:417-426.

77. Joy TR, Hegele RA. Narrative review: statin-related myopathy. *Ann Intern Med* 2009;150(12):858.

78. Armitage J. Safety of statins in clinical practice. *Lancet* 2007;370:1781-1790.

79. Venero CV, Thompson PD. Managing statin myopathy. *Endocrinol Metab Clin North Am* 2009;38:121-136.

80. Abd TT, Jacobson TA. Statin-induced myopathy: a review and update. *Expert Opin Drug Saf* 2011;10:373-387.

81. Warren JD, Blumbergs PC, Thompson PD. Rhabdomyolysis: a review. *Muscle Nerve* 2002;25:332-347.

82. Bruckert E, Hayem G, Dejager S, et al. Mild to moderate muscular symptoms with high-dosage statin therapy in hyperlipidemic patients—the PRIMO study. *Cardiovasc Drugs Ther* 2005;19(6):403-414.

83. Hansen KE, Hildebrand JP, Ferguson EE, Stein JH. Outcomes in 45 patients with statin-associated myopathy. *Arch Intern Med* 2005;165(22):2671-2676.

84. Phillips PS, Haas RH, Bannykh S, et al. Statin-associated myopathy with normal creatine kinase levels. The Scripps Mercy Clinical Research Center. *Ann Intern Med* 2002;137:581-585.

85. Mohaupt MG, Karas RH, Babiychuk EB, et al. Association between statin-associated myopathy and skeletal muscle damage. *CMAJ* 2009;181(1-2):E11-E18.

86. Grable-Esposito P, Katzberg HD, Greenberg SA, et al. Immune-mediated necrotizing myopathy associated with statins. *Muscle Nerve* 2010;41(2):185-190.

87. Gupta A, Thompson PD. The relationship of vitamin D deficiency to statin myopathy. *Atherosclerosis* 2011;215(1):23-29. Epub 2010 Dec 5.

88. Grundy S. Can statins cause chronic low-grade myopathy? *Ann Intern Med* 2002;137:617-618.

89. Thompson PD, Clarkson P, Karas RH. Statin-associated myopathy. *JAMA* 2003;289(13):1681-1690.

90. McGowan MD. There is no evidence for an increase in acute coronary syndromes after short-term abrupt discontinuation of statins in stable cardiac patients. *Circulation* 2004;110:2333-2335.

91. Backes JM, Moriarty PM, Ruisinger JF, Gibson CA. Effects of once weekly rosuvastatin among patients with a prior statin intolerance. *Am J Cardiol* 2007;100:554-555.

92. Backes JM, Venero CV, Gibson CA, et al. Effectiveness and tolerability of every-other-day rosuvastatin dosing in patients with prior statin intolerance. *Ann Pharmacother* 2008;42:341-346.

93. Lu Z, Kou W, Du B, et al. Chinese Coronary Secondary Prevention Study Group. Effect of Xuezhikang, an extract from red yeast Chinese rice, on coronary events in a Chinese population with previous myocardial infarction. *Am J Cardiol* 2008;101(12):1689-1693.

94. Becker DJ, Gordon RY, Halbert SC, et al. Red yeast rice for dyslipidemia in statin-intolerant patients: a randomized trial. *Ann Intern Med* 2009;150(12):830-839, W147-W149.

95. Halbert SC, French B, Gordon RY, et al. Tolerability of red yeast rice (2,400 mg twice daily) versus pravastatin (20 mg twice daily) in patients with previous statin intolerance. *Am J Cardiol* 2010;105(2):198-204.

96. Eckel R. Approach to the patient who is intolerant of statin therapy. *J Clin Endocrinol Metab* 2010;95(5):2015-2022.

97. Sattar N, Preiss D, Murray HM, et al. Statins and risk of incident diabetes: a collaborative meta-analysis of randomized statin trials. *Lancet* 2010;375(9716):735-742.

98. Knopp RH, Brown WV, Dujovne CA, et al. Effects of fenofibrate on plasma lipoproteins in hypercholesterolemia and combined hyperlipidemia. *Am J Med* 1987;83(5B):50-59.

99. Ginsberg HN, Elam MB, Lovato LC, et al. ACCORD Study Group. Effects of combination lipid therapy in type 2 diabetes mellitus. *N Engl J Med* 2010;362(17):1563-1574.

100. Boden WE, Probstfield JL, Anderson T, et al, for the AIM-HIGH Investigators. Niacin in patients with low HDL cholesterol levels receiving intensive statin therapy. *N Engl J Med* 2011;365:2255-2267.

101. Davidson MH, Dillon MA, Gordon B, et al. Colesevelam hydrochloride (cholestagel): a new potent bile acid sequestrant associated with a low incidence of gastrointestinal side effects. *Arch Intern Med* 1999;159:1893-1900.

102. Donovan JM, Stypinski D, Stiles MR, Olson TA, Burke SK. Drug interactions with colesevelam hydrochloride, a novel, potent lipid-lowering agent. *Cardiovasc Drugs Ther* 2000;14(6):681-690.

103. Knapp HH, Schrott H, Ma P, et al. Efficacy and safety of combination simvastatin and colesevelam in patients with primary hypercholesterolemia. *Am J Med* 2001;110(5):352-360.

104. Bays HE, Goldberg RB, Truitt KE, Jones MR. Colesevelam hydrochloride therapy in patients with type 2 diabetes mellitus treated with metformin: glucose and lipid effects. *Arch Intern Med* 2008;168(18):1975-1983.

105. Lipid Research Clinics Program. The Lipid Research Clinics Coronary Primary Prevention Trial results. I: Reduction in the incidence of coronary heart disease. *JAMA* 1984;251:351-364.

106. Brensike JF, Levy RI, Kelsey SF, et al. Effects of therapy with cholestyramine on progression of coronary arteriosclerosis: results of the NHLBI Type II Coronary Intervention Study. *Circulation* 1984;69:313-324.

107. Watts GF, Lewis B, Brunt JNH, et al. Effects on coronary artery disease of lipid-lowering diet, or diet plus cholestyramine, in the St. Thomas' Atherosclerosis Regression Study (STARS). *Lancet* 1992;339:563-569.

108. Brown G, Albers JJ, Fisher LD, et al. Regression of coronary artery disease as a result of intensive lipid-lowering therapy in men with high levels of apolipoprotein B. *N Engl J Med* 1990;323:1289-1298.

109. Reference deleted in proofs.

110. Garcia-Calvo M, Lisnock J, Bull HG, et al. The target of ezetimibe is Niemann-Pick C1-Like 1 (NPC1L1). *Proc Natl Acad Sci U S A* 2005;102(23):8132-8137.

111. von Bergmann K, Sudhop T, Lutjohann D. Cholesterol and plant sterol absorption: recent insights. *Am J Cardiol* 2005;96(1A):10D-14D.

112. Zema MJ. Colesevelam HCl and ezetimibe combination therapy provides effective lipid-lowering in difficult-to-treat patients with hypercholesterolemia. *Am J Ther* 2005;12(4):306-310.

113. Gagne C, Gaudet D, Bruckert E. Ezetimibe Study Group. Efficacy and safety of ezetimibe coadministered with atorvastatin or simvastatin in patients with homozygous familial hypercholesterolemia. *Circulation* 2002;105(21):2469-2475.

114. Baigent C, Landray MJ, Reith C, et al. SHARP Investigators. The effects of lowering LDL cholesterol with simvastatin plus ezetimibe in patients with chronic kidney disease (Study of Heart and Renal Protection): a randomised placebo-controlled trial. *Lancet* 2011;377:2181-2192.

115. Califf RM, Lokhnygina Y, Cannon CP, et al. An update on the IMProved reduction of outcomes: Vytorin Efficacy International Trial (IMPROVE-IT) design. *Am Heart J* 2010;159(5):705-709.

116. Zetia (ezetimibe) package insert. Available at http://www.merck.com/product/usa/pi_circulars/z/zetia/zetia_pi.pdf. Accessed June 25, 2012.

117. Thompson GR, Grundy SM. History and development of plant sterol and stanol esters for cholesterol-lowering purposes. *Am J Cardiol* 2005;96(Suppl):3D-9D.

118. Grundy SM. Stanol esters as a component of maximal dietary therapy in the National Cholesterol Education Program Adult Treatment Panel III Report. *Am J Cardiol* 2005; 96(Suppl):47D-50D.

119. O'Neill FH, Sanders TA, Thompson GR. Comparison of efficacy of plant stanol ester and sterol ester: short-term and longer-term studies. *Am J Cardiol* 2005;96(1A):29D-36D.

120. Miettinen TA, Gylling H. Effect of statins on noncholesterol sterol levels: implications for use of plant stanols and sterols. *Am J Cardiol* 2005;96(1A):40D-46D.

121. Plat J, van Onselen EN, van Heugten MM, Mensink RP. Effects on serum lipids, lipoproteins and fat soluble antioxidant concentrations of consumption frequency of margarines and shortenings enriched with plant stanol esters. *Eur J Clin Nutr* 2000;54:671-677.

122. Cater NB, Garcia-Garcia AB, Vega GL, Grundy SM. Responsiveness of plasma lipids and lipoproteins to plant stanol esters. *Am J Cardiol* 2005;96(Suppl):23D-28D.

123. Law M. Plant sterol and stanol margarines and health. *Br Med J* 2000;320:861-864.

124. Wilund KR, Yu L, Xu F, et al. No association between plasma levels of plant sterols and atherosclerosis in mice and men. *Arterioscler Thromb Vasc Biol* 2004;24:2326-2332.

125. Katan MB, Grundy SM, Jones P, et al. Stresa Workshop Participants. Efficacy and safety of plant stanols and sterols in the management of blood cholesterol levels. *Mayo Clin Proc* 2003;78:965-978.

126. Alpha Tocopherol, β-Carotene Prevention Study Group. The effect of vitamin E and beta carotene on the incidence of lung cancer and other cancers in male smokers. *N Engl J Med* 1994;330:1029-1035.

CH
24

DRUGS FOR ELEVATED LOW-DENSITY LIPOPROTEIN CHOLESTEROL

Therapy to Manage Low High-Density Lipoprotein Cholesterol and Elevated Triglycerides

Michael H. Davidson

RATIONALE FOR COMBINATION THERAPY, 434

Lack of Achievement of Non–High-Density Lipoprotein
Goals, 434
Residual Risk for Statin Therapy, 434

COMBINED DYSLIPIDEMIA, 435

Non–High-Density Lipoprotein Cholesterol Reduction, 435
Therapy to Modify High-Density Lipoprotein, 435
Statin-Fibrate Combination, 436
Statin-Niacin Combination, 436
Statin–Omega-3 Fatty Acids Combination, 437

CHOLESTERYL ESTER TRANSFER PROTEIN
INHIBITION, 438

CONCLUSION, 440

REFERENCES, 440

As the population becomes more obese and the prevalence of diabetes and metabolic syndrome increases, low-density lipoprotein cholesterol (LDL-c) is increasingly losing its value as a predictor for cardiovascular (CV) risk. In addition, targeting LDL-c treatment to less than 70 mg/dL has achieved significant cardiovascular disease (CVD) benefits, but a high residual risk continues, especially if other lipid parameters, such as triglyceride (TG) and high-density lipoprotein cholesterol (HDL-c) levels remain abnormal. Identifiable residual risk factors include low HDL-c and elevated TGs, LDL particle number, apolipoprotein (Apo) B, high-sensitivity C-reactive protein (hs-CRP), and lipoprotein-associated phospholipase A2 (Lp-PLA2). Although additional therapeutic intervention beyond statin therapy to modify these residual risk factors has not yet been proven to reduce CV events, ample evidence suggests that patients with these abnormalities remain at increased risk despite having LDL-c and non–HDL-c at goal (<70 mg/dL and <100 mg/dL, respectively), according to the National Cholesterol Education Program Adult Treatment Panel III (NCEP ATP III) 2004 update. Statin combination therapy with niacin, fibrates, and prescription omega-3 fatty acids provides additional improvements in non–HDL-c and HDL-c. Clinical trials are underway to evaluate the effects of niacin in combination with a statin on CV outcomes. Cholesteryl ester transfer protein (CETP) inhibitors, which increase HDL-c, are also in late-phase development, with the potential to address the residual risk for patients with low HDL.

Rationale for Combination Therapy

Lipid treatment options to reduce coronary heart disease (CHD) risk have focused on lifestyle changes and LDL-c–lowering therapy, most commonly with statins, as recommended by the ATP III.[1] However, studies show that a significant proportion of patients who receive statin therapy do not achieve all optimal lipid levels, particularly those patients with mixed dyslipidemia.[2-4] Substantial residual risk of CV events may exist in patients with abnormal TGs and HDL-c after statin treatment has been initiated. Specifically, the clinical benefit of having a TG level below 150 mg/dL on statin treatment has been demonstrated in an acute coronary syndrome (ACS) population.[2] The Pravastatin or Atorvastatin Evaluation and Infection Therapy–Thrombolysis in Myocardial Infarction 22 (PROVE-IT–TIMI 22) trial observed a significant 1.6% reduction in the incidence of death, myocardial infarction (MI), and recurrent ACS for each 10 mg/dL (0.113 mol/L) decrement in TG levels after adjusting for LDL-c.[2] Statin trials demonstrate that for patients with elevated TGs or low HDL-c, risk for a future CHD event is increased by 40% to 70% (Figures 25-1 and 25-2).[3,4]

Currently available statins and other lipid-altering drugs used as monotherapy often do not reach optimal levels in all lipid parameters; therefore, the combination of statins and other lipid-altering drugs that target TG and HDL-c levels can potentially fill this unmet need in patients with mixed dyslipidemia.

Lack of Achievement of Non–High-Density Lipoprotein Goals

Many patients with CHD have therapeutic needs that exceed the simple reductions in LDL-c obtained by using statins. The ATP III has acknowledged the increasing evidence of an independent association between hypertriglyceridemia and CHD by issuing guidelines that identify non–HDL-c as a secondary target for therapy in patients with elevated TG levels.[1] This association is likely related to the atherogenicity of some species of TG-rich lipoproteins, particularly small very-low-density lipoprotein (VLDL) and intermediate-density lipoprotein particles. Elevation of these "remnant" lipoproteins has been shown to contribute to atherosclerosis in mice.[5] Evidence exists that genetic dyslipidemias characterized by increased concentrations of remnant lipoproteins are associated with the development of premature CHD, and remnant lipoprotein levels strongly predict the progression of atherosclerosis.[6] In addition, in both observational studies and during treatment in clinical trials, levels of ApoB, reflecting the total number of circulating atherogenic particles (LDL plus VLDL), are better associated with CHD risk than with LDL-c concentration.[7]

Residual Risk for Statin Therapy

With the recognition that additional event reduction can be obtained by more intensive LDL-c reductions in some patients who are at very high risk for CHD events, the ATP III recommended the therapeutic optional goal for LDL-c less than 70 mg/dL and non–HDL-c less than 100 mg/dL.[6] Cholesterol-lowering therapy with statins has been established as an effective method for reducing death and MI among patients with CHD. However, a significant number of individuals who receive statin therapy continue to have high residual risk. An important clinical challenge exists to reduce residual CHD risk with optimal therapies without increasing adverse effects. Combination therapy appears most appropriate for patients with a high rate of events on optimal statin therapy. In addition to lifestyle modification, the use of combination therapy in CHD is an acknowledged strategy in optimal management to prevent or delay the morbidity and mortality associated with CHD and its risk factors. Current recommendations for CHD prevention and treatment advise the use of combination drug therapy for high-risk patients, including those with combined hyperlipidemia and diabetic dyslipidemia.[8]

In light of the residual risk of CHD events in statin trials within certain subgroups, combination therapy appears most appropriate in patients with a high rate of events despite optimal statin therapy. The updated ATP III guidelines recommend an optional LDL-c goal of less than 70 mg/dL in patients at very high risk, including those with established CVD in conjunction with multiple major risk factors, severe or poorly controlled risk factors, multiple metabolic syndrome components, or ACS.[6] In a national survey of compliance with the ATP III guidelines, 75% of patients with CHD met the definition of "very high risk," yet only 18% had an LDL-c level below 70 mg/dL, and only 4% had an LDL-c level below 70 mg/dL and a non–HDL-c level below 100 mg/dL when TGs were above 200 mg/dL.[9] These data substantiate the use of more aggressive statin therapy and implementation of combination therapy to reduce residual risks with statins.

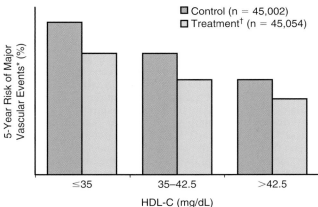

Low HDL-C and Risk for CVD in Statin Trials: CTT Meta-Analysis

□ Control (n = 45,002)
□ Treatment[†] (n = 45,054)

FIGURE 25-1 Low levels of high-density lipoprotein cholesterol (*HDL-c*) remains a significant risk factor in patients on statin therapy. *Combined outcome of nonfatal MI, CHD death, nonfatal or fatal stroke, or coronary revascularization. †Event rate per 1 mmol/L (39 mg/dL) reduction in LDL-c. CHD, coronary heart disease; CVD, cardiovascular disease; CTT, Cholesterol Treatment Trialists; LDL-C, low-density–lipoprotein cholesterol; MI, myocardial infarction.

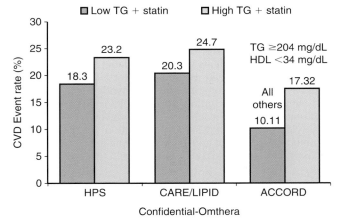

Statin Monotherapy Does Not Eliminate the CVD Risk Associated With High TGs

□ Low TG + statin   □ High TG + statin

TG ≥204 mg/dL
HDL <34 mg/dL

Confidential-Omthera

FIGURE 25-2 Statin monotherapy does not eliminate the cardiovascular disease risk associated with high triglycerides. ACCORD, Action to Control Cardiovascular Risk in Diabetes trial; CARE/LIPID, Cholesterol and Recurrent Events trial/Long-Term Intervention with Pravastatin in Ischemic Disease; CVD, cardiovascular disease; HDL, high-density lipoprotein; HPS, Heart Protection Study; TGs, triglycerides.

Combined Dyslipidemia

Non–High-Density Lipoprotein Cholesterol Reduction

The ATP III identified non–HDL-c as a secondary therapeutic target for individuals with elevated TGs of 200 mg/dL or more.[1] Non–HDL-c goals are set 30 mg/dL above the LDL-c goal for a patient's risk category (Table 25-1), a level based on the Friedewald formula,[10] in which VLDL cholesterol (VLDL-c) levels are estimated to be one fifth of the TG concentration. Because TG concentrations below 150 mg/dL are considered normal, a VLDL-c concentration below 30 mg/dL is within the normal range. As TG levels increase, the fraction of non–HDL-c accounted for by LDL-c declines.

Non–HDL-c correlates well with ApoB concentration and is therefore a good proxy for the total number of circulating atherogenic particles.[11] Consistent with this relationship, population studies have shown non–HDL-c to be a somewhat stronger predictor of CVD and mortality risk than LDL-c.[12]

Therapy to Modify High-Density Lipoprotein

The success of LDL-c reduction to improve cardiovascular outcomes is now well recognized. Heart failure hospitalizations have dropped 29.5% nationally over the past decade, largely because fewer MIs resulted in a decrease in the development of heart failure. Although the reasons for this decline are many, better risk factor modification, especially LDL-c control with statins, is believed to be a major contributor.

Yet, despite optimal LDL-c management, patients with low HDL-c remain at increased risk for cardiovascular events. Low HDL-c is a powerful risk factor, equivalent to elevated LDL-c for premature

TABLE 25-1	Additive Effects of Fibrates, Niacin, and Omega-3 Fatty Acids on the Various Biomarkers and Lipoprotein Subfractions Associated with Cardiovascular Risk		
	OMEGA-3 FATTY ACIDS	**FENOFIBRATE/ FENOFIBRIC ACID**	**NIACIN**
LDL-c	↑	—	↓
Non-HDL	↓	↓	↓
Triglycerides	↓↓	↓↓	↓
ApoB	↓	↓	↓↓
ApoA1	—	↑	↑↑
LDL-P	↓	—	↓
LDL size	↑	↑	↑
VLDL-P	↓	↓	↓
VLDL size	↓	↑↓	NA
HDL-P	—	↑	↑
HDL size	—		↑
Lp-PLA2	↓	NA	↑A
hs-CRP	—	↓	NA
Homocysteine	—	↑↑	↑
RLP-C	↓	↓	↓
ApoCIII	↓	↓	↓

ApoA1, apolipoprotein A1; ApoB, apolipoprotein B; ApoCIII, apolipoprotein CIII; HDL, high-density lipoprotein; HDL-p, high-density lipoprotein particle number; hs-CRP, high-sensitivity C-reactive protein; LDL-c, low-density lipoprotein cholesterol; LDL-p, low-density lipoprotein particle number; Lp-PLA2, lipoprotein-associated phospholipase A2; NA, not applicable; RPL-C, remnant lipoprotein cholesterol; VLDL, very-low-density lipoprotein; VLDL-p, very-low-density lipoprotein particle number.

CHD, and high HDL-c provides protection from cardiovascular mortality. Therefore, logic presumes that therapeutic approaches to raise HDL-c should reduce events.

To date, however, efforts to increase HDL-c by pharmacologic means have not shown a clinical benefit. Estrogen, torcetrapib, and most recently niacin raised HDL-c in trials; not only did these agents fail to provide a clinical benefit, they may have caused harm. Although off-target effects may have been responsible, profound confusion remains as to why raising HDL-c has not achieved the expected benefits.

The *HDL hypothesis*, as yet unproven, suggests that the benefits of modifying HDL are mediated through several atheroprotective mechanisms. Most importantly, HDL removes excess cholesterol from peripheral tissues and delivers it to the liver for elimination via the bile into the gut, a process known as *reverse cholesterol transport* (RCT). Because free cholesterol cannot be metabolized in humans on its own, this RCT process represents an important mechanism for regulating cholesterol pools and maintaining cholesterol homeostasis.

The key role that HDL plays in mediating the RCT process is regarded as the primary mechanism by which HDL affects atherosclerosis. HDL functionality may be more important than absolute HDL-c levels, and recent data indicate that HDL has both proinflammatory and antiinflammatory properties. However, no large trials have yet confirmed this hypothesis. The view that raising HDL-c will result in a CV benefit is likely overly simplistic. On the horizon are new CETP-modulating drugs that do not share the off-target toxicity of torcetrapib. The dal-VESSEL and dal-PLAQUE trials of dalcetrapib recently demonstrated its vascular safety.[13] In the Determining the Efficacy and Tolerability of CETP Inhibition With Anacetrapib (DEFINE) trial, the cardiovascular toxicity associated with torcetrapib was ruled out with anacetrapib.[14] Large outcomes trials are now underway to evaluate the clinical benefits of these drugs in populations with high CV risk. Despite disappointment and confusion, the quest to establish the value of modifying HDL continues, and it is hoped this promising target of therapy will yield the results that address a very important unmet medical need.

Statin-Fibrate Combination

Fibrates are an important class of drugs for the management of dyslipidemia. This class of drugs is generally well tolerated but is infrequently associated with several safety issues. By activating peroxisome proliferator activated receptor α (PPARα), fibrates result in the regulation of several genes important in lipid metabolism. These include increasing the expression of lipoprotein lipase and reducing the production of ApoC-III, an inhibitor of lipoprotein lipase activity, both of which enhance the lipolysis and elimination of TG-rich particles. In addition, increases in the production of apolipoprotein AI (ApoA-I) and ApoA-II contribute to an increase in HDL-c. Fibrates may reversibly increase creatinine and homocysteine but are not associated with an increased risk for renal failure in clinical trials. In patients with combined dyslipidemia, fibrate-statin combination therapy can be used to promote reductions in LDL and TGs and simultaneous increases in HDL-c.

Fibrates are associated with a slightly increased risk (<1.0%) for myopathy, cholelithiasis, and venous thrombosis. In clinical trials with patients who did not have elevated TGs and/or low HDL levels, fibrates are associated with an increase in non-CV mortality. In combination with statins, gemfibrozil generally should be avoided. The preferred option is fenofibrate, which is not associated with an inhibition of statin metabolism.[3] Clinicians are advised to measure serum creatinine before fibrate use and to adjust the dose accordingly for renal impairment. Routine monitoring of creatinine is not required, but if a patient has a clinically important increase in creatinine, and other potential causes of creatinine increase have been excluded, consideration should be given to discontinuing fibrate therapy or reducing the dose.[15] The active metabolite of fenofibrate, fenofibric acid, has been approved for clinical use in combination with a statin.

A total of 2715 patients were randomly assigned to 12-week treatment with either fenofibric acid 135 mg monotherapy; low-, moderate-, or high-dose statin (rosuvastatin, simvastatin, or atorvastatin) monotherapy; or fenofibric acid plus a low- or moderate-dose statin. Fenofibric acid plus low-dose statin combination therapy resulted in significantly greater improvements in HDL-c, TG, non–HDL-c, VLDL-c, total cholesterol, ApoB, and hs-CRP compared with low-dose statin monotherapy. The safety of combination fenofibric acid 135 mg with a statin was similar to monotherapy for each drug, and no cases of rhabdomyolysis were reported. Outcome studies are underway to evaluate whether the beneficial effects of a combination of fenofibrate and statins on lipoproteins translates into a reduction in the residual risk for patients on statin monotherapy with elevated TGs and low HDL-c.[16]

The Action to Control Cardiovascular Risk in Diabetes (ACCORD) trial is the most recent study to compare the combination of a statin (simvastatin) and fenofibrate with a statin alone in an all-comer diabetes population.[17] Although designed primarily to compare the effects of more intensive and less intensive glucose control, the study also compared intensive and standard blood pressure control in 4733 of the patients (n = 10,251), and it investigated the impact of adding fenofibrate to a statin on the lipid profile and CV outcomes in the remaining 5518 patients.

In the lipid arm of ACCORD, 2765 patients were randomized to receive simvastatin plus fenofibrate, and 2753 patients were to receive simvastatin plus placebo. The impact on the lipid profile was as predicted, with a slight decrease in mean total cholesterol, no change in mean LDL-c, a modest increase in HDL-c (modest increases in HDL-c are seen in studies in which patients have high levels of TGs), and a significant decrease in TGs from about 160 mg/dL to 120 mg/dL in the fenofibrate group.

In terms of the primary macrovascular outcome—CV death, nonfatal MI, and nonfatal stroke—no difference was reported between the groups in the proportion of patients with events, the time to event, or the total events between the two arms of the trial. In addition, no difference was noted between the two groups in terms of major prespecified secondary macrovascular outcomes, including major CV events, nonfatal MI, stroke, and death from any cause.

As expected from previous trials with fibrates, a potential but not statistically positive benefit was observed in patients with high levels of TGs and low levels of HDL (which represented just 20% of the study population), with a 31% risk reduction in this patient population ($P = .064$). It is important to bear in mind that even on a statin, the population with a combination of high TGs and low HDL-c had a 70% higher event rate than those who did not meet this criteria (456 events [17.3%] vs. 2284 events [10.1%]), which represents a very high residual risk. The fibrate worked well in this population based on the absolute risk reduction (485 [12.4%] events with the combination vs. 456 [17.3%] with the statin alone). The addition of a fibrate thus seems to provide a substantial benefit in patients with high TGs and low HDL-c. In terms of number needed to treat, 20 patients with type 2 diabetes and atherogenic dyslipidemia would need to be treated for 5 years to prevent a single CV event. This compares favorably with results from other trials with fibrates, including the Helsinki Heart Study (HHS), Bezafibrate Infarction Prevention (BIP) study, Veterans Affairs High-Density Lipoprotein Cholesterol Intervention Trial (VAHIT), and Fenofibrate Intervention and Event Lowering in Diabetes (FIELD), which all show substantial risk reductions in this population.[18]

Statin-Niacin Combination

Niacin, or nicotinic acid, is a soluble B vitamin that has favorable effects on all major lipid subfractions but has limited use because of its side-effect profile. The specific mechanism of action of niacin is not well understood, but it appears to reduce ApoB secretion, thereby lowering both VLDL and LDL, increasing ApoA-I, and lowering lipoprotein A [Lp(a)]. However, in contrast to previous dogma, data now suggest that niacin also increases the secretion of HDL ApoA-I by upregulating both adenosine triphosphate–binding cassette transporter (ABCA1) and ApoA-I gene expression in the liver.[19] This results in the expression of very large HDL particles that are more slowly catabolized because of their increased size. Niacin was one of the first lipid-altering drugs to demonstrate a reduction in CHD events in the Coronary Drug Project.[20] At present, niacin is the most effective HDL-raising therapy. Although the mechanism by which niacin raises HDL is not well understood, the predominant hypothesis was that niacin inhibits the holoparticle uptake of HDL, resulting in delayed catabolism. More recent data, however, suggest that niacin may increase ApoA-1 production.[21] Niacin has been demonstrated to lower LDL by 10% to 20%, TGs by 20% to 40%, and Lp(a) by 10% to 30%, and it raises HDL by 15% to 30%.

Statin-niacin combination therapy has been used to reduce residual CV risk. Niacin is often added to a statin in patients with combined hyperlipidemia, especially if the HDL is low or Lp(a) is high. Although statins have demonstrated an approximate reduction in CHD events by 30%, combination therapy with statins and niacin has resulted in reductions of 75%. This significant reduction in CHD events suggests that other effects of niacin—such as TG lowering, Lp(a) lowering, and HDL raising—may also contribute to the benefits.

Adding niacin to a statin is a likely combination because niacin has the most significant effects on raising HDL. A number of trials[19] have demonstrated the safety of this combination and its efficacy in inhibiting the progression of atherosclerosis. Most trials have used either immediate-release niacin or extended-release niacin. Because of the safety data of extended-release niacin in combination with a statin, there has been increased interest in the use of combination therapy to maximize risk reduction in patients with dyslipidemia.

In the HDL Atherosclerosis Treatment Study (HATS), the group treated with simvastatin (10 to 20 mg/day) plus niacin (2 to 4 g/day) showed a significant risk reduction of 90% for composite CV endpoints—death from coronary causes, confirmed MI or stroke, or revascularization—compared with those taking placebo (P = .03).[22] In addition, a 0.4% regression in coronary stenosis was reported with simvastatin-niacin combination therapy, but progression was seen in other treatment groups receiving antioxidants alone, simvastatin plus niacin plus antioxidants, or placebo (P < .001).[23] Studies to evaluate statin-niacin combination therapy have consistently demonstrated the efficacy in increasing HDL-c and reducing TG and LDL-c.[24-27] Additional studies to compare statin monotherapy with statin-niacin combination therapy indicate that statins and niacin have additive effects on HDL-c. Angiographic studies further support the effect of statin-niacin combination therapy in impeding the progression of CHD.[22]

As demonstrated by the Arterial Biology for the Investigation of the Treatment Effects of Reducing Cholesterol (ARBITER) 2 trial, adding extended-release niacin to statin therapy increased HDL-c by 21% and slowed the progression of atherosclerosis, as measured by change in carotid intima media thickness (CIMT), compared with statin therapy alone in patients with known CHD and low HDL-c levels.[28] The ARBITER 6-HALTS (HDL and LDL Treatment Strategies) trial[29] was designed to compare the effects of LDL-c lowering with ezetimibe or HDL-c raising with niacin in combination with a statin on CIMT. Patients with CHD or a CHD equivalent, receiving stable statin treatment, with LDL-c below 100 mg/dL and HDL-c below 50 mg/dL for men or 55 mg/dL for women were randomly assigned to ezetimibe (10 mg/day) or extended-release niacin (target dose, 2000 mg/day). The primary endpoint was change in mean CIMT, analyzed according to a last observation carried forward method. The original study was terminated early on the basis of a prespecified interim analysis that showed superiority of niacin over ezetimibe on change in CIMT. Niacin and ezetimibe both produced the expected, and approximately equal, reductions in non–HDL-c, but niacin raised HDL-c by 18.4%. Niacin (n = 154) resulted in significant reduction (regression) in mean CIMT (−0.0102 ± 0.0026 mm; P < .001) and maximal CIMT (−0.0124 ±

0.0036 mm; P = .001), whereas ezetimibe (n = 161) did not reduce mean CIMT (−0.0016 ± 0.0024 mm; P = .88) or maximal CIMT (−0.0005 ± 0.0029 mm; P = .88) compared with baseline. A significant difference was observed that favored niacin for both mean CIMT (P = .016) and maximal CIMT (P = .01). By lowering non–HDL-c and raising HDL-c, niacin induces regression of CIMT in high-risk patients with low HDL-c, whereas an LDL-c–lowering strategy with ezetimibe in combination with a statin stops progression.

The Atherothrombosis Intervention in Metabolic Syndrome with Low HDL Cholesterol/High Triglyceride and Impact on Global Health Outcomes (AIM-HIGH) trial was a multicenter clinical trial carried out at approximately 90 sites in the United States and Canada.[30] AIM-HIGH was meant to test whether adding high-dose, extended-release niacin to a statin (simvastatin) is better than a statin alone in reducing long-term CV events in participants whose LDL-c was controlled and who had a history of CVD, low levels of HDL cholesterol, and high levels of TGs. The National Heart, Lung, and Blood Institute (NHLBI) of the National Institutes of Health (NIH) stopped the AIM-HIGH clinical trial 18 months earlier than planned. The trial found that adding high-dose, extended-release niacin to statin treatment in people with heart and vascular disease did not reduce the risk of CV events, including heart attacks and stroke.

It is unclear why the HDL-c–raising effects of niacin did not reduce CV events compared with aggressive treatment to LDL-c targets. Niacin treatment has different effects on the cholesterol and particle measures of LDL and HDL, and it significantly raises HDL-c but without increasing HDL particle number (HDL-p). In addition, it modestly reduces LDL-c, but it usually lowers LDL particle number (LDL-p) much more. The AIM-HIGH trial assessed the efficacy of increasing HDL-c and correcting other non-LDL lipid abnormalities with niacin in CHD patients with optimally treated LDL-c, but the trial design precluded assessment of the potential benefit of LDL-p lowering.

Statin–Omega-3 Fatty Acids Combination

Omega-3 fatty acids, or fish oils, are essential fatty acids thought to inhibit VLDL and TG synthesis in the liver, although the exact molecular mechanisms are not well understood. Omega-3 fatty acids significantly reduce TG levels and increase LDL-c levels in patients with high TG levels. Dietary supplementation with the n-3 polyunsaturated fatty acids (PUFAs) eicosapentaenoic acid (EPA) and docosahexaenoic acid (DHA) lowers the risk of death, nonfatal coronary events, and stroke after MI.[31] PUFAs reduce TG levels by 20% to 30% in most patients, but they reduce TGs by up to 50% in patients with severe hypertriglyceridemia (TG >750 mg/dL [>8.47 mmol/L]).[32,33] Studies of combination therapy with n-3 PUFAs and pravastatin 40 mg/day[34] or simvastatin 20 mg/day[35] demonstrated LDL-c reductions of 13% to 24% and TG reductions of 27% to 30%, respectively. Similarly, combination therapy with atorvastatin 10 mg resulted in significant reductions of the concentration of small, dense LDL particles and increases in HDL-c compared with monotherapy.[36]

A highly purified pharmaceutical grade omega-3 fatty acid marine fish oil formulation contains high concentrations of EPA (440 mg) and DHA (260 mg), along with 4 mg (6 IU) vitamin E in each 1-g capsule. Prescription omega-3 fatty acid marine oils are indicated for the treatment of hypertriglyceridemia, and they significantly reduce serum TGs by 19% to 55% at doses of 4 capsules per day when administered over periods from 6 weeks to several years. In the Combination of Prescription Omega-3 With Simvastatin (COMBOS) trial, median percentage decreases in non–HDL-c were significantly greater with combination therapy, using simvastatin 40 mg and omega-3-acid ethyl esters 4 g/day, compared with placebo plus simvastatin (9.0% vs. 2.2% respectively; P < .001). In addition, combination therapy significantly lowered TG (29.5%) and VLDL-c (27.5%) levels, raised HDL-c (3.4%), and lowered total cholesterol/HDL-c ratio (9.6%; P ≤ .001 vs. placebo for all); however, LDL-c increased by 3.5%.[37]

In a post hoc analysis of data from the COMBOS study, the predictors of the LDL-c response to prescription omega-3-acid ethyl esters (P-OM3) therapy was the baseline LDL-c. The median LDL-c response in the P-OM3 group was +9.5% (first tertile, <80.4 mg/dL), −0.9% (second tertile), and −6.4% (third tertile, ≥99.0 mg/dL). Non-HDL-c, VLDL-c, HDL-c, and TG responses did not vary significantly by baseline LDL-c tertile. The reductions in VLDL-c concentrations were greater than the increases in LDL-c, where present, resulting in a net decrease in the concentration of cholesterol carried by atherogenic particles (non–HDL-c) in all baseline LDL-c tertiles. In conclusion, these results suggest that the increase in LDL-c that occurred with the addition of P-OM3 to simvastatin therapy in patients with mixed dyslipidemia was confined predominantly to those with low LDL-c levels while receiving simvastatin monotherapy. In addition, LDL-p and ApoB are reduced with P-OM3 in combination with a statin. These data suggest that the increase in LDL-c with omega-3 therapy is an increase in LDL-p size rather than particle number.[37] Compared with placebo, P-OM3 reduced mean VLDL particle (VLDL-p) size and increased LDL-p size ($P = .006$ for both) without altering HDL-p size.

The doses of EPA and DHA obtainable from typical consumption of fatty fish and unprocessed marine oil products (~30% omega-3 fatty acids) are insufficient for the treatment of severe hypertriglyceridemia. This has prompted the development of concentrated forms of omega-3 fatty acids. Prescription omega-3-acid ethyl esters (Lovaza), produced by ethanol extraction and distillation of omega-3 fatty acids, contain 84% EPA plus DHA ethyl esters and are approved by the U.S. Food and Drug Administration (FDA) as an adjunct to diet for the treatment of severe hypertriglyceridemia in adults.[38] Subsequently, a product has been developed that undergoes an additional manufacturing step to hydrolyze and distill the ethyl esters into omega-3 free fatty acids (FFAs).

The Epanova Compared to Lovaza in a Pharmacokinetic Single-Dose Evaluation (ECLIPSE) study assessed the relative bioavailability of a single 4-g oral dose of the FFA omega-3 product compared with ethyl ester omega-3 in 54 healthy volunteers, and it furthermore examined the effect of low-fat and high-fat diet on relative bioavailability. Significantly higher plasma EPA and DHA levels (peak concentrations and areas under the curve) were observed with omega-3 FFA compared with omega-3 ethyl ester in both the low-fat and high-fat diet conditions.[39] Most notably, in the low-fat diet condition, the single dose of the omega-3 FFA resulted in an area under the curve (AUC) for EPA plus DHA that was four times higher than that in the omega-3 ethyl ester condition. Unlike the triglyceride and ethyl ester forms of omega-3 fatty acids, the FFA form does not require pancreatic lipase hydrolysis; thus, as shown in ECLIPSE, it has greater bioavailability, particularly when consumed in conjunction with a low-fat diet after a single dose.

A concern with some triglyceride-lowering therapies is their potential LDL-c–elevating effect.[38,40] Fibrates and fish oil increase LDL-c by as much as 35% to 45% when administered to patients with severe hypertriglyceridemia; this is due in part to an increased rate of conversion of VLDL to LDL[41-44] and results in an increase in LDL-p and a rise in LDL-c concentration. Reducing the substrate for CETP may also play a role, because this enzyme catalyzes the exchange of triglyceride from VLDL for cholesteryl ester from LDL and HDL particles.[45] Thus, reducing the triglyceride concentration tends to result in larger, more cholesterol-rich LDL and HDL particles.[46] A highly purified form of EPA—ethyl eicosapentate, or AMR101—contains at least 96% EPA ethyl ester and no DHA. The Multi-Center, Placebo-Controlled, Randomized, Double-Blind, 12-Week Study with an Open-Label Extension (MARINE) trial[11,47] examined doses of 2 and 4 g/day of AMR101 among 229 diet-stable patients with very high TGs (≥500 and ≤2000 mg/dL), with or without background statin therapy). The study resulted in TG reductions of 19.7% ($P < .005$) and 33.1% ($P < .0001$), respectively, but AMR101 did not significantly increase placebo-corrected LDL-c levels (+5.2% and −2.3%, respectively).

When TG and LDL-c responses to AMR101 are examined against results from trials of omega-3 EPA plus DHA ethyl ester, which have been shown to increase LDL-c by 0.7% to 46%, the increase in LDL-c with 2 g/day AMR101 is in line with the expected change in LDL-c with a 20% decrease in TG, but the LDL-c response to 4 g/day AMR101 (a 2.3% reduction) is lower than predicted and should be explored further. Median baseline LDL-c concentration, which has been reported to be inversely associated with the change in LDL-c during treatment,[40] was 86.0 mg/dL in MARINE. A systematic review of the individual effects of EPA and DHA on serum LDL-c and other lipoprotein lipid concentrations[48] reported that whereas both EPA and DHA reduced TG, DHA was associated with increases in LDL-c that were directly and significantly associated with the baseline TG concentration. In four of the six studies, these elevations were not observed after EPA treatment. DHA, and not EPA, also appears to increase HDL and LDL particle size.[49-52]

These results are consistent with previous head-to-head comparisons of pure EPA to DHA, which demonstrated that EPA supplementation resulted in less TG lowering and HDL-c raising than DHA, and DHA increased LDL-c more than EPA, although this increase in LDL-c was found to be associated with a greater increase in LDL-p, albeit in a limited dataset. Further research is needed to investigate the effects of EPA versus DHA on LDL-p and its clinical significance.

Cholesteryl Ester Transfer Protein Inhibition

A newer approach for elevating HDL-c is through the inhibition of CETP, a very large protein that plays an important role in cholesterol metabolism; it is responsible for the transfer of cholesteryl esters from HDL to VLDLs and LDLs (Figure 25-3), and it has a hydrophobic tunnel across the molecule that can accommodate neutral lipid. CETP is a shuttle-type structure, promoting an equal mass gradient transfer of TG for cholesterol ester between HDL and ApoB lipoproteins. CETP appears to equilibrate lipoprotein concentrations of TGs and cholesterol ester by moving TGs from where they are high (VLDL) to where they are low (HDL and LDL) in exchange for an equal mass gradient of cholesterol ester. Animals that lack CETP have very high HDL and very low LDL. Therefore, the role of CETP is important in modulating HDL size by redistributing cholesterol ester from TG-rich particles into HDL. The TG-enriched HDL is further acted upon by hepatic lipase to

CETP Mechanism of Action: The Shuttle Model

CETP operates by a carrier mechanism, accepting neutral lipids (TG and cholesteryl ester) from a donor particle, shuttling them through the aqueous phase, and delivering them to an acceptor lipoprotein.

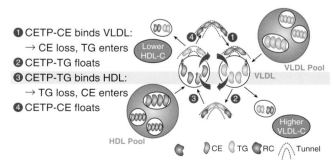

❶ CETP-CE binds VLDL:
 → CE loss, TG enters
❷ CETP-TG floats
❸ CETP-TG binds HDL:
 → TG loss, CE enters
❹ CETP-CE floats

FIGURE 25-3 Cholesteryl ester transfer protein (*CETP*) mechanism of action: the shuttle model. HDL-C, high-density lipoprotein cholesterol; RC, reverse cholesterol transport; TG, triglyceride; VLDL, very-low-density lipoprotein.

form a smaller, dense HDL that is more rapidly catabolized. Therefore, inhibiting CETP by maintaining HDL-p will reduce HDL catabolism. CETP is also involved in transporting TGs in exchange for cholesterol ester from TG-rich particles to LDL, therefore LDL becomes TG enriched and is further hydrolyzed by the lipases to form a small, dense LDL. Many aspects of CETP affect the atherogenicity of the lipoprotein particle. CETP attaches to the VLDL; takes in TG, for which it exchanges cholesterol ester, shuttling the TG over to the HDL; and goes back and forth between these two particles. There is binding of the CETP to HDL to transport these various constituents from one lipoprotein to the other (see Figure 25-3).[53]

Animal studies with mice and rabbits demonstrated the potency of CETP inhibition in modulating HDL-c. Rabbits treated with the CETP inhibitor torcetrapib showed increases in HDL from about 57 to 207 mg/dL. The effect of torcetrapib on the kinetics of CETP binding to HDL was analyzed, as were the inhibitor effects attributed to the formation of a nonproductive complex between CETP and HDL. Studies in humans established that CETP inhibition was effective in increasing HDL-c and decreasing LDL-c beyond reductions seen with atorvastatin alone. Concurrent atorvastatin treatment with torcetrapib was shown to reduce ApoB-100 levels by enhancing VLDL ApoB-100 clearance and reducing production of intermediate-density lipoproteins and LDL ApoB-100.[54]

Despite the impressive effects of CETP inhibition by torcetrapib in raising HDL-c levels, results from clinical trials raise skepticism over its therapeutic use. The Investigation of Lipid Level Management Using Coronary Ultrasound to Assess Reduction of Atherosclerosis by CETP Inhibition and HDL Elevation (ILLUSTRATE) trial assessed the effect of torcetrapib 60 mg plus atorvastatin compared with atorvastatin monotherapy on the progression of atherosclerosis in 1188 patients with CHD. Atorvastatin in an initial dose of 10 mg was titrated at 2-week intervals to 20, 40, or 80 mg to achieve target LDL-c levels. After 24 months, an approximate 61% relative increase was noted in HDL-c along with a 20% relative decrease in LDL-c.[54]

In another study, disease progression in 910 patients, as measured by repeated intravascular ultrasonography of the percent change of atheroma volume, was not significant in the treatment groups (0.19% in the atorvastatin-only group and 0.12% in the torcetrapib-atorvastatin group, $P = .72$). In addition, no statistical difference was seen in the change in 10 mm of the most diseased subsegment (reduction of 3.3 mm^3 in the atorvastatin-only group and 4.2 mm^3 in the torcetrapib-atorvastatin group; $P = .12$).[55] In addition, torcetrapib was associated with an increase in systolic blood pressure of 4.6 mm Hg and an increase in all-cause mortality, resulting in the discontinuation of the trial.

The Investigation of Lipid Level Management to Understand its Impact in Atherosclerotic Events (ILLUMINATE) trial was a phase 3 trial with approximately 15,000 patients at high risk for CHD randomized to treatment with torcetrapib (60 mg) plus atorvastatin versus atorvastatin alone (10 to 80 mg). The trial was stopped because of significant increases in all-cause mortality in the torcetrapib-atorvastatin versus atorvastatin groups (82 vs. 51 deaths, respectively).[54]

Although torcetrapib increased the mortality rate in the ILLUMINATE trial, cautious optimism remains that CETP inhibition might be a viable option to raise HDL-c and lower LDL-c to reduce CV risk. The ILLUSTRATE trial[56] showed that the greater the HDL-c increase during treatment, the greater the reduction in the percent atheroma volume. This finding suggests a positive benefit with torcetrapib on atherosclerosis, which was offset by the adverse effect on blood pressure and vascular toxicity. This was not supported by the Rating Atherosclerotic Disease Change by Imaging With a New Cholesteryl-Ester-Transfer Protein Inhibitor (RADIANCE) 1 and 2 trials. A better understanding has also been gained of the off-target effects of torcetrapib that is not shared by at least two other CETP inhibitors, dalcetrapib and anacetrapib. In early human trials, torcetrapib was shown to increase blood pressure by 2 to 3 mm Hg and, in later trials such as ILLUMINATE,

the increase in blood pressure levels of high-risk patients was approximately 4 to 5 mm Hg.[54] An investigation discovered that torcetrapib, but not dalcetrapib, stimulated aldosterone production in a human adrenal cell line and stimulated 11-β-hydroxylase, an enzyme in steroid production.[53] The steroidogenic effect of torcetrapib in humans may explain the increased rate of sepsis and cancer in the ILLUMINATE trial. Torcetrapib and angiotensin II share a number of common properties centered on *CYP11B2* gene expression, which torcetrapib simulates, possibly explaining the aldosterone and steroidogenic effect that led to the off-target toxicity.

Dalcetrapib also has a different mechanism than torcetrapib in regard to CETP inhibition. Dalcetrapib binds to CETP and induces a conformational change in the CETP molecule that hinders its ability then to bind to HDL in the plasma.[53] Instead, torcetrapib binds to CETP and results in a triple complex of torcetrapib and HDL. Also, dalcetrapib does not increase blood pressure in humans.

Anacetrapib also does not share the increase in aldosterone production in the adrenal cell line as with torcetrapib. Anacetrapib is a more potent CETP inhibitor than dalcetrapib and increases HDL-c by 50% to 75% and lowers LDL-c by approximately 30% at 100 mg/day. The DEFINE study demonstrated the CV safety of anacetrapib 100 mg/day in 1800 patients at high CV risk over the course of 18 months of therapy. In this study, anacetrapib increased HDL-c by 108% and decreased LDL-c by 39%, with no difference in major coronary events in the anacetrapib group compared with placebo; in addition, there was even a suggestion of benefit with a significant reduction in revascularizations.[14]

Clinical trials to evaluate the effects of dalcetrapib on CV outcome are presently underway. Dal-OUTCOMES is a multicenter, randomized, double-blind, placebo-controlled trial designed to test the hypothesis that CETP inhibition with dalcetrapib reduces CV morbidity and mortality in patients with ACS. The study randomized approximately 15,600 patients to receive daily doses of dalcetrapib 600 mg or matching placebo, beginning 4 to 12 weeks after an index ACS event; no prespecified boundaries were set for HDL-c levels at entry. The primary efficacy measure is time to first occurrence of CHD, death, nonfatal acute MI, unstable angina requiring hospital admission, resuscitated cardiac arrest, or atherothrombotic stroke. The trial will continue until 1600 primary endpoint events have occurred, all evaluable patients have been monitored for at least 2 years, and 80% of evaluable subjects have been followed for at least 2.5 years.[57]

To summarize, CETP plays an important role in reverse cholesterol transport and the maintenance of cholesterol homeostasis. CETP inhibition may reduce the risk of atherosclerosis in patients with dyslipidemia by significantly increasing HDL-c. Animal models support the antiatherosclerotic effects of CETP inhibition. In light of recent data,[4] the significance of targeting HDL-c in addition to LDL-c for the control of CV risk is evident, as clinical trial evidence demonstrates that low HDL-c is associated with increased risk for morbidity and mortality related to coronary artery disease (CAD). A number of strategies can be used to increase HDL-c levels, including pharmacologic management focused on the use of statins, statin combination therapy, and investigational drugs that target HDL-c metabolism, reverse cholesterol transport, and CETP inhibition; however, a reduction in clinical CVD events as a result of these strategies has not as yet been shown. In light of data documenting the off-target toxicity of torcetrapib on aldosterone and steroid production, two other CETP inhibitors without the off-target effects are progressing in phase 3 clinical trials. Dalcetrapib is being evaluated for morbidity and mortality benefits in an ACS population, and anacetrapib will be evaluated by a 30,000-patient outcome trial in high-risk patients (REVEAL HPS-3 TIMI-55, ClinicalTrials.gov NCT01252953). Targeting HDL-c may become an integral component of the management of CAD, and continued testing of investigational therapies aimed at increasing HDL-c levels may result in additional options for reducing risk for CAD.

Conclusion

The prevalence of diabetes and metabolic syndrome is rapidly increasing throughout the world. Consequently, LDL-c is losing its value as a sole predictor for CV risk, especially in patients with high TGs and low HDL-c. Non–HDL-c is the lipid parameter that incorporates both LDL-c and TGs into a target that more appropriately reflects risk in a patient population with mixed dyslipidemia.

Although the efficacy of additional therapeutic intervention beyond statin therapy to modify these residual risk factors has not yet been proven, there is ample evidence that patients with diabetes and metabolic syndrome remain at increased risk despite an LDL-c and non–HDL-c at goal (<70 and <100 mg/dL, respectively) according to the NCEP ATP III 2004 update.[10] Statin combination therapy with niacin, fibrates, and P-OM3 provides additional improvements in non–HDL-c and HDL-c. In addition, CETP inhibitors that increase HDL-c are also in late-phase development to potentially address the residual risk for patients with low HDL-c.

REFERENCES

1. Expert Panel on Detection, Evaluation, and Treatment of High Blood Cholesterol in Adults. Executive summary of the Third Report of the National Cholesterol Education Program (NCEP) Expert Panel on Detection, Evaluation, and Treatment of High Blood Cholesterol in Adults (Adult Treatment Panel III). *JAMA* 2001;285:2486-2497.

2. Miller M, Cannon CP, Murphy SA, et al. PROVE IT-TIMI 22 Investigators. Impact of triglyceride levels beyond low-density lipoprotein cholesterol after acute coronary syndrome in the PROVE IT–TIMI 22 trial. *J Am Coll Cardiol* 2008;51:724-730.

3. Davidson MH. Reducing residual risk for patients on statin therapy: the potential role of combination therapy. *Am J Cardiol* 2005;96(Suppl):3K-13K.

4. Baigent C, Blackwell L, Emberson J, et al. Cholesterol Treatment Trialists' (CTT) Collaboration. Efficacy and safety of more intensive lowering of LDL cholesterol: a meta-analysis of data from 170,000 participants in 26 randomised trials. *Lancet* 2010;376(9753):1670-1681.

5. Breslow JL. Mouse models of atherosclerosis. *Science* 1996;272:685-688.

6. Grundy SM, Cleeman JI, Merz CN, et al. Implications of recent clinical trials for the National Cholesterol Education Program Adult Treatment Panel III guidelines. *Circulation* 2004;110:227-239.

7. Sniderman AD, Furberg CK, Keech A, et al. Apolipoproteins versus lipids as indicators of coronary risk and as targets for statin therapy. *Lancet* 2003;361:777-780.

8. Brunzell JD, Davidson M, Furberg CD, et al. American Diabetes Association; American College of Cardiology Foundation. Lipoprotein management in patients with cardiometabolic risk: consensus statement from the American Diabetes Association and the American College of Cardiology Foundation. *Diabetes Care* 2008;31:811-822.

9. Davidson, MH, Maki KC, Pearson TA, et al. Results of the National Cholesterol Education Program (NCEP) Evaluation Project Utilizing Novel E-Technology (NEPTUNE) II survey: implications for treatment under the recent NCEP Writing Group recommendations. *Am J Cardiol* 2005;96:556-563.

10. Friedewald WT, Levy RI, Fredrickson DS. Estimation of the concentration of low-density lipoprotein cholesterol in plasma, without use of the preparative ultracentrifuge. *Clin Chem* 1972;18:499-502.

11. Ballantyne CM, Andrews TC, Hsia JA, Kramer JH, Shear C. ACCESS Study Group. Correlation of non–high-density lipoprotein cholesterol with apolipoprotein B: effect of 5-hydroxymethylglutaryl coenzyme A reductase inhibitors on non–high-density lipoprotein cholesterol levels. *Am J Cardiol* 2001;88:265-269.

12. Robinson JG, Wang S, Smith BJ, Jacobson TA. Meta-analysis of the relationship between non–high-density lipoprotein cholesterol reduction and coronary heart disease risk. *J Am Coll Cardiol* 2009;53:316-322.

13. Fayad ZA, Mani V, Woodward M, et al, for the dal-PLAQUE Investigators. Safety and efficacy of dalcetrapib on atherosclerotic disease using novel non-invasive multimodality imaging (dal-PLAQUE): a randomised clinical trial. *Lancet* 2011;378(9802):1547-1559.

14. Cannon CP, Shah S, Dansky HM, et al. DEFINE Investigators. Safety of anacetrapib in patients with or at high risk for coronary heart disease. *N Engl J Med* 2010;363:2406-2415.

15. Davidson MH, Armani A, McKenney JM, Jacobson TA. Safety considerations with fibrate therapy. *Am J Cardiol* 2007;99(6A):3C-18C.

16. Jones PH, Cusi K, Davidson MH, et al. Efficacy and safety of fenofibric acid co-administered with low- or moderate-dose statin in patients with mixed dyslipidemia and type 2 diabetes mellitus: results of a pooled subgroup analysis from three randomized, controlled, double-blind trials. *Am J Cardiovasc Drugs* 2009;10:e73-e84.

17. Ginsberg HN, Elam MB, Lovato LC, et al. ACCORD Study Group. Effects of combination lipid therapy in type 2 diabetes mellitus. *N Engl J Med* 2010;362:1563-1574.

18. Sacks FM, Carey VJ, Fruchart JC. Combination lipid therapy in type 2 diabetes. *N Engl J Med* 2010;363:692-694.

19. Lamon-Fava S, Diffenderfer MR, Barrett PH, et al. Extended-release niacin alters the metabolism of plasma apolipoprotein (Apo) A-I and ApoB-containing lipoproteins. *Arterioscler Thromb Vasc Biol* 2008;28:1672-1678.

20. Canner PL, Berge KG, Wenger NK, et al. Fifteen year mortality in Coronary Drug Project patients: long-term benefit with niacin. *J Am Coll Cardiol* 1986;8:1245-1255.

21. Brown G, Albers JJ, Fisher LD, et al. Regression of coronary artery disease as a result of intensive lipid-lowering therapy in men with high levels of apolipoprotein B. *N Engl J Med* 1990;323(19):1289-1298.

22. Brown B, Brockenbrough A, Zhao X-Q, et al. Very intensive lipid therapy with lovastatin, niacin, and colestipol for prevention of death and myocardial infarction: a 10-year Familial Atherosclerosis Treatment Study (FATS) follow-up. *Circulation* 1998;98:I-635. Abstract 3341.

23. Brown BG, Zhao XQ, Chait A, et al. Simvastatin and niacin, antioxidant vitamins, or the combination for the prevention of coronary disease. *N Engl J Med* 2001;345:1583-1592.

24. Yim BT, Chong PH. Niacin-ER and lovastatin treatment of hypercholesterolemia and mixed dyslipidemia. *Ann Pharmacother* 2003;37:106-115.

25. Kashyap ML, McGovern ME, Berra K, et al. Long-term safety and efficacy of a once-daily niacin/lovastatin formulation for patients with dyslipidemia. *Am J Cardiol* 2002;89:672-678.

26. Hunninghake DB, McGovern ME, Koren M, et al. A dose-ranging study of a new, once-daily, dual-component drug product containing niacin extended-release and lovastatin. *Clin Cardiol* 2003;26:112-118.

27. Bays HE, Dujovne CA, McGovern ME, et al. Comparison of once daily, niacin extended-release/lovastatin with standard doses of atorvastatin and simvastatin (the ADvicor Versus Other Cholesterol-Modulating Agents Trial Evaluation [ADVOCATE]). *Am J Cardiol* 2003;91:667-672.

28. Taylor AJ, Villines TC, Devine PJ, et al. Extended-release niacin or ezetimibe and carotid intima-media thickness. *N Engl J Med* 2009;361:2113-2122.

29. Villines TC, Stanek EJ, Devine PJ, et al. The ARBITER 6-HALTS Trial (Arterial Biology for the Investigation of the Treatment Effects of Reducing Cholesterol 6–HDL and LDL Treatment Strategies in Atherosclerosis). *J Am Coll Cardiol* 2010;55:2721-2726.

30. ClinicalTrials.gov. Niacin plus statin to prevent vascular events (AIM HIGH). Accessed 2010 August at www.clinicaltrials.gov/ct2/show/NCT00120289?term=AIM-HIGH&rank=3.

31. GISSI-Prevenzione Investigators. Dietary supplementation with n-3 polyunsaturated fatty acids and vitamin E after myocardial infarction: results of the GISSI-Prevenzione trial. *Lancet* 1999;354:447-455.

32. O'Keefe JH, Harris WS. From Inuit to implementation: omega-3 fatty acids come of age. *Mayo Clinic Proc* 2000;75:607-614.

33. Harris WS, Ginsberg HN, Arunakul N, et al. Safety and efficacy of omacor in severe hypertriglyceridemia. *J Cardiovasc Risk* 1997;4:385-391.

34. Contacos C, Barter PJ, Sullivan DR. Effect of pravastatin and omega-3 fatty acids on plasma lipids and lipoproteins in patients with combined hyperlipidemia. *Arterioscler Thromb* 1993;13:1755-1762.

35. Nordøy A, Bønaa KH, Nilsen H, et al. Effects of simvastatin and omega-3 fatty acids on plasma lipoproteins and lipid peroxidation in patients with combined hyperlipidaemia. *J Intern Med* 1998;243:163-170.

36. Nordøy A, Hansen JB, Brox J, Svensson B. Effects of atorvastatin and omega-3 fatty acids on LDL subfractions and postprandial hyperlipemia in patients with combined hyperlipemia. *Nutr Metab Cardiovasc Dis* 2001;11:7-16.

37. Maki KC, Dicklin MR, Davidson MH, Doyle RT, Ballantyne CM. COMBination of prescription Omega-3 with Simvastatin (COMBOS) Investigators. Baseline lipoprotein lipids and low-density lipoprotein cholesterol response to prescription omega-3 acid ethyl ester added to Simvastatin therapy. *Am J Cardiol* 2010;105(10):1409-1412.

38. Lovaza (omega-3-acid ethyl esters) package insert. Available at http://us.gsk.com/products/assets/us_lovaza.pdf. Accessed June 25, 2012.

39. Kling DF, Johnson J, Rooney M, Davidson M. Omega-3 free fatty acids demonstrate more than 4-fold greater bioavailability for EPA and DHA compared with omega-3-acid ethyl esters in conjunction with a low-fat diet: the ECLIPSE study. *J Clin Lipidol* 2011;105:231.

40. Maki KC, Dicklin MR, Davidson MH, et al. Baseline lipoprotein lipids and low-density lipoprotein cholesterol response to prescription omega-3 acid ethyl ester added to simvastatin therapy. *Am J Cardiol* 2010;105:1409-1412.

41. Maki KC. Fibrates for the treatment of the metabolic syndrome. *Curr Atheroscler Rep* 2004;6:45-51.

42. Maki KC, Dicklin MR, Lawless AL, Reeves MS. Omega-3 fatty acids for the treatment of elevated triglycerides. *Clin Lipidol* 2009;4:425-437.

43. Chan DC, Watts GF, Barrett PHR, et al. Regulatory effects of HMG CoA reductase inhibitors and fish oils on Apo B-100 kinetics in insulin resistant obese male subjects with dyslipidemia. *Diabetes* 2002;51:2377-2386.

44. Chan DC, Watts GF, Mori TA, et al. Randomized controlled trial of the effect of n-3 fatty acid supplementation on the metabolism of apolipoprotein B-100 and chylomicron remnants in men with visceral obesity. *Am J Clin Nutr* 2003;77:300-307.

45. Packard CJ. Triacylglycerol-rich lipoproteins and the generation of small, dense, low-density lipoprotein. *Biochem Soc Trans* 2003;31:1066-1069.

46. Davidson MH, Maki KC, Bays H, et al. Effects of prescription omega-3-acid ethyl esters on lipoprotein particle concentrations, apolipoproteins AI and CIII, and lipoprotein-associated phospholipase A2 mass in statin-treated subjects with hypertriglyceridemia. *J Clin Lipidol* 2009;3:332-340.

47. Bays HE, Ballantyne CM, Kastelein JJ, et al. Eicosapentaenoic acid ethyl ester (AMR101) therapy in patients with very high triglyceride levels (from the Multicenter, plAcebo-controlled, Randomized, double-blINd, 12-week study with an open-label Extension [MARINE] trial). *Am J Cardiol* 2011;108:682-690.

48. Jacobson TA, Soni PN, Glickstein SA, Rowe JD. Effects of eicosapentaenoic acid and docosahexaenoic acid on low-density lipoprotein cholesterol: a critical review. *J Clin Lipidol* 2011;105:200-201.

49. Mori TA, Burke V, Puddey IB, et al. Purified eicosapentaenoic acid and docosahexaenoic acids have differential effects on serum lipids and lipoproteins, LDL particle size, glucose, and insulin in mildly hyperlipidemic men. *Am J Clin Nutr* 2000;71:1085-1094.

50. Woodman RJ, Mori TA, Burke V, et al. Docosahexaenoic acid but not eicosapentaenoic acid increases LDL particle size in treated hypertensive type 2 diabetic patients. *Diabetes Care* 2003;26:253.

51. Breslow JL. n-3 fatty acids and cardiovascular disease. *Am J Clin Nutr* 2006;83(Suppl):1477S-1482S.

52. Cottin SC, Sanders TA, Hall WL. The differential effects of EPA and DHA on cardiovascular risk factors. *Proc Nutr Soc* 2011;70:215-231.

53. Davidson MH. Update on CETP inhibition. *J Clin Lipidol* 2010;4:394-398.

54. Barter P. Lessons learned from the Investigation of Lipid Level Management to Understand its Impact in Atherosclerotic Events (ILLUMINATE) trial. *Am J Cardiol* 2009;104(Suppl):10E-15E.

55. Nicholls SJ. High-density lipoprotein and progression rate of atherosclerosis in intravascular ultrasound trials. *Am J Cardiol* 2009;104(Suppl):16E-21E.

56. Nicholls SJ, Tuzcu EM, Brennan DM, Tardif JC, Nissen SE. Cholesteryl ester transfer protein inhibition, high-density lipoprotein raising, and progression of coronary atherosclerosis: insights from ILLUSTRATE (Investigation of Lipid Level Management Using Coronary Ultrasound to Assess Reduction of Atherosclerosis by CETP Inhibition and HDL Elevation). *Circulation* 2008;118:2506-2514.

57. Schwartz GG, Olsson AG, Ballantyne CM, et al. dal-OUTCOMES Committees and Investigators. Rationale and design of the dal-OUTCOMES trial: efficacy and safety of dalcetrapib in patients with recent acute coronary syndrome. *Am Heart J* 2009;158:e896-e901.

CH
25

THERAPY TO MANAGE LOW HIGH-DENSITY LIPOPROTEIN CHOLESTEROL AND ELEVATED TRIGLYCERIDES

Cardiovascular Disease and Lifestyle Modification

Frank M. Sacks and Kathy McManus

DIETARY FATS AND BLOOD LIPIDS, 442

High-Carbohydrate, Low-Fat Diets to Reduce
   Low-Density Lipoprotein Cholesterol and Blood
   Pressure, 442
The DASH Diet, 442
Low-Fat Diets, Low Saturated Fat, and Cardiovascular Disease:
   Clinical Trials and Epidemiology, 443
Moderate Unsaturated Fat Diets, 444

Reduced-Carbohydrate, Higher Unsaturated Fat, and Protein
   Diets: A New Twist to the DASH Dietary Approach, 445
Type of Carbohydrate, 445
Fish Oil to Prevent Coronary Heart Disease, 445

OBESITY, 446

Clinical Assessment of Obesity, 446
Goals for Weight Loss and Management, 448

Determination of Calorie Levels for Weight Loss, 448
2010 Dietary Guidelines, 448
Healthy Eating Patterns, 448
Physical Activity, 450
Overall Effect of Diet and Lifestyle, 450

REFERENCES, 452

Because of the difficulty many patients have in improving their diet, physicians may be tempted to lose faith in a nonpharmacologic approach to the treatment of cardiovascular disease (CVD). This chapter describes the strong scientific base that supports healthy nutrition and regular exercise and provides practical approaches to illustrate how patients can achieve positive lifestyle modification.

Epidemiologic observations worldwide show a pattern of CVD prevalence that points directly at poor nutrition, too much food, and erosion of a healthy lifestyle as the causes of high rates of CVD worldwide. Very low rates of CVD still exist in parts of Mediterranean countries and Japan and China, where traditional diets and lifestyles are maintained. During the transition to a developed economy typical of North America and Europe, the incidence of CVD and diabetes increases rapidly, as has been evident worldwide and most notably in South Asia and Latin America.

Although drug therapy for hyperlipidemia has had huge success in decreasing CVD, national guidelines rightfully still call for nutrition and exercise for primary prevention.[1-3] For secondary prevention, nutrition and drug therapy should be used together. Diet and drug treatments are additive in improving risk factors such as low-density lipoprotein cholesterol (LDL-c), blood pressure, and insulin resistance and in reducing CVD. Improved diet quality reduces CVD, even when body weight remains excessive.[4,5] However, weight loss has its own benefits: it can raise high-density lipoprotein cholesterol (HDL-c), lower triglyceride (TG) levels, improve insulin sensitivity, and lower blood pressure. When adopted intensively and taken to their full potential, diet and weight loss may eliminate the need for drug therapy for hyperlipidemia, hypertension, or type 2 diabetes, and it may simplify the ever more complex multidrug regimens necessary to control these conditions.

Dietary Fats and Blood Lipids

Saturated fats, trans (unsaturated) fats from partially hydrogenated vegetable oils, and cholesterol increase blood LDL-c levels.[6,7] Saturated fat and cholesterol are present mainly in dairy fat and red meat, whereas trans fats are present in most fried foods and baked products in the United States. Trans fatty acids are also present in dairy and meat fat, formed in the ruminant gut by bacteria during digestion. All guidelines call for reduction in these dietary lipids. When saturated fats, trans fats, and cholesterol are reduced in the diet, LDL-c decreases in proportion to the magnitude of the dietary changes. This happens with whatever nutrients replace them, which is the rationale for traditional guidelines that recommend a low-fat, carbohydrate-rich diet as a pragmatic way to reduce unhealthy fats. The remaining question is whether nutrients and foods other than those rich in carbohydrates could replace the unhealthy fats; other possible replacements are unsaturated fats and oils and protein. Beneficial potentials of unsaturated fats have

been established, and new mechanisms are still being discovered.[8,9] Moreover, dietary protein improves CVD risk factors.[10,11] The effects on blood lipids and blood pressure of approaches that emphasize either carbohydrate, unsaturated fat, or protein were compared in the Optimal Macronutrient Intake (OMNI) Heart trial, which is discussed later in this chapter.[10]

High-Carbohydrate, Low-Fat Diets to Reduce Low-Density Lipoprotein Cholesterol and Blood Pressure

Low-fat, high-carbohydrate diets reduce LDL-c generally by a modest amount, 5% to 10%, in proportion to adherence.[6,7] Very-low-fat, low-cholesterol diets can reduce LDL-c more, but acceptability by the general public may be limited; in addition, very-low-fat diets may be deficient in essential fatty acids. Low-fat, high-carbohydrate diets reduce LDL-c as well as reduce HDL-c and raise TGs (Figure 26-1).[6,7] Because the LDL/HDL ratio is unchanged, CVD risk cannot be assumed to decrease on a low-fat diet. In fact, replacing saturated and trans fats with monounsaturated and polyunsaturated fats, rather than carbohydrate, is more strongly associated with improved lipid risk factors and reduced CVD in epidemiologic studies and clinical trials.[6,7,12] Furthermore, the type of carbohydrate-containing foods that replace saturated fat–rich foods influences risk factors and coronary heart disease (CHD).[13] In addition, some carbohydrate-rich foods raise blood glucose less than others, and it is these that possess the favorable effects.[13]

The DASH Diet

The Dietary Approaches to Stop Hypertension (DASH) study attempted to combine information from epidemiology and animal studies on possible new dietary means to prevent and treat hypertension.[14] Although weight loss and dietary sodium reduction had long been shown to lower blood pressure, population studies suggested that other nutrients may also have beneficial effects. The DASH research group designed a dietary pattern rich in fruits and vegetables and low-fat dairy products that included nuts and whole grains and was low in red meat and sugar-containing desserts and beverages. The DASH diet substantially reduced blood pressure and extended the potential for nutritional control of hypertension.[14] When the DASH diet was combined with reduced sodium, the beneficial effects were even stronger (Figure 26-2).[15] In the typical older patient population in clinical practice, the DASH diet with low sodium content reduced systolic blood pressure by 15 mm Hg in those with mild hypertension and 10 mm Hg in those with above-average blood pressure (120 to 139 mm Hg),[16] now termed *prehypertension*. Older patients responded to the DASH diet and low sodium more than younger patients, which

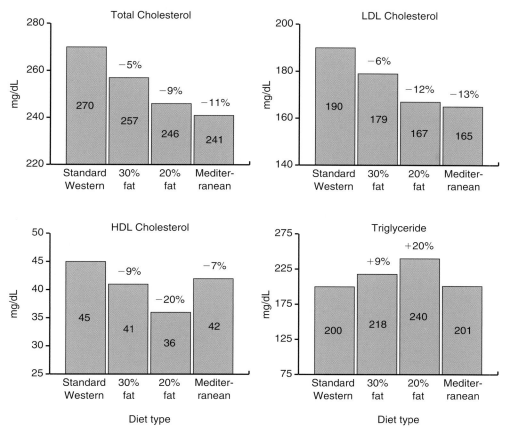

FIGURE 26-1 Effect of cholesterol-lowering diets on blood lipid risk factors. HDL, high-density lipoprotein; LDL, low-density lipoprotein. *(Modified from Sacks FM, Katan M. Randomized clinical trials on the effects of dietary fat and carbohydrate on plasma lipoproteins and cardiovascular disease. Am J Med 2002;113[Suppl 9B]:13S-24S.)*

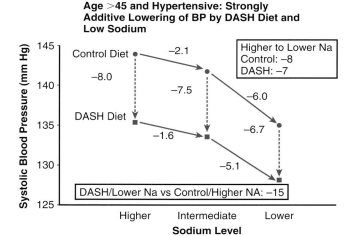

FIGURE 26-2 Effect of the low-sodium Dietary Approaches to Stop Hypertension *(DASH)* diet on systolic blood pressure in older patients with mild hypertension. BP, blood pressure. *(Data from Sacks FM, Bray GA, Carey VJ, et al. Comparison of weight-loss diets with different compositions of fat, protein, and carbohydrates. N Engl J Med 2009;360:859-873.)*

flattened the relation between blood pressure and age to such an extent that little change in blood pressure with age would be expected in those who optimize their diet.[17]

The DASH diet also reduced LDL-c, as would be predicted from its low content of saturated fat and cholesterol.[18] However, HDL-c also decreased predictably by approximately the same percentage

as LDL-c, and the ratio did not change. Interestingly, TGs did not increase on the DASH diet, as they often do on a high-carbohydrate diet. Perhaps this is because of the relatively good type of carbohydrates consumed, those with a low glycemic index, which cause reduced blood glucose response.[19] Overall, predicted CVD risk was reduced on the DASH diet because of its benefits of lower blood pressure and LDL-c outweighing the reduced HDL-c.[18] With low sodium, CVD risk on the DASH diet improved more. DASH is considered the benchmark dietary pattern recommended by the U.S. Dietary Goals Committee.[1] More and more, dietary patterns and the component foods, rather than specific nutrients, are being used as the basis of dietary recommendations as reviewed recently.[20]

Low-Fat Diets, Low Saturated Fat, and Cardiovascular Disease: Clinical Trials and Epidemiology

Low-fat diets never had a satisfactory test in a randomized clinical trial with clinical endpoints. The Women's Health Initiative (WHI) was an attempt to test this diet in a trial of 160,000 women in the United States. These women were randomized to either a low-fat, high-carbohydrate diet recommended to be rich in fruits and vegetables or to a no-intervention comparison group and were followed for 7.5 years. No effect on CVD endpoints or cancer occurred.[21] Although the WHI set a goal for reducing total fat to 20%, it was clear from lack of HDL reduction or TG increase, both biomarkers of dietary fat reduction, that the participants were able to reduce fat only minimally. Previous small-scale trials did not find reduction in CVD with low-fat diets.[7] In a small group of patients with CHD, Ornish and colleagues used a very low-fat vegetarian diet as a major part of an overall lifestyle change that included intensive exercise,[22] and meals were provided to the patients. Coronary stenosis improved in the treated group, although the study was not large enough to evaluate an effect on clinical events. A less intensive program of low-fat diet and exercise in Heidelberg, Germany, also found benefits on coronary stenosis.[23] Epidemiologic data generally have not found a relation between amount of total fat and CHD.[24] Even more, the amount of dietary saturated fat, which has proven effects on LDL-c and atherogenesis, does not predict CHD in many epidemiologic studies.[25-26] This has provided grist for recent controversy on saturated fat and CHD and the advisability of low-fat diets. In fact, implicit in the traditional, multiple-variable statistical models that evaluate saturated fat are the replacement foods and nutrients in the specific populations studied. If most people who eat a small amount of saturated and total fat instead eat high-carbohydrate junk food, saturated fat gains the illusion of neutrality. A newer epidemiologic approach developed by Willett and colleagues tests specific exchanges of foods and nutrients in the population.[27] This technique effectively resolved the controversy by showing that low saturated fat intake is predictive of low CHD rates only if healthful low–glycemic index carbohydrates or polyunsaturated fats are increased.[12,13,28] A low-fat dietary pattern can be based on healthy foods—such as whole grains, fruits and vegetables, low-fat dairy products, and fish and lean meats—or it can have plenty of high-carbohydrate, high-calorie foods such as refined flour products, desserts, and sugar-containing drinks. The type of low-fat diet may be important to its success or failure for risk factor improvement.

Effects of standard low-fat, high-carbohydrate diets on CVD risk factors and CHD are as follows:

- Reduction of LDL-c concentration
- Reduction of HDL-c concentration
- No effect on the LDL/HDL cholesterol ratio
- Increase in TG levels (usually)
- Improvement in coronary stenosis (with an intensive exercise program)
- No reduction in CHD in epidemiologic studies or small-scale, short-duration trials
- No reduction in CVD in the definitive WHI

A low-fat diet that truly expresses a healthful dietary pattern has not been tested in a large, randomized trial with clinical CHD outcomes, although epidemiologic studies suggest that it would be beneficial.

Moderate Unsaturated Fat Diets

Replacing saturated fat with unsaturated fat has a long history of CVD prevention. In the 1950s and 1960s, an era lacking effective and well-tolerated CVD prevention drugs, polyunsaturated vegetable oils from corn, soybeans, and safflower seeds were used essentially as medicine to lower blood cholesterol. These polyunsaturated oils are the most potent LDL-lowering nutrients, and several clinical trials have demonstrated significant reductions in CVD from their use.[7] A unique type of unsaturated oil is rapeseed oil (Canola), which is mainly monounsaturated fat but also has omega-3 fatty acid and α-linolenic acid (ALA) components. The Lyon Heart Study used rapeseed oil with a Mediterranean diet in a secondary prevention study and found a reduction in CVD.[29] ALA, also prevalent in soybean oil and some vegetable products, is strongly protective against CHD in epidemiologic studies.[30] However, a recent trial showed supplements of ALA given to elderly patients after myocardial infarction (MI) did not reduce CHD compared with a placebo.[31] An explanation suggested by Campos and colleagues is that ALA reduces CHD only when it is increased from a very low dietary level, as exists in many countries, which can be studied by epidemiology.[32,33] Finally, olive oil and high-monounsaturated varieties of sunflower and safflower oils have primarily monounsaturated oils. This class of vegetable oil improves risk factors, although they have not been tested in a clinical end-point trial.

Whatever unsaturated fat is used to replace saturated and trans fats, whether unhydrogenated liquid vegetable oils—such as rapeseed, olive, sunflower, safflower, peanut, or soybean oil—or from nuts, total fat intake can be made to remain the same, or it can be increased to replace some carbohydrate. It is uncertain whether polyunsaturated or monounsaturated fat is superior for preventing CHD, although current evidence favors polyunsaturated oils.[12] Polyunsaturated fats have slightly more effect than monounsaturated fat in lowering LDL levels[6,7] and perhaps in reducing serum inflammatory markers.[8,9] Any type of fat raises HDL-c and lowers TGs compared with carbohydrate. However, the type of carbohydrate food may relate to its metabolic effects.[19] Diets high in unsaturated fats improve the lipid profile compared with saturated fat as well as carbohydrate.

Randomized trials definitively show the benefits of polyunsaturated fats. Three of four[34-37] randomized trials showed significant benefits on coronary disease rates (Table 26-1). In addition to lowering LDL, polyunsaturated fats may reduce the vascular inflammatory response and may limit the propensity of LDL particles to bind to vascular cells and deposit their cholesterol in vascular intima.[8,9] In monkeys, polyunsaturated fats from vegetable oils actually reduced coronary atherosclerosis.[38] Polyunsaturated fats from vegetable oils also have antiarrhythmogenic actions, although this property has not been tested in a clinical trial.[39] Thus, much evidence exists for the use of polyunsaturated oils to replace saturated fats to prevent coronary disease.

Monounsaturated fat has a weaker direct relationship to coronary disease prevention compared with polyunsaturated fat. A clinical trial that specifically raised monounsaturated fats to prevent CHD has not been performed. Monkey models of atherosclerosis do not show a benefit of monounsaturated fats;[38] however, in humans, monounsaturated fats are nearly as effective as polyunsaturated fats to decrease LDL and preserve HDL and TG levels.[6,7] Monounsaturated oils, particularly olive oil, have been an integral part of the centuries-old traditional Mediterranean diet, which has been associated with very low CVD rates.[40] Thus, there are reasons

TABLE 26-1	Clinical Trials of Diet Therapy with Polyunsaturated Vegetable Oils to Reduce Coronary Events: Substitution of Polyunsaturated Fat for Saturated Fat				
STUDY	N	DIETARY FAT	DURATION (YEARS)	Δ CHOLESTEROL*	Δ CVD†
Finnish Mental Hospital	676	34%	6	−15%‡	−43%‡
Oslo	412	39%	5	−14%‡	−25%‡
Medical Research Council soy oil	393	46%	4	−15%‡	−12%
Los Angeles	846	40%	8	−13%‡	−34%‡

Cardiovascular disease (CVD) is defined as myocardial infarction or sudden death for the Finnish, Oslo, and MRC trials and myocardial infarction, sudden death, or stroke for the Los Angeles trial. Trials with at least 2 years of average follow-up were included.
*Percentage change in serum cholesterol in the treatment group compared with the change in the control group.
†Percentage difference in coronary event rates in the treatment compared with the control group.
‡$P \leq .05$.

to advocate increased intake of unsaturated oils from a variety of sources, both monounsaturated and polyunsaturated.

Reduced-Carbohydrate, Higher Unsaturated Fat, and Protein Diets: A New Twist to the DASH Dietary Approach

The DASH diet, considered the benchmark diet for health in the United States,[1] is low in fat and high in carbohydrate. Although it reduced blood pressure and LDL-c, it reduced HDL-c also and did not affect TG levels.[18] In view of the favorable evidence on the effects of unsaturated fats on HDL and TGs, it was hypothesized that the DASH diet could be improved in its overall effects on CVD risk factors by replacing some of the carbohydrate with unsaturated fats. In addition, higher protein intake, replacing carbohydrate, was predictive of reductions in blood pressure and CVD in epidemiologic studies, and small-scale studies found favorable effects on lipid risk factors. The OMNI Heart study designed three healthful diets: one high in carbohydrate, similar to the DASH diet; another high in unsaturated fat; and a third high in protein from mixed sources.[10] All three were low in saturated fat and cholesterol and high in fruits, vegetables, nuts, and low-fat dairy products, thereby building on the dietary approach of DASH. All three diets substantially improved blood pressure and LDL-c; however, lowering carbohydrate intake by raising either unsaturated fat or protein further reduced blood pressure and TG levels. The unsaturated-fat diet raised HDL-c, whereas the protein diet lowered LDL-c and HDL-c (Table 26-2). Taken together, moderate reduction in carbohydrate intake, from 58% to 48% of total calories, produced 11% to 13% further reduction in estimated CVD risk beyond the 20% effect of the DASH-type diet. Several publications described in detail this dietary approach to advise physicians, dietitians, and patients.[17,41,42]

Effects of reduced-carbohydrate, high–unsaturated-fat diets on CVD are as follows:

- Reduction in blood pressure
- Reduction in LDL-c concentration
- Preservation of HDL-c concentration
- Reduction in the LDL-c/HDL-c ratio
- Decrease in TG levels compared with low-fat diets
- Reduction in CVD events (polyunsaturated fats)

The effects of increased protein and lower carbohydrate intakes are as follows (CVD was not directly studied in a randomized trial):

- Lowered blood pressure
- Lowered LDL-c
- Lowered HDL-c
- Lowered TGs
- Lowered CVD risk (in epidemiologic studies)

Type of Carbohydrate

The usual mix of carbohydrates in the Western diet contains large amounts of refined polysaccharides, such as in bread and baked goods, and sugars in juices and soda. These have a high glycemic index, causing glucose and insulin to rise substantially.[19] Other types of carbohydrates, those found in whole grains and vegetables, have a lower glycemic index because the digestion and absorption of the glucose occur more slowly and cause less of a rise in blood glucose and hence a lower rise in insulin. The low glycemic index of grains and vegetables is partly explained by the fiber content of these foods but also by the intrinsic digestibility of the food. These foods also cause less of a rise in plasma TG levels than the more commonly eaten carbohydrates that are higher on the glycemic index. Some of the concerns about a low-fat diet can be set aside if a patient truly eats foods with a low glycemic index, rather than the ubiquitous, less desirable high-carbohydrate foods that all too often are a major part of low-fat diets. As mentioned, a diet of low–glycemic index, carbohydrate-rich foods was predictive of reduced CHD when these replaced saturated fat in a meta-analysis,[13] whereas diets with carbohydrates high on the glycemic index were not.

Fish Oil to Prevent Coronary Heart Disease

In the early 1980s, two lines of evidence coalesced to engender widespread excitement on the potentially cardioprotective effects of omega-3 fatty acids from fish oil (EPA, DHA). Populations that eat large amounts of fatty fish had low rates of CVD, and in many epidemiologic studies, n-3 polyunsaturated fatty acid (PUFA) intake and blood levels are inversely related to CVD, a finding confirmed by randomized trials.[43-45] For example, The Diet and Reinfarction Trial (DART) tested the effect of increased intake of fatty fish or fish oil (1.5 g/day) for 2 years in 2033 Welsh men who had had an acute MI.[46] This small amount of fatty fish or fish oil significantly reduced coronary and total mortality rates; however, nonfatal MI was not significantly affected. These results have been reinforced by the Groupo Italiano per lo Studio della Sopravvivenza nell'Infarto Myocardico (GISSI) Prevenzione trial, which tested 1 g/day of n-3 PUFAs in 11,324 Italian patients surviving a recent MI.[47] In both trials the death rate began to lessen in the fish oil group as early as 3 months after treatment was started, and a Japanese trial of primary prevention of CVD with fish oil showed striking reductions in nonfatal CVD events.[48] Thus, relatively low doses of fish oil, 1 to 2 g/day, may be cardioprotective because of several mechanisms yet to be specifically determined.

Omega-3 fatty acids are metabolized to prostaglandins, leukotrienes, and resolvins that are antithrombotic, antiinflammatory, and vasodilating. However, the most established clinical benefit of fish oil is the reduction of blood TG levels. A large dose is necessary, and 10 to 15 capsules (1 g) of fish oil that contain between 20% and 50% omega-3 fatty acids are required. A prescription version of fish oil that is 90% omega-3 fatty acids is available, which requires fewer capsules. Use of fish oil for hypertriglyceridemia is discussed in Chapter 25.

Fish oil and other PUFAs have potential antiarrhythmic effects, increasing the depolarization threshold of ion channels.[39] Reduction in fatal CHD events has been reported in epidemiologic

TABLE 26-2	Beneficial Effects on Blood Pressure and Blood Lipids of Replacing Carbohydrate with Protein or Unsaturated Fat (OMNI Heart Study)			
		Mean Change from Baseline		
FACTOR	BASELINE	CARBOHYDRATES	PROTEIN	UNSATURATED FAT
LDL (mg/dL)	157	−20	−24	−22
HDL (mg/dL)	50	−1	−3	0
Triglyceride (mg/dL)	102	0	−16	−9
Systolic BP (mm Hg)	146	−13	−16	−16
Risk reduction		16%	21%	20%

BP, blood pressure; HDL, high-density lipoprotein; LDL, low-density lipoprotein; OMNI, Optimum Macronutrient Intake trial.

studies, often attributed to reduced sudden death.[43-45] However, a broader view of the benefits of omega-3 fatty acids is necessary because sudden death cannot account for all CVD event reductions, nonfatal as well as fatal, found in epidemiologic studies and clinical trials. Clinical trials that tested fish oil in patients with cardiac arrhythmias did not confirm protection against ventricular tachyarrhythmias in those with implanted defibrillators[49-51] or against atrial fibrillation.[52]

Effects of fish oil intake are as follows:

- Large doses (>5 g/day omega-3 fatty acids)
  - Reduction in blood TGs
  - Reduction in blood pressure
  - Prevention of thrombosis
- Small doses (1 to 2 g/day omega-3 fatty acids)
  - Prevention of CVD events, fatal and nonfatal

Obesity

The obesity epidemic continues to plague the United States. More than one third of U.S. adults—more than 72 million people—and 17% of U.S. children are obese.[53] From 1980 through 2008, obesity rates for adults have doubled, and rates for children have tripled.[53] The sex-specific prevalence of obesity was 32% of men and 36% of women from 2007 through 2008, and 25% of men and 31% of women aged 20 to 34 years were obese compared with 40% and 42% of 55- to 64-year-olds. After age 64 years, the prevalence of obesity declines; the rate is 26% in men and women 75 years and older. The prevalence of obesity is greater among non-Hispanic blacks and Mexican Americans than among non-Hispanic whites.[54] The health consequences of obesity are significant and include a higher risk of CHD, type 2 diabetes, high blood pressure, high total cholesterol and TG levels, sleep apnea, liver and gallbladder disease, and reproductive health complications. Obesity was estimated to cost $79 billion in 1998 in the Unites States. By 2008, the cost was estimated to have risen to $147 billion.[55]

The debate regarding what diet is most effective for treating obesity and overweight has been informed in the past 3 years by large, long-term randomized trials. In the past few years, a number of longer term trials (≥2 years) have published data examining not just weight loss but sustainability of lost weight. Sacks and colleagues[56] conducted a randomized trial in 811 overweight or obese people and concluded that reduced calorie diets result in clinically meaningful weight loss regardless of which macronutrients they emphasize. After 2 years, weight loss remained similar in those who were assigned to a diet with 15% protein and those assigned to a diet with 25% protein (3.0 and 3.6 kg, respectively); in those assigned to a diet with 20% fat and those assigned to a diet with 40% fat (3.3 kg for both groups); and in those assigned to a diet with 65% carbohydrate and those assigned to a diet with 35% carbohydrate (2.9 and 3.4 kg, respectively) (P > .20 for all comparisons; Figure 26-3). Participation in group counseling sessions was strongly predictive of weight loss at 2 years, and conclusions were that weight-loss diets can be tailored to individual patients on the basis of their personal and cultural preferences and may therefore have the best chance for long-term success.

Shai and colleagues conducted a randomized trial in 322 overweight or obese people that found that a Mediterranean diet or a low-carbohydrate, high-protein Atkins diet produced similar weight loss after 2 years and slightly more than a low-fat diet.[57] The Atkins diet group had the most weight loss early in the trial but also had the most weight regain. Finally, Foster and colleagues compared the effects of an Atkins diet with a low-fat diet in a 2-year randomized trial and found no difference.[58]

The Look AHEAD (Action for Health in Diabetes) was a multicenter randomized clinical trial to compare the effects of an intensive lifestyle intervention and diabetes support and education on incidence of major CVD events in overweight and obese individuals with type 2 diabetes mellitus. Averaged over 4 years,

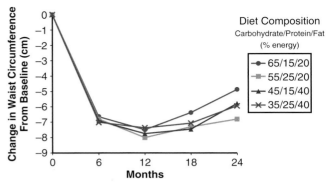

Pounds Lost in Completers

FIGURE 26-3 Reduction in waist circumference in overweight or obese subjects. *(From Sacks FM, Bray GA, Carey VJ, et al. Comparison of weight-loss diets with different compositions of fat, protein, and carbohydrates. N Engl J Med 2009;360(9):859-873.)*

the intensive lifestyle intervention produced better weight loss and improvements in fitness, glycemic control, and CVD risk factors.[59]

These long-term diet interventions support the accomplishment of weight loss sustained over an extended period (2 years and more) in overweight and obese individuals by several dietary and behavioral approaches. Dietary patterns influenced weight gain during 20 years in large cohorts of middle-aged and older U.S. women and men.[60] Foods associated with weight gain were potato chips, potatoes, sugar-sweetened beverages, and red meats. Foods associated with weight loss were vegetables, whole grains, fruits, nuts, and yogurt.

Clinical Assessment of Obesity

Body mass index (BMI), expressed as weight in kilograms divided by height in meters squared (kg/m^2), is commonly used to classify overweight. BMI does not measure percentage of body fat. The BMI of an individual who weighs 180 pounds and is 67 inches tall is calculated as follows:

$$180 \text{ lb} \div 2.2 \text{ kg/lb} = 81.8 \text{ kg}$$

$$67 \text{ in} \times 2.54 = 170.2 \text{ cm} = 1.7 \text{ m}$$

$$\text{BMI} = 81.8 \text{ kg} \div (1.7)^2 = 28.3 \text{ kg/m}^2$$

A BMI table is shown in Table 26-3.

An expert panel convened by the National Heart, Lung, and Blood Institute (NHLBI) in cooperation with the National Institute of Diabetes and Digestive and Kidney Diseases (NIDDK) identified the following categories for BMI:[61]

Obesity Class	BMI (kg/m^2)
Underweight	<18.5
Normal	18.5 to 24.9
Overweight	25.0 to 29.9
Obesity (type I)	30.0 to 34.9
Obesity (type II)	35.0 to 39.9
Extreme obesity (type III)	≥40

The presence of excess fat in the abdomen out of proportion to total body fat is an independent predictor of risk factors and morbidity. Waist circumference is positively correlated with abdominal fat content, and it provides a clinically acceptable measurement for assessing a patient's abdominal fat content before and during weight loss treatment.[61] High risk for the development of hypertension, diabetes, and CVD is associated in women with a waist circumference more than 35 inches (>88 cm)

TABLE 26-3   Body Mass Index (BMI) Table

BMI HEIGHT (in)	19	20	21	22	23	24	25	26	27	28	29	30	31	32	33	34	35
									WEIGHT (lb)								
58	91	96	100	105	110	115	119	124	129	134	138	143	148	153	158	162	167
59	94	99	104	109	114	119	124	128	133	138	143	148	153	158	163	168	173
60	97	102	107	112	118	123	128	133	138	143	148	153	158	163	168	174	179
61	100	106	111	116	122	127	132	137	143	148	153	158	164	169	174	180	185
62	104	109	115	120	126	131	136	142	147	153	158	164	169	175	180	186	191
63	107	113	118	124	130	135	141	146	152	158	163	169	175	180	186	191	197
64	110	116	122	128	134	140	145	151	157	163	169	174	180	186	192	197	204
65	114	120	126	132	138	144	150	156	162	168	174	180	186	192	198	204	210
66	118	124	130	136	142	148	155	161	167	173	179	186	192	198	204	210	216
67	121	127	134	140	146	153	159	166	172	178	185	191	198	204	211	217	223
68	125	131	138	144	151	158	164	171	177	184	190	197	203	210	216	223	230
69	128	135	142	149	155	162	169	176	182	189	196	203	209	216	223	230	236
70	132	139	146	153	160	167	174	181	188	195	202	209	216	222	229	236	243
71	136	143	150	157	165	172	179	186	193	200	208	215	222	229	236	243	250
72	140	147	154	162	169	177	184	191	199	206	213	221	228	235	242	250	258
73	144	151	159	166	174	182	189	197	204	212	219	227	235	242	250	257	265
74	148	155	163	171	179	186	194	202	210	218	225	233	241	249	256	264	272
75	152	160	168	176	184	192	200	208	216	224	232	240	248	256	264	272	279
76	156	164	172	180	189	197	205	213	221	230	238	246	254	263	271	279	287

BMI HEIGHT (in)	36	37	38	39	40	41	42	43	44	45	46	47	48	49	50	51	52	53	54
										WEIGHT (lb)									
58	172	177	181	186	191	196	201	205	210	215	220	224	229	234	239	244	248	253	258
59	178	183	188	193	198	203	208	212	217	222	227	232	237	242	247	252	257	262	267
60	184	189	194	199	204	209	215	220	225	230	235	240	245	250	255	261	266	271	276
61	190	195	201	206	211	217	222	227	232	238	243	248	254	259	264	269	275	280	285
62	196	202	207	213	218	224	229	235	240	246	251	256	262	267	273	278	284	289	295
63	203	208	214	220	225	231	237	242	248	254	259	265	270	278	282	287	293	299	304
64	209	215	221	227	232	238	244	250	256	262	267	273	279	285	291	296	302	308	314
65	216	222	228	234	240	246	252	258	264	270	276	282	288	294	300	306	312	318	324
66	223	229	235	241	247	253	260	266	272	278	284	291	297	303	309	315	322	328	334
67	230	236	242	249	255	261	268	274	280	287	293	299	306	312	319	325	331	338	344
68	236	243	249	256	262	269	276	282	289	295	302	308	315	322	328	335	341	348	354
69	243	250	257	263	270	277	284	291	297	304	311	318	324	338	338	345	351	358	365
70	250	257	264	271	278	285	292	299	306	313	320	327	334	341	348	355	362	369	376
71	257	265	272	279	286	293	301	308	315	322	329	338	343	351	358	365	372	379	386
72	265	272	279	287	294	302	309	316	324	331	338	346	353	361	368	375	383	390	397
73	272	280	288	295	203	310	318	325	333	340	348	355	363	371	378	386	393	401	408
74	280	287	295	303	311	319	326	334	342	350	358	365	373	381	389	396	404	412	420
75	287	295	303	311	319	327	335	343	351	359	367	375	383	391	399	407	415	423	431
76	295	304	312	320	328	336	344	353	361	369	377	385	394	402	410	418	426	435	443

To use the table, find the appropriate height in the left column labeled "Height." Move across to a given weight. The number at the top of the column is the body mass index (BMI) at that height and weight. Pounds have been rounded off.

and in men more than 40 inches (>102 cm). These waist circumference cutoff points lose their incremental predictive power in patients with a BMI of 35 kg/m² or more because these patients exceed the cutoff.[61]

Assessments for obesity should include height, weight, and waist circumference, and medical examination should rule out other physiologic causes and assess overall risk status. In addition to a medical evaluation, a psychologic assessment may be beneficial. This may include assessment for barriers to treatment such as eating disorders, addictions, depression, and other mental disorders.

The nutrition assessment consists of an evaluation of current eating patterns, including number and timing of meals and snacks, food preparation methods, and frequency of eating away from home. A history of weight and dieting should be assessed along with weight changes after the age of 18 years. An assessment of motivation for weight loss, readiness for change based on the Stages of Change model,[62] and barriers to treatment that include knowledge support systems, financial concerns, and physical limitations should be ascertained. In addition, physical activity level—including type of exercise, duration, and intensity—and the patient's commitment to a program should be determined.

Goals for Weight Loss and Management

The general goals of weight loss and management are to 1) prevent further weight gain, 2) reduce body weight, 3) maintain lost weight over the long term, and 4) reduce risk factors associated with obesity. Recommendations for weight loss from the NHLBI Expert Panel[61] include 1) loss of 10% of baseline weight over 6 months; 2) for a BMI of 27 to 35, a weight loss of 0.5 to 1 lb/wk or 300 to 500 kcal/day; 3) for BMI over 35, a weight loss of 1 to 2 lb/wk or 500 to 1000 kcal/day, and 4) exercise 30 minutes five times per week. Good evidence from randomized clinical trials shows that overweight (BMI 25.0 to 29.9 kg/m²) and obese (BMI ≥30 kg/m²) people can successfully reduce health risks with a weight loss of 10% of baseline weight. With success, further weight loss can be attempted if warranted through further assessment.

Determination of Calorie Levels for Weight Loss

The focus of diet intervention for weight loss in overweight or obese patients is a low-calorie diet. There is no eating plan that produces weight loss without a planned reduction in calories, and many equations are available to determine caloric needs. Most include 1) determining the basal metabolic rate (BMR), 2) adding in activity calories, 3) adding the BMR to the activity calories for maintenance calories, and, when weight loss is necessary, 4) subtracting calories for weight loss.

A review in the *Journal of the American Dietetic Association* showed that the Mifflin-St. Jeor equation was the most reliable equation to predict BMR[63] and did so within 10% of the measured metabolic rate. After determining BMR, the next step is to determine activity calories. The activity calories are based on examining the percentage increase in calories associated with different types of daily activities.[64] Step three is to determine maintenance calories, which is done by adding basal calories from the equation to activity calories. Step four is the determination of weight-loss calories by subtracting 500 kcal/day for weight loss of 1 lb/wk or 250 kcal/day for weight loss of 0.5 lb/wk from the daily maintenance calories.

For example, a 50-year-old woman who is 5 feet, 3 inches tall and weighs 72.7 kg has a low activity level. The Mifflin-St. Jeor formula is used below to determine the calories needed for weight loss.

Step 1: calculate BMR:

$$[10 \times \text{weight in kg } (72.7)] + [6.25 \times \text{height in cm } (160 \text{ cm})] - [5 \times \text{age } (50)] - 161$$

$$727 + 1000 - 250 - 161$$

$$\text{BMR} = 1316$$

Step 2: determine activity calories:

1.00	Sedentary
1.12	Low active
1.27	Active
1.45	Very active

Step 3: calories for weight maintenance:

Multiply BMR by activity calories: $1316 \times 1.2 = 1579$ kcal

Step 4: For weight loss of 0.5 lb/wk, subtract 250 kcal from weight maintenance calories:

$$1579 - 250 = 1329 \text{ kcal for weight loss}$$

A simpler method to determine a calorie level for a weight-loss diet is to select a standard calorie level that has been used in many clinical trials on weight loss. Diets containing 1200 to 1600 kcal/day can be selected for most women; a diet between 1500 and 1800 kcal/day can be chosen for men. The higher levels may be appropriate for women who weigh 165 lb or more or those who exercise regularly.

2010 Dietary Guidelines

To address the current calorie imbalance in the United States, the U.S. Department of Agriculture and U.S. Department of Health and Human Services 2010 Dietary Guidelines encourage individuals to become more conscious of what they eat and what they do.[1] This means increasing awareness of what, when, why, and how much they eat, deliberately making better choices regarding what and how much they consume, and seeking ways to be more physically active. The guidelines identify several behaviors and practices that have been shown to help people manage their food and beverage intake and calorie expenditure and ultimately manage body weight. The behaviors with the strongest evidence related to body weight include:

- Focusing on the total number of calories consumed
- Monitoring food intake
- When eating out, choosing smaller portions or lower calorie options
- Preparing, serving, and consuming smaller portions of foods and beverages, especially those high in calories
- Eating a nutrient-dense breakfast
- Limiting "screen time" (television, video games, computer) to no more than 1 to 2 hours per day

Healthy Eating Patterns

The DASH and OMNI Heart diets have been described earlier in this chapter. The DASH Sodium trial[15] studied levels of sodium in diets of people without hypertension. More than 400 participants were randomly assigned to eat either a standard diet or DASH diet. Within the assigned diet, participants ate foods with high, intermediate, and low levels of sodium for 30 consecutive days. Results showed the lower the sodium intake, the greater the reduction of systolic blood pressure in both groups. An example of the DASH Sodium diet plan is shown in Table 26-4.

THE MEDITERRANEAN DIET

Another model of a healthful eating pattern is the traditional Mediterranean diet, which reflects food patterns that were typical of Crete, much of the rest of Greece, and southern Italy in the 1960s. The selection of this specific time and these geographic

TABLE 26-4 DASH Sodium Diet at 2000 Calories

2300-mg SODIUM MENU	SODIUM (mg)	SUBSTITUTION TO REDUCE SODIUM TO 1500 mg	SODIUM (mg)
Breakfast			
¾ cup bran flakes cereal	220	¾ cup shredded wheat cereal	1
1 medium banana	1		
1 cup low-fat milk	107		
1 slice whole wheat bread	149		
1 tsp soft (tub) margarine	26	1 tsp unsalted soft (tub) margarine	0
1 cup orange juice	5		
Lunch			
¾ cup chicken salad	179	Remove salt from the recipe	120
2 slices whole wheat bread	299		
1 Tbsp Dijon mustard	373	1 Tbsp regular mustard	175
Salad:			
½ cup fresh cucumber slices	1		
½ cup tomato wedges	5		
1 Tbsp sunflower seeds	0		
1 tsp Italian dressing, low calorie	43		
½ cup fruit cocktail, juice pack	5		
Dinner	26		
	1		
	107		
3 oz beef, eye of round	35		
2 Tbsp beef gravy, fat free	165		
1 cup green beans, sautéed with ½ tsp canola oil	12		
1 small baked potato	14		
1 Tbsp sour cream, fat free	21		
1 Tbsp grated natural cheddar cheese, reduced fat	67	1 Tbsp natural cheddar cheese, reduced fat, low sodium	1
1 Tbsp chopped scallions	1		
1 small whole wheat roll	148		
1 tsp soft (tub) margarine	26	1 tsp unsalted soft (tub) margarine	0
1 small apple	1		
1 cup low-fat milk	107		
Snacks			
½ cup almonds, unsalted	0		
½ cup raisins	4		
½ cup fruit yogurt, fat free, no sugar added	86		
Totals	2101		1507

	Sodium Level	
NUTRIENTS PER DAY	**2300 mg**	**1500 mg**
Calories	2062	2037
Total fat	63 g	59 g
Calories from fat	28%	26%
Saturated fat	13 g	12 g
Calories from saturated fat	6%	5%
Cholesterol	155 mg	155 mg
Sodium	2101 mg	1507 mg

areas is based on the evidence that adult life expectancy for populations in these areas was among the highest in the world, and rates of CHD, major cancers, and some other diet-related chronic diseases were among the lowest in the world. The Mediterranean diet of the early 1960s is described by the following broad characteristics:

- An abundance of minimally processed plant foods, including vegetables, fruit, grains, beans, potatoes, nuts, and seeds
- Olive oil as the principal fat
- Cheese and yogurt eaten daily in low to moderate amounts
- Fresh fruit as daily dessert and sweets containing sugar or honey eaten a few times per month
- Red meat eaten infrequently
- Wine in moderation with meals

In the traditional Mediterranean diet, the percentage of calories from fat varies from 28% to 40% depending on the region. Most of the fat is monounsaturated, with saturated fat being less than 8% of total calories. The Mediterranean pyramid illustrated in Figure 26-4 is designed to convey a general sense of the relative proportions and frequency of consumption of foods that contribute to this overall dietary pattern. At the base of the pyramid, the diet features many different types of grains, bread, pasta, rice, bulgur (cracked wheat), and potatoes. Daily consumption of fruits, vegetables, beans, legumes, and nuts is encouraged, along with olive oil and moderate amounts of cheese and yogurt. Fish, poultry, and eggs are the main protein sources, and red meat is limited to a few times a month.

A Mediterranean-style diet can be successfully imported into the American diet by using the main principles but substituting foods readily available and acceptable to the American palate. Table 26-5 illustrates 1500- and 1800-kcal menus patterned after the Mediterranean diet. The 1500-kcal meal plan can be used for a general weight-loss plan for many adults, whereas an 1800-kcal meal plan is designed for weight maintenance.

Overall, the main objective in selecting healthful diets is to choose those that will reduce risk of chronic disease and that are palatable and acceptable for long-term health. The Mediterranean diet, OMNI Heart diet, and DASH Sodium diet are approaches to eating that have proven acceptable and healthy.

Physical Activity

Physical activity can be defined as an athletic, recreational, or occupational activity that works the muscles and uses more energy than is used at rest.[65] Examples may include activities such as swimming, ice skating, walking, or daily activities such as cleaning and gardening. The term *physical activity* is commonly used interchangeably with *exercise*; however, exercise is a planned and structured physical activity such as playing on a sports team, lifting weights, or taking a yoga class. It can be useful to think in terms of physical activity, rather than exercise, and to stress that physical activity can be any body movement that uses energy and enhances health.

There are three components of physical activity: duration, frequency, and intensity. *Duration* indicates the length of time that the activity is performed; for example, 30 minutes of running or 2 hours of house cleaning. *Frequency* is the number of times the activity is done, such as three times per week. *Intensity* indicates how much work is required to perform the activity. For instance, cycling at a pace greater than 20 mph is a more intense activity than cycling at a pace less than 10 mph because it takes more energy to achieve the faster speed. When increasing physical activity, it is recommended that only one of these factors be increased at a time to facilitate habitual physical activity and reduce the risk of injury.

The American Heart Association (AHA) and the American College of Sports Medicine (ACSM) recommend that all healthy adults aged 18 to 65 years take part in moderate-intensity aerobic physical activity for at least 30 minutes, 5 days per week.[66] Alternatively, 20 minutes of vigorous-intensity aerobic activity 3 days per week, or a combination of intensities, is also adequate. For example, a person may walk briskly for 30 minutes on 2 days and jog for 20 minutes on 2 days to meet the recommendations for physical activity. In addition to aerobic activity, the AHA/ACSM guidelines suggest that healthy adults engage in muscle-strengthening activity twice a week to promote good health and physical independence. Specifically, muscle-strengthening activity that includes all the major muscle groups should include 8 to 10 exercises on each of 2 nonconsecutive days. A weight resistance that allows 8 to 12 repetitions of each exercise should be used to improve both strength and endurance.

The benefits of physical activity include a reduction in the risk of CVD, stroke, hypertension, osteoporosis, type 2 diabetes mellitus, depression, and colon and breast cancers.[66] It is unclear at this point how the individual components of intensity, duration, and frequency affect health outcomes, although there is some evidence to indicate that vigorous-intensity activity may have a greater effect on reducing CVD.

The number of calories burned during physical activity varies depending on body weight, metabolism, current fitness level, exercise intensity, and environmental conditions. Table 26-6 gives examples of calories used during 1 hour of various physical activities for three body weights; a person who weighs more burns more calories per minute than someone who weighs less. For comparison purposes, it is important to note that 3500 kcal of energy is equal to 1 lb of weight. Therefore, if an energy deficit of 3500 calories is achieved through physical activity or diet over the course of 1 week, this ideally would result in 1 lb of weight loss. Calorie expenditures for various physical activities can be found in Table 26-6.[67]

Overall Effect of Diet and Lifestyle

With full adherence, diet and exercise have very strong potential for major improvements in risk factors, dyslipidemia, high blood pressure, diabetes, and obesity (Box 26-1).[68]

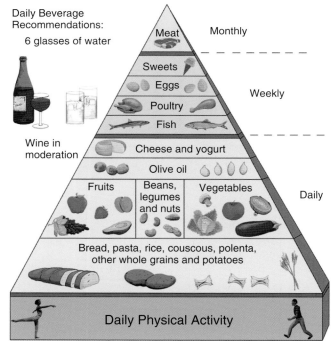

FIGURE 26-4 The traditional Mediterranean diet pyramid, developed in collaboration with the Nutrition Department of Harvard School of Public Health and the Oldways Preservation and Exchange Trust of Boston.

TABLE 26-5 Mediterranean-Style Sample Menus

1500 kcal/day

Breakfast

1 cup oatmeal

½ cup nonfat milk

½ cup strawberries

2 Tbsp pecans

Lunch

4 oz turkey breast with lettuce, tomato

1 Tbsp light mayonnaise

2 slices whole wheat bread

1 pear

Snack

1 cup baby carrots

2 Tbsp hummus

Dinner

5 oz broiled salmon

1 cup whole wheat couscous

1 cup fresh asparagus, cooked in 1 Tbsp olive oil with fresh garlic

Calories		1498
Protein		100 g (26%)
Carbohydrate		163 g (41%)
Fat		58 g (33%)
	Saturated	8.5 g
	Monounsaturated	26.5 g
	Polyunsaturated	13.5 g
	Cholesterol	173 mg
Fiber:		35 g

1800 kcal/day

Breakfast

Omelet cooked in 1 Tbsp olive oil

½ cup egg substitute with ¼ cup chopped green peppers and onions

2 slices whole wheat toast

1 orange

Lunch

2 cups mixed salad greens with

½ cup chickpeas

¼ cup corn

¼ cup tabbouleh

1 Tbsp oil and vinegar dressing

1 small whole wheat pita

2 Tbsp almonds

1 apple

Snack

½ cup nonfat plain yogurt

½ oz dry roasted walnuts

Dinner

5 oz baked chicken breast

1 baked sweet potato

1 cup fresh spinach, stir-fried in

1 Tbsp olive oil

Calories		1810
Protein		47 g (20%)
Carbohydrate		249 g (48%)
Fat		56 g (22%)
	Saturated	18 g
	Monounsaturated	20 g
	Polyunsaturated	18 g
	Cholesterol	300 mg
Fiber:		25 g

Percent values are percent of total calories.

Box 26-1 Major Reduction in Cardiovascular Disease Risk from Modest Improvements in Lifestyle: The Nurses' Health Study

Primary Prevention of Cardiovascular Disease: Five Attributes to Define Low Risk in the Nurses' Health Study

1. Diet in upper 40% of population
   - Good fat: Low saturated and trans fats, high polyunsaturated fat, high fish oil
   - Good carbohydrates: Low glycemic load, high fiber (whole grains)
   - High folate (vegetables, fruit)
2. Not currently smoking
3. Moderate alcoholic beverage drinking (1 drink every other day to daily)
4. Regular exercise (0.5 h daily; e.g., 2 mph walking)
5. BMI <25 kg/m² (optimal, <21 kg/m²)

Three Low-Risk Attributes*
1. Good diet
2. No smoking
3. Regular exercise

Four Low-Risk Attributes†
1. Good diet
2. No smoking
3. Regular exercise
4. BMI <25 kg/m²

Five Low-Risk Attributes
All the above, plus moderate alcohol‡

*With this lifestyle, 51% of coronary events and strokes could be avoided, but only 13% of nurses practiced this.

†With this lifestyle, 60% of events could be avoided, but only 7% of nurses practiced this.

‡With this lifestyle, 74% of cardiovascular disease events and 82% of coronary events could be avoided, but only 3% of nurses practiced this.

BMI, body mass index.

Modified from Stampfer MJ, Hu FB, Manson JE, et al. Primary prevention of coronary heart disease in women through diet and lifestyle. *N Engl J Med* 2000;343:16-22.

TABLE 26-6   Energy Expenditures

PHYSICAL ACTIVITY (1-HOUR DURATION)	Body Weight and Calories Burned (kcal)			
	130 lb	155 lb	180 lb	205 lb
Aerobics, general	384	457	531	605
Basketball, shooting baskets	266	317	368	419
Bowling	177	211	245	279
Cleaning, dusting	148	176	204	233
Cycling, 10-11.9 mph	354	422	490	558
Gardening	236	281	327	372
Running, 12-min mile	472	563	654	745
Running, 9-min mile	649	774	899	1024
Running, 7-min mile	826	985	1144	1303
Stretching, hatha yoga	236	281	327	372
Swimming laps, freestyle, slow	413	493	572	651
Walking, 3 mph	195	232	270	307
Weight lifting, light workout	177	211	245	279

REFERENCES

1. U.S. Department of Agriculture and U.S. Department of Health and Human Services. *Dietary Guidelines for Americans: 2010*, 7th ed. 2010, Washington, DC, U.S. Government Printing Office.
2. Lloyd-Jones DM, Hong Y, Labarthe D, et al. Defining and setting national goals for cardiovascular health promotion and disease reduction: the American Heart Association's strategic Impact Goal through 2020 and beyond. *Circulation* 2010;121:586-613.
3. Lichtenstein AH, Appel LJ, Brands M, et al. Diet and lifestyle recommendations revision 2006: a scientific statement from the American Heart Association Nutrition Committee. *Circulation* 2006;114:82-96.
4. He J, Ogden LG, Vupputuri S, et al. Dietary sodium intake and subsequent risk of cardiovascular disease in overweight adults. *JAMA* 1999;282:2027-2034.
5. Stampfer MJ, Hu FB, Manson JE, et al. Primary prevention of coronary heart disease in women through diet and lifestyle. *N Engl J Med* 2000;343:16-22.
6. Mensink RP, Katan MB. Effect of dietary fatty acids on serum lipids and lipoproteins: a meta-analysis of 27 trials. *Arterioscler Thromb* 1992;12:911-919.
7. Sacks FM, Katan M. Randomized clinical trials on the effects of dietary fat and carbohydrate on plasma lipoproteins and cardiovascular disease. *Am J Med* 2002;113(Suppl 9B): 13S-24S.
8. Ferrucci L, Cherubini A, Bandinelli S, et al. Relationship of plasma polyunsaturated fatty acids to circulating inflammatory markers. *J Clin Endocrinol Metab* 2006;91:439-446.
9. Sacks FM, Campos H. Polyunsaturated fatty acids, inflammation, and cardiovascular disease: time to widen our view of the mechanisms. *J Clin Endocrinol Metab* 2006; 91:398-400.
10. Appel LJ, Sacks FM, Carey V, et al. The effects of protein, fat and carbohydrate intake on blood pressure and serum lipids: results of the OmniHeart Randomized Trial. *JAMA* 2005;294:2455-2464.
11. He J, Gu D, Wu X, et al. Effect of soybean protein on blood pressure. *Ann Intern Med* 2005;143:1-9.
12. Jakobsen MU, O'Reilly EJ, Heitmann BL, et al. Major types of dietary fat and risk of coronary heart disease: a pooled analysis of 11 cohort studies. *Am J Clin Nutr* 2009;89: 1425-1432.
13. Jakobsen MU, Dethlefsen C, Joensen AM, et al. Intake of carbohydrates compared with intake of saturated fatty acids and risk of myocardial infarction: importance of the glycemic index. *Am J Clin Nutr* 2010;91:1764-1768.
14. Appel LJ, Moore TJ, Obarzanek E, et al. The effect of dietary patterns on blood pressure: results from the Dietary Approaches to Stop Hypertension trial. *N Engl J Med* 1997;11: 1117-1124.
15. Sacks FM, Svetkey LP, Vollmer WM, et al. Effects on blood pressure of reduced dietary sodium and the Dietary Approaches to Stop Hypertension (DASH) diet. *N Engl J Med* 2001;344:3-10.
16. Bray GA, Vollmer WM, Sacks FM, et al. A further subgroup analysis of the effects of the DASH diet and three dietary sodium levels on blood pressure: results of the DASH-Sodium Trial. *Am J Cardiol* 2004;94:222-227.
17. Sacks FM, Campos H. Dietary therapy in hypertension. *N Engl J Med* 2010;362:2102-2112.
18. Obarzanek E, Sacks FM, Vollmer WM, et al. Effects on blood lipids of a blood pressure lowering diet: the Dietary Approaches to Stop Hypertension (DASH) Trial. *Am J Clin Nutr* 2001;74:80-89.
19. Ludwig DS. The glycemic index: physiological mechanisms relating to obesity, diabetes, and cardiovascular disease. *JAMA* 2002;287:2414-2423.
20. Mozaffarian D, Appel LJ, Van Horn L. Components of a cardioprotective diet: new insights. *Circulation* 2011;123:2870-2891.

21. Howard BV, Van Horn L, Judith Hsia J, et al. Low-fat dietary pattern and risk of cardiovascular disease: the Women's Health Initiative Randomized Controlled Dietary Modification Trial. *JAMA* 2006;295:655-666.
22. Ornish D, Brown SE, Scherwitz LW, et al. Can lifestyle changes reverse coronary heart disease? The Lifestyle Heart Trial. *Lancet* 1990;336:129-133.
23. Schuler G, Hambrecht R, Schlierf G, et al. Regular physical exercise and low-fat diet: effects on progression of coronary artery disease. *Circulation* 1992;86:1-11.
24. Ascherio A. Epidemiologic studies on dietary fats and coronary heart disease. *Am J Med* 2002;113(Suppl 9B):9S-12S.
25. Siri-Tarino PW, Sun Q, Hu FB, Krauss RM. Meta-analysis of prospective cohort studies evaluating the association of saturated fat with cardiovascular disease. *Am J Clin Nutr* 2010;91:502-509.
26. Micha R, Mozaffarian D. Saturated fat consumption and effects on cardiometabolic risk factors and coronary heart disease, stroke, and diabetes mellitus: a fresh look at the evidence. *Lipids* 2010;45:893-905.
27. Willett WC. *Nutritional epidemiology*, 2nd ed. 1998, New York, Oxford University Press.
28. Mozaffarian D, Micha R, Wallace S. Effects on coronary heart disease of increasing polyunsaturated fat in place of saturated fat: a systematic review and meta-analysis of randomized controlled trials. *PLoS Med* 2010;7:e1000252.
29. de Lorgeril M, Renaud S, Mamelle N, et al. Mediterranean alpha-linolenic acid–rich diet in secondary prevention of coronary heart disease. *Lancet* 1994;343:1454-1459.
30. Baylin A, Kabagambe EK, Ascherio A, Spiegelman D, Campos H. Adipose tissue alpha-linolenic acid and nonfatal acute myocardial infarction in Costa Rica. *Circulation* 2003; 107:1586-1591.
31. Kromhaut D, Giltay EJ, Gelejinse JM; Alpha Omega Trial Group. N-3 fatty acids and cardiovascular events after myocardial infarction. *N Engl J Med* 2010;363:2015-2026.
32. Campos H, Balin A, Willett WC. Alpha-linolenic acid and risk of nonfatal acute myocardial infarction. *Circulation* 2008;118:339-345.
33. Petrova S, Dimitrov P, Willett WC, Campos H. The global availability of n-3 fatty acids. *Public Health Nutr* 2011;31:1-8.
34. Dayton S, Pearce ML, Hashimoto S, et al. A controlled clinical trial of a diet high in unsaturated fat in preventing complications of atherosclerosis. *Circulation* 1969;40 (Suppl II):II1-II63.
35. Leren P. The Olso Diet-Heart Study: eleven-year report. *Circulation* 1970;42:935-942.
36. Turpeinen O, Karvonen MJ, Pekkarinen M, et al. Dietary prevention of coronary heart disease: the Finnish Mental Hospital Study. *Int J Epidemiol* 1979;8:99-118.
37. Controlled trial of soy-bean oil in myocardial infarction. *Lancet* 1968;ii:693-700.
38. Rudel LL, Parks JS, Hedrick CC, et al. Lipoprotein and cholesterol metabolism in diet-induced coronary artery atherosclerosis in primates: role of cholesterol and fatty acids. *Prog Lipid Res* 1998;37:353-370.
39. Kang JX, Leaf A. Effect of long-chain polyunsaturated fatty acids on the contraction of neonatal rat cardiac myocytes. *Proc Natl Acad Sci U S A* 1994;91:9886-9890.
40. Keys A. *Seven countries: a multivariate analysis of death and coronary heart disease*. 1980, Cambridge, MA, Harvard University Press.
41. DeSouza RJ, Swain JF, Appel LJ, Sacks FM. Alternatives for macronutrient intake and chronic disease: a comparison of OmniHeart diets with popular diets and with dietary recommendations. *Am J Clin Nutr* 2008;88:1-11.
42. Swain JF, McCarron PB, Hamilton EF, Sacks FM, Appel LJ. Characteristics of the dietary patterns tested in the Optimal Macronutrient Intake Trial to Prevent Heart Disease (Omni Heart): options for a heart-healthy diet. *J Am Diet Assoc* 2008;108:257-265.
43. Mozaffarian D, Rimm EB. Fish intake, contaminants, and human health: evaluating the risks and the benefits. *JAMA* 2006;296:1885-1899.
44. Leon H, Shibata MC, Sivakumaran S, et al. Effect of fish oil on arrhythmias and mortality: systematic review. *Br Med J* 2008;337:a2931.
45. Wang C, Harris WS, Chung M, et al. n-3 Fatty acids from fish or fish-oil supplements, but not α-linolenic acid, benefit cardiovascular disease outcomes in primary- and secondary-prevention studies: a systematic review. *Am J Clin Nutr* 2006;84:5-17.
46. Burr ML, Fehily AM, Gilbert JF, et al. Effects of changes in fat, fish, and fibre intakes on death and myocardial reinfarction: diet and reinfarction trial (DART). *Lancet* 1989;2: 757-761.
47. GISSI-Prevention Investigators. Dietary supplementation with n-3 polyunsaturated fatty acids and vitamin E after myocardial infarction: results of the GISSI-Prevenzione trial. *Lancet* 1999;354:447-455.
48. Yokoyama M. Effects of eicosapentaenoic acid (EPA) on major cardiovascular events in hypercholesterolemic patients: the Japan EPA Lipid Intervention Study (JELIS). Presented at the American Heart Association Scientific Sessions, November 14, 2005.
49. Raitt MH, Connor WE, Morris C, et al. Fish oil supplementation and risk of ventricular tachycardia and ventricular fibrillation in patients with implantable defibrillators: a randomized controlled trial. *JAMA* 2005;293:2884-2891.
50. Leaf A, Albert CM, Josephson M, et al. Fatty Acid Antiarrhythmia Trial Investigators. Prevention of fatal arrhythmias in high-risk subjects by fish oil n-3 fatty acid intake. *Circulation* 2005;112:2762-2768.
51. Brouwer IA, Raitt MH, Dullemeijer C, et al. Effect of fish oil on ventricular tachyarrhythmia in three studies in patients with implantable cardioverter defibrillators. *Eur Heart J* 2009;30:820-826.
52. Kowey PR, Reiffel JA, Ellenbogen KA, Naccarelli GV, Pratt CM. Efficacy and safety of prescription omega-3 fatty acids for the prevention of recurrent symptomatic atrial fibrillation: a randomized controlled trial. *JAMA* 2010;304:2363-2372.
53. Centers for Disease Control and Prevention. Vital Signs: State-specific Obesity Prevalence among Adults—United States, 2009. *MMWR*. Available at http://www.cdc.gov/mmwr/preview/mmwrhtml/mm59e0803a1.htm#tab.
54. Ogden CL, Carroll MD. Prevalence of Overweight, Obesity, and Extreme Obesity Among Adults: United States, Trends 1976-1980 through 2007-2008. Centers for Disease Control and Prevention Health-E Stats.
55. Finkelstein EA, Trogdon JG, Cohen JW, Dietz W. Annual medical spending attributable to obesity: payer- and service-specific estimates. *Health Aff (Millwood)* 2009;28(5): w822-w831.

56. Sacks FM, Bray GA, Carey VJ, et al. Comparison of weight-loss diets with different compositions of fat, protein, and carbohydrates. *N Engl J Med* 2009;360(9):859-873.

57. Shai I, Schwarzfuchs D, Henkin Y, et al, for the Dietary Intervention Randomized Controlled Trial (DIRECT) Group. Weight loss with a low-carbohydrate, Mediterranean, or low-fat diet. *N Engl J Med* 2008;359:229-241.

58. Foster GD, Wyatt HR, Hill JO, et al. Weight and metabolic outcomes after 2 years on a low-carbohydrate versus low-fat diet: a randomized trial. *Ann Intern Med* 2010;153: 147-157.

59. Wing RR; Look Ahead Research Group. Long-term effects of a lifestyle intervention on weight and cardiovascular risk factors in individuals with type 2 diabetes mellitus: four-year results of the Look Ahead trial. *Arch Intern Med* 2010;170:1566-1575.

60. Mozaffarian D, Hao T, Rimm EB, Willett WC, Hu FB. Changes in diet and lifestyle and long-term weight gain in women and men. *N Engl J Med* 2011;364:2392-2404.

61. Pi-Sunyer FX, et al. Clinical Guidelines on the Identification, Evaluation, and Treatment of Overweight and Obesity in Adults: the Evidence Report. NIH Publication No. 98-4083. Sept 1998, Washington, DC, National Institutes of Health.

62. Prochaska JO, Velicer WF. The transtheoretical model of health behavior change. *Am J Health Promot* 1997;12(1):38-48.

63. Frankenfield D, Roth-Yousey L, Compher C; Evidence Analysis Working Group. Comparison of predictive equations for resting metabolic rate in healthy nonobese and obese adults: a systematic review. *J Am Diet Assoc* 2005;105(5):775-789.

64. Zello GA. Dietary reference intakes for the macronutrients and energy: considerations for physical activity. *Appl Physiol Nutr Metab* 2006;31:74-79.

65. National Heart, Lung, and Blood Institute. Diseases and Conditions Index. What is Physical Activity? Accessed 2011 Apr 25 at www.nhlbi.nih.gov/health/dci/Diseases/phys/phys_what.html.

66. Haskell WL, Lee I, Pate RR, et al. Physical activity and public health: updated recommendations for adults from the American College of Sports Medicine and the American Heart Association. *Med Sci Sports Exerc* 2007;3908:1423-1434.

67. Adapted from activity list accessed 2011 Apr 26 at www.nutristrategy.com/activitylist4.htm.

68. Stampfer MJ, Hu FB, Manson JE, et al. Primary prevention of coronary heart disease in women through diet and lifestyle. *N Engl J Med* 2000;343:16-22.

CARDIOVASCULAR DISEASE AND LIFESTYLE MODIFICATION

Steps Beyond Diet and Drug Therapy for Severe Hypercholesterolemia

Bruce R. Gordon and Lisa Cooper Hudgins

DEFINITION OF THE TARGET POPULATION, 454

DESCRIPTION OF THE PATIENT POPULATION, 454

Homozygous Familial Hypercholesterolemia, 454
Patients with Low-Density Lipoprotein Cholesterol
    Concentrations of More than 200 mg/dL and Coronary
    Artery Disease, 455
Patients with Low-Density Lipoprotein Cholesterol
    Concentrations of More than 300 mg/dL Without Coronary
    Artery Disease, 455

EXTRACORPOREAL THERAPIES FOR THE TREATMENT OF
SEVERE HYPERCHOLESTEROLEMIA, 455

Technical Aspects, 455
Risks of Low-Density Lipoprotein Apheresis, 457
Benefits of Low-Density Lipoprotein Apheresis, 457
Benefits of Low-Density Lipoprotein Apheresis Beyond
    Reducing Low-Density Lipoprotein Concentrations, 458

LOW-DENSITY LIPOPROTEIN APHERESIS: FAILURE TO
TREAT INDIVIDUALS WHO MAY BENEFIT, 458

SURGICAL PROCEDURES, 458

Portacaval Shunt, 458
Liver Transplantation, 459
Partial Ileal Bypass, 460
Gene Therapy, 460

CONCLUSIONS AND RECOMMENDATIONS FOR
THERAPY, 461

REFERENCES, 461

A small subset of patients with hypercholesterolemia have an inadequate lipid-lowering response to maximal diet and drug treatment and should be considered for additional therapy to come as close as possible to the therapeutic targets of the National Cholesterol Education Program (NCEP). The development of new classes of lipid-modifying drugs should increase the number of patients who achieve lipid goals. Most candidates for treatment beyond diet and drugs are patients with familial hypercholesterolemia (FH), including all individuals with homozygous FH and patients with heterozygous FH who do not attain NCEP goals.

Traditional treatment options alone or in combination include plasmapheresis, low-density lipoprotein apheresis (LDLA), portacaval shunt, liver transplantation, and partial ileal bypass (PIB) surgery. Plasmapheresis is a nonspecific extracorporeal procedure that removes all plasma proteins, including high-density lipoprotein (HDL), from the blood. A superior method that specifically lowers LDL cholesterol (LDL-c) in these patients is LDLA. Methods for performing LDLA include dextran sulfate cellulose adsorption, immunoadsorption, heparin-induced extracorporeal precipitation (HELP), and perfusion through whole blood–compatible columns. Time-averaged LDL lowering of 40% to 50% is achieved with weekly or biweekly LDLA therapy. The U.S. Food and Drug Administration (FDA) has approved LDLA for patients who, despite maximal tolerated diet and drug therapy, have an LDL-c concentration greater than 300 mg/dL without coronary artery disease (CAD) or an LDL-c concentration greater than 200 mg/dL with CAD. Systems that use dextran sulfate cellulose adsorption, such as the Liposorber System (Kaneka, Osaka, Japan) and the HELP Plasmat Futura System (B. Braun Medical Inc., Bethlehem, PA), are available in the United States. The gap between FDA-approved LDL-c levels for initiating LDLA and those levels established as clinical LDL-c targets has grown, and newer guidelines target LDL-c levels of 70 mg/dL or less in many individuals with CAD.

Surgical procedures for lowering LDL-c are more invasive than LDLA and should only be considered if LDLA therapy does not provide adequate LDL-c lowering or if it is technically difficult to perform. Portacaval shunts have been used to achieve LDL-c lowering of approximately 40% in patients with homozygous FH, but concerns about long-term hepatic and endocrine complications have limited its usefulness. Liver transplantation can achieve near-normal LDL-c levels but is associated with the need for long-term immunosuppressive therapy. Improvements in surgical techniques and immunosuppressive therapies have made liver transplantation an increasingly attractive option. PIB surgery has slowed the progression of CAD, but it has appreciable morbidity and is not appropriate for patients with homozygous FH. Gene

transfer has been unsuccessfully tested in a small number of patients, and at present it is not a therapeutic option. LDLA is beneficial in patients with refractory hypercholesterolemia and CAD and is the therapy of choice for patients who require treatment beyond diet and drugs. The rapidity of clinical improvement in patients who receive LDLA suggests mechanisms in addition to the regression of plaque. Whole blood–compatible systems for LDLA are simpler than standard LDLA to perform. These systems have been used extensively in Europe but have not been introduced in the United States.

Definition of the Target Population

Because nondietary, nonpharmacologic therapy for hypercholesterolemia entails a major commitment from the patient and medical community, and in some instances substantial risk, clear guidelines for considering such therapy are necessary. All patients should have therapeutic lifestyle changes (TLCs) instituted and should be treated with maximum combination lipid-lowering drug therapy that includes, as tolerated, a 3-hydroxy-3-methylglutaryl coenzyme A (HMG-CoA) reductase inhibitor, a bile acid binder, and nicotinic acid. The usefulness of ezetimibe in this population is less clear, but it has continued to be used for lack of better alternatives. Some patients will also be treated with promising experimental pharmacologic therapies such as mipomersen, an apolipoprotein B (ApoB) antisense drug.[1] Criteria for additional therapy should include the degree of LDL-c elevation and whether the patient has CAD or multiple risk factors for CAD. The FDA has approved LDLA for the management of patients with CAD and LDL-c concentrations of more than 200 mg/dL or patients without CAD but an LDL-c concentration of more than 300 mg/dL. Individuals with extremely high triglyceride concentrations or secondary causes of hypercholesterolemia are generally not candidates for the therapies described in this chapter.

Description of the Patient Population

Homozygous Familial Hypercholesterolemia

The clearest indication for nondietary, nondrug therapy is in patients with homozygous FH. The classic form of this disorder is caused by the inheritance of two mutant genes at the LDL receptor locus. The clinical expression for classical homozygous FH occurs in approximately 1 person in 1 million. The defect in LDL receptor function causes a marked elevation in the plasma concentration of LDL-c, which typically exceeds 500 mg/dL but can reach as high as 1000 mg/dL.[2] HDL cholesterol (HDL-c) concentrations tend to be substantially below normal. Clinical features include the presence of xanthomas, severe aortic root disease that includes aortic stenosis, and the premature onset of CAD. Angina pectoris, myocardial infarction (MI), or sudden death frequently occurs between the ages of 5 and 20 years. Mabuchi and colleagues[3] followed 10 patients with homozygous FH for a period of approximately 14 years. During that time, 6 of the patients died from sudden death or heart failure at an average age of 26 years. Similar observations were reported in patients from South Africa.[4]

The severity of the clinical expression depends to a great extent on the percentage of functioning LDL receptors. In the study by Goldstein and Brown[5] of 57 homozygotes, more than one fourth of receptor-absent patients died before the age of 25 years compared with 1 of 26 individuals with residual LDL receptor activity. Because of the very high risk of premature CAD and the poor response to diet and drug therapy, all patients with homozygous FH require alternative therapy. It is possible that some individuals who phenotypically appear to have homozygous FH have one gene expressing a defective ApoB that will result in decreased clearance of LDL-c.

Patients with Low-Density Lipoprotein Cholesterol Concentrations of More than 200 mg/dL and Coronary Artery Disease

The majority of patients in this group will have the heterozygous form of FH. This disorder has a prevalence of approximately 1 in 500 persons and is typically manifested by the occurrence of premature CAD by the fifth decade for men and the sixth decade for women. Clinically similar syndromes are produced by defects in the LDL receptor and defective ApoB structure with impaired receptor binding. The presence of both CAD and elevated LDL-c concentrations greatly increases the risk of subsequent coronary events; therefore patients with CAD require intensive LDL-c concentration control. The reinfarction rate found in seven secondary prevention trials reviewed by Pekkanen and colleagues[6] was approximately 6% annually compared with a 1% to 2% rate of first infarction in four primary prevention trials. Trials in patients with marked hypercholesterolemia[7,8] have reported regression or a lower rate of progression of coronary lesions when the elevated LDL-c concentration is lowered with diet and drugs. Coupled with the impressive results from the trials that used the statins, a very persuasive case can be made for the aggressive treatment of subjects with FH to achieve LDL-c targets set forth by the NCEP.

Patients with Low-Density Lipoprotein Cholesterol Concentrations of More than 300 mg/dL Without Coronary Artery Disease

The decision whether to use nondietary, nondrug therapy for primary prevention in asymptomatic adults is never as easy as it is in homozygotes. The risk of premature CAD is most apparent in patients with FH because of the presence of lifelong elevated LDL-c concentrations. In addition, the presence of risk factors other than LDL-c helps determine which patients are most likely to develop CAD. For example, a lipoprotein A [Lp(a)] concentration of more than 20 mg/dL has been recognized as an independent risk factor in patients with FH.[9,10] The use of noninvasive screening procedures for CAD, such as quantitation of coronary artery calcium, provides additional guidance for determining whether patients with elevated LDL-c will develop clinically significant disease.[11]

Based on current FDA guidelines, it is reasonable to consider nondietary, nondrug therapy for primary prevention in patients with an LDL-c concentration of more than 300 mg/dL despite diet and maximal tolerated lipid-lowering drug therapy.

Extracorporeal Therapies for the Treatment of Severe Hypercholesterolemia

The first report of plasma exchange for FH was published by de Gennes and colleagues[12] in 1967. In 1975 Thompson and colleagues[13] described the use of plasmapheresis with an automated cell separator to treat patients with homozygous FH. Plasmapheresis therapy has been shown to improve the survival of treated homozygotes compared with their untreated control siblings.[14]

The nonselectivity of plasmapheresis led to the development of LDLA for the specific removal of ApoB-containing lipoproteins from the blood. The use and clinical acceptance of the procedure have increased worldwide, including approval in 1996 by the FDA, and it is most useful in patients who respond incompletely to diet and lipid-lowering drug therapy because of drug intolerance or extremely high baseline LDL-c concentrations. The specific removal of ApoB-containing lipoproteins using heparin agarose beads was first described in 1976 by Lupien and colleagues.[15] Methods for performing LDLA include HELP[16] columns that contain immobilized antibodies to LDL,[17] and columns that contain dextran sulfate cellulose.[18,19] Whole blood–compatible systems that use columns containing either a modified polyacrylate gel (DALI System; Fresenius AG, St. Wendel, Germany)[20] or dextran sulfate (Liposorber-D, Kaneka)[21] single- or double-column technologies have been developed and are available outside the United States.

LDLA will lower both LDL-c and Lp(a). An immunoadsorption system has been developed that specifically targets Lp(a) for patients in whom elevated Lp(a) is the primary problem, but it is not widely available.

Technical Aspects

Fortunately, venous access from an antecubital fossa vein is most often sufficient for LDLA because of the lower blood flow rates required (50 to 100 mL/min) compared with hemodialysis (400 mL/min). If access from antecubital fossa veins provides insufficient blood flow, the placement of a catheter, fistula, or graft may be necessary.

Some form of anticoagulation is necessary for all extracorporeal procedures. Heparin and acid citrate dextrose (ACD) are the anticoagulants most commonly used in extracorporeal therapies. Heparin is typically used for extracorporeal procedures that involve a membrane to separate whole blood into plasma and cells or in the whole blood–compatible system. Typically, a heparin bolus of approximately 30 to 60 U/kg is administered, followed by a continuous infusion of approximately 1000 U/h. ACD has the advantage of rapid metabolism and produces little residual effect after the procedure. Side effects as a result of ACD administration include symptoms of hypocalcemia, which may include perioral tingling, hypotension, or, very rarely, tetany.

Most forms of LDLA require the separation of blood into cells and plasma before the plasma is processed to specifically remove ApoB-containing lipoproteins. Whole blood–compatible systems use direct adsorption of lipoproteins on columns and thereby eliminate the requirement for cell separation. For systems that require cell separation, either a membrane or centrifuge is used to separate blood into plasma and cellular elements. Membrane separation of blood is simpler and requires less extracorporeal volume, but it is less efficient than centrifugal techniques.

Most patients are treated with LDLA at a treatment frequency of approximately every 2 weeks. This is based on the rebound of the LDL-c and on the observation that most patients prefer to be treated no more often than every other week. At a treatment frequency of every 2 weeks, reduction in pretreatment LDL-c level is usually stepwise until a new plateau is reached.

Cholesterol reduction can be quantified by measuring the achievement using either acute or time-averaged lowering (Figure

456

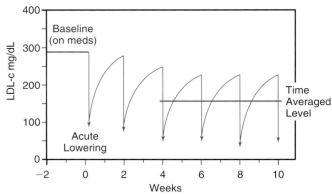

FIGURE 27-1 Acute and time-averaged lowering of low-density lipoprotein cholesterol (*LDL-c*) for LDL apheresis treatments. The acute lowering is the difference in pretreatment and posttreatment levels as a percentage of the pretreatment level. The time-averaged level is determined by measuring a "rebound" following a treatment.

27-1). The acute lowering is the difference between preprocedure and postprocedure lipid values as a percent of the initial value and is a function of the amount of plasma or blood processed during a single treatment. LDLA procedures process 1.5 to 2.0 plasma or blood volumes and reduce LDL-c concentrations short term by 70% to 80%. For a blood flow of 50 to 80 mL/min, it takes about 3 hours to process 1.5 to 2.0 plasma or blood volumes.

Although acute lowering is helpful in determining treatment efficiency, the time-averaged lipid value is a better indicator of the lipid concentration to which the patient's arteries are exposed over an extended period. The time-averaged lowering is related to the treatment frequency and rate of rebound. The time-averaged lipid value is estimated by the formula 0.73 (pre–LDL-c − post–LDL-c) plus post LDL-c, or it can be directly determined by measuring LDL-c daily after a treatment. The time-averaged LDL-c lowering is usually between 40% and 50%.

LDLA has been reported to maintain or increase HDL-c concentrations over time.[22] The mechanism for this effect is unknown, but the increase in HDL-c is seen most frequently in subjects with homozygous FH. In contrast, plasmapheresis lowers HDL-c through nonspecific depletion of all plasma constituents including HDL-c.

LOW-DENSITY LIPOPROTEIN APHERESIS USING DEXTRAN SULFATE CELLULOSE COLUMNS

Dextran sulfate cellulose selectively binds ApoB-containing lipoproteins on the basis of a charge attraction. Dextran sulfate cellulose columns were initially provided by the manufacturer as single, large-volume, nonregenerable columns that could be attached to any cell separator. Limited LDL-binding capacity resulted in the development of dual regenerable columns in a system that included a hollow-fiber primary cell separator (Figure 27-2). Plasma is alternately perfused through each 150-mL column, permitting the regeneration of the off-line column with hypertonic sodium chloride solution; a computerized unit controls the process. After passing through the adsorbent column, the plasma is recombined with the cells and returned to the patient. The advantage of this system is the almost unlimited LDL-binding capacity as a result of the on-line regeneration of the columns. The columns are discarded after each treatment.

LOW-DENSITY LIPOPROTEIN APHERESIS USING IMMUNOADSORPTION COLUMNS

Immunoadsorption for the performance of LDLA has been used to treat patients for approximately 25 years. Polyclonal monospecific or monoclonal antibodies to ApoB are immobilized on a support, typically sepharose beads, and are packed into glass

Dextran Sulfate Cellulose and Immunoadsorption Systems

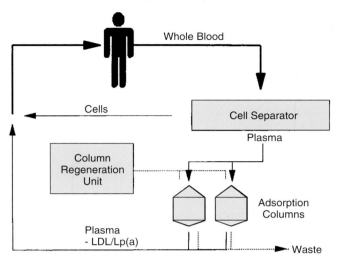

FIGURE 27-2 Schematic representation of dextran sulfate cellulose and immunoadsorption low-density lipoprotein (*LDL*) apheresis systems. Lp(a), lipoprotein A.

columns. Each patient has two columns, which are reused during each procedure and reused from one procedure to the next because of the expense. Online regeneration of the columns is controlled by a column regeneration unit (see Figure 27-2). Typically, the columns are eluted with an acid solution, neutralized with a buffer solution, and then rinsed with saline. The procedure requires storage of the columns between treatments. All ApoB-containing lipoproteins are removed: LDL, very-low-density lipoprotein (VLDL), and Lp(a). Because the columns are reused multiple times, they must be monitored for loss of activity that may occur after several months. In addition, sensitization of the patient to small quantities of shed antibody has been demonstrated.[23] Because of the cumbersome requirement of storing columns between uses, immunoadsorption LDLA is used less commonly than the other methods described in this chapter. A variant of this technique primarily removes circulating Lp(a) for patients in whom elevated Lp(a) levels are thought to be the primary problem.

LOW-DENSITY LIPOPROTEIN APHERESIS USING HEPARIN-INDUCED EXTRACORPOREAL LOW-DENSITY LIPOPROTEIN PRECIPITATION

HELP LDLA specifically removes LDL, VLDL, and Lp(a) while minimally affecting HDL. HELP differs from other procedures in that it removes a substantial quantity of fibrinogen. The technique is based on the precipitation of positively charged LDL and other β-lipoproteins when heparin is added at a pH just above 5.0 (Figure 27-3). A few other plasma proteins precipitate to some extent with heparin, most notably fibrinogen. An anion exchange column removes excess heparin, and the plasma is treated with bicarbonate dialysis and ultrafiltration to return the pH to normal and remove excess fluid. The entire process is controlled by a microprocessor.

LOW-DENSITY LIPOPROTEIN APHERESIS USING WHOLE BLOOD–COMPATIBLE SYSTEMS

Potential cost savings and simplicity of use make a whole blood–compatible system very attractive for the performance of LDLA. Two systems are most commonly used: the DALI System and Liposorber-D (Figure 27-4). A comparison between the whole blood–compatible systems and classic techniques for performing

HELP System

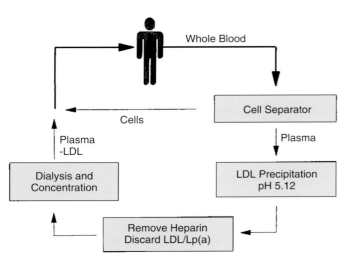

LDL Apheresis Using the DALI or Liposorber-D Systems

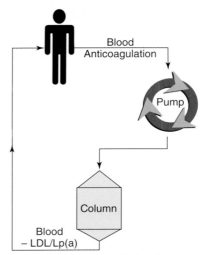

FIGURE 27-3 Schematic representation of the heparin-induced extracorporeal low-density lipoprotein (*LDL*) precipitation (*HELP*) apheresis system. Lp(a), lipoprotein A.

FIGURE 27-4 Schematic representation of whole-blood low-density lipoprotein (*LDL*) apheresis. Lp(a), lipoprotein A.

FACTOR	DALI	LIPOSORBER-D	LIPOSORBER	IMMUNOADSORPTION	HELP
Setup time (approximate)	30 min	30 min	60 min	60 min	60 min
Reusable	No	No	No	Yes	No
Plasma/blood	Whole blood	Whole blood	Plasma	Plasma	Plasma
Principle	Polyacrylate	Dextran sulfate	Dextran sulfate	Antibodies	Heparin precipitation

TABLE 27-1 Comparison of LDL Apheresis Methods

DALI, direct adsorption of lipoproteins; Liposorber-D, dextran sulfate–based whole-blood perfusion system; Liposorber, dextran sulfate cellulose column–based system; Immunoadsorption, low-density lipoprotein (LDL) apheresis using columns containing immobilized antibodies on a support; HELP, heparin-induced extracorporeal precipitation.

LDLA is shown in Table 27-1. The DALI system uses a modified polyacrylate gel immobilized on a solid support. The mechanism of ApoB binding is an electrostatic interaction between the positive charges of the ApoB and the negatively charged carbohydrate moieties on the polyanionic gel. The Liposorber-D system is based on binding of ApoB-containing lipoproteins to dextran sulfate. The matrix has been modified to permit the safe interaction between whole blood and the column.

The initial two-center study of the DALI procedure[20] reported on 12 hypercholesterolemic patients treated once each with columns containing 480 mL polyacrylate gel. No side effects were observed. A follow-up study reported the use of this technology in the therapy of three hypercholesterolemic subjects with atherosclerosis.[24] The acute reduction in lipids was 66% for LDL-c, 63% for Lp(a), and 29% for triglycerides. HDL and fibrinogen were lowered minimally. No clinically significant adverse events occurred, and the changes in biochemical and hematologic parameters were minor. The authors noted that the setup time for the procedure was only 30 minutes as opposed to 1 hour or more for other forms of LDLA. The clinical experience in 10 subjects treated with the Liposorber D system[21] demonstrated an LDL cholesterol reduction of 62%. No significant side effects were observed. Recently a whole blood, dual-column system has been tested[25] and was found better able to lower LDL-c acutely compared with the single-column technique (79.7% vs. 68.2%).

Risks of Low-Density Lipoprotein Apheresis

Adverse reactions as a result of LDLA have been few. The extracorporeal volume is well tolerated even in patients with severe CAD

and in children as young as 3 years.[26] Hypotension requiring infusion of saline occurs in less than 5% of treatments, and unusual side effects include angina, hemolysis, and allergic or anaphylactic reactions. In immunoadsorption treatments, possible causes of adverse reactions include complement activation and sensitization of the patient to column constituents. An anaphylactoid reaction during dextran sulfate LDLA has been described in patients taking angiotensin-converting enzyme (ACE) inhibitors.[27] The mechanism is related to release of bradykinin during LDLA with concomitant decreased degradation of kinins by ACE inhibitors. The DALI system also activates the kallikrein-kinin system. The best approach is to switch patients from ACE inhibitors to angiotensin II receptor–blocking drugs before the initiation of LDLA. Treatments with immunoadsorption LDLA or the HELP system are not associated with this clinical problem. For systems utilizing whole blood–compatible columns, the long-term effects of whole blood interactions with the column, such as cell activation, are unknown.

Benefits of Low-Density Lipoprotein Apheresis

Regression of tendon xanthoma and improvement in CAD have been demonstrated in patients with severe hypercholesterolemia when the LDL-c concentration is lowered through LDLA protocols. In the LDL Apheresis Regression Study (LARS),[28] angiographic evidence for regression of CAD was observed in 10 of 30 patients treated with LDLA and lipid-lowering drugs despite a baseline LDL concentration of 311 mg/dL. The HELP-LDL Apheresis Multicenter Study[29] was a 2-year investigation in 51 patients treated with weekly LDLA and lipid-lowering drugs. Computer-assisted analysis of paired angiograms from 33 evaluable patients revealed that 23 patients had regression, 1 had little change, and 9 patients had progression. The German Multicenter LDL Apheresis Trial[30] was a four-center, 3-year prospective trial of 32 patients with FH. All patients who had symptomatic CAD demonstrated improvements in their symptoms by the end of the study. Improvement in electro-cardiographic (ECG) stress testing was demonstrated in 17 patients. Analysis of the paired angiograms did not reveal regression of disease, although definite progression of disease was observed in only five patients over 3 years.

An important study was the LDL-Apheresis Atherosclerosis Regression Study (LAARS), a prospective 2-year, randomized, single-center study in men with hypercholesterolemia and CAD.[31] This trial demonstrated that the addition of biweekly LDLA to treatment with simvastatin improved regional myocardial perfusion and decreased myocardial ischemia; it is interesting to note that little change was seen in the coronary angiograms. Peripheral vascular disease was also found to improve in LAARS, as shown by standardized techniques including B-mode ultrasound.

Studies using intravascular ultrasound demonstrate that the angiogram may miss changes that occur in the blood vessel wall rather than in the blood vessel lumen. The Low-Density Lipoprotein-Apheresis Coronary Morphology and Reserve Trial (LACMART) used intravascular ultrasound to compare change in coronary artery disease in 18 patients with FH randomized to 1 year of either drug therapy or LDLA combined with drug therapy.[32] Favorable changes in coronary artery minimal luminal diameter and plaque burden were observed in subjects who received LDLA plus drug compared with subjects receiving drug alone. LDLA with the Liposorber system decreased the rate of restenosis in patients with elevated Lp(a) concentrations who had undergone coronary angioplasty.[33]

A multicenter study in the United States demonstrated the ability of LDLA to decrease the number of clinical events in patients with CAD.[34] The rate of clinical events per 1000 patient-months decreased from 9.14 for the 5-year period before the initiation of LDLA to 4.72 during the LDLA period (P = .037). An analysis of data from the U.S. LDLA Registry, established at the time of FDA approval of LDLA, confirmed the decrease in clinical events in a larger number of patients. In 1998, Mabuchi and colleagues[35] reported long-term outcome data in a study of 130 heterozygous FH patients with CAD, in which LDLA combined with drug therapy produced a reduction in coronary events during a 6-year period. The rate of coronary events in the LDLA-plus-drug group (n = 87) was 10% compared with 36% in the drug-alone group (n = 43).

Benefits of Low-Density Lipoprotein Apheresis Beyond Reducing Low-Density Lipoprotein Concentrations

The rapidity of clinical responses in some patients receiving LDLA has suggested effects in addition to LDL lowering and regression of plaque. Several mechanisms may contribute to this observation, including decreased blood viscosity with improved blood rheology[36] and downregulation of leukocyte and endothelial adhesion molecules.[37] Tamai and colleagues[38] measured forearm blood flow while infusing acetylcholine before and after a single LDLA treatment and found that vasodilation responses were significantly augmented. The reductions in LDL and oxidized LDL correlated with the increase in acetylcholine-induced vasodilation.

Low-Density Lipoprotein Apheresis: Failure to Treat Individuals Who May Benefit

In the United States, LDLA is available at roughly 70 centers that treat approximately 325 patients—a fraction of the eligible patient

population. Reasons for lack of penetration for this therapy include its complexity, cost, and time commitment. It is hoped that efforts to establish a registry for patients with FH will help solve this problem.

Surgical Procedures
Portacaval Shunt

In 1963 a portacaval diversion was used to treat a child with a glycogen storage disease.[39] The observation by Starzl and colleagues that the hyperlipidemia in patients with glycogen storage disease was improved by portacaval shunting[40] provided the basis for using the procedure, starting in 1973, to treat severe forms of hypercholesterolemia.[41] The majority of reported cases were in patients who had homozygous FH[42-44] with a few cases of severe heterozygous FH also reported.

TECHNIQUE

With the exception of the earliest procedures, all patients received end-to-side portacaval anastomoses, in which the portal vein is severed and connected with sutures to the suprarenal inferior vena cava, causing portal blood to completely bypass the liver (Figure 27-5). The liver retains arterial flow through the hepatic artery.

CHOLESTEROL LOWERING

Table 27-2 shows the consistent and substantial total cholesterol and LDL-c lowering in 17 LDL-receptor–negative patients. Nine were from Starzl's series[43] and eight were treated at our center, four of whom had shunt surgery at the University of Pittsburgh and metabolic studies at the Rockefeller University. All but one patient showed at least a 25% reduction. The cholesterol level plateaued at about 6 months and was sustained in all patients for the period of follow-up (4 months to 27 years), with no evidence of shunt closure. The HDL concentrations increased in every subject in our series (average, 36%) but had a more variable response in Starzl's series. Triglyceride concentrations, usually normal in this disease, decreased in all subjects except one. Two patients with heterozygous FH reported by Starzl and colleagues[43] had a similar lipid response to portacaval shunting. Less successful lowering was

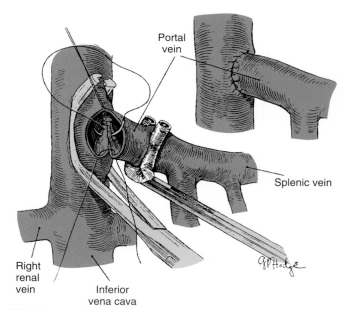

FIGURE 27-5 End-to-side portacaval shunt. (From Zuidema GD, Cameron JL, Zeppa R. Portal hypertension. In Nora PF, editor: Operative surgery: principles and techniques. 1980, Philadelphia, Lea & Febiger, p 694.)

TABLE 27-2	Effect of Portacaval Shunt Surgery on Lipid Profiles in Familial Homozygous Hypercholesterolemia			
	Average % Change (Range)			
	STARZL		**ROGOSIN INSTITUTE**	
Total cholesterol	−37	(−23 to −55)	−42	(−31 to −50)
LDL cholesterol	−36	(−21 to −44)	−43	(−36 to −50)
HDL cholesterol	−22	(−66 to +26)	+36	(+15 to +50)
Triglycerides	−19	(−63 to +80)	−35	(−12 to −63)

Data were obtained from 17 LDL receptor–negative patients before and at least 4 months after shunting, performed at ages 2 through 21 years; 9 patients were reported in Starzl TE, Chase HP, Ahrens EH Jr, et al. Portacaval shunt in patients with familial hypercholesterolemia. *Ann Surg* 1983;198:273-283, data from 8 patients are from our unpublished observations. HDL, high-density lipoprotein; LDL, low-density lipoprotein.

TABLE 27-3	Summary of Liver and Heart-Liver Transplantation for the Treatment of Homozygous Familial Hypercholesterolemia		
		LIVER TRANSPLANT	**HEART-LIVER TRANSPLANT**
Number of subjects		28	6
Date of surgery		1985 to 2011	1984 to 1996
Age at surgery (y)		1 to 21	6 to 46
Length of follow-up (y)		0.1 to 18	0.5 to 9
Preoperative cholesterol (mg/dL)		480 to 1170	700 to 1160
Follow-up cholesterol (mg/dL)		98 to 196	174 to 221
Number of deaths		1 at 2 years	3 at 1 month and 4 at 7 years
Number with retransplants		2	2
Number on statin therapy		8	2

Data from references 50 to 71 and unpublished data of four patients from the Rogosin Institute. Includes four patients with prior ileal bypass or portacaval shunt surgery or both. Follow-up cholesterol data exclude four patients with heterozygote living-related donors.

reported when the shunt was not fully patent, or when collateral vessels were not completely tied off at the time of surgery.[44]

The hypocholesterolemic effect is coincidental with a marked decrease in cholesterol, bile acid, and LDL ApoB synthesis and a decrease in cholesterol pool size.[45,46] Exogenous cholesterol absorption remains unchanged. In a 21-year-old receptor-negative homozygote patient, a liver biopsy 3 months after portacaval shunt revealed a marked decrease in the size of the hepatocytes, content of lipid and glycogen, and of both rough and smooth endoplasmic reticula.[47] HMG-CoA reductase activity was decreased by 56%, and receptor-independent binding of LDL was significantly increased. These changes in the liver after a portacaval shunt have been attributed to loss of the first pass of portal blood containing high concentrations of hepatotropic substances, with the most important being insulin.[41] However, many other synthetic functions of the liver, including the production of albumin, are unaffected.

RISKS AND BENEFITS

Portacaval shunt surgery is generally well tolerated even in patients with symptomatic cardiac disease. The patient is typically discharged 3 to 4 days after surgery, with a single surgical follow-up visit 2 weeks later. In two of the larger series combined, one perioperative death occurred among 25 patients, most of whom had valvular or coronary disease at the time of surgery.[43,44] An NIH-sponsored registry of 45 shunted hypercholesterolemic patients reported three deaths within 30 days of surgery.[42]

The most feared adverse effect of the shunt is encephalopathy and intellectual deterioration; however, except for a single reported case of a brief period of coma 9 months after surgery in a 2-year-old child, no encephalopathy has been reported.[42-44] At our center, an adult heterozygote and four prepubertal homozygotes tested before and 1.5 to 2.5 years after surgery showed no changes in electroencephalogram, intelligence quotient, and other psychologic parameters. One underwent portacaval shunt surgery at age 4 years and is now a fully employed, healthy, 30-year-old college graduate. Another died suddenly at age 9 years of an MI 4.5 years after shunt surgery. At autopsy, he had mild cerebroventricular dilation and slightly thickened leptomeninges but no astrocyte proliferation or other changes typical of hepatic encephalopathy.

For the follow-up periods reported, generally longer than 5 years, no evidence of progressive hepatic dysfunction has been found. However, mildly elevated serum levels of liver enzymes and ammonia may occur[43] along with slight prolongations of prothrombin time and partial thromboplastin time. The acceleration in linear growth in children after shunting, previously attributed to improved health,[43] may be due to alterations in sex hormones. Two of our shunted prepubertal male patients had rapid growth, accelerated bone age, and increased serum testosterone; one female patient developed amenorrhea, high testosterone and insulin

levels, ovarian cysts, and other characteristics of the polycystic ovary syndrome. Menstrual irregularities and increased serum testosterone have been reported after portacaval shunt in postmenarchal females, although a survey of pituitary and thyroid function, including testosterone before and 4 to 6 months after surgery, did not show changes.[48] Clearly, the long-term effects of portacaval shunt surgery on liver function, growth, and sexual maturation need to be much better defined.

The follow-up of patients undergoing portacaval shunting has demonstrated that xanthomas regress and cardiac disease can improve. Starzl and colleagues[43] reported two cases of improved aortic stenosis 13 and 16 months after surgery, respectively. Coronary angiography in seven patients performed 7 months to 7 years after the procedure suggested improvement in one patient and disease stabilization in four.[43,49] However, coronary disease often progresses unless this surgery is combined with LDLA to sufficiently lower LDL-c.

TREATMENT GUIDELINES

Because of the uncertain long-term hepatic and endocrine effects, portacaval shunt surgery should be reserved as adjunct therapy to LDLA in patients with elevated LDL-c levels and significant cardiovascular disease. Portacaval shunt surgery is also an option for young children with significant valvular or coronary disease, or both, who are not large enough for treatment with LDLA and are not candidates for liver transplantation. The surgery should be performed before major clinical deterioration, at a time when the benefits of the surgery outweigh the risks of the operative procedure.

Liver Transplantation

The first liver transplantation for homozygous FH was performed in a 6-year-old patient by Starzl in 1984.[50] Because of diffuse coronary atherosclerosis, heart transplantation was performed at the same time. Table 27-3 summarizes the results for six homozygous FH patients treated with combined heart-liver transplants (ages 6 to 46 years) and for 28 patients with liver-only transplants (ages 1 to 21 years).[50-71] This includes four of our patients who were transplanted at ages that ranged from 3 to 18 years. The longest reported follow-up has been 9 years after combined heart-liver transplant[50] and 18 years after liver-only transplant (personal communication)[52]; 12 patients were followed up for at least 4 years. Four patients previously had ileal bypass surgery or portacaval shunts, or both, which made the liver transplant surgery more technically difficult.[53,54] Eight patients aged 1 to 15 years had normal coronary and aortic valves at the time of liver transplantation and were well 6 months to 6 years later.[55-58,65,68,70] Four of these young patients each received a transplant from a heterozygote parent and thus required statin therapy to lower LDL into the normal range. Statin therapy was continued after transplantation in four other patients with cardiac disease, including three siblings,[56,58,71] and ezetimibe was used in one.[66]

CHOLESTEROL LOWERING

After liver transplantation, most homozygous FH patients meet or exceed NCEP guidelines (total cholesterol, <225 mg/dL) within a few weeks. These excellent results were sustained over time and occurred despite treatment with steroids, cyclosporine, and other immunosuppressant agents that can increase lipid concentrations. After transplant, Lp(a) has also been reported to decrease[59] and HDL-c may increase.

RISKS AND BENEFITS

Of the six homozygous FH patients receiving heart and liver transplants, one died within 1 month of surgery after repeat heart-liver transplantation,[53] another died 4 years later from noncompliance with immunotherapy (personal communication),[55] and a third died 7 years later, probably as a result of chronic rejection of the heart.[60] Of the 28 patients with liver-only transplants, one death occurred from MI 2 years after surgery.[61] Four patients required another liver transplant because of infectious hepatitis, hepatic artery thrombosis, chronic hepatic rejection, or MI. One 13-year-old patient had an MI immediately after liver transplant surgery and required coronary artery bypass grafting.[62] One patient with coronary artery stenosis at transplant required two stent placements 1 and 2 years after transplantation and kidney transplantation for renal failure because of possible tacrolimus toxicity.[67] The benefits for the vascular system have not been systematically documented, although five reports documented the absence of progression[55,59,62] and regression.[63,66] Growth and development occurred normally.

TREATMENT GUIDELINES

For the treatment of some homozygous FH patients, the benefits of the sizable and sustained reduction in the level of LDL-c may outweigh the risks of transplant surgery, chronic rejection, and immunosuppressive therapy. The general outcome from liver transplantation continues to improve, with the most recent 5-year survival in the pediatric age group near 90% overall and higher for those with metabolic liver disorders.[72] However, in practical terms, liver transplantation may not be a treatment option because waiting lists may be long for cadaver livers, and many family members, including parents, have partial defects of the LDL receptor and therefore are not optimal liver donors. Until more information becomes available on the long-term health of liver transplant recipients, liver transplantation should be reserved for the homozygous FH patient with established cardiovascular disease or evidence of progression despite maximum treatment with LDLA and drugs.

It is important to note that the liver transplant surgery should be performed before the vascular or valvular disease progresses to an unstable state. In the case of life-threatening heart failure, liver and heart transplantation can be combined, but not without increased surgical complications and mortality risk.

Partial Ileal Bypass

In 1963, the PIB surgical procedure was introduced for the management of hypercholesterolemia,[73] and today more than 600 PIB procedures have been performed for this purpose.[74,75] The procedure lowers serum cholesterol by increasing the fecal loss of cholesterol and bile acids. A reduction in the absorption of cholesterol and bile acids stimulates an increase in hepatic cholesterol synthesis, but it also stimulates LDL receptor expression and the hepatic conversion of cholesterol to replenish the depleted bile acid reservoir.[76] Its use has been best evaluated in patients with heterozygous FH, and the lack of LDL receptors in homozygous FH may explain the minimal clinical response to PIB in this disorder.[77,78]

TECHNIQUE

The PIB operation for lowering cholesterol bypasses the distal 200 cm or the distal third of the small intestine, whichever is greater. The ileum is divided, the proximal segment is anastomosed to the side of the cecum, and the closed distal segment is tacked to the cecum. This procedure is different from the procedure for weight loss, which includes a more extensive 90% jejunal-ileal bypass.

CHOLESTEROL LOWERING

The Program on the Surgical Control of the Hyperlipidemias (POSCH)[74,79,80] randomized 421 middle-aged survivors of MI with an LDL-c of at least 140 mg/dL to cholesterol-lowering therapy with PIB. The study began in 1975, before the general availability of HMG-CoA reductase inhibitors. At 5 years, surgery resulted in a 23% decrease in total cholesterol, a 38% decrease in LDL-c, a 4% increase in HDL-c, and a 20% increase in triglycerides. The responses were generally sustained for as long as surgical bypass was maintained, up to 20 years, and synergy with statins has been reported.[75]

RISKS AND BENEFITS

The operative and perioperative mortality rates are extremely low in PIB surgery, and the principal side effect is more frequent and looser stools. During the first 5 years of follow-up, 6% to 8% of the surgically treated patients in the POSCH trial reported watery or frothy stools compared with 0% to 1% of control subjects. The average weight loss was 5.3 kg. Of PIB patients, 13.5% had at least one symptom of bowel obstruction (the majority occurred within the first year), but only 3.6% required surgical intervention. Surgically treated patients had a higher incidence of kidney stones (4% vs. 0.7% per year) and gallstones (17% vs. 5%). Twenty-three (6%) of the POSCH patients underwent reversal of surgery between 2 and 11 years after surgery, usually because of diarrhea.

The POSCH trial demonstrated that lipid lowering by PIB resulted in less progression and regression of coronary and peripheral vascular atherosclerosis compared with controls at 3, 5, 7, and 10 years after surgery.[79] Overall mortality rate was reduced by 20% at 18 years of follow-up,[80] and no increase in colorectal cancer was reported.

Gene Therapy

Progress in molecular biology has provided hope for fixing the basic error in patients with severe FH through a technique called *gene transfer*. In a single therapeutic trial, liver tissue from five patients, aged 7 to 41 years, with homozygous FH was harvested; the normal LDL receptor gene was transduced with a recombinant retrovirus into the cells, and the hepatocytes were reinfused into each patient through the mesenteric vein.[81] At 4 months a liver biopsy and in situ hybridization using an RNA probe specific for the recombinant-derived LDL receptor transcript revealed relatively few hepatocytes containing the transgene. In addition, only two of five subjects showed significant reductions in LDL-c (19% and 23%, respectively).

Although this attempt demonstrated the feasibility of correcting the LDL receptor abnormality in a limited number of hepatocytes, it was clear that better methods of gene therapy were necessary to correct this disorder. More appealing is intravenous delivery of the gene targeted specifically to the intact liver. To be effective, normal genes must be incorporated into hepatocytes at physiologic levels for a prolonged period and without immunorejection. Fortunately, other viral vectors and nonviral approaches for gene transfer may be applicable.[82] Marked and sustained reduction in LDL-c and atherosclerosis has been recently achieved in LDL receptor–deficient mice injected intravenously with novel, less immunogenic, liver-specific viral vectors, such as adeno-associated virus 8,[83] lentivirus,[84] and a helper-dependent adenovirus depleted of immunogenic viral genes.[85]

Conclusions and Recommendations for Therapy

The treatment of patients with hypercholesterolemia who respond inadequately to diet and lipid-lowering drug therapy remains a challenge. Patients with homozygous FH are the clearest candidates for additional therapy because of their poor response to standard treatments. LDLA has been the most commonly used treatment modality and is the safest alternative; this therapy should be initiated as early as possible. Generally an age of 3 years or a body weight of 15 kg is the lower limit because of difficulties with vascular access and the approximate 200 mL of blood in the extracorporeal circuit. An additional 10% to 20% cholesterol lowering can be achieved with the addition of a statin and ezetimibe. Liver transplantation, or combined heart-liver transplantation when heart function is severely impaired, should be considered if LDLA plus medication is technically difficult or inadequate at controlling the LDL-c concentration and progression of atherosclerosis. Liver transplant is often limited by donor availability, and when it is unfeasible or unacceptable, combination therapy with portacaval shunting, LDLA, and medication may lower LDL-c sufficiently to prevent progression of atherosclerosis. Plasmapheresis is an alternative when LDLA is not available. Gene therapy is not in use in clinical trials at present but is in active study in animal models.

The most frequent indication for LDLA is in the adult patient with heterozygous FH who has CAD and LDL-c concentrations higher than 200 mg/dL despite maximal diet and drug therapy. The use of nondietary, nonpharmacologic therapy as primary prevention in heterozygous patients without CAD but with LDL-c concentrations of more than 300 mg/dL, and who are inadequately responsive to standard measures, is more problematic. The standard risk factors should be used to segregate a small subset of individuals at the highest risk for the development of atherosclerosis in whom additional therapy is reasonable. The best alternative is LDLA, but if this is not possible, PIB is also an option. Particularly for these patients, the decision to provide these therapies must be individualized.

REFERENCES

1. Raal FJ, Santos RD, Blom DJ, et al. Mipomersen, an apolipoprotein B synthesis inhibitor, for lowering of LDL cholesterol concentrations in patients with homozygous familial hypercholesterolaemia: a randomised, double-blind, placebo-controlled trial. *Lancet* 2010;375:959-961.
2. Goldstein JL, Hobbs HH, Brown MS. Familial hypercholesterolemia. In Scriver CR, Beaudet AL, Sly WS, et al (eds): *The metabolic and molecular bases of inherited disease*, 8th ed. 2001, New York, McGraw-Hill, pp 2863-2913.
3. Mabuchi H, Koizumi J, Shimizu M, et al. Development of coronary heart disease in familial hypercholesterolemia. *Circulation* 1989;79:225-332.
4. Haitis B, Baker SG, Meyer TE, et al. Natural history and cardiac manifestations of homozygous familial hypercholesterolemia. *Q J Med* 1990;76:731-740.
5. Goldstein JL, Brown MS. The LDL receptor defect in familial hypercholesterolemia: implications for pathogenesis and therapy. *Med Clin North Am* 1982;66:335-362.
6. Pekkanen J, Linn S, Heiss G, et al. Ten-year mortality from cardiovascular disease in relation to cholesterol level among men with and without preexisting cardiovascular disease. *N Engl J Med* 1990;322:1700-1707.
7. Brown G, Albers JJ, Fisher LD, et al. Regression of coronary artery disease as a result of intensive lipid-lowering therapy in men with high levels of apolipoprotein B. *N Engl J Med* 1990;323:1289-1298.
8. Kane JP, Malloy MJ, Ports TA, et al. Regression of coronary atherosclerosis during treatment of familial hypercholesterolemia with combined drug regimens. *JAMA* 1990;264:3007-3012.
9. Seed M, Hoppichler F, Reaveley D, et al. Relation of serum lipoprotein(a) concentration and apolipoprotein(a) phenotype to coronary heart disease in patients with familial hypercholesterolemia. *N Engl J Med* 1990;322:1494-1499.
10. Wiklund O, Angelin B, Olofsson SO, et al. Apolipoprotein(a) and ischaemic heart disease in familial hypercholesterolaemia. *Lancet* 1990;335:1360-1363.
11. Arad Y, Kenneth J, Goodman KJ, et al. Coronary calcification, coronary disease risk factors, C-reactive protein, and atherosclerotic cardiovascular disease events: the St. Francis Heart Study. *J Am Coll Cardiol* 2005;46:158-165.
12. de Gennes JL, Touraine R, Maunand B, et al. Homozygous cutaneotendinous forms of hypercholesterolemic xanthomatosis in an exemplary familial case: trial of plasmapheresis as an heroic treatment. *Bull Mem Soc Hosp (Paris)* 1967;118:1377-1402.
13. Thompson GR, Lowenthal R, Myant NB. Plasma exchange in the management of homozygous familial hypercholesterolaemia. *Lancet* 1975;1:1208-1211.
14. Thompson GR, Miller JP, Breslow JL. Improved survival of patients with homozygous familial hypercholesterolaemia treated with plasma exchange. *Br Med J* 1985;291:1671-1673.
15. Lupien PJ, Moorjani S, Awad J. A new approach to the management of familial hypercholesterolaemia: removal of plasma cholesterol based on the principle of affinity chromatography. *Lancet* 1976;1:1261-1264.
16. Schuff-Werner P, Armstrong VW, Eisenhauer TH, et al. Treatment of severe hypercholesterolemia by heparin-induced extracorporeal LDL precipitation (HELP). *Contrib Infus Ther* 1988;23:118-126.
17. Stoffel W, Borberg H, Greve V. Application of specific extracorporeal removal of low density lipoprotein in familial hypercholesterolaemia. *Lancet* 1981;2:1005-1007.
18. Yokoyama S, Hayashi R, Satani M, et al. Selective removal of low density lipoprotein by plasmapheresis in familial hypercholesterolemia. *Arteriosclerosis* 1985;5:613-622.
19. Gordon BR, Kelsey SF, Bilheimer DW, et al. Treatment of refractory familial hypercholesterolemia by low-density lipoprotein apheresis using an automated dextran sulfate cellulose adsorption system. *Am J Cardiol* 1992;70:1010-1016.
20. Bosch T, Schmidt B, Kleophas W, et al. LDL hemoperfusion—a new procedure for LDL-apheresis: first clinical application of an LDL adsorber compatible with human whole blood. *Artif Organs* 1997;21:977-982.
21. Otto C, Kern P, Bambauer R, et al. Efficacy and safety of a new whole-blood low-density lipoprotein apheresis system (Liposorber-D) in severe hypercholesterolemia. *Artif Organs* 2003;27:1116-1122.
22. Parker TS, Gordon BR, Saal SD, et al. Plasma high density lipoprotein is increased in man when low density lipoprotein (LDL) is lowered by LDL-pheresis. *Proc Natl Acad Sci U S A* 1986;83:777-781.
23. Gordon BR, Sloan BJ, Parker TS, et al. Humoral immune response following extracorporeal immunoadsorption therapy of patients with hypercholesterolemia. *Transfusion* 1990;30:318-321.
24. Bosch T, Lennertz A, Kordes B, et al. Low density lipoprotein hemoperfusion by direct adsorption of lipoproteins from whole blood (DALI apheresis): clinical experience from a single center. *Ther Apher* 1999;3:209-213.
25. Hequet O, Le QH, Rigal D, et al. The first results demonstrating efficiency and safety of a double-column whole blood method of LDL-apheresis. *Transfus Apher Sci* 2010;42:3-10.
26. Hudgins LC, Kleinman B, Scheur A, et al. Long-term safety and efficacy of low-density lipoprotein apheresis in childhood for homozygous familial hypercholesterolemia. *Am J Cardiol* 2008;102:1199-1204.
27. Olbricht CJ, Schaumann D, Fischer D. Anaphylactoid reactions, LDL apheresis with dextran sulphate, and ACE inhibitors. *Lancet* 1992;340:908-909.
28. Tatami R, Inoue N, Itoh H, et al. Regression of coronary atherosclerosis by combined LDL apheresis and lipid-lowering drug therapy in patients with familial hypercholesterolemia: a multicenter study. *Atherosclerosis* 1992;95:1-13.
29. Schuff-Werner P, Gohlke H, Bartmann U, et al. The HELP-LDL Apheresis Multicenter Study, an angiographically assessed trial on the role of LDL apheresis in the secondary prevention of coronary heart disease. II. Final evaluation of the effect of regular treatment on LDL-cholesterol plasma concentrations and the course of coronary heart disease. *Eur J Clin Invest* 1994;24:724-732.
30. Borberg H, Oette K. Experience with and conclusions from three different trials on low density lipoprotein apheresis. In Agishi T, Kawamura A, Mineshima M, editors: *Therapeutic plasmapheresis (XII)*. Zeist, The Netherlands, 1993, VSP, pp 13-20.
31. Kroon AA, Aengevaeren WRM, van der Werf T, et al. LDL-Apheresis Atherosclerosis Regression Study (LAARS): effect of aggressive versus conventional lipid-lowering treatment on coronary atherosclerosis. *Circulation* 1996;93:1826-1835.
32. Matsuzaki M, Hiramori K, Imaizumi T, et al. Intravascular ultrasound evaluation of coronary plaque regression by low density lipoprotein-apheresis in familial hypercholesterolemia: the Low Density Lipoprotein-Apheresis Coronary Morphology and Reserve Trial (LACMART). *J Am C Cardiol* 2002;40:220-227.
33. Daida H, Young JL, Yokoi H, et al. Prevention of restenosis after percutaneous transluminal coronary angioplasty by reducing lipoprotein(a) levels with low-density lipoprotein apheresis. *Am J Cardiol* 1994;73:1037-1040.
34. Gordon BR, Kelsey SF, Bilheimer DW, et al. Long-term effects of LDL apheresis using an automated dextran sulfate cellulose adsorption system. *Am J Cardiol* 1998;81:407-411.
35. Mabuchi H, Koizumi J, Shimizu M, et al. Long-term efficacy of low density lipoprotein apheresis on coronary heart disease in familial hypercholesterolemia. *Am J Cardiol* 1998;82:1489-1495.
36. Brunner R, Widder RA, Walter P, et al. Change in hemorrheological and biochemical parameters following membrane differential filtration. *Int J Artif Organs* 1995;18:794-798.
37. Uno H, Ueki Y, Murashima J, et al. Removal of LDL from plasma by adsorption reduces adhesion molecules on mononuclear cells in patients with arteriosclerotic obliterans. *Atherosclerosis* 1995;116:93-102.
38. Tamai O, Matsuoka H, Itabe H, et al. Single LDL apheresis improves endothelium-dependent vasodilation in hypercholesterolemic humans. *Circulation* 1997;95:76-82.
39. Starzl TE, Marchioro TL, Sexton AW, et al. The effect of portacaval transposition on carbohydrate metabolism: experimental and clinical observations. *Surgery* 1965;57:687-697.
40. Starzl TE, Putnam CW, Porter KA, et al. Portal diversion for the treatment of glycogen storage disease in humans. *Ann Surg* 1973;178:525-539.

41. Starzl TE, Chase HP, Putnam CW, et al. Portacaval shunt in hyperlipoproteinaemia. *Lancet* 1973;2:940-944.

42. Mitchell SC. Portacaval shunt in familial hypercholesterolaemia. *Lancet* 1983;1:193.

43. Starzl TE, Chase HP, Ahrens EH Jr, et al. Portacaval shunt in patients with familial hypercholesterolemia. *Ann Surg* 1983;198:273-283.

44. Forman MB, Baker SG, Mieny CJ, et al. Treatment of homozygous familial hypercholesterolaemia with portacaval shunt. *Atherosclerosis* 1982;41:349-361.

45. McNamara DJ, Ahrens EF Jr, Kolb R, et al. Treatment of familial hypercholesterolemia by portacaval anastomosis: effect on cholesterol metabolism and pool size. *Proc Natl Acad Sci U S A* 1983;80:564-568.

46. Bilheimer DW, Goldstein JL, Grundy SM, et al. Reduction in cholesterol and low density lipoprotein synthesis after portacaval shunt surgery in a patient with homozygous familial hypercholesterolemia. *J Clin Invest* 1975;56:1420.

47. Hoeg JM, Demosky SJ Jr, Schaefer EJ, et al. The effect of portacaval shunt on hepatic lipoprotein metabolism in familial hypercholesterolemia. *J Surg Res* 1985;39:369-377.

48. Kalk WJ, Russel D, Seftel HC, et al. Pituitary and thyroid function before and after portacaval anastomosis in patients with normal livers. *J Clin Endocrinol Metab* 1980;51:1450-1453.

49. Reeves F, Gosselin F, Herbert Y, et al. Long term follow-up after portacaval shunt and internal mammary coronary bypass graft in homozygous familial hypercholesterolemia: report of two cases. *Can J Cardiol* 1990;6:171-174.

50. Starzl TE, Bilheimer DW, Bahnson HT, et al. Heart-liver transplantation in a patient with familial hypercholesterolemia. *Lancet* 1984;1:1382-1383.

51. Valdivielso P, Escolar JL, Cuevas-Mons V, et al. Lipids and lipoprotein changes after heart and liver transplantation in a patient with homozygous familial hypercholesterolemia. *Ann Intern Med* 1988;108:204-206.

52. Sokal EM, Ulla L, Harvengt C, et al. Liver transplantation for familial hypercholesterolemia before the onset of cardiovascular complications. *Transplantation* 1992;55:432-433.

53. Bahnson HT. Transplant of other organs with the heart. *Cardiovasc Clin* 1990;20:237.

54. Lopez-Santamaria M, Migliazza L, Gamez M, et al. Liver transplantation in patients with homozygotic familial hypercholesterolemia previously treated by end-to-side portacaval shunt and ileal bypass. *J Pediatr Surg* 2000;35:630-633.

55. Castilla Cabezas JA, Lopez-Cillero P, Jimenez J, et al. Role of orthotopic liver transplant in the treatment of homozygous familial hypercholesterolemia. *Rev Esp Enferm Dig* 2000;92:601-608.

56. Shirahata Y, Ohkohchi N, Kawagishi N, et al. Living-donor liver transplantation for homozygous familial hypercholesterolemia from a donor with heterozygous hypercholesterolemia. *Transpl Int* 2003;16:276-279.

57. Moyle M, Tate B. Homozygous familial hypercholesterolemia presenting with cutaneous xanthomas: response to liver transplantation. *Austr J Derm* 2004;45:226-228.

58. Khalifeh M, Faraj W, Heaton N, et al. Successful living-related liver transplantation for familial hypercholesterolemia in the Middle East. *Transpl Int* 2005;17:735-739.

59. Barbir M, Khaghani A, Kehely A, et al. Normal levels of lipoproteins including lipoprotein (a) after liver-heart transplantation in a patient with homozygous familial hypercholesterolemia. *Q J Med* 1992;85:807-812.

60. Starzl TE. The little drummer girls. In *The puzzle people*. 1992, Pittsburgh, University of Pittsburgh Press, pp 327-331.

61. Shroti M, Fernando BS, Sudhindran S, et al. Long-term outcome of liver transplantation for familial hypercholesterolemia. *Transplant Proc* 2003;35:381-382.

62. Brush JE Jr, Leon MB, Starzl TE, et al. Successful treatment of angina pectoris with liver transplantation and bilateral internal mammary bypass graft surgery in familial hypercholesterolemia. *Am Heart J* 1988;116:1365-1367.

63. Revell SP, Noble-Jamieson G, Johnston P, et al. Liver transplantation for homozygous familial hypercholesterolaemia. *Arch Dis Child* 1995;73:456-458.

64. Cefalu AB, Barraco G, Noto D, et al. Six novel mutations of the LDL receptor gene in FH kindred of Sicilian and Paraguayan descent. *Int J Mol Med* 2006;17:539-546.

65. Kawagishi N, Satoh K, Enomoto Y, et al. Two cases in one family of living donor liver transplantation for homozygous familial hypercholesterolemia. *J Gastroenterol* 2006;41:501-502.

66. Schmidt HH, Tietge UJ, Buettner J, et al. Liver transplantation in a subject with familial hypercholesterolemia carrying the homozygous p.W577R LDL-receptor gene mutation. *Clin Transplant* 2008;22:180-184.

67. Popescu I, Habib N, Dima S, et al. Domino liver transplantation using a graft from a donor with familial hypercholesterolemia: seven-yr follow-up. *Clin Transplant* 2009;23:565-570.

68. Kakaei F, Nikeghbalian S, Kazemi K, et al. Liver transplantation for homozygous familial hypercholesterolemia: two case reports. *Transplant Proc* 2009;41:2939-2941.

69. Liu C, Niu DM, Loong CC, et al. Domino liver graft from a patient with familial hypercholesterolemia. *Pediatr Transplant* 2010;14:E30-E33.

70. Maiorana A, Nobili V, Calandra S, et al. Preemptive liver transplantation in a child with familial hypercholesterolemia. *Pediatr Transplant* 2010;15:E25-E29.

71. Kucukkartallar T, Yankol Y, Kanmaz T, et al. Liver transplantation as a treatment option for three siblings with homozygous familial hypercholesterolemia. *Pediatr Transplant* 2011;15:281-284.

72. Kamath BM, Olthoff KM. Liver transplantation in children: update 2010. *Pediatr Clin North Am* 2010;57:401-414.

73. Buchwald H. Surgical operation to lower circulating cholesterol. *Circulation* 1963;28:649.

74. Buchwald H, Varco RL, Matts JP, et al. Effect of partial ileal bypass surgery on mortality and morbidity from coronary heart disease in patients with hypercholesterolemia. *N Engl J Med* 1990;323:946-955.

75. Ohri SK, Keane PF, Swift I, et al. Reappraisal of partial ileal bypass for the treatment of familial hypercholesterolemia. *Am J Gastroenterol* 1989;84:740-743.

76. Moore RB, Frantz ID Jr, Buchwald H. Changes in cholesterol pool size, turnover rate, and fecal bile acid and sterol excretion after partial ileal bypass in hypercholesterolemic patients. *Surgery* 1969;65:98-108.

77. Deckelbaum, RJ, Lees RS, Small, DM, et al. Failure of complete bile diversion and oral bile acid therapy in the treatment of homozygous familial hypercholesterolemia. *N Engl J Med* 1977;296:465-470.

78. Miettinen TA. Comparison of cholestyramine, ileal by-pass and portacaval shunt in the treatment of familial hypercholesterolemia. In Gotto AM Jr, Smith LC, Allen B, editors: *Atherosclerosis V*. 1980, New York, Springer-Verlag, pp 470-473.

79. Buchwald H, Varco RL, Boen JR, et al. Effective lipid modification by partial ileal bypass reduced long-term coronary heart disease mortality and morbidity: five year post trial follow-up report from the POSCH. *Arch Intern Med* 1998;158:1253-1261.

80. Buchwald H, Williams SE, Matts JP, et al. Overall mortality in the program on the surgical control of the hyperlipidemias. *J Am Coll Surg* 2002;195:327-331.

81. Grossman M, Rader DJ, Muller DWM, et al. A pilot study of ex vivo gene therapy for homozygous familial hypercholesterolemia. *Nat Med* 1995;1:1148-1154.

82. Vaessen SF, Twisk J, Kastelein JJ. Gene therapy in disorders of lipoprotein metabolism. *Curr Gene Ther* 2007;7:35-47.

83. Kassim SH, Li H, Vandenberghe LH, et al. Gene therapy in a humanized mouse model of familial hypercholesterolemia leads to marked regression of atherosclerosis. *PLoS One* 2010;5:e13424.

84. Kankkonen HM, Vahakangas E, Marr RA, et al. Long-term lowering of plasma cholesterol levels in LDL-receptor–deficient WHHL rabbits by gene therapy. *Mol Ther* 2004;9:548-556.

85. Nomura S, Merched A, Nour E, et al. Low-density lipoprotein receptor gene using helper-dependent adenovirus produces long-term protection against atherosclerosis in a mouse model of familial hypercholesterolemia. *Gene Therapy* 2004;11:1540-1548.

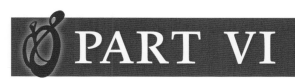

CHAPTER **28**

Initial Evaluation and Approach to the Patient with Hypertension

Marie Krousel-Wood and Suzanne Oparil

OVERVIEW AND DEFINITIONS, 463

EVALUATION OF THE PATIENT, 463

History, 463
Present Illness, 464
Family History, 465
Past Medical History, 465
Review of Systems, 465

Personal History, 465
Physical Examination, 465
Blood Pressure Measurement, 466
Laboratory Evaluation, 466
Overview of Treatment of the Hypertensive Patient, 467
Resistant Hypertension, 467

ADHERENCE TO ANTIHYPERTENSIVE MEDICATIONS, 468

LIFESTYLE MODIFICATIONS: OVERVIEW, 468

Practical Approaches to Encouraging Lifestyle
    Modifications, 469

CONCLUSION, 472

REFERENCES, 472

Overview and Definitions

Hypertension is defined as a systolic blood pressure (SBP) of 140 mm Hg or higher, a diastolic blood pressure (DBP) of 90 mm Hg or higher, or current use of antihypertensive medications. Hypertension persists as a major public health problem that affects 76.4 million U.S. adults—more than one third of the adult population.[1-3] The aging of the population and, more importantly, an increase in the prevalence of obesity have contributed to the rising prevalence of hypertension, which is higher than the Healthy People 2020 goal of 26.9%.[4-6] As a result of the age-related rise in blood pressure (BP), hypertension commonly occurs in middle-aged and older adults; adults aged 50 years and older have a lifetime risk for hypertension of 90%.[7]

Hypertension is a major risk factor for coronary heart disease, stroke, renal failure, all-cause mortality, and shortened life expectancy.[8] The positive association between SBP and DBP and cardiovascular outcomes is strong, continuous, graded, and etiologically significant.[9] Hypertension is heterogeneous in its pathophysiology, and its effect on target organs is also a function of associated risk factors that include diabetes mellitus, dyslipidemia, and tobacco abuse. The current classification of BP in the adult population proposed by the Joint National Committee on Prevention, Evaluation, Diagnosis and Treatment of Hypertension (JNC 7)[1] is provided in Table 28-1. This classification is based on the average of two or more seated BP readings, properly measured with well-maintained equipment, at each of two or more visits to the office or clinic.

Most patients with hypertension can be evaluated and treated in the ambulatory care setting; however, a small minority require urgent or emergency treatment based on the clinical presentation of acute or accelerated hypertension-related target organ damage rather than BP values per se (see Chapter 32). Although adult hypertensive emergencies are usually associated with very high BP, often in excess of 220/110 mm Hg, patients with much lower BP also require emergency treatment in the presence of serious complications such as preeclampsia or eclampsia, hypertensive encephalopathy, or acute renal failure.

Evaluation of the Patient

The purpose of diagnosing and treating hypertension is to prevent the development of target organ damage, cardiovascular and cerebrovascular disease, and chronic kidney disease (CKD). To do this effectively, it is important to estimate the patient's global cardiovascular risk and, in particular, to identify other modifiable risk factors such as dyslipidemia, smoking, and diabetes. Most contemporary guidelines for hypertension management stress the need to consider the likely impact of all risk factors before making clinical management decisions, and they recommend a system of evaluating combined risk factor effects.[10-13] For example, the British National Institute for Health and Clinical Excellence guidelines recommend using a formal estimation of cardiovascular risk to discuss prognosis and health care options with hypertensive patients, both for increased BP and for other modifiable risk factors.[11] Figure 28-1 and Boxes 28-1 and 28-2 show the pertinent elements of the history and physical assessment of the hypertensive patient.

History

The patient history should provide clues as to whether the patient truly has hypertension, whether it is primary or secondary, and whether it has resulted in target organ damage or cardiovascular disease outcomes. Patients should be queried about other modifiable risk factors—such as diabetes, smoking, or dyslipidemia—that would affect their prognosis and therefore possibly alter the treatment plan. A variety of cardiovascular risk estimation systems have been developed and adapted for the primary care setting.[10,14-18] These vary in complexity and ease of use; current trends favor simpler systems of risk estimation and management, with minimal requirement for laboratory testing.[19] Of these, the Framingham Risk Score has been assessed and validated in the broadest range of populations and has the most years of follow-up. A newer version of the Framingham Risk Score predicts 10-year risk of specific cardiovascular disease endpoints—coronary heart disease, stroke, heart failure, and peripheral

TABLE 28-1   Classification of Blood Pressure for Adults

CLASSIFICATION	SBP (MM HG)		DBP (MM HG)
Normal	<120	and	<80
Prehypertension	120-139	or	80-89
Stage 1 hypertension	140-159	or	90-99
Stage 2 hypertension	≥160	or	≥100

BP, blood pressure; DBP, diastolic blood pressure; SBP, systolic blood pressure.
Data from Chobanian AV, Bakris GL, Black HR, et al. Seventh report of the Joint National Committee on Prevention, Detection, Evaluation, and Treatment of High Blood Pressure. *Hypertension* 2003;42(6):1206-1252.

vascular disease (PAD)—as well as global cardiovascular disease risk.[14] An online and downloadable risk calculator is available at www.nhlbi.nih.gov/guidelines/cholesterol and www.framingham heartstudy.org. Electronic risk estimation that can be automated and linked to the patient's electronic medical record is gaining in popularity and facilitates the use of cardiovascular disease risk assessment in primary care.

Present Illness

It is important to determine when the patient first became aware of having hypertension. Sudden or very recent onset or exacerbation of hypertension may increase the likelihood of a secondary cause. Ask about past physical examinations and

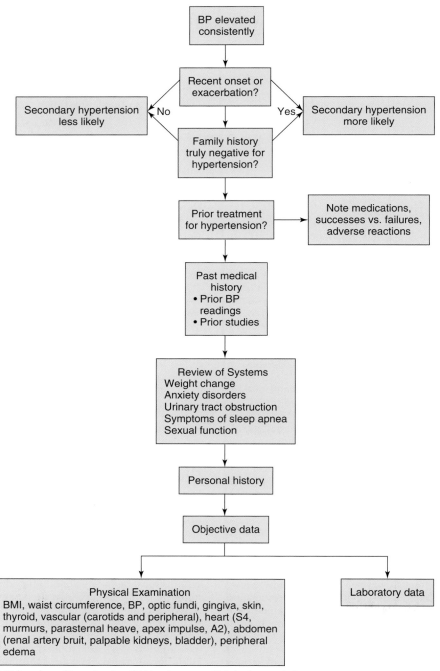

FIGURE 28-1   Flowchart for initial workup of hypertension. BP, blood pressure; BMI, body mass index.

Box 28-1 Elements of the Personal History for Hypertension

Dietary intake of salt, processed foods, and fruits and vegetables
Smoking history
Alcohol consumption (specific amounts and type)
Caffeine intake (coffee, tea, cola beverages, pills)
Use of pressor agents (nasal sprays, cold remedies)
Licorice intake, with a focus on licorice of British, French, or Belgian origin; certain laxative abuse and chewing tobacco (rare causes)
Use or abuse of organic, herbal, and health food remedies
Use of nonsteroidal antiinflammatory drugs
Exercise type, frequency, and duration
Occupational history; note stress levels
Marital history
Educational history if not defined by occupation

Box 28-2 Selected Causes of Secondary Hypertension

Chronic kidney disease
Coarctation of the aorta
Cushing syndrome and other glucocorticoid excess states, including long-term steroid therapy
Drug-induced or drug-related (includes nonsteroidal antiinflammatory drugs; illicit pressor agents such as cocaine; sympathomimetic agents, such as nasal decongestants and diet drugs, cyclosporine and tacrolimus, erythropoietin, and licorice; and alternative agents, such as ephedra [Ma huang] and bitter orange)
Primary aldosteronism and other mineralocorticoid excess states
Renovascular hypertension
Sleep apnea
Pheochromocytoma
Thyroid/parathyroid disease

Modified from Chobanian AV, Bakris GL, Black HR, et al. Seventh report of the Joint National Committee on Prevention, Detection, Evaluation, and Treatment of High Blood Pressure. *Hypertension* 2003;42(6):1206-1252.

determine what BP readings were obtained by other health care providers. Obtain a history of previous hypertension evaluation, with particular attention to data that may have already been collected and need not be duplicated. If the patient has been previously treated for hypertension, a detailed list of medications used, their effect or lack thereof, and any adverse effects is very useful. Importantly, patients who report multiple pharmacologically improbable and often bizarre "allergies" to medications may be having anxiety syndromes or panic attacks rather than true hypertension. Anxiety-induced hypertension may not respond to antihypertensive therapy. These patients require anxiolytic agents and care from a specialist in treating anxiety disorders.

Family History

Family history should be extended to both maternal and paternal grandparents, aunts and uncles, and siblings and children. Seek information on strokes, premature cardiac death, and kidney failure in addition to heart failure and hypertension.

Past Medical History

Medical records should be reviewed for BP readings taken at the time of hospitalizations or procedures, for imaging studies of the brain or kidneys, and for laboratory data that may reveal evidence of CKD or decreased serum potassium levels. Particular attention should be paid to pregnancy history in women because preeclampsia and other forms of pregnancy-related hypertension predict both sustained hypertension and increased cardiovascular disease risk later in life. Computed tomography (CT) or magnetic resonance imaging (MRI) scans taken because of headaches might provide evidence of hypertension-associated brain lesions.

Review of Systems

The review of systems should focus on clues to possible secondary causes of hypertension, target organ damage, and prior cardiovascular disease events. Details of prior hospitalizations should be queried. Recent weight gain may be associated with new-onset hypertension; if the patient is able to lose the weight, the loss offers the opportunity to control the BP without medication. Inadvertent weight loss may be a clue to hyperthyroidism or pheochromocytoma. A history of "spells" characterized by sweating, palpitations, and headache suggests the possibility of pheochromocytoma but may also be a manifestation of anxiety unrelated to hypertension or cardiovascular disease. A history of anxiety or depression is important because anxiolytic or antidepressant medications may adversely affect BP and response to antihypertensive medications, and patients with panic attacks and anxiety-induced BP elevations may not respond to conventional antihypertensive therapy. Furthermore, depression is associated with low adherence to antihypertensive medications and may be an important barrier to hypertension management.[20,21]

Daytime sleepiness or a history of loud snoring, especially when associated with apneic spells, is strongly suggestive of obstructive sleep apnea, a condition known to be associated with treatment-resistant hypertension.[22] The patient's bed partner may be a good source of information on snoring, but a formal sleep study is needed to confirm the diagnosis and develop treatment strategies.

Personal History

Detailed information about lifestyle that includes diet, physical activity, smoking, and alcohol consumption is needed to establish a basis for the lifestyle modification component of antihypertensive therapy (see Box 28-1). High intake of alcohol and caffeine-containing beverages—including coffee, tea, and soft drinks—can increase BP and make treatment more difficult. Patients should be queried about use of medications or dietary supplements that can elevate BP (see Box 28-1). Prominent among these are pain medications, particularly nonsteroidal antiinflammatory drugs (NSAIDs). Because many patients do not regard over-the-counter preparations as true "medicines," it is important to ask specifically about pain and pain treatments, as well as herbal preparations, dietary supplements, and weight-loss preparations. Nasal decongestants and cold remedies have sympathomimetic effects that can elevate BP significantly. Immunosuppressive drugs and many agents used in cancer treatment also elevate BP.

The social history includes information about education, job status, marital history, and living situation, and it can provide valuable information about psychosocial stresses that can elevate BP and impair response to treatment. In extreme stress situations—such as the 2011 tsunami in Japan and the destructive tornadoes in the United States—hypertension and related cardiovascular disease events can appear de novo in epidemic fashion. Getting to know your patient's social situation and expressing empathy are critical to developing trust and initiating a successful strategy for managing BP and cardiovascular risk over the long term.

Physical Examination

To begin, the patient's weight and height should be measured, and the body mass index (BMI) should be calculated. Measuring the waist circumference provides additional predictive information regarding metabolic syndrome and coronary heart disease risk. Examination of the skin for café-au-lait spots, neurofibromatomata, hair pattern changes, factitious lesions, and signs of domestic violence may reveal clues to diagnoses of secondary causes of hypertension. In addition, the optic fundi should be examined for retinal hemorrhages, exudates, papilledema, and arteriovenous crossing defects, all evidence of microvascular and macrovascular disease.

This is particularly important for patients with very high BP and for those in whom hypertensive emergency is suspected. The eyes, facial features, and body habitus may also give clues to hyperthyroidism, hypothyroidism, and Cushing syndrome. Gingival hypertrophy should be looked for, because antecedent gingival hypertrophy is a relative contraindication to treatment with dihydropyridine calcium channel blockers.

Next, the carotid arteries should be examined by auscultation and palpation, looking for evidence of vascular disease. The thyroid should be palpated and the neck inspected for jugular venous distention indicative of volume overload and heart failure.

Moving to the trunk, the lungs should be examined for signs of heart failure, and the heart should be examined carefully for evidence of abnormalities of rate or rhythm, murmurs, and signs of heart failure. The abdominal examination should include careful auscultation for renal artery and abdominal aortic bruits and palpation for masses, enlarged kidneys indicative of polycystic kidney disease, and a distended urinary bladder indicative of urinary outflow obstruction. A distended bladder may cause increased sympathetic discharge and BP elevation.

The lower extremities should be palpated for edema and pulses; the radial and femoral arteries should be palpated simultaneously to detect a pulse delay suggestive of aortic coarctation. The femoral arteries should be examined by auscultation to look for evidence of vascular disease. Measurement of BP in the leg as well as in the arm can be used to calculate the ankle brachial index (ABI), an indirect measure of PAD and a predictor of all-cause mortality and cardiovascular disease mortality, and to detect aortic coarctation.[23,24]

Neurologic examination should be performed as a baseline because stroke is a frequent complication of hypertension and also to document residual deficits in patients with previous stroke. Cognitive function should be assessed, particularly in elderly patients; cognitive decline and dementia are important complications of hypertension in the elderly.

Blood Pressure Measurement

The diagnosis and treatment of hypertension are critically dependent on accurate assessment of BP. JNC 7 and American Heart Association (AHA) guidelines for auscultatory measurement of office BP are outlined in Box 28-3.[1,16] The patient should be seated comfortably with feet on the floor and back supported. The patient should be at rest for at least 10 minutes and should not have consumed tobacco or caffeine in the previous 30 minutes. The possibility that the patient may have recently used illicit vasoactive drugs should be assessed. The bare arm should

be fitted with a cuff of correct size and supported at heart level. The cuff should be inflated until either the radial or brachial pulse disappears from the palpating fingertip. The pressure should then be reduced by a few mm Hg per second, until the first Korotkoff sound is heard. Disappearance of the sound usually marks the diastolic pressure. BP should be measured in both arms and with the patient standing at the first office visit. The arm with the higher readings should be used for future examinations to minimize inconsistency in visit-to-visit measurements.

Semiautomated devices that use an oscillometric method of BP determination are increasingly being used in hypertension studies and in office practice. If the instrument has been validated and the correct procedures for patient positioning have been followed, these devices eliminate observer error and free staff time. Check www.dableducational.org to determine whether your instrument has been validated.

Although office BP measurement remains the gold standard for assessing treatment responses in randomized, controlled trials, home BP measurements taken by the patient or a friend or family member are increasingly being used for monitoring treatment.[25-27] Engaging hypertensive patients in self-monitoring of BP has the advantage of involving them in their own care and is cost effective. Ambulatory BP monitoring (ABPM), in which BP is measured and recorded at frequent intervals throughout the day (usually every 15 or 30 minutes), has been shown to provide important prognostic information in untreated patients and is now required by some guidelines to make a diagnosis of hypertension.[11] ABPM is indicated for the diagnosis of "white coat hypertension," in which BP is elevated in the office but is normal or controlled in the out-of-office setting, and masked hypertension, in which BP is normal or controlled in the office but elevated in other settings. ABPM is useful in diagnosing episodic hypertension and treatment resistance. The disadvantages of ABPM include high cost and inconvenience to the patient.

Laboratory Evaluation

In the absence of specific clues to secondary hypertension from the history and physical examination, the basic initial laboratory evaluation should be simple (Box 28-4). A baseline electrocardiogram (ECG) should be part of the initial evaluation of every hypertensive patient to assess target organ damage. If left ventricular hypertrophy is evident, it should be confirmed by echocardiogram. Urinalysis, measurement of serum creatinine, and calculation of estimated glomerular filtration rate (eGFR) using the four-part Modification of Diet in Renal Disease equation are useful for assessing damage to the kidney as a target organ. These measures are particularly important in older patients with long-standing hypertension, among whom CKD is a growing problem that may require modification of antihypertensive treatment regimens, such as administration of more potent diuretics. Measurement of albuminuria and calculation of the albumin/creatinine ratio in morning-voided spot-urine samples has predictive value for both renal and cardiovascular disease, particularly in patients with diabetes.

Serum potassium measurement may provide important clues to secondary hypertension such as that seen with hyperaldosteronism. Elevated serum glucose should lead to further testing given

---

 Box 28-3 Office Measurement of Blood Pressure

Regularly inspect and validate equipment.
Train and regularly retrain people who take blood pressure.
Properly prepare and position the patient. Patient should be:
- Seated quietly in a chair with feet on floor for at least 5 minutes
- Arm at heart level
- No caffeine, exercise, or smoking for at least 30 minutes before

Use an appropriately sized cuff that encircles at least 80% of the arm.
Inflate the cuff to 20 to 30 mm Hg above the point at which palpated radial or brachial pulse disappears.
Deflate the cuff at about 2 mm Hg/second.
The first Korotkoff sound denotes systolic pressure; disappearance of the sounds denotes diastolic pressure.
On the first visit, take readings in both arms. Note and record the arm with the higher pressure, and use this arm for all subsequent readings. Note that the higher systolic and diastolic blood pressure may be found in different arms.
Take standing blood pressure, especially before titrating doses upward.

Modified from Chobanian AV, Bakris GL, Black HR, et al. Seventh report of the Joint National Committee on Prevention, Detection, Evaluation, and Treatment of High Blood Pressure. *Hypertension* 2003;42(6):1206-1252.

 Box 28-4 Routine Laboratory Tests

Twelve-lead electrocardiogram
Urinalysis (check for microalbuminuria in patients with diabetes)
Blood glucose level
Hematocrit
Serum potassium level
Serum creatinine level and estimated glomerular filtration rate
Lipoprotein profile
Urinary albumin level

the important interaction between hypertension and diabetes. Although not specifically part of the hypertensive workup, an assessment of the lipoprotein profile should be made because of risk factor clustering. Assays of plasma renin activity and plasma and urinary aldosterone levels are not recommended for the initial evaluation of the hypertensive patient; however, these assays may play a role in the diagnosis of secondary or resistant hypertension, as discussed in Chapter 31.

Overview of Treatment of the Hypertensive Patient

Once the initial evaluation of the patient has been completed, decisions on the choice of therapy must be made. The JNC 7 algorithm (Figure 28-2) is a useful guide for most hypertensive patients. Lifestyle modifications discussed in the remainder of this chapter should be initiated and maintained in all hypertensive patients. For those who require pharmacologic treatment, compelling indications such as heart failure, recent MI, high coronary disease risk, diabetes, CKD, and recurrent stroke prevention should first be identified because a compelling indication may drive the selection of antihypertensive medication. If there is no such indication, treatment is based on the stage of hypertension. Once treatment has begun, regular follow-up should be

scheduled, and the frequency of follow-up visits depends on the level of BP control and on the presence of other cardiovascular risk factors or target organ damage.

Resistant Hypertension

If the patient fails to achieve goal BP despite treatment with full doses of three or more antihypertensive agents of different classes, one of which is a diuretic, the diagnosis is resistant hypertension.[22,28] Although the cause of resistant hypertension is almost always multifactorial, common factors include lifestyle characteristics such as obesity, high alcohol intake, and excess sodium intake; drug-related causes, such as with sympathomimetic agents or NSAIDs; and secondary causes of hypertension that may include primary aldosteronism, CKD, renal artery stenosis, and obstructive sleep apnea (see Boxes 28-2 and 28-5). The most frequent cause of resistant hypertension is volume overload. A recent National Health and Nutrition Examination Survey (NHANES) reported that in treated hypertensive U.S. adults, apparent treatment-resistant hypertension has increased in prevalence from 15.9% (1998 through 2004) to 28.0% (2005 through 2008).[28,29] In this nationwide survey, four or more health care visits per year, obesity, CKD, and a Framingham 10-year coronary risk score above 20% were associated with apparent treatment-resistant hypertension.

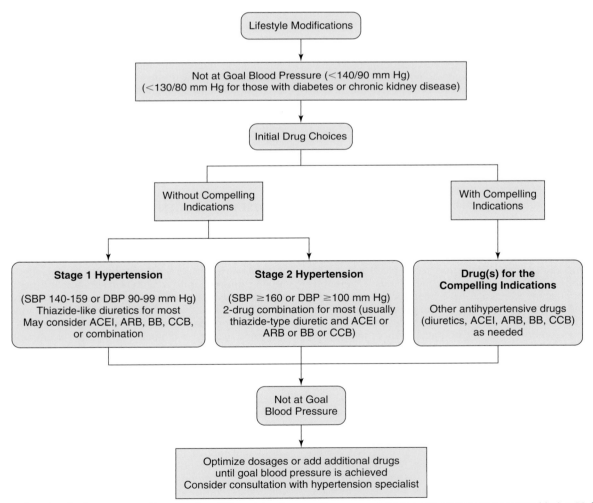

FIGURE 28-2 Algorithm for the treatment of hypertension. ACEI, angiotensin-converting enzyme inhibitor; ARB, angiotensin II receptor blocker; BB, β-adrenergic receptor blocker; CCB, calcium channel blocker; DBP, diastolic blood pressure; SBP, systolic blood pressure. *(Modified from Chobanian AV, Bakris GL, Black HR, et al. National High Blood Pressure Coordinating Committee. Seventh report of the Joint National Committee on Prevention, Detection, Evaluation, and Treatment of High Blood Pressure. Hypertension 2003;42:1206-1252.)*

CH
28

Box 28-5 Causes of Resistant Hypertension

Volume overload
- Excess sodium intake
- Volume retention from kidney disease
- Inadequate diuretic therapy

Drug-induced hypertension or other causes
- Inadequate drug dosage
- Inappropriate combinations
- Drug-induced hypertension (see Boxes 28-1 and 28-2)

Associated conditions
- Obesity
- Excess alcohol intake

Secondary causes of hypertension (see Box 28-2)

Modified from Chobanian AV, Bakris GL, Black HR, et al. Seventh report of the Joint National Committee on Prevention, Detection, Evaluation, and Treatment of High Blood Pressure. *Hypertension* 2003;42(6):1206-1252.

Box 28-6 Barriers to Medication Adherence[32,34,35]

Patient-Specific Barriers
Forgetfulness
Beliefs and perceptions
Lack of knowledge about hypertension
Lack of social support
Quality of life
Dependent care

Disease-Specific Barriers
Asymptomatic nature of disease
Depression/depressive symptoms
Comorbidities

Medication-Specific Barriers
Side effects
Complexity of medication regimen
Cost of medications
Complementary and alternative medicine use

Logistic Barriers
Frequency of health care visits
Filling prescription medications
Access to health care

Adherence to Antihypertensive Medications

According to the NHANES, 50.1% of all adult hypertensive patients in the United States have controlled BP, and among those treated for hypertension, only 69% have controlled BP.[2] Most patients with hypertension require pharmacologic therapy to achieve goal BP, and continuous adherence to antihypertensive medications over time is needed to achieve and maintain BP control. In evaluating patients who do not reach goal BP, it is important to consider poor adherence to prescribed regimens, prescription of an inadequate number and insufficient doses of antihypertensive medications (i.e., therapeutic inertia), or inappropriate combinations of medications.[21,28] Many patients do not take their medications as prescribed or at all. Low adherence and decline in adherence to prescribed drugs over time are key contributors to uncontrolled BP in patients with new-onset or established hypertension and are associated with adverse outcomes and higher health care costs.[21,30-33] In a recent nationwide study, 27% of participants with hypertension and CKD were not taking antihypertensive medications as prescribed.[33] In a meta-analysis, adherent versus nonadherent patients had a 3.44 higher odds ratio (95% confidence interval [CI], 1.60 to 7.37) for hypertension control.[31]

Assessing patient adherence to antihypertensive medications in outpatient settings is an important first step to understanding the effectiveness of the treatments prescribed, identifying barriers to treatment, and improving BP control. There is no gold standard for measuring adherence in the office or clinic; however, available techniques include validated self-report tools, electronic adherence monitoring, pharmacy fill rates, and pill counts.[34] Numerous barriers to medication adherence have been identified and may be categorized into patient-specific, disease-specific, medication-specific, and logistical barriers,[33,35,36] which provide a useful framework to facilitate communication with patients about medication adherence (Box 28-6).

Interventions aimed at improving adherence have been classified into several broad groups: *patient educational interventions*, such as didactic teaching; *patient behavioral interventions*, including patient motivation, drug packaging, support, reminders, and simplification of dosing; *provider interventions*; and *complex or combined patient interventions*—that is, educational interventions coupled with behavioral interventions.[37] Multiple strategies to improve medication adherence have been investigated, but no single intervention has emerged as superior. Systematic reviews of clinical trials have found that patient behavioral interventions,[38-41] provider education interventions,[42-44] and combination patient interventions[42,43] improved adherence; the effects of patient educational interventions alone on medication adherence have been inconclusive. Because several barriers may influence

medication adherence and no single intervention has been identified as the gold standard for improving adherence, a patient-centered approach that tailors interventions to overcome patient-specific barriers is warranted.[44] Consideration should be given to engaging nonphysician health care providers, particularly those with skills in pharmaceutical counseling or behavioral interventions, to implement adherence interventions. Use of these providers has proven effective in improving medication adherence and limiting the demands placed on the physician's time in busy clinics.[45,46]

Physicians and other health care providers should consider low medication adherence as a factor contributing to poor BP control and should communicate the importance of medication adherence to their patients, consider strategies to overcome barriers to medication adherence, and actively engage patients to improve adherence.

Lifestyle Modifications: Overview

Adopting a healthy lifestyle is a critical component of the prevention and management of hypertension. Despite the availability of effective medical therapy for treatment of hypertension, the BP control rate for adults with hypertension in the United States is only 50.1%.[2] In addition to treatment resistance and poor medication adherence, an unhealthy lifestyle is an important contributor to poor BP control. Well-established dietary risk factors for high BP include low potassium intake, excess salt intake, high alcohol consumption, excess weight, and suboptimal consumption of fruits, vegetables, and low-fat dairy products.[47] Evidence from clinical research studies that include randomized controlled trials has demonstrated that lifestyle modification, alone or in combination with antihypertensive medication, decreases BP and enhances the efficacy of antihypertensive medications, and it decreases cardiovascular risk.[1,47-51]

The major recommendations for lifestyle modifications in the JNC 7 report include maintaining a normal body weight; consuming a diet rich in fruits, vegetables, and low-fat dairy products; reducing dietary sodium intake; engaging in regular physical activity; and limiting consumption of alcohol (Table 28-2).[50-56] Increasing dietary potassium lowers BP and should be part of the management plan for prevention and treatment of hypertension.[57-59] An Institute of Medicine report on the dietary intakes for electrolytes and water provides recommendations for potassium and

TABLE 28-2 Lifestyle Modifications for the Management of Hypertension

CATEGORY	RECOMMENDATION FOR MODIFICATION	APPROXIMATE SYSTOLIC BLOOD PRESSURE REDUCTION RANGE
Weight	Maintain normal body weight (BMI 18.5-24.9 kg/m^2)	5-20 mm Hg/10 kg weight loss
Physical activity	Engage in regular aerobic physical activity, such as brisk walking at least 30 min/day most days of the week	4-9 mm Hg
Diet plan	Consume a diet rich in fruits, vegetables, and low-fat dairy products with a reduced content of saturated and total fat	8-14 mm Hg
Dietary sodium	Reduce dietary sodium intake to ≤100 mmol/day (2.4 g sodium or 6 g sodium chloride)	2-8 mm Hg
Dietary potassium	Increase dietary potassium intake to 120 mmol/day (4.7 g)	2-7 mm Hg
Alcohol consumption	Limit consumption to ≤2 drinks per day (1 oz or 30 mL ethanol, such as 24 oz beer, 10 oz wine, or 3 oz 80-proof whiskey) in most men and no more than one drink per day (0.5 oz ethanol) in lighter weight people and women	2-4 mm Hg

The effects of implementing these modifications are dose and time dependent and could be higher for some individuals.
From Chobanian AV, Bakris GL, Black HR, et al. Seventh report of the Joint National Committee on Prevention, Detection, Evaluation, and Treatment of High Blood Pressure. *Hypertension* 2003;42(6):1206-1252.

sodium intake.[60] The recommended intake for potassium is 4.7 g (120 mmol) per day, which contrasts with an average intake of approximately 2.0 to 3.0 g of potassium per day in U.S. adults. An adequate intake for sodium was set at 1.5 g/day (65 mmol) for young adults, 1.3 g/day for those between 56 and 70 years, and 1.2 g/day for those 71 years of age and older. An upper intake level for sodium was set at 2.3 g (100 mmol) per day, and a recent position statement from the American Society of Hypertension on dietary approaches to lower BP endorses these recommendations.[47]

Practical Approaches to Encouraging Lifestyle Modifications

Individual changes in lifestyle are achievable, provided the approaches are practical, address barriers, and are relevant to the patient. Sustaining individual behavior change over the long term is challenging given the powerful cultural forces, societal norms, and commercial interests that foster a sedentary lifestyle, a suboptimal diet, and overconsumption of calories.[47] Physicians and other health care providers, by example and by advice, have a powerful influence on their patients' willingness to make lifestyle changes. Translating scientific evidence for behavior change into clinical practice presents unique challenges in the management of the patient with hypertension, in part because of the asymptomatic and chronic nature of the condition and the limited duration and scope of routine office visits. Nevertheless, simple assessments such as measurement of height and weight to calculate BMI, provision of basic advice such as "eat less, move more," and encouragement of lifestyle modifications are feasible in clinic practices. Several factors influence the success of physician- and provider-directed attempts to achieve lifestyle changes: organizational structure of the office, the skills of the provider and staff, and the availability of patient management algorithms that include locally available resources.[47]

Other factors are associated with adherence to recommendations for the management of hypertension. The conceptual framework presented in Figure 28-3 outlines the link between the risk factors for low adherence to prescribed regimens, poor clinical outcomes, and increased cost and resource utilization.[35] Not surprisingly, patients value their quality of life in general and how they feel specifically. Emphasizing improvements in quality of life associated with lifestyle modifications will likely improve adherence to recommendations and ultimately improve clinical outcomes. Simplifying the behavior change and minimizing the side effects of the therapeutic regimen will likely lead to greater adherence.

BARRIERS TO LIFESTYLE MODIFICATIONS

To be effective in encouraging lifestyle modifications, physicians and other health care providers must first understand risk factors for, and barriers to, following the recommendations. Two broad categories of barriers contribute to poor adherence: *system-specific barriers*—that is, general access, health care, and environmental barriers—and *patient-specific barriers*. System-specific barriers include inadequate access to the proper foods and exercise facilities because of high cost, low availability, or lack of transportation to grocery stores and community recreational facilities. Other system barriers are poor access to health care facilities and poor access to providers for evaluation and management of hypertension in addition to limited physician and other health care provider knowledge of the lifestyle recommendations, including practical approaches to adhering to the recommendations. Environmental factors such as climate and unsafe neighborhoods also contribute to poor adherence.

Patient-specific barriers include limited knowledge of their disease and of the importance of lifestyle modifications in its management and lack of motivation to change behaviors. Other patient-specific barriers include the presence of concomitant illnesses, such as arthritis or pulmonary disease, that may decrease quality of life, limit ability to engage in exercise regimens, and increase the complexity of treatment. Furthermore, the patient's cultural and religious background may not support changes in dietary choices or increases in physical activity. These barriers alone or in combination may trigger patient use of unconventional or alternative therapies that may negatively affect patient adherence to lifestyle modifications. A better understanding of these barriers and their relevance to a particular patient is important in counseling patients regarding practical approaches to behavior change.

APPROACHES TO INCREASING THE ADOPTION OF LIFESTYLE MODIFICATIONS

In overcoming barriers to lifestyle changes, two general strategies for the management of high BP and its complications are helpful: a system-driven, population-based strategy and a patient-driven, targeted strategy. The system-driven, population-based approach strives to achieve a downward shift in the distribution of BP in the general population. Examples of this approach include providing ready access to healthier lifestyle options for the general population by decreasing sodium content, saturated fat, and caloric density in processed foods; providing caloric information at the point of purchase in restaurants and stores; enriching foods with

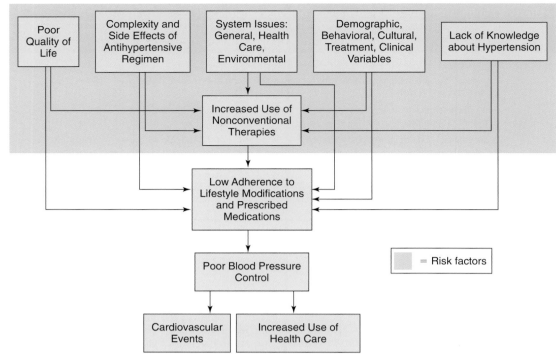

FIGURE 28-3 Factors associated with patient adherence to antihypertensive therapeutic regimens. *(Modified from Krousel-Wood MA, Thomas S, Muntner P, et al. Medication adherence: a key factor in achieving blood pressure control and good clinical outcomes in hypertensive patients.* Curr Opin Cardiol *2004;19:357-362.)*

minerals such as potassium; having government and employer incentives that promote healthy lifestyles; and providing safe and convenient opportunities for exercise in communities.[1,47,58]

The clinic visit provides an opportunity to implement the targeted patient-driven approach. In this setting, providers can explore patient-specific barriers to adherence and tailor recommendations to the individual patient. Advice by itself is not effective. One key to influencing lifestyle modification is assessing patients' readiness to change and matching the interaction to the patients' readiness to adopt healthy lifestyles.

Readiness for Change

Assessing a patient's readiness for change is based, in part, on stages of change.[61] Using these stages, patient readiness to follow lifestyle recommendations is classified in four stages: 1) the *precontemplation stage* ("I won't"); 2) the *contemplation stage* ("I might" in 6 months); 3) the *preparation stage* ("I will" in 30 days); and 4) the *action stage* ("I am" in less than 6 months).

Drawing from motivational interviewing strategies,[62] the Antihypertensive and Lipid-Lowering Treatment to Prevent Heart Attack Trial (ALLHAT) Dissemination Committee suggested physicians and other providers use the acronym PICM—for *permission, interest, confidence,* and *match*—in approaching patients regarding lifestyle recommendations.

Permission: Ask the patient's permission to talk about lifestyle changes.

Interest: Assess the patient's readiness for change. Discern how interested the patient is in adopting lifestyle modifications on a scale of 1 to 10 (higher score indicating greater interest).

Confidence: Ask how sure the patient is that he or she can manage the behavior.

Match: Match the health care provider's message to the interest and confidence of the patient.

For example, in the office setting, if a patient states that his interest level in adopting lifestyle changes is a 6 on a scale of 1 to 10, the physician should proceed in eliciting change statements, such as "What would it take for you to be a 7 or 8?" If a patient expresses low interest in changing behaviors, the physician should ask the

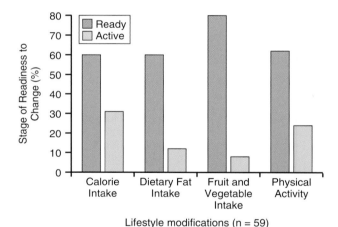

FIGURE 28-4 Stage of readiness by lifestyle modification. *(Modified from Taylor WC, Hepworth JT, Lees E, et al. Readiness to change physical activity and dietary practices and willingness to consult healthcare providers.* Health Res Policy Systems *2004;2:2.)*

patient, "Would you be willing to listen to me about why I want you to change?"

In Figure 28-4, readiness for change for physical activity and three dietary practices are shown for 59 adult minority patients from three community health centers.[63] Readiness to change and interest in communicating with health care providers, separate dimensions in this study, were significantly related for physical activity but not for dietary practices. Patients who were ready for change or who were actively engaged in physical activity were significantly more interested in discussing physical activity than those classified as not ready to increase physical activity. The goal is to move patients along a continuum of change because movement toward readiness to change is a key step toward successful adoption of a healthier lifestyle. Physicians and other health care providers may want to use a simple tool to assess patients' readiness and confidence to change for different lifestyle modifications. Such a tool is available online at www.hindawi.com/journals/apm/2011/215842. This tool may help identify which lifestyle behaviors to target first and how to set patient-specific goals and assess progress over time.[64]

TIPS FOR SUCCESS IN ADOPTING HEALTHIER DIETARY PRACTICES

One way to boost a patient's interest and confidence in adopting healthier dietary practices is to provide simple guidelines for making better choices that can be easily integrated into his or her routine. Understanding the nutritional content of the food the patient eats is an important first step in choosing food that is lower in sodium, fat, and calorie content and higher in minerals such as potassium and calcium. Reading labels on food products and relating the nutritional content to the lifestyle recommendations prior to purchasing the products facilitates adherence. Foods that are lower in sodium and fat are available, but the patient should realize that terms such as "reduced fat" and "fat free" are not synonymous; neither are the terms "low sodium" and "sodium free" (Tables 28-3 and 28-4). Patients should also be aware of the serving size when they are looking for the caloric content of the foods they buy. For example, the calories per serving of most cereals are approximately 110; however, for cereal A the serving size may be 1/4 cup, and for cereal B the serving size may be 1 cup. The patient may be surprised that eating a cup of cereal A would result in his or her consuming 440 calories. Choosing snacks that are high in potassium—fresh bananas, tomatoes, sweet potatoes, and leafy green vegetables—can increase adherence to the potassium recommendation.

Patients should be encouraged to switch from processed foods, such as canned foods and frozen dinners, to unprocessed fresh and fresh-frozen foods. Processing of food has a dramatic effect on its mineral content. For example, the sodium content of processed canned peas (23.6 mmol/100 g) is much higher than the corresponding content of fresh or fresh-frozen peas (0.1 mmol/100 g). In contrast, the potassium content of fresh or fresh-frozen peas (8.1 mmol/100 g) is much higher than the corresponding content in canned peas (2.5 mmol/100 g). A patient should keep a simple log of the foods and drinks that he or she has consumed. These logs provide valuable feedback to the patient and health care provider. For example, a patient may bring in a log of foods and drinks consumed over a 2-week period, indicating consumption of six 12-ounce sodas (nondiet) per day. This information might prompt a conversation with the patient regarding the sugar, sodium, and calorie content of soda and the benefits of switching to water or other lower calorie beverages. Some patients may benefit from keeping a more detailed dietary log aimed at identifying the calorie, sodium, and potassium content of the products.

Several recommendations may assist overweight or obese patients in reducing their intake of calories. Patients can limit their consumption of fatty foods by reading labels and choosing fat-free, low-fat, and lower calorie options. If patients frequently eat out, modifications can be made in the preparation of foods, such as switching from fried to grilled meats and asking for steamed vegetables in lieu of fried or baked potatoes. Food and drinks with high sugar content should be avoided, and patients can gradually reduce portion sizes and resist the urge to "supersize" food orders. Fresh fruits and vegetables can be used to replace higher calorie snacks such as chips and cookies. Patients seeking structured diets can adopt meal plans such as the Dietary Approaches to Stop Hypertension (DASH) diet plan, available online at www.nih.gov/news/pr/apr97/Dash.htm (see Chapter 26). The DASH diet and similar diets are safe and can be used in the general population. However, because of the high potassium, phosphorus, and protein content, these diets are not recommended for people with CKD.[47]

Tips for success in reducing dietary sodium intake are also available. Patients should be encouraged to buy fresh or fresh-frozen foods and to read food labels carefully and choose reduced-salt options. High-sodium foods such as nuts, chips, luncheon meats, most fast foods, most canned foods, pickles, and olives should be avoided. Patients should be encouraged to substitute pepper, lemon juice, garlic, spices, mustard, herbs, and salt substitutes for table salt and to avoid, or at least limit, the use of salt shakers. At restaurants, those seeking to reduce sodium and calorie content should ask for food preparation modifications, such as having the sauce or salad dressing placed on the side of the serving plate to limit the amount consumed.

TIPS FOR SUCCESS IN INCREASING PHYSICAL ACTIVITY

Engaging in a regular exercise program is the best way to increase and maintain moderate-intensity physical activity for at least 30 minutes most days of the week (at least 5). The 30 minutes may be accumulated in 10-minute sessions spread out over a 24-hour period. Warm-up and cool-down activities should be part of the routine, along with wearing properly fitted socks and shoes and clothing appropriate for exercise. If patients do little or no exercise, they should be instructed to start slowly, with lower intensity and shorter duration activities, building up to 30 minutes 5 days a week. Suitable regimens include use of a home-based exercise videotape regularly (30 min/day at least 5 day/week), participation in a swimming program for 90 minutes per day at least 4 days per week, walking for 1 hour at least 3 days per week, or playing tennis for 2 hours every other day. Patients who choose a plan that has realistic goals, fits into their schedules, and is appropriate for their budget are more likely to adhere to the program. In addition to engaging in a formal exercise program, many other practical approaches can be incorporated into a person's daily routine: using the stairs instead of an elevator for going up or down one or two floors, parking further from the entrances of buildings to increase walking, and getting up to change the television channel instead of using the remote control.

GENERAL TIPS FOR ADOPTING HEALTHIER LIFESTYLES

Arranging for social support and a periodic review of progress with a knowledgeable counselor helps with adoption and maintenance of healthy lifestyles. Engaging a family member or friend in the effort is often of great benefit. Counselors trained in behavior change techniques provide valuable insight into patient-specific strategies for lifestyle modification. As more individuals desire

TABLE 28-3	Label Language for Fat
Fat free	<0.5 g per serving
Low saturated fat	≤1 g per serving
Low fat	≤3 g per serving
Reduced fat	At least 25% less fat than regular version
Light in fat	Half the fat compared with regular version

TABLE 28-4	Label Language for Sodium
Sodium free	<5 mg per serving
Very low sodium	≤35 mg per serving
Low sodium	≤140 mg per serving
Low sodium meal	≤140 mg per 3.5 oz serving
Light sodium	At least 50% less sodium per serving than regular version
Reduced or less sodium	At least 25% less sodium per serving than the regular version
Unsalted/no added salt	No salt added during processing

healthy dietary options and practical approaches for increasing physical activity, the demand and supply of opportunities for the general population to achieve this goal will increase, creating continuous feedback between system-driven population approaches and patient-driven targeted approaches. As more people adopt healthier lifestyles, the demand and supply of affordable low-fat foods, low-carbohydrate options, and fresh or fresh-frozen fruits and vegetables for the general population should increase.

Conclusion

After completing the initial evaluation of the patient, decisions on the choice of therapy must be made. The JNC 7 algorithm can serve as a guide for most patients. For those who require pharmacologic treatment, we recommend first identifying any compelling indications, such as heart failure or recent MI, that may drive the choice of the antihypertensive medication. If there is no compelling indication, treatment is based on the stage of hypertension.

All patients should be encouraged to initiate and maintain the lifestyle modifications discussed in this chapter, because lifestyle modifications such as weight loss, increased physical activity, and dietary changes have been shown to improve BP control. Timely adoption of these modifications can reduce hypertension-related target-organ damage and interrupt the costly cycle of this prevalent, chronic disorder. Careful attention to patient adherence to prescribed medications is needed. As more patients integrate healthier choices into their daily routine and adhere to antihypertensive medications as prescribed, we should achieve better BP control rates overall, bringing us closer to the Healthy People 2020 goal.[6]

REFERENCES

1. Chobanian AV, Bakris GL, Black HR, et al. Seventh report of the Joint National Committee on Prevention, Detection, Evaluation, and Treatment of High Blood Pressure. *Hypertension* 2003;42(6):1206-1252.
2. Egan BM, Zhao Y, Axon RN. US trends in prevalence, awareness, treatment, and control of hypertension, 1988-2008. *JAMA* 2010;303(20):2043-2050.
3. Roger VL, Go AS, Lloyd-Jones DM, et al. American Heart Association Statistics Committee and Stroke Statistics Subcommittee. Heart disease and stroke statistics—2011 update: a report from the American Heart Association. *Circulation* 2011;123(4):e18-e209.
4. Cutler JA, Sorlie PD, Wolz M, et al. Trends in hypertension prevalence, awareness, treatment, and control rates in United States adults between 1988-1994 and 1999-2004. *Hypertension* 2008;52(5):818-827.
5. Fields LE, Burt VL, Cutler JA, et al. The burden of adult hypertension in the United States 1999 to 2000: a rising tide. *Hypertension* 2004;44(4):398-404.
6. U.S. Department of Health and Human Services, Office of Disease Prevention and Promotion. Healthy People 2020. 2011, Washington, DC. Accessed 2011 Dec 13 at http://healthypeople.gov/2020/topicsobjectives2020/default.aspx.
7. Vasan RS, Beiser A, Seshadri S, et al. Residual lifetime risk for developing hypertension in middle-aged women and men: the Framingham Heart Study. *JAMA* 2002;287(8):1003-1010.
8. Kearney PM, Whelton M, Reynolds K, et al. Global burden of hypertension: analysis of worldwide data. *Lancet* 2005;365(9455):217-223.
9. Lewington S, Clarke R, Qizilbash N, Peto R, Collins R. Age-specific relevance of usual blood pressure to vascular mortality: a meta-analysis of individual data for one million adults in 61 prospective studies. *Lancet* 2002;360(9349):1903-1913.
10. Cooney MT, Dudina A, D'Agostino R, Graham IM. Cardiovascular risk-estimation systems in primary prevention: Do they differ? Do they make a difference? Can we see the future? *Circulation* 2010;122(3):300-310.
11. Krause T, Lovibond K, Caulfield M, McCormack T, Williams B; Guideline Development Group. Management of hypertension: summary of NICE guidance. *Br Med J* 2011;343:d4891-d4896.
12. Mancia G, Laurent S, Agabiti-Rosei E, et al. Reappraisal of European guidelines on hypertension management: a European Society of Hypertension Task Force document. *J Hypertens* 2009;27:2121-2158.
13. National Heart, Lung and Blood Institute. Clinical Practice Guidelines. Accessed 2011 Dec 13 at http://www.nhlbi.nih.gov/guidelines/index.htm.
14. D'Agostino RB Sr, Vasan RS, Pencina MJ, et al. General cardiovascular risk profile for use in primary care: the Framingham Heart Study. *Circulation* 2008;117:743-753.
15. Conroy RM, Pyorala K, Fitzgerald AP, et al. Estimation of ten-year risk of fatal cardiovascular disease in Europe: the SCORE project. *Eur Heart J* 2003;24:987-1003.
16. Hippisley-Cox J, Coupland C, Vinogradova Y, et al. Predicting cardiovascular risk in England and Wales: prospective derivation and validation of QRISK2. *Br Med J* 2008;336:1475-1482.
17. Ridker PM, Buring JE, Rifai N, Cook NR. Development and validation of improved algorithms for the assessment of global cardiovascular risk in women: the Reynolds Risk Score. *JAMA* 2007;297:611-619.

18. Ridker PM, Paynter NP, Rifai N, Gaziano JM, Cook NR. C-reactive protein and parental history improve global cardiovascular risk prediction: the Reynolds Risk Score for men. *Circulation* 2008;118:2243-2251.
19. Graham IM, Stewart M, Hertog MG. Factors impeding the implementation of cardiovascular prevention guidelines: findings from a survey conducted by the European Society of Cardiology. *Eur J Cardiovasc Prev Rehabil* 2006;13:839-845.
20. Krousel-Wood M, Islam T, Muntner P, et al. Association of depression with antihypertensive medication adherence in older adults: cross-sectional and longitudinal findings from CoSMO. *Ann Behav Med* 2010;40(3):248-257.
21. Krousel-Wood M, Joyce C, Holt E, et al. Predictors of decline in medication adherence: results from the Cohort Study of Medication Adherence among Older Adults. *Hypertension* 2011;58:804-810.
22. Calhoun DA, Jones D, Textor S, et al. Resistant hypertension: diagnosis, evaluation, and treatment—a scientific statement from the American Heart Association Professional Education Committee of the Council for High Blood Pressure Research. *Circulation* 2008;117(25):e510-e526.
23. Resnick HE, Lindsay RS, McDermott MM, et al. Relationship of high and low ankle brachial index to all-cause and cardiovascular disease mortality: the Strong Heart Study. *Circulation* 2004;109(6):733-739.
24. Hirsch AT, Haskal ZJ, Hertzer NR, et al. ACC/AHA guidelines for the management of patients with peripheral arterial disease (lower extremity, renal, mesenteric, and abdominal aortic): a collaborative report from the American Associations for Vascular Surgery/Society for Vascular Surgery, Society for Cardiovascular Angiography and Interventions, Society for Vascular Medicine and Biology, Society of Interventional Radiology, and the ACC/AHA Task Force on Practice Guidelines (writing committee to develop guidelines for the management of patients with peripheral arterial disease)—summary of recommendations. *J Vasc Interv Radiol* 2006;17(9):1383-1397.
25. Pickering TG, Hall JE, Appel LJ, et al. Recommendations for blood pressure measurement in humans and experimental animals: Part 1. Blood pressure measurement in humans: a statement for professionals from the subcommittee of professionl and public education of the American Heart Association Council on High Blood Pressure Education of the American Heart Association Council on High Blood Pressure Research. *Hypertension* 2005;45:142-161.
26. Ghuman N, Campbell P, White WB. Role of ambulatory and home blood pressure recording in clinical practice. *Curr Cardiol Rep* 2009;11(6):414-421.
27. Pickering TG, White WB, Giles TD, et al. When and how to use self (home) and ambulatory blood pressure monitoring. *J Am Soc Hypertens* 2010;4(2):56-61.
28. Egan BM, Zhao Y, Axon RN, Brzezinski WA, Ferdinand KC. Uncontrolled and apparent treatment resistant hypertension in the United States, 1988 to 2008. *Circulation* 2011;124(9):1046-1058.
29. Persell SD. Prevalence of resistant hypertension in the United States, 2003-2008. *Hypertension* 2011;57(6):1076-1080.
30. Caro JJ, Salas M, Speckman JL, Raggio G, Jackson JD. Persistence with treatment for hypertension in actual practice. *CMAJ* 1999;160(1):31-37.
31. DiMatteo MR, Giordani PJ, Lepper HS, Croghan TW. Patient adherence and medical treatment outcomes: a meta-analysis. *Med Care* 2002;40(9):794-811.
32. Esposti LD, Saragoni S, Benemei S, et al. Adherence to antihypertensive medications and health outcomes among newly treated hypertensive patients. *Clinicoecon Outcomes Res* 2011;3:47-54.
33. Krousel-Wood MA, Muntner P, Islam T, Morisky DE, Webber LS. Barriers to and determinants of medication adherence in hypertension management: perspective of the cohort study of medication adherence among older adults. *Med Clin North Am* 2009;93(3):753-769.
34. Hawkshead J, Krousel-Wood MA. Techniques of measuring medication adherence in hypertensive patients in outpatient settings: advantages and limitations. *Dis Manag Health Outcomes* 2007;15:109-118.
35. Krousel-Wood M, Thomas S, Muntner P, Morisky D. Medication adherence: a key factor in achieving blood pressure control and good clinical outcomes in hypertensive patients. *Curr Opin Cardiol* 2004;19(4):357-362.
36. Ogedegbe G, Harrison M, Robbins L, Mancuso CA, Allegrante JP. Barriers and facilitators of medication adherence in hypertensive African Americans: a qualitative study. *Ethn Dis* 2004;14:3-12.
37. Krousel-Wood M, Hyre A, Muntner P, Morisky DE. Methods to improve medication adherence in hypertensive patients: current status and future directions. *Curr Opin Cardiol* 2005;20:296-300.
38. Conn VS, Hafdahl AR, Cooper PS, et al. Interventions to improve medication adherence among older adults: meta-analysis of adherence outcomes among randomized controlled trials. *Gerontologist* 2009;49(4):447-462.
39. Roter DL, Hall JA, Merisca R, et al. Effectiveness of interventions to improve patient compliance: a meta-analysis. *Med Care* 1998;36(8):1138-1161.
40. Schroeder K, Fahey T, Ebrahim S. How can we improve adherence to blood pressure–lowering medication in ambulatory care? Systematic review of randomized controlled trials. *Arch Intern Med* 2004;164(7):722-732.
41. Wetzels GE, Nelemans P, Schouten JS, Prins MH. Facts and fiction of poor compliance as a cause of inadequate blood pressure control: a systematic review. *J Hypertens* 2004;22(10):1849-1855.
42. McDonald HP, Garg AX, Haynes RB. Interventions to enhance patient adherence to medication prescriptions: scientific review. *JAMA* 2002;288(22):2868-2879.
43. Takiya LN, Peterson AM, Finley RS. Meta-analysis of interventions for medication adherence to antihypertensives. *Ann Pharmacother* 2004;38(10):1617-1624.
44. Krousel-Wood M, Hyre A, Muntner P, Morisky D. Methods to improve medication adherence in patients with hypertension: current status and future directions. *Curr Opin Cardiol* 2005;20(4):296-300.
45. Cutrona SL, Choudhry NK, Stedman M, et al. Physician effectiveness in interventions to improve cardiovascular medication adherence: a systematic review. *J Gen Intern Med* 2010;25(10):1090-1096.

46. Morgado MP, Morgado SR, Mendes LC, Pereira LJ, Castelo-Branco M. Pharmacist interventions to enhance blood pressure control and adherence to antihypertensive therapy: review and meta-analysis. *Am J Health Syst Pharm* 2011;68(3):241-253.

47. Appel LJ, Giles TD, Black HR, et al. ASH position paper: dietary approaches to lower blood pressure. *J Am Soc Hypertens* 2010;4(2):79-89.

48. Chen ST, Maruthur NM, Appel LJ. The effect of dietary patterns on estimated coronary heart disease risk: results from the Dietary Approaches to Stop Hypertension (DASH) trial. *Circ Cardiovasc Qual Outcomes* 2010;3(5):484-489.

49. Maruthur NM, Wang NY, Appel LJ. Lifestyle interventions reduce coronary heart disease risk: results from the PREMIER Trial. *Circulation* 2009;119(15):2026-2031.

50. Chobanian AV, Hill M. National Heart, Lung, and Blood Institute Workshop on Sodium and Blood Pressure: a critical review of current scientific evidence. *Hypertension* 2000;35(4):858-863.

51. He J, Whelton PK, Appel LJ, Charleston J, Klag MJ. Long-term effects of weight loss and dietary sodium reduction on incidence of hypertension. *Hypertension* 2000;35(2):544-549.

52. Sacks FM, Svetkey LP, Vollmer WM, et al. Effects on blood pressure of reduced dietary sodium and the Dietary Approaches to Stop Hypertension (DASH) diet. DASH-Sodium Collaborative Research Group. *N Engl J Med* 2001;344(1):3-10.

53. The Trials of Hypertension Prevention Collaborative Research Group. Effects of weight loss and sodium reduction intervention on blood pressure and hypertension incidence in overweight people with high-normal blood pressure. *Arch Intern Med* 1997;157(6):657-667.

54. Vollmer WM, Sacks FM, Ard J, et al. Effects of diet and sodium intake on blood pressure: subgroup analysis of the DASH-sodium trial. *Ann Intern Med* 2001;135(12):1019-1028.

55. Whelton SP, Chin A, Xin X, He J. Effect of aerobic exercise on blood pressure: a meta-analysis of randomized, controlled trials. *Ann Intern Med* 2002;136(7):493-503.

56. Xin X, He J, Frontini MG, Ogden LG, Motsamai OI, Whelton PK. Effects of alcohol reduction on blood pressure: a meta-analysis of randomized controlled trials. *Hypertension* 2001;38(5):1112-1117.

57. Cook NR, Obarzanek E, Cutler JA, et al. Joint effects of sodium and potassium intake on subsequent cardiovascular disease: the Trials of Hypertension Prevention follow-up study. *Arch Intern Med* 2009;169(1):32-40.

58. Geleijnse JM, Kok FJ, Grobbee DE. Blood pressure response to changes in sodium and potassium intake: a metaregression analysis of randomised trials. *J Hum Hypertens* 2003;17(7):471-480.

59. Whelton PK, He J, Appel LJ, et al. Primary prevention of hypertension: clinical and public health advisory from the National High Blood Pressure Education Program. *JAMA* 2002;288(15):1882-1888.

60. Panel on Dietary Reference Intakes for Electrolytes and Water. Dietary Reference Intakes for Water, Potassium, Sodium, Chloride, and Sulfate. Institute of Medicine of the National Academies. 2005, Washington, DC, National Academies Press.

61. Prochaska JO, Velicer WF. The transtheoretical model of health behavior change. *Am J Health Promot* 1997;12(1):38-48.

62. Miller WR, Rollnick S. *Motivational interviewing: preparing people for change*, 2nd ed. 2002, New York, The Guilford Press.

63. Taylor WC, Hepworth JT, Lees E, et al. Readiness to change physical activity and dietary practices and willingness to consult healthcare providers. *Health Res Policy Syst* 2004;2(1):2.

64. Gillespie ND, Lenz TL. Implementation of a tool to modify behavior in a chronic disease management program. *Adv Prev Med* 2011:215842.

INITIAL EVALUATION AND APPROACH TO THE PATIENT WITH HYPERTENSION

CHAPTER 29 Pharmacologic Management of Hypertension

Joseph J. Saseen

OVERVIEW, 474

PRINCIPLES OF TREATMENT, 474

Evidence-Based Treatment, 474
Blood Pressure Goals, 474

SELECTING DRUG THERAPY, 474

Uncomplicated Hypertension, 475
Patients with Compelling Indications, 475

OVERVIEW OF DRUG CLASSES, 476

Angiotensin-Converting Enzyme Inhibitors, 478
Angiotensin Receptor Blockers, 478

Calcium Channel Blockers, 479
Diuretics: Thiazides, 480
β-Blockers, 481
Aldosterone Antagonists, 482
Other Agents, 482

IMPLEMENTING DRUG THERAPY, 484

Need for 24-Hour Coverage, 484
Monotherapy Versus Combination Therapy, 484
Effects of Patient Characteristics on Blood Pressure
 Lowering, 484
Monitoring, 484

Adherence, 486
Step-Down Therapy, 486

SPECIAL POPULATIONS, 486

Elderly Patients, 486
African-American Patients, 487

REFERENCES, 487

Overview

The pharmacologic management of hypertension has evolved significantly over the past few decades. In the past, thiazide diuretics and β-blockers were highly recommended as the only first-line therapies due to landmark evidence that demonstrated reduced risks of cardiovascular (CV) events.[1-3] However, newer drug therapies have been introduced that include angiotensin-converting enzyme (ACE) inhibitors, angiotensin II receptor blockers (ARBs), and calcium channel blockers (CCBs). These agents have been evaluated in outcomes-based trials and have been established as effective in preventing CV events. Moreover, newer evidence from outcomes trials has clarified the role of other agents, such as β-blockers and α-antagonists, in the treatment of hypertension.[4,5]

Many important considerations influence the pharmacologic treatment of hypertension. These include selection of individual agents and drug classes and the choice of either monotherapy or combination therapy approaches when initiating therapy. Ongoing assessment of drug effectiveness and monitoring for adverse drug effects are also needed. Clinicians have the option of titrating and changing therapy through additions and/or modifications to achieve goal blood pressure (BP) values. Promoting and optimizing adherence to treatment are also essential to treat patients with hypertension optimally. All of these aspects of treatment are covered in this chapter.

Principles of Treatment

Evidence-Based Treatment

The prevailing guiding principle of hypertension management is to treat with the intent of reducing risk of CV events and thereby reducing CV morbidity and mortality. Outcomes trials have clearly established that a variety of antihypertensive drug therapies reduce risk of CV events.[6-8] Moreover, results of comparative outcomes-based clinical trials[9] and clinical trials in patients with concomitant cardiovascular disease (CVD) have enhanced the ability of clinicians to implement evidence-based drug therapy to manage hypertension.

Blood Pressure Goals

Most contemporary guidelines endorse a BP goal of less than 140/90 mm Hg for most patients with hypertension and less than 130/80 mm Hg for patients with diabetes or chronic kidney disease (CKD).[8,10] Controversy surrounds whether this lower goal should extend to patients with coronary artery disease (CAD), noncoronary atherosclerotic vascular disease (ischemic stroke, peripheral arterial disease), and those with a 10-year risk of coronary heart disease according to a Framingham risk score of 10% or lower.[10] The latter recommendation appeared in a 2007 American Heart Association (AHA) scientific statement but was modified and later rescinded in the recent American College of Cardiology Foundation (ACCF)/AHA/American Medical Association (AMA) Physician Consortium for Performance Improvement 2011 Performance Measures for Adults with Coronary Artery Disease and Hypertension Task Force report.[11] Based on the lack of available trials that directly compare the clinical outcomes of CAD patients treated to different BP targets, and on the heterogeneity of outcomes in trials in which coronary patients with baseline BP below 140/90 mm Hg were treated with antihypertensive drugs, the Task Force recommended a more conservative BP goal below 140/90 mm Hg as a performance measure. They acknowledged that lower targets may be appropriate in some patients with CAD or other conditions but that it is unclear how such patients could be reliably identified for purposes of performance measurement.

Furthermore, current evidence has challenged whether aggressive BP goals—that is, those below 130/80 mm Hg—provide additional clinical benefit compared with the standard BP goal of less than 140/90 mm Hg in other patient groups, including those with uncomplicated hypertension,[12,13] diabetes,[14] CKD,[15] and concomitant diabetes and CAD.[16] Regardless of which goal clinicians select, BP reduction to a target goal is a clinically acceptable therapeutic strategy. Achieving target BP goals generally requires a combination of drug therapy and lifestyle modification.

Selecting Drug Therapy

Clinicians should select antihypertensive drug therapy that has been proven to reduce risk of CV events in addition to lowering BP. They should also consider the baseline CV risk of the hypertensive patient. Identifying whether the patient has compelling indications for a specific drug therapy, as summarized in Figure 29-1, is the first step in selecting appropriate antihypertensive treatment. Clinicians should then consider effectiveness in lowering BP, minimizing risk for adverse events, and other patient-specific characteristics to help further guide and narrow selection of an individual drug, especially when more than one drug therapy option is identified.

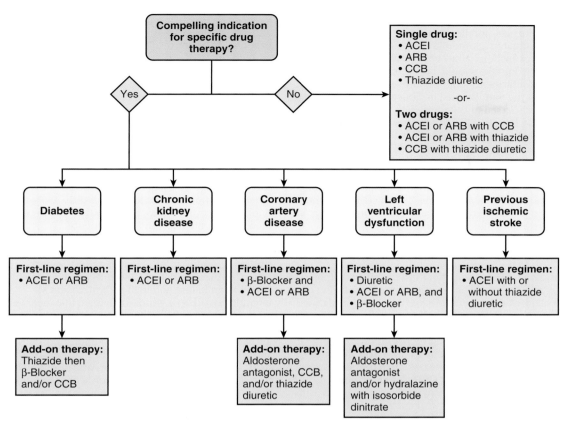

FIGURE 29-1 Hypertension treatment algorithm based on Joint National Committee (JNC-7) guidelines and the 2007 American Heart Association scientific statement.[8,10] First-line regimens are therapies proven to reduce the risk of cardiovascular events in the given patient situation. ACEI, angiotensin-converting enzyme inhibitor; ARB, angiotensin receptor blocker; CCB, calcium channel blocker.

Uncomplicated Hypertension

Many pharmacotherapeutic approaches are appropriate as first-line treatment options for patients with hypertension who have no comorbid condition that would dictate selection of specific antihypertensive drug therapy. Most guidelines have identified the following five drug classes as first-line choices for patients with uncomplicated hypertension: 1) thiazide diuretics, 2) β-blockers, 3) ACE inhibitors, 4) ARBs, or 5) CCBs.[8] All these agents have been proven to reduce CV events in patients with hypertension. Moreover, the Seventh Report of the Joint National Committee on Prevention, Detection, Evaluation, and Treatment of High Blood Pressure (JNC-7) recommends thiazide diuretics for most patients, if single-drug therapy is used, or as the first component of a two-drug combination. This recommendation was based on a number of randomized controlled trials, including the Anti-hypertensive and Lipid-Lowering Treatment to Prevent Heart Attack Trial (ALLHAT), which compared thiazide diuretic therapy to placebo or to other active treatments.[17] Some guidelines and scientific statements have relegated β-blockers to the ranks of second-line therapy options in uncomplicated hypertension,[10,18-20] based on evidence that indicates that although β-blockers reduce risk of CV events in hypertensive patients more effectively than placebo, they are not as effective as thiazide diuretics, ACE inhibitors, ARBs, or CCBs.[4]

Patients with Compelling Indications

Compelling indications represent comorbid medical conditions other than hypertension for which specific antihypertensive drug therapy reduces risk of CV events and/or disease progression. Patients with compelling indications are at high risk for CV events and should receive other CV risk-reduction modalities—antiplatelet

therapy, dyslipidemia therapy, smoking cessation, and obesity management—in addition to specific, targeted antihypertensive treatment.

DIABETES

Many patients with diabetes, either type 1 or type 2, have hypertension and require antihypertensive drug therapy. Most of these patients require at least two or three drugs to attain BP control. Many guidelines and expert statements recommend that patients with diabetes and hypertension be treated with either an ACE inhibitor or an ARB as first-line therapy[21,22] because this has been proven to reduce the risk of CV events and kidney disease progression in patients with diabetes.[23-25]

Other antihypertensive drugs should be added to ACE inhibitor or ARB therapy as needed to control BP. In particular, a diuretic is typically recommended as the first add-on therapy. Results from the Action in Diabetes and Vascular Disease: Preterax and Diamicron MR Controlled Evaluation Post Trial Observational Study (ADVANCE) support the combination of an ACE inhibitor with a thiazide in reducing microvascular and macrovascular disease in patients with diabetes.[26] Other data support the use of CCB therapy in patients with diabetes.[24,25,27,28] CCBs do not have adverse metabolic effects and do not affect glycemic control in diabetes. Their use as an add-on therapy is typically effective and safe. Therefore, clinicians may choose a CCB over a thiazide diuretic as the first add-on therapy to treat patients with hypertension and diabetes. The American Society of Hypertension (ASH) recommends the use of dual CCB therapy, a dihydropyridine with a nondihydropyridine, as a possible option in diabetic patients with hypertension that is difficult to control, because this approach has been shown to provide additive antihypertensive effects.[21,29]

When a diuretic is needed as add-on therapy in a patient with diabetes, a thiazide diuretic is typically recommended in patients with an estimated glomerular filtration rate (eGFR) of 30 mL/min/1.73 m² or higher.[22] However, if eGFR is below 30 mL/min/1.73 m², a loop diuretic should be considered.[22] Moreover, the ASH identifies chlorthalidone as the suggested thiazide diuretic, because it is the diuretic used in clinical trials, and it forms the basis for the cardiovascular outcome data.[21]

β-Blockers are also beneficial in the treatment of hypertension in patients with diabetes.[30,31] A β-blocker should be considered as the third or perhaps fourth add-on agent for BP control in these patients.[21] There is a risk of hyperglycemia with β-blocker therapy, but it is small and varies depending on the type of β-blocker used. For example, the Glycemic Effects in Diabetes Mellitus: Carvedilol-Metoprolol Comparison in Hypertensives (GEMINI) trial demonstrated that carvedilol had no significant effect on glucose in patients with diabetes, but metoprolol did.[32]

CHRONIC KIDNEY DISEASE

The JNC-7 considers CKD a compelling indication for either an ACE inhibitor or ARB therapy.[8] For the purposes of identifying this compelling indication, CKD in general stage 3 or higher is defined as 1) an eGFR below 60 mL/min/1.73 m² (correlating to a serum creatinine >1.3 mg/dL in women or >1.5 mg/dL in men), or 2) albuminuria (>300 mg/day or >200 mg/g creatinine).[8] In general, this is stage 3 or higher CKD. Treatment with an ACE inhibitor or ARB has been proven to reduce the rate of kidney disease progression and to lower BP in patients with CKD and proteinuria.

Diuretics are generally needed in hypertensive patients with CKD for both BP control and volume regulation. A thiazide or thiazide-like diuretic is recommended in CKD patients with an eGFR of 30 mL/min/1.73 m² or higher.[22] When eGFR is below the 30 mL/min/1.73 m² threshold, or when the patient develops volume overload and edema, a loop diuretic should be used.[22]

CORONARY ARTERY DISEASE

Patients with CAD—that is, a prior history of myocardial infarction (MI), chronic stable angina, or acute coronary syndrome—are at high risk for recurrent CV events and CV death. CAD is considered a compelling indication for specific antihypertensive therapy that is proven to reduce risk of CV disease outcomes.[33-36] β-Blocker treatment is the cornerstone of drug therapy for patients with hypertension and CAD because of proven long-term benefits.[33-36] In patients with acute MI, β-blocker therapy reduces risk of death by more than 20%.[37] In patients with CAD, β-blocker therapy reduces stimulation of the myocardium, balances myocardial oxygen supply and demand, and treats ischemic symptoms. Along with β-blocker therapy, patients should be treated with an ACE inhibitor or ARB to further reduce the risk of CV events, likely by preventing adverse cardiac remodeling.[33-36] These benefits are present even if BP reduction is not needed.[10,38]

Add-on therapy to a β-blocker plus ACE inhibitor (or ARB) regimen may both lower BP and reduce risk of CV events in patients with CAD. Thiazide or thiazidelike diuretics are proven add-on therapies. A CCB is also appropriate to treat ischemic symptoms. If added to a β-blocker, a dihydropyridine CCB should be chosen to avoid risk of excessive bradycardia, and even heart block, that is seen with β-blocker–nondihydropyridine CCB combinations. If a β-blocker cannot be used because of a contraindication or intolerable side effects, a nondihydropyridine CCB would be preferable owing to its ability to lower heart rate and reduce myocardial oxygen demand.

LEFT VENTRICULAR DYSFUNCTION

Antihypertensive drug therapy has been studied extensively in patients with left ventricular (LV) dysfunction or systolic heart failure, and it has been shown to improve LV function and to reduce related CV events, such as heart failure hospitalizations and CV death, at least in part by mechanisms other than BP lowering. Treatment with a "standard regimen" of a diuretic, ACE inhibitor or ARB, and an appropriate β-blocker has been proven to reduce the risk of CV events in patients with LV dysfunction.[8,10,39] Diuretic therapy, most often with a loop diuretic, relieves or prevents fluid overload in addition to lowering BP and preventing CV events; ACE inhibitor (or ARB) and β-blocker therapies are used to reduce risk of CV events and risk of death. For patients with intolerance to ACE inhibitor therapy, an ARB is an acceptable alternative.[40-43] Use of β-blocker therapy in combination with ACE inhibitor (or ARB) therapy both reduces risk of CV events and death and increases ejection fraction.[39] However, β-blocker therapy should be initiated using recommended starting doses (low doses) titrated up appropriately to a target dose. Only metoprolol, carvedilol, and bisoprolol have been studied sufficiently to recommend their use in patients with LV dysfunction.[39]

Beyond a standard regimen of a diuretic, ACE inhibitor or ARB, and an appropriate β-blocker, several add-on therapies have been studied.[39] Addition of an aldosterone antagonist is proven to further reduce the risk of CV events in patients with both mild and severe heart failure and in those with recent MI.[44-46] Another option is to add an ARB to a standard regimen that includes an ACE inhibitor.[47] However, most clinicians prefer to add an aldosterone antagonist ahead of an ARB to a standard regimen that includes an ACE inhibitor, because the addition of an ARB has only been shown to reduce the risk of certain CV events, namely hospitalized heart failure, not death.[47] Lastly, for African-American patients, addition of hydralazine in combination with isosorbide dinitrate is an option that has been shown to reduce the risk of CV events.[48]

PREVIOUS ISCHEMIC STROKE

History of stroke, specifically ischemic stroke, is a compelling indication for the use of a diuretic, with or without an ACE inhibitor, to reduce risk of a second stroke.[8,49,50] A meta-analysis of seven randomized controlled trials showed that diuretics alone and in combination with ACE inhibitors, but not β-blockers or ACE inhibitors used alone, reduced risk of recurrent stroke, MI, and total CV events; however, no effect was seen on mortality rate. CCBs and ARBs were not evaluated in any of the included trials.

The Protection Against Recurrent Stroke Study (PROGRESS) confirmed that recurrent stroke can be reduced in patients with a history of ischemic stroke when a thiazide-type diuretic is added to an ACE inhibitor.[51] Reduction in recurrent stroke was seen with this combination, even when pretreatment BP was below 140/90 mm Hg; however, recurrent stroke was not reduced with ACE inhibitor monotherapy in this study.

ARB therapy in patients with a history of stroke has not definitively been shown to reduce risk of recurrent stroke or CV events. The Morbidity and Mortality After Stroke: Eprosartan Compared with Nitrendipine for Secondary Prevention (MOSES) study demonstrated better reductions in recurrent stroke with ARB therapy compared with a dihydropyridine CCB, suggesting that CV endpoints are reduced with ARB therapy in patients with prior stroke.[52] However, in the Prevention Regimen for Effectively Avoiding Second Strokes (PROFESS) trial, patients with a history of ischemic stroke had similar rates of recurrent stroke and CV events with ARB therapy compared with placebo[53]; therefore the role of ARB therapy in secondary prevention of ischemic stroke has not been established.

Overview of Drug Classes

Many classes of drugs are available for the treatment of hypertension. The most frequently used antihypertensive drug classes are ACE inhibitors, ARBs, CCBs, and thiazide or thiazidelike diuretics. β-Blockers, aldosterone antagonists, and α-blockers are also commonly used as add-on therapy or for patients with compelling indications. These drug classes are summarized in Table 29-1.

PHARMACOLOGIC MANAGEMENT OF HYPERTENSION

TABLE 29-1   Overview of Commonly Used Antihypertensive Drug Classes

CLASS	MECHANISM OF ACTION	ROLE IN THERAPY	AVOID USE	SITUATIONS WITH POTENTIALLY FAVORABLE EFFECTS	SITUATIONS WITH POTENTIALLY UNFAVORABLE EFFECTS
ACE inhibitors	Inhibition of ACE results in decreased production of angiotensin II, which causes decreased vasoconstriction, decreased aldosterone secretion, and sodium and water retention. Also results in decreased breakdown of bradykinin and other vasoactive peptides, which results in vasodilation and allergic responses.	First-line or add-on therapy for uncomplicated hypertension. First-line therapy for compelling indications of diabetes, chronic kidney disease, coronary artery disease, left ventricular dysfunction, or previous ischemic stroke	Pregnancy, bilateral renal artery stenosis, history of angioedema	Low-normal potassium, prediabetes, albuminuria	High-normal potassium or hyperkalemia, volume depletion
Angiotensin receptor blockers	Blockade at the angiotensin II type 1 receptor results in decreased angiotensin II effects, which causes decreased vasoconstriction, decreased aldosterone secretion, and sodium and water retention.	First-line or add-on therapy for uncomplicated hypertension. First-line therapy for compelling indications of diabetes, chronic kidney disease, coronary artery disease, or left ventricular dysfunction. Commonly used as an alternative for patients with intolerance to ACE inhibitors	Pregnancy, bilateral renal artery stenosis	Low-normal potassium, prediabetes	High-normal potassium or hyperkalemia, volume depletion
Dihydropyridine calcium channel blockers	Blocking of cellular calcium entry through the L-type channel results in reduced total peripheral resistance through arterial vasodilation.	First-line or add-on therapy for uncomplicated hypertension. Add-on therapy for diabetes or coronary artery disease	Left ventricular dysfunction (all except amlodipine and felodipine)	Reynaud syndrome, elderly patients with isolated systolic hypertension, cyclosporine-induced hypertension	Peripheral edema, high-normal heart rate or tachycardia
Nondihydropyridine calcium channel blockers	Decreased cellular calcium entry through the L-type channel results in reduced total peripheral resistance through arterial vasodilation. Decreased myocardial contractility results in negative inotropic effects, and blocked AV nodal conduction results in decreased heart rate.	First-line or add-on therapy for uncomplicated hypertension. Add-on therapy for diabetes. Alternative to β-blockers in coronary artery disease	Second- or third-degree heart block, left ventricular dysfunction	Reynaud syndrome, migraine headache, arrhythmias, high-normal heart rate or tachycardia	Peripheral edema, low-normal heart rate
Thiazide diuretics	Initial transient effects cause natriuresis, resulting in reductions in cardiac output and decreased blood volume. Long-term persistent effects result in decreased peripheral vascular resistance.	First-line or add-on therapy for uncomplicated hypertension. First-line therapy for compelling indications of left ventricular dysfunction or previous ischemic stroke. Add-on therapy for diabetes or coronary artery disease	Prior anaphylactic and/or Stevens-Johnson–type reactions to sulfa-type drugs (less extreme reactions are not an absolute contraindication), gout, hyponatremia, hypokalemia	Osteoporosis or at increased risk for osteoporosis, high-normal potassium	Gout, prediabetes, low-normal potassium, elevated fasting glucose
β-Blockers	Blockade of β-1 receptors results in reduced cardiac output and reduced heart rate. Also inhibits renin release, decreases adrenergic central nervous system effects, and reduces catecholamine release/response.	Add-on therapy for uncomplicated hypertension. First-line therapy for compelling indications of coronary artery disease or left ventricular dysfunction. Add-on therapy for diabetes	Second- or third-degree heart block, acute decompensated heart failure, severe bronchospastic disease	Migraine headache, tachyarrhythmia, high-normal heart rate or tachycardia, hyperthyroidism, essential tremor, preoperative hypertension	Bronchospastic disease, chronic obstructive pulmonary disease, symptoms of hypoglycemia, high physical activity
Aldosterone antagonists	Blockade of aldosterone receptor results in decreased vasoconstriction and decreased sodium/water retention.	Add-on therapy for resistant hypertension. Add-on therapy for coronary artery disease or left ventricular dysfunction	Hypotension, dehydration, hyperkalemia	Low-normal potassium, chronic kidney disease	High-normal potassium

ACE, angiotensin-converting enzyme.

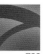

Angiotensin-Converting Enzyme Inhibitors

ACE inhibitors may be used as a first-line therapy for uncomplicated hypertension and are included in all first-line regimens for patients with compelling indications (Table 29-2).[8] They inhibit angiotensin-converting enzyme and result in decreased production of angiotensin II and decreased breakdown of bradykinin; thus they promote vasodilation.[54] ACE inhibitor use is not accompanied by unfavorable compensatory changes such as sodium and water retention or increased heart rate. However, adding a thiazide, even in small doses, to ACE inhibitor therapy enhances the antihypertensive efficacy of the ACE inhibitor, because diuretic-induced sodium depletion activates the renin-angiotensin-aldosterone system and makes BP more angiotensin II dependent.[55] Similarly, addition of either a dihydropyridine or a nondihydropyridine CCB enhances the BP-lowering effects of the ACE inhibitor.[55] β-Blockers can also be given together with ACE inhibitors, although the incremental effect on BP lowering is minor. β-Blockade in this combination may be beneficial, because it blunts the reactive rise in plasma renin activity that accompanies ACE inhibitor therapy.

ACE inhibitor therapy has benefits beyond BP lowering. Long-term ACE inhibitor therapy delays the onset of type 2 diabetes.[56] Further, ACE inhibitor therapy can restore endothelial function in patients with endothelial dysfunction, and it can remodel blood vessels, and in the process, it improves vascular compliance.[57] By blocking the effects of angiotensin II, ACE inhibitor therapy inhibits constriction of the efferent arteriole in the glomerulus. This pharmacologic effect has been used to explain the benefits of ACE inhibitors in slowing progression of kidney disease[58,59]; however, it is unclear whether these renal benefits of ACE inhibitors are independent of BP lowering.[60]

ACE inhibitors are effective in lowering BP in most patients but are generally less effective as monotherapy in salt-sensitive, low-renin forms of hypertension—such as that often found in African-American, diabetic, and elderly hypertensive patients—unless administered in higher than usual doses.[61] However, BP responses to ACE inhibitor therapy are variable, and some individuals in these groups experience significant BP reductions with usual doses. The dose-response curve for BP reduction is steep at low doses of ACE inhibitors but typically flattens at moderate to high doses. The antihypertensive effects of ACE inhibitors are linked to the patient's volume status. When volume losses occur, both intentional (diuretic therapy) and unintentional (sweating/exercise), major decreases in BP and deterioration in renal function to the point of acute renal failure can result from ACE inhibitor therapy.

Adverse effects associated with ACE inhibitors include cough, angioedema, and a distinctive form of functional renal insufficiency.[62] A dry cough can occur with ACE inhibitor therapy, likely owing to the decreased breakdown of peptide mediators, including substance P and bradykinin. If cough occurs with an ACE inhibitor, it is unlikely that switching to another ACE inhibitor will relieve this symptom, as it appears to be a class effect. If a patient experiences angioedema, future treatment with an ACE inhibitor is contraindicated. Under these circumstances, an ARB is a reasonable alternative,[63] although angioedema has rarely been reported with ARBs.

The occurrence of functional renal insufficiency with an ACE inhibitor does not preclude future use of ACE inhibitor therapy, unless high-grade bilateral renal artery stenosis is present. Initiation of ACE inhibitor therapy often reduces GFR, owing to the decrease in angiotensin II–induced constrictor effects on the efferent arteriole. This effect is typically limited to an increase in serum creatinine of less than 30% and is not a reason to discontinue therapy.[64]

Angiotensin Receptor Blockers

ARBs are first-line options for treatment of uncomplicated hypertension and are a reasonable alternative to ACE inhibitor therapy for many patients with compelling indications (Table 29-3). The ARBs blunt the effects of angiotensin II via direct blockade of the angiotensin II type 1 receptor; they have no effect on generation of angiotensin II or breakdown of bradykinin or substance P. ARBs differ in bioavailability, rate of absorption, volume of distribution, and metabolism—that is, whether it metabolizes cytochrome (CY) P450—but these pharmacokinetic differences are of little practical consequence.[65] Duration of receptor occupancy, a surrogate for the BP-lowering effect of the ARB class, is most relevant when low doses of ARBs are used. All ARBs are eliminated through some combination of renal and hepatic clearance. This distinguishes the ARBs from ACE inhibitors, which are predominantly renally cleared.

Most ARBs are indicated for once-daily dosing, but at low doses, they may lose efficacy at the end of a dose interval, thereby necessitating twice-daily dosing. Similar to ACE inhibitors, certain patient groups are generally more responsive (high-renin and young hypertensive patients) or less responsive (low-renin, salt-sensitive, volume-expanded individuals, such as African Americans) to ARB monotherapy. Also similar to the ACE inhibitors, the effectiveness of an ARB in lowering BP is increased with addition of a diuretic or a CCB. On the basis of experience with ACE inhibitors, it can be expected that addition of a β-blocker to an ARB would have a minimal additional effect on BP but might be indicated to treat a compelling indication.

The Ongoing Telmisartan Alone and in Combination with Ramipril Global Endpoint Trial (ONTARGET) compared the effects of ARB-based therapy to ACE inhibitor–based therapy and combination therapy with ARBs and ACE inhibitors on CV events in patients at high risk of CVD, the majority of whom had

TABLE 29-2	Summary of ACE Inhibitors in Hypertension		
DRUG	**DOSE RANGE (MG/DAY)***	**DAILY DOSES**	**SPECIAL CONSIDERATIONS†**
Benazepril (Lotensin)	10-80	1 or 2	Risk of hyperkalemia is increased in severe chronic kidney disease or when combined with a potassium-sparing diuretic, aldosterone antagonist, angiotensin recepter blocker, direct renin inhibitor, or potassium supplements
Captopril (Capoten)	75-450	2 or 3	
Enalapril (Renitec, Vasotec)	5-40	1 or 2	Can cause acute kidney failure in patients with severe bilateral renal artery stenosis, severe stenosis in an artery to a solitary kidney, volume depletion, or severe heart failure
Fosinopril (Monopril)	10-80	1 or 2	
Lisinopril (Prinivil, Zestril)	10-80	1	Usually results in small increases in serum creatinine (typically less than 30% from baseline)
Moexipril (Univasc)	7.5-30	1	
Perindopril (Aceon)	4-16	1 or 2	*Never use* in pregnancy
Quinapril (Accupril)	10-80	1 or 2	*Never use* with history of angioedema
Ramipril (Altace)	2.5-20	1 or 2	Starting dose can be halved in patients at risk for orthostatic hypotension
Trandolapril (Mavik)	1-8	1 or 2	Can increase lithium concentrations

*Lists the typical starting and maximum daily doses for the management of hypertension.
†Apply to all drugs in table.

TABLE 29-3 **Summary of Angiotensin Receptor Blockers in Hypertension**

DRUG	DOSE RANGE (MG/DAY)	DAILY DOSES	SPECIAL CONSIDERATIONS†
Azilsartan medoxomil (Edarbi)	80	1	Risk of hyperkalemia is increased in severe CKD or in combination with a potassium-sparing diuretic, aldosterone antagonist, ACEI, direct renin inhibitor, or potassium supplements
Candesartan cilexetil (Atacand)	16-32	1	
Eprosartan mesylate (Teveten)	600-800	1 or 2	Can cause acute kidney failure in patients with severe bilateral renal artery stenosis or severe stenosis in an artery to a solitary kidney
Irbesartan (Avapro)	150-300	1	
Losartan potassium (Cozaar)	50-100	1 or 2	Usually results in small increases in serum creatinine (typically less than 30% from baseline)
Olmesartan medoxomil (Benicar)	20-40	1	*Never use* in pregnancy
Telmisartan (Micardis)	40-80	1	Starting dose can be halved in patients at risk for orthostatic hypotension
Valsartan (Diovan)	80-320	1	Can increase lithium concentrations

*Lists the typical starting and maximum daily doses for the management of hypertension.
†Apply to all drugs in table.
ACEI, angiotensin-converting enzyme inhibitors; CKD, chronic kidney disease.

TABLE 29-4 **Summary of Calcium Channel Blockers in Hypertension**

DRUG	DOSE RANGE (MG/DAY)*	DAILY DOSES	SPECIAL CONSIDERATIONS
Dihydropyridines			
Amlodipine (Norvasc)	2.5-10	1	Short-acting dihydropyridines (i.e., immediate-release nifedipine, immediate-release nicardipine) are not listed because they should not be used to manage hypertension
Felodipine (Plendil)	2.5-10	1	
Isradipine SR (Dynacirc SR)	5-20	1	
Nicardipine, sustained-release (Cardene SR)	60-120	2	Dihydropyridines are more potent arterial vasodilators than nondihydropyridines
Nifedipine, long-acting (Adalat CC, Nifedical XL, Procardia XL)	30-120	1	Concurrent use with an angiotensin-converting enzyme inhibitor or angiotensin receptor blocker can minimize peripheral edema
Nisoldipine (Sular)	17-34	1	
Nondihydropyridines			
Diltiazem, sustained-release and extended-release (Cardizem CD, Cardizem LA, Cartia XT, Dilacor XR, Diltia XT, Tiazac, Taztia XT)	120-540	1	Preferentially use extended-release, once-daily products
			Risk of heart block is increased when used in combination with β-blockers or digoxin
Verapamil, sustained-release (Calan SR, Isoptin SR, Verelan)	120-480	1 or 2	Most diltiazem and verapamil products are not interchangeable on an equipotent mg-per-mg basis because of different release mechanisms and bioavailability
Verapamil, controlled-onset, extended-release (Covera HS)	180-480	1	Cardizem LA, Covera HS, and Verelan PM have delayed drug release for several hours after dosing
Verapamil, sustained-release, slow-onset (Verelan PM)	100-400	1	When dosed in the evening, these can provide chronotherapeutic drug delivery
			Can inhibit cytochrome p450 3A4 metabolism and interact with many drugs
			Can increase cyclosporine concentrations

*Dose range lists the typical starting and maximum daily doses for the management of hypertension. The dosage range for diltiazem varies based on the product; refer to manufacturer recommendations for exact dose.

hypertension.[66] The main finding was that the ACE inhibitors and ARBs were equally effective for lowering BP and preventing CV events, but the combination produced minimal additional BP lowering and no benefit in preventing CV events compared with either monotherapy. Further, adverse events occurred more frequently with the combination than with either drug therapy alone. Accordingly, ACE inhibitors with ARB combinations are not recommended for the treatment of uncomplicated hypertension.

ARBs are firmly established as an alternative and are arguably on par with ACE inhibitors for the compelling indications of diabetes, CKD, CAD (post MI), and LV dysfunction.[8,33,34,36,39,43,67-70] However, results of outcome trials of ARBs for prevention of recurrent stroke are conflicting.[52,53]

ARBs have a low rate of adverse effects and result in high adherence and persistence rates in patients with uncomplicated hypertension.[71] Cough does not occur with ARBs, and angioedema is rarely a problem. Data from the prospective, randomized, placebo-controlled Telmisartan Randomized Assessment Study in ACE Intolerant Subjects with Cardiovascular Disease (TRANSCEND) trial indicate that patients with angioedema on ACE inhibitor therapy will not experience angioedema with an ARB.[63]

Calcium Channel Blockers

The CCBs include two main subclasses of compounds: the *dihydropyridines* and the *nondihydropyridines*. These can be further subdivided into the *benzothiazepines*, such as diltiazem, and *phenylalkylamines*, such as verapamil. Although all CCBs block L-type calcium channels, and all have vasodilator effects, these subclasses have distinctly different structures and pharmacologic characteristics (Table 29-4).[55] CCBs can be used as first-line therapy for uncomplicated hypertension, and they have a compelling indication as add-on therapy for patients with diabetes and CAD.[8] Several other uses are possible for dihydropyridine CCBs, such as cyclosporine-induced hypertension and Raynaud phenomenon, and for nondihydropyridine CCBs, including atrial fibrillation and migraine headache prevention. Because CCBs are not associated with metabolic side effects, patients who experience such effects from other antihypertensive drugs can be safely treated with CCBs.

Dihydropyridine CCBs are potent arterial vasodilators that can elicit activation of the sympathetic nervous system and result in reflex tachycardia. Nondihydropyridine CCBs are less potent arterial vasodilators but have major effects on the heart, and they have clinically significant negative inotropic effects; second-generation dihydropyridine CCBs, such as amlodipine or felodipine, are selective for the vasculature and have little, if any, effect on cardiac contractility. CCBs do not have adverse metabolic effects.

The adverse effects of CCBs are predictable based on their pharmacologic properties.[72] With all CCBs, blockade of L-type calcium channels can decrease lower esophageal sphincter pressure and cause gastroesophageal reflux. Typically this is not a treatment-limiting effect. All CCBs can slow gastrointestinal transit time and increase risk of constipation; verapamil has the highest incidence of this adverse effect. Rarely CCBs can cause gingival hyperplasia or polyuria. Because of their potent arterial dilation, dihydropyridine CCBs frequently cause flushing, headache, and peripheral edema; the peripheral edema is caused by a selective decrease in arteriolar resistance, whereby precapillary hydrostatic pressures increase and favor a fluid shift into the interstitial compartment. CCB-related edema is dose dependent and is more common in women and older people. Peripheral edema can be a treatment- or dose-limiting side effect of dihydropyridine CCBs that can be slow to resolve without intervention but is mitigated by reducing the dihydropyridine dose, by adding an ACE inhibitor or ARB, and by encouraging the patient to elevate the lower extremities whenever possible. Diuretic therapy is relatively ineffective in reducing CCB-induced edema and is not recommended as a management strategy. For bothersome peripheral edema that does not resolve with dose reduction or addition of ACE inhibitor or ARB therapy, the CCB must be discontinued.

Nondihydropyridine CCBs can cause atrioventricular (AV) block and resultant bradycardia, particularly when administered in high doses or with sympatholytic drugs such as β-blockers, and they are contraindicated in patients with LV dysfunction because of the risk of heart failure exacerbation as a result of their negative inotropic effects. Verapamil and diltiazem inhibit the CYP450 3A4 isoenzyme system and can result in drug interactions, such as with cyclosporine and simvastatin.

The availability of sustained-release delivery systems for CCBs, particularly the dihydropyridines, has enhanced their use because of a reduced side-effect profile and more sustained BP reduction. Short-acting dihydropyridine CCBs reduce BP abruptly, activating the sympathetic nervous system and potentially inciting coronary ischemia. This process does not occur with long-acting dihydropyridine CCBs, which lower BP gradually and smoothly.

All patient groups are to some degree responsive to CCB monotherapy. Low-renin, salt-sensitive, volume-expanded patients, such as diabetic and African-American patients, are more often responsive to a CCB than to an ACE inhibitor or a β-blocker. Elderly patients are also highly responsive to the vasodilator and BP-lowering effects of CCBs; however, these are generalizations that may not reliably predict the magnitude of BP reduction in individual patients.

Diuretics: Thiazides

Thiazide and thiazide-like diuretics are widely used in the treatment of hypertension (Table 29-5). They are recommended as first-line agents for uncomplicated hypertension and in patients with compelling indications such as LV dysfunction, although loop diuretics are commonly needed in this situation, and previous ischemic stroke. Thiazide and thiazide-like diuretics have been shown in numerous controlled clinical trials to decrease hypertension-associated morbidity and mortality.[1-3,8] They are particularly effective in lowering BP in African Americans and the elderly. Diuretics combine well with nearly every other antihypertensive drug class[73,74] and are available in fixed-dose combinations with most other drug classes.

The effects of a thiazide or thiazide-like diuretic on BP can be divided into three sequential phases: 1) short-term, 2) long-term, and 3) chronic.[73] In the *short-term phase*, the first 2 to 4 weeks, reductions in BP are related to decreases in cardiac output and plasma volume. At this time, there is an increase in plasma renin activity and a transient increase in peripheral vascular resistance. During the *long-term phase* of diuretic therapy, cardiac output and plasma volume return to pretreatment levels, but BP is still decreased because of a persistent decrease in peripheral vascular resistance despite the increase in plasma renin activity. The *chronic* antihypertensive effect of thiazide diuretics is more closely

TABLE 29-5	Summary of Diuretics in Hypertension		
DRUG	**DOSE RANGE (MG/DAY)***	**DAILY DOSES**	**SPECIAL CONSIDERATIONS**
Thiazides			
Chlorthalidone (Hydone, Hygroton, Thalitone)	12.5-50	1	Most effective diuretic class for lowering blood pressure in most patients
Hydrochlorothiazide (Aquazide H, Carozide, Diaqua, Esidrix, Ezide, Hydro Par, HydroDIURIL. Hydrocot, Hydrokraft, Loqua, Oretic)	12.5-50	1	Usual doses mitigate adverse metabolic effects Chlorthalidone is 1.5 to 2 times more potent than hydrochlorothiazide Additional benefits in osteoporosis by retaining calcium
Indapamide (Lozol)	1.25-5	1	Patients with prediabetes have an increased risk of progressing to type 2 diabetes Can increase lithium concentrations
Loop			
Furosemide (Lasix, Delone, Furocot, Lo-Aqua)	20-600	2	May be preferred over thiazides in patients with severe CKD or chronic heart failure
Torsemide (Demadex)	5-10	1	
Potassium Sparing			
Amiloride (Midamor)	5-20	1	Primarily used to minimize thiazide-associated hypokalemia
Triamterene (Dyrenium)	37.5-75	1	Trimaterene should only be used in combination with hydrochlorothiazide when used for hypertension Does not significantly lower blood pressure unless used with another diuretic Risk of hyperkalemia is increased in severe CKD or when combined with an aldosterone antagonist, ACE inhibitor, ARB, direct renin inhibitor, or potassium supplements

*Lists the typical starting and maximum daily doses for the management of hypertension.
ACE, angiotensin-converting enzyme; ARB, angiotensin receptor blocker; CKD, chronic kidney disease.

related to a persistent reduction in total peripheral resistance than to volume reduction.[73]

Hydrochlorothiazide (HCTZ) is the most frequently used thiazide diuretic in the United States, although chlorthalidone is the diuretic that was used in many of the landmark clinical outcomes trials.[1-3,17] The pharmacokinetic and pharmacodynamic profile of chlorthalidone is distinctly different from that of HCTZ. On a milligram-per-milligram basis, chlorthalidone is 1.5 to 2 times more potent than HCTZ.[75] In recommended doses, chlorthalidone is more effective in lowering systolic BP (SBP) than hydrochlorothiazide, as evidenced by 24-hour ambulatory BPs.[76] This likely is because chlorthalidone has a longer half-life than HCTZ (50 to 60 hours vs. 9 to 10 hours).[73] Further, the 24-hour BP-lowering effect of HCTZ in doses of 12.5 to 25 mg/day, those most commonly used in clinical practice, is inferior to other antihypertensive drug classes—including ACE inhibitors, ARBs, CCBs, and even β-blockers. Moreover, HCTZ 12.4 to 25 mg/day is also inferior to HCTZ 50 mg/day.[77]

The thiazide diuretics have a number of adverse metabolic effects that include hypokalemia, hypomagnesemia, glucose intolerance, hypercholesterolemia, and hyperuricemia. These adverse effects are dose dependent and were most prominent in the early years of thiazide use, when high doses (100 to 200 mg/day) were frequently used. In currently used doses, these adverse effects are less troublesome and can be minimized by concomitant administration of a potassium supplement; a potassium-sparing diuretic; or an ACE inhibitor, ARB, or aldosterone antagonist. In ALLHAT,

patients treated with chlorthalidone had a significantly higher incidence of progression to type 2 diabetes than patients treated with lisinopril or amlodipine, a trend consistently seen in other clinical trials.[17,56] However, elevated blood glucose levels and new-onset diabetes in the context of chlorthalidone treatment were not associated with an increase in risk of CVD events in that trial.[28,78,79] Nevertheless, clinicians should be aware that thiazide diuretic therapy can push patients at very high risk for dysglycemia (patients with prediabetes) into type 2 diabetes at a higher rate than other antihypertensive drug classes.

The loop diuretics do not reduce BP as well as thiazides, particularly when dosed once a day. Loop diuretics should be reserved for patients who require treatment of volume overload or edema in addition to BP lowering, and they are more appropriate and effective than thiazide diuretics in lowering BP and controlling volume in patients who have severe CKD (eGFR <30/min/1.73 m^2).[73]

β-Blockers

β-Blockers can be divided into four subclasses based on their pharmacologic effects (Table 29-6).[58] *Cardioselective β-blockers*— such as atenolol, bisoprolol, metoprolol, and nebivolol—selectively block β$_1$-receptors when used in approved doses. *Nonselective β-blockers* also block β$_2$-receptors in the lung and sometimes result in bronchoconstriction. *β-Blockers with intrinsic sympathomimetic activity* block β$_1$- and sometimes β$_2$-receptors but also keep them partially activated; these agents have little to no role in clinical

TABLE 29-6   Summary of β-Blockers in Hypertension

DRUG	DOSE RANGE (MG/DAY)*	DAILY DOSES	SPECIAL CONSIDERATIONS
Cardioselective			
Atenolol (Tenormin)	25-100	1 or 2	Blocks β$_1$ receptors with low to moderate doses but some may block β$_2$ receptors with high doses
Betaxolol (Kerlone)	5-20	1	Can be used in asthma or COPD in low to moderate doses
Bisoprolol (Zebeta)	2.5-20	1	Nebivolol can result in vasodilation and fewer side effects because of nitric oxide effects
Metoprolol tartrate (Lopressor)	100-450	2	Can cause rebound hypertension if stopped abruptly
Metoprolol succinate extended release (Toprol XL)	25-400	1	Adverse metabolic effects (dyslipidemia, hyperglycemia) are minimal
			Can cause angina if used with cocaine
Nebivolol (Bystolic)	5-40	1	Risk of heart block is increased when used in combination with nondihydropyridine CCBs or digoxin
Nonselective			
Nadolol (Corgard)	20-320	1	Blocks both β$_1$ and β$_2$ receptors at all doses
Propranolol (Inderal)	40-640	2	Should not be used in asthma or COPD
Propranolol, long-acting (Inderal LA, Innopran XL)	60-640	1	Nonselective β-blockade may be beneficial for use in noncardiovascular conditions (e.g., hyperthyroidism, essential tremor, migraine headache)
			Can cause rebound hypertension if stopped abruptly
Timolol (Blocadren)	20-60	2	Adverse metabolic effects (dyslipidemia, hyperglycemia) are minimal
			Can cause angina if used with cocaine
			Risk of heart block is increased when used in combination with nondihydropyridine CCBs or digoxin
Intrinsic Sympathomimetic Activity			
Acebutolol (Sectral)	400-1200	2	*Never use* in patients with coronary artery disease
Penbutolol (Levatol)	20-80	1	Keeps β-receptors partially stimulated while maintaining blockade
			Can cause rebound hypertension if stopped abruptly
Pindolol (Visken)	10-60	2	Adverse metabolic effects (dyslipidemia, hyperglycemia) are minimal
			Can cause angina if used with cocaine
			Risk of heart block is increased when used in combination with nondihydropyridine CCBs or digoxin
Mixed α-/β-Blockers			
Carvedilol (Coreg)	12.5-50	2	Blocks β$_1$, β$_2$, and α-receptors, resulting in additional peripheral vasodilation
Carvedilol phosphate (Coreg CR)	20-80	1	Do not use in asthma or COPD
			Can cause rebound hypertension if stopped abruptly
Labetalol (Normodyne, Trandate)	200-2400	2	Lowest risk of all β-blockers of causing angina when used with cocaine
			Risk of heart block is increased when used in combination with nondihydropyridine CCBs or digoxin

*Lists the typical starting and maximum daily doses for the management of hypertension.
CCB, calcium channel blocker; COPD, chronic obstructive pulmonary disease.

practice and are contraindicated in patients with CAD. The *mixed α-/β-blockers*, carvedilol and labetalol, block peripheral $α_1$-receptors and both $β_1$- and $β_2$-receptors. These agents share the pharmacologic properties of nonselective β-blockers but have a lower degree of α-blockade than pure α-blockers, and their α-blocking effects become attenuated with chronic use.

Use of β-blockers for hypertension has declined over the past several years owing to their limited efficacy in preventing CV outcomes in randomized trials and their adverse-effect profiles. Escalating doses of β-blockers can induce salt and water retention, making diuretics a needed adjunctive form of therapy. Abrupt discontinuation of a β-blocker, particularly when administered in high doses, may be followed by adrenergically mediated rebound hypertension[55]; therefore a stepwise reduction in dose is needed when discontinuing therapy. β-Blockers administered with either verapamil or diltiazem can cause sharp reductions in heart rate and risk of heart block, and this combination should be used with caution. Erectile dysfunction, hyperglycemia, and dyslipidemia have been reported with β-blockers, but these can be minimized by use of low to moderate doses.[80,81] The metabolic side effects, hyperglycemia and dyslipidemia, are less frequent with low doses of traditional β-blockers, vasodilating β-blockers (nebivolol), and mixed α-/β-blockers (e.g., carvedilol) than with high doses of traditional β-blockers.[32]

For patients with uncomplicated hypertension, β-blockers are considered a first-line option in the JNC-7 guidelines[8] but are considered add-on therapy in newer guidelines and scientific statements.[10,18] β-Blockers have a compelling indication for treatment of CAD, especially post MI, and also come with a high coronary disease risk and a higher risk of LV dysfunction.[8] They also have a compelling indication as add-on therapy in diabetes.[8] These drugs may be helpful for patients with high adrenergic drive, essential tremor, tachycardia, or arrhythmias but should not supplant appropriate first-line agents—ACE inhibitors, ARBs, CCBs, and diuretics—that have been proven to be more effective in reducing risk of CV events in patients with uncomplicated hypertension.[4,10] β-Blockers are useful as add-on therapy in hypertensive patients with tachycardic responses to other antihypertensive drug classes, such as dihydropyridine CCBs or arterial vasodilators.

Aldosterone Antagonists

The two clinically available aldosterone antagonists are spironolactone and eplerenone (Table 29-7). These agents are particularly useful in the treatment of resistant hypertension, and indications for their use in patients with CAD (after MI) and heart failure are compelling.[8]

Spironolactone is a nonselective steroid receptor agonist/antagonist that has progestogenic and antiandrogenic effects in addition to its aldosterone receptor–blocking activity. These side effects can lead to painful gynecomastia and erectile dysfunction in men and to menstrual irregularities in women. The gynecomastia is dose dependent, may be unilateral or bilateral, and may be accompanied by the appearance of discrete breast masses. Gynecomastia is generally reversible with discontinuation of the drug, but the time required for reversal can be prolonged. The onset of

action for spironolactone is characteristically slow, with a peak response at 48 hours or more after the first dose. This may be caused by a requirement of several days of spironolactone dosing for its active metabolites to reach steady-state plasma/tissue levels. In contrast, no active metabolites have been identified for eplerenone. Spironolactone has been used extensively with or without a thiazide diuretic in the treatment of uncomplicated hypertension and more recently as add-on therapy in patients with resistant hypertension.[82]

Eplerenone is highly selective for blockade of the aldosterone receptor and has a much lower incidence of progestogenic and antiandrogenic side effects, including gynecomastia, than spironolactone.[83] Eplerenone can be safely substituted for spironolactone in the patient with gynecomastia. The BP-lowering effect of eplerenone is less than that of spironolactone, and there is less experience with it in the treatment of uncomplicated hypertension.

Hyperkalemia (>5.5 mEq/L) can occur with either of the aldosterone antagonists and is the major limiting factor for use of these agents. Hyperkalemia occurs most typically when aldosterone antagonists are administered to patients with CKD and/or in combination with other agents known to increase serum potassium, such as ACE inhibitors and ARBs.

Other Agents

Several classes of available drugs are effective in lowering BP and are approved for the treatment of hypertension but have not been shown in clinical trials to reduce the risk of CV events (see Table 29-8). These agents are not generally recommended as first-line treatment but may be used as add-on therapy for uncomplicated hypertension and in hypertensive patients with comorbid conditions that are responsive to them.

α-BLOCKERS

Peripheral $α_1$-adrenergic-blocking drugs, or α-blockers, are effective in reducing BP.[55] At therapeutic doses, these agents block peripheral α-adrenergic receptors and result in arterial vasodilation. Initiating therapy at a low dose followed by dose escalation is necessary to minimize the risk of first-dose orthostatic hypotension or syncope. This occurs with all α-blockers, particularly in volume-contracted patients, but it is less common with the longer–half-life agents (doxazosin, terazosin). Because the stimulation of peripheral α-receptors that normally occurs to maintain BP when a person assumes the upright posture is attenuated or absent when α-blocker therapy is used, orthostatic hypotension can occur. α-Blockers can also trigger compensatory renal sodium retention and volume expansion; thus they should be given with a diuretic, unless doses are kept very low. Dizziness, headache, and drowsiness are other common side effects of α-blockers.

Since early termination of the doxazosin treatment arm in ALLHAT, α-blockers have not been recommended as a first-line antihypertensive treatment in the United States.[5,8] However, α-blockers provide symptomatic relief for patients with benign prostatic hyperplasia (BPH) by improving both BPH symptom score and urinary flow.

TABLE 29-7	Summary of Aldosterone Antagonists in Hypertension		
DRUG	**DOSE RANGE (MG/DAY)***	**DAILY DOSES**	**SPECIAL CONSIDERATIONS**
Eplerenone (Inspra)	50-100	1 or 2	Contraindicated if estimated creatinine clearance is <50 mL/min, serum creatinine >1.8 mg/dL in women or >2 mg/dL in men, or in type 2 diabetes with microalbuminuria
Spironolactone (Aldactone)	25-50	1 or 2	Often used as add-on therapy in resistant hypertension
			Risk of hyperkalemia is increased in severe CKD or when combined with a potassium-sparing diuretic, ACE inhibitor, ARB, direct renin inhibitor, or potassium supplements

*Lists the typical starting and maximum daily doses for the management of hypertension.
ACE, angiotensin-converting enzyme; ARB, angiotensin receptor blocker; CKD, chronic kidney disease.

TABLE 29-8   Summary of Other Antihypertensive Drugs

CLASS	DRUG	DOSE RANGE (MG/DAY)*	DAILY DOSES	SPECIAL CONSIDERATIONS
α_1-Blockers	Doxazosin (Cardura) Prazosin (Minipress) Terazosin (Hytrin)	1-16 2-20 1-20	1 2 or 3 1 or 2	High risk of orthostatic hypotension, especially with first dose Patients should rise from sitting or lying down slowly to minimize orthostatic hypotension risk Additional symptomatic benefits in benign prostatic hyperplasia
Direct renin inhibitor	Aliskiren (Tekturna)	150-300	1	Can cause hyperkalemia in patients with CKD and diabetes or in those receiving a potassium-sparing diuretic, aldosterone antagonist, ACE inhibitor, or ARB Can cause acute kidney failure in patients with severe bilateral renal artery stenosis or severe stenosis in an artery to a solitary kidney Usually results in small increases in serum creatinine (typically <30% from baseline) *Never use* in pregnancy Starting dose can be halved in patients at risk for orthostatic hypotension
Central α_2 agonists	Clonidine (Catapres, Kapvay, Nexiclon) Clonidine patch (Catapres-TTS) Methyldopa (Aldomet)	0.2-2.4 0.1 to 0.6 500-3000	2 Once weekly 2-4	Can cause rebound hypertension if stopped abruptly Optimally used with a diuretic to diminish fluid retention Clonidine patch should be replaced once per week
Rauwolfia alkaloid	Reserpine	0.05-0.25	1	Optimally used with a diuretic to diminish fluid retention
Direct arterial vasodilators	Minoxidil (Loniten) Hydralazine (Apresoline)	2.5-100 20-300	1 or 2 2-4	Optimally used with a diuretic and β-blocker to mitigate fluid retention and reflex tachycardia

*Lists the typical starting and maximum daily doses for the management of hypertension.
ACE, angiotensin-converting enzyme; ARB, angiotensin receptor blocker; CKD, chronic kidney disease.

ARTERIAL VASODILATORS

Hydralazine and minoxidil are direct arterial vasodilators that lower BP but cause compensatory tachycardia and sodium retention. When used for chronic hypertension, these agents should be used in combination with both a diuretic and β-blocker or nondihydropyridine CCB to mitigate these side effects. These agents are often used as add-on therapy to manage resistant hypertension, particularly in patients with severe CKD.

Hydralazine has a dose-dependent increased risk of drug-induced lupus with long-term use,[55] and it must be given multiple times daily, which can compromise adherence. Because of its long track record of safety in pregnant women, hydralazine is recommended for the treatment of gestational hypertension,[84] and in combination with isosorbide dinitrate, it is recommended for the treatment of heart failure in African-American patients.[39,48]

One undesirable adverse effect of minoxidil use is hypertrichosis, particularly in women. Hair growth begins within 3 to 6 weeks of starting therapy; it occurs over the temples and eyebrows initially, then it spreads to areas between the eyebrows and hairline or sideburn regions and finally to the trunk, extremities, and scalp. Hypertrichosis usually disappears within a few weeks of discontinuing minoxidil, although in some cases the process is prolonged.

CENTRAL α-AGONISTS

Central α-agonists stimulate α_2-receptors in the brain and result in decreased sympathetic nervous outflow and decreased peripheral arterial resistance.[55] They lower BP effectively and quickly but can also cause rebound hypertension when stopped abruptly after chronic use. Central α-agonists often result in sodium and water retention; thus it may be desirable to use these drugs in combination with a diuretic.

Clonidine is the most commonly prescribed central α-agonist. It is limited by dose-dependent anticholinergic side effects such as drowsiness, dry mouth, and constipation. Clonidine is also available in a transdermal delivery system, which offers potential advantages but can cause skin irritation. Transdermal clonidine is particularly useful in the management of the labile hypertensive patient who requires multiple medications, the hospitalized patient who cannot take medications by mouth, and the patient prone to early-morning surges in BP. Clonidine overdose can produce paradoxical hypertension when the depressor effects of central α_2-adrenergic–receptor stimulation are exceeded by the pressor effects of peripheral α_2-adrenergic–receptor stimulation, resulting in a predominantly vasoconstrictive response.

Methyldopa is a central α-agonist used almost exclusively in gestational hypertension and in the management of chronic hypertension in pregnancy because of its long history of safety.[84] Methyldopa offers no advantage over clonidine in hypertension management other than producing fewer anticholinergic side effects, and it has been associated with hepatotoxicity.

DIRECT RENIN INHIBITOR

Aliskiren is the only direct renin inhibitor currently available. It binds directly to the catalytic site of renin and prevents it from cleaving angiotensinogen to generate angiotensin I, thus attenuating downstream events in the renin-angiotensin-aldosterone cascade and resulting in BP lowering.[85] It has a long half-life and provides a 24-hour antihypertensive effect with once-daily dosing. Most of the cautions and adverse effects seen with ACE inhibitors and ARBs apply to aliskiren, and it should never be used in pregnancy. Similar to ACE inhibitors, angioedema has been reported in patients treated with aliskiren, and small increases in creatinine and serum potassium can be seen with its use, similar to ACE inhibitors and ARBs.

Aliskiren is approved as monotherapy or in combination therapy for hypertension. However, because it represents a new drug class and has not been shown to prevent CV events, it is not preferred as first-line therapy. Aliskiren has demonstrated efficacy in lowering BP when used in combination with a thiazide, ACE inhibitor, ARB, or CCB, but it has not been well studied in combination with maximum doses of these agents. The Aliskiren in the Evaluation of Proteinuria in Diabetes (AVOID) trial demonstrated that the combination of aliskiren with losartan resulted in a reduction in proteinuria compared with losartan alone in patients with type 2 diabetes.[86] Aliskiren may also have a potential renoprotective role in this patient group.

RAUWOLFIA ALKALOIDS

Reserpine depletes norepinephrine from sympathetic nerve endings and blocks transport of norepinephrine into storage granules, thereby reducing norepinephrine release into the synapse after nerve stimulation. Reserpine can also deplete catecholamines in the brain and the myocardium, which can lead to dose-dependent sedation, depression, and decreased cardiac output. Reserpine lowers BP by reducing sympathetic tone and peripheral vascular resistance, and it is rarely used in the treatment of hypertension, in part because of perceived side effects. Its strong sympatholytic effect results in increased parasympathetic activity, which can manifest as nasal stuffiness, increased gastric acid secretion, diarrhea, and bradycardia. Side effects limited use of this agent several decades ago, when doses as high as 0.75 mg daily were used. However, if used in doses of 0.10 to 0.25 mg daily, these side effects are minimal. The most effective use of reserpine is in combination with a thiazide diuretic, which can mitigate related sodium and water retention.

Implementing Drug Therapy

Need for 24-Hour Coverage

Self-monitoring of BP and/or ambulatory BP monitoring can be used to assess 24-hour control.[87] The failure of an antihypertensive drug to reduce BP over 24 hours can relate to its short half-life, the way it is formulated, biologic factors that dictate patient responsiveness, or a combination of these factors. Importantly, failure to maintain its antihypertensive effect for 24 hours can expose the patient to the full brunt of the next day's early-morning surge in BP and the attendant risk of an early-morning ischemic event.[88]

Once-daily medications effective for 24 hours or longer are preferred agents for treating hypertension. Within each major drug class, clinicians have the option of drugs that have half-lives long enough to allow once-daily dosing and provide complete 24-hour antihypertensive effects. It is important to note, however, that some drugs approved for once-daily dosing have relatively short half-lives. These short–half-life agents might lose their BP-lowering effects near the end of the dosing interval when dosed once daily. They typically are indicated with the option of either once- or twice-daily dosing, so dosing these agents twice daily should be considered.

Monotherapy Versus Combination Therapy

MONOTHERAPY

The historic approach to initiating antihypertensive drug treatment is with monotherapy, generally with a stepped-care approach that involves starting with one drug followed by the sequential addition of agents until the goal BP is attained. The stepped-care approach was established based on initiating therapy with either a diuretic or a β-blocker. Substitution therapy involves the replacement of one antihypertensive drug class with another and is most appropriate if the first drug class chosen either does not lower BP to goal or is associated with adverse effects. Monotherapy with a substitution or stepped-care approach is appropriate for patients with stage 1 hypertension, in whom it is expected that a single drug may be sufficient for BP control.

COMBINATION THERAPY

Most patients with hypertension will require at least two drugs to attain their BP goal. Initial therapy with two antihypertensive drugs, either as separate tablets or in fixed-dose combinations, is recommended for patients with stage 2 hypertension and for some patients with stage 1 hypertension who are at high risk for CV disease.[8,10,89-92]

It is reasonable for clinicians to strongly consider adding more than one antihypertensive drug for patients who are far from their BP goal (i.e., more than 20/10 mm Hg away). In the Avoiding Cardiovascular Events Through Combination Therapy in Patients Living With Systolic Hypertension (ACCOMPLISH) trial, two different two-drug regimens were compared head-to-head long term in patients with hypertension and additional CV risk factors.[89] In both treatment groups, goal BP attainment rates were greater than 70%, demonstrating the efficacy of initial two-drug therapy. This approach results in a more rapid yet safe attainment of goal BP values compared with starting with monotherapy.[90]

Combinations with complementary mechanisms of action generally have additive effects in lowering BP, but combinations of drugs from the same or very similar drug classes are not generally more effective than monotherapy.[66] Thiazide diuretics are additive with most other antihypertensive drug classes, including ACE inhibitors, ARBs, and β-blockers.[73] Other combinations that are considered additive are CCBs, particularly dihydropyridines, with an ACE inhibitor or ARB. All of these combinations are available as fixed-dose combination products (Table 29-9). By decreasing pill burden, fixed-dose combinations have the advantage of increasing adherence to therapy.[91,93]

The approach of using low to moderate doses of two or more drugs in combination is generally preferred over using high doses of individual drugs. This minimizes risk of dose-related adverse effects that might compromise long-term adherence. With most antihypertensive drug classes, other than ACE inhibitors and ARBs, higher doses are associated with a higher risk of adverse effects.[94]

Effects of Patient Characteristics on Blood Pressure Lowering

The selection of a drug to treat patients with uncomplicated hypertension (without compelling indications) is influenced by anticipated efficacy in lowering BP and the likelihood of treatment-related complications. Individual patient responses to antihypertensive drugs may vary considerably because of patient-specific characteristics, such as race and age. For example, in the Veterans Administration Cooperative Trial, 1292 patients were randomly administered drugs—atenolol, captopril, clonidine, diltiazem, prazosin, or hydrochlorothiazide—from six different antihypertensive medication classes.[95] The CCB (diltiazem), the ACE inhibitor (captopril), and the β-blocker (atenolol) worked best in blacks, young white men, and older white men, respectively.[95] Thus, if no compelling indication exists for certain specific drugs or drug classes, it is appropriate to consider individual patient characteristics when selecting antihypertensive drug therapy.

Monitoring

Ongoing monitoring of patients on antihypertensive drug therapy should include assessments of efficacy in reducing BP, treatment-related complications, and progression to development of hypertension-associated target-organ damage. After implementing drug therapy or increasing doses of drug therapy, 2 to 4 weeks is a reasonable time frame in which to assess effectiveness (BP lowering) and presence of treatment-related complications (adverse effects). BP should be checked within 1 to 7 days if patients are in hypertensive urgency. Monitoring parameters for common antihypertensive drugs are listed in Table 29-10.

TABLE 29-9 Fixed-Dose Combination Products for Hypertension

COMBINATION	DRUGS	STRENGTHS (MG/MG)
ACE inhibitor with thiazide	Benazepril/hydrochlorothiazide (Lotensin HCT)	5/6.25, 10/12.5, 20/12.5, 20/25
	Captopril/hydrochlorothiazide (Capozide)	25/15, 25/25, 50/15, 50/25
	Enalapril/hydrochlorothiazide (Vaseretic)	5/12.5, 10/25
	Lisinopril/hydrochlorothiazide (Prinzide, Zestoretic)	10/12.5, 20/12.5, 20/25
	Moexipril/hydrochlorothiazide (Uniretic)	7.5/12.5, 15/25
	Quinapril/hydrochlorothiazide (Accuretic)	10/12.5, 20/12.5, 20/25
ARB with thiazide	Candesartan cilexitil/hydrochlorothiazide (Atacand HCT)	16/12.5, 32/12.5
	Eprosartan mesylate/hydrochlorothiazide (Teveten HCT)	600/12.5, 600/25
	Irbesartan/hydrochlorothiazide (Avalide)	75/12.5, 150/12.5, 300/12.5
	Losartan potassium/hydrochlorothiazide (Hyzaar)	50/12.5, 100/25
	Olmesartan medoxomil/hydrochlorothiazide (Benicar HCT)	20/12.5, 40/12.5, 40/25
	Telmisartan/hydrochlorothiazide (Micardis HCT)	40/12.5, 80/12.5
	Valsartan/hydrochlorothiazide (Diovan HCT)	80/12.5, 160/12.5
β-Blocker with thiazide	Atenolol/chlorthalidone (Tenoretic)	50/25, 100/25
	Bisoprolol/hydrochlorothiazide (Ziac)	2.5/6.25, 5/6.25, 10/6.25
	Propranolol hydrochloride/hydrochlorothiazide (Inderide)	40/25, 80/25
	Propranol LA/hydrochlorothiazide (Inderide LA)	80/50, 120/50, 160/50
	Metoprolol tartrate/hydrochlorothiazide (Lopressor HCT)	50/25, 100/25
	Nadolol/bendroflumethiazide (Corzide)	40/5, 80/5
	Timolol maleate/hydrochlorothiazide (Timolide)	10/25
ACE inhibitor with CCB	Amlodipine besylate/benazepril hydrocholoride (Lotrel)	2.5/10, 5/10, 10/20
	Enalapril maleate/felodipine (Lexxel)	5/5
	Trandolapril/verapamil ER (Tarka)	2/180, 1/240, 2/240, 4/240
ARB with CCB	Amlodipine/olmesartan medoxomil (Azor)	5/20, 10/20, 5/40, 10/40
	Telmisartan/amlodipine (Twynsta)	40/5, 40/10, 80/5, 80/10
	Valsartan/amlodipine (Exforge)	5/160, 10/160, 5/320,10/320
ARB with direct renin inhibitor	Aliskiren/valsartan (Valturna)	150/160, 300/320
Direct renin inhibitor with thiazide	Aliskiren/hydrochlorothiazide (Tekturna HCT)	150/12.5, 150/25, 300/12.5, 300/25
Direct renin inhibitor with CCB	Aliskiren/amlodipine (Tekamlo)	150/5, 150/10, 300/5, 300/10
ARB with CCB with thiazide	Amlodipine/valsartan/hydrochlorothiazide (Exforge HCT)	5/160/12.5, 5/160/25, 10/160/12.5, 10/160/25, 10/320/25
	Olmesartan medoxomil/amlodipine/hydrochlorothiazide (Tribenzor)	20/5/12.5, 40/5/12.5, 40/5/25, 40/10/12.5, 40/10/25

ACE, angiotensin-converting enzyme; ARB, angiotensin receptor blocker; CCB, calcium channel blocker.

TABLE 29-10 Monitoring and Adverse Effects with Antihypertensive Drug Therapy

DRUG CLASS	MONITORING PARAMETERS	ADVERSE EFFECTS
Diuretic	BP, BUN/serum creatinine, serum electrolytes (potassium, magnesium, sodium), uric acid (for thiazides especially)	Electrolyte depletion (hypokalemia, hyponatremia, hypomagnesemia), hyperkalemia with potassium-sparing agents, dehydration and orthostatic hypotension, exacerbation of gout (mostly thiazides)
Aldosterone antagonist	BP, BUN/serum creatinine, serum potassium	Hyperkalemia, especially in chronic kidney disease; dehydration and orthostatic hypotension; hyponatremia; gynecomastia with spironolactone
ACE inibitor	BP, BUN/serum creatinine, serum potassium	Dry cough, hyperkalemia, renal failure in those with bilateral renal artery stenosis, angioedema
ARB	BP, BUN/serum creatinine, serum potassium	Hyperkalemia, renal failure in those with bilateral renal artery stenosis
Dihydropyridine CCB	BP, heart rate	Tachycardia, peripheral edema, headache, flushing, worsening GERD
Nondihydropyridine CCB	BP, heart rate	Heart block, constipation, peripheral edema, worsening GERD
β-Blocker	BP, heart rate	Exercise intolerance, fatigue, heart block, exacerbation of peripheral arterial disease, erectile dysfunction, masking signs and symptoms of hypoglycemia

ACEI, angiotensin-converting enzyme inhibitors; ARB, angiotensin II receptor blocker; BP, blood pressure; BUN, blood urea nitrogen; CCB, calcium channel blocker; GERD, gastroesophageal reflux disease.

Monitoring BP, usually with office BP measurements, is the primary method for determining effectiveness of antihypertensive therapy and achievement of BP goals. Home self-measurement of BP and 24-hour ambulatory BP (ABP) measurement are also used. Self-monitoring of BP provides a larger number of readings and thus adds to the precision of BP determination in a given patient over time. Self-monitoring is particularly useful for assessment of BP in patients with "white coat" hypertension.[96] Office BP measurements are generally higher than self-monitored BP or ABP measurements,[87] such that the upper limit of normal clinic BP is below 140/90 mm Hg; of self-monitored BP, it is 135/85 mm Hg; and of 24-hour ABP, it is below 130/80 mm Hg.

The overarching reason to treat hypertension is to reduce the risk of hypertension-associated target-organ damage and CVD events; thus periodic evaluation for occurrence of such complications is prudent. Importantly, development of complications might represent a compelling indication for specific pharmacotherapy (see Figure 29-1). Screening and treatment for concomitant CVD risk factors should be carried out in all patients with hypertension. Low-dose aspirin should be considered for hypertensive patients with Framingham risk scores of 10% or higher or for patients with atherosclerotic vascular disease. Managing dyslipidemia with a statin-based regimen should always be considered, specifically in the case of elevated low-density lipoprotein (LDL) cholesterol.

Adherence

Because hypertension is typically asymptomatic, hence the nickname "the silent killer," clinicians should proactively promote adherence with drug therapy. Patients should be informed of the risks of uncontrolled hypertension and the long-term benefits of drug therapy in reducing risk of CV events. High adherence with antihypertensive drug therapy is associated with a lower risk of CV events in patients with hypertension.[97]

Clinician-patient communication regarding realistic expectations for BP-lowering effectiveness and side effects of antihypertensive treatment is critical. For example, patients started on single-drug therapy should be informed that dosage increases and addition of a second or third drug are frequently needed to attain BP goals.[80,81,98] Patients should be reassured that routine monitoring, including self-measurements of BP, can easily assess effectiveness and detect side effects of treatment. Importantly, the availability of several affordable drug therapy options allows clinicians flexibility for titrating and modifying therapy.

Multiple strategies have been identified to improve adherence with antihypertensive drug therapy.[8] Many of these involve designing and modifying regimens that are adaptable. It is easier for patients to adhere to once-daily regimens than to those that require multiple daily doses. Use of affordable medications, such as generic or brand-name drugs included in the patient's insurance plan, can impact a patient's ability to sustain adherence to drug therapy. Lastly, use of fixed-dose combination products can improve adherence and under some circumstances may decrease patients' overall drug costs.

Step-Down Therapy

Decreasing the number and/or dosage of antihypertensive drugs may be considered after BP has been effectively controlled for at least 1 year.[99] If attempted, this should be done in a deliberate, slow, and progressive manner. Continued clinical surveillance is necessary with this step-down therapy approach, because BP can rise again to hypertensive levels, sometimes months or years after medication is discontinued; this occurs frequently when previously successful lifestyle modifications are not sustained.[100]

Special Populations
Elderly Patients

Hypertension is the most frequent modifiable risk factor for mortality in the elderly (age 65 years or older). Known benefits of treating hypertension in older patients, primarily those in their seventh decade, have been demonstrated in the Systolic Hypertension in the Elderly Program (SHEP), Stroke Prevention Trial in Sickle Cell Anemia (STOP), and Systolic Hypertension in Europe (Syst-EUR) trials.[2,3,101] Further, the Hypertension in the Very Elderly Trial (HYVET) clearly established that treating hypertension with drug therapy in patients 80 years of age or older reduces the risk of CV events, and particularly mortality, compared with placebo.[7]

ISOLATED SYSTOLIC HYPERTENSION

Both SBP and diastolic BP (DBP) increase until age 55 to 60 years, after which DBP stabilizes and then declines; SBP continues to rise until the eighth or ninth decade. Thus, most elderly hypertensive patients have elevated SBP and normal DBP, a pattern referred to as *isolated systolic hypertension* (ISH). In the elderly ISH is caused by increases in arterial stiffness and early-wave reflections, both of which cause a selective increase in SBP, and ISH is a major risk factor for CV death in the elderly.

Clinical assessment of ISH can be confounded by a widened auscultatory gap, which may lead to underestimation of SBP; therefore it is important to inflate the cuff to above 200 mm Hg when measuring BP in the elderly. People at advanced ages are prone to develop pseudohypertension, a phenomenon related to calcified, noncompressible arteries, in which cuff BP can significantly overestimate true intraarterial BP. This finding can be diagnosed by manually inflating the BP cuff above SBP, whereupon brachial or radial artery pulses should be obliterated. If these arteries remain palpable, a positive Osler sign, the patient likely has a component of pseudohypertension.

BLOOD PRESSURE GOALS

The once-common notion that ISH is a physiologic consequence of aging that preserves organ perfusion and does not require treatment has been dispelled by results of randomized controlled trials. The SHEP and Syst-EUR trials have clearly documented benefit of BP reduction in older patients.[3,101] Treatment of ISH in older patients with a SBP of 160 mm Hg or higher is supported by strong evidence, whereas evidence for treatment of ISH patients with a baseline SBP of 140 to 159 mm Hg is less strong.[102]

The JNC-7 recommends that goal BP values in older patients follow the same treatment principles as those in younger adult patients,[8] treating to a goal BP below 140/90 mm Hg for most patients and below 130/80 mm Hg in patients with diabetes or CKD. However, patient-specific adjustments based on tolerability of treatment and overall health status are reasonable. In patients 80 years of age or older, HYVET provides the only controlled long-term data; the BP goal in this study was below 150/80 mm Hg,[7] therefore some clinicians may cite this evidence as a reason to target a BP goal of less than 150/80 mm Hg in the very elderly. In 2011, the ACCF/AHA published an expert consensus document regarding hypertension in the elderly.[103] This consensus document recommends a target SBP of 140 mm Hg or lower for all patients age 55 and older. However, they state that although an achieved SBP of less than 140 mm Hg is appropriate for patients aged 55 to 79 years, an achieved SBP of 140 to 145 mm Hg can be acceptable in patients aged 80 and older, if tolerated. This recommendation for patients 80 years or older is based on the SBP values achieved in HYVET.

ORTHOSTATIC HYPOTENSION

In the elderly and in patients with hypertensive crisis, BP should be lowered gradually to avoid sudden excessive reductions in cerebral or coronary blood flow. In the elderly patient with long-standing hypertension, rapid BP reduction may be poorly tolerated because of diminished cerebral or coronary artery autoregulatory ability.[55] If BP drops below the autoregulatory range, symptoms of cerebral hypoperfusion—such as dizziness, fatigue, and forgetfulness—may arise. Concern about an "excessive" BP drop in the elderly or otherwise vulnerable patient should not, however, preclude attempting to reach recommended BP goals within a relatively short time (weeks rather than months).

Elderly patients, especially the very elderly and those with ISH, are at high risk for *orthostatic hypotension*, defined as an SBP decrease of more than 20 mm Hg after 3 minutes of standing. Orthostatic hypotension can happen with any antihypertensive agent in the very elderly but is particularly problematic with diuretics and α-blockers.[8,103] Use of low initial doses of antihypertensive medications and gradual dosage titration, as well as avoidance of volume depletion, will minimize the risk of orthostatic hypotension. For patients 80 years or older, it is recommended that therapy be initiated with a single drug followed by addition of a second drug if needed, even with stage 2 hypertension.[103]

SELECTING DRUG THERAPY

First-line agents such as ACE inhibitors, ARBs, CCBs, and thiazide diuretics should be the primary agents used to treat elderly patients with hypertension.[103] Thiazide diuretics and CCBs decrease CV events and can be used as first-line therapy in the elderly,[104] and ACE inhibitors or ARBs are also recommended first-line agents. β-Blockers may be less effective in elderly patients and have not been shown to reduce all-cause mortality rates when used as monotherapy.[4,103] However, β-blockers are useful to treat compelling indications and as add-on therapy after first-line drugs.[103] Central α-agonists and peripheral α-blockers often result in troubling side effects, such as dry mouth and orthostatic hypotension, and therefore should be used with caution in elderly patients.

African-American Patients

The prevalence of hypertension and risk of associated complications such as target-organ disease that includes end-stage renal disease, LV hypertrophy, and heart failure are high among African-American patients with hypertension. The treatment of hypertension in this population is complex and includes socioeconomic and behavioral issues and health care beliefs that typically influence the success or failure of a particular regimen.[19] Black patients as a group respond somewhat less well than nonblacks to monotherapy with β-blockers, ACE inhibitors, and ARBs. This may be related to their tendency to have a salt-sensitive, low-renin form of hypertension.[105] However, when higher doses of ACE inhibitors and ARBs are used, significant BP lowering is seen. Blacks and nonblacks generally respond equally well to diuretics and CCBs.

The International Society on Hypertension in Blacks (ISHIB) published a consensus statement, "Management of High Blood Pressure in African Americans," in 2010.[19] This statement considers two distinct black populations: *primary-prevention patients*—those without target-organ damage, preclinical CV disease, or overt CV disease—and *secondary-prevention patients*, who have target-organ damage, preclinical CV disease, and/or a history of CV disease. Goal BPs recommended by ISHIB are more aggressive than the JNC-7 recommendations: a target below 135/85 mm Hg is recommended for primary prevention, and BP below 130/80 mm Hg is recommended for secondary prevention. The ISHIB consensus statement provides several general recommendations for therapy in blacks[19]: initiation of drug therapy with a monotherapy approach, with preferential selection of either a diuretic or CCB, is recommended when BP is 10 mm Hg or less above goal; initiation of therapy with a two-drug combination is recommended when BP is 10 to 15 mm Hg or more above goal. Further, the combination of a CCB with an ACE inhibitor or ARB or of a thiazide diuretic with an ACE inhibitor or ARB is recommended.

REFERENCES

1. MRC Working Party. Medical Research Council trial of treatment of hypertension in older adults: principal results. *Br Med J* 1992;304(6824):405-412.
2. Dahlof B, Lindholm LH, Hansson L, et al. Morbidity and mortality in the Swedish Trial in Old Patients with Hypertension (STOP-Hypertension). *Lancet* 1991;338(8778):1281-1285.
3. SHEP Cooperative Research Group. Prevention of stroke by antihypertensive drug treatment in older persons with isolated systolic hypertension: final results of the Systolic Hypertension in the Elderly Program (SHEP). *JAMA* 1991;265(24):3255-3264.
4. Wiysonge C, Bradley H, Mayosi B, et al. Beta-blockers for hypertension. *Cochrane Database Syst Rev* 2007;(1):CD002003.
5. Diuretic versus alpha-blocker as first-step antihypertensive therapy: final results from the Antihypertensive and Lipid-Lowering Treatment to Prevent Heart Attack Trial (ALLHAT). *Hypertension* 2003;42(3):239-246.
6. Turnbull F. Effects of different blood-pressure–lowering regimens on major cardiovascular events: results of prospectively-designed overviews of randomised trials. *Lancet* 2003;362(9395):1527-1535.
7. Beckett NS, Peters R, Fletcher AE, et al. Treatment of hypertension in patients 80 years of age or older. *N Engl J Med* 2008;358(18):1887-1898.
8. Chobanian AV, Bakris GL, Black HR, et al. Seventh report of the Joint National Committee on Prevention, Detection, Evaluation, and Treatment of High Blood Pressure. *Hypertension* 2003;42(6):1206-1252.
9. Saseen JJ, MacLaughlin EJ, Westfall JM. Treatment of uncomplicated hypertension: are ACE inhibitors and calcium channel blockers as effective as diuretics and beta-blockers? *J Am Board Fam Pract* 2003;16(2):156-164.
10. Rosendorff C, Black HR, Cannon CP, et al. Treatment of hypertension in the prevention and management of ischemic heart disease: a scientific statement from the American Heart Association Council for High Blood Pressure Research and the Councils on Clinical Cardiology and Epidemiology and Prevention. *Circulation* 2007;115(21):2761-2788.
11. Drozda J Jr, Messer JV, Spertus J, et al. ACCF/AHA/AMA-PCPI 2011 performance measures for adults with coronary artery disease and hypertension: a report of the American College of Cardiology Foundation/American Heart Association Task Force on Performance Measures and the American Medical Association-Physician Consortium for Performance Improvement. *Circulation* 2011;124(2):248-270.
12. Mitka M. Aggressively treating hypertension remains strategy of uncertain benefit. *JAMA* 2009;302(10):1047-1048.
13. Arguedas JA, Perez MI, Wright JM. Treatment blood pressure targets for hypertension. *Cochrane Database Syst Rev* 2009;(3):CD004349.
14. Cushman WC, Evans GW, Byington RP, et al. Effects of intensive blood-pressure control in type 2 diabetes mellitus. *N Engl J Med* 2010;362(17):1575-1585.
15. Appel LJ, Wright JT Jr, Greene T, et al. Intensive blood-pressure control in hypertensive chronic kidney disease. *N Engl J Med* 2010;363(10):918-929.
16. Cooper-DeHoff RM, Gong Y, Handberg EM, et al. Tight blood pressure control and cardiovascular outcomes among hypertensive patients with diabetes and coronary artery disease. *JAMA* 2010;304(1):61-68.
17. ALLHAT Officers and Coordinators for the ALLHAT Collaborative Research Group. Major outcomes in high-risk hypertensive patients randomized to angiotensin-converting enzyme inhibitor or calcium channel blocker vs diuretic: the Antihypertensive and Lipid-Lowering Treatment to Prevent Heart Attack Trial (ALLHAT). *JAMA* 2002;288(23):2981-2997.
18. National Collaborating Centre for Chronic Conditions. *Hypertension: management of hypertension in adults in primary care: partial update*. London: Royal College of Physicians, 2006.
19. Flack JM, Sica DA, Bakris G, et al. Management of high blood pressure in blacks: an update of the International Society on Hypertension in Blacks consensus statement. *Hypertension* 2010;56(5):780-800.
20. Aronow WS, Fleg JL, Pepine CJ, et al. ACCF/AHA 2011 expert consensus document on hypertension in the elderly: a report of the American College of Cardiology Foundation Task Force on Clinical Expert Consensus Documents. *Circulation* 2011;124(5);e175.
21. Bakris GL, Sowers JR. ASH position paper: treatment of hypertension in patients with diabetes—an update. *J Clin Hypertens (Greenwich)* 2008;10(9):707-713; discussion 714-715.
22. Standards of medical care in diabetes—2011. *Diabetes Care* 2011;34(Suppl 1):S11-S61.
23. Heart Outcomes Prevention Evaluation Study Investigators. Effects of ramipril on cardiovascular and microvascular outcomes in people with diabetes mellitus: results of the HOPE study and MICRO-HOPE substudy. *Lancet* 2000;355(9200):253-259.
24. Estacio RO, Jeffers BW, Hiatt WR, et al. The effect of nisoldipine as compared with enalapril on cardiovascular outcomes in patients with non–insulin-dependent diabetes and hypertension. *N Engl J Med* 1998;338(10):645-652.
25. Tatti P, Pahor M, Byington RP, et al. Outcome results of the Fosinopril Versus Amlodipine Cardiovascular Events Randomized Trial (FACET) in patients with hypertension and NIDDM. *Diabetes Care* 1998;21(4):597-603.
26. Patel A, MacMahon S, Chalmers J, et al. Effects of a fixed combination of perindopril and indapamide on macrovascular and microvascular outcomes in patients with type 2 diabetes mellitus (the ADVANCE trial): a randomised controlled trial. *Lancet* 2007;370(9590):829-840.
27. Tuomilehto J, Rastenyte D, Birkenhager WH, et al; Systolic Hypertension in Europe Trial Investigators. Effects of calcium-channel blockade in older patients with diabetes and systolic hypertension. *N Engl J Med* 1999;340(9):677-684.
28. Whelton PK, Barzilay J, Cushman WC, et al. Clinical outcomes in antihypertensive treatment of type 2 diabetes, impaired fasting glucose concentration, and normoglycemia: Antihypertensive and Lipid-Lowering Treatment to Prevent Heart Attack Trial (ALLHAT). *Arch Intern Med* 2005;165(12):1401-1409.
29. Saseen JJ, Carter BL, Brown TE, et al. Comparison of nifedipine alone and with diltiazem or verapamil in hypertension. *Hypertension* 1996;28(1):109-114.
30. UK Prospective Diabetes Study Group. Efficacy of atenolol and captopril in reducing risk of macrovascular and microvascular complications in type 2 diabetes: UKPDS 39. *Br Med J* 1998;317(7160):713-720.
31. Holman RR, Paul SK, Bethel MA, et al. Long-term follow-up after tight control of blood pressure in type 2 diabetes. *N Engl J Med* 2008;359(15):1565-1576.
32. Bakris GL, Fonseca V, Katholi RE, et al. Metabolic effects of carvedilol vs metoprolol in patients with type 2 diabetes mellitus and hypertension: a randomized controlled trial. *JAMA* 2004;292(18):2227-2236.
33. Anderson JL, Adams CD, Antman EM, et al. ACC/AHA 2007 guidelines for the management of patients with unstable angina/non–ST-elevation myocardial infarction: a report of the American College of Cardiology/American Heart Association Task Force on Practice Guidelines (Writing Committee to Revise the 2002 Guidelines for the Management of Patients with Unstable Angina/Non–ST-Elevation Myocardial Infarction)

PHARMACOLOGIC MANAGEMENT OF HYPERTENSION

developed in collaboration with the American College of Emergency Physicians, the Society for Cardiovascular Angiography and Interventions, and the Society of Thoracic Surgeons. Endorsed by the American Association of Cardiovascular and Pulmonary Rehabilitation and the Society for Academic Emergency Medicine. *J Am Coll Cardiol* 2007; 50(7):e1-e157.

34. Antman EM, Hand M, Armstrong PW, et al. 2007 focused update of the ACC/AHA 2004 guidelines for the management of patients with ST-elevation myocardial infarction: a report of the American College of Cardiology/American Heart Association Task Force on Practice Guidelines: developed in collaboration with the Canadian Cardiovascular Society. Endorsed by the American Academy of Family Physicians: 2007 Writing Group to Review New Evidence and Update the ACC/AHA 2004 Guidelines for the Management of Patients with ST-Elevation Myocardial Infarction, Writing on Behalf of the 2004 Writing Committee. *Circulation* 2008;117(2):296-329.

35. Fraker TD Jr, Fihn SD, Gibbons RJ, et al. 2007 Chronic angina focused update of the ACC/AHA 2002 guidelines for the management of patients with chronic stable angina: a report of the American College of Cardiology/American Heart Association Task Force on Practice Guidelines Writing Group to develop the focused update of the 2002 guidelines for the management of patients with chronic stable angina. *Circulation* 2007;116(23):2762-2772.

36. Smith SC Jr, Allen J, Blair SN, et al. AHA/ACC guidelines for secondary prevention for patients with coronary and other atherosclerotic vascular disease: 2006 update endorsed by the National Heart, Lung, and Blood Institute. *J Am Coll Cardiol* 2006;47(10):2130-2139.

37. Freemantle N, Cleland J, Young P, et al. Beta blockade after myocardial infarction: systematic review and meta regression analysis. *Br Med J* 1999;318(7200):1730-1737.

38. Thompson AM, Hu T, Eshelbrenner CL, et al. Antihypertensive treatment and secondary prevention of cardiovascular disease events among persons without hypertension: a meta-analysis. *JAMA* 2011;305(9):913-922.

39. Hunt SA, Abraham WT, Chin MH, et al. 2009 focused update incorporated into the ACC/AHA 2005 guidelines for the diagnosis and management of heart failure in adults: a report of the American College of Cardiology Foundation/American Heart Association Task Force on Practice Guidelines: developed in collaboration with the International Society for Heart and Lung Transplantation. *Circulation* 2009;119(14):e391-e479.

40. Cohn JN, Tognoni G. A randomized trial of the angiotensin-receptor blocker valsartan in chronic heart failure. *N Engl J Med* 2001;345(23):1667-1675.

41. Pitt B, Poole-Wilson PA, Segal R, et al. Effect of losartan compared with captopril on mortality in patients with symptomatic heart failure: randomised trial—the Losartan Heart Failure Survival Study ELITE II. *Lancet* 2000;355(9215):1582-1587.

42. Pitt B, Segal R, Martinez FA, et al. Randomised trial of losartan versus captopril in patients over 65 with heart failure (Evaluation of Losartan in the Elderly Study, ELITE). *Lancet* 1997;349(9054):747-752.

43. Granger CB, McMurray JJ, Yusuf S, et al. Effects of candesartan in patients with chronic heart failure and reduced left-ventricular systolic function intolerant to angiotensin-converting–enzyme inhibitors: the CHARM-Alternative trial. *Lancet* 2003;362(9386): 772-776.

44. Pitt B, Zannad F, Remme WJ, et al; Randomized Aldactone Evaluation Study Investigators. The effect of spironolactone on morbidity and mortality in patients with severe heart failure. *N Engl J Med* 1999;341(10):709-717.

45. Pitt B, Remme W, Zannad F, et al. Eplerenone, a selective aldosterone blocker, in patients with left ventricular dysfunction after myocardial infarction. *N Engl J Med* 2003;348(14):1309-1321.

46. Zannad F, McMurray JJ, Krum H, et al. Eplerenone in patients with systolic heart failure and mild symptoms. *N Engl J Med* 2011;364(1):11-21.

47. McMurray JJ, Ostergren J, Swedberg K, et al. Effects of candesartan in patients with chronic heart failure and reduced left-ventricular systolic function taking angiotensin-converting–enzyme inhibitors: the CHARM-Added trial. *Lancet* 2003;362(9386):767-771.

48. Taylor AL, Ziesche S, Yancy C, et al. Combination of isosorbide dinitrate and hydralazine in blacks with heart failure. *N Engl J Med* 2004;351(20):2049-2057.

49. Furie KL, Kasner SE, Adams RJ, et al. Guidelines for the prevention of stroke in patients with stroke or transient ischemic attack: a guideline for healthcare professionals from the American Heart Association/American Stroke Association. *Stroke* 2011;42(1):227-276.

50. Rashid P, Leonardi-Bee J, Bath P. Blood pressure reduction and secondary prevention of stroke and other vascular events: a systematic review. *Stroke* 2003;34(11):2741-2748.

51. PROGRESS Collaborative Group. Randomised trial of a perindopril-based blood-pressure–lowering regimen among 6,105 individuals with previous stroke or transient ischaemic attack. *Lancet* 2001;358(9287):1033-1041.

52. Schrader J, Luders S, Kulschewski A, et al. Morbidity and mortality after stroke, eprosartan compared with nitrendipine for secondary prevention: principal results of a prospective randomized controlled study (MOSES). *Stroke* 2005;36(6):1218-1226.

53. Yusuf S, Diener HC, Sacco RL, et al. Telmisartan to prevent recurrent stroke and cardiovascular events. *N Engl J Med* 2008;359(12):1225-1237.

54. Sica DA. Pharmacotherapy review: angiotensin-converting enzyme inhibitors. *J Clin Hypertens (Greenwich)* 2005;7(8):485-488.

55. Kaplan NM. *Kaplan's clinical hypertension*, 9th ed. 2006, Philadelphia, Lippincott, Williams & Wilkins.

56. Elliott WJ, Meyer PM. Incident diabetes in clinical trials of antihypertensive drugs: a network meta-analysis. *Lancet* 2007;369(9557):201-207.

57. Vanhoutte PM. Endothelial dysfunction and inhibition of converting enzyme. *Eur Heart J* 1998;19(Suppl J):J7-J15.

58. Wright JT Jr, Bakris G, Greene T, et al. Effect of blood pressure lowering and antihypertensive drug class on progression of hypertensive kidney disease: results from the AASK trial. *JAMA* 2002;288(19):2421-2431.

59. Lewis EJ, Hunsicker LG, Bain RP, et al; the Collaborative Study Group. The effect of angiotensin-converting–enzyme inhibition on diabetic nephropathy. *N Engl J Med* 1993;329(20):1456-1462.

60. Casas JP, Chua W, Loukogeorgakis S, et al. Effect of inhibitors of the renin-angiotensin system and other antihypertensive drugs on renal outcomes: systematic review and meta-analysis. *Lancet* 2005;366(9502):2026-2033.

61. Weir MR, Gray JM, Paster R, et al; the Trandolapril Multicenter Study Group. Differing mechanisms of action of angiotensin-converting enzyme inhibition in black and white hypertensive patients. *Hypertension* 1995;26(1):124-130.

62. Schoolwerth AC, Sica DA, Ballermann BJ, et al. Renal considerations in angiotensin-converting–enzyme inhibitor therapy: a statement for healthcare professionals from the Council on the Kidney in Cardiovascular Disease and the Council for High Blood Pressure Research of the American Heart Association. *Circulation* 2001;104(16): 1985-1991.

63. Yusuf S, Teo K, Anderson C, et al. Effects of the angiotensin-receptor blocker telmisartan on cardiovascular events in high-risk patients intolerant to angiotensin-converting enzyme inhibitors: a randomised controlled trial. *Lancet* 2008;372(9644):1174-1183.

64. Bakris GL, Williams M, Dworkin L, et al; National Kidney Foundation Hypertension and Diabetes Executive Committees Working Group. Preserving renal function in adults with hypertension and diabetes: a consensus approach. *Am J Kidney Dis* 2000;36(3): 646-661.

65. Sica DA. Angiotensin receptor blockers and drug-drug interactions. *Expert Opin Drug Saf* 2005;4(1):139-140.

66. Yusuf S, Teo KK, Pogue J, et al. Telmisartan, ramipril, or both in patients at high risk for vascular events. *N Engl J Med* 2008;358(15):1547-1559.

67. Brenner BM, Cooper ME, de Zeeuw D, et al. Effects of losartan on renal and cardiovascular outcomes in patients with type 2 diabetes and nephropathy. *N Engl J Med* 2001;345(12):861-869.

68. Lewis EJ, Hunsicker LG, Clarke WR, et al. Renoprotective effect of the angiotensin-receptor antagonist irbesartan in patients with nephropathy due to type 2 diabetes. *N Engl J Med* 2001;345(12):851-860.

69. Lindholm LH, Ibsen H, Dahlof B, et al. Cardiovascular morbidity and mortality in patients with diabetes in the Losartan Intervention For Endpoint reduction in hypertension study (LIFE): a randomised trial against atenolol. *Lancet* 2002;359(9311):1004-1010.

70. Haller H, Ito S, Izzo JL Jr, et al. Olmesartan for the delay or prevention of microalbuminuria in type 2 diabetes. *N Engl J Med* 2011;364(10):907-917.

71. Kronish IM, Woodward M, Sergie Z, et al. Meta-analysis: impact of drug class on adherence to antihypertensives. *Circulation* 2011;123(15):1611-1621.

72. Sica DA. Calcium channel blockers: a more expansive treatment role. *J Clin Hypertens (Greenwich)* 2005;7(4 Suppl 1):2-4.

73. Ernst ME, Moser M. Use of diuretics in patients with hypertension. *N Engl J Med* 2009;361(22):2153-2164.

74. Wright JT Jr, Dunn JK, Cutler JA, et al. Outcomes in hypertensive black and nonblack patients treated with chlorthalidone, amlodipine, and lisinopril. *JAMA* 2005;293(13): 1595-1608.

75. Carter BL, Ernst ME, Cohen JD. Hydrochlorothiazide versus chlorthalidone: evidence supporting their interchangeability. *Hypertension* 2004;43(1):4-9.

76. Ernst ME, Carter BL, Goerdt CJ, et al. Comparative antihypertensive effects of hydrochlorothiazide and chlorthalidone on ambulatory and office blood pressure. *Hypertension* 2006;47(3):352-358.

77. Messerli FH, Makani H, Benjo A, et al. Antihypertensive efficacy of hydrochlorothiazide as evaluated by ambulatory blood pressure monitoring: a meta-analysis of randomized trials. *J Am Coll Cardiol* 2011;57(5):590-600.

78. Barzilay JI, Davis BR, Cutler JA, et al. Fasting glucose levels and incident diabetes mellitus in older nondiabetic adults randomized to receive 3 different classes of antihypertensive treatment: a report from the Antihypertensive and Lipid-Lowering Treatment to Prevent Heart Attack Trial (ALLHAT). *Arch Intern Med* 2006;166(20):2191-2201.

79. Black HR, Davis B, Barzilay J, et al. Metabolic and clinical outcomes in nondiabetic individuals with the metabolic syndrome assigned to chlorthalidone, amlodipine, or lisinopril as initial treatment for hypertension: a report from the Antihypertensive and Lipid-Lowering Treatment to Prevent Heart Attack Trial (ALLHAT). *Diabetes Care* 2008;31(2):353-360.

80. Grimm RH Jr, Flack JM, Grandits GA, et al. Long-term effects on plasma lipids of diet and drugs to treat hypertension. Treatment of Mild Hypertension Study (TOMHS) Research Group. *JAMA* 1996;275(20):1549-1556.

81. Grimm RH Jr, Grandits GA, Prineas RJ, et al. Long-term effects on sexual function of five antihypertensive drugs and nutritional hygienic treatment in hypertensive men and women. Treatment of Mild Hypertension Study (TOMHS). *Hypertension* 1997;29(1 Pt 1):8-14.

82. Calhoun DA, Jones D, Textor S, et al. Resistant hypertension: diagnosis, evaluation, and treatment—a scientific statement from the American Heart Association Professional Education Committee of the Council for High Blood Pressure Research. *Circulation* 2008;117(25):e510-e526.

83. Zillich AJ, Carter BL. Eplerenone: a novel selective aldosterone blocker. *Ann Pharmacother* 2002;36(10):1567-1576.

84. Report of the National High Blood Pressure Education Program Working Group on High Blood Pressure in Pregnancy. *Am J Obstet Gynecol* 2000;183(1):S1-S22.

85. Staessen JA, Li Y, Richart T. Oral renin inhibitors. *Lancet* 2006;368(9545):1449-1456.

86. Parving HH, Persson F, Lewis JB, et al. Aliskiren combined with losartan in type 2 diabetes and nephropathy. *N Engl J Med* 2008;358(23):2433-2446.

87. Pickering TG, White WB. ASH position paper: home and ambulatory blood pressure monitoring—when and how to use self (home) and ambulatory blood pressure monitoring. *J Clin Hypertens (Greenwich)* 2008;10(11):850-855.

88. Smolensky MH. Chronobiology and chronotherapeutics: applications to cardiovascular medicine. *Am J Hypertens* 1996;9(4 Pt 3):11S-21S.

89. Jamerson K, Weber MA, Bakris GL, et al. Benazepril plus amlodipine or hydrochlorothiazide for hypertension in high-risk patients. *N Engl J Med* 2008;359(23): 2417-2428.

90. Brown MJ, McInnes GT, Papst CC, et al. Aliskiren and the calcium channel blocker amlodipine combination as an initial treatment strategy for hypertension control (ACCELERATE): a randomised, parallel-group trial. *Lancet* 2011;377(9762):312-320.

91. Gupta AK, Arshad S, Poulter NR. Compliance, safety, and effectiveness of fixed-dose combinations of antihypertensive agents: a meta-analysis. *Hypertension* 2010;55(2): 399-407.

92. Bangalore S, Shahane A, Parkar S, et al. Compliance and fixed-dose combination therapy. *Curr Hypertens Rep* 2007;9(3):184-189.

93. Bangalore S, Kamalakkannan G, Parkar S, et al. Fixed-dose combinations improve medication compliance: a meta-analysis. *Am J Med* 2007;120(8):713-719.

94. Law MR, Wald NJ, Morris JK, et al. Value of low dose combination treatment with blood pressure lowering drugs: analysis of 354 randomised trials. *Br Med J* 2003;326(7404):1427.

95. Materson BJ, Reda DJ, Cushman WC, et al. Single-drug therapy for hypertension in men: a comparison of six antihypertensive agents with placebo. The Department of Veterans Affairs Cooperative Study Group on Antihypertensive Agents. *N Engl J Med* 1993;328(13):914-921.

96. Staessen JA, Den Hond E, Celis H, et al. Antihypertensive treatment based on blood pressure measurement at home or in the physician's office: a randomized controlled trial. *JAMA* 2004;291(8):955-964.

97. Mazzaglia G, Ambrosioni E, Alacqua M, et al. Adherence to antihypertensive medications and cardiovascular morbidity among newly diagnosed hypertensive patients. *Circulation* 2009;120(16):1598-1605.

98. Grimm RH Jr, Grandits GA, Cutler JA, et al. Relationships of quality-of-life measures to long-term lifestyle and drug treatment in the Treatment of Mild Hypertension Study. *Arch Intern Med* 1997;157(6):638-648.

99. Finnerty FA Jr. Stepped-down therapy versus intermittent therapy in systemic hypertension. *Am J Cardiol* 1990;66(19):1373-1374.

100. Whelton PK, Appel LJ, Espeland MA, et al. Sodium reduction and weight loss in the treatment of hypertension in older persons: a randomized controlled Trial of Nonpharmacologic Interventions in the Elderly (TONE). TONE Collaborative Research Group. *JAMA* 1998;279(11):839-846.

101. Staessen JA, Fagard R, Thijs L, et al; Systolic Hypertension in Europe (Syst-Eur) Trial Investigators. Randomised double-blind comparison of placebo and active treatment for older patients with isolated systolic hypertension. *Lancet* 1997;350(9080):757-764.

102. Chaudhry SI, Krumholz HM, Foody JM. Systolic hypertension in older persons. *JAMA* 2004;292(9):1074-1080.

103. Aronow WS, Fleg JL, Pepine CJ, et al. ACCF/AHA 2011 expert consensus document on hypertension in the elderly: a report of the American College of Cardiology Foundation Task Force on Clinical Expert Consensus Documents. *Circulation* 2011;123(21):2434-2506.

104. Staessen JA, Wang J, Bianchi G, et al. Essential hypertension. *Lancet* 2003;361(9369):1629-1641.

105. Saunders E, Weir MR, Kong BW, et al. A comparison of the efficacy and safety of a betablocker, a calcium channel blocker, and a converting enzyme inhibitor in hypertensive blacks. *Arch Intern Med* 1990;150(8):1707-1713.

PHARMACOLOGIC MANAGEMENT OF HYPERTENSION

Endocrine Causes of Hypertension

William F. Young Jr.

PHEOCHROMOCYTOMA, 490

Presentation, 490
Diagnosis, 490
Principles of Treatment, 490

PRIMARY ALDOSTERONISM, 494

Diagnosis, 495
Principles of Treatment, 496
Pharmacologic Treatment, 497

OTHER FORMS OF MINERALOCORTICOID EXCESS, 497

Hyperdeoxycorticosteronism, 497
Apparent Mineralocorticoid Excess
　Syndromes, 498

THYROID AND PARATHYROID DISEASE, 499

Thyroid Dysfunction, 499
Primary Hyperparathyroidism, 499
Acromegaly, 499

REFERENCES, 500

Hypertension may be the initial manifestation of many endocrine disorders (Box 30-1). Although endocrine causes of hypertension are uncommon, an accurate diagnosis provides clinicians with a unique treatment opportunity: to render a surgical cure or to achieve a dramatic response with pharmacologic therapy. This chapter reviews the therapeutic approaches to endocrine disorders ranging from the classic adrenal causes of hypertension, such as pheochromocytoma and primary aldosteronism, to pituitary-dependent hypertension, such as Cushing syndrome and acromegaly.

Pheochromocytoma

Catecholamine-producing tumors that arise from chromaffin cells of the adrenal medulla and the sympathetic ganglia are termed *pheochromocytomas* and *catecholamine-secreting paragangliomas* (or *extraadrenal pheochromocytomas*), respectively. Because clinical presentations of these disorders and the therapeutic approaches to them are similar, the term *pheochromocytoma* is often used to refer to both adrenal pheochromocytomas and catecholamine-secreting paragangliomas.

Presentation

Although catecholamine-secreting tumors are rare (annual incidence of 2 to 8 cases per 1 million persons), it is important to suspect, confirm, localize, and resect these tumors because 1) the associated hypertension is curable with surgical removal of the tumor, 2) the risk of a lethal paroxysm exists, 3) at least 10% of the tumors are malignant, and 4) 15% to 25% are familial, and detection of this tumor in the proband may result in early diagnosis in other family members.[1,2] These tumors occur with equal frequency in men and women, primarily in the third, fourth, and fifth decades. Patients harboring catecholamine-secreting tumors may be asymptomatic and may come to medical attention with an incidentally discovered adrenal mass on computerized imaging. However, symptoms are usually present and result from the pharmacologic effects of excessive levels of catecholamines or cosecreted peptide hormones (Box 30-2). The resultant hypertension may be sustained or paroxysmal. Episodic symptoms may occur in spells, or paroxysms, that can be extremely variable in presentation.

SYNDROMIC PHEOCHROMOCYTOMA

Approximately 15% to 25% of patients with catecholamine-secreting tumors have associated germline mutations, inherited mutations present in all cells of the body, in genes known to cause genetic disease.[1,3-10] The familial neurocristopathic syndromes associated with adrenal pheochromocytoma include multiple endocrine neoplasia (MEN) type 2A, MEN 2B, neurofibromatosis type 1,

von Hippel–Lindau disease, and familial paraganglioma (Table 30-1).[3,10,11] Another syndrome associated with catecholamine-secreting tumors that does not appear to be inherited is the so-called *Carney triad:* gastric leiomyosarcoma, pulmonary chondroma, and extraadrenal pheochromocytoma.[12]

More genetic causes of pheochromocytoma and paraganglioma are yet to be discovered. For example, truncating germline mutations in the transmembrane-encoding gene *TMEM127* on chromosome 2q11 were recently shown to be present in approximately 30% of affected patients with familial disease and in about 3% of patients with apparently sporadic pheochromocytomas without a known genetic cause.[9] *TMEM127* is a negative regulator of mammalian target of rapamycin (mTOR) effector proteins.

Diagnosis

The diagnostic approach to catecholamine-producing tumors is divided into two series of studies (Figure 30-1). First, the diagnosis of a catecholamine-producing tumor must be suspected and then confirmed biochemically by increased concentrations of fractionated metanephrines (metanephrine and normetanephrine) and catecholamines (norepinephrine, epinephrine, and dopamine) in the urine or plasma. The 24-hour urinary excretion rates of fractionated metanephrines and catecholamines are the tests of choice to detect catecholamine-secreting tumors (see Figure 30-1).[1,13] Measurement of the concentrations of plasma-fractionated metanephrines is also useful in case-detection testing for pheochromocytoma.

The next step is to localize the catecholamine-producing tumor to guide the surgical approach. Computer-assisted abdominal and pelvic imaging, either magnetic resonance imaging (MRI) or computed tomography (CT), is the first localization test. About 95% of these tumors are in the abdomen or pelvis, with approximately 85% of them in the adrenal glands. If the findings on abdominal imaging are negative, scintigraphic localization with [123I]metaiodobenzylguanidine ([123I]-MIBG) is indicated. Thorough discussions of the diagnostic investigation of catecholamine-producing tumors may be found elsewhere.[1,10,11,13-16]

Principles of Treatment

The treatment of choice for pheochromocytoma is surgical resection. Most of the tumors are benign and can be totally excised. However, preoperatively, the long- and short-term effects of excess circulating catecholamines should be reversed.

PREOPERATIVE MANAGEMENT

Combined α- and β-adrenergic blockade is required preoperatively to control blood pressure and prevent intraoperative hypertensive crises. α-Adrenergic blockade should be started 7 to 10

Box 30-1 Endocrine Causes of Hypertension

Adrenal Dependent
Pheochromocytoma
Primary aldosteronism
Hyperdeoxycorticosteronism
  Congenital adrenal hyperplasia
    11β-Hydroxylase deficiency
    17α-Hydroxylase deficiency
  Deoxycorticosterone-producing tumor
  Primary cortisol resistance
Cushing syndrome

**Apparent Mineralocorticoid Excess (AME)/
11β-Hydroxysteroid Dehydrogenase Deficiency**
Genetic
  Type I AME
  Type II AME
Acquired
  Licorice or carbenoxolone ingestion (type I AME)
  Cushing syndrome (type II AME)

Thyroid Dependent
Hypothyroidism
Hyperthyroidism

Parathyroid Dependent
Hyperparathyroidism

Pituitary Dependent
Acromegaly
Cushing syndrome

Box 30-2 Signs and Symptoms Associated with Catecholamine-Secreting Tumors

Spell Related
Headache
Palpitation
Diaphoresis
Epigastric and chest pain
Pallor
Nausea
Dyspnea
Anxiety
Hypertension
Tremor

Chronic
Hypertension
Orthostatic hypotension
Grade II to IV retinopathy
Tremor
Fever
Weight loss
Congestive heart failure: dilated or hypertrophic cardiomyopathy
Hyperglycemia
Constipation
Painless hematuria (associated with urinary bladder paraganglioma)
Ectopic hormone secretion—dependent symptoms (e.g., CRH/ACTH, GHRH, PTH-RP, VIP)

Not Typical of Pheochromocytoma
Flushing

ACTH, adrenocorticotropic hormone; CRH, corticotropin-releasing hormone; GHRH, growth hormone–releasing hormone; PTH-RP, parathyroid hormone–related peptide; VIP, vasoactive intestinal polypeptide.

TABLE 30-1   Autosomal Dominant Syndromes Associated with Pheochromocytoma and Paraganglioma

SYNDROME	GENE	TYPICAL TUMOR LOCATION	ASSOCIATED NEOPLASMS AND CONDITIONS
SDHD (familial paraganglioma type 1)*	SDHD	Skull base, neck, occasionally abdomen and chest	Gastrointestinal stromal tumors
SDHAF2 (familial paraganglioma type 2)*	SDHAF2	Skull base, neck	None recognized
SDHC (familial paraganglioma type 3)	SDHC	Skull base, neck, occasionally abdomen and chest	None recognized
SDHB (familial paraganglioma type 4)	SDHB	Abdomen, pelvis, occasionally skull base, neck, chest	Malignant paraganglioma, renal cell carcinoma, gastrointestinal stromal tumor
MEN 2A	RET	Adrenal medulla, bilaterally	Medullary thyroid cancer in all patients, primary hyperparathyroidism in 20%, cutaneous lichen amyloidosis in 5%
MEN 2B	RET	Adrenal medulla, bilaterally	Medullary thyroid cancer in all patients, mucocutaneous neuromas (typically involving the tongue, lips, and eyelids) in most patients, skeletal deformities (e.g., kyphoscoliosis or lordosis), joint laxity, myelinated corneal nerves, intestinal ganglioneuromas (Hirschsprung disease)
Neurofibromatosis type 1	NF1	Adrenal-periadrenal	Neurofibromas, multiple café au lait spots, axillary and inguinal freckling, iris hamartomas (Lisch nodules), bony abnormalities, central nervous system gliomas, macrocephaly, and cognitive deficits
von Hippel–Lindau disease	VHL	Adrenal medulla, bilaterally	Hemangioblastoma (involving the cerebellum, spinal cord, or brain stem), retinal angioma, clear-cell renal cell carcinoma, pancreatic neuroendocrine tumors, endolymphatic sac tumors of the middle ear, serous cystadenomas of the pancreas, papillary cystadenomas of the epididymis and broad ligament

*Associated with maternal imprinting.
MEN, multiple endocrine neoplasia; SDH, succinate dehydrogenase.

---

days preoperatively to allow expansion of the contracted blood volume. A liberal salt diet is advised during the preoperative period. After adequate α-adrenergic blockade has been achieved, β-adrenergic blockade is initiated, usually about 3 days preoperatively. Echocardiography performed preoperatively may be helpful in detecting catecholamine cardiomyopathy.

α-Adrenergic Blockade

Phenoxybenzamine is an irreversible long-acting α-adrenergic blocking agent (Table 30-2). The effects of daily administration are cumulative for nearly 1 week, and approximately 25% of an oral dose is absorbed. Phenoxybenzamine is available in 10-mg capsules. The initial dosage is 10 mg orally one to two times a day,

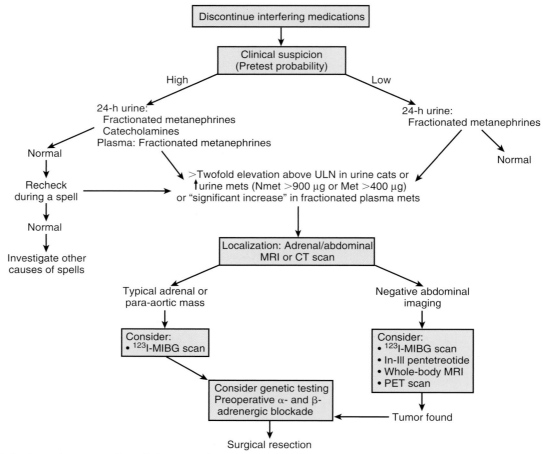

FIGURE 30-1 Evaluation and treatment of catecholamine-producing tumors. Clinical suspicion is triggered by paroxysmal symptoms, especially hypertension; hypertension that is intermittent, unusually labile, or resistant to treatment; family history of pheochromocytoma or associated conditions; or an incidentally discovered adrenal mass. CT, computed tomography; mets, metabolic equivalents; ^{123}I-MIBG, ^{123}I-metaiodobenzylguanidine; MRI, magnetic resonance imaging; PET, positron emission tomography; ULN, upper limit of normal. (*Modified from Young WF Jr. Pheochromocytoma: 1926-1993.* Trends Endocrinol Metab *1993;4:122-127.*)

TABLE 30-2	**Orally Administered Drugs Used to Treat Pheochromocytoma**	
DRUG	**DOSAGE (mg/day*)** **INITIAL TO MAXIMUM**	**SIDE EFFECTS**
α-Adrenergic–Blocking Agents		
Phenoxybenzamine	20-100†	Postural hypotension, tachycardia, miosis, nasal congestion, diarrhea, inhibition of ejaculation, fatigue
Prazosin	1-20‡	First-dose effect, dizziness, drowsiness, headache, fatigue, palpitations, nausea
Terazosin	1-20†	First-dose effect, asthenia, blurred vision, dizziness, nasal congestion, nausea, peripheral edema, palpitations, somnolence
Doxazosin	1-20	First-dose effect, orthostasis, peripheral edema, fatigue, somnolence
Combined α- and β-Adrenergic–Blocking Agent		
Labetalol	200-1200†	Dizziness, fatigue, nausea, nasal congestion, impotence
Calcium Channel Blockers		
Nicardipine, sustained release	60-120†	Edema, dizziness, headache, flushing, nausea, dyspepsia
Catecholamine Synthesis Inhibitor		
α-Methyl-ρ-L-tyrosine (metyrosine)	1000-4000‡	Sedation, diarrhea, anxiety, nightmares, crystalluria, galactorrhea, extrapyramidal symptoms

*Given once daily unless otherwise indicated.
†Given in two doses daily.
‡Given in three or four doses daily.

and the dosage is increased by 10 to 20 mg every 2 to 3 days as needed to control blood pressure and spells. The average dosage is 20 to 100 mg/day. The target blood pressure is less than 120/80 mm Hg seated, with systolic blood pressure greater than 90 mm Hg standing. These target blood pressure readings may be modified on the basis of age and comorbid disease. Side effects include postural hypotension, tachycardia, miosis, nasal congestion, inhibition of ejaculation, diarrhea, and fatigue. Prazosin, terazosin, and doxazosin are selective α₁-adrenergic blocking agents. Because these agents have a more favorable side-effect profile, they may be preferable to phenoxybenzamine when long-term pharmacologic treatment is indicated (e.g., for mild, metabolically active metastatic pheochromocytoma). However, phenoxybenzamine is the drug preferred for preoperative preparation because it provides nonselective α-adrenergic blockade of long duration. Effective α-adrenergic blockade permits expansion of blood volume, which is usually severely decreased because of excessive adrenergic vasoconstriction.

β-Adrenergic Blockade

A β-adrenergic antagonist should be administered only after α-adrenergic blockade is effective because β-adrenergic blockade alone may increase the severity of the hypertension through unopposed α-adrenergic stimulation. Preoperative β-adrenergic blockade is indicated to control the tachycardia associated with both the high concentrations of circulating catecholamines and the α-adrenergic blockade. Caution is indicated if the patient has asthma or congestive heart failure. A chronic excess level of catecholamines can produce myocardiopathy, and β-adrenergic blockade can result in acute pulmonary edema. Noncardioselective β-adrenergic blockers, such as propranolol and nadolol, or cardioselective β-adrenergic blockers, such as atenolol and metoprolol, may be used. Mechanisms of action, routes of metabolism, dosages, and side effects of β-adrenergic blockers are discussed in Chapter 29. When initiating treatment with a β-adrenergic blocker, the drug should be started at a low dose. For example, propranolol is usually started at a dose of 10 mg orally every 6 hours at least 4 to 7 days after the initiation of α-adrenergic blockade. The dose is increased as necessary to control the tachycardia with a target heart rate of 80 beats/min.

Labetalol exhibits both selective α_1-adrenergic and nonselective β-adrenergic blocking activities in a ratio of approximately 1:3 (see Table 30-2). Paradoxical hypertensive responses in patients with pheochromocytoma treated with labetalol have been reported, presumably because of incomplete α-adrenergic blockade. Therefore, the safety of labetalol as primary therapy is controversial.

Catecholamine Synthesis Inhibitor

Occasionally, α- and β-adrenergic blocking agents may be ineffective or poorly tolerated, and an alternative medical approach is needed. α-Methyl-p-L-tyrosine (metyrosine) inhibits the synthesis of catecholamines by blocking the rate-limiting enzyme tyrosine hydroxylase. It is absorbed rapidly from the gastrointestinal tract, and most of it is excreted unchanged in the urine. Metyrosine is available as 250-mg capsules, and the initial dosage is 250 mg orally four times a day. The total dosage may be increased by 500 mg/day, every 1 or 2 days, to a maximum of 4 g/day (1 g four times per day) as needed for blood pressure control. Side effects include sedation, somnolence, depression, diarrhea, anxiety, nightmares, crystalluria and urolithiasis, galactorrhea, and extrapyramidal manifestations. Therefore, this agent should be used only after other agents have been ineffective or when an ablative procedure for metastatic disease is planned, such as radiofrequency ablation (RFA) of hepatic metastases or cyroablation of bony metastases. The extrapyramidal effects of phenothiazines or haloperidol may be potentiated, and their concomitant use with metyrosine should be avoided. High fluid intake to avoid crystalluria is suggested for any patient taking more than 2 g daily. Metyrosine is especially useful for patients who cannot be treated with combined α- and β-adrenergic blockade for cardiopulmonary reasons.

Calcium Channel Blockers

Calcium channel blockers (CCBs), which block norepinephrine-mediated calcium transport into vascular smooth muscle, have been used successfully at several medical centers to preoperatively prepare patients with pheochromocytoma. Nicardipine is the most commonly used CCB in this setting. It is given orally to control blood pressure preoperatively and is given as an intravenous (IV) infusion intraoperatively. When CCBs are used as the primary mode of antihypertensive therapy, they appear to be just as effective as α- and β-adrenergic blockade.

ACUTE HYPERTENSIVE CRISES

Acute hypertensive crises may occur before or during surgery and should be treated with nitroprusside, phentolamine, or nicardipine administered intravenously (Table 30-3; see also Chapter 32). Sodium nitroprusside is an ideal vasodilator for intraoperative management of hypertensive episodes because of its rapid onset of action and short duration of effect. It is administered as an IV infusion at 0.5 to 5.0 μg/kg body weight/min and adjusted every few minutes for target blood pressure response; to keep the steady-state thiocyanate concentration below 1 mmol/L, the rate of a prolonged infusion should be no more than 3 μg/kg/min. Phentolamine is a short-acting, nonselective α-adrenergic blocker available in lyophilized form in 5-mg vials. An initial test dose of 1 mg is administered and followed by repeat 5-mg boluses or continuous infusion if necessary. The response to phentolamine is maximal 2 to 3 minutes after a bolus injection and lasts 10 to 15 minutes. Nicardipine infusion is initiated at 5 mg/h, and the infusion rate may be increased by 2.5 mg/h every 15 minutes up to a maximum of 15 mg/h.

ANESTHESIA AND SURGERY

Resection of a catecholamine-secreting tumor is a high-risk surgical procedure, and an experienced surgeon and anesthesiologist are required. The last oral doses of α- and β-adrenergic blockers can be administered orally early in the morning on the day of the operation. Fentanyl, ketamine, and morphine should be avoided because they can potentially stimulate catecholamine release from a pheochromocytoma. Also, parasympathetic nervous system blockade with atropine should be avoided because of the associated tachycardia. Anesthesia may be induced with IV injection of propofol, etomidate, or barbiturates in combination with synthetic opioids. Most anesthetic gases can be used, but halothane and desflurane should be avoided. Cardiovascular and hemodynamic variables must be monitored closely, and continuous measurement of intraarterial pressure and heart rhythm is required. If the patient

TABLE 30-3	Intravenously Administered Drugs Used to Treat Pheochromocytoma
AGENT	**DOSAGE RANGE**
For Hypertension	
Phentolamine	Initiate with a 1-mg intravenous IV test dose, followed by 2- to 5-mg IV boluses as needed or continuous infusion.
Nitroprusside	Infusion rates of 2 μg/kg/min are suggested as safe; rates >4 μg/kg/min may lead to cyanide toxicity within 3 hours. Doses >10 μg/kg/min are rarely required; maximal dose should not exceed 800 μg/min.
Nicardipine	Initiate therapy at 5 mg/h; infusion rate may be increased by 2.5 mg/h up to a maximum of 15 mg/h.
For Cardiac Arrhythmia	
Lidocaine	Initiate therapy with a bolus of 1-1.5 mg/kg (75-100 mg); additional boluses of 0.5-0.75 mg/kg (25-50 mg) can be given q5-10min if needed, up to a maximum of 3 mg/kg. Loading is followed by a maintenance infusion of 2-4 mg/min (30-50 μg/kg/min), adjusted for effect, in the setting of altered metabolism (e.g., heart failure, liver congestion) and as guided by blood level monitoring.
Esmolol	A loading dose of 0.5 mg/kg/min is infused followed by a maintenance infusion of 0.05 mg/kg/min for the next 4 min. Depending on the desired ventricular response, the maintenance infusion may then be continued at 0.05 mg/kg/min or increased stepwise (e.g., by 0.1-mg/kg/min increments to a maximum of 0.2 mg/kg/min), with each step being maintained for ≥4 min.

IV, intravenous.

has congestive heart failure or decreased cardiac reserve, monitoring of pulmonary capillary wedge pressure is indicated. Surgical survival rates are 98% to 100%, and the preoperative and perioperative treatment approach outlined here is the same for adults and children.[15]

The laparoscopic approach to the adrenal gland is the procedure of choice for patients with solitary intraadrenal pheochromocytomas less than 8 to 10 cm in diameter. The average length of hospitalization for patients who undergo laparoscopic adrenalectomy for pheochromocytoma is 1 to 2 days. If the pheochromocytoma is in the adrenal gland, the entire gland should be removed. Laparoscopic adrenalectomy for pheochromocytoma should be converted to open adrenalectomy for difficult dissection, invasion, adhesions, or surgeon inexperience. If bilateral adrenalectomy is planned preoperatively, the patient should receive glucocorticoid stress coverage while awaiting transfer to the operating room. Glucocorticoid coverage should be initiated in the operating room if unexpected bilateral adrenalectomy is necessary. Cortical-sparing bilateral adrenalectomies have been used to treat patients with MEN 2 and von Hippel–Lindau disease. However, in MEN 2 patients, there is a concern with leaving residual adrenal medullary tissue behind because it increases the risk of recurrent pheochromocytoma. An anterior midline abdominal surgical approach is indicated for abdominal paragangliomas, whereas those of the neck, chest, and urinary bladder require specialized approaches.

Hypotension may occur after surgical resection of the pheochromocytoma, and it should be treated with fluids and IV pressor agents as needed. Postoperative hypotension is less frequent in patients who have had adequate preoperative α-adrenergic blockade combined with a diet high in sodium content. If both adrenal glands were manipulated during surgery, adrenocortical insufficiency should be considered as a potential cause of postoperative hypotension. Because hypoglycemia can occur in the immediate postoperative period, blood glucose levels should be monitored, and fluid given intravenously should contain 5% dextrose.

Blood pressure is usually normal by the time of hospital discharge, but some patients remain hypertensive for up to 4 to 8 weeks postoperatively. Long-standing, persistent hypertension does occur and may be related to inadvertent ligation of a polar renal artery, resetting of baroreceptors, hemodynamic changes, structural changes of the blood vessels, altered sensitivity of the vessels to pressor substances, functional or structural renal changes, or coincident primary hypertension.

LONG-TERM POSTOPERATIVE FOLLOW-UP

Approximately 1 to 2 weeks after surgery, fractionated metanephrines and catecholamines should be measured by collecting a 24-hour urine specimen. If the levels are normal, the resection of the pheochromocytoma should be considered complete. Increased levels of fractionated catecholamines and metanephrines detected postoperatively are consistent with residual tumor, either a second primary lesion or occult metastases. If bilateral adrenalectomy was performed, life-long glucocorticoid and mineralocorticoid replacement therapy is prescribed, and 24-hour urinary excretion of fractionated metanephrines and catecholamines or plasma-fractionated metanephrines should be checked annually for life. Annual biochemical testing assesses for metastatic disease, tumor recurrence in the adrenal bed, or delayed appearance of multiple primary tumors. Recurrence rates are highest for patients with familial disease and/or paraganglioma. Follow-up imaging with CT or MRI is not needed unless the fractionated metanephrines and/or catecholamine levels become elevated or the original tumor was associated with minimal catecholamine excess.

Clinicians should consider genetic testing for patients with one or more of the following: paraganglioma, pheochromocytoma diagnosed at a young age (<30 years), a family history of pheochromocytoma, or any sign that suggests a genetic cause, such as retinal angiomas, axillary freckling, café au lait spots, cerebellar tumor, medullary thyroid carcinoma, and hyperparathyroidism. In addition, all first-degree relatives of a patient with pheochromocytoma or paraganglioma should have biochemical testing, such as a 24-hour urine test for fractionated metanephrines and catecholamines. If mutation testing in a patient is positive, first-degree relatives should have stepwise (parents and children first) germline screening.

MALIGNANT PHEOCHROMOCYTOMA

Distinguishing between benign and malignant catecholamine-secreting tumors on the basis of clinical, biochemical, or histopathologic characteristics is difficult. The only cure for malignant pheochromocytoma is complete surgical resection. Malignancy is rare in patients with a familial adrenal syndrome, but it is common in those with familial paraganglioma caused by mutations in *SDHB*. Although the mean 5-year survival rate for patients with malignant pheochromocytoma is less than 50%, the prognosis is variable: approximately 50% of patients have an indolent form of the disease, with a life expectancy of more than 20 years, and the other 50% have rapidly progressive disease, with death occurring within 1 to 3 years. Metastatic sites include local tissue, liver, bone, lung, and lymph nodes; if possible, metastatic lesions should be resected. Skeletal metastatic lesions that are painful or threaten structural function can be treated with external radiotherapy or cyroablation therapy. External radiotherapy can also be used to treat unresectable soft tissue lesions.

Local tumor irradiation with therapeutic doses of ^{131}I-MIBG has produced partial and temporary responses in approximately one third of patients. Thrombotic therapy for large unresectable liver metastases and RFA for small (<3 cm) liver metastases are options to be considered. In selected cases, long-acting octreotide has been beneficial. If the tumor is considered aggressive, and the patient's quality of life is affected, combination chemotherapy may be considered.[17] Treatment with tyrosine kinase inhibitors has resulted in short-term tumor regression.[18] Management of a patient who has malignant pheochromocytoma can be frustrating because curative options are limited. Clearly, innovative prospective protocols are needed to identify new treatment options for this neoplasm.

PHEOCHROMOCYTOMA IN PREGNANCY

Pheochromocytoma in pregnancy can cause the death of both the fetus and the mother. The treatment of hypertensive crisis is the same as that for nonpregnant patients, with the exception that nitroprusside should be avoided in the pregnant patient. Although some controversy exists about the most appropriate management, pheochromocytomas should be resected if diagnosed during the first two trimesters of pregnancy. The preoperative preparation is the same as that for nonpregnant patients. If medical therapy is chosen, or if the patient is in the third trimester, cesarean section and removal of the pheochromocytoma in the same operation are indicated. Spontaneous labor and delivery should be avoided.

Primary Aldosteronism

Hypertension, suppressed plasma renin activity (PRA), and increased adrenal aldosterone secretion characterize the syndrome of primary aldosteronism, first described in 1955.[1,19] Aldosterone-producing adenoma (APA) and bilateral idiopathic hyperaldosteronism (IHA) are the most common subtypes of primary aldosteronism (Box 30-3). Although the etiology of IHA is yet to be determined, a subset of APAs are associated with somatic mutations of the gene that encodes an inwardly rectifying potassium channel (*KCNJ5*).[20] A much less common form, unilateral hyperplasia, or primary adrenal hyperplasia (PAH), is caused by micronodular or macronodular hyperplasia of the zona glomerulosa of one adrenal gland.[21] Familial hyperaldosteronism (FH) is also rare, and three types have been described: FH types I, II, and

III.[22] *FH type I*, or *glucocorticoid-remediable aldosteronism* (GRA), is autosomal dominant in inheritance and is associated with variable degrees of hyperaldosteronism, high levels of hybrid steroids (18-hydroxycortisol and 18-oxocortisol), and suppression with exogenous glucocorticoids. *FH type II* refers to the familial occurrence of APA or IHA or both.[22,23] *FH type III* refers to severe congenital primary aldosteronism associated with bilateral zona glomerulosa hyperplasia because of germline mutations in the *KCNJ5* gene.[20,24]

Diagnosis

CASE DETECTION

In the past, clinicians would not consider the diagnosis of primary aldosteronism unless the patient presented with spontaneous hypokalemia, and then the diagnostic evaluation would require discontinuing antihypertensive medications for at least 2 weeks.[1] The spontaneous "hypokalemia/no antihypertensive drug" diagnostic approach resulted in predicted prevalence rates of less than 0.5% of hypertensive patients.[1,21] However, it is now recognized that most patients with primary aldosteronism are not hypokalemic and that case detection can be completed with a simple blood test (plasma aldosterone concentration [PAC]/plasma renin activity [PRA] ratio) while the patient is taking antihypertensive drugs.[21,25] Using the PAC/PRA ratio as a case-detection test, followed by aldosterone suppression confirmatory testing, has

resulted in much higher prevalence estimates (5% to 10% of all patients with hypertension) for primary aldosteronism.[1,21,25,26] Patients with hypertension and hypokalemia, regardless of the presumed cause (e.g., diuretic treatment), and most patients with treatment-resistant hypertension should undergo screening for primary aldosteronism with a PAC/PRA ratio (cutoff is laboratory dependent; Figure 30-2). A high PAC/PRA ratio is a positive screening test result, a finding that warrants confirmatory testing.

CONFIRMING THE DIAGNOSIS

Confirmatory testing is completed with sodium suppression testing: oral sodium loading, saline suppression test, captopril stimulation test, or fludrocortisone suppression testing.[25] At the Mayo Clinic, we prefer the high-sodium diet for 3 to 4 days with 24-hour urine collection (day 3 to 4) for aldosterone, sodium, and creatinine.[21] When the 24-hour urinary sodium is more than 200 mEq, confirming adequate sodium loading, patients with primary aldosteronism demonstrate autonomous aldosterone production with urinary aldosterone levels higher than 12 μg/24 h (>33 nmol/day). During oral sodium loading, it is important to monitor serum electrolytes and blood pressure daily and to increase potassium supplementation and antihypertensive medications as indicated.

SUBTYPE EVALUATION

Unilateral adrenalectomy in patients with APA or PAH results in normalization of hypokalemia; hypertension is improved in all patients and is cured in approximately 30% to 60%.[27-30] In IHA, unilateral or bilateral adrenalectomy seldom corrects the hypertension; IHA and GRA should therefore be treated medically. For patients who want to pursue a surgical cure, the accurate distinction between the subtypes of primary aldosteronism is a critical step (Figure 30-3); the subtype evaluation may require one or more tests, the first of which is imaging the adrenal glands with CT. When a solitary hypodense (Hounsfield unit score <10) unilateral macroadenoma (>1 cm but <2 cm) and normal contralateral adrenal morphology are found on CT in a young patient (<40 years) with primary aldosteronism, unilateral adrenalectomy is a reasonable therapeutic option. However, in many cases, CT

> **Box 30-3 Subtypes of Primary Aldosteronism**

Aldosterone-producing adenoma (APA)
Idiopathic hyperaldosteronism (IHA)
Primary adrenal hyperplasia (unilateral adrenal hyperplasia)
Aldosterone-producing adrenocortical carcinoma
Ectopic aldosterone-producing tumor (e.g., ovarian tumor)
Familial hyperaldosteronism (FH)
   Glucocorticoid-remediable aldosteronism (FH type I)
   FH type II (APA and/or IHA)
   FH type III (germline mutations in *KCNJ5*)

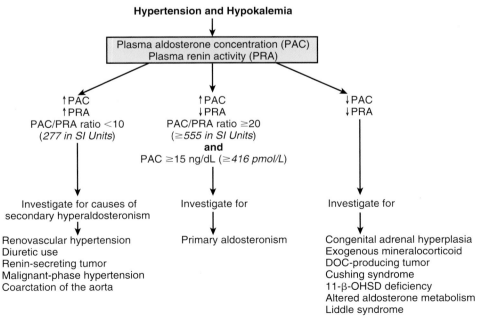

FIGURE 30-2 Use of the plasma aldosterone concentration (*PAC*)/plasma renin activity (*PRA*) ratio to differentiate among different causes of hypertension and hypokalemia. DOC, deoxycorticosterone; OHSD, hydroxysteroid dehydrogenase. (*Modified from Young WF Jr, Hogan MJ. Renin-independent hypermineralocorticoidism. Trends Endocrinol Metab 1994;5:97-106.*)

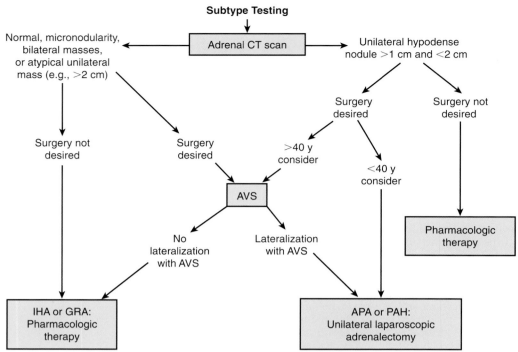

FIGURE 30-3 Subtype evaluation of primary aldosteronism. APA, aldosterone-producing adenoma; AVS, adrenal venous sampling; CT, computed tomography; GRA, glucocorticoid-remediable aldosteronism; IHA, idiopathic hyperaldosteronism; PAH, primary adrenal hyperplasia. *(Modified from Young WF Jr, Hogan MJ. Renin-independent hypermineralocorticoidism.* Trends Endocrinol Metab *1994;5:97-106.)*

may show normal-appearing adrenals, minimal unilateral adrenal limb thickening, unilateral microadenomas (≤1 cm), or bilateral macroadenomas. However, adrenal CT is not accurate in distinguishing between APA and IHA.[31-33] In one study of 203 patients with primary aldosteronism who were evaluated with both CT and adrenal venous sampling, CT was accurate in only 53% of patients; based on CT findings, 42 patients (22%) would have been incorrectly excluded as candidates for adrenalectomy, and 48 (25%) might have had unnecessary or inappropriate surgery.[32] In a systematic review of 38 studies in a total of 950 patients with primary aldosteronism, adrenal CT/MRI results did not agree with adrenal venous sampling findings in 359 (38%) of 950 patients; based on CT/MRI, 19% of patients would have undergone noncurative surgery, and 19% would have been offered medical therapy instead of curative adrenalectomy.[33] Thus, adrenal venous sampling is the standard test to distinguish between unilateral and bilateral disease in patients with primary aldosteronism.[32-34] Adrenal venous sampling is an intricate procedure because the right adrenal vein is small and may be difficult to locate and cannulate; the success rate depends on the proficiency of the angiographer.[35] A review of 47 reports found that the success rate for cannulating the right adrenal vein in 384 patients was 74%.[36] With experience, and by focusing the expertise to one or two radiologists at a referral center, the adrenal venous sampling success rate can be as high as 96%.[32,34,37]

Patients with APAs have more severe hypertension, have more frequent hypokalemia, higher plasma (>25 ng/dL, >694 pmol/L) and urinary (>30 µg/day, >83 nmol/day) levels of aldosterone, and are younger (<50 years) than those with IHA. However, these factors are not absolute predictors of unilateral versus bilateral adrenal disease. Some centers and clinical practice guidelines recommend that adrenal venous sampling be performed in all patients who have the diagnosis of primary aldosteronism.[25,33] The use of adrenal venous sampling should be based on patient preference, age, comorbidities, and clinical probability of finding an APA.[21,32] A more practical approach is the selective use of adrenal venous sampling, as outlined in Figure 30-3.

Principles of Treatment

The treatment goal is to prevent the morbidity and mortality associated with hypertension, hypokalemia, and cardiovascular damage. The cause of the primary aldosteronism helps to determine the appropriate treatment. Normalization of blood pressure should not be the only goal in managing the patient with primary aldosteronism. In addition to the kidney and colon, mineralocorticoid receptors are present in the heart, brain, and blood vessels. Excessive secretion of aldosterone is associated with increased risk of cardiovascular disease and morbidity. This issue was addressed in a retrospective study that compared 124 patients with primary aldosteronism with 465 patients with apparent essential hypertension who were matched for age, gender, and blood pressure (mean, 175/107 mm Hg).[38] The patients with primary aldosteronism had significantly higher rates of stroke (12.9% vs. 3.4% in those with essential hypertension), nonfatal myocardial infarction (4.0% vs. 0.6%), and atrial fibrillation (7.3% vs. 0.6%). The rate of cardiovascular complications appeared to be similar in those with an adrenal adenoma and adrenal hyperplasia. In addition, aldosterone excess can induce adverse cardiovascular effects independent of blood pressure.[39] Therefore, normalization of circulating aldosterone or aldosterone-receptor blockade should be part of the management plan for all patients with primary aldosteronism.

In addition, clinicians must understand that most patients with long-standing primary aldosteronism have some degree of renal insufficiency that is masked by the glomerular hyperfiltration associated with aldosterone excess.[40-42] The true degree of renal insufficiency may only become evident after effective pharmacologic or surgical therapy.[40-42]

SURGICAL TREATMENT OF ALDOSTERONE-PRODUCING ADENOMA AND UNILATERAL HYPERPLASIA

Unilateral laparoscopic adrenalectomy is an excellent treatment option for patients with APA or unilateral hyperplasia.[25,43] Although blood pressure control improves in nearly 100% of patients post-operatively, average long-term cure rates of hypertension after unilateral adrenalectomy for APA range from 30% to 60%.[28,30] Persistent hypertension following adrenalectomy is correlated directly with having more than one first-degree relative with hypertension, use of more than two antihypertensive agents pre-operatively, older age, increased serum creatinine level, and duration of hypertension, and it is most likely due to coexistent primary hypertension.[28,30]

Laparoscopic adrenalectomy is the preferred surgical approach, and it is associated with shorter hospital stays and less long-term morbidity than the conventional open approach.[43] Because APAs are small and may be multiple, the entire adrenal gland should be removed. To decrease the surgical risk, hypokalemia should be corrected with potassium supplements and/or a mineralocorti-coid receptor antagonist preoperatively. The mineralocorticoid receptor antagonist and potassium supplements should be discontinued postoperatively. PAC should be measured 1 to 2 days after the operation to confirm a biochemical cure, serum potassium levels should be monitored weekly for 4 weeks after surgery, and a generous sodium diet should be followed to avoid the hyperkalemia of hypoaldosteronism that may occur because of the chronic suppression of the renin-angiotensin-aldosterone system. In approximately 5% of APA patients, clinically significant hyperkalemia may develop after surgery, and short-term fludrocortisone supplementation may be required.[44] Typically, the hypertension that was associated with aldosterone excess resolves in 1 to 3 months postoperatively.

RFA of aldosterone-producing adenomas has been reported.[45] However, this treatment approach should not be used until long-term studies document both safety and efficacy.

Pharmacologic Treatment

IHA and GRA should be treated medically. In addition, APA patients may be treated medically if the medical treatment includes mineralocorticoid receptor blockade.[21,25] A sodium-restricted diet (<100 mEq/day), maintenance of ideal body weight, tobacco avoidance, and regular aerobic exercise contribute significantly to the success of pharmacologic treatment.

For more than 4 decades, spironolactone has been the drug of choice to treat primary aldosteronism. It is available as 25-, 50-, and 100 mg-tablets. The dosage is 12.5 to 25 mg/day initially and is increased to 400 mg/day if necessary to achieve a high-normal serum potassium concentration without the aid of oral potassium chloride supplementation. Hypokalemia responds promptly, but hypertension may take as long as 4 to 8 weeks to be corrected. After several months of therapy this dosage often can be decreased to as little as 12.5 to 50 mg/day; dosage titration is based on a goal serum potassium level in the high-normal range. Serum potassium and creatinine should be monitored frequently during the first 4 to 6 weeks of therapy, especially in patients with renal insufficiency or diabetes mellitus. Spironolactone increases the half-life of digoxin, and for patients taking this drug, the dosage may need to be adjusted when treatment with spironolactone is started. Concomitant therapy with salicylates should be avoided because salicylates interfere with the tubular secretion of an active metabolite and decrease the effectiveness of spironolactone. However, spironolactone is not selective for the mineralocorticoid receptor. For example, antagonism at the testosterone receptor may result in painful gynecomastia, erectile dysfunction, and decreased libido in men; agonist activity at the progesterone receptor results in menstrual irregularity in women.

Eplerenone is a steroid-based antimineralocorticoid that acts as a competitive and selective mineralocorticoid receptor antagonist; it was approved by the Food and Drug Administration (FDA) for the treatment of uncomplicated essential hypertension in 2003. The 9,11-epoxide group in eplerenone results in a marked reduction of the molecule's progestational and antiandrogenic actions compared with spironolactone; eplerenone has 0.1% of

the binding affinity to androgen receptors and less than 1% of the binding affinity to progesterone receptors compared with spironolactone. A multicenter, randomized, double-blind, active-controlled, and parallel-group trial comparing the efficacy of eplerenone versus spironolactone for the treatment of primary aldosteronism found that spironolactone had a statistically significant greater antihypertensive effect.[46] Eplerenone is available as 25- and 50-mg tablets. For primary aldosteronism, it is reasonable to start with a dose of 25 mg twice daily (the dosage is twice daily because of the shorter half-life of eplerenone compared with spironolactone), and it should be titrated upward for a target high-normal serum potassium concentration without the aid of potassium supplements. The maximum dose approved by the FDA for hypertension is 100 mg/day. Potency studies with eplerenone show a 50% less milligram-per-milligram potency when compared with spironolactone. As with spironolactone, it is important to follow blood pressure, serum potassium, and serum creatinine levels closely. Side effects with eplerenone include dizziness, headache, fatigue, diarrhea, hypertriglyceridemia, and elevated liver enzyme levels.

Patients with IHA frequently require a second antihypertensive agent to achieve good blood pressure control. Hypervolemia is a major reason for resistance to drug therapy, and low doses of a thiazide, such as 12.5 to 50 mg of hydrochlorothiazide daily, or a related sulfonamide diuretic are effective in combination with the mineralocorticoid receptor antagonist. Because these agents often lead to further hypokalemia, serum potassium levels should be monitored. In addition to these therapies, aldosterone synthase inhibitors are in development and may prove to be good treatment options for patients with primary aldosteronism.[47]

PHARMACOLOGIC TREATMENT OF GLUCOCORTICOID-REMEDIABLE ALDOSTERONISM

Before initiating treatment, GRA should be confirmed with genetic testing. In the GRA patient, long-term treatment with physiologic doses of a glucocorticoid normalizes blood pressure and corrects hypokalemia. The clinician should be cautious about iatrogenic Cushing syndrome with excessive doses of glucocorticoids, especially with the use of dexamethasone in children. The smallest effective dose of shorter acting agents, such as prednisone or hydrocortisone, should be prescribed in relation to body surface area (e.g., hydrocortisone 10 to 12 mg/m^2/day). Target blood pressure in children should be guided by age-specific blood pressure percentiles. Children should be monitored by pediatricians with expertise in glucocorticoid therapy, with careful attention paid to preventing retardation of linear growth by overtreatment. Treatment with mineralocorticoid receptor antagonists in these patients may be just as effective and avoids the potential disruption of the hypothalamic-pituitary-adrenal axis and risk of iatrogenic side effects. In addition, glucocorticoid therapy or mineralocorticoid receptor blockade may even have a role in normotensive GRA patients.

Other Forms of Mineralocorticoid Excess

The spectrum of effects of excess mineralocorticoid in patients with low PRA includes hyperdeoxycorticosteronism, Cushing syndrome, and apparent mineralocorticoid excess (see Box 30-1). These diagnoses should be considered when PAC and PRA are low in patients with hypertension and hypokalemia (see Figure 30-2).

Hyperdeoxycorticosteronism

CONGENITAL ADRENAL HYPERPLASIA

Congenital adrenal hyperplasia (CAH) is caused by enzymatic defects in adrenal steroidogenesis that result in deficient secretion of cortisol. The lack of inhibitory feedback by cortisol on the hypothalamus and pituitary produces an adrenocorticotropic hormone (ACTH)–driven buildup of cortisol precursors relative to the enzymatic deficiency. A deficiency of both 11-β-hydroxylase and 17-α-hydroxylase causes hypertension and hypokalemia because of hypersecretion of the mineralocorticoid 11-deoxycorticosterone (DOC). The mineralocorticoid effect of increased circulating levels of DOC also decreases PRA and aldosterone secretion. These defects are autosomal recessive in inheritance and typically are diagnosed in childhood; however, partial enzymatic defects have been shown to cause hypertension in adults.

11-β-Hydroxylase Deficiency

Approximately 5% of all cases of CAH are due to 11-β-hydroxylase deficiency; the prevalence in whites is 1 in 100,000. In addition to high levels of DOC and 11-deoxycortisol, the substrate mass effect results in increased levels of adrenal androgens. Girls come to medical attention in childhood with hypertension, hypokalemia, and virilization; in boys, pseudoprecocious puberty is apparent. Approximately two thirds of patients have mild to moderate hypertension; markedly increased levels of DOC, 11-deoxycortisol, and adrenal androgens confirm the diagnosis. Glucocorticoid replacement normalizes the steroid abnormalities and hypertension. Replacement options in adults include dexamethasone (0.5 to 0.75 mg/day), prednisone (5 mg in the morning and 2.5 mg in the evening), or hydrocortisone (20 mg in the morning and 10 mg in the evening). For screening, family members should have the cosyntropin stimulation test for cortisol and 11-deoxycortisol.

17-α-Hydroxylase Deficiency

The 17-α-hydroxylase deficiency form of CAH is rare; only 120 cases have been reported. The deficiency results in decreased production of cortisol and sex hormones. Genetic 46,XY males are seen initially with either pseudohermaphroditism or as phenotypic females, and 46,XX females present with primary amenorrhea. Therefore, a person with this form of CAH may not come to medical attention until puberty. The biochemical findings include low concentrations of plasma adrenal androgens, plasma 17-α-hydroxyprogesterone, aldosterone, and cortisol and increased plasma concentrations of DOC, corticosterone, and 18-hydroxycorticosterone, which suppress PRA. As with 11-β-hydroxylase deficiency, glucocorticoid replacement corrects the steroid abnormalities and hypertension, although sex steroids also need to be replaced. For screening, family members should have the cosyntropin stimulation test for cortisol and 17-hydroxypregnenolone.

DEOXYCORTICOSTERONE-PRODUCING TUMOR

DOC-producing adrenal tumors are usually large and malignant. Some of them secrete androgens and estrogens in addition to DOC, which may cause virilization in women and feminization in men. A high level of plasma DOC or urinary tetrahydrodeoxycorticosterone and a large adrenal tumor seen on CT confirm the diagnosis. Optimal treatment is complete surgical resection.

PRIMARY CORTISOL RESISTANCE

Increased cortisol secretion and plasma cortisol concentrations without evidence of Cushing syndrome are found in patients with primary cortisol resistance, a rare familial syndrome. The syndrome is characterized by hypokalemic alkalosis, hypertension, increased plasma concentrations of DOC, and increased adrenal androgen secretion, which are probably caused by several defects in glucocorticoid receptors and in the steroid-receptor complex. The treatment for the mineralocorticoid-dependent hypertension is blockade of the mineralocorticoid receptor with spironolactone or suppression of ACTH secretion with dexamethasone at the dosages outlined in the preceding sections on primary aldosteronism and CAH, respectively.

Apparent Mineralocorticoid Excess Syndromes

Cortisol can be a potent mineralocorticoid. The microsomal enzyme 11-β-hydroxysteroid dehydrogenase (11-β-OHSD; EC 1.1.1.146) is responsible for the renal metabolism of cortisol to the metabolically inactive cortisone. Deficiency of this enzyme results in a high intrarenal concentration of cortisol and hypertension, hypokalemia, suppressed PRA, and low aldosterone levels. An increased ratio of urinary cortisol to cortisone confirms the diagnosis.

Two types of defects have been described in the renal metabolism of cortisol. *Type I apparent mineralocorticoid excess* (AME) syndrome refers to deficiency in the 11-β-OHSD enzyme. *Type II AME* is due to a deficiency in the ring A reduction metabolic pathway. Treatment includes blockade of the mineralocorticoid receptor with spironolactone or suppression of endogenous cortisol secretion with dexamethasone. The congenital forms are rare autosomal recessive disorders, but the acquired forms are more common and include licorice-induced hypertension and Cushing syndrome.

CUSHING SYNDROME

Hypertension occurs in 75% to 80% of patients with Cushing syndrome. The mechanisms of hypertension include increased production of DOC, increased vascular reactivity to catecholamines, and cortisol inactivation overload with stimulation of the mineralocorticoid receptor. Deficient cortisol ring A reduction caused by overload of metabolizing enzymes results in a functional type II AME in patients with severe hypercortisolism. Cushing syndrome is a symptom complex that results from prolonged exposure to supraphysiologic concentrations of glucocorticoids. The source of excess glucocorticoids may be exogenous (iatrogenic) or endogenous. Endogenous Cushing syndrome is caused by 1) hypersecretion of corticotropin (ACTH), referred to as *ACTH-dependent Cushing syndrome*, or 2) primary adrenal hypersecretion of glucocorticoids, referred to as *ACTH-independent Cushing syndrome*. The overall treatment program for patients with Cushing syndrome includes the resolution of hypercortisolism, the concomitant treatment of the complications of the syndrome (hypertension, osteoporosis, and diabetes mellitus), and, after definitive treatment, the management of glucocorticoid withdrawal and hypothalamic-pituitary-adrenal axis recovery.

Presentation

Typical signs and symptoms of Cushing syndrome include weight gain with central obesity; facial rounding and plethora; dorsocervical fat pads; easy bruising; fine "cigarette paper" skin; poor wound healing; purple striae; proximal muscle weakness; emotional and cognitive changes that include irritability, crying, depression, and restlessness; hypertension; osteoporosis; opportunistic and fungal infections, such as mucocutaneous candidiasis, tinea versicolor, and pityriasis; altered reproductive function; and hirsutism.

Diagnosis

Accurate diagnosis of Cushing syndrome and subtype is essential to direct the appropriate treatment program. Because of the known manifestations of the disorder, hypercortisolism must be suspected and then confirmed with measurements of the serum and 24-hour urine concentrations of cortisol and midnight salivary cortisol. Autonomous hypercortisolism is confirmed with the low-dose dexamethasone suppression test (dexamethasone 0.5 mg orally q6h for 2 days); a 24-hour urinary cortisol excretion of 20 mg or greater confirms the diagnosis. The plasma ACTH concentration classifies the subtype of hypercortisolism as either ACTH dependent ("normal" to high levels of ACTH) or ACTH independent (undetectable ACTH).

MRI of the pituitary gland should be performed in patients with ACTH-dependent Cushing syndrome. If a pituitary tumor is not found with computerized imaging, further evaluation is indicated, with imaging of the lung and inferior petrosal sinus sampling for ACTH with ovine corticotropin-releasing hormone stimulation.

In patients with ACTH-independent hypercortisolism, the high-dose dexamethasone suppression test shows no suppression in urinary cortisol excretion. In these patients, computerized imaging of the adrenal glands usually indicates the type of adrenal disease.

PRINCIPLES OF TREATMENT

For patients with pituitary-dependent disease, selective pituitary adenomectomy by transsphenoidal surgery is the treatment of choice. The long-term surgical cure rate for ACTH-secreting microadenomas is approximately 80%. If pituitary adenomectomy is not curative, bilateral adrenalectomy and pituitary irradiation are adjunctive treatment options. For patients with primary adrenocortical disease or ectopic ACTH production, surgical extirpation of an adrenal adenoma or carcinoma or the source of ectopic ACTH production is the treatment of choice. For patients with ACTH-independent bilateral macronodular or micronodular hyperplasia, bilateral adrenalectomy is the preferred treatment. Pharmacologic therapy is reserved for patients not cured with these surgical approaches.

The hypertension associated with Cushing syndrome should be treated until a surgical cure is obtained. Spironolactone at dosages used to treat primary aldosteronism is effective in reversing the hypokalemia. Second-step agents, such as thiazide diuretics, may be added for optimal control of blood pressure. The hypertension associated with the hypercortisolism usually resolves over several weeks after the surgical cure, and antihypertensive agents can be tapered and withdrawn.

Thyroid and Parathyroid Disease

Dysfunction of the thyroid and parathyroid glands may be the sole cause of hypertension or may contribute significantly to underlying primary hypertension.

Thyroid Dysfunction

PRESENTATION AND DIAGNOSIS

Hyperthyroidism is the clinical syndrome that occurs when excessive amounts of circulating thyroid hormones interact with thyroid hormone receptors on peripheral tissues. This results in increased metabolic activity and increased sensitivity to circulating catecholamines. Thyrotoxic patients usually have high cardiac output and increased systolic blood pressure.

Hypothyroidism is the syndrome resulting from deficiency of thyroid hormones, which causes many metabolic processes to slow down. The frequency of hypertension, usually diastolic, is increased threefold in hypothyroid patients.

The clinical suspicion of thyroid gland dysfunction is confirmed with laboratory tests. Increased blood levels of thyroid hormones (thyroxine and triiodothyronine) and low serum levels of thyroid-stimulating hormone (TSH) are the hallmarks of hyperthyroidism. The diagnosis of hypothyroidism is based on low serum levels of thyroid hormone and increased serum levels of TSH.

PRINCIPLES OF TREATMENT

The initial management of patients with hypertension who have hyperthyroidism includes a β-adrenergic blocker, such as atenolol, to treat hypertension, tachycardia, and tremor. The definitive treatment of hyperthyroidism is cause specific. For example, patients with autoimmune hyperthyroidism (Graves disease) should have thyroid gland ablation with iodine-131. For patients with hyperthyroidism caused by multinodular goiter (Plummer disease), ^{131}I is

usually not curative, and subtotal thyroidectomy is the treatment of choice. Finally, if the hyperthyroidism is associated with acute thyroid inflammation, such as with subacute thyroiditis, temporary treatment (~3 months) with a β-adrenergic inhibitor may be all that is needed.

Treatment of thyroid hormone deficiency decreases blood pressure in most patients with hypertension. Synthetic levothyroxine is the treatment of choice for hypothyroidism. The initial dosage of levothyroxine is based on body weight (1.6 mg/kg/day), but the daily dosage requirement may be lower in older patients (<1.0 mg/kg/day). In patients older than 50 years or in those with cardiac disease, the initial dosage of levothyroxine should be lower, a total of 25 to 50 mg/day, and it should be increased every 2 weeks by 25 mg until the target dosage is achieved. Clinical and biochemical reevaluations should be completed at 2-month intervals, until the serum TSH concentration has normalized.

Primary Hyperparathyroidism

PRESENTATION AND DIAGNOSIS

Hypercalcemia is associated with an increased frequency of hypertension.[48] The most common cause of hypercalcemia is primary hyperparathyroidism. The frequency of hypertension in patients with primary hyperparathyroidism varies from 10% to 60%.[48] In most cases, the disease is caused by a benign, solitary parathyroid adenoma. However, when associated with the MEN syndromes, the hyperparathyroidism is usually due to hyperplasia of all four parathyroid glands.

Most patients with primary hyperparathyroidism are asymptomatic, and the focus of the presentation may be the side effects of chronic hypercalcemia: polyuria and polydipsia, constipation, osteoporosis, renal lithiasis, peptic ulcer disease, and hypertension. The hallmarks of primary hyperparathyroidism are hypercalcemia, hypophosphatemia, and an increased serum concentration of parathyroid hormone. In patients with hypercalcemia, measurement of the serum concentration of parathyroid hormone is the most specific way to diagnose primary hyperparathyroidism. If the serum concentration of parathyroid hormone is not increased, the clinical data should be reviewed, and nonparathyroid causes of hypercalcemia should be investigated; these include pheochromocytoma, hyperthyroidism, cancer, multiple myeloma, vitamin D intoxication, and sarcoidosis.

PRINCIPLES OF TREATMENT

The treatment of hyperparathyroidism is surgical. This involves neck exploration, identification of all four parathyroid glands, and, in sporadic cases, removal of the single adenoma; in the case of MEN, subtotal resection (3.5 glands) of the hyperplastic glands is therapeutic.

Acromegaly

PRESENTATION AND DIAGNOSIS

Chronic growth hormone (GH) excess from a GH-producing pituitary tumor results in the clinical syndrome of acromegaly. The effects of chronic excess of GH include acral and soft tissue overgrowth, progressive dental malocclusion, degenerative arthritis related to chondral and synovial tissue overgrowth within joints, low-pitched sonorous voice, excessive sweating and oily skin, perineural hypertrophy leading to nerve entrapment (e.g., carpal tunnel syndrome), cardiac dysfunction, and hypertension, the latter occurring in 20% to 40% of the patients.[49]

A patient with acromegaly has a characteristic appearance that includes coarsening of facial features, prognathism, frontal bossing, spadelike hands, and wide feet. Often, the patient has a history of progressive increase in shoe, glove, ring, or hat size. These changes may occur slowly and may go unrecognized by the patient, family, and physician.

The diagnosis of acromegaly depends on two criteria: a GH level that is not suppressed to less than 1 mg/L after an oral glucose load (75 to 100 g) and an increased serum concentration of insulinlike growth factor I. The laboratory assessment of acromegaly is supplemented with MRI of the pituitary.

PRINCIPLES OF TREATMENT

Treatment is indicated for all patients who have signs and symptoms of acromegaly and biochemical confirmation of the syndrome. The goals of treatment are to prevent the long-term consequences of GH excess, remove the pituitary neoplasm, and preserve normal pituitary tissue and function. Pituitary surgery is the treatment of choice; if necessary, it is supplemented with medical therapy and/or irradiation. The hypertension of acromegaly is most effectively treated by curing the excess of GH.[49] If a surgical cure is not possible, the hypertension usually responds well to diuretic therapy.

REFERENCES

1. Young WF. Endocrine hypertension: then and now. *Endocr Pract* 2010;16:1-52.
2. Young WF Jr. Pheochromocytoma: 1926-1993. *Trends Endocrinol Metab* 1993;4(4):122-127.
3. Klein RD, Jin L, Rumilla K, Young WF Jr, Lloyd RV. Germline *SDHB* mutations are common in patients with apparently sporadic sympathetic paragangliomas. *Diagn Mol Pathol* 2008;17(2):94-100.
4. Hao HX, Khalimonchuk O, Schraders M, et al. *SDH5*, a gene required for flavination of succinate dehydrogenase, is mutated in paraganglioma. *Science* 2009;325(5944):1139-1142.
5. Neumann HP, Erlic Z, Boedeker CC, et al. Clinical predictors for germline mutations in head and neck paraganglioma patients: cost reduction strategy in genetic diagnostic process as fall-out. *Cancer Res* 2009;69(8):3650-3656.
6. Bayley JP, Kunst HP, Cascon A, et al. *SDHAF2* mutations in familial and sporadic paraganglioma and phaeochromocytoma. *Lancet Oncol* 2010;11(4):366-372.
7. Burnichon N, Briere JJ, Libe R, et al. *SDHA* is a tumor suppressor gene causing paraganglioma. *Hum Mol Genet* 2010;19(15):3011-3020.
8. Cerecer-Gil NY, Figuera LE, Llamas FJ, et al. Mutation of *SDHB* is a cause of hypoxia-related high-altitude paraganglioma. *Clin Cancer Res* 2010;16(16):4148-4154.
9. Qin Y, Yao L, King EE, et al. Germline mutations in *TMEM127* confer susceptibility to pheochromocytoma. *Nat Genet* 2010;42(3):229-333.
10. Ricketts CJ, Forman JR, Rattenberry E, et al. Tumor risks and genotype-phenotype-proteotype analysis in 358 patients with germline mutations in *SDHB* and *SDHD*. *Hum Mutat* 2010;31(1):41-51.
11. Carney JA. Carney triad: a syndrome featuring paragangliomic, adrenocortical, and possibly other endocrine tumors. *J Clin Endocrinol Metab* 2009;94(10):3656-3662.
12. Young WF Jr. Paragangliomas: clinical overview. *Ann N Y Acad Sci* 2006;1073:21-29.
13. Perry CG, Sawka AM, Singh R, et al. The diagnostic efficacy of urinary fractionated metanephrines measured by tandem mass spectrometry in detection of pheochromocytoma. *Clin Endocrinol (Oxf)* 2007;66(5):703-708.
14. Brown ML, Zayas GE, Abel MD, Young WF Jr, Schaff HV. Mediastinal paragangliomas: the Mayo Clinic experience. *Ann Thorac Surg* 2008;86(3):946-951.
15. Waguespack SG, Rich T, Grubbs E, et al. A current review of the etiology, diagnosis, and treatment of pediatric pheochromocytoma and paraganglioma. *J Clin Endocrinol Metab* 2010;95(5):2023-2037.
16. Freel EM, Stanson AW, Thompson GB, et al. Adrenal venous sampling for catecholamines: a normal value study. *J Clin Endocrinol Metab* 2010;95(3):1328-1332.
17. Huang H, Abraham J, Hung E, et al. Treatment of malignant pheochromocytoma/paraganglioma with cyclophosphamide, vincristine, and dacarbazine: recommendation from a 22-year follow-up of 18 patients. *Cancer* 2008 15;113(8):2020-2028.
18. Joshua AM, Ezzat S, Asa SL, et al. Rationale and evidence for sunitinib in the treatment of malignant paraganglioma/pheochromocytoma. *J Clin Endocrinol Metab* 2009;94(1):5-9.
19. Young WF Jr, Hogan MJ. Renin-independent hypermineralocorticoidism. *Trends Endocrinol Metab* 1994;5(3):97-106.
20. Choi M, Scholl UI, Yue P, et al. K+ channel mutations in adrenal aldosterone-producing adenomas and hereditary hypertension. *Science* 2011;331(6018):768-772.
21. Young WF. Primary aldosteronism: renaissance of a syndrome. *Clin Endocrinol (Oxf)* 2007;66(5):607-618.
22. Quack I, Vonend O, Rump LC. Familial hyperaldosteronism I-III. *Horm Metab Res* 2010;42(6):424-428.
23. Sukor N, Mulatero P, Gordon RD, et al. Further evidence for linkage of familial hyperaldosteronism type II at chromosome 7p22 in Italian as well as Australian and South American families. *J Hypertens* 2008;26(8):1577-1582.
24. Geller DS, Zhang J, Wisgerhof MV, et al. A novel form of human mendelian hypertension featuring nonglucocorticoid-remediable aldosteronism. *J Clin Endocrinol Metab* 2008;93(8):3117-3123.
25. Funder JW, Carey RM, Fardella C, et al. Case detection, diagnosis, and treatment of patients with primary aldosteronism: an Endocrine Society clinical practice guideline. *J Clin Endocrinol Metab* 2008;93(9):3266-3281.
26. Mulatero P, Stowasser M, Loh KC, et al. Increased diagnosis of primary aldosteronism, including surgically correctable forms, in centers from five continents. *J Clin Endocrinol Metab* 2004;89(3):1045-1050.
27. Meyer A, Brabant G, Behrend M. Long-term follow-up after adrenalectomy for primary aldosteronism. *World J Surg* 2005;29(2):155-159.
28. Sawka AM, Young WF, Thompson GB, et al. Primary aldosteronism: factors associated with normalization of blood pressure after surgery. *Ann Intern Med* 2001;135(4):258-261.
29. Rossi GP, Bolognesi M, Rizzoni D, et al. Vascular remodeling and duration of hypertension predict outcome of adrenalectomy in primary aldosteronism patients. *Hypertension* 2008;51(6):1366-1371.
30. Sukor N, Gordon RD, Ku YK, Jones M, Stowasser M. Role of unilateral adrenalectomy in bilateral primary aldosteronism: a 22-year single center experience. *J Clin Endocrinol Metab* 2009;94(7):2437-2445.
31. Young WF Jr. Primary aldosteronism—one picture is not worth a thousand words. *Ann Intern Med* 2009;151(5):357-358.
32. Young WF, Stanson AW, Thompson GB, et al. Role for adrenal venous sampling in primary aldosteronism. *Surgery* 2004;136(6):1227-1235.
33. Kempers MJ, Lenders JW, van Outheusden L, et al. Systematic review: diagnostic procedures to differentiate unilateral from bilateral adrenal abnormality in primary aldosteronism. *Ann Intern Med* 2009;151(5):329-337.
34. Young WF, Stanson AW. What are the keys to successful adrenal venous sampling (AVS) in patients with primary aldosteronism? *Clin Endocrinol (Oxf)* 2009;70(1):14-17.
35. Vonend O, Ockenfels N, Gao X, et al. Adrenal venous sampling: evaluation of the German Conn's Registry. *Hypertension* 2011;57(5):990-995. Epub 2011 Mar 7.
36. Young WF Jr, Klee GG. Primary aldosteronism: diagnostic evaluation. *Endocrinol Metab Clin North Am* 1988;17(2):367-395.
37. Daunt N. Adrenal vein sampling: how to make it quick, easy, and successful. *Radiographics* 2005;25(Suppl 1):S143-S158.
38. Milliez P, Girerd X, Plouin PF, et al. Evidence for an increased rate of cardiovascular events in patients with primary aldosteronism. *J Am Coll Cardiol* 2005;45(8):1243-1248.
39. Stowasser M, Sharman J, Leano R, et al. Evidence for abnormal left ventricular structure and function in normotensive individuals with familial hyperaldosteronism type I. *J Clin Endocrinol Metab* 2005;90(9):5070-5076.
40. Reincke M, Rump LC, Quinkler M, et al. Risk factors associated with a low glomerular filtration rate in primary aldosteronism. *J Clin Endocrinol Metab* 2009;94(3):869-875.
41. Sechi LA, Di Fabio A, Bazzocchi M, Uzzau A, Catena C. Intrarenal hemodynamics in primary aldosteronism before and after treatment. *J Clin Endocrinol Metab* 2009;94(4):1191-1197.
42. Kuo CC, Wu VC, Tsai CW, Wu KD. Relative kidney hyperfiltration in primary aldosteronism: a meta-analysis. *J Renin Angiotensin Aldosterone Syst* 2011;12(2):113-122. Epub 2011 Mar 24.
43. Assalia A, Gagner M. Laparoscopic adrenalectomy. *Br J Surg* 2004;91(10):1259-1274.
44. Huang WT, Chau T, Wu ST, Lin SH. Prolonged hyperkalemia following unilateral adrenalectomy for primary hyperaldosteronism. *Clin Nephrol* 2010;73(5):392-397.
45. Liu SY, Ng EK, Lee PS, et al. Radiofrequency ablation for benign aldosterone-producing adenoma: a scarless technique to an old disease. *Ann Surg* 2010;252(6):1058-1064.
46. Parthasarathy HK, Menard J, White WB, et al. A double-blind, randomized study comparing the antihypertensive effect of eplerenone and spironolactone in patients with hypertension and evidence of primary aldosteronism. *J Hypertens* 2011;29(5):980-990.
47. Amar L, Azizi M, Menard J, et al. Aldosterone synthase inhibition with LCI699: a proof-of-concept study in patients with primary aldosteronism. *Hypertension* 2010;56(5):831-838.
48. Heyliger A, Tangpricha V, Weber C, Sharma J. Parathyroidectomy decreases systolic and diastolic blood pressure in hypertensive patients with primary hyperparathyroidism. *Surgery* 2009;146(6):1042-1047.
49. Berg C, Petersenn S, Lahner H, et al. Cardiovascular risk factors in patients with uncontrolled and long-term acromegaly: comparison with matched data from the general population and the effect of disease control. *J Clin Endocrinol Metab* 2010;95(8):3648-3656.

CHAPTER 31

Resistant Hypertension

Maria Czarina Acelajado and David A. Calhoun

PSEUDORESISTANCE, 501

DIAGNOSIS, 501

Ambulatory Blood Pressure Monitoring, 501

CARDIOVASCULAR RISK, 502

SECONDARY CAUSES OF HYPERTENSION, 502

Obstructive Sleep Apnea And Resistant Hypertension, 502

Primary Aldosteronism And Resistant Hypertension, 504

INTERFERING SUBSTANCES, 504

Dietary Sodium, 504

PHARMACOLOGIC TREATMENT, 504

Diuretics, 505

Mineralocorticoid Receptor Antagonists, 505

Other Antihypertensive Agents, 507

Other Treatment Modalities, 507

Role of the Hypertension Specialist, 508

REFERENCES, 508

Resistant hypertension (RHTN) is defined as blood pressure (BP) that remains above goal in spite of concurrent use of three antihypertensive agents from different classes, prescribed at optimal doses, one of which is ideally a diuretic.[1] Patients whose BP is controlled by four or more antihypertensive medications are also considered to have RHTN. Important risk factors for the development of RHTN include older age, obesity, chronic kidney disease (CKD), diabetes, obstructive sleep apnea (OSA), consumption of a high-salt diet, African-American race, and female gender.[1]

The prevalence of RHTN is not known precisely but is substantial. In a 14-year retrospective review of patients referred to a hypertension specialty clinic, the overall prevalence of RHTN was 18% and was noted to increase over time.[2] Another review of a primary care network in the Southeastern United States showed that as many as 16.2% of hypertensive patients met the criteria for having RHTN based on the definition of needing three or more medications to achieve control. Of these, 12.7% had BP above 140/90 mm Hg while taking three or more antihypertensive medications, and the remaining 3.5% had controlled BP but were taking four or more medications.[3] Prospective data from large outcome trials have estimated the prevalence of RHTN to be 20% to 30%.[4,5] The prevalence of RHTN is expected to rise, mainly because of the aging population and the increasing prevalence of obesity, sleep apnea, diabetes, and CKD.[6]

Pseudoresistance

The term *resistant hypertension* is not synonymous with *uncontrolled hypertension* (Box 31-1). The latter may include patients whose BP is not controlled because of improper BP measurement technique, poor adherence to medications, or presence of a "white coat effect," in which the office BP readings are higher than those obtained elsewhere, such as in the home or workplace. These causes of *pseudoresistance* should be sought out and corrected.

Nonadherence may be difficult to detect, particularly in patients who come to medical attention with BP above goal but insist that they are taking their medications as directed. A retrospective review found that 16% of patients with RHTN who were seen at a hypertension clinic were nonadherent to their medications.[7] In a prospective trial involving 41 patients with RHTN, 20% were found to be nonadherent to the antihypertensive regimen using electronic compliance monitoring.[8] In this study, monitoring compliance alone reduced the mean BP from 156/106 to 145/97 mm Hg without changes in the antihypertensive drug regimen, and a third of the patients achieved goal BP (<140/90 mm Hg) after 2 months. Most cases of nonadherence stem from forgetfulness, adverse reactions to medications, and patient perception that the drug did not work. Given these considerations, simplifying the antihypertensive drug regimen may be of benefit, such as by using long-acting medications dosed once daily and reducing the pill burden by using fixed-dose combinations. Furthermore, inquiring about the occurrence of adverse reactions and correcting patient misperceptions about their medications during the clinic visit are part of good patient care.

Diagnosis

Although RHTN is usually diagnosed based on traditional clinic BP readings, home BP monitoring is increasingly used to gauge BP control and screen for the so-called white coat effect—the rise in BP induced by an alerting reaction to a physician's visit. As in the clinic, patients should check their BP at home while seated quietly in a chair, with the feet flat, legs uncrossed, the back supported, the arm resting on a tabletop or a countertop at the level of the heart.[9] An appropriately sized cuff should be applied on a bare arm. Two to three readings should be taken, both in the morning and at night. Patients should be counseled to refrain from talking during the BP measurement and to wait at least 30 minutes after eating, smoking, and exercise before the BP is taken, as these actions can affect the results. Automated oscillometric devices that measure the BP from the brachial artery are preferred for home use because this is easier for patients and has been found to be as reliable as the auscultatory method, the standard technique used in the clinic. Although deemed less reliable, wrist monitors may have potential in morbidly obese patients, whose arms cannot be used for BP measurement, but routine use of wrist monitors must be evaluated further.[9]

Home BP measurements are used increasingly to supplement office BP readings and to assist in making rational therapeutic decisions. Whereas office BP measurements have inherent weaknesses—the foremost being the infrequent or one-time measurements, which may not reflect a patient's usual BP—they can be improved by increasing the number of readings per visit; attempting to eliminate terminal digit preference by avoiding rounded-off values, which are commonly rounded off to the nearest 5 or 10; and reporting the BP value in multiples of 2, corresponding to the line markings on most sphygmomanometers. Taken together, out-of-office and clinic BPs give the clinician an overall picture of the patient's BP and enable the making of rational therapeutic decisions to achieve the BP goal.

Ambulatory Blood Pressure Monitoring

Twenty-four-hour ambulatory BP monitoring (ABPM) measures out-of-office BP values over a 24-hour period, which provides an even better assessment of BP and its diurnal pattern. Measurement of 24-hour ABPM permits detection of a normal *dipping pattern*—a 10% to 20% nocturnal decline in BP compared with daytime values—or the absence of such, referred to as a *nondipping pattern:* the morning BP surge, a rise in BP after awakening, along with BP variability. Abnormalities in all these parameters have been linked to increased cardiovascular (CV) risk in hypertensive patients, especially those with RHTN.[10,11] The risk for cardiovascular events is more tightly correlated to 24-hour ABPM than office BP. In 86 patients with uncontrolled diastolic BP (DBP >100 mm Hg) while on a three-drug antihypertensive regimen that included a diuretic, the highest CV risk—defined as presence of target organ damage, such as left ventricular hypertension (LVH), and retinopathy or elevations in serum creatinine and fatal and nonfatal CV events

CH
31

within the follow-up period, which averaged 49 months—was found in those in the highest tertile of ambulatory DBP (>97 mm Hg) at baseline, even when the analysis excluded patients with previous CV events.[12] This was achieved in spite of similar baseline office BP values between the tertiles of ambulatory DBP, showing that ABPM better identified those RHTN patients at higher risk.

The high cost of 24-hour ABPM makes it impractical to use in monitoring response to therapy in office practice, at least in the U.S. health care system. In present practice, it does not supersede the use of office and home BP measurements to guide medical treatment in patients with RHTN. ABPM is useful in evaluating patients with RHTN and making therapeutic decisions if home and office BPs are not sufficient for clinical decision making. This can occur when white coat hypertension or masked hypertension— that is, when office BPs are normal and out-of-office BPs are elevated—are suspected but difficult to assess using home or workplace BP measurements, as when the self-measured and/or home BP values are borderline (125/75 mm Hg to 135/85 mm Hg). ABPM may also help the clinician evaluate the effects of complex antihypertensive regimens, particularly in ruling out nocturnal hypotension resulting from polypharmacy. Furthermore, there may be an increasing role for 24-hour ABPM in the diagnosis of hypertension in the future; the recent draft guidelines of the National Institute for Health and Clinical Excellence (NICE) in the United Kingdom espouse the use of 24-hour ABPM to confirm the diagnosis of hypertension, with an option to use home monitoring if 24-hour ABPM is not tolerated, rather than to rely solely on clinic BP to make the diagnosis.[13] If this is supported by appropriate legislation or changes in insurance payment policies, the recommendation could pave the way for greater use of 24-hour ABPM in confirming the diagnosis of hypertension.

Cardiovascular Risk

An early study demonstrated that patients with RHTN had greater risk for a CV event—such as myocardial infarction (MI), stroke, transient ischemic attack (TIA), or progressive heart failure— compared with patients whose BP was controlled over an average follow-up of 49 months.[12] These findings were mirrored in another study, which showed that patients with RHTN confirmed by 24-hour ABPM had a higher risk for stroke, heart failure, and MI than patients without RHTN.[14] Moreover, there is a greater incidence of target organ damage—such as left ventricular hypertrophy, retinopathy, nephropathy, and carotid intimal disease—in patients with RHTN.[15-17] Patients with RHTN have higher pulse wave velocities (PWVs) than patients with controlled BP, signifying that these patients have greater arterial stiffness, another marker of increased CV risk.[18] Lastly, patients with RHTN have a higher incidence of comorbidities that include diabetes, obesity, and OSA, all of which are associated with increased CV risk.[19-21]

Secondary Causes of Hypertension

Secondary hypertension is more common in the subset of patients with RHTN than in the general hypertensive population (Box 31-2).[1] In particular, primary aldosteronism and OSA are more

common in patients with RHTN than in those without RHTN. Likewise, CKD—which may be the cause or the result of long-standing, poorly controlled hypertension—and renal artery stenosis are common in patients with RHTN, but their exact prevalence is not known.

Screening strategies for the presence of secondary causes of hypertension in patients with RHTN are summarized in Table 31-1. Kidney function is usually assessed through measurement of serum creatinine, calculation of the estimated glomerular filtration rate (eGFR), and a spot urine specimen to check for proteinuria. Kidney function should be evaluated in every RHTN patient because the findings have implications for both the choice of medications and the BP goal (<130/80 mm Hg in patients with CKD and proteinuria). Furthermore, given the high prevalence of primary aldosteronism and OSA in patients with RHTN, every RHTN patient should have a plasma aldosterone/renin ratio measurement at baseline and a clinical scoring test for OSA, such as the Berlin Questionnaire or the Epworth Sleepiness Scale. Confirmatory tests may be performed once a positive screening test is obtained (see Table 31-1). For the other secondary causes, screening may be done as clinically warranted. Referrals to appropriate specialists should be made when the screening and/or confirmatory tests suggest or confirm the presence of the disease (see Table 31-1).

Obstructive Sleep Apnea and Resistant Hypertension

The Wisconsin Sleep Cohort Study showed a direct linear relationship between severity of obstructive sleep apnea, severity of hypertension, and risk of developing hypertension.[22] In this population-based study, the likelihood of developing hypertension increased with increasing severity of OSA; those with moderate to severe OSA, defined as an apnea-hypopnea index (AHI) above 15 events per hour, were 2.89 times more likely to have an elevated BP at the 4-year follow-up examination compared with those with no apneic or hypopneic events at baseline. In general, every additional episode of apnea or hypopnea per hour of sleep was associated with a twofold rise in systolic BP (SBP).

OSA is strongly and independently correlated with RHTN. An early study in patients with RHTN confirmed by 24-hour ABPM who underwent overnight polysomnography (PSG) irrespective of sleep-related symptoms showed that OSA, defined as AHI above 10 events per hour, was highly prevalent and affected as many as 83% of study participants.[19] A more recent study from the same group confirmed the finding of a higher prevalence of OSA in patients with RHTN compared with those who had controlled hypertension.[23] In a different study design, in which patients with OSA were selected and evaluated in terms of BP control, more severe OSA was associated with uncontrolled BP, although not necessarily RHTN, even in the presence of reasonably aggressive treatment (82% of patients with uncontrolled BP were taking more than two antihypertensive medications).[24] Of note, OSA is more

TABLE 31-1 Secondary Causes of Hypertension

SECONDARY CAUSE	SCREENING TESTS	CONFIRMATORY TESTS	TREATMENT
More Common			
Primary aldosteronism	Aldosterone/renin ratio	Oral sodium loading Isotonic saline infusion Fludrocortisone suppression test Captopril suppression test	Depends on etiology Surgical (unilateral adrenalectomy) Medical management (mineralocorticoid antagonists) Referral to appropriate specialist
Obstructive sleep apnea	Berlin Questionnaire Epworth Sleepiness Scale Polysomnography	Polysomnography	Continuous positive airway pressure machine Surgery (uvulopalatopharyngoplasty) Referral to appropriate specialist
Renal parenchymal disease	Kidney function tests (serum creatinine, estimated glomerular filtration rate) Renal ultrasound	Determine etiology of renal failure	Depends on etiology Referral to appropriate specialist
Renal artery stenosis	Renal Doppler MR angiography CT angiography	Renal artery angiography	Angioplasty ± stenting Referral to appropriate specialist
Uncommon			
Cushing syndrome	Urine cortisol Late-night salivary cortisol Dexamethasone suppression tests	Low-dose dexamethasone suppression test Plasma ACTH Pituitary imaging or adrenal CT scan	Depends on etiology (surgery, medical adrenalectomy, radiation) Referral to appropriate specialist
Pheochromocytoma	Plasma metanephrines Urine metanephrines	Nuclear imaging (e.g., MIBG scan)	Surgical removal of tumor Referral to appropriate specialist
Hyperparathyroidism	Serum calcium level Parathyroid hormone level	Parathyroid hormone level	Depends on etiology Referral to appropriate specialist
Coarctation of the aorta	2D echocardiogram	Transesophageal echocardiogram MR imaging Cardiac catheterization	Angioplasty and stenting of coarctation Surgery Referral to appropriate specialist
Intracranial tumor	Brain imaging studies (e.g., cranial CT, MR imaging)	Depends on findings of screening	Depends on etiology of tumor Referral to appropriate specialist

2D, two-dimensional; ACTH, adrenocorticotrophic hormone; CT, computed tomography; MIBG, iodine-131 or iodine-123-metaiodobenzylguanidine; MR, magnetic resonance.
From Acelajado MC, Calhoun DA, Oparil S. Reduction of blood pressure in patients with treatment-resistant hypertension. *Expert Opin Pharmacother* 2009;10:2959-2971.

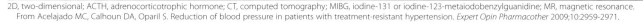

common (96% vs. 65%; P = .014), and also more severe, in men than in women (mean AHI, 32.2 ± 4.5 events/h vs. 14.0 ± 3.1 events/h; P = .004) despite similar age, body mass index, and BP readings.[23]

The close association between OSA and RHTN has been attributed to increased sympathetic nervous system activity brought about by intermittent episodes of hypoxia during sleep.[25] Recent work, however, has suggested that the rostral fluid shift that occurs overnight may contribute in a major way to the high prevalence of OSA in RHTN.[26] In patients with OSA, the rostral fluid shift, as evidenced by changes in neck and calf circumferences before and after sleep, was greater in patients with RHTN compared with patients with controlled BP, evidenced by a greater increase in neck circumference and reduction in calf circumference (P = .02 and .001, respectively) in those with RHTN.

Continuous positive airway pressure (CPAP) is the treatment of choice for poor sleep quality in patients with OSA, but it produces only modest reductions in BP in the general population of hypertensive patients with OSA. A meta-analysis of studies of patients with OSA and hypertension showed a mean BP reduction of 2.5/1.8 mm Hg with CPAP use, and benefit was greater in patients with a higher baseline BP, those who were more obese, and those with more severe OSA.[27] A meta-analysis of placebo-controlled CPAP trials that used ABPM confirmed this finding, with a decrease in 24-hour ambulatory mean arterial pressure (MAP) of only 1.69 mm Hg (95% confidence interval [CI], −2.69 to −0.69) with CPAP use, and the greatest BP reductions occurred at night (night-time SBP decline of 2.82 mm Hg; 95% CI, −5.48 to −0.18; P = .03).[28]

The above results suggest that patients with more severe forms of hypertension, such as RHTN, may have greater benefit from CPAP treatment. In an observational study, patients with OSA and RHTN who were on CPAP therapy were shown to have a greater reduction in BP following initiation of CPAP compared with those who had OSA without RHTN at 1 year of follow-up; mean difference in MAP was −5.8 mm Hg in patients with RHTN (P = .03) and −0.8 mm Hg in patients without RHTN (P = .53).[29] Interestingly, in this study, only the level of the baseline BP and diuretic use, and not baseline AHI or hours of CPAP use, predicted the decline in BP after initiation of CPAP. In a prospective study involving 33 patients with OSA and RHTN, CPAP significantly reduced 24-hour SBP by 5.2 mm Hg and nighttime SBP by 6.1 mm Hg,[30] and the percentage of patients with a dipping nocturnal BP pattern increased from 9.1% to 36.4% after CPAP was initiated. Furthermore, in a study that compared CPAP treatment to conventional antihypertensive therapy in patients with RHTN and OSA, use of CPAP for more than 5.8 hours per night was associated with a 24-hour ambulatory BP decline of 10/7 mm Hg, and an increase in the percentage of patients with a nocturnal dipping pattern (51.7% vs. 24.1%) was seen in the third month of treatment.[31]

Counseling patients with RHTN to obtain adequate nighttime sleep is prudent because sleep deprivation raises BP and worsens BP control in hypertensive patients.[32] Although OSA is likely the most significant contributor to shortened sleep times in patients with RHTN because of the multiple apneic and hypopneic episodes that disrupt sleep, it has been shown that, independent of OSA, patients with RHTN have lower sleep efficiency compared with normotensive patients or hypertensive patients with controlled BP.[33] In one study, RHTN patients were matched for AHI with controls who were normotensive or who had controlled BP, and those with RHTN had a shorter total sleep time (by 33.8 and 37.2 minutes, respectively; P = .02 for both) and a shorter rapid-eye movement (REM) sleep time (by 9.6 minutes [P = .06] and 11.6 minutes [P = .04], respectively). Although these findings do not establish causality, they suggest that sleep deprivation, independent of OSA, may contribute to antihypertensive treatment resistance and, conversely, that RHTN may result in poor-quality sleep. It remains to be seen whether measures to promote better sleep will translate into better BP control and better CV outcomes for patients with RHTN.

Primary Aldosteronism and Resistant Hypertension

Primary aldosteronism (PA), which is common in RHTN, is characterized by excess production of aldosterone by the adrenal glands and suppressed secretion of renin by the kidneys. The prevalence of PA is screened by using aldosterone-renin ratio and confirmed by fludrocortisone testing; it is much higher (14% to 21%) in patients with RHTN than in the unselected hypertensive population (5% to 10%).[34-36] For example, among 88 patients with RHTN who were consecutively referred to the hypertension clinic of the University of Alabama at Birmingham, 18 patients (20%) were confirmed to have PA based on a high 24-hour urinary aldosterone excretion (>12 µg) paired with a suppressed plasma renin activity level (<1 ng/mL/h) with a high-sodium diet (urinary sodium excretion >200 mEq/day). Other investigators have demonstrated a similar prevalence of PA in patients with RHTN.[37-39]

The presence of excess aldosterone likely contributes to treatment resistance and augments CV risk in patients with RHTN. Excess aldosterone, acting via nongenomic mechanisms on mineralocorticoid receptors, influences cell volume, oxidation-reduction state, and vascular function; this results in endothelial dysfunction, vascular stiffness, fibrosis, increased oxidative stress, and inflammation. Clinically, these become manifest as a greater incidence of target organ damage (LVH, proteinuria, and retinal hemorrhages) in hypertensive patients with PA compared with hypertensive patients without biochemical evidence of PA. The higher prevalence of PA and the increased CV risk in patients with RHTN underscore the importance of screening for PA in patients with RHTN.

Hypokalemia, previously believed to be a prerequisite for the diagnosis of PA, is now considered to be a late manifestation of the disorder, and its absence should not be used to exclude the diagnosis. In 20 patients with RHTN and biochemical evidence of PA, the serum potassium levels ranged from 3.7 to 4.7 mmol/L.[40] In another study that involved 216 patients with hypertension, 71% of whom had RHTN, 71% of the patients with PA had normal potassium levels (range, 3.7 to 4.2 mmol/L).[41] Clearly, given the high prevalence of PA in patients with RHTN, the absence of hypokalemia should not deter the physician from screening for PA.

Both PA and OSA are common in patients with RHTN. In a prospective evaluation of 114 patients with RHTN, increased prevalence of both PA, confirmed by 24-hour urine aldosterone excretion, and OSA, screened for using the Berlin Questionnaire, was reported.[42] In those who were classified as being at high risk for having OSA, a diagnosis of PA was twice as likely as in patients who were at low risk for OSA based on the Berlin Questionnaire. A subsequent study showed that plasma aldosterone concentration was correlated to the AHI in patients with RHTN, a finding not seen in those with controlled hypertension.[43] Conversely, severity of sleep apnea was found to be related to the degree of aldosterone excess in patients with RHTN and hyperaldosteronism.[44] These findings support the hypothesis that aldosterone excess, OSA, and RHTN may be causally related and that both OSA and PA contribute to the treatment resistance of the hypertension. Hence, in a patient with RHTN, it is important to screen for these conditions and provide appropriate treatment as needed as an adjunct to usual antihypertensive therapy.

Interfering Substances

The concomitant intake of substances known to raise BP may complicate the management of RHTN. Nonsteroidal antiinflammatory drugs (NSAIDs) and selective cyclooxygenase (COX)-2 inhibitors are the most common offenders.[45] Other substances known to interfere with BP control are listed in Box 31-3. The physician should inquire about intake of these substances during the interview, and patients should be counseled about their use.

Dietary Sodium

Excessive dietary sodium contributes significantly to treatment resistance. In a randomized, crossover study that involved 12 patients with RHTN who consumed either a low-sodium diet (50 mmol/day) or a high-sodium diet (250 mmol/day), those who received the low-sodium diet for 1 week had a mean office systolic and diastolic BP reduction of 22.7/9.1 mm Hg (P = .0008) compared with those who had a high sodium intake (P = .0065).[46] Ambulatory BP readings mirrored the office BPs: 24-hour averages in those who consumed a low-sodium diet were 20.1/9.8 mm Hg lower than those who had high sodium intake (P = .0002 for both). Twenty-four-hour urinary sodium excretion confirmed that the patients were ingesting the appropriate diets, with mean values of 46.1 and 252.2 mmol/day, respectively. Plasma renin activity (PRA) increased (+1.85 ng/mL/h; P = .0042), and brain natriuretic peptide (BNP) decreased (−23.2 pg/mL; P = .0041) in participants with the low sodium intake, consistent with reductions in intravascular volume. Because all patients included were taking hydrochlorothiazide in a stable dose (25 mg/day), these results provide convincing evidence that persistent fluid retention contributes to treatment resistance and that this is attributable, in part, to the increased sodium in the diet.

The above data show that dietary sodium reduction should be integrated into the management of patients with RHTN. Given that most patients tend to underestimate their daily sodium intake and that meaningful reductions in dietary sodium may be difficult to attain, referral to a nutritionist for expert dietary advice may be warranted.

Pharmacologic Treatment

After screening for potentially correctable causes of uncontrolled BP—such as pseudoresistance, interfering substances, and secondary causes—the patient's antihypertensive regimen should be evaluated. The definition of RHTN presumes that these patients are taking a minimum of three medications, prescribed at optimal doses, and it recognizes that the patient's age, the presence of comorbidities such as CKD or congestive heart failure, and the

Box 31-3 Substances that Can Interfere with Blood Pressure Control

Nonsteroidal antiinflammatory drugs (nonselective and COX-2 selective drugs)
Sympathomimetic agents (weight-loss pills, decongestants, cocaine)
Amphetamine and amphetamine-like substances, including modafinil
Exogenous steroids (glucocorticoids and mineralocorticoids)
Ketoconazole
Antidepressants (MAO inhibitors, tricyclic antidepressants)
Anxiolytics, such as buspirone
Alcohol
Caffeine
Oral contraceptive pills and exogenous estrogen, including danazol
Immunosuppressants, particularly cyclosporine
Erythropoietin
Antiemetics (metoclopramide, alizapride)
Natural licorice, usually found in oral tobacco products
Ephedra (Ma huang)

COX, cyclooxygenase; MAO, monoamine oxidase.

presence of adverse reactions may limit the maximal dose that can be given. The physician also needs to determine whether the combination is rational and whether it incorporates medications with complementary mechanisms of action to maximize efficacy while reducing the possibility of adverse events. In our practice, the combination of a renin-angiotensin system (RAS) blocker, such as an angiotensin-converting enzyme (ACE) inhibitor or angiotensin II–receptor blocker (ARB), a calcium channel blocker (CCB), and a thiazide diuretic is most frequently used in patients without contraindications to these agents. As discussed below, our choice for a fourth antihypertensive agent is a mineralocorticoid receptor antagonist in patients with RHTN, even without evidence of aldosterone excess. Choosing a fifth, sixth, or seventh agent is often challenging and should be tailored to the patient's profile.

Diuretics

Patients with RHTN with or without evidence of aldosterone excess have been shown to be fluid overloaded despite treatment with an RAS blocker and a diuretic. This has been demonstrated by increased levels of BNP and elevated right and left ventricular end-diastolic volumes in patients with RHTN, regardless of aldosterone status (Figure 31-1).[47]

In patients with RHTN who were seen at one of two university-based hypertension clinics, a suboptimal antihypertensive drug regimen, most notably a result of inadequate use of diuretics (inappropriately low doses, inappropriate agents, no use at all, was the most common cause of apparent treatment resistance (54% of cases).[7] When appropriate changes were made—adding a diuretic, increasing diuretic dose, or switching to another diuretic class that was appropriate based on the patient's kidney function—BP goal was attained in 65% of patients. These findings highlight the important role of volume excess in driving treatment resistance in these patients.

Among the diuretics, thiazide-type agents are preferred because of extensive evidence from randomized controlled outcome trials that they decrease risk for CV death and morbidity and also because of their wide availability and low cost. Chlorthalidone is preferred by many hypertension specialists, because it is the agent used in major outcome trials that showed benefit. In the Antihypertensive and Lipid-Lowering Treatment to Prevent Heart Attack Trial (ALLHAT), chlorthalidone was comparable to amlodipine and lisinopril in reducing CV mortality rates, and it was superior to the other agents in preventing some secondary outcomes, such as heart failure.[4] Compared to hydrochlorothiazide, the thiazide diuretic most widely available in fixed-dose antihypertensive drug combinations in the United States, chlorthalidone is more effective in reducing SBP, as evidenced by 24-hour ABPM.[48] Chlorthalidone at 25 mg/day lowered 24-hour mean SBP by 12.4 (±1.8) mm Hg, which was greater than the effect achieved by hydrochlorothiazide at 50 mg/day (7.4 ± 1.7 mm Hg; $P = .054$; Figure 31-2). Chlorthalidone is more potent, has a longer duration of action, and produces greater BP reductions than hydrochlorothiazide.

Mineralocorticoid Receptor Antagonists

In our referral practice, low-dose spironolactone (12.5 to 25 mg/day) reduced BP significantly—by 25/12 mm Hg—after 6 months of treatment in patients with RHTN who were receiving a triple-drug antihypertensive regimen that included an RAS blocker (ACE inhibitor or ARB) and a diuretic in full doses (Figure 31-3).[49] At the end of the 6-month follow-up, the number of antihypertensive medications prescribed decreased significantly from baseline (4 to 3.5; $P < .05$). BP responses were similar in patients with or without primary aldosteronism and in African-American and Caucasian patients.

Similarly, spironolactone in higher doses (25 to 100 mg/day) given as a fourth or fifth antihypertensive agent to 175 patients with RHTN for an average of 7 months produced office and 24-hour ambulatory BP reductions of 14/7 mm Hg and 16/9 mm Hg, respectively ($P < .001$).[50] Greater BP response to spironolactone was seen in patients with a higher waist circumference, lower aortic PWV (less arterial stiffness), and lower serum potassium levels. Neither the serum aldosterone nor the PRA predicted the response to spironolactone. In the 31 patients in whom the spironolactone dose was titrated to 100 mg/day, the BP-lowering effect was not different from that seen in patients who were receiving 25 or 50 mg/day. Importantly, this effect was seen in the presence of conventional diuretic therapy (100% of study patients).

In the Anglo-Scandinavian Cardiac Outcomes Trial (ASCOT), spironolactone was given as a fourth-line antihypertensive agent, in addition to a mean of 2.9 antihypertensive drugs, to 1411 patients with uncontrolled BP. Mean BP fell by 21.9/9.5 mm Hg ($P < .001$) during spironolactone therapy at a median dose of 25 mg/day and with a mean treatment duration of 1.3 years.[51] In another study, spironolactone at 25 to 50 mg/day lowered BP by 21.7/8.5 mm Hg when given in addition to a three-drug antihypertensive regimen that included an RAS blocker and a thiazide diuretic (bendroflumethiazide at 2.5 mg/day, given to 80.4% of patients).[52] Those who achieved the largest BP reduction after addition of spironolactone (BP decline of >30 mm Hg in 40.3% of study patients) tended to lose more weight (mean, 0.75 kg), but the change from baseline was not significant.

The above studies demonstrate that spironolactone produces robust BP reductions when added to a regimen that includes an RAS blocker (ACE inhibitor or ARB). Compared with dual RAS

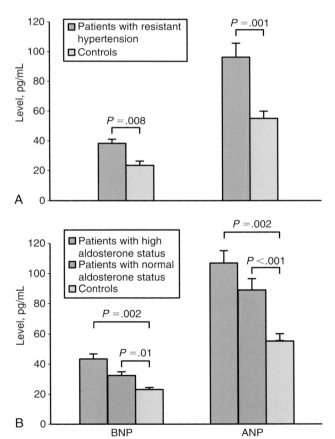

FIGURE 31-1 Atrial natriuretic peptide (*ANP*) and brain natriuretic peptide (*BNP*) levels in patients with resistant hypertension (RHTN) compared with controls and in patients with RHTN and normal or high aldosterone status compared with controls. Note the significant incremental increase in ANP and BNP levels from controls, to patients with RHTN and normal aldosterone status, to patients with RHTN and high aldosterone status. (*Data from Gaddam KK, Nishizaka MK, Pratt-Ubunama MN, et al. Characterization of resistant hypertension: association between resistant hypertension, aldosterone, and persistent intravascular volume expansion. Arch Intern Med 2008;168:1159-1164.*)

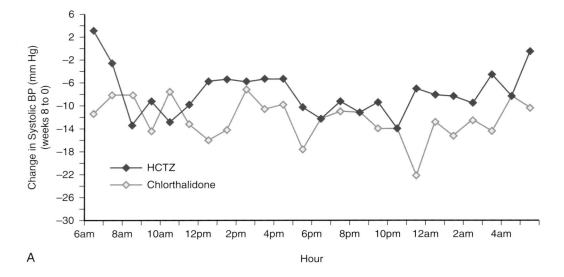

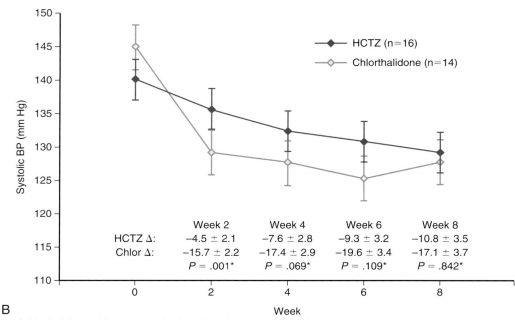

FIGURE 31-2 Effects of chlorthalidone (*Chlor*) versus hydrochlorothiazide (*HCTZ*) on blood pressure (*BP*) in hypertensive patients. **A,** Changes in mean 24-hour systolic ambulatory BP. **B,** Changes in mean office systolic BP. The reduction in mean 24-hour systolic ambulatory BP was greater with chlorthalidone use (12.4 ± 1.8 mm Hg) compared with hydrochlorothiazide (7.4 ± 1.7 mm Hg; *P* = .054), primarily because of its effect of reducing nighttime systolic BP.

blockade with an ACE inhibitor plus an ARB, spironolactone 25 mg/day added to a single RAS blocker, either an ACE inhibitor or an ARB, produces greater BP reductions in patients with RHTN and normal renal function.[53] Twenty-four-hour BP reduction in patients who were given spironolactone plus an ACE inhibitor or ARB for 12 weeks was 20.8/8.8 mm Hg compared with a BP reduction of 12.9/7.1 mm Hg achieved with dual RAS blockade (*P* < .0001). As a result, BP control (<140/90 mm Hg) was achieved in more patients who were given spironolactone (56.4%) versus dual RAS blockade (20.5%).

The fluid retention induced by aldosterone excess is reversed effectively by spironolactone. In 37 patients with RHTN and hyperaldosteronism, treatment with spironolactone (25 mg/day and force-titrated to 50 mg/day after 4 weeks) significantly reduced right and left ventricular end-diastolic volumes, left atrial volume, and left ventricular mass on cardiac magnetic resonance imaging (MRI) within 3 months. These effects persisted at 6 months of treatment, independent of office systolic BP and BNP.[54] In contrast, in patients with RHTN and normal aldosterone status, spironolactone lowered office systolic BP and reduced left ventricular mass

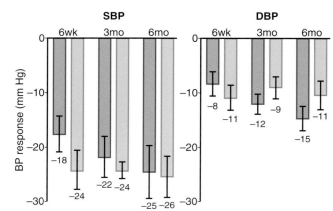

FIGURE 31-3 Effect of low-dose spironolactone on blood pressure (*BP*) in patients with resistant hypertension, with (*blue bars*) or without (*yellow bars*) primary aldosteronism. DBP, diastolic blood pressure; SBP, systolic blood pressure. (*Data from Nishizaka MK, et al. Efficacy of low-dose spironolactone in subjects with resistant hypertension. Am J Hypertens 2003;16:925-930.*)

index without a change in right or left ventricular end-diastolic volume, left atrial volume, or BNP. These results suggest that in patients with aldosterone excess, treatment with spironolactone reduces BP by producing large reductions in intravascular volume, whereas in those with normal aldosterone levels, spironolactone decreases BP by promoting vasodilation and decreasing peripheral resistance.

Beyond causing sodium retention and increased BP, aldosterone excess and mineralocorticoid receptor activation in the setting of a high-sodium diet induce endothelial dysfunction, oxidative stress, inflammation, and fibrosis, thereby promoting cardiovascular remodeling and renal injury in patients with hypertension.[55] As previously mentioned, significant dietary sodium reduction is difficult to achieve and maintain for most patients, and in this setting, mineralocorticoid receptor antagonists may be particularly important in mitigating the target organ damage induced by consumption of a high-sodium diet and the presence of excess aldosterone.

In patients with RHTN, spironolactone has benefits that extend beyond BP lowering. Vascular stiffness, as measured by the augmentation index and PWV, has been shown to be reduced with the administration of spironolactone (50 mg/day) in previously untreated patients with essential hypertension.[56] This effect was seen even after correcting for the decrease in BP seen with spironolactone treatment.

A preliminary open-label study of 12 patients with RHTN and moderate to severe OSA (AHI ≥15 events/hour) who were maintained on thiazide diuretic therapy showed that OSA severity was decreased, as assessed by full-night PSG, after 8 weeks of treatment with spironolactone (25 mg/day initially, then force-titrated to 50 mg/day after 4 weeks).[57] The AHI, hypoxic index, supine AHI, and AHI during REM sleep were all decreased significantly compared with baseline, regardless of aldosterone status (Figure 31-4). Furthermore, neck circumference and BNP showed statistically nonsignificant reductions during treatment. The results suggest that more effective diuresis brought about by aldosterone blockade in addition to thiazide treatment, evidenced by higher posttreatment PRA and creatinine values and a tendency toward lower BNP values, reduces the severity of OSA, possibly by decreasing pharyngeal edema, thereby lowering upper airway resistance.

Spironolactone is safe and is relatively well tolerated in RHTN patients. Adverse reactions to spironolactone are uncommon and occur in 4% to 7% of patients, usually at doses greater than 50 mg/day, and are generally mild in severity.[49-51] These include gynecomastia or breast discomfort, particularly in men; reduction in libido; and increases in serum potassium, all of which are reversible after discontinuation of treatment or reduction of spironolactone dose. Increases in serum creatinine occur, but progression to overt kidney failure is seldom seen.

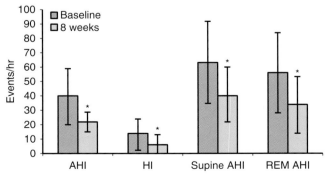

FIGURE 31-4 Changes in the apnea-hypopnea index (*AHI*), hypoxic index (*HI*), supine AHI, and AHI during rapid-eye movement (*REM*) sleep in patients with resistant hypertension who received spironolactone for 8 weeks. (*Data from Gaddam K, Pimenta E, Thomas SJ, et al. Spironolactone reduces severity of obstructive sleep apnoea in patients with resistant hypertension: a preliminary report. J Hum Hypertens 2010;24:532-537.*)

Other Antihypertensive Agents

Doxazosin is an α_1-adrenergic receptor blocker that causes vasodilation and decreased peripheral vascular resistance. Although it is not recommended as a first-line antihypertensive agent because of the absence of outcome benefit in randomized controlled trials (see Chapter 29),[58] it is useful in reducing BP when added to multidrug antihypertensive regimens in patients with RHTN. A retrospective review of patients with RHTN who were given doxazosin (mean dose, 6.9 mg/day) as part of a four- to eight-drug antihypertensive regimen—usually as a fifth agent in addition to a diuretic, RAS blocker, CCB, and β-blocker—showed that its addition lowered BP by 33/19 mm Hg, enabling 76% of study patients to achieve the BP goal below 140/90 mm Hg.[59] In another study, doxazosin at a mean dose of 4 mg/day produced reductions in BP of 16/7 mm Hg after 6 months when added to a three-drug antihypertensive regimen, and it effectively controlled BP to a goal of less than 140/90 mm Hg in 23% of patients.[60] In ASCOT, addition of doxazosin as a third antihypertensive agent in those with uncontrolled BP reduced BP by 11.7/6.9 mm Hg, and as many as 29.7% of the doxazosin-treated participants achieved the target BP.[61] Doxazosin was well tolerated in these studies, and the development of overt heart failure was not seen.

Amiloride, which directly blocks the epithelial sodium channel (ENaC), has also been used in patients with RHTN. Administration of the combination of amiloride and hydrochlorothiazide at 2.5 and 25 mg daily to 38 patients with RHTN and low plasma renin activity (17 of whom had primary aldosteronism) lowered the BP by 31/15 mm Hg.[62] Amiloride was associated with clinically insignificant increases in serum potassium and creatinine but was otherwise well tolerated.

Other Treatment Modalities

RENAL SYMPATHETIC DENERVATION

The persistence of BP elevation in patients with RHTN who are receiving maximal recommended antihypertensive regimens has led investigators to look for other treatment modalities that could be used to lower BP. It has long been established that renal sympathetic nerves play a role in the pathogenesis of hypertension.[63] Efferent renal sympathetic nerves stimulate renin release, promote sodium reabsorption, and reduce renal blood flow, all of which contribute to the elevated BP. Afferent signals from the kidney modulate central sympathetic outflow and contribute directly to neurogenic hypertension. Nonselective surgical sympathectomy has been used to lower BP in the past, but postprocedural complications—anhidrosis, sexual and urinary dysfunction, orthostatic hypotension, and tachycardia, to name a few—prolonged postoperative recovery, and the unpredictability of the results led to the abandonment of this practice, particularly once effective and well-tolerated antihypertensive drugs became available. With the advent of catheter-based radiofrequency ablation techniques, there has been a resurgence of interest in selectively interrupting renal sympathetic nerves to reduce BP.[64]

Selective catheterization of the renal artery and the subsequent application of low-power radiofrequency treatments along the length of both main renal arteries to denervate both kidneys have been shown to be effective in reducing BP in patients with RHTN.[65-68] In a multicenter, prospective, randomized trial that involved 106 patients with uncontrolled BP (SBP >160 mm Hg, >150 mm Hg in diabetics) in spite of use of three or more antihypertensive medications, renal sympathetic denervation reduced office BP by 32/12 ± 23/11 mm Hg at 6-month follow-up ($P < .001$ for both), an effect that was not seen in the control group, who had maintained previous antihypertensive treatment alone and in whom BP was decreased by only 1/0 ± 21/10 mm Hg ($P = .77$ and .83, respectively).[67] Complications that arose from the procedure included a femoral artery pseudoaneurysm that was reduced by manual compression, back pain (one patient), urinary tract infection (one patient), and paresthesias (one patient), and one patient had a postprocedural drop in BP that necessitated reduction in antihypertensive medications. Furthermore, seven patients had transient intraprocedural bradycardia that required atropine, but with no serious sequelae noted. During the 6-month follow-up, no evidence of development of renal artery stenosis or aneurysmal dilation was reported in the patients who underwent the procedure. Renal sympathetic denervation is a promising therapy for hypertensive patients who are resistant to conventional medical treatment and for those whose medication choices are limited by adverse effects or intolerance.

BAROREFLEX ACTIVATION THERAPY

Electrical stimulation of the baroreceptors using an implantable device (Rheos; CVRx, Minneapolis, MN) has been evaluated for the treatment of patients with RHTN. Increased baroreceptor firing leads to decreased sympathetic drive and increased parasympathetic tone, which result in decreases in peripheral vascular resistance, heart rate, stroke volume, and blood pressure.[69] The Rheos device, an implanted impulse generator with leads that tunnel subcutaneously and attach to both carotid sinuses, was evaluated in a randomized, placebo-controlled, double-blind phase III clinical trial that involved 265 patients with RHTN who were taking an average of 5.2 antihypertensive medications at baseline.[70] Patients randomized to baroreflex activation therapy had up to a 35 mm Hg drop in systolic BP at the 12-month follow-up and a reduction of up to 40% in the incidence of serious adverse events related to hypertensive urgency. The incidence of adverse events related to the procedure was comparable to that reported in endarterectomy trials but did not meet prespecified criteria (82.5%) for event-free rates (trial achieved 74.8%). More studies are needed to evaluate the risk/benefit ratio of baroreflex stimulation in patients with RHTN.

Role of the Hypertension Specialist

Patients with RHTN often benefit from a referral to a hypertension specialist. In a review of 20 patients with RHTN who were referred to a hypertension clinic and managed by a team that consisted of a certified hypertension specialist, nurse practitioner, nutritionist, and a pharmacist, clinic BP decreased by 15.7/6.6 mm Hg ($P =$ .0041 and .03, respectively) from the time of the first visit (average follow-up, 134 days).[71] A goal BP below 140/90 mm Hg was achieved in 40% of patients without a significant increase in the number of antihypertensive medications, but with modification of the treatment regimen of most patients, with greater use of diuretics and spironolactone and reductions in use of centrally acting agents (from 30% to 5%).

In a university-based hypertension clinic, 52% of patients with RHTN who were referred for evaluation achieved target BP during follow-up (<140/90 mm Hg for uncomplicated patients and <130/85 mm Hg for those with diabetes or CKD).[7] Overall average BP decreased from 169/94 mm Hg to 142/82 mm Hg at the end of the study. A suboptimal medical regimen was the cause for treatment resistance in the majority of cases, and BP improved after diuretics were added or the dose was increased, or if the diuretic prescribed was changed to the correct diuretic class based on the patient's kidney function.

It is recommended that patients with RHTN whose BP remains above goal for 6 months after appropriate treatment modifications be referred to a hypertension specialist for further evaluation and management.[1] Furthermore, referrals to the appropriate specialist should be made if a secondary cause for persistently elevated BP is suspected or found.

REFERENCES

1. Calhoun DA, Jones D, Textor S, et al. Resistant hypertension: diagnosis, evaluation and treatment. A scientific statement from the American Heart Association Professional Education Committee of the Council for High Blood Pressure Research. *Hypertension* 2008;51:1403-1419.
2. Leotta G, Rabbia F, Canade A, et al. Characteristics of the patients referred to a hypertension unit between 1989 and 2003. *J Hum Hypertens* 2008;22:119-121.
3. Egan BM, Zhao Y, Rehman SU, et al. Treatment resistant hypertension in a community-based practice network. *J Clin Hypertens* 2009;OR-12:A6 (abstract).
4. The ALLHAT Officers and Coordinators for the ALLHAT Collaborative Research Group. Major outcomes in high-risk hypertensive patients randomized to angiotensin-converting enzyme inhibitor or calcium channel blocker vs. diuretic. *JAMA* 2002;288:2981-2977.
5. Dahlof B, Devereux RB, Kjeldsen SE, et al., for the LIFE Study Group. Cardiovascular morbidity and mortality in the Losartan Intervention for Endpoint reduction in hypertension study (LIFE): a randomized trial against atenolol. *Lancet* 2002;359:995-1003.
6. Goodfriend TL, Calhoun DA. Resistant hypertension, obesity, sleep apnea, and aldosterone: theory and therapy. *Hypertension* 2004;40:518-524.
7. Garg JP, Elliott WJ, Folker A, Izhar M, Black HR. Resistant hypertension revisited: a comparison of two university based cohorts. *Am J Hypertens* 2005;18:619-626.
8. Burnier M, Schneider MP, Chiolero A, Fallab-Stubi CL, Brunner HR. Electronic compliance monitoring in resistant hypertension: the basis for rational therapeutic decisions. *J Hypertens* 2001;19:335-341.
9. Pickering TG, Miller NH, Ogedegbe G, et al. Call to action on use and reimbursement for home blood pressure monitoring. A joint scientific statement from the American Heart Association, American Society of Hypertension, and Preventive Cardiovascular Nurses Association. *Hypertension* 2008;52:10-29.
10. Ben-Dov IZ, Kark JD, Ben-Ishay D, et al. Predictors of all-cause mortality in clinical ambulatory monitoring: unique aspects of blood pressure during sleep. *Hypertension* 2007;49:1213-1214.
11. Muxfeldt ES, Cardoso CR, Salles GF. Prognostic value of nocturnal blood pressure reduction in resistant hypertension. *Arch Intern Med* 2009;169:874-880.
12. Redon J, Campos C, Narciso ML, et al. Prognostic value of ambulatory blood pressure monitoring in refractory hypertension: a prospective study. *Hypertension* 1998;31:712-718.
13. National Institute for Health and Clinical Excellence. The clinical management of hypertension in adults. Clinical guideline (draft for consultation). National Clinical Guidelines Centre. Accessed July 27 2011 at www.nice.org.uk/nicemedia/live/12167/53225/53225.pdf.
14. Pierdomenico SD, Lapenna D, Bucci A, et al. Cardiovascular outcome in treated hypertensive patients with responder, masked, false resistant, and true resistant hypertension. *Am J Hypertens* 2005;18:1422-1428.
15. Castelpoggi CH, Pereira VS, Fiszman R, et al. A blunted decrease in nocturnal blood pressure is independently associated with increased aortic stiffness in patients with resistant hypertension. *Hypertens Res* 2009;32:591-596.
16. Cuspidi C, Macca G, Sampieri L, et al. High prevalence of cardiac and extracardiac target organ damage in refractory hypertension. *J Hypertens* 2001;2063-2070.
17. Cuspidi C, Vaccarella A, Negri F, Sala C. Resistant hypertension and left ventricular hypertrophy: an overview. *J Am Soc Hypertens* 2010;4:319-324.
18. Rosa J, Strauch B, Petrak O, et al. Relationship between clinical, 24-hour, average daytime and nighttime blood pressure and measures of arterial stiffness in patients with essential hypertension. *Physiol Res* 2008;57:303-306.
19. Logan AG, Perlikowski SM, Mente A, et al. High prevalence of unrecognized sleep apnoea in drug-resistant hypertension. *J Hypertens* 2001;19:2271-2277.
20. Bramlage P, Pittrow D, Wittchen HU, et al. Hypertension in overweight and obese primary care patients is highly prevalent and poorly controlled. *Am J Hypertens* 2004;17:904-910.
21. Martell N, Rodriguez-Cerrillo M, Grobbee DE, et al. High prevalence of secondary hypertension and insulin resistance in patients with refractory hypertension. *Blood Press* 2003;12:149-154.
22. Young T, Peppard P, Palta M, et al. Population-based study of sleep-disordered breathing as a risk factor for hypertension. *Arch Intern Med* 1997;157(15):1746-1752.
23. Ruttanaumpawan P, Nopmaneejumruslers C, Logan AG, et al. Association between refractory hypertension and obstructive sleep apnea. *J Hypertens* 2009;27:1439-1445.
24. Lavie P, Hoffstein V. Sleep apnea syndrome: a possible contributing factor to resistant hypertension. *Sleep* 2001;24:721-725.
25. Gilmartin GS, Lynch M, Tamisier R, Weiss JW. Chronic intermittent hypoxia in humans during 28 nights results in blood pressure elevation and increased muscle sympathetic nerve activity. *Am J Physiol Heart Circ Physiol* 2010;299:H925-H931.
26. Friedman O, Bradley TD, Chan CT, Parkes R, Logan AG. Relationship between overnight rostral fluid shift and obstructive sleep apnea in drug-resistant hypertension. *Hypertension* 2010;56:1077-1082.
27. Bazzano LA, Khan Z, Reynolds K, He J. Effect of nocturnal nasal continuous positive airway pressure on blood pressure in obstructive sleep apnea. *Hypertension* 2007;50:417-423.
28. Haentjens P, Van Meerhaeghe A, Moscariello A, et al. The impact of continuous positive airway pressure on blood pressure in patients with obstructive sleep apnea syndrome: evidence from a meta-analysis of placebo-controlled randomized trials. *Arch Intern Med* 2007;167:757-765.
29. Denaika TA, Kinasewitz GT, Tawk MM. Effects of nocturnal continuous positive airway pressure therapy in patients with resistant hypertension and obstructive sleep apnea. *J Clin Sleep Med* 2009;5:103-107.
30. Martinez-Garcia MA, Gomez-Aldaravi R, Soler-Cataluna JJ, et al. Positive effect of CPAP treatment on the control of difficult-to-treat hypertension. *Eur Respir J* 2007;29:951-957.
31. Lozano L, Tovar JL, Sampol G, et al. Continuous positive airway pressure treatment in sleep apnea patients with resistant hypertension: a randomized, controlled trial. *J Hypertens* 2010;28:2161-2168.
32. Lusardi P, Zoppi A, Preti P, et al. Effects of insufficient sleep on blood pressure in hypertensive patients: a 24-h study. *Am J Hypertens* 1999;12:63-68.
33. Friedman O, Bradley TD, Ruttanaumpawan P, Logan AG. Independent association of drug-resistant hypertension to reduced sleep duration and efficiency. *Am J Hypertens* 2010;23:174-179.
34. Rossi GP, Bernini G, Caliumi C, et al.; PAPY Study Investigators. A prospective study of the prevalence of primary aldosteronism in 1,125 hypertensive patients. *J Am Coll Cardiol* 2006;48:2293-2300.
35. Mosso L, Carvajal C, Gonzalez A, et al. Primary aldosteronism and hypertensive disease. *Hypertension* 2003;42:161-165.

36. Strauch B, Zelinka T, Hampf M, Bernhardt R, Widimsky J Jr. Prevalence of primary hyperal-dosteronism in moderate to severe hypertension in the Central Europe region. *J Hum Hypertens* 2003;17:329-352.

37. Eide K, Torjesen PA, Drolsum A, et al. Low-renin status in therapy resistant hypertension: a clue to efficient treatment. *J Hypertens* 2004;22:2219-2226.

38. Gallay BJ, Ahmad S, Xu L, et al. Screening for primary aldosteronism without discontinuing hypertensive medications: plasma aldosterone-renin ratio. *Am J Kidney Dis* 2001;37(4): 699-705.

39. Umpierrez GE, Cantey P, Smiley D, et al. Primary aldosteronism in diabetic subjects with resistant hypertension. *Diabetes Care* 2007;30:1699-1703.

40. Benchetrit S, Bernheim J, Podjarny E. Normokalemic hyperaldosteronism in patients with resistant hypertension. *Isr Med Assoc J* 2002;4:17-20.

41. Rayner BL, Opie LH, Davidson JS. The aldosterone/renin ratio as a screening test for primary aldosteronism. *S Afr Med J* 2000;90:394-400.

42. Calhoun DA, Nishizaka MK, Zaman MA, Harding SM. Aldosterone excretion among subjects with resistant hypertension and symptoms of sleep apnea. *Chest* 2004;125:112-117.

43. Pratt-Ubunama MN, Nishizaka MK, Boedefeld RA, et al. Plasma aldosterone is related to severity of obstructive sleep apnea in subjects with resistant hypertension. *Chest* 2007;131:453-459.

44. Gonzaga CC, Gaddam KK, Ahmed MI, et al. Severity of obstructive sleep apnea is related to aldosterone status in subjects with resistant hypertension. *J Clin Sleep Med* 2010;6:363-368.

45. Ishiguro C, Fukita T, Omori T, et al. Assessing the effects of non-steroidal anti-inflammatory drugs on anti-hypertensive drug therapy using postmarketing surveillance database. *J Epidemiol* 2008;18(3):119-124.

46. Pimenta E, Gaddam KK, Oparil S, et al. Effects of dietary sodium reduction on blood pressure in subjects with resistant hypertension: results from a randomized trial. *Hypertension* 2009;54:475-481.

47. Gaddam KK, Nishizaka MK, Pratt-Ubunama MN, et al. Characterization of resistant hypertension: association between resistant hypertension, aldosterone, and persistent intravascular volume expansion. *Arch Intern Med* 2008;168:1159-1164.

48. Ernst ME, Carter BL, Goerdt CJ, et al. Comparative antihypertensive effects of hydrochlorothiazide and chlorthalidone on ambulatory and office blood pressure. *Hypertension* 2006;47:352-358.

49. Nishizaka MK, Zaman MA, Calhoun DA. Efficacy of low-dose spironolactone in subjects with resistant hypertension. *Am J Hypertens* 2003;16:925-930.

50. De Souza F, Muxfeldt E, Fiszman R, Salles G. Efficacy of spironolactone therapy in patients with true resistant hypertension. *Hypertension* 2010;55:147-152.

51. Chapman N, Dobson J, Wilson S, et al., on behalf of the Anglo-Scandinavian Cardiac Outcomes Trial investigators. Effect of spironolactone on blood pressure in subjects with resistant hypertension. *Hypertension* 2007;49:839-845.

52. Lane DA, Shah S, Beevers DG. Low-dose spironolactone in the management of resistant hypertension: a surveillance study. *J Hypertens* 2007;25:891-894.

53. Alvarez-Alvarez B, Abad-Cardiel M, Fernandez-Cruz A, Martell-Claros N. Management of resistant arterial hypertension: role of spironolactone versus double blockade of the renin-angiotensin-aldosterone system. *J Hypertens* 2010;11;2329-2335.

54. Gaddam K, Corros C, Pimenta E, et al. Rapid reversal of left ventricular hypertrophy and intracardiac volume overload in patients with resistant hypertension and hyperaldosteronism: a prospective clinical study. *Hypertension* 2010;55:1137-1142.

55. Marney AM, Brown NJ. Aldosterone and end-organ damage. *Clin Sci* 2007;113:267-278.

56. Mahmud A, Feely J. Aldosterone-to-renin ratio, arterial stiffness and response to aldosterone antagonism in essential hypertension. *Am J Hypertens* 2005;18:50-55.

57. Gaddam K, Pimenta E, Thomas SJ, et al. Spironolactone reduces severity of obstructive sleep apnoea in patients with resistant hypertension: a preliminary report. *J Hum Hypertens* 2010;24(8):532-537.

58. ALLHAT Collaborative Research Group. Major cardiovascular events in hypertensive patients randomized to doxazosin vs chlorthalidone: the Antihypertensive and Lipid Lowering treatment to prevent Heart Attack Trial (ALLHAT). *JAMA* 2000;283: 1967-1975.

59. Ceral J, Solar M. Doxazosin: safety and efficacy in the treatment of resistant arterial hypertension. *Blood Press* 2009;18:74-77.

60. Rodilla E, Costa JA, Perez-Lahiguera F, et al. Spironolactone and doxazosin treatment in patients with resistant hypertension. *Rev Esp Cardiol* 2009;62:158-166.

61. Chapman N, Chang CL, Dahlof B, et al., on behalf of the ASCOT investigators. Effect of doxazosin gastrointestinal therapeutic system as third-line antihypertensive therapy on blood pressure and lipids in the Anglo-Scandinavian Cardiac Outcomes Trial. *Circulation* 2008;118:42-48.

62. Eide IK, Torjesen PA, Drolsum A, Babovic A, Lilledahl NP. Low-reinin status in therapy-resistant hypertension: a cue to efficient treatment. *J Hypertens* 2004;22:2217-2226.

63. Sobotka PA, Mahfoud F, Schlaich MP, et al. Sympatho-renal axis in chronic disease. *Clin Res Cardiol* 2011;100(12):1049-1057. Epub 2011 Jun 19.

64. Schlaich MP, Krum H, Esler MD. New therapeutic approaches to resistant hypertension. *Curr Hypertens Rep* 2010;12:296-302.

65. Krum H, Schlaich M, Whitbourn R, et al. Catheter-based renal sympathetic denervation for resistant hypertension: a multicentre safety and proof-of-principle cohort study. *Lancet* 2009;373:1275-1281.

66. Schlaich MP, Sobotka PA, Krum H, Lambert E, Esler MD. Renal sympathetic-nerve ablation for uncontrolled hypertension. *N Engl J Med* 2009;361:932-934.

67. Esler MD, Krum H, Sobotka PA, et al., for the Symplicity HTN-2 Investigators. Renal sympathetic denervation in patients with treatment-resistant hypertension (the Symplicity HTN-2 Trial): a randomised controlled trial. *Lancet* 2010;376:1903-1909.

68. Symplicity HTN-1 Investigators. Catheter-based renal sympathetic denervation for resistant hypertension: durability of blood pressure reduction out to 24 months. *Hypertension* 2011;57:911-917.

69. Filippone JD, Bisognano JD. Baroreflex stimulation in the treatment of hypertension. *Curr Opin Nephrol Hypertens* 2007;16:403-407.

70. Bisognano JD, Bakris G, Nadim MK, et al. Baroreflex activation therapy lowers blood pressure in patients with resistant hypertension: results from the double blind, randomized, placebo-controlled Rheos pivotal trial. *J Am Coll Cardiol* 2011;58:765-773.

71. Nasir JM, Durning SJ, Durrance KA, Denton GD. Effect of a multidisciplinary clinic for the treatment of refractory hypertension. *South Med J* 2006;99:780.

Hypertensive Crisis

Brigitte M. Baumann and Raymond R. Townsend

OVERVIEW, 510

DEFINITIONS, 510

Hypertensive Urgency, 510
Hypertensive Emergency, 510
Hypertensive Crisis, 510
Malignant and Accelerated Hypertension, 510

EPIDEMIOLOGY AND ETIOLOGY, 510

PATHOPHYSIOLOGY, 510

Patient Evaluation, 511

MANAGEMENT OF HYPERTENSIVE EMERGENCY, 513

Cardiovascular Presentations, 513
Neurologic Presentations, 515
Renal Presentations, 517
Catecholaminergic Presentations, 517

Pediatric Hypertensive Emergencies, 518
Obstetric Presentations: Preeclampsia and Eclampsia, 518
Hemorrhage and Post–Vascular Surgery Presentations, 518

FOLLOW-UP AND PROGNOSIS, 519

CAVEATS TO THERAPY IN HYPERTENSIVE EMERGENCY CARE, 519

REFERENCES, 519

Overview

The prevalence of hypertension in American adults aged 18 years and older increased from 24% to 29% from the early 1990s to 2008.[1] Worldwide, approximately 1 billion individuals are currently affected, and a projected 1.6 billion will be affected by 2025.[2] Of these individuals, a minority will experience an acute and dramatic rise in blood pressure (BP) that results in a hypertensive crisis.[3] Some will come to medical attention with a marked elevation in BP only, and others will be seen with both BP elevation and end organ damage. The latter group is considered as having a hypertensive emergency, and rapid BP control is essential to prevent further morbidity and mortality. This chapter discusses the definitions, epidemiology, pathophysiology, evaluation, and management of hypertensive emergencies.

Definitions

Hypertensive Urgency

A *hypertensive urgency* occurs when a patient comes to medical attention with severe hypertension (systolic blood pressure [SBP] ≥180 mm Hg or a diastolic blood pressure [DBP] ≥120 mm Hg) but does not have associated acute end organ damage of the central nervous system (CNS), cardiovascular system, or kidneys.[4] BP must be reduced over hours to days, which may occur in a closely monitored outpatient setting.

Hypertensive Emergency

Both hypertensive urgencies and emergencies are associated with markedly elevated BPs; however, a *hypertensive emergency* differs from *hypertensive urgency* in two important respects. First, the hallmark of a hypertensive emergency is the presence of acute end organ damage and, less so, a high degree of BP elevation. End organ damage is often the result of the acute rise in BP. Second, unlike patients who present with hypertensive urgencies, those seen with hypertensive emergencies require immediate therapy to reduce BP within minutes to hours to prevent further morbidity and mortality.[4]

Hypertensive Crisis

The term *hypertensive crisis* encompasses both hypertensive urgencies and emergencies and is more reflective of the high degree of BP elevation. Common causes and presentations of hypertensive crisis are presented in Box 32-1.

Malignant and Accelerated Hypertension

Malignant hypertension and *accelerated hypertension* are older terms that are less commonly used. These have been replaced by the above terms in national guidelines.[4]

Epidemiology and Etiology

Approximately 3% to 5% of patients who come to the emergency department because of symptoms of extreme hypertension will have a hypertensive crisis; of those, up to one third will have a hypertensive emergency.[5,6] Men are more likely than women to come to medical attention with a hypertensive emergency, although the risk is also increased in women who are postmenopausal.[6] Racial and ethnic factors mirror the prevalence of poorly controlled hypertension, with non-Hispanic blacks having the highest risk for a hypertensive emergency, followed by non-Hispanic whites and, lastly, Hispanics.[7] Other risk factors for the development of hypertensive crisis include older age, increasing degrees of obesity, prior history of heart failure, hypertensive or coronary heart disease, the need for multiple antihypertensive medications, and a history of nonadherence to medications.[8,9] The development of hypertensive crisis has also been linked to several social and socioeconomic factors, including cigarette smoking, lack of a primary care physician, and lack of medical insurance.[9,10]

Hypertensive emergency more commonly affects adults, but it can occur at any age. It can affect neonates with congenital renal artery hypoplasia, children with acute glomerulonephritis, pregnant teenage girls with eclampsia, middle-aged or older patients with treatment nonadherence, or elderly people with atherosclerotic renal artery stenosis. Such individuals are not typically accustomed to significant elevations in BP and may come to medical attention with signs and symptoms of hypertensive emergency at much lower BP levels than patients with long-standing, poorly controlled hypertension, in whom severe elevation in BP can be tolerated with less risk of target organ damage.

Pathophysiology

The development of hypertensive emergency centers on dysregulation of pressure-dependent blood flow in critical vascular beds—the cerebral, cardiac, and renal circulations—which can deteriorate into frank vasculitis and ischemia. Although blood vessels normally autoregulate blood flow over a substantial range of mean arterial pressure (MAP; Figure 32-1), when the range of autoregulatory capacity is exceeded, vasoconstriction no longer compensates adequately, and a superperfusion of the tissue occurs, leading to target organ damage. Vessels take on a "sausage string" appearance that results from areas of intense vasoconstriction alternating with areas of vascular exhaustion and dilation.

The flip side of this pathophysiology is equally important. Chronic hypertension results in functional and structural changes in the arterial walls, which shift the vascular autoregulatory curve to the right (see Figure 32-1). This permits patients with hypertension to maintain organ perfusion at higher MAP levels. The purposeful lowering of MAP with medication during a hypertensive emergency into a range appropriate for a normotensive individual risks reducing the pressure below the autoregulatory capacity of

Box 32-1 Presentations and Causes of Hypertensive Crisis

General

Abrupt increase in blood pressure in patients with chronic hypertension

Ingestion of drugs, particularly sympathomimetic agents such as cocaine, amphetamines, phenycyclidine hydrochloride (PCP), lysergic acid diethylamide (LSD), diet pills, and tricyclic antidepressants

Withdrawal from antihypertensive agents, usually centrally acting agents such as clonidine and β-antagonists

Ingestion of tyramine-containing foods or other sympathomimetics combined with monoamine oxidase inhibitor therapy

Pheochromocytoma

Vasculitis

Autonomic hyperactivity in the presence of Guillain-Barré or spinal cord syndromes

Cardiac

Myocardial infarction and unstable angina

Acute pulmonary edema

Acute aortic dissection

Renal

Renovascular hypertension

Chronic parenchymal renal disease with increasing creatinine

Scleroderma renal crisis and other collagen vascular diseases

Acute glomerulonephritis

Renin-secreting tumor

Neurologic

Stroke, intracerebral hemorrhage, subarachnoid hemorrhage

Head injury

Encephalopathy

Obstetric/Gynecologic

Eclampsia

Postsurgical

Post—coronary artery bypass grafting

Post—carotid artery repair

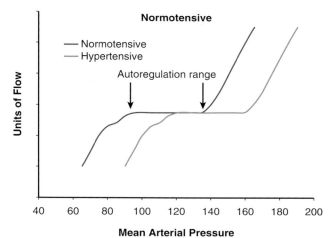

FIGURE 32-1 Shown are two curves, normotensive (*blue line*) and hypertensive (*yellow line*). Both groups maintain steady flow over a range of pressure labeled as "autoregulation" and depicted for the normotensive patient. The autoregulation curve is shifted rightward in the chronic hypertensive patients. Although this protects them from excessive flow, until higher pressures are reached (compared with the normotensive patient), reduction of mean arterial pressure in the hypertensive patients to levels near the lower end of the autoregulatory curve in normotensive patients risks tissue ischemia because of the adaptation to chronically elevated pressure.

the hypertension-adapted circulation, reducing tissue perfusion, and precipitating ischemia and even infarction. This process often appears pathophysiologically as *fibrinoid necrosis* of the vascular media and intima. This leads to thrombosis and fibrin deposition in the vessel wall, with manifestations such as retinal hemorrhage or cotton-wool spots and papilledema, heart failure, and kidney function compromise.

Many potential factors in addition to the physical elevation of the BP itself contribute to hypertensive emergency.[11] Among locally produced factors are prostaglandins, free radicals, mitogenic and chemoattractant factors, proliferation factors, and cytokines. Endothelial damage, smooth muscle proliferation, and platelet aggregation contribute to the tissue injury seen in these patients. Among the systemic factors are increases in renin and angiotensin II, catecholamines, endothelin, and vasopressin levels. Pressure natriuresis occurs in this setting and leads to hypovolemia, which potentiates the further release of vasoconstrictor substances such as renin and catecholamines. These factors increase BP, aggravate endothelial damage, and ultimately lead to tissue ischemia and damage. One study showed a possible association of a polymorphism of the angiotensin-converting enzyme (ACE) and the DD

genotype with hypertensive emergencies in men, suggesting a genetic facet to hypertensive emergency.[12] Despite the impressive array of pathogenic factors, treatment remains largely empiric in most situations, with a limited number of reliable and potent antihypertensive agents. People who survive a hypertensive emergency continue to show poorer endothelial function and stiffer vessels compared with healthy controls and those with hypertension who have never had a hypertensive emergency.[13]

Patient Evaluation

The initial evaluation of patients with severely elevated BP should be targeted to rapidly identify those who come to medical attention with a hypertensive emergency. Unlike patients who come in with isolated severe BP elevation and have hours to days to attain adequate BP control, patients who are seen initially with acute end organ damage need emergency therapy within minutes to prevent further morbidity. To this end, a focused history and a directed physical examination should direct initial ancillary testing, which will facilitate the selection of appropriate antihypertensive agents.

HISTORY, PHYSICAL EXAMINATION, AND ANCILLARY TESTING

Patients should be questioned about prior history of hypertension, its severity, and previous end organ damage. Use of prescription drugs, over-the-counter medications, and herbal supplements should be queried, as outlined in Box 32-2. *Ephedra sinica*, a Chinese medicinal herb also known as *Ma huang*, contains ephedrine and stimulates the nervous and endocrine systems to generate an acute rise in BP.[14] Although *Ephedra* was banned by the U.S. Food and Drug Administration (FDA) in 2006, it can still be obtained outside the United States and from Internet sources as a diet aid or stimulant. The "legal" or "ephedrine-free" supplement, *Citrus aurantium*, also known as *bitter orange*, is available in the United States and has hemodynamic effects similar to *Ephedra*.[14,15] Ingestion of large amounts of real licorice, an herbal remedy used to treat peptic ulcers, may also lead to a hypertensive crisis. Real licorice contains triterpene glycosides, including glycyrrhizic acid, which increase sodium retention by potentiating mineralocorticoid activity. Long-term use leads to a gradual increase in BP; when large doses are ingested within a short time, an acute rise in BP may occur.[16]

The physical examination should be directed toward the identification of end organ damage and additional factors that could affect medical management. First, several BP measurements should be obtained with an appropriate size cuff in both arms and in a leg if peripheral pulses are markedly reduced. BP assessments

TABLE 32-1   Ancillary Testing for Patients with Severely Elevated Blood Pressure

ANCILLARY TEST	FINDINGS
CBC and a peripheral smear	Microangiopathic hemolytic anemia
Chemistry panel	Evidence of electrolyte abnormalities, such as hypokalemia from aldosterone activation or hyperkalemia from renal insufficiency
Electrocardiogram	Myocardial ischemia, MI, and LV hypertrophy Electrolyte abnormalities: flattened or inverted T waves or U waves (hypokalemia) or peaked T waves (hyperkalemia)
Urinalysis with microscopic examination of the urinary sediment	May reveal significant proteinuria, red blood cells, and/or cellular casts suggestive of renal parenchymal disease
Urine drug screen	To screen for illicit sympathomimetic drug use
Chest radiograph	May reveal pulmonary edema or a widened mediastinum, raising suspicion of an aortic dissection
Noncontrast CT of the head in patients with focal neurologic findings or an altered sensorium	To rule out a hemorrhagic CVA, mass lesion, or an ischemic event

CBC, complete blood count; CT, computed tomography, CVA, cerebrovascular accident; LV left ventricular; MI, myocardial infarction.

Box 32-2 Historic Data to Obtain in a Patient with Severely Elevated Blood Pressure

Past Medical History

Is there a history of high blood pressure? If so, what is the baseline blood pressure?

Is there a history of end-organ damage, such as cerebrovascular accident, myocardial infarction, renal disease, congestive heart failure, or aortic dissection?

Is there a prior history of preeclampsia or eclampsia?

Is the patient postpartum? (Eclampsia may occur up to 8 weeks postpartum.)

Medications

Is the patient compliant with medication regimens?

Have there been recent changes in medications, such as cessation of one drug or initiation of a new drug?

Does that patient use over-the-counter medications or herbal supplements, such as diet aids or cold preparations (phenylpropanolamine, Ephedra [Ma huang], pseudoephedrine)?

Did the patient abruptly cease taking a β-blocker or centrally acting agent such as clonidine? (Guanfacine hydrochloride may also lead to rebound hypertension but is less likely to result in hypertensive emergency compared with clonidine.)

Is the patient currently taking a monoamine oxidase inhibitor?

Has the patient overindulged in foods known to trigger hypertensive events, such as real licorice or tyromine-containing foods?

Social History

Does the patient use illicit drugs, such as cocaine, amphetamines, lysergic acid diethylamide (LSD), or phencyclidine hydrochloride (PCP)?

Box 32-3 Symptoms and Physical Findings

Symptoms

Chest pain (myocardial ischemia/infarction, aortic dissection)

Back pain (aortic dissection)

Shortness of breath (acute pulmonary edema secondary to left ventricular failure)

Headache (intracerebral or subarachnoid hemorrhage or hypertensive encephalopathy)

Confusion or history of confusion reported by caregivers (hypertensive encephalopathy)

Focal weakness, dysarthria (cerebrovascular accident)

Nausea, vomiting (if associated with headache, these may be early signs of hypertensive encephalopathy)

Seizures (hypertensive encephalopathy or eclampsia)

Profuse diaphoresis and palpitations (pheochromocytoma)

Blurry vision (papilledema)

Physical Examination

Blood pressure discrepancy between arms (if >20 mm Hg, consider aortic dissection)

Orthostatic blood pressure drop (to identify volume depletion)

Funduscopic Examination

Grade III retinopathy: flame-shaped hemorrhages, cotton-wool spots, yellow-white exudates

Grade IV retinopathy: papilledema with blurring of the disc margins, retinal hemorrhages, exudates

Pulmonary Examination

Crackles suggestive of pulmonary edema

Cardiac Examination

Auscultation for new murmurs

Aortic insufficiency as a result of aortic dissection

Mitral regurgitation as a result of ischemic rupture of papillary muscle

Elevated jugular venous pressure

S3 gallop

Abdominal Examination

Systolic or diastolic abdominal bruit suggestive of renovascular disease

Neurologic Examination

Focal findings that include visual field deficits and subtle cerebellar disturbances indicative of an ischemic or hemorrhagic cerebrovascular accident

Confusion or flapping tremor (hypertensive encephalopathy, a diagnosis of exclusion)

should be attempted with the patient supine and standing, if the medical condition allows, to identify orthostatic changes and volume depletion. In addition to orthostatic BP measurements, other assessments of fluid status, including an examination of the patient's mucous membranes and skin turgor, should be undertaken. Urine output should be closely monitored to assist with fluid management. Anuria, oliguria, or hematuria may reflect acute renal injury and should be immediately addressed. The remainder of the physical examination should be focused on the pulmonary, cardiovascular, and neurologic systems as outlined in Box 32-3.

Suggested ancillary testing for the determination of acute end organ damage is provided in Table 32-1. In patients with focal neurologic findings or an altered sensorium, a noncontrast computed tomography (CT) of the head should be obtained to rule out a hemorrhagic cerebrovascular accident (CVA) and may provide evidence of a mass lesion or an ischemic event.[17] Magnetic resonance imaging (MRI) may be used to further identify cerebral pathology, but given the increased time needed to conduct this imaging study and the limited access of health

care providers to the patient, this is best undertaken when the patient has been stabilized and BP treatment has been initiated. Additional diagnostic testing may be needed to identify less common causes of hypertensive emergency. For example, patients who come to medical attention with significant tachycardia and sweating, signs of catecholamine excess, should undergo plasma metanephrine or urine metanephrine and catecholamine testing based on the degree of clinical suspicion for pheochromocytoma.[18,19]

Management of Hypertensive Emergency

The goal in patient management is a gradual and controlled reduction of MAP by 20% to 25% within 1 hour of arrival to the emergency department, with additional reductions over the next several hours to days.[4] Selection of antihypertensive agents should be based on the clinical manifestations of disease and individual patient characteristics. Patients should be managed either in the emergency department, if presenting de novo, or in another intensive care setting to allow close monitoring and frequent adjustments in antihypertensive therapy. In patients whose BP is labile or difficult to control, continuous BP monitoring via an arterial line may be needed. The goal is to achieve the fine balance of minimizing end organ damage via initial BP reduction while concurrently avoiding hypoperfusion of cerebral, coronary, and renovascular beds. The two primary exceptions to this rule apply to patients with suspected acute aortic dissection, in whom the risk of morbidity and mortality as a result of inadequate BP and heart rate control outweighs the risk of hypoperfusion syndromes. Secondly, aggressive BP control in patients seen with neurologic hypertensive emergencies, particularly those with ischemic CVAs, remains controversial.[20-22]

Dosing of agents used in hypertensive crisis and the typical indications for their use are outlined in Table 32-2. Because available parenteral drugs have differential effects on the various target organs that may be involved in hypertensive crisis, the approach outlined in the following sections is recommended. A final general management principle includes careful consideration of the patient's fluid status. Natriuresis as a result of hypertension presents with subtle or overt volume depletion.[23] Initiation of a vasodilator may lead to a precipitous drop in BP; therefore the initial management of these patients may include the administration of intravenous (IV) isotonic sodium chloride solution. Restoration of intravascular volume results in a downregulation of the renin-angiotensin-aldosterone system (RAAS), promoting a break in the hypertensive cycle.

Cardiovascular Presentations

Hypertensive emergencies that involve the heart and aorta include acute coronary syndromes, left ventricular (LV) failure and acute pulmonary edema, and aortic dissection. Nitroglycerin, nitroprusside, and nicardipine are the three drugs most commonly used, sometimes in combination, in these settings. All three drugs can cause reflex tachycardia, but their coronary arterial dilator effects usually offset the increased cardiac oxygen demand. Although nicardipine has not been widely studied in acute myocardial ischemia, there are plausible grounds for its use, particularly in the setting of no-reflow phenomenon, which often accompanies percutaneous coronary intervention (PCI) for acute ST-elevation myocardial infarction (MI).[24] There is no target BP for hypertensive emergencies that involve cardiac ischemia/infarction or pulmonary edema, and the goal of therapy is to improve cardiac perfusion. Typically, a 10% to 15% reduction in BP results in a dramatic improvement in perfusion and in symptoms.

ACUTE CORONARY SYNDROMES

Acute coronary syndromes involved in hypertensive emergencies include unstable angina and acute myocardial ischemia and MI. Reduction of elevated systemic BP decreases myocardial work, wall tension, and oxygen demand. Although no conclusive evidence demonstrates that acute treatment is beneficial, it is theorized that reduction of systemic BP may limit myocardial necrosis in the early phase of infarction.[25] Coronary syndromes are typically

managed with IV nitroglycerin, which decreases LV preload and increases coronary artery perfusion.[25] Because it is a weak arteriolar dilator at lower doses, its ability to reduce BP is less than that of other vasodilators such as nitroprusside. Nitroprusside should not be given in isolation because of the potential for sympathetic reflex tachycardia, which may further increase myocardial oxygen demand. Instead, nitroprusside should be administered in conjunction with a β-blocker, which will control the heart rate and may provide additional BP reduction.

LEFT VENTRICULAR FAILURE AND ACUTE PULMONARY EDEMA

Acute LV failure may be precipitated by severe hypertension because of increased cardiac workload. The goal of therapy is to reduce cardiac workload so that the myocardium can maintain a cardiac output sufficient to meet the demands of the peripheral circulation. This may be accomplished by preload and afterload reduction and by diuresis.[26] Nitroglycerin is a first-line agent with a primary effect on preload reduction. Sodium nitroprusside, a balanced vasodilator, decreases both preload and afterload and may be used on its own or in conjunction with nitroglycerin.[26] The ACE inhibitor enalaprilat has been shown to be effective and well tolerated in acute pulmonary edema,[27] although in the prehospital setting sublingual nitroglycerin is preferred over enalaprilat.[28] In most instances, a loop-blocking diuretic is given along with the above agents.

Newer agents include clevidipine, a third-generation dihydropyridine calcium channel blocker (CCB) that has been shown to reduce BP without unexpected hypotension or adverse events in a small group of acute heart failure patients.[29] Investigational agents such as relaxin, a natural human peptide that affects multiple vascular control pathways, and rolofylline, an adenosine α_1-receptor antagonist, have not been shown to be superior to placebo in patients with acute heart failure.[30,31] Drugs that increase cardiac workload via a reflex tachycardia (hydralazine) or those that decrease myocardial contractility (β-blockers given alone) should be avoided.[26] Similarly, positive inotropes should be avoided in this setting. Two factors that have been associated with increased mortality rate include the use of inotropes and a delay of more than 6 hours from time of presentation in the initiation of vasoactive therapy.[32,33]

AORTIC DISSECTION

Of all hypertensive emergencies, acute aortic dissection carries with it the highest mortality rate if treatment is delayed. Patients with aortic arch dissections (type A) typically come to medical attention with tearing back or chest pain, and those with dissections of the descending aorta (type B) come in with back and abdominal pain. Signs suggestive of an acute aortic dissection include a difference in brachial artery pressure of at least 20 mm Hg, new pulse deficits, and a new aortic regurgitation murmur. Patients with connective tissue disorders that weaken the media of the arterial wall, such as Marfan syndrome or Ehlers-Danlos syndrome, are at increased risk.[34,35] Incidence of aortic dissection is also increased in patients who are pregnant and in those who use cocaine or methamphetamines.[36,37] Men are two times more likely than women to have an aortic dissection, and more than one third of all cases are missed on initial evaluation.[37]

Regardless of the type of dissection, immediate initiation of BP and heart rate control is needed to decrease the shearing forces on the aortic wall. SBP should be rapidly reduced to between 100 and 120 mm Hg. A short-acting β-blocker, such as esmolol, is typically initiated and followed by an infusion of sodium nitroprusside. The use of a β-blocker helps prevent reflex tachycardia that results from the vasodilating and BP-reducing effects of sodium nitroprusside. Use of a vasodilator alone is contraindicated because it may result in an increase in the velocity of ventricular contraction and cause further propagation of the dissection. Other therapeutic

TABLE 32-2   Parenteral Antihypertensive Agents Used in Hypertensive Emergencies

AGENT	DOSING	ONSET	DURATION OF EFFECT	USE	ADVERSE EFFECTS/ CONTRAINDICATIONS*
ACE Inhibitor					
Enalaprilat	1.25 mg	10-15 min	Up to 6 h	Renal emergencies	Angioedema; difficult to predict responses; occasional dramatic fall in blood pressure noted Contraindicated in pregnant patients
α-Blocker					
Phentolamine	1-5 mg over 1 min, repeat every 5-10 min	1 min	<10 min	Use with suspected catecholamine excess	Tachycardia, headache, angina
β-Blockers					
Esmolol	0.2-0.5 mg/kg over 1 min, then 0.05 mg/kg/min for 4 min, then increase dose 0.05 mg/kg at 5-min intervals up to 0.2 mg/kg/min	1-2 min	10 min	Postoperative presentations, coronary ischemia, thoracic aorta dissection	Heart block, bronchospasm, heart failure
Labetalol	0.5-2 mg/min; alternatively, 20-80 mg IV bolus q5-10min; up to 300 mg total dose	5 min	Up to 6 h	Postoperative, neurologic, and coronary presentations; after α-blockade in patients with adrenergic crisis	Heart failure, scalp tingling, flushing Avoid in patients with depressed left ventricular function, greater than first-degree heart block, asthma
Calcium Antagonists					
Clevidipine	1-2 mg/h; maximum infusion 21 mg/h	2-4 min	5-15 min	Role not yet defined; used perioperatively in heart failure and renal patients; limited experience in the pediatric population	Cleviprex contains approximately 0.2 g of lipid per mL (2.0 kcal) Lipid intake restrictions may be necessary for patients with significant disorders of lipid metabolism Contraindicated in patients with severe aortic stenosis
Nicardipine	5-15 mg/h; increase by 1-2.5 mg/kg q15min	5-10 min	1 h, up to 4 h	Postoperative presentations	Tachycardia, headache, nausea, and vomiting; phlebitis at infusion site if peripheral vein is used for >24 h Avoid in patients with coronary ischemia (increase in heart rate may worsen ischemia)
Dopamine Agonist					
Fenoldopam	0.1-0.3 µg/kg/min	<5 min	30 min	Renal presentations (does not impair GFR) Used as alternative to nitroprusside, especially postoperatively	Tachycardia, headache, flushing; may reduce potassium; less effective after 48 h Contraindicated in patients with glaucoma
Vasodilators					
Diazoxide	50-150 mg bolus; 15-30 mg/min continuous infusion	2-5 min	3-12 h	Used rarely	Tachycardia, angina, nausea, increased glucose Not used for coronary presentations or with aortic dissection because of heart rate increase
Hydralazine	10-20 mg bolus at 1 mg/min	10-20 min	3-8 h	Eclampsia	Increased heart rate limits value in cardiac presentations and may worsen angina Increased intracranial pressure limits value in neurologic presentations
Nitroglycerin	5-100 µg/min (titrate q5min)	2-5 min	5-10 min	Acute MI, pulmonary edema, cocaine use with coronary ischemia	Headache (severe), nausea, vomiting
Nitroprusside	0.3-10 µg/kg/min	<1 min	1-10 min	Encephalopathy, pulmonary edema Most hypertensive emergencies managed with this drug	Headache, nausea, vomiting Cyanide and thiocyanate toxicity is more likely with reduced renal function, rate >2 µg/kg/min, and prolonged (>24-48 h) duration of therapy Avoid in pregnant patients

Continued

TABLE 32-2 Parenteral Antihypertensive Agents Used in Hypertensive Emergencies—cont'd

AGENT	DOSING	ONSET	DURATION OF EFFECT	USE	ADVERSE EFFECTS/ CONTRAINDICATIONS*
Ganglionic Blocker					
Trimethaphan	0.5-5 mg/min	1-5 min	5-10 min	Aortic dissection Uncommonly used because of frequent instability in BP effect; mostly supplanted by nitroprusside	Urine retention, ileus, respiratory arrest
Miscellaneous					
Magnesium sulfate	1 g/min infusion; up to 4 g; maximum dose over the first 15 min is 6 g for the treatment of seizures Intramuscular has slower onset and lasts longer; goal serum concentration is 4-6 mEq/L	<1 min	30 min	Eclampsia	Sweating, flushing, respiratory and cardiac arrest

*All agents in this table have hypotension as an adverse effect.
BP, blood pressure; ACE, angiotensin-converting enzyme; GFR, glomerular filtration rate; IV, intravenous; MI, myocardial infarction.

agents that have been used include nicardipine and fenoldopam, both of which are less toxic alternatives to sodium nitroprusside.[38] Labetalol, a combined α- and β-adrenergic antagonist, is an excellent alternative, but because of its longer duration of action, it may be more difficult to titrate.

Definitive management depends on the type of dissection; thus an imaging study is required to delineate the origin and extension of the dissection. A widened mediastinum on chest radiography is present in only 25% of cases, and unless it is obtained at the bedside in parallel with other management, it may delay time to a definitive imaging study.[39] Because of its increased availability, rapid completion time, and high sensitivity and specificity, CT angiography (CTA) has emerged as the first-line diagnostic study (Figure 32-2). If CTA is inconclusive, an MRI or a transesophageal echocardiogram (TEE) should be obtained. Ascending aortic dissections require surgical repair, whereas dissections that involve the descending aorta are generally managed medically. Surgical intervention may be needed for distal dissections that are leaking or ruptured or that compromise blood flow to a vital organ. In patients with complicated type B dissections, early stent-graft implantation has resulted in more favorable aortic remodeling and reduced late complications (see Chapter 40).[40]

Neurologic Presentations

Differentiating neurologic emergencies can be challenging, but it is necessary because of critical differences in management. Patients with acute ischemic and hemorrhagic cerebrovascular syndromes typically come to medical attention with focal neurologic signs, and the diagnosis is typically confirmed with CT or MRI (Figure 32-3). Subarachnoid hemorrhage (SAH) may also be evident on imaging, but if it is not present, a lumbar puncture may be required. Hypertensive encephalopathy is typically a diagnosis of exclusion; however, unlike patients with hypertensive neurologic emergencies, those with hypertensive encephalopathy improve rapidly with aggressive BP management.

ISCHEMIC CEREBROVASCULAR SYNDROMES

Although BP control in patients with a history of ischemic CVA has been shown to be beneficial in reducing long-term morbidity and mortality rates, BP reduction in the acute setting remains controversial. Several studies have documented clinical deterioration in patients after the initiation of BP treatment, and others have demonstrated worse outcomes in patients with increasingly elevated BP levels.[41-44] Most studies have shown that BP variability in the acute stroke setting is a risk factor for increased morbidity and mortality rates.[42,45] This finding underscores the delicate balance

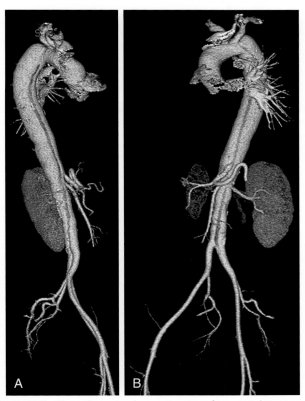

FIGURE 32-2 Three-dimensional reconstruction of computed tomographic angiography of the chest and abdomen showing a chronic Stanford type B aortic dissection. **A,** Impression of the true lumen and extension of the dissection flap to the aortic bifurcation. **B,** The right kidney is supplied by the true lumen of the dissection and has atrophied. Note the normal-sized left kidney supplied by the false lumen.

between reaching sufficient BP control and maintaining adequate cerebral perfusion in patients with neurologic cerebrovascular syndromes.

Current guidelines recommend that BP in patients with acute ischemic CVAs should not be reduced, unless their hypertension is severe (systolic >220 mm Hg or diastolic >120 mm Hg) or they have a concomitant hypertensive emergency with high risk of morbidity and mortality, such as with myocardial ischemia, aortic dissection, hypertensive encephalopathy, or preeclampsia/

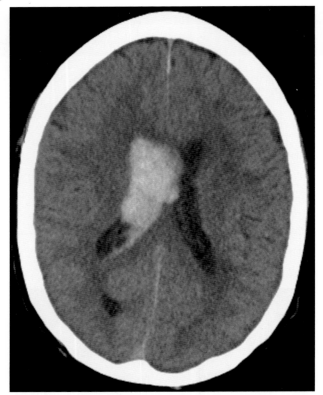

FIGURE 32-3 This patient presented with a severe headache and severely elevated blood pressure (195/115 mm Hg). Axial noncontrast computed tomography shows acute intracerebral hemorrhage of the right caudate nucleus with mass effect, midline shift, and intraventricular extension.

eclampsia.[21,22] If antihypertensive treatment is initiated, the mean arterial BP should be lowered by no more than 15%, and the DBP should not be lowered beyond 110 mm Hg within the first 24 hours.[22] After the first 24 hours, patients with known hypertension may be started back on their BP medications.[22] However, the utility of this approach is questionable; a trial demonstrated that continuation of antihypertensive drugs did not reduce 2-week death or dependency, cardiovascular event rate, or death at 6 months after an acute stroke.[46] In patients with extracranial or intracranial stenoses, a slower BP reduction (over 7 to 10 days) is recommended given the increased risk for cerebral hypoperfusion. For all ischemic cerebrovascular events, IV labetalol, nicardipine, and transdermal nitroglycerin may be used to control BP in patients who are eligible to receive recombinant tissue plasminogen activator (thrombolysis). Sodium nitroprusside should not be used because of the theoretical risk of increased intracranial pressure (ICP) and platelet dysfunction.[22]

HEMORRHAGIC CEREBROVASCULAR SYNDROMES

Acute BP control is also controversial in patients with hemorrhagic cerebrovascular syndromes, such as intracerebral hemorrhage and SAH. It is postulated that BP reduction may decrease bleeding and hematoma expansion, but this potential benefit must be weighed against the risk of further reducing cerebral blood flow if cerebral perfusion is already impaired by elevated ICP.[47]

INTRACEREBRAL HEMORRHAGE

According to current guidelines, aggressive BP control should only be considered in patients with SBP above 200 mm Hg or MAP above 150 mm Hg.[47] In patients with SBP above 180 mm Hg or MAP above 130 mm Hg and evidence or suspicion of elevated ICP,

monitoring of ICP should be considered, and BP reduction should be initiated using intermittent or continuous IV medication to keep cerebral perfusion pressure in the range of 61 to 80 mm Hg. In patients with SBP above 180 mm Hg or MAP above 130 mm Hg who have no evidence of elevated ICP, a modest reduction of BP using IV agents may be considered (target MAP of 110 mm Hg or target BP of 160/90 mm Hg).[47] Although BP control has been shown to decrease hematoma expansion, clinically significant improvement in 90-day death and dependency has not been demonstrated.[48] Agents for use in patients with intracranial hemorrhage (ICH) include labetalol, nicardipine, esmolol, enalapril, hydralazine, and nitroglycerin.[47]

SUBARACHNOID HEMORRHAGE

As with ICH, BP reduction in the setting of SAH is also controversial. To date, no well-controlled studies have examined whether BP control in acute SAH influences rebleeding; therefore no consensus guidelines for BP control exist. If BP is severely elevated, a short-acting, continuous-infusion IV agent with a reliable dose/response relation and a favorable safety profile—such as nicardipine, labetalol, or esmolol—may be initiated.[49]

Nimodipine, an oral CCB, is approved for use in patients with SAH.[47] It is thought that the reduction in morbidity and improvement in functional outcome with nimodipine use may have been due to cerebral protection, rather than an effect on the cerebral vasculature, because no reduction was demonstrated in angiographic vasospasm in patients taking this medication.[50]

HYPERTENSIVE ENCEPHALOPATHY

Patients with chronic, uncontrolled hypertension are more likely to experience hypertensive encephalopathy, but this condition may also occur in previously normotensive patients who have an acute and rapid rise in BP. Patients with renal insufficiency are also at greater risk than those with normal renal function. Patients with hypertensive encephalopathy typically come to medical attention with a generalized, severe headache followed by confusion, lethargy, and somnolence. Other clinical features include restlessness, agitation, nausea, vomiting, and visual disturbances. Physical examination is notable for funduscopic changes, and most patients have papilledema. Patients with neurologic changes should undergo laboratory evaluation and imaging to exclude other causes such as CVA, intracranial mass, and uremic encephalopathy; in addition, MRI may reveal edema of the white matter.[51] Reversible posterior leukoencephalopathy syndrome occurs when edema is localized to the parietooccipital regions (Figure 32-4). When localized to the pontine area of the brain, it is referred to as *hypertensive brain stem encephalopathy.*

Unlike other neurologic hypertensive emergencies, treatment of hypertensive encephalopathy requires immediate BP control—that is, reduction of MAP by approximately 20% or reduction in DBP to levels not lower than 100 mm Hg within the first 1 to 2 hours—and withdrawal of exacerbating factors, such as erythropoietin.[51] More aggressive BP reduction, especially in the elderly or in patients with poorly controlled hypertension, may lead to cerebral hypoperfusion and possibly even stroke.[51] The patient's symptoms and neurologic status should improve as the BP is brought under control. Agents that interrupt the renin-angiotensin system, such as β-blockers and ACE inhibitors, are preferred. Nicardipine and fenoldopam may also be used as second-line agents. Vasodilators such as sodium nitroprusside and hydralazine stimulate renin secretion and are less likely to be efficacious.[52] Sodium nitroprusside and nitroglycerin also have the potential to increase ICP.[51] Clonidine is also not recommended because it is a CNS depressant, which may make it difficult to monitor the patient's neurologic status. IV benzodiazepines or anticonvulsants such as phenytoin or fosphenytoin should be used in patients who come to medical attention with seizures, and further reduction in BP may occur with the administration of these agents.[53]

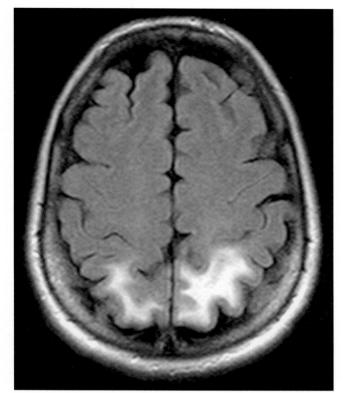

FIGURE 32-4 Axial fluid-attenuated inversion recovery T2-weighted magnetic resonance imaging showing bilateral symmetric vasogenic edema involving the subcortical white matter in the posterior parietooccipital lobes. No mass effect is present.

Renal Presentations

Hematuria or a worsening of renal function characterizes kidney involvement in hypertensive emergency. Gross hematuria is less common than microscopic hematuria, and its presence should trigger a urologic evaluation once BP is stabilized. Acute renal failure can both cause and result from elevated BP, and severe hypertension often accompanies acute renal failure. Consequently, a urinalysis and measurement of serum creatinine should be undertaken in the initial evaluation of patients with extreme BP increases. Hypertensive emergencies characterized by kidney involvement may occur in the course of essential hypertension or in settings of thrombotic thrombocytopenic purpura and scleroderma.[54,55] Kidney failure is often accompanied by increased serum lactate dehydrogenase (from microangiopathic hemolysis) and activation of the RAAS.[56]

Not uncommonly—and in our experience, more so in African-American patients—successful treatment of hypertensive emergencies in patients with reduced renal function results in further renal function impairment. This worsening of renal function is often transient and can occur even when the BP is correctly titrated downward in a controlled and gradual fashion. Moreover, worsening renal function can result in the need for acute dialysis. When this happens, many patients can discontinue dialysis during long-term follow-up, if BP remains well controlled, although in some the need for dialysis is permanent.[56,57] Therapy in hypertensive emergencies that involve renal presentations should reduce systemic vascular resistance while preserving renal blood flow. The dopamine agonist fenoldopam and the CCBs nicardipine and clevidipine can be effective in this situation. Nitroprusside is also effective, but it carries a risk of cyanide and thiocyanate toxicity. Compared with nitroprusside, fenoldopam improves natriuresis and creatinine clearance in patients with elevated BP and impaired renal function.[58]

Catecholaminergic Presentations

Four classic settings exist in which an excess of catecholamines can result in a hypertensive emergency: 1) acute withdrawal of antihypertensive therapy, 2) pheochromocytoma, 3) sympathomimetic drug use, and 4) autonomic dysfunction.

ACUTE WITHDRAWAL OF ANTIHYPERTENSIVE THERAPY

The most common withdrawal syndrome is associated with the abrupt discontinuation of oral clonidine, but it may also occur in patients using transdermal clonidine. This rebound phenomenon is thought to be due to the rapid return of catecholamine secretion following cessation of α-agonist therapy. Patients who are on concomitant β-blocker therapy are even more susceptible to rebound hypertension following clonidine withdrawal because β-blockade results in unopposed α-mediated vasoconstriction. These patients come to medical attention with anxiety, palpitations, sweating, nausea, headache, and severe rebound hypertension. A withdrawal syndrome as a result of sudden cessation of β-blockers may also occur. Withdrawal of short-acting β-adrenergic antagonists such as propanolol may lead to an increase in adrenergic activity because of the upregulation of β-adrenergic receptors. In most patients, BP will be only moderately elevated, and withdrawal generally does not result in hypertensive crisis, thus differentiating β-adrenergic antagonist withdrawal syndrome from clonidine withdrawal.[59] However, patients with underlying cardiac disease may have accelerated angina or myocardial ischemia or may die after abrupt withdrawal of a β-adrenergic antagonist. In both cases, BP is best controlled by readministering the withdrawn drug. If this is not possible, or if the patient requires additional BP treatment, phentolamine, sodium nitroprusside, or labetalol should be initiated. Acute coronary syndromes as a result of β-blocker withdrawal should be managed with reinitiation of β-blockade in addition to standard therapy that includes aspirin, nitroglycerin, and percutaneous interventions or thrombolytic therapy, as appropriate.

PHEOCHROMOCYTOMA

Although the condition is rare, the diagnosis of pheochromocytoma is important because at least 10% of tumors are malignant, patients may present with life-threatening hypertension, and with surgical removal, affected patients may be cured of disease.[60] Some cases are associated with familial syndromes, such as multiple endocrine neoplasia (MEN) type 2B, neurofibromatosis, and von Hippel–Lindau disease; therefore, examination of the skin for neurofibromas, port wine stains, and café-au-lait spots may aid in the diagnosis. Patients typically report episodes of headaches, diaphoresis, and palpitations in association with severe hypertension. Attacks vary in frequency; some are as infrequent as once a month or less but may be so frequent as to occur several times a day, with each attack lasting minutes to several hours.

To exclude a diagnosis of pheochromocytoma, patients should have fractionated metanephrines and catecholamines measured by a 24-hour urine collection. This testing has both high sensitivity and specificity (98%) and results in few false-positive test results. If clinical suspicion is very high, the clinician could proceed directly to measuring plasma fractionated metanephrines (see Chapter 30).[18,19] In uncertain cases, measurement of plasma catecholamines should be reserved as a second-line test mainly because of its low specificity (85% to 89%), which falls to 77% in patients older than 60 years.[61] The high rate of false-positive test results from plasma measurements may result in unnecessary radiologic imaging and surgical procedures to locate the mass.

To avoid interference with the interpretation of urine catecholamine testing, tricyclic antidepressants should not be given. Initiation of antihypertensive agents is appropriate if needed for BP control. First-line agents include IV phentolamine, which achieves α-adrenergic blockade, or sodium nitroprusside. Administration of a β-blocker in isolation is contraindicated because β-blocker therapy can result in unopposed α-adrenergic vasoconstriction, which may result in further BP elevation. Nicardipine has been used as a second-line agent and, intraoperatively, is associated with low morbidity and mortality rates (see Chapter 30).[62]

SYMPATHOMIMETIC DRUGS

The effects of cocaine, amphetamines, phencyclidine hydrochloride (PCP), and lysergic acid diethylamide (LSD) are primarily the result of α-adrenergic stimulation. Cocaine use, in particular, results in increased myocardial oxygen demand because of increased heart rate and systemic arterial pressure and decreased myocardial oxygen supply as a result of vasoconstriction and accelerated atherosclerosis of the epicardial coronary arteries. Appropriate agents to aid in BP control include a direct vasodilator (phentolamine, nitroprusside, nitroglycerin) or a benzodiazepine.[63] The use of an α- and β-blocking agent, such as labetalol, may also be considered, especially in light of new evidence that β-blockers given to patients with cocaine-associated chest pain significantly, and safely, reduced SBP acutely, and maintenance β-blocker therapy reduced cardiovascular mortality rate by 71%.[64]

Patients receiving monoamine oxidase (MAO) inhibitor therapy who have consumed tyramine-containing foods—fermented cheeses, smoked or aged meats, avocados, alcoholic beverages—may also experience a hyperadrenergic state. The rise in BP is due to a decrease in intestinal tyramine metabolism and an increase in tyramine absorption. Elevated tyramine competes with tyrosine for transport across the blood-brain barrier. Once transported into synaptic vesicles, tyramine displaces norepinephrine into the extracellular space, resulting in a sympathetic surge and elevated BP. Selective MAO-B inhibitors, such as selegiline, and selective and reversible inhibitors of MAO-A, such as moclobemide, do not carry the risk of hypertensive crisis that results from consuming tyramine-containing foods.[65] Options for BP control, based on mechanism of action rather than clinical evidence, include phentolamine or nitroprusside.

AUTONOMIC DYSFUNCTION

Autonomic dysfunction that results from spinal cord injury, severe head injury, or Guillain-Barré syndrome is best controlled with phentolamine or sodium nitroprusside.

Pediatric Hypertensive Emergencies

Hypertension in children is defined as either an SBP or DBP in the 95th percentile or above, measured on three or more occasions. In a child, severe BP elevations (>99th percentile +5 mm Hg) accompanied by acute end organ damage constitute a hypertensive emergency, although this is rare in children and occurs in less than 1% of all emergency department visits.

Children who have preexisting hypertension as a result of chronic kidney disease are at a higher risk of hypertensive emergency, particularly if their BP is poorly controlled or if they are noncompliant with their antihypertensive management. Children who have no prior history of hypertension are at increased risk if they have a history of umbilical vein or artery catheterization, have a recent skin or upper respiratory infection (poststreptococcal glomerulonephritis), or are victims of domestic violence (traumatic brain injury leading to a hypertensive crisis). Adolescents at increased risk include those who abuse sympathomimetic drugs and pregnant teenage girls, who have the highest risk for preeclampsia and eclampsia. Evaluation and ancillary testing are similar to those of adults, with a focus on acute renal injury because the kidney is the most common organ to be affected in younger children. Unfortunately, no large published trials are available to evaluate hypertensive management in children. Nevertheless, the goals are the same as for adults: a 25% reduction in BP over the first 8 hours and control of life-threatening complications, such as seizures and respiratory failure as a result of

pulmonary edema. Labetalol, hydralazine, and nicardipine are commonly used agents for pediatric hypertensive emergencies.[66]

Obstetric Presentations: Preeclampsia and Eclampsia

Obstetric hypertensive emergencies are usually diagnosed at lower BP levels than hypertensive emergencies in nonpregnant patients. Preeclampsia and eclampsia should not be considered as separate disease states but rather as processes along a continuum. Patients with preeclampsia come to medical attention with elevated BP (SBP ≥140 mm Hg and DBP ≥90 mm Hg) and proteinuria (excretion of ≥0.3 g/day of protein), typically after the twentieth week of gestation. The majority of these women are normotensive prior to pregnancy. When preeclampsia is accompanied by new-onset grand mal seizures, the disease has progressed to eclampsia. Patients at higher risk for the development of preeclampsia and eclampsia include nonwhite, nulliparous women from low socioeconomic backgrounds. It is important to note that eclampsia can occur from 20 weeks of gestation to 8 weeks postpartum.[67]

The definitive treatment for both severe preeclampsia and eclampsia is delivery of the infant and placenta.[68] However, this may not be feasible because of fetal immaturity or maternal instability. Control of BP is required to prevent stroke, which accounts for 15% to 20% of deaths that result from eclampsia. Therapy should be initiated at an SBP of 150 mm Hg or greater and a DBP of 105 to 110 mm Hg or greater.[69] Magnesium sulfate is the standard therapy for prophylaxis and treatment of seizures and hypertensive encephalopathy in eclamptic patients, with a loading dosage of 4 to 6 g over 15 to 20 minutes. The goal is to prevent further seizures and the complications that can ensue, including maternal neuronal death, rhabdomyolysis, metabolic acidosis, respiratory infections, and respiratory failure. An additional benefit of antenatal magnesium sulfate therapy is that it appears to confer a neuroprotective benefit to the child; several studies demonstrate a decreased risk of cerebral palsy and severe motor dysfunction with this therapy.[70]

BP control can be achieved with either hydralazine or labetalol. Hydralazine is preferred (in 5- to 10-mg boluses q20min as needed) because of its long-standing safety record. Because its use may be accompanied by reflex tachycardia, labetalol (starting with a 10- to 20-mg bolus) may be used as an alternative first-line agent or to control the reflex tachycardia that results from hydralazine administration. Second-line agents include CCBs such as IV nicardipine. Data to support a specific target BP in these patients are limited. Ideally, mean arterial BP should not be reduced more than 25% over 2 hours, and the BP goal ranges between 130 to 150 mm Hg systolic and 80 to 100 mm Hg diastolic, as specified in current guidelines.[71]

Several antihypertensive agents are contraindicated in pregnancy. The ganglion-blocking agent trimethaphan increases the risk of meconium ileus. ACE inhibitors, angiotensin II receptor antagonists, and direct renin inhibitors should not be used because of the increased risk of fetal cardiac and renal abnormalities. Sodium nitroprusside should be avoided because of possible fetal cyanide toxicity, but it may be used as the agent of last resort. Because hypovolemia may be present in patients with pregnancy-induced hypertension, diuretics should be avoided (see Chapter 34).

Hemorrhage and Post–Vascular Surgery Presentations

Bleeding that does not respond to direct pressure and occurs in association with severe BP elevation can be a hypertensive emergency. Common bleeding sites are the nose, urinary tract, and surgical sites, especially in the post–vascular surgery patient. The bleeding is usually witnessed by the patient, which often induces substantial anxiety, thus contributing to the BP elevation.

Consequently, it may be wise both to lower the BP acutely and to provide judicious anxiolytic therapy.

In postoperative situations, particularly after coronary artery bypass graft (CABG) surgery or carotid endarterectomy, bleeding from vascular anastomoses is a significant concern. In the post-CABG patient, nitroglycerin is an effective and rational way to manage BP. Post–carotid endarterectomy patients frequently have labile BP that can last for days. One possible cause is disruption of the baroreceptor reflex from trauma or damage to the carotid sinus or vagus nerve during surgery. Hypertension in this period can lead to the *hyperperfusion syndrome* and neck hematoma, particularly in patients undergoing percutaneous stenting procedures. This hyperperfusion syndrome is seen in patients with high-grade carotid artery stenosis, especially with bilateral disease, presumably because of a maximal dilation of the arteries distal to the stenosis to maintain perfusion when autoregulatory mechanisms are lost. After the stenosis is relieved by surgery or stenting, there is hyperperfusion of that hemisphere, with increased risk of ICH and seizures.[72] In the largest series of carotid vascular repair reported so far, the incidence of hyperperfusion syndrome was about 1.5%, with complete neurologic recovery usually seen in less than 24 hours.[72]

Clevidipine, a third-generation dihydropyridine CCB, was specifically designed for the treatment of acute hypertension because it has a rapid onset and offset of action. It has been studied in post–vascular surgery patients, and when compared with nitroglycerin, sodium nitroprusside, and nicardipine, the composite safety endpoint of 30-day death, MI, stroke, or renal dysfunction did not differ among treatment groups. Clevidipine was more effective than nitroglycerin or sodium nitroprusside in maintaining BP control, and a trend toward lower mortality rate was seen in the clevidipine group in these studies.[73]

Follow-up and Prognosis

Patients with hypertensive emergency typically require several days of hospitalization to allow BP control and to transition to oral antihypertensive agents. Discharge planning should be focused on the prevention of recurrent episodes. For patients who come to the hospital in hypertensive crisis as a result of illicit drug use, counseling should be initiated during the hospitalization and ongoing counseling should be arranged. Nonadherence or abrupt withdrawal of medications should be carefully investigated because it is often due to several factors. Patients may stop medications because they can no longer afford them or because they no longer have access to a primary care physician because of a lack of medical insurance coverage. Health care providers should be sensitive to these issues and must familiarize themselves with medication costs. If finances are a concern and the patient requires combination therapy, multiple medications in lieu of a combination agent should be prescribed to lower out-of-pocket costs. Generic medications and low-cost 30-day supply medications should be used liberally.

All patients should have a follow-up appointment scheduled prior to hospital discharge. Those who have had frequent hypertensive crises and those who require complex antihypertensive regimens or additional secondary diagnostic evaluation should be referred to a hypertension specialist.

Few available data address patient outcomes after hypertensive crisis. In developing countries, in-hospital death rates for treated patients are as high as 45%.[74] Long-term prognosis is also lacking, and one study demonstrated a 60% mortality rate at 3 years. The most common causes of death are renal failure (40%), CVA (24%), MI (11%), and heart failure (10%).[75]

Caveats to Therapy in Hypertensive Emergency Care

- Prior to initiating antihypertensive therapy, establish the goals of therapy. Smaller titrations of medications may be considered,

especially in patients who come to medical attention with neurovascular syndromes, in which a slower BP reduction is preferable to a large and rapid reduction.
- In the acute setting, there is no role for "routine" administration of diuretics. Patients with a hypertensive emergency other than acute pulmonary edema tend to be volume depleted, and diuresis may exacerbate the BP elevation. Once effective BP reduction has been achieved, salt and water retention is often evident, which jeopardizes continued BP control. At that point diuretic therapy tends to be more rational and effective, which typically occurs after the first 24 to 48 hours of management.
- In patients who are seen with aortic dissection, rapid BP reduction is essential to decrease morbidity and mortality. In all other scenarios, a more conservative BP reduction is ideal.
- A key element in prevention of future episodes is adequate care and follow-up after hospitalization.

REFERENCES

1. Egan BM, Zhao Y, Axon RN. US trends in prevalence, awareness, treatment, and control of hypertension, 1988-2008. *JAMA* 2010;303(20):2043-2050.
2. Kearney PM, Whelton M, Reynolds K, et al. Global burden of hypertension: analysis of worldwide data. *Lancet* 2005;365:217-223.
3. Gudbrandsson T. Malignant hypertension: a clinical follow-up study with special reference to renal and cardiovascular function and immunogenetic factors. *Acta Med Scand* 1981;650(Suppl):1-62.
4. Chobanian AV, Bakris GL, Black HR, et al. Seventh report of the Joint National Committee on Prevention, Detection, Evaluation, and Treatment of High Blood Pressure. *Hypertension* 2003;42:1206-1252.
5. Karras DJ, Ufberg JW, Heilpern KL, et al. Elevated blood pressure in urban emergency department patients. *Acad Emerg Med* 2005;12:835-843.
6. Zampaglione B, Pascale C, Marchisio M, Cavallo-Perin P. Hypertensive urgencies and emergencies: prevalence and clinical presentation. *Hypertension* 1996;27(1):144-147.
7. Fryar CD, Hirsch R, Eberhardt MS, Yoon SS, Wright JD. Hypertension, high serum total cholesterol, and diabetes: racial and ethnic prevalence differences in U.S. adults, 1999-2006. *NCHS Data Brief* 2010;(36):1-8.
8. Saguner AM, Dür S, Perrig M, et al. Risk factors promoting hypertensive crises: evidence from a longitudinal study. *Am J Hypertens* 2010;23(7):775-780.
9. Tisdale JE, Huang MB, Borzak S. Risk factors for hypertensive crisis: importance of outpatient blood pressure control. *Fam Pract* 2004;21:420-424.
10. Van den Born BJ, Koopmans RP, Groeneveld JO, et al. Ethnic disparities in the incidence, presentation, and complications of malignant hypertension. *J Hypertens* 2006;24:2299-2304.
11. Beilin LJ, Goldby FS, Mohring J. High arterial pressure versus humoral factors in the pathogenesis of the vascular lesions of malignant hypertension. *Clin Sci Mol Med* 1977;52(2):111-117.
12. Sunder-Plassmann G, Kittler H, Eberle C, et al. Angiotensin converting enzyme DD genotype is associated with hypertension crisis. *Crit Care Med* 2002;30(10):2236-2241.
13. Shantsila A, Dwivedi G, Shantsila E, et al. Persistent macrovascular and microvascular dysfunction in patients with malignant hypertension. *Hypertension* 2011;57(3):490-496.
14. McBride BF, Karapanos AK, Krudysz A, et al. Electrocardiographic and hemodynamic effects of a multicomponent dietary supplement containing ephedra and caffeine: a randomized controlled trial. *JAMA* 2004;291(2):216-221.
15. Bui LT, Nguyen DT, Ambrose PJ. Blood pressure and heart rate effects following a single dose of bitter orange. *Ann Pharmacother* 2006;40(1):53-57.
16. Miettinen HE, Piippo K, Hannila-Handelberg T, et al. Licorice-induced hypertension and common variants of genes regulating renal sodium reabsorption. *Ann Med* 2010;42(6):465-474.
17. Fischbein NJ, Wijman CA. Nontraumatic intracranial hemorrhage. *Neuroimaging Clin N Am* 2010;20(4):469-492.
18. Kudva YC, Sawka AM, Young WF Jr. Clinical review 164: the laboratory diagnosis of adrenal pheochromocytoma—the Mayo Clinic experience. *J Clin Endocrinol Metab* 2003;88(10):4533-4539.
19. de Jong WH, Eisenhofer G, Post WJ, et al. Dietary influences on plasma and urinary metanephrines: implications for diagnosis of catecholamine-producing tumors. *J Clin Endocrinol Metab* 2009;94(8):2841-2849.
20. Sandset EC, Bath PM, Boysen G, et al.; SCAST Study Group. The angiotensin-receptor blocker candesartan for treatment of acute stroke (SCAST): a randomised, placebo-controlled, double-blind trial. *Lancet* 2011;377(9767):741-750.
21. Potter JF, Robinson TG, Ford GA, et al. Controlling hypertension and hypotension immediately post-stroke (CHHIPS): a randomised, placebo-controlled, double-blind pilot trial. *Lancet Neurol* 2009;8(1):48-56.
22. Adams HP Jr, del Zoppo G, Alberts MJ, et al. Guidelines for the early management of adults with ischemic stroke: a guideline from the American Heart Association/American Stroke Association Stroke Council, Clinical Cardiology Council, Cardiovascular Radiology and Intervention Council, and the Atherosclerotic Peripheral Vascular Disease and Quality of Care Outcomes in Research Interdisciplinary Working Groups: the American Academy of Neurology affirms the value of this guideline as an educational tool for neurologists. *Stroke* 2007;38(5):1655-1711.
23. van Paassen P, de Zeeuw D, de Jong PE, Navis G. Renin inhibition improves pressure natriuresis in essential hypertension. *J Am Soc Nephrol* 2000;11(10):1813-1818.
24. Rezkalla SH, Dharmashankar KC, Abdalrahman IB, Kloner RA. No-reflow phenomenon following percutaneous coronary intervention for acute myocardial infarction: incidence, outcome, and effect of pharmacologic therapy. *J Interv Cardiol* 2010;23(5):429-436.

25. Anderson JL, Adams CD, Antman EM, et al. ACC/AHA 2007 guidelines for the management of patients with unstable angina/non–ST-elevation myocardial infarction: a report of the American College of Cardiology/American Heart Association Task Force on Practice Guidelines (Writing Committee to Revise the 2002 Guidelines for the Management of Patients with Unstable Angina/Non–ST-Elevation Myocardial Infarction): developed in collaboration with the American College of Emergency Physicians, American College of Physicians, Society for Academic Emergency Medicine, Society for Cardiovascular Angiography and Interventions, and Society of Thoracic Surgeons. *J Am Coll Cardiol* 2007;50:e1-e157.

26. Nieminen MS, Böhm M, Cowie MR, et al.; ESC Committee for Practice Guideline (CPG). Executive summary of the guidelines on the diagnosis and treatment of acute heart failure: the Task Force on Acute Heart Failure of the European Society of Cardiology. *Eur Heart J* 2005;26(4):384-416.

27. Wagner F, Yeter R, Bisson S, Siniawski H, Hetzer R. Beneficial hemodynamic and renal effects of intravenous enalaprilat following coronary artery bypass surgery complicated by left ventricular dysfunction. *Crit Care Med* 2003;31(5):1421-1428.

28. Hirschl MM, Schreiber W, Woisetschläger C, Kaff A, Raab H. [Sublingual nitroglycerin or intravenous enalaprilat in preclinical treatement of hypertensive patients with pulmonary edema]. *Z Kardiol* (in German) 1999;88(3):208-214.

29. Peacock FW 4th, Varon J, Ebrahimi R, Dunbar L, Pollack CV Jr. Clevidipine for severe hypertension in acute heart failure: a VELOCITY trial analysis. *Congest Heart Fail* 2010;16(2):55-59.

30. Teerlink JR, Metra M, Felker GM, et al. Relaxin for the treatment of patients with acute heart failure (Pre-RELAX-AHF): a multicentre, randomised, placebo-controlled, parallel-group, dose-finding phase IIb study. *Lancet* 2009;373(9673):1429-1439.

31. Massie BM, O'Connor CM, Metra M, et al.; PROTECT Investigators and Committees. Rolofylline, an adenosine A1-receptor antagonist, in acute heart failure. *N Engl J Med* 2010;363(15):1419-1428.

32. Costanzo MR, Johannes RS, Pine M, et al. The safety of intravenous diuretics alone versus diuretics plus parenteral vasoactive therapies in hospitalized patients with acutely decompensated heart failure: a propensity score and instrumental variable analysis using the Acutely Decompensated Heart Failure National Registry (ADHERE) database. *Am Heart J* 2007;154(2):267-277.

33. Peacock WF, Emerman C, Costanzo MR, et al. Early vasoactive drugs improve heart failure outcomes. *Congest Heart Fail* 2009;15(6):256-264.

34. Mimoun L, Detaint D, Hamroun D, et al. Dissection in Marfan syndrome: the importance of the descending aorta. *Eur Heart J* 2011;32(4):443-449.

35. Wako E, LeDoux D, Mitsumori L, Aldea GS. The emerging epidemic of methamphetamine-induced aortic dissections. *J Card Surg* 2007;22(5):390-393.

36. Nienaber CA, Fattori R, Mehta RH, et al.; International Registry of Acute Aortic Dissection. Gender-related differences in acute aortic dissection. *Circulation* 2004;109(24):3014-3021.

37. Niclauss L, Delay D, von Segesser LK. Type A dissection in young patients. *Interact Cardiovasc Thorac Surg* 2011;12(2):194-198.

38. Kim KH, Moon IS, Park JS, Koh YB, Ahn H. Nicardipine hydrochloride injectable phase IV open-label clinical trial: study on the anti-hypertensive effect and safety of nicardipine for acute aortic dissection. *J Int Med Res* 2002;30(3):337-345.

39. Hagan PG, Nienaber CA, Isselbacher EM, et al. The International Registry of Acute Aortic Dissection (IRAD): new insights into an old disease. *JAMA* 2000;283(7):897-903.

40. Tsagakis K, Pacini D, Di Bartolomeo R, et al. Multicenter early experience with extended aortic repair in acute aortic dissection: is simultaneous descending stent grafting justified? *J Thorac Cardiovasc Surg* 2010;140(6 Suppl):S116-S120.

41. Castillo J, Leira R, García MM, et al. Blood pressure decrease during the acute phase of ischemic stroke is associated with brain injury and poor stroke outcome. *Stroke* 2004;35(2):520-526.

42. Oliveira-Filho J, Silva SC, Trabuco CC, et al. Detrimental effect of blood pressure reduction in the first 24 hours of acute stroke onset. *Neurology* 2003;61(8):1047-1051.

43. Keezer MR, Yu AY, Zhu B, Wolfson C, Côté R. Blood pressure and antihypertensive therapy as predictors of early outcome in acute ischemic stroke. *Cerebrovasc Dis* 2008;25(3):202-208.

44. Sare GM, Ali M, Shuaib A, Bath PM; VISTA Collaboration. Relationship between hyperacute blood pressure and outcome after ischemic stroke: data from the VISTA collaboration. *Stroke* 2009;40(6):2098-2103.

45. Yong M, Diener HC, Kaste M, Mau J. Characteristics of blood pressure profiles as predictors of long-term outcome after acute ischemic stroke. *Stroke* 2005;36(12):2619-2625.

46. Robinson TG, Potter JF, Ford GA, et al.; COSSACS Investigators. Effects of antihypertensive treatment after acute stroke in the Continue or Stop Post-Stroke Antihypertensives Collaborative Study (COSSACS): a prospective, randomised, open, blinded-endpoint trial. *Lancet Neurol* 2010;9(8):767-775.

47. Morgenstern LB, Hemphill JC 3rd, Anderson C, et al.; on behalf of the American Heart Association Stroke Council and Council on Cardiovascular Nursing. Guidelines for the Management of Spontaneous Intracerebral Hemorrhage. A Guideline for Healthcare Professionals From the American Heart Association/American Stroke Association. *Stroke* 2010;41(9):2108-2129.

48. Arima H, Anderson CS, Wang JG, et al.; Intensive Blood Pressure Reduction in Acute Cerebral Haemorrhage Trial investigators. Lower treatment blood pressure is associated with greatest reduction in hematoma growth after acute intracerebral hemorrhage. *Hypertension* 2010;56:852-858.

49. Bederson JB, Connolly ES Jr, Batjer HH, et al.; American Heart Association. Guidelines for the management of aneurysmal subarachnoid hemorrhage: a statement for healthcare professionals from a special writing group of the Stroke Council, American Heart Association. *Stroke* 2009;40(3):994-1025.

50. Allen GS, Ahn HS, Preziosi TJ, et al. Cerebral arterial spasm: a controlled trial of nimodipine in patients with subarachnoid hemorrhage. *N Engl J Med* 1983;308:619-624.

51. Gardner CJ, Lee K. Hyperperfusion syndromes: insight into the pathophysiology and treatment of hypertensive encephalopathy. *CNS Spectr* 2007;12(1):35-42.

52. Blumenfeld JD, Laragh JH. Management of hypertensive crises: the scientific basis for treatment decisions. *Am J Hypertens* 2001;14(11 Pt 1):1154-1167.

53. Delanty N, Vaughan CJ, French JA. Medical causes of seizures. *Lancet* 1998;352:383-390.

54. Curtis JJ, Luke RG, Dustan HP, et al. Remission of essential hypertension after renal transplantation. *N Engl J Med* 1983;27;309(17):1009-1015.

55. Ruggenenti P, Remuzzi G. Malignant vascular disease of the kidney: nature of the lesions, mediators of disease progression, and the case for bilateral nephrectomy. *Am J Kidney Dis* 1996;27(4):459-475.

56. Shavit L, Reinus C, Slotki I. Severe renal failure and microangiopathic hemolysis induced by malignant hypertension: case series and review of literature. *Clin Nephrol* 2010;73(2):147-152.

57. Bakir AA, Bazilinski N, Dunea G. Transient and sustained recovery from renal shutdown in accelerated hypertension. *Am J Med* 1986;80:172-176.

58. Shusterman NH, Elliott WJ, White WB. Fenoldopam, but not nitroprusside, improves renal function in severely hypertensive patients with impaired renal function. *Am J Med* 1993;95:161-168.

59. Teichert M, de Smet PA, Hofman A, Witteman JC, Stricker BH. Discontinuation of beta-blockers and the risk of myocardial infarction in the elderly. *Drug Saf* 2007;30(6):541-549.

60. Strong VE, Kennedy T, Al-Ahmadie H, et al. Prognostic indicators of malignancy in adrenal pheochromocytomas: clinical, histopathologic, and cell cycle/apoptosis gene expression analysis. *Surgery* 2008;143(6):759-768.

61. Sawka AM, Jaeschke R, Singh RJ, Young WF Jr. A comparison of biochemical tests for pheochromocytoma: measurement of fractionated plasma metanephrines compared with the combination of 24-hour urinary metanephrines and catecholamines. *J Clin Endocrinol Metab* 2003;88(2):553-558.

62. Lebuffe G, Dosseh ED, Tek G, et al. The effect of calcium channel blockers on outcome following the surgical treatment of phaeochromocytomas and paragangliomas. *Anaesthesia* 2005;60(5):439-444.

63. Baumann BM, Perrone J, Hornig SE, Shofer FS, Hollander JE. Randomized, double-blind, placebo-controlled trial of diazepam, nitroglycerin, or both for treatment of patients with potential cocaine-associated acute coronary syndromes. *Acad Emerg Med* 2000;7(8):878-885.

64. Rangel C, Shu RG, Lazar LD, et al. Beta-blockers for chest pain associated with recent cocaine use. *Arch Intern Med* 2010;170(10):874-879.

65. Yamada M, Yasuhara H. Clinical pharmacology of MAO inhibitors: safety and future. *Neurotoxicology* 2004;25(1-2):215-221.

66. Flynn JT, Tullus K. Severe hypertension in children and adolescents: pathophysiology and treatment. *Pediatr Nephrol* 2009;24(6):1101-1112.

67. Minnerup J, Kleffner I, Wersching H, et al. Late onset postpartum eclampsia: it is really never too late—a case of eclampsia 8 weeks after delivery. *Stroke Res Treat* 2010. pii:798616. Epub 2009 Sep 1.

68. Lucas MJ, Leveno KJ, Cunningham FG. A comparison of magnesium sulfate with phenytoin for the prevention of eclampsia. *N Engl J Med* 1995;333:201-205.

69. ACOG Practice bulletin no. 33: diagnosis and management of preeclampsia and eclampsia. *Obstet Gynecol* 2002;99(1):159-167.

70. Costantine MM, Weiner SJ. Eunice Kennedy Shriver National Institute of Child Health and Human Development Maternal–Fetal Medicine Units Network. Effects of antenatal exposure to magnesium sulfate on neuroprotection and mortality in preterm infants: a meta-analysis. *Obstet Gynecol* 2009;114(2 Pt 1):354-364.

71. Visintin C, Mugglestone MA, Almerie MQ, et al.; Guideline Development Group. Management of hypertensive disorders during pregnancy: summary of NICE guidance. *Br Med J* 2010;341:c2207.

72. Brantley HP, Kiessling JL, Milteer HB Jr, Mendelsohn FO. Hyperperfusion syndrome following carotid artery stenting: the largest single-operator series to date. *J Invasive Cardiol* 2009;21(1):27-30.

73. Aronson S, Dyke CM, Stierer KA, et al. The ECLIPSE trials: comparative studies of clevidipine to nitroglycerin, sodium nitroprusside, and nicardipine for acute hypertension treatment in cardiac surgery patients. *Anesth Analg* 2008;107(4):1110-1121.

74. Arodiwe EB, Ike SO, Nwokediuko SC. Case fatality among hypertension-related admissions in Enugu, Nigeria. *Niger J Clin Pract* 2009;12(2):153-156.

75. Lip GY, Beevers M, Beevers DG. Complications and survival of 315 patients with malignant-phase hypertension. *J Hypertens* 1995;13:915-924.

Hypertension in Pregnancy

Alice Wang, Ellen W. Seely, and S. Ananth Karumanchi

OVERVIEW, 521

EPIDEMIOLOGY AND RISK FACTORS, 521

PATHOPHYSIOLOGY, 521

Preeclampsia, 521
Chronic Hypertension, 523
Gestational Hypertension, 523

DIAGNOSIS, 523

TREATMENT, 524

Prevention, 524
Treatment of Hypertension in Pregnancy, 524
Acute Management of Severe Hypertension in Pregnancy, 525
Prevention and Management of Eclampsia, 525

IMPLICATIONS FOR LATER CARDIOVASCULAR
DISEASE, 525

CONCLUSIONS, 526

REFERENCES, 526

Overview

Hypertensive disorders during pregnancy are classified into four categories, as recommended by the National High Blood Pressure Education Program Working Group on High Blood Pressure in Pregnancy: 1) chronic hypertension, 2) preeclampsia-eclampsia, 3) preeclampsia superimposed on chronic hypertension, and 4) gestational hypertension.[1] *Chronic hypertension* is defined as blood pressure (BP) that exceeds 140/90 mm Hg before pregnancy or before 20 weeks' gestation. *Preeclampsia* is defined as the new onset of hypertension and proteinuria after 20 weeks' gestation.[2] *Gestational hypertension* is transient hypertension of pregnancy that is identified in the latter half of the pregnancy.

Epidemiology and Risk Factors

Hypertension complicates 7% to 10% of all pregnancies.[1] In women of childbearing age, the prevalence of chronic hypertension varies according to age, race, and body mass index (BMI). It was estimated that in the United States, from 1999 through 2004, 1% to 4% of women aged 18 to 29 years and 5% to 15% of women aged 30 to 39 years had chronic hypertension.[3] According to the U.S. Nationwide Inpatient Survey, 1.7% of pregnancies in 2004 were complicated by chronic hypertension.[4] Accurate estimates of the incidence of preeclampsia and gestational hypertension are more difficult to obtain because of the diagnostic variability in the classification of the diseases. Based on the incidence of preeclampsia and gestational hypertension in the control groups in large randomized clinical trials, the incidence of preeclampsia in the United States has been extrapolated to be between 3% and 6%, and the incidence of gestational hypertension is extrapolated to be 5% to 6%.[4,5] The incidence of preeclampsia is also subject to geographic variability because of differences in maternal characteristics, such as age at delivery.

Death from preeclampsia is grossly dissimilar among countries. In places where access to health care is limited, preeclampsia is a leading cause of maternal mortality, with estimates of more than 60,000 maternal deaths per year.[6] In developed countries, maternal lives are saved at the cost of premature delivery of the neonate.[7]

The risk factors for preeclampsia are varied (Table 33-1). Genetic factors are at least partially responsible, as both a maternal and paternal family history of the disease predisposes to preeclampsia.[8] A woman's risk for severe preeclampsia is increased twofold to fourfold if she has a first-degree relative with a history of preeclampsia.[9] There is a sevenfold risk of recurrence of preeclampsia for women who have had the condition in a previous pregnancy.[10] However, most cases of preeclampsia occur in healthy nulliparous women.[11] Associations between preeclampsia and nulliparity,[10] change in paternity from a previous pregnancy,[12] short or long interpregnancy interval (less than 2 years or more than 10 years),[13] use of barrier contraception,[14] and conception by intracytoplasmic sperm injection[15] implicate a possible immunogenic exposure to paternal antigen as a predisposing factor. Multiple gestation is an additional risk factor, and triplet gestation carries an even greater risk than twin gestation; this suggests that increased placental mass may also play a role.[10] Classic cardiovascular (CV) risk factors are also associated with an increased risk for preeclampsia; these include maternal age greater than 40 years, insulin resistance, obesity, systemic inflammation, and preexisting hypertension.[10,16-18] The increased prevalence of chronic hypertension and other comorbid medical illnesses in women older than 35 years may explain the increased frequency of preeclampsia among older women. Paradoxically, the only known factor associated with reduced risk for preeclampsia is cigarette smoking, which is directly associated with fetal growth restriction.[19]

Pathophysiology

Preeclampsia

The exact cause of preeclampsia is not known, but placental dysfunction is necessary for the development of the disease. Because delivery of the placenta is curative, preeclampsia is postulated to originate in the placenta[20] with subsequent widespread maternal endothelial dysfunction. Upon pathologic examination, placentas from women with severe preeclampsia usually have infarcts, atherosis, thrombosis, and signs of chronic inflammation.[21] In preeclampsia, the invasion of the cytotrophoblasts is incomplete, with cytotrophoblast cells present only in the superficial layers of the decidua.[22] The spiral arteries fail to be invaded or remodeled, resulting in high-resistance vessels. Decreased placental perfusion is reflected by abnormal uterine artery Doppler waveforms.[23]

In preeclampsia, placental antiangiogenic factors, specifically soluble fms-related tyrosine kinase 1 (sFlt-1), are upregulated and released into the circulation; these factors disrupt the maternal endothelium, resulting in hypertension, proteinuria, and other systemic manifestations of preeclampsia (Figure 33-1). Also, sFlt-1 is a truncated splice variant of the membrane-bound vascular endothelial growth factor (VEGF) receptor fms-related tyrosine kinase 1 (Flt-1), also called *VEGFR1*, and sFlt-1 acts by binding VEGF and placental growth factor (PlGF) in the circulation and preventing interaction with their endogenous receptors.[24] In addition, sFlt-1 antagonizes the stabilizing effect of VEGF on endothelial cells in mature blood vessels in the kidney, liver, and brain. Several investigators have confirmed that the increase in maternal circulating sFlt-1 precedes the onset of clinical disease[25-27] and is correlated with disease severity.[27,28] Animals given systemic exogenous sFlt-1 develop a preeclampsia-like syndrome that includes hypertension; proteinuria; and glomerular endotheliosis,[29] the pathognomonic renal lesion of preeclampsia, in which the endothelial cells of the glomerulus swell and endothelial fenestrations are lost.[30]

In addition to sFlt-1, other antiangiogenic factors, such as endostatin and soluble endoglin, are also altered in preeclampsia.[31] Soluble endoglin (sEng), a truncated form of endoglin (ENG)—a cell-surface receptor for transforming growth factor β1 (TGF-β1), which binds and antagonizes TGF-β1—is upregulated in preeclampsia. Levels of sEng are significantly increased in preeclamptic placentas.[32] As with sFlt-1, circulating sEng levels are elevated weeks prior to preeclampsia onset.[32] Soluble endoglin worsens the vascular damage mediated by sFlt-1 in pregnant animals, inducing a severe preeclampsia-like syndrome with features of the *hemolysis, elevated liver enzymes, low platelets* (HELLP) syndrome.[33] Overexpression of both sFlt-1 and sEng in rodents produces a phenotype that resembles reversible posterior leukoencephalopathy in

TABLE 33-1	Major Risk Factors for Preeclampsia
RISK FACTOR	**OR or RR (95% CI)**
Antiphospholipid antibody syndrome	9.7 (4.3-21.7)[10]
Renal disease	7.8 (2.2-28.2)[122]
Prior preeclampsia	7.2 (5.8-8.8)[10]
Nulliparity	5.4 (2.8-10.3)[123]
Chronic hypertension	3.8 (3.4-4.3)[124]
Diabetes mellitus	3.6 (2.5-5.0)[10]
High altitude	3.6 (1.1-11.9)[125]
Multiple gestations	3.5 (3.0-4.2)[126]
Strong family history of cardiovascular disease (heart disease or stroke in ≥2 first-degree relatives)	3.2 (1.4-7.7)[127]
Systemic lupus erythematosus	3.0 (2.7-3.3)[128]
Obesity	2.5 (1.7-3.7)[129]
Family history of preeclampsia in first-degree relative	2.3-2.6 (1.8-3.6)[8,9]
Advanced maternal age (>40 years)	1.68 (1.23-2.29) nulliparas 1.96 (1.34-2.87) multiparas[10]
Excessive gestational weight gain (>35 lb)	1.88 (1.74-2.04)[130]

CI, confidence interval; OR, odds ratio; RR, relative risk.
From Maynard SE, Karumanchi SA, Thadhani R. Hypertension and kidney disease in pregnancy. In Taal MW, Chertow GM, Marsden PA, et al, editors. *Brenner & Rector's the kidney*, ed 9, Philadelphia, 2002, Elsevier.

women with eclampsia and includes focal vasospasm, hypertension, and increased vascular permeability associated with brain edema.[34]

The renin-angiotensin-aldosterone axis is also affected in preeclampsia. Unlike normal pregnant women, whose vasculature demonstrates decreased responsiveness to vasoactive peptides such as angiotensin II and epinephrine, the vasculature in women who develop preeclampsia is hyperresponsive to these hormones.[35] Studies have identified agonistic angiotensin II type 1 (AT1) receptor autoantibodies in women with preeclampsia.[36] When AT1 receptor autoantibodies obtained from preeclamptic women are injected into pregnant mice, the mice develop hypertension and proteinuria and have increased levels of both sFlt-1 and sEng.[37]

Whether placental ischemia/hypoxia is a cause or consequence of preeclampsia is not clear. In pregnant primates and rats, surgical constriction of uterine blood flow[38,39] has been shown to induce hypertension and proteinuria. Women with preeclampsia and those residing at high altitudes share similar alterations in placental hypoxia-inducible factor (HIF) and HIF targets.[40] In populations living at high altitudes, the rates of preeclampsia are increased twofold to fourfold.[10] In vitro, primary trophoblast cells cultured from first-trimester placentas have upregulated expression and secretion of soluble Flt-1 protein when exposed to hypoxia.[41]

Because normal placentation requires the development of fetal immune tolerance by the mother, immune maladaption has been proposed as an explanation for the pathogenesis of preeclampsia. It has been observed that preeclampsia occurs more often in women during first pregnancies, in those using barrier contraceptive methods that reduce maternal exposure to paternal antigens in sperm,[14] after a change in paternity,[42] and after a long interpregnancy interval.[43] These observations suggest that in preeclampsia, there may be a disordered maternal immune response to paternally derived fetal antigens. Furthermore, immunocompromised women with untreated human immunodeficiency virus (HIV) have a very low incidence of preeclampsia. Once the immune system of a woman with HIV has been reconstituted after starting antiretroviral therapy, the risk of preeclampsia returns to that of the general population.[44]

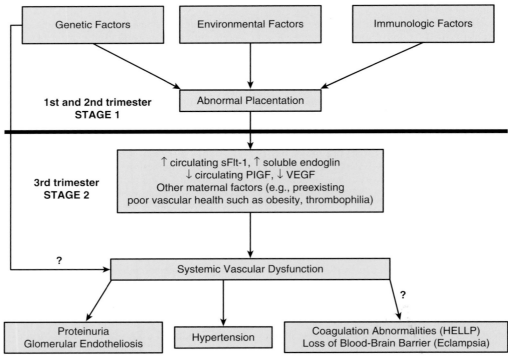

FIGURE 33-1 The pathogenesis of preeclampsia. HELLP, hemolysis, elevated liver enzymes, low platelets syndrome; PlGF, serum placental growth factor; sFlt-1, soluble fms-related tyrosine kinase 1; VEGF, vascular endothelial growth factor.

Placental oxidative stress, the excess production of damaging reactive oxygen species, is also thought to contribute to endothelial dysfunction in preeclampsia, as supported by several animal models and human trials.[45] In women with preeclampsia, increased circulating fetal DNA and syncytiotrophoblast debris are evident in the maternal circulation.[46-48] This proinflammatory debris consists of syncytiotrophoblast membrane microparticles and cytokeratin fragments. In preeclampsia, production of enzymatic antioxidants is decreased,[49-51] superoxide generation is increased,[52,53] placental levels of lipid peroxidation are higher,[54] and production and secretion of isoprostanes are increased.[54]

Chronic Hypertension

Chronic hypertension may be either essential (90%) or secondary to some identifiable underlying disorder, such as renal disease (polycystic kidneys, renal artery stenosis), endocrine disorders (adrenocorticosteroid or mineralocorticoid excess, pheochromocytoma), or coarctation of the aorta. The majority of women with uncomplicated chronic hypertension are expected to have successful pregnancies; however, these women are more likely to be hospitalized for hypertension and are more likely to undergo cesarean delivery.[55] Women with chronic hypertension have a threefold higher risk of placental abruption[56] and have a significantly higher risk of developing preeclampsia; 20% to 25% of women with chronic hypertension develop preeclampsia during pregnancy. Although superimposed preeclampsia may not be associated with worse perinatal outcomes compared with preeclampsia, superimposed preeclampsia has been associated with greater intervention-related events that include delivery at less than 34 weeks' gestation, cesarean delivery, and neonatal intensive care unit admission.[57]

Gestational Hypertension

Gestational hypertension refers to hypertension with onset in the latter part of pregnancy (>20 weeks' gestation) without proteinuria, followed by normalization of the BP postpartum. Of women who initially come to medical attention with apparent gestational hypertension, about one third progress to preeclampsia. Women with gestational hypertension usually have good pregnancy outcomes but may be at risk for chronic hypertension later in life.

Diagnosis

New-onset hypertension is diagnosed in a pregnant woman who was normotensive prior to 20 weeks' gestation as a systolic blood pressure (SBP) greater than 140 mm Hg and a diastolic blood pressure (DBP) greater than 90 mm Hg on two successive measurements 4 to 6 hours apart. *Proteinuria* is defined as 300 mg or more of protein in a 24-hour urine sample or 1+ dipstick proteinuria on two occasions at least 6 hours apart.[58] Determining whether elevated BP identified during pregnancy is due to chronic hypertension or preeclampsia can be a challenge, especially when no prior BP measurements are available. New-onset or worsening hypertension after 20 weeks' gestation should lead to a careful evaluation for other manifestations of preeclampsia. Criteria proposed by the National Institutes of Health (NIH) Working Group Report to help clarify chronic hypertension with superimposed preeclampsia include a significant increase in BP (30 mm Hg systolic, 15 mm Hg diastolic) in association with new-onset proteinuria and hyperuricemia or features of HELLP syndrome.[58]

Women with suspected or diagnosed preeclampsia should be hospitalized for careful evaluation. If severe hypertension or preeclampsia is diagnosed in the first or early second trimester, gestational trophoblastic disease and/or molar pregnancy should be excluded. Symptoms of preeclampsia include visual changes, headache, epigastric pain as a result of hepatic swelling and stretching of the liver capsule, edema, and rapid weight gain. Preeclampsia, a systemic vascular disorder, can affect multiple organs. Complications of preeclampsia that affect the developing fetus include iatrogenic prematurity,[59] fetal intrauterine growth restriction (IUGR), oligohydramnios, bronchopulmonary dysplasia,[60] and increased rate of perinatal mortality.[61] Maternal complications include placental abruption, seizures, intracerebral hemorrhage, pulmonary edema as a result of capillary leak or myocardial dysfunction, acute renal failure with proteinuria greater than 4 to 5 g/day, hepatic swelling, infarction or rupture, and disseminated intravascular coagulation. HELLP syndrome, a variant of preeclampsia, occurs in approximately 20% of women with severe preeclampsia.[62] Approximately 20% of women with HELLP syndrome develop disseminated intravascular coagulation, which carries a poor prognosis for both mother and fetus.[62] However, 10% to 15% of women who have HELLP syndrome have neither hypertension nor proteinuria.[63]

Perhaps the most frightening complication of preeclampsia is eclampsia, defined by the presence of seizures. In eclampsia, brain edema and pathologic vasoconstriction leads to the characteristic white matter changes of reversible posterior leukoencephalopathy syndrome (RPLS), also observed in hypertensive encephalopathy and with cytotoxic immunosuppressive therapies.[64] Pregnant patients who come to medical attention with seizures or severe headache may have RPLS diagnosed by computed tomography (CT) or magnetic resonance imaging (MRI) scans.[65]

Laboratory tests such as liver function tests, quantification of urine protein, and serum creatinine are helpful in the evaluation for preeclampsia and HELLP (Box 33-1). Usually low in pregnancy, uric acid is more likely to be in the upper nonpregnant range or elevated in women with preeclampsia; it has been used as a diagnostic aid and as a predictor of adverse outcomes in preeclampsia, but its predictive value is generally modest.[66,67] Urinalysis or spot urine specimens for protein/creatinine ratios may be used as a screen for proteinuria. Abnormal results should be quantified with a 24-hour urine collection when time permits. The normal range for protein excretion in pregnancy is up to 300 mg/day in a 24-hour urine collection. The degree of proteinuria in preeclampsia can vary widely and is a poor predictor of adverse maternal and fetal outcomes.[68] Elevated levels of hepatic transaminases may occur in the absence of epigastric or right upper quadrant pain. A complete blood count (CBC) and peripheral blood smear should also be obtained to rule out HELLP. Ultrasonography is often used to assess the status of the fetus, specifically for growth restriction and for evidence of impaired umbilical artery blood flow.

Currently, no single laboratory test can provide a reliable diagnosis of preeclampsia. Some women come to medical attention with so-called *atypical preeclampsia,* with neither hypertension nor proteinuria, and they progress to unexpectedly severe disease.[69] Measurement of circulating angiogenic protein ratios may help distinguish preeclampsia from hypertension or proteinuria from other causes, such as diabetes or systemic lupus erythematosus.[70,71] However, not all patients with preeclampsia have been reported to have altered sFlt-1 and PlGF.[72] It is unclear whether the subset of preeclamptic patients with low levels of sFlt-1 has an alternative,

---

> **Box 33-1 Laboratory Tests in the Evaluation of the Pregnant Hypertensive Patient**
>
> Twenty-four-hour urine protein or urinalysis or spot urine specimen for protein/creatinine ratio
> Complete blood count
> Blood chemistry levels:
> - Electrolytes
> - Blood urea nitrogen
> - Creatinine
> - Uric acid
> - Transaminases
> - Total protein
> - Calcium, magnesium
>
> Ultrasound/Doppler for evaluation of growth restriction

nonangiogenic form of the disease. Alternatively, women with underlying vascular disease may develop preeclamptic signs and symptoms at relatively lower levels of sFlt-1.[73] Future prospective studies and clinical trials will define how to best utilize these angiogenic proteins as clinical biomarkers.

Treatment

Prevention

Interventions that could prevent preeclampsia would revolutionize prenatal care. However, no such intervention has yet been identified. Prevention of disease may require a fuller understanding of the underlying etiology of the disease. Sodium restriction and/or diuretics were once popular strategies until a meta-analysis revealed no difference in the incidence of the disease as a result of these therapies.[74] Low-dose aspirin has been extensively studied for disease prevention. In multiple large randomized, placebo-controlled trials that included more than 30,000 women, administration of low-dose aspirin (60 to 100 mg/day) failed to reduce the incidence of preeclampsia in healthy nulliparous women or high-risk women.[5,75,76] However, a meta-analysis of 27 studies with more than 10,000 women found a significant reduction in preeclampsia, gestational hypertension, IUGR, and preterm birth with low-dose aspirin prophylaxis started at 16 weeks or earlier in those at moderate or high risk for preeclampsia.[77] A 2007 Cochrane meta-analysis of 59 trials with more than 37,000 women found a 17% reduction in risk of preeclampsia associated with use of antiplatelet agents, with a significant increase in absolute risk reduction in women at high risk for the disease (number needed to treat [NNT] = 19) compared with those at moderate risk (NNT = 119).[78] Because of the conflicting data from the large randomized studies and meta-analyses, the use of aspirin for the prevention of preeclampsia remains controversial.

A small trial explored the benefit of dietary supplementation with L-arginine, a precursor of nitric oxide, for 10 to 12 weeks in pregnant women with mild chronic hypertension and found no significant difference in maternal and neonatal complications, but it was associated with a reduced need for antihypertensive medications.[79] Supplementation with vitamin C or E during pregnancy also did not reduce the risk of preeclampsia in nulliparous women; neither did it decrease the risk of IUGR nor the risk of death or other serious outcomes in their infants.[80-82] Dietary calcium supplementation also failed to reduce the incidence of preeclampsia or improve fetal outcomes.[83] Because vitamin D deficiency may be a risk factor for preeclampsia,[84] vitamin D trials are currently under way. No effective therapies to prevent preeclampsia are available.

Treatment of Hypertension in Pregnancy

Although the greatest risk to the patient with chronic hypertension who becomes pregnant is development of superimposed pre-eclampsia, no evidence suggests that pharmacologic treatment of mild hypertension can reduce the incidence of preeclampsia. Pharmacologic treatment of mild hypertension in pregnant women merely increases the likelihood of IUGR[85]; therefore the threshold for initiating antihypertensive therapy is higher for pregnant women than for the general hypertensive population. When maternal BP exceeds 160/105 mm Hg, drug treatment is recommended.[58] DBP greater than 110 mm Hg has been associated with an increased risk of placental abruption and IUGR, and SBP greater than 160 mm Hg increases the risk of maternal intracerebral hemorrhage. Physicians should have a lower threshold for starting antihypertensive medication (>139/89 mm Hg) in women with preexisting end-organ damage from chronic hypertension, and they should establish a lower target BP.[86]

Very few large, randomized, controlled multicenter studies of antihypertensive therapy in pregnancy have been done. Recommendations for use of antihypertensive agents in pregnancy are summarized in Table 33-2. The central adrenergic inhibitor methyldopa remains a popular drug choice because of its long record of use and apparent safety, including evidence from a 7.5-year follow-up study of infants whose mothers had received the drug.[87] β-Adrenergic blocking agents have been associated with an increased incidence of fetal growth restriction in some studies. Many clinicians currently use labetalol, a combined α- and β-adrenergic blocker,[88,89] because it appears to have fewer adverse effects on fetal growth compared with atenolol or propanolol.[90] Also used as medication to inhibit labor, nifedipine is a long-acting oral calcium channel blocker used by many clinicians to titrate maternal BP. All major antihypertensive agents can be used cautiously,[91] with the exception of angiotensin-converting enzyme (ACE) inhibitors and angiotensin II receptor blockers (ARBs; both pregnancy category D), because they are associated with fetal

TABLE 33-2	Antihypertensive Medications in Pregnancy	
DRUG*	**ADVANTAGES**	**DISADVANTAGES**
Methyldopa (PO; B)	Extensive safety data	Short duration of action and bid or tid dosing
Labetalol (IV or PO; C)	Appears to be safe; labetalol is preferred over other β-blockers because of a theoretical beneficial effect of α-blockade on uteroplacental blood flow	Short duration of action and bid or tid dosing
Long-acting nifedipine (PO; C)	Appears to be safe; available in a slow-release preparation that allows once-daily dosing	
Hydralazine (PO or IV; C)	Extensive clinical experience	Increased risk of maternal hypotension and placental abruption when used acutely
Metoprolol (C)	Potential for once-daily dosing using long-acting formulation	Safety data less extensive than for labetalol
Generally Avoided		
Diuretics	No clear evidence of adverse fetal effects	May impair pregnancy-associated expansion in plasma volume
Atenolol		May impair fetal growth
Nitroprusside		Risk of fetal cyanide poisoning if used for >4 h
Contraindicated		
ACE inhibitors		Multiple fetal anomalies
Angiotensin receptor antagonists		Similar risks as ACE inhibitors

*FDA pregnancy use designations for the individual drugs are shown in parentheses.
ACE, angiotensin-converting enzyme; IV, intravenous; PO, oral.
From Maynard SE, Karumanchi SA, Thadhani R. Hypertension and kidney disease in pregnancy. In Taal MW, Chertow GM, Marsden PA, et al, editors. *Brenner & Rector's the kidney*, ed 9, Philadelphia, Elsevier.

renal dysgenesis or fetal death when used in the second and third trimesters and with increased risk of CV and central nervous system malformations when used in the first trimester.[92] Because of this association, women of childbearing age who are on ACE inhibitors or ARBs should be switched to another class of agent before conception when planning pregnancy. No clinical data are available on the use of renin inhibitors such as aliskerin (category D) during pregnancy.

Women who require antihypertensive medication after delivery may breastfeed. Although antihypertensive medications are excreted into breast milk, drug levels are low and are considered to confer low risk given the benefits of breastfeeding. The American Academy of Pediatrics considers most antihypertensive medications—including methyldopa, labetalol, captopril, diltiazem, verapamil, hydrochlorothiazide, and hydralazine—to be compatible with breastfeeding. Because of case reports of bradycardia in breast-fed infants whose mothers were taking atenolol, this agent should be used with caution in nursing mothers.[93]

Acute Management of Severe Hypertension in Pregnancy

The goal for acute treatment of severe hypertension in pregnancy should be the gradual lowering of SBP to less than 160 mm Hg and DBP to less than 105 mm Hg to prevent maternal cerebrovascular and CV complications while maintaining uteroplacental blood flow. Antihypertensive medications used during pregnancy are listed in Table 33-2. Intravenous hydralazine and labetalol and oral nifedipine are commonly used for the treatment of severe hypertension in pregnancy. A meta-analysis of 21 studies that compared hydralazine with labetalol or nifedipine for acute management of hypertension in pregnancy suggested an increased risk for maternal hypotension and oliguria, placental abruption, and lower Apgar scores with hydralazine.[94] Labetalol should not be given to women with asthma, congestive heart failure, or sympathetic crises related to the use of cocaine and/or amphetamines. Sodium nitroprusside should be avoided when possible because it can generate cyanide ions, which can reach toxic and potentially lethal levels for the fetus.[95]

Women with established preeclampsia must be observed very closely, either as an inpatient or as an outpatient, in a comprehensive home-monitoring program. Close fetal monitoring is essential to follow fetal growth rate and to monitor amniotic fluid levels. Depending on the gestational age and maternal status, early delivery should be considered for sustained maternal SBP greater than 160 mm Hg or DBP greater than 105 mm Hg. In addition, delivery should be considered if there is retinal edema or vasospasm and right upper quadrant tenderness. In severe maternal disease, delivery is often at the cost of fetal death. When preeclampsia develops early in the third trimester, attempts are often made to prolong the pregnancy to allow for further fetal growth and maturation with immediate delivery if either maternal or fetal deterioration should occur. When the pregnancy is near term, induction of labor is the therapy of choice, but when severe preeclampsia develops early in gestation, termination of pregnancy is considered. Curative therapy of preeclampsia requires delivery of the placenta.[96]

Prevention and Management of Eclampsia

Cerebrovascular complications, including stroke and cerebral hemorrhage, are responsible for the majority of eclampsia-related deaths.[97] When a mother has an eclamptic seizure, fetal bradycardia secondary to the transient hypoxic event is common but resolves with maintenance of the maternal airway and administration of oxygen. Women with severe preeclampsia or eclampsia are often treated with magnesium sulfate prophylaxis to prevent the development or recurrence of seizures.[96] Although magnesium sulfate is not given to treat hypertension, it is the therapy of choice to prevent recurrence of seizures and is superior to phenytoin or

diazepam in preventing eclampsia.[98-100] Until the introduction of magnesium sulfate therapy in the 1930s, nearly 30% of women with eclampsia died. Magnesium sulfate has a relatively wide margin of safety; however, it is helpful to monitor serum magnesium levels in patients receiving magnesium sulfate because respiratory depression may occur at levels in excess of 8 mEq/L. Magnesium is cleared almost exclusively by renal excretion, and women with renal insufficiency may develop hypermagnesemia. Women receiving magnesium sulfate should be monitored for respiratory depression, adequate urine output, and cardiac arrhythmias by electrocardiogram (ECG) for evidence of widened QRS or prolonged QT intervals. In addition, magnesium sulfate can interfere with uterine contractions, and many patients who receive magnesium sulfate require oxytocin (Pitocin) for augmentation of labor. Parenteral magnesium promptly crosses the placenta to achieve equilibrium in fetal serum, and the neonate may be depressed at birth if there is severe hypermagnesemia. It is also important to note that up to one third of eclampsia cases can occur postpartum, even up to 6 weeks after delivery.[101] Magnesium sulfate seizure prophylaxis is usually continued for at least 24 hours postpartum.

Implications for Later Cardiovascular Disease

Epidemiologic studies have shown possible long-term CV consequences for women who have new-onset hypertension in pregnancy. Within 7 years of a pregnancy complicated by preeclampsia, approximately 20% of the women will develop hypertension or microalbuminuria.[102] An average of 14 years after a pregnancy complicated by preeclampsia, more than 50% of women will have hypertension, three to four times the risk found in women without preeclampsia.[103] For both preeclampsia and gestational hypertension, the overall long-term risk of CV and cerebrovascular disease is twice that of age-matched controls.[104,105] Women who have had a history of preterm (<34 weeks) preeclampsia have even higher risk of death from cardiovascular disease (CVD), four to eight times the risk of women who had a normal pregnancy.[103,106,107] Severe preeclampsia, recurrent preeclampsia, preeclampsia with preterm birth, and preeclampsia with IUGR are most strongly associated with future adverse CV outcomes. Based on these and other data, the American Heart Association has recognized preeclampsia, gestational diabetes, and pregnancy-induced hypertension as risk factors for CVD in women.[108]

Many CV risk factors—chronic hypertension, diabetes, obesity, renal disease, and metabolic syndrome—are common to both preeclampsia and CVD. Approximately 50% of the elevated risk for future hypertension after preeclampsia can be explained by shared risk factors[109]; therefore pregnancy could be viewed as a physiologic stress test that may reveal a subclinical CVD phenotype.[110,111] However, an increase in long-term CV mortality is present even for healthy women with no prior CV risk factors who develop preeclampsia. Thus, preeclampsia may lead to subtle vascular damage or persistent endothelial dysfunction that may be associated with long-term CV risk.

The mechanisms that account for increased risk of CVD in women with a history of preeclampsia are not yet well understood. Some of the abnormalities observed in the setting of preeclampsia—or which precede its development, such as endothelial dysfunction, angiotensin II sensitivity, and elevations in antiangiogenic factors—have been shown to persist months to years after a preeclamptic pregnancy. Women with prior new-onset hypertension in pregnancy demonstrate increased sensitivity and increased pressor responsiveness to infused angiotensin II postpartum.[112] Markers of endothelial activation, including VCAM-1 and ICAM-1, appear to be elevated more than 15 years after pregnancy complicated by preeclampsia, independent of BMI and smoking status.[113]

Although levels of sFlt-1 decline after delivery of the placenta, a persistent antiangiogenic milieu may predispose women to CVD. Some studies have shown that levels of sFlt-1 are higher in women with a history of preeclampsia an average of 18 months postpartum, independent of BMI, BP, and smoking.[114-116] The source of sFlt-1 in nonpregnant women may be peripheral blood mononuclear cells, because monocytes in women with preeclampsia produce elevated levels of sFlt-1 compared with those from control subjects.[117,118] Persistent alterations in levels of antiangiogenic proteins may explain both the elevated CVD risk and the lower risk of malignancy[103] and higher risk of acquired hypothyroidism[119] in women with a history of preeclampsia. Patients with chronic kidney disease (CKD) or a history of myocardial infarction or stroke also have elevated levels of sFlt-1.[118] High sFlt-1 levels are also associated with carotid intima-media thickness and progression of atherosclerosis in hypertensive subjects.[120] Pulmonary and systemic vascular dysfunction have been recently described in young offspring of mothers with preeclampsia, but the mechanisms responsible for these phenotypes are unknown.[121]

Women with preeclampsia should have outpatient follow-up after hospital discharge to ensure normalization of BP and to assess biochemical abnormalities. As preeclampsia resolves with placenta delivery, antihypertensive therapy can usually be discontinued. Women with persistent hypertension require ongoing reassessment of BP and appropriate treatment. Although it is well established that women with a history of preeclampsia have a higher long-term risk of CVD, the independent contribution of preeclampsia to CVD remains unknown.[111]

Conclusions

Given both the short- and long-term morbidity as a result of hypertension in pregnancy, it is imperative that research to further our understanding of the pathogenesis of preeclampsia be undertaken. Antihypertensive medications do not modify the progression to preeclampsia; however, they do decrease the maternal risk for potential cerebral vascular events. Antiseizure prophylaxis with magnesium sulfate therapy is now the standard of care and is superior to phenytoin or diazepam in preventing recurrent seizures. For worsening preeclampsia, delivery of the placenta is the only cure. A history of prior preeclampsia or gestational hypertension, especially when associated with preterm delivery or fetal growth restriction, carries long-term CVD risk.

REFERENCES

1. Report of the National High Blood Pressure Education Program Working Group on High Blood Pressure in Pregnancy. *Am J Obstet Gynecol* 2000;183(1):S1-S22.
2. World Health Report: *Make Every Mother and Child Count.* 2005, Geneva, World Health Organization.
3. Cutler JA, Sorlie PD, Wolz M, et al. Trends in hypertension prevalence, awareness, treatment, and control rates in United States adults between 1988-1994 and 1999-2004. *Hypertension* 2008;52(5):818-827.
4. Wallis AB, Saftlas AF, Hsia J, Atrash HK. Secular trends in the rates of preeclampsia, eclampsia, and gestational hypertension, United States, 1987-2004. *Am J Hypertens* 2008;21(5):521-526.
5. Sibai BM, Caritis SN, Thom E, et al. Prevention of preeclampsia with low-dose aspirin in healthy, nulliparous pregnant women. The National Institute of Child Health and Human Development Network of Maternal-Fetal Medicine Units. *N Engl J Med* 1993;329(17):1213-1218.
6. MacKay AP, Berg CJ, Atrash HK. Pregnancy-related mortality from preeclampsia and eclampsia. *Obstet Gynecol* 2001;97(4):533-538.
7. Wang A, Rana S, Karumanchi SA. Preeclampsia: the role of angiogenic factors in its pathogenesis. *Physiology (Bethesda)* 2009;24:147-158.
8. Esplin MS, Fausett MB, Fraser A, et al. Paternal and maternal components of the predisposition to preeclampsia. *N Engl J Med* 2001;344(12):867-872.
9. Carr DB, Epplein M, Johnson CO, Easterling TR, Critchlow CW. A sister's risk: family history as a predictor of preeclampsia. *Am J Obstet Gynecol* 2005;193(3 Pt 2):965-972.
10. Duckitt K, Harrington D. Risk factors for pre-eclampsia at antenatal booking: systematic review of controlled studies. *Br Med J* 2005;330(7491):565.
11. World Health Organization survey. Royal College of Obstetricians and Gynaecologists Proceedings. 2003.
12. Tubbergen P, Lachmeijer AM, Althuisius SM, et al. Change in paternity: a risk factor for preeclampsia in multiparous women? *J Reprod Immunol* 1999;45(1):81-88.
13. Skjaerven R, Wilcox AJ, Lie RT. The interval between pregnancies and the risk of preeclampsia. *N Engl J Med* 2002;346(1):33-38.
14. Klonoff-Cohen HS, Savitz DA, Cefalo RC, McCann MF. An epidemiologic study of contraception and preeclampsia. *JAMA* 1989;262(22):3143-3147.
15. Wang JX, Knottnerus AM, Schuit G, et al. Surgically obtained sperm and risk of gestational hypertension and pre-eclampsia. *Lancet* 2002;359(9307):673-674.
16. Yogev Y, Chen R, Hod M, et al, for the HAPO Study Cooperative Research Group. Hyperglycemia and Adverse Pregnancy Outcome (HAPO) study: preeclampsia. *Am J Obstet Gynecol* 2010;202(3):255.e1-e7.
17. Wolf M, Kettyle E, Sandler L, et al, Obesity and preeclampsia: the potential role of inflammation. *Obstet Gynecol* 2001;98(5 Pt 1):757-762.
18. Conde-Agudelo A, Althabe F, Belizan JM, Kafury-Goeta AC. Cigarette smoking during pregnancy and risk of preeclampsia: a systematic review. *Am J Obstet Gynecol* 1999;181(4):1026-1035.
19. England LJ, Levine RJ, Qian C, et al. Smoking before pregnancy and risk of gestational hypertension and preeclampsia. *Am J Obstet Gynecol* 2002;186(5):1035-1040.
20. Matsuo K, Kooshesh S, Dinc M, et al. Late postpartum eclampsia: report of two cases managed by uterine curettage and review of the literature. *Am J Perinatol* 2007;24(4):257-266.
21. Salafia CM, Pezzullo JC, Lopez-Zeno JA, et al. Placental pathologic features of preterm preeclampsia. *Am J Obstet Gynecol* 1995;173(4):1097-1105.
22. Zhou Y, Damsky CH, Chiu K, Roberts JM, Fisher SJ. Preeclampsia is associated with abnormal expression of adhesion molecules by invasive cytotrophoblasts. *J Clin Invest* 1993;91(3):950-960.
23. North RA, Ferrier C, Long D, Townend K, Kincaid-Smith P. Uterine artery Doppler flow velocity waveforms in the second trimester for the prediction of preeclampsia and fetal growth retardation. *Obstet Gynecol* 1994;83(3):378-386.
24. Kendall RL, Thomas KA. Inhibition of vascular endothelial cell growth factor activity by an endogenously encoded soluble receptor. *Proc Natl Acad Sci U S A* 1993;90(22):10705-10709.
25. Sibai BM, Gordon T, Thom E, et al. Risk factors for preeclampsia in healthy nulliparous women: a prospective multicenter study. The National Institute of Child Health and Human Development Network of Maternal-Fetal Medicine Units. *Am J Obstet Gynecol* 1995;172(2 Pt 1):642-648.
26. McKeeman GC, Ardill JE, Caldwell CM, Hunter AJ, McClure N. Soluble vascular endothelial growth factor receptor-1 (sFlt-1) is increased throughout gestation in patients who have preeclampsia develop. *Am J Obstet Gynecol* 2004;191(4):1240-1246.
27. Levine RJ, Maynard SE, Qian C, et al. Circulating angiogenic factors and the risk of preeclampsia. *N Engl J Med* 2004;350(7):672-683.
28. Chaiworapongsa T, Romero R, Espinoza J, et al. Evidence supporting a role for blockade of the vascular endothelial growth factor system in the pathophysiology of preeclampsia. Young Investigator Award. *Am J Obstet Gynecol* 2004;190(6):1541-1547; discussion 1547-1550.
29. Conrad KP, Jeyabalan A, Danielson LA, Kerchner LJ, Novak J. Role of relaxin in maternal renal vasodilation of pregnancy. *Ann N Y Acad Sci* 2005;1041:147-154.
30. Stillman IE, Karumanchi SA. The glomerular injury of preeclampsia. *J Am Soc Nephrol* 2007;18(8):2281-2284.
31. Hirtenlehner K, Pollheimer J, Lichtenberger C, et al. Elevated serum concentrations of the angiogenesis inhibitor endostatin in preeclamptic women. *J Soc Gynecol Investig* 2003;10(7):412-417.
32. Levine RJ, Lam C, Qian C, et al. Soluble endoglin and other circulating antiangiogenic factors in preeclampsia. *N Engl J Med* 2006;355(10):992-1005.
33. Roque H, Paidas MJ, Funai EF, Kuczynski E, Lockwood CJ. Maternal thrombophilias are not associated with early pregnancy loss. *Thromb Haemost* 2004;91(2):290-295.
34. Maharaj AS, Walshe TE, Saint-Geniez M, et al. VEGF and TGF-beta are required for the maintenance of the choroid plexus and ependyma. *J Exp Med* 2008;205(2):491-501.
35. Gant NF, Daley GL, Chand S, Whalley PJ, MacDonald PC. A study of angiotensin II pressor response throughout primigravid pregnancy. *J Clin Invest* 1973;52(11):2682-2689.
36. Wallukat G, Homuth V, Fischer T, et al. Patients with preeclampsia develop agonistic autoantibodies against the angiotensin AT1 receptor. *J Clin Invest* 1999;103(7):945-952.
37. Zhou CC, Zhang Y, Irani RA, et al. Angiotensin receptor agonistic autoantibodies induce pre-eclampsia in pregnant mice. *Nat Med* 2008;14(8):855-862.
38. Makris A, Thornton C, Thompson J, et al. Uteroplacental ischemia results in proteinuric hypertension and elevated sFLT-1. *Kidney Int* 2007;71(10):977-984.
39. Granger JP, LaMarca BB, Cockrell K, et al. Reduced uterine perfusion pressure (RUPP) model for studying cardiovascular-renal dysfunction in response to placental ischemia. *Methods Mol Med* 2006;122:383-392.
40. Rajakumar A, Brandon HM, Daftary A, Ness R, Conrad KP. Evidence for the functional activity of hypoxia-inducible transcription factors overexpressed in preeclamptic placentae. *Placenta* 2004;25(10):763-769.
41. Nagamatsu T, Fujii T, Kusumi M, et al. Cytotrophoblasts up-regulate soluble fms-like tyrosine kinase-1 expression under reduced oxygen: an implication for the placental vascular development and the pathophysiology of preeclampsia. *Endocrinology* 2004;145(11):4838-4845.
42. Finnerty FA Jr, Buchholz JH, Guillaudeu RL. The blood volumes and plasma protein during levarterenol-induced hypertension. *J Clin Invest* 1958;37(3):425-429.
43. Baylis C. The mechanism of the increase in glomerular filtration rate in the twelve-day pregnant rat. *J Physiol* 1980;305:405-414.
44. Wimalasundera RC, Larbalestier N, Smith JH, et al. Pre-eclampsia, antiretroviral therapy, and immune reconstitution. *Lancet* 2002;360(9340):1152-1154.
45. Hladunewich MA, Derby GC, Lafayette RA, et al. Effect of L-arginine therapy on the glomerular injury of preeclampsia: a randomized controlled trial. *Obstet Gynecol* 2006;107(4):886-895.
46. Fiore G, Florio P, Micheli L, et al. Endothelin-1 triggers placental oxidative stress pathways: putative role in preeclampsia. *J Clin Endocrinol Metab* 2005;90(7):4205-4210.
47. Goodman RP, Killam AP, Brash AR, Branch RA. Prostacyclin production during pregnancy: comparison of production during normal pregnancy and pregnancy complicated by hypertension. *Am J Obstet Gynecol* 1982;142(7):817-822.
48. Fitzgerald DJ, Entman SS, Mulloy K, FitzGerald GA. Decreased prostacyclin biosynthesis preceding the clinical manifestation of pregnancy-induced hypertension. *Circulation* 1987;75(5):956-963.
49. Staff AC, Berge L, Haugen G, et al. Dietary supplementation with L-arginine or placebo in women with pre-eclampsia. *Acta Obstet Gynecol Scand* 2004;83(1):103-107.

50. Battistini B, Dussault P. The many aspects of endothelins in ischemia-reperfusion injury: emergence of a key mediator. *J Invest Surg* 1998;11(5):297-313.

51. Schiff E, Ben-Baruch G, Peleg E, et al. Immunoreactive circulating endothelin-1 in normal and hypertensive pregnancies. *Am J Obstet Gynecol* 1992;166(2):624-628.

52. Scalera F, Schlembach D, Beinder E. Production of vasoactive substances by human umbilical vein endothelial cells after incubation with serum from preeclamptic patients. *Eur J Obstet Gynecol Reprod Biol* 2001;99(2):172-178.

53. Greenberg SG, Baker RS, Yang D, Clark KE. Effects of continuous infusion of endothelin-1 in pregnant sheep. *Hypertension* 1997;30(6):1585-1590.

54. Walsh SW, Vaughan JE, Wang Y, Roberts LJ 2nd. Placental isoprostane is significantly increased in preeclampsia. *Faseb J* 2000;14(10):1289-1296.

55. Rey E, Couturier A. The prognosis of pregnancy in women with chronic hypertension. *Am J Obstet Gynecol* 1994;171(2):410-416.

56. Ananth CV, Savitz DA, Williams MA. Placental abruption and its association with hypertension and prolonged rupture of membranes: a methodologic review and meta-analysis. *Obstet Gynecol* 1996;88(2):309-318.

57. Tuuli MG, Rampersad R, Stamilio D, Macones G, Odibo AO. Perinatal outcomes in women with preeclampsia and superimposed preeclampsia: do they differ? *Am J Obstet Gynecol* 2011;204(6):508.

58. National High Blood Pressure Education Program Working Group Report on High Blood Pressure in Pregnancy. *Am J Obstet Gynecol* 1990;163(5 Pt 1):1691-1712.

59. Zhang J, Villar J, Sun W, et al. Blood pressure dynamics during pregnancy and spontaneous preterm birth. *Am J Obstet Gynecol* 2007;197(2):162, e1-e6.

60. Hansen AR, Barnes CM, Folkman J, McElrath TF. Maternal preeclampsia predicts the development of bronchopulmonary dysplasia. *J Pediatr* 2010;156(4):532-536.

61. Sibai B, Dekker G, Kupferminc M. Pre-eclampsia. *Lancet* 2005;365(9461):785-799.

62. Sibai BM, Ramadan MK, Usta I, et al. Maternal morbidity and mortality in 442 pregnancies with hemolysis, elevated liver enzymes, and low platelets (HELLP syndrome). *Am J Obstet Gynecol* 1993;169(4):1000-1006.

63. Sibai BM. Biomarker for hypertension-preeclampsia: are we close yet? *Am J Obstet Gynecol* 2007;197(1):1-2.

64. Hinchey J, Chaves C, Appignani B, et al. A reversible posterior leukoencephalopathy syndrome. *N Engl J Med* 1996;334(8):494-500.

65. Schwartz RB, Feske SK, Polak JF, et al. Preeclampsia-eclampsia: clinical and neuroradiographic correlates and insights into the pathogenesis of hypertensive encephalopathy. *Radiology* 2000;217(2):371-376.

66. Thangaratinam S, Ismail KM, Sharp S, Coomarasamy A, Khan KS. Accuracy of serum uric acid in predicting complications of pre-eclampsia: a systematic review. *BJOG* 2006;113(4):369-378.

67. Lim KH, Friedman SA, Ecker JL, Kao L, Kilpatrick SJ. The clinical utility of serum uric acid measurements in hypertensive diseases of pregnancy. *Am J Obstet Gynecol* 1998;178(5):1067-1071.

68. Thangaratinam S, Coomarasamy A, O'Mahony F, et al. Estimation of proteinuria as a predictor of complications of pre-eclampsia: a systematic review. *BMC Med* 2009; 7:10.

69. Sibai BM, Stella CL. Diagnosis and management of atypical preeclampsia-eclampsia. *Am J Obstet Gynecol* 2009;200(5):481, e1-e7.

70. Qazi U, Lam C, Karumanchi SA, Petri M. Soluble Fms-like tyrosine kinase associated with preeclampsia in pregnancy in systemic lupus erythematosus. *J Rheumatol* 2008; 35(4):631-634.

71. Cohen A, Lim KH, Lee Y, et al. Circulating levels of the antiangiogenic marker soluble FMS-like tyrosine kinase 1 are elevated in women with pregestational diabetes and preeclampsia: angiogenic markers in preeclampsia and preexisting diabetes. *Diabetes Care* 2007;30(2):375-377.

72. Powers RW, Roberts JM, Cooper KM, et al. Maternal serum soluble fms-like tyrosine kinase 1 concentrations are not increased in early pregnancy and decrease more slowly postpartum in women who develop preeclampsia. *Am J Obstet Gynecol* 2005;193(1):185-191.

73. Levine RJ, Qian C, Maynard SE, et al. Serum sFlt1 concentration during preeclampsia and mid trimester blood pressure in healthy nulliparous women. *Am J Obstet Gynecol* 2006;194(4):1034-1041.

74. Collins R, Yusuf S, Peto R. Overview of randomised trials of diuretics in pregnancy. *Br Med J (Clin Res Ed)* 1985;290(6461):17-23.

75. CLASP (Collaborative Low-dose Aspirin Study in Pregnancy) Collaborative Group. CLASP: a randomised trial of low-dose aspirin for the prevention and treatment of pre-eclampsia among 9364 pregnant women. *Lancet* 1994;343(8898):619-629.

76. Caritis S, Sibai B, Hauth J, et al. Low-dose aspirin to prevent preeclampsia in women at high risk. National Institute of Child Health and Human Development Network of Maternal-Fetal Medicine Units. *N Engl J Med* 1998;338(11):701-705.

77. Bujold E, Roberge S, Lacasse Y, et al. Prevention of preeclampsia and intrauterine growth restriction with aspirin started in early pregnancy: a meta-analysis. *Obstet Gynecol* 2010;116(2 Pt 1):402-414.

78. Duley L, Henderson-Smart DJ, Meher S, King JF. Antiplatelet agents for preventing pre-eclampsia and its complications. *Cochrane Database Syst Rev* 2007;(2):CD004659.

79. Neri I, Monari F, Sgarbi L, et al. L-arginine supplementation in women with chronic hypertension: impact on blood pressure and maternal and neonatal complications. *J Matern Fetal Neonatal Med* 2010;23(12):1456-1460.

80. Neithardt AB, Dooley SL, Borensztajn J. Prediction of 24-hour protein excretion in pregnancy with a single voided urine protein-to-creatinine ratio. *Am J Obstet Gynecol* 2002;186(5):883-886.

81. Briley AL, Poston L, Shennan AH. Vitamins C and E and the prevention of preeclampsia. *N Engl J Med* 2006;355(10):1065-1066; author reply 1066.

82. Poston L, Briley AL, Seed PT, Kelly FJ, Shennan AH. Vitamin C and vitamin E in pregnant women at risk for pre-eclampsia (VIP trial): randomised placebo-controlled trial. *Lancet* 2006;367(9517):1145-1154.

83. Levine RJ, Hauth JC, Curet LB, et al. Trial of calcium to prevent preeclampsia. *N Engl J Med* 1997;337(2):69-76.

84. Bodnar LM, Catov JM, Simhan HN, et al. Maternal vitamin D deficiency increases the risk of preeclampsia. *J Clin Endocrinol Metab* 2007;92(9):3517-3522.

85. Nakhai-Pour HR, Rey E, Bérard A. Antihypertensive medication use during pregnancy and the risk of major congenital malformations or small-for-gestational-age newborns. *Birth Defects Res B Dev Reprod Toxicol* 2010;89(2):147-154.

86. Magee LA, von Dadelszen P. The management of severe hypertension. *Semin Perinatol* 2009;33(3):138-142.

87. Cockburn J, Moar VA, Ounsted M, Redman CW. Final report of study on hypertension during pregnancy: the effects of specific treatment on the growth and development of the children. *Lancet* 1982;1(8273):647-649.

88. Villar J, Abalos E, Nardin JM, Merialdi M, Carroli G. Strategies to prevent and treat preeclampsia: evidence from randomized controlled trials. *Semin Nephrol* 2004;24(6):607-615.

89. Podymow T, August P, Umans JG. Antihypertensive therapy in pregnancy. *Semin Nephrol* 2004;24(6):616-625.

90. Lardoux H, Gerard J, Blazquez G, Chouty F, Flouvat B. Hypertension in pregnancy: evaluation of two beta blockers atenolol and labetalol. *Eur Heart J* 1983;4(Suppl G):35-40.

91. Abalos E, Duley L, Steyn DW, Henderson-Smart DJ. Antihypertensive drug therapy for mild to moderate hypertension during pregnancy. *Cochrane Database Syst Rev* 2007;(1):CD002252.

92. Cooper WO, Hernandez-Diaz S, Arbogast PG, et al. Major congenital malformations after first-trimester exposure to ACE inhibitors. *N Engl J Med* 2006;354(23):2443-2451.

93. American Academy of Pediatrics Committee on Drugs. Transfer of drugs and other chemicals into human milk. *Pediatrics* 2001;108(3):776-789.

94. Magee LA, Cham C, Waterman EJ, Ohlsson A, von Dadelszen P. Hydralazine for treatment of severe hypertension in pregnancy: meta-analysis. *Br Med J* 2003;327(7421):955-960.

95. Sass N, Itamoto CH, Silva MP, Torloni MR, Atallah AN. Does sodium nitroprusside kill babies? A systematic review. *Sao Paulo Med J* 2007;125(2):108-111.

96. ACOG practice bulletin. Diagnosis and management of preeclampsia and eclampsia. *Obstet Gynecol* 2002;99(1):159-167.

97. Sibai BM. Diagnosis, prevention, and management of eclampsia. *Obstet Gynecol* 2005;105(2):402-410.

98. Altman D, Carroli G, Duley L, et al. Do women with pre-eclampsia, and their babies, benefit from magnesium sulphate? The Magpie Trial: a randomised placebo-controlled trial. *Lancet* 2002;359(9321):1877-1890.

99. Duley L, Henderson-Smart D. Magnesium sulphate versus phenytoin for eclampsia. *Cochrane Database Syst Rev* 2003;(4):CD000128.

100. Lucas MJ, Leveno KJ, Cunningham FG. A comparison of magnesium sulfate with phenytoin for the prevention of eclampsia. *N Engl J Med* 1995;333(4):201-205.

101. Gorton E, Whitfield HN. Renal calculi in pregnancy. *Br J Urol* 1997;80(Suppl 1):4-9.

102. Lyons HA. Centrally acting hormones and respiration. *Pharmacol Ther B* 1976;2(4):743-751.

103. Bellamy L, Casas JP, Hingorani AD, Williams DJ. Pre-eclampsia and risk of cardiovascular disease and cancer in later life: systematic review and meta-analysis. *Br Med J* 2007;335(7627):974.

104. Buhling KJ, Elze L, Henrich W, et al. The usefulness of glycosuria and the influence of maternal blood pressure in screening for gestational diabetes. *Eur J Obstet Gynecol Reprod Biol* 2004;113(2):145-148.

105. Davison JM, Shiells EA, Philips PR, Lindheimer MD. Influence of humoral and volume factors on altered osmoregulation of normal human pregnancy. *Am J Physiol* 1990;258(4 Pt 2):F900-F907.

106. Lykke JA, Langhoff-Roos J, Sibai BM, et al. Hypertensive pregnancy disorders and subsequent cardiovascular morbidity and type 2 diabetes mellitus in the mother. *Hypertension* 2009;53(6):944-951.

107. Ray JG, Vermeulen MJ, Schull MJ, Redelmeier DA. Cardiovascular health after maternal placental syndromes (CHAMPS): population-based retrospective cohort study. *Lancet* 2005;366(9499):1797-1803.

108. Mosca L, Benjamin EJ, Berra K, et al. Effectiveness-based guidelines for the prevention of cardiovascular disease in women—2011 update: a guideline from the American Heart Association. *Circulation* 2011;123(11):1243-1262.

109. Romundstad PR, Magnussen EB, Smith GD, Vatten LJ. Hypertension in pregnancy and later cardiovascular risk: common antecedents? *Circulation* 2010;122(6):579-584.

110. Sattar N, Greer IA. Pregnancy complications and maternal cardiovascular risk: opportunities for intervention and screening? *Br Med J* 2002;325(7356):157-160.

111. Rich-Edwards JW, McElrath TF, Karumanchi SA, Seely EW. Breathing life into the lifecourse approach: pregnancy history and cardiovascular disease in women. *Hypertension* 2010;56(3):331-334.

112. Saxena AR, Karumanchi SA, Brown NJ, et al. Increased sensitivity to angiotensin II is present postpartum in women with a history of hypertensive pregnancy. *Hypertension* 2010;55(5):1239-1245.

113. Sattar N, Ramsay J, Crawford L, Cheyne H, Greer IA. Classic and novel risk factor parameters in women with a history of preeclampsia. *Hypertension* 2003;42(1):39-42.

114. Wolf M, Hubel CA, Lam C, et al. Preeclampsia and future cardiovascular disease: potential role of altered angiogenesis and insulin resistance. *J Clin Endocrinol Metab* 2004;89(12):6239-6243.

115. Germain AM, Romanik MC, Guerra I, et al. Endothelial dysfunction: a link among preeclampsia, recurrent pregnancy loss, and future cardiovascular events? *Hypertension* 2007;49(1):90-95.

116. Saxena AR, Karumanchi SA, Brown NJ, et al. Increased sensitivity to angiotensin II is present postpartum in women with a history of hypertensive pregnancy. *Hypertension* 2010;55(5):1239-1245.

117. Rajakumar A, Michael HM, Rajakumar PA, et al. Extra-placental expression of vascular endothelial growth factor receptor-1, (Flt-1) and soluble Flt-1 (sFlt-1), by peripheral blood mononuclear cells (PBMCs) in normotensive and preeclamptic pregnant women. *Placenta* 2005;26(7):563-573.

118. Di Marco GS, Reuter S, Hillebrand U, et al. The soluble VEGF receptor sFlt1 contributes to endothelial dysfunction in CKD. *J Am Soc Nephrol* 2009;20(10):2235-2245.

119. Levine RJ, Vatten LJ, Horowitz GL, et al. Pre-eclampsia, soluble fms-like tyrosine kinase 1, and the risk of reduced thyroid function: nested case-control and population based study. *Br Med J* 2009;339:b4336.

120. Shin S, Lee SH, Park S, et al. Soluble Fms-like tyrosine kinase-1 and the progression of carotid intima-media thickness. *Circ J* 2010:74(10):2211-2215.

121. Jayet PY, Rimoldi SF, Stuber T, et al. Pulmonary and systemic vascular dysfunction in young offspring of mothers with preeclampsia. *Circulation* 2010;122(5):488-494.

122. Mostello D, Catlin TK, Roman L, Holcomb WL Jr, Leet T. Preeclampsia in the parous woman: who is at risk? *Am J Obstet Gynecol* 2002;187(2):425-429.

123. Eskenazi B, Fenster L, Sidney S. A multivariate analysis of risk factors for preeclampsia. *JAMA* 1991;266(2):237-241.

124. Zetterstrom K, Lindeberg SN, Haglund B, Hanson U. Maternal complications in women with chronic hypertension: a population-based cohort study. *Acta Obstet Gynecol Scand* 2005;84(5):419-424.

125. Palmer SK, Moore LG, Young D, et al. Altered blood pressure course during normal pregnancy and increased preeclampsia at high altitude (3100 meters) in Colorado. *Am J Obstet Gynecol* 1999;180(5):1161-1168.

126. Krotz S, Fajardo J, Ghandi S, Patel A, Keith LG. Hypertensive disease in twin pregnancies: a review. *Twin Res* 2002;5(1):8-14.

127. Ness RB, Markovic N, Bass D, Harger G, Roberts JM. Family history of hypertension, heart disease, and stroke among women who develop hypertension in pregnancy. *Obstet Gynecol* 2003;102(6):1366-1371.

128. Clowse MEB, Jamison M, Myers E, James AH. A national study of the complications of lupus in pregnancy. *Am J Obstet Gynecol* 2008;199(2):127.

129. Weiss JL, Malone FD, Emig D, et al. Obesity, obstetric complications and cesarean delivery rate—a population-based screening study. *Am J Obstet Gynecol* 2004;190(4):1091-1097.

130. DeVader SR, Neeley HL, Myles TD, Leet TL. Evaluation of gestational weight gain guidelines for women with normal prepregnancy body mass index. *Obstet Gynecol* 2007;110(4):745-751.

CHAPTER 34

Management of Hypertension in Children and Adolescents

Joseph T. Flynn and Bonita E. Falkner

OVERVIEW, 529

DEFINITIONS OF HIGH BLOOD PRESSURE IN CHILDREN, 529

CONFIRMATION OF ELEVATED BLOOD PRESSURE, 529

PRIMARY VERSUS SECONDARY HYPERTENSION IN CHILDHOOD, 529

Approach to Therapy, 534

SUMMARY, 536

REFERENCES, 536

Overview

Hypertension may occur at any time during childhood, from the newborn period through adolescence. Because measurement of blood pressure (BP) in children during routine health care visits has become common practice, and as a result of the rising rates of childhood obesity, more cases of hypertension in the young are being identified. The prevalence of hypertension in asymptomatic children and adolescents is approximately 3.5%,[1,2] with higher rates of hypertension seen among obese children and adolescents; therefore hypertension is a common chronic health issue in childhood. Because secondary causes of hypertension can be detected more frequently in hypertensive children than in adults, the approach to evaluation of hypertension in the young differs from that in adults. Childhood hypertension also has some similarities to hypertension in adults. Children with primary, or essential, hypertension commonly have the same risk factors for cardiovascular (CV) disease as adults, and they can benefit from interventions to control BP. Clinical factors that are important in making treatment decisions regarding hypertensive children and adolescents include whether 1) the hypertension is primary or secondary to an underlying cause, 2) other CV risk factors or comorbidities are present, and 3) target organ damage is evident.

Definitions of High Blood Pressure in Children

The level of BP that is considered elevated in a child varies depending on age and body size. *Hypertension* is defined as an average systolic and/or diastolic BP at or above the 95th percentile for sex, age, and height on three or more occasions.[3] Reference BP levels in children at the various BP percentiles are provided in Tables 34-1 and 34-2. In young people 18 years or older, recommendations of the Joint National Committee on Prevention, Detection, Evaluation, and Treatment of High Blood Pressure (JNC) should be followed; it defines *hypertension* as a BP reading above 140/90 mm Hg on two or more office visits.[4]

Prehypertension in children is defined as average systolic and/or diastolic BP at or above the 90th percentile and below the 95th percentile for sex, age, and height; *normal* BP is defined as average BP below the 90th percentile. The definition of *prehypertension* is the same in adolescents as in adults, namely a BP reading above 120/80 mm Hg. This is because by 12 years of age in both boys and girls, the 90th percentile for systolic and diastolic BP is above the adult prehypertension threshold of 120/80 mm Hg.[3] For all children and adolescents, the severity of hypertension should be staged once an individual is diagnosed with hypertension (Table 34-3). Staging the severity of hypertension is helpful in guiding subsequent evaluation and management. Figure 34-1 provides an algorithm that outlines recommended BP monitoring, evaluation, and management for children with prehypertension and hypertension with and without obesity.

Confirmation of Elevated Blood Pressure

BP in childhood is more labile than in adulthood, and even children with secondary causes of hypertension demonstrate significant variability in office BP readings. In addition, the phenomenon of regression to the mean is commonly observed. Thus, it is crucial to confirm that the child's BP is truly elevated before making the diagnosis of hypertension, embarking on a diagnostic evaluation, or considering pharmacologic therapy. A first step in verifying the diagnosis of hypertension is to ensure that BP is being measured correctly. The National High Blood Pressure Education Program Working Group recommends auscultation as the preferred method of BP measurement in the young; the organization has specifically stated that elevated readings obtained with oscillometric devices should be repeated by auscultation.[3] Data from pediatric hypertension clinics demonstrate that BP readings obtained with oscillometric devices are frequently not consistent with BP measurements obtained by auscultation,[5] confirming the recommendations of the Working Group. In children the BP cuff size must be appropriate for the size of the child to ensure an accurate reading. The bladder of the cuff should encircle 80% to 100% of the arm circumference, or else the reading may be falsely elevated. Concurrent with the childhood obesity epidemic, arm sizes of children have increased, so that more adolescents will require use of a large adult or thigh cuff to obtain an accurate BP reading.[6] Even children referred for evaluation of suspected hypertension should have additional office BP measurements to verify the diagnosis.[7] Ambulatory BP monitoring (ABPM) is very useful for confirmation of hypertension and to identify patients with "white coat" hypertension.[8]

Primary Versus Secondary Hypertension in Childhood

Young children are more likely to have secondary hypertension, whereas in adolescents, primary hypertension accounts for the majority of cases.[9] Renal diseases are the most frequent causes of secondary hypertension in asymptomatic children. In children and adolescents with primary hypertension, the prevalence of a family history of hypertension has been reported to be in excess of 80%.[9] Obesity is more common among pediatric patients with primary hypertension than among those with secondary hypertension, and it is associated with an earlier age of onset of hypertension independent of family history.[10]

Evaluation of the hypertensive child or adolescent begins with a comprehensive medical history and physical examination. Table 34-4 lists history and physical exam findings suggestive of secondary hypertension in children. The history should include questions about over-the-counter, prescription, and illicit drug use because many substances commonly used by adolescents can cause or exacerbate hypertension and complicate treatment. Examples of these substances are listed in Table 34-5.

Text continued on page 533

TABLE 34-1   Systolic BP Levels for Boys by Age and Height Percentile

AGE (Y)	BP PERCENTILE	SYSTOLIC BP (MM HG) PERCENTILE OF HEIGHT							DIASTOLIC BP (MM HG) PERCENTILE OF HEIGHT						
		5TH	10TH	25TH	50TH	75TH	90TH	95TH	5TH	10TH	25TH	50TH	75TH	90TH	95TH
1	50th	80	81	83	85	87	88	89	34	35	36	37	38	39	39
	90th	94	95	97	99	100	102	103	49	50	51	52	53	53	54
	95th	98	99	101	103	104	106	106	54	54	55	56	57	58	58
	99th	105	106	108	110	112	113	114	61	62	63	64	65	66	66
2	50th	84	85	87	88	90	92	92	39	40	41	42	43	44	44
	90th	97	99	100	102	104	105	106	54	55	56	57	58	58	59
	95th	101	102	104	106	108	109	110	59	59	60	61	62	63	63
	99th	109	110	111	113	115	117	117	66	67	68	69	70	71	71
3	50th	86	87	89	91	93	94	95	44	44	45	46	47	48	48
	90th	100	101	103	105	107	108	109	59	59	60	61	62	63	63
	95th	104	105	107	109	110	112	113	63	63	64	65	66	67	67
	99th	111	112	114	116	118	119	120	71	71	72	73	74	75	75
4	50th	88	89	91	93	95	96	97	47	48	49	50	51	51	52
	90th	102	103	105	107	109	110	111	62	63	64	65	66	66	67
	95th	106	107	109	111	112	114	115	66	67	68	69	70	71	71
	99th	113	114	116	118	120	121	122	74	75	76	77	78	78	79
5	50th	90	91	93	95	96	98	98	50	51	52	53	54	55	55
	90th	104	105	106	108	110	111	112	65	66	67	68	69	69	70
	95th	108	109	110	112	114	115	116	69	70	71	72	73	74	74
	99th	115	116	118	120	121	123	123	77	78	79	80	81	81	82
6	50th	91	92	94	96	98	99	100	53	53	54	55	56	57	57
	90th	105	106	108	110	111	113	113	68	68	69	70	71	72	72
	95th	109	110	112	114	115	117	117	72	72	73	74	75	76	76
	99th	116	117	119	121	123	124	125	80	80	81	82	83	84	84
7	50th	92	94	95	97	99	100	101	55	55	56	57	58	59	59
	90th	106	107	109	111	113	114	115	70	70	71	72	73	74	74
	95th	110	111	113	115	117	118	119	74	74	75	76	77	78	78
	99th	117	118	120	122	124	125	126	82	82	83	84	85	86	86
8	50th	94	95	97	99	100	102	102	56	57	58	59	60	60	61
	90th	107	109	110	112	114	115	116	71	72	72	73	74	75	76
	95th	111	112	114	116	118	119	120	75	76	77	78	79	79	80
	99th	119	120	122	123	125	127	127	83	84	85	86	87	87	88
9	50th	95	96	98	100	102	103	104	57	58	59	60	61	61	62
	90th	109	110	112	114	115	117	118	72	73	74	75	76	76	77
	95th	113	114	116	118	119	121	121	76	77	78	79	80	81	81
	99th	120	121	123	125	127	128	129	84	85	86	87	88	88	89
10	50th	97	98	100	102	103	105	106	58	59	60	61	61	62	63
	90th	111	112	114	115	117	119	119	73	73	74	75	76	77	78
	95th	115	116	117	119	121	122	123	77	78	79	80	81	81	82
	99th	122	123	125	127	128	130	130	85	86	86	88	88	89	90
11	50th	99	100	102	104	105	107	107	59	59	60	61	62	63	63
	90th	113	114	115	117	119	120	121	74	74	75	76	77	78	78
	95th	117	118	119	121	123	124	125	78	78	79	80	81	82	82
	99th	124	125	127	129	130	132	132	86	86	87	88	89	90	90
12	50th	101	102	104	106	108	109	110	59	60	61	62	63	63	64
	90th	115	116	118	120	121	123	123	74	75	75	76	77	78	79
	95th	119	120	122	123	125	127	127	78	79	80	81	82	82	83
	99th	126	127	129	131	133	134	135	86	87	88	89	90	90	91
13	50th	104	105	106	108	110	111	112	60	60	61	62	63	64	64
	90th	117	118	120	122	124	125	126	75	75	76	77	78	79	79
	95th	121	122	124	126	128	129	130	79	79	80	81	82	83	83
	99th	128	130	131	133	135	136	137	87	87	88	89	90	91	91
14	50th	106	107	109	111	113	114	115	60	61	62	63	64	65	65
	90th	120	121	123	125	126	128	128	75	76	77	78	79	79	80
	95th	124	125	127	128	130	132	132	80	80	81	82	83	84	84
	99th	131	132	134	136	138	139	140	87	88	89	90	91	92	92
15	50th	109	110	112	113	115	117	117	61	62	63	64	65	66	66
	90th	122	124	125	127	129	130	131	76	77	78	79	80	80	81
	95th	126	127	129	131	133	134	135	81	81	82	83	84	85	85
	99th	134	135	136	138	140	142	142	88	89	90	91	92	93	93

Continued

TABLE 34-1   Systolic BP Levels for Boys by Age and Height Percentile—cont'd

AGE (Y)	BP PERCENTILE	SYSTOLIC BP (MM HG) PERCENTILE OF HEIGHT							DIASTOLIC BP (MM HG) PERCENTILE OF HEIGHT						
		5TH	10TH	25TH	50TH	75TH	90TH	95TH	5TH	10TH	25TH	50TH	75TH	90TH	95TH
16	50th	111	112	114	116	118	119	120	63	63	64	65	66	67	67
	90th	125	126	128	130	131	133	134	78	78	79	80	81	82	82
	95th	129	130	132	134	135	137	137	82	83	83	84	85	86	87
	99th	136	137	139	141	143	144	145	90	90	91	92	93	94	94
17	50th	114	115	116	118	120	121	122	65	66	66	67	68	69	70
	90th	127	128	130	132	134	135	136	80	80	81	82	83	84	84
	95th	131	132	134	136	138	139	140	84	85	86	87	87	88	89
	99th	139	140	141	143	145	146	147	92	93	93	94	95	96	97

BP, blood pressure.

TABLE 34-2   Systolic BP Levels for Girls by Age and Height Percentile

AGE (Y)	BP PERCENTILE	SYSTOLIC BP (MM HG) PERCENTILE OF HEIGHT							DIASTOLIC BP (MM HG) PERCENTILE OF HEIGHT						
		5TH	10TH	25TH	50TH	75TH	90TH	95TH	5TH	10TH	25TH	50TH	75TH	90TH	95TH
1	50th	83	84	85	86	88	89	90	38	39	39	40	41	41	42
	90th	97	97	98	100	101	102	103	52	53	53	54	55	55	56
	95th	100	101	102	104	105	106	107	56	57	57	58	59	59	60
	99th	108	108	109	111	112	113	114	64	64	65	65	66	67	67
2	50th	85	85	87	88	89	91	91	43	44	44	45	46	46	47
	90th	98	99	100	101	103	104	105	57	58	58	59	60	61	61
	95th	102	103	104	105	107	108	109	61	62	62	63	64	65	65
	99th	109	110	111	112	114	115	116	69	69	70	70	71	72	72
3	50th	86	87	88	89	91	92	93	47	48	48	49	50	50	51
	90th	100	100	102	103	104	106	106	61	62	62	63	64	64	65
	95th	104	104	105	107	108	109	110	65	66	66	67	68	68	69
	99th	111	111	113	114	115	116	117	73	73	74	74	75	76	76
4	50th	88	88	90	91	92	94	94	50	50	51	52	52	53	54
	90th	101	102	103	104	106	107	108	64	64	65	66	67	67	68
	95th	105	106	107	108	110	111	112	68	68	69	70	71	71	72
	99th	112	113	114	115	117	118	119	76	76	76	77	78	79	79
5	50th	89	90	91	93	94	95	96	52	53	53	54	55	55	56
	90th	103	103	105	106	107	109	109	66	67	67	68	69	69	70
	95th	107	107	108	110	111	112	113	70	71	71	72	73	73	74
	99th	114	114	116	117	118	120	120	78	78	79	79	80	81	81
6	50th	91	92	93	94	96	97	98	54	54	55	56	56	57	58
	90th	104	105	106	108	109	110	111	68	68	69	70	70	71	72
	95th	108	109	110	111	113	114	115	72	72	73	74	74	75	76
	99th	115	116	117	119	120	121	122	80	80	80	81	82	83	83
7	50th	93	93	95	96	97	99	99	55	56	56	57	58	58	59
	90th	106	107	108	109	111	112	113	69	70	70	71	72	72	73
	95th	110	111	112	113	115	116	116	73	74	74	75	76	76	77
	99th	117	118	119	120	122	123	124	81	81	82	82	83	84	84
8	50th	95	95	96	98	99	100	101	57	57	57	58	59	60	60
	90th	108	109	110	111	113	114	114	71	71	71	72	73	74	74
	95th	112	112	114	115	116	118	118	75	75	75	76	77	78	78
	99th	119	120	121	122	123	125	125	82	82	83	83	84	85	86
9	50th	96	97	98	100	101	102	103	58	58	58	59	60	61	61
	90th	110	110	112	113	114	116	116	72	72	72	73	74	75	75
	95th	114	114	115	117	118	119	120	76	76	76	77	78	79	79
	99th	121	121	123	124	125	127	127	83	83	84	84	85	86	87
10	50th	98	99	100	102	103	104	105	59	59	59	60	61	62	62
	90th	112	112	114	115	116	118	118	73	73	73	74	75	76	76
	95th	116	116	117	119	120	121	122	77	77	77	78	79	80	80
	99th	123	123	125	126	127	129	129	84	84	85	86	86	87	88
11	50th	100	101	102	103	105	106	107	60	60	60	61	62	63	63
	90th	114	114	116	117	118	119	120	74	74	74	75	76	77	77
	95th	118	118	119	121	122	123	124	78	78	78	79	80	81	81
	99th	125	125	126	128	129	130	131	85	85	86	87	87	88	89

Continued

TABLE 34-2   Systolic BP Levels for Girls by Age and Height Percentile—cont'd

AGE (Y)	BP PERCENTILE	SYSTOLIC BP (MM HG) PERCENTILE OF HEIGHT							DIASTOLIC BP (MM HG) PERCENTILE OF HEIGHT						
		5TH	10TH	25TH	50TH	75TH	90TH	95TH	5TH	10TH	25TH	50TH	75TH	90TH	95TH
12	50th	102	103	104	105	107	108	109	61	61	61	62	63	64	64
	90th	116	116	117	119	120	121	122	75	75	75	76	77	78	78
	95th	119	120	121	123	124	125	126	79	79	79	80	81	82	82
	99th	127	127	128	130	131	132	133	86	86	87	88	88	89	90
13	50th	104	105	106	107	109	110	110	62	62	62	63	64	65	65
	90th	117	118	119	121	122	123	124	76	76	76	77	78	79	79
	95th	121	122	123	124	126	127	128	80	80	80	81	82	83	83
	99th	128	129	130	132	133	134	135	87	87	88	89	89	90	91
14	50th	106	106	107	109	110	111	112	63	63	63	64	65	66	66
	90th	119	120	121	122	124	125	125	77	77	77	78	79	80	80
	95th	123	123	125	126	127	129	129	81	81	81	82	83	84	84
	99th	130	131	132	133	135	136	136	88	88	89	90	90	91	92
15	50th	107	108	109	110	111	113	113	64	64	64	65	66	67	67
	90th	120	121	122	123	125	126	127	78	78	78	79	80	81	81
	95th	124	125	126	127	129	130	131	82	82	82	83	84	85	85
	99th	131	132	133	134	136	137	138	89	89	90	91	91	92	93
16	50th	108	108	110	111	112	114	114	64	64	65	66	66	67	68
	90th	121	122	123	124	126	127	128	78	78	79	80	81	81	82
	95th	125	126	127	128	130	131	132	82	82	83	84	85	85	86
	99th	132	133	134	135	137	138	139	90	90	90	91	92	93	93
17	50th	108	109	110	111	113	114	115	64	65	65	66	67	67	68
	90th	122	122	123	125	126	127	128	78	79	79	80	81	81	82
	95th	125	126	127	129	130	131	132	82	83	83	84	85	85	86
	99th	133	133	134	136	137	138	139	90	90	91	91	92	93	93

BP, blood pressure.

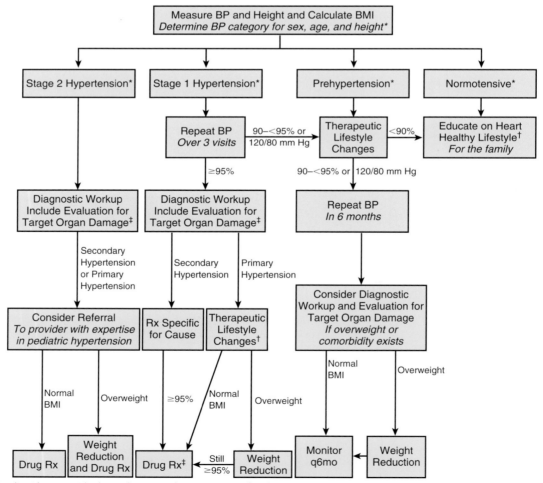

FIGURE 34-1   An algorithm to guide the evaluation and management of prehypertension and stage 1 and stage 2 hypertension. *See Tables 34-1 to 34-5 for blood pressure classification. †Diet modification and physical activity. ‡Children and adolescents with stage 1 and 2 hypertension should receive an echocardiogram to evaluate for target organ damage. Also consider an echocardiogram in children with diabetes or other risk factors. BMI, body mass index; BP, blood pressure; Rx, treatment.

TABLE 34-3 Classification of Hypertension in Pediatric Patients

BLOOD PRESSURE CLASSIFICATION	CHILDREN AND ADOLESCENTS <18 YEARS	ADOLESCENTS ≥18 YEARS
Normal	SBP and DBP <90th percentile	SBP <120 mm Hg and DBP <80 mm Hg
Prehypertension	SBP or DBP 90th to 95th percentile or BP >120/80 even if <90th percentile	SBP 120 to 139 mm Hg or DBP 80 to 89 mm Hg
Stage 1 hypertension	SBP or DBP ≥95th to 99th percentile + 5 mm Hg	SBP 140 to 159 mm Hg or DBP 90 to 99 mm Hg
Stage 2 hypertension	SBP or DBP >99th percentile + 5 mm Hg	SBP ≥160 mm Hg or DBP ≥100 mm Hg

DBP, diastolic blood pressure; SBP, systolic blood pressure.
Modified from National High Blood Pressure Education Program Working Group on High Blood Pressure in Children and Adolescents. The fourth report on the diagnosis, evaluation, and treatment of high blood pressure in children and adolescents. *Pediatrics* 2004;114(2 Suppl 4):555-576; and Chobanian AV, Bakris GL, Black HR, et al. The seventh report of the Joint National Committee on Prevention, Detection, Evaluation, and Treatment of High Blood Pressure: the JNC 7 report. *JAMA* 2003;289(19):2560-2572.

TABLE 34-4 History and Physical Examination Findings Suggestive of Secondary Hypertension

FINDING	SUGGESTS
Present in History	
Known UTI or UTI symptoms	Reflux nephropathy
Joint pains, rash, fever	Vasculitis, SLE
Acute onset of gross hematuria	Glomerulonephritis, renal venous thrombosis
Renal trauma	Renal infarct, renal artery stenosis
Abdominal radiation	Radiation nephritis, renal artery stenosis
Renal transplant	Transplant renal artery stenosis
Precocious puberty	Adrenal disorder
Muscle cramping, constipation	Hyperaldosteronism
Excessive sweating, headache, pallor, and/or flushing	Pheochromocytoma
Illicit drug use	Drug-induced hypertension
Present on Examination	
BP >140/100 mm Hg at any age	Secondary hypertension
Leg BP < arm BP	Aortic coarctation
Poor growth, pallor	Chronic renal disease
Turner syndrome	Aortic coarctation
Café-au-lait spots	Renal artery stenosis
Delayed leg pulses	Aortic coarctation
Precocious puberty	Adrenal disorder
Bruits over upper abdomen	Renal artery stenosis
Edema	Renal disease
Excessive sweating	Pheochromocytoma
Excessive pigmentation	Adrenal disorder
Striae in a male	Drug-induced hypertension

BP, blood pressure; SLE, systemic lupus erythematosus; UTI, urinary tract infection.

TABLE 34-5 Substances that May Elevate Blood Pressure in Childhood

PRESCRIPTION MEDICATIONS	NONPRESCRIPTION MEDICATIONS	OTHERS
Calcineurin inhibitors (e.g., cyclosporine, tacrolimus)	Caffeine	Cocaine
COX-2 inhibitors (e.g., celecoxib, others)	Ephedrine	DHEA
Erythropoietin	Nonsteroidal antiinflammatory drugs*	Ethanol
Glucocorticoids	Pseudoephedrine	Heavy metals (lead, mercury)
Migraine medications (e.g., ergotamine, sumatriptan)		Herbal preparations (e.g., Ephedra, *Glycyrrhiza*)
Oral contraceptives		MDMA (ecstasy)
Phenylpropanolamine		Tobacco
Pseudoephedrine		
Stimulant medications* (e.g., dexedrine, methylphenidate, amphetamine derivatives)		
Tricyclic antidepressants*		

*Cause elevated blood pressure relatively infrequently compared with the other agents in the table.
COX, cyclooxygenase; DHEA, dehydroepiandosterone; MDMA, 3,4-methylenedioxy-N-methylamphetamine.

Pediatric patients with confirmed hypertension should undergo a diagnostic evaluation tailored to confirm or exclude secondary causes and to identify other CV risk factors.[3] Several reports confirm the frequent detection of dyslipidemia in children and adolescents with high BP, especially among those who are obese.[11,12] The typical pattern is normal to slightly elevated total cholesterol with low high-density lipoprotein (HDL) cholesterol and elevated triglycerides. This pattern is similar to the dyslipidemia that occurs in type 2 diabetes and may reflect a component of insulin resistance, even in nonobese patients with hypertension. Obese adolescents with hypertension may also have impaired glucose tolerance; together, these findings are consistent with the metabolic syndrome.[12] Identification of multiple CV risk factors in children or adolescents is indicative of a greater risk for premature CV disease, and it calls for more intensive management.

Target organ damage in hypertensive children is an indication for use of antihypertensive medications.[3] Left ventricular hypertrophy (LVH) is the most easily detectable target organ effect of hypertension in adolescents. The prevalence of LVH in hypertensive children and adolescents has been reported to be as high as 30% to 40%, when ascertained by echocardiography and pediatric criteria are applied.[13,14] Although the adverse effects of LVH seen in adults, such as sudden cardiac death, have not been demonstrated in hypertensive children, LVH is an important finding that indicates a need for treatment to control BP and monitoring to prevent progression of LVH. In both adolescents and children, echocardiography, rather than electrocardiography (ECG), is the preferred method to detect LVH. Left ventricular mass should be indexed to height to correct for age and the effects of obesity.[3]

Other target organ effects of high BP have been investigated in children and adolescents. Reports from these studies describe an association of retinal arteriole dimension with BP level in healthy children,[15] and in some hypertensive children and adolescents, an increase in carotid intimal-medial thickness (cIMT),[16,17] microalbuminuria,[18,19] and subtle neurocognitive deficits are seen, particularly in the domain of executive function.[20,21] However, more data are needed before carotid imaging, urine microalbumin testing, and neurocognitive assessment can be recommended for routine clinical use in the young.

Approach to Therapy

NONPHARMACOLOGIC APPROACHES

Weight loss, aerobic exercise, and dietary modifications have all been shown to reduce BP in children and adolescents and are considered primary treatment,[3] especially in those with obesity-related hypertension. Studies in obese children have demonstrated that modest weight loss not only decreases BP but also improves other CV risk factors, such as dyslipidemia and insulin resistance.[22,23] Although weight loss in obese children is difficult and frequently unsuccessful, identifying a medical complication of obesity, such as hypertension, can sometimes provide the necessary motivation for patients and families to make the appropriate lifestyle changes. In this context, family-based interventions should be considered because they have been shown to be reasonably successful in the long term.[24]

Aerobic forms of exercise are generally included in the management of hypertension in the young. Many children are already participating in one or more appropriate activities and may only need to increase the frequency and/or intensity of these. Increases in physical activity have clear benefit in contributing to weight control and can also result in improvements in insulin resistance, endothelial function, and other atherogenic risk factors.[25] The combination of increased physical activity and improved fitness along with decreases in body fat may also forestall the development of type 2 diabetes in at-risk individuals. At the very least, the amount of time spent in sedentary activities such as television viewing should be restricted to fewer than 2 hours per day.[26]

Cessation of regular exercise is generally followed by a rise in BP to preexercise levels. Furthermore, exercise alone is unlikely to control BP and should be combined with dietary changes for best results in terms of BP reduction and weight control. The combination of dietary changes and exercise training may also improve vascular function.[26]

Dietary modification has received consideration for both treatment and prevention of hypertension in children and adolescents. Nutrients that have been examined include the obvious—such as sodium, potassium, and calcium—and also include folate, caffeine, and other substances. The typical dietary sodium intake of most children and adolescents in the United States far exceeds nutritional requirements, largely because of consumption of processed foods and fast foods. Results of studies that tested the effects of reduced sodium intake on BP are not as clear in children as they have been in adults. However, a meta-analysis of 10 separate studies that investigated the effect of a change in sodium intake on BP in children found that a 54% reduction in sodium intake was associated with a 2.47 mm Hg reduction in systolic BP.[27] A high salt intake increases thirst,[27,28] and high dietary sodium intakes of children have been linked to the obesity epidemic through increased consumption of sweetened drinks.[28,29] These findings suggest that limitation of dietary sodium intake could have an important role in treatment of obese adolescents with hypertension.

Other nutrients that have been examined in patients with hypertension include potassium and calcium, both of which have been shown to have antihypertensive effects. A 2-year trial of potassium and calcium supplementation in hypertensive, salt-sensitive Chinese children demonstrated that this combination significantly reduced systolic BP,[30] suggesting that a diet low in sodium and

enriched in potassium and calcium may be more effective in the treatment of hypertension than a diet that only restricts sodium intake. An example of such a diet is the Dietary Approaches to Stop Hypertension (DASH) diet, which is high in fruits, vegetables, and low-fat dairy foods. The DASH diet has been shown to lower BP in adults with hypertension, even in those receiving antihypertensive medication.[31] A recent pilot study demonstrated that the DASH eating plan can also reduce BP in children and adolescents with modest BP elevation (>90th percentile).[32] It is logical to apply a DASH diet tailored to children and adolescents to the treatment of childhood hypertension. The DASH diet also incorporates higher intake of fiber and other micronutrients and lower saturated fat intake, which may confer further benefit given the frequent presence of dyslipidemia in hypertensive adolescents.

Nonpharmacologic approaches are generally recommended as first-line treatment of hypertension in the young, especially in those who are obese. To be most effective, these measures need to be implemented in a systematic manner, with extensive family involvement and long-term support. They should be instituted even if there is an indication for initiation of antihypertensive medications because successful lifestyle intervention will complement pharmacologic treatment.

USE OF ANTIHYPERTENSIVE MEDICATIONS

In addition to lifestyle modification, antihypertensive medications are needed in some hypertensive children and adolescents to achieve the desired BP. There are potential benefits of initiating drug therapy early in life for children with hypertension.[33] However, data on the risks and benefits of long-term antihypertensive drug therapy in the pediatric age group are still limited, and making decisions on the optimal timing for drug treatment continues to be difficult. It is recommended that a definite indication for initiating pharmacologic therapy be present before antihypertensive medication is prescribed in a child or adolescent.[3] Specific indications are:

- Stage 2 hypertension (see Table 34-5)
- Symptomatic hypertension
- Secondary hypertension
- Hypertensive target organ damage
- Diabetes mellitus (types 1 and 2)
- Persistent hypertension despite nonpharmacologic measures

Most of the above represent situations in which BP reduction is likely to be of benefit in treatment of a concomitant condition; for example, reduction of BP in patients with diabetes is an important strategy to slow the development of diabetic nephropathy, and reduction of BP in patients with chronic kidney disease (CKD) slows the rate of progression toward end-stage renal disease. Hypertensive children who either do not comply with or do not respond to a reasonable trial (6 to 12 months) of nonpharmacologic measures should be prescribed antihypertensive medications because of their risk of developing hypertensive target organ damage. Repeat assessment for LVH and other forms of hypertensive target organ damage may be helpful in determining how long to continue lifestyle measures alone.

An important issue related to use of antihypertensive medications in the young is the availability of evidence-based information on efficacy and safety. Given the relatively low incidence of hypertension in childhood, it is not surprising that in the past, industry-sponsored trials were not conducted in pediatric populations, and most drugs had to be used empirically. The passage of the Food and Drug Administration Modernization Act (FDAMA) in 1997, which was followed by additional legislation—including the Best Pharmaceuticals for Children Act, Pediatric Research Equity Act, and the FDA Amendments Act of 2007—has led to many pediatric clinical trials of antihypertensive medications and has increased the number of such medications with specific labeling for treatment of hypertension in children.

Currently, little guidance exists as to what class of antihypertensive agent should be chosen as the initial agent in hypertensive adolescents. Although adult clinical practice guidelines have clear recommendations based on clinical trial evidence, a similar evidence base is lacking for pediatric patients. Clinical trials designed to compare different classes of antihypertensive agents have not been conducted in the young. Until data are available to differentiate the advantages and disadvantages of different classes of antihypertensive medications in adolescents, it is reasonable to consider several classes of agents—including diuretics, β-blockers, angiotensin-converting enzyme (ACE) inhibitors, angiotensin receptor blockers (ARBs), and calcium channel blockers (CCBs)—as potentially acceptable first-line agents.

Some clinical situations exist in which specific classes of antihypertensive agents are indicated. ACE inhibitors or ARBs are preferred in children with CKD because of the beneficial effects of these drugs on slowing deterioration in renal function.[34] In hypertensive adolescents with metabolic syndrome, the potential adverse effects of thiazide diuretics and some β-blocking agents on glucose metabolism should be kept in mind, and alternatives should be considered as the first-choice medication.[35]

The most frequently used first-line medications in the treatment of hypertensive children are either ACE inhibitors or CCBs. Clinical trial data on efficacy and safety in hypertensive children and adolescents are now available for nearly all ACE inhibitors. Suspension preparations of some ACE inhibitors were studied, and instructions for their preparation can be found in the FDA-approved labels. The side effects of ACE inhibitors—cough, rash, and neutropenia—are rarely seen in children; these drugs are usually well tolerated, and many formulations have the advantage of once-a-day dosing. ACE inhibitors are effective in controlling BP and also have beneficial effects on renal and cardiac function. Importantly, as noted above, ACE inhibitors provide the benefit of renal protection in children with diabetes or CKD.[34] Because of vasodilator effects on the efferent arteriole, ACE inhibitors can reduce glomerular filtration and should be used with caution in patients with renal artery stenosis, a solitary kidney, or a transplanted kidney. ACE inhibitors are contraindicated during pregnancy because of possible teratogenic effects on the fetus[36]; these agents may be prescribed for children, but this must be done with appropriate counseling regarding contraception in adolescent girls who are or may become sexually active.

ARBs also block the renin-angiotensin system and have benefits similar to those of ACE inhibitors. Pediatric clinical trial data are now available on several ARBs, and experience is developing with use of ARBs in treatment of hypertension in children and adolescents.[37-41] They generally have been as effective as other classes of agents in reducing BP and did not cause hyperkalemia or other significant adverse effects. However, no ARB has been labeled for use in children younger than 6 years because of concerns about safety in this age group. As with some ACE inhibitors, suspension formulations for several ARBs have been studied—including losartan, candesartan, and valsartan—and instructions for their preparation are included in the FDA-approved labels for these agents. Overall, ARBs appear to be safe and effective agents for treating hypertension in children and adolescents, although the pregnancy precaution for ACE inhibitors applies to ARBs as well.

Several of the dihydropyridine CCBs are useful in the treatment of hypertensive children, whereas the nondihydropyridine CCBs do not have such a role. Clinical trial data on the efficacy and safety of several of the newer CCB compounds support their use in treatment of childhood hypertension.[42] CCBs can be used in children as initial therapy or as second- or third-line medications when more than one drug is needed to control BP. When CCBs are needed for BP control in chronic hypertension, long-acting preparations are preferred.

β-Adrenergic blockers (BBs) are one of the oldest classes of antihypertensive medications that have been used in pediatric hypertension. These drugs lower BP by blocking stimulation of β1- and β2-adrenergic receptors by the sympathetic nervous system, thus affecting one of the more important underlying mechanisms of hypertension. Many different BBs that have varying affinities for adrenoceptors are available.[43] However, clinical trial data on efficacy and safety of BBs in hypertensive children are limited. Considerable data are available on the use of propranolol in children, because it is one of the oldest available BBs; but this information has largely been from studies of children with various cardiac conditions or portal hypertension. Of the newer BBs, extended-release metoprolol has pediatric clinical trial data that demonstrate efficacy and safety.[44] BBs are good choices for treatment of hypertension in nonasthmatic children, but these drugs may not be well tolerated by athletes because of reduced exercise capacity.

Based on clinical trial data, diuretics are generally recommended as initial drug therapy in adults with uncomplicated hypertension. Similar data are not available in children, so unless there is clinical evidence of fluid retention in a hypertensive child, diuretics are usually not the first step in drug treatment. Thiazide diuretics may cause hypokalemia in children, resulting in a need for potassium supplements. Taking the potassium supplements is extremely unpleasant for children and may lead to adherence problems. However, a low-dose diuretic can be useful as a second or third drug in children who require multiple drugs to achieve BP control. They may be especially useful as add-on therapy when the initial agent is an ACE inhibitor or ARB.

Most hypertensive children and adolescents are asymptomatic or have nonspecific symptoms that may not be ascribed to elevated BP.[45] Absence of symptoms in an otherwise healthy child can make adherence to a daily medication schedule difficult. Adolescents often do not remember to take their medications and do not like to be perceived as different from their peers. The likelihood of adherence will improve if BP control can be achieved with a single once-daily agent. Adverse effects of the chosen drug should also be considered. When more than one agent is needed to achieve the desired BP, available combination preparations may improve adherence.

A "stepped care" approach (Figure 34-2) is recommended for use of antihypertensive medications in hypertensive children and adolescents.[3] Stepped care allows individualization of therapy and ongoing assessment of efficacy and adverse effects. Given the new FDA-approved pediatric labeling for many antihypertensive agents, most clinicians are able to prescribe agents labeled for pediatric use. Suggested initial and maximal doses of various antihypertensive agents are given in Table 34-6.

Treatment goals for hypertensive children and adolescents take into consideration the presence of concomitant disease.[3] For patients with uncomplicated primary hypertension and no

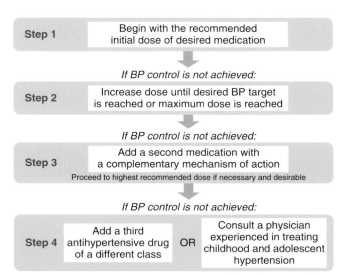

FIGURE 34-2 Stepped approach to pharmacologic management of hypertension in adolescents. BP, blood pressure.

TABLE 34-6   Suggested Doses of Antihypertensive Medications for Use in Children and Adolescents

CLASS	DRUG	STARTING DOSE	INTERVAL	MAXIMUM DOSAGE*
Aldosterone receptor antagonists (ARAs)	Eplerenone	25 mg	qd, bid	100 mg/day
	Spironolactone†	1 mg/kg	qd, bid	3.3 mg/kg up to 100 mg/day
Angiotensin-converting enzyme (ACE) inhibitors	Benazepril†	0.2 mg/kg up to 10 mg	qd	0.6 mg/kg up to 40 mg/day
	Captopril†	0.3-0.5 mg/kg	bid, tid	6 mg/kg up to 450 mg/day
	Enalapril†	0.08 mg/kg	qd	0.6 mg/kg up to 40 mg/day
	Fosinopril	0.1 mg/kg up to 10 mg	qd	0.6 mg/kg up to 40 mg/day
	Lisinopril†	0.07 mg/kg up to 5 mg	qd	0.6 mg/kg up to 40 mg/day
	Quinapril	5-10 mg	qd	80 mg/day
Angiotensin-receptor blockers	Candesartan	1-6 years, 0.2 mg/kg	qd	1-6 years, 0.4 mg/kg
		6-17 years, BW <50 kg, 4-8 mg		6-17 years, BW <50 kg, 16 mg
		6-17 years, BW >50 kg, 8-16 mg		6-17 years, BW >50 kg, 32 mg
	Losartan†	0.75 mg/kg up to 50 mg	qd	1.4 mg/kg up to 100 mg/day
	Olmesartan	BW 20-34 kg, 10 mg	qd	BW 20-34 kg, 20 mg
		≥35 kg, 20 mg		≥35 kg, 40 mg
	Valsartan†	<6 years, 5 to 10 mg	qd	<6 years, 80 mg
		6-17 years, 1.3 mg/kg up to 40 mg		6-17 years, 2.7 mg/kg up to 160 mg/day
α- and β-Adrenergic antagonists	Labetalol†	2-3 mg/kg	bid	10-12 mg/kg up to 1.2 mg/day
	Carvedilol	0.1 mg/kg up to 12.5 mg	bid	0.5 mg/kg up to 25 mg
β-Adrenergic antagonists	Atenolol†	0.5-1 mg/kg	qd, bid	2 mg/kg up to 100 mg/day
	Bisoprolol/HCTZ	0.04 mg/kg up to 2.5/6.25 mg	qd	10/6.25 mg/day
	Metoprolol	1-2 mg/kg	bid	6 mg/kg up to 200 mg/day
	Propranolol	1 mg/kg	bid, tid	16 mg/kg up to 640 mg/day
Calcium channel blockers	Amlodipine†	0.06 mg/kg	qd	0.3 mg/kg up to 10 mg/day
	Felodipine	2.5 mg	qd	10 mg/day
	Isradipine†	0.05-0.15 mg/kg	tid, qid	0.8 mg/kg up to 20 mg/day
	Extended-release nifedipine	0.25-0.5 mg/kg	qd, bid	3 mg/kg up to 120 mg/day
Central α-agonist	Clonidine†	5-10 µg/kg	bid, tid	25 µg/kg up to 0.9 mg/day
Diuretics	Amiloride	5-10 mg	qd	20 mg/day
	Chlorthalidone	0.3 mg/kg	qd	2 mg/kg up to 50 mg/day
	Furosemide	0.5-2.0 mg/kg	qd, bid	6 mg/kg/day
	HCTZ	0.5-1 mg/kg	qd	3 mg/kg up to 50 mg/day
Vasodilators	Hydralazine	0.25 mg/kg	tid, qid	7.5 mg/kg up to 200 mg/day
	Minoxidil	0.1-0.2 mg/kg	bid, tid	1 mg/kg up to 50 mg/day

*The maximum recommended adult dose should never be exceeded.
†Information on preparation of a stable extemporaneous suspension is available for these agents.
BW, body weight; HCTZ, hydrochlorothiazide.

hypertensive target organ damage, goal BP should be below the 95th percentile for age, gender, and height, whereas for those with secondary hypertension, diabetes, or hypertensive target organ damage, goal BP should be below the 90th percentile for age, gender, and height. These goals are consistent with current recommendations for therapy of hypertension in adults that recommend treatment to a lower BP goal in patients with complicated hypertension, such as those with diabetes or renal disease.[4] The European Society of Hypertension has recently issued updated guidelines for management of childhood hypertension that recommend an even lower goal, below the 75th percentile, for patients with CKD.[46]

Treatment of hypertension does not end when medications are prescribed. Management of a hypertensive child requires follow-up at regular intervals to ensure that the desired BP goal has been reached, assess adherence to therapy, and monitor for medication-related adverse effects. Hypertensive adolescents can be encouraged to monitor their BP at home using an appropriate device in order to increase their involvement in treatment and improve adherence. Continuation of lifestyle modification should also be encouraged to achieve and maintain BP control. Laboratory studies should be repeated periodically, especially fasting lipid and glucose studies in obese adolescents and electrolyte, blood urea nitrogen (BUN), and creatinine measurements in those treated with diuretics, ACE inhibitors, or ARBs. Adolescent girls treated with ACE inhibitors or ARBs should receive ongoing counseling to avoid pregnancy and to use effective contraception if sexually active because of the risks for fetal injury associated with these drugs.

Summary

Hypertension and prehypertension are common childhood health problems, and the prevalence of childhood hypertension appears to be increasing as a consequence of the childhood obesity epidemic. Key steps in the management of children and adolescents with hypertension include first verifying the diagnosis and then conducting an evaluation to distinguish primary from secondary hypertension and to identify other cardiovascular and metabolic risk factors and target-organ damage. Lifestyle modifications that include changes in diet, physical activity, and weight control are appropriate for all children and adolescents with high BP, particularly those who are overweight or sedentary. Specific indications for using pharmacologic therapy to achieve goal BP levels include stage 2 hypertension, secondary hypertension, symptomatic hypertension, CKD, and diabetes.

REFERENCES

1. McNiece KL, Poffenbarger TS, Turner JL, et al. Prevalence of hypertension and pre-hypertension among adolescents. *J Pediatrics* 2007;150(6):640-644, 644.e1.
2. Hansen HS, Froberg K, Hyldebrandt N, Nielsen JR. A controlled study of eight months of physical training and reduction of blood pressure in children: the Odense schoolchild study. *Br Med J* (Clinical research ed) 1991;303(6804):682-685.

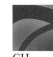

3. National High Blood Pressure Education Program Working Group on High Blood Pressure in Children and Adolescents. The fourth report on the diagnosis, evaluation, and treatment of high blood pressure in children and adolescents. *Pediatrics* 2004;114(2 Suppl 4):555-576.

4. Chobanian AV, Bakris GL, Black HR, et al. The seventh report of the Joint National Committee on Prevention, Detection, Evaluation, and Treatment of High Blood Pressure: the JNC 7 report. *JAMA* 2003;289(19):2560-2572.

5. Podoll A, Grenier M, Croix B, Feig DI. Inaccuracy in pediatric outpatient blood pressure measurement. *Pediatrics* 2007;119(3):e538-e543.

6. Prineas RJ, Ostchega Y, Carroll M, Dillon C, McDowell M. US demographic trends in mid-arm circumference and recommended blood pressure cuffs for children and adolescents: data from the National Health and Nutrition Examination Survey 1988-2004. *Blood Press Monit* 2007;12(2):75-80.

7. Swinford RD, Portman RJ. Evaluation of the hypertensive pediatric patient. In Flynn JT, Ingelfinger JR, Portman RJ, editors: *Pediatric hypertension*, 2nd ed. 2011, Humana Press, New York, pp 499-516.

8. Swartz SJ, Srivaths PR, Croix B, Feig DI. Cost-effectiveness of ambulatory blood pressure monitoring in the initial evaluation of hypertension in children. *Pediatrics* 2008;122(6):1177-1181.

9. Flynn JT, Alderman MH. Characteristics of children with primary hypertension seen at a referral center. *Pediatr Nephrol* 2005;20(7):961-966.

10. Robinson RF, Batisky DL, Hayes JR, Nahata MC, Mahan JD. Body mass index in primary and secondary pediatric hypertension. *Pediatr Nephrol* 2004;19(12):1379-1384.

11. Boyd GS, Koenigsberg J, Falkner B, Gidding S, Hassink S. Effect of obesity and high blood pressure on plasma lipid levels in children and adolescents. *Pediatrics* 2005;116(2):442-446.

12. Weiss R, Dziura J, Burgert TS, et al. Obesity and the metabolic syndrome in children and adolescents. *N Engl J Med* 2004;350(23):2362-2374.

13. Hanevold CD, Pollock JS, Harshfield GA. Racial differences in microalbumin excretion in healthy adolescents. *Hypertension* 2008;51(2):334-338.

14. Brady TM, Fivush B, Flynn JT, Parekh R. Ability of blood pressure to predict left ventricular hypertrophy in children with primary hypertension. *J Pediatr* 2008;152(1):73-78, 78.e1.

15. Mitchell P, Cheung N, de Haseth K, et al. Blood pressure and retinal arteriolar narrowing in children. *Hypertension* 2007;49(5):1156-1162.

16. Lande MB, Carson NL, Roy J, Meagher CC. Effects of childhood primary hypertension on carotid intima media thickness: a matched controlled study. *Hypertension* 2006;48(1):40-44.

17. Sorof JM, Alexandrov AA, Dardwell G, Portman JR. Carotid artery intimal-medial thickness and left ventricular hypertrophy in children with elevated blood pressure. *Pediatrics* 2003;111:61-66.

18. Assadi F. Effect of microalbuminuria lowering on regression of left ventricular hypertrophy in children and adolescents with essential hypertension. *Pediatric Cardiology* 2007;28(1):27-33.

19. Lubrano R, Travasso E, Raggi C, et al. Blood pressure load, proteinuria and renal function in pre-hypertensive children. *Pediatr Nephrol* 2009;24(4):823-831.

20. Lande MB, Kaczorowski JM, Auinger P, Schwartz GJ, Weitzman M. Elevated blood pressure and decreased cognitive function among school-age children and adolescents in the United States. *J Pediatr* 2003;143(6):720-724.

21. Lande MB, Adams H, Falkner B, et al. Parental assessments of internalizing and externalizing behavior and executive function in children with primary hypertension. *J Pediatr* 2009;154(2):207-212.

22. Williams CL, Hayman LL, Daniels SR, et al. Cardiovascular health in childhood: a statement for health professionals from the Committee on Atherosclerosis, Hypertension, and Obesity in the Young (AHOY) of the Council on Cardiovascular Disease in the Young, American Heart Association. *Circulation* 2002;106(1):143-160.

23. Reinehr T, Andler W. Changes in the atherogenic risk factor profile according to degree of weight loss. *Arch Dis Child* 2004;89(5):419-422.

24. Kalarchian MA, Levine MD, Arslanian SA, et al. Family-based treatment of severe pediatric obesity: randomized, controlled trial. *Pediatrics* 2009;124(4):1060-1068.

25. Farpour-Lambert NJ, Aggoun Y, Marchand LM, et al. Physical activity reduces systemic blood pressure and improves early markers of atherosclerosis in pre-pubertal obese children. *J Am Coll Cardiol* 2009;54(25):2396-2406.

26. Ribeiro MM, Silva AG, Santos NS, et al. Diet and exercise training restore blood pressure and vasodilatory responses during physiological maneuvers in obese children. *Circulation* 2005;111(15):1915-1923.

27. He FJ, MacGregor GA. Importance of salt in determining blood pressure in children: meta-analysis of controlled trials. *Hypertension* 2006;48(5):861-869.

28. He FJ, Macgregor GA. Response to salt intake in children: increasing concerns? *Hypertension* 2006;48:861-869.

29. He FJ, Marrero NM, MacGregor GA. Salt intake is related to soft drink consumption in children and adolescents: a link to obesity? *Hypertension* 2008;51(3):629-634.

30. Mu JJ, Liu ZQ, Liu WM, et al. Reduction of blood pressure with calcium and potassium supplementation in children with salt sensitivity: a 2-year double-blinded placebo-controlled trial. *J Hum Hypertens* 2005;19(6):479-483.

31. Appel LJ, Moore TJ, Obarzanek E, et al. A clinical trial on the effects of dietary patterns on blood pressure. DASH Collaborative Research Group. *N Engl J Med* 1997;336(16):1117-1124.

32. Couch SC, Saelens BE, Levin L, et al. The efficacy of a clinic-based behavioral nutrition intervention emphasizing a DASH-type diet for adolescents with elevated blood pressure. *J Pediatrics* 2008;152(4):494-501.

33. Portman RJ, Nesbitt S. Would preemptive therapy in childhood prevent cardiovascular disease? *J Clin Hypertens (Greenwich)* 2007;9(10):739-741.

34. Shatat IF, Flynn JT. Hypertension in children with chronic kidney disease. *Adv Chronic Kidney Dis* 2005;12(4):378-384.

35. Puri M, Flynn JT. Management of hypertension in children and adolescents with the metabolic syndrome. *J Cardiometab Syndr* 2006;1:259-268.

36. Cooper WO, Hernandez-Diaz S, Arbogast PG, et al. Major congenital malformations after first-trimester exposure to ACE inhibitors. *N Engl J Med* 2006;354(23):2443-2451.

37. Shahinfar S, Cano F, Soffer BA, et al. A double-blind, dose-response study of losartan in hypertensive children. *Am J Hypertens* 2005;18(2 Pt 1):183-190.

38. Schaefer F, van de Walle J, Zurowska A, et al. Efficacy, safety and pharmacokinetics of candesartan cilexetil in hypertensive children from 1 to less than 6 years of age. *J Hypertens* 2010;28(5):1083-1090.

39. Flynn JT, Meyers KE, Neto JP, et al. Efficacy and safety of the angiotensin receptor blocker valsartan in children with hypertension aged 1 to 5 years. *Hypertension* 2008;52(2):222-228.

40. Trachtman H, Hainer JW, Sugg J, et al; Candesartan in Children with Hypertension (CINCH) Investigators. Efficacy, safety, and pharmacokinetics of candesartan cilexetil in hypertensive children aged 6 to 17 years. *J Clin Hypertens (Greenwich)* 2008;10:743-750.

41. Hazan L, Hernández Rodriguez OA, Bhorat AE, et al. A double-blind, dose-response study of the efficacy and safety of olmesartan medoxomil in children and adolescents with hypertension. *Hypertension* 2010;55(6):1323-1330.

42. Flynn JT. Management of hypertension in the young: role of antihypertensive medications. *J Cardiovasc Pharmacol* 2011;58(2):111-120.

43. Manrique C, Giles TD, Ferdinand KC, Sowers JR. Realities of newer beta-blockers for the management of hypertension. *J Clin Hypertens (Greenwich)* 2009;11(7):369-375.

44. Batisky DL, Sorof JM, Sugg J, et al. Efficacy and safety of extended release metoprolol succinate in hypertensive children 6 to 16 years of age: a clinical trial experience. *J Pediatr* 2007;150(2):134-139, 139.e1.

45. Croix B, Feig DI. Childhood hypertension is not a silent disease. *Pediatr Nephrol* 2006;21(4):527-532.

46. Lurbe E, Cifkova R, Cruickshank JK, et al. Management of high blood pressure in children and adolescents: recommendations of the European Society of Hypertension. *J Hypertens* 2009;27(9):1719-1742.

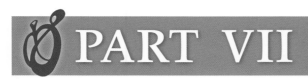

PART VII

OTHER VASCULAR CONDITIONS

CHAPTER **35**   **Peripheral Artery Disease**

Todd S. Perlstein and Marc Z. Krichavsky

OVERVIEW, 539

MEDICAL THERAPY OF PERIPHERAL ARTERY DISEASE, 539

CARDIOVASCULAR RISK REDUCTION, 539

Antiplatelet Therapy, 539
Anticoagulant Therapy, 541
Lipid-Lowering Drugs, 541
Antihypertensive Therapy, 542
Angiotensin-Converting Enzyme Inhibitor Therapy, 542
β-Blocker Therapy, 542
Smoking Cessation Therapy, 542

DIABETES, 543

INTERMITTENT CLAUDICATION, 543

Pentoxifylline, 543
Cilostazol, 543

PERIOPERATIVE MEDICAL THERAPY FOR NONCARDIAC VASCULAR SURGERY, 544

β-Blockers, 544
Statin Therapy, 544
Antiplatelet Therapy, 544

INTERVENTIONAL MANAGEMENT OF PERIPHERAL ARTERY DISEASE, 544

Indications for Revascularization, 545
Procedural Considerations, 546

AORTOILIAC DISEASE, 546

FEMORAL-POPLITEAL DISEASE, 547

INFRAPOPLITEAL DISEASE, 549

THERAPEUTIC ANGIOGENESIS, 549

CONCLUSIONS, 549

REFERENCES, 550

Overview

This chapter focuses on the medical and endovascular management of atherosclerotic peripheral artery disease (PAD). The American Heart Association (AHA) Symposium on Atherosclerotic Peripheral Vascular Disease recommended that the term *peripheral artery disease* be used to refer to disease that affects the upper or lower extremities.[1] This chapter focuses on the more prevalent lower extremity PAD.

PAD affects 5.9% of adults older than 40 years. The prevalence of PAD increases with age and the number of risk factors and afflicts 29% of adults who either are older than 70 years or are older than 50 years but smoke or have diabetes.[2-5] The risk factors for PAD are generally the same as those for coronary artery disease (CAD). Among traditional risk factors, smoking and diabetes are most strongly associated with PAD, but kidney disease is notable among nontraditional risk factors.[6] Most patients with PAD are asymptomatic, a minority have intermittent claudication, and critical limb ischemia (CLI) affects only 1% to 2% of patients. Regardless of symptom status, patients with PAD have a high risk of cardiovascular (CV) morbidity and mortality (Figure 35-1).[4] Myocardial infarction (MI), stroke, and death are more common than limb events in patients with PAD; therefore PAD patients require aggressive secondary prevention interventions such as smoking cessation and antihypertensive, antiplatelet, and cholesterol-lowering therapies to prevent CV events. First-line therapy for intermittent claudication is a supervised exercise program. Revascularization is generally reserved for patients with severe claudication that does not respond to exercise or medical therapy and for those with CLI. The location and characteristics of obstructive disease determine the best revascularization strategy, with more complex and more distal lesions often better suited for surgical reconstruction. Rapidly evolving technology has expanded the types of lesions amenable to percutaneous intervention and has lowered the threshold for this therapy. Therapeutic angiogenesis continues to hold great promise, although as yet unrealized, for patients in whom mechanical revascularization is not possible.

Medical Therapy of Peripheral Artery Disease

Medical therapy in PAD has two goals: the prevention of CV events and improvement in lower extremity outcomes (Figure 35-2). The detection of PAD and application of preventive therapies have the potential to be of great public health benefit (Table 35-1).

Cardiovascular Risk Reduction

Antiplatelet Therapy

A secondary analysis of the Physicians' Health Study suggests that aspirin may prevent the development of PAD requiring revascularization but not stable PAD that causes intermittent claudication.[7] This seeming discrepancy is consistent with the concept that antiplatelet therapy is most effective at preventing unstable disease as a result of thrombosis and is less effective at preventing more stable disease resulting from progressive atherosclerosis.[8]

Two large, placebo-controlled trials have examined the role of low-dose aspirin (100 mg) in the primary prevention of CV events in patients with asymptomatic PAD and no other symptomatic atherosclerotic vascular disease: the Aspirin for Asymptomatic Atherosclerosis (AAA) trial and the Prevention of Progression of Arterial Disease and Diabetes (POPADAD) trial, which enrolled patients with both PAD and diabetes.[9,10] Both the POPADAD trial (hazard ratio [HR], 0.98; 95% confidence interval [CI], 0.76 to 1.26) and the AAA trial (HR, 1.03; 95% CI, 0.84 to 1.27) found that aspirin did not reduce the risk of major adverse CV events. However, each trial had significant limitations, including a higher than recommended cutoff for ankle brachial index (ABI) to define the

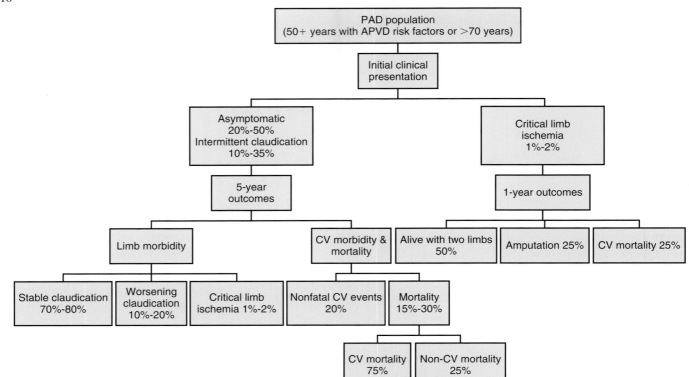

FIGURE 35-1 The natural history of peripheral artery disease (*PAD*). All patients with PAD are at high risk of cardiovascular (*CV*) morbidity and mortality. In patients with asymptomatic PAD or intermittent claudication, limb morbidity is less common than cardiovascular morbidity and mortality. Critical limb ischemia has a severe prognosis. (*Modified from Hirsch AT, Haskal ZJ, Hertzer NR, et al. ACC/AHA 2005 practice guidelines for the management of patients with peripheral arterial disease (lower extremity, renal, mesenteric, and abdominal aortic). Circulation 2006;113[11]:e463-e654.*)

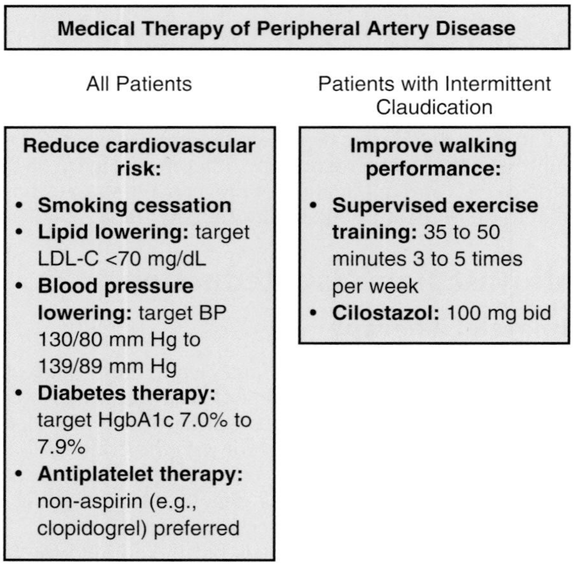

Medical Therapy of Peripheral Artery Disease	
All Patients	**Patients with Intermittent Claudication**
Reduce cardiovascular risk: • **Smoking cessation** • **Lipid lowering:** target LDL-C <70 mg/dL • **Blood pressure lowering:** target BP 130/80 mm Hg to 139/89 mm Hg • **Diabetes therapy:** target HgbA1c 7.0% to 7.9% • **Antiplatelet therapy:** non-aspirin (e.g., clopidogrel) preferred	**Improve walking performance:** • **Supervised exercise training:** 35 to 50 minutes 3 to 5 times per week • **Cilostazol:** 100 mg bid

FIGURE 35-2 Summary of the authors' recommendation for medical therapy in peripheral artery disease (PAD). All patients with PAD should receive intensive risk factor modifications. The preference for nonaspirin antiplatelet therapy is based on the CAPRIE trial and on the meta-analysis of Robless et al.[13] BP, blood pressure; HgbA1c, hemoglobin A1c; LDL-C, low-density lipoprotein cholesterol. (*Data from Robless P, Mikhailidis DP, Stansby G. Systematic review of antiplatelet therapy for the prevention of myocardial infarction, stroke or vascular death in patients with peripheral vascular disease. Br J Surg 2001;88[6]:787-800; and A randomised, blinded trial of clopidogrel versus aspirin in patients at risk of ischaemic events [CAPRIE]. CAPRIE Steering Committee. Lancet 1996;348[9038]: 1329-1339.*)

presence of PAD, much lower than expected event rates, and poor adherence to assigned aspirin therapy in the AAA trial. These limitations do not allow dismissing the effect aspirin may have in preventing CV events in patients with asymptomatic PAD.[11] A recent meta-analysis highlighted the inadequacy of the data to address the use of aspirin therapy in PAD.[11,12] The 2011 update of the American College of Cardiology (ACC)/AHA guidelines for the management of PAD give the use of antiplatelet therapy to reduce the risk of MI, stroke, or vascular death in asymptomatic PAD a higher recommendation if the ABI is 0.90 or below (class IIa, level of evidence [LOE] C) than if the ABI is between 0.91 and 0.99 (class IIb, LOE A).[5]

Robless and colleagues[13] performed a meta-analysis of randomized, controlled trials of antiplatelet therapy exclusively in patients with *symptomatic* PAD. There were 24 placebo-controlled trials of antiplatelet therapy in a total of 6036 patients with intermittent claudication and 10 placebo-controlled trials of antiplatelet therapy with a total of 1765 patients undergoing revascularization. The primary outcome examined was the composite of MI, stroke, or CV death. Antiplatelet therapy was associated with a 22% risk reduction (odds ratio [OR], 0.78; 95% CI, 0.63 to 0.96) in patients with claudication, a 24% risk reduction (OR, 0.76; 95% CI, 0.54 to 1.05) in patients who underwent surgical revascularization, and a 27% risk reduction (OR, 0.73; 95% CI, 0.23 to 2.31) in patients who underwent percutaneous balloon angioplasty. Similar results were obtained by the contemporaneous Antithrombotic Trialists' Collaboration meta-analysis, which included 9214 patients with PAD enrolled in 42 trials.[14] Robless and colleagues' meta-analysis also included five trials involving 6929 patients with PAD that compared other antiplatelet agents—clopidogrel, ticlopidine, or dipyridamole-aspirin in combination—to aspirin therapy. The non–aspirin-treated patients had fewer CV events (6.6%) compared with aspirin-treated

TABLE 35-1 Potential U.S. Population Benefit of Peripheral Artery Disease Detection and Treatment

PREVENTIVE THERAPY GOAL	PAD POPULATION NOT MEETING GOAL	INDIVIDUAL THERAPY RELATIVE RISK REDUCTION	POPULATION RELATIVE RISK REDUCTION	CUMULATIVE RELATIVE RISK	POTENTIAL MACE PREVENTED/5 YEARS
LDL-c <70 mg/dL	95%	20%	19%	0.81	269,800
Antiplatelet therapy	39%	12%	5%	0.77	326,600
BP <140/90 mm Hg	46%	20%	9%	0.70	426,000
Smoking cessation	29%	40%	12%	0.62	539,600

BP, blood pressure; LDL-c, low-density lipoprotein cholesterol; MACE, major cardiac event; PAD, peripheral artery disease.
Modified from Pande RL, Hiatt WR, Zhang P, et al. A pooled analysis of the durability and predictors of treatment response of cilostazol in patients with intermittent claudication. *Vasc Med* 2010;15(3):181-188.

patients (8.4%), resulting in a 24% risk reduction (OR, 0.76; 95% CI, 0.64 to 0.91) compared with aspirin therapy. The majority of those comparative data came from the Clopidogrel Versus Aspirin in Patients at Risk of Ischemic Events (CAPRIE) study, a trial of clopidogrel versus aspirin in the prevention of a composite outcome cluster of ischemic stroke, MI, or vascular death in patients with symptomatic atherosclerotic vascular disease.[15] In the 6452 patients with PAD in CAPRIE, clopidogrel was associated with an absolute 1.1% (0.4% to 1.7%) and a relative 23.8% (8.9% to 36.2%) risk reduction compared with aspirin. The more recent Clopidogrel for High Atherothrombotic Risk and Ischemic Stabilization, Management, and Avoidance (CHARISMA) trial of aspirin plus clopidogrel versus aspirin alone estimated a 15% (HR, 0.85; 95% CI, 0.66 to 1.08) reduction in risk for MI, stroke, or CV death for the combined therapy in patients with symptomatic PAD.[16] In addition, Robless et al. found that the nonaspirin antiplatelet agents tended to be associated with a lower risk of major bleeding events compared with aspirin therapy (OR, 0.73; 95% CI, 0.51 to 1.06).[13] In total, a review of the evidence suggests that nonaspirin (i.e., clopidogrel) monotherapy may be the most effective antiplatelet therapy in symptomatic PAD.[11,12] The 2011 American College of Cardiology Foundation (ACCF)/AHA guidelines for the management of PAD recommend antiplatelet therapy to reduce the risk of MI, stroke, and vascular death in patients with symptomatic PAD (class I, LOE A).[5] The individual antiplatelet agents aspirin and clopidogrel are recommended with a lower level of evidence (class I, LOE B). The combination of aspirin and clopidogrel as an alternative to either alone may be considered, but the efficacy is not well established (class IIb, LOE C).

Anticoagulant Therapy

Few data address the role of oral anticoagulant therapy in PAD. A meta-analysis of oral anticoagulation in patients with CAD found that moderate- to high-intensity oral anticoagulation (international normalized ratio [INR] ≥2.0) plus aspirin significantly reduced the composite of MI, stroke, or death compared with aspirin alone (OR, 0.56; 95% CI, 17% to 77%) but at a twofold increased risk of major bleeding events.[17] No evidence supported the use of low-intensity (INR <2.0) oral anticoagulation. The Warfarin Antiplatelet Vascular Evaluation (WAVE) trial subsequently compared moderate-intensity (INR 2.0 to 3.0) oral anticoagulation with warfarin and antiplatelet therapy to antiplatelet therapy alone in the prevention of MI, stroke, revascularization, and CV death in patients with symptomatic atherosclerotic peripheral vascular disease, in which 82% of the patients had lower extremity PAD.[18] Warfarin anticoagulation combined with antiplatelet therapy did not significantly reduce the risk of MI, stroke, or death (RR, 0.92; 95% CI, 0.73 to 1.16) or MI, stroke, death, or revascularization (RR, 0.91; 95% CI, 0.74 to 1.12), and life-threatening bleeding was 3.4-fold more common in the combined-treatment group. The 2011 ACCF/AHA guidelines for the management of PAD recommend against the use of warfarin in addition to antiplatelet therapy to reduce the risk of adverse CV ischemic events in PAD (class III, LOE B).[5]

Lipid-Lowering Drugs

No large clinical trial of cholesterol-lowering therapy has been performed exclusively in patients with PAD; therefore the evidence supporting the use of cholesterol-lowering therapy in PAD is derived from PAD cohort studies or PAD subgroup analyses of clinical trials.

HMG-CoA REDUCTASE INHIBITOR (STATIN) THERAPY

The landmark Scandinavian Simvastatin Survival Study (4S) and West of Scotland Coronary Prevention Study (WOSCOPS) included only 253 and 193 people with PAD, respectively.[19,20] Of note, a secondary analysis of the 4S trial found that simvastatin therapy reduced the risk of new or worsening claudication.[21] The Heart Protection Study (HPS), which randomized 20,536 adults with either known vascular disease or diabetes to simvastatin 40 mg or placebo, was the first cholesterol-lowering trial to enroll a substantial number of people with peripheral vascular disease (both PAD and other types) and without diagnosed CAD.[22] Among the 6748 individuals with peripheral vascular disease, simvastatin therapy significantly reduced the risk of major vascular events (relative RR, 22%; 95% CI, 15% to 29%). In addition, simvastatin therapy reduced the risk of peripheral vascular events (relative RR, 16%; 95% CI, 5% to 25%) among all participants.[23] The relative reduction was similar in patients with or without PAD at baseline, but the higher event rate in patients with preexisting PAD translated into a larger absolute risk reduction (20 per 1000 vs. 3 per 1000) in patients with PAD compared with those without PAD.[23] Thus, statin therapy is effective at reducing both coronary and noncoronary vascular events in patients with PAD.

A revision of the National Cholesterol Education Program Adult Treatment Panel III (NCEP ATP III) guidelines recommended that patients with PAD be designated as either high risk or very high risk.[24] Individuals with PAD are considered to be at very high risk in the presence of multiple major risk factors, severe and poorly controlled risk factors, or multiple components of the metabolic syndrome. For most patients with PAD, the LDL-cholesterol (LDL-c) goal is less than 100 mg/dL, and a target of less than 70 mg/dL is to be considered in those deemed to be at very high risk. The ACC/AHA guidelines for the management of PAD concur with these recommendations, and the 2011 ACCF/AHA secondary prevention guidelines recommend that an adequate dose of statin is one that reduces LDL-c to less than the target level *and* achieves a 30% or more lowering of LDL-c.[4,5,25]

NONSTATIN LIPID-LOWERING THERAPY

Statin-induced myalgias are particularly relevant in the care of patients with PAD given the high burden of leg symptoms in that population.[26] Clinicians caring for patients with PAD should be familiar with the ACC/AHA/National Heart, Lung, and Blood Institute (NHLBI) clinical advisory on the use and safety of statin therapy.[27] The 2011 ACCF/AHA secondary prevention guidelines recommend that LDL-c–lowering therapy with bile acid seques-trants or niacin is reasonable (class IIa, LOE B), or ezetimibe may be considered (class IIB, LOE B) in patients who either do not toler-ate statins or do not achieve LDL-c goals on maximal statin therapy.[25] Fibrates should be started in addition to statin therapy in patients who have triglycerides above 500 mg/dL to prevent acute pancreatitis (class I, LOE C). For patients with elevated cholesterol (non–high-density lipoprotein [HDL]) while on adequate statin, niacin, or fibrate therapy may be reasonable (class IIb, LOE B). Of note, both niacin and fibrates may be particularly effective at pre-venting CV events in high-risk patients, characterized by high tri-glycerides and low HDL cholesterol (HDL-c).[28,29]

Antihypertensive Therapy

Treatment of high blood pressure with antihypertensive drug therapy effectively reduces the risk of stroke, MI, heart failure, and death.[30] The Joint National Commission (JNC) currently recom-mends that individuals with hypertension be treated to a target blood pressure below 140/90 mm Hg and that those at particularly high risk for CV events be treated to a target blood pressure below 130/80 mm Hg. The ACC/AHA guidelines for the treatment of PAD recommend a treatment goal below 140/90 mm Hg in general for patients with PAD and below 130/80 mm Hg for those with diabe-tes or chronic renal disease (class I, LOE A).[4,5] However, no clinical trial has definitively shown that targeting a blood pressure below 130/80 mm Hg is more effective at preventing CV events than tar-geting a blood pressure below 140/90 mm Hg. With regard to PAD, in a small subgroup of the Appropriate Blood Pressure Control in Diabetes (ABCD) study of 950 subjects with type 2 diabetes, inten-sive treatment to a mean blood pressure of 128/75 mm Hg was associated with a markedly reduced risk of CV events compared with placebo treatment that achieved blood pressure of 137/81 mm Hg.[31] However, no difference was reported in event rates between treatment strategies in the entire study population, so the PAD subgroup analysis should be considered hypothesis generating.

The more aggressive BP target for diabetes has come under scrutiny. A meta-analysis of antihypertensive trials in type 2 diabe-tes and impaired fasting glucose by Bangalore and colleagues revealed that the risk of CV death and MI was not improved by achieving a systolic blood pressure (SBP) below 130 mm Hg com-pared with achieving an SBP below 135 mm Hg, and it suggested that the optimal BP in patients with diabetes may be between 130 and 135 mm Hg systolic and 80 to 85 mm Hg diastolic.[32] Similarly, trial data do not support that targeting BP below 130/80 mm Hg in patients with chronic kidney disease lessens the risk of CV disease.[33] In fact, an achieved blood pressure below 130/80 mm Hg was associated with a higher incidence of adverse events. Thus, the available data do not support targeting a blood pressure below 130/80 mm Hg in PAD patients with diabetes or chronic kidney disease.

Angiotensin-Converting Enzyme Inhibitor Therapy

The 2005 ACC/AHA guidelines for the treatment of PAD and its 2011 update state that the use of angiotensin-converting enzyme (ACE) inhibitors is reasonable for symptomatic (class IIa, LOE B) and asymptomatic (class IIb, LOE C) patients with PAD to reduce the risk of adverse CV events. Support for the use of ACE inhibitors to reduce CV risk in patients with PAD comes principally from the Heart Outcomes Prevention Evaluation (HOPE) study.[4,34] In the HOPE study, 9297 subjects at high risk for atherosclerotic events, on the basis of existing atherosclerosis and/or diabetes but without LV dysfunction, were randomized to either ramipril or placebo and were followed for a mean of 5 years. Ramipril therapy was associ-ated with a 22% (95% CI, 14% to 30%) relative reduction in the risk of MI, stroke, or CV death—a benefit observed in patients with both

symptomatic and asymptomatic PAD.[35] Several other placebo-controlled trials have randomized subjects at high risk for CV events to ACE inhibitor or angiotensin receptor blocker (ARB) therapy, and overall these trials demonstrate a reduction in the risk of MI, stroke, and death.[36-41] Of these trials, in the only one with an active comparator group, the Comparison of Amlodipine Versus Enalapril to Limit Occurrences of Thrombosis (CAMELOT) trial, subjects were randomized to placebo, enalapril, or amlodipine.[41] Amlodipine achieved an event rate risk reduction that tended to be greater than enalapril (HR, 0.81; 95% CI, 0.63 to 1.04) and was significantly less than placebo (HR, 0.69; 95% CI, 0.54 to 0.88), whereas the risk reduction achieved by enalapril compared with placebo was not statistically significant (HR, 0.85; 95% CI, 0.67 to 1.07). These results suggest that caution must be taken in interpret-ing the placebo-controlled trials of ACE inhibitor therapy.

β-Blocker Therapy

Concerns have been raised that β-adrenergic blockers might impair walking capacity in patients with PAD. These concerns are based on β2-receptor–mediated vasodilation, glycogenolysis, and gluconeogenesis, which may cause noncardioselective β-blockers such as propanolol to adversely affect skeletal muscle performance during exercise.[42] Radack and Deck conducted a meta-analysis of randomized controlled trials that examined the effect of β-blockers on walking capacity or endurance time.[43] The results of the analysis strongly suggested that β-blockers do not adversely affect walking capacity in PAD, a conclusion subsequently confirmed by Para-vastu and colleagues.[42] A recent comparison of nebivolol with hydrochlorothiazide in hypertensive patients with intermittent claudication did not find that nebivolol impaired walking perfor-mance.[44] Also, β-blockers do not impair quality of life in patients with PAD and concomitant chronic obstructive pulmonary disease (COPD).[45] β-Blocker therapy should not be withheld from patients with PAD and an indication for administration.

Smoking Cessation Therapy

Cigarette smoking is the most important risk factor for the develop-ment and progression of PAD.[46] Active smokers have more severe PAD, worse claudication, and reduced exercise capacity compared with former smokers.[47,48] These differences are independent of the ABI, suggesting that smoking adversely affects leg muscle perfor-mance by mechanisms beyond reduction of blood flow. Cessation of smoking increases the chance of improvement in ankle pres-sure and exercise tolerance in intermittent claudication.[49] Contin-ued smoking accelerates the progression of PAD and increases the risk of CLI, loss of graft patency, and amputation.[50] Smoking cessa-tion is associated with twofold greater 5- and 10-year survival among patients with symptomatic PAD, a survival benefit that becomes evident within 1 year of smoking cessation.[51,52] Approxi-mately one third of patients with PAD are interested in quitting smoking immediately and are receptive to a formal smoking cessation program.[53] An intensive smoking cessation intervention that includes counseling and pharmacologic aids for smoking cessation greatly increases short-term quit rates.

Pharmacologic aids for smoking cessation include nicotine replacement, bupropion hydrochloride (Zyban), and varenicline (Chantix). Bupropion is a weak inhibitor of the neuronal uptake of norepinephrine and dopamine but has no effect on serotonin. Varenicline stimulates dopamine, which results in reduced crav-ings and fewer withdrawal symptoms, and it also blocks nicotine receptors. Eisenberg and colleagues conducted a meta-analysis of 69 double-blind, placebo-controlled randomized trials of smoking cessation with biochemically validated outcomes that included a total of 32,908 participants. Bupropion, varenicline, and nicotine replacement therapy were found to approximately double the odds of smoking cessation compared with placebo (Figure 35-3).[54] In addition, varenicline was associated with twice the smoking cessation rate of bupropion when compared in head-to-head trials.

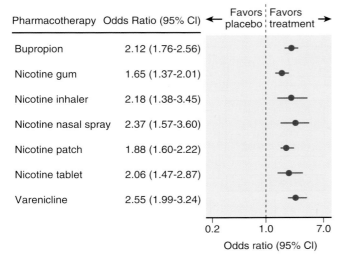

Pharmacotherapy	Odds Ratio (95% CI)
Bupropion	2.12 (1.76-2.56)
Nicotine gum	1.65 (1.37-2.01)
Nicotine inhaler	2.18 (1.38-3.45)
Nicotine nasal spray	2.37 (1.57-3.60)
Nicotine patch	1.88 (1.60-2.22)
Nicotine tablet	2.06 (1.47-2.87)
Varenicline	2.55 (1.99-3.24)

FIGURE 35-3 Pharmacotherapies for smoking cessation and their clinical efficacy. Data were adjusted for mean age, sex, and mean number of cigarettes per day. CI, confidence interval. (*From Eisenberg MJ, Filion KB, Yavin D, et al. Pharmacotherapies for smoking cessation: a meta-analysis of randomized controlled trials. CMAJ 2008;179[2]:135-144.*)

Box 35-1 Class I Recommendations for Smoking Cessation in Patients with Peripheral Artery Disease

1. Patients who are smokers or former smokers should be asked about status of tobacco use at every visit. (*Level of Evidence*: A)
2. Patients should be assisted with counseling and with developing a plan for quitting that may include pharmacotherapy and/or referral to a smoking cessation program. (*Level of Evidence*: A)
3. Individuals with lower extremity peripheral artery disease who smoke cigarettes or use other forms of tobacco should be advised by each of their clinicians to stop smoking, and they should be offered behavioral and pharmacologic treatment. (*Level of Evidence*: C)
4. In the absence of some contraindication or other compelling clinical indication, physicians should offer one or more pharmacologic therapies that include varenicline, bupropion, and nicotine replacement therapy. (*Level of Evidence*: A)

From Rooke TW, Hirsch AT, Misra S, et al. 2011 ACCF/AHA focused update of the guideline for the management of patients with peripheral artery disease (updating the 2005 guideline). *Vasc Med* 2011;16(6):452-476.

The absolute smoking cessation rates ranged from 13% to 26%, indicating that the majority of patients treated with smoking cessation pharmacotherapy are not successful in quitting smoking. The current 2005 ACC/AHA guidelines for the treatment of PAD and recommendations for smoking cessation in patients with PAD are summarized in Box 35-1.[5]

Diabetes

No clinical trial has tested whether intensive hypoglycemic therapy improves CV outcomes in patients with PAD and diabetes. The ACC/AHA guidelines for the treatment of PAD recommend targeting a hemoglobin A1c to less than 7% to reduce microvascular complications and potentially improve CV outcomes (class IIa, LOE C).[4] Since that guideline was published, three large clinical trials have tested whether intensive blood glucose lowering improves CV outcomes. Collectively, these trials did not show that intensive glucose lowering lessens the risk for CV events in diabetes.[55] The AHA/ACC 2011 secondary prevention guidelines accordingly downgraded this recommendation (class IIb, LOE C).[25] Lifestyle modifications that include daily physical activity, weight management, blood pressure control, and lipid management are recommended for all patients with diabetes (class I, LOE B).

Intermittent Claudication

Quality of life is significantly affected by intermittent claudication and can be improved by relief of symptoms and increased walking distance.[56,57] Supervised exercise training should be considered first-line therapy for eligible patients with claudication. In a meta-analysis of 21 studies, Gardner and Poehlman[58] found that supervised exercise improves pain-free walking time by 180% and maximal walking time by 120% in patients with intermittent claudication. A meta-analysis of randomized controlled trials concluded that exercise improved maximal walking capacity by an average of 150% (range, 75% to 230%) compared with nonsupervised exercise programs.[59] The improvement in walking capacity achieved by exercise training exceeds that of pharmacotherapy and compares favorably with revascularization.[4] The Claudication: Exercise Versus Endoluminal Revascularization (CLEVER) study found that supervised exercise training achieved a greater improvement in peak walking time but less improvement in PAD-specific quality of life than did stent revascularization in patients with aortoiliac PAD and claudication; both treatments did far better than optimal medical therapy alone.[60] The ACC/AHA guidelines for PAD recommend that a program of supervised exercise training be the initial treatment modality for patients with intermittent claudication (class I, LOE A; Figure 35-4). It is recommended that the program consist of at least 30- to 45-minute sessions three times per week for a minimum of 12 weeks. Treadmill and track walking are most beneficial, and the workload should elicit claudication symptoms of moderate severity within 3 to 5 minutes. After a brief rest period, the exercise-rest pattern is repeated. An initial standard treadmill test performed with 12-lead electrocardiographic (ECG) monitoring before initiation of the exercise training program can identify ischemic, arrhythmic, and hemodynamic instability to ensure safety of the program.

Pentoxifylline

Pentoxifylline, a methylxanthine derivative, was the first drug approved by the U.S. Food and Drug Administration (FDA) for management of intermittent claudication. The proposed mechanisms by which it might benefit claudication include decreases in blood viscosity, platelet adhesion, and fibrinogen and improvement of red blood cell deformability. The largest trial to examine the effect of pentoxifylline in intermittent claudication, the Scandinavian Study Group trial with 150 patients, failed to demonstrate a significant improvement in pain-free or maximal walking distance compared with placebo. A meta-analysis of clinical trials found that pentoxifylline has a slight but significant beneficial effect on intermittent claudication, but whether a significant benefit is achieved is controversial.[61,62]

Cilostazol

Cilostazol, a phosphodiesterase (PDE) type 3 inhibitor, was the second drug approved by the FDA for intermittent claudication. Its two main physiologic effects are vasodilation and inhibition of platelet aggregation, but it is unclear how it improves intermittent claudication. A patient-level meta-analysis of nine trials found that cilostazol significantly improved maximal walking distance on average of 42.1 meters compared with placebo (*P* < .0001).[63] Despite concerns about the potential increase in mortality associated with the use of PDE type 3 inhibitors, no effect on mortality rate was demonstrated (HR, 0.95; 95% CI, 0.68 to 1.35). In the only head-to-head comparison, cilostazol improved intermittent claudication significantly more than both pentoxifylline and placebo therapy, but pentoxifylline was not different compared with placebo.[62] The most common adverse effects, which are generally mild in severity, are headache, diarrhea, abnormal stools, infection,

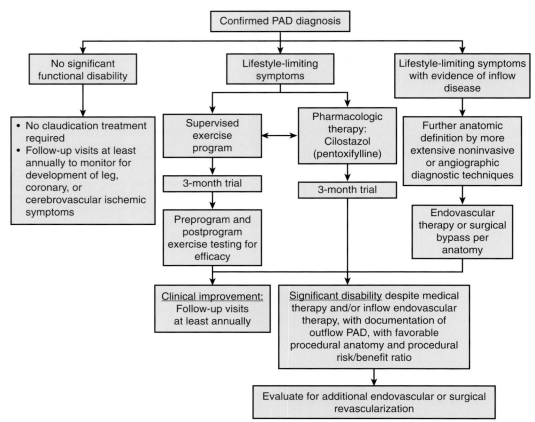

FIGURE 35-4 Management strategy for peripheral artery disease (*PAD*). *(Modified from Hirsch AT, Haskal ZJ, Hertzer NR, et al. ACC/AHA 2005 practice guidelines for the management of patients with peripheral arterial disease (lower extremity, renal, mesenteric, and abdominal aortic). Circulation 2006;113[11]:e463-e654.)*

rhinitis, and peripheral edema.[64] Cilostazol is contraindicated in patients with congestive heart failure and severe hepatic or renal impairment, and it should be taken in lower doses in patients also taking diltiazem, omeprazole, or other inhibitors of the cytochrome (CY) P450 isoenzymes CYP2C19 and CYP3A4.

Perioperative Medical Therapy for Noncardiac Vascular Surgery

Patients undergoing noncardiac vascular surgery are at increased risk for perioperative adverse CV events. Major predictors of cardiac complications include unstable coronary syndromes, decompensated heart failure, high-degree atrioventricular block, ventricular tachycardia or uncontrolled supraventricular arrhythmia, and severe valvular disease.[65] β-Blocker, statin, and antiplatelet drugs are medical therapies commonly used to lessen cardiac risk in vascular surgery.

β-Blockers

Optimally applied preoperative and postoperative β-blockade reduces the risk of MI and death associated with noncardiac vascular surgery. Optimal application of β-blocker therapy entails initiating therapy at least 7 days prior to surgery, using a long-acting β-blocker, targeting heart rate below 60 beats/min preoperatively and below 80 beats/min intraoperatively and postoperatively, and being careful to avoid hypotension in the postoperative period.[66] The ACC/AHA perioperative guidelines recommend that perioperative β-blockade be continued after surgery in patients receiving β-blockers for indications such as angina or arrhythmia (class I, LOE C) and in patients undergoing vascular surgery who have evidence of coronary ischemia on preoperative testing (class I,

LOE B).[67] β-Blockers are also recommended for patients whose preoperative assessment identified CAD or who have a higher risk of CV complications defined by the presence of multiple clinical risk factors (class II, LOE B). Patients undergoing vascular surgery who either are at low cardiac risk or have evidence of extensive ischemia on stress imaging (five or more segments on dobutamine stress echocardiography) may not derive benefit from β-blocker therapy.[68,69]

Statin Therapy

Withdrawal of statin therapy in the perioperative period is associated with a marked increase in the risk of MI and death.[70] Preoperative initiation of high-intensity, long-acting statin therapy reduces the risk of MI and death in patients at high CV risk undergoing vascular surgery.[71-73] Higher intensity statin therapy is associated with a reduced risk of postoperative MI and CV death compared with low-intensity statin therapy.[74]

Antiplatelet Therapy

The role of antiplatelet therapy in preventing cardiac complications of noncardiac vascular surgery is not well studied.[75] A decision analysis suggested that aspirin therapy would offer a small (0.73%) decrease in perioperative mortality rate at the expense of a 2.46% increased rate of hemorrhage complications.[76]

Interventional Management of Peripheral Artery Disease

Advances in surgical and endovascular techniques have allowed for a significant expansion of the number of patients and the scope of conditions that can be treated with revascularization therapies. However, it bears emphasis that despite this exciting evolution in the treatment armamentarium for PAD, management of the systemic disease of atherosclerosis with aggressive lifestyle modification and medical therapy remains critical to preventing future CV events and prolonging the lives of patients.

Patients with lower extremity arterial disease are often equally focused on relief of the pain that reduces their quality of life. They also fear future limb outcomes such as ulcerations, tissue loss, and amputations. Patients with intermittent claudication or CLI have a worse quality of life as measured by objective scales than patients with advanced heart failure or COPD.[77] Revascularization plays a critical role in improving quality of life and in preventing these dreaded limb outcomes.

Indications for Revascularization

The AHA and ACC endorse revascularization of PAD in patients with CLI and in those with lifestyle-limiting claudication that results in significant disability despite a trial of exercise and/or medical therapy.[4]

Surgical revascularization has long been the standard therapy for arterial reconstruction, but because of relatively high perioperative CV morbidity and mortality rates in PAD patients, it has been reserved for patients with CLI or severe claudication. The durability of aortofemoral bypass and infrainguinal bypass with autologous saphenous vein continues to be the standard to which endovascular therapies are compared.[78]

A paucity of well-designed randomized trials are available that examine the role and efficacy of endovascular interventions. A randomized trial that compared balloon angioplasty with medical therapy for unilateral claudication demonstrated a superior pain-free walking distance, higher ABI, and improved vessel patency rates with balloon angioplasty.[79] A meta-analysis of intervention with percutaneous transluminal angioplasty (PTA) versus exercise therapy in patients with claudication demonstrated similar quality of life and superior functional capacity with a better ABI in the revascularization group.[80] In the Bypass Versus Angioplasty in Severe Ischemia of the Leg (BASIL) trial, 452 patients with CLI and infrainguinal disease were randomized to percutaneous or surgical revascularization. In the initial results published in 2005, the two strategies demonstrated equivalent primary endpoints of amputation-free survival (57% vs. 52%; P = not significant) after 3 years of follow-up.[81] Subsequent analyses observed that among patients who survived more than 2 years, patients who underwent surgical revascularization had an increased overall survival of 7.3 months (P = .02).[82]

Patient and physician preference for minimally invasive therapies and advances in endovascular techniques that offer durability comparable to surgical revascularization have led to substantial increases in the number of endovascular procedures performed by cardiologists, vascular surgeons, and interventional radiologists.[83] The choice of endovascular versus surgical revascularization is determined by anatomic considerations and patient comorbidities that may influence the risk/benefit balance of a particular approach. The Trans-Atlantic Inter-Society Consensus Document (TASC) has classified lesions into four groups of suitability for endovascular versus surgical revascularization based on the location, length of diseased arterial segment, and presence of occlusive versus stenotic disease (Figure 35-5).[78] The overlap between endovascular and surgical categories reflects the rapidly changing landscape of what can be approached endovascularly and the difficulty of stratifying all variables of an individual patient's anatomy into an all-inclusive algorithm.

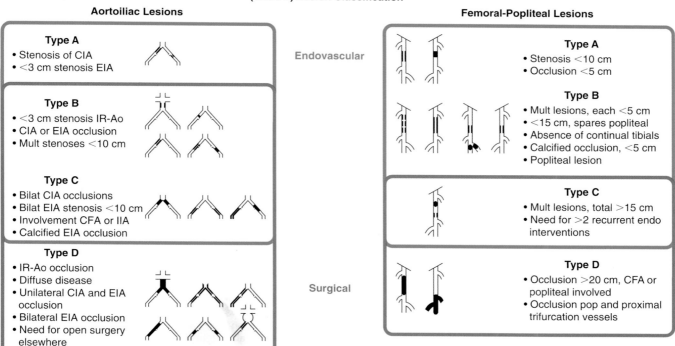

Trans-Atlantic Inter-Society Consensus (TASC II) Lesion Classification

Aortoiliac Lesions

Type A
- Stenosis of CIA
- <3 cm stenosis EIA

Type B
- <3 cm stenosis IR-Ao
- CIA or EIA occlusion
- Mult stenoses <10 cm

Type C
- Bilat CIA occlusions
- Bilat EIA stenosis <10 cm
- Involvement CFA or IIA
- Calcified EIA occlusion

Type D
- IR-Ao occlusion
- Diffuse disease
- Unilateral CIA and EIA occlusion
- Bilateral EIA occlusion
- Need for open surgery elsewhere

Endovascular

Surgical

Femoral-Popliteal Lesions

Type A
- Stenosis <10 cm
- Occlusion <5 cm

Type B
- Mult lesions, each <5 cm
- <15 cm, spares popliteal
- Absence of continual tibials
- Calcified occlusion, <5 cm
- Popliteal lesion

Type C
- Mult lesions, total >15 cm
- Need for >2 recurrent endo interventions

Type D
- Occlusion >20 cm, CFA or popliteal involved
- Occlusion pop and proximal trifurcation vessels

FIGURE 35-5 The Trans-Atlantic Inter-Society Consensus (TASC) statement provides recommendations for surgical or endovascular revascularization based on location and severity of peripheral artery disease. Endovascular intervention is an appropriate first-line strategy for TASC A and B lesions, and surgical revascularization is preferred for TASC D lesions. Disease falling into TASC C category may be approached by either strategy. CFA, common femoral artery; CIA, common iliac artery; EIA, external iliac artery; IIA, internal iliac artery; IR-Ao, infrarenal aorta. *(From Norgren L, Hiatt WR, Dormandy JA, et al. Inter-Society Consensus for the Management of Peripheral Arterial Disease [TASC II]. J Vasc Surg 2007;45[Suppl S]:S5-S67.)*

CH
35

Procedural Considerations

Careful planning prior to endovascular revascularization procedures can improve the likelihood of success of the procedure and can help avoid potential complications. Noninvasive diagnostic testing should be obtained prior to any invasive procedures. Arterial ultrasound, segmental Doppler pressure measurements, computed tomographic angiography (CTA), and magnetic resonance angiography (MRA) allow better appreciation of the location and extent of the arterial disease. This can help determine anatomic suitability for endovascular revascularization and can help assess the best vascular access approach to successfully treat a particular patient. Strategic selection of the access site can be the difference between success and failure of a particular procedure. Proximal aortoiliac disease is often best approached by ipsilateral retrograde common femoral artery access. Obstructive lesions near and below the inguinal ligament (external iliac, common femoral, superficial femoral, profunda femoris, and popliteal arteries) are typically approached by retrograde access in the contralateral common femoral artery. Diagnostic assessment and treatment of the target vessel are then performed "up and over" the iliac bifurcation. Distal infrapopliteal disease—that is, disease that affects the anterior tibial, posterior tibial, and peroneal arteries—is often best approached by ipsilateral antegrade access. Frequently, more than one vascular access site is required; for example, bilateral common femoral access is used to treat disease of the aortic bifurcation, and upper extremity access is achieved via the radial or brachial arteries to approach a common iliac occlusion from both "above and below." Although 5-Fr sheaths are typically adequate for diagnostic angiography, most interventional procedures require at least a 6-Fr sheath, with larger access required for some specialized devices, larger diameter stents, and covered stents.

Use of periprocedural antiplatelet medications and anticoagulation is largely extrapolated from the literature on coronary intervention. Typically, patients are given aspirin (325 mg) prior to the procedure, and in cases of a planned intervention, patients are given clopidogrel (300- to 600-mg load, 75 mg/day). Systemic intravenous (IV) heparin is given in a weight-based dose to achieve an activated clotting time of 250 to 300 seconds, although direct thrombin inhibitors such as bivalirudin are also being increasingly used; glycoprotein IIb/IIIa inhibitors are not commonly used in peripheral interventions. Guidewires used in peripheral interventions vary from 0.014- to 0.035-inch systems, depending on the size of the vessel being treated and the amount of support needed to deliver the necessary balloon or stent. As a general principle, the lowest profile system of guidewires, balloons, and stents needed to successfully complete the procedure should be selected. Angioplasty balloons are available as compliant, noncompliant, and cutting balloons, and drug-coated balloons deliver a variety of investigational drugs and proangiogenic factors. Major categories of stents include balloon-expandable, self-expanding, covered, and drug-eluting stents (DESs). The choice of a stent typically depends on the vascular territory being treated and, to some degree, operator preference. Adjunctive techniques such as atherectomy, vascular brachytherapy, and cryotherapy are available and are useful in particular niche situations. The advantages and disadvantages of these technologies are discussed in the following sections.

Aortoiliac Disease

Obstructive lesions that affect the distal aorta and common iliac, internal, and external iliac arteries are collectively referred to as *in-flow disease*. Patients with aortoiliac occlusive disease come to medical attention with classic calf claudication or less typical symptoms such as buttock or thigh discomfort and erectile dysfunction. When multilevel disease is present that includes aortoiliac disease amenable to endovascular revascularization, treatment of the proximal aortoiliac disease alone will often relieve symptoms and is therefore suggested as an initial strategy (Figure 35-6).

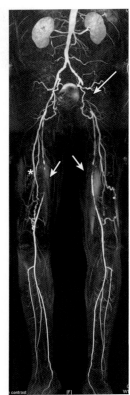

FIGURE 35-6 Multilevel peripheral artery disease with aortoiliac (inflow) and superficial femoral artery (infrainguinal) occlusive disease. Magnetic resonance angiogram depicts occlusion of the left external iliac artery and bilateral superficial femoral artery. Note extensive bilateral collaterals from the profunda femoris artery, which reconstitute distal superficial femoral arteries and allow perfusion of relatively unaffected infrapopliteal vessels.

Head-to-head comparisons of endovascular versus surgical revascularization of iliac disease are largely limited to balloon angioplasty versus bypass surgery. These trials showed equivalent endpoints for the two strategies,[84] although stents offer greater long-term durability than balloon angioplasty. A meta-analysis of 2000 endovascular iliac procedures found a 43% improvement in 4-year patency in stented lesions as opposed to lesions treated with balloon angioplasty only.[85] In the Safety and Efficacy of Express LD to Treat Stenosed or Occlusive Atherosclerotic Disease in Iliac Arteries (MELODIE) trial, the 2-year primary and assisted patencies of a dedicated iliac balloon-expandable stent were 87.8% and 98.2%, respectively.[86] The strategy of primary stent placement versus provisional stent placement in the case of a suboptimal angioplasty result has been investigated in a number of clinical trials. In focal, nonocclusive lesions, the two strategies were equivalent, with no difference in durability reported at a mean of 5.6 years follow-up, and the operators were able to avoid using a stent in 63% of the procedures.[87] Nevertheless, the majority of aortoiliac interventions performed today involve stent placement, and endovascular treatment is now considered first-line revascularization therapy in most cases of aortoiliac disease, with procedural success rates (>90%) and long-term patency (74% to 87% at 3 years) equivalent to surgical revascularization.[84]

A number of studies have investigated the ideal type of stent. Balloon-expandable stents have superior radial strength, have less foreshortening, and allow for more precise placement compared with self-expanding nitinol stents. Aortoiliac bifurcation disease is typically treated with simultaneously deployed balloon-expandable stents (Figure 35-7). Nitinol self-expanding stents are more flexible and deliverable, and they conform better to tortuous and ectatic vessels and areas where external compression and flexion may be

FIGURE 35-7   Occlusive aortoiliac disease successfully treated with simultaneously deployed balloon-expandable stents. **A,** Digital subtraction angiogram reveals occlusion of the distal aorta and bilateral common iliac arteries in a patient with claudication and absent femoral pulses. **B,** After aortoiliac stenting, flow is reconstituted. Balloon-expandable stents are preferred at the iliac bifurcation because of their superior radial strength and precision of deployment compared with self-expanding nitinol stents.

a concern, such as in the external iliac artery as it approaches the inguinal ligament (Figure 35-8). The Cordis Randomized Iliac Stent Project (CRISP) trial found no difference in long-term patency between two types of self-expanding stents, nitinol versus stainless steel.[88] Covered stents have traditionally been helpful in treatment of iliac aneurysms, arteriovenous (AV) fistulas, and hemodialysis access salvage, and they are potentially lifesaving in cases of iliac perforation or rupture; however, they may have more expanded applications in obstructive atherosclerotic disease. Covered stents are traditionally lined with a layer of polytetrafluoroethylene (PTFE) on the intimal surface, although other materials have also been investigated. They have been manufactured for both balloon-expandable self-expanding stent platforms. The potential advantage of covered stents is the physical barrier provided by the PTFE, which prevents ingrowth of tissue through the open cells in the stent struts as a result of neointimal hyperplasia or disease progression. Notably, hyperplasia and restenosis can still occur at the distal and proximal edges of the stents. In a nonrandomized retrospective study of 54 patients with iliac bifurcation disease treated with simultaneous "kissing" stents, covered stents had a superior primary patency (92% vs. 62%; $P = .02$) at 29.5 months' follow-up compared with bare-metal stents.[89] The Viabahn stent (W.L. Gore, Newark, DE) is a self-expanding covered stent that is FDA approved for endovascular use, and its role in lower extremity interventions will be further studied in the randomized iCast Atrium Registry Ultrasound Study (ICARUS).

Femoral-Popliteal Disease

The superficial femoral artery (SFA) is unique in that it runs the length of the thigh without any significant side branches and is subject to a range of forces that alter the flow dynamics, including extension, flexion, contraction, torsion, and compression. As a result, the SFA is one of the arteries most commonly affected in patients with risk factors that predispose them to PAD. Patients with

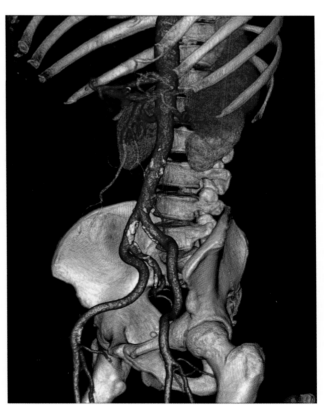

FIGURE 35-8   Arterial segments in areas subjected to tortuosity, bending, and torsion are suitable for treatment with flexible self-expanding stents. This image depicts an oblique view of computed tomographic angiographic reconstruction of the iliac vessels. The tortuous course of the external iliac arteries exiting the pelvis lends itself to treatment with self-expanding stents.

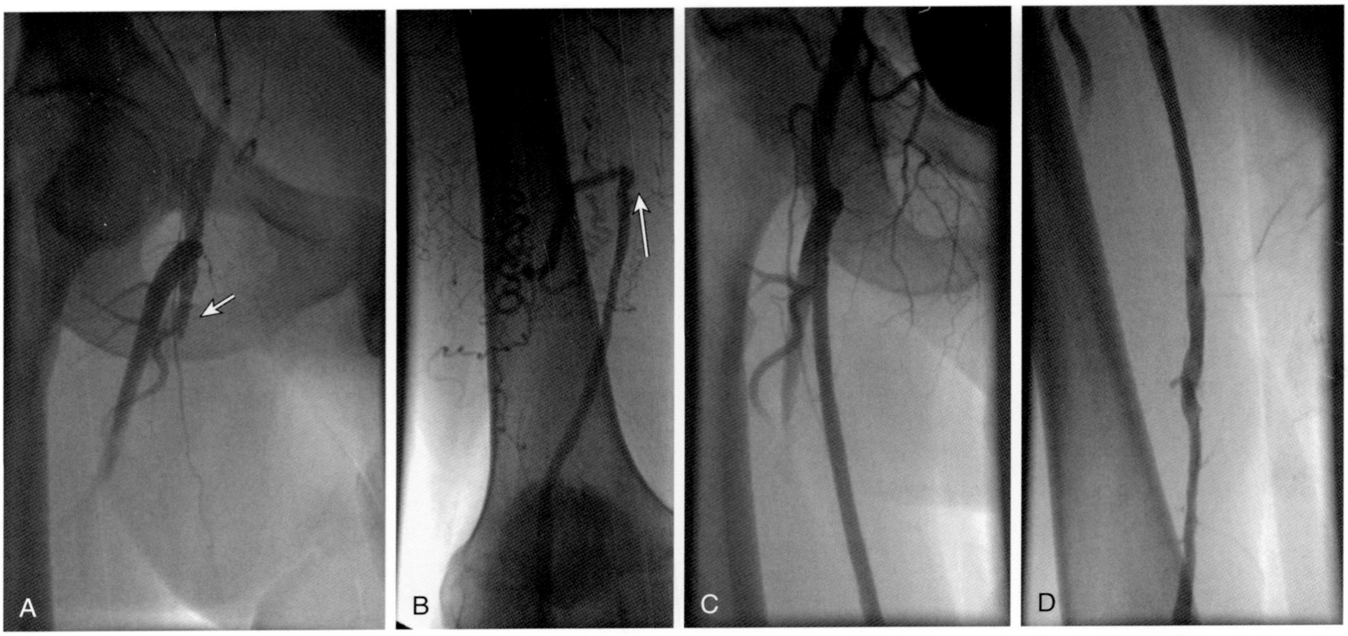

FIGURE 35-9 Long-segment occlusion of the superficial femoral artery. With advances in endovascular tools, extensive disease of the infrainguinal vessels can now be treated with percutaneous interventions. **A,** Angiogram of the right common femoral and profunda femoris arteries shows proximal occlusion of the superficial femoral artery (*arrow*). **B,** The superficial femoral artery reconstitutes above the knee via collaterals from the profunda femoris (*arrow*). **C** and **D,** After stenting with self-expanding stents, the vessel is reconstituted.

SFA disease often present with long occlusions and collateral networks from the profunda femoris artery that prevent CLI but provide insufficient perfusion for exercise. The same forces are responsible for the Achilles heel of SFA interventions: difficulty crossing long-segment occlusions and high restenosis rates. The development of hydrophilic wires, reentry devices, low-profile angioplasty balloons, and self-expanding nitinol stents has dramatically increased the number of SFA lesions that may be approached endovascularly (Figure 35-9).

The decision to perform balloon angioplasty instead of stenting depends on anatomic considerations in the SFA; this is in contradistinction with the iliac artery, in which primary stenting is typically the first-line therapy. Two randomized trials compared angioplasty versus stenting of the SFA with divergent results. In one trial, stents were associated with superior durability and functional outcomes compared with PTA alone in long-segment lesions.[90] However, in the case of shorter, nonocclusive lesions (<10 cm), balloon angioplasty has similar durability to stent placement, with provisional stenting reserved for dissections or other suboptimal angioplasty results (Figure 35-10).[91]

Only self-expanding stents are used in the SFA because of the extrinsic forces to which the vessel is subjected. Stent fractures remain a concern, particularly in long lesions with overlapping stents, with fracture rates that range from 2% to 28% depending on stent composition and architecture.[92] Covered stents lined with PTFE, such as the Viabahn stent (W.L. Gore) or Fluency stent (Bard Medical, Murray Hill, NJ), are being investigated for use in the SFA and in the iliac artery. Preliminary 1-year interim data from the Viabahn Versus Bare Nitinol Stent in the Treatment of Long Lesion (≥8 cm) Superficial Femoral Artery Occlusive Disease (VIBRANT) study suggested lower rates of stent fracture in Viabahn compared with traditional nitinol self-expanding stents.[93] Stents placed in areas of active joint flexion, such as the common femoral and popliteal arteries, may be particularly prone to stent fracture. Novel stent architecture designs have provided some optimism for endovascular treatment of this disease subset. One example is the Supera stent (IDEV Technologies, Webster, TX), a nitinol stent constructed of six braided nitinol filaments interwoven to maximize radial strength and compliance and to minimize incidence of stent fracture. In a registry of 177 patients with complex femoral-popliteal

disease, including disease that extended into the popliteal artery in nearly half of the cases, the primary and secondary patency rates were 76.1% and 91.9%, respectively, and the stent fracture rate was 0.0% at 24-month follow-up. These novel stents will require further refinement and investigation, and balloon angioplasty or surgical revascularization with endarterectomy and/or patch angioplasty remains the current standard of care for most patients with common femoral and popliteal disease.[94]

Given the length of stents required to treat SFA disease and the subsequent risk of restenosis, investigators have hoped to translate the use of DESs from the coronary to the peripheral circulation. In one study, 480 subjects with symptomatic above-the-knee femoral-popliteal disease of moderate length (<140 mm) were randomized to primary treatment with a Zilver PTX paclitaxel-eluting, polymer-free, nitinol, self-expanding stent (Cook Medical, Bloomington, IN) versus PTA with provisional stenting. Primary DES placement had superior event-free survival (90.4% vs. 82.6%; P < .004) and primary patency (83.1% vs. 32.8%; P < .001) versus PTA at a 12-month follow-up. In addition, a secondary randomization to provisional DES versus bare-metal stent was done following unsatisfactory PTA as defined by a flow-limiting dissection, residual stenosis greater than 30%, or transluminal mean gradient greater than 5 mm Hg. Similarly, DES was favored in both event-free survival and 12-month patency (89.9% vs. 73.0%; P < .01).[95] However, not all trials have favored DES. The Sirolimus-Eluting Versus Bare Nitinol Stent for Obstructive Superficial Femoral Artery Disease (SIROCCO II) trial randomized 57 patients to a polymer-based, sirolimus-eluting SMART stent (Cordis Johnson & Johnson, Warren, NJ) versus a bare-metal stent and found no significant advantage for DES versus bare-metal stent with regard to luminal late loss, binary restenosis rates, clinical outcomes, or adverse outcomes at 6-month follow-up.[96] The technique of drug elution into the arterial wall to prevent restenosis has been applied to balloon angioplasty. Prolonged inflation of a drug-coated balloon allows elution of a hydrophilic drug into the intima with a goal of preventing restenosis without stent placement. The Local Taxan with Short Time Exposure for Reduction of Restenosis in Distal Arteries (THUNDER) trial investigated using angioplasty balloons coated with paclitaxel and found significantly lower rates of restenosis and less need for repeat revascularization compared with traditional angioplasty

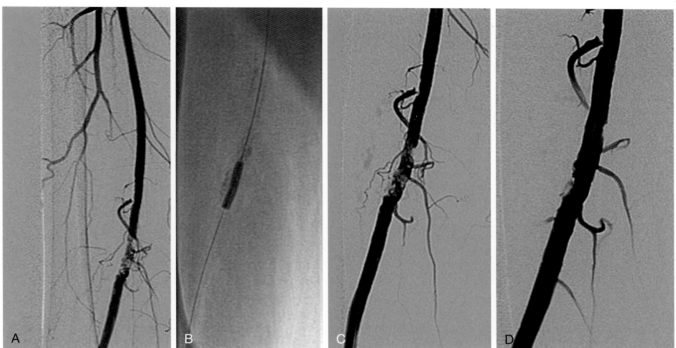

FIGURE 35-10 Short-segment stenosis of the superficial femoral artery is amenable to balloon angioplasty with stenting reserved for suboptimal results. **A,** Angiography demonstrates a severe, focal, calcified stenosis of the mid right superficial femoral artery. **B,** This lesion was initially treated with balloon angioplasty. **C,** Appearance of dissection and plaque recoil after balloon angioplasty. **D,** After placement of a self-expanding nitinol stent.

(17% vs. 44%; P = .01), but it did not compare drug-coated angioplasty stenting to a primary stenting strategy (DES or bare metal).[97] Similar results were noted in the Femoral Paclitaxed (FemPac) trial, which compared standard balloon angioplasty to another balloon-paclitaxel platform.[98] The heterogeneity of these results may reflect differences between these trials that include drug type, presence of polymer, stent architecture, patient population, and clinical endpoints. It seems likely that the next generation of stents for the femoral-popliteal anatomy will be drug eluting, and further investigation will be important in clarifying their role.

Infrapopliteal Disease

Revascularization of PAD that affects the arteries below the knee is primarily indicated for wound healing or limb salvage in cases of CLI. Patency rates are variable and depend on the length of diseased segment and distal artery patency. However, the goal of care in these patients is focused more on wound healing, avoidance of amputation, and relief of pain as opposed to vessel patency. Once the high metabolic demands of a healing wound are satisfied, tibial vessel patency is less crucial to maintain intact pedal tissues. Balloon angioplasty is typically the standard of care for infrapopliteal disease (Figure 35-11). In comparison to bypass surgery, balloon angioplasty offers equivalent limb salvage (75.3% vs. 76.0%) and amputation-free survival (37.7% vs. 37.3%) rates, and it is significantly less invasive in this patient population with multiple medical comorbidities.[99] Small case series using coronary DES for tibial disease in CLI have been reported with encouraging results,[100] but larger randomized trials such as the Percutaneous Transluminal Angioplasty and Drug-Eluting Stents for Intrapopliteal Lesions in Critical Limb Ischemia (PADI) trial are still ongoing and will provide further guidance in this lesion subset.[101]

Therapeutic Angiogenesis

Promoting angiogenesis using genetic protein, stem cell–based therapies is a promising option for the treatment of peripheral vascular disease that is unresponsive to medical and surgical therapy.[102] Unlike traditional revascularization, which focuses on mechanical macrovascular solutions, angiogenesis seeks to improve the microcirculation by stimulating new capillary and collateral arterial vessel formation. Isner and Baumgartner reported the first administration of an angiogenic growth factor, plasmid phVEGF, to a patient with PAD, and they reported encouraging results from a small, uncontrolled trial.[103] Subsequent controlled trials, however, did not detect a benefit of VEGF administration to patients with CLI.[104,105] Intramuscular administration of fibroblast growth factor-1 (FGF-1) to patients with CLI reduced the need for amputations in the Therapeutic Angiogenesis Leg Ischemia Study for Management of Arteriopathy and Non-Healing Ulcer (TALISMAN) trial, although the primary endpoint of ulcer healing was not met.[106] The subsequent phase III NVIFGF Gene Therapy on Amputation-Free Survival in Critical Limb Ischemia (TAMARIS) trial did not confirm a benefit of FGF-1 on amputation-free survival in patients with CLI.[107] Intramuscular injection of hepatocyte growth factor (HGF) plasmid vector to patients with CLI increased transcutaneous partial pressure of oxygen compared with placebo but did not improve the ABI, nor did it provide pain relief, promote wound healing, or prevent major amputation.[108] A phase I study of hypoxia-inducible factor-1α (HIF-1α) hinted at potential benefit for limb salvage in CLI; however, the subsequent larger controlled trial did not find that intramuscular administration of HIF-1α was effective for patients with PAD and intermittent claudication.[109] Although clinical trial results to date have been disappointing, the dream of therapeutic angiogenesis for the treatment of CLI may still yet be realized.[102]

Conclusions

Endovascular therapies continue to improve and allow for minimally invasive therapy of more complex vascular disease. New catheter, wire, balloon, and stent designs along with bioabsorbable materials and drug-delivery systems promise to further improve both acute results and long-term patency. Biologic approaches such as therapeutic angiogenesis may augment or in some cases supplant mechanical approaches to revascularization the same as

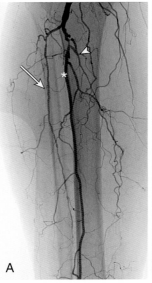
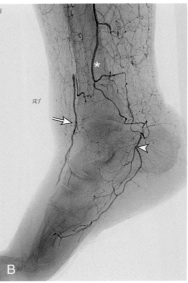
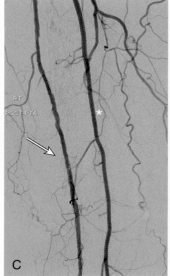
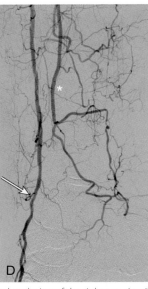

FIGURE 35-11 Infrapopliteal angioplasty for limb salvage in a patient with critical limb ischemia. **A,** Diffuse disease and distal occlusion of the right anterior tibial artery (*arrow*). The posterior tibial artery is occluded proximally (*arrowhead*). The peroneal artery (*asterisk*), which does not provide direct flow to the foot, is patent with proximal stenosis. **B,** Pedal circulation and reconstitution of the anterior tibial artery as the dorsalis pedis artery (*arrow*) and posterior tibial artery as the plantar artery (*arrowhead*) via collaterals from the peroneal artery (*asterisk*). **C** and **D,** After balloon angioplasty, brisk flow is noted in the anterior tibial artery (**C,** *arrow*) and dorsalis pedal artery (**D,** *arrow*). The peroneal artery (*asterisks*) continues to supply collaterals to the posterior tibial and plantar vessels, which were not targeted for revascularization. This intervention allowed complete and durable healing of a large foot ulcer.

stents or bypass surgery. Rigorous evaluations of these new therapies in prospective randomized trials are needed to guide and inform our use of these technologies. In addition to efficacy and safety, cost-effectiveness analyses will be critical to guide our adoption and utilization of new techniques. Although technical innovations will continue to expand the boundaries of surgical and minimally invasive endovascular therapies, medical therapy remains the foundation of treatment of systemic atherosclerosis as the underlying cause of PAD. Development of novel pharmacotherapies and recognition of the benefit of supervised exercise therapy by payer organizations are essential for noninvasive management of patients with intermittent claudication. Arterial revascularization, increasingly by endovascular techniques, is a complementary and invaluable tool for the relief of pain, improvement in quality of life, and prevention of tissue loss and amputation in selected subsets of patients. The optimal care of the underlying disease processes and clinical manifestations of PAD is best provided in a collaborative fashion by vascular specialists with expertise in medical management, exercise therapy, and endovascular and surgical revascularization.

REFERENCES

1. Hiatt WR, Goldstone J, Smith SC Jr, et al. Atherosclerotic Peripheral Vascular Disease Symposium II: nomenclature for vascular diseases. *Circulation* 2008;118(25):2826-2829.
2. Pande RL, Perlstein TS, Beckman JA, Creager MA. Secondary prevention and mortality in peripheral artery disease: National Health and Nutrition Examination Study, 1999 to 2004. *Circulation* 2011;124(1):17-23.
3. Hirsch AT, Criqui MH, Treat-Jacobson D, et al. Peripheral arterial disease detection, awareness, and treatment in primary care. *JAMA* 2001;286(11):1317-1324.
4. Hirsch AT, Haskal ZJ, Hertzer NR, et al. ACC/AHA 2005 practice guidelines for the management of patients with peripheral arterial disease (lower extremity, renal, mesenteric, and abdominal aortic). *Circulation* 2006;113(11):e463-e654.
5. Rooke TW, Hirsch AT, Misra S, et al. 2011 ACCF/AHA focused update of the guideline for the management of patients with peripheral artery disease (updating the 2005 guideline). *Vasc Med* 2011;16(6):452-476.
6. Fowkes FG, Housley E, Riemersma RA, et al. Smoking, lipids, glucose intolerance, and blood pressure as risk factors for peripheral atherosclerosis compared with ischemic heart disease in the Edinburgh Artery Study. *Am J Epidemiol* 1992;135(4):331-340.
7. Goldhaber SZ, Manson JE, Stampfer MJ, et al. Low-dose aspirin and subsequent peripheral arterial surgery in the Physicians' Health Study. *Lancet* 1992;340(8812):143-145.
8. Ridker PM, Manson JE, Buring JE, Goldhaber SZ, Hennekens CH. The effect of chronic platelet inhibition with low-dose aspirin on atherosclerotic progression and acute thrombosis: clinical evidence from the Physicians' Health Study. *Am Heart J* 1991;122(6):1588-1592.
9. Belch J, MacCuish A, Campbell I, et al. The prevention of progression of arterial disease and diabetes (POPADAD) trial: factorial randomised placebo controlled trial of aspirin and antioxidants in patients with diabetes and asymptomatic peripheral arterial disease. *Br Med J* 2008;337:a1840.
10. Fowkes FG, Price JF, Stewart MC, et al. Aspirin for prevention of cardiovascular events in a general population screened for a low ankle brachial index: a randomized controlled trial. *JAMA* 2010;303(9):841-848.
11. McDermott MM, Criqui MH. Aspirin and secondary prevention in peripheral artery disease: a perspective for the early 21st century. *JAMA* 2009;301(18):1927-1928.
12. Berger JS, Krantz MJ, Kittelson JM, Hiatt WR. Aspirin for the prevention of cardiovascular events in patients with peripheral artery disease: a meta-analysis of randomized trials. *JAMA* 2009;301(18):1909-1919.
13. Robless P, Mikhailidis DP, Stansby G. Systematic review of antiplatelet therapy for the prevention of myocardial infarction, stroke or vascular death in patients with peripheral vascular disease. *Br J Surg* 2001;88(6):787-800.
14. Collaborative meta-analysis of randomised trials of antiplatelet therapy for prevention of death, myocardial infarction, and stroke in high risk patients. *Br Med J* 2002;324(7329):71-86.
15. A randomised, blinded trial of clopidogrel versus aspirin in patients at risk of ischaemic events (CAPRIE). CAPRIE Steering Committee. *Lancet* 1996;348(9038):1329-1339.
16. Cacoub PP, Bhatt DL, Steg PG, Topol EJ, Creager MA. Patients with peripheral arterial disease in the CHARISMA trial. *Eur Heart J* 2009;30(2):192-201.
17. Anand SS, Yusuf S. Oral anticoagulant therapy in patients with coronary artery disease: a meta-analysis. *JAMA* 1999;282(21):2058-2067.
18. Anand S, Yusuf S, Xie C, et al. Oral anticoagulant and antiplatelet therapy and peripheral arterial disease. *N Engl J Med* 2007;357(3):217-227.
19. Randomised trial of cholesterol lowering in 4444 patients with coronary heart disease: the Scandinavian Simvastatin Survival Study (4S). *Lancet* 1994;344(8934):1383-1389.
20. Shepherd J, Cobbe SM, Ford I, et al. Prevention of coronary heart disease with pravastatin in men with hypercholesterolemia. West of Scotland Coronary Prevention Study Group. *N Engl J Med* 1995;333(20):1301-1307.
21. Pedersen TR, Kjekshus J, Pyorala K, et al. Effect of simvastatin on ischemic signs and symptoms in the Scandinavian Simvastatin Survival Study (4S). *Am J Cardiol* 1998;81(3):333-335.
22. MRC/BHF Heart Protection Study of cholesterol lowering with simvastatin in 20,536 high-risk individuals: a randomised placebo-controlled trial. *Lancet* 2002;360(9326):7-22.
23. Randomized trial of the effects of cholesterol-lowering with simvastatin on peripheral vascular and other major vascular outcomes in 20,536 people with peripheral arterial disease and other high-risk conditions. *J Vasc Surg* 2007;45(4):645-654; discussion 653-654.
24. Grundy SM, Cleeman JI, Merz CN, et al. Implications of recent clinical trials for the National Cholesterol Education Program Adult Treatment Panel III guidelines. *Circulation* 2004;110(2):227-239.
25. Smith SC Jr, Benjamin EJ, Bonow RO, et al. AHA/ACCF secondary prevention and risk reduction therapy for patients with coronary and other atherosclerotic vascular disease: 2011 update: a guideline from the American Heart Association and American College of Cardiology Foundation. *Circulation* 2011;124(22):2458-2473.

26. McDermott MM, Mehta S, Greenland P. Exertional leg symptoms other than intermittent claudication are common in peripheral arterial disease. *Arch Intern Med* 1999;159(4): 387-392.

27. Pasternak RC, Smith SC Jr, Bairey-Merz CN, et al. ACC/AHA/NHLBI Clinical Advisory on the Use and Safety of Statins. *Circulation* 2002;106(8):1024-1028.

28. Sacks FM, Carey VJ, Fruchart JC. Combination lipid therapy in type 2 diabetes. *N Engl J Med* 2010;363(7):692-694; author reply 694-695.

29. Canner PL, Furberg CD, McGovern ME. Benefits of niacin in patients with versus without the metabolic syndrome and healed myocardial infarction (from the Coronary Drug Project). *Am J Cardiol* 2006;97(4):477-479.

30. Chobanian AV, Bakris GL, Black HR, et al. The Seventh Report of the Joint National Committee on Prevention, Detection, Evaluation, and Treatment of High Blood Pressure: the JNC 7 report. *JAMA* 2003;289(19):2560-2572.

31. Mehler PS, Coll JR, Estacio R, et al. Intensive blood pressure control reduces the risk of cardiovascular events in patients with peripheral arterial disease and type 2 diabetes. *Circulation* 2003;107(5):753-756.

32. Bangalore S, Kumar S, Lobach I, Messerli FH. Blood pressure targets in subjects with type 2 diabetes mellitus/impaired fasting glucose: observations from traditional and bayesian random-effects meta-analyses of randomized trials. *Circulation* 2011;123(24): 2799-2810.

33. Upadhyay A, Earley A, Haynes SM, Uhlig K. Systematic review: blood pressure target in chronic kidney disease and proteinuria as an effect modifier. *Ann Intern Med* 2011; 154(8):541-548.

34. Yusuf S, Sleight P, Pogue J, et al. Effects of an angiotensin-converting-enzyme inhibitor, ramipril, on cardiovascular events in high-risk patients. The Heart Outcomes Prevention Evaluation Study Investigators. *N Engl J Med* 2000;342(3):145-153.

35. Ostergren J, Sleight P, Dagenais G, et al. Impact of ramipril in patients with evidence of clinical or subclinical peripheral arterial disease. *Eur Heart J* 2004;25(1):17-24.

36. Fox KM. Efficacy of perindopril in reduction of cardiovascular events among patients with stable coronary artery disease: randomised, double-blind, placebo-controlled, multicentre trial (the EUROPA study). *Lancet* 2003;362(9386):782-788.

37. Braunwald E, Domanski MJ, Fowler SE, et al. Angiotensin-converting-enzyme inhibition in stable coronary artery disease. *N Engl J Med* 2004;351(20):2058-2068.

38. Yusuf S, Diener HC, Sacco RL, et al. Telmisartan to prevent recurrent stroke and cardiovascular events. *N Engl J Med* 2008;359(12):1225-1237.

39. Yusuf S, Teo K, Anderson C, et al. Effects of the angiotensin-receptor blocker telmisartan on cardiovascular events in high-risk patients intolerant to angiotensin-converting enzyme inhibitors: a randomised controlled trial. *Lancet* 2008;372(9644):1174-1183.

40. Yusuf S, Teo KK, Pogue J, et al. Telmisartan, ramipril, or both in patients at high risk for vascular events. *N Engl J Med* 2008;358(15):1547-1559.

41. Nissen SE, Tuzcu EM, Libby P, et al. Effect of antihypertensive agents on cardiovascular events in patients with coronary disease and normal blood pressure: the CAMELOT study: a randomized controlled trial. *JAMA* 2004;292(18):2217-2225.

42. Paravastu SC, Mendonca DA, da Silva A. Beta blockers for peripheral arterial disease. *Eur J Vasc Endovasc Surg* 2009;38(1):66-70.

43. Radack K, Deck C. Beta-adrenergic blocker therapy does not worsen intermittent claudication in subjects with peripheral arterial disease: a meta-analysis of randomized controlled trials. *Arch Intern Med* 1991;151(9):1769-1776.

44. Diehm C, Pittrow D, Lawall H. Effect of nebivolol vs. hydrochlorothiazide on the walking capacity in hypertensive patients with intermittent claudication. *J Hypertens* 2011;29(7):1448-1456.

45. van Gestel YR, Hoeks SE, Sin DD, et al. Beta-blockers and health-related quality of life in patients with peripheral arterial disease and COPD. *Int J Chron Obstruct Pulmon Dis* 2009;4:177-183.

46. Conen D, Everett BM, Kurth T, et al. Smoking, smoking status, and risk for symptomatic peripheral artery disease in women: a cohort study. *Ann Intern Med* 2011;154(11): 719-726.

47. Gardner AW. The effect of cigarette smoking on exercise capacity in patients with intermittent claudication. *Vasc Med* 1996;1(3):181-186.

48. Cahan MA, Montgomery P, Otis RB, et al. The effect of cigarette smoking status on six-minute walk distance in patients with intermittent claudication. *Angiology* 1999; 50(7):537-546.

49. Quick CR, Cotton LT. The measured effect of stopping smoking on intermittent claudication. *Br J Surg* 1982;69(Suppl):S24-S26.

50. Lassila R, Lepantalo M. Cigarette smoking and the outcome after lower limb arterial surgery. *Acta Chir Scand* 1988;154(11-12):635-640.

51. Faulkner KW, House AK, Castleden WM. The effect of cessation of smoking on the accumulative survival rates of patients with symptomatic peripheral vascular disease. *Med J Aust* 1983;1(5):217-219.

52. Jonason T, Bergstrom R. Cessation of smoking in patients with intermittent claudication: effects on the risk of peripheral vascular complications, myocardial infarction and mortality. *Acta Med Scand* 1987;221(3):253-260.

53. Hennrikus D, Joseph AM, Lando HA, et al. Effectiveness of a smoking cessation program for peripheral artery disease patients: a randomized controlled trial. *J Am Coll Cardiol* 2010;56(25):2105-2112.

54. Eisenberg MJ, Filion KB, Yavin D, et al. Pharmacotherapies for smoking cessation: a meta-analysis of randomized controlled trials. *CMAJ* 2008;179(2):135-144.

55. Skyler JS, Bergenstal R, Bonow RO, et al. Intensive glycemic control and the prevention of cardiovascular events: implications of the ACCORD, ADVANCE, and VA diabetes trials: a position statement of the American Diabetes Association and a scientific statement of the American College of Cardiology Foundation and the American Heart Association. *Circulation* 2009;119(2):351-357.

56. Spronk S, White JV, Bosch JL, Hunink MG. Impact of claudication and its treatment on quality of life. *Semin Vasc Surg* 2007;20(1):3-9.

57. Mays RJ, Casserly IP, Kohrt WM, et al. Assessment of functional status and quality of life in claudication. *J Vasc Surg* 2011;53(5):1410-1421.

58. Gardner AW, Poehlman ET. Exercise rehabilitation programs for the treatment of claudication pain: a meta-analysis. *JAMA* 1995;274(12):975-980.

59. Bendermacher BL, Willigendael EM, Teijink JA, Prins MH. Supervised exercise therapy versus non-supervised exercise therapy for intermittent claudication. *Cochrane Database Syst Rev* 2006(2):CD005263.

60. Murphy TP, Hirsch AT, Ricotta JJ, et al. The Claudication: Exercise Vs. Endoluminal Revascularization (CLEVER) study: rationale and methods. *J Vasc Surg* 2008;47(6): 1356-1363.

61. Hood SC, Moher D, Barber GG. Management of intermittent claudication with pentoxifylline: meta-analysis of randomized controlled trials. *CMAJ* 1996;155(8):1053-1059.

62. Dawson DL, Cutler BS, Hiatt WR, et al. A comparison of cilostazol and pentoxifylline for treating intermittent claudication. *Am J Med* 2000;109(7):523-530.

63. Pande RL, Hiatt WR, Zhang P, et al. A pooled analysis of the durability and predictors of treatment response of cilostazol in patients with intermittent claudication. *Vasc Med* 2010;15(3):181-188.

64. Chapman TM, Goa KL. Cilostazol: a review of its use in intermittent claudication. *Am J Cardiovasc Drugs* 2003;3(2):117-138.

65. Fleisher LA, Beckman JA, Brown KA, et al. 2009 ACCF/AHA focused update on perioperative beta blockade incorporated into the ACC/AHA 2007 guidelines on perioperative cardiovascular evaluation and care for noncardiac surgery: a report of the American College of Cardiology Foundation/American Heart Association Task Force on Practice Guidelines. *Circulation* 2009;120(21):e169-e276.

66. Feringa HH, Bax JJ, Boersma E, et al. High-dose beta-blockers and tight heart rate control reduce myocardial ischemia and troponin T release in vascular surgery patients. *Circulation* 2006;114(1 Suppl):I344-I349.

67. Fleischmann KE, Beckman JA, Buller CE, et al. 2009 ACCF/AHA focused update on perioperative beta blockade: a report of the American College Of Cardiology Foundation/American Heart Association Task Force on Practice Guidelines. *Circulation* 2009;120(21): 2123-2151.

68. Lindenauer PK, Pekow P, Wang K, et al. Perioperative beta-blocker therapy and mortality after major noncardiac surgery. *N Engl J Med* 2005;353(4):349-361.

69. Boersma E, Poldermans D, Bax JJ, et al. Predictors of cardiac events after major vascular surgery: role of clinical characteristics, dobutamine echocardiography, and beta-blocker therapy. *JAMA* 2001;285(14):1865-1873.

70. Schouten O, Hoeks SE, Welten GM, et al. Effect of statin withdrawal on frequency of cardiac events after vascular surgery. *Am J Cardiol* 2007;100(2):316-320.

71. Schouten O, Bax JJ, Dunkelgrun M, et al. Statins for the prevention of perioperative cardiovascular complications in vascular surgery. *J Vasc Surg* 2006;44(2):419-424.

72. Schouten O, Boersma E, Hoeks SE, et al. Fluvastatin and perioperative events in patients undergoing vascular surgery. *N Engl J Med* 2009;361(10):980-989.

73. Le Manach Y, Ibanez Esteves C, Bertrand M, et al. Impact of preoperative statin therapy on adverse postoperative outcomes in patients undergoing vascular surgery. *Anesthesiology* 2011;114(1):98-104.

74. Feringa HH, Bax JJ, Schouten O, Poldermans D. Ischemic heart disease in renal transplant candidates: towards non-invasive approaches for preoperative risk stratification. *Eur J Echocardiogr* 2005;6(5):313-316.

75. Fleisher LA, Eagle KA. Clinical practice: lowering cardiac risk in noncardiac surgery. *N Engl J Med* 2001;345(23):1677-1682.

76. Neilipovitz DT, Bryson GL, Nichol G. The effect of perioperative aspirin therapy in peripheral vascular surgery: a decision analysis. *Anesth Analg* 2001;93(3):573-580.

77. Ware JE Jr. The status of health assessment 1994. *Annu Rev Public Health* 1995;16: 327-354.

78. Norgren L, Hiatt WR, Dormandy JA, et al. Inter-Society Consensus for the Management of Peripheral Arterial Disease (TASC II). *J Vasc Surg* 2007;45(Suppl S):S5-S67.

79. Whyman MR, Fowkes FG, Kerracher EM, et al. Randomised controlled trial of percutaneous transluminal angioplasty for intermittent claudication. *Eur J Vasc Endovasc Surg* 1996;12(2):167-172.

80. Spronk S, Bosch JL, Veen HF, den Hoed PT, Hunink MG. Intermittent claudication: functional capacity and quality of life after exercise training or percutaneous transluminal angioplasty—systematic review. *Radiology* 2005;235(3):833-842.

81. Adam DJ, Beard JD, Cleveland T, et al. Bypass versus angioplasty in severe ischaemia of the leg (BASIL): multicentre, randomised controlled trial. *Lancet* 2005;366(9501): 1925-1934.

82. Bradbury AW, Adam DJ, Bell J, et al. Bypass versus Angioplasty in Severe Ischaemia of the Leg (BASIL) trial: an intention-to-treat analysis of amputation-free and overall survival in patients randomized to a bypass surgery-first or a balloon angioplasty-first revascularization strategy. *J Vasc Surg* 2010;51(5 Suppl):5S-17S.

83. Goodney PP, Beck AW, Nagle J, Welch HG, Zwolak RM. National trends in lower extremity bypass surgery, endovascular interventions, and major amputations. *J Vasc Surg* 2009;50(1):54-60.

84. White CJ, Gray WA. Endovascular therapies for peripheral arterial disease: an evidence-based review. *Circulation* 2007;116(19):2203-2215.

85. Bosch JL, Hunink MG. Meta-analysis of the results of percutaneous transluminal angioplasty and stent placement for aortoiliac occlusive disease. *Radiology* 1997; 204(1):87-96.

86. Stockx L, Poncyljusz W, Krzanowski M, et al. Express LD vascular stent in the treatment of iliac artery lesions: 24-month results from the MELODIE trial. *J Endovasc Ther* 2010;17(5):633-641.

87. Klein WM, van der Graaf Y, Seegers J, et al. Dutch iliac stent trial: long-term results in patients randomized for primary or selective stent placement. *Radiology* 2006;238(2): 734-744.

88. Ponec D, Jaff MR, Swischuk J, et al. The Nitinol SMART stent vs Wallstent for suboptimal iliac artery angioplasty: CRISP-US trial results. *J Vasc Interv Radiol* 2004;15(9):911-918.

89. Sabri SS, Choudhri A, Orgera G, et al. Outcomes of covered kissing stent placement compared with bare metal stent placement in the treatment of atherosclerotic occlusive disease at the aortic bifurcation. *J Vasc Interv Radiol* 2010;21(7):995-1003.

90. Schillinger M, Sabeti S, Loewe C, et al. Balloon angioplasty versus implantation of nitinol stents in the superficial femoral artery. *N Engl J Med* 2006;354(18):1879-1888.

91. Krankenberg H, Schluter M, Steinkamp HJ, et al. Nitinol stent implantation versus percutaneous transluminal angioplasty in superficial femoral artery lesions up to

10 cm in length: the femoral artery stenting trial (FAST). *Circulation* 2007;116(3):285-292.

92. Schlager O, Dick P, Sabeti S, et al. Long-segment SFA stenting—the dark sides: in-stent restenosis, clinical deterioration, and stent fractures. *J Endovasc Ther* 2005;12(6):676-684.

93. Ansel G. Interim results of the VIBRANT trial. In: *Vascular interventional advances*. 2009, Las Vegas.

94. Scheinert D, Grummt L, Piorkowski M, et al. A novel self-expanding interwoven nitinol stent for complex femoropopliteal lesions: 24-month results of the SUPERA SFA registry. *J Endovasc Ther* 2011;18(6):745-752.

95. Dake MD, Ansel GM, Jaff MR, et al. Paclitaxel-eluting stents show superiority to balloon angioplasty and bare metal stents in femoropopliteal disease: twelve-month Zilver PTX randomized study results. *Circ Cardiovasc Interv* 2011;4(5):495-504.

96. Duda SH, Bosiers M, Lammer J, et al. Sirolimus-eluting versus bare nitinol stent for obstructive superficial femoral artery disease: the SIROCCO II trial. *J Vasc Interv Radiol* 2005;16(3):331-338.

97. Tepe G, Zeller T, Albrecht T, et al. Local delivery of paclitaxel to inhibit restenosis during angioplasty of the leg. *N Engl J Med* 2008;358(7):689-699.

98. Werk M, Langner S, Reinkensmeier B, et al. Inhibition of restenosis in femoropopliteal arteries: paclitaxel-coated versus uncoated balloon: femoral paclitaxel randomized pilot trial. *Circulation* 2008;118(13):1358-1365.

99. Soderstrom MI, Arvela EM, Korhonen M, et al. Infrapopliteal percutaneous transluminal angioplasty versus bypass surgery as first-line strategies in critical leg ischemia: a propensity score analysis. *Ann Surg* 2010;252(5):765-773.

100. Grant AG, White CJ, Collins TJ, et al. Infrapopliteal drug-eluting stents for chronic limb ischemia. *Catheter Cardiovasc Interv* 2008;71(1):108-111.

101. Martens JM, Knippenberg B, Vos JA, et al. Update on PADI trial: percutaneous transluminal angioplasty and drug-eluting stents for infrapopliteal lesions in critical limb ischemia. *J Vasc Surg* 2009;50(3):687-689.

102. Pacilli A, Faggioli G, Stella A, Pasquinelli G. An update on therapeutic angiogenesis for peripheral vascular disease. *Ann Vasc Surg* 2010;24(2):258-268.

103. Isner JM, Pieczek A, Schainfeld R, et al. Clinical evidence of angiogenesis after arterial gene transfer of phVEGF165 in patient with ischaemic limb. *Lancet* 1996;348(9024):370-374.

104. Kusumanto YH, Hospers GA, Mulder NH, Tio RA. Therapeutic angiogenesis with vascular endothelial growth factor in peripheral and coronary artery disease: a review. *Int J Cardiovasc Intervent* 2003;5(1):27-34.

105. Rajagopalan S, Mohler ER 3rd, Lederman RJ, et al. Regional angiogenesis with vascular endothelial growth factor in peripheral arterial disease: a phase II randomized, double-blind, controlled study of adenoviral delivery of vascular endothelial growth factor 121 in patients with disabling intermittent claudication. *Circulation* 2003;108(16):1933-1938.

106. Nikol S, Baumgartner I, Van Belle E, et al. Therapeutic angiogenesis with intramuscular NV1FGF improves amputation-free survival in patients with critical limb ischemia. *Mol Ther* 2008;16(5):972-978.

107. Belch J, Hiatt WR, Baumgartner I, et al. Effect of fibroblast growth factor NV1FGF on amputation and death: a randomised placebo-controlled trial of gene therapy in critical limb ischaemia. *Lancet* 2011;377(9781):1929-1937.

108. Powell RJ, Simons M, Mendelsohn FO, et al. Results of a double-blind, placebo-controlled study to assess the safety of intramuscular injection of hepatocyte growth factor plasmid to improve limb perfusion in patients with critical limb ischemia. *Circulation* 2008;118(1):58-65.

109. Sneider EB, Nowicki PT, Messina LM. Regenerative medicine in the treatment of peripheral arterial disease. *J Cell Biochem* 2009;108(4):753-761.

CHAPTER 36

Cerebrovascular Disease

Piotr Sobieszczyk

ATHEROSCLEROTIC CAROTID ARTERY DISEASE AND
STROKE, 553

Risk of Stroke, 553
Prevalence of Carotid Artery Disease, 553

MEDICAL THERAPY OF ATHEROSCLEROTIC CAROTID
ARTERY DISEASE, 555

Smoking Cessation, 555
Antihypertensive Therapy, 555

Lipid-Lowering Therapy, 556
Antiplatelet Therapy, 557

REVASCULARIZATION FOR CAROTID ARTERY
DISEASE, 558

Surgical Revascularization, 559
Endovascular Therapy for Carotid Artery Stenosis, 562
Should Asymptomatic Carotid Artery Stenosis Be
Revascularized? 565

Carotid Artery Disease and Coronary Artery Bypass Graft
Surgery, 566

REFERENCES, 568

Stroke is the fourth leading cause of death in the United States and accounts for approximately 1 in 18 deaths every year.[1] Both men and women are affected equally, and 6 of every 10 deaths from cerebrovascular accidents (CVAs) occur in women. For survivors, stroke becomes a cause of long-term disability. The annual incidence of new CVA approaches 610,000, and an estimated 185,000 patients have recurrent stroke.[1] A large number of cerebral infarcts go unrecognized, and their prevalence increases with age. Silent ischemic events occur in 11% of patients between the ages of 55 and 64 years, with rates reaching 32% among septuagenarians.[1] The economic dimensions of cerebrovascular disease are vast, with health care expenditures related to stroke treatment estimated to be $68.9 billion in 2009.[2]

Carotid artery disease has long been recognized as an important cause of cerebrovascular events. Atherosclerosis is the predominant cause of carotid artery narrowing and occlusion (Figure 36-1). Stroke occurs via the mechanism of artery-to-artery embolism: rupture of a plaque or friable lesion releases embolic debris. The risk of CVA increases with lesion severity. Hemispheric malperfusion can rarely occur in patients with severe, nearly occlusive stenosis and concomitant disease in the remaining cervical vessel. Such events are usually triggered by conditions of relative systemic hypotension, such as during cardiopulmonary bypass. Other causes of carotid disease, such as carotid artery dissection, fibromuscular dysplasia, or Takayasu arteritis, are infrequent yet important to recognize because their management differs from that of atherosclerotic disease.

Since the introduction of modern surgical endarterectomy by Eastcott in 1954, therapy for symptomatic and asymptomatic atherosclerotic carotid artery disease has undergone a tremendous, yet somewhat circular, evolution. After years of debate over the benefits of carotid endarterectomy (CEA) for stroke prevention, landmark trials in the 1980s and 1990s convincingly showed the benefit of revascularization in symptomatic patients. The benefit of prophylactic revascularization in asymptomatic patients with moderate to severe carotid stenosis was less tangible, yet the strategy was embraced, resulting in a significant increase in carotid artery surgeries. The next stage in the evolution of carotid artery therapy involved the intense and partisan debate over the merits of less invasive revascularization by carotid artery stenting (CAS), which is especially attractive for patients with advanced cardiovascular disease. Recent trials point to equipoise between these two revascularization strategies. Today, the success of medical therapy in stroke prevention returns the debate to its origin: should asymptomatic patients be revascularized at all, or should medical therapy be continued until the onset of symptoms? The hardest clinical decision does not revolve around the type of revascularization therapy but rather whether revascularization is needed at all.

Atherosclerotic Carotid Artery Disease and Stroke

Risk of Stroke

Ischemic stroke is responsible for 88% of all CVAs, and intracerebral and subarachnoid hemorrhage account for 9% and 3% of all strokes, respectively.[3] Carotid artery disease is a well-established cause of ischemic stroke, but the degree of its contribution is difficult to determine. Data from several studies allow a reasonable estimate of the role carotid artery disease plays in the burden of CVA.

A population study conducted in the 1980s in Olmstead County, Minnesota, attributed 18% of new ischemic strokes to combined intracranial and extracranial large vessel disease, but the specific contribution of extracranial carotid artery disease was not characterized. Data from the Northern Manhattan Stroke Study (NOMASS) suggest that 7% of all new ischemic strokes are related to carotid artery stenosis of 60% or more. The incidence of stroke related to carotid artery disease varies with ethnic background. In the 1990s, the incidence of cerebral infarction caused by carotid artery disease was 17 per 100,000 (95% confidence interval [CI], 8 to 26) among African Americans, 9 per 100,000 (95% CI, 5 to 13) for Hispanics, and 5 per 100,000 (95% CI, 2 to 8) for whites.[4] Data from the Brain Attack Surveillance in Corpus Christi (BASIC) Project suggest that among patients who come to medical attention with a transient ischemic attack (TIA), carotid artery disease exceeding 70% stenosis is present in 9.5% of patients.[5] In this population study, however, only 55% of patients with TIA underwent carotid ultrasound imaging. Similar observations were made in a series of 438 patients admitted with acute stroke in the NOMASS study; extracranial carotid artery disease was identified as the cause of CVA in 9% of patients, and intracranial atherosclerosis was responsible for 8% of the events. Lacunar strokes represented 30% of the events, and a cardioembolic etiology was identified in 21% of patients, with the remaining 31% categorized as cryptogenic and 1% due to other causes.[6] With the definition of *cerebrovascular event* widened to include TIA and CVA, analysis of consecutive patients seen over a period of 2 years at a community hospital revealed that carotid artery stenosis of 50% of more was identified in 33% of white patients and 15% of black patents (*P* = .001). Extracranial carotid artery disease was identified as the cause of stroke in 8% of patients, and intracranial atherosclerotic disease was identified in another 8%.[7] It thus appears that atherosclerotic cerebrovascular disease is responsible for 16% to 17% of all ischemic cerebrovascular events, and extracranial carotid disease accounts for half of these.

Prevalence of Carotid Artery Disease

The prevalence of atherosclerotic carotid artery disease depends on its definition. Carotid artery stenosis of 50% or more detected

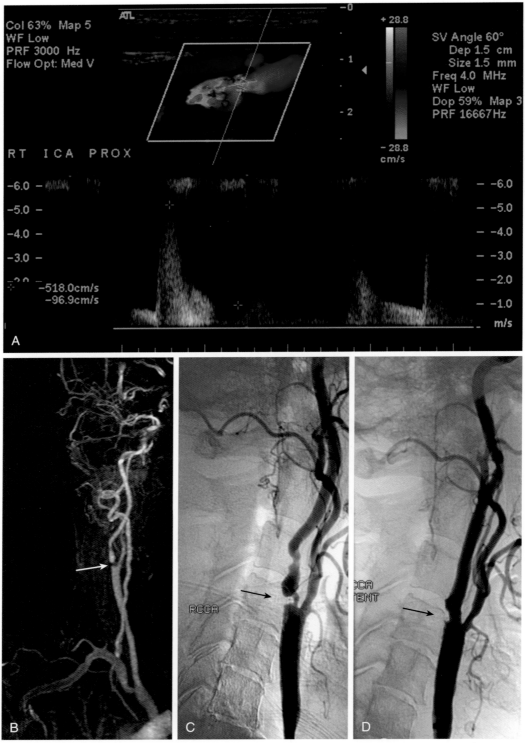

FIGURE 36-1 Atherosclerotic carotid artery stenosis is examined with several imaging modalities. **A,** Carotid ultrasound image of the right internal carotid artery (ICA). Elevated velocities above 500 cm/s are consistent with a high-grade (>90%) stenosis. **B,** Magnetic resonance angiography of the same artery with a severe proximal right ICA stenosis (*arrow*). **C,** Digital subtraction angiogram obtained as part of carotid stenting procedure confirms the location and severity of stenosis (*arrow*). RCCA, right common carotid artery. **D,** The right ICA after deployment of a self-expanding stent.

by ultrasound has been traditionally considered to be clinically relevant. In the Framingham Heart Study, carotid artery disease thus defined was present in 7% of women and 9% of men older than 66 years.[8] Similar prevalence was reported among subjects 65 years and older enrolled in the Cardiovascular Health Study. Moderate carotid artery stenosis of 50% to 74% was present in 7% of

men and 5% of women, whereas severe stenosis (75% to 100%) was present in 2.3% of men and 1.1% of women. These statistics are supported by a meta-analysis composed of 40 studies that reported on prevalence of asymptomatic carotid artery disease. The pooled prevalence of stenosis between 50% and 70% was 4.2% (95% CI, 3.1% to 5.7%), and pooled prevalence of severe stenosis (70% or greater) was 1.7% (95% CI, 0.7% to 3.9%). The prevalence of carotid artery disease was lower in women, and it increased with age.[9]

The traditional definition of clinically significant carotid artery disease has evolved. The importance of "subclinical" carotid artery disease characterized by thickening of the intimal layer has been underscored by evidence from the Atherosclerosis Risk in Communities (ARIC) study, suggesting that atherosclerotic plaque without hemodynamically significant stenosis is predictive of future stroke.[10] The prevalence of this subclinical disease is much higher; in the NOMASS study, 62% of subjects had carotid plaque thickness of 0.9 mm detected by carotid ultrasound.[11] Intensive risk factor modification is therefore appropriate for patients with subclinical carotid artery disease.

Medical Therapy of Atherosclerotic Carotid Artery Disease

Medical therapy plays a fundamental role in the primary and secondary prevention of cerebrovascular and cardiovascular events in patients with carotid artery disease. Because cumulative, long-term effects of atherosclerotic risk factors lead to progression of carotid stenosis, primary prevention has been focused on aggressive risk factor modification.[12] Data extrapolated from large-scale studies to examining the cardiovascular effects of risk factor reduction support the efficacy of these interventions in primary stroke prevention. The importance of medical therapy for prevention of recurrent stroke in patients with carotid artery stenosis has been well documented in randomized clinical trials. It is important to recognize that the absolute population effect of medical intervention in stroke prevention is bound to be much larger than that of much more popular revascularization procedures applied to a small number of patients at risk.

A majority of the trials that have examined the efficacy of non-invasive therapies for stroke prevention included a heterogeneous population. Despite the fact that most of these trials excluded patients at risk of cardioembolic stroke, the etiology of the stroke was nonetheless not exclusively tied to carotid artery disease. Despite these limitations, the fact that many of the risk factors are shared among patients with cerebral ischemic events from carotid artery disease and those with other etiologies allows extrapolation of these results and application of their conclusions to patients with carotid artery disease.

Epidemiologic studies suggest that, despite an aging population, the incidence of ischemic stroke has been declining. Although a direct relationship is difficult to prove, control of hypertension along with antiplatelet and lipid-lowering therapies are likely in large part responsible for these observations. A comparison of stroke rates in the Oxford Community Stroke Project conducted between 1981 and 1984 with event rates in the Oxford Vascular Study conducted in the same location between 2002 to 2004 showed that despite a 33% increase in those aged 75 years or older, the number of new ischemic strokes fell by 29% ($P = .0002$). There was a concurrent substantial reduction in the proportion of smokers, mean cholesterol levels, and mean systolic and diastolic blood pressures, as well as a substantial increase in the use of antiplatelet, lipid-lowering, and antihypertensive therapies.[13] Despite the unequivocal benefits of risk factor modification in patients with carotid artery disease, medical therapy is vastly under-utilized. Among patients who underwent CEA or coronary revascularization, the proportion of patients with optimal control of blood pressure and dyslipidemia increased only from 22% before surgery to 33% after revascularization ($P = .05$).[14]

Although intensive medical therapy is imperative for all patients with atherosclerotic extracranial cerebrovascular disease, the practitioner must establish whether the patient has had symptoms of cerebral ischemia or whether he or she remains asymptomatic. Patients in the former category have much higher rates of recurrent events and should be considered for revascularization in addition to intense medical therapy.

Smoking Cessation

Cigarette smoking is a major independent risk factor for recurrent stroke. The overall relative risk of ischemic stroke associated with smoking is 1.9 (95% CI, 1.71 to 2.16).[15] Survivors of CVA or TIA who stop smoking reduce the relative rate of stroke recurrence by 50%.[16] Data from the Framingham Heart Study suggest that the risk of first stroke decreases significantly after 2 years of abstinence, and after 5 years, it reaches the risk of nonsmokers.[17] In the Framingham study, the odds ratio (OR) for development of moderate carotid artery stenosis was 1.08 (95% CI, 1.03 to 1.13) for every 5 pack-years of smoking.[12] The conclusions from the NOMASS study were even more condemning: the relative risk of developing a 60% or greater stenosis was 1.5 among smokers.[18] Moreover, the severity of carotid artery stenosis is directly related to the duration and amount of nicotine use.[19] Accordingly, the multisocietal guidelines on management of cervical carotid and vertebral artery disease consider smoking cessation a class I recommendation (level of evidence B).[20]

Antihypertensive Therapy

Data from the Framingham study firmly established that systolic hypertension is associated with increased risk of carotid artery stenosis.[12] Independently of the direct effect of hypertension on stroke risk, an increase of 20 mm Hg in systolic blood pressure raised the odds ratio for developing moderate carotid artery stenosis to 2.11 (95% CI, 1.51 to 2.97). It is also clear that the risk of stroke increases continuously with rising blood pressure, and the association is particularly strong for systolic blood pressure.[21] The direct relationship between blood pressure lowering and risk of stroke as a result of carotid artery stenosis has not been studied in large-scale randomized trials, and evidence supporting the benefit of blood pressure control comes from studies that enroll more heterogeneous patients.

A meta-analysis of 42 randomized trials to assess cerebrovascular outcomes in patients with hypertension documented a relative risk reduction in the stroke rate of 0.71 with blood pressure–lowering therapy (95% CI, 0.63 to 0.81; $P < .001$).[22]

The benefit of antihypertensive therapy is particularly effective in the elderly. The Systolic Hypertension in the Elderly Program (SHEP) documented a 36% reduction in the incidence of stroke (95% CI, 18% to 50%; $P = .003$) among hypertensive patients older than 60 years.[23] The Systolic Hypertension in Europe (Syst-Eur) trial confirmed these findings. This study evaluated the effect of blood pressure lowering in 4695 patients older than 60 years who were randomized to placebo or active treatment with a combination of calcium channel blocker (CCB), diuretic, and angiotensin-converting enzyme (ACE) inhibitor. Patients in the active treatment group had a 42% risk reduction for any stroke (95% CI, 18% to 60%; $P = .003$).[24] Another trial examined the effect of blood pressure control with diuretic and ACE inhibitor therapy in a group of 3845 octogenarians. Patients in the active arm showed a trend toward a 30% reduction in the risk of fatal or nonfatal stroke (95% CI, −1 to 51; $P = .6$) and a 39% reduction in the risk of death from stroke (95% CI, 1 to 61; $P = .05$).[25]

It appears that all of the major classes of antihypertensive agents are effective in reducing the risk of stroke, provided they effectively lower the blood pressure. When compared with placebo, treatment with thiazide diuretic therapy was associated with a relative risk ratio of 0.68 (95% CI, 0.57 to 0.71), β-blockers yielded a risk ratio of 0.83 (95% CI, 0.72 to 0.97), ACE inhibitors resulted in a risk ratio of 0.65 (95% CI, 0.52 to 0.82), and CCBs carried a risk ratio of 0.58 (95% CI, 0.41 to 0.84).[26] Diuretic therapy may be of particular benefit in the African-American population.[27] Nevertheless, there is no convincing evidence that any class of antihypertensive agents is superior in reducing the risk of stroke.

The impact of the intensity of blood pressure lowering on stroke risk reduction is uncertain. A target blood pressure below that recommended by guidelines has been shown to further reduce the risk of stroke by 23%, with evidence that every decrement in blood pressure yields a further lowering of the stroke risk.[28] However, the largest trial to evaluate the benefits of different blood pressure targets did not find a difference in the stroke risk among patients who achieved progressively lower blood pressure.[29]

Current guidelines published jointly by the American Heart Association (AHA), American College of Cardiology (ACC), the American Stroke Association (ASA), and many other societies involved in the care of patients with cerebrovascular disease recommend that patients with asymptomatic extracranial atherosclerosis and hypertension receive therapy to reach blood pressure below 140/90 mm Hg.[20]

The benefit of blood pressure control is also clear among patients who have already had a TIA or CVA. Data gathered from therapeutic interventions in 15,527 symptomatic patients showed that antihypertensive therapy significantly reduced recurrent stroke rates (OR, 0.74; 95% CI, 0.67 to 0.83).[30] Diuretics, CCBs, and renin-angiotensin system inhibitors are commonly used in symptomatic patients without convincing evidence of superiority of one class over the other. The Prevention Regimen for Effectively Avoiding Second Strokes (PRoFESS) study group compared the benefit of the angiotensin receptor blocker (ARB) telmisartan to placebo in 20,332 patients with ischemic stroke.[31] After 2.5 years of therapy, telmisartan did not reduce the risk of recurrent stroke, but aggressive blood pressure control in the placebo group resulted in a minimal difference in systolic blood pressure between the groups. The Morbidity and Mortality After Stroke, Eprosartan Compared with Nitrendipine for Secondary Prevention (MOSES) trial compared the effect of eprosartan, an ARB, to nitrendipine, a CCB, in 1405 hypertensive patients with CVA or TIA. Both agents effectively reduced systolic blood pressure, but eprosartan significantly reduced the risk of recurrent ischemic cerebrovascular events.[32] The subsequent Perindopril Protection Against Recurrent Stroke Study (PROGRESS) showed that treatment with the ARB perindopril was effective in reducing the risk of recurrent stroke by 28% (95% CI, 17% to 38%; $P < .0001$), and combined therapy with an ARB and diuretic reduced the risk of stroke by 43% (95% CI, 30% to 54%).[33] Thus, although many guidelines favor the combination of an ACE inhibitor or ARB with a diuretic, the actual blood pressure lowering may be more important than the agents used to accomplish it.

Lipid-Lowering Therapy

Most epidemiologic studies confirm the association between elevated cholesterol levels and the risk of ischemic stroke, although the relationship is weaker than that between hyperlipidemia and myocardial infarction (MI). The largest body of evidence comes from the Multiple Risk Factor Intervention Trial (MRFIT), which enrolled 350,000 men aged 35 to 57 years with elevated total cholesterol level in the absence of diabetes or documented coronary artery disease. The risk of death from ischemic stroke directly correlated with severity of hyperlipidemia, and those with a total cholesterol level in excess of 278 mg/dL had an adjusted 2.57 relative risk of death from ischemic stroke.[34] Among smokers, the risk of ischemic stroke was increased if total cholesterol exceeded 270 mg/dL.[35]

The effect of elevated cholesterol levels on the risk of ischemic stroke crosses ethnic and gender lines. In the Asia Pacific Cohort Studies Collaboration (APCSC) the risk of ischemic stoke rose by 25% for every 1 mmol/L increase in total cholesterol (95% CI, 13% to 40%).[36] This relationship between cholesterol levels and the risk of ischemic stroke has also been established among women.[37,38]

The relationship between the serum cholesterol levels and carotid artery disease is particularly strong. Data from the Framingham study suggest that every rise of 10 mg/dL (0.26 mmol/L) in total cholesterol level is associated with an OR of 1.1 for progression from minimal to moderate carotid artery stenosis.[12] A rise in low-density lipoprotein (LDL) level of 1.55 mmol/L (60 mg/dL) leads to a 1.26-fold increase in the maximum internal carotid

artery plaque thickness.[11] The Atherosclerosis Risk in Communities study has confirmed this positive association between intima-media thickness of the carotid artery and the LDL levels and documented a negative association with the high-density lipoprotein (HDL) cholesterol levels.[39]

The rupture of atherosclerotic carotid plaque is related to its composition, with larger lipid cores conveying a higher risk of rupture and thromboembolic event.[40] In patients with atherosclerotic plaque in the carotid artery, the OR for the presence of a lipid-rich core was 2.76 (95% CI, 1.01 to 7.51) and 4.63 (95% CI, 1.56 to 13.75) in the middle and highest tertiles of total cholesterol level, respectively.[41] It follows that lipid-lowering therapy would likely reduce the risk of stroke by reducing progression or inducing regression of atherosclerotic changes in the carotid artery and by stabilizing the plaque and reducing its vulnerability to rupture. Progression of carotid intima thickness is indeed inversely related to the magnitude of LDL cholesterol (LDL-c) reduction.[42] The beneficial effect of statin therapy on progression of atherosclerotic carotid artery disease is evident even among low-risk patients with subclinical atherosclerosis.[43] Statin therapy has been shown to modulate the inflammatory changes noted in the carotid artery plaque. In a randomized study, 90-day therapy with simvastatin abolished 18F-fluorodeoxyglucose (FDG) uptake in the carotid plaques, suggesting that statin therapy attenuates inflammation within carotid artery plaque.[44] In patients with carotid artery stenosis, the effect of 6-month therapy with atorvastatin to a target LDL-c below 100 mg/dL enhanced plaque echogenicity and reduced the levels of the vascular calcification inhibitors osteopontin and osteoprotegrin, suggesting a transformation to a more stable and less vulnerable plaque.[45] In a prospective study, Spence and colleagues[46] evaluated the effect of intensive statin therapy on the incidence of carotid plaque–related microembolization detected on transcranial Doppler examination. After initiation of high-dose statin therapy, irrespective of the index LDL-c levels, the detection of microemboli declined from 12.3% of patients to 3.7% ($P < .001$). This observation corresponded to a decline in the combined rate of stroke, death, MI, or carotid revascularization because of ischemic symptoms during the study from 17.6% to 5.6% ($P < .001$).

Not surprisingly, lipid-lowering therapy with statins has become a cornerstone of therapy for patients with atherosclerotic carotid artery disease. Data from a meta-analysis that combined more than 90,000 patients with mean baseline LDL-c levels of 149 mg/dL (3.79 mmol/L) suggest that statin therapy can reduce the risk of ischemic stroke by 22% (relative risk [RR], 0.78; 99% CI, 0.70 to 0.87; $P < .0001$) for each decrease in LDL-c level of 1 mmol/L (39 mg/dL).[47] Each 10% reduction in the LDL-c level yielded a 15.6% reduction (95% CI, 6.7% to 23.6%) in the risk of stroke.[42] A larger analysis of more than 160,000 patients documented that each 1 mmol/L (39 mg/dL) decrease in the LDL-c level resulted in a 21.1% reduction (95% CI, 6.3 to 33.5; $P = .009$) in the risk of CVA.[48] After 5 years of treatment with statin therapy, these reductions translated into 8 fewer patients suffering from a CVA per 1000 patients with preexisting coronary artery disease and 5 fewer CVA events per 1000 study participants who did not have established coronary artery disease.[47]

Data from randomized trials to compare carotid artery surgery with medical therapy for primary stroke prevention suggest that patients treated with statins have lower long-term stroke rates compared with those not receiving lipid-lowering therapy, regardless of whether they were randomized to the CEA arm or medical therapy.[49]

Large randomized trials also confirm the beneficial effect of statin therapy in secondary prevention of stroke or TIA. The Stroke Prevention by Aggressive Reductions in Cholesterol Levels (SPARCL) trial showed that lipid-lowering therapy with atorvastatin administered at a daily dose of 80 mg reduced recurrent stroke by 16% among patients with a prior ischemic event of noncardioembolic etiology. Secondary analysis suggested that patients with carotid artery stenosis derived particular benefit from this therapy with a 33% reduction in their risk of CVA or TIA (HR, 0.66; 95% CI, 50% to 89%; P = .005).[50] The optimal LDL-c target appears to mirror that aimed for in patients with coronary artery disease. Data from the SPARCL trial suggest that LDL-c below 70 mg/dL resulted in an additional 28% reduction in stroke risk compared with patients with an LDL-c level of 100 mg/dL.[51] Data emerging from trials to examine the effects of intense versus "standard" LDL-c lowering also suggest that reaching a target of 100 mg/dL or less achieved a 16% relative risk reduction in stroke.[48]

The effects of other lipid-lowering therapies on the risk of ischemic stroke have not been well established. The Fenofibrate Intervention and Event Lowering in Diabetes (FIELD) study evaluated the effect of fenofibrate therapy on cardiovascular events in people with diabetes and did not find any reduction in stroke rates.[52] Similar findings were reported in the Bezafibrate Infarction Prevention (BIP) study, which enrolled patients with established coronary artery disease and low HDL-c levels.[53] The Action to Control Cardiovascular Risk in Diabetes (ACCORD) trial randomized patients with type 2 diabetes who were at high risk for cardiovascular events to therapy with either simvastatin or a combination of simvastatin and fenofibrate. This trial failed to show any additive benefit to fenofibrate therapy. After a mean follow-up of 4.7 years, the annual stroke rate was 0.36 in the monotherapy arm and 0.38 in the combined therapy arms (hazard ratio [HR] 1.05; 95% CI, 0.71 to 1.56).[54]

The prematurely terminated National Institutes of Health (NIH)-sponsored Atherothrombosis Intervention in Metabolic Syndrome With Low HDL/High Triglycerides: Impact on Global Health Outcomes (AIM-HIGH) trial investigated the effect of combined therapy with a statin and high-dose nicotinic acid compared with statin monotherapy in patients with a history of cardiovascular disease, low HDL-c, and elevated triglyceride levels. During the 32-month follow-up, 29 strokes occurred in the dual-therapy group, and 18 strokes occurred in the monotherapy group.[55] Nine of the strokes in the nicotinic acid arm occurred after cessation of therapy. Although the increased risk of stroke with niacin therapy has not been shown in prior studies, its benefit on stroke reduction is unlikely.

The optimal LDL-c level in patients with moderate to severe carotid artery disease will be addressed in the upcoming report of the National Cholesterol Education Program Adult Treatment Panel IV (NCEP ATP IV). The ATP III guidelines, updated in 2004, recommend that patients with atherosclerotic carotid artery disease be treated as patients with coronary artery disease, with an LDL-c goal below 100 mg/dL and an optional goal below 70 mg/dL.[56] This recommendation is supported by current ACC/AHA/ASA guidelines.[20]

Antiplatelet Therapy

Antiplatelet therapy has not been proven to prevent cerebrovascular ischemia in patients with asymptomatic carotid artery disease. Nevertheless, asymptomatic patients should be treated with aspirin (81 to 325 mg daily) to reduce ischemic events in other arterial beds. The Asymptomatic Cervical Bruit (ACB) study was designed to investigate the effect of aspirin on stroke rates in asymptomatic patients with a 50% or greater carotid artery stenosis. This small study was significantly underpowered (372 patients were enrolled), and the event rates after nearly 2 years of follow-up were similar: 12.3% in the placebo group and 11% in the aspirin group (P = .61).[57]

No other randomized trials have examined the role of antiplatelet therapy in asymptomatic patients with cervical carotid artery disease. The ACC/AHA/ASA guidelines give a class I (level of evidence A) recommendation for aspirin therapy for asymptomatic patients with carotid artery disease to prevent MI and other ischemic cardiovascular events.[20]

In contrast, the role of antiplatelet therapy has been well studied and established in patients with symptomatic cerebrovascular disease.[58] Among patients with symptomatic carotid artery disease, aspirin achieved a modest relative risk reduction in recurrent stroke risk of 13%.[59] Clopidogrel therapy was evaluated in the

Clopidogrel Versus Aspirin in Patients at Risk of Ischemic Events (CAPRIE) trial to reduce the relative risk of composite outcome of MI, CVA, or vascular death in patients with prior cerebral ischemic events. In a subgroup of patients enrolled after suffering a stroke, clopidogrel achieved a nonsignificant risk reduction of 7.3% (95% CI, −5.7 to 18.7) compared with aspirin therapy.[60]

Evidence from small studies suggests that dual antiplatelet therapy may be of particular benefit in patients with recently symptomatic carotid artery stenosis of 50% or more, but evidence from larger trials is less convincing. Micromebolic signals (MES) detected during a 1-hour transcranial Doppler recording are markers of future stroke or TIA. The Clopidogrel and Aspirin for Reduction of Emboli in Symptomatic Carotid Stenosis (CARESS) study enrolled recently symptomatic patients with carotid artery stenosis of 50% or more and examined the effect of aspirin and clopidogrel therapy on the frequency of MES. The proportion of patients with detected microemboli after 7 days of therapy with aspirin and clopidogrel was reduced by 44% (95% CI, 13.8 to 58.0; P = .0046) compared with patients treated with aspirin alone.[61] The Clopidogrel Plus Aspirin Versus Aspirin Alone for Reducing Embolization in Patients with Acute Symptomatic Cerebral or Carotid Artery Stenosis (CLAIR) study examined a similar patient population and showed that treatment with aspirin and clopidogrel achieved a relative risk reduction of 42.4% (95% CI, 4.6 to 65.2; P = .025) in the presence of MES compared with aspirin monotherapy.[62]

Evidence from larger randomized clinical trials of dual antiplatelet therapy is less convincing (Table 36-1). Combined aspirin and clopidogrel therapy was examined in the Aspirin and Clopidogrel Compared with Clopidogrel Alone After Recent Ischemic Stroke or Transient Ischemic Attack in High-Risk Patients (MATCH) trial of secondary stroke prevention and failed to show overall benefit compared with clopidogrel monotherapy, although in a subgroup of patients treated within 1 week of the index event, a trend was seen in reduction of stroke that favored dual antiplatelet therapy.[63] The Fast Assessment of Stroke and Transient Ischemic Attack to Prevent Early Recurrence (FASTER) study yielded similar conclusions; in patients who had a recent cerebrovascular event, clopidogrel and aspirin therapy were associated with a 90-day recurrent event rate of 7.1%, compared with 10.8% in patients treated with aspirin alone (95% CI, 0.3 to 1.2).[64] Secondary analysis of patients with CVA or TIA within 30 days of enrollment in the Clopidogrel for High Atherothrombotic Risk and Ischemic Stabilization, Management, and Avoidance (CHARISMA) trial that compared dual antiplatelet therapy to aspirin showed only a trend toward lower rates of recurrent cerebrovascular events (4.9% vs. 6.1%; 95% CI, 0.62 to 1.03).[65] Inconclusive benefit and higher risk of bleeding associated with clopidogrel and aspirin therapy, especially among the elderly, tempered the enthusiasm initially associated with this therapy.

The efficacy of combining aspirin and dipyridamole to prevent recurrent stroke was investigated in the European Stroke Prevention Study (ESPS)-2 and the European/Australasian Stroke Prevention in Reversible Ischemia Trial (ESPRIT).[66,67] ESPS-2 randomized 6602 patients with a TIA or CVA within 90 days of enrollment in a 2 × 2 factorial design to treatment with placebo, aspirin alone (50 mg daily), dipyridamole alone, or a combination of aspirin and dipyridamole. During a 2-year follow-up, the recurrent stroke rate was 15.8% in the placebo group, 12.9% in the aspirin-alone group, 13.2% in the dipyridamole-alone group, and 9.9% in the group receiving combination therapy; the difference among all four groups reached statistical significance (P < .001). The risk of recurrent stroke was reduced by 18% with aspirin therapy compared with placebo (P = .013), 16.3% with dipyridamole (P = .039), and 37% with combination therapy (P < .001). Combined therapy reduced the relative risk of stroke by 23.1% compared with aspirin alone (P = .006) and by 24.7% compared with dipyridamole alone (P = .002). Dual therapy was associated with higher rates of bleeding and dipyridamole-related headaches. The latter side effect has consistently limited the use of dipyridamole in general practice.

TABLE 36-1   Results of Contemporary Trials of Antiplatelet Therapy for Secondary Stroke Prevention

TRIAL	PATIENTS (N)	THERAPY	FOLLOW-UP DURATION	Recurrent CVA and TIA (%)			Major Bleeding Complications (%)		
				EXPERIMENTAL ARM	CONTROL ARM	STATISTICAL SIGNIFICANCE	ACTIVE ARM	COMPARISON ARM	STATISTICAL SIGNIFICANCE
ESPS-2 1996[66]	3298	ASA vs. placebo	24 mo	12.9	15.8	$P = .013$	3.33	1.3	$P < .001$
ESPS-2 1996[66]	3303	DPA vs. placebo	24 mo	13.2	15.8	$P = .039$	1.45	1.3	$P < .001$
CAPRIE 1996[60] CVA subgroup	6431	Clopidogrel vs. ASA	23 mo	9.74	10.6	NS	1.38	1.55	$P = $ NS
MATCH 2004[63]	7599	ASA + clopidogrel vs. clopidogrel	18 mo	8	9	$P = .353$	2.6	1.3	ARI, 1.3%; 95% CI, 0.6-1.9
CHARISMA 2010[65] CVA subgroup	2163	ASA + clopidogrel vs. ASA	27 mo	4.9	6.1	95% CI, 0.62-1.03	1.9	1.7	95% CI, 0.71-1.73
FASTER 2007[64]	392	ASA + clopidogrel vs. ASA	90 days	7.1	10.8	RR, 0.7; 95% CI, 0.3-1.2	3.0	0	$P = .03$
ESPS-2 1996[66]	3299	ASA + DPA vs. ASA	24 mo	9.9	12.9	$P = .006$	3.6	3.3	$P = $ NS
ESPRIT 2006[67]	2739	ASA + DPA vs. ASA	3.5 y	7	8.4	HR, 0.84; 95% CI, 0.64-1.1	2.6	3.8	HR, 0.67; 95% CI, 0.44-1.03
PRoFESS 2008[68]	20,332	ASA + DPA vs. clopidogrel	2.5 y	9	8.8	HR, 1.01; 95% CI, 0.92-1.11	4.1	3.6	95% CI, 1.0-1.32

ARI, absolute risk increase; ASA, aspirin; CI, confidence interval; CVA, cerebrovascular accident; DPA, dipyridamole; HR, hazard ratio; NS, not significant; RR, risk ratio; TIA, transient ischemic attack.

Patients enrolled in the dipyridamole arms were much more likely to stop their medication compared with those in aspirin or placebo arms, and 8% of patients treated with dipyridamole stopped their therapy because of headaches.

ESPRIT enrolled patients who had a cerebrovascular event of presumed arterial origin, although only 10% had a greater than 50% stenosis in one or both carotid arteries. Whereas combination therapy was effective in reducing the combined endpoint of vascular events, the rates of recurrent stroke were not statistically different (7% vs. 8.4%; 95% CI, 0.64 to 1.1). A high percentage of patients in combined therapy were unable to continue therapy because of dipyridamole-induced headaches: after 5 years of follow-up, only 66% of patients in the combined-therapy arm were able to continue their medication compared with 84% in the aspirin-alone arm. The disappointing results of combined dipyridamole and aspirin therapy in secondary prevention were further reinforced by the PRoFESS study. This trial enrolled 20,332 patients with prior stroke and randomized them to either extended-release dipyridamole (200 mg) and aspirin (25 mg) or clopidogrel monotherapy.[68] After 2.5 years of follow-up, 9% of patients receiving combined therapy had another stroke, an event that occurred in 8.8% of patients treated with clopidogrel (HR, 1.01; 95% CI, 0.92 to 1.11); combined therapy was also more likely to cause major bleeding (4.1% vs. 3.6%; HR 1.16; 95% CI, 1.00 to 1.32).

Compared with monotherapy, cumulative experience with dual antiplatelet therapy—aspirin and clopidogrel or aspirin and dipyridamole—points toward a significant reduction in recurrent stroke, from 5.0% to 3.3% (RR, 0.67; 95% CI, 0.49 to 0.93).[69] This benefit did come at the cost of a trend in increased rates of major bleeding, which occurred in 0.9% of patients receiving dual therapy versus 0.4% in those treated with monotherapy (RR, 2.09; 95% CI, 0.86 to 5.06).

The data on other antiplatelet agents are less robust. In the Cilostazol for Prevention of Secondary Stroke (CSPS)-2 trial, cilostazol reduced the risk of recurrent stroke (HR, 0.74; 95% CI, 0.56 to 0.98) and caused less bleeding than aspirin. Terutroban, a thromboxane A2 receptor antagonist, failed to show superiority to aspirin in preventing recurrent cerebral ischemic events.[70] Other antiplatelet agents, such as prasugrel and ticagrelor, have been noted to have higher risks of bleeding, and their role in management of carotid artery disease has not been defined. Nevertheless, the issue of clopidogrel resistance in patients with pharmacologic inhibition of cytochrome P450 or its genetic polymorphisms opens the door for other, more potent antiplatelet agents with more favorable safety profiles.

The role of vitamin K antagonists in secondary prevention of stroke of arterial origin was examined in the Stroke Prevention in the Reversible Ischemia Trial (SPIRIT) and ESPRIT.[71,72] These studies convincingly established that warfarin therapy provided no benefit irrespective of the intensity of anticoagulation, and it increased the risk of intracranial hemorrhage. The Warfarin-Aspirin Recurrent Stroke Study (WARSS) to compare warfarin therapy with aspirin in patients with recent stroke included a subgroup of patients with carotid artery disease. Although this trial excluded patients who qualified for revascularization, warfarin was not superior to aspirin during a 2-year course of therapy.[73] Current societal guidelines recommend aspirin monotherapy (75 to 325 mg), clopidogrel monotherapy, or aspirin and dipyridamole therapy for symptomatic patients with carotid artery disease (class I, level of evidence B).[20]

Revascularization for Carotid Artery Disease

In 2005, 135,701 CEA (Figure 36-2) and stenting procedures (Figure 36-3) were performed in the United States, and 92% of these interventions were performed in asymptomatic patients.[74] The total

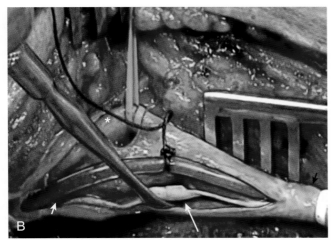

FIGURE 36-2 Carotid artery bifurcation exposed during carotid endarterectomy. The *black arrow* points to the distal common carotid artery (CCA), and the *asterisk* marks the external carotid artery. The *short white arrow* points to the proximal internal carotid artery (ICA). An arteriotomy opens the distal CCA and proximal ICA, and a shunt is seen directing blood flow around the exposed artery. The atherosclerotic plaque and the intima are being removed (*long white arrow*).

number of carotid revascularization procedures has been declining, from 388.1 procedures per 100,000 Medicare beneficiaries in 1998 to 345.8 per 100,000 in 2004. Within this period, the number of surgical procedures declined by 17%, but the number of carotid stenting procedures more than doubled.

Surgical Revascularization

CAROTID ENDARTERECTOMY FOR SYMPTOMATIC CAROTID ARTERY STENOSIS

Patients who come to medical attention after a TIA or nondisabling stroke have an increased risk of major and fatal stroke. Population-based studies in the United Kingdom reported that the risk of stroke after a TIA is 8% to 9% at 7 days and 12% at 30 days.[75,76] Among health maintenance organization patients who came to the emergency department with a TIA, the 90-day risk of stroke was 10.5%.[5] The timing of revascularization in symptomatic patients is an important determinant of future outcomes because the benefit of revascularization is greatest when offered within 2 weeks after the index event, and it diminishes steadily thereafter. That is, early revascularization reduces the risk of recurrent ischemic cerebrovascular events.[77,78] Unfortunately, as few as 6% of symptomatic patients undergo timely revascularization.[77]

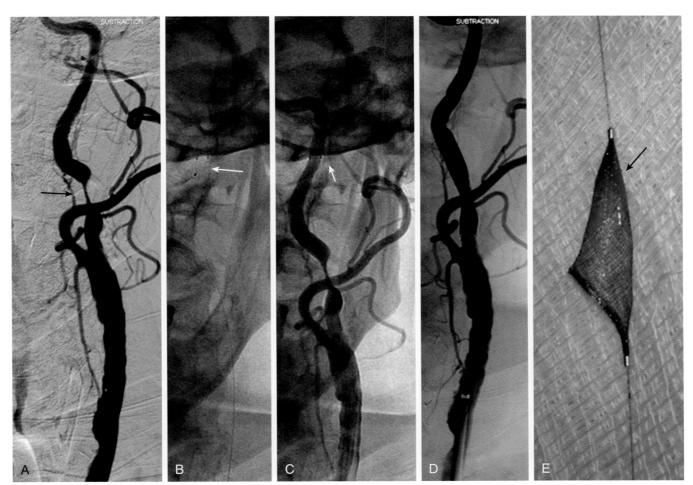

FIGURE 36-3 Serial steps during carotid artery stenting. **A,** A digital subtraction angiogram of a severely stenosed internal carotid artery (ICA; *arrow*). The external carotid artery crosses over and partly obscures the ICA stenosis. **B,** A filter distal embolic protection device positioned in the mid-distal ICA (*arrow*), distal to the stenosis. The net of the filter allows blood flow but traps any embolic debris released from the lesion during stent deployment. **C,** Cine angiogram confirming lesion location and filter position (*arrow*) just before stent deployment. **D,** Completion angiogram. A stent is deployed in the ICA without residual stenosis. **E,** Filter embolic protection after its retrieval. Note the dark yellow plaque debris trapped in its apex.

The North American Symptomatic Carotid Endarterectomy Trial (NASCET) conclusively demonstrated the benefit of CEA in patients with carotid artery stenosis of 50% or greater who had symptoms of a stroke or TIA in the preceding 6 to 12 months. The absolute risk of stroke was reduced by 8% per year,[79] and the most profound benefit occurred in patients with a 70% to 90% stenosis. In addition, NASCET provided a lasting definition for assessing angiographic carotid artery stenosis and allowed standardization of carotid ultrasound velocities in relationship to angiographic stenosis severity (Figure 36-4).

The European Carotid Surgery Trial (ECST) enrolled patients with ischemic symptoms attributed to the ipsilateral carotid stenosis. The angiographic definition of *stenosis* in the trial differed from the NASCET definition and used the more difficult to reproduce carotid bifurcation dimensions as the basis of the calculation. As a result, the ECST stenosis estimates were routinely higher than those calculated using the NASCET-derived method. The trial enrolled 2518 patients and reported interim results when 3-year follow-up results were available for 2200 of them.[80] The trial concluded that patients with ECST-defined stenosis of 0% to 29% had very low event rates with surgery or medical therapy and that the benefit of CEA was outweighed by perioperative complications. The benefit of surgery in patients with ECST-defined stenosis of 30% to 69% remained uncertain, and patients continued to be followed. In the group with 70% to 99% stenosis, however, surgery provided a measurable benefit. In the surgical arm, 7.5% of patients had a stroke or died in the perioperative period, but the risk of subsequent ipsilateral stroke during follow-up was 2.8%. In comparison, 16.8% of patients treated medically developed an ipsilateral stroke. Thus once the up-front surgical risk was excluded, surgery provided a sixfold decrease in the risk of ipsilateral stroke

($P < .0001$). After 3 years, the total risk of surgical death and any stroke was 12.3% in the surgical arm and 21.9% in the medical arm ($P < .01$). Final results of the trial were published in 1998 and reported on a total cohort of 3024 patients.[81] In the final analysis, only patients with an ECST-defined stenosis of 80% (90% among women) derived sufficient long-term benefit to overcome the 7% perioperative risk of death and stroke (see Table 36-1).

In 1991, the Veterans Administration 309 trial (VA 309) reported a nonsignificant trend that favored surgical intervention among patients with symptomatic carotid stenosis.[82] The trial was stopped early because of publication of the NASCET and ECST results. Rothwell and colleagues[83] reanalyzed all the prerandomization angiograms in the ECST trial and recalculated the stenosis using the NASCET criteria. Pooling the data on the 6092 patients from the NASCET, ECST, and VA 309 trial data, they showed that surgery increased the 5-year risk of stroke in patients with NASCET stenosis of less than 30%; it offered no benefit for patients with stenosis in the 30% to 49% range (absolute risk reduction [ARR], 3.2%, $P = .6$); it was of marginal benefit in patients with 50% to 69% stenosis (ARR, 4.6%; $P = .04$); but it was strikingly beneficial in patients with carotid artery stenosis of 70% to 99% (ARR, 16%; $P < .001$). Thus the benefit of revascularization in symptomatic patients with angiographic carotid artery stenosis of 50% or more (70% by noninvasive imaging) was firmly established.

The benefit of carotid artery revascularization in symptomatic patients is clear, yet the importance of concomitant medical therapy cannot be understated. Hackam and colleagues calculated a potential cumulative effect of combining five therapies for prevention of recurrent events in patients who had a stroke or TIA. The combination of aspirin, statin, antihypertensive agent, exercise, and dietary modification could result in an 80% relative risk reduction, translating into a number needed to treat (NNT) of 5 to avoid one death.[83a]

The ACC/AHA/ASA guidelines recommend CEA (class I, level of evidence B) for patients with a 70% or greater carotid artery stenosis who have had an ipsilateral nondisabling CVA or TIA in the preceding 6 months, provided they have an average or low surgical risk and an anticipated rate of perioperative stroke or death below 6%.[20] For the first time, CAS (discussed further below) is considered an equivalent alternative in this group of patients, provided they are suitable for endovascular procedures, and the periprocedural risk of stroke and death falls below 6%. Furthermore, it is reasonable to favor CEA over CAS in older patients, especially in those with complex arterial geometry.

CAROTID ENDARTERECTOMY FOR ASYMPTOMATIC CAROTID ARTERY STENOSIS

Three early trials examined the role of CEA in primary prevention of ipsilateral stroke in patients with asymptomatic carotid artery disease. These trials—Carotid Artery Surgery Asymptomatic Narrowing Operation Versus Aspirin (CASANOVA),[84] Mayo Asymptomatic Carotid Endarterectomy (MACE),[85] and VA[86] trials—failed to show any benefit to surgical therapy in long-term stroke prevention. The lasting contribution of the MACE trial may be the observation of higher perioperative TIA and MI rates compared with the medical arm, likely related to the absence of therapy in the surgical arm (Table 36-2).

Surgical revascularization was subsequently tested again in two randomized landmark trials. The Asymptomatic Carotid Atherosclerosis Study (ACAS), conducted between 1987 and 1993, and the Asymptomatic Carotid Surgery Trial (ACST), conducted between 1993 and 2003, demonstrated a small but significant benefit of CEA over the best medical therapy available at the time. These two trials have shaped the treatment of patients with moderate and severe asymptomatic carotid artery disease over the last two decades, and they continue to fuel a heated debate.

ACAS enrolled 1662 patients with carotid artery stenosis of 60% or more and randomized them to either medical therapy that consisted of aspirin or CEA.[87] Women represented 34% of the

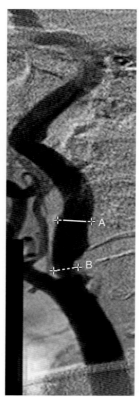

FIGURE 36-4 An illustration of the North American Symptomatic Carotid Endarterectomy Trial (NASCET) criteria for calculating the severity of carotid artery stenosis. The severity of the angiographic stenosis is defined by the equation $[(1 - B)/A] \times 100\%$, where B defines the diameter of the minimal residual lumen in the internal carotid artery (ICA), and A is the diameter of the ICA lumen distal to the stenosis at the point where the walls of the vessel become parallel.

TABLE 36-2 Summary of the Results of Randomized Surgical Trials Comparing Carotid Endarterectomy to Best Available Medical Therapy

TRIAL	PATIENTS (N)	STENOSIS SEVERITY (%)	MEAN FOLLOW-UP (Y)	Ipsilateral Stroke		P VALUE	PERIOPERATIVE CVA AND DEATH (%)
				MEDICAL (%)	CEA (%)		
Symptomatic Carotid Artery Disease							
NASCET, 1991[79]	659	70-99	1.5	26	9	<.001	5.8
NASCET, 1991[79]	858	50-69	1.5	22.2	15.7	.045	6.7
ECST, 1991, 1998[80,81]	576	>80*	3	26.5	14.9	<.001	7
VA 309, 1991[82]	129	70-99	1	26	7.9	.004	NA
Pooled NASCET/ ECST/VA, 2003[83]	1095	>70	5	ARR = 16		<.001	7.1
Asymptomatic Carotid Artery Stenosis							
CASANOVA,1991[84]	410	50-90	3	11.3	10.7	.48	4.62
VA, 1993[86]	444	50-99	4	8.6	4.7	.06	NA
ACAS, 1995[87]	1662	50-99	2.7	11	4.8	.006	2.3
ACST, 2004[88]	3120	≥70	3.4	6.4	11.8	<.001	3.1

*The 80% stenosis in ECST was calculated using the ECST protocol, which overestimated stenosis severity compared with the NASCET criteria.
ARR, absolute risk reduction; CEA, carotid endarterectomy; CVA, cerebrovascular accident; NA, not applicable.

enrolled subjects. After a median follow-up of 2.7 years, the aggregate 5-year risk of ipsilateral stroke and any perioperative stroke or death was 11% in the medical therapy arm and 5.1% in the surgical arm, representing a 53% relative risk reduction (95% CI, 22% to 72%). The absolute risk reduction achieved by CEA was 5.9% with an NNT of 17. Additional analysis suggested that 59 strokes would be prevented by 1000 successful carotid surgeries. Interestingly, no relationship was found between the severity of carotid artery stenosis and the risk of stroke or benefit of revascularization.

The ACST collaborative group enrolled 3120 asymptomatic patients with carotid artery stenosis of 70% or more who were randomized to immediate CEA or indefinite deferral.[88] Patients in the latter group were managed medically and underwent surgery at a rate of 4% per year. Perioperative death and stroke occurred in 3.1% of patients (95% CI, 2.3 to 4.1). Patients were monitored for up to 5 years, with a mean follow-up of 3.4 years. The combined endpoint of perioperative stroke and death and any nonoperative stroke occurred in 6.4% of patients in the immediate intervention arm and in 11.8% of patients treated medically ($P < .0001$). This endpoint of any stroke was different from the endpoint used in the ACAS trial, which adjudicated ipsilateral stroke. The rate of fatal or disabling stroke was 3.5% versus 6.1% ($P = .004$), and the rate was 2.1% versus 4.2% for fatal strokes ($P = .006$) in the surgical and medical arms, respectively.

Mirroring the results of ACAS, the severity of carotid artery stenosis did not correlate with the risk of stroke or benefit of surgical intervention: the 5-year risk of stroke among patients with carotid artery stenosis less than 80% was 2.1% in the surgical arm and 9.5% in the medical arm; for those with a stenosis greater than 80%, the risk was 3.2% and 9.6%, respectively. The benefit of carotid artery surgery became evident after 2 years of follow-up. The relative risk reduction attributed to CEA was 46%, and absolute risk reduction was 5.4% or 1% per year. This risk reduction translated to an NNT of 19 and the prevention of 53 strokes per 1000 carotid surgeries.

The evolution of medical therapy during the decade of enrollment was reflected in the increasing use of statins and antihypertensive agents. Statin therapy was used in 17% of patients enrolled between 1993 and 1996 and in 58% of patients enrolled from 2000 through 2003. At last follow-up, 90% of patients were treated with antiplatelet agents, 81% of patients received antihypertensive therapy, and only 70% of patients were treated with statins.

Women, who made up 34% of the study population, benefited from CEA only after the perioperative events of stroke and death were excluded. Even after the data from ACAS and ACST were combined to analyze event rates in a greater number of women, the trend toward benefit of CEA was not significant (OR, 1.04; 95% CI, 0.7 to 1.6).[89]

The 10-year follow-up of ACST showed that the benefit of CEA extended beyond the initial follow-up period.[49] After 10 years, the combined endpoint of operative stroke and death and nonoperative stroke occurred in 13.4% of patients in the surgical arm and in 17.9% of patients in the deferred arm. Thus, after 10 years, the relative risk reduction was 26%, with an absolute risk reduction of 4.6% or 0.46% per year. This 10-year analysis revealed also that the stroke risk for women younger than 75 years was finally lowered by CEA from 16% in the medical arm to 10.2% in the surgical arm, an absolute risk reduction of 0.58% per year.

ACAS resulted in the embracing of CEA in patients with asymptomatic carotid artery stenosis, provided that the perioperative morbidity and mortality rates were less than the 3% mandated by guidelines. Within a few years of publication of the ACAS trial, the number of carotid surgeries in the United States increased by 94% to 150,000 carotid surgeries per year.[90] However, in the United Kingdom, the number of operations needed to prevent one disabling or fatal stroke was not judged to be cost effective, and the number of surgeries remained constant.[91]

Subsequent analysis of the trial engendered controversy regarding the wide application of its results. Only 9% of the enrolled patients completed the 5 years of follow-up, which questioned the interpretation of the Kaplan-Meier estimates of 5-year risk. The relative risk reduction in the combined rate of major ipsilateral stroke or any perioperative stroke or death was reduced by 43% at 5 years, but the relative reduction during the first 4.5 years was near nil, and the result was driven by just three outcome events. Thus, 5-year prognosis is an important determinant in selection of asymptomatic patients for CEA, and the average absolute risk reduction of disabling stroke as a result of CEA was 0.5%.[91] The benefit of endarterectomy did not extend to women, who were underrepresented in this study. Among the 281 women treated with surgery, 15 met an endpoint compared with 14 events recorded in the 287 women treated medically, yielding an odds ratio of 1.10 (95% CI, 0.52 to 1.32). Women developed perioperative complications at a rate of 3.6% compared with 1.7% observed in men. Thus, although men had a relative risk reduction of 66%, the benefit of surgery was not statistically significant in women, who achieved a relative risk reduction of 17% (95% CI, 96% to 65%). Similar outcomes were noted in the 5-year follow-up of ACAST. Among the 539 women treated with endarterectomy, 31 had a perioperative stroke or operative death compared with 34 who had a perioperative stroke or died in the group of 327 women treated medically, with an odds ratio of 0.90 (95% CI, 0.55 to 1.49).

The rigorous site-selection process raised concerns about the generalizability of the study results. Participating surgeons were required to document performance of at least 12 carotid surgeries per year with a perioperative mortality rate in their last 50 cases less than 3% in a symptomatic and 5% in symptomatic patients. Only 70% of sites were accepted into the study.[92] As a result, the perioperative rate of stroke and death in the trial was 1.5% (95% CI, 0.6% to 2.4%), and mortality rate was 0.14% (95% CI, 0% to 0.4%). Indeed, subsequent audits of CEA in asymptomatic patients, performed in 10 states in the United States between 1995 and 1996, revealed 30-day death or stroke rates of 5.9%, which declined to 5.4% for surgeries performed between 1998 and 1999.[93] A meta-analysis of 46 CEA series performed in asymptomatic patients within 5 years after the publication of ACAS documented a much higher mortality rate of 1.11% and combined stroke and death rate of 4.3%.[91] The benefit asymptomatic patients derive from carotid artery surgery depends on a low perioperative risk achieved in randomized trials, which may be hard to reproduce in routine clinical practice.

Both trials failed to convincingly show benefit from surgical endarterectomy in patients older than 75 years. In the ACAS trial, patients older than 80 years were excluded from the study, and the number of patients between 75 and 80 years was small. In the ACST study, CEA did not confer any benefit in older patients, even after excluding the perioperative events.

CEA in asymptomatic patients may thus lower the long-term risk of stroke at the price of the higher short-term risk of procedure-related death and stroke. As the stroke rates decline with intensive medical therapy, the long-term risk and benefit ratio of these interventions must be carefully assessed in each patient.

Endovascular Therapy for Carotid Artery Stenosis

The impetus for development of CAS techniques was provided by the relatively high cardiovascular complication rates associated with CEA in patients considered to be at high risk for such surgery because of medical comorbidities or anatomic challenges. Anatomic features that increase the risk of CEA include internal carotid artery lesions located above the angle of the jaw, cervical scarring as a result of radiation therapy (Figure 36-5), an immobile neck, or restenosis after prior CEA surgery (Figure 36-6). CAS evolved from plain angioplasty to a platform of self-expanding stents combined with various embolic protection devices. After heated debates over the last decade, technological advances and a series of rigorous trials led to acceptance of endovascular therapy as an acceptable standard of care for an ever-increasing subset of patients with asymptomatic and symptomatic carotid artery disease.

The U.S. Food and Drug Administration (FDA) approved CAS for patients considered at high risk for CEA in 2004. In May 2011, the FDA expanded the indications to include symptomatic and asymptomatic patients irrespective of surgical risk.

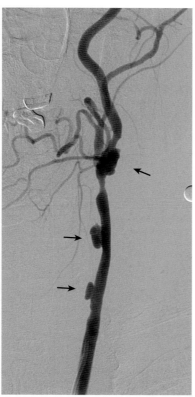

FIGURE 36-5 Carotid artery disease in a patient with a transient ischemic attack and history of high-dose radiation therapy to the neck for nasopharyngeal malignancy. The common carotid and internal carotid arteries have areas of moderate stenosis, focal ulceration, and aneurysm formation (*arrows*). Carotid artery stenting may be a better form of revascularization in a scarred neck.

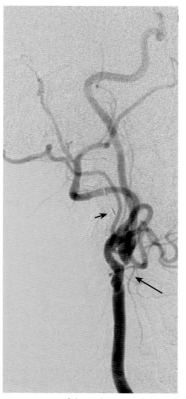

FIGURE 36-6 Severe stenosis of the right internal carotid artery (*long arrow*) in a patient with prior carotid endarterectomy (CEA). Note the surgical staples (*short arrow*). CEA restenosis confirms a higher risk of perioperative complications, and carotid artery stenting is usually the preferred form of revascularization.

CAROTID ARTERY STENTING IN SYMPTOMATIC AND ASYMPTOMATIC PATIENTS AT HIGH SURGICAL RISK: DATA FROM LARGE REGISTRIES

Early evaluations of modern endovascular therapies with self-expanding stents and embolic protection devices consisted primarily of FDA-mandated and manufacturer-sponsored nonrandomized registries. The scrutiny of the FDA led to creation of quality registries with prospective data collection and independent event adjudication that encompassed more than 10,000 primarily asymptomatic high-risk patients. These registries enrolled only patients considered at high risk for CEA, and their outcomes were compared with objective performance criteria (OPC). This criterion was based on historic outcomes of high-risk patients undergoing CEA, with 30-day stroke and death rates as high as 11% among patients with high-risk medical comorbidities, and 15% for those with high-risk anatomic features (CEA restenosis, prior neck radiation, prior neck surgery, high cervical lesion). Enrollment criteria required that asymptomatic patients have 80% or greater carotid stenosis, and symptomatic lesions had to have 50% or greater stenosis. The majority of patients enrolled in these registries were asymptomatic. Data from carotid stenting registries that enroll patients at high risk for surgery suggest that this revascularization strategy can be performed with complication rates below the 6% required for symptomatic patients and 3% for asymptomatic patients who are at an acceptable risk for CEA.

The largest of these high-risk registries were the Carotid Acculink/Accunet Post-Approval Trial to Uncover Unanticipated or Rare Events (CAPTURE)-1 (3500 patients), the Emboshield and Xact Post Approval Carotid Stent Trial (EXACT; 2145 patients), CAPTURE-2 (3388 patients), and the Stenting and Angioplasty With Protection in Patients at High Risk for Endarterectomy (SAPPHIRE) World-wide Registry (2001 patients). The CAPTURE registries evaluated the Acculink stent and Accunet filter distal embolic protection device (DEP; Abbot Vascular, Santa Clara, CA), the first CAS platform approved by the FDA. The EXACT registry evaluated the Xact stent and Emboshield DEP (Abbot Vascular), and in the SAPPHIRE registry, patients were treated with the Precise stent and Angioguard DEP (both Cordis/Johnson & Johnson, Warren, NJ).

In the CAPTURE-1 registry, 14% of enrolled patients were symptomatic.[94] The primary endpoint of 30-day death, any stroke, or MI occurred in 6.3%. In the CAPTURE-2 and EXACT registries published 2 years later, the primary endpoint of 30-day death or stroke occurred in 3.4% of patients (95% CI, 2.9% to 4.0%) in the CAPTURE-2 and in 4.1% of patients in the EXACT registry (95% CI, 3.3% to 5.0%).[95] When these two registries were combined, the overall primary endpoint occurred in 5.3% of symptomatic patients younger than 80 years (95% CI, 3.6% to 7.4%) and in 2.9% of asymptomatic patients in the same age group (95% CI, 2.4% to 3.4%). Patients older than 80 years had higher event rates: 10.5% among symptomatic patients (95% CI, 6.3% to 16.0%) and 4.4% among asymptomatic participants (95% CI, 3.3% to 5.7%). This combined analysis showed that in high-risk nonoctogenarians, carotid stenting could meet the AHA requirements for perioperative event rates among symptomatic and asymptomatic normal-risk patients. Further analysis of these registries identified a strong correlation between operator experience and event rates: operators who performed 72 stenting procedures had consistently low 30-day event rates (<3%).

The SAPPHIRE Worldwide Registry captured data on 2001 high-risk patients, 28% of whom were symptomatic. The 30-day combined adverse-event rate occurred in 4.4% of all patients (death, 1.1%; stroke, 3.2%; MI, 0.7%).[96]

CAROTID ARTERY STENTING IN PATIENTS AT HIGH SURGICAL RISK: DATA FROM RANDOMIZED TRIALS

The SAPPHIRE study was the first randomized trial to compare CAS using a nitinol self-expanding stent and DEP (Precise stent/Angioguard DEP, Cordis/Johnson & Johnson) with CEA in patients at high surgical risk. This multicenter, randomized, noninferiority study enrolled symptomatic patients with carotid artery stenosis of 50% or more and asymptomatic patients with carotid artery stenosis of 80% or more as determined by ultrasound. A third of the enrolled patients were symptomatic. The primary endpoint consisted of combined death, stroke, and MI within 30 days of revascularization and death and ipsilateral stroke occurring between days 31 and 1 year. All patients had to be considered suitable for CEA despite their high-risk features. Patients who were not suitable candidates for surgery (n = 406) were enrolled in a stenting registry, and those not amenable to endovascular intervention (n = 7) were enrolled in a surgical registry. Among 334 patients who were randomized, the primary event occurred at 1 year in 12.2% of patients who underwent stenting and in 20.1% of patients who were treated surgically (P = .004). In the immediate perioperative period, death, stroke, or MI occurred in 4.8% of patients in the CAS arm and in 9.8% of patients in the CEA arm (P = .09). The primary outcome was influenced heavily by higher rates of perioperative MI, 3.0% versus 7.5% (P = .07). The symptom status did not impact the comparison between the two treatment strategies. The SAPPHIRE investigators subsequently reported the 3-year results, which confirmed that the long-term outcomes were not different between patients treated with CEA or CAS.[97]

The results of this trial confirmed the noninferiority of CAS in this patient group. On the basis of the SAPPHIRE trial, the FDA approved CAS in 2004 for symptomatic and asymptomatic patients at high risk of perioperative complications because of medical comorbidities or anatomic features. Because of ongoing concerns about the efficacy CAS, the Center for Medicare and Medicaid Services limited reimbursement of CAS to high-risk symptomatic patients with carotid artery stenosis of 70% or greater. Coverage was subsequently extended for treatment of symptomatic patients with 50% or greater stenosis and asymptomatic patients with stenosis of 80% or more, provided that they were enrolled in either postapproval registry studies or randomized controlled trials. This has led to a substantial increase in CAS procedures.[98] At the same time, enrollment in the postapproval registries provided valuable technical and clinical information about patients most likely to benefit from these procedures.

CAROTID ARTERY STENTING IN NORMAL-RISK SYMPTOMATIC PATIENTS

Three randomized trials compared CAS to CEA in patients with symptomatic carotid artery disease and standard surgical risk. The Endarterectomy Versus Angioplasty in Patients with Symptomatic Severe Carotid Stenosis (EVA-3S) trial, a noninferiority study, randomized standard surgical risk patients within 4 months of TIA or nondisabling stroke as a result of carotid artery stenosis of 60% or more.[99] The primary endpoint of this French study was a composite of any stroke or death within 30 days after revascularization. The trial was stopped early, after enrollment of 527 of the planned 872 patients, because of concerns about safety and futility. The primary endpoint was observed in 9.6% of patients in the endovascular arm and in 3.9% of patients in the surgical arm (P = .01). The prespecified secondary endpoint was a composite of any periprocedural stroke or death and any nonprocedural ipsilateral stroke during the subsequent 4 years. The secondary endpoint was observed in 11.1% of CAS patients and in 6.2% of CEA patients (HR, 1.97; CI, 1.06 to 3.67; P = .03).[99] Thus, the risk of stroke after the immediate periprocedural period was very low in both groups, suggesting durability of both procedures. The failure of CAS in this trial stemmed from high periprocedural complications, an observation that critics attributed to the controversial trial design.

Another noninferiority study, the Stent-Supported Percutaneous Angioplasty of the Carotid Artery Versus Endarterectomy (SPACE) trial, was conducted in Germany, Austria, and Switzerland. The trial aimed to enroll standard surgical-risk patients who suffered a TIA or nondisabling stroke within 6 months of randomization and had an ipsilateral 70% or greater carotid artery stenosis. The trial was stopped after enrollment of 1183 patients, when it was determined that the 2500 patients required to achieve sufficient statistical power could not be enrolled because of funding limitations and slow enrollment. The primary endpoint of ipsilateral stroke and death within 30 days of revascularization was noted in 6.84% of patients undergoing stenting and in 6.34% of patients treated with CEA (absolute difference, 0.51%; 90% CI, −1.89% to 2.91%). The trial failed to demonstrate noninferiority of endovascular therapy. After 2 years of follow-up, the rates of ipsilateral stroke did not differ between the two groups: they were 9.5% with CAS versus 8.8% in the CEA arm (HR, 1.1; 95% CI, 0.75 to 1.61).[100] Longer term follow-up from the EVA-3S and SPACE trials showed low rates of ipsilateral stroke, suggesting excellent durability of both forms of revascularization.

The third study, the International Carotid Stenting Study (ICSS), randomized 1713 patients with recently symptomatic carotid artery stenosis exceeding 50% to treatment with CAS or endarterectomy.[101] The primary endpoint of the study was fatal or disabling stroke in any territory after 3 years of follow-up. The interim safety analysis of this trial adjudicated the 120-day rate of stroke, death, or periprocedural MI. The rate of disabling stroke or death was not statistically different in the two groups and occurred in 4.0% of patients in the stenting arm and in 3.2% of patients in the endarterectomy arm (HR, 1.28; 95% CI, 0.77 to 2.11). However, the incidence of any stroke, death, or MI was higher in the stenting arm compared with the endarterectomy group and occurred in 8.5% compared with 5.2% of patients, respectively (HR, 1.69; 95% CI, 1.16 to 2.45; P = .006). It appears that the difference in short-term outcomes may have rested on higher rates of nondisabling stroke noted in the CAS arm. Only longer follow-up will determine whether this observation has a lasting clinical significance.

One of the major criticisms of these trials was the relative inexperience of the operators performing carotid stenting procedures. In the CAPTURE-2 registry, operator and site experience were shown to be the most important determinants of periprocedural outcomes. A threshold of 72 cases appears to be needed to achieve death and stroke rates below 3%.[102] In the EVA-3S trial, lifetime experience of at least 12 CAS procedures was required, but operators were allowed to participate in the trial if they had performed five carotid stenting procedures and 30 interventions in noncarotid supraaortic vessels. Alternatively, investigators who did not fulfill these requirements were allowed to perform carotid stenting procedures in the presence of an experienced tutor, and vascular surgeons were required to have performed at least 25 carotid CEA operations in the 12 months preceding enrollment. Operators whose procedural experience exceeded 50 carotid stenting procedures performed only 16% of stenting procedures in the trial, and 39% of the procedures were performed by physicians in training.[103] This inexperience may have accounted for a high rate of conversion from endovascular to surgical therapy, which reached 5%. In the SPACE study, performance of a minimum of 25 carotid stenting procedures was required for participation in the trial. However, during the trial, this requirement was altered to allow operators with 10-case experience to participate under supervision of a proctor. Vascular surgeons who performed CEAs had to demonstrate acceptable mortality and morbidity rates in the previous 25 consecutive CEA operations. In ICSS, operators were required to document performance of 50 stenting procedures with 10 of them required to be carotid interventions; however, proctoring was allowed for operators who did not meet these requirements.[104]

Data from the trials suggest that operator experience may not have been related to periprocedural outcomes. In the EVA-3S trial, the periprocedural risk of stroke or death was 12.2% when the procedure was performed by operators with 50-case experience and 11% when performed by operators with less experience. Additional concerns about the trials revolved around adequate postprocedural dual antiplatelet therapies and inconsistent use of DEP devices (used in 27% of the procedures in the SPACE trial).

One of the valuable lessons to emerge over the last 5 years from the U.S.-based registries and the European trials is the notion that just as some patients are at high risk of perioperative complications associated with CEA, there are indeed patients who have a higher risk of complications with CAS. These limitations are not physiologic but are rather anatomic and "geometrical." Patients with unfavorable aortic arch anatomy and tortuous carotid vessels may frustrate even a keen operator attempting to advance catheters to the carotid artery (Figure 36-7). Complex manipulations in atherosclerotic vessels do increase the risk of a periprocedural ischemic event. Similarly, lesion characteristics such as filling defects, complex ulcerated plaques, and thrombus increase the risk of embolic events during stent deployment or balloon dilation. Although patients with characteristics that represent high surgical risk are routinely excluded from comparative studies, features considered high risk for CAS have not been subjected to the same level of scrutiny.

CAROTID ARTERY STENTING IN NORMAL-RISK SYMPTOMATIC AND ASYMPTOMATIC PATIENTS: CREST

The Carotid Revascularization Endarterectomy Versus Stenting Trial (CREST) included both symptomatic and asymptomatic standard-risk patients enrolled in the United States and Canada. The initial trial design allowed enrollment of only symptomatic patients within 6 months of cerebrovascular events who had 50% or more carotid artery stenosis on angiography or 70% or more stenosis on ultrasound, magnetic resonance angiography (MRA), or computed tomographic angiography (CTA). After 5 years of enrollment, the design was altered to include asymptomatic patients with angiographic evidence of 60% or more stenosis, ultrasound evidence of 70% or more stenosis, or 80% or more stenosis diagnosed by MRA or CTA. The primary composite endpoint was specified as any stroke, MI, or death in the periprocedural period or any ipsilateral stroke within 4 years. A total of 2502 patients were randomized and followed for a median of 2.5 years. Over 85% of the enrolled patients had carotid stenosis of 70% or more, and 47% of patients were asymptomatic. Octogenarians comprised 9% of the study population.

The primary endpoint did not differ between the two treatment groups and occurred in 7.2% of patients in the endovascular arm and 6.8% in the surgical arm (HR with stenting, 1.11; 95% CI, 0.81 to 1.51; P = .51). This result held true regardless of gender or symptom status. Additional analysis showed that the 4-year rate of ipsilateral stroke or death was 6.4% in the stenting arm and 4.7% in the CEA arm (HR, 1.37; P = .03). Among asymptomatic patients, the 4-year rate of stroke or death was 4.5% in the stenting arm and 2.7% in the surgical arm (HR, 1.86; P = .07). Among symptomatic patients, the rates were 8.0% in the CAS arm compared with 6.4% in the surgical group (HR, 1.5; P = .03).

Periprocedural risk of death did not differ between the two arms (0.7% vs. 0.3%; P = .18); the risk of MI was higher in the surgical arm (1.1% vs. 2.3%; P = .03), and risk of any stroke was higher in the stent group (4.1% vs. 2.3%; P = .01). However, the higher rate of periprocedural stroke in the CAS arm was driven by higher rates of minor strokes (3.2% vs. 1.7%; P = .01), whereas the rates of major disabling stroke did not differ. The importance of the higher rates of nondisabling strokes should not be ignored; after all, the goal of any revascularization strategy is to prevent any neurologic events. Interestingly, although the overall rate of residual neurologic deficit from minor strokes detected on the NIH stroke scale was higher at 30 days after the procedure (1.2% in the CAS arm vs. 0.6% in the CEA arm), this difference was no longer detected at 6 months (0.6% vs. 0.6%). The trial also showed that a minor stroke did not impact the patient's survival during the trial. Beyond the periprocedural period, both revascularization strategies provided durable stroke prevention: the incidence of ipsilateral stroke was 2.0 in the CAS arm and 2.4 in the CEA group (P = .85).

The significance of periprocedural MI, defined as twofold or higher elevation of creatine kinase or troponin with associated

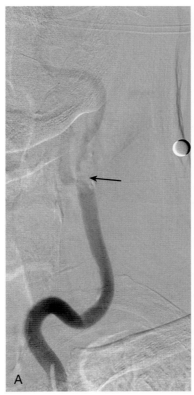
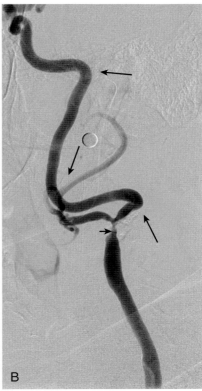

FIGURE 36-7 Tortuosity of the aortic arch and carotid vessels may create a high carotid artery stenting risk in which excessive catheter manipulations increase the risk of periprocedural complications. **A,** Tortuosity in the proximal common carotid artery. The *arrow* points to a stenosis in the carotid bifurcation. **B,** Moderately tortuous internal carotid artery with several bends of variable acuity (*arrows*). Both vessels were stented successfully, but excessive carotid tortuosity may be best treated surgically.

symptoms or electrocardiographic (ECG) evidence of ischemia, has been evaluated in a post hoc analysis. Patients with a diagnosis of perioperative MI had a higher mortality during the follow-up compared with patients who did not have an MI (HR, 3.4; 95% CI, 1.67 to 6.92, $P < .001$). Indeed, even patients with positive biomarkers and without symptoms or ECG evidence of coronary ischemia fared worse than patients without serologic evidence of myocardial injury (death HR, 3.57; 95% CI, 1.46 to 8.68; $P = .005$). MI or isolated biomarker elevation were confirmed to be independent predictors of death.[105] Thus, patients with perioperative MI or "silent" troponin elevation were three to four times more likely to die during the follow-up. The inherent limitations of a post hoc analysis and the small number of patients with MI or troponin elevation (62 patients in a cohort of 2502) do not permit firm conclusions about the significance of these observations on long-term differences between CAS and CEA. The observed events likely identify a group of patients with advanced systemic atherosclerosis whose life expectancy is influenced primarily by ischemic events outside the cerebrovascular bed.

Results of CREST led to FDA approval of CAS as equivalent therapy for patients with symptomatic and asymptomatic carotid artery disease irrespective of their surgical risk. The ACC/AHA/ASA guidelines give CAS a class I recommendation (evidence level B, as compared with level A for CEA) as appropriate revascularization therapy in symptomatic patients with an angiographic carotid stenosis of 50% or more (≥70% on noninvasive imaging). A class IIb recommendation was given for CAS in selected asymptomatic patients with 70% or greater carotid artery stenosis detected by ultrasound.[20]

Should Asymptomatic Carotid Artery Stenosis Be Revascularized?

CEA is recommended for severe but asymptomatic carotid artery disease based on the outcomes of three trials conducted between 1983 and 2003: the Veterans' Affairs Cooperative Study (VACS), the

Asymptomatic Carotid Atherosclerosis Study (ACAS), and the Asymptomatic Carotid Surgery Trial (ACST). The common thread in these trials was an overall reduction of approximately 1% in the average annual absolute risk of stroke among patients who underwent CEA.

The influence of advances in medical therapy on temporal changes in stroke risk among patients with asymptomatic carotid artery stenosis is evident from the results of ACAS and ACST. In ACAS, published in 1995, the annual rate of ipsilateral stroke in the medically treated arm was 2.2%. The rate of ipsilateral stroke decreased to 1.1% by the time the 5-year results of ACST were published in 2004, and they were further reduced to 0.7% 5 years later, when the 10-year follow-up results of ACST were published in 2010. Thus, in the 15 years since the publication of ACAS, the rate of stroke ipsilateral to the carotid artery stenosis declined by 60% in patients treated medically. The annual rates of any stroke similarly declined, from 3.5% per year to 2.4% and 1.4%, respectively.[106] Intensive use of modern medical therapy in patients with asymptomatic carotid artery stenosis of more than 50% severity can lower the annual rate of any ipsilateral ischemic stroke to 0.34%.[107]

These results may have changed attitudes toward carotid revascularization in asymptomatic patients. In 1997 a consortium of Canadian neurologists recommended against CEA in asymptomatic patients.[108] The European Stroke Initiative recommended medical treatment for asymptomatic patients with hemodynamically significant carotid artery stenosis.[109] The uncertainty regarding revascularization of asymptomatic patients is further reflected by results of a poll conducted by the *New England Journal of Medicine*. Asked how an otherwise healthy patient with 70% to 80% asymptomatic carotid artery stenosis should be managed, 50% of health care practitioners favored medical therapy.[110]

Carotid endarterectomy, when performed in high-volume centers and on patients with acceptable surgical risk, can be associated with low perioperative event rates. Contemporary series suggest perioperative stroke, death, and MI rates of 0.96%, 0.56%, and 0.22%, respectively.[111] When combined with results from ACST, such data suggest an average annual risk of stroke of 1% after CEA. Yet, the Second Manifestation of Arterial Disease (SMART) study suggested that among asymptomatic patients with established atherosclerotic vascular disease, the annual risk of stroke among patients with carotid artery stenosis over 50% is 0.8%. Indeed, the hazard ratio for ischemic stroke was similar whether the index stenosis was 50% to 69% (HR, 0.6; 95% CI, 0.1 to 4.1) or 70% to 99% (HR, 0.7; 95% CI, 0.2 to 3.0).[112] Only 45% of patients in this study were treated with lipid-lowering therapy, and 63% received antiplatelet therapy. Perhaps not surprisingly, patients in this study were more likely to die of vascular causes than they were to develop an ischemic stroke. These observations question the benefit of widespread revascularization, surgical or percutaneous, for primary stroke prevention.

There are undoubtedly subsets of patients with asymptomatic carotid artery disease who may benefit from revascularization. Neither ACAS nor ACST identified any patient characteristics that portended a higher risk of cerebrovascular events. Neither age older than 75 years, severity of carotid stenosis, or contralateral carotid occlusion were associated with higher stroke risk. In clinical practice, patients who have evidence of rapid progression of stenosis on serial ultrasound examinations despite appropriate medical therapy may represent a high-risk cohort. Progression of carotid artery stenosis has been shown to be a significant predictor of CVA and TIA.[113] Similarly, plaque-specific characteristics may help identify lesions, which portend a higher stroke risk. However, no perfect test is available to identify which carotid lesion carries a higher risk of embolization or occlusion and thus should be targeted for revascularization. The baseline severity of the asymptomatic stenosis did not correlate with the subsequent stroke risk in ACAS or ACST and did not predict the risk of stroke in a cohort of 1004 asymptomatic veterans followed over a period of 10 years.[113] Even the presence of contralateral occlusion does not seem to increase the risk of stroke in medically treated asymptomatic patients.[114] The prospective Asymptomatic Carotid Stenosis and Risk of Stroke (ACSRS) study showed that the stenosis severity did correlate with the risk of stroke; thus asymptomatic patients with a 50% to 69% stenosis determined by the ECST criteria carried a 0.8% annual risk of ipsilateral stroke, whereas among patients with 70% to 89% stenosis and 90% to 99% stenosis, that annual risk was 1.4% and 2.4%, respectively.[115] Although commonly relied on in clinical practice to identify high-risk patients, the severity of a carotid artery lesion may not be the most reliable predictor of future ischemic events attributable to that lesion.

Several markers of plaque vulnerability have been proposed. Multiple ultrasonographic plaque characteristics have been evaluated and graded according to their lucency, measurement of plaque area, or assessment of the juxtaluminal black area; all have been shown to correlate with increased rate of ischemic events.[116,117] Carotid plaque echolucency can be quantified by computer measurement of the gray values of all the plaque pixels to form a gray-scale median (GSM) score. This score can be used to determine plaque vulnerability and its propensity to cause ischemic events. Patients with a high GSM score have more echogenic plaque, with an annual risk of stroke of 0.6%, and those with a GSM score less than 15 had a 3.5% annual stroke risk.[117] This score has also been associated with plaque vulnerability. In the Tromsø study, plaque echogenicity was assessed by carotid ultrasound in asymptomatic patients with variable degrees of carotid artery stenosis. The adjusted relative risk of cerebrovascular events in patients with echolucent plaques was 4.6 (95% CI, 1.1 to 18.9), and a statistically significant linear relationship was found between the degree of plaque lucency and the risk of cerebrovascular events.[118]

Spence investigated whether detection of MES by transcranial Doppler in patients with carotid artery stenosis exceeding 60% might identify a group of patients at higher risk of subsequent stroke. Among 319 patients followed up for 2 years, those with evidence of microemboli on the index exam were more likely to have a stroke during the first year of follow-up (15.6%; 95% CI, 4.1 to 79 vs. 1%; 95% CI, 1.01 to 1.36; P < .0001).[119] The predictive value of transcranial Doppler was reaffirmed by the investigators of the international Asymptomatic Carotid Emboli Study (ACES) project.[120] This study enrolled 467 patients with asymptomatic carotid artery stenosis of 70% or more. Embolic signals were detected at baseline in 16.5% of patients, and their presence imparted a hazard ratio for ipsilateral stroke and TIA of 2.54 (95% CI, 1.2 to 5.36; P = .015) compared with those without detectable MES. For ipsilateral stroke alone, the hazard ratio was 5.57 (95% CI, 1.61 to 19.32; P = .007). The annual risk of ipsilateral stroke for those with MES was 3.62%, and it was 0.7% in those without. This study not only suggests that the transcranial Doppler exam is a valuable risk-stratifying tool, but it also underscores the low risk of stroke in a majority of patients with asymptomatic carotid artery stenosis who qualify for consideration of revascularization. The combination of ultrasonic plaque echolucency and transcranial Doppler detection of microemboli in predicting ischemic events was evaluated in a subgroup of 435 subjects in ACES.[121] A total of 435 subjects underwent a baseline ultrasound assessment of plaque morphology and transcranial Doppler examination. An echolucent plaque was present in 37.7% of carotid lesions, and 6.3% of subjects had both echolucent plaque and detectable microemboli. Plaque lucency alone was associated with an increased risk of ipsilateral stroke (HR, 6.43; 95% CI, 1.36 to 30.44; P = .019), but the combination of plaque lucency and detectable microembolic signals identified patients whose risk of ipsilateral stroke was even higher, with a hazard ratio of 10.61 (95% CI, 2.98 to 37.82; P = .0003). This association remained significant when adjusted for cardiovascular risk factors, severity of the carotid stenosis, and antiplatelet and statin therapy. Three-dimensional assessment of carotid artery plaque in patients with 60% or greater stenosis suggested that presence of plaque ulceration also confers a higher risk of ischemic events and may identify patients who could benefit from revascularization.[122]

Transcranial Doppler examination is a labor-intensive and time-consuming technique with limited application as a large-volume clinical tool. Despite many series that support its predictive value, some studies have not found transcranial Doppler exam able to predict event-free survival among patients with asymptomatic carotid artery disease.[123]

The refinement of magnetic resonance plaque imaging techniques has resulted in some evaluation of this technique to identify a high-risk subgroup of patients. In a prospective trial, serial MRI evaluation of asymptomatic patients with carotid artery stenosis of 50% to 80% detected on ultrasound revealed that patients with a thinner and ruptured fibrous cap, intraplaque hemorrhage, or large lipid core had higher rates of ipsilateral stroke compared with patients without these features.[124] The presence of intraplaque hemorrhage detected by MRI has been associated with a threefold increase in the risk of ipsilateral ischemic events (RR, 3.6; 95% CI, 2.5 to 4.7; P < .001).[125]

Carotid Artery Disease and Coronary Artery Bypass Graft Surgery

The management of concurrent carotid and coronary artery disease is controversial. The clinical approach to patients with coronary artery disease that requires surgical revascularization and who also have carotid artery stenosis rests on the principle that the symptomatic arterial bed should be treated first. In modern practice, synchronous coronary and carotid revascularization is reserved for patients who have symptoms of both cerebral and coronary ischemia or those with severe carotid artery disease and high risk of neurologic complications from coronary artery bypass surgery. Although single-center observational studies document acceptable outcomes from combined revascularization, community-based experience has been less encouraging. No large-scale randomized studies are available to guide clinical management of these complex patients.

Every year in the United States, about 5000 combined carotid and coronary revascularizations are performed during the same hospitalization.[126] Simultaneous coronary artery bypass grafting (CABG) surgery and CEA has been proposed to lower the perioperative incidence of stroke in two groups of patients: those with symptomatic coronary artery disease requiring CABG who also have cerebrovascular symptoms as a result of carotid artery stenosis and those with asymptomatic but high-grade carotid lesions.

The cause of neurologic events at the time of coronary artery bypass surgery is multifactorial, and indiscriminate carotid revascularization is unlikely to reduce the risk of perioperative CVA or TIA. As many as 60% of strokes that occur with coronary artery bypass surgery are embolic and related to plaque embolization from aortic cross-clamping. Cerebral hypoperfusion during cardiopulmonary bypass or during heart repositioning during off-pump surgery accounts for 8% of perioperative strokes; 3% are lacunar, 1% are thrombotic, 1% are hemorrhagic, and an additional 10% are presumed to be caused by multiple etiologies.[127] Aortic arch disease is likely the most common source of embolic events, and even mild aortic arch atheroma imparts a fourfold increase in the risk of perioperative stroke.[128]

Cerebral hypoperfusion during cardiopulmonary bypass as a result of severe, albeit asymptomatic, carotid artery stenosis has been proposed as a potential mechanism of intraoperative cerebral ischemia. It is unclear whether carotid artery disease is the actual culprit or merely a marker for other conditions associated with a high risk of perioperative stroke, such as aortic arch atheroma. The prevalence of hemodynamically significant carotid artery disease (>50%) in patients with severe coronary artery disease requiring surgical revascularization is estimated at 12% to 17%, and it decreases to 6% to 8.5% for patients with carotid artery stenosis greater than 80%.[129-132] Unilateral carotid artery occlusion has been observed in 0.6% of patients undergoing coronary artery surgery, and bilateral occlusion has been observed in 0.04%.[133]

The risk of perioperative stroke in patients without significant carotid artery disease is well below 2% but increases to 3% in patients with 50% to 99% unilateral stenosis and to 5% in those with bilateral stenosis. However, this relationship may underscore a higher risk of stroke imparted by diffuse atherosclerosis evidenced by carotid artery disease, rather than validate a causal relationship between perioperative stroke and carotid atherosclerosis, and few studies focus on whether the stroke occurred ipsilateral to the diseased carotid artery.

Systematic review of the literature documented that stroke after CABG surgery occurs in 1.7% of patients, but in 66% of patients, the event manifests after the first postoperative day. This observation suggests that malperfusion as a result of intraoperative hypotension was not the primary cause.[134] Interestingly, as many as 85% of CABG-related strokes occurred in patients with no significant carotid artery disease.[135]

Patients with unilateral carotid occlusion had a 7% to 11% risk of perioperative stroke. However, 50% of patients who developed postoperative stroke did not have any carotid artery disease, and 60% to 80% of infarctions documented on neuroimaging could not be attributed to carotid artery lesions.[134,136] Thus prophylactic endarterectomy in an asymptomatic patient would only reduce 40% to 50% of stroke risk at the time of CABG.

Another retrospective analysis reported much higher rates of peri-CABG stroke. Patients with symptomatic or asymptomatic 50% to 99% carotid artery stenosis or occlusion incurred a 7.4% risk of stroke (95% CI, 4.8 to 9.9), which increased to 9.1% (95% CI, 4.8 to 16) in those with 80% to 99% stenosis or occlusion. Asymptomatic patients without contralateral occlusion had a lower risk of stroke: 3.8% (95% CI, 2.0 to 4.8) with a 50% to 99% stenosis and 2.0% (95% CI, 1.0 to 5.7) in those with 70% to 99% stenosis. The prevalence of perioperative ipsilateral stroke in patients with unilateral asymptomatic 50% to 99% stenosis was 2.0% (95% CI, 1.0 to 3.8), and the risk did not increase with worsening lesion severity of 70% to 99% or 80% to 99%. Patients with bilateral asymptomatic 50% to 99% stenosis or 50% to 99% stenosis and contralateral occlusion had a 6.5% risk of perioperative stroke. The risk of stroke in patients with bilateral 80% to 99% stenosis undergoing combined CABG/CEA was 5.7% in the hemisphere ipsilateral to the nonoperated contralateral stenosis. Thus no compelling evidence supports prophylactic CEA/CABG in patients with unilateral asymptomatic stenosis. This approach may be considered in patients with severe bilateral asymptomatic disease, but such a strategy would only benefit 1% to 2% of all cardiac surgical patients.[137] Other retrospective series suggest that the risk of perioperative stroke in asymptomatic patients with carotid artery stenosis of 75% or more is not different than in those with less severe disease (3.4% vs. 3.6%; $P = 1.0$).[138]

Strategies of combined CABG and CEA or staged surgeries have shown some benefit in reducing the risk of perioperative stroke. Systematic reviews have been hindered by variable proportions of symptomatic and asymptomatic patients and various permutations of staging coronary and cerebral revascularization. In general, the 30 day risk of stroke from combined CEA and CABG has been shown to be as high as 4.6%, whereas staged CEA followed by CABG had a 2.7% risk of stroke. CABG followed by CEA carried a 6.3% risk of stroke, and CAS followed by CABG was found to carry a 4.2% risk of stroke.[135] However, the combined rates of stroke, death, and MI were prohibitively high with any strategy: synchronous CABG and CEA had a 30-day risk of death or stroke of 8.2%, compared with a 6.1% risk in patients undergoing CEA followed by CABG and a 7.3% risk in patients undergoing the procedures in reversed order. Interestingly, the stroke risk was relatively high (9.1%) in patents undergoing CABG after CAS, although this may be due to data that predate refinement of stenting techniques and wide adoption of DEP devices. Indeed, a later review of the National Inpatient Sample of 27,084 patients undergoing carotid and coronary revascularization during the same admission showed that combined CEA and CABG carried an inpatient death and stroke rate of 8.6%; among patients undergoing CAS followed by coronary surgery, that risk was somewhat lower, at 6.9%.[126] The decision-making process behind selecting the type of carotid revascularization and its timing was not elucidated in this retrospective analysis. Only 4% of patients in this sample had symptomatic carotid artery disease, and 14.2% of them suffered stroke or death when treated with synchronous CABG and CEA—a high price to pay in patients with no baseline cerebrovascular symptoms.

Evidence suggests that the sequence of carotid and coronary revascularization may not be important. In a retrospective review of CEA and CABG surgeries performed between 1998 and 2007 during the same hospitalization, a strategy of simultaneous revascularization and revascularization on different days resulted in similar mortality rates (4.2% and 4.5%, respectively) and neurologic complications (3.5% and 3.9%, respectively).[139] Patients who underwent staged revascularization had a higher rate of postoperative complications but represented a group with higher baseline morbidity.

The advent of CAS has prompted many to investigate the safety of CAS in preparation for coronary artery bypass surgery. A strategy of CAS in asymptomatic patients with 80% or greater stenosis with subsequent coronary artery bypass surgery 14 to 30 days later has been shown to be safe, with a combined rate of stroke and death of 4.8% at 30 days after cardiac surgery.[140] Stroke occurred in 3.1% of patients, half of them after the carotid stenting procedure and before the cardiac surgery. Only 40% of patients in this series were treated with embolic protection during the stenting procedures. Perioperative stroke, MI, and death rates as low as 2.4% have been reported in other series of patients undergoing CAS before coronary revascularization.[141]

CAS before CABG is still performed quite infrequently and comprises about 3% of combined revascularization procedures.[126] In retrospective studies of concurrent carotid and coronary revascularization performed in the United States between 2000 and 2005, a carotid stenting strategy has been shown to be more common in a group with a higher burden of comorbidities and was shown to convey a lower risk of perioperative stroke compared with end-arterectomy (2.4% vs. 3.9%; $P < .001$).[126]

Cumulative experience suggests that CAS before CABG has a similar risk of perioperative stroke (4.2%) and combined MI, stroke, and death (9.4%) as does CEA performed before CABG.[142] These results reflect outcomes after carotid stenting in patients who are predominantly asymptomatic with unilateral carotid artery stenosis but who may carry a higher burden of medical comorbidities, which influenced the decision to proceed with CAS over CEA.

Several smaller series suggest that these combined revascularization strategies can be achieved with lower risk. Among patients undergoing CABG, CAS was performed an average of 28 days before surgery if patients had a recent CVA or TIA attributable to a carotid artery stenosis of 70% or greater. The risk of major stroke occurring within 30 days after CABG was 1.5%, but minor stroke occurred in 7% of patients, exclusively before coronary revascularization.[143]

Most of the data on perioperative stroke predate the universal acceptance of aggressive medical therapy. Retrospective studies suggest that medical therapy may be superior to combined surgical revascularization strategies, reporting a 15.1% perioperative stroke risk in patients undergoing CEA-CABG versus 0% ($P = .004$) in patients who receive optimal medical therapy during the perioperative period.[144]

In the absence of a randomized trial, it is impossible to determine whether combined revascularization consistently reduces the risk of perioperative stroke. In patients with severe bilateral carotid artery disease in whom coronary artery surgery can be delayed, CAS and completion of 4 weeks of clopidogrel may be a reasonable alternative.

The decision to combine revascularization strategies should consider whether the patient is symptomatic and whether the disease is unilateral or bilateral. In patients with neurologic symptoms, carotid revascularization should be considered before or simultaneously with coronary revascularization, but the first approach appears to be associated with fewer complications. CAS in these patients may carry a higher risk of perioperative stroke, although the available data may reflect a higher comorbidity index in patients undergoing stenting procedures. In patients with asymptomatic disease, medical therapy of carotid disease should be considered in the perioperative period, especially in patients with acute coronary syndromes, in whom cardiac surgery should not be delayed. Carotid revascularization in asymptomatic patients should be reserved for patients with bilateral high-grade disease. CAS may be an attractive alternative to CEA in this group of patients.

The safety of synchronous CABG and CEA in patients with asymptomatic high-grade carotid artery stenosis will be evaluated in the randomized Coronary Artery Bypass Graft Surgery in Patients with Asymptomatic Carotid Stenosis (CABACS) trial, which started enrollment of 1160 patients in 2010.[145]

REFERENCES

1. Roger VL, Go AS, Lloyd-Jones DM, et al. Heart disease and stroke statistics—2012 update: a report from the American Heart Association. *Circulation* 2012;125:e2-e220.
2. Lloyd-Jones D, Adams R, Carnethon M, et al. Heart disease and stroke statistics—2009 update: a report from the American Heart Association Statistics Committee and Stroke Statistics Subcommittee. *Circulation* 2009;119:e21-e181.
3. Rosamond W, Flegal K, Furie K, et al. Heart disease and stroke statistics—2008 update: a report from the American Heart Association Statistics Committee and Stroke Statistics Subcommittee. *Circulation* 2008;117:e25-e146.
4. White H, Boden-Albala B, Wang C, et al. Ischemic stroke subtype incidence among whites, blacks, and Hispanics: the Northern Manhattan Study. *Circulation* 2005;111:1327-1331.
5. Lisabeth LD, Ireland JK, Risser JM, et al. Stroke risk after transient ischemic attack in a population-based setting. *Stroke* 2004;35:1842-1846.
6. Sacco RL, Kargman DE, Gu Q, Zamanillo MC. Race-ethnicity and determinants of intracranial atherosclerotic cerebral infarction. The Northern Manhattan Stroke Study. *Stroke* 1995;26:14-20.
7. Wityk RJ, Lehman D, Klag M, et al. Race and sex differences in the distribution of cerebral atherosclerosis. *Stroke* 1996;27:1974-1980.
8. Fine-Edelstein JS, Wolf PA, O'Leary DH, et al. Precursors of extracranial carotid atherosclerosis in the Framingham study. *Neurology* 1994;44:1046-1050.
9. de Weerd M, Greving JP, de Jong AW, Buskens E, Bots ML. Prevalence of asymptomatic carotid artery stenosis according to age and sex: systematic review and metaregression analysis. *Stroke* 2009;40:1105-1113.
10. Chambless LE, Folsom AR, Clegg LX, et al. Carotid wall thickness is predictive of incident clinical stroke: the Atherosclerosis Risk in Communities (ARIC) study. *Am J Epidemiol* 2000;151:478-487.
11. Sacco RL, Roberts JK, Boden-Albala B, et al. Race-ethnicity and determinants of carotid atherosclerosis in a multiethnic population. The Northern Manhattan Stroke Study. *Stroke* 1997;28:929-935.
12. Wilson PW, Hoeg JM, D'Agostino RB, et al. Cumulative effects of high cholesterol levels, high blood pressure, and cigarette smoking on carotid stenosis. *N Engl J Med* 1997;337:516-522.
13. Rothwell PM, Coull AJ, Giles MF, et al. Change in stroke incidence, mortality, case-fatality, severity, and risk factors in Oxfordshire, UK from 1981 to 2004 (Oxford Vascular Study). *Lancet* 2004;363:1925-1933.
14. Cheng EM, Asch SM, Brook RH, et al. Suboptimal control of atherosclerotic disease risk factors after cardiac and cerebrovascular procedures. *Stroke* 2007;38:929-934.
15. Shinton R, Beevers G. Meta-analysis of relation between cigarette smoking and stroke. *Br Med J* 1989;298:789-794.
16. Wannamethee SG, Shaper AG, Whincup PH, Walker M. Smoking cessation and the risk of stroke in middle-aged men. *JAMA* 1995;274:155-160.
17. Wolf PA, D'Agostino RB, Kannel WB, Bonita R, Belanger AJ. Cigarette smoking as a risk factor for stroke: the Framingham study. *JAMA* 1988;259:1025-1029.
18. Mast H, Thompson JL, Lin IF, et al. Cigarette smoking as a determinant of high-grade carotid artery stenosis in Hispanic, black, and white patients with stroke or transient ischemic attack. *Stroke* 1998;29:908-912.
19. Tell GS, Rutan GH, Kronmal RA, et al; Cardiovascular Health Study (CHS) Collaborative Research Group. Correlates of blood pressure in community-dwelling older adults: the Cardiovascular Health Study. *Hypertension* 1994;23:59-67.
20. Brott TG, Halperin JL, Abbara S, et al. 2011 ASA/ACCF/AHA/AANN/AANS/ACR/ASNR/CNS/SAIP/SCAI/SIR/SNIS/SVM/SVS guideline on the management of patients with extracranial carotid and vertebral artery disease: executive summary. A report of the American College of Cardiology Foundation/American Heart Association Task Force on practice guidelines, and the American Stroke Association, American Association of Neuroscience Nurses, American Association of Neurological Surgeons, American College of Radiology, American Society of Neuroradiology, Congress of Neurological Surgeons, Society of Atherosclerosis Imaging and Prevention, Society for Cardiovascular Angiography and Interventions, Society of Interventional Radiology, Society of NeuroInterventional Surgery, Society for Vascular Medicine, and Society for Vascular Surgery. *Stroke* 2011;42:e420-e463.
21. Lewington S, Clarke R, Qizilbash N, Peto R, Collins R. Age-specific relevance of usual blood pressure to vascular mortality: a meta-analysis of individual data for one million adults in 61 prospective studies. *Lancet* 2002;360:1903-1913.
22. Psaty BM, Lumley T, Furberg CD, et al. Health outcomes associated with various antihypertensive therapies used as first-line agents: a network meta-analysis. *JAMA* 2003;289:2534-2544.
23. Prevention of stroke by antihypertensive drug treatment in older persons with isolated systolic hypertension: final results of the Systolic Hypertension in the Elderly Program (SHEP). SHEP Cooperative Research Group. *JAMA* 1991;265:3255-3264.
24. Staessen JA, Fagard R, Thijs L, for the Systolic Hypertension in Europe (Syst-Eur) Trial Investigators. Randomised double-blind comparison of placebo and active treatment for older patients with isolated systolic hypertension. *Lancet* 1997;350:757-764.
25. Beckett NS, Peters R, Fletcher AE, et al. Treatment of hypertension in patients 80 years of age or older. *N Engl J Med* 2008;358:1887-1898.
26. Wright JM, Musini VM. First-line drugs for hypertension. *Cochrane Database Syst Rev* 2009:CD001841.
27. Major outcomes in high-risk hypertensive patients randomized to angiotensin-converting enzyme inhibitor or channel blocker vs diuretic: the Antihypertensive and Lipid-Lowering Treatment to Prevent Heart Attack Trial (ALLHAT). *JAMA* 2002;288:2981-2997.
28. Turnbull F. Effects of different blood-pressure–lowering regimens on major cardiovascular events: results of prospectively-designed overviews of randomised trials. *Lancet* 2003;362:1527-1535.
29. Hansson L, Zanchetti A, Carruthers SG, et al, for the HOT Study Group. Effects of intensive blood-pressure lowering and low-dose aspirin in patients with hypertension: principal results of the Hypertension Optimal Treatment (HOT) randomised trial. *Lancet* 1998;351:1755-1762.
30. Rashid P, Leonardi-Bee J, Bath P. Blood pressure reduction and secondary prevention of stroke and other vascular events: a systematic review. *Stroke* 2003;34:2741-2748.
31. Yusuf S, Diener HC, Sacco RL, et al. Telmisartan to prevent recurrent stroke and cardiovascular events. *N Engl J Med* 2008;359:1225-1237.
32. Schrader J, Luders S, Kulschewski A, et al. Morbidity and mortality after stroke, eprosartan compared with nitrendipine for secondary prevention: principal results of a prospective randomized controlled study (MOSES). *Stroke* 2005;36:1218-1226.
33. Randomised trial of a perindopril-based blood-pressure–lowering regimen among 6,105 individuals with previous stroke or transient ischaemic attack. *Lancet* 2001;358:1033-1041.
34. Iso H, Jacobs DR Jr, Wentworth D, Neaton JD, Cohen JD. Serum cholesterol levels and six-year mortality from stroke in 350,977 men screened for the multiple risk factor intervention trial. *N Engl J Med* 1989;320:904-910.
35. Leppala JM, Virtamo J, Fogelholm R, Albanes D, Heinonen OP. Different risk factors for different stroke subtypes: association of blood pressure, cholesterol, and antioxidants. *Stroke* 1999;30:2535-2540.
36. Zhang X, Patel A, Horibe H, et al. Cholesterol, coronary heart disease, and stroke in the Asia Pacific region. *Int J Epidemiol* 2003;32:563-572.
37. Horenstein RB, Smith DE, Mosca L. Cholesterol predicts stroke mortality in the Women's Pooling Project. *Stroke* 2002;33:1863-1868.

38. Kurth T, Everett BM, Buring JE, et al. Lipid levels and the risk of ischemic stroke in women. *Neurology* 2007;68:556-562.

39. Sharrett AR, Patsch W, Sorlie PD, et al. Associations of lipoprotein cholesterols, apolipoproteins A-I and B, and triglycerides with carotid atherosclerosis and coronary heart disease. The Atherosclerosis Risk in Communities (ARIC) Study. *Arterioscler Thromb* 1994;14:1098-1104.

40. Falk E, Shah PK, Fuster V. Coronary plaque disruption. *Circulation* 1995;92:657-671.

41. Wasserman BA, Sharrett AR, Lai S, et al. Risk factor associations with the presence of a lipid core in carotid plaque of asymptomatic individuals using high-resolution MRI: the multi-ethnic study of atherosclerosis (MESA). *Stroke* 2008;39:329-335.

42. Amarenco P, Labreuche J, Lavallee P, Touboul PJ. Statins in stroke prevention and carotid atherosclerosis: systematic review and up-to-date meta-analysis. *Stroke* 2004; 35:2902-2909.

43. Crouse JR 3rd, Raichlen JS, Riley WA, et al. Effect of rosuvastatin on progression of carotid intima-media thickness in low-risk individuals with subclinical atherosclerosis: the METEOR Trial. *JAMA* 2007;297:1344-1353.

44. Tahara N, Kai H, Ishibashi M, et al. Simvastatin attenuates plaque inflammation: evaluation by fluorodeoxyglucose positron emission tomography. *J Am Coll Cardiol* 2006;48:1825-1831.

45. Kadoglou NP, Gerasimidis T, Moumtzouoglou A, et al. Intensive lipid-lowering therapy ameliorates novel calcification markers and GSM score in patients with carotid stenosis. *Eur J Vasc Endovasc Surg* 2008;35:661-668.

46. Spence JD, Coates V, Li H, et al. Effects of intensive medical therapy on microemboli and cardiovascular risk in asymptomatic carotid stenosis. *Arch Neurol* 2010;67:180-186.

47. Baigent C, Keech A, Kearney PM, et al. Efficacy and safety of cholesterol-lowering treatment: prospective meta-analysis of data from 90,056 participants in 14 randomised trials of statins. *Lancet* 2005;366:1267-1278.

48. Amarenco P, Labreuche J. Lipid management in the prevention of stroke: review and updated meta-analysis of statins for stroke prevention. *Lancet Neurol* 2009;8:453-463.

49. Halliday A, Harrison M, Hayter E, et al. 10-year stroke prevention after successful carotid endarterectomy for asymptomatic stenosis (ACST-1): a multicentre randomised trial. *Lancet* 2010;376:1074-1084.

50. Sillesen H, Amarenco P, Hennerici MG, et al. Atorvastatin reduces the risk of cardiovascular events in patients with carotid atherosclerosis: a secondary analysis of the Stroke Prevention by Aggressive Reduction in Cholesterol Levels (SPARCL) trial. *Stroke* 2008;39:3297-3302.

51. Amarenco P, Goldstein LB, Szarek M, et al. Effects of intense low-density lipoprotein cholesterol reduction in patients with stroke or transient ischemic attack: the Stroke Prevention by Aggressive Reduction in Cholesterol Levels (SPARCL) trial. *Stroke* 2007; 38:3198-3204.

52. Keech A, Simes RJ, Barter P, et al. Effects of long-term fenofibrate therapy on cardiovascular events in 9795 people with type 2 diabetes mellitus (the FIELD study): randomised controlled trial. *Lancet* 2005;366:1849-1861.

53. Secondary prevention by raising HDL cholesterol and reducing triglycerides in patients with coronary artery disease: the Bezafibrate Infarction Prevention (BIP) study. *Circulation* 2000;102:21-27.

54. Ginsberg HN, Elam MB, Lovato LC, et al. Effects of combination lipid therapy in type 2 diabetes mellitus. *N Engl J Med* 2010;362:1563-1574.

55. The AIM-HIGH Investigators. Niacin in patients with low HDL cholesterol levels receiving intensive statin therapy. *N Engl J Med* 2011;365:2255-2267.

56. Grundy SM, Cleeman JI, Merz CN, et al. Implications of recent clinical trials for the National Cholesterol Education Program Adult Treatment Panel III guidelines. *Circulation* 2004; 110:227-239.

57. Cote R, Battista RN, Abrahamowicz M, et al. Lack of effect of aspirin in asymptomatic patients with carotid bruits and substantial carotid narrowing: the Asymptomatic Cervical Bruit Study Group. *Ann Intern Med* 1995;123:649-655.

58. Collaborative meta-analysis of randomised trials of antiplatelet therapy for prevention of death, myocardial infarction, and stroke in high risk patients. *Br Med J* 2002;324:71-86.

59. Algra A, van Gijn J. Cumulative meta-analysis of aspirin efficacy after cerebral ischaemia of arterial origin. *J Neurol Neurosurg Psychiatry* 1999;66:255.

60. CAPRIE Steering Committee. A randomised, blinded trial of clopidogrel versus aspirin in patients at risk of ischaemic events (CAPRIE). *Lancet* 1996;348:1329-1339.

61. Markus HS, Droste DW, Kaps M, et al. Dual antiplatelet therapy with clopidogrel and aspirin in symptomatic carotid stenosis evaluated using Doppler embolic signal detection: the Clopidogrel and Aspirin for Reduction of Emboli in Symptomatic Carotid Stenosis (CARESS) trial. *Circulation* 2005;111:2233-2240.

62. Wong KS, Chen C, Fu J, et al. Clopidogrel plus aspirin versus aspirin alone for reducing embolisation in patients with acute symptomatic cerebral or carotid artery stenosis (CLAIR study): a randomised, open-label, blinded-endpoint trial. *Lancet Neurol* 2010;9: 489-497.

63. Diener HC, Bogousslavsky J, Brass LM, et al. Aspirin and clopidogrel compared with clopidogrel alone after recent ischaemic stroke or transient ischaemic attack in high-risk patients (MATCH): randomised, double-blind, placebo-controlled trial. *Lancet* 2004;364: 331-337.

64. Kennedy J, Hill MD, Ryckborst KJ, et al. Fast assessment of stroke and transient ischaemic attack to prevent early recurrence (FASTER): a randomised controlled pilot trial. *Lancet Neurol* 2007;6:961-969.

65. Hankey GJ, Johnston SC, Easton JD, et al. Effect of clopidogrel plus ASA vs. ASA early after TIA and ischaemic stroke: a substudy of the CHARISMA trial. *Int J Stroke* 2011;6:3-9.

66. Diener HC, Cunha L, Forbes C, et al. European Stroke Prevention Study. 2. Dipyridamole and acetylsalicylic acid in the secondary prevention of stroke. *J Neurol Sci* 1996;143:1-13.

67. Halkes PH, van Gijn J, Kappelle LJ, Koudstaal PJ, Algra A. Aspirin plus dipyridamole versus aspirin alone after cerebral ischaemia of arterial origin (ESPRIT): randomised controlled trial. *Lancet* 2006;367:1665-1673.

68. Sacco RL, Diener HC, Yusuf S, et al. Aspirin and extended-release dipyridamole versus clopidogrel for recurrent stroke. *N Engl J Med* 2008;359:1238-1251.

69. Geeganage CM, Diener HC, Algra A, et al. Dual or mono antiplatelet therapy for patients with acute ischemic stroke or transient ischemic attack: systematic review and meta-analysis of randomized controlled trials. *Stroke* 2012;43(4):1058-1066.

70. Bousser MG, Amarenco P, Chamorro A, et al. Terutroban versus aspirin in patients with cerebral ischaemic events (PERFORM): a randomised, double-blind, parallel-group trial. *Lancet* 2011;377:2013-2022.

71. Halkes PH, van Gijn J, Kappelle LJ, Koudstaal PJ, Algra A. Medium intensity oral anticoagulants versus aspirin after cerebral ischaemia of arterial origin (ESPRIT): a randomised controlled trial. *Lancet Neurol* 2007;6:115-124.

72. The Stroke Prevention in Reversible Ischemia Trial (SPIRIT) Study Group. A randomized trial of anticoagulants versus aspirin after cerebral ischemia of presumed arterial origin. *Ann Neurol* 1997;42:857-865.

73. Mohr JP, Thompson JL, Lazar RM, et al. A comparison of warfarin and aspirin for the prevention of recurrent ischemic stroke. *N Engl J Med* 2001;345:1444-1451.

74. McPhee JT, Schanzer A, Messina LM, Eslami MH. Carotid artery stenting has increased rates of postprocedure stroke, death, and resource utilization than does carotid endarterectomy in the United States, 2005. *J Vasc Surg* 2008;48:1442-1450, 1450 e1.

75. Lovett JK, Dennis MS, Sandercock PAG, et al. Very early risk of stroke after a first transient ischemic attack. *Stroke* 2003;34:e138-e140.

76. Coull AJ, Lovett JK, Rothwell PM. Population based study of early risk of stroke after transient ischaemic attack or minor stroke: implications for public education and organisation of services. *Br Med J* 2004;328:326.

77. Fairhead JF, Mehta Z, Rothwell PM. Population-based study of delays in carotid imaging and surgery and the risk of recurrent stroke. *Neurology* 2005;65:371-375.

78. Marnane M, Ni Chroinin D, Callaly E, et al. Stroke recurrence within the time window recommended for carotid endarterectomy. *Neurology* 2011;77:738-743.

79. Barnett HJ, Taylor DW, Eliasziw M, et al, for the North American Symptomatic Carotid Endarterectomy Trial Collaborators. Benefit of carotid endarterectomy in patients with symptomatic moderate or severe stenosis. *New Engl J Med* 1998;339:1415-1425.

80. European Carotid Surgery Trialists' Collaborative Group. MRC European Carotid Surgery Trial: interim results for symptomatic patients with severe (70-99%) or with mild (0-29%) carotid stenosis. *Lancet* 1991;337:1235-1243.

81. Randomised trial of endarterectomy for recently symptomatic carotid stenosis: final results of the MRC European Carotid Surgery Trial (ECST). *Lancet* 1998;351: 1379-1387.

82. Mayberg MR, Wilson SE, Yatsu F, et al, for the Veterans Affairs Cooperative Studies Program 309 Trialist Group. Carotid endarterectomy and prevention of cerebral ischemia in symptomatic carotid stenosis. *JAMA* 1991;266:3289-3294.

83. Rothwell PM, Eliasziw M, Gutnikov SA, et al. Analysis of pooled data from the randomised controlled trials of endarterectomy for symptomatic carotid stenosis. *Lancet* 2003; 361:107-116.

83a. Hackam DG, Spence JD. Combining multiple approaches for the secondary prevention of vascular events after stroke: a quantitative modeling study. *Stroke* 2007;38:1881.

84. Carotid surgery versus medical therapy in asymptomatic carotid stenosis. The CASANOVA Study Group. *Stroke* 1991;22:1229-1235.

85. Results of a randomized controlled trial of carotid endarterectomy for asymptomatic carotid stenosis. Mayo Asymptomatic Carotid Endarterectomy Study Group. *Mayo Clinic Proc* 1992;67:513-518.

86. Hobson RW 2nd, Weiss DG, Fields WS, et al, for The Veterans Affairs Cooperative Study Group. Efficacy of carotid endarterectomy for asymptomatic carotid stenosis. *N Engl J Med* 1993;328:221-227.

87. Executive Committee for the Asymptomatic Carotid Atherosclerosis Study. Endarterectomy for asymptomatic carotid artery stenosis. *JAMA* 1995;273:1421-1428.

88. Halliday A, Mansfield A, Marro J, et al. Prevention of disabling and fatal strokes by successful carotid endarterectomy in patients without recent neurological symptoms: randomised controlled trial. *Lancet* 2004;363:1491-1502.

89. Rothwell PM. ACST: Which subgroups will benefit most from carotid endarterectomy? *Lancet* 2004;364:1122-1123; author reply 1125-1126.

90. Tu JV, Hannan EL, Anderson GM, et al. The fall and rise of carotid endarterectomy in the United States and Canada. *N Engl J Med* 1998;339:1441-1447.

91. Rothwell PM, Goldstein LB. Carotid endarterectomy for asymptomatic carotid stenosis. *Stroke* 2004;35:2425-2427.

92. Moore WS, Young B, Baker WH, et al, for the ACAS Investigators. Surgical results: a justification of the surgeon selection process for the ACAS trial. *J Vasc Surg* 1996;23: 323-328.

93. Kresowik TF, Bratzler DW, Kresowik RA, et al. Multistate improvement in process and outcomes of carotid endarterectomy. *J Vasc Surg* 2004;39:372-380.

94. Gray WA, Yadav JS, Verta P, et al. The CAPTURE registry: results of carotid stenting with embolic protection in the post approval setting. *Catheter Cardiovasc Interv* 2007;69:341-348.

95. Gray WA, Chaturvedi S, Verta P. Thirty-day outcomes for carotid artery stenting in 6320 patients from 2 prospective, multicenter, high-surgical-risk registries. *Circ Cardiovasc Interv* 2009;2:159-166.

96. Massop D, Dave R, Metzger C, et al. Stenting and angioplasty with protection in patients at high-risk for endarterectomy: SAPPHIRE Worldwide Registry first 2,001 patients. *Catheter Cardiovasc Interv* 2009;73:129-136.

97. Gurm HS, Yadav JS, Fayad P, et al. Long-term results of carotid stenting versus endarterectomy in high-risk patients. *N Engl J Med* 2008;358:1572-1579.

98. Patel MR, Greiner MA, DiMartino LD, et al. Geographic variation in carotid revascularization among Medicare beneficiaries, 2003-2006. *Arch Intern Med* 2010;170:1218-1225.

99. Mas JL, Trinquart L, Leys D, et al. Endarterectomy Versus Angioplasty in Patients with Symptomatic Severe Carotid Stenosis (EVA-3S) trial: results up to 4 years from a randomised, multicentre trial. *Lancet Neurol* 2008;7:885-892.

100. Eckstein HH, Ringleb P, Allenberg JR, et al. Results of the Stent-Protected Angioplasty versus Carotid Endarterectomy (SPACE) study to treat symptomatic stenoses at 2 years: a multinational, prospective, randomised trial. *Lancet Neurol* 2008;7:893-902.

101. Ederle J, Dobson J, Featherstone RL, et al. Carotid artery stenting compared with endarterectomy in patients with symptomatic carotid stenosis (International Carotid Stenting Study): an interim analysis of a randomised controlled trial. *Lancet* 2010; 375:985-997.

102. Gray WA, Rosenfield KA, Jaff MR, et al. Influence of site and operator characteristics on carotid artery stent outcomes: analysis of the CAPTURE 2 (Carotid ACCULINK/ACCUNET Post Approval Trial to Uncover Rare Events) clinical study. *JACC Cardiovasc Interv* 2011; 4:235-246.

103. Roffi M, Sievert H, Gray WA, et al. Carotid artery stenting versus surgery: adequate comparisons? *Lancet Neurol* 2010;9:339-341; author reply 341-342.

104. Ringleb PA, Hacke W. [Stent and surgery for symptomatic carotid stenosis. SPACE study results]. *Der Nervenarzt* 2007;78:1130-1137.

105. Blackshear JL, Cutlip DE, Roubin GS, et al. Myocardial infarction after carotid stenting and endarterectomy: results from the carotid revascularization endarterectomy versus stenting trial. *Circulation* 2011;123:2571-2578.

106. Naylor AR. Time to rethink management strategies in asymptomatic carotid artery disease. *Nat Rev Cardiol* 2011;9(2):116-124.

107. Marquardt L, Geraghty OC, Mehta Z, Rothwell PM. Low risk of ipsilateral stroke in patients with asymptomatic carotid stenosis on best medical treatment: a prospective, population-based study. *Stroke* 2010;41:e11-e17.

108. Perry JR, Szalai JP, Norris JW. Consensus against both endarterectomy and routine screening for asymptomatic carotid artery stenosis. Canadian Stroke Consortium. *Arch Neurol* 1997;54:25-28.

109. Olsen TS, Langhorne P, Diener HC, et al. European Stroke Initiative Recommendations for Stroke Management—update 2003. *Cerebrovasc Dis* 2003;16:311-337.

110. Klein A, Solomon CG, Hamel MB. Clinical decisions: management of carotid stenosis—polling results. *New Engl J Med* 2008;358:e23.

111. Woo K, Garg J, Hye RJ, Dilley RB. Contemporary results of carotid endarterectomy for asymptomatic carotid stenosis. *Stroke* 2010;41:975-979.

112. Goessens BM, Visseren FL, Kappelle LJ, Algra A, van der Graaf Y. Asymptomatic carotid artery stenosis and the risk of new vascular events in patients with manifest arterial disease: the SMART study. *Stroke* 2007;38:1470-1475.

113. Bertges DJ, Muluk V, Whittle J, et al. Relevance of carotid stenosis progression as a predictor of ischemic neurological outcomes. *Arch Intern Med* 2003;163:2285-2289.

114. Baker WH, Howard VJ, Howard G, Toole JF. Effect of contralateral occlusion on long-term efficacy of endarterectomy in the asymptomatic carotid atherosclerosis study (ACAS). ACAS Investigators. *Stroke* 2000;31:2330-2334.

115. Nicolaides AN, Kakkos SK, Griffin M, et al. Severity of asymptomatic carotid stenosis and risk of ipsilateral hemispheric ischaemic events: results from the ACSRS study. *Eur J Vasc Endovasc Surg* 2005;30:275-284.

116. Geroulakos G, Ramaswami G, Nicolaides A, et al. Characterization of symptomatic and asymptomatic carotid plaques using high-resolution real-time ultrasonography. *Br J Surg* 1993;80:1274-1277.

117. Nicolaides AN, Kakkos SK, Kyriacou E, et al. Asymptomatic internal carotid artery stenosis and cerebrovascular risk stratification. *J Vasc Surg* 2010;52:1486-1496, e1-e5.

118. Mathiesen EB, Bønaa KH, Joakimsen O. Echolucent plaques are associated with high risk of ischemic cerebrovascular events in carotid stenosis: the Tromsø study. *Circulation* 2001;103:2171-2175.

119. Spence JD, Tamayo A, Lownie SP, Ng WP, Ferguson GG. Absence of microemboli on transcranial Doppler identifies low-risk patients with asymptomatic carotid stenosis. *Stroke* 2005;36:2373-2378.

120. Markus HS, King A, Shipley M, et al. Asymptomatic embolisation for prediction of stroke in the Asymptomatic Carotid Emboli Study (ACES): a prospective observational study. *Lancet Neurol* 2010;9:663-671.

121. Topakian R, King A, Kwon SU, et al. Ultrasonic plaque echolucency and emboli signals predict stroke in asymptomatic carotid stenosis. *Neurology* 2011;77:751-758.

122. Madani A, Beletsky V, Tamayo A, Munoz C, Spence JD. High-risk asymptomatic carotid stenosis: ulceration on 3D ultrasound vs TCD microemboli. *Neurology* 2011;77:744-750.

123. Abbott AL, Chambers BR, Stork JL, et al. Embolic signals and prediction of ipsilateral stroke or transient ischemic attack in asymptomatic carotid stenosis: a multicenter prospective cohort study. *Stroke* 2005;36:1128-1133.

124. Takaya N, Yuan C, Chu B, et al. Association between carotid plaque characteristics and subsequent ischemic cerebrovascular events: a prospective assessment with MRI—initial results. *Stroke* 2006;37:818-823.

125. Singh N, Moody AR, Gladstone DJ, et al. Moderate carotid artery stenosis: MR imaging-depicted intraplaque hemorrhage predicts risk of cerebrovascular ischemic events in asymptomatic men. *Radiology* 2009;252:502-508.

126. Timaran CH, Rosero EB, Smith ST, et al. Trends and outcomes of concurrent carotid revascularization and coronary bypass. *J Vasc Surg* 2008;48:355-360; discussion 360-361.

127. Likosky DS, Marrin CA, Caplan LR, et al. Determination of etiologic mechanisms of strokes secondary to coronary artery bypass graft surgery. *Stroke* 2003;34:2830-2834.

128. Djaiani G, Fedorko L, Borger M, et al. Mild to moderate atheromatous disease of the thoracic aorta and new ischemic brain lesions after conventional coronary artery bypass graft surgery. *Stroke* 2004;35:e356-e358.

129. Schwartz LB, Bridgman AH, Kieffer RW, et al. Asymptomatic carotid artery stenosis and stroke in patients undergoing cardiopulmonary bypass. *J Vasc Surg* 1995;21:146-153.

130. Ricotta JJ, Faggioli GL, Castilone A, Hassett JM, for the Buffalo Cardiac-Cerebral Study Group. Risk factors for stroke after cardiac surgery. *J Vasc Surg* 1995;21:359-363; discussion 364.

131. Berens ES, Kouchoukos NT, Murphy SF, Wareing TH. Preoperative carotid artery screening in elderly patients undergoing cardiac surgery. *J Vasc Surg* 1992;15:313-321; discussion 322-323.

132. Salasidis GC, Latter DA, Steinmetz OK, Blair JF, Graham AM. Carotid artery duplex scanning in preoperative assessment for coronary artery revascularization: the association between peripheral vascular disease, carotid artery stenosis, and stroke. *J Vasc Surg* 1995;21:154-160; discussion 161-162.

133. Brener BJ, Brief DK, Alpert J, et al. A four-year experience with preoperative noninvasive carotid evaluation of two thousand twenty-six patients undergoing cardiac surgery. *J Vasc Surg* 1984;1:326-338.

134. Naylor AR, Mehta Z, Rothwell PM, Bell PR. Carotid artery disease and stroke during coronary artery bypass: a critical review of the literature. *Eur J Vasc Surg* 2002;23:283-294.

135. Naylor AR. Does the risk of post-CABG stroke merit staged or synchronous reconstruction in patients with symptomatic or asymptomatic carotid disease? *J Cardiovasc Surg* 2009;50:71-81.

136. Barbut D, Grassineau D, Lis E, et al. Posterior distribution of infarcts in strokes related to cardiac operations. *Ann Thorac Surg* 1998;65:1656-1659.

137. Naylor AR, Bown MJ. Stroke after cardiac surgery and its association with asymptomatic carotid disease: an updated systematic review and meta-analysis. *Eur J Vasc Surg* 2011;41:607-624.

138. Mahmoudi M, Hill PC, Xue Z, et al. Patients with severe asymptomatic carotid artery stenosis do not have a higher risk of stroke and mortality after coronary artery bypass surgery. *Stroke* 2011;42:2801-2805.

139. Gopaldas RR, Chu D, Dao TK, et al. Staged versus synchronous carotid endarterectomy and coronary artery bypass grafting: analysis of 10-year nationwide outcomes. *Ann Thorac Surg* 2011;91:1323-1329; discussion 1329.

140. Van der Heyden J, Suttorp MJ, Bal ET, et al. Staged carotid angioplasty and stenting followed by cardiac surgery in patients with severe asymptomatic carotid artery stenosis: early and long-term results. *Circulation* 2007;116:2036-2042.

141. Ribichini F, Tomai F, Reimers B, et al. Clinical outcome after endovascular, surgical or hybrid revascularisation in patients with combined carotid and coronary artery disease: the Finalised Research In ENDovascular Strategies Study Group (FRIENDS). *EuroIntervention* 2010;6:328-335.

142. Naylor AR, Mehta Z, Rothwell PM. A systematic review and meta-analysis of 30-day outcomes following staged carotid artery stenting and coronary bypass. *Eur J Vasc Surg* 2009;37:379-387.

143. Van der Heyden J, Van Neerven D, Sonker U, et al. Carotid artery stenting and cardiac surgery in symptomatic patients. *JACC Cardiovasc Interv* 2011;4:1190-1196.

144. Li Y, Walicki D, Mathiesen C, et al. Strokes after cardiac surgery and relationship to carotid stenosis. *Arch Neurol* 2009;66:1091-1096.

145. Knipp SC, Scherag A, Beyersdorf F, et al. Randomized comparison of synchronous CABG and carotid endarterectomy vs. isolated CABG in patients with asymptomatic carotid stenosis: the CABACS trial. *Int J Stroke* 2011 Nov 22 [Epub ahead of print].

CHAPTER 37 Renal Artery Stenosis

Ido Weinberg and Michael R. Jaff

OVERVIEW, 571

CLINICAL MANIFESTATIONS, 571

NATURAL HISTORY OF RENAL ARTERY STENOSIS, 571

DIAGNOSIS OF RENAL ARTERY STENOSIS, 571

TREATMENT OF ATHEROSCLEROTIC RENAL ARTERY STENOSIS, 574

Medical Therapy, 574
Which Patients Should Be Revascularized? 574
Catheter-Based Intervention, 575

Surveillance of Renovascular Disease, 577
Catheter-Based Renal Artery Sympathetic Denervation, 578

CONCLUSION, 578

REFERENCES, 578

Overview

Atherosclerotic renal artery stenosis (ARAS) is common, although renal artery stenosis (RAS) may be due to etiologies other than atherosclerosis, including fibromuscular dysplasia (FMD), segmental arterial mediolysis (SAM), dissection, or arteritis. Any consideration of the treatment of RAS must take into account the underlying cause; however, atherosclerosis is by far the most common etiology. ARAS has been found to affect 6.8% of patients in the Cardiovascular Health Study, a population-based study of the elderly.[1] It is even more prevalent in at-risk populations, including patients with poorly controlled hypertension (HTN) and systemic atherosclerosis.[2,3] Atherosclerotic renovascular disease is found in 18% to 20% of patients with coronary artery disease and in 59% of patients with peripheral artery disease.[4,5] FMD, which is likely underreported, is present in 10% of patients with renovascular HTN.[6]

Clinical Manifestations

ARAS has been implicated as a cause of HTN, deterioration of renal function, and cardiac disturbance syndromes (recurrent unexplained congestive heart failure, refractory angina, and "flash" pulmonary edema). HTN related to underlying RAS should be suspected in individuals who either are young, suggesting a nonatherosclerotic etiology, or are older than 55 years at the time of onset of HTN. Resistant HTN—defined as the inability to achieve goal blood pressure of 140/90 mm Hg or lower despite the use of three antihypertensive medications at maximum tolerable doses and in appropriate combinations—is another important clinical clue for underlying RAS.[7] Other significant clinical clues, which should prompt an investigation for ARAS, are listed in Box 37-1.

The pathophysiologic mechanism for renovascular HTN in the face of unilateral ARAS has been well described. The kidney ipsilateral to the stenosis responds by secreting renin, which promotes sodium retention and vasoconstriction via the renin-angiotensin-aldosterone pathway. This causes an increase in blood pressure, and the contralateral kidney reacts by invoking a pressure natriuresis. Sodium excretion is followed by extracellular volume contraction, which in turn causes the affected kidney to secrete more renin because its perfusion pressure is further reduced. Eventually, the nonstenotic kidney cannot compensate any further, resulting in progressive HTN.[8]

Chronic kidney disease (CKD) in patients with ARAS may result from long-standing systemic HTN, renal ischemia, recurrent atheromatous embolization from the aorta, and contrast nephropathy as a result of multiple imaging studies.[9] There is no known linear relationship between the degree of ARAS and HTN or renal dysfunction.[10] Notwithstanding, ARAS is found more often in patients with end-stage renal disease (ESRD) than in the general population.[11] ARAS progresses over time, leading to more severe stenosis and ipsilateral renal atrophy.[12] As the baseline severity of ARAS worsens, the rate of progression to renal artery occlusion increases.[13]

Natural History of Renal Artery Stenosis

The natural history of ARAS is incompletely understood. In some studies, mortality rate and changes in serum creatinine over time were not correlated with baseline degree of stenosis.[14,15] In contrast, other studies have found that the severity of the stenosis predicted progression of disease, progression to occlusion, and renal atrophy.[12,13] However, the consequences of RAS in FMD are different, and patients with FMD usually do not come to medical attention with renal dysfunction but rather with isolated HTN.[16]

Diagnosis of Renal Artery Stenosis

Noninvasive diagnosis and later surveillance of RAS can be reliably performed with several modalities. Renal artery duplex ultrasonography (RADUS), magnetic resonance angiography (MRA), and computed tomographic angiography (CTA) are all part of the modern diagnostic armamentarium for RAS. Indications for renal artery imaging include clinical suspicion of RAS, as outlined in Box 37-1, and surveillance following revascularization.[17] Typically, ARAS presents as ostial stenosis, representing plaque from the abdominal aorta draped into the origin of the renal artery. Nonatherosclerotic causes of RAS demonstrate other classic angiographic appearances. For example, FMD is most often found in the mid and distal segments of the renal artery and, depending on the type of FMD, has a characteristic beaded appearance.

RADUS is an ideal noninvasive test to confirm or refute the diagnosis of RAS because it is accurate, inexpensive, and painless (Figure 37-1). In a prospective series that compared 102 RADUS exams to contrast angiography, the sensitivity of duplex ultrasonography was 98%, specificity was 99%, positive predictive value was 99%, and negative predictive value was 97%.[18] Renal artery Doppler ultrasound (DUS) has also been shown to be accurate in the diagnosis and surveillance of renal artery FMD, albeit only in a small series. It may identify the typical beaded appearance of the medial fibroplasia variant and suggests mid or distal renal artery involvement by peak systolic velocity (PSV) measurements.[19]

The principles of diagnosis of ARAS with RADUS are based on the use of the PSV within the renal artery, as well as the ratio of the PSV measured in the aorta at the level of the superior mesenteric artery and the PSV at the level of the renal artery origin, known as the *renal/aortic ratio* (RAR). Categories of RAS detected by RADUS include 0% to 59% stenosis, 60% to 99% stenosis, and occlusion (Table 37-1). A PSV greater than 200 cm/s with poststenotic turbulence and an RAR above 3.5 suggest a 60% to 99% stenosis. A typical parvus et tardus waveform in the distal main renal artery or parenchymal branches suggests a proximal stenosis, but it is not accurate as an indirect measure of main RAS. RADUS requires technical competence, with the need for highly skilled technologists and physicians to perform and interpret the results. Limitations of RADUS include difficulty visualizing the renal arteries because of overlying bowel gas or morbid obesity, the challenge of identifying polar (accessory) renal arteries, and difficulty identifying distal renal artery disease.[20]

Box 37-1 Clinical Clues to the Diagnosis of Renal Artery Stenosis

Factors Related to Hypertension
New-onset hypertension (<40 or >55 years)
Resistant hypertension
Exacerbation of previously well-controlled hypertension
Hypertensive emergency

Factors Related to Comorbidities
Hypertension and/or chronic kidney disease and multivessel coronary
  artery disease
Hypertension and peripheral artery disease

Factors Related to Renal Function
Azotemia after therapy with ACE inhibitors or angiotensin receptor
  blockers
Unexplained azotemia
Discrepancy in renal size

Other Clues
Systolic and diastolic epigastric bruit, particularly with radiation to one
  flank

ACE, angiotensin-converting enzyme.

TABLE 37-1 Duplex Ultrasound Criteria for Renal Artery Stenosis

RENAL ARTERY	PEAK SYSTOLIC VELOCITY	RENAL/AORTIC RATIO*
Native Artery		
Normal	<200 cm/s	<3.5
1%-59% stenosis	<200 cm/s	<3.5
60%-99% stenosis	>200 cm/s plus poststenotic turbulence	>3.5
Occlusion	No detectable flow in the renal artery	
Stented Artery		
0%-59%	<240 cm/s without PST	
60%-99%	>300 cm/s	>4.3
Occlusion	No detectable flow in the renal artery	

*The renal/aortic ratio cannot be used if the aortic peak systolic velocity is >100 cm/s or <40 cm/s.
PST, post-stenotic turbulence.

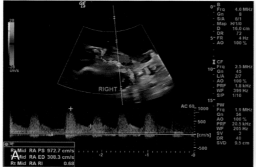 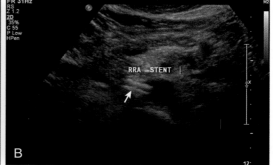

FIGURE 37-1   **A,** Right renal artery (*RRA*) stenosis demonstrated by color-enhanced renal artery duplex ultrasonography with peak systolic velocity measured at 972 cm/s. **B,** Grayscale ultrasound image of a left renal artery stent.

CTA and MRA represent important axial imaging strategies for assessment of the renal arteries because they provide excellent three-dimensional images of the renal arteries, including identification of accessory (polar) renal arteries, and they also offer important visualization of the abdominal aorta and kidneys. CTA and MRA can accurately identify and assess the progression of other pathologies within the renal artery, including aneurysms, which may occur in arteries affected by atherosclerosis and FMD.[19]

CTA and MRA also have some inherent disadvantages. CTA is challenged by the presence of arterial calcification that may obscure the arterial lumen, whereas MRA is not affected by calcium. MRA has a tendency to overestimate the severity of arterial stenosis and cannot visualize the arterial lumen within metallic stents. CTA and MRA are also limited in their ability to assess distal RAS, which is more typical in FMD than in ARAS.[21] CTA mandates the use of iodinated contrast and external-beam radiation, which makes it an unattractive method for serial surveillance of ARAS. MRA, on the other hand, is not appropriate for patients with claustrophobia or metallic implants such as pacemakers, defibrillators, and renal artery metallic stents. Gadolinium-based contrast agents commonly used in MRA are associated with a risk of nephrogenic systemic sclerosis in patients with CKD. Many believe that gadolinium is required to accurately evaluate the status of the renal arteries; therefore both CTA and MRA have limited use in the presence of CKD, a prevalent condition in patients suspected to have ARAS. A meta-analysis found much higher diagnostic value for both CTA and MRA in the diagnosis of

ARAS.[23] Receiver operating characteristic (ROC) curves were 0.99 for CTA, 0.99 for gadolinium-enhanced MRA, and 0.97 for non–gadolinium-enhanced MRA, indicating high sensitivity with low false-positive rates. Because both CTA and MRA may prompt invasive procedures, the low false-positive rates seen with these tests are reassuring.

The accuracy of MRA was reinforced by another meta-analysis performed to determine the need for and diagnostic accuracy of gadolinium-based contrast agents with MRA of the renal arteries.[21] The criterion for accuracy was whether MRA could detect the difference between greater than 50% and 50% or less stenosis. A total of 998 patients, in whom MRA was compared with catheter angiography, were included. The sensitivity and specificity for noncontrast MRA were 94% and 85%, respectively. For contrast-enhanced MRA, the sensitivity and specificity were higher at 97% and 93%, respectively.

Despite its sound theoretical basis, captopril renal scintigraphy does not offer acceptable sensitivity for the diagnosis of ARAS, nor has it been consistently shown to predict clinical outcomes.[24] It is especially inaccurate in patients with bilateral renal artery disease and for those with impaired renal function, both likely scenarios in ARAS.

Catheter-based angiography is still considered the gold standard in the diagnosis of ARAS. Angiography has the ability to acquire multiple images at various angles, and it reliably identifies accessory vessels and other anatomic variants, plus it allows concomitant revascularization, should it be necessary (Figure 37-2).

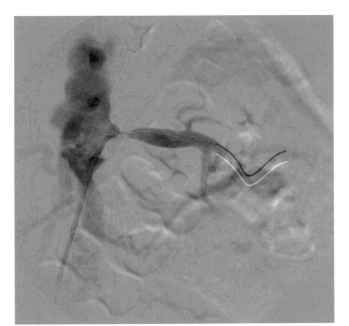

FIGURE 37-2 Severe atherosclerotic stenosis at the ostium of the left renal artery demonstrated on digital subtraction angiography.

Angiography is considered to be the most accurate diagnostic approach for FMD, because it can accurately evaluate the distal portions of the vessel.[19] Furthermore, intravascular ultrasound (IVUS) and translesional pressure measurements are often needed to evaluate the significance of a stenosis in renal artery FMD, because this is often difficult to assess angiographically.[16] The need for IVUS to assess lesion significance was demonstrated in a small trial that reported the correlation between DUS findings suggestive of FMD, catheter-based angiography, IVUS, and clinical outcomes after percutaneous transluminal renal angioplasty (PTRA) in 20 patients. Interestingly, DUS correlated with IVUS findings and favorable clinical outcome, whereas angiography alone would not have categorized at least five patients as having FMD (Figure 37-3).[25]

Choosing the correct imaging study for a particular patient depends on multiple variables (Figure 37-4). First, the indication for imaging should affect the imaging modality used. Although RADUS is an excellent choice for screening for RAS and for surveillance following endovascular revascularization, it may not offer complete anatomic information. Furthermore, although the typical anatomy of FMD may be visualized with RADUS, CTA and MRA are better suited to establish the diagnosis of FMD. Second, the need to image multiple vascular beds may dictate the choice of diagnostic modality. RADUS provides information on discrete vascular beds such as the renal, carotid, and peripheral arteries. However, clinicians frequently suspect involvement of other vascular beds. For instance, dynamic compromise of renal artery

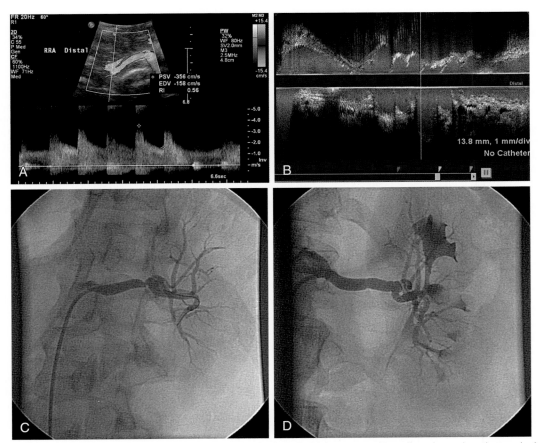

FIGURE 37-3 **A,** Right renal artery (*RRA*) stenosis as a result of fibromuscular dysplasia (FMD) demonstrated by color-enhanced renal artery duplex ultrasonography. The area of turbulence and stenosis is in the distal segment of the artery, in contrast to the ostial location of atherosclerotic lesions. **B,** RRA stenosis as a result of medial fibroplasia demonstrated by intravascular ultrasound. The black void in the artery lumen represents the catheter-related artifact. The bright border of the arterial wall has the characteristic beaded appearance of FMD. **C,** Intimal variant of FMD before percutaneous transluminal renal angioplasty. The lesion is a focal stenosis in the distal left renal artery. **D,** Intimal FMD in the same patient following percutaneous transluminal renal angioplasty.

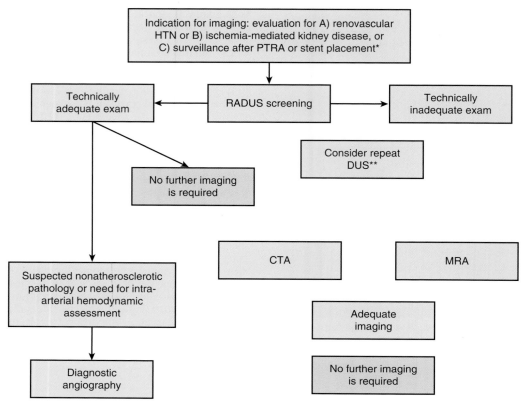

FIGURE 37-4 Diagnostic algorithm for evaluation of atherosclerotic renal artery stenosis. Choosing between magnetic resonance angiography (*MRA*) and computed tomographic angiography (*CTA*) depends on local expertise, availability, and patient characteristics that include metallic implants, claustrophobia, body habitus, and contrast allergies. *No further imaging is indicated when adequate image quality is consistent with clinical suspicion. **If bowel gas was present during first exam. DUS, Doppler ultrasound; PTRA, percutaneous transluminal renal angioplasty; RADUS, renal artery duplex ultrasonography.

perfusion emanating from an aortic dissection requires imaging of the entire aorta. Similarly, CTA and MRA offer clear advantages when aortitis or arteritis is suspected, and more global involvement of the aorta and its branches must be assessed.

Third, patient characteristics should influence the choice of diagnostic imaging. Allergy to iodinated contrast, CKD, the presence of a pacemaker, patient body habitus, and patient preference (e.g., claustrophobia) are examples of such characteristics. Finally, local technical expertise also plays a critical role in the choice of imaging modality.

Treatment of Atherosclerotic Renal Artery Stenosis

Medical Therapy

Optimal medical therapy is the backbone of treatment for ARAS, whether intervention is required or not. Patients with atherosclerotic involvement of the renal arteries must receive comprehensive therapy to reduce cardiovascular risk, not just to control blood pressure.[26] Medical therapy includes lipid-lowering therapy, smoking cessation, glycemic control in the face of diabetes mellitus, and antiplatelet medications despite the lack of evidence to demonstrate benefit specifically in patients with ARAS.

The association of statin use with death and renal outcomes has been examined in a retrospective analysis of 104 patients with ARAS who were followed for up to 134 months.[27] At baseline, patients who received statins had better renal function but were receiving a larger number of antihypertensive and antiplatelet agents. By the end of surveillance, patients in the statin group were less likely to die or double their serum creatinine, and fewer were likely to progress to ESRD.

Blood pressure reduction must target Joint National Committee VII goals, typically below 140/90 mm Hg or below 130/80 mm Hg for patients with diabetes or CKD.[28] Angiotensin-converting enzyme (ACE) inhibitors are of particular benefit for patients with ARAS, and their use is supported by societal guidelines.[5] Angiotensin receptor antagonists can be used as an alternative. An analysis of outcomes in a retrospective evaluation of 190 patients treated with either revascularization or medical therapy showed better survival for patients treated with ACE inhibition over a mean follow-up of over 54 months.[29] This effect was seen in both groups of patients, whether they were revascularized or not. However, clinicians must be aware of the risks of administering ACE inhibitors in patients with global renal ischemia (bilateral severe stenosis or stenosis to a solitary functioning kidney). These patients are at risk of developing progressive azotemia and therefore must have close monitoring of their renal function. Other classes of antihypertensive agents that may be effective in patients with ARAS include β-blockers, diuretics, and calcium channel blockers.[5] The goals of blood pressure control in patients with renal artery FMD are identical to those with ARAS.

Patients with ARAS are empirically treated with daily aspirin (81 mg); however, this practice is not based on evidence from large-scale randomized trials. All patients with medically treated RAS should be monitored for adverse effects of pharmacotherapy, loss of blood pressure control, deterioration in renal function, or progressive renal atrophy. All may be indications for intervention in the appropriate clinical setting.

Which Patients Should Be Revascularized?

It is the experience of many clinicians that renal artery stenting halts the progression of deterioration in renal function and improves blood pressure control. Current guidelines suggest that treatment of ARAS should be offered only to symptomatic patients. Revascularization therapy should also be considered in patients with hemodynamically significant RAS and accelerated, resistant, or malignant HTN; high blood pressure with an unexplained unilateral small kidney; and HTN with intolerance of medical therapy. Other indications for revascularization include progressive CKD over the previous 3 to 6 months with bilateral RAS or ARAS of a solitary functioning kidney, unstable angina in the setting of severe HTN, recurrent unexplained congestive heart failure, or sudden unexplained pulmonary edema.[5] However, not all patients respond favorably to treatment, and renal artery intervention should not be offered to all patients with ARAS.

Unfortunately, identifying patients who are more likely to respond to revascularization is not straightforward. First, a hemodynamically significant RAS, typically greater than 70%, must be identified by noninvasive imaging studies. If the indication for revascularization is preservation of renal function, particularly in patients with preexisting CKD, it must be confirmed that the etiology of the CKD is ischemic and potentially reversible in nature. Conventionally, patients with CKD over many years do not respond as well to endovascular renal artery stent revascularization (ERASR) as do patients with rapidly deteriorating renal function over the previous 8 to 12 weeks. In a retrospective analysis of 59 patients with ARAS greater than 60% followed up for a mean of 627 days, including 314 days prior to the procedure, the slope of the deterioration in renal function for at least 3 months prior to the procedure was associated with favorable outcomes.[30] The potential for improvement in renal function may also be deduced from renal mass. Patients with atrophic kidneys, typically less than 7 cm in pole-to-pole length, are generally not considered candidates for ERASR, whereas patients with global renal ischemia with renal length greater than 8 cm may experience clinical benefit.[24,31] ERASR for unilateral RAS may be particularly successful if the nonstenotic kidney has intrinsic renal parenchymal disease.[32,33]

Several other predictors of clinical improvement after renal artery stenting have been identified in small clinical studies. Cortical thinning may be an important ultrasonographic marker of progressive intrinsic renal disease and may point to a potential lack of clinical benefit of ERASR.[34] The renal resistive index (RRI) is an ultrasound-derived measure designed to evaluate the status of parenchymal renal arterial perfusion. The resistive index is calculated by the following equation:

$$[1 - (EDV/PSV)] \times 100$$

where *EDV* refers to end diastolic velocity and PSV refers to peak systolic velocity. RRI is measured in the renal cortex and medulla and in both the superior and inferior poles of the kidney. An RRI above 0.8 suggests intrinsic parenchymal disease, which is unlikely to benefit from treatment of the upstream RAS. An RRI below 0.8, on the other hand, may suggest better clinical outcomes after renal artery revascularization,[35] although the predictive utility of this index has been challenged in more recent publications.[36]

Other preprocedural, noninvasive measures may serve to predict the success of ERASR. Elevated serum brain natriuretic peptide (BNP) identifies patients likely to have favorable clinical outcomes after revascularization,[37] whereas preprocedural proteinuria seems to correlate with poor outcome.[38] However, the Safety and Effectiveness Study of the Herculink Elite Renal Stent to Treat Renal Artery Stenosis (HERCULES) represented the largest cohort of patients in whom BNP levels were prospectively compared with blood pressure response following ERASR, and it failed to demonstrate a predictive value for preprocedural BNP in 202 patients with uncontrolled HTN and ARAS.[39]

Measurements acquired during angiography may aid in predicting the clinical benefit of ERASR. Hemodynamic significance of a lesion can be inferred from the translesional pressure gradient.[33,40] In one study, a hyperemic systolic gradient of 21 mm Hg or more was the single best predictor of a sustained blood pressure response 12 months after ERASR (sensitivity, 82%; specificity, 84%; accuracy, 84%).[40] In a second study of individuals with moderate to severe ARAS undergoing ERASR, baseline stenosis severity was not predictive of clinical outcomes, whereas responders were predicted by measuring a provoked translesional pressure gradient following administration of dopamine.[33] The fractional flow reserve is another angiographic measure that has been shown to add predictive value in ERASR patients in an elegant trial performed in 17 individuals.[41] An elevated renal frame count predicted response in a retrospective analysis of 17 hypertensive patients undergoing ERASR.[42]

Many of the aforementioned predictors of outcome have not been validated in conjunction with other metrics; therefore it is currently unknown how reliable these factors may be in clinical practice, either alone or in combination with other clinical signals.

Catheter-Based Intervention

Endovascular therapies for the primary treatment of ARAS have all but replaced open surgical procedures. Treating ARAS with PTRA has been heralded by an early report that described long-term (42 months) improvement in blood pressure control and stabilization or improvement in renal function in 10 patients with HTN and azotemia.[43] The mechanism underlying ARAS is often bulky, atheromatous, aortorenal plaque, and PTRA does not provide durable patency, because the artery tends to develop profound elastic recoil and restenosis. ERASR, on the other hand, offers an acute procedural success rate of up to 98%,[44] which is higher than the success rate reported with PTRA. The procedural success rate of 57% was reported in a prospective randomized study in 40 patients who underwent PTRA, and it was 88% in 41 patients who underwent ERASR.[45] Primary patency at 6 months after PTRA ranged from only 29% in this study to 84% in another retrospective cohort of 104 patients who underwent PTRA.[46] A meta-analysis compared studies of ERASR and PTRA from 1995 to 1998.[47] The restenosis rate was lower following stent placement compared with PTRA (17% vs. 26%; P < .001) after a mean follow-up of 17 and 19 months, respectively.

More recent data support the superiority of ERASR over PTRA for ARAS in prospective multicenter trials. The Evaluation of the Safety and Effectiveness of Renal Artery Stenting After Unsuccessful Balloon Angioplasty (ASPIRE-2) study was a prospective, multicenter, nonrandomized trial that reported 2-year outcomes of a balloon-expandable stent (Cordis/Johnson & Johnson, New Brunswick, NJ) in 208 patients with ARAS and uncontrolled HTN in whom PTRA failed, with failure defined as flow-limiting dissection, residual stenosis of 50% or more, or a persistent translesional pressure gradient of more than 5 mm Hg. Blood pressure was statistically lower at 2 years of follow-up.[48]

In the Stenting in Renal Dysfunction Caused by Atherosclerotic Renal Artery Stenosis (STAR) trial, only 3.2% of patients treated with renal artery stents had restenosis by the end of follow-up.[49] The aforementioned HERCULES trial offers the most contemporary report of ERASR for HTN. A balloon-expandable stent (Abbott Vascular, Santa Clara, CA) was used to treat 241 lesions, and restenosis was noted in 10.5% of patients at 9 months.[39]

Endovascular treatment of ARAS should always be accompanied by optimal medical therapy, although no data are available to establish which periprocedural medical therapy improves short- and long-term success of the procedure.[50] It must also be kept in mind that renal artery interventions are not without risk, and complications can be related to arterial access and include hematoma, retroperitoneal hemorrhage, and pseudoaneurysm. Systemic complications include deterioration of renal function, from either contrast-induced acute tubular necrosis or atheroembolization; renal artery dissection, perforation, or occlusion; and death.[48,49,51-54] Although reported complication rates up to 28.3% have been described,[53] serious adverse effects are usually far less common. For example, the serious adverse event rate at 30 days in the HERCULES trial was only 1.5%.[39]

Deteriorating renal function after intervention should receive specific attention. One potential contributor to reduced renal function after PTRA and ERASR is renal artery atheroembolization. Because no specific biomarker or noninvasive method allows quantification of embolization during procedures, the presence of emboli is inferred from our knowledge of their existence after manipulations in other vascular beds and from functional deterioration in some patients after seemingly successful procedures. By use of distal embolic protection (DEP) devices, the presence of such embolic debris has been demonstrated in more than 50% of patients.[55] The Randomized Comparison of Safety and Efficacy of Renal Stenting Trial (RESIST) was a prospective study that used a 2 × 2 factorial design to compare DEP to no DEP and abciximab to placebo in 100 patients undergoing ERASR. Although DEP alone did not show benefit, the combination of a DEP device with abciximab, a potent antiplatelet agent, demonstrated stabilization of renal function.[56] Because atheroemboli likely originate from the bulky aortic atherosclerotic plaque, meticulous attention to procedural technique during an ERASR procedure should reduce the likelihood of atheroembolization. Several techniques have been developed to achieve this, including the *no-touch* or *telescoping* technique, in which a guidewire is deployed in the abdominal aorta, followed by advancement of a catheter toward the renal artery ostium; the wire is removed before direct engagement of the guide catheter into the renal artery ostium.[57]

Three prospective trials to examine the efficacy of PTRA or ERASR compared with medical treatment for ARAS have raised significant concerns regarding the benefit of ERASR. Despite the prospective, multicenter nature of these trials, they all suffer from inherent flaws that impair our ability to draw conclusions. A comparison of the most contemporary trials comparing catheter-based treatment with medical treatment for ARAS is presented in Table 37-2.

The Dutch Renal Artery Stenosis Intervention Cooperative (DRASTIC) trial examined the efficacy of PTRA in 106 patients with ARAS for treatment of HTN.[53] In this study, 106 patients who had HTN and ARAS with serum creatinine concentration below 2.3 mg/dL (200 µmol/L) were randomized to PTRA or medical treatment. An intention-to-treat analysis performed at the end of the trial did not reveal a difference in blood pressure control between the two groups. However, several factors make it difficult to draw robust conclusions from this trial; among these is the inclusion of patients without hemodynamically significant ARAS,[33] lack of stenting, and a high crossover rate.

The previously mentioned STAR trial was a prospective, non-blinded, randomized trial that compared medical treatment with medical treatment plus ERASR in 140 patients with ARAS and CKD.[49] The primary endpoint was a decrease of more than 20% in creatinine clearance after 2 years, with ARAS defined as greater than 50% stenosis. A statistically insignificant excess of events was seen in the medically treated group (22% vs. 16%), thereby suggesting that medical therapy is as effective as ERASR in patients with CKD and ARAS. However, multiple flaws must be noted in the design of the STAR trial. Many patients were identified by noninvasive methods as having RAS greater than 50% without hemodynamic or independent core laboratory verification of stenosis severity. The low rate of clinical events at the end of follow-up may have resulted from the lenient definition of hemodynamically significant ARAS. Furthermore, 18 of the 64 patients randomized to the stent group ultimately did not receive a stent because of mild to moderate RAS found with angiography. Although a per-protocol analysis did not change the conclusion, compared with the intention-to-treat analysis, this observation highlights a central flaw in the trial design.[30]

The Angioplasty and Stent for Renal Artery Lesions (ASTRAL) trial is the largest randomized trial of ARAS management to date.[54] ASTRAL was a prospective, randomized comparison of optimal medical therapy alone or in combination with stent deployment in 806 patients with ARAS. The primary endpoint was comparison of renal function in the two arms. During a median follow-up of 34 months, renal function remained unchanged, and blood pressure decreased symmetrically in both treatment groups. No difference was found between the two strategies in the intention-to-treat or per-protocol analysis. Despite this, patients in the revascularization arm of the study required fewer antihypertensive medications to control blood pressure than those in the medication-only group (P = .03). The rate of progression of renal impairment trended to be lower in the revascularization group, as shown by the slope of the reciprocal of the serum creatinine level (-0.07×10^{-3} L/µmol per year in the revascularization group, compared with -0.13×10^{-3} L/µmol in the medical therapy group; P = .06). Complications were unusually high in the stented group and included two deaths and three lower extremity amputations, prompting the authors

TABLE 37-2 Comparison of Recent Renal Artery Intervention Studies

	DRASTIC[53]	ASPIRE-2[48]	STAR[49]	ASTRAL[54]
Year of publication	2000	2005	2009	2009
Primary endpoint	Blood pressure reduction	Patency/serious adverse events	Renal function	Renal function
Inclusion	HTN, ARAS >50%, Cr <2.3 mg/dL	HTN, failure of PTRA for ARAS ≥70% and residual stenosis ≥50%	Cl$_{Cr}$ <80 mL/min, ARAS >50%	ARAS*
No. of patients (treatment/ intervention)	56/50	208†	64/74	403/403
Mean follow-up (mo)	12	24‡	33.6	24
Rate of stenting in intervention arm (%)	3.4	100	98.4	95
Rate of any complication (%)	28.3	19.4	15.7	29
Inclusion of patients later found not to have significant ARAS	+	−	+	+
Outcome in revascularization arm	Improved BP control, fewer medications needed to control HTN	Beneficial impact on HTN	No improvement in renal function compared with medical arm	Trend toward slower renal function decline, fewer medications needed to control HTN

*ARAS was suspected if HTN or unexplained renal dysfunction was evident.
†Total number of patients (prospective multicenter registry).
‡No mean available; 79% of the patients were followed up for 24 months.
ARAS, atherosclerotic renal artery stenosis; BP, blood pressure; Cl$_{Cr}$, creatinine clearance; Cr, creatinine; HTN, hypertension; PTRA, percutaneous transluminal renal angioplasty.

to conclude that the risks of ERASR outweighed the benefits. However, ASTRAL also has serious methodologic drawbacks. Only 59% of enrolled patients had baseline ARAS greater than 70%, and "borderline lesions" were not assessed for hemodynamic significance. Patients were recruited into ASTRAL only if their treating physicians were unsure about their potential to benefit from the procedure. It is likely that many patients who may have qualified for randomization were not recruited and simply underwent ERASR. This group would include patients with unilateral ARAS and HTN and patients with global renal ischemia and mild CKD, for whom the investigators felt that they knew which therapy was best. The annual enrollment per center was very low, averaging two patients. Operator inexperience is supported by a low procedural technical success rate of 79% and the previously mentioned high complication rate of 8%. Finally, similar to the other trials, 25% of patients in both the medical and angiographic group had a creatinine clearance of over 50 mL/min. These patients do not fit the profile of patients with ARAS and ischemic nephropathy and thus should not have been included in the trial.

Two other ongoing trials aim to examine the benefit of ERASR for ARAS. The first is the Cardiovascular Outcomes of Renal Artery Lesions (CORAL) trial,[58] which will represent the largest prospective randomized trial ever performed in patients with ARAS. CORAL is a U.S. National Institutes of Health (NIH)-funded trial that has completed recruitment and is now in the follow-up phase. Patients with HTN and ARAS—defined as greater than 80% stenosis by angiography or a measured translesional pressure gradient above 20 mm Hg—were randomized to stent with embolic protection or optimal medical therapy. Midway through trial enrollment, the use of embolic protection was made optional at the discretion of the investigator. The primary endpoint of the trial is event-free survival from cardiovascular and renal adverse events.

The second trial—a Randomized, Multicenter, Prospective Study Comparing Best Medical Treatment Versus Best Medical Treatment Plus Renal Artery Stenting in Patients with Hemodynamically Relevant Atheroslerotic Renal Artery Stenosis (RADAR)—aims to randomize patients with hemodynamically significant ARAS to best medical treatment and best medical treatment with ERASR. Patients will be included if they have an estimated glomerular filtration rate (eGFR) greater than 10 mL/min and RAS of 70% or more or an elevated resistive index.[59]

Patients with FMD-associated RAS are frequently treated with catheter-based interventions. Indications for endovascular therapy include new-onset HTN and HTN with intolerance to medications.[16] In contrast to ARAS, stenotic lesions in FMD often respond favorably to PTRA alone. A recently published meta-analysis reported the results of 47 trials of PTRA in patients with FMD and HTN.[60] Of the 997 reported procedures, only eight arteries were treated with a stent. The overall procedural success rate was 88.2%, and blood pressure response was reported to occur in 45.7% of patients, although considerable heterogeneity existed between trials regarding definitions of "cured" HTN and duration of follow-up. Blood pressure response was less favorable with increasing age and increasing duration of HTN, and the major and minor complication rates were 6.3% and 5.3%, respectively. Restenosis in patients with FMD is usually a result of inadequate angioplasty in the first intervention and is classically managed with repeat PTRA.[19,61] A stent may be used for resistant cases, to manage complications, and to exclude renal artery aneurysms. Complementing PTRA with IVUS may ensure more accurate diagnosis of culprit lesions and may help direct the intervention to the stenosed segment.[16]

Surveillance of Renovascular Disease

Patients diagnosed with ARAS should be followed longitudinally, whether they undergo revascularization or management primarily with medical therapy. RADUS remains the most useful tool for surveillance and is also useful in surveillance of stented renal arteries because the entire renal artery can be imaged despite the presence of a metallic endoprosthesis (see Figure 37-1).

Surveillance protocols vary depending on the etiology of the stenosis, because the natural history, distribution, and extrarenal manifestations differ among various disease processes.

An acceptable protocol for surveillance of ARAS is based on the clinical scenario and anatomic findings. If the stenosis is 60% or less, the ipsilateral kidney is normal in size, and the contralateral renal artery is widely patent, an examination is performed in 6 months; if the condition unchanged, annual RADUS is reasonable. Patients with global renal ischemia should have an examination in 6 months, and if the condition is unchanged from the prior exam, subsequent annual studies are reasonable. Factors that may prompt more frequent testing include deterioration in blood pressure control, progressive renal dysfunction, or renal atrophy.

Surveillance following ERASR should incorporate both clinical and imaging data. The natural history of in-stent restenosis and the criteria for its diagnosis should be well characterized prior to establishment of surveillance. Neither of these factors has been adequately analyzed in the medical literature.

First, there are currently no studies to evaluate surveillance of stented renal arteries. A single-center, retrospective analysis of 1150 ERASR procedures performed over 10 years found an overall need for reintervention in 11% of patients. Most of the repeat procedures occurred within the first 2 years and were triggered by recurrent HTN.[62] In the same trial, a restenosis rate of 54% was reported, although criteria used to make this diagnosis were lenient, including a PSV of 180 cm/s or more. Another 4-year retrospective follow-up study of patients who underwent balloon-expandable stent deployment reported only clinical outcomes.[63] Whereas sustained blood pressure control was noted, no data have been offered regarding its correlation with restenosis, nor have survival curves been presented. Second, the criteria for in-stent restenosis are still not entirely clear. Suggested criteria for detecting in-stent restenosis greater than 60% include a PSV of 300 cm/s or more with poststenotic turbulence and/or an RAR of 4.3 or more. A PSV below 240 cm/s accurately excludes significant stenosis.[64]

In another study, a comparison was conducted between duplex ultrasound findings in 31 renal arteries with in-stent restenosis and 30 stenotic native renal arteries. Stenosis was angiographically validated in both groups.[65] The mean PSV was higher in the stented group (452 vs. 360 cm/s; $P = .002$), and the RAR was 6.0 versus 4.0 in patients with in-stent restenosis versus native RAS ($P = .02$). ROC curves revealed that a PSV of 395 cm/s yielded a sensitivity of 83%, specificity of 88%, and accuracy of 87% for detecting restenosis of 70% or more. An RAR of 5.1 yielded an accuracy of 88%. Based on these results and convention, patients are usually followed by DUS soon after stent placement, at 6 and 12 months, and annually thereafter.

FMD primarily affects the renal and, to a lesser degree, the extracranial carotid arteries.[66] Other vascular beds should be examined as part of a comprehensive approach to patients with renal artery FMD, specifically the extracranial carotid arteries. As in ARAS, the natural history of renal artery FMD should dictate the frequency of patient surveillance. Understanding disease progression is hindered by the difficulty in assessing true lesion significance without intraarterial pressure or IVUS measurements.[16] In an angiographic surveillance study of 51 renal arteries with FMD followed for up to 10 years, 16% of arteries demonstrated either progression or new evidence of disease in those arteries previously unaffected. No disease progression was noted in patients older than 40 years.[67] A retrospective comparison of 71 patients with incidentally discovered renal artery FMD and 49 patients with normal renal arteries reported that after a mean follow-up of 4.4 years, patients with FMD were more likely to develop HTN (26% vs. 6%; $P < .01$).[68]

Another retrospective analysis reviewed the records of 29 women with HTN who underwent 38 PTRA procedures for renal artery FMD.[69] Pressure gradients across the affected arteries were not recorded, but patients were followed 1 month after the procedure and every 6 months thereafter with RADUS. After 3 months, 72% of patients responded to treatment as evidenced by improvement or resolution of HTN. The 5-year primary patency was 66%, and assisted primary patency was 87%. None of the patients had CKD.

Postprocedural surveillance for FMD is conventionally recommended soon after the procedure and at 6 and 12 months and yearly thereafter.[16,19] Importantly, restenosis is not always an adequate indication to prompt reintervention, because correlation between imaging and clinical presentation may be poor. The natural history of FMD after the intervention was reported in a prospective follow-up of 27 patients undergoing 31 procedures.[70] One patient required a stent as a result of a dissection. At a mean of 10 months, seven patients developed restenosis, including the patient with the stent; HTN was cured in 74% of patients, but correlation between clinical and imaging outcomes was poor. Outcomes of PTRA in patients with FMD types other than medial fibroplasia have been reported in small series with higher rates of restenosis and periprocedural complications.[71]

Catheter-Based Renal Artery Sympathetic Denervation

A novel intervention with the potential to become an important management tool for patients with medication-resistant HTN is catheter-based renal artery sympathetic denervation. Given the increasing prevalence of treatment-resistant HTN in the general population,[72] novel nonpharmacologic approaches may have a significant impact on management of HTN. Renal artery sympathetic denervation uses radiofrequency energy delivered via the renal artery to disrupt renal afferent and efferent nerves. Its therapeutic effect relies on the central role of the sympathetic nervous system in the pathogenesis of HTN.[73] Denervation therapy has been tested in the Renal Denervation in Patients with Uncontrolled Hypertension (Symplicity HTN-2) trial. Blood pressure response was compared between hypertensive patients undergoing renal sympathetic denervation and controls.[74] Patients were enrolled if they had baseline systolic blood pressure at or above 160 mm Hg (≥150 mm Hg in patients with diabetes) despite compliance with three or more antihypertensive drugs. At 6 months, both systolic and diastolic blood pressures were lower in the treatment group (a decrease of 32/12 vs. 1/0 mm Hg; $P < .0001$). Moreover, a larger proportion of treated patients were able to reduce the number of antihypertensive medications required to control blood pressure (20% vs. 8%; $P = .04$). No serious complications were recorded with the procedure, and blood pressure control following sympathetic denervation was shown to be durable for 2 years.[75] In addition to the obvious benefit of blood pressure reduction, renal denervation may offer other systemic benefits that include improved glycemic control.[76] A large-scale, multicenter, randomized trial in the United States has begun recruitment.

Conclusion

ARAS is prevalent and has potential serious medical consequences, and treatment options include medical and interventional therapies. Despite clear understanding of the pathophysiology of renin-mediated HTN and encouraging nonrandomized data that favor intervention, results of randomized trials to compare ERASR with medical treatment have been disappointing. The key component for clinical efficacy most likely lies in proper patient selection. Although some indications for intervention remain unequivocal, no clinically useful tool is available to predict which patients will derive benefit from revascularization, such as improved blood pressure control or preservation of renal function. Renal artery FMD is also common, probably underrecognized, and offers unique diagnostic and management challenges when compared with other etiologies in patients with ARAS. Renal artery sympathetic denervation is an exciting and novel approach for treatment-resistant primary HTN, but it requires more study in large randomized trials.

REFERENCES

1. Hansen KJ, Edwards MS, Craven TE, et al. Prevalence of renovascular disease in the elderly: a population-based study. *J Vasc Surg* 2002;36:443-451.
2. Davis RP, Pearce JD, Craven TE, et al. Atherosclerotic renovascular disease among hypertensive adults. *J Vasc Surg* 2009;50:564-570.
3. Olin JW, Melia M, Young JR, Graor RA, Risius B. Prevalence of atherosclerotic renal artery stenosis in patients with atherosclerosis elsewhere. *Am J Med* 1990;88:46N-51N.
4. Rihal CS, Textor SC, Breen JF, et al. Incidental renal artery stenosis among a prospective cohort of hypertensive patients undergoing coronary angiography. *Mayo Clin Proc* 2002;77:309-316.
5. Hirsch AT, Haskal ZJ, Hertzer NR, et al. ACC/AHA 2005 Practice Guidelines for the management of patients with peripheral arterial disease (lower extremity, renal, mesenteric, and abdominal aortic). *Circulation* 2006;113:e463-e654.
6. Safian RD, Textor SC. Renal-artery stenosis. *N Engl J Med* 2001;344:431-442.
7. Textor SC. Current approaches to renovascular hypertension. *Med Clin North Am* 2009;93:717-732.
8. Garovic VD, Textor SC. Renovascular hypertension and ischemic nephropathy. *Circulation* 2005;112:1362-1374.
9. Manske CL, Sprafka JM, Strony JT, Wang Y. Contrast nephropathy in azotemic diabetic patients undergoing coronary angiography. *Am J Med* 1990;89:615-620.
10. Chrysochou C, Kalra PA. Epidemiology and natural history of atherosclerotic renovascular disease. *Prog Cardiovasc Dis* 2009;52:184-195.
11. Guzman RP, Zierler RE, Isaacson JA, Bergelin RO, Strandness DE Jr. Renal atrophy and arterial stenosis: a prospective study with duplex ultrasound. *Hypertension* 1994;23:346-350.
12. Caps MT, Zierler RE, Polissar NL, et al. Risk of atrophy in kidneys with atherosclerotic renal artery stenosis. *Kidney Int* 1998;53:735-742.
13. Schreiber MJ, Pohl MA, Novick AC. The natural history of atherosclerotic and fibrous renal artery disease. *Urol Clin North Am* 1984;11:383-392.
14. Iglesias JI, Hamburger RJ, Feldman L, Kaufman JS. The natural history of incidental renal artery stenosis in patients with aortoiliac vascular disease. *Am J Med* 2000;109:642-647.
15. Williamson WK, Abou-Zamzam AM Jr, Moneta GL, et al. Prophylactic repair of renal artery stenosis is not justified in patients who require infrarenal aortic reconstruction. *J Vasc Surg* 1998;28:14-20.
16. Slovut DP, Olin JW. Fibromuscular dysplasia. *N Engl J Med* 2004;350:1862-1871.
17. Dworkin LD, Cooper CJ. Clinical practice: renal-artery stenosis. *N Engl J Med* 2009;361:1972-1978.
18. Olin JW, Piedmonte MR, Young JR, et al. The utility of duplex ultrasound scanning of the renal arteries for diagnosing significant renal artery stenosis. *Ann Intern Med* 1995;122:833-838.
19. Olin JW, Sealove BA. Diagnosis, management, and future developments of fibromuscular dysplasia. *J Vasc Surg* 2011;53:826-836.
20. Das CJ, Neyaz Z, Thapa P, Sharma S, Vashist S. Fibromuscular dysplasia of the renal arteries: a radiological review. *Int Urol Nephrol* 2007;39:233-238.
21. Tan KT, van Beek EJ, Brown PW, et al. Magnetic resonance angiography for the diagnosis of renal artery stenosis: a meta-analysis. *Clin Radiol* 2002;57:617-624.
22. Reference deleted in proofs.
23. Vasbinder GB, Nelemans PJ, Kessels AG, et al. Diagnostic tests for renal artery stenosis in patients suspected of having renovascular hypertension: a meta-analysis. *Ann Intern Med* 2001;135:401-411.
24. Soulez G, Therasse E, Qanadli SD, et al. Prediction of clinical response after renal angioplasty: respective value of renal Doppler sonography and scintigraphy. *AJR Am J Roentgenol* 2003;181:1029-1035.
25. Gowda MS, Loeb AL, Crouse LJ, Kramer PH. Complementary roles of color-flow duplex imaging and intravascular ultrasound in the diagnosis of renal artery fibromuscular dysplasia: should renal arteriography serve as the "gold standard"? *J Am Coll Cardiol* 2003;41:1305-1311.
26. Reich SB. Renal-artery stenosis. *N Engl J Med* 2001;345:221.
27. Silva VS, Martin LC, Franco RJ, et al. Pleiotropic effects of statins may improve outcomes in atherosclerotic renovascular disease. *Am J Hypertens* 2008;21:1163-1168.
28. Chobanian AV, Bakris GL, Black HR, et al. The seventh report of the Joint National Committee on Prevention, Detection, Evaluation, and Treatment of High Blood Pressure: the JNC 7 report. *JAMA* 2003;289:2560-2572.
29. Losito A, Errico R, Santirosi P, et al. Long-term follow-up of atherosclerotic renovascular disease: beneficial effect of ACE inhibition. *Nephrol Dial Transplant* 2005;20:1604-1609.
30. Muray S, Martin M, Amoedo ML, et al. Rapid decline in renal function reflects reversibility and predicts the outcome after angioplasty in renal artery stenosis. *Am J Kidney Dis* 2002;39:60-66.
31. Bommart S, Cliche A, Therasse E, et al. Renal artery revascularization: predictive value of kidney length and volume weighted by resistive index. *AJR Am J Roentgenol* 2010;194:1365-1372.
32. White CJ. Catheter-based therapy for atherosclerotic renal artery stenosis. *Circulation* 2006;113:1464-1473.
33. White CJ. Optimizing outcomes for renal artery intervention. *Circ Cardiovasc Interv* 2010;3:184-192.
34. Beland MD, Walle NL, Machan JT, Cronan JJ. Renal cortical thickness measured at ultrasound: is it better than renal length as an indicator of renal function in chronic kidney disease? *AJR Am J Roentgenol* 2010;195:W146-W149.
35. Radermacher J, Chavan A, Bleck J, et al. Use of Doppler ultrasonography to predict the outcome of therapy for renal-artery stenosis. *N Engl J Med* 2001;344:410-417.
36. Zeller T, Frank U, Muller C, et al. Predictors of improved renal function after percutaneous stent-supported angioplasty of severe atherosclerotic ostial renal artery stenosis. *Circulation* 2003;108:2244-2249.
37. Silva JA, Chan AW, White CJ, et al. Elevated brain natriuretic peptide predicts blood pressure response after stent revascularization in patients with renal artery stenosis. *Circulation* 2005;111:328-333.

38. Chrysochou C, Cheung CM, Durow M, et al. Proteinuria as a predictor of renal functional outcome after revascularization in atherosclerotic renovascular disease (ARVD). *QJM* 2009;102:283-288.

39. Jaff MR, Textor SC; HERCULES Executive Committee and Investigators. Does elevated brain natriuretic peptide (BNP) predict outcomes for patients with uncontrolled hypertension in renal artery stenting? Results from the HERCULES trial. Presented at the Society for Cardiovascular Angiography and Intervention 2011 Scientific Session. Baltimore, May 6, 2011.

40. Leesar MA, Varma J, Shapira A, et al. Prediction of hypertension improvement after stenting of renal artery stenosis: comparative accuracy of translesional pressure gradients, intravascular ultrasound, and angiography. *J Am Coll Cardiol* 2009;53:2363-2371.

41. Mitchell JA, Subramanian R, White CJ, et al. Predicting blood pressure improvement in hypertensive patients after renal artery stent placement: renal fractional flow reserve. *Catheter Cardiovasc Interv* 2007;69:685-689.

42. Mahmud E, Smith TW, Palakodeti V, et al. Renal frame count and renal blush grade: quantitative measures that predict the success of renal stenting in hypertensive patients with renal artery stenosis. *JACC Cardiovasc Interv* 2008;1:286-292.

43. Ying CY, Tifft CP, Gavras H, Chobanian AV. Renal revascularization in the azotemic hypertensive patient resistant to therapy. *N Engl J Med* 1984;311:1070-1075.

44. Simon JF. Stenting atherosclerotic renal arteries: time to be less aggressive. *Cleve Clin J Med* 2010;77:178-189.

45. van de Ven PJ, Kaatee R, Beutler JJ, et al. Arterial stenting and balloon angioplasty in ostial atherosclerotic renovascular disease: a randomized trial. *Lancet* 1999;353:282-286.

46. Plouin PF, Darne B, Chatellier G, et al. Restenosis after a first percutaneous transluminal renal angioplasty. *Hypertension* 1993;21:89-96.

47. Leertouwer TC, Gussenhoven EJ, Bosch JL, et al. Stent placement for renal arterial stenosis: where do we stand? A meta-analysis. *Radiology* 2000;216:78-85.

48. Rocha-Singh K, Jaff MR, Rosenfield K; ASPIRE-2 Trial Investigators. Evaluation of the safety and effectiveness of renal artery stenting after unsuccessful balloon angioplasty: the ASPIRE-2 study. *J Am Coll Cardiol* 2005;46:776-783.

49. Bax L, Woittiez AJ, Kouwenberg HJ, et al. Stent placement in patients with atherosclerotic renal artery stenosis and impaired renal function: a randomized trial. *Ann Intern Med* 2009;150:840-848.

50. Balk E, Raman G, Chung M, et al. Effectiveness of management strategies for renal artery stenosis: a systematic review. *Ann Intern Med* 2006;145:901-912.

51. Plouin PF, Chatellier G, Darne B, Raynaud A. Blood pressure outcome of angioplasty in atherosclerotic renal artery stenosis: a randomized trial. Essai multicentrique medicaments vs angioplastie (EMMA) study group. *Hypertension* 1998;31:823-829.

52. Webster J, Marshall F, Abdalla M, et al. Randomised comparison of percutaneous angioplasty versus continued medical therapy for hypertensive patients with atheromatous renal artery stenosis. Scottish and Newcastle Renal Artery Stenosis Collaborative Group. *J Hum Hypertens* 1998;12:329-335.

53. van Jaarsveld BC, Krijnen P, Pieterman H, et al. Dutch Renal Artery Stenosis Intervention Cooperative Study Group. The effect of balloon angioplasty on hypertension in atherosclerotic renal-artery stenosis. *N Engl J Med* 2000;342:1007-1014.

54. Wheatley K, Ives N, Gray R, et al. ASTRAL Investigators. Revascularization versus medical therapy for renal-artery stenosis. *N Engl J Med* 2009;361:1953-1962.

55. Henry M, Henry I, Klonaris C, et al. Renal angioplasty and stenting under protection: the way for the future? *Catheter Cardiovasc Interv* 2003;60:299-312.

56. Cooper CJ, Haller ST, Colyer W, et al. Embolic protection and platelet inhibition during renal artery stenting. *Circulation* 2008;117:2752-2760.

57. Feldman RL, Wargovich TJ, Bittl JA. No-touch technique for reducing aortic wall trauma during renal artery stenting. *Catheter Cardiovasc Interv* 1999;46:245-248.

58. Cooper CJ, Murphy TP, Matsumoto A, et al. Stent revascularization for the prevention of cardiovascular and renal events among patients with renal artery stenosis and systolic hypertension: rationale and design of the CORAL trial. *Am Heart J* 2006;152:59-66.

59. Schwarzwalder U, Hauk M, Zeller T. RADAR: a randomized, multi-centre, prospective study comparing best medical treatment versus best medical treatment plus renal artery stenting in patients with hemodynamically relevant atherosclerotic renal artery stenosis. *Trials* 2009;10:60.

60. Trinquart L, Mounier-Vehier C, Sapoval M, Gagnon N, Plouin PF. Efficacy of revascularization for renal artery stenosis caused by fibromuscular dysplasia: a systematic review and meta-analysis. *Hypertension* 2010;56:525-532.

61. Sos TA, Pickering TG, Sniderman K, et al. Percutaneous transluminal renal angioplasty in renovascular hypertension due to atheroma or fibromuscular dysplasia. *N Engl J Med* 1983;309:274-279.

62. Stone PA, Campbell JE, Aburahma AF, et al. Ten-year experience with renal artery in-stent stenosis. *J Vasc Surg* 2011;53:1026-1031.

63. Dorros G, Jaff M, Mathiak L, He T; Multicenter Registry Participants. Multicenter Palmaz stent renal artery stenosis revascularization registry report: four-year follow-up of 1,058 successful patients. *Catheter Cardiovasc Interv* 2002;55(2):182-188.

64. Galin I, Trost B, Kang J, Lookstein R, Jaff MR. Validation of renal duplex ultrasound in detecting renal artery stenosis post stenting. Presented at the Annual Scientific Session of the American College of Cardiology. Chicago, March 2008.

65. Chi YW, White CJ, Thornton S, Milani RV. Ultrasound velocity criteria for renal in-stent restenosis. *J Vasc Surg* 2009;50:119-123.

66. Olin JW, Froehlich JB, Gu X, et al. Clinical features and presenting symptoms and signs of fibromuscular dysplasia: a report of the Fibromuscular Dysplasia Patient Registry. Presented at the FMD Society Annual Scientific Sessions, Cleveland, May 2011.

67. Meaney TF, Dustan HP, McCormack LJ. Natural history of renal arterial disease. *Radiology* 1968;91:881-887.

68. Cragg AH, Smith TP, Thompson BH, et al. Incidental fibromuscular dysplasia in potential renal donors: long-term clinical follow-up. *Radiology* 1989;172:145-147.

69. Davies MG, Saad WE, Peden EK, et al. The long-term outcomes of percutaneous therapy for renal artery fibromuscular dysplasia. *J Vasc Surg* 2008;48:865-871.

70. Birrer M, Do DD, Mahler F, Triller J, Baumgartner I. Treatment of renal artery fibromuscular dysplasia with balloon angioplasty: a prospective follow-up study. *Eur J Vasc Endovasc Surg* 2002;23:146-152.

71. Barrier P, Julien A, Guillaume C, et al. Technical and clinical results after percutaneous angioplasty in non-medial fibromuscular dysplasia: outcome after endovascular management of unifocal renal artery stenoses in 30 patients. *Cardiovasc Intervent Radiol* 2010;33:270-277.

72. Egan BM, Zhao Y, Axon RN, Brzezinski WA, Ferdinand KC. Uncontrolled and apparent treatment resistant hypertension in the United States, 1988 to 2008. *Circulation* 2011;124:1046-1058.

73. Schlaich MP, Krum H, Sobotka PA, Esler MD. Renal denervation and hypertension. *Am J Hypertens* 2011;24:635-642.

74. Esler MD, Krum H, Sobotka PA, et al, for the Symplicity HTN-2 Investigators. Renal sympathetic denervation in patients with treatment-resistant hypertension (the Symplicity HTN-2 trial): a randomized controlled trial. *Lancet* 2010;376:1903-1909.

75. Symplicity HTN-1 Investigators. Catheter-based renal sympathetic denervation for resistant hypertension: durability of blood pressure reduction out to 24 months. *Hypertension* 2011;57:911-917.

76. Mahfoud F, Schlaich M, Kindermann I, et al. Effect of renal sympathetic denervation on glucose metabolism in patients with resistant hypertension: a pilot study. *Circulation* 2011;123:1940-1946.

CHAPTER 38 # Pulmonary Embolism and Deep Vein Thrombosis

Samuel Z. Goldhaber and Gregory Piazza

EPIDEMIOLOGY AND RISK FACTORS, 580

PATHOPHYSIOLOGY AND NATURAL HISTORY, 582

DIAGNOSIS, 582

Deep Vein Thrombosis, 582
Pulmonary Embolism, 583

MANAGEMENT, 586

Spectrum of Disease: Superficial Venous Thrombosis, Deep Vein
  Thrombosis, and Pulmonary Embolism, 586

Anticoagulation, 587
Basic Versus Advanced Therapy for Venous
  Thromboembolism, 589

PREVENTION, 591

Prevention of Venous Thromboembolism in Patients with
  Cancer, 591
Implementation of in-Hospital Prophylaxis, 592
Hip Replacement, Knee Replacement, and Hip Fracture, 592
Mechanical Prophylaxis, 592

CONCLUSIONS, 593

REFERENCES, 593

Venous thromboembolism (VTE), defined as deep vein thrombosis (DVT) and pulmonary embolism (PE), is the third most common cardiovascular disorder after myocardial infarction (MI) and stroke.[1] Yet until the past decade, VTE was not fully embraced by the community of cardiovascular medicine clinicians as a high-priority issue. However, a dramatic shift in thinking has occurred, and PE and DVT have become accepted as essential considerations in the care rendered by cardiovascular medicine specialists. Therefore, VTE-related clinical problems are being referred with increasing frequency to cardiologists for both hospitalized patients and outpatients.

New therapies are emerging as novel oral anticoagulants undergo rigorous clinical trials for VTE prophylaxis and treatment. Major ongoing studies will also provide new information, such as the role of peripherally administered thrombolysis for patients with submassive PE, the utility of rapid-turnaround genetic testing to determine the optimal starting dose for warfarin, and the role of catheter-directed pharmacomechanical therapy for patients with massive femoral or iliofemoral DVT.

Epidemiology and Risk Factors

The incidence of VTE rises sharply after 60 years of age in both men and women. The 2008 U.S. Surgeon General's Call to Action to Prevent Deep Vein Thrombosis and Pulmonary Embolism estimates that 100,000 to 180,000 deaths occur annually from PE in the United States alone.[2] In the United States, the Longitudinal Investigation of Thromboembolism Etiology (LITE) was composed of 21,680 participants with VTE.[3] The VTE age-standardized incidence was 1.92 per 1000 person-years, and the 28-day case fatality rate was 11% after a first VTE episode. Cancer-associated VTE had a high 28-day case fatality rate of 25%, and the 90-day mortality rate associated with PE approached 15%, exceeding that of MI.

In registries, approximately half of the VTE cases are idiopathic and unprovoked, whereas the other half are secondary to risk factors, both environmental and genetic. Acquired risk factors are far more common than inherited thrombophilias. Advanced age, malignancy, immobility, and recent trauma, surgery, or hospitalization are well-recognized risk factors. The lupus anticoagulant, antiphospholipid antibodies, and anticardiolipin antibodies are potent acquired risk factors for VTE, and VTE is an important health concern for women. Pregnancy, oral contraceptives that contain estrogen, and hormone replacement therapy are important VTE risk factors. Among women of childbearing age, oral contraceptive use remains the most frequent risk factor for VTE.[4] One of the most intriguing ways to estimate the future risk of VTE is to use the new web-based QThrombosis algorithm (www.QThrombosis.org), created in the United Kingdom from routinely collected data from general practices.[5] Details are in Table 38-1.

Chronic medical conditions such as heart failure, chronic obstructive pulmonary disease (COPD), and systemic inflammatory disorders such as inflammatory bowel disease (IBS)[6] also contribute to the risk of VTE. C-reactive protein, a marker of inflammation, is an independent risk factor for VTE.[7] Metabolic syndrome is also a probable risk factor for VTE.[8] Cigarette smoking, overweight and obesity, and physical activity are other modifiable VTE risk factors.[9-12]

The media publicize the danger of long-haul air travel as a risk factor for PE and DVT. Consequently, the public often construes prolonged travel as the sole or most important VTE risk factor. Long-haul air travel, usually defined as at least 4 to 6 hours of flight time, is on rare occasions considered the most likely precipitant of VTE. An overview of 14 studies found that travel is associated with a nearly threefold higher risk for VTE, with an apparent dose-response relationship of 18% higher risk for each 2-hour increase in travel duration.[13] In the Registry of Patients with Venous Thromboembolism (RIETE), travel-related VTE occurred most often in patients who had at least one of the following risk factors: high body mass index (BMI), previous VTE, hormone use, and thrombophilia.[14]

Cancer predisposes to VTE, and those with stomach and pancreatic cancer are considered at very high risk for developing VTE. Lymphoma and lung, gynecologic, bladder, and testicular cancer are considered high risk for associated VTE. Based on a retrospective study from the Mayo Clinic, active cancer appears to be associated with arm, intraabdominal, or bilateral leg DVT, but not PE.[15] Khorona and colleagues[16] have developed a predictive model for chemotherapy-associated VTE (Table 38-2).

The genetic influence on VTE is highlighted by a nationwide epidemiologic study in Sweden.[17] Among 45,362 hospitalized patients with VTE, 2393 affected siblings were identified, with a familial standardized incidence ratio of 2.45 overall. Familial risk was highest between 10 and 19 years of age, with a standardized incidence ratio of 4.77; the risk decreased at 60 to 69 years of age to a standardized incidence ratio of 2.08. The environmental association was much weaker. Spouses had a low familial risk, with a standardized incidence ratio of 1.07. This study highlights the value of obtaining sibling history as a predictor of the risk of VTE.

Inherited thrombophilias are frequently suspected in patients seen with VTE at a young age, multiple family members with VTE, idiopathic or recurrent VTE, or recurrent spontaneous abortions. Major inherited thrombophilias include factor V Leiden, *prothrombin gene mutation 20210*, and deficiencies of protein C, protein S, or antithrombin. Prevalence of inherited thrombophilias varies by population, but testing for hypercoagulable states should be reserved for patients in whom a high suspicion is present and in whom the results of the evaluation will affect therapy.[18] Even individuals with homozygous *factor V Leiden*

TABLE 38-1   The QThrombosis Adjusted Hazard Ratios for Final Models in the Derivation Cohort (n = 2,314,701)

	Women			Men		
	EVENTS (N)	ADJUSTED HR (95% CI)	P VALUE	EVENTS (N)	ADJUSTED HR (95% CI)	P VALUE
Smoking Status						
Nonsmoker	4533	1.00		3148	1.00	
Ex-smoker	1689	1.07 (1.01-1.15)	.030	2238	1.06 (0.995-1.13)	.070
Light smoker	443	1.22 (1.09-1.37)	.001	618	1.22 (1.09-1.35)	<.001
Moderate smoker	558	1.17 (1.05-1.29)	.003	592	1.37 (1.22-1.52)	<.001
Heavy smoker	375	1.34 (1.18-1.52)	<.001	562	1.49 (1.33-1.66)	<.001
Medical History						
Varicose veins	407	1.40 (1.24-1.58)	<.001	172	1.38 (1.18-1.63)	<.001
Congestive cardiac failure	206	1.40 (1.2-1.62)	<.001	168	1.33 (1.13-1.57)	.001
Chronic renal disease	46	1.60 (1.17-2.19)	.003	62	1.92 (1.50-2.44)	<.001
Any cancer	573	1.85 (1.69-2.03)	<.001	505	2.18 (1.97-2.41)	<.001
Chronic obstructive airway disease	360	1.41 (1.24-1.62)	<.001	429	1.62 (1.45-1.80)	<.001
Inflammatory bowel disease	87	1.45 (1.15-1.82)	.002	94	1.5 (1.18-1.91)	.001
Hospital admission in past 6 months	244	1.86 (1.63-2.14)	<.001	209	1.93 (1.64-2.27)	<.001
Current Medications						
Antipsychotic drugs	187	1.55 (1.32-1.81)	<.001	121	1.84 (1.51-2.23)	<.001
Tamoxifen	97	1.48 (1.19-1.84)	<.001	NA	NA	NA
Oral contraceptives	229	1.33 (1.12-1.58)	.001	NA	NA	NA
Hormone replacement therapy	447	1.20 (1.08-1.34)	.001	NA	NA	NA

CI, confidence interval; HR, hazard ratio; NA, not applicable.

TABLE 38-2   Khorana Predictive Model for Chemotherapy-Associated Venous Thromboembolism

PATIENT CHARACTERISTIC	RISK SCORE
Site of Primary Cancer	
Very high risk (stomach, pancreas)	2
High risk (lung, lymphoma, gynecologic, bladder, testicular)	1
Laboratory Measurements	
Prechemotherapy platelet count $\geq 350 \times 10^9$/L	1
Hemoglobin <10 g/dL or use of red cell growth factors	1
Prechemotherapy leukocyte count >11×10^9/L	1
Body mass index ≥ 35 kg/m^2	1

TOTAL SCORE	RISK CATEGORY	RISK OF SYMPTOMATIC VENOUS THROMBOEMBOLISM
0	Low	0.3%-0.8%
1 or 2	Intermediate	1.8%-2.0%
≥ 3 or higher	High	6.7%-7.7%

From Khorana AA, Kuderer NM, Culakova E, et al. Development and validation of a predictive model for chemotherapy-associated thrombosis. Blood 2008;111:4902-4907.

and/or homozygous *prothrombin G20210A* or double heterozygous carriers of *factor V Leiden* and *prothrombin G20210A* do not have a high risk of recurrent VTE.[19]

Quality of hospital care influences the likelihood of survival from acute PE, and the death rate among hospitalized patients appears to be higher for those admitted during weekends. Among hospitals in the Northeast region of Italy, 26,560 PE cases were reviewed over an 11-year period.[20] Weekend admissions were associated with higher rates of in-hospital death than weekday admissions, even after adjusting for baseline characteristics that included comorbidities. The mortality rate was 28% for weekend admissions compared with 24.8% for weekday admissions.

The focus of studying VTE has been in acute-care hospitals; few studies have addressed the development of DVT and PE in rehabilitation facilities. Therefore, a prospective observational study of 24 rehabilitation facilities in Italy was undertaken to determine the frequency of symptomatic VTE during rehabilitation facility hospitalizations that had a median duration of 26 days.[21] Overall, 2.4% of 3039 patients had symptomatic VTE, and the median time to VTE from admission to the long-term care unit was 13 days. Multivariable analysis showed that previous VTE increased the likelihood of a new VTE by a hazard ratio of 5.67, and cancer had a hazard ratio of 2.26 for new VTE. The overall in-hospital mortality rate was 15.1%. Lack of prophylaxis against VTE conferred a hazard ratio of 1.64 for death (Table 38-3).

TABLE 38-3	Multivariate Analysis to Correlate Prognostic Variables and in-Hospital Death in a Study of Rehabilitation Hospitals			
VARIABLE	CLASSIFICATION	HR	95% CI	P VALUE
Age (years)	>75 vs. ≤75	1.80	1.46-2.22	<.001
Gender	Male vs. female	1.37	1.13-1.66	<.01
Previous VTE	Yes vs. no	1.10	0.74-1.62	.64
Rankin score	≥4 vs. <4	3.46	2.20-5.43	<.001
Medical disease	Yes vs. no	0.59	0.32-1.07	.08
Recent surgery	Yes vs. no	0.12	0.06-0.23	<.001
Cancer	Yes vs. no	3.64	3.02-4.39	<.001
Time free from prophylaxis	Yes vs. no	1.64	1.36-1.98	<.001

CI, confidence interval; HR, hazard ratio; VTE, venous thromboembolism.

Pathophysiology and Natural History

DVT results from a combination of pathophysiologic states of endothelial injury, stasis, and hypercoagulability. Although thrombosis may develop in the deep veins of the upper extremity and pelvis, the most common site for DVT is in the deep veins of the lower extremity. Thrombi usually originate from the deep venous system of the lower extremities and pelvis, embolize through the inferior vena cava (IVC) and right heart, and obstruct the pulmonary arterial tree, thereby causing hemodynamic and gas-exchange abnormalities.[22] DVT can also cause paradoxical embolism to the arterial circulation.[23]

Direct physical obstruction of the pulmonary arteries in addition to hypoxemia and release of potent pulmonary arterial vasoconstrictors increase pulmonary vascular resistance and right ventricular (RV) afterload.[24] Acute RV pressure overload may result in RV hypokinesis and dilation, tricuspid regurgitation, and ultimately right heart failure. Patients with acute PE and RV failure may decompensate and develop systemic arterial hypotension, cardiogenic shock, and cardiac arrest. Increased diastolic pressure causes deviation of the interventricular septum toward the left ventricle (LV) and impairs LV preload. RV pressure overload may also result in increased wall stress and ischemia by increasing myocardial oxygen demand while simultaneously limiting its supply (Figure 38-1). Mismatch between myocardial oxygen demand and supply as a result of pressure overload may result in RV infarction. Gas-exchange abnormalities in patients with acute PE are most often due to a combination of ventilation/perfusion mismatch, increases in total dead space, and right-to-left shunting.

DVT may result in the debilitating long-term complications of postthrombotic syndrome of the legs in 25% to 50% of patients with VTE.[25] These include chronic calf discomfort, especially when standing, as well as brownish skin pigmentation changes, particularly of the medial malleolus. Rarely, ulceration that requires surgical skin grafting may ensue. Although postthrombotic syndrome is never life threatening, it can cause a marked decrease in the quality of life and is responsible for increased health care costs in affected patients. Those with severe postthrombotic syndrome may be forced to stop working as a result of their disability. Furthermore, no specific cure is available for this complication of VTE. The main risk factors for postthrombotic syndrome are persistent leg symptoms 1 month after acute DVT, anatomically extensive DVT, recurrent ipsilateral DVT, obesity, and older age. Subtherapeutic dosing of initial oral anticoagulation therapy for DVT treatment may also be linked to subsequent postthrombotic syndrome.

Chronic thromboembolic pulmonary hypertension[26] occurs in about 2% to 4% of patients who have PE. This condition usually causes dyspnea, initially with exertion and eventually at rest. Persistent macrovascular obstruction and vasoconstriction ensue,

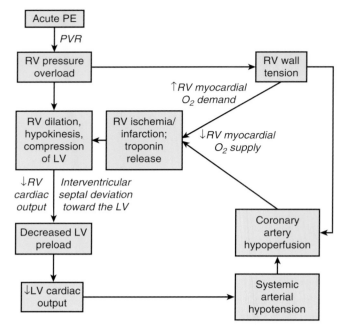

FIGURE 38-1 The pathophysiology of right ventricular (RV) dysfunction as a result of acute pulmonary embolism (PE). PVR, pulmonary vascular resistance; LV, left ventricular.

and a small vessel arteriopathy develops that is characterized by medial hypertrophy, intimal proliferation, and microvascular thrombosis. Patients develop progressive pulmonary hypertension and worsening right heart failure, which can be fatal. Patients generally come to medical attention in their 40s, although the diagnosis may be overlooked, because many patients do not have a history of clinically overt PE. A typical mode of death is sudden cardiac death during exertion.

Diagnosis

Deep Vein Thrombosis

CLINICAL PRESENTATION

Patients with lower extremity DVT may report a cramping or pulling sensation of the calf or thigh that worsens with ambulation. Physical examination findings include warmth, edema, erythema, and palpation tenderness of the extremity. DVT may also develop in the upper extremities, especially in the setting of chronically indwelling central venous catheters and in syndromes of thoracic outlet obstruction. Upper extremity DVT is also a recognized complication of pacemaker and internal cardiac defibrillator placement.

Clinical Likelihood Assessment

The Wells score for DVT[27] is the best known clinical probability assessment tool for clinically suspected DVT. It is a straightforward point-score system with a maximum of eight score points, with one point each given for 1) cancer, 2) paralysis or recent plaster cast, 3) bed rest longer than 3 days or surgery in the previous 4 weeks, 4) pain on palpation of deep veins, 5) swelling of the entire leg, 6) an affected calf more than 3 cm larger in diameter than the unaffected calf, 7) pitting edema of affected side, and 8) dilated superficial veins. Two points are subtracted if an alternative diagnosis is at least as probable as DVT. Low probability is no points, intermediate clinical probability is one to two points; and three or more points is considered high clinical probability of DVT.

Laboratory Testing

Plasma D-dimer is a degradation product of cross-linked fibrin and serves as a nonspecific marker of endogenous fibrinolysis. It is

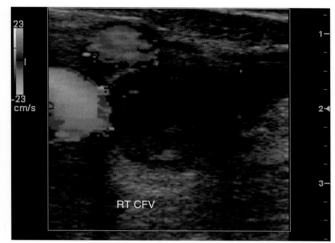

FIGURE 38-2 Color Doppler ultrasound image demonstrating absence of blood flow in the right common femoral vein (*RT CFV, arrow*) consistent with the diagnosis of deep vein thrombosis in a 35-year-old woman who came to medical attention at 38 weeks of pregnancy with right leg swelling and pain.

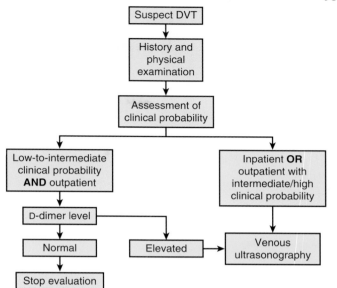

FIGURE 38-3 Overall diagnostic algorithm for evaluation of suspected deep vein thrombosis (*DVT*).

elevated in VTE and in many other systemic illnesses and conditions such as MI, heart failure, infection, surgery, and pregnancy. D-dimer has the greatest utility in evaluation of outpatients or emergency department patients with suspected VTE because many inpatients will have elevated levels as a result of other conditions. D-dimer offers the greatest accuracy for suspected DVT when used in combination with an assessment of clinical likelihood. In patients with low or intermediate clinical probability, a negative D-dimer can exclude the diagnosis of DVT without further testing, such as with ultrasonography. Among patients with intermediate-to-high clinical suspicion for DVT, further evaluation is often warranted despite negative D-dimer results.[28] Intermediate clinical probability is a "gray zone" concerning whether a negative D-dimer suffices to exclude DVT. In Europe, the tendency is to use D-dimer as a screening laboratory test prior to ordering a venous ultrasound for intermediate clinical probability patients. In the United States, the tendency is to go directly to venous ultrasonography when DVT is suspected in patients with intermediate clinical probability. Patients with a high clinical probability should not be tested with D-dimer but should undergo imaging to detect VTE.

Imaging

Venous ultrasonography is the initial imaging test of choice for evaluation of suspected lower or upper extremity DVT. The inability to compress a vein is diagnostic of DVT (Figure 38-2). Anatomic constraints limit ultrasonographic evaluation of the pelvic veins and upper extremity veins proximal to the clavicle.

Alternative imaging modalities for evaluation of suspected DVT include computed tomography (CT), magnetic resonance (MR), and contrast venography. These techniques are generally reserved for imaging venous segments inadequately assessed by venous ultrasonography.

Overall Diagnostic Algorithm

An overall algorithm for evaluation of suspected DVT combines an assessment of clinical probability, D-dimer testing, and noninvasive imaging when appropriate (Figure 38-3). Contrast venography is almost never needed for DVT diagnosis.

Pulmonary Embolism

CLINICAL PRESENTATION

The clinical presentation of acute PE varies widely. Dyspnea without any obvious explanation is the most frequently reported symptom. Severe dyspnea, cyanosis, or syncope suggests massive PE, whereas pleuritic pain, cough, or hemoptysis may indicate a smaller, peripherally located PE. On physical examination, tachypnea is the most common sign. PE patients may also exhibit signs of RV failure such as tachycardia, distended neck veins, tricuspid regurgitation, and an accentuated sound of pulmonic valve closure (P2).

Four decision rules are commonly used to assess the clinical likelihood of PE: 1) the Wells rule,[29] 2) the revised Geneva score,[30] 3) the simplified Wells rule,[31] and 4) the simplified revised Geneva score. Of these four rules, the Wells rule and the revised Geneva score are the two most popular and are commonly used (Table 38-4). In a prospective cohort study of 807 consecutive patients with suspected acute PE, all four clinical decision rules showed similar performance for exclusion of acute PE when used in combination with a normal D-dimer result.[32]

Laboratory Testing

D-Dimer testing is most helpful in patients with suspected PE who come to medical attention as outpatients or come in to the emergency department. Because of its high negative predictive value, the D-dimer enzyme-linked immunosorbent assay (ELISA) can be used to exclude PE in outpatients with low to moderate pretest probability without the need for further costly testing. Inpatients should proceed directly to imaging as the initial test for PE because many will already have elevated D-dimer levels as a result of comorbid illness.[33]

Electrocardiogram

The electrocardiogram (ECG) may demonstrate findings suggestive of RV strain as a result of PE, such as right bundle branch block or T-wave inversion in leads V1 through V4. The ECG is sometimes entirely normal. The only abnormality often is nonspecific, such as sinus tachycardia; however, the ECG may suggest alternative diagnoses, such as MI, pericarditis, or pericardial tamponade.

Chest Radiography

Like the ECG, the chest radiograph may suggest alternative diagnoses such as pneumonia or pneumothorax. A normal or near-normal chest radiograph in a patient with otherwise unexplained dyspnea or hypoxemia suggests PE. The majority of patients with PE will have some abnormality, such as cardiomegaly or pleural effusion, on radiography.

CH
38

TABLE 38-4	Clinical Decision Rules to Assess the Clinical Likelihood of Pulmonary Embolism		
		Points	
CLINICAL DECISION RULE		ORIGINAL VERSION	SIMPLIFIED VERSION
Wells Rule			
Previous PE or DVT		1.5	1
Heart rate >100 beats/min		1.5	1
Surgery or immobilization within previous 4 weeks		1.5	1
Hemoptysis		1	1
Active cancer		1	1
Clinical signs of DVT		3	1
Alternative diagnosis less likely than PE		3	1
Clinical Probability			
PE unlikely		≤4	≤1
PE likely		>4	>1
Revised Geneva Score			
Previous DVT or PE		3	1
Heart rate 75 to 94 beats/min ≥95 beats/min		3 5	1 2
Surgery or fracture within previous 30 days		2	1
Hemoptysis		2	1
Active cancer		2	1
Unilateral lower limb pain		3	1
Pain on lower limb deep venous palpation and unilateral edema		4	1
Age >65 years		1	1
Clinical Probability			
PE unlikely		≤5	≤2
PE likely		>5	>2

DVT, deep vein thrombosis; PE, pulmonary embolism.

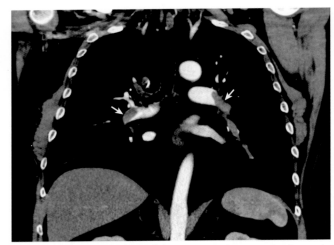

FIGURE 38-4 Contrast-enhanced chest computed tomography demonstrating bilateral main pulmonary artery emboli (*arrows*) in a 60-year-old man with acute-onset shortness of breath and chest pain.

Chest Computed Tomography for Diagnosis and Risk Stratification

Contrast-enhanced chest CT has emerged as the dominant diagnostic imaging technique to detect suspected PE (Figure 38-4).[34] Although chest CT angiography can be combined with CT venography to search for the source of PE, this approach appears to be low yield, and it does not generally justify the incremental radiation exposure or cost.[35] State-of-the-art CT scan resolution is excellent and can detect PEs as small as 1 mm; whether an isolated, tiny, subsegmental PE is of clinical importance remains undetermined.[36] Increasing attention is focused on procedures to minimize and reduce the radiation dose. For example, breast shielding in women can substantially reduce radiation exposure.[37]

After PE is detected on chest CT, the same imaging test can be used to assess RV enlargement, a predictor of poor clinical outcome. Detection of *RV enlargement* on chest CT, defined as an RV/LV diameter ratio of greater than 0.9, predicts increased 30-day mortality.[38] Chest CT is especially useful because these ratios are acquired during the initial diagnostic scan and require no additional imaging (Figure 38-5). In a multicenter study of 457 patients, 303 had RV enlargement on chest CT. In-hospital death or clinical deterioration occurred in 44 patients with RV enlargement and in 8 patients without (14.5% vs. 5.2%, respectively; *P* < .004).[39]

Measuring the ratio of the RV/LV dimensions on chest CT scan is a surrogate method of assessing the ratio of RV/LV volume. CT scan software can analyze three-dimensional (3D) volumes of the RV and LV. This requires manually outlining the endocardial contours on the transverse sections comprising the minimal and maximal expanse of the ventricles. In a study of 260 PE patients undergoing 3D volume measurement, 57 (22%) had adverse outcomes, including 20 (7.7%) who died. In this study, 3D ventricular volume measurement predicted early death in patients with acute PE independent of clinical risk factors and comorbidities.[40]

Echocardiography for Diagnosis and Risk Stratification

Although insensitive for diagnosis, transthoracic echocardiography (TTE) is superb for detecting RV dysfunction in the setting of pressure overload and serves to risk stratify patients with proven acute PE (Figure 38-6). Echocardiography remains the imaging technique of choice for detection of RV dysfunction in the setting of PE and identification of submassive PE patients. Echocardiography should be performed in patients with acute PE and clinical evidence of RV failure, elevated levels of cardiac biomarkers, or unexpected clinical decompensation. Characteristic echocardiographic findings in patients with submassive PE include RV dilation and hypokinesis, interventricular septal flattening and paradoxical motion toward the LV, abnormal transmitral Doppler flow profile (represented by the A wave making a greater contribution to LV diastole than the E wave), tricuspid regurgitation, pulmonary hypertension as identified by a peak tricuspid regurgitant jet velocity greater than 2.6 m/s, and loss of inspiratory collapse of the IVC. The finding of severe free wall hypokinesis and apical sparing (McConnell sign) is specific for acute PE. In a study of 141 PE patients, the troponin I values and echocardiographic data were correlated with 30-day mortality. Patients with elevated troponin levels and RV enlargement were at significantly greater risk for death after PE than patients with only one or neither adverse prognostic marker.[41] Transesophageal echocardiography (TEE) may be useful for diagnosis of proximal PE, especially in critically ill patients who cannot safely be transported.

Lung Scanning

Ventilation-perfusion lung scans are usually obtained only in patients with major renal impairment, anaphylaxis with intravenous (IV) iodinated contrast, or who are pregnant. A high probability scan in the setting of moderate to high clinical suspicion virtually guarantees the diagnosis, and a normal scan excludes it. However, most patients have nondiagnostic scans.

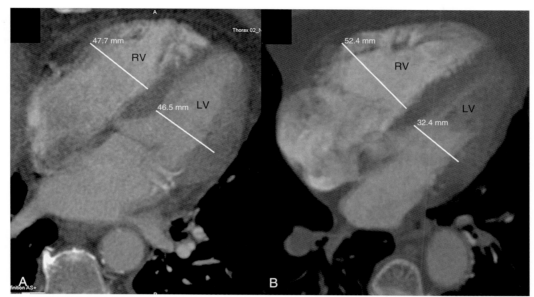

FIGURE 38-5 **A,** Contrast-enhanced chest computed tomography (CT) demonstrating a mild increase in the right ventricular (*RV*)/left ventricular (*LV*) diameter ratio (1.0; normal ratio = ≤0.9) in a 52-year-old woman with acute pulmonary embolism (PE). **B,** Contrast-enhanced chest CT demonstrates severe RV enlargement (RV diameter/LV diameter ratio = 1.6) in a 64-year-old man with acute PE.

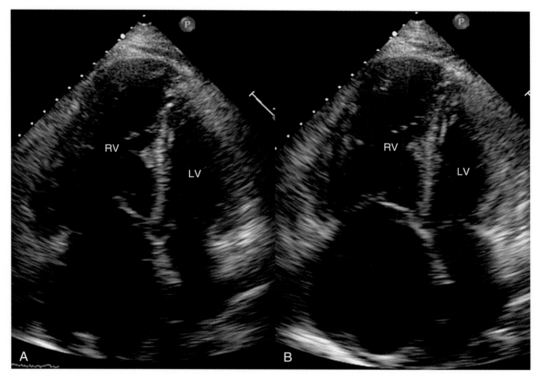

FIGURE 38-6 **A,** Transthoracic echocardiogram, apical four-chamber view, demonstrates marked diastolic right ventricular (*RV*) dilation compared with the left ventricle (*LV*) in a 45-year-old man with colon cancer and acute pulmonary embolism. **B,** In systole, a minimal decrease in RV chamber size is observed, consistent with severe RV hypokinesis.

Magnetic Resonance Imaging

In the Prospective Investigation of Pulmonary Embolism Diagnosis (PIOPED) III, MR angiography showed low sensitivity for detection of PE,[42] and MR was technically inadequate in 25% of the 371 studies performed. If technically inadequate studies are included, only 57% of PEs (59 of 104) were identified with MR in PIOPED III; therefore, until further technological improvements evolve, MR

does not have a role for the diagnosis of PE unless massive PE is suspected and no other modality can be used for imaging.

Overall Diagnostic Algorithm

Diagnostic algorithms that integrate an assessment of clinical probability with appropriate use of D-dimer testing and imaging allow management decisions to be made efficiently and safely in the

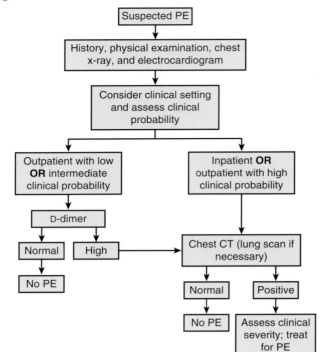

FIGURE 38-7 An integrated diagnostic algorithm for patients with suspected pulmonary embolism (*PE*). CT, computed tomography.

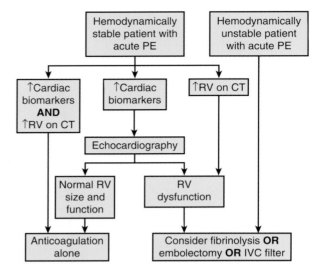

FIGURE 38-8 An algorithm for risk stratification of patients with acute pulmonary embolism (*PE*). CT, computed tomography; IVC, inferior vena cava; RV, right ventricle.

TABLE 38-5	Simplified Pulmonary Embolism Severity Index	
VARIABLE		**POINTS***
Age >80 years		1
History of cancer		1
History of chronic cardiopulmonary disease		1
Pulse ≥110 beats/min		1
Systolic blood pressure <100 mm Hg		1
Arterial oxyhemoglobin saturation (SaO_2) <90%		1

*A total point score is obtained by adding the points; a score of zero indicates low risk, and a score of 1 or more indicates high risk.

majority of patients with suspected PE (Figure 38-7).[43] It appears that a completely noninvasive diagnostic approach can be undertaken for nearly all patients with suspected PE.[44] Invasive contrast pulmonary angiography is reserved for PE patients in whom catheter-assisted pharmacomechanical intervention is anticipated.

OVERALL RISK STRATIFICATION OF PULMONARY EMBOLISM

The American Heart Association (AHA) issued a comprehensive scientific statement on VTE and provided definitions of massive and submassive PE. *Massive PE* is defined as presentation with sustained hypotension, specifically, a low blood pressure not due to another cause, including systolic blood pressure less than 90 mm Hg for at least 15 minutes or a low blood pressure that requires inotropic support; or pulselessness or persistent profound bradycardia (heart rate <40 beats/min) with signs or symptoms of shock. *Submassive PE* is defined as PE with RV dysfunction or myocardial necrosis without hypotension.[45]

Although the clinical presentation of hemodynamic instability differentiates massive from nonmassive PE, detection of RV dysfunction is required to identify normotensive patients with submassive PE. RV dysfunction in patients with PE has been associated with increased 30-day mortality and risk of VTE recurrence.[24] Clinical examination, ECG, cardiac biomarkers, chest CT, and echocardiography are important tools for detection of RV dysfunction (Figure 38-8).

Physical examination findings of RV failure and ECG evidence of RV strain are rapid and inexpensive indicators of submassive PE. Elevations in cardiac biomarkers—including troponin, brain natriuretic peptide (BNP), and heart fatty acid–binding protein (H-FABP)—are associated with RV dysfunction and identify patients with submassive PE.[46] It appears that highly sensitive troponin T assays—which are not approved by the U.S. Food and Drug Administration (FDA) but are available in Europe—may improve risk stratification of PE compared with conventional troponin T assays.[47] For clinical assessment, both the simplified PE Severity

Index (Table 38-5) and the European Society of Cardiology prognostic model (Table 38-6) successfully predict 30-day mortality after acute PE.[48]

Management

Spectrum of Disease: Superficial Venous Thrombosis, Deep Vein Thrombosis, and Pulmonary Embolism

Superficial venous thrombosis can lead to DVT. In a prospective cross-sectional cohort study, 844 consecutive patients were identified with symptomatic superficial venous thrombosis that was at least 5 cm on compression ultrasonography. At the time of diagnosis, 210 patients (25%) also had DVT or symptomatic PE. Among 586 superficial venous thrombosis patients without VTE who underwent a subsequent 3-month follow-up, 58 (10.2%) developed thromboembolic complications, including 46 (8.3%) with symptomatic VTE.[49]

In a randomized trial of 3002 patients with superficial venous thrombosis, fondaparinux (2.5 mg daily for 45 days) was compared with placebo. The primary efficacy endpoint was a composite of death, symptomatic VTE, or extension/recurrence of superficial venous thrombosis. The primary endpoint occurred in 13 (0.9%) in the fondaparinux group compared with 88 (5.9%) in the placebo group (P < .001). Symptomatic VTE occurred in 0.2% of the fondaparinux group versus 1.3% in the placebo group;

TABLE 38-6	European Society of Cardiology Prognostic Model		
	Risk Markers		
PE-RELATED EARLY MORTALITY RISK	**CLINICAL (SHOCK OR HYPOTENSION)**	**RV DYSFUNCTION**	**MYOCARDIAL INJURY**
High (>15%)	+	+	+
Intermediate (3%-15%)	−	+	±
Low (<1%)	−	−	±

Modified from Torbicki A, Perrier A, Konstantinides S, et al. Guidelines I the diagnosis and management of acute pulmonary embolism. Eur Heart J 2008;29:2296-2315.

therefore, 88 patients would need to be treated to prevent one PE or DVT.[50]

DVT encompasses a wide spectrum of disease, including phlegmasia cerulea dolens and iliofemoral, femoral, popliteal, isolated calf, and upper extremity DVT. Phlegmasia cerulea dolens and iliofemoral DVT may result in postthrombotic syndrome if not treated with advanced therapy such as fibrinolysis or thrombectomy. Whether femoral DVT warrants advanced therapy to prevent postthrombotic syndrome remains uncertain. Superior vena cava syndrome may complicate upper extremity DVT in the setting of chronic, indwelling venous foreign bodies, such as pacemaker or defibrillator leads. Patients with leg DVT should be treated with graduated compression stockings (GCS) 30 to 40 mm Hg below the knee, to decrease the likelihood of postthrombotic syndrome.[51]

Acute PE is composed of a number of clinical syndromes, including massive PE, submassive PE, and PE with normal blood pressure and preserved RV function. The term *massive PE* describes a condition seen in a subset of PE patients who present with syncope, hypotension, cardiogenic shock, or cardiac arrest. Normotensive patients with acute PE and evidence of RV dysfunction have submassive PE and have an increased risk of adverse events and early mortality.[46] *Pulmonary infarction syndrome* describes a condition in patients who usually come to medical attention with painful pleurisy and have a distal wedge-shaped infiltrate on chest radiograph or CT scan. This syndrome is a consequence of distal embolization. Although adequate pain control may be difficult to achieve, the syndrome usually has a favorable prognosis.

Anticoagulation

Anticoagulation is the cornerstone of therapy for patients with VTE regardless of whether advanced therapies are also pursued. The current therapeutic armamentarium (Box 38-1) includes unfractionated heparin, low-molecular-weight heparins, fondaparinux, warfarin, and direct factor Xa or IIa inhibitors.

UNFRACTIONATED HEPARIN

Patients with VTE, especially PE but also iliofemoral DVT, may be clinically unstable. Therefore, they initially are suitable candidates for immediate anticoagulation with IV unfractionated heparin (UFH), which can be discontinued and rapidly reversed; UFH is therefore preferred for patients who might undergo advanced therapies for VTE such as fibrinolysis, catheter-based intervention, surgery, or IVC filter placement. UFH is administered as a bolus followed by continuous infusion and is titrated to a goal of activated partial thromboplastin time (aPTT) two to three times the upper limit of normal, or approximately 60 to 80 seconds. A standard initial dose of UFH in patients with normal liver function is an 80 U/kg bolus followed by a continuous IV infusion of 18 U/kg/h.

Heparin-Induced Thrombocytopenia

Heparin-induced thrombocytopenia (HIT) occurs when heparin-dependent platelet-activating antibodies recognize platelet factor 4 (PF4) bound to heparin. HIT is much more likely to cause VTE

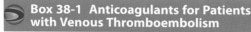

Box 38-1 Anticoagulants for Patients with Venous Thromboembolism

Parenteral Anticoagulants (Initial Therapy)

Unfractionated heparin: Ideal for patients who are unstable, or for those who have an adverse prognosis, because of easy "on/off" control of anticoagulation in the event that thrombolysis or embolectomy is required

Low-molecular-weight heparin: Ideal for stable patients with a good prognosis in whom advanced therapy is not being considered

Fondaparinux: Ideal for stable patients with a good prognosis; used off-label to treat stable patients with suspected or proven HIT

Argatroban: Ideal for patients with kidney disease and HIT or suspected HIT

Lepirudin/bivalirudin: Ideal for patients with liver disease and HIT or suspected HIT

Oral Anticoagulants

Warfarin: The only FDA-approved oral agent for anticoagulation of PE and DVT

Dabigatran: Not FDA approved for VTE treatment

Rivaroxaban: Not FDA approved for VTE treatment

Apixaban: Not FDA approved for VTE treatment

DVT, deep vein thrombosis; FDA, Food and Drug Administration; HIT, heparin-induced thrombocytopenia; PE, pulmonary embolism; VTE, venous thromboembolism.

than cause arterial thrombosis. Pathologic immunoglobulin G activates platelets via Fc receptors, which results in the release of microparticles that generate thrombin. The platelet count falls 5 to 10 days after starting heparin, typically to less than half the baseline platelet count and usually in the 40,000 to 70,000 range. Risk factors for HIT include longer versus shorter exposure to heparin; IV, rather than subcutaneous, heparin exposure; UFH rather than low-molecular-weight heparin (LMWH); surgery, especially cardiac surgery; and female gender, especially with prophylactic doses of heparin.[52] ELISA testing quantifies anti-PF4/heparin antibody levels. Plasma is incubated in a PF4/heparin-coated microwell. Antibody levels are measured in optical density (OD) units. The higher the OD, the more likely the diagnosis of HIT with thrombosis and the more likely the diagnosis of acute PE (Figure 38-9).[53] Of note, those with pathogenic platelet-activating antibodies indicative of HIT comprise a small subset of those with an anti-PF4/heparin immune response. Widespread detection of anti-PF4/heparin antibodies with commercially available ELISA has promoted an overdiagnosis phenomenon.[54] Three direct thrombin inhibitors have been FDA approved for treating HIT or suspected HIT, and all are administered as continuous IV infusions and are dose adjusted using the aPTT; the target PTT is usually 60 to 80 seconds. All increase the international normalized ratio (INR), which makes assessment of the desired warfarin dose challenging because the INR decreases after these agents are discontinued. Argatroban is metabolized by the liver and is best used in patients with kidney disease; lepirudin and bivalirudin are metabolized by the kidney and are best used in patients with liver disease. Bivalirudin is only approved by the FDA for use in patients undergoing cardiac catheterization or percutaneous coronary intervention; however, it is often used off-label for any acutely ill patient with HIT or suspected HIT, but the dose must be adjusted downward for patients with kidney disease.

CH
38

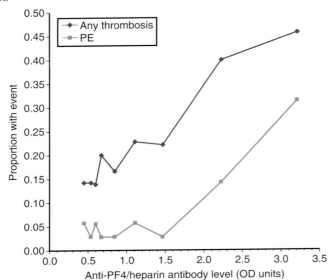

FIGURE 38-9 Association of anti–platelet factor 4 (*PF4*)/heparin antibody level with any arterial or venous thrombosis and pulmonary embolism (*PE*). The proportion with any thrombosis by 30 days and the proportion with PE are shown as a function of anti-PF4/heparin antibody level. Increases in anti-PF4/heparin antibody level were significantly associated with greater proportions of any thrombosis and PE by 30 days.

LOW-MOLECULAR-WEIGHT HEPARIN

LMWH is best suited for initial anticoagulant therapy among patients with an excellent prognosis who appear clinically stable, have normal or near-normal RV function, and have no elevation in troponin level. LMWH is dosed according to weight and is administered subcutaneously, and it does not require routine dose adjustment or laboratory monitoring. LMWH is at least as safe and effective as UFH for immediate anticoagulation and transition to oral anticoagulation after acute VTE. In contrast to UFH, which is mostly eliminated by the liver, LMWHs are cleared renally.

Cancer patients with VTE have a high risk of VTE recurrence, especially if they are anticoagulated with warfarin. Therefore, LMWH as monotherapy is generally recommended for at least the first 3 months of therapy. This approach will halve the rate of recurrent VTE compared with using LMWH as a bridge to warfarin.[55] Whether cancer patients should remain on indefinite-duration LMWH monotherapy or be switched to warfarin after an initial 3 to 6 months of therapy remains uncertain.[56]

FONDAPARINUX

Fondaparinux, a synthetic pentasaccharide, does not cause HIT; this differentiates fondaparinux from UFH and LMWH. Fondaparinux is FDA approved for initial therapy of DVT and PE as a bridge to warfarin therapy. In addition, fondaparinux is often used off-label to anticoagulate clinically stable VTE patients with suspected or proven HIT. Fondaparinux is administered once daily, and its half-life is 17 hours. The dosing regimen is simple and straightforward; it is supplied in prefilled syringes of 2.5 (for VTE prophylaxis), 5.0, 7.5, and 10 mg. The recommended VTE treatment dose for patients with normal renal function is 5.0 mg for patients who weigh less than 50 kg, 7.5 mg for patients 50 kg to 100 kg, and 10 mg for patients who weigh more than 100 kg.

WARFARIN

Marketed since 1954, warfarin achieves its anticoagulant effect by producing hemostatically defective vitamin K–dependent coagulant proteins: factors II, VII, IX, and X. Warfarin is a challenging drug to use effectively and safely because it has a widely variable anticoagulant response. Warfarin has multiple drug-drug and drug-food interactions, and it has a slow onset and offset of action of 4 to 7 days.

Laboratory monitoring is performed by measuring the prothrombin time (PT), which assesses depression of vitamin K–dependent clotting factors. Commercial PT reagents vary markedly in their responsiveness to warfarin-induced reduction in clotting factors; therefore, laboratory results are now standardized using the INR. The target INR for treatment of VTE is usually between 2.0 and 3.0; high INRs predispose to bleeding complications, whereas low INRs are associated with recurrent VTE. All patients taking warfarin should wear a medical alert bracelet or jewelry item that will inform emergency medical personnel responding to trauma that warfarin reversal should be considered to help prevent catastrophic bleeding. Two registries have provided data to help identify patients at high risk for bleeding (Box 38-2).[57,58] Warfarin-related bleeding can be reversed with oral vitamin K,[59] fresh frozen plasma, prothrombin complex concentrate, or recombinant factor VIIa.

The warfarin dose should be reduced when managing debilitated, frail, or elderly patients. In contrast, because green vegetables contain vitamin K and lower the INR, higher than average doses of warfarin may be necessary for patients who eat these vegetables frequently. Concomitant medications with antiplatelet effects—such as aspirin and other nonsteroidal antiinflammatory agents, high-dose acetaminophen,[60] fish oil supplements, vitamin E, and alcohol—may increase the bleeding risk without increasing the INR.

Centralized anticoagulation clinics, usually staffed by nurses or pharmacists, have improved the quality and safety of warfarin dosing. These clinics use databases devoted to warfarin management, in which patients' INRs and warfarin doses can be readily tracked. An excellent anticoagulation clinic will maintain an overall time within the therapeutic INR range of at least 60%.

Point-of-care INR testing devices provide the INR result within 2 minutes by using a drop of whole blood obtained from a fingertip puncture. Appropriately selected patients can be taught to self-test their INRs, and especially motivated patients can even be taught to self-dose their warfarin. Patients who self-test appreciate the added convenience and time savings of self-testing, and they usually appreciate the additional control they have over their own medical care. A trial at one center of 737 patients found that self-managed patients had fewer bleeding complications.[61] However, a larger trial of 2922 patients at 28 centers did not find that self-testing improved efficacy or safety of anticoagulation.[62]

Genetic determinants of warfarin dose-response include *CYP2C9* variant alleles, which impair the hydroxylation of S-warfarin and result in extremely low warfarin dose requirements, and variants in the gene that encodes vitamin K epoxide reductase complex 1, *VKORC1*. Variability in the INR response to warfarin appears more strongly associated with *VKORC1* than with *CYP2C9*.[63] A multiple regression model using the predictors of *CYP2C9*, *VKORC1*, age, sex, and drug interactions explains about half of the variance in warfarin dose.[64]

Use of a pharmacogenetic algorithm for initiating warfarin dosing appears to be of greatest benefit among those patients who require very high (≥7 mg) or very low doses (≤3 mg) of warfarin.[65] This approach may be cost effective when initiating warfarin in patients at high risk for hemorrhage.[66] The largest randomized trial to date studied 206 patients who received either pharmacogenetic-guided or standard warfarin dosing. The primary endpoint, reduction in out-of-range INRs, was not achieved in the group undergoing rapid-turnaround genetic testing.[67] An observational study using historic controls found that, compared with conventional warfarin dosing, rapid-turnaround genetic testing reduced hospitalization rates, including the risk of hospitalization for bleeding or thromboembolism.[68] Thus, clinical equipoise exists. Therefore, the National Heart, Lung and Blood Institute (NHLBI) sponsored two large randomized trials on rapid-turnaround genetic testing; one is the Clarification of Optimal Anticoagulation Through Genetics (COAG, ClinicalTrials.gov identifier NCT00839657). More than 1200 patients will be randomized to a genotype-guided versus clinical-guided warfarin dosing algorithm. The primary endpoint is the percentage of time participants spend within the therapeutic INR range; results are expected in 2014. The other, the Genetics Informatics Trial (GIFT) of Warfarin to Prevent DVT (ClinicalTrials.gov identifier NCT01006733), with a planned 1600 patients, should also yield results in 2014.

For patients receiving warfarin, withholding anticoagulation for 4 to 5 days is generally required to allow warfarin to wash out. When patients undergo elective surgery or common outpatient procedures, such as colonoscopy with possible excision of colonic polyps, warfarin must be temporarily discontinued. One approach, so-called *bridging*, uses a strategy of prescribing LMWH preoperatively while the warfarin effect dissipates. However, when anticoagulation is temporarily interrupted for an invasive procedure, the rate of thromboembolism is low among VTE patients, even when bridging is not implemented.[69] This is true especially for patients whose VTE event occurred more than 3 months prior to the planned invasive procedure and who do not have major thrombophilic conditions such as antiphospholipid antibody syndrome. The prescription of LMWH for several days preoperatively increases the likelihood of bleeding complications; in addition, the complexity of the dosing protocols to bridge frequently leads to misunderstandings and miscommunication about the intended dosing regimen; therefore, the practice of routine bridging for VTE patients is falling into disfavor.

DIRECT FACTOR XA AND FACTOR IIA INHIBITORS

Two new oral anticoagulants, dabigatran[70] and rivaroxaban,[71] are administered in fixed doses without any need for laboratory coagulation monitoring.[72] They are noninferior to warfarin and will likely be approved for VTE treatment. The Efficacy and Safety of Dabigatran Compared to Warfarin for 6 Month Treatment of Acute Symptomatic Venous Thromboembolism (RE-COVER, ClinicalTrials.gov identifier NCT00291330) trial compared dabigatran 150 mg twice daily to warfarin for 2539 patients with acute DVT.[70] A total of 30 (2.4%) of the 1274 patients randomly assigned to receive dabigatran had recurrent VTE compared with 27 (2.1%) of the 1265 patients randomly assigned to warfarin. The hazard ratio with dabigatran was 1.10 (95% confidence interval [CI], 0.65 to 1.84). Major bleeding episodes occurred in 20 patients assigned to dabigatran (1.6%) and in 24 patients assigned to warfarin (1.9%; hazard ratio [HR] with dabigatran, 0.82; 95% CI, 0.45 to 1.48).

The Oral Direct Factor Xa Inhibitor Rivaroxaban in Patients with Acute Symptomatic Deep-Vein Thrombosis Without Symptomatic Pulmonary Embolism (Einstein-DVT) evaluation comprised two studies.[72a] The first compared rivaroxaban and warfarin for acute DVT treatment. The second, conducted in parallel, was composed of patients who had completed at least 6 months of anticoagulation and whose physicians were uncertain whether to continue long-term anticoagulation. These patients were randomized to receive rivaroxaban or placebo. The primary efficacy outcome for both studies was recurrent VTE. The study of rivaroxaban for acute DVT included 3449 patients; 1731 were given rivaroxaban, and 1718 were given enoxaparin as a "bridge" to a vitamin K antagonist. Rivaroxaban had noninferior efficacy with respect to the primary outcome, resulting in 36 events (2.1%) versus 51 events with an enoxaparin–vitamin K antagonist (3.0%; HR, 0.68; 95% CI, 0.44 to 1.04; *P* < .001). In the continued-treatment study, which included 602 patients in the rivaroxaban group and 594 in the placebo group, rivaroxaban had superior efficacy that resulted in 8 events (1.3%) versus 42 (7.1%) with placebo (HR, 0.18; 95% CI, 0.09 to 0.39; *P* < .001).

Basic Versus Advanced Therapy for Venous Thromboembolism

Approximately two thirds of PE patients have an excellent prognosis when initially assessed. These patients often do not come to the attention of the cardiovascular medicine specialist, but they are ideal candidates for treatment with basic therapy with anticoagulation alone. In specially selected low-risk patients with PE, those who have reliable and frequent home health care services coupled with strong family and social support, outpatient management in the context of a well-funded clinical trial (mostly in Europe) was noninferior to hospitalization.[73]

Advanced therapy for patients with anatomically large DVT of the femoral or iliofemoral veins consists of pharmacomechanical therapy with catheter-assisted low-dose thrombolysis and mechanical disruption of thrombus. In a 2011 Scientific Statement of the AHA, this approach was considered "reasonable as first-line therapy to prevent postthrombotic syndrome in selected patients at low risk of bleeding complications." The AHA also recommends that all DVT patients wear 30 to 40 mm Hg knee-high GCS for at least 2 years.[45]

For patients with massive PE, the AHA scientific statement recommends fibrinolysis for those with an "acceptable risk of bleeding complications." The AHA considers catheter embolectomy with fragmentation and surgical embolectomy reasonable procedures for patients with massive PE and contraindications to fibrinolysis. For patients with submassive PE, the AHA recommends consideration of fibrinolysis for those with severe RV dysfunction, major myocardial necrosis, or worsening respiratory insufficiency coupled with a low risk of bleeding. For patients with submassive PE, the AHA states that catheter or surgical embolectomy "may be considered."[45]

DEEP VEIN THROMBOSIS

Advanced therapy is often appropriate for young, otherwise healthy patients with proximal upper extremity or iliofemoral DVT and severe symptoms. Fibrinolysis should be catheter directed to gain access to the obstructed deep venous system.[74] The NHLBI-sponsored Acute Venous Thrombosis: Thrombus Removal with Adjunctive Catheter-Directed Thrombolysis (ATTRACT [ClinicalTrials.gov identifier NCT00790335]) trial will determine whether catheter-based fibrinolytic therapy can safely prevent postthrombotic syndrome and improve quality of life in patients with proximal DVT. Surgical thrombectomy can be considered in patients with massive or severely symptomatic DVT in whom fibrinolysis has failed or is contraindicated.

ADVANCED THERAPY FOR PULMONARY EMBOLISM

Consensus guidelines[45,75] recommend advanced therapy for patients with massive PE. The U.S. FDA has approved recombinant tissue plasminogen activator (100 mg) administered as a continuous infusion over 2 hours for fibrinolysis of acute massive PE.[24] The use of fibrinolysis in patients with submassive PE remains controversial.[46] However, the Pulmonary Embolism in Thrombolysis Study (PEITHO [ClinicalTrials.gov identifier NCT00639743]) is randomizing 1000 patients to tenecteplase or placebo; results should be available in 2013.[76]

The goals of fibrinolysis are rapid reduction in RV pressure overload, stabilization of hemodynamics, and normalization of gas exchange. In addition to rapidly improving RV function, fibrinolysis may help prevent the development of chronic thromboembolic pulmonary hypertension.[77] All patients being considered for fibrinolysis require meticulous screening for contraindications that make the bleeding risk prohibitive. Intracranial hemorrhage is the most feared and severe complication of fibrinolytic therapy. Even in experienced centers, major bleeding from fibrinolytic therapy is problematic, especially outside the context of a clinical trial.[78] Of 104 patients who received alteplase for acute PE but were not part of a clinical trial, major bleeding occurred in 20 patients (19%). The principal site of bleeding was unknown in 9 patients (45%), gastrointestinal in 6 (30%), retroperitoneal in 3 (15%), intracranial in 1 (5%), and splenic in 1 (5%). Independent predictors of major hemorrhage were the administration of catecholamines for systemic arterial hypotension, comorbidities such as cancer and diabetes mellitus, and an elevated INR before fibrinolysis.

For patients in whom major contraindications to fibrinolytic therapy are present, or in whom an initial trial of fibrinolysis has failed, alternative options such as catheter-assisted embolectomy or surgical embolectomy may be considered. Catheter-assisted embolectomy is an emerging technique that usually, but not always, combines low-dose "local" fibrinolysis with thrombus fragmentation or aspiration, called *pharmacomechanical therapy*. In a systematic review of 594 patients from 35 studies, clinical success was achieved in 87% of patients undergoing catheter-assisted embolectomy, with relatively low rates of minor and major procedural complications.[79] One promising catheter-based approach is the use of catheter-directed, ultrasound-accelerated thrombolysis, which appears to reduce clot burden rapidly and reverse RV enlargement.[80]

Surgical embolectomy is indicated for patients in whom fibrinolysis or catheter-based techniques have failed or are contraindicated, as well as for those with paradoxical embolism, persistent right heart thrombi, or a "clot in transit." Surgical embolectomy[81] requires a median sternotomy and cardiopulmonary bypass and is most successful in patients with large, centrally located thrombi.[82,83]

DURATION OF ANTICOAGULATION

Determination of optimal duration of anticoagulation for VTE requires an assessment of the patient's long-term risk of VTE recurrence after treatment of the initial episode (Figure 38-10).[75,84] A population-based strategy recommends limited-duration anticoagulation of 3 to 6 months for provoked VTE and indefinite-duration anticoagulation for patients with low bleeding risk and unprovoked (idiopathic) VTE. Patients with malignancy and VTE comprise a population with a substantially increased risk of VTE recurrence; therefore, such patients are generally prescribed prolonged anticoagulation as long as the cancer is active, which may be difficult or impossible to determine. Although not endorsed by evidence-based guidelines, an individualized approach incorporating D-dimer testing or lower extremity venous imaging after completion of standard therapy for VTE has been evaluated to determine optimal duration of anticoagulation.[86]

After the first 6 months of anticoagulation, most patients who continue indefinite-duration anticoagulation with warfarin will continue standard-intensity anticoagulation with a target INR between 2.0 and 3.0.[87] Another option, proven effective and safe, is low-intensity anticoagulation with a target INR between 1.5 and 2.0.[88] With this option, patients have been successfully managed with INRs obtained only once every 2 months.

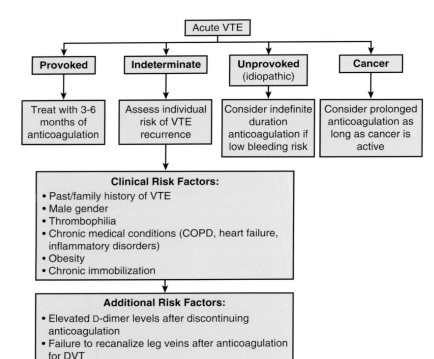

FIGURE 38-10 An approach to optimizing duration of anticoagulation in patients with venous thromboembolism (*VTE*). COPD, chronic obstructive pulmonary disease; DVT, deep vein thrombosis.

INFERIOR VENA CAVA FILTERS

IVC filter insertion is used for patients with massive or submassive PE in whom fibrinolysis and embolectomy are contraindicated or unavailable. IVC filters are also indicated for patients in whom standard anticoagulation is contraindicated, such as those with active bleeding. IVC filters reduce the risk of PE in the short term but appear to increase the risk of DVT in the long term. IVC filter insertion does not arrest the thrombotic process and may be associated with vascular access site and other complications, such as fracture and fragment embolization.[89] Retrievable IVC filters provide a safe and effective alternative to permanent filters and may be removed up to several months after insertion in patients with transient contraindications to anticoagulation.

A proliferation in the use of IVC filters has been seen,[89a] and from 1985 through 2006, some 803,000 vena cava filters were inserted—285,000 in patients with PE, 360,000 in patients with DVT only, and 158,000 in patients who had neither. The largest proportional increases in the use of vena cava filters since the introduction of retrievable filters was in patients at risk of PE who had neither PE nor DVT. The trend toward increased use in this group began before retrievable filters were introduced, with a threefold increase between 2001 and 2006. Increased use of permanent and retrievable vena cava filters in the United States indicates liberalization of indications.

Most retrievable filters are not retrieved, nor is any attempt made to retrieve them. In a study of 144 patients with retrievable filters at a community hospital, retrieval was attempted in only 14 (10%) of 144 patients at an average of 4.6 months.[89b] Retrieval was successful in 10 (71%) of 14 patients. Nonbleeding complications of IVC filters occurred in 12 (8.3%) of 144 patients, and half of those complications occurred after 3 months of insertion. Three patients (2.1%) had IVC thrombosis, 1 patient (1.3%) had a new DVT, 6 patients (4.2%) had a new DVT alone, 1 patient (0.7%) had a new DVT with a new PE, and 2 patients (1.3%) had filter migration. In 2010, the FDA stated that it was "concerned that these retrievable IVC filters, intended for short-term placement, are not always removed once a patient's risk for PE subsides. Known long-term risks associated with IVC filters include but are not limited to lower limb deep vein thrombosis, filter fracture, filter migration, filter embolization, and IVC perforation."[90]

The 2011 AHA scientific statement recommends IVC filters for PE patients who have 1) contraindications to anticoagulation, 2) recurrent PE despite adequate anticoagulation, and 3) very poor cardiopulmonary reserve, "including those with massive PE."[45]

Prevention

Pharmacologic thromboprophylaxis with UFH, LMWH, or fondaparinux reduces VTE incidence in both general surgical[91] and acutely ill general medical[92-94] hospitalized patients. VTE thromboprophylaxis also reduces all-cause mortality in surgical patients.[95] However, no evidence of a mortality benefit is associated with pharmacologic VTE prophylaxis for hospitalized general medical patients. Therefore, an international, multicenter, randomized, double-blind study to compare the overall mortality rate in acutely ill medical patients treated with enoxaparin versus placebo in addition to graduated elastic stockings (LIFENOX) was undertaken to evaluate the impact of pharmacologic thromboprophylaxis on all-cause mortality in acutely ill medical patients randomized to enoxaparin (40 mg/day) plus GCS versus placebo plus GCS.[96] The primary efficacy outcome was all-cause mortality 30 days after randomization. The primary safety outcome was major bleeding during the treatment period and up to 48 hours after. In total, 8307 patients received GCS plus enoxaparin (n = 4171) or GCS plus placebo (n = 4136). All-cause mortality rates at day 30 were 4.9% in the enoxaparin group compared with 4.8% in the placebo group (risk ratio [RR], 1.0; 95% CI, 0.8 to 1.2; $P =$ .83). Major bleeding rates were 0.4% and 0.3% in enoxaparin and placebo groups, respectively (RR, 1.4; 95% CI, 0.7 to 3.1; $P =$ .35).

Thus, no reduction was seen in all-cause mortality associated with the use of enoxaparin and GCS compared with GCS alone.

Despite lack of reduction in all-cause mortality among hospitalized medically ill patients, VTE prophylaxis is the standard of care to prevent DVT and PE. The American College of Chest Physicians' guidelines recommend "that every hospital develop a formal strategy that addresses the prevention of VTE."[97] It is estimated that in the United States alone, about 8 million medical patients and 4 million surgical patients are hospitalized annually with a moderate or high risk of VTE.[98] Modeling studies suggest that 2 of every 100 acutely ill hospitalized medical patients in the United States are afflicted annually with VTE.[99] Over the ensuing 5 years, the VTE from a single year generates an estimated cumulative 50,000 VTE-related deaths, 28,000 recurrent DVTs, 6700 recurrent PEs, 140,000 cases of postthrombotic syndrome, and 5000 cases of chronic thromboembolic pulmonary hypertension.[100]

In an individual patient data meta-analysis of enoxaparin versus UFH for VTE prevention in medical patients, enoxaparin (40 mg) reduced VTE by about one third compared with UFH at 5000 U two or three times daily.[101] Compared with placebo, anticoagulant prophylaxis with either LMWH or UFH more than halved the frequency of symptomatic PE.[102]

One caveat is that patients may not receive the prescribed injectable anticoagulant, even while they are hospitalized. One study identified 250 consecutive patients prescribed VTE prophylaxis with UFH or LMWH.[103] Medication adherence was greater with LMWH (95%) than with UFH three times daily (88%) or two times daily (87%; $P < .001$). Patients who were prescribed LMWH more often received all scheduled doses (77%) compared with UFH three times (54%) or two times daily (45%; $P < .001$). The most common reason for omitted doses was patient refusal, which explained 44% of UFH and 39% of LMWH orders that were not administered. Future educational initiatives that explain the rationale of VTE prophylaxis to patients may provide the motivation necessary to improve medication adherence during hospitalization.[104]

Although the use of VTE prophylaxis should be virtually universal among hospitalized patients, there appears to be a failure-to-prophylax syndrome worldwide.[105] The Venous Thromboembolism Risk and Prophylaxis in the Acute Hospital Care Setting (ENDORSE) study is a multinational cross-sectional study that enrolled 68,183 patients from 358 hospitals, 45% surgical and 55% medical. Half were judged to have at least moderate risk for developing VTE. Of the at-risk surgical patients, 58% received guideline-recommended prophylaxis compared with 40% of at-risk medical patients. Accordingly, the incidence of VTE among hospitalized medical patients remains unacceptably high.[106] The ENDORSE investigators found that establishing hospital-wide VTE prophylaxis protocols and performing local audits to assess implementation of VTE prevention policies increased the proportion of patients who received prophylaxis.[107]

Prevention of Venous Thromboembolism in Patients with Cancer

The Prevention of Venous and Arterial Thromboembolism in Cancer Patients Undergoing Chemotherapy with a Low Molecular Weight Heparin (PROTECHT) investigators studied nadroparin (3800 U once daily) versus placebo for prevention of VTE in 1150 ambulatory patients receiving chemotherapy with metastatic or locally advanced solid cancer. Nadroparin nearly halved the rate of VTE, from 3.9% to 2.0%.[108] The Evaluation of AVE5026 in the Prevention of Venous Thromboembolism in Cancer Patients Undergoing Chemotherapy (SAVE ONCO) studied semuloparin (20 mg once daily) versus placebo in patients with metastatic or locally advanced cancers.[109] Semuloparin was initiated with a new chemotherapy course and was continued until the regimen was changed. Thromboembolic events were reduced from 3.4% in the placebo group to 1.2% in the semuloparin group ($P < .001$), and major bleeding did not differ between the groups (1.2% vs. 1.1%).

Implementation of in-Hospital Prophylaxis

Among the most effective DVT prevention strategies are an array of computerized decision-support systems,[110] such as the multi-screen electronic alert currently used at Brigham and Women's Hospital to augment VTE prophylaxis.[111] Electronic alert systems maintain effectiveness over time, generally halve the rate of VTE,[112] and are cost effective.[113] Electronic alerts to prevent VTE among hospitalized patients appear to be more effective than "human" alerts—that is, a hospital staff member informing the attending physician that a particular patient is at high risk for VTE but is not receiving prophylaxis.[114]

Hip Replacement, Knee Replacement, and Hip Fracture

More than 800,000 Americans undergo hip or knee replacement annually, and controversy has erupted between proponents of the American College of Chest Physicians (ACCP) guidelines and those of the American Association of Orthopedic Surgeons (AAOS) over VTE prophylaxis in high-risk orthopedic surgery.[115] The AAOS emphasizes that PE prevention is the ultimate goal of prophylaxis. However, intensive anticoagulation to prevent asymptomatic DVT can cause wound hematoma, infection, and additional pain, cost, and prolonged hospitalization. Until recently, the AAOS endorsed aspirin as one method of achieving VTE prophylaxis. In contrast, the ACCP stated that aspirin is ineffective for VTE prophylaxis.

This controversy prompted both the AAOS and ACCP to reexamine the data. On September 24, 2011, the AAOS radically revised its guidelines and stopped specifically endorsing aspirin (Box 38-3).[116] Meanwhile, the ACCP reexamined the evidence and included aspirin as a legitimate prophylaxis strategy against VTE in high-risk orthopedic surgery in its new guidelines issued in 2012. This reassessment was based on the Pulmonary Embolism Prevention (PEP) trial, which enrolled 13,356 patients undergoing surgery for hip fracture and 4088 patients undergoing elective total hip or knee replacement.[117] PEP was initially considered methodologically flawed, but it has been recently reexamined and validated as having good methodology. The use of aspirin is attractive for several reasons; it is inexpensive, is administered orally, does not require laboratory monitoring, and is associated with low bleeding rates. In PEP, the study treatment was 160 mg aspirin daily or placebo. Among hip fracture patients, the aspirin group had a 43% reduction in PE and a 29% reduction in symptomatic DVT; aspirin prevented four fatal PEs per 1000 patients. Among elective total hip or knee replacement patients, aspirin reduced the VTE rate by 19%.

Despite this positive reassessment of aspirin, the vast majority of VTE experts recommend non–aspirin-based VTE pharmacoprophylaxis. Alternative pharmacoprophylactic regimens include LMWH, fondaparinux (2.5 mg once daily), or warfarin. Novel oral anticoagulants have also been licensed globally for VTE prevention in hip and knee replacement surgery. For example, in July 2011, the FDA approved the direct factor Xa inhibitor rivaroxaban in a dose of 10 mg daily as VTE prophylaxis for 35 days after hip replacement[118,119] and for 12 days after knee replacement surgery.[120,121] In May 2011, the European Union approved the direct factor Xa inhibitor apixaban in a dose of 2.5 mg twice daily for 32 to 38 days after hip replacement[122] and for 10 to 14 days after total knee replacement.[123]

Mechanical Prophylaxis

Mechanical prophylactic measures, including GCS and intermittent pneumatic compression devices, should be considered in

Box 38-3 American Academy of Orthopedic Surgeons Guidelines for Venous Thromboembolism Prevention in Elective Hip and Knee Replacement

1. We recommend against routine postoperative duplex venous ultrasonography screening. (Grade of recommendation: Strong)
2. Current evidence is not clear about whether factors other than a history of previous venous thromboembolism (VTE) increase the risk of VTE in patients undergoing elective hip or knee arthroplasty; therefore, we cannot recommend for or against routinely assessing these patients for additional risk factors. (Grade of recommendation: Inconclusive)
3. Patients should be assessed for known bleeding disorders such as hemophilia and for active liver disease, which further increase the risk for bleeding and bleeding-associated complications. (Grade of recommendation: Consensus)
4. We suggest that patients discontinue antiplatelet agents (e.g., aspirin, clopidogrel) before undergoing elective hip or knee arthroplasty. (Grade of recommendation: Moderate)
5. We suggest the use of pharmacologic agents and/or mechanical compressive devices for the prevention of VTE in patients undergoing elective hip or knee arthroplasty and who are not at elevated risk beyond that of the surgery itself for VTE or bleeding. (Grade of recommendation: Moderate)
6. Current evidence is unclear about which prophylactic strategies are optimal or suboptimal; therefore, we are unable to recommend for or against specific prophylactics in these patients. (Grade of recommendation: Inconclusive)
7. Patients undergoing elective hip or knee arthroplasty who have also had a previous VTE should receive pharmacologic prophylaxis and be treated with mechanical compressive devices. (Grade of recommendation: Consensus)
8. Patients undergoing elective hip or knee arthroplasty who also have a known bleeding disorder (e.g., hemophilia) and/or active liver disease should be treated with mechanical compressive devices to prevent VTE. (Grade of recommendation: Consensus)
9. Patients should undergo early mobilization following elective hip and knee arthroplasty. Early mobilization is low in cost, poses minimal risk to the patient, and is consistent with current practice. (Grade of recommendation: Consensus)
10. We suggest the use of neuraxial anesthesia—such as intrathecal, epidural, and spinal anesthesia—for patients undergoing elective hip or knee arthroplasty to help limit blood loss, even though evidence suggests that neuraxial anesthesia does not affect the occurrence of venous thromboembolic disease. (Grade of recommendation: Moderate)
11. Current evidence does not provide clear guidance about whether inferior vena cava filters prevent pulmonary embolism in patients undergoing elective hip and knee arthroplasty who also have a contraindication to chemoprophylaxis and/or known residual VTE disease. Therefore, we are unable to recommend for or against the use of such filters. (Grade of recommendation: Inconclusive)

From the American Academy of Orthopaedic Surgeons. Preventing venous thromboembolic disease in patients undergoing elective hip and knee arthroplasty: evidence-based guideline and evidence report. Available at http://www.aaos.org/research/guidelines/VTE/VTE_full_guideline.pdf.

at-risk patients who are not candidates for pharmacologic thromboprophylaxis. Intermittent pneumatic compression appears to be cost effective in general surgery.[124] Nevertheless, thigh-high GCS failed to reduce the frequency of proximal DVT in a large randomized, controlled trial of patients who had had a major stroke.[125] In a separate trial of VTE prophylaxis after major abdominal surgery, the addition of fondaparinux (2.5 mg/day) to intermittent pneumatic compression reduced the VTE rate by 70% compared with intermittent pneumatic compression alone.[126]

UNCONVENTIONAL PROPHYLAXIS

Vitamin E

The Women's Health Study randomized 39,876 women to receive a prophylactic dose of 600 U of vitamin E or placebo.[127] After a median follow-up of 10 years, a 21% reduction in VTE was reported among women assigned to vitamin E therapy. The reduction was most striking among women with VTE before randomization (44% reduction) and in women with either the factor V Leiden mutation or the prothrombin gene mutation (49% reduction).

Statins

In the Justification for the use of Statins in Primary Prevention: an Intervention Trial Evaluating Rosuvastatin (JUPITER), 17,802 apparently healthy men and women with both low-density lipoprotein (LDL) cholesterol levels below 130 mg/dL and high-sensitivity C-reactive protein (hs-CRP) levels of 2.0 mg/dL or higher were randomized to receive rosuvastatin (20 mg/day) or placebo.[1] The prespecified endpoint of symptomatic VTE was reduced by 43% in the rosuvastatin group ($P = .007$). Notably, statins do not increase bleeding risk.

DURATION OF PROPHYLAXIS AND EXTENSION OF PROPHYLAXIS AFTER HOSPITAL DISCHARGE

After initial, short-term, in-hospital VTE prophylaxis of about 1 week, 3 weeks of extended enoxaparin prophylaxis is FDA approved following abdominal or pelvic cancer surgery[128] and following hip replacement surgery.[129]

The risk of VTE persists after hospital discharge for both postoperative and acutely ill medical patients. However, no study has demonstrated that an extended duration of VTE prophylaxis in this patient population yields a net clinical benefit.

In the Extended Clinical Prophylaxis in Acutely Ill Medical Patients (EXCLAIM) trial, 5963 subjects were given open-label enoxaparin (40 mg once daily) for an average of 10 days prior to randomization to either continued enoxaparin or to placebo injection for an additional 28 days.[130] Compared with placebo, extended enoxaparin prophylaxis in the EXCLAIM trial population significantly reduced the rate of VTE from 4.0% to 2.5%. Most of this benefit reflected a fourfold reduction in symptomatic proximal DVT. However, compared with placebo, extended enoxaparin prophylaxis significantly increased the rate of major bleeding, from 0.3% to 0.8%.

The Multicenter, Randomized, Parallel Group Efficacy and Safety Study for the Prevention of Venous Thromboembolism in Hospitalized Medically Ill Patients Comparing Rivaroxaban with Enoxaparin (MAGELLAN) compared extended prophylaxis with oral rivaroxaban (10 mg once daily) with a 6- to 14-day course of subcutaneous enoxaparin (40 mg once daily) in 8101 medically ill patients. At day 10, the primary efficacy outcome, a composite of VTE and VTE-related death, occurred in 2.7% in both groups. However, at day 35, the primary efficacy endpoint was significantly lower with extended rivaroxaban than with enoxaparin (4.4% and 5.7%, respectively; HR, 0.77; 95% CI, 0.62 to 0.96; $P = .02$), and the efficacy benefit of rivaroxaban was offset by an increase in treatment-related major bleeding and clinically relevant nonmajor bleeding with rivaroxaban compared with enoxaparin, both at 1 to 10 days (2.8% and 1.2%, respectively) and at 11 to 35 days (1.4% and 0.5%, respectively).

In the Study of Apixaban for the Prevention of Thrombosis-Related Events in Patients With Acute Medical Illness (ADOPT) trial, 6528 medically ill hospitalized patients were randomized to oral apixaban, 2.5 mg twice daily for 30 days, or to subcutaneous enoxaparin, 40 mg once daily for 6 to 14 days. The primary efficacy outcome was the 30-day composite of VTE-related death, PE, symptomatic DVT, or asymptomatic proximal leg DVT as detected by systematic bilateral compression ultrasonography on days 5 through 14 and 30. The primary efficacy outcome occurred in 2.71% of patients randomized to receive apixaban and in 3.06% of those given enoxaparin plus placebo ($P = .44$). Major bleeding at day 30 occurred in 0.47% in the apixaban group and 0.19% in the enoxaparin group ($P = .04$). In medically ill patients, an extended course of thromboprophylaxis with apixaban was not superior to a shorter course of enoxaparin.

TABLE 38-7	Padua Prediction Score: Risk Assessment Model with High Risk of Venous Thromboembolism Defined as ≥4 Points	
BASELINE FEATURES		**SCORE**
Active cancer		3
Prior venous thromboembolism		3
Reduced mobility		3
Thrombophilia		3
Recent trauma/surgery		2
Age ≥70 years		1
Heart or respiratory failure		1
Acute myocardial infarction or ischemic stroke		1
Acute infection or rheumatologic disorder		1
Obesity (body mass index ≥30)		1
Ongoing hormonal treatment		1

The contemporary clinical trial results for extended VTE prophylaxis in medically ill patients suggest that improved predictive models are needed to identify a more narrow range of patients at risk for VTE after hospital discharge. In the International Medical Prevention Registry on Venous Thromboembolism (IMPROVE) registry, the most important risk factors for VTE were previous VTE, known thrombophilia, cancer, age older than 60 years, lower limb paralysis, immobilization for more than 1 week, and admission to an intensive care unit.[131] Another promising approach to identify medical patients at the highest risk of developing VTE is the Padua Prediction Score risk assessment model.[132] In this model, medical patients at high risk of VTE are given four or more score points (Table 38-7).

Conclusions

The ultimate goal is eradication of hospital-acquired VTE. Evidence-based trials indicate that implementation of VTE prophylaxis efforts should be focused on acutely ill medical patients, many of whom are not receiving guideline-mandated pharmacotherapy. Efforts to prevent VTE among hospitalized patients are improving but are not yet adequate.[133] Electronic systems can be improved to alert care providers about high-risk patients who are not receiving protective measures, and it is crucial to ensure that the prescribed medication orders are being adhered to by patients and care providers. However, more research is needed to identify the optimal medical patients who will benefit from extended VTE prophylaxis after hospital discharge.

REFERENCES

1. Glynn RJ, Danielson E, Fonseca FA, et al. A randomized trial of rosuvastatin in the prevention of venous thromboembolism. *N Engl J Med* 2009;360(18):1851-1861.
2. The surgeon general's call to action to prevent deep vein thrombosis and pulmonary embolism. 2008, U.S. Department of Health and Human Services. Available at www.surgeongeneral.gov/library/calls/deepvein. Accessed Oct 1, 2011.
3. Cushman M, Tsai AW, White RH, et al. Deep vein thrombosis and pulmonary embolism in two cohorts: the longitudinal investigation of thromboembolism etiology. *Am J Med* 2004;117(1):19-25.
4. Blanco-Molina A, Trujillo-Santos J, Tirado R, et al. Venous thromboembolism in women using hormonal contraceptives: findings from the RIETE Registry. *Thromb Haemost* 2009;101(3):478-482.
5. Hippisley-Cox J, Coupland C. Development and validation of risk prediction algorithm (QThrombosis) to estimate future risk of venous thromboembolism: prospective cohort study. *Br Med J* 2011;343:d4656.
6. Novacek G, Weltermann A, Sobala A, et al. Inflammatory bowel disease is a risk factor for recurrent venous thromboembolism. *Gastroenterology* 2010;139(3):779-787, 787.e1.
7. Folsom AR, Lutsey PL, Astor BC, Cushman M. C-reactive protein and venous thromboembolism: a prospective investigation in the ARIC cohort. *Thromb Haemost* 2009;102(4):615-619.

CH
38

PULMONARY EMBOLISM AND DEEP VEIN THROMBOSIS

8. Ageno W, Dentali F, Grandi AM. New evidence on the potential role of the metabolic syndrome as a risk factor for venous thromboembolism. *J Thromb Haemost* 2009;7(5): 736-738.

9. Severinsen MT, Kristensen SR, Johnsen SP, et al. Smoking and venous thromboembolism: a Danish follow-up study. *J Thromb Haemost* 2009;7(8):1297-1303.

10. Goldhaber SZ, Grodstein F, Stampfer MJ, et al. A prospective study of risk factors for pulmonary embolism in women. *JAMA* 1997;277(8):642-645.

11. Stein PD, Beemath A, Olson RE. Obesity as a risk factor in venous thromboembolism. *Am J Med* 2005;118(9):978-980.

12. Kabrhel C, Varraso R, Goldhaber SZ, Rimm E, Camargo CA Jr. Physical inactivity and idiopathic pulmonary embolism in women: prospective study. *Br Med J* 2011; 343:d3867.

13. Chandra D, Parisini E, Mozaffarian D. Meta-analysis: travel and risk for venous thromboembolism. *Ann Intern Med* 2009;151(3):180-190.

14. Tsoran I, Saharov G, Brenner B, et al. Prolonged travel and venous thromboembolism findings from the RIETE registry. *Thromb Res* 2010;126(4):287-291.

15. Tafur AJ, Kalsi H, Wysokinski WE, et al. The association of active cancer with venous thromboembolism location: a population-based study. *Mayo Clin Proc* 2011; 86(1):25-30.

16. Khorana AA, Kuderer NM, Culakova E, Lyman GH, Francis CW. Development and validation of a predictive model for chemotherapy-associated thrombosis. *Blood* 2008; 111(10):4902-4907.

17. Zoller B, Li X, Sundquist J, Sundquist K. Age- and gender-specific familial risks for venous thromboembolism: a nationwide epidemiological study based on hospitalizations in Sweden. *Circulation* 2011;124(9):1012-1020.

18. Dalen JE. Should patients with venous thromboembolism be screened for thrombophilia? *Am J Med* 2008;121(6):458-463.

19. Lijfering WM, Middeldorp S, Veeger NJ, et al. Risk of recurrent venous thrombosis in homozygous carriers and double heterozygous carriers of factor V Leiden and prothrombin G20210A. *Circulation* 2010;121(15):1706-1712.

20. Gallerani M, Imberti D, Ageno W, Dentali F, Manfredini R. Higher mortality rate in patients hospitalised for acute pulmonary embolism during weekends. *Thromb Haemost* 2011; 106(1):83-89.

21. Scannapieco G, Ageno W, Airoldi A, et al. Incidence and predictors of venous thromboembolism in post–acute care patients: a prospective cohort study. *Thromb Haemost* 2010;104(4):734-740.

22. Tapson VF. Acute pulmonary embolism. *N Engl J Med* 2008;358(10):1037-1052.

23. Maron BA, Shekar PS, Goldhaber SZ. Paradoxical embolism. *Circulation* 2010;122(19): 1968-1972.

24. Piazza G, Goldhaber SZ. Fibrinolysis for acute pulmonary embolism. *Vasc Med* 2010;15(5):419-428.

25. Kahn SR. The post thrombotic syndrome. *Thromb Res* 2011;127(Suppl 3):S89-S92.

26. Piazza G, Goldhaber SZ. Chronic thromboembolic pulmonary hypertension. *N Engl J Med* 2011;364(4):351-360.

27. Wells PS, Anderson DR, Bormanis J, et al. Value of assessment of pretest probability of deep-vein thrombosis in clinical management. *Lancet* 1997;350(9094):1795-1798.

28. Bounameaux H, Perrier A, Righini M. Diagnosis of venous thromboembolism: an update. *Vasc Med* 2010;15(5):399-406.

29. Wells PS, Anderson DR, Rodger M, et al. Derivation of a simple clinical model to categorize patients' probability of pulmonary embolism: increasing the model's utility with the SimpliRED D-dimer. *Thromb Haemost* 2000;83(3):416-420.

30. Le Gal G, Righini M, Roy PM, et al. Prediction of pulmonary embolism in the emergency department: the revised Geneva score. *Ann Intern Med* 2006;144(3):165-171.

31. Gibson NS, Sohne M, Kruip MJ, et al. Further validation and simplification of the Wells clinical decision rule in pulmonary embolism. *Thromb Haemost* 2008;99(1):229-234.

32. Douma RA, Mos IC, Erkens PM, et al. Performance of 4 clinical decision rules in the diagnostic management of acute pulmonary embolism: a prospective cohort study. *Ann Intern Med* 2011;154(11):709-718.

33. Righini M, Perrier A, De Moerloose P, Bounameaux H. D-Dimer for venous thromboembolism diagnosis: 20 years later. *J Thromb Haemost* 2008;6(7):1059-1071.

34. Hunsaker AR, Lu MT, Goldhaber SZ, Rybicki FJ. Imaging in acute pulmonary embolism with special clinical scenarios. *Circ Cardiovasc Imaging* 2010;3(4):491-500.

35. Hunsaker AR, Zou KH, Poh AC, et al. Routine pelvic and lower extremity CT venography in patients undergoing pulmonary CT angiography. *AJR Am J Roentgenol* 2008; 190(2):322-326.

36. Carrier M, Righini M, Wells PS, et al. Subsegmental pulmonary embolism diagnosed by computed tomography: incidence and clinical implications: a systematic review and meta-analysis of the management outcome studies. *J Thromb Haemost* 2010;8(8): 1716-1722.

37. Hurwitz LM, Yoshizumi TT, Goodman PC, et al. Radiation dose savings for adult pulmonary embolus 64-MDCT using bismuth breast shields, lower peak kilovoltage, and automatic tube current modulation. *AJR Am J Roentgenol* 2009;192(1):244-253.

38. Lu MT, Cai T, Ersoy H, et al. Interval increase in right-left ventricular diameter ratios at CT as a predictor of 30-day mortality after acute pulmonary embolism: initial experience. *Radiology* 2008;246(1):281-287.

39. Becattini C, Agnelli G, Vedovati MC, et al. Multidetector computed tomography for acute pulmonary embolism: diagnosis and risk stratification in a single test. *Eur Heart J* 2011;32(13):1657-1663.

40. Kang DK, Thilo C, Schoepf UJ, et al. CT signs of right ventricular dysfunction: prognostic role in acute pulmonary embolism. *JACC Cardiovasc Imaging* 2011;4(8):841-849.

41. Scridon T, Scridon C, Skali H, et al. Prognostic significance of troponin elevation and right ventricular enlargement in acute pulmonary embolism. *Am J Cardiol* 2005; 96(2):303-305.

42. Stein PD, Chenevert TL, Fowler SE, et al. Gadolinium-enhanced magnetic resonance angiography for pulmonary embolism: a multicenter prospective study (PIOPED III). *Ann Intern Med* 2010;152(7):434-443, W142-W143.

43. Agnelli G, Becattini C. Acute pulmonary embolism. *N Engl J Med* 2010;363(3):266-274.

44. Moores LK, King CS, Holley AB. Current approach to the diagnosis of acute nonmassive pulmonary embolism. *Chest* 2011;140(2):509-518.

45. Jaff MR, McMurtry MS, Archer SL, et al. Management of massive and submassive pulmonary embolism, iliofemoral deep vein thrombosis, and chronic thromboembolic pulmonary hypertension: a scientific statement from the American Heart Association. *Circulation* 2011;123(16):1788-1830.

46. Piazza G, Goldhaber SZ. Management of submassive pulmonary embolism. *Circulation* 2010;122(11):1124-1129.

47. Lankeit M, Friesen D, Aschoff J, et al. Highly sensitive troponin T assay in normotensive patients with acute pulmonary embolism. *Eur Heart J* 2010;31(15):1836-1844.

48. Lankeit M, Gomez V, Wagner C, et al. A strategy combining imaging and laboratory biomarkers in comparison to a simplified clinical score for risk stratification of patients with acute pulmonary embolism. *Chest* 2012;141(4):916-922.

49. Decousus H, Quere I, Presles E, et al. Superficial venous thrombosis and venous thromboembolism: a large, prospective epidemiologic study. *Ann Intern Med* 2010;152(4): 218-224.

50. Decousus H, Prandoni P, Mismetti P, et al. Fondaparinux for the treatment of superficial-vein thrombosis in the legs. *N Engl J Med* 2010;363(13):1222-1232.

51. Musani MH, Matta F, Yaekoub AY, et al. Venous compression for prevention of postthrombotic syndrome: a meta-analysis. *Am J Med* 2010;123(8):735-740.

52. Warkentin TE, Eikelboom JW. Who is (still) getting HIT? *Chest* 2007;131(6):1620-1622.

53. Baroletti S. Thrombosis in suspected heparin-induced thrombocytopenia occurs more often with high antibody levels. *Am J Med* 2012;125(1):44-49.

54. Warkentin TE. HIT paradigms and paradoxes. *J Thromb Haemost* 2011;9(Suppl 1):105-117.

55. Lee AY, Levine MN, Baker RI, et al. Low-molecular-weight heparin versus a coumarin for the prevention of recurrent venous thromboembolism in patients with cancer. *N Engl J Med* 2003;349(2):146-153.

56. Agnelli G, Verso M. Management of venous thromboembolism in patients with cancer. *J Thromb Haemost* 2011;9(Suppl 1):316-324.

57. Decousus H, Tapson VF, Bergmann JF, et al. Factors at admission associated with bleeding risk in medical patients: findings from the IMPROVE investigators. *Chest* 2011; 139(1):69-79.

58. Nieto JA, Solano R, Ruiz-Ribo MD, et al. Fatal bleeding in patients receiving anticoagulant therapy for venous thromboembolism: findings from the RIETE registry. *J Thromb Haemost* 2010;8(6):1216-1222.

59. Crowther MA, Garcia D, Ageno W, et al. Oral vitamin K effectively treats international normalised ratio (INR) values in excess of 10: results of a prospective cohort study. *Thromb Haemost* 2010;104(1):118-121.

60. Hughes GJ, Patel PN, Saxena N. Effect of acetaminophen on international normalized ratio in patients receiving warfarin therapy. *Pharmacotherapy* 2011;31(6):591-597.

61. Menendez-Jandula B, Souto JC, Oliver A, et al. Comparing self-management of oral anticoagulant therapy with clinic management: a randomized trial. *Ann Intern Med* 2005;142(1):1-10.

62. Matchar DB, Jacobson A, Dolor R, et al. Effect of home testing of international normalized ratio on clinical events. *N Engl J Med* 2010;363(17):1608-1620.

63. Schwarz UI, Ritchie MD, Bradford Y, et al. Genetic determinants of response to warfarin during initial anticoagulation. *N Engl J Med* 2008;358(10):999-1008.

64. Wadelius M, Chen LY, Lindh JD, et al. The largest prospective warfarin-treated cohort supports genetic forecasting. *Blood* 2009;113(4):784-792.

65. Klein TE, Altman RB, Eriksson N, et al. Estimation of the warfarin dose with clinical and pharmacogenetic data. *N Engl J Med* 2009;360(8):753-764.

66. Eckman MH, Rosand J, Greenberg SM, Gage BF. Cost-effectiveness of using pharmacogenetic information in warfarin dosing for patients with nonvalvular atrial fibrillation. *Ann Intern Med* 2009;150(2):73-83.

67. Anderson JL, Horne BD, Stevens SM, et al. Randomized trial of genotype-guided versus standard warfarin dosing in patients initiating oral anticoagulation. *Circulation* 2007;116(22):2563-2570.

68. Epstein RS, Moyer TP, Aubert RE, et al. Warfarin genotyping reduces hospitalization rates results from the MM-WES (Medco-Mayo Warfarin Effectiveness study). *J Am Coll Cardiol* 2010;55(25):2804-2812.

69. McBane RD, Wysokinski WE, Daniels PR, et al. Periprocedural anticoagulation management of patients with venous thromboembolism. *Arterioscler Thromb Vasc Biol* 2010; 30(3):442-448.

70. Schulman S, Kearon C, Kakkar AK, et al. Dabigatran versus warfarin in the treatment of acute venous thromboembolism. *N Engl J Med* 2009;361(24):2342-2352.

71. Bauersachs R, Berkowitz SD, Brenner B, et al. Oral rivaroxaban for symptomatic venous thromboembolism. *N Engl J Med* 2010;363(26):2499-2510.

72. Bauer KA. Recent progress in anticoagulant therapy: oral direct inhibitors of thrombin and factor Xa. *J Thromb Haemost* 2011;9(Suppl 1):12-19.

72a. The EINSTEIN Investigators. Oral rivaroxaban for symptomatic venous thromboembolism. *N Engl J Med* 2010;363:2499-2510.

73. Aujesky D, Roy PM, Verschuren F, et al. Outpatient versus inpatient treatment for patients with acute pulmonary embolism: an international, open-label, randomised, non-inferiority trial. *Lancet* 2011;378(9785):41-48.

74. Karthikesalingam A, Young EL, Hinchliffe RJ, et al. A systematic review of percutaneous mechanical thrombectomy in the treatment of deep venous thrombosis. *Eur J Vasc Endovasc Surg* 2011;41(4):554-565.

75. Kearon C, Kahn SR, Agnelli G, et al. Antithrombotic therapy for venous thromboembolic disease: American College of Chest Physicians Evidence-Based Clinical Practice Guidelines (8th edition). *Chest* 2008;133(6 Suppl):454S-545S.

76. The Steering Committee. Single-bolus tenecteplase plus heparin compared with heparin alone for normotensive patients with acute pulmonary embolism, who have evidence of right ventricular dysfunction and myocardial injury: rationale and design of the Pulmonary Embolism Thrombolysis (PEITHO) Trial. *Am Heart J* 2012;163(1):33-38.e1.

77. Kline JA, Steuerwald MT, Marchick MR, Hernandez-Nino J, Rose GA. Prospective evaluation of right ventricular function and functional status 6 months after acute submassive

pulmonary embolism: frequency of persistent or subsequent elevation in estimated pulmonary artery pressure. *Chest* 2009;136(5):1202-1210.

78. Fiumara K, Kucher N, Fanikos J, Goldhaber SZ. Predictors of major hemorrhage following fibrinolysis for acute pulmonary embolism. *Am J Cardiol* 2006;97(1):127-129.

79. Kuo WT, Gould MK, Louie JD, et al. Catheter-directed therapy for the treatment of massive pulmonary embolism: systematic review and meta-analysis of modern techniques. *J Vasc Interv Radiol* 2009;20(11):1431-1440.

80. Engelhardt TC, Taylor AJ, Simprini LA, Kucher N. Catheter-directed ultrasound-accelerated thrombolysis for the treatment of acute pulmonary embolism. *Thromb Res* 2011;128(2):149-154.

81. Aklog L, Williams CS, Byrne JG, Goldhaber SZ. Acute pulmonary embolectomy: a contemporary approach. *Circulation* 2002;105(12):1416-1419.

82. Stein PD, Alnas M, Beemath A, Patel NR. Outcome of pulmonary embolectomy. *Am J Cardiol* 2007;99(3):421-423.

83. Fukuda I, Taniguchi S, Fukui K, et al. Improved outcome of surgical pulmonary embolectomy by aggressive intervention for critically ill patients. *Ann Thorac Surg* 2011;91(3):728-732.

84. Goldhaber SZ, Piazza G. Optimal duration of anticoagulation after venous thromboembolism. *Circulation* 2011;123(6):664-667.

85. Reference deleted in proofs.

86. Douketis J, Tosetto A, Marcucci M, et al. Patient-level meta-analysis: effect of measurement timing, threshold, and patient age on ability of D-dimer testing to assess recurrence risk after unprovoked venous thromboembolism. *Ann Intern Med* 2010;153(8):523-531.

87. Kearon C, Ginsberg JS, Kovacs MJ, et al. Comparison of low-intensity warfarin therapy with conventional-intensity warfarin therapy for long-term prevention of recurrent venous thromboembolism. *N Engl J Med* 2003;349(7):631-639.

88. Ridker PM, Goldhaber SZ, Danielson E, et al. Long-term, low-intensity warfarin therapy for the prevention of recurrent venous thromboembolism. *N Engl J Med* 2003;348(15):1425-1434.

89. Nicholson W, Nicholson WJ, Tolerico P, et al. Prevalence of fracture and fragment embolization of Bard retrievable vena cava filters and clinical implications including cardiac perforation and tamponade. *Arch Intern Med* 2010;170(20):1827-1831.

89a. Stan DD, Matta F, Hull RD. Increasing use of vena cava filters for prevention of pulmonary embolism. *Am J Med* 2011;124:655-661.

89b. Jariva M, Younas F, Moinuddin I, et al. Outcomes with retrievable inferior vena cava filters. *J Invasive Cardiol* 2010;28:235-239.

90. Inferior Vena Cava (IVC) Filters: Initial Communication. Risk of Adverse Events with Long Term Use. Posted 8/9/2010. Available at www.fda.gov/Safety/MedWatch/SafetyInformation/SafetyAlertsforHumanMedicalProducts/ucm221707.htm. Accessed Oct 1, 2011.

91. Prevention of fatal postoperative pulmonary embolism by low doses of heparin: an international multicentre trial. *Lancet* 1975;2(7924):45-51.

92. Cohen AT, Davidson BL, Gallus AS, et al. Efficacy and safety of fondaparinux for the prevention of venous thromboembolism in older acute medical patients: randomised placebo controlled trial. *Br Med J* 2006;332(7537):325-329.

93. Leizorovicz A, Cohen AT, Turpie AG, et al. Randomized, placebo-controlled trial of dalteparin for the prevention of venous thromboembolism in acutely ill medical patients. *Circulation* 2004;110(7):874-879.

94. Samama MM, Cohen AT, Darmon JY, et al; Prophylaxis in Medical Patients with Enoxaparin Study Group. A comparison of enoxaparin with placebo for the prevention of venous thromboembolism in acutely ill medical patients. *N Engl J Med* 1999;341(11):793-800.

95. Collins R, Scrimgeour A, Yusuf S, Peto R. Reduction in fatal pulmonary embolism and venous thrombosis by perioperative administration of subcutaneous heparin: overview of results of randomized trials in general, orthopedic, and urologic surgery. *N Engl J Med* 1988;318(18):1162-1173.

96. Kakkar AK, Cimminiello C, Goldhaber SZ, et al. Low-molecular-weight heparin and mortality in acutely ill medical patients. *N Engl J Med* 2012;565:2463-2472.

97. Geerts WH, Bergqvist D, Pineo GF, et al. Prevention of venous thromboembolism: American College of Chest Physicians evidence-based clinical practice guidelines (8th edition). *Chest* 2008;133(6 Suppl):381S-453S.

98. Anderson FA Jr, Zayaruzny M, Heit JA, Fidan D, Cohen AT. Estimated annual numbers of US acute-care hospital patients at risk for venous thromboembolism. *Am J Hematol* 2007;82(9):777-782.

99. Piazza G, Fanikos J, Zayaruzny M, Goldhaber SZ. Venous thromboembolic events in hospitalised medical patients. *Thromb Haemost* 2009;102(3):505-510.

100. Fanikos J, Piazza G, Zayaruzny M, Goldhaber SZ. Long-term complications of medical patients with hospital-acquired venous thromboembolism. *Thromb Haemost* 2009;102(4):688-693.

101. Laporte S, Liotier J, Bertoletti L, et al. Individual patient data meta-analysis of enoxaparin vs. unfractionated heparin for venous thromboembolism prevention in medical patients. *J Thromb Haemost* 2011;9(3):464-472.

102. Dentali F, Douketis JD, Gianni M, Lim W, Crowther MA. Meta-analysis: anticoagulant prophylaxis to prevent symptomatic venous thromboembolism in hospitalized medical patients. *Ann Intern Med* 2007;146(4):278-288.

103. Fanikos J, Stevens LA, Labreche M, et al. Adherence to pharmacological thromboprophylaxis orders in hospitalized patients. *Am J Med* 2010;123(6):536-541.

104. Piazza G, Nguyen TN, Morrison R, et al. Patient education program for venous thromboembolism prevention in hospitalized patients. *Am J Med* 2012;125(3):258-264.

105. Cohen AT, Tapson VF, Bergmann JF, et al. Venous thromboembolism risk and prophylaxis in the acute hospital care setting (ENDORSE study): a multinational cross-sectional study. *Lancet* 2008;371(9610):387-394.

106. Piazza G, Goldhaber SZ. Improving clinical effectiveness in thromboprophylaxis for hospitalized medical patients. *Am J Med* 2009;122(3):230-232.

107. Anderson FA Jr, Goldhaber SZ, Tapson VF, et al. Improving practices in US hospitals to prevent venous thromboembolism: lessons from ENDORSE. *Am J Med* 2010;123(12):1099-1106, e8.

108. Agnelli G, Gussoni G, Bianchini C, et al. Nadroparin for the prevention of thromboembolic events in ambulatory patients with metastatic or locally advanced solid cancer receiving chemotherapy: a randomised, placebo-controlled, double-blind study. *Lancet Oncol* 2009;10(10):943-949.

109. Agnelli G, George DJ, Kakkar AK, et al. Semuloparin for thromboprophylaxis in patients receiving chemotherapy for cancer. *N Engl J med* 2012;366:601-609.

110. Piazza G, Goldhaber SZ. Computerized decision support for the cardiovascular clinician: applications for venous thromboembolism prevention and beyond. *Circulation* 2009;120(12):1133-1137.

111. Fiumara K, Piovella C, Hurwitz S, et al. Multi-screen electronic alerts to augment venous thromboembolism prophylaxis. *Thromb Haemost* 2010;103(2):312-317.

112. Lecumberri R, Marques M, Diaz-Navarlaz MT, et al. Maintained effectiveness of an electronic alert system to prevent venous thromboembolism among hospitalized patients. *Thromb Haemost* 2008;100(4):699-704.

113. Lecumberri R, Panizo E, Gomez-Guiu A, et al. Economic impact of an electronic alert system to prevent venous thromboembolism in hospitalised patients. *J Thromb Haemost* 2011;9(6):1108-1115.

114. Piazza G, Rosenbaum EJ, Pendergast W, et al. Physician alerts to prevent symptomatic venous thromboembolism in hospitalized patients. *Circulation* 2009;119(16):2196-2201.

115. Eikelboom JW, Karthikeyan G, Fagel N, Hirsh J. American Association of Orthopedic Surgeons and American College of Chest Physicians guidelines for venous thromboembolism prevention in hip and knee arthroplasty differ: what are the implications for clinicians and patients? *Chest* 2009;135(2):513-520.

116. Guideline on Preventing Venous Thromboembolic Disease in Patients Undergoing Elective Hip and Knee Arthroplasty. Available at www.aaos.org/research/guidelines/VTE/VTE_guideline.asp. Accessed Oct 1, 2011.

117. Prevention of pulmonary embolism and deep vein thrombosis with low dose aspirin: Pulmonary Embolism Prevention (PEP) trial. *Lancet* 2000;355(9212):1295-1302.

118. Eriksson BI, Borris LC, Friedman RJ, et al. Rivaroxaban versus enoxaparin for thromboprophylaxis after hip arthroplasty. *N Engl J Med* 2008;358(26):2765-2775.

119. Kakkar AK, Brenner B, Dahl OE, et al. Extended duration rivaroxaban versus short-term enoxaparin for the prevention of venous thromboembolism after total hip arthroplasty: a double-blind, randomised controlled trial. *Lancet* 2008;372(9632):31-39.

120. Lassen MR, Ageno W, Borris LC, et al. Rivaroxaban versus enoxaparin for thromboprophylaxis after total knee arthroplasty. *N Engl J Med* 2008;358(26):2776-2786.

121. Turpie AG, Lassen MR, Davidson BL, et al. Rivaroxaban versus enoxaparin for thromboprophylaxis after total knee arthroplasty (RECORD4): a randomised trial. *Lancet* 2009;373(9676):1673-1680.

122. Lassen MR, Gallus A, Raskob GE, et al. Apixaban versus enoxaparin for thromboprophylaxis after hip replacement. *N Engl J Med* 2010;363(26):2487-2498.

123. Lassen MR, Raskob GE, Gallus A, et al. Apixaban versus enoxaparin for thromboprophylaxis after knee replacement (ADVANCE-2): a randomised double-blind trial. *Lancet* 2010;375(9717):807-815.

124. Nicolaides A, Goldhaber SZ, Maxwell GL, et al. Cost benefit of intermittent pneumatic compression for venous thromboembolism prophylaxis in general surgery. *Int Angiol* 2008;27(6):500-506.

125. Dennis M, Sandercock PA, Reid J, et al. Effectiveness of thigh-length graduated compression stockings to reduce the risk of deep vein thrombosis after stroke (CLOTS trial 1): a multicentre, randomised controlled trial. *Lancet* 2009;373(9679):1958-1965.

126. Turpie AG, Bauer KA, Caprini JA, et al. Fondaparinux combined with intermittent pneumatic compression vs. intermittent pneumatic compression alone for prevention of venous thromboembolism after abdominal surgery: a randomized, double-blind comparison. *J Thromb Haemost* 2007;5(9):1854-1861.

127. Glynn RJ, Ridker PM, Goldhaber SZ, Zee RY, Buring JE. Effects of random allocation to vitamin E supplementation on the occurrence of venous thromboembolism: report from the Women's Health Study. *Circulation* 2007;116(13):1497-1503.

128. Bergqvist D, Agnelli G, Cohen AT, et al. Duration of prophylaxis against venous thromboembolism with enoxaparin after surgery for cancer. *N Engl J Med* 2002;346(13):975-980.

129. Bergqvist D, Benoni G, Björgell O, et al. Low-molecular-weight heparin (enoxaparin) as prophylaxis against venous thromboembolism after total hip replacement. *N Engl J Med* 1996;335(10):696-700.

130. Hull RD, Schellong SM, Tapson VF, et al. Extended-duration venous thromboembolism prophylaxis in acutely ill medical patients with recently reduced mobility: a randomized trial. *Ann Intern Med* 2010;153(1):8-18.

131. Spyropoulos AC, Anderson FA Jr, Fitzgerald G, et al. Predictive and associative models to identify hospitalized medical patients at risk for VTE. *Chest* 2011;140(3):706-714.

132. Barbar S, Noventa F, Rossetto V, et al. A risk assessment model for the identification of hospitalized medical patients at risk for venous thromboembolism: the Padua Prediction Score. *J Thromb Haemost* 2010;8(11):2450-2457.

133. Stein PD, Matta F, Dalen JE. Is the campaign to prevent VTE in hospitalized patients working? *Chest* 2011;139(6):1317-1321.

CHAPTER 39

Treatment of Pulmonary Arterial Hypertension

Alexander R. Opotowsky and Michael J. Landzberg

CURRENT STATE OF DIAGNOSIS, 596

EPIDEMIOLOGIC ASSOCIATIONS, 596

CURRENT PATHOBIOLOGIC PARADIGM OF PULMONARY ARTERIAL HYPERTENSION, 596

DIAGNOSIS AND RISK STRATIFICATION, 596

CURRENT STATE OF THERAPY, 599

Prostanoids, 599
Endothelin Receptor Antagonism, 601
Phosphodiesterase Inhibition, 601
Atrial Septostomy, 602
Transplantation for Idiopathic Pulmonary Arterial Hypertension, 602

MEDICAL THERAPY ALGORITHMS, 602

NEW PATHOBIOLOGIC AND CARE PARADIGMS, 604

PREGNANCY AND CONTRACEPTION, 604

REFERENCES, 604

Current State of Diagnosis

The previous classification of "primary" pulmonary hypertension (PPH), or pulmonary hypertension of unknown etiology, used in earlier editions of this text covered a relatively small percentage of pulmonary hypertensive disorders. A newer classification of *pulmonary arterial hypertension* (PAH)—either familial, occurring in approximately 6% of PAH cases, or sporadic, nonfamilial *idiopathic pulmonary arterial hypertension* (iPAH)—has expanded the clinical entity to include various disorders that share common physiologic, hemodynamic, pathologic, and anatomic features. Similarities among these syndromes have been sufficient to allow standardized study populations for testing mechanisms of disease and the application of therapeutics.

PAH describes a small subset of all cases of *pulmonary hypertension* (PH), defined as a mean pulmonary artery (PA) pressure of 25 mm Hg or greater. Other more common causes with distinct physiology include PH as a result of left heart disease and PH associated with parenchymal lung disease and hypoxemia (Table 39-1). Treatment for PH in that situation is usually focused on the underlying cause, although research is ongoing to determine whether pulmonary vasodilators may also be beneficial in those populations. Treatment of these diseases is not discussed in detail in this chapter.

Epidemiologic Associations

Multicenter registries established from 1981 through the present[1,2] have reported the incidence of iPAH in the United States and Europe to be 1 to 2 million per year. A number of established exposures or concomitant conditions are associated with PAH (Box 39-1). Among the more important of these are scleroderma, especially of the limited type (CREST syndrome: calcinosis, Raynaud phenomenon, esophageal involvement, sclerodactyly, and telangiectasia), with estimated prevalence of PAH at 12% to 14%; human immunodeficiency virus (HIV), with an estimated cumulative incidence of 0.5%; and portal hypertension, with estimated prevalence between 0.25% and 2%.[3-5] An association with female gender, typically 2:1 prevalence or greater, remains unexplained and is true for iPAH and PAH associated with many other triggers. The tremendous differences in therapy and outcomes for patients with severe pulmonary hypertension associated with valvular or myopathic heart disease or proximal or distal chronic thromboembolic disease (i.e., non-PAH pulmonary hypertension) mandate a thorough search for treatable secondary etiologies (see Table 39-1).

Analyses of epidemiologic databases have suggested similar survival of untreated patients with severe PAH regardless of etiology. Median survival between 2.8 and 3.4 years has been reported for the affected adult patient (Figure 39-1). Survival correlates with variables relating to right ventricular (RV) function—typically assessed by hemodynamic measures of systemic cardiac output, mixed venous oxygen saturation, and right atrial pressure—and physical capacity, measured by 6-minute walk distance.[6] A notable exception is Eisenmenger syndrome, in which 10-year survival rates range from 58% to 80%, depending on patient age at the time of diagnosis.[7] The reasons for the greater survival seen in those with severe PAH associated with Eisenmenger syndrome or shunt-related pulmonary hypertension with associated cyanosis are unclear, but evidence suggests that increased pulmonary afterload is better tolerated when it is shared between right and left heart chambers.

Current Pathobiologic Paradigm of Pulmonary Arterial Hypertension

An important concept in the pathophysiology of PAH is that exposure to specific triggers in an individual with an underlying genetic predisposition initiates a cascade of events that lead to the development of PAH. Although various potential triggers have been identified, current understanding of the vascular biology of this disease continues to hold that abnormalities of the pulmonary vascular endothelium are central to the pathophysiologic process. Endothelial injury may initiate a cascade that includes endothelial dysfunction, growth factor and cytokine imbalance, coagulation abnormalities, and platelet-endothelial cell-leukocyte imbalances. Imbalance of vasomodulators that include mitogens, vasoconstrictors, and vasodilators such as endothelin, prostacyclin, and nitric oxide and their controlling substances contributes to inflammation (Figure 39-2). These, in turn, lead to pulmonary vasoconstriction, vascular smooth muscle cell proliferation, thrombosis in situ, and further vascular injury.

Diagnosis and Risk Stratification

People with PAH typically come to medical attention either because of symptoms such as dyspnea, angina, chest fullness or pain, bloating, volume retention, or syncope; through incidental discovery during evaluation for other disease; or during screening for PAH among families or patients with identified risks. Typically, diagnosis may be suggested by evidence on physical examination of RV failure or a loud pulmonary component of the second heart sound. Transthoracic echocardiography (TTE) plays a major role in confirming clinical findings and is an important screening tool in high-risk groups such as those with cirrhosis or scleroderma. RV and PA pressures ascertained by measure of Doppler-based tricuspid velocities are often used as the sole indicator of PH, but echocardiography provides an array of other parameters that should be included in any assessment of patients with suspected PH or PAH. These include markers of RV dilation or dysfunction, such as low tricuspid annular plane systolic excursion; markers

TABLE 39-1	Causes of Secondary PH and Potential Studies to Elucidate the Diagnosis
SECONDARY CAUSES OF PH	**POSSIBLE DIAGNOSTIC STUDIES**
Chronic thromboembolic PH	V/Q scan, CT, or direct angiography
Pulmonary vein obstruction	MRI, CT, catheterization
Congenital heart disease	Echocardiography, MRI
Left atrial hypertension	Echocardiography, BNP, invasive hemodynamic measurements
Pulmonary airway disease	PFTs, arterial blood gas measurement
Hypoventilation	Sleep apnea testing
Interstitial lung disease	PFTs, arterial blood gas measurement, chest CT
Rheumatologic disease	Serology, tissue biopsy, chest CT
Cirrhosis of the liver	LFTs, ultrasound, CT, biopsy
Peripheral pulmonary stenosis	V/Q scan, angiography, MRI
Hemoglobinopathies	CBC and smear, electrophoresis

BNP, brain natriuretic peptide; CBC, complete blood count; CT, computed tomography; LFT, liver function test; MRI, magnetic resonance imaging; PFT, pulmonary function test; PH, pulmonary hypertension; V/Q, ventilation/perfusion.

Box 39-1 Exposures and Conditions Associated with Pulmonary Arterial Hypertension

Stimulants
Anorexigens (dexedrine, aminorex, fenfluramine)
Catecholamines (cocaine, pheochromocytoma)
Portal hypertension/cirrhosis
Connective tissue diseases (scleroderma, mixed connective tissue disease, systemic lupus, rheumatoid arthritis)
Infection (HIV, schistosomiasis)
Large-volume or high-pressure intracardiac or intravascular shunting
Myeloproliferative disorders
Sickle cell disease, hemoglobinopathies, and platelet diseases
Toxin ingestion (e.g., L-tryptophan, toxic oil)

of increased pulmonary vascular resistance, such as rapid acceleration time or mid-systolic notching of the right ventricular outflow tract (RVOT) pulse wave Doppler envelope; or indirect markers of increased RV afterload, such as systolic flattening of the ventricular septum.[8] Although echocardiography does reliably assess systolic ventricular function, it can only estimate pressures and diastolic cardiac function. Thus, confirmatory testing relies on hemodynamic assessment at cardiac catheterization. Typically, this includes measurement of right- and left-sided pressures, flow, and resistance, which assists in diagnosis and prognostic assessment; limited angiography may also be indicated. Hemodynamic testing should include maneuvers to test reactivity of pulmonary flow and resistance to acute administration of pulmonary vasodilator agents. Reactivity of the pulmonary arterial bed is typically tested by inhalation of nitric oxide with or without oxygen, inhalation or intravenous (IV) administration of specific prostanoids, or IV administration of acetylcholine or adenosine. Catheterization should be performed in regional specialty centers to decrease associated risk and improve reliability of diagnosis and testing. In general, a catheter-based measure of mean PA pressure over 25 mm Hg (or systolic PA pressure more than one-third to one-half systemic levels) defines pulmonary hypertension. The clinical significance of exercise-induced PH remains less well defined but is suggested when mean PA pressure rises to more than 30 mm Hg on exertion.

Response to acute administration of pulmonary vasodilator therapy has classically been described as a decrease of 20% or more in mean PA pressure with stability or improvement in pulmonary blood flow, but various definitions are used in clinical practice. Such a response is observed in 10% to 20% of tested patients, potentially reflecting a subset of patients with an earlier, or less lethal, phase of disease. A positive vasodilator response was initially believed to correlate with improved functional and survival outcomes in response to therapy with calcium channel blockers (CCBs).[9] Recent data suggest a weaker predictive value of the cutoff of a 20% reduction in PA pressure, which has led to the suggestion of adding an absolute fall of mean PA pressure to 40 mm Hg or less to classify a responder. This more stringent definition of response enhances prediction of improvement with CCB therapy.[10] In the past, acute vasodilator responsiveness was

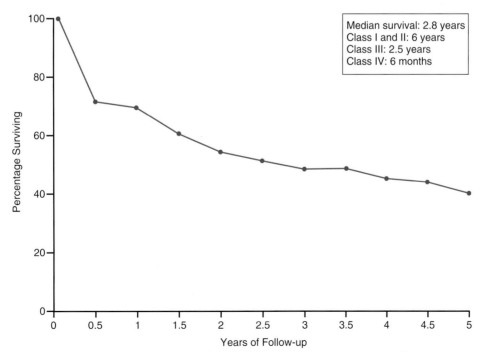

Median survival: 2.8 years
Class I and II: 6 years
Class III: 2.5 years
Class IV: 6 months

FIGURE 39-1 Untreated survival rates (by World Health Organization functional class) with severe pulmonary arterial hypertension. *(Modified from D'Alonzo GE, Barst RJ, Ayres SM. Survival in patients with PPH: results from a National Prospective Registry. Ann Intern Med 1991;115:343-349.)*

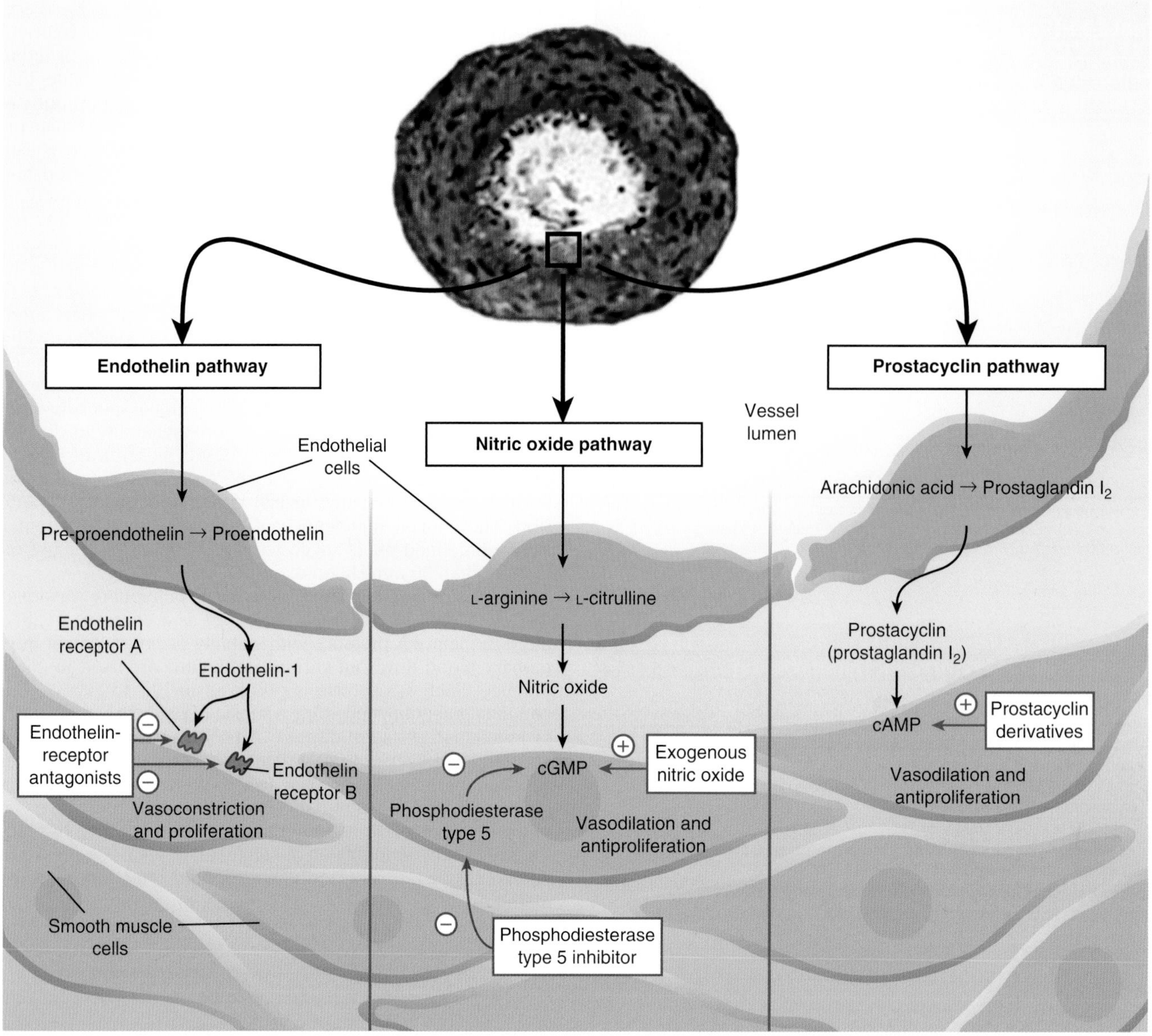

FIGURE 39-2 Current vascular inflammation and constriction model of idiopathic pulmonary arterial hypertension. cAMP, cyclic adenosine monophosphate; cGMP, cyclic guanosine monophosphate. *(From Humbert M, Sitbon O, Simmoneau G. Treatment of pulmonary arterial hypertension. N Engl J Med 2004;14:1425-1436.)*

critical to risk stratification and choice of therapy, and it still carries significance for both aspects of care. However, favorable long-term effects on PA pressure, functional capacity, and survival have been documented with newer agents—such as prostanoids, endothelin antagonists, and phosphodiesterase (PDE)-5 inhibitors—among patients who do not demonstrate acute vasodilator responsiveness, which raises new hope for such patients.

Accurate differential diagnosis and identification of treatable etiologies for PAH mandate additional patient testing dictated by particular clinical scenarios. Pulmonary disease should be evaluated with chest radiography; pulmonary function testing that includes a measure of diffusion capacity; high-resolution chest computed tomography (CT) scan, typically with angiography and pulmonary embolism protocol; or a ventilation/perfusion (V/Q) scan. Additional tests should include serologic testing for autoimmune connective tissue disease, liver and renal function measurements, complete blood count (CBC) assessment, and HIV testing when appropriate. Abdominal ultrasound, with or without flow assessment in the portal veins; liver-spleen scintigraphy; and sleep testing may also be needed to complete the evaluation (see Table 39-1). Such testing may suggest disease-specific

therapies that include oxygen administration, positive airway pressure ventilation, alternative organ therapy or transplantation, surgical pulmonary endarterectomy,[11] and balloon pulmonary angioplasty.[12,13]

Functional capacity is assessed by a formal measure of 6-minute walking capacity or cardiopulmonary exercise testing with a measure of maximal oxygen consumption[14] and has become a routine prognostic tool, both for initial survival prediction and to predict response to therapy. The 6-minute walk test is also a convenient way to follow changes in functional capacity over time. Subjective assessment of functional capacity using the New York Hospital Association (NYHA) classification or the modified World Health Organization (WHO) functional classification (Box-39-2) correlates with outcomes in both untreated and treated patients and has been used to define populations in randomized, controlled trials (RCTs).[15] Dyspnea (Borg) scales have been used in RCTs, although their individual additive prognostic potential remains unclear. Serologic testing of biomarkers, including troponins and natriuretic peptides, remains under investigation but appears to reflect disease severity and prognosis, as it does in heart failure and other conditions.

> **Box 39-2 World Health Organization Functional Classification of Pulmonary Hypertension**
>
> Class I: Patients with pulmonary hypertension but without resulting limitation of physical activity. Ordinary physical activity does not cause undue dyspnea or fatigue, chest pain, or near syncope.
>
> Class II: Patients with pulmonary hypertension that results in slight limitation of physical activity. They are comfortable at rest, but ordinary physical activity causes undue dyspnea or fatigue, chest pain, or near syncope.
>
> Class III: Patients with pulmonary hypertension that results in marked limitation of physical activity. They are comfortable at rest, but less than ordinary activity causes undue dyspnea or fatigue, chest pain, or near syncope.
>
> Class IV: Patients with pulmonary hypertension that leaves them unable to carry out any physical activity without symptoms. These patients manifest signs of right heart failure, and dyspnea and/or fatigue may even be present at rest. Discomfort is increased by any physical activity.

Current State of Therapy

CCBs were the first widely accepted therapeutic agents for patients with PAH. Their use was predicated on the vasoconstrictor model of PAH, envisioning PAH being due in large part to dysregulation of vasoconstriction in small pulmonary arteries and characterized by lamellar intimal fibrosis, medial hypertrophy, and neovascular plexiform lesions. To date, no randomized comparison trial has tested the effect and risk of different types of CCBs, although nifedipine has remained the prototype therapy for the small percentage of patients who are responders to acute administration of vasodilator agents during cardiac catheterization. The clinical effect typically requires drug doses much higher than those commonly used to treat systemic arterial hypertension. Such dosage requirements are unpredictable and may be accompanied by considerable adverse effects. Dose-response testing is therefore typically performed with indwelling PA pressure monitoring to identify eventual effective target dosage. Most centers recommend achieving this target dose in a graded fashion to minimize adverse effects as the systemic vasculature accommodates to the drug effect. More recent, uncontrolled databases suggest that CCBs may be even less effective than previously thought,[10] which may require a change to a more stringent definition of "acute vasodilator responsiveness" to better define the population in whom this class of medication will be effective. With the advent of several classes of oral selective pulmonary vasodilators, the role of isolated CCB therapy is unclear, and their clinical use varies widely. CCB therapy can have a negative inotropic effect and is generally believed to be contraindicated in patients who come to medical attention with substantial right atrial pressure elevation or a marked decrease in cardiac output given their potential.

The benefit of what is referred to as *conventional PAH therapy*— including warfarin, oxygen, digoxin, and diuretics—is unclear. Warfarin's benefit has been extrapolated from subset analyses of retrospective single-center studies and is based on pathologic data from lung biopsies and postmortem examinations that confirm thrombosis in situ within the pulmonary vasculature. Warfarin therapy is generally advised, with a target international normalized ratio (INR) of 2.0 to 3.0, depending on individual patient risk of bleeding. Recent multicenter RCTs of other therapeutic agents for PAH have noted the use of oral anticoagulants at the time of inclusion in 51% to 86% of enrolled patients.

Short-term administration of digoxin has beneficial hemodynamic effects in PAH.[16] However, long-term digoxin administration for patients with right heart dysfunction as a result of PAH has not been studied. The use of short-term digoxin therapy in this scenario has been declining; digoxin administration at the time of inclusion in recent multicenter RCTs was noted in 18% to 53% of subjects. Diuretic therapy, which may assist in volume control, is likewise unstudied in the chronic state. Its use has been documented in

49% to 70% of patients during recent multicenter RCTs of other therapies for PAH. Use of oxygen is unsupported, other than that defined for appropriate patients with chronic lung disease and hypoxemia.

Over the past decade, the vasoconstriction monolayer model of PAH has been replaced with the vascular wall inflammation paradigm discussed earlier, along with several other mechanisms of initial injury and progression of disease. The introduction of novel therapies reflects this change in thought regarding the pathobiology of this disease. For the majority of affected patients, modern treatment focuses on mediators of chemotaxis, cellular proliferation, and differentiation and regulation of vasoactive peptides and growth factors. These mediators currently include prostanoids (IV, inhaled, and oral), endothelin antagonists, and PDE inhibitors.

Prostanoids

The earliest multicenter randomized clinical trials focused on use of IV prostacyclin (epoprostenol). Patients treated with epoprostenol and conventional therapy showed improved survival and better exercise tolerance, increased cardiac output, and decreased pulmonary vascular resistance compared with controls treated with conventional therapy alone.[17] These results have been confirmed both in patients with iPAH and in those with PAH associated with scleroderma, and longer term benefit was demonstrated in multiple subsequent studies (Figure 39-3).[18] However, the personal and financial costs of epoprostenol use are protean, necessitating continuous administration via a commercially available personal pump attached by tubing to a centrally placed, indwelling venous catheter and daily personal admixture of the drug. Common drug side effects include flushing, headache, peculiar jaw pain with the first bite of each meal, bone and muscle pain, local and systemic infection, nausea, diarrhea, hypotension, tachyphylaxis, and potentially life-threatening rebound PH upon drug withdrawal. Typical dosing begins at 0.5 to 2.0 ng/kg/min, with adjustments based on effect and tachyphylaxis, typically every 3 to 10 days although often with more rapid titration upon initiation. Eventual plateauing of the dose may occur, without need for dosage augmentation. Periodic invasive hemodynamic assessment is required to ensure adequacy of dosage and avoidance of overdose. This medication is currently approved by the U.S. Food and Drug Administration (FDA) for PAH patients in WHO functional class III or IV. Pharmaceutical cost ranges from approximately $33,000 to $75,000 annually, and drug benefit is limited, with improved 6-minute walk distance of 20 to 30 meters and extension of survival to 63% at 3 years. Predictors of survival at the start of therapy have included functional class (poor prognosis if initial 6-minute walk <250 m), cardiac index, mean right atrial pressure (poor prognosis if ≥12 mm Hg), and mean PA pressure; predictors of survival after 1 year of therapy include improvement in cardiac index and decrease in right atrial pressure.

Multicenter randomized clinical trials, all of which have required right heart catheterization for entry, have shown favorable effects for other prostanoids. The treprostinil study evaluated subcutaneous (SC) administration of a tricyclic benzidine analogue of prostacyclin.[19] This 12-week, double-blind RCT included 470 patients (81% women) with a mean age of 44 years and diverse etiology of PAH: 271 patients had iPAH, 90 had connective tissue disease, and 109 had congenital heart disease. Functional capacity was WHO functional class II in 12% of patients, class III in 81%, and class IV in 7%, with a mean baseline 6-minute walk distance of 327 meters. Study drug was started at 1.25 ng/kg/min with weekly dosage increases. Endpoints included improvement in 6-minute walking distance and hemodynamic parameters. At the trial's conclusion, there was only a 10-meter difference in 6-minute walk distance between the study groups. However, this difference increased as final tolerated drug dosage increased, with a 36.1 ± 10 meter increase when study drug dosage was more than 13.8 ng/kg/min. Benefits persisted at 18 months of therapy, with

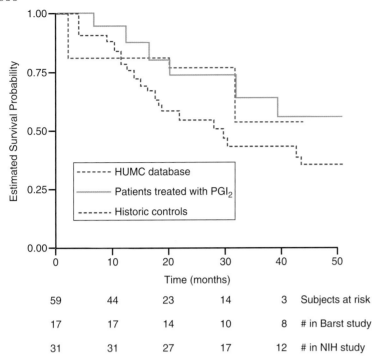

Time (months)

59	44	23	14	3	Subjects at risk
17	17	14	10	8	# in Barst study
31	31	27	17	12	# in NIH study

FIGURE 39-3 Survival in severe pulmonary arterial hypertension treatment with epoprostenol. HUMC, Hackensack University Medical Center; NIH, National Institutes of Health; PGI₂, prostacyclin. (*Modified from Shapiro SM, Oudiz RJ, Cao T, et al. Primary pulmonary hypertension: improved long-term effects and survival with continuous intravenous epoprostenol infusion. J Am Coll Cardiol 1997;30:343-349.*)

the most common side effect being pain at the infusion site. Other side effects were similar to those seen for epoprostenol. Further studies have demonstrated that IV treprostinil (Remodulin) is also effective in improving 6-minute walk distance.[20] This medication (both IV and SC) is currently FDA approved for patients with PAH and in WHO functional class of II to IV "to diminish symptoms associated with exercise." It has the benefit of being a more stable compound that requires a smaller mechanical pump with less demanding storage requirements and, as noted earlier, can be administered subcutaneously. Local injection site pain has been frequent, although various strategies have been designed to reduce this side effect. The cost of annual therapy has been estimated at $93,000.

The Arterial Pulmonary Hypertension and Beraprost European Trial (ALPHABET) evaluated beraprost, an oral prostacyclin analog.[21] This 12-week, double-blind RCT enrolled 130 patients with a mean age of 45 years. Women made up 62% of this group, and the causes of PAH were again diverse: 63 patients had iPAH, 13 had connective tissue disease, 24 had congenital heart disease, 21 had portal hypertension, and 9 were HIV positive. Functional capacity at enrollment included those in WHO functional class II (50%) and III (50%), with a mean baseline 6-minute walk of 373 meters. Study drug was started at a dose of 20 µg administered orally four times a day with weekly dosage increases. The maximal and median daily doses of beraprost were 480 µg and 320 µg, respectively. The endpoints measured at 12 weeks included the 6-minute walk distance, hemodynamic parameters, and Borg dyspnea index. At the end of the trial, there was nearly a 30-meter difference in 6-minute walk distance between the study groups. This difference was more pronounced in patients with iPAH compared with those with other types of PAH. Continued drug benefit after 1 year of therapy was lost in a subsequent trial, and this agent is currently not FDA approved for use in PAH.[22]

The Aerosolized Iloprost Randomized (AIR) study investigated iloprost, an inhaled prostacyclin analogue.[23] This was a double-blind randomized trial, with enrollment based on baseline 6-minute walk (mean distance, 323 m). The study drug was started at 2.5 to 5.0 µg inhaled six to nine times a day with overnight breaks and dosage adjustments over the first 8 days. The combined endpoint assessed at 12 weeks was defined as 10% improvement of 6-minute walk distance and improved WHO

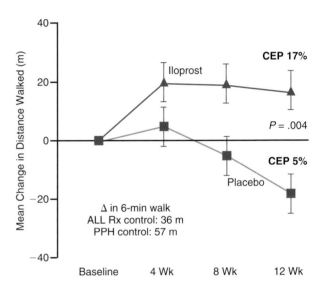

FIGURE 39-4 Functional capacity in severe pulmonary arterial hypertension: treatment with iloprost. CEP, combined endpoint; PPH, primary pulmonary hypertension; Rx, medication. (*Modified from Olschewski H, Simonneau G, Galie N, et al. Inhaled iloprost in severe pulmonary hypertension. N Engl J Med 2002;347:322-329.*)

functional class, hemodynamic parameters, Borg dyspnea score, and quality of life (QOL). Among the 203 patients who were enrolled, 67% were women, 102 had iPAH, 35 had connective tissue disease, 57 had chronic thromboembolic PAH, and 9 had developed anorexigen-related PAH. The mean age at enrollment was 51 years, and the WHO functional capacity class at enrollment was either III (59%) or IV (41%). At trial's end, 17% of the iloprost-treated patients, compared with 4% of placebo-treated patients, achieved the primary endpoint. A 36-meter difference in 6-minute walk distance was reported between the study groups (Figure 39-4). This difference was more pronounced in patients with iPAH compared with those with other recognized triggers of PAH. Iloprost was approved by the FDA in 2004 for patients with PAH and WHO functional class III or IV symptoms.

Inhaled treprostinil was studied in the Treprostinil Sodium Inhalation Used in the Management of Pulmonary Arterial Hypertension (TRIUMPH) study of 235 PAH patients (56% with iPAH or familial PAH [fPAH], 33% with connective tissue disease, and 11% with other causes) who were already on oral PAH therapy (70% bosentan, 30% sildenafil) for an average of almost 2 years prior to starting inhaled treprostinil.[24] The average age was 33 years, and 81.2% of the study subjects were women. The vast majority of patients were in WHO functional class III (98%) with the remainder in class IV, and the baseline 6-minute walk distance was 348 meters. After 12 weeks, an increase in walking distance of 20 meters was reported compared with placebo ($P = .0004$). Subjects with walk distances in the bottom quartile at baseline had the greatest improvement (mean increase, 49 m). Improvements were noted in NT-pro–brain natriuretic peptide (BNP) levels and QOL but not in functional class or time to clinical worsening. Compared with placebo, side effects that were significantly more common among treprostinil subjects included cough (54% vs. 29%), headache (41% vs. 23%), and flushing (15% vs. <1%). Inhaled treprostinil (Tyvaso) was FDA approved in 2009 for treatment of PAH to improve exercise ability in patients with functional class III and iPAH, fPAH, or PAH associated with connective tissue disease.

No pulmonary vasodilator therapies are currently approved for WHO class III PH associated with lung disease or hypoxemia, although it is unclear how to approach patients with clinically suspected coexisting PAH. It should be noted that inhaled therapy, whether treprostinil or iloprost, is often chosen as first-line therapy for patients with clinically important parenchymal lung disease and coexisting elevation or pulmonary vascular resistance believed to be out of proportion to the degree of lung disease. Inhaled therapy is often chosen because of the belief that it is less likely to cause worsening V/Q mismatch in such patients; however, the utility of this approach is controversial and is under active study.

Endothelin Receptor Antagonism

Endothelin and its receptors play complex roles in the regulation of endothelial function, systemic arterial pressure, and pulmonary vascular function.[25,26] Endothelin-1 is a 21-chain amino acid peptide that appears to play a major role in the pathophysiology of PAH. Two main receptors for endothelin-1, endothelin type A (ETA) and type B (ETB) receptors, have quite distinct physiologic effects.[26,27] Activation of ETA causes vasoconstriction, whereas activation of ETB elicits a more complex response that includes a major vasodilatory effect. Activation of ETB receptors also appears more likely to cause liver aminotransferase elevation, thus theoretical considerations suggest a benefit to more specific ETA antagonism compared with nonselective ET receptor blockade. Both FDA-approved ET-receptor antagonists are teratogenic and have a propensity to cause peripheral edema.

The Bosentan Randomized Trial of Endothelin Antagonist Therapy (BREATHE) was comprised a series of trials to assess the safety and efficacy of a combined ETA and ETB antagonist, bosentan, in the treatment of iPAH and other forms of PAH. The BREATHE-1 study was a double-blind randomized trial, with enrollment based on baseline 6-minute walk distance (mean distance, 335 m).[28] Study drug was started at 62.5 mg administered orally twice daily for 4 weeks and then increased to either 125 or 250 mg twice daily for 12 weeks. The primary endpoints measured at 16 weeks included the 6-minute walk distance, hemodynamic parameters, Borg dyspnea score, and WHO functional class. A total of 213 patients were enrolled in the study: 79% were women, 151 had iPAH, and 62 had connective tissue disease. The mean age at enrollment was 48 years, and baseline functional capacity was class III (92%) or IV (8%). At the end of the trial, a 44-meter difference in 6-minute walk distance was reported between the study groups (Figure 39-5). Benefits persisted during long-term follow-up, and the most common side effects were liver function test (LFT) abnormalities that mandated monthly LFT checks for patients prescribed this drug and mild, likely

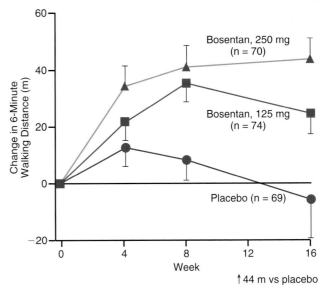

FIGURE 39-5 Functional capacity in severe pulmonary arterial hypertension: treatment with bosentan. *(Modified from Rubin LJ, Badesch DB, Barst RJ, et al. Bosentan therapy for pulmonary arterial hypertension. N Engl J Med 2002;346:896-903.)*

dilutional, anemia. The FDA subsequently approved bosentan use in patients with PAH in functional class III or IV. Annual cost of bosentan therapy currently exceeds $40,000.[29]

The Ambrisentan in Pulmonary Arterial Hypertension, Randomized, Double-Blind, Placebo-Controlled, Multicenter Efficacy Studies (ARIES-1 and ARIES-2) were concurrent studies of ambrisentan, a more specific oral ETA receptor antagonist. The trials were conducted in patients with iPAH or PAH associated with anorexigen use, HIV infection, or connective tissue disease,[30] and the majority of subjects were in functional class II or III (38% and 55%, respectively). Ambrisentan was used in doses between 1 and 10 mg, and the primary endpoint was change in 6-minute walk distance after 12 weeks. The placebo-corrected increase in walk distance for 5- and 10-mg doses of ambrisentan were 31 and 51 meters, respectively (both $P < .01$ vs. placebo), and a concomitant decrease in plasma BNP concentration was noted for the subset of 110 subjects in whom this marker was measured. Peripheral edema occurred in approximately one fourth of ambrisentan-treated subjects in the ARIES-1 trial, and dose-dependent nasal congestion was seen in 3% to 10.4% of patients. For the 280 subjects who completed an open-label 48-week extension, the increase in walk distance was maintained (average, 39 m compared with baseline). Of note, none of the subjects treated with ambrisentan developed a threefold elevation in aminotransferase levels. Ambrisentan (5 or 10 mg orally once daily, starting with 5 mg) was approved by the FDA in 2007 for treatment of PAH. In March 2011, the FDA removed the warning regarding potential hepatotoxicity and concluded that monthly LFT monitoring was not indicated. The cost of the drug for a year of therapy approaches $55,000.

Phosphodiesterase Inhibition

PDE inhibition, particularly inhibition of PDE-5, blocks metabolism of cyclic guanosine monophosphate (cGMP), enhances cGMP-mediated relaxation and growth inhibition of vascular smooth muscle cells in the lungs of patients with iPAH, and potentially improves clinical outcomes. Recent trials have led to FDA approval of such therapy for patients with PAH.

Sildenafil citrate, an oral inhibitor of PDE-5, was evaluated in a double-blind randomized trial, with enrollment based on baseline 6-minute walk (mean distance, 344 m).[31] After 12 weeks of therapy with 20, 40, or 80 mg three times daily, investigators assessed 6-minute walk distance, hemodynamic parameters, Borg dyspnea score, and WHO functional class in 277 patients. In this trial, 75% of subjects were women, 175 had iPAH, 87 had connective tissue disease, and 18 patients had repaired congenital systemic pulmonary shunts. The mean age at enrollment was 49 years, and baseline functional capacity class was either II (39%), III (58%), or IV (3%). At the trial's conclusion, a 45- to 50-meter difference in 6-minute walk distance was noted between the sildenafil-treated groups and those who received a placebo, with no statistically significant differences among the different dosages. Hemodynamics (cardiac index and pulmonary vascular resistance) improved more dramatically with higher doses. Clinical benefits persisted during 1 year of follow-up, and the most common side effects were flushing, dyspepsia, and diarrhea. The FDA subsequently approved sildenafil use in patients with PAH. The current cost per year of therapy is approximately $13,000.[29]

Tadalafil is a longer-acting PDE-5 inhibitor with once-daily oral dosing. The Pulmonary Arterial Hypertension and Response to Tadalafil (PHIRST) study randomized 405 patients whose etiology ranged from idiopathic, familial, or anorexigen-induced PAH to connective tissue disease and congenital heart disease to placebo or varying doses (2.5 to 40 mg) of tadalafil for 16 weeks with a primary endpoint of improvement in 6-minute walk distance.[32] The majority of subjects were functional class III (approximately 65%) with the remainder being mainly class II (approximately 30%). Of note, just over half of the subjects were already treated with bosentan. Significant dose-dependent improvement in walking distance was noted in groups treated with 10, 20, and 40 mg, but only the 40-mg dose met the prespecified value of statistical significance; it increased walking distance by 33 meters compared with placebo ($P < .01$). The improvement in 6-minute walk distance in treatment-naïve patients appeared larger than the improvement seen in those treated with bosentan (44 vs. 23 m); that improvement appeared to be sustained in a large subset of patients followed up for over 44 weeks. The most common adverse event likely related to tadalafil was headache, seen in 20% to 40% of subjects. A small number of patients developed more severe adverse events that included retinal artery occlusion, priapism, and hypotension. In May 2009, the FDA approved a 40-mg daily dose of tadalafil (Adcirca) to improve exercise capacity in patients with PAH. The average annual cost of therapy ranges between $10,000 and $12,000.

The role of combination therapy in the treatment of PAH is unclear.[33,34] Almost all current therapies, with the exception of inhaled treprostinil, have been approved based on placebo-controlled studies. Current clinical practice usually includes starting a single agent, with the choice based on the type of PH, functional class, and comorbidities. A significant subset of patients has shown inadequate symptomatic improvement with a given therapy, and many practitioners opt to add a second agent with a different physiologic mechanism. For example, a patient with functional class IV symptoms may be started on IV epoprostenol with uptitration of the dose until further increases are not tolerated because of adverse effects. A second agent with a different mechanism, either an endothelin receptor blocker or PDE inhibitor, may be prescribed. Few rigorously conducted studies support such an approach, and it seems that randomized controlled study data for such decisions will be difficult to obtain. On the other end of the spectrum, patients with functional class II or III symptoms may be started on one type of oral therapy. If they show inadequate improvement over the course of several months, clinicians may then opt to add a second agent; current published expert guidelines for PAH therapies support this approach (Figure 39-6).[35]

The TRIUMPH study suggests that combined therapy may add a modest additional benefit when inhaled treprostinil is added to bosentan or sildenafil.[24] The results of published studies thus far have been variable, but combination therapies are a subject of active investigation that should result in clinical data that will allow an evidence-based approach to this practice.

Atrial Septostomy

The rationale for an atrial septostomy as therapy for patients with iPAH is based on the suggestion that the presence of an atrial septal defect or patent foramen ovale appears to confer a benefit in patients with iPAH.[36] It has been suggested that, in the setting of severe PH, RV dysfunction, and low cardiac output, an intraatrial defect with right-to-left shunting preserves forward cardiac output but at the expense of systemic arterial hypoxemia. One cohort study reported a survival benefit in patients treated with atrial septostomy compared with historic control subjects.[37] Procedure-related morbidity and mortality rates in early studies have been high, although these were substantially lower in expert hands. Randomized studies have not been performed, making such therapy a reasonable option only at centers with considerable expertise and only for patients in whom alternative therapy as a bridge to transplantation is unavailable.

Transplantation for Idiopathic Pulmonary Arterial Hypertension

Single-lung, double-lung, and heart-lung transplantation have been used for patients with severe PAH, with a 5-year survival of approximately 50%. Procedural morbidity and mortality rates are much higher for transplantation for PAH compared with that for other forms of lung disease. Until QOL indexes or survival benefit is improved with changes in surgical techniques and medical support, transplantation should be reserved for selected patients with PAH that is refractory to medical therapy.

Medical Therapy Algorithms

In the United States, prescription of current IV and nonparenteral therapies for PAH focuses on FDA-approved therapies administered to patients in particular WHO functional classes in which the approved medications were tested. Thus, prostanoids are used for functional class IV patients, and bosentan, ambrisentan, treprostinil, iloprost, sildenafil, or tadalafil is used for those in functional class III (see Figure 39-6). If patients do not respond to initial diagnostic acute vasodilator challenge, and hence are not candidates for CCB therapy, our recommendations for therapy include the following:

- WHO functional class II: Start with an oral therapy: sildenafil, tadalafil, bosentan, or ambrisentan. Alternative therapy includes inhaled or SC treprostinil. Inhaled therapy is often preferred in patients with concomitant parenchymal lung disease.
- WHO functional class III: Start with an oral or inhaled agent, but consider primary IV therapy in specific patients. Options include bosentan, ambrisentan, sildenafil, or tadalafil or inhaled iloprost or treprostinil.
- WHO functional class IV: Start with IV prostanoid epoprostenol with treprostinil as an alternative. An inhaled prostanoid (iloprost or treprostinil) can be used if the patient is intolerant of IV therapy. Consider additional oral therapy 4 to 12 weeks later if substantive clinical improvement is absent.

These recommendations are based on FDA-approved medications, with several other options, such as beraprost, available in other countries. Patients in functional class IV whose symptoms do not improve to class II after several months of therapy and those with persistently elevated right atrial (RA) pressure or low systemic cardiac output are typically referred for consideration for lung or heart-lung transplantation.[15] Worsening of functional class, new symptoms of neurohormonal activation, or a decrease in 6-minute walk time over 10% of baseline with worsening dyspnea typically prompt a full reassessment for potential causes of deterioration and adjustment of therapy.

Historically, PAH patients were often dissuaded from substantial aerobic activity. Such activity is often accompanied by hypoxemia and can trigger symptoms ranging from dyspnea to syncope.

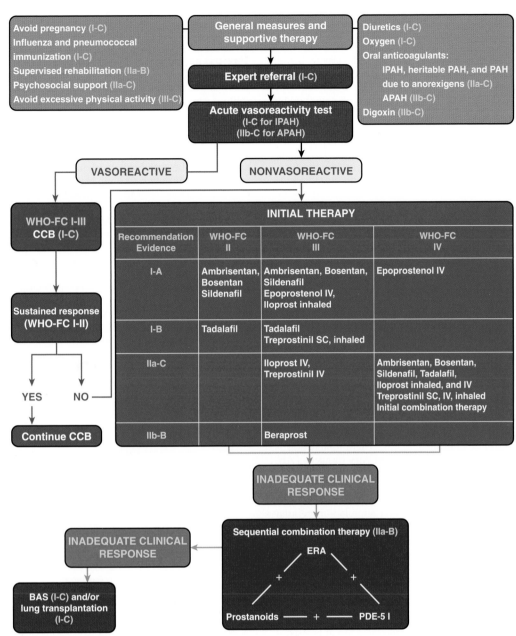

FIGURE 39-6 A proposed treatment algorithm. APAH, associated pulmonary arterial hypertension; BAS, balloon atrial septostomy; CCB, calcium channel blocker; ERA, endothelin receptor antagonist; IPAH, idiopathic pulmonary arterial hypertension; IV, intravenous; PAH, pulmonary arterial hypertension; PDE-5 I, phosphodiesterase 5 inhibitor; SC, subcutaneous; WHO-FC, World Health Organization functional class. *(From Galie N, Hoeper MM, Humbert M, et al. Guidelines for the diagnosis and treatment of pulmonary hypertension: the Task Force for the Diagnosis and Treatment of Pulmonary Hypertension of the European Society of Cardiology [ESC] and the European Respiratory Society [ERS], endorsed by the International Society of Heart and Lung Transplantation [ISHLT]. Eur Heart J 2009;30[20]:2493-2537.)*

However, a European study published in 2006 demonstrated the safety and impressive positive impact of an intensive exercise program on 15 of 30 PAH patients randomized to a 3-week inpatient exercise program followed by a 12-week continued home program. The study population was similar to that enrolled in randomized trials of medical therapy (mean age 50 years, 67% female, mostly WHO functional class III) except for a somewhat higher average 6-minute walk distance at baseline (approximately 425 m). In the intensive exercise group, 6-minute walk distance improved compared with placebo by 111 meters ($P < .0001$), an improvement more than double what has generally been seen in drug studies. QOL and WHO functional class notably improved.[38] Although a 3-week inpatient stay may not be a realistic option for most patients in the current health care system, this study confirms that monitored exercise training is generally a safe and effective approach to improving function and QOL in patients

with PAH. Restriction of aerobic exercise no longer has a prominent role in PAH care.

Therapies tested to support left ventricular (LV) contractile function, decreased muscular remodeling, neurohormonal activation, and inflammation and to reduce alveolar hypoxia have not been adequately studied in patients with PAH. Therefore the role of β-blockers, nesiritide, angiotensin-converting enzyme (ACE) inhibitors, angiotensin receptor blockers (ARBs), and spironolactone in the therapeutic armamentarium for PAH is uncertain. Effects of situational stress reduction, nutrition support, and treatment of sleep-disordered breathing have yet to be rigorously studied in this population. The nuances of combination or transition therapies, as well as elucidation of markers of responsiveness to such therapies, are topics of current investigation. Use of implanted continuous hemodynamic recording devices to monitor PA pressure has been described and appears to predict 6-minute walk distance and symptomatic response to changes in therapy, although the ability of such data to facilitate clinical benefit has yet to be demonstrated.[39]

Patients should be counseled to practice safe airline travel. Most commercial airlines are pressurized to an equivalent of 1800 to 2400 meters above sea level, with hypobaric hypoxia typically seen at 1500 to 2000 meters. Frequent rests and concomitant oxygen use are recommended for patients with PAH. Other prudent precautions include budgeting of energy to personal goals while promoting improved aerobic fitness and conditioning and excellent skin, dental, and overall infection control strategies along with episodic laboratory checks of renal and hepatic function and CBCs. Patients with PAH should be vigilant regarding the use of even simple, over-the-counter agents with potential for alterations in renal or hepatic function, and they must be educated on their disease and its management.

New Pathobiologic and Care Paradigms

Increasing evidence supports the involvement of genetically inherited abnormalities in endothelial cell apoptosis and growth potential, with links of familial and sporadic iPAH to bone morphogenetic protein receptor BMPR2, a member of the tumor growth factor (TGF)-β superfamily. Additional links have been identified to angiopoietin-1, endoglin, and ALK-1, which encodes a BMP receptor. The role of testing for mutations in these genes is unclear. Even testing a patient's family members poses real challenges because these mutations have far from complete penetrance.[40-43]

Increasing data suggest that the hallmark lesion of PAH and other forms of PAH, the plexiform lesion, is a response phenomenon to local hypoxia or inflammation and represents a tumorlike proliferation of endothelial cells. This proliferation is monoclonal in iPAH and polyclonal in secondary forms of PAH. To date, the functional significance of these lesions and their components and the temporal control of vascular growth remain elusive.[44]

Markers of cellular inflammation, matrix stimulation, cellular growth, and platelet and coagulant activity can now be studied in circulation and in situ. Alterations of fractalkine (chemokine ligand 1), RANTES, interleukin-1β, interleukin-6, soluble ICAM and VCAM, P-selectin, E-selectin, von Willebrand factor, serotonin, and plasminogen activator inhibitor 1 have been noted in biopsy samples and in serum of patients with PAH. But the need remains to further characterize, as well as correlate, changes in these factors with disease severity or progression.[45,46]

Endothelial cell (EC) activation abnormalities are at the heart of current understanding of and therapeutic approaches to PAH. Successful use of long-term nitric oxide (NO) administration has been demonstrated, although randomized clinical trials remain to be orchestrated, and such therapy is unlikely to be cost effective because of the method in which NO is currently used and marketed. Abnormalities in VEGF have been described in patients with PAH, but it is unclear where these abnormalities lie in the activation of the overall inflammation and constriction scheme.

The role of serotonin as a trigger for development of PAH was highlighted by the effect of Phen-fen (dexfenfluramine and phentermine) and other anorexigens on pulmonary artery smooth muscle (sM) cell 5-hydroxytriptamine (5HT)-2A and 5HT-1B receptors.[47] A unified theory of serotonin activation remains to be clearly defined, and therapeutic trials of serotonin receptor blockers and serotonin transporters have been suggested. Other abnormalities in sM cell components in patients with PAH may include dysfunctional voltage-dependent potassium channels, which can be altered with anorexigenic agents such as aminorex, dexfenfluramine, and phentermine.

Increased extracellular matrix (ECM) production is another hallmark of PAH, with abnormalities of serine elastase that cause elevations in basic fibroblast growth factor (bFGF) that lead to changes in matrix metalloproteinases (MMPs), production of tenascin, and phosphorylation of growth factor receptors and sM cell proliferation.[48]

Pregnancy and Contraception

The risk of pregnancy-related death for women with PAH is substantial. Despite the use of modern pulmonary vasoactive agents, mortality rates in the modern era are only slightly lower than previously reported rates of 30% to 50%,[49,50] and the risk persists for weeks after delivery. Thus, women with severe PAH are strongly counseled against pregnancy, and methods of contraception should be reviewed in detail. For women who come to medical attention during pregnancy, maternal risk of termination may be similar, if not greater, depending on the timing of the presentation. Warfarin-based teratogenic risk may be substantial at doses typically used in PAH therapy, although thromboembolism during pregnancy in this hypercoaguable population could be catastrophic. Any patient continuing pregnancy should be closely monitored by regional centers of expertise, with access to all levels of supportive maternal and fetal care. Reliable and judicious contraception based on patient education remains a hallmark of appropriate care, although appropriateness and effectiveness of individual therapies—in particular, hormonal contraception—remains untested in this population. Tubal ligation, similar to any noncardiopulmonary surgery, may carry substantial morbid and mortal risks in patients with PAH and should not be undertaken without consideration of alternatives.

REFERENCES

1. Newman JH, Fanburg BL, Archer SL, et al. Pulmonary arterial hypertension: future directions: report of a National Heart, Lung and Blood Institute/Office of Rare Diseases workshop. *Circulation* 2004;109(24):2947-2952.
2. The International Primary Pulmonary Hypertension Study (IPPHS). *Chest* 1994;105(2 Suppl):37S-41S.
3. Yamane K, Ihn H, Asano Y, et al. Clinical and laboratory features of scleroderma patients with pulmonary hypertension. *Rheumatology (Oxford)* 2000;39(11):1269-1271.
4. Speich R, Jenni R, Opravil M, Pfab M, Russi EW. Primary pulmonary hypertension in HIV infection. *Chest* 1991;100(5):1268-1271.
5. Hadengue A, Benhayoun MK, Lebrec D, Benhamou JP. Pulmonary hypertension complicating portal hypertension: prevalence and relation to splanchnic hemodynamics. *Gastroenterology* 1991;100(2):520-528.
6. D'Alonzo GE, Barst RJ, Ayres SM, et al. Survival in patients with primary pulmonary hypertension: results from a national prospective registry. *Ann Intern Med* 1991;115(5):343-349.
7. Oya H, Nagaya N, Uematsu M, et al. Poor prognosis and related factors in adults with Eisenmenger syndrome. *Am Heart J* 2002;143(4):739-744.
8. Arkles JS, Opotowsky AR, Ojeda J, et al. Shape of the right ventricular Doppler envelope predicts hemodynamics and right heart function in pulmonary hypertension. *Am J Respir Crit Care Med* 2011;183(2):268-276.
9. Rich S, Kaufmann E, Levy PS. The effect of high doses of calcium-channel blockers on survival in primary pulmonary hypertension. *N Engl J Med* 1992;327(2):76-81.
10. Sitbon O, Humbert M, Jais X, et al. Long-term response to calcium channel blockers in idiopathic pulmonary arterial hypertension. *Circulation* 2005;111(23):3105-3111.
11. Moser KM, Auger WR, Fedullo PF. Chronic major-vessel thromboembolic pulmonary hypertension. *Circulation* 1990;81(6):1735-1743.
12. Kreutzer J, Landzberg MJ, Preminger TJ, et al. Isolated peripheral pulmonary artery stenoses in the adult. *Circulation* 1996;93(7):1417-1423.
13. Feinstein JA, Goldhaber SZ, Lock JE, Ferndandes SM, Landzberg MJ. Balloon pulmonary angioplasty for treatment of chronic thromboembolic pulmonary hypertension. *Circulation* 2001;103(1):10-13.
14. Wensel R, Opitz CF, Anker SD, et al. Assessment of survival in patients with primary pulmonary hypertension: importance of cardiopulmonary exercise testing. *Circulation* 2002;106(3):319-324.
15. McLaughlin VV, Shillington A, Rich S. Survival in primary pulmonary hypertension: the impact of epoprostenol therapy. *Circulation* 2002;106(12):1477-1482.
16. Rich S, Seidlitz M, Dodin E, et al. The short-term effects of digoxin in patients with right ventricular dysfunction from pulmonary hypertension. *Chest* 1998;114(3):787-792.
17. Barst RJ, Rubin LJ, Long WA, et al.; the Primary Pulmonary Hypertension Study Group. A comparison of continuous intravenous epoprostenol (prostacyclin) with conventional therapy for primary pulmonary hypertension. *N Engl J Med* 1996;334(5):296-302.
18. Shapiro SM, Oudiz RJ, Cao T, et al. Primary pulmonary hypertension: improved long-term effects and survival with continuous intravenous epoprostenol infusion. *J Am Coll Cardiol* 1997;30(2):343-349.
19. Simonneau G, Barst RJ, Galie N, et al. Continuous subcutaneous infusion of treprostinil, a prostacyclin analogue, in patients with pulmonary arterial hypertension: a double-blind, randomized, placebo-controlled trial. *Am J Respir Crit Care Med* 2002;165(6):800-804.
20. Tapson VF, Gomberg-Maitland M, McLaughlin VV, et al. Safety and efficacy of IV treprostinil for pulmonary arterial hypertension: a prospective, multicenter, open-label, 12-week trial. *Chest* 2006;129(3):683-688.

21. Galie N, Humbert M, Vachiery JL, et al. Effects of beraprost sodium, an oral prostacyclin analogue, in patients with pulmonary arterial hypertension: a randomized, double-blind, placebo-controlled trial. *J Am Coll Cardiol* 2002;39(9):1496-1502.

22. Barst RJ, McGoon M, McLaughlin V, et al. Beraprost therapy for pulmonary arterial hypertension. *J Am Coll Cardiol* 2003;41(12):2119-2125.

23. Olschewski H, Simonneau G, Galie N, et al. Inhaled iloprost for severe pulmonary hypertension. *N Engl J Med* 2002;347(5):322-329.

24. McLaughlin VV, Benza RL, Rubin LJ, et al. Addition of inhaled treprostinil to oral therapy for pulmonary arterial hypertension: a randomized controlled clinical trial. *J Am Coll Cardiol* 2010;55(18):1915-1922.

25. Shao D, Park JE, Wort SJ. The role of endothelin-1 in the pathogenesis of pulmonary arterial hypertension. *Pharmacol Res* 2011;63(6):504-511.

26. Schneider MP, Boesen EI, Pollock DM. Contrasting actions of endothelin ET(A) and ET(B) receptors in cardiovascular disease. *Ann Rev Pharmacol Toxicol* 2007;47:731-759.

27. Ivy D, McMurtry IF, Yanagisawa M, et al. Endothelin B receptor deficiency potentiates ET-1 and hypoxic pulmonary vasoconstriction. *Am J Physiol Lung Cellular Molecular Physiol* 2001;280(5):L1040-L1048.

28. Rubin LJ, Badesch DB, Barst RJ, et al. Bosentan therapy for pulmonary arterial hypertension. *N Engl J Med* 2002;346(12):896-903.

29. Archer SL, Michelakis ED. Phosphodiesterase type 5 inhibitors for pulmonary arterial hypertension. *N Engl J Med* 2009;361(19):1864-1871.

30. Galie N, Olschewski H, Oudiz RJ, et al. Ambrisentan for the treatment of pulmonary arterial hypertension: results of the ambrisentan in pulmonary arterial hypertension, randomized, double-blind, placebo-controlled, multicenter, efficacy (ARIES) study 1 and 2. *Circulation* 2008;117(23):3010-3019.

31. Galie N, Ghofrani HA, Torbicki A, et al. Sildenafil citrate therapy for pulmonary arterial hypertension. *N Engl J Med* 2005;353(20):2148-2157.

32. Galie N, Brundage BH, Ghofrani HA, et al. Tadalafil therapy for pulmonary arterial hypertension. *Circulation* 2009;119(22):2894-2903.

33. Meis T, Behr J. Pulmonary hypertension: role of combination therapy. *Curr Vasc Pharmacol* 2011;9(4):457-464.

34. Abraham T, Wu G, Vastey F, et al. Role of combination therapy in the treatment of pulmonary arterial hypertension. *Pharmacotherapy* 2010;30(4):390-404.

35. Galie N, Hoeper MM, Humbert M, et al. Guidelines for the diagnosis and treatment of pulmonary hypertension: the Task Force for the Diagnosis and Treatment of Pulmonary Hypertension of the European Society of Cardiology (ESC) and the European Respiratory Society (ERS), endorsed by the International Society of Heart and Lung Transplantation (ISHLT). *Eur Heart J* 2009;30(20):2493-2537.

36. Rozkovec A, Montanes P, Oakley CM. Factors that influence the outcome of primary pulmonary hypertension. *Br Heart J* 1986;55(5):449-458.

37. Sandoval J, Gaspar J, Pulido T, et al. Graded balloon dilation atrial septostomy in severe primary pulmonary hypertension: a therapeutic alternative for patients nonresponsive to vasodilator treatment. *J Am Coll Cardiol* 1998;32(2):297-304.

38. Mereles D, Ehlken N, Kreuscher S, et al. Exercise and respiratory training improve exercise capacity and quality of life in patients with severe chronic pulmonary hypertension. *Circulation* 2006;114(14):1482-1489.

39. Frantz RP, Benza RL, Kjellstrom B, et al. Continuous hemodynamic monitoring in patients with pulmonary arterial hypertension. *J Heart Lung Transplant* 2008;27(7):780-788.

40. Du L, Sullivan CC, Chu D, et al. Signaling molecules in nonfamilial pulmonary hypertension. *N Engl J Med* 2003;348(6):500-509.

41. Newman JH, Wheeler L, Lane KB, et al. Mutation in the gene for bone morphogenetic protein receptor II as a cause of primary pulmonary hypertension in a large kindred. *N Engl J Med* 2001;345(5):319-324.

42. Trembath RC, Thomson JR, Machado RD, et al. Clinical and molecular genetic features of pulmonary hypertension in patients with hereditary hemorrhagic telangiectasia. *N Engl J Med* 2001;345(5):325-334.

43. Machado RD, Eickelberg O, Elliott CG, et al. Genetics and genomics of pulmonary arterial hypertension. *J Am Coll Cardiol* 2009;54(1 Suppl):S32-S42.

44. Lee SD, Shroyer KR, Markham NE, et al. Monoclonal endothelial cell proliferation is present in primary but not secondary pulmonary hypertension. *J Clin Invest* 1998;101(5):927-934.

45. Dorfmuller P, Zarka V, Durand-Gasselin I, et al. Chemokine RANTES in severe pulmonary arterial hypertension. *Am J Respir Crit Care Med* 2002;165(4):534-539.

46. Welsh CH, Hassell KL, Badesch DB, Kressin DC, Marlar RA. Coagulation and fibrinolytic profiles in patients with severe pulmonary hypertension. *Chest* 1996;110(3):710-717.

47. MacLean MR, Herve P, Eddahibi S, Adnot S. 5-hydroxytryptamine and the pulmonary circulation: receptors, transporters and relevance to pulmonary arterial hypertension. *Br J Pharmacol* 2000;131(2):161-168.

48. Cowan KN, Jones PL, Rabinovitch M. Elastase and matrix metalloproteinase inhibitors induce regression, and tenascin-C antisense prevents progression, of vascular disease. *J Clin Invest* 2000;105(1):21-34.

49. Weiss BM, Zemp L, Seifert B, et al. Outcome of pulmonary vascular disease in pregnancy: a systematic overview from 1978 through 1996. *J Am Coll Cardiol* 1998;31(7):1650-1657.

50. Bedard E, Dimopoulos K, Gatzoulis MA. Has there been any progress made on pregnancy outcomes among women with pulmonary arterial hypertension? *Eur Heart J* 2009;30(3):256-265.

CH
39

TREATMENT OF PULMONARY ARTERIAL HYPERTENSION

ABDOMINAL AORTIC ANEURYSMS, 606

Surgical Management, 606
Medical Management, 607

THORACIC AORTIC ANEURYSMS, 608

Surgical Management, 608
Medical Management, 613

AORTIC DISSECTION, 613

Definitive Therapy, 614
Long-Term Therapy and Late Follow-up, 616

INTRAMURAL HEMATOMA, 617

PENETRATING ATHEROSCLEROTIC ULCER, 617

THORACIC AORTIC ATHEROEMBOLISM, 617

REFERENCES, 618

Abdominal Aortic Aneurysms

Surgical Management

The paramount concern in managing abdominal aortic aneurysms (AAAs) is their tendency to rupture. The mortality rate from rupture is quite high: among the participants in the U.K. Small Aneurysm Trial who had a ruptured abdominal aneurysm, 25% died before reaching a hospital, and 51% died in the hospital without undergoing surgery. The operative mortality rate for the 13% who underwent emergent surgery was 46% compared with 4% to 6% for elective surgery, yielding an overall 30-day survival of just 11%.[1] To prevent the associated mortality risk, elective surgical repair is the therapy of choice for aneurysms considered to be at significant risk of rupture.

It is well established that the risk of rupture increases with aneurysm size. The U.K. Small Aneurysm Trial found that aneurysms smaller than 4.0 cm have a 0.3% annual risk of rupture, those 4.0 to 4.9 cm have a 1.5% annual risk of rupture, and those 5.0 to 5.9 cm have a 6.5% annual risk of rupture.[2] For aneurysms 6.0 to 6.9 cm, the risk of rupture is 10%, which then rises sharply to 33% for aneurysms 7.0 cm or larger. Although abdominal aneurysms are less prevalent among women, when present they rupture three times more frequently than they do in men and at a smaller aortic diameter (mean diameter: 5 cm in women vs. 6 cm in men). Rupture is also more common among current smokers and in those with hypertension.

Because 80% of AAAs expand over time, with as many as 15% to 20% expanding rapidly (≥0.5 cm/y), the risk of rupture may concomitantly increase with time. Accordingly, the ability to predict rates of aortic aneurysm expansion would be useful in estimating the risk of future rupture. Although the mean rate of AAA expansion is thought to approximate 0.4 cm per year, the rates of expansion within a population are extremely variable; expansion rates even vary within one individual over time. Baseline aneurysm size is perhaps the best predictor of aneurysm expansion rate; larger aneurysms expand more rapidly than smaller ones, probably as a consequence of the LaPlace law. A rapid rate of expansion apparently also predicts aneurysm rupture, especially with abdominal aneurysms 5 cm or greater in diameter; therefore many surgeons consider both large size and rapid expansion to be indications for repair.

The goal of treating AAAs is to prolong life by preventing rupture. The decision to operate must weigh the natural history of the aneurysm and life expectancy of the patient against the anticipated morbidity and mortality of the proposed surgical procedure. Operative mortality rate is 4% to 6% overall for elective aneurysm repair and as low as 2% in low-risk patients. However, operative mortality rate rises to 19% for urgent aortic repair, and, as previously noted, it reaches 50% for repair of a ruptured aneurysm. Aneurysm size remains the primary indicator for repair of asymptomatic aneurysms. For many years, debate has surrounded the minimum aneurysm diameter that necessitates surgery. Two large-scale clinical trials have investigated this question. The U.K. Small

Aneurysm Trial randomized 1090 patients aged 60 to 76 years with small aortic aneurysms (diameter, 4.0 to 5.5 cm) to either early elective surgery or regular ultrasonographic surveillance.[3] They found no long-term difference in survival between the early-surgery group and the surveillance group, although after 8 years, total mortality was slightly lower in the early-surgery group. However, because the operative mortality rate in this trial was 5.8%, some practitioners have questioned whether there may have been a survival benefit from early surgery had the operative mortality rate been lower. A similar trial, the Aneurysm Detection and Management (ADAM) Veterans Affairs Cooperative Study,[4] has suggested otherwise. In ADAM, 1136 patients with small asymptomatic aneurysms (diameter, 4.0 to 5.4 cm) were randomized to undergo immediate surgical repair or surveillance at 6-month intervals by ultrasonography or computed tomography (CT) scanning. Despite a remarkably low operative mortality rate of 2.1%, after a mean follow-up of 5 years, no difference was reported in survival between the two groups. Collectively, these trials suggest that surgery is not indicated in most instances for patients with asymptomatic aneurysms less than 5.5 cm. However, it should be recognized that the subjects randomized to the surveillance arms of these trials are subject to careful clinical follow-up, with both medical management and regular surveillance imaging to monitor the aneurysm; such careful follow-up does not always take place in general practice settings outside a trial. Another important limitation is that these two study populations consisted almost entirely of men (U.K. Small Aneurysm Trial, 78% male; ADAM, 99% male), and because the risk of aneurysm rupture is greater and occurs at smaller diameters in women than in men, these results may not apply equally to women.[5] Indeed, recognizing that aneurysms tend to rupture at smaller sizes in women, the Joint Council of the American Association for Vascular Surgery and Society for Vascular Surgery has formally recommended that women undergo elective repair at an aortic diameter of 4.5 to 5.0 cm.[6]

Surgical repair of AAAs consists of opening the aneurysm and inserting a synthetic prosthesis, usually fabricated of Dacron or expanded polytetrafluoroethylene (ePTFE; Gore-Tex). Sometimes, a simple tube graft is all that is necessary, although frequently the operation must be carried distally into one or both iliac arteries to excise the aneurysm completely. In the case of large aneurysms, much of the aneurysm wall may be left in situ, called the *intrasaccular approach of Creech*, thereby reducing the need for extensive dissection and thus decreasing aortic cross-clamping time.

A less invasive alternative to open surgery for repair of AAAs is the use of percutaneously implanted expanding endovascular stent-grafts (see Figure 40-1). The device consists of a collapsible prosthetic tube graft that is inserted remotely, such as via the femoral artery, and advanced transluminally across the aneurysm under fluoroscopic guidance; the device is then secured at both its proximal and distal ends with an expandable stent-attachment system. For aortic aneurysm repair, the stent-graft serves to bridge the region of the aneurysm, thereby excluding it from the circulation while allowing aortic blood flow to continue distally through the prosthetic stent-graft lumen. In some cases, stent-grafts are

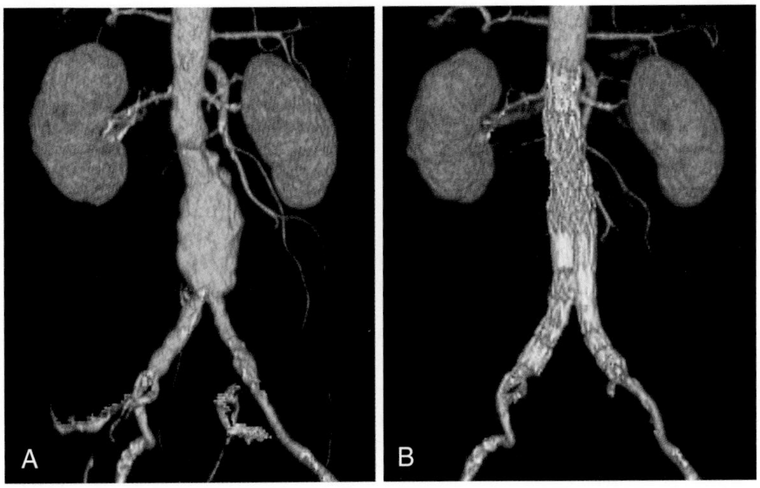

FIGURE 40-1 **A,** An infrarenal abdominal aortic aneurysm measuring approximately 6 cm. **B,** The aneurysm was treated with an endovascular stent-graft, which excluded the aneurysm sac from the circulation and caused it to thrombose.

bifurcated, with two arms on the distal end designed to extend into the common iliac arteries, when these vessels are aneurysmal as well. The rate of successful stent-graft implantation in several series over the past decade has ranged from 78% to 99%, with several recent large series reporting rates of 98%. Despite these favorable results, only 30% to 60% of patients with AAAs have aneurysm anatomy suitable for endovascular repair. One of the major technical difficulties associated with the stent-graft technique that has yet to be overcome is the frequent occurrence of endoleaks, which are seen angiographically as persistent contrast flow into the aneurysm sac because of failure to completely exclude the aneurysm from the aortic circulation. If left untreated, such leaks may leave the patient at continued risk for aneurysm expansion or rupture; these often necessitate secondary interventions.

Several randomized controlled trials (RCTs) have defined the short- and mid-term outcomes of endovascular aneurysm repair. The Dutch Randomized Endovascular Aneurysm Management (DREAM) trial compared open repair with endovascular repair in 345 patients with an abdominal aneurysm 5 cm or larger in diameter who were suitable candidates for either technique. The 30-day operative mortality rate was significantly lower in the endovascular repair group than in the open repair group, at 1.2% versus 4.6%, respectively.[7] The Endovascular Aneurysm Repair (EVAR) trial randomized 1082 patients similar to those above and found a significant and nearly identical reduction in operative mortality rate: 1.7% in the endovascular repair group versus 4.7% in the open repair group.[8] Collectively, these trials generated enthusiasm because they demonstrated a clear early mortality benefit for endovascular repair.

However, despite their favorable early success rates, longitudinal studies of endovascular stent-graft repair have reported failure rates of approximately 3% per year, 1% for rupture and 2% for conversion to open repair, compared with failure rates of 0.3% for open repair.[9] Not surprisingly, the mid-term outcomes have been far less encouraging. Indeed, in the DREAM trial, the 2-year cumulative survival rates were actually no different for endovascular versus open repair, at 89.7% and 89.6%, respectively.[10] Moreover, in the EVAR trial, at 4 years a persistent reduction was noted in aneurysm-related deaths in the endovascular stent-graft group (4% vs. 7%; *P* = .04), but no difference was reported between the two groups in all-cause mortality.[11] At 6 to 10 years, even the early benefit with respect to aneurysm-related death was lost, at least partially as a result of late endograft rupture.[12] These trials indicate that endovascular aneurysm repair offers no late advantage over open repair among those who are good candidates for either procedure.

Because of the lack of overall long-term benefit of stent-grafting compared with open repair, the use of stent-grafts for endovascular repair of AAAs has generally been limited to a subset of patients, typically older patients or those at high operative risk. However,

even the role of endovascular stent-grafting in this setting is now uncertain. In the recently published EVAR-2 trial, patients with large AAAs who were considered physically ineligible for open repair because of high risk of death or complications were randomized to endovascular stent-graft repair versus no intervention and were followed for up to 8 years.[13] The investigators found that endovascular repair was associated with a significantly lower rate of aneurysm-related mortality, primarily through prevention of late aneurysm rupture, but no difference was seen in overall mortality compared with nonintervention controls. Thus, the role for endovascular stent-graft repair in such a high-risk population remains uncertain.[14]

Medical Management

Risk factor modification is fundamental in the medical management of AAAs. Most patients with AAAs are cigarette smokers, and given the increased risk of aneurysm rupture among active smokers, the habit must be discontinued. In addition, hypertension should be carefully controlled.

β-Blockers had long been considered an important therapy for reducing the risk of aneurysm expansion and rupture, and early animal studies appeared to support such a role. In humans, however, the data have been disappointing. Several trials have shown that treatment with propranolol has no significant impact on the rate of growth of smaller aneurysms (<4 cm in diameter), and any benefit in larger aneurysms was not clinically significant.[15] Moreover, in most trials, patients tolerated β-blockers poorly, leading to diminished quality of life (QOL) scores and high rates of discontinuation of β-blocker therapy.[16] The lack of definitive benefit and the poor tolerance of these agents have led the Society of Vascular Surgery to state in its 2009 guidelines that "the use of β-blockers to reduce the risk of AAA expansion and rupture is not recommended."[17] Nevertheless, it is still reasonable to use β-blockers in aneurysm patients when there are other indications for their use.

A variety of evidence supports the idea that the renin-angiotensin system plays a role in the pathogenesis of AAAs, and evidence in animal studies suggests that treatment with angiotensin-converting enzyme (ACE) inhibitors may slow the growth of aortic aneurysms in the rat elastase–induced aneurysm model.[18] Angiotensin receptor blockers (ARBs) have been similarly beneficial in some animal models but not in others, although this may reflect the methods used to induce the aortic aneurysms.[16] In a population-based case-control study of patients 65 years of age or older admitted to the hospital with a primary diagnosis of AAA (ruptured or nonruptured), Hackam and colleagues[19] found that the use of ACE inhibitors within the 3 to 12 months prior to admission was associated with a significantly lower risk of aneurysm rupture (odds ratio

[OR], 0.82; 95% confidence interval [CI], 0.74 to 0.90). However, they found no risk reduction associated with the use of β-blockers or ARBs. These findings are encouraging, but several other studies of aortic aneurysms have not found evidence of benefit from ACE inhibitor therapy.[16] Randomized, controlled clinical trials are needed to demonstrate a causal relationship between ACE inhibitor use and improved outcomes.

Inflammation plays an important role in the pathogenesis of AAAs. Statins are known to have antiinflammatory effects in addition to their lipid-lowering effects; there has therefore been hope that they may improve outcomes in patients with aneurysms. Evidence in animal models suggests that statins significantly suppress matrix metalloproteinase (MMP)-9 levels and reduce the rate of aneurysm expansion.[20] Indeed, these appeared to hold considerable promise when a nonrandomized study of 130 patients with AAAs showed significantly lower rates of aneurysm growth among those treated with statins ($P < .001$).[21] However, much of the data suggesting a benefit of statin therapy is considered to be of poor quality, and a recent meta-analysis that included seven trials with quality data found no evidence of an association between statin therapy and lower aneurysm growth rates.[22] No RCTs of statin therapy for aneurysms are available, and given that most patients with AAAs merit treatment with statins for other atherosclerotic vascular disease, such trials may no longer even be possible.

Another pharmacologic approach to the inhibition of proteolysis is through the use of tetracyclines, which weakly inhibit MMPs through a mechanism unrelated to their antibiotic activity. In animal models of AAA, treatment with either doxycycline or tetracycline derivatives without antibiotic activity reduced aortic wall production of MMP-9, led to preservation of medial elastin, and reduced aneurysmal expansion. In one murine model, doxycycline administration reduced aneurysm growth by 33% to 66% at circulating doxycycline levels similar to those achieved in humans at standard doses.[23] The early data in human trials are encouraging. In a recent trial, Lindeman and colleagues found that 2 weeks of preoperative treatment with oral doxycycline resulted in reduced MMP-9 levels, a 72% reduction of the aortic wall neutrophils, and a 95% reduction of the aortic wall cytotoxic T-cell content within aneurysm wall tissue resected at surgery.[24] In a relatively small trial of 92 subjects, roxithromycin therapy for 28 days reduced the rate of aneurysm expansion by 44% in the first year of follow-up, but only by 5% in the second year.[25] Other approaches to targeting the aortic wall inflammatory process include treatment with macrolide immunosuppressants. In a rat model, treatment with rapamycin following aneurysm induction significantly reduced the rate of aneurysm expansion by 40% and reduced levels of MMP-9 in the aortic wall by 54% compared with controls.[26] However, in the absence of randomized clinical trial data, treatment of patients with antibiotics or immunosuppressants to slow aneurysm growth cannot yet be recommended.

Thoracic Aortic Aneurysms

The etiology and management of thoracic aortic aneurysms (TAAs) differ depending on the segment of the aorta involved. Aneurysms of the ascending thoracic aorta most often result from medial degeneration, which occurs to some extent with aging and is accelerated by hypertension. At younger ages, medial degeneration is classically associated with Marfan syndrome or other connective tissue disorders, such as Ehlers-Danlos syndrome type IV (vascular type) or Loeys-Dietz syndrome. Medial degeneration is also evident histologically in the ascending aorta among those with a congenitally bicuspid aortic valve and a dilated aorta and in those with a familial TAA syndrome. Aneurysms in the aortic arch are often contiguous with aneurysms of the ascending or descending aorta and may be due to medial degeneration, atherosclerotic disease, prior trauma, or infections. The predominant cause of aneurysms of the descending thoracic aorta is atherosclerosis.

The natural history of TAAs is that they grow over time and that the risk of aortic dissection or rupture increases with increasing aortic diameter. The rate of aortic rupture increases when aneurysms reach a diameter of 5 cm, whereupon the risk significantly increases; risk increases further still at diameters of 6 cm or greater. Based on a longitudinal observational study from Yale,[26a] in a multivariate logistic regression analysis of the predictors of dissection or rupture, compared with smaller aneurysms, the relative risk associated with an aneurysm diameter of 5.0 to 5.9 cm was 2.5, and with a diameter of 6 cm or larger, the relative risk was 5.2.

The therapeutic goals of management of patients with TAAs are therefore to use medication and lifestyle modification to try to reduce the rate of aortic growth, reduce the risk of aneurysm rupture or dissection, and intervene and repair the affected aortic segment in a timely fashion when benefits of intervention are believed to outweigh the risks.

Surgical Management

The optimal timing of surgical repair of TAAs remains uncertain for several reasons. First, the data available on the natural history of thoracic aneurysms are limited, especially with respect to the outcomes of surgical intervention. Second, with the high incidence of coexisting cardiovascular disease in this population, many patients die of other cardiovascular diseases before their aneurysms ever rupture. Finally, significant risks are associated with thoracic aortic surgery, particularly in the arch and descending aorta, that in many cases may outweigh the potential benefits of aortic repair. Consequently, no uniform accepted thresholds have been established for aortic repair.

Many of the recommendations that follow are based on the 2010 American College of Cardiology (ACC)/American Heart Association (AHA) guidelines for the diagnosis and management of patients with thoracic aortic disease.[27] According to these guidelines, for sporadic or degenerative aneurysms of the aortic root or ascending thoracic aorta, surgery is recommended when the aortic diameter is 5.5 cm or greater. However, those with Marfan syndrome or Ehlers-Danlos syndrome type IV are believed to be at increased risk of aortic dissection; therefore the threshold for surgery in those patients is reduced to 5 cm. This threshold may be as low as 4 to 5 cm in good surgical candidates, in the presence of a family history of aortic rupture or dissection at a diameter less than 5 cm, or if there is significant aortic regurgitation. Similarly, for those with an underlying bicuspid aortic valve, aortic repair is recommended when the diameter of the root or ascending aorta is 5 cm or greater.

Those with Loeys-Dietz syndrome are prone to death at a young age from aortic dissection at relatively small aortic diameters, so the threshold for surgical repair is lowered accordingly. In such patients surgery is recommended when the aortic root reaches an internal diameter of 4.2 cm or greater on transesophageal echocardiography (TEE) or an external diameter of 4.4 to 4.6 cm or greater by CT or magnetic resonance imaging (MRI).

Ascending thoracic aortic replacement is also recommended in cases that show rapid growth, considered to be 0.5 cm per year or more. However, it should be noted that erroneous measurements on an imaging study often suggest rapid growth of this magnitude, so before the decision to operate is based on this finding, two sets of the same kind of images (e.g., two computed tomographic angiograms) must be compared side by side, with one reader making equivalent measurements of each.

Importantly, these recommendations are based on the assumption that the patient is of average size. Clearly, the range of "normal" aortic diameters varies directly with patient size; in larger patients, the threshold for surgery should be raised, and in smaller patients, the threshold should be reduced. Two methods have been most widely adopted for correcting aortic size threshold for body size. The first is from the work of Svensson and colleagues, who recommended that for patients with Marfan syndrome or for those with a bicuspid aortic valve, if the maximal cross-sectional area in

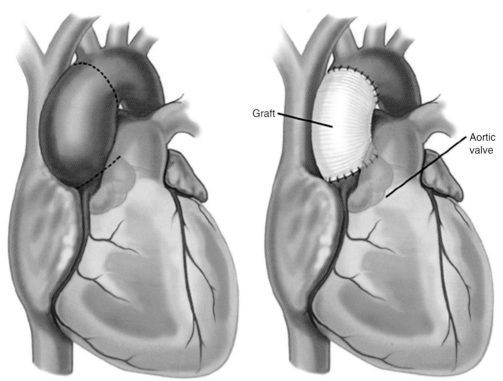

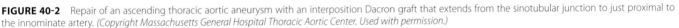

FIGURE 40-2   Repair of an ascending thoracic aortic aneurysm with an interposition Dacron graft that extends from the sinotubular junction to just proximal to the innominate artery. *(Copyright Massachusetts General Hospital Thoracic Aortic Center. Used with permission.)*

square centimeters of the ascending aorta or root divided by the patient's height in meters exceeds a ratio of 10, surgical repair is reasonable.[28,29] Alternatively, Davies and colleagues[30] created an aortic size index that equals aortic diameter (in centimeters) divided by body surface area (in meters squared) and stratifies patients into low-, intermediate-, and high-risk groups to guide the timing of surgery.

For asymptomatic patients with isolated aneurysms of the aortic arch, surgical repair is recommended at an aortic diameter of 5.5 cm or larger. Aneurysms of the arch often accompany ascending TAAs; if patients are to undergo repair of the ascending aorta, it is reasonable to perform concomitant hemiarch or total arch repair at smaller arch diameters.

Repair of descending TAAs carries a greater risk. Consequently, the threshold diameters for surgery are larger. For patients with degenerative aneurysms, surgery is recommended at an aortic diameter of 6.0 to 6.5 cm or greater, whereas for those at increased risk of dissection or rupture, such as those with Marfan syndrome or a chronic dissection, surgery is recommended at a diameter of 5.5 to 6.0 cm.[31] However, these various threshold diameters should serve only as a general guideline, and the timing of intervention must be individualized based on patient-specific factors such as age, comorbidities, aneurysm etiology, family history, body size, and the rate of aortic growth.

For an isolated aneurysm of the ascending aorta, the aneurysm is resected and replaced with a simple interposition prosthetic Dacron graft (Figure 40-2) by using cardiopulmonary bypass. Repair of aortic root aneurysms is more complex, however, because the three aortic valve cusps are suspended within the aortic root. Historically, surgery to replace the aortic root required a composite graft consisting of a Dacron tube with a prosthetic aortic valve sewn into one end, also known as the *Bentall procedure,* prior to the repair. After the aortic root and valve have been resected, the valved conduit is sewn directly to the aortic annulus, and the coronary arteries are then reimplanted into the Dacron graft as buttons (Figure 40-3). However, for those with structurally normal aortic valve leaflets, this procedure necessitates replacing their normal native valve with a prosthetic valve, which carries

both short- and long-term risks. Fortunately, for root aneurysms, it is now possible to excise the aortic root tissue while sparing the aortic valve and then resuspending the native valve within the graft. This procedure was first introduced in 1979 by Sir Magdi Yacoub with a remodeling technique and subsequently modified by Tirone David in 1988 with a reimplantation technique (see Figure 40-4). The original reimplantation technique, often referred to as *David-I,* used a straight tube graft, whereas a subsequent modification, referred to as *David-V,* uses a graft that bulges at the level of the valve to mimic the sinuses of Valsalva. "Valsalva grafts" are now commercially available to simplify the David-V procedure. The repair appears to be quite durable, with less than 2% developing significant aortic regurgitation at 8 to 10 years.[32,33]

When younger patients have a dilated aortic root but the aortic valve cannot be spared, an alternative to a composite aortic graft is a pulmonary autograft, also known as the *Ross procedure.* This involves replacing the patient's native aortic valve and root with the patient's own pulmonary root, which is transplanted into the aortic position. The pulmonary root is then replaced with a cryopreserved homograft root. Another surgical alternative to a composite graft is the use of cryopreserved aortic allografts (cadaveric aortic root and proximal ascending aorta). However, these approaches are generally not favored because their durability is often limited by late autograft root dilation or late structural valvular deterioration, respectively.[34]

Ascending TAAs often extend into the proximal aortic arch, but the mid and distal arch is preserved. In such cases surgeons will often perform a hemiarch repair, in which the proximal portion of the lesser curvature of the arch is resected, and the distal end of the ascending aortic graft is beveled for an anastomosis to the underside of the arch (Figure 40-5). The hemiarch repair requires a brief period of hypothermic circulatory arrest, but the arrest times are short enough that antegrade cerebral perfusion is not necessary, and outcomes are quite good.

Aneurysms of the aortic arch can be successfully surgically excised, but the procedure remains particularly challenging. Neurologic damage is a major cause of morbidity and mortality from aortic arch repair and typically results from embolization of

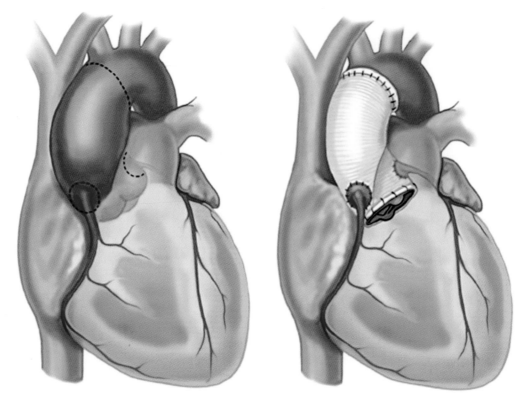

FIGURE 40-3 Repair of an aortic root aneurysm with a composite aortic graft. The native coronary arteries are removed from the native aorta as buttons, and the native aortic valve is excised along with the aneurysm; the composite aortic graft is then sewn into place, and the coronary artery buttons are reattached to the Dacron graft. *(Copyright Massachusetts General Hospital Thoracic Aortic Center. Used with permission.)*

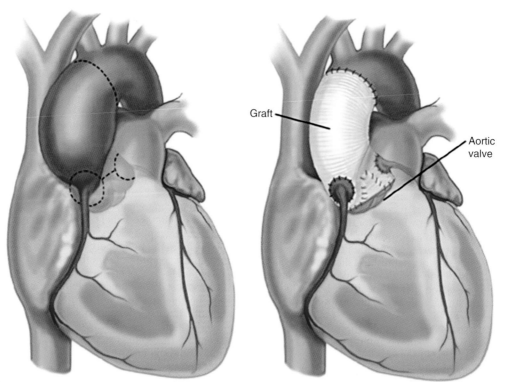

FIGURE 40-4 Valve-sparing root repair for an aortic root aneurysm. When the aortic root walls are excised, the native aortic valve is spared and then resuspended within the Dacron graft in an anatomic configuration. As in Figure 40-3, the coronary arteries are reimplanted as buttons. *(Copyright Massachusetts General Hospital Thoracic Aortic Center. Used with permission.)*

atherosclerotic debris or global ischemic injury during antegrade circulatory arrest. The brachiocephalic vessels must be removed from the aortic arch before its resection and must then be reimplanted into the prosthetic tube graft arch after its interposition. Traditionally, the surgical procedure involved removing and then reimplanting the brachiocephalic vessels en bloc (i.e., as an island of native aortic tissue containing the three branch vessels), after which normal cerebral perfusion is restored. More recently, however, surgical techniques have been introduced to reduce the hypothermic circulatory arrest times and limit embolic events by placing a multilimbed prosthetic arch graft, to which each arch vessel is in turn individually anastomosed (Figure 40-6).

Three methods of cerebral protection have been used for aortic arch surgery. The traditional method has been to use profound hypothermic circulatory arrest with arrest of cerebral perfusion.

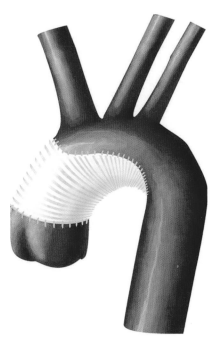

FIGURE 40-5 Ascending thoracic aortic replacement with hemiarch repair. The underside of the aortic arch is repaired with a beveled graft, which remodels a dilated proximal aortic arch without the complexity or risk of a total arch repair. *(From Sundaram B, Quint LE, Patel HJ, Deeb GM. CT findings following thoracic aortic surgery. Radiographics 2007;27:1583-1594.)*

The hypothermia is intended to reduce the cerebral metabolic rate by cooling to 10° to 13° C. However, the simplicity of the technique is offset by the high incidence of stroke and temporary neurologic dysfunction. In 1990, the use of retrograde cerebral perfusion via a superior vena cava cannula was introduced as an adjunct for cerebral protection during hypothermic arrest. It was originally suggested that this technique would improve outcomes by providing nutrients and oxygen to the brain and by flushing out both air and particulate matter that would otherwise embolize from the cerebral and carotid arteries. More extensive studies have shown that there is, in fact, no metabolic benefit to the brain from retrograde cerebral perfusion, and several studies have shown no improvement in outcomes. More recently, a technique of selective antegrade cerebral perfusion was introduced in which perfusion cannulae inserted directly into the cerebral vessels allow perfusion of the brain through all but brief periods during the procedure. Indeed, the use of the multilimbed prosthetic aortic graft makes selective antegrade cerebral perfusion easier and more effective. This technique allows for a longer period of safe circulatory arrest, which is of greater importance in more complex arch procedures. The available data suggest that selective antegrade cerebral perfusion does not reduce the risk of stroke but does significantly reduce the incidence of temporary neurologic dysfunction.[35,36] The persistent stroke risk may be due to the fact that direct cannulation of the brachiocephalic arteries can cause embolization of debris. To overcome this, many surgeons now prefer antegrade cerebral perfusion via cannulation of the right axillary artery,[37] which has been associated with significantly improved outcomes,[36] or with the use of a trifurcated graft anastomosed to the brachiocephalic arteries.[38] Historically, for aortic arch repair, the rates of stroke were as high 4% to 11%, but with the use of these modern techniques in experienced hands, the rates are as low as 2% to 9%.[39]

Unfortunately, many of the patients with aortic arch aneurysms are elderly, and they have a large burden of atherosclerosis; this

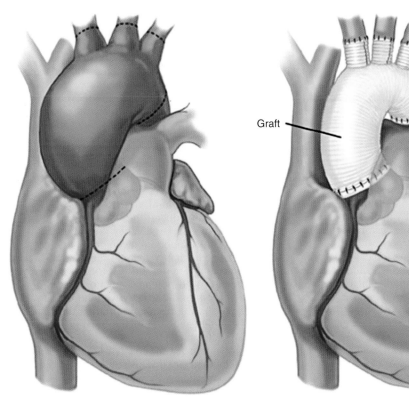

FIGURE 40-6 Total aortic arch repair with an arch graft and three prefabricated branches made to anastomose to the brachiocephalic arteries. *(Copyright Massachusetts General Hospital Thoracic Aortic Center. Used with permission.)*

Graft

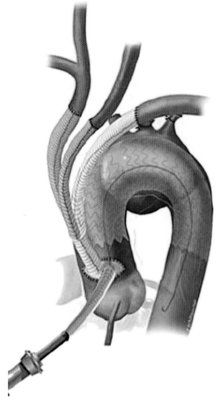

FIGURE 40-7 Hybrid procedure to treat an aortic arch aneurysm. First, a trifurcated graft is placed from the proximal ascending thoracic aorta to bypass the three arch vessels. Second, an endovascular stent-graft is placed from across the aortic arch, excluding the arch aneurysm from the circulation. *(From Milewski RK, Szeto WY, Pochettino A, et al. Have hybrid procedures replaced open aortic arch reconstruction in high-risk patients? A comparative study of elective open arch debranching with endovascular stent graft placement and conventional elective open total and distal aortic arch reconstruction. J Thorac Cardiovasc Surg 2010;140:590-597.)*

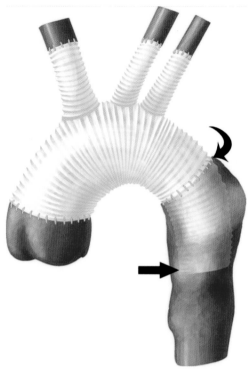

FIGURE 40-8 An elephant trunk procedure. A total aortic arch repair is performed, as in Figure 40-5, but in this case, attached to the distal end of the arch graft (*curved arrow*) is a Dacron sleeve that is left hanging freely (*straight arrow*) within the lumen of the descending thoracic aorta to facilitate a subsequent repair of the dilated descending thoracic aorta. *(From Sundaram B, Quint LE, Patel HJ, Deeb GM. CT findings following thoracic aortic surgery. Radiographics 2007;27:1583-1594.)*

places them at significant increased risk for stroke and death from open arch repair. In recent years, a hybrid procedure has been introduced as a potential alternative for arch repair in high-risk patients. This involves two steps, the first of which is an open de-branching of the aortic arch that involves anastomosis of the proximal end of a trifurcated graft to the proximal ascending thoracic aorta and the three distal branches to each of the brachiocephalic arteries. The second step is a covered thoracic endovascular stent-graft that is then advanced retrograde across the aortic arch and deployed with its landing zones proximal and distal to the arch, thus excluding the diseased arch from the circulation (Figure 40-7). This technique met with technical success and favorable outcomes. Although open repair is still clearly the technique of choice in favorable surgical candidates, the hybrid debranching–stent grafting procedure is a reasonable option in older high-risk candidates.[40]

Many of the patients who undergo surgical repair of a TAA have multiple aortic segments involved. Such widespread aneurysmal dilation of the aorta presents a particular challenge to the surgeon and often precludes surgery. Although it is possible to successfully replace virtually the entire diseased thoracic aorta, attempts to replace the ascending arch and descending thoracic aorta in one surgery carry increased risks. An alternative strategy is the use of a staged procedure, known as the *elephant trunk technique,* in which the ascending aorta and arch are replaced initially, and beyond the distal anastomosis, an extra length of Dacron graft is left dangling freely within the lumen of the proximal descending thoracic aorta (Figure 40-8). This "trunk" facilitates the subsequent repair of the descending thoracic aorta in one of

two ways: if open surgical repair is performed, the trunk permits easy cross-clamping of the proximal descending thoracic aorta; alternatively, thoracic endovascular stent-grafting (see below) may be performed,[41] in which the trunk provides an ideal proximal landing zone.

Elective surgical repair of ascending and descending TAAs in large centers is associated with mortality rates of 1% to 4% and 4% to 9%, respectively. Major complications include stroke and hemorrhage. A catastrophic complication of resection of descending TAAs is postoperative paraplegia secondary to interruption of the blood supply to the spinal cord. The incidence of paraplegia has been as high as 13% to 17%, but in most modern series it is 3% to 5%. A number of methods have been proposed to reduce the likelihood of paraplegia, although none has proved to be consistently safe and effective. One of the more promising techniques involves regional hypothermic protection of the spinal cord with epidural cooling during surgical repair of the aorta, which has reduced the frequency of spinal cord complications to 3% in one large series compared with a historic control of 20%. Other important techniques that may also reduce the risk of spinal cord injury include the reimplantation of patent critical intercostal arteries, the use of intraoperative somatosensory- or motor-evoked potential monitoring, maintenance of distal aortic perfusion during surgery with the use of atriofemoral (left heart) bypass to the distal aorta during the proximal anastomosis, and the maintenance of high arterial pressure during the first several days after surgery.

An alternative approach to the surgical management of descending thoracic aneurysms is the use of a transluminally placed endovascular stent-graft. This technique has the advantage of being far less invasive than surgery with potentially fewer postoperative complications and a lower morbidity rate. However, the aortic anatomy has to be favorable, with adequate proximal and distal landing zones, so not all patients are reasonable candidates for stent-grafting. A multicenter, prospective, nonrandomized phase II study of the Gore Tag thoracic aortic endoprosthesis (W.L. Gore & Associates, Flagstaff, AZ) was conducted at 17 academic centers and enrolled 142 selected patients. Device implantation was successful in 98%. The 30-day event rates for stroke, temporary or permanent paraplegia, and death were 3%, 3%, and 2%, respectively—far lower than event rates in an open surgical control population.[42] In a follow-up report of the same trial, at 5 years, aneurysm-related mortality rate was only 3% for the thoracic endovascular aortic repair (TEVAR) group versus 12% for open surgery controls.[43] Yet despite the lower aneurysm-related mortality rate, at 5 years no difference was reported in all-cause mortality, likely reflecting the fact that the TEVAR patients tended to be older, with numerous comorbidities. As with open surgical repair, spinal cord ischemia can occur during TEVAR, so protective techniques should be used, such as spinal cord drainage and elevation of systemic arterial pressure during the early postoperative period.

An important limitation to TEVAR is that even after successful deployment of an endograft in the thoracic aorta, endoleaks may appear. Type I endoleaks are the most common variety and result from blood leaking into the aneurysm sac via the proximal or distal endograft attachment site. Type II endoleaks occur when blood flows retrograde through a branch artery, such as an intercostal artery, located between the stent-graft's landing zones. Type III endoleaks occur because of a mechanical device failure, such as a tear in the fabric of the graft or separation in the junction of two stent components. The average prevalence of endoleaks at 30 days is 10%. New endoleaks may also arise late after successful stent-graft deployment. Consequently, TEVAR patients require at least annual surveillance imaging with computed tomographic angiography (CTA) to monitor for endoleaks, to confirm that the aneurysm sac is not expanding, and to confirm stent-graft integrity. Because type I and III endoleaks allow blood at systemic pressure to enter the aneurysm sac, attempts are usually made to repair them via additional endovascular techniques. Type II endoleaks are usually only observed, provided there is no evidence of aneurysm sac expansion.[44]

Medical Management

The long-term impact of medical therapy on aneurysm growth and survival in patients with typical atherosclerotic thoracic aneurysms has not been well investigated. However, a study of the efficacy of β-blockers in adult patients with Marfan syndrome found that therapy significantly slowed the rate of aortic dilation, reduced adverse clinical endpoints (death, aortic dissection, aortic regurgitation, and aortic root >6 cm), and significantly lowered mortality rates.[45] Although the study examined only the effect of β-blockade in patients with Marfan syndrome, it follows logically that medical therapy to reduce the rate of rise of left ventricular pressure (dP/dt) and control blood pressure would be beneficial in the treatment of TAAs of other etiologies as well; β-blockade has therefore become a mainstay of therapy.

Dietz and colleagues demonstrated in a mouse model of Marfan syndrome that TAAs are associated with an excessive activity of transforming growth factor (TGF)-β, and that TGF-β antibodies are able to block abnormal aortic growth. It turns out that losartan, an FDA-approved antihypertensive medication, has similar anti–TGF-β activity, and in the same mouse models, losartan also blocked abnormal aortic growth, and it did so more effectively than β-blockers.[46] In addition, in nonrandomized human studies, losartan blunted aortic growth in Marfan patients whose aortas had grown despite β-blocker therapy.[47] To formally address this question, a large, multicenter, randomized, placebo-controlled trial of losartan in Marfan syndrome was well underway at the time of this writing. Of note, evidence also suggests that ACE inhibitors may slow growth of aortic root aneurysms in humans with Marfan syndrome,[48] although research on these agents is quite limited.

It should be noted that losartan has not yet been proven to be of benefit in Marfan syndrome, let alone in TAAs of other etiologies. Therefore, at present, it cannot be recommended over β-blockers, which also have not proven to be effective among non-Marfan aneurysm patients. However, an aneurysm patient with sufficient blood pressure to permit two agents to be used may be prudently considered for the combination of a β-blocker with losartan, with the goal to control and maintain the blood pressure in the range of 110/70 to 125/80 mm Hg.

Aortic Dissection

A detailed discussion of the diagnostic imaging of aortic dissection is beyond the scope of this text, but it is important to recognize how the specific findings of the imaging studies affect therapeutic decision making. The primary goal of imaging is to diagnose the presence of aortic dissection or other acute aortic syndrome and the extent of aortic involvement, in effect distinguishing type A from type B. In addition, identifying the presence of concomitant hemopericardium is critical because its presence indicates that blood has been leaking from the ascending thoracic aorta, so rupture may be imminent, thus making the need for surgical repair a true emergency. Identifying the presence and severity of aortic insufficiency and evaluating the structure and function of the aortic valve will inform the surgeon as to whether the valve needs to be resuspended, repaired, or replaced. If the aortic dissection is diagnosed initially by CTA, data on aortic valve function would not be provided; however, a follow-up TEE is routinely obtained in the operating room before initiation of cardiopulmonary bypass. Moreover, the intraoperative TEE can guide the surgeon in assessing the success of any aortic valve repair. Finally, it is important to look for evidence of distal malperfusion (see discussion below) at presentation because even if the patient has a type A aortic dissection, the presence of malperfusion may necessitate distal intervention immediately before or immediately after ascending thoracic aortic replacement.

The goal of therapy for acute aortic dissection is to prevent its potentially lethal complications, particularly aortic rupture and malperfusion. When aortic dissection is strongly suspected, patients should immediately be placed in an acute care setting for hemodynamic stabilization and monitoring of blood pressure, cardiac rhythm, and urine output. The goal of medical therapy is to reduce dP/dt and any systemic hypertension with antihypertensive medications and to control pain, usually with intravenous (IV) morphine sulfate. The use of long-acting medications should be avoided in patients who are surgical candidates because such drugs may complicate intraoperative arterial pressure management. Initial therapeutic goals include the elimination of pain and reduction of systolic blood pressure to 100 to 120 mm Hg (mean of 60 to 75 mm Hg) or the lowest level commensurate with adequate perfusion of vital organs, specifically the heart, brain, and kidneys.

Sodium nitroprusside is very effective for the acute reduction of arterial pressure. It is initially infused at 20 μg/min with the dosage titrated upward, as high as 800 μg/min, according to the blood pressure response. However, when used alone, sodium nitroprusside can actually cause an increase in dP/dt, which in turn may potentially contribute to propagation of the dissection. Therefore, concomitant β-blocking treatment is essential. For patients with acute or chronic renal insufficiency, IV fenoldopam may be preferable to sodium nitroprusside.

To reduce dP/dt acutely, an IV β-blocker should be administered in incremental doses until evidence of satisfactory β-blockade is noted, usually indicated by a heart rate of 60 to 80 beats/min in the acute setting. Because propranolol was the first generally available β-blocker, it has been used most widely to treat aortic dissection, but other β-blockers are also effective. Propranolol should be administered in IV doses of 1 mg every 3 to 5 minutes until the desired effect is achieved, although the maximum initial dose should not exceed 0.15 mg/kg, or approximately 10 mg. To maintain adequate β-blockade as evidenced by the heart rate, additional propranolol should be given intravenously every 4 to 6 hours, or it should be administered as a continuous infusion.

Labetalol, which acts as both an α- and β-adrenergic receptor blocker, can be especially useful in the setting of aortic dissection because it effectively lowers both dP/dt and arterial pressure. The initial dose of labetalol is 20 mg, administered intravenously over 2 minutes, followed by additional doses of 40 to 80 mg every 10 to 15 minutes, up to a maximum total dose of 300 mg, until the heart rate and blood pressure have been controlled. Maintenance dosing can then be achieved with a continuous IV infusion, starting at 2 mg/min and titrating up to 5 to 10 mg/min.

The ultra–short-acting β-blocker esmolol may be particularly useful in patients with labile arterial pressure, especially if surgery is planned, because this drug can be abruptly discontinued if necessary. It is administered as a 500 μg/kg IV bolus followed by continuous infusion at 50 μg/kg/min and titrated up to 200 μg/kg/min. Esmolol can also be useful as a means to test β-blocker safety and tolerance in patients with a history of obstructive pulmonary disease who may be at uncertain risk for bronchospasm from β-blocker administration. In such patients, a cardioselective β-blocker, such as atenolol or metoprolol, can be considered.

When contraindications exist to the use of β-blockers—including severe sinus bradycardia, second- or third-degree atrioventricular block, congestive heart failure, or bronchospasm—other agents to reduce arterial pressure and dP/dt should be considered. Calcium channel antagonists, which are effective in managing hypertensive crisis, are used on occasion in the treatment of aortic dissection. The combined vasodilator and negative inotropic effects of both diltiazem and verapamil make these agents well suited for the treatment of aortic dissection. Moreover, these agents may be administered intravenously.

Refractory hypertension may result when a dissection compromises one or both of the renal arteries, thereby causing the release of large amounts of renin. In this situation, the most efficacious antihypertensive may be the ACE inhibitor enalaprilat, which is initially administered by IV in doses of 0.625 to 1.25 mg every 6 hours and then titrated upward if necessary to a maximum of 5 mg every 6 hours. Alternatively, interventional therapy to restore normal renal perfusion is the more definitive way to manage hypertension in such cases.

In the event that a patient with suspected aortic dissection has significant hypotension, rapid volume expansion should be considered given the possible presence of cardiac tamponade or aortic rupture. However, before initiating aggressive treatment of such hypotension, the clinician should take care to exclude the possibility of *pseudohypotension*, which occurs when arterial pressure is being measured in an extremity where the circulation is selectively compromised by the dissection. If vasopressors are absolutely required for refractory hypotension, norepinephrine (Levophed) or phenylephrine (Neo-Synephrine) is preferred. Dopamine should be reserved for improving renal perfusion and should be used only at very low doses, given that it may raise dP/dt.

Definitive Therapy

Patients with type A aortic dissection are at high risk of death from rupture into the pericardium, leading to cardiac tamponade, pulseless electrical activity, and death. Consequently, definitive management of type A aortic dissection involves open surgery to replace the dissected ascending thoracic aorta. Occasional patients with proximal dissection who refuse surgery or for whom surgery is contraindicated, such as by age or prior debilitating illness, may be treated successfully with medical therapy with a 30-day survival rate of up to 42%.[49] On the other hand, patients sustaining acute type B dissection are at much lower risk of early death from complications of the dissection than are those with proximal dissection. A large retrospective series has shown, by multivariate analysis, that medical therapy provides an outcome equivalent to that of surgical therapy in patients with uncomplicated distal dissection. As a consequence, medical therapy for such patients is favored. An important exception is that when distal dissection is complicated by vital organ or limb ischemia, uncontrolled pain, or rapid expansion, medical therapy yields poor results and surgery is therefore recommended.

The usual objectives of definitive surgical therapy include resection of the most severely damaged segment of aorta, excision of the intimal tear when possible, and obliteration of entry into the false lumen by suturing the edges of the dissected aorta both proximally and distally. After the diseased segment that contains the intimal tear is resected—typically a segment of the ascending aorta in proximal dissections or the proximal descending aorta in distal dissections—aortic continuity is reestablished by interposing a prosthetic sleeve graft between the two ends of the aorta.

Importantly, several studies have demonstrated that the immediate and long-term survival of patients treated surgically was not significantly affected by failure to excise the intimal tear. Some patients with proximal dissection have an intimal tear located in the aortic arch. Because surgical repair of the arch may increase the morbidity and mortality associated with the procedure, and because resection of the tear may not necessarily improve survival,[50] many surgeons elect not to repair the arch if the sole purpose of surgery is resection of the intimal tear. However, with improvements in surgical technique during the past decade, several groups suggest that even these challenging lesions can be resected with favorable results.

When aortic regurgitation complicates aortic dissection, simple decompression of the false lumen is sometimes all that is required to allow resuspension of the aortic leaflets and restoration of valvular competence. More often, however, preservation of the aortic valve requires approximation of the two layers of dissected aortic wall and resuspension of the commissures with pledgeted sutures. In this setting, the use of intraoperative TEE may be particularly helpful to the surgeon in guiding aortic valve repair.[51] This resuspension technique has had favorable results with a fairly low incidence of recurrent aortic regurgitation in long-term follow-up. Preserving the aortic valve in this fashion may avoid the complications associated with prosthetic valve replacement, especially the requirement for oral anticoagulation, which may pose an added risk in patients prone to future aortic rupture.

Prosthetic aortic valve replacement is sometimes necessary, however, either because attempts at valve repair are unsuccessful or in the setting of preexisting valvular disease or Marfan syndrome. Many surgeons are aggressive about replacing the aortic valve if it appears that even moderate aortic regurgitation will remain after the leaflets are resuspended, and they choose to avoid the risk of having to replace the aortic valve at some later date in a second operation through a diseased aorta. When the proximal aorta is fragile or badly torn, most surgeons use a composite prosthetic graft, such as those described earlier, for replacement of both the ascending aorta and the aortic valve together. The operative procedure for aortic dissection is technically demanding because the wall of the diseased aorta is often friable, and the repair must be performed with meticulous care. Use of Teflon felt to buttress the wall and prevent sutures from tearing through the fragile aorta is essential.

Intervention for type B aortic dissection is generally reserved for patients with acute complications, which include malperfusion, refractory hypertension, refractory pain, and an enlarging aortic aneurysm. Malperfusion may manifest as mesenteric, renal, or limb ischemia, and it is usually caused by either static or dynamic obstruction (Figure 40-9). *Static obstruction* results from the extension of the dissection flap into a branch artery, leading to narrowing or occlusion of the branch true lumen. *Dynamic obstruction* arises when the dissected distal aorta has few or no reentry sites and, consequently, the false lumen expands but then cannot decompress in diastole. The false lumen then becomes distended and markedly compresses the true lumen in the distal aorta, which restricts the volume and pressure of flow to arterial branches supplied by the true lumen. Mesenteric ischemia is the major cause

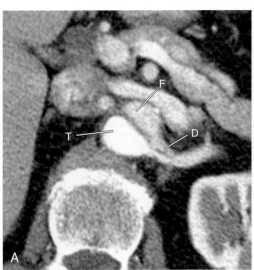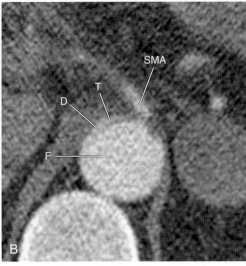

FIGURE 40-9 Causes of malperfusion in aortic dissection. **A,** Static obstruction, in which the dissection flap (*D*), which separates the true (*T*) and false (*F*) lumens, extends into the left renal artery. **B,** Dynamic obstruction, in which the large false lumen dramatically compresses the true lumen, which is now barely visible anterior to the dissection flap and impairs flow to the superior mesenteric artery (*SMA*). *(Copyright Massachusetts General Hospital Thoracic Aortic Center. Used with permission.)*

of death in type B aortic dissection, so clinical vigilance should be high, and its appearance should prompt timely intervention.

The traditional approach for managing complicated type B dissections had been open surgery with fenestration and an interposition graft, but this was associated with a high early mortality rate of about 18% to 31%. More recently, percutaneous interventions have quickly become the preferred techniques for dealing with complications. One percutaneous approach is to directly address the specific distal complication, such as by stenting open a narrowed branch artery to relieve static obstruction or by fenestrating the dissection flap to relieve dynamic obstruction (Figure 40-10). The favored percutaneous approach is to address the distal complications by addressing the proximal cause of the dissection, which is the site of intimal tear; a covered endovascular stent-graft is delivered retrograde to the proximal part of the dissected aorta, where it is deployed and seals off the proximal entry tear, which in turn decompresses the false lumen distally (Figure 40-11). Early studies of endovascular stent-grafting to treat complicated type B dissections showed excellent success in relieving acute complications and producing favorable 1-year survival. In nonrandomized trials, percutaneous interventions have been shown to be effective and are associated with a mortality rate significantly below that of open repair.[52,53] However, in some cases, the false lumen distal to the covered stent-graft does not fully decompress, so newer techniques are now being investigated to extend the stent-graft distally, and uncovered stents are used as scaffolding to obliterate the false lumen in the abdominal aorta. The technique was initially given the acronym PETTICOAT, for *provisional extension to induce complete attachment.* Introduced by Nienaber and colleagues,[54] it is now being studied in the Study of Thoracic Aortic Type B Dissection Using Endoluminal Repair (STABLE) trial, an international clinical trial to evaluate the Zenith Dissection Endovascular System (Cook Medical, Bloomington, IN) for the treatment of type B thoracic aortic dissections.

Given the success of endovascular stent-grafting in the management of complicated type B aortic dissection, some have proposed that it may be beneficial to stent-graft uncomplicated type B dissections prophylactically to prevent life-threatening distal complications and perhaps reduce late aortic growth by eliminating flow to the false lumen. The Investigation of Stent Grafts in Aortic Dissection (INSTEAD) trial was the first large, randomized prospective trial to investigate this possibility,[55] but it found that compared with optimal medical therapy, endovascular stent-grafting conferred no benefit over the first 2 years of follow-up. However, in this trial, patients were enrolled between 2 and 34 weeks following their

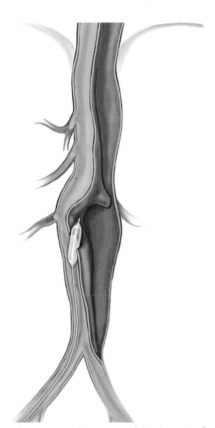

FIGURE 40-10 Percutaneous fenestration of the dissection flap in a type B aortic dissection complicated by dynamic obstruction and malperfusion. A wire is advanced retrograde from the femoral artery to the visceral segment of the abdominal aorta; the wire pierces the dissection flap, a balloon-tipped catheter is advanced over the wire, and the balloon is inflated to rip a hole in the dissection flap. Several holes are created with the goal of decompressing the distended false lumen. *(Copyright Massachusetts General Hospital Thoracic Aortic Center. Used with permission.)*

acute type B dissection, making it unlikely that the stent-graft could prevent the most serious complications, which typically occur within the first 2 weeks. Moreover, the patients treated with optimal medical therapy fared remarkably well in this trial, with a mortality rate of only 4% at 2 years compared with 11% in the

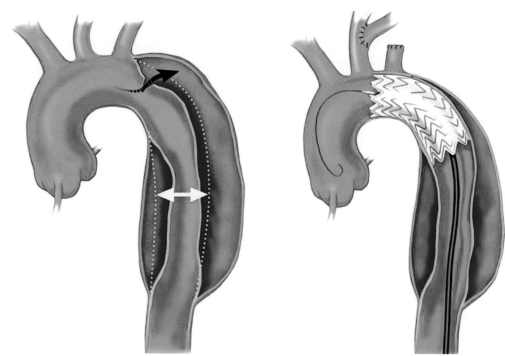

FIGURE 40-11 Thoracic endovascular stent-graft for managing a complicated type B aortic dissection. To reduce the risk of neurologic complications, surgeons often first perform a left subclavian to carotid artery bypass to maintain perfusion of the left subclavian artery after graft deployment. A covered endovascular stent-graft is then deployed in the proximal descending thoracic aorta, with the goal of covering over the entry tear, through which blood flows into the false lumen, thus decompressing the false lumen and promoting its thrombosis. *(Copyright Massachusetts General Hospital Thoracic Aortic Center. Used with permission.)*

TEVAR group (*P* = .15). Indeed, the survival in the group treated with optimal medical therapy was far better than the historic 1-year survival rate of about 85% for medically managed type B dissections.[56] It must be recognized that with a 2-year mortality rate of only 4%, it would have been hard for an intervention of any kind to outperform medical therapy. Fortunately, a second randomized study, the Acute Dissection Stent-Grafting or Best Medical Treatment (ADSORB) trial, is now under way in Europe. It has a design similar to INSTEAD, except that patients will be enrolled at days 0 through 14 after acute uncomplicated type B dissections, so it may reveal whether any benefit can be gained from early endovascular stent-grafting.

Those with uncomplicated type B dissections are best managed medically. As described above, the primary management goal is to reduce dP/dt and control blood pressure. Although IV agents are initially preferred, once the hemodynamics are controlled and the patient has remained stable for perhaps 12 to 24 hours, oral agents should be started. Over time the doses of these oral agents should be titrated upward as IV agents are weaned off. The patient should remain in an intensive care unit (ICU) setting until IV agents have been discontinued for at least 6 to 12 hours without any significant spikes in blood pressure.

In most cases hypertension is brought under control over the course of the first 1 to 3 days. However, severe hypertension occurs early in the hospitalization for acute type B aortic dissection, even among those without a history of significant hypertension. In some cases refractory hypertension may be due to malperfusion of one or both kidneys, in which case intervention may be indicated. However, in a prior retrospective analysis, my group found that although almost two thirds of patients with distal dissections required the administration of four or more antihypertensive medications to control refractory hypertension early in their hospitalization, they had no evidence of malperfusion. Moreover, in these cases the hypertension typically improved 5 to 7 days after onset of the dissection, allowing for a reduction in antihypertensive therapy without the need for intervention.[57] The etiology for this acute early hypertensive response is uncertain but

may reflect a marked increase in sympathetic tone triggered by the severe inflammation of the aortic wall that accompanies dissection.

Another goal in the medical management of type B dissection is to monitor the patient vigilantly for any evidence of branch arterial compromise, the most lethal consequence of which is mesenteric ischemia. Unfortunately, the clinical features of mesenteric ischemia may initially be subtle and therefore go unrecognized; by the time these features have become clinically obvious, organ damage may be irreversible. Adding to the diagnostic challenge is the fact that in as many as half of such cases,[58] imaging studies such as CTA may not be interpreted as showing evidence of malperfusion. Consequently, it is imperative to maintain a strong clinical suspicion for mesenteric ischemia and have a low threshold for surgical or percutaneous intervention when any evidence of malperfusion exists.

Long-Term Therapy and Late Follow-up

Long-term medical therapy to control hypertension and reduce dP/dt is indicated for all patients who have sustained an aortic dissection, regardless of whether their in-hospital definitive treatment was surgical or medical. Indeed, one study found that late aneurysm rupture after aortic dissection was 10 times more common in patients with poorly controlled hypertension than in those with controlled blood pressure, which dramatically demonstrates the importance of aggressive lifelong antihypertensive therapy. Systolic blood pressure should be maintained at or below 130 mm Hg; the preferred agents are β-blockers or, if contraindicated, other agents with a negative inotropic and hypotensive effect, such as verapamil or diltiazem. ACE inhibitors and ARBs are attractive antihypertensive agents for treating aortic dissection, and they may be of particular benefit in patients with some degree of renal ischemia as a consequence of the dissection.

Up to 29% of late deaths following surgery result from rupture of either the dissecting aneurysm or another aneurysm at a remote site. Moreover, the incidence of subsequent aneurysm formation at a site remote from the surgical repair is 17% to 25%, and these remote aneurysms account for many of the rupture-related deaths. Many such aneurysms occur from dilation of the residual false lumen in the more distal aortic segments not resected at the time of surgery. Because the dissected aneurysm wall is relatively thin and consists of only the outer half of the original aortic wall, these aneurysms rupture more frequently than do typical atherosclerotic thoracic aneurysms. Thus, an aggressive approach to treating such late-appearing aneurysms may be indicated.

The high incidence of late aneurysm formation and rupture emphasizes both the diffuse nature of the aortic disease process in this population and the tremendous importance of careful follow-up. The primary goal of long-term surveillance is the early detection of aortic lesions that might require subsequent surgical intervention. The clinician must remain watchful for the appearance of new aneurysms or rapid aneurysm expansion, progression or recurrence of dissection, aortic regurgitation, and peripheral vascular compromise.

Follow-up evaluation of patients after aortic dissection should include serial aortic imaging with CT, MRI, or TEE. We generally prefer CT for serial monitoring of these patients because it is completely noninvasive and provides excellent anatomic detail that may be exceedingly helpful in evaluating interval changes. Patients are at highest risk immediately after hospitalization and during the first 2 years, with the risk progressively declining thereafter. It is therefore important to have more frequent early follow-up; for example, patients can be seen and imaged at 1, 3, 6, and 12 months initially following the dissection, after which time they can often be reimaged at 12-month intervals, assuming they are otherwise stable.

Intramural Hematoma

Intramural hematoma is an acute aortic syndrome. Essentially, a hemorrhage is contained within the medial layer of the aortic wall, but unlike classic aortic dissection, no tear is evident in the intima, and no active communication is apparent between the hematoma and the aortic lumen. The natural history of intramural hematoma, however, remains less well defined than that of classic aortic dissection. A review of 160 patients from 11 studies reporting outcomes of aortic intramural hematoma found that proximal intramural hematoma was associated with mortality rates of 47% when managed medically and 24% when managed surgically.[59] On the other hand, distal intramural hematoma was associated with a mortality rate of 13% with medical management compared with 15% with surgical repair. These rates are remarkably similar to those for classic aortic dissection.[49] Consequently, most treatment centers currently accept a general management strategy for aortic intramural hematoma similar to that used for classic aortic dissection; proximal aortic involvement is treated surgically, and distal aortic involvement is managed medically. Physicians should have a low threshold for proceeding to surgery in patients with distal disease if symptoms persist or evidence of progression is seen. Medical management should therefore include serial imaging studies to monitor progression or regression of the intramural hematoma.

Several recent reports have suggested that the outcomes associated with proximal intramural hematoma may be more benign than with classic aortic dissection, with a large proportion of patients surviving with medical therapy alone. For example, Song and coworkers[60] reported in-hospital mortality rates for medically managed proximal and distal intramural hematomas of only 7% and 1%, respectively, both of which are substantially lower than the previously reported rates of 47% and 13%, respectively. But the patient population in this study may not be comparable. In fact, in Song and colleagues' series, 29% of apparent aortic dissection cases were diagnosed as intramural hematoma, a proportion about double what other investigators have reported. This series may have thus identified and included more subtle cases of intramural hematoma, which would go undetected in

other hospitals and are likely to be associated with a lower risk of progression or rupture. There may be a continuum of risk for intramural hematoma, rather than an absolute risk. The morphologic features that distinguish intramural hematoma from classic aortic dissection, such as the absence of a patent false lumen, suggest that intramural hematomas are somewhat less likely to rupture. However, factors that increase aortic wall stress, such as large aortic diameters and thick hematomas, could increase the risk of rupture or dissection. Indeed, one recent study of acute intramural hematoma[61] found that a maximum aortic diameter of 50 mm or larger independently predicted progression, whereas in another study of patients with distal intramural hematoma managed medically,[62] both a maximum aortic diameter of 40 mm or larger and a maximum aortic wall thickness of 10 mm or larger independently predicted progression. These findings confirm that some patients with intramural hematoma may be at considerably lower risk than others, suggesting that baseline differences in patient characteristics could substantially influence outcomes. However, until further studies better define patients at very low risk, our group still recommends the strategy of routine aortic surgery for proximal intramural hematoma.[63]

Penetrating Atherosclerotic Ulcer

The natural history of a penetrating atherosclerotic ulcer remains largely unclear and likely differs significantly between patients presenting with symptoms (i.e., acute aortic syndrome) and those seen without symptoms (i.e., an incidental finding). At present, no consensus prevails regarding a definitive treatment strategy. Certainly, patients who are hemodynamically unstable or who have evidence of pseudoaneurysm formation or transmural rupture should undergo urgent surgical repair. Continued or recurrent pain, distal embolization, and progressive aneurysmal dilation are also indications for surgery. However, it remains unclear whether otherwise stable patients with distal penetrating atherosclerotic ulcers should undergo surgery, or if they can be safely managed medically, as in the case of classic aortic dissection. In one study of 26 patients with penetrating atherosclerotic ulcer,[64] no difference was reported in the 1- and 5-year survival rates between surgical and medical management strategies, suggesting that surgery may not improve the otherwise poor prognosis. Transluminal placement of an endovascular stent-graft may become a lower risk alternative to surgery in such patients.

Ganaha and coworkers[65] examined the outcomes of 31 patients with penetrating atherosclerotic ulcers, of whom 17 were managed medically, 8 underwent surgical repair, and 6 underwent stent-grafting for evidence of aortic rupture or impending rupture. Importantly, no significant difference was noted in early survival among the three strategies. The authors compared patients with a progressive in-hospital course—defined as aortic rupture, hematoma expansion, or appearance of a distinct false lumen—to those with a stable course. Uncontrolled pain and an enlarging pleural effusion were both highly predictive of a progressive course. CT findings associated with a progressive, rather than a stable, course included maximal diameter of the ulcer (21 vs. 12 mm, respectively), maximal depth of the ulcer (14 vs. 7 mm, respectively), and an ulcer located in the proximal third of the descending aorta rather than more distal. With these various markers, about half of the patients in the study would have been considered low risk for a progressive course. Our group recommends treating patients with such uncomplicated conditions with antihypertensive medications and close monitoring with serial imaging studies, similar to the management of a patient with a distal aortic dissection.

Thoracic Aortic Atheroembolism

Atherosclerotic disease of the aortic arch is commonly found in patients who present with acute stroke. Moreover, the presence of arch atheromas has been shown to be a risk factor for recurrent stroke and other embolic events. In a meta-analysis by Macleod and colleagues,[66] among those with aortic arch atheromas, the odds ratio of stroke was 3.76 (95% CI, 2.57 to 5.51), and plaques of 4 mm or greater in thickness were most strongly associated with risk of stroke or other vascular embolic events.

Because atheromas appear to be a combination of atherosclerotic plaques and superimposed thrombus, anticoagulant therapy makes intuitive sense. However, historically, some health care providers have been reluctant to use warfarin in patients with aortic atheroma because of concern that plaque hemorrhage could release debris and trigger atheroembolic syndrome. However, the risk of clinical atheroembolic syndrome during warfarin therapy in such patients appears to be quite low, with only one episode among 134 at-risk patients with complex aortic plaques treated in the Stroke Prevention in Atrial Fibrillation (SPAF) trial.[67] Moreover, in this trial, warfarin was not only safe, it was effective; the stroke rate was only 4% at 1 year in the adjusted-dose warfarin group (INR, 2.0 to 3.0) compared with 16% in the group treated with a fixed, low dose of warfarin (INR, 1.2 to 1.5) plus aspirin (relative risk reduction, 75%; $P = .02$). Among a similarly sized nonrandomized trial of oral anticoagulation versus antiplatelet therapy, a significantly lower embolic rate was seen among those treated with anticoagulation: 0% versus 22% (OR, 0.06; 95% CI, 0.003 to 1.2; $P = .016$).[67a] These two reports suggest that among patients with large aortic arch atheromas, warfarin is not harmful and may reduce stroke rates. However, because these were small, nonrandomized trials, their findings are insufficient to justify the routine use of warfarin in high-risk patients. Fortunately, the Aortic Arch–Related Cerebral Hazard (ARCH) trial was initiated.[68] Designed as an ongoing, open-label, randomized study of patients with nondisabling stroke or peripheral emboli who have aortic arch atheromas of 4 mm or greater in thickness, patients are to be randomized to oral anticoagulation (target INR, 2.0 to 3.0) versus daily aspirin (75 mg) plus clopidogrel (75 mg) and followed longitudinally every 4 months for evidence of recurrent vascular events. Results are expected in 2014, but in anticipation of the outcomes of this key trial, the recent ACC/AHA guidelines have made a class IIb recommendation (level of evidence C), stating that "oral anticoagulation therapy with warfarin (INR, 2.0 to 3.0) or antiplatelet therapy may be considered in stroke patients with aortic arch atheroma of 4.0 mm or greater to prevent recurrent stroke."[27]

Another reasonable approach to reducing the risk of thromboembolism in those with aortic atheromas is the use of statin therapy to halt or reverse the atherosclerotic process. Indeed, statins have been shown to reduce both primary and secondary stroke rates in a variety of populations. In an observational study of 519 patients with large aortic plaques on TEE, statin use was associated with a relative risk reduction for ischemic stroke of 59%.[69] Once again, randomized, controlled clinical trials are needed to prove that statins reduce event rates; however, such studies may be difficult to perform because most patients with stroke or significant aortic plaques will have other indications for statin therapy. One alternative approach is to compare high-dose statin therapy to low-dose statin therapy rather than to placebo. Indeed, evidence from a randomized prospective trial of patients with asymptomatic aortic plaques suggests that, compared with low-dose therapy, high-dose atorvastatin is associated with a significant reduction in plaque volume.[70] The recent ACC/AHA guidelines make a class IIa (level of evidence C) recommendation that "treatment with a statin is a reasonable option for patients with aortic arch atheroma to reduce the risk of stroke."[27]

Surgical aortic arch endarterectomy has been attempted for patients with thromboembolism originating from aortic arch atheroma, and early case reports described success. However, in a large series of 3404 patients undergoing cardiac surgery, 268 (8%) had arch atheromas 5 mm or larger with protruding elements by TEE, and aortic arch endarterectomy was performed in 43 (16%) at the discretion of the surgeon. Unfortunately, the performance of endarterectomy was associated with a threefold higher rate of perioperative stroke than no endarterectomy—35% versus 12% ($P < .0001$).[71] Covered endovascular stent-grafts offer the potential

advantage of shielding severely diseased aortic segments to prevent further embolization, but treatment of arch atheromas would require a hybrid procedure with debranching plus stent-grafting. Moreover, the endovascular manipulation may itself produce periprocedural embolization. Thus, no evidence justifies prophylactic endarterectomy or aortic arch stent-grafting for patients with protruding atheromas.

REFERENCES

1. Brown LC, Powell JT. Risk factors for aneurysm rupture in patients kept under ultrasound surveillance. UK Small Aneurysm Trial Participants. *Ann Surg* 1999;230:289-296.
2. Lederle FA, Johnson GR, Wilson SE, et al. Rupture rate of large abdominal aortic aneurysms in patients refusing or unfit for elective repair. *JAMA* 2002;287:2968-2972.
3. The United Kingdom Small Aneurysm Trial Participants. Long-term outcomes of immediate repair compared with surveillance of small abdominal aortic aneurysms. *N Engl J Med* 2002;346:1445-1452.
4. Lederle FA, Wilson ES, Johnson GR, et al. Immediate repair compared with surveillance of small abdominal aortic aneurysms. *N Engl J Med* 2002;346:1437-1444.
5. Thompson RW. Detection and management of small aortic aneurysms. *N Engl J Med* 2002;346:1484-1486.
6. Brewster DC, Cronenwett JL, Hallett JW Jr, et al. Guidelines for the treatment of abdominal aortic aneurysms. Report of a subcommittee of the Joint Council of the American Association for Vascular Surgery and Society for Vascular Surgery. *J Vasc Surg* 2003;37:1106-1117.
7. Prinssen M, Verhoeven EL, Buth J, et al.; Dutch Randomized Endovascular Aneurysm Management (DREAM) Trial Group. A randomized trial comparing conventional and endovascular repair of abdominal aortic aneurysms. *N Engl J Med* 2004;351:1607-1618.
8. Greenhalgh RM, Brown LC, Kwong GP, et al. Comparison of endovascular aneurysm repair with open repair in patients with abdominal aortic aneurysm (EVAR trial 1), 30-day operative mortality results: randomised controlled trial. *Lancet* 2004;364:843-848.
9. Lederle FA. Abdominal aortic aneurysm—open versus endovascular repair. *N Engl J Med* 2004;351:1677-1679.
10. Blankensteijn JD, de Jong SE, Prinssen M, et al.; Dutch Randomized Endovascular Aneurysm Management (DREAM) Trial Group. Two-year outcomes after conventional or endovascular repair of abdominal aortic aneurysms. *N Engl J Med* 2005;352:2398-2405.
11. EVAR trial participants. Endovascular aneurysm repair versus open repair in patients with abdominal aortic aneurysm (EVAR trial 1): randomised controlled trial. *Lancet* 2005;365:2179-2186.
12. The United Kingdom EVAR Trial Investigators. Endovascular versus open repair of abdominal aortic aneurysm. *N Engl J Med* 2010;362:1863-1871.
13. The United Kingdom EVAR Trial Investigators. Endovascular repair of aortic aneurysm in patients physically ineligible for open repair. *N Engl J Med* 2010;362:1872-1880.
14. Rooke TM , Hirsch AT, Misra S, et al. 2011 ACCF/AHA focused update of the guideline for the management of patients with peripheral artery disease (updating the 2005 guideline). *J Am Coll Cardol* 2011;58:2020-2045.
15. The Propranolol Aneurysm Trial Investigators. Propranolol for small abdominal aortic aneurysms: results of a randomized trial. *J Vasc Surg* 2002;35:72-79.
16. Baxter BT, Terrin MC, Dahlman RL. Medical management of small abdominal aortic aneurysms. *Circulation* 2008;117:1883-1889.
17. Chaikof EL, Brewster DC, Dalman RL, et al. The care of patients with an abdominal aortic aneurysm: the Society for Vascular Surgery practice guidelines. *J Vasc Surg* 2009;50(Suppl):S2-S49.
18. Liao S, Miralles M, Kelley BJ, et al. Suppression of experimental abdominal aortic aneurysms in the rat by treatment with angiotensin-converting enzyme inhibitors. *J Vasc Surg* 2001;33:1057-1064.
19. Hackam DG, Thiruchelvam D, Redelmeier DA. Angiotensin-converting enzyme inhibitors and aortic rupture: a population-based case-control study. *Lancet* 2006;368:659-665.
20. Kalyanasundaram A, Elmore JR, Manazer JR, et al. Simvastatin suppresses experimental aortic aneurysm expansion. *J Vasc Surg* 2006;43:117-124.
21. Sukhija R, Aronow WS, Sandhu R, et al. Mortality and size of abdominal aortic aneurysm at long-term follow-up of patients not treated surgically and treated with and without statins. *Am J Cardiol* 2006;97:279-280.
22. Twine CP, Williams IM. Systematic review and meta-analysis of the effects of statin therapy on abdominal aortic aneurysms. *Br J Surg* 2011;98:346-353.
23. Prall AK, Longo M, Mayhan WG, et al. Doxycycline in patients with abdominal aortic aneurysms and in mice: comparison of serum levels and effect on aneurysm growth in mice. *J Vasc Surg* 2002;35:923-929.
24. Lindeman JHN, Abdul-Hussien H, van Bockel JH, et al. Clinical trial of doxycycline for matrix metalloproteinase-9 inhibition in patients with an abdominal aneurysm: doxycycline selectively depletes aortic wall neutrophils and cytotoxic T cells. *Circulation* 2009;119:2209-2216.
25. Vammen S, Lindholt JS, Ostergaard L, et al. Randomized double-blind trial of roxithromycin for prevention of abdominal aortic aneurysm expansion. *Br J Surg* 2001;88:1066-1072.
26. Lawrence DM, Singh RS, Franklin DP, et al. Rapamycin suppresses experimental aortic aneurysm growth. *J Vasc Surg* 2004;40:334-338.
26a. Coady MA, Rizzo JA, Hammond GL, et al. Surgical intervention criteria for thoracic aortic aneurysms: a study of growth rates and complications. *Ann Thorac Surg* 1999;67:1922–1926.
27. Hiratzka LF, Bakris GL, Beckman JA, et al. 2010 ACCF/AHA/AATS/ACR/ASA/SCA/SCAI/SIR/STS/SVM Guidelines for the Diagnosis and Management of Patients with Thoracic Aortic Disease: Executive Summary. *Circulation* 2010;121:e266-e369.
28. Svensson LG, Khitin L. Aortic cross-sectional area/height ratio timing of aortic surgery in asymptomatic patients with Marfan syndrome. *J Thorac Cardiovasc Surg* 2002;123:360-361.

29. Svensson LG, Kim KH, Lytle BW, et al. Relationship of aortic cross-sectional area to height ratio and the risk of aortic dissection in patients with bicuspid aortic valves. *J Thorac Cardiovasc Surg* 2003;126:892-893.

30. Davies RR, Gallo A, Coady MA, et al. Novel measurement of relative aortic size predicts rupture of thoracic aortic aneurysms. *Ann Thorac Surg* 2006;81:169-177.

31. Coady MA, Ikonomidis JS, Cheung AT, et al. Surgical management of descending thoracic aortic disease: open and endovascular approaches: a scientific statement from the American Heart Association. *Circulation* 2010;121:2780-2804.

32. David TE, Ivanov J, Armstrong S, et al. Aortic valve-sparing operations in patients with aneurysms of the aortic root or ascending aorta. *Ann Thorac Surg* 2002;74: S1758-S1761.

33. Miller CD. Valve-sparing aortic root replacement: current state of the art and where are we headed? *Ann Thorac Surg* 2007;83:S736-S739.

34. Isselbacher EM. Contemporary reviews in cardiovascular medicine: thoracic and abdominal aortic aneurysms. *Circulation* 2005;111:816-828.

35. Hagl C, Ergin MA, Galla JD, et al. Neurologic outcome after ascending aorta–aortic arch operations: effect of brain protection technique in high-risk patients. *J Thorac Cardiovasc Surg* 2001;121:1107-1121.

36. Immer FF, Moser B, Krahenbuhl ES, et al. Arterial access through the right subclavian artery in surgery of the aortic arch improves neurologic outcome and mid-term quality of life. *Ann Thorac Surg* 2008;85:1614-1618.

37. Kulik A, Castner CF, Kouchoukos NT. Outcomes after total aortic arch replacement with right axillary artery cannulation and a presewn multibranched graft. *Ann Thorac Surg* 2011;92:889-897.

38. Spielvogel D, Etz CD, Silovitz D, et al. Aortic arch replacement with a trifurcated graft. *Ann Thorac Surg* 2007;83:S791-S795.

39. Kazui T, Washiyama N, Muhammad BAH, et al. Improved results of atherosclerotic arch aneurysm operations with a refined technique. *J Thorac Cardiovasc Surg* 2001; 121:491-499.

40. Milewski RK, Szeto WY, Pochettino A, et al. Have hybrid procedures replaced open aortic arch reconstruction in high-risk patients? A comparative study of elective open arch debranching with endovascular stent graft placement and conventional elective open total and distal aortic arch reconstruction. *J Thorac Cardiovasc Surg* 2010;140:590-597.

41. Greenberg RK, Haddad F, Svensson L, et al. Hybrid approaches to thoracic aortic aneurysms: the role of endovascular elephant trunk completion. *Circulation* 2005;112: 2619-2626.

42. Makaroun MS, Dillavou ED, Kee ST, et al. Endovascular treatment of thoracic aortic aneurysms: results of the phase II multicenter trial of the GORE TAG thoracic endoprosthesis. *J Vasc Surg* 2005;41:1-9.

43. Makaroun MS, Dillavou ED, Wheatley GH, et al, for the Gore TAG Investigators. Five-year results of endovascular treatment with the Gore TAG device compared with open repair of thoracic aortic aneurysms. *J Vasc Surg* 2008;47:912-918.

44. Ricotta JJ. Endoleak management and postoperative surveillance following endovascular repair of thoracic aortic aneurysms. *J Vasc Surg* 2010;52:91S-99S.

45. Shores J, Berger KR, Murphy EA, et al. Progression of aortic dilatation and the benefit of long-term β-adrenergic blockade in Marfan's syndrome. *N Engl J Med* 1994;330: 1335-1341.

46. Habashi JP, Judge DP, Holm TM, et al. Losartan, an AT1 antagonist, prevents aortic aneurysm in a mouse model of Marfan syndrome. *Science* 2006;312:117-121.

47. Brooke BS, Habashi JP, Judge DP, et al. Angiotensin II blockade and aortic-root dilation in Marfan's syndrome. *N Engl J Med* 2008;358:2787-2795.

48. Ahimastos AA, Anuradha Aggarwal A, D'Orsa KM, et al. Effect of perindopril on large artery stiffness and aortic root diameter in patients with Marfan syndrome: a randomized controlled trial. *JAMA* 2007;298:1539-1547.

49. Hagan PG, Nienaber CA, Isselbacher EM, et al. The International Registry of Acute Aortic Dissection (IRAD): new insights into an old disease. *J Am Med Assoc* 2000;283:897-903.

50. Sabik JF, Lytle BW, Blackstone EH, et al. Long-term effectiveness of operations for ascending aortic dissections. *J Thorac Cardiovasc Surg* 2000;119:946-962.

51. Movsowitz HD, Levine RA, Hilgenberg AD, et al. Transesophageal echocardiographic description of the mechanisms of aortic regurgitation in acute type A aortic dissection: implications for aortic valve repair. *J Am Coll Cardiol* 2000;36:884-890.

52. Fattori R, Tsai TT, Myrmel T. Complicated acute type B dissection: is surgery still the best option? Report from the International Registry of Acute Aortic Dissection. *J Am Coll Cardiol Intv* 2008;1;395-402.

53. Zeeshan A, Woo EY, Bavaria JE, et al. Thoracic endovascular aortic repair for acute complicated type B aortic dissection: superiority relative to conventional open surgical and medical therapy. *J Thorac Cardiovasc Surg* 2010;140:S109-S115.

54. Nienaber CA, Kische S, Zeller T, et al. Provisional extension to induce complete attachment after stent-graft placement in type B aortic dissection: the PETTICOAT concept. *J Endovasc Ther* 2006;13:738-746.

55. Nienaber C, Rousseau H, Eggebrecht H, et al. Randomized comparison of strategies for type B aortic dissection: the INvestigation of STEnt grafts in Aortic Dissection (INSTEAD) trial. *Circulation* 2009;120:2519-2528.

56. Umaña JP, Lai DT, Mitchell RS, et al. Is medical therapy still the most optimal treatment strategy for patients with acute type B aortic dissections? *J Thorac Cardiovasc Surg* 2002;124:896-910.

57. Januzzi JL, Sabatine MS, Choi JC, et al. Refractory systemic hypertension following type B aortic dissection. *Am J Cardiol* 2001;88:686-688.

58. Neri E, Sassi S, Massetti M, et al. Nonocclusive intestinal ischemia in patients with acute aortic dissection. *J Thorac Cardiovasc Surg* 2002;36:738-745.

59. Sawhney NS, DeMaria AN, Blanchard DG. Aortic intramural hematoma: an increasingly recognized and potentially fatal entity. *Chest* 2001;120:1340-1346.

60. Song J-K, Kim H-S, Song JM, et al. Outcomes of medically treated patients with aortic intramural hematoma. *Am J Med* 2002;113:181-187.

61. Kaji S, Nishigami K, Akasaka T, et al. Prediction of progression or regression of type A aortic intramural hematoma by computed tomography. *Circulation* 1999;100(19 Suppl): II281-II286.

62. Sueyoshi E, Imada T, Sakamoto I, et al. Analysis of predictive factors for progression of type B aortic intramural hematoma with computed tomography. *J Vasc Surg* 2002; 35:1179-1183.

63. Isselbacher EM. Intramural hematoma of the aorta: should we let down our guard? *Am J Med* 2002;113:244-246.

64. Tittle SL, Lynch RJ, Cole PE, et al. Midterm follow-up of penetrating ulcer and intramural hematoma of the aorta. *J Thorac Cardiovasc Surg* 2002;123:1051-1059.

65. Ganaha F, Miller DC, Sugimoto K, et al. Prognosis of aortic intramural hematoma with and without penetrating atherosclerotic ulcer: a clinical and radiological analysis. *Circulation* 2002;106:342-348.

66. Macleod MR, Amarenco P, Davis SM, et al. Atheroma of the aortic arch: an important and poorly recognized factor in the etiology of stroke. *Lancet Neurol* 2004;3:408-414.

67. The Stroke Prevention in Atrial Fibrillation Investigators Committee on Echocardiography. Transesophageal echocardiographic correlates of thromboembolism in high risk patients with nonvalvular atrial fibrillation. *Ann Intern Med* 1998:639-647.

67a. Ferrari E, Vidal R, Chevallier T, Baudouy M. Atherosclerosis of the thoracic aorta and aortic debris as a marker of poor prognosis: benefit of oral anticoagulants. *J Am Coll Cardiol* 1999;33:1317–1322.

68. U.S. National Institutes of Health. Aortic Arch Related Cerebral Hazard Trial. Available at http://clinicaltrials.gov/ct2/show/results/NCT00235248.

69. Tunick PA, Nayar AC, Goodkin GM, et al. Effect of treatment on the incidence of stroke and other emboli in 519 patients with severe thoracic aortic plaque. *Am J Cardiol* 2002;90:1320-1325.

70. Yonemura A, Momiyama Y, Fayad ZA, et al. Effect of lipid-lowering therapy with atorvastatin on atherosclerotic aortic plaques: a 2 year follow-up by noninvasive MRI. *Eur J Cardiovasc Prev Rehabil* 2009;16:222-228.

71. Stern A, Tunick PA, Culliford AT, et al. Protruding aortic arch atheromas: risk of stroke during heart surgery with and without aortic arch endarterectomy. *Am Heart J* 1999;138:746-752.

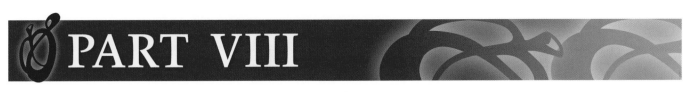

PART VIII

OTHER CARDIOVASCULAR CONDITIONS

CHAPTER 41

Pharmacologic Options for Treating Cardiovascular Disease During Pregnancy

Sharon C. Reimold and Lisa W. Forbess

HYPERTENSION, 621

EDEMA, 623

VALVULAR HEART DISEASE, 623

THROMBOEMBOLIC DISEASE DURING PREGNANCY, 624

Fibrinolysis, 626

ISCHEMIC HEART DISEASE, 626

LIPID DISORDERS, 627

HEART FAILURE, 627

CARDIAC ARRHYTHMIAS, 628

MARFAN SYNDROME, 629

PULMONARY HYPERTENSION, 629

ANTIBIOTIC PROPHYLAXIS, 630

REFERENCES, 630

Pregnancy leads to an expansion of blood volume and altered pharmacokinetics of therapeutic agents. In addition, cardiovascular therapies may have effects on the fetus by crossing the blood-placenta barrier and on the newborn through excretion in breast milk. Physicians caring for pregnant and lactating patients with cardiovascular disorders should understand the hemodynamic changes associated with pregnancy, as well as the pharmacokinetics of various drugs, to make rational and safe decisions regarding pharmacologic therapy during pregnancy, delivery, and the early postpartum period.

Increases in human chorionic somatomammotropin lead to an increase in red blood cell (RBC) formation and subsequently to an increase in RBC mass in pregnancy. An increase in estrogen levels leads to activation of the renin-angiotensin axis. Activation of the renin-angiotensin axis leads to sodium and water retention and results in an increase in extracellular volume. The combined impact of these two changes is to increase blood volume by 30% to 50% over baseline during pregnancy.[1] This increase in blood volume begins before the end of the first trimester and levels off by the middle of the third trimester. Increases in extracellular volume are proportionally larger than increases in RBC volume and represent one cause of the *anemia of pregnancy*.[1] This "physiologic anemia" can be partially corrected with iron supplementation.[2]

During pregnancy, the cardiovascular system must adapt to the increased hemodynamic load. Cardiac output increases throughout pregnancy by increases in heart rate and stroke volume. To accomplish these changes, small increases occur in left and right ventricular diastolic volumes. Impedance to left ventricular (LV) ejection is also decreased because estrogen produces an increase in aortic compliance and a decrease in systemic vascular resistance. The fall in systemic vascular resistance is multifactorial. Gestational hormone activity; increasing circulating levels of prostaglandins, atrial natriuretic peptides, and endothelial nitric oxide; and the creation of a low-resistance placental circulation in the pregnant uterus all contribute to a fall in systemic vascular resistance.[2-4] The systolic pressure begins to fall during the first trimester, nadirs in midpregnancy, and returns to normal before term. Diastolic pressure decreases more than systolic pressure,

thus causing a widened pulse pressure. Decreased blood pressure may be most pronounced during the second trimester and must be considered when prescribing therapies for cardiovascular disorders.

The pharmacokinetics of drugs are altered because of changes in gastrointestinal (GI) and renal function during pregnancy. Decreases in GI motility may lead to decreased and delayed GI absorption. This decreased motility is quite heterogeneous. Increases in fatty tissue and decreased maternal hepatic enzyme activity may decrease the metabolism of some pharmacologic agents. In addition, the distribution of the increased cardiac output is altered in pregnancy; a large amount of flow is distributed to the uterus to allow fetal growth and development, and renal blood flow increases during pregnancy, with a 30% to 80% increase in glomerular filtration rate. Therefore drugs may be eliminated more rapidly during pregnancy than in the nonpregnant state. Metabolic considerations for drug dosing in pregnancy are listed in Table 41-1.

The ability of a pharmacologic agent to cross the placental barrier must be considered. Early in pregnancy, the fetal blood-brain barrier is not developed; therefore agents that cross the placental barrier may affect general fetal development, specifically fetal central nervous system (CNS) development. Some drug therapies are associated with significant adverse effects that include death, developmental malformations, and abnormal growth. Data on the safety of pharmacologic agents in pregnancy are paramount, but for many agents, clinical data from patients are limited. Recommendations for safety are often extrapolated from available animal data. The text *Drugs in Pregnancy and Lactation: A Reference Guide to Fetal and Neonatal Risk* is a useful reference for physicians caring for pregnant patients.[5] Table 41-2 lists the classification of cardioactive drugs and the most common risks associated with their use during pregnancy and lactation.

Hypertension

For a full discussion of the treatment of hypertension in pregnancy, see Chapter 39.

TABLE 41-1   Factors Leading to Altered Pharmacokinetics in Pregnancy

ALTERED SYSTEMS	IMPACT OF CHANGES
Gastrointestinal motility	Decreased motility and absorption are caused by elevated estrogens.
Hepatic enzyme activity	Enzyme activity may be decreased in pregnancy, leading to slower metabolism.
Increased volume of distribution and increased levels of fatty tissue	Increases result in altered protein binding and volume of distribution of some agents (e.g., digoxin).
Increased renal blood flow	Increased glomerular filtration rate may lead to increased drug clearance.
Altered distribution of cardiac output	Proportion of cardiac output dedicated to the uterus is increased, and impact on the fetal-placental unit is dependent on the ability of the agent to cross the placental barrier and migrate through fetal tissues.

TABLE 41-2   Risk of Cardiac Drugs to the Fetus and Newborn

DRUG	PLACENTAL TRANSFER	RISK FACTORS*	FETAL EFFECTS	BREASTFEEDING RISK
Adenosine	?	C_M	No adverse effects reported	No data
Alteplase	No	C_M	Risk of hemorrhage; limited data with no fetal risk	Compatible
Amiodarone	Yes	C_M	Hypothyroidism, premature birth, hypotonia, large fontanelle	No
Amlodipine	Unknown	C_M	No studies	No data
Argatroban	Unknown	B_M	No human data; poor oral absorption suggests low risk	Unknown
Aspirin	Yes	C_M/D third trimester, full dose	Risk of hemorrhage	Potential toxicity
Atenolol	Yes	D_M	Low birth weight	Yes
Atorvastatin	?	X_M	No data	No data, potential toxicity
Bosentan	?	X_M	No data	Potential toxicity
Captopril	Yes	D_M	Teratogenic when used in second and third trimesters; produces renal defects and hypocalvaria, perhaps as a result of fetal hypotension and decreased renal blood flow	Yes
Carvedilol	?	C_M/D if used in the second or third trimesters	No human data	Unknown
Clopidogrel	?	B_M	No human data	Unknown
Dabigatran	?	C	No human data	Unknown
Danaparoid	?	B_M	No human data	Unknown
Digitalis	Yes	C	Low birth weight	Yes
Diltiazem	Yes	C_M	No adequate human studies	Yes
Dofetilide	?	C_M	No human data; teratogenic in animals at doses 2-4 times human doses	Unknown
Dronedarone	?	X	No human data; teratogenic in animals at maximum recommended human dose	Unknown
Enalapril	Yes	D_M	Teratogenic when used in second and third trimesters; produces renal defects and hypocalvaria, perhaps as a result of fetal hypotension and decreased renal blood flow	Yes
Enoxaparin	No	B_M	Thrombocytopenia, bleeding	Yes
Eplerenone	?	B_M	No data	No data
Epoprostenol	?	B_M	No data	Probably compatible
Fondaparinux	?	B_M	No human data	Unknown
Furosemide	Yes	C_M	Decreased Na^+, K^+, glucose	Yes
Hydralazine	Yes	C_M	Lupus-like syndrome	Yes
Hydrochlorothiazide	Yes	D_M	Decreased Na^+, K^+, glucose	Yes; can suppress lactation
Iloprost	?	C_M	No human data; teratogenic in animals	No data
Isoproterenol	?	C_M	Tachycardia; no adequate human studies	No data

TABLE 41-2   Risk of Cardiac Drugs to the Fetus and Newborn—cont'd

DRUG	PLACENTAL TRANSFER	RISK FACTORS*	FETAL EFFECTS	BREASTFEEDING RISK
Labetalol	Yes	C_M/D_M	Growth retardation	Yes
Lidocaine	Yes	C_M	Bradycardia and central nervous system toxic effects	No data
Losartan	?	C_M/D second and third trimesters	For risks, see Captopril	Probably compatible
Metoprolol	Yes	B_M	No obvious risk; no long-term data	Yes
Mexiletine	Yes	C_M	Bradycardia, small infants, low Apgar score, hypoglycemia	Yes
Nifedipine	Yes	C_M	No adequate human studies; use with care	Yes
Nitroglycerin	?	B/C	No adequate human studies	No data
Prasugrel	?	B	No human data	No data
Procainamide	Yes	C_M	None	Yes
Propranolol	Yes	C_M	Growth retardation, prematurity, hypoglycemia, bradycardia, respiratory depression	Yes
Quinidine	Yes	C_M	Thrombocytopenia	Yes
Sildenafil	?	B_M	No human data	No data
Sodium nitroprusside	Yes	C_M	Potentially toxic; no adequate human studies	No
Spironolactone	?	C_M	Limited human data; teratogenic in animals (feminization and reproductive abnormalities in rats)	Limited data; probably compatible
Streptokinase	Yes	C_M	No adequate human studies	No data
Torsemide	?	B_M	No teratogenicity	Unknown
Unfractionated heparin	No	C_M	Thrombocytopenia, acute distress	Yes
Verapamil	Yes	C_M	No adequate human studies	Yes
Warfarin	Yes	D_M	Abortion, hemorrhage	Yes

*Subscript M indicates that the manufacturer has rated the risk.
Question marks = unknown.
Category B risk factors: Either animal reproduction studies have not demonstrated a fetal risk, but no controlled studies in pregnant women are available, or animal reproduction studies have shown an adverse effect (other than a decrease in fertility) that was not confirmed in controlled studies in women in the first trimester, and there is no evidence of a risk in later trimesters.
Category C risk factors: Either studies in animals have revealed adverse effects on the fetus, and no controlled studies in pregnant women are available, or studies in women and animals are not available. Drugs should be given only if the potential benefit justifies the potential risk to the fetus.
Category D risk factors: Positive evidence of human fetal risk exists, but the benefits from use in pregnant women may be acceptable despite the risk, such as if the drug is needed for a life-threatening situation, for which safer drugs cannot be used or are ineffective.
Category X risk factors: Studies in animals or humans have shown fetal abnormalities and/or there is evidence of human/fetal risk from a variety of investigational or marketing experience. In addition, the risk are felt to outweigh the benefits.
Data from drug packaging information and Briggs GG, Freeman RK, Yaffee SJ. *Drugs in pregnancy and lactation.* Philadelphia, 2008, Williams & Wilkins.

Edema

Peripheral edema is common in pregnancy and may be seen in patients with or without underlying cardiovascular disorders. Routine treatment of edema with diuretics is not recommended, but compression stockings may be useful for women with bothersome edema. These stockings also decrease venous stasis and may be helpful in patients who have a history of venous thromboembolism. Diuretics should be used sparingly in pregnancy because they may interfere with the normal physiologic volume expansion of pregnancy. Loop diuretics are indicated in the management of edema associated with congestive heart failure, nephrosis, cirrhosis, or preeclampsia. In general, diuretics should not be used as first-line antihypertensive agents and are recommended only in combination with antiadrenergic agents and vasodilators. Furosemide is generally the diuretic of choice, although it crosses the placenta and may result in increased fetal urine production.[6] Furosemide is excreted in breast milk but does not appear to affect the infant adversely.[6] Thiazide diuretics cross the placenta and can cause fetal bradycardia and fetal or neonatal jaundice, thrombocytopenia, hypoglycemia, hemolytic anemia, and hyponatremia.[7] Although thiazide diuretics have been used to suppress milk production, the American Academy of Pediatrics (AAP) classifies thiazide diuretics as compatible with breastfeeding.[6,7] Data are

inadequate regarding the use of potassium-sparing diuretics in pregnancy, but it is known that spironolactone can adversely affect sexual differentiation in males and is contraindicated in pregnancy,[7] yet the AAP classifies spironolactone as compatible with breastfeeding.[6]

Valvular Heart Disease

As the heart enlarges with pregnancy, most women develop a small amount of mitral and tricuspid regurgitation. This amount of regurgitation is only slightly more than physiologic and generally does not produce any symptoms, nor does it require therapy. Women with preexisting aortic or mitral regurgitation related to structural heart disease tend to tolerate pregnancy well because of the decreased systemic vascular resistance of pregnancy, which serves as a natural vasodilator. However, patients with severe aortic or mitral regurgitation may experience difficulty in handling the increased volume load imposed on the heart by pregnancy. In these patients, optimal therapy may include valve repair or replacement prior to pregnancy. Angiotensin-converting enzyme (ACE) inhibitors and angiotensin II receptor blockers (ARBs) are commonly used in nonpregnant patients with severe mitral or aortic regurgitation to decrease the afterload on the LV. Both ACE inhibitors and ARBs cross the placenta and appear to rise to toxic levels in the fetus; they mainly affect the developing urogenital tract but also cause a number of other abnormalities (see Table 41-2).[8,9] Although limited data suggest that ACE inhibitor exposure in the first trimester may not be harmful,[10,11] without definitive proof of safety early in pregnancy, both ACE inhibitors and ARBs should be discontinued before conception whenever possible and avoided throughout pregnancy. During pregnancy, hydralazine and nitrates can be used as a substitute for ACE inhibitors and ARBs. In symptomatic patients, medical therapies include bed rest, nitrates, digoxin, salt restriction, and administration of loop diuretics. Symptomatic patients may benefit from invasive hemodynamic monitoring during labor and delivery, but epidural anesthesia can be administered safely.[12]

Patients with mild to moderate aortic stenosis have few cardiovascular complications with pregnancy. However, severe aortic stenosis is poorly tolerated in pregnancy and may lead to hospitalization, atrial arrhythmias, congestive heart failure, and premature delivery. Fetal outcome is also affected, with a higher incidence of preterm birth, intrauterine growth retardation (IUGR), and neonatal respiratory distress syndrome.[13,14] Medical therapy for symptomatic aortic stenosis is limited to diuretics and bed rest. Patients refractory to medical therapy must be treated surgically or with palliative balloon valvuloplasty; the latter seems to be associated with a lower risk of fetal loss and is the preferred treatment.[15] There are many reports of successful aortic valve replacement during pregnancy, but unfortunately, surgical valve replacement is associated with a fetal mortality rate of up to 30%.[16] During labor, epidural anesthesia must be used cautiously to avoid hypotension and reflex tachycardia, and invasive hemodynamic monitoring is recommended for labor and delivery. Vaginal delivery is preferred with assisted second stage of labor, and general anesthesia is the preferred technique for cesarean section.[17] Postpartum hemorrhage can be catastrophic for women with severe aortic stenosis, and it must be managed aggressively.

Patients with rheumatic mitral stenosis may first develop symptoms during pregnancy. As heart rate increases during the second trimester, the diastolic filling period decreases and left atrial pressure increases. These changes may lead to atrial distension, which may be associated with dyspnea and the development of atrial fibrillation (AF). By slowing the heart rate and improving diastolic filling time, left atrial filling pressures may be reduced by the use of β-adrenergic blocking agents. Use of $β_1$-selective agents is preferred because of the lack of interference with $β_2$-mediated uterine relaxation.[18] Restriction of physical activity is also important in controlling heart rate and symptoms. AF may be poorly tolerated during pregnancy, and in a hemodynamically unstable patient, it should be promptly treated with cardioversion. Rapid restoration of sinus rhythm decreases left atrial pressure and congestive symptoms, but the risk of thromboembolic complications must be considered prior to cardioversion.

Pregnancy is a hypercoagulable state because of the increased levels of factors I, II, VII, VIII, IX, and X, and this may increase the risk of thromboembolism in patients with severe mitral stenosis, even in the absence of AF. Clinically overt left atrial thrombus has been reported in the absence of AF in three patients: one patient had a left middle cerebral artery stroke, one patient had partial occlusion of the mitral valve orifice, and another patient had worsening of heart failure.[17,19] For patients who come to medical attention with AF, digoxin and β-blockers can be used safely to control the ventricular response. If digoxin and β-blockers do not adequately control the ventricular rate, verapamil can be added. Verapamil is not teratogenic and appears relatively safe, although maternal hypotension has been reported after an intravenous (IV) bolus of verapamil.[6] There is less experience with diltiazem, but a Michigan Medicaid surveillance study suggests an association between diltiazem and congenital cardiovascular defects.[6] Short-term use of IV diltiazem to control ventricular rate may be considered safe and effective; in addition, full-dose anticoagulation is indicated for these patients, and proceeding with early cardioversion is recommended. To rule out the presence of left atrial

thrombus, transesophageal echocardiography (TEE) should be performed.

Patients who have symptoms related to mitral stenosis prior to the end of the first trimester (the beginning of volume expansion for these patients) are unlikely to tolerate pregnancy well. Percutaneous valvuloplasty at an experienced center or surgical commissurotomy should be considered for these patients. Percutaneous balloon mitral valvuloplasty during pregnancy has been reported in hundreds of patients with good outcomes,[12,17] but the procedure should be avoided in the first trimester to avoid fetal radiation during organogenesis, and it should be reserved for patients who are refractory to medical therapy. Mitral valve surgery should only be considered for medically refractory patients who are not suitable candidates for percutaneous valvuloplasty because the risks to both mother and fetus are significantly greater. In a review of the outcomes of cardiovascular surgery in 161 pregnant women, maternal mortality rate was reported to be 9%, and fetal or neonatal mortality rate was 29%.[15] Vaginal delivery with assisted second stage of labor can be permitted, with cesarian section reserved for obstetric indications. Invasive hemodynamic monitoring is recommended with use of epidural anesthesia.[20] In addition, β-blocking agents, and occasionally diuretics, may be used to decrease the left atrial filling pressures at the time of delivery. The autotransfusion of blood from the uterus shortly after delivery is associated with an increase in left atrial filling pressures (increases of approximately 10 mm Hg might be expected) and can precipitate pulmonary edema.

Isolated valvular pulmonic stenosis (PS), even when severe, is typically well tolerated throughout pregnancy. Although the number of reported pregnancies complicated by isolated PS is small, severe PS does not seem to adversely affect maternal or fetal outcome. Balloon valvuloplasty should be considered in symptomatic patients. Pulmonic stenosis is frequently associated with more complex congenital heart disease, which is reviewed in Chapter 42.

Thromboembolic Disease During Pregnancy

Anticoagulation is indicated during pregnancy for the prevention and treatment of venous thromboembolism in patients with mechanical heart valves and for the prevention of complications in women with thrombophilia or recurrent late pregnancy loss. Pregnancy is a hypercoagulable state because of the increased production of clotting factors and an acquired resistance to the endogenous anticoagulant activated protein C.[21] In addition, a reduction in protein S and the cofactor for protein C and a decrease in fibrinolysis occur.[21] This prothrombotic state, along with lower extremity venous stasis caused by an enlarging uterus, increases the likelihood of deep venous thrombosis (DVT) during pregnancy. Venous thromboembolism is five to six times more common in pregnant women compared with nonpregnant women, and pulmonary embolism remains a leading cause of maternal death throughout the United States. Acquired or hereditary thrombophilia occurs in almost two thirds of women with a history of recurrent miscarriages, preeclampsia, IUGR, abruptio placentae, or stillbirths associated with microvascular thrombosis in placental blood vessels.[21,22] Heritable thrombophilia includes factor V Leiden and prothrombin gene *20210A* mutations, antithrombin III, protein C and S deficiencies, dysfibrinogenemias, and hyperhomocystinemia. Acquired disorders include anticardiolipin antibodies and the lupus anticoagulant. The magnitude of risk for thromboembolism during pregnancy varies according to the specific thrombophilia. Because thrombophilic disorders can be seen in up to 20% of normal pregnancies, screening is recommended for selected women with unexplained late or recurrent fetal losses of unclear etiology. Anticoagulation strategies are controversial, but prophylaxis is recommended for those at increased risk, and therapeutic anticoagulation is recommended for those at highest risk.

The antithrombotics currently available for the prevention and treatment of thromboembolism and valve thrombosis include unfractionated heparin (UFH), low-molecular-weight heparins (LMWHs), heparinoids, coumarin derivatives, and aspirin. The direct thrombin inhibitors, such as hirudin, cross the placenta and have not been evaluated during pregnancy. In evaluating an anticoagulant strategy, two potential fetal complications of treatment must be considered: teratogenicity and bleeding. Neither UFH nor LMWH crosses the placenta; therefore these do not have the potential to cause fetal bleeding or teratogenicity. Numerous studies have shown that UFH and LMWH therapy are safe for the fetus. In contrast, coumarin derivatives cross the placenta and carry the potential for fetal bleeding and teratogenicity. Coumarin's effect on the fetus is most marked during the first trimester and causes a warfarin embryopathy, other fetopathic effects, and spontaneous abortions. The fetal warfarin embryopathy consists of nasal hypoplasia, which can result in nasal bridge depression, upper airway obstruction, and/or stippled epiphyses.[23] Significant CNS abnormalities—including microcephaly, optic atrophy, and hydrocephalus—have been reported, as have spontaneous abortions, stillbirths, and neonatal deaths.[23] The exposure period of greatest risk for warfarin embryopathy and spontaneous abortion is between the sixth and twelfth weeks of gestation. However, the period of risk for the development of CNS abnormalities is controversial, but it may be throughout pregnancy. One cohort study reported a higher incidence of neurodevelopmental problems in children exposed to coumarin in the second and third trimesters.[24] The ongoing exposure to coumarin may result in cerebral microhemorrhages, which can lead to abnormal brain development. Dabigatran, a new oral and reversible direct thrombin inhibitor and an alternative to warfarin in patients with AF, has not been studied in pregnancy.

A systematic review of the literature on anticoagulation management during pregnancy in women with mechanical heart valves documented the risk of warfarin embryopathy to be 6.4% in 1234 pregnancies.[25] When warfarin was discontinued, with heparin substituted prior to 6 weeks' gestation and continued through 12 weeks, the risk of warfarin embryopathy was eliminated entirely. Warfarin use throughout pregnancy was associated with the lowest risk of valve thrombosis, 3.9%, which increased to 9.2% with substitution of heparin from week 6 to week 12. Warfarin use between 6 and 12 weeks was associated with a 33.9% spontaneous abortion rate compared with a rate of 14.7% when heparin was used before week 6. It is noteworthy that 46% of the patients studied had first-generation valves, typically cage-and-ball valves or Bjork-Shiley single-tilting disc valves, and only 7.1% had newer bileaflet valves. The authors concluded that use of heparin in the first trimester eliminates the fetal warfarin embryopathy and lowers the spontaneous abortion rate but subjects the woman to an increased risk of valve thrombosis and thromboembolism.

In clinical practice, the use of warfarin during pregnancy varies. Many clinicians, particularly in the United States, avoid warfarin entirely throughout pregnancy. Other clinicians reintroduce warfarin after the first trimester and discontinue its use at approximately 36 weeks, to avoid major maternal and fetal bleeding during late pregnancy and around the time of delivery. Some have suggested that high-risk patients and those with first-generation mechanical mitral valves, a history of AF, previous thromboembolism, or significant LV dysfunction should be maintained on warfarin from weeks 0 through 6 and then again from 12 through 35 weeks or even throughout pregnancy. An INR of 2.5 to 3.5 is recommended for these patients. Some have also suggested adding low-dose aspirin to the regimen because it has been shown to decrease the incidence of valve thrombosis in nonpregnant patients, albeit with a slight increase in bleeding risk.[26,27]

If the mother is fully anticoagulated with warfarin at the onset of labor, fresh-frozen plasma should be administered. Warfarin can usually be restarted on the first postpartum day. Overlap therapy with IV UFH may be needed until warfarin becomes effective, depending on the maternal indication for anticoagulation. Warfarin is safe to administer to women who are breastfeeding, and it does not alter clotting mechanisms in the infant.[28] The AAP has classified warfarin and dicumarol as safe to use by women who are breastfeeding.[28]

UFH has been used extensively for treating thrombotic disorders associated with pregnancy. Potential complications of its use include hemorrhage, thrombocytopenia, and osteopenia. Significant osteopenia may occur in up to one third of women treated with long-term UFH.[29] Thrombocytopenia is a less common adverse effect, but it may affect up to 10% of patients. Approximately 3% of nonpregnant patients treated with UFH acquire heparin-induced thrombocytopenia (HIT), an immunoglobulin G (IgG)–mediated thrombocytopenia frequently complicated by extension of preexisting venous thromboembolism or new arterial thrombosis.[30] This represents a serious complication of heparin therapy and requires monitoring of the platelet count throughout the course of treatment. Long-term therapy with heparin during pregnancy is feasible via subcutaneous injection or continuous IV infusion.[31,32] Subcutaneous UFH may have to be administered at doses as high as 10,000 to 20,000 U every 8 to 12 hours. Current recommendations for heparin therapy vary according to the level of risk for each patient. Dosing of UFH requires adjustment throughout pregnancy, and higher doses may be needed if subcutaneous heparin is used for the prevention of prosthetic valve–related thrombosis. The most recent American College of Cardiology (ACC)/American Heart Association (AHA)/European Society of Cardiology (ESC) guidelines recommend achieving a target activated partial thromboplastin time (aPTT) of two to three times control for women with mechanical heart valves.[7,33,34] In a 1992 review, Elkayam[2] advocated adjustment of heparin dosing to a minimum aPTT of 2.5 times control, with monitoring of a predose (trough) level to determine a possible need for dosing every 8 hours to prevent a drop to subtherapeutic levels. Subcutaneous UFH should be discontinued 24 hours prior to elective induction of labor. Intravenous UFH can be initiated and then discontinued 4 to 6 hours prior to the expected time of delivery.[35]

For patients in whom subcutaneous UFH therapy is ineffective, continuous infusion of UFH may be used. Placement of a semipermanent indwelling line makes this feasible.[36] Small infusion pumps are available and may be loaded with prefilled heparin cartridges. Monitoring of this therapy requires measurement of aPTT and adjustment of doses as needed.

For many physicians, LMWH has become the preferred agent for the prevention and treatment of venous thromboembolism during pregnancy and for the management of women with mechanical heart valves because it offers several advantages over UFH. LMWHs have approximately 92% bioavailability compared with 30% for UFH, and they have a longer half-life compared with UFH. Moreover, LMWHs have a more predictable anticoagulant response and a lower incidence of HIT, osteopenia, and bleeding complications.

Increasing data have been collected regarding the use of LMWH in pregnancy.[37-42] In one review of 486 pregnancies in which LMWH was used, symptomatic osteoporosis was observed in only one patient treated with LMWH.[41] Only three patients had a thromboembolic event during therapy, and rare allergic reactions were noted along with minor bleeding in 2.7% of the population. In pregnancy, LMWHs are frequently administered twice a day for the prevention of thrombosis in high-risk patients. Enoxaparin is most commonly administered subcutaneously at 1 mg/kg twice a day, with the dose adjusted during pregnancy as maternal weight and clearance increase. Dalteparin can be dosed at 100 U/kg every 12 hours. Monitoring of factor Xa levels is recommended at 2-week intervals during pregnancy, with measurements performed 4 to 6 hours after the last dose; doses of LMWH should be adjusted to achieve target factor Xa levels.[17,42] It is important to note that the recommendation for monitoring anti–factor Xa levels is unique to pregnancy and is due to the changing pharmacokinetics and dynamics that occur over the course of pregnancy.

Pregnancy in a patient with a mechanical heart valve poses difficult issues with respect to anticoagulation. Pregnant women are at particularly high risk for thromboembolic complications, with incidence ranging from 7.5% to 23%.[43-45] Most events occur as valve thrombosis, with an associated mortality rate of 40%.[43,44,46] The highest risk patients are those with older, higher profile mechanical mitral valves, such as the Bjork-Shiley or Starr-Edwards caged-ball valve, and those with AF or LV dysfunction.[25,45]

The use of LMWH during pregnancy for management of patients with prosthetic heart valves remains controversial because of an early warning by the manufacturer and the Food and Drug Administration (FDA) in July 2001 regarding safety. In 2004, labeling approved by the FDA specifically indicated that use of LMWH for thrombotic prophylaxis in pregnant women with mechanical prosthetic heart valves had not been adequately studied. Several case reports and small series describe the use of LMWH in pregnant women with prosthetic heart valves, some of which have noted treatment failures despite adequate anti–factor Xa levels.[42,47] Further review has shown that many of the complications were associated with an inadequate dose, lack of monitoring, or subtherapeutic anti-Xa levels.[45] A randomized, open-label trial was to compare enoxaparin with warfarin and UFH in pregnant women with prosthetic valves, but the trial was terminated after enrollment of only 12 patients as a result of two deaths from prosthetic valve thrombosis in the enoxaparin group. Both were high-risk patients who had a subtherapeutic anti-Xa level less than the recommended 0.3 to 1.0 IU/mL. Oran and colleagues[49] reviewed the risks of maternal and fetal complications in pregnant women with prosthetic heart valves treated with LMWH. Valve thrombosis occurred in 7 (8.6%) of 81 pregnancies, and the overall thromboembolic rate was 12.4% (10 of 81 patients). However, 9 of the 10 received fixed-dose LMWH.[48] Among 51 pregnancies in which anti–factor Xa levels were monitored, only one patient was reported to have had a thromboembolic complication, and the live-birth rate was 87.7%. The 2008 American College of Chest Physicians (ACCP) recommendations for women with mechanical heart valves outline four possible regimens: 1) adjusted-dose LMWH twice daily throughout pregnancy (grade 1c recommendation), adjusted to achieve the manufacturer's peak anti–factor Xa level 1 to 1.2 U/mL 4 hours after subcutaneous injection (grade 2c recommendation); 2) adjusted-dose UFH throughout pregnancy, administered subcutaneously every 12 hours in doses adjusted to keep the midinterval aPTT at at least twice control or to attain an anti-Xa heparin level of 0.35 to 0.70 U/mL (grade 1c recommendation); 3) UFH or LMWH until the thirteenth week, with warfarin substitution until close to delivery, when UFH or LMWH is resumed; and 4) in women at very high risk of thromboembolism, including those with older-generation prostheses in the mitral position or a history of thromboembolism, in which case vitamin K antagonists are suggested throughout pregnancy, with replacement by UFH or LMWH close to delivery after a comprehensive review of the potential risks and benefits with the patient (grade 2c recommendation). The recommended INR is 3.0, with a range from 2.5 to 3.5. For women at the highest risk of thromboembolism, the addition of low-dose aspirin (75 to 100 mg) is recommended.[50] The 2008 ACC/AHA guidelines recommend low-dose aspirin in the second and third trimesters of pregnancy in addition to warfarin or heparin (a class IIa recommendation).[33] In a review of the management of prosthetic valves in pregnancy, Elkayam and Bitar[45] modified the recommendations of the seventh ACCP consensus by differentiating between patients at higher and lower risk and by advocating monitoring trough levels of heparin activity in addition to peak levels. In higher risk patients, UFH should be adjusted to maintain aPTT at 2.5 to 3.5 times control, and LMWH should be adjusted to a predose anti-Xa level of approximately 0.7U/mL. In lower risk patients, UFH should be adjusted to an aPTT of 2.0 to 3.0 times control, and LMWH should be adjusted to a predose anti-Xa level of approximately 0.6 U/mL.

Fibrinolysis

Although pregnancy has been perceived as an absolute contraindication to fibrinolysis, fibrinolytic agents have been used in pregnant patients for a variety of indications, including iliac vein thrombosis, acute myocardial infarction (MI), massive pulmonary embolism, stroke, renal vein thrombosis, and prosthetic valve thrombosis.[45,51-54] Fibrinolytic agents, such as streptokinase and tissue plasminogen activator (tPA), have been used in pregnancy for acute MI and pulmonary embolism complicated by hemodynamic instability or right ventricular (RV) dysfunction.[55-57] These agents have been used during the first trimester without overt developmental abnormalities, and no known congenital defects are associated with the use of fibrinolytic agents. However, the risks associated with these agents include significant bleeding, peripheral embolization, premature labor, and death, and a few cases of placental abruption and neonatal intracranial hemorrhage have been reported.[58] Depending on the case, however, the benefits may outweigh the risks. The high molecular weight of tPA precludes transfer to the fetus, but streptokinase does cross the placenta in small amounts but has minimal fibrinolytic effects.

Ischemic Heart Disease

Unstable angina and acute MI may develop in pregnancy through a variety of mechanisms, including spontaneous coronary artery dissection, atherosclerotic coronary artery disease (CAD), or use of a toxin such as cocaine. Women who develop atherosclerotic CAD in pregnancy tend to be patients with a high burden of cardiovascular risk, such as from diabetes, smoking, hypertension, lipid disorders, or a family history of premature CAD. Development of acute MI is associated with maternal and fetal death because fetal demise frequently occurs simultaneously with maternal death. Mortality rates from MI appear to be higher in late pregnancy, but this may be attributable to the increased hemodynamic demands on the heart during this period. Optimal delivery of such a patient requires coordination and planning by the cardiologist, obstetrician, pediatrician, and anesthesiologist.[59,60]

In general, treatment of MI in pregnancy is unchanged from that of the nonpregnant patient. Primary percutaneous coronary intervention (PCI) is recommended as first-line treatment given the risk of fibrinolysis. Both thrombolytic therapy and PCI have been performed successfully in acute coronary syndromes during pregnancy.[56,57,61,62] Angiography aids in defining the etiology of the syndrome, such as dissection or thrombosis. Although primary concerns have focused on the risks of contrast agents and radiation on the fetus, radiation shielding can be performed to decrease the radiation exposure. Expected exposure ranges from less than 0.01 to 0.1 Gy, depending on the complexity of the procedure.[58] Coronary artery stenting may be used to treat a coronary artery dissection or atheromatous lesion.[62] Few data are available on the use of antiplatelet agents in pregnancy, such as clopidogrel or platelet IIb/IIIa inhibitors. Isolated case reports that demonstrate successful use of these agents in pregnancy may be found.[62-64] However, these agents should be used only with the understanding that there is an increased risk of maternal and fetal bleeding; the safety of drug-eluting stents in pregnant subjects is unknown. The need for long-term dual antiplatelet therapy is problematic during pregnancy, and bare-metal stenting is recommended.[64] Coronary artery bypass during pregnancy carries a high risk to the fetus, with an estimated mortality rate of 20%, whereas the maternal risk is similar to that of nonpregnant patients.[64,65]

Antianginal therapy during pregnancy includes β-adrenergic blocking agents, calcium channel blockers (CCBs), heparin, and nitrates.[6,66,67] The risks of β-adrenergic blocking agents have been previously described (see Table 40-2), and a limited number of reports exist on the use of nitroglycerin during pregnancy, especially during the first trimester. Transdermal nitroglycerin patches have been used as tocolytic agents, but hypotension and headaches are common side effects of nitrate use, as they are in nonpregnant individuals.

CCBs have been used for the treatment of hypertension, arrhythmias, and ischemia. Specifically, diltiazem has been used successfully to treat ischemia, but it is associated with adverse fetal effects in experimental animals.[68] More experience has been gained by using verapamil to treat supraventricular arrhythmias,[69] although verapamil may be associated with hypotension in the mother but otherwise appears to be safe for the mother and fetus; in addition, nifedipine has been used for the treatment of hypertension in pregnancy. The aforementioned CCBs are considered compatible with breastfeeding by the AAP. No reports on the use of amlodipine in human pregnancy or lactation are available.

Previous recommendations suggested avoiding aspirin during pregnancy because of the potential risk of premature closure of the ductus arteriosus. However, a meta-analysis by Imperiale and a large randomized trial (Collaborative Low-Dose Aspirin Study in Pregnancy [CLASP]) found no increased risk of fetal or maternal side effects with aspirin doses of 60 to 150 mg daily.[35,70] High doses of aspirin (325 to 650 mg/day) should be avoided throughout pregnancy because aspirin may affect maternal and fetal homeostasis and may cause cardiovascular septal defects, IUGR, and premature ductus arteriosus closure, which may lead to persistent pulmonary hypertension in the neonate.[6] Low-dose aspirin may be beneficial in patients with antiphospholipid antibodies, those at high risk for developing preeclampsia, those with recurrent late pregnancy loss, and patients at high risk for prosthetic valve thrombosis.[4,35,50] We recommend low-dose aspirin throughout pregnancy in patients with known obstructive CAD. Although aspirin is excreted into breast milk in low concentrations, no adverse effects on platelet function in the nursing infant exposed to aspirin have been reported, but it is a potential risk.[6,7,50] The AAP advises cautious use of aspirin during lactation.[5] The use of cholesterol-lowering drugs is an integral part of therapy in patients with CAD and is addressed below.

Lipid Disorders

An increasing number of young women have been diagnosed with lipid disorders. Patients with severe hyperlipidemia and other cardiac risk factors—such as hypertension, diabetes, and a family history of premature CAD—may be treated with lipid-lowering agents to decrease the risk of subsequent cardiac events. Few data are available on the use of statin agents during pregnancy,[71-73] although some animal data demonstrate developmental abnormalities with high-dose fluvastatin and atorvastatin.[7] Reports of exposure to lovastatin and simvastatin during pregnancy are available from postmarketing surveillance and include data on 134 patients with variable exposure to these agents.[7,71,73] Pregnancy outcomes were not markedly different from those of a normal population, but the number of patients was adequate only to exclude a threefold to fourfold increase in adverse outcomes. Because the risks of statin drugs during pregnancy are unclear and the benefits of treatment of these disorders during pregnancy are unknown, the current recommendations are to stop these agents prior to conception and avoid them throughout pregnancy.

Bile acid sequestrants, such as cholestyramine and colestipol, are used in the treatment of type IIa hyperlipidemia associated with low-density lipoprotein (LDL) elevation. Although few data are available on fetal effects, these drugs are not absorbed and therefore should not be teratogenic. However, a theoretical risk to the fetus is present from the reduced maternal absorption of fat-soluble vitamins. Given the lack of data, current recommendations are to avoid these drugs throughout pregnancy. There are no reports of bile acid sequestrant use in lactation, but these drugs are considered compatible with breastfeeding.[6]

Very little information is available on the use of niacin, gemfibrozil, fenofibrate, or ezetimibe in human pregnancy. Animal studies with high-dose gemfibrozil, fenofibrate, and ezetimibe demonstrate toxic fetal effects.[6] In general, discontinuation of lipid-lowering drugs is not believed to put the mother at risk; given the lack of data on fetal effects, these drugs should be discontinued prior to conception and avoided throughout pregnancy and lactation.

Heart Failure

Peripartum cardiomyopathy (PPCM) is defined as the development of dilated cardiomyopathy from the last month of pregnancy through the first 6 months after delivery, when other causes of heart failure have been excluded.[2] The echocardiographic criteria for a diagnosis of PPCM include an LV ejection fraction (LVEF) less than 45% or fractional shortening of less than 30% and an LV end-diastolic dimension greater than 2.7 cm/m^2.[74] This diagnosis is associated with mortality rates that range from 9% to 50%, depending on the series,[2,12,75-77] and worsening heart failure, arrhythmia, and thromboembolic events are frequent causes of death. The outcome for PPCM appears to be better than the outcome for idiopathic dilated cardiomyopathy unrelated to pregnancy, with approximately 50% of patients with PPCM demonstrating marked improvement in ventricular function and clinical symptoms compared with 10% in idiopathic dilated cardiomyopathy.[77] The long-term outlook of PPCM is variable—some patients return to normal functional capacity with normal heart size and function, some have persistent LV dilation and/or dysfunction, and some ultimately die or receive cardiac transplantation.[78]

Treatment of PPCM is similar to that for congestive heart failure of any etiology; bed rest and sodium and fluid restriction are recommended initially, and medical therapy may include digoxin, diuretics, and afterload reduction. Digoxin has been used extensively in pregnancy to treat supraventricular arrhythmias, although it may have to be administered at high daily doses prior to delivery (0.25 to 0.50 mg/day orally) because of its increased bioavailability. Digoxin is relatively safe for both the fetus and the mother and may be used safely during breastfeeding.[79,80] Diuretics should be used sparingly to avoid a decrease in placental perfusion, and furosemide is the diuretic of choice. Spironolactone should be avoided because its antiandrogenic effects may cause fetal endocrine dysfunction and may interfere with reproductive tract formation. No data are available on the use of eplerenone.

Afterload reduction is advantageous for many patients with heart failure, but ACE inhibitors and ARBs should be avoided until after delivery because they are teratogenic. Very low concentrations of ACE inhibitors have been detected in breast milk, but both captopril and enalapril are considered compatible with breastfeeding by the AAP. Hydralazine, with or without use of nitrates, is another treatment option for vasodilation during pregnancy. There is extensive experience with hydralazine in pregnancy, with no significant adverse maternal or fetal outcomes seen,[81] although a higher incidence of development of a lupuslike syndrome in the mother is present. Although it is excreted in breast milk in low concentrations, hydralazine may be used by the nursing mother. Doses may start at 10 mg orally three or four times per day and may be increased up to 50 mg three or four times per day in the pregnant patient. Addition of β-blockers can be considered, especially in the setting of arrhythmia. However, because the use of β-blockers is associated with low birth weight, and the benefit of β-blockers in heart failure is a long-term benefit, it is prudent to initiate β-blockade after delivery. No human data are available on the use of carvedilol in pregnancy; it is best reserved for postpartum medical management. No data are available on the use of nesiritide in pregnant or lactating patients.

Patients with PPCM have a high rate of thromboembolism, which may complicate up to 53% of cases.[82] Anticoagulation is recommended for patients, particularly for those with an ejection fraction less than 35%.[77,83] During pregnancy, LMWH or UFH would be preferred over warfarin; postpartum, warfarin can be initiated.

For the hemodynamically unstable patient, the first priority is reestablishing adequate maternal circulation with inotropic or mechanical support as needed. If cardiac output is inadequate to support the fetus, or if the supportive therapy for the mother puts the fetus at risk, prompt delivery is recommended. Women develop PPCM in the last month of pregnancy; therefore delivery occurs near term with a good chance for fetal survival. Following delivery, the medical regimen should be altered to include β-blockers and ACE inhibitors as tolerated. Cardiac transplantation has also been performed successfully for these patients postpartum.

Subsequent pregnancies in patients with PPCM are associated with adverse outcomes that include worsening heart failure, transplantation, and death. Elkayam and colleagues[84] surveyed cardiologists to assess the outcomes of subsequent pregnancies in patients with PPCM. This group of 44 women had 60 subsequent pregnancies and were divided into those patients with recovery of LV function with LVEF above 50% (n = 28) and persistent LV dysfunction with LVEF below 50% (n = 16) prior to the subsequent pregnancy. Echocardiographic data demonstrated a reduction in the ejection fraction in patients from both groups during the subsequent pregnancy. Development of heart failure symptoms was more likely in those patients with LV dysfunction (44%) than in those patients with normal LV function prior to the pregnancy (21%). Three deaths were reported in the patients with persistent LV dysfunction. The volume overload associated with pregnancy may unmask abnormal contractile reserve associated with PPCM.[85] Although death in patients with normalization of LV function is rare, there is risk for a significant and persistent decline in LV function. LV dysfunction is seen in approximately 20% of patients, with persistent LV dysfunction in approximately half.[86,87] Patients should be counseled on the risk of subsequent pregnancy and on the safest and most effective contraceptive method. For patients who decide to proceed with another pregnancy, ACE inhibitors and ARBs should be discontinued because of teratogenicity, and an isosorbide dinitrate–hydralazine combination should be initiated. A follow-up echocardiogram should be performed to reassess LV function 3 months after the change in therapy,[88] and a baseline brain natriuretic protein (BNP) level may also be useful. Early termination of an unintentional pregnancy should be considered, particularly in women with persistent LV dysfunction.

Cardiac Arrhythmias

Cardiac rhythm disorders are common during pregnancy and range from sinus tachycardia and premature atrial and ventricular beats to ventricular tachycardia. Rhythm disorders may become apparent for the first time during pregnancy. In addition, patients with underlying rhythm disorders may have an exacerbation of the disturbance during pregnancy. These rhythm disorders may become apparent as volume expansion occurs, and atrial expansion may lead to increased atrial irritability and may precipitate AF or supraventricular tachycardia. Anemia, thyroid disorders, and extrinsic precipitants such as caffeine, sympathomimetic amines, and alcohol may lead to rhythm disorders during pregnancy and in the nonpregnant state. Occasionally, patients experience arrhythmias only when pregnant.

Inappropriate sinus tachycardia may be present in some patients. The typical patient has sinus tachycardia out of proportion to the stage of pregnancy in the absence of thyroid disease, anemia, cardiac dysfunction, or infection. This may be associated with maternal anxiety and high sympathetic tone. Patients with inappropriate sinus tachycardia may experience dyspnea at low workloads, but appropriate volume and salt expansion may limit the symptoms produced by this disorder. Treatment with β-adrenergic blocking agents is effective for this disorder but should be prescribed only for severe cases, given the relatively benign nature of this condition.

Atrial premature contractions may be associated with symptoms but rarely need to be treated in pregnancy. For patients with supraventricular tachycardia, vagal maneuvers should be attempted first; if such maneuvers are not effective, IV adenosine may be administered.[89-91] Given at 3 to 6 mg intravenously, it is highly effective for the termination of such arrhythmias. Adenosine has a short half-life, making it a safe drug for use in pregnancy, and no fetal complications related to adenosine have been reported. In addition, β-adrenergic blocking agents and verapamil have been used to terminate supraventricular arrhythmias.[92,93]

Some patients have recurrent episodes of supraventricular tachycardia that warrant suppressive antiarrhythmic therapy. In the absence of preexcitation, atrioventricular (AV) node–blocking agents may be used. Digoxin has been used extensively in pregnancy without reported significant side effects, although the volume of distribution of digoxin is increased during pregnancy, which may lead to an increased dosage requirement (0.25 to 0.50 mg/day). Verapamil and β-adrenergic blocking agents have also been used to suppress supraventricular tachycardia.

AF and atrial flutter may develop in pregnancy. For patients with significant structural heart disease, development of AF or atrial flutter can result in acute hemodynamic decompensation. Patients without hypotension, chest discomfort, or dyspnea can be treated with AV node–blocking agents such as digoxin, β-blockers, diltiazem, or verapamil to achieve rate control. For patients who need antiarrhythmic therapy to facilitate conversion, conventional and contemporary agents are available. The most experience is available with quinidine, which has been used in pregnancy for more than 50 years. Quinidine toxicity in the mother can lead to severe nausea, vomiting, diarrhea, light-headedness, and tinnitus. Cardiac effects include hypotension, torsades de pointes, and sudden death. Quinidine crosses the placenta and leads to similar fetal and maternal serum levels. Although neonatal thrombocytopenia has been reported, this agent is classified as relatively safe in pregnancy.[7,69,94] Quinidine also has oxytocic properties at high doses but rarely results in pregnancy loss. It is excreted in breast milk but does not cause major problems for the nursing infant.

Procainamide has also been used for the treatment of atrial and ventricular arrhythmias and is not associated with any developmental abnormalities.[94] Excreted in breast milk, procainamide and its primary metabolite, N-acetylprocainamide, are not associated with adverse short-term effects.[95] Little is known about the long-term impact of this agent on the development of antinuclear antibodies or lupuslike syndromes in the child.

Flecainide and propafenone, both class Ic agents, are useful in managing ventricular and supraventricular tachycardias and appear to be relatively safe during pregnancy.[6,93,96] More experience has been gained with flecainide than propafenone because it has been successfully used in the treatment of fetal tachycardias. All class Ic agents should be avoided in patients with prior MI or cardiomyopathy because of the risk of death reported in the Cardiac Arrhythmia Suppression Trial (CAST).[97] Sotalol is a class II agent with non–cardiac-selective β-receptor antagonist properties and is generally considered safe. Sotalol has been used during pregnancy for the treatment of hypertension and has become a first- or second-line agent in the treatment of fetal tachycardia.[96] The greatest concern with sotalol is the proarrhythmic risk to both the mother and the fetus. Ibutilide and dofetilide are class III antiarrhythmics that have been released for the acute conversion of atrial flutter and AF in nonpregnant patients. There are no reports of their use in pregnancy, and they should be avoided; dofetilide has been shown to be teratogenic in animal studies.[5] Amiodarone has gained increasing popularity as an antiarrhythmic agent in the United States, largely because of its increased efficacy over other agents and its relative freedom from proarrhythmic risk. It is widely used in the conversion of AF and atrial flutter, for maintenance of sinus rhythm, and in the treatment of ventricular tachycardia. However, amiodarone contains iodine and leads to increased circulating iodine levels.[98] The elevated iodine levels may produce neonatal hypothyroidism; therefore use of amiodarone in pregnancy is restricted to severe or life-threatening cases. Although many women have an increase in ventricular premature beats during pregnancy, few develop nonsustained or sustained ventricular tachycardia. The initial evaluation of ventricular tachycardia should include an evaluation for structural heart disease. Patients without structural heart disease and ventricular tachycardia have low risk for mortality and morbidity and often can be treated with β-blocking agents. Patients with structural heart disease—such as RV dysplasia, hypertrophic cardiomyopathy, CAD, PPCM, or long QT syndrome—who have ventricular tachycardia are at higher risk for serious arrhythmias.

For hemodynamically tolerated ventricular tachycardia, treatment should begin with lidocaine or procainamide. Lidocaine is also used in pregnancy as a local anesthetic, and it crosses the placenta and readily appears in the fetal circulation. It has been associated with CNS depression in the newborn if high levels are achieved. Nonetheless, it remains appropriate therapy for acute treatment of ventricular tachycardia. Amiodarone therapy is usually avoided unless the arrhythmia is severe or life-threatening. Type Ic agents such as flecainide and propafenone are contraindicated for patients with structural heart disease. Some of these patients may have to be treated with chronic suppressive antiarrhythmic therapy or with implantable devices, depending on the nature of their underlying disorder. The newer implantable devices are smaller and may be implanted in the prepectoral position, and minimal fetal radiation exposure is required for successful placement of a device during pregnancy.

Rarely, cardiopulmonary resuscitation is needed during pregnancy,[99] although effective delivery of chest compressions may be difficult. Positioning the patient on her left side may optimize blood return from the periphery. If the arrest occurs prior to fetal viability, efforts should be directed toward maternal resuscitation. If the arrest occurs after this time, the focus of the resuscitation is on both the mother and the fetus, which should be delivered rapidly by cesarean section.

Marfan Syndrome

Marfan syndrome is an autosomal dominant disorder produced by mutations in the fibrillin gene. Patients with this syndrome may have ocular, musculoskeletal, and cardiac abnormalities. The most common cardiovascular disorders include myxomatous mitral valve disease with mitral regurgitation, aortic regurgitation, and aortic root enlargement. Patients with Marfan syndrome are at increased risk for aortic dissection during pregnancy.[100] Patients at highest risk for this complication are those with significant aortic root enlargement (>4.0 cm) prior to pregnancy.[100] Elective surgical repair of a dilated aortic root larger than 4.5 cm is recommended prior to conception.[33] Even patients without significant aortic root dilation before pregnancy are at a higher risk for this complication than are patients without Marfan syndrome, and they should be counseled accordingly.

The use of β-adrenergic blocking agents is associated with a decreased rate of aortic root dilation and a decrease in the progression of aortic regurgitation. These agents also attenuate the risk of aortic dissection during pregnancy. For these reasons, patients with Marfan syndrome should be treated with a β-blocker throughout pregnancy. Preconception counseling is crucial for these patients to examine maternal risk and optimize the medical therapy for women at acceptable risk for pregnancy.

Pulmonary Hypertension

Women with significant pulmonary hypertension are at extremely high risk for maternal morbidity and mortality and fetal demise. The increased risk of maternal mortality is seen throughout pregnancy and in the first few weeks following delivery. Pregnancy in women with Eisenmenger syndrome is associated with maternal mortality rates from 36% to 39%.[12,101,102] The increased cardiac output and decreased systemic vascular resistance of pregnancy can result in increased right-to-left shunting with worsening cyanosis in patients with this syndrome (see Chapter 42). Primary pulmonary hypertension is also associated with a high maternal mortality rate, with recent series reporting rates from 30% to 40%[2,103] and older series reporting rates up to 50%.[102] Death frequently occurs in the early postpartum period and is associated with pulmonary hypertensive crisis, in situ pulmonary artery thrombosis, progressive RV failure, arrhythmias, and sudden death.[2] Recognition of this high maternal mortality rate has led physicians to recommend effective contraception, tubal ligation, and, in the event of pregnancy, early termination.[104]

In more recent years, maternal mortality rates have decreased to the 25% range with improvements in prepregnancy counseling and multidisciplinary management throughout pregnancy, delivery, and the postpartum period.[105-107] For patients with pulmonary hypertension who opt to continue a pregnancy, early and prolonged bed rest may be important,[101] and supplemental oxygen may be helpful. Medical therapy includes anticoagulation because in situ thrombosis is a mechanism of maternal demise. Anticoagulation is recommended throughout gestation and in the early postpartum period. LMWH or UFH can be used, although no consensus has been reached on the use and choice of targeted therapy, nor has agreement been reached on the use of anticoagulation or mode and timing of delivery in women who wish to continue with pregnancy.[49] The phosphodiesterase-5 inhibitors sildenafil and tadalafil are administered orally, whereas prostacyclin (epoprostenol) and the prostacyclin analogues iloprost and treprostinil are given via nebulizer or continuous subcutaneous or IV infusion. Numerous case reports have described successful use of these therapies in pregnancy, during labor and delivery, and in the early postpartum period.[103,105,106,108-112] Endothelin receptor antagonists (bosentan, sitaxsentan, ambrisentan) are contraindicated in pregnancy and have shown teratogenicity in animal studies (FDA category X).[5]

Symptomatic deterioration often occurs in the second or third trimester and may warrant hospitalization. Patients can come to medical attention with fatigue, exertional dyspnea, syncope, chest pain, palpitations, cough, hemoptysis, and leg edema. Premature rupture of membranes is common and should be anticipated.[2,109] Avoidance of increases in pulmonary vascular resistance and maintenance of RV preload and contractility are essential in the management of labor and delivery in these patients.[113] Mode of delivery is controversial; some recommend vaginal delivery under epidural anesthesia, reserving cesarean section for obstetric indications because of the associated greater morbidity and mortality.[114] Others recommend elective cesarean section in the middle of the third trimester to avoid the maximal increase in cardiac output seen in the latter weeks of pregnancy and to avoid the hemodynamic effects of pushing. Oxygen should be administered to minimize hypoxemia, and inhaled nitric oxide or IV or inhaled prostaglandins may be used to lower pulmonary vascular resistance. The increased risk of maternal death persists for the first few weeks after delivery, and monitoring in an intensive care unit is recommended for the first several days following delivery.

Kiely and colleagues[105] reported a consecutive series of 10 pregnancies in 9 patients from 2002 through 2009 using a multidisciplinary approach. For patients in World Health Organization (WHO) functional class III who are not on treatment, inhaled iloprost was recommended. For patients in WHO functional class II, inhaled iloprost was recommended starting in the second trimester. If a patient deteriorated, parenteral prostacyclin was initiated, and more recent patients were offered sildenafil. Anticoagulation with LMWH was used throughout pregnancy, and patients were evaluated every 4 weeks until week 28, then every 2 weeks, and then weekly. Delivery via cesarean section at 34 weeks' gestation with epidural anesthesia, cardiac monitoring, oximetry, and arterial and central venous monitoring was recommended. The patients were observed in a critical care unit for 7 days postpartum. No fetal deaths occurred, and only one maternal death was reported in a postpartum patient who discontinued medical therapy against medical advice 4 weeks after delivery and refused admission despite clinical deterioration.

Antibiotic Prophylaxis

Antibiotic prophylaxis of bacterial endocarditis is no longer recommended by the AHA for a variety of dental, respiratory, GI, and genitourinary tract procedures, unless the patient is in a high-risk category.[115] The 2007 AHA recommendations for prophylaxis prior to dental procedures are for patients at high risk for endocarditis and include those with prosthetic cardiac valves; a prior history of endocarditis; surgically constructed systemic-pulmonary shunts; unrepaired cyanotic congenital heart disease; repair of congenital heart disease with prosthetic material or device, whether placed surgically or by catheter intervention, within the 6 months prior to the procedure; repaired congenital defects with residual defects at or near a device or prosthetic patch; and a history of cardiac transplantation and cardiac valvulopathy.

Few cases of endocarditis have been associated with delivery. Bacteremia after vaginal delivery was believed to be uncommon, with a reported frequency of 1% to 5%[17,116,117] compared with rates of 60% to 90% for dental procedures. For this reason, antibiotic prophylaxis was not recommended in the 1998 ACC/AHA practice guidelines for uncomplicated vaginal or abdominal delivery, unless bacteremia or active infection is suspected.[118] For high-risk patients, prophylaxis during vaginal delivery remains optional. Many disagree with these guidelines, arguing that complications are usually unexpected and that giving antibiotics after a complication puts the high-risk cardiac patient at risk. Moreover, recent reports have demonstrated a significantly higher rate of bacteremia following labor and delivery, ranging from 14% to 19%.[119-121] In addition, a recent review of cases of endocarditis complicating pregnancy found significant fetal and maternal mortality rates of 15% and 22%, respectively.[122] Given the recent finding of a higher incidence of bacteremia, the relative low cost of antibiotic prophylaxis, and the major morbidity and mortality of endocarditis, many institutions routinely give prophylactic antibiotics to high-risk patients with valvular and congenital heart disease prior to delivery.[17] A typical regimen would be ampicillin 2.0 g intramuscularly (IM) or by IV plus gentamicin 1.5 mg/kg (not to exceed 120 mg) given at initiation of labor or within 30 minutes of a cesarean section, followed by 1 g ampicillin IM or IV or 2 g oral amoxicillin 6 hours later. For penicillin-allergic patients, vancomycin 1.0 g IV is recommended.[118] For moderate-risk patients, a single dose of ampicillin 2 g or vancomycin 1 g is recommended. Practitioners should realize that routine antimicrobial prophylaxis does have its downside: cost considerations, resultant changes in skin flora with high rates of colonization by resistant staphylococci, and the potential for adverse effects on neonates with resistant bacterial infections must be taken into account when instituting practice guidelines.

REFERENCES

1. Elkayam U. Pregnancy and cardiovascular disease. In Braunwald E editor. *Heart disease: a textbook of cardiovascular medicine*. Philadelphia, 1992, WB Saunders, pp 1790-1809.
2. Elkayam U. Pregnancy and cardiovascular disease. In Zipes DP, Libby P, Bonow RO, et al, editors. *Heart disease: a textbook of cardiovascular medicine*. Philadelphia, 2005, WB Saunders, pp 1965-1983.
3. Elkayam U, Gleicher N. Hemodynamics and cardiac function during normal pregnancy and the puerperium. In Elkayam U, Gleicher N, editors. *Cardiac problems in pregnancy*. New York, 1998, Wiley-Liss, pp 3-21.
4. Roberts JM, Pearson GD, Cutler JA, et al. Summary of the NHLBI Working Group on Research on Hypertension During Pregnancy. *Hypertens Pregnancy* 2003;22: 109-127.
5. Briggs GG, Freeman RK, Yaffee SJ, editors. *Drugs in pregnancy and lactation: a reference guide to fetal and neonatal risk*. Philadelphia, 2011, Lippincott, Williams & Wilkins.
6. Briggs GG, Freeman RK, Yaffe SJ. *Drugs in pregnancy and lactation*. Philadelphia, 2005, Lippincott, Williams & Wilkins, pp 705-707.
7. Qasqas SA, McPherson C, Frishman WH, et al. Cardiovascular pharmacotherapeutic considerations during pregnancy and lactation. *Cardiol Rev* 2004;12:240-261.
8. Duminy PC, Burger PD. Fetal abnormality associated with the use of captopril during pregnancy. *S Afr Med J* 1981;60:805.
9. Ferris TF, Weir EK. Effect of captopril on uterine blood flow and prostaglandin E synthesis in the pregnant rabbit. *J Clin Invest* 1983;71:809-815.
10. From the Centers for Disease Control and Prevention. Postmarketing surveillance for angiotensin-converting enzyme inhibitor use during the first trimester of pregnancy—United States, Canada, and Israel, 1987-1995. *JAMA* 1997;277:1193-1194.
11. Lip GY, Churchill D, Beevers M, et al. Angiotensin-converting-enzyme inhibitors in early pregnancy. *Lancet* 1997;350:1446-1447.
12. Klein LL, Galan HL. Cardiac disease in pregnancy. *Obstet Gynecol Clin North Am* 2004;31:429-459, viii.
13. Hameed A, Karaalp IS, Tummala PP, et al. The effect of valvular heart disease on maternal and fetal outcome of pregnancy. *J Am Coll Cardiol* 2001;37:893-899.
14. Silversides CK, Colman JM, Sermer M, et al. Early and intermediate-term outcomes of pregnancy with congenital aortic stenosis. *Am J Cardiol* 2003;91:1386-1389.
15. Weiss BM, von Segesser LK, Alon E, et al. Outcome of cardiovascular surgery and pregnancy: a systematic review of the period 1984-1996. *Am J Obstet Gynecol* 1998;179:1643-1653.
16. Chambers CE, Clark SL. Cardiac surgery during pregnancy. *Clin Obstet Gynecol* 1994;37:316-323.
17. Elkayam U, Bitar F. Valvular heart disease and pregnancy part I: native valves. *J Am Coll Cardiol* 2005;46:223-230.
18. Hurst AK, Hoffman K, Fishman WH. The use of β-adrenergic blocking agents in pregnancy and lactation. In Elkayam U, Gleicher N, editors. *Cardiac problems in pregnancy*. New York, 1998, Wiley-Liss, pp 351-390.
19. Hameed A, Akhter MW, Bitar F, et al. Left atrial thrombosis in pregnant women with mitral stenosis and sinus rhythm. *Am J Obstet Gynecol* 2005;193:501-504.
20. Hemmings GT, Whalley DG, O'Connor PJ, et al. Invasive monitoring and anaesthetic management of a parturient with mitral stenosis. *Can J Anaesth* 1987;34:182-185.
21. Doyle NM, Monga M. Thromboembolic disease in pregnancy. *Obstet Gynecol Clin North Am* 2004;31:319-344, vi.
22. Kujovich JL. Thrombophilia and pregnancy complications. *Am J Obstet Gynecol* 2004; 191:412-424.
23. Pettifor JM, Benson R. Congenital malformations associated with the administration of oral anticoagulants during pregnancy. *J Pediatr* 1975;86:459-462.
24. Wesseling J, Van Driel D, Heymans HS, et al. Coumarins during pregnancy: long-term effects on growth and development of school-age children. *Thromb Haemost* 2001;85: 609-613.
25. Chan WS, Anand S, Ginsberg JS. Anticoagulation of pregnant women with mechanical heart valves: a systematic review of the literature. *Arch Intern Med* 2000;160:191-196.
26. Turpie AG, Gent M, Laupacis A, et al. A comparison of aspirin with placebo in patients treated with warfarin after heart-valve replacement. *N Engl J Med* 1993;329: 524-529.
27. Cappelleri JC, Fiore LD, Brophy MT, et al. Efficacy and safety of combined anticoagulant and antiplatelet therapy versus anticoagulant monotherapy after mechanical heart-valve replacement: a meta-analysis. *Am Heart J* 1995;130:547-552.
28. McKenna R, Cole ER, Vasan U. Is warfarin sodium contraindicated in the lactating mother? *J Pediatr* 1983;103:325-327.
29. Barbour LA, Kick SD, Steiner JF, et al. A prospective study of heparin-induced osteoporosis in pregnancy using bone densitometry. *Am J Obstet Gynecol* 1994;170:862-869.
30. Warkentin TE, Levine MN, Hirsh J, et al. Heparin-induced thrombocytopenia in patients treated with low-molecular-weight heparin or unfractionated heparin. *N Engl J Med* 1995;332:1330-1335.
31. Henny CP, ten Cate H, Buller HR, et al. Ambulatory heparin treatment. *Lancet* 1982;1:615.
32. Rabinovici J, Mani A, Barkai G, et al. Long-term ambulatory anticoagulation by constant subcutaneous heparin infusion in pregnancy: case report. *Br J Obstet Gynaecol* 1987; 94:89-91.
33. Bonow RO, Carabello BA, Chatterjee K, et al. 2008 focused update incorporated into the ACC/AHA 2006 guidelines for the management of patients with valvular heart disease: a report of the American College of Cardiology/American Heart Association Task Force on Practice Guidelines (Writing Committee to revise the 1998 guidelines for the management of patients with valvular heart disease). Endorsed by the Society of Cardiovascular Anesthesiologists, Society for Cardiovascular Angiography and Interventions, and Society of Thoracic Surgeons. *J Am Coll Cardiol* 2008; 52:e1-e142.
34. Brill-Edwards P, Ginsberg JS, Johnston M, et al. Establishing a therapeutic range for heparin therapy. *Ann Intern Med* 1993;119:104-109.
35. Bates SM, Greer IA, Hirsh J, et al. Use of antithrombotic agents during pregnancy: the Seventh ACCP Conference on Antithrombotic and Thrombolytic Therapy. *Chest* 2004;126:627S-644S.
36. Nelson DM, Stempel LE, Fabri PJ, et al. Hickman catheter use in a pregnant patient requiring therapeutic heparin anticoagulation. *Am J Obstet Gynecol* 1984;149:461-462.
37. Dulitzki M, Pauzner R, Langevitz P, et al. Low-molecular-weight heparin during pregnancy and delivery: preliminary experience with 41 pregnancies. *Obstet Gynecol* 1996;87: 380-383.
38. Fejgin MD, Lourwood DL. Low molecular weight heparins and their use in obstetrics and gynecology. *Obstet Gynecol Surv* 1994;49:424-431.
39. Hurst AK, Hoffman K, Frishman W. The use of β-adrenergic blocking agents in pregnancy and lactation. In Elkayam U, Gleicher N, editors. *Cardiac problems in pregnancy*. New York, 1998, Wiley-Liss, pp 357-372.
40. Nelson-Piercy C, Letsky EA, de Swiet M. Low-molecular-weight heparin for obstetric thromboprophylaxis: experience of sixty-nine pregnancies in sixty-one women at high risk. *Am J Obstet Gynecol* 1997;176:1062-1068.
41. Sanson BJ, Lensing AW, Prins MH, et al. Safety of low-molecular-weight heparin in pregnancy: a systematic review. *Thromb Haemost* 1999;81:668-672.
42. Yinon Y, Siu SC, Warshafsky C, et al. Use of low molecular weight heparin in pregnant women with mechanical heart valves. *Am J Cardiol* 2009;104:1259-1263.
43. Danik S, Fuster V. Anticoagulation in pregnant women with prosthetic heart valves. *Mt Sinai J Med* 2004;71:322-329.
44. Salazar E, Izaguirre R, Verdejo J, et al. Failure of adjusted doses of subcutaneous heparin to prevent thromboembolic phenomena in pregnant patients with mechanical cardiac valve prostheses. *J Am Coll Cardiol* 1996;27:1698-1703.

45. Elkayam U, Bitar F. Valvular heart disease and pregnancy: part II: prosthetic valves. *J Am Coll Cardiol* 2005;46:403-410.
46. Sbarouni E, Oakley CM. Outcome of pregnancy in women with valve prostheses. *Br Heart J* 1994;71:196-201.
47. Greer I, Hunt BJ. Low molecular weight heparin in pregnancy: current issues. *Br J Haematology* 2004;128.
48. Reference deleted in proofs.
49. Oran B, Lee-Parritz A, Ansell J. Low molecular weight heparin for the prophylaxis of thromboembolism in women with prosthetic mechanical heart valves during pregnancy. *Thromb Haemost* 2004;92:747-751.
50. Bates SM, Greer IA, Pabinger I, et al. Venous thromboembolism, thrombophilia, antithrombotic therapy, and pregnancy: American College of Chest Physicians Evidence-Based Clinical Practice Guidelines (8th Edition). *Chest* 2008;133:844S-886S.
51. Patel RK, Fasan O, Arya R. Thrombolysis in pregnancy. *Thromb Haemost* 2003;90:1216-1217.
52. Song JY, Valentino L. A pregnant patient with renal vein thrombosis successfully treated with low-dose thrombolytic therapy: a case report. *Am J Obstet Gynecol* 2005;192:2073-2075.
53. Johnson DM, Kramer DC, Cohen E, et al. Thrombolytic therapy for acute stroke in late pregnancy with intra-arterial recombinant tissue plasminogen activator. *Stroke* 2005;36:e53-e55.
54. Acharya G, Singh K, Hansen JB, et al. Catheter-directed thrombolysis for the management of postpartum deep venous thrombosis. *Obstet Gynecol Surv* 2005;60:427-428.
55. Cowan NC, de Belder MA, Rothman MT. Coronary angioplasty in pregnancy. *Br Heart J* 1988;59:588-592.
56. Ludwig H. Results of streptokinase therapy in deep venous thrombosis during pregnancy. *Postgrad Med J* 1973;49:65.
57. Pfeifer GW. The use of thrombolytic therapy in obstetrics and gynaecology. *Australas Ann Med* 1970;19:28-31.
58. Roth A, Elkayam U. Acute myocardial infarction associated with pregnancy. *Ann Intern Med* 1996;125:751-762.
59. Hands ME, Johnson MD, Saltzman DH, et al. The cardiac, obstetric, and anesthetic management of pregnancy complicated by acute myocardial infarction. *J Clin Anesth* 1990;2:258-268.
60. Hankins GD, Wendel GD Jr, Leveno KJ, et al. Myocardial infarction during pregnancy: a review. *Obstet Gynecol* 1985;65:139-146.
61. Delclos GL, Davila F. Thrombolytic therapy for pulmonary embolism in pregnancy: a case report. *Am J Obstet Gynecol* 1986;155:375-376.
62. Sebastian C, Scherlag M, Kugelmass A, et al. Primary stent implantation for acute myocardial infarction during pregnancy: use of abciximab, ticlopidine, and aspirin. *Cathet Cardiovasc Diagn* 1998;45:275-279.
63. Babic Z, Gabric ID, Pintaric H. Successful primary percutaneous coronary intervention in the first trimester of pregnancy. *Catheter Cardiovasc Interv* 2011;77:522-525.
64. Roth A, Elkayam U. Acute myocardial infarction associated with pregnancy. *J Am Coll Cardiol* 2008;52:171-180.
65. Parry AJ, Westaby S. Cardiopulmonary bypass during pregnancy. *Ann Thorac Surg* 1996;61:1865-1869.
66. Butters L, Kennedy S, Rubin PC. Atenolol in essential hypertension during pregnancy. *Br Med J* 1990;301:587-589.
67. Cotton DB, Jones MM, Longmire S, et al. Role of intravenous nitroglycerin in the treatment of severe pregnancy-induced hypertension complicated by pulmonary edema. *Am J Obstet Gynecol* 1986;154:91-93.
68. Lubbe WF. Use of diltiazem during pregnancy. *N Z Med J* 1987;100:121.
69. Rotmensch HH, Elkayam U, Frishman W. Antiarrhythmic drug therapy during pregnancy. *Ann Intern Med* 1983;98:487-497.
70. Low dose aspirin in pregnancy and early childhood development: follow up of the collaborative low dose aspirin study in pregnancy. CLASP collaborative group. *Br J Obstet Gynaecol* 1995;102:861-868.
71. Mevacor package insert. Merck Sharp & Dome, 1993.
72. Pravachol package insert. Bristol-Myers Squibb Company, 1995.
73. Zocor package insert. Merck & Company, 1995.
74. Hibbard JU, Lindheimer M, Lang RM. A modified definition for peripartum cardiomyopathy and prognosis based on echocardiography. *Obstet Gynecol* 1999;94:311-316.
75. Elkayam U, Akhter MW, Singh H, et al. Pregnancy-associated cardiomyopathy: clinical characteristics and a comparison between early and late presentation. *Circulation* 2005;111:2050-2055.
76. Pearson GD, Veille JC, Rahimtoola S, et al. Peripartum cardiomyopathy: National Heart, Lung, and Blood Institute and Office of Rare Diseases (National Institutes of Health) workshop recommendations and review. *JAMA* 2000;283:1183-1188.
77. Tidswell M. Peripartum cardiomyopathy. *Crit Care Clin* 2004;20:777-788, xi.
78. Cole P, Cook F, Plappert T, et al. Longitudinal changes in left ventricular architecture and function in peripartum cardiomyopathy. *Am J Cardiol* 1987;60:871-876.
79. American Academy of Pediatrics Committee on Drugs. The transfer of drugs and other chemicals into human milk. *Pediatrics* 1994;93:137-150.
80. Finley JP, Waxman MB, Wong PY, et al. Digoxin excretion in human milk. *J Pediatr* 1979;94:339-340.
81. Tamari I, Eldar M, Rabinowitz B, et al. Medical treatment of cardiovascular disorders during pregnancy. *Am Heart J* 1982;104:1357-1363.
82. Lampert MB, Lang RM. Peripartum cardiomyopathy. *Am Heart J* 1995;130:860-870.
83. Lang RM, Lampert MB, Poppas A, et al. Perpartal cardiomyopathy. In Elkayam U, Gleicher N, editors. *Cardiac problems in pregnancy*. New York, 1998, Wiley-Liss, pp 87-100.
84. Elkayam U, Tummala PP, Rao K, et al. Maternal and fetal outcomes of subsequent pregnancies in women with peripartum cardiomyopathy. *N Engl J Med* 2001;344:1567-1571.
85. Reimold SC, Rutherford JD. Peripartum cardiomyopathy. *N Engl J Med* 2001;344:1629-1630.
86. Elkayam U, Tummala PP, Rao K, et al. Maternal and fetal outcomes of subsequent pregnancies in women with peripartum cardiomyopathy. *N Engl J Med* 2001;344:1567-1571.
87. Elkayam U. Pregnant again after peripartum cardiomyopathy: to be or not to be? *Eur Heart J* 2002;23:753-756.
88. Elkayam U. Clinical characteristics of peripartum cardiomyopathy in the United States diagnosis, prognosis, and management. *J Am Coll Cardiol* 2011;58:659-670.
89. Harrison JK, Greenfield RA, Wharton JM. Acute termination of supraventricular tachycardia by adenosine during pregnancy. *Am Heart J* 1992;123:1386-1388.
90. Mason BA, Ricci-Goodman J, Koos BJ. Adenosine in the treatment of maternal paroxysmal supraventricular tachycardia. *Obstet Gynecol* 1992;80:478-480.
91. Podolsky SM, Varon J. Adenosine use during pregnancy. *Ann Emerg Med* 1991;20:1027-1028.
92. Gowda RM, Khan IA, Mehta NJ, et al. Cardiac arrhythmias in pregnancy: clinical and therapeutic considerations. *Int J Cardiol* 2003;88:129-133.
93. Joglar JA, Page RL. Antiarrhythmic drugs in pregnancy. *Curr Opin Cardiol* 2001;16:40-45.
94. Little BB, Gilstrap LC 3rd. Cardiovascular drugs during pregnancy. *Clin Obstet Gynecol* 1989;32:13-20.
95. Pittard WB 3rd, Glazier H. Procainamide excretion in human milk. *J Pediatr* 1983;102:631-633.
96. Oudijk MA, Ruskamp JM, Ambachtsheer BE, et al. Drug treatment of fetal tachycardias. *Paediatr Drugs* 2002;4:49-63.
97. Echt DS, Liebson PR, Mitchell LB, et al. Mortality and morbidity in patients receiving encainide, flecainide, or placebo. The Cardiac Arrhythmia Suppression Trial. *N Engl J Med* 1991;324:781-788.
98. McKenna WJ, Harris L, Rowland E, et al. Amiodarone therapy during pregnancy. *Am J Cardiol* 1983;51:1231-1233.
99. Lee RV, Rodgers BD, White LM, et al. Cardiopulmonary resuscitation of pregnant women. *Am J Med* 1986;81:311-318.
100. Pyeritz RE. Maternal and fetal complications of pregnancy in the Marfan syndrome. *Am J Med* 1981;71:784-790.
101. Gleicher N, Midwall J, Hochberger D, et al. Eisenmenger's syndrome and pregnancy. *Obstet Gynecol Surv* 1979;34:721-741.
102. Weiss BM, Zemp L, Seifert B, et al. Outcome of pulmonary vascular disease in pregnancy: a systematic overview from 1978 through 1996. *J Am Coll Cardiol* 1998;31:1650-1657.
103. Stewart R, Tuazon D, Olson G, et al. Pregnancy and primary pulmonary hypertension: successful outcome with epoprostenol therapy. *Chest* 2001;119:973-975.
104. McLaughlin VV, Archer SL, Badesch DB, et al. ACCF/AHA 2009 expert consensus document on pulmonary hypertension: a report of the American College of Cardiology Foundation Task Force on Expert Consensus Documents and the American Heart Association Developed in Collaboration with the American College of Chest Physicians; American Thoracic Society, Inc.; and the Pulmonary Hypertension Association. *J Am Coll Cardiol* 2009;53:1573-1619.
105. Kiely DG, Condliffe R, Webster V, et al. Improved survival in pregnancy and pulmonary hypertension using a multiprofessional approach. *Br J Obstet Gynecol* 2010;117:565-574.
106. Bonnin M, Mercier FJ, Sitbon O, et al. Severe pulmonary hypertension during pregnancy: mode of delivery and anesthetic management of 15 consecutive cases. *Anesthesiology* 2005;102:1133-1137; discussion 1135A-1136A.
107. Bedard E, Dimopoulos K, Gatzoulis MA. Has there been any progress made on pregnancy outcomes among women with pulmonary arterial hypertension? *Eur Heart J* 2009;30:256-265.
108. Decoene C, Bourzoufi K, Moreau D, et al. Use of inhaled nitric oxide for emergency Cesarean section in a woman with unexpected primary pulmonary hypertension. *Can J Anaesth* 2001;48:584-587.
109. Monnery L, Nanson J, Charlton G. Primary pulmonary hypertension in pregnancy; a role for novel vasodilators. *Br J Anaesth* 2001;87:295-298.
110. Nootens M, Rich S. Successful management of labor and delivery in primary pulmonary hypertension. *Am J Cardiol* 1993;71:1124-1125.
111. Weiss BM, Maggiorini M, Jenni R, et al. Pregnant patient with primary pulmonary hypertension: inhaled pulmonary vasodilators and epidural anesthesia for cesarean delivery. *Anesthesiology* 2000;92:1191-1194.
112. Easterling TR, Ralph DD, Schmucker BC. Pulmonary hypertension in pregnancy: treatment with pulmonary vasodilators. *Obstet Gynecol* 1999; 93:494-498.
113. Mangano DT. Anaesthesia for the pregnant cardiac patient. In Shnider SM, Levinson G, editors. *Anaesthesia for obstetrics*. Baltimore, 1983, Williams & Wilkins, pp 502-508.
114. McLaughlin VV, Genthner DE, Panella MM, et al. Reduction in pulmonary vascular resistance with long-term epoprostenol (prostacyclin) therapy in primary pulmonary hypertension. *N Engl J Med* 1998; 338:273-277.
115. Wilson W, Taubert KA, Gewitz M, et al. Prevention of infective endocarditis: guidelines from the American Heart Association: a guideline from the American Heart Association Rheumatic Fever, Endocarditis, and Kawasaki Disease Committee, Council on Cardiovascular Disease in the Young, and the Council on Clinical Cardiology, Council on Cardiovascular Surgery and Anesthesia, and the Quality of Care and Outcomes Research Interdisciplinary Working Group. *Circulation* 2007;116:1736-1754.
116. McFaul PB, Dornan JC, Lamki H, et al. Pregnancy complicated by maternal heart disease: a review of 519 women. *Br J Obstet Gynaecol* 1988;95:861-867.
117. Sugrue D, Blake S, Troy P, et al. Antibiotic prophylaxis against infective endocarditis after normal delivery—is it necessary? *Br Heart J* 1980;44:499-502.
118. Bonow RO, Carabello B, de Leon AC, et al. ACC/AHA guidelines for the management of patients with valvular heart disease: executive summary. A report of the American College of Cardiology/American Heart Association Task Force on Practice Guidelines (Committee on Management of Patients with Valvular Heart Disease). *J Heart Valve Dis* 1998;7:672-707.
119. Boggess KA, Watts DH, Hillier SL, et al. Bacteremia shortly after placental separation during cesarean delivery. *Obstet Gynecol* 1996;87:779-784.
120. Petanovic M, Zagar Z. The significance of asymptomatic bacteremia for the newborn. *Acta Obstet Gynecol Scand* 2001;80:813-817.
121. Furman B, Shoham-Vardi I, Bashiri A, et al. Clinical significance and outcome of preterm prelabor rupture of membranes: population-based study. *Eur J Obstet Gynecol Reprod Biol* 2000;92:209-216.
122. Campuzano K, Roque H, Bolnick A, et al. Bacterial endocarditis complicating pregnancy: case report and systematic review of the literature. *Arch Gynecol Obstet* 2003;268:251-255.

CHAPTER 42   Care for Adults with Congenital Heart Disease

Michael J. Landzberg, Giuseppe Martucci, and Mary Mullen

ISSUES FOR THE CARE PROVIDER, 632

Endocarditis, 632

LEFT-TO-RIGHT SHUNTING: GENERAL PRINCIPLES, 632

CYANOSIS, 633

Major Cyanotic Organ Complications, 634
Cardiopulmonary Exercise, 634
Neurologic Effects, 634
Recommendations for Management of the Cyanotic
    Patient, 635

PREGNANCY, 635

Recommendations, 636

NONCARDIAC SURGERY, 636

Recommendations, 636

ARRHYTHMIA MANAGEMENT, 636

Exercise and Athletic Participation, 636
Transplantation, 637

GUIDELINES FOR MANAGEMENT OF PATIENTS WITH
SPECIFIC CONGENITAL CARDIAC LESIONS, 637

Atrial Septal Defects, 637
Patent Foramen Ovale, 639
Bicuspid Aortic Valve, 640
Pulmonary Stenosis, 640

Aortic Coarctation, 641
Tetralogy of Fallot, 643
Patent Ductus Arteriosus, 645
Ventricular Septal Defects, 646
Post–Myocardial Infarction Ventricular Septal Rupture, 647
Perimembranous Ventral Septal Defect Closure, 647
Postoperative Residual Defects, Collaterals, and
    Fenestrations, 647

REFERENCES, 649

Adult congenital heart disease (ACHD) remains a unique and challenging illness in a population in need of lifelong cardiac follow-up and care. In the United States, this rapidly expanding group is estimated to exceed its pediatric counterparts, with more than 1 million persons estimated to have ACHD.[1,2] Included in the ACHD population are young and older adults who remain unrepaired; those who have undergone palliative procedures, such as systemic-pulmonary or cavopulmonary shunts; and patients who have undergone complete surgical and transcatheter repair with or without known residua (Table 42-1).[3]

An increase in ACHD patient complexity continues to be observed. The significant upward shift in median age of the entire ACHD population is accompanied by improved survival of patients with complicated anomalies—tetralogy of Fallot, single ventricle, transposition of the great arteries—who have greater health care needs, use more resources, and require increased understanding by general and specialty caregivers.[4,5] Intensity of general comorbidity and cardiovascular medical illness has increased as longstanding atrial, ventricular, and pulmonary vascular volume abnormalities have contributed to increased incidence of arrhythmias, ventricular failure, pulmonary vascular disease, and thrombosis along with general medical illnesses such as diabetes, chronic renal insufficiency, and obesity. Close interaction between pediatric and adult cardiologists, interventional cardiologists, cardiac surgeons, and primary physicians, assisted by specially trained ACHD clinicians and centers adhering to established care guidelines, appears necessary for successful care of ACHD patients within all levels of regional and local care.[6,7]

Issues for the Care Provider

Endocarditis

Despite improvements in antibiotic therapy and diagnostic strategies, many adults with CHD remain at lifelong risk from infective endocarditis. Potential for infection occurs in the setting of structural cardiac lesions that generate turbulent blood flow or those that present abnormal or sequestered tissue surfaces that favor growth of microorganisms. Transient bacteremia allows colonization of fibrin/platelet meshwork on the endocardial or prosthetic surface. Unrepaired defects at greatest risk include high-velocity lesions such as ventricular septal defects (VSDs) and left-sided stenotic or regurgitant valves. Infective endocarditis is rare in low-pressure lesions such as mild valvular pulmonary stenosis (VPS) or in secundum atrial septal defect. After complete surgical repair, endocarditis risk may be significantly decreased, unchanged, or

increased as a result of placement of a prosthetic valve or conduit. A 30-year follow-up study addressed the risk of infective endocarditis after surgery for congenital heart defects[8]; the highest incidence was found in patients after repair of aortic valve stenosis, with 20.6% having an episode of endocarditis after 30 years. No cases were reported after repair of patent ductus arteriosus, secundum atrial septal defect, or pulmonary valve stenosis.

A high index of suspicion for the presence of infective endocarditis in adults with CHD should be maintained because of significantly varied clinical presentations. Patients may have definitive microbiologic data or may show the classic manifestations of fever, weight loss, night sweats, splinter hemorrhages, Janeway lesions, and Osler nodes. Other patients may pose diagnostic challenges. Algorithms that combine clinical criteria with echocardiography may assist evaluation.[7,9] Transthoracic echocardiography (TTE) may demonstrate vegetations, abscesses, new prosthetic valve dehiscence, or valvar regurgitation. Transesophageal echocardiography (TEE) has a higher sensitivity for the presence of vegetations and may improve diagnostic accuracy.[7] Empiric antibiotic therapy is often initiated in the acutely ill patient while microbiologic data are pending.[10] Therapy for active or presumed infection by common bacterial pathogens is discussed in Chapter 43.

Patients and other medical care providers should be educated about decreasing the risk for infective endocarditis by promotion of optimal gum health for all patients and through the use of established guidelines for antibiotic prophylaxis prior to undergoing dental, gastrointestinal, or genitourinary procedures in selected patients.[11] Cardiologists are often asked about the necessity of closing a small VSD or patent ductus arteriosus to reduce the chance of developing endocarditis. In the modern antibiotic era, surgical or transcatheter correction of a small, hemodynamically insignificant VSD or patent ductus arteriosus with the primary intent to decrease or eliminate the risk of subacute bacterial endocarditis (SBE) risk is not recommended.[12]

Left-to-Right Shunting: General Principles

Patients with the potential for left-to-right intravascular recirculation of systemic arterial blood into the systemic venous circulation pose challenges for health care providers because of the risk of volume overload and the development of congestive symptoms. These shunts depend on both the presence of a physical passage between the arterial and venous circulations and a differential resistance to flow within these circuits. Capacitance and resistance

TABLE 42-1   Palliative Surgical Procedures and Surgical Repairs

NAME	PROCEDURE	INDICATION	LONG-TERM COMPLICATIONS
Palliation			
Blalock-Taussig shunt	Anastomosis of divided subclavian artery to right or left pulmonary artery	Tetralogy of Fallot, single-ventricle or pulmonary stenosis	Pulmonary vascular disease, pulmonary artery distortion, ventricular volume overload, decreased ventricular function
Waterston shunt	Ascending aorta to right pulmonary artery anastomosis	Tetralogy of Fallot, single-ventricle or pulmonary stenosis	Same as for Blalock-Taussig shunt
Potts shunt	Ascending aortaright pulmonary artery anastomosis	Tetralogy of Fallot, single-ventricle or pulmonary stenosis	Same as for Blalock-Taussig shunt
Classic Glenn anastomosis	Superior vena cava–right pulmonary artery anastomosis	Single-ventricle physiology	Pulmonary arteriovenous malformations, cyanosis
Bidirectional Glenn	Superior vena cava–right pulmonary artery anastomosis, pulmonary arteries in continuity	Single-ventricle physiology	Cyanosis
Repair			
Mustard procedure	Atrial baffle	D-transposition of the great arteries	Arrhythmias, decreased systemic RV function, baffle leak or obstruction, abnormal atrial volume conduction
Senning operation	Atrial baffle	D-transposition of the great arteries	Same as for Mustard procedure
Rastelli operation	Intraventricular repair and RV–pulmonary artery conduit	D-transposition of the great arteries, ventricular septal defect, LV outflow tract obstruction	Conduit obstruction, myocardial dysfunction, arrhythmia
Fontan procedure	Atriopulmonary or total cavopulmonary connection for separation of systemic and pulmonary circulations	Tricuspid atresia, single-ventricle physiology	Arrhythmia, thrombus, protein-losing enteropathy, atrial distortion, abnormal volume conduction, baffle leak
Ross operation	Aortic valve replacement with native pulmonary valve, pulmonary homograft	Aortic stenosis, aortic regurgitation	Pulmonary regurgitation, homograft obstruction, aortic regurgitation
Konno operation	Aortoventriculoplasty	Tunnel subaortic stenosis	Recurrent subaortic stenosis
Arterial switch operation	Anatomiccorrection with coronary transfer	D-transposition of the great arteries	Supravalvular PS, supravalvular aortic stenosis, dilation of neoaortic root
Damus-Kaye-Stansel operation	Arterial-level repair without coronary transfer	Double-outlet RV (Taussig-Bing–type subaortic stenosis, D-transposition of the great arteries, coronary pattern not appropriate for transfer)	Native aortic regurgitation, thrombosis in coronary arterial blind pouch
Takeuchi procedure	Intrapulmonary baffle of anomalous coronary artery from the pulmonary artery	Anomalous left coronary artery from the pulmonary artery	Baffle obstruction or leak, supravalvular PS

LV, left ventricle; PS, pulmonary stenosis; RV, right ventricle.

to filling in the most proximal downstream chamber or vessel to the existing shunt are the most important determinants of direction and extent of flow. Increased left-to-right shunt flow depends on decreased vascular or ventricular compliance or increased pressure and increased systemic vascular resistance, such as may occur in the setting of aging, stress, heart failure, and certain hypermetabolic states. Decreased shunting may result from a fall in systemic arterial resistance that occurs in pregnancy, sepsis, and endocrinologic illness. The results of acute volume loss can be mixed based on the effects of decreased blood pressure versus increased systemic vascular resistance. Assessment of chronic shunting is better performed once such conditions have been corrected. Regardless of the nature and extent of intravascular shunting, and even with predominant left-to-right shunting, the potential for right-to-left passage of even a minute quantity of blood at some phase of the cardiac cycle typically exists. Therefore, precautions should be taken, such as reduction of intravenous (IV) catheter particulate matter by vigilant attention to best care practices or by rigorous filtering.

Cyanosis

Cyanosis is the dark blue discoloration of skin and mucous membranes caused by increased amounts of reduced or abnormal hemoglobin in cutaneous blood vessels. Underlying pathology, extent of skin pigmentation, keratinization, and capillary density may influence the degree of cyanosis. In addition, cyanosis may fluctuate as a result of alterations in hematologic parameters and changes in cardiovascular, pulmonary, and renal function. Sequelae of long-term cyanosis occur in virtually every organ system and may have profound consequences.

In general, clinically evident cyanosis is seen at an arterial saturation of approximately 85%, although in patients with dark skin pigmentation, cyanosis may not be recognized until oxygen saturation is considerably lower. Cyanosis most frequently encountered by the physician caring for adults with CHD is caused by right-to-left intravascular shunting of systemic venous blood into the systemic arterial circulation. This situation depends on either physical obstruction of pulmonary blood flow or elevation of pulmonary vascular resistance. Increased pulmonary vascular resistance may be transient and reactive to secondary stimuli that include oxygen, acetylcholine, prostaglandin (PGE_1), prostacyclin (PGI_2), endothelin antagonism, phosphodiesterase (PDE) inhibition, or nitric oxide or it may be more "fixed," with increased arteriolar muscularity, intimal hyperplasia, and decreased numbers of intraacinar arteries.[13] Major congenital lesions that may occur with cyanosis in adulthood include unoperated lesions, such as tetralogy of Fallot and its variants, and Ebstein anomaly as well as in patients with single-ventricle physiology, either repaired or after a palliative procedure. In addition, patients with unrepaired left-to-right shunt lesions may come to medical attention with cyanosis secondary to reversed shunting in the presence of elevated resistance or Eisenmenger syndrome.[14]

Major Cyanotic Organ Complications

MUSCULOSKELETAL CHANGES

The presence of clubbing is a significant accompaniment to central cyanosis. This is a flattening of the nail beds, which causes loss of the normal 160-degree angle between the base of the nail and the adjoining skin.[15] Clubbing is a component of hypertrophic osteoarthropathy, a clinical syndrome that also includes periostosis and joint swelling. The severity of clubbing varies with extent of cyanosis; in the setting of differential cyanosis, it is found only in the cyanotic region. Histologic findings associated with clubbing include dilation and thickening of vascular walls, an increase in blood vessel–associated connective tissue, and the development of multiple, tiny, arteriovenous connections.[15] In addition, increased thickness of the periosteum is observed along with increased bone resorption.

HEMATOLOGIC CHANGES

Arterial oxygen content in cyanotic individuals is maintained by compensatory changes in cardiac output, hemoglobin concentration, and 2,3-diphosphoglycerate (2,3-DPG) levels. Increased production of erythropoietin is triggered by tissue hypoxia, which produces an increase in erythrocyte mass and blood volume. This improves oxygen-carrying capacity by increasing hemoglobin; however, extreme elevations in hematocrit may result in symptoms of hyperviscosity.[16] Such syndromes may manifest as headache, visual changes, mild parasthesias, fatigue, or musculoskeletal symptomatology. Iron deficiency as a result of reduced deformability of microcytic red blood cells also contributes to increased blood viscosity.[17] In addition, diminished iron stores affect tissue oxygen delivery, as evidenced by a more right-shifted oxyhemoglobin dissociation curve.

Cyanotic patients may be divided into two categories, compensated and decompensated erythrocytosis.[18] Patients with *compensated erythrocytosis* are iron replete, have stable volume status and hematocrit, are in multiorgan system balance, and do not have symptoms of hyperviscosity. Patients with *decompensated erythrocytosis* are iron deficient and have continually rising hematocrits, often as a result of episodic, identifiable, and correctable influences: dehydration, acute increase in right-to-left shunting or pulmonary resistance, heart failure, infection, or central nervous system events. These patients have symptoms previously attributed solely to hyperviscosity, and they may be treated by phlebotomy, which could further worsen iron deficiency. Correction of the underlying influence, coupled with repletion of iron stores, remains the primary treatment. Isovolumic phlebotomy is advised only for symptoms in patients with hematocrit typically greater than 65% to 70% when adequately hydrated and after correction of potential precipitating factors and, on occasion, prior to surgery or catheterization. Phlebotomy is not advised for an isolated elevation of the hematocrit in compensated patients without symptoms. Iron repletion in cyanotic patients frequently further increases serum hemoglobin, although it has been shown to improve functional capacity and quality of life.[19,20] Optimal achieved hemoglobin for such patients has only been theorized, and guidelines for phlebotomy to restore a reasonable hematocrit below 65% in this setting are lacking.

An increased tendency for perioperative bleeding has long been recognized in patients with cyanotic CHD, and numerous abnormalities of hemostasis have been reported in this population. These have included prolonged prothrombin time, thrombocytopenia, impaired platelet aggregation, and shortened platelet survival. In some individuals, the problem may be compounded by deficiency of vitamin K–dependent clotting factors because of

altered hepatic function in the setting of passive congestion secondary to chronic heart failure. The use of anticoagulants and antiplatelet agents in the cyanotic patient has been controversial; however, no data exist to support the increased risk of bleeding associated with long-term anticoagulation. Long-term anticoagulation therapy is typically prescribed if other standard indications such as atrial fibrillation or a mechanical prosthetic heart valve are present.

RENAL CHANGES

Abnormalities of renal function are frequently recognized in patients with cyanotic heart disease. Urinalysis results that suggest glomerulopathy have been noted to occur in up to one third of the population of adults with cyanotic CHD.[21] Associated renal pathology takes the form of altered glomerular architecture, including focal glomerular sclerosis, congestion, mesangial hypercellularity, and disorders of renal function. Cyanotic patients have been shown to exhibit a decreased glomerular filtration rate (GFR), proteinuria, and impaired water handling. Renal dysfunction may be compounded by the use of long-term diuretic therapy or associated decreased ventricular function. Reduction of concomitant risks for acute renal dysfunction, such as ensuring adequate hydration, and dosing medications based on estimates of GFR are advised.

Gout has long been associated with cyanotic heart disease. Cyanotic patients have been found to have increased serum uric acid levels as a result of decreased fractional urate excretion rather than increased production. Cornerstones of symptomatic management of acute gouty arthritis in cyanotic patients include the use of colchicine (0.5 to 0.6 mg orally every 1 to 2 hours) and corticosteroids (40 to 60 mg/day orally). Nonsteroidal antiinflammatory agents are generally not preferred as first-line agents because of potential deleterious effects on renal function. Maintenance therapy with allopurinol (100 mg orally every day or every other day) may be required for recurrent episodes; according to recommendations, in settings of an acute decrease in renal function, the allopurinol dose should be reduced rather than discontinued.

Cardiopulmonary Exercise

Decreased ventricular function has been described in cyanotic patients with persistence after repair in some groups, although causation remains unclear.[22] Contributing factors include age at repair, extent of cyanosis, and the presence of pressure or volume overload. Potential mechanisms for ventricular dysfunction secondary to cyanosis may involve myocardial hypoxia, with oxygen demand exceeding supply, as well as altered coronary perfusion as a result of erythrocytosis, resulting in myocardial necrosis and fibrosis.

Cyanotic patients have been noted to have increased dyspnea on exertion and decreased exercise tolerance. Patients with single-ventricle physiology have been shown to have significant exercise limitations as determined by decreased exercise time, total work performed, peak heart rate, peak oxygen uptake, and arterial oxygen saturation.[23] In healthy individuals, oxygen demand and CO_2 production are closely matched by circulatory and respiratory changes during exercise. Right-to-left shunting produces changes in both oxygen uptake and ventilation. During exercise, cyanotic patients show decreased oxygen uptake and a delay in establishment of a steady state. In addition, cyanotic patients exhibit higher exercise ventilation than control patients.[24] Presumably, this occurs as a result of increased pCO_2 and hydrogen ion concentration in the systemic arterial system from right-to-left shunting.

Neurologic Effects

A variety of neurologic effects are associated with the presence of chronic cyanosis because of right-to-left shunt lesions. The ability of blood flow to bypass the pulmonary circulation leads to the possibility of embolization to the cerebral circulation of substances that might have been filtered in the lungs. Cyanotic patients are therefore at risk for both brain abscesses from septic embolization and ischemic strokes precipitated by migration of thrombus, air, or foreign particles.[25] The physician should have a low threshold for obtaining brain imaging in a patient with a fever, headache, or fixed and localizing neurologic signs. It is important to note that the differential diagnosis in a cyanotic patient with transient neurologic symptoms includes transient ischemic attacks (TIAs), infection, and hyperviscosity.

Long-standing cyanotic CHD has been associated with intellectual impairment,[26] poor school performance, and difficulties with social adaptation that include persistence of a dependent lifestyle. However, confounding variables in establishing the effect of cyanosis on social and intellectual functioning include the possible contributions of cardiac surgery and circulatory arrest, the psychologic effects of chronic illness, and the influences of parental and societal attitudes given the severity of illness. Throughout a patient's life, every potential response to understand and limit these effects should be made to bolster the patient's independence and self-confidence.

Recommendations for Management of the Cyanotic Patient

It is important to recognize and correct any secondary situations that may provoke increased cyanosis regardless of underlying congenital pathology. Infection, dehydration, and erythrocytosis may all increase cyanosis. Other precipitants include worsening ventricular function, ischemic myocardial changes, increased atrioventricular (AV) valvular regurgitation, increased pulmonary vascular resistance, and alteration in renal or hepatic function. It is also important to avoid routinely resorting to phlebotomy for increased cyanosis without a search for other correctable causes. Anemia or iron deficiency may cause profound fatigue and worsening symptoms. In addition to alleviation of intercurrent illness, therapeutics must be based on a thorough understanding of the underlying pathology causing cyanosis.

In general, steps should be taken to increase the amount of oxygen in the blood. This may be achieved by improving oxygen-carrying capacity by increasing the hematocrit, administering oxygen if oxygen saturation is low, improving ventilation if pCO_2 is high, and judiciously choosing methods to optimize volume status. Tissue perfusion and oxygen extraction help determine oxygen content of mixed systemic venous blood. Abnormalities of both decreased tissue perfusion with profound dehydration and increased oxygen extraction with systemic ventricular failure may lead to decreased oxygen content of mixed systemic venous blood. In the setting of intracardiac shunting, these changes may account for acute or chronic increases in cyanosis. Thus, depending on the clinical situation, patients may need either volume expansion or diuresis.

Augmentation of pulmonary blood flow should use methods to decrease pulmonary vascular resistance if it is elevated. Appropriate measures may include administering oxygen, eliminating acidosis, and using specific pulmonary vasomodulators such as nitric oxide, endothelin antagonists, PDE antagonists, or inhaled or parenteral prostanoids.[27] The use of home oxygen therapy has been suggested to improve pulmonary blood flow in patients with irreversible pulmonary vascular disease, although few data are available from longer term studies.[28] Only open-label trials have been performed, with therapies that include continuous IV prostacyclin[29-31] and continuous inhaled nitric oxide.[32] The use of oral endothelin antagonism with a combined endothelin receptor antagonist has been demonstrated in randomized controlled studies to improve functional ability and hemodynamics in symptomatic patients with Eisenmenger syndrome.[18,33] Discussion of the use of such agents in patients with Eisenmenger syndrome has

been recommended in national guidelines, and studies of additional or combined advanced pulmonary arterial hypertension therapy for these patients is encouraging.[34]

Cyanosis may be lessened by improvement in ventricular function. This will occur upon optimizing forward cardiac output and improving mixed venous O_2 saturation. In addition, the use of angiotensin-converting enzyme (ACE) inhibitors even in patients with intracardiac shunting[35] may help maximize ventricular function, particularly in patients with AV valvular regurgitation, in which afterload reduction enhances output. In the critically ill patient, the use of IV agents such as isoproterenol, milrinone, dobutamine, and sodium nitroprusside may prove efficacious, although these agents have not been studied formally.

Concern arises about the ability of cyanotic patients to tolerate the reduction of partial pressure of oxygen produced during commercial airline flights. However, recent cohort series suggest experience to the contrary, with no longer term adverse outcomes associated with air travel.[36,37] Similar to native residents of high altitudes, patients with congenital cyanotic heart disease have been shown to have a decreased ventilatory response to acute hypoxia. This has been shown to return to normal after surgery to correct the cyanosis. We recommend minimization of cyanosis prior to flights if travel is desired or necessary. Metabolic demands and stress should be reduced, with baggage and transportation assistance coordinated with early airport arrival. Adequate preflight and in-transport rest, proper nutrition, and adequate hydration are emphasized. Use of supplemental oxygen, available on most commercial flights, should be discussed and is recommended for symptomatic patients.

Pregnancy

Reproductive issues are of major concern for the growing population of young women with corrected or palliated CHD. Successful counseling and planning for childbearing for women with CHD is currently the rule, with limited exceptions. In advising such patients, the cardiologist must be familiar with the physiology of existing cardiac lesions in the gravid state and with contemporary guidelines for genetic screening of cardiac defects. Optimal care is provided in a comprehensive center by a team of specialists that includes cardiologists, high-risk obstetricians, anesthesiologists, fetal echocardiographers, and geneticists.

Hemodynamic changes that occur in pregnancy may have significant consequences for the patient with CHD. Increased blood volume, stroke volume, and heart rate lead to augmented cardiac output in the antepartum period. Decline in systemic vascular resistance as a result of hormonal influences may result in increased right-to-left shunting. The physiologic anemia of pregnancy may exacerbate preexisting difficulties with tissue oxygen delivery. Labor and delivery are accompanied by hemodynamic shifts from pain, uterine contractions, anesthesia effects, and bleeding.

Pregnancy outcomes for women with specific congenital heart defects and their offspring have been detailed in a number of published reports.[38-40] However, most existing data regarding risks and success of pregnancy in CHD are anecdotal and may have changed with newer therapeutics. Ongoing efforts are directed at the development of tools for risk stratification of pregnancy-related complications in women with cardiac defects. The retrospective Cardiac Disease in Pregnancy (CARPREG) cohort study examined 276 pregnancies in 221 women with heart disease who received obstetric care at three major institutions from 1986 through 1994. Multivariate analysis identified five independent predictors of maternal cardiac events,[41] which included 1) prior cardiac events, 2) prior arrhythmia, 3) New York Hospital Association (NYHA) functional class greater than II or cyanosis during the baseline antenatal visit, 4) left heart obstruction, and 5) myocardial dysfunction. Maternal NYHA class above II or cyanosis during the initial visit independently predicted neonatal complications such as prematurity, respiratory distress syndrome, and low birth weight. In addition, a higher proportion of pregnancies that ended in miscarriage was found in each of these two groups. Additive peripartum risk was seen with maternal subpulmonary ventricular dysfunction and in women with significant AV valve regurgitation or prosthesis in an analysis of separate large congenital heart disease–specific pregnancy databases and similar risk scale assessment.[42,43] Of note, none of the above databases included patients with severe pulmonary hypertension. However, most centers that care for patients with severe fixed pulmonary hypertension (primary or secondary, with or without intracardiac shunting) would argue that such patients remain at prohibitive maternal risk of morbidity and mortality, even despite modern advanced pulmonary arterial hypertension therapy.[44,45] Functional parameters, such as exercise endurance and heart rate variability, may add further predictive ability regarding maternal outcomes in these populations.[46]

Recommendations

If possible, women of childbearing age who have CHD should undergo a comprehensive preconception evaluation that includes determination of ventricular function, assessment of left heart obstruction, examination for right-to-left shunting, review of arrhythmias, and testing of functional ability. Analysis of current medications should identify those contraindicated during pregnancy, with particular attention to warfarin and ACE inhibitors. Genetic counseling that includes karyotype examination or fluorescence in situ hybridization (FISH) for microdeletion of chromosome 22 should be provided for patients with CHD, not only for those with identified hereditary defects. Patients are advised that cardiac fetal echocardiography at 16 to 20 weeks' gestation may allow early identification of potential fetal cardiac malformations.

Throughout pregnancy, patients should be monitored at regular intervals and in conjunction with obstetricians, maternal-fetal medicine clinicians, and anesthesiologists knowledgeable in the care of adults with CHD. In our practice, we evaluate patients at least once during each trimester of pregnancy. Causes of increased cyanosis should be investigated, and heart failure should be promptly treated. Strategies that may be used during labor and delivery, if necessary, include the use of early epidural anesthesia to control pain and avoidance of major alterations in systemic vascular resistance, provision of supplemental oxygen, and use of techniques designed to decrease volume shifts. The need for cardiac monitoring and/or pulmonary artery catheters, as well as the shortening of the second stage of labor, should be evaluated on an individual case basis. Vigilance should be heightened in the first 48 hours postpartum—and at times, up to several weeks—with particular attention to fluid management, hemodynamic status, pulmonary vascular resistance, and potential for thromboembolism. The use of anticoagulant therapy to prevent thrombotic complications in the third trimester and postpartum in patients with right-to-left shunts is controversial. American Heart Association (AHA) guidelines do not recommend endocarditis prophylaxis for uncomplicated vaginal deliveries or cesarean section, although many centers deviate from this guideline in practice.[7]

Noncardiac Surgery

The primary cardiologist is often asked to assist in the management of adults with CHD who are undergoing noncardiac surgery, and recommendations must be individualized for particular patients and surgeries. A retrospective cohort study examined perioperative morbidity and mortality for 276 adults and children with CHD undergoing noncardiac surgical procedures.[47] Major risk factors associated with complications included the presence of cyanosis, congestive heart failure (CHF), and poor general health. Noncardiac surgical procedures in patients with Eisenmenger syndrome are associated with increased risk for complications.[48]

Recommendations

The primary cardiologist should actively assist in perioperative management decisions. Anesthetic induction regimens should be chosen with regard to their effects of maintaining oxygen saturation, for hemodynamic stability of ventricular function, and for loading conditions.[30,49] Basic tenets of operative management for patients with shunts include avoiding acute increases or decreases in systemic vascular resistance, which may have important effects on shunt flow and systemic perfusion. Particular vigilance to avoid deep venous thrombosis (DVT) and paradoxical embolism is warranted, and all IV devices should be guarded with meticulous caution via best care principles to avoid embolization of gaseous or particulate matter. Appropriate preoperative sedation and postoperative pain control should use agents that do not lower systemic venous resistance. Because hypovolemia will increase shunting and decrease arterial oxygen saturation, patients should be carefully monitored for postural blood pressure swings that result in increased cyanosis. Scrupulous attention should be paid to control of blood loss and monitoring of the postoperative hematocrit.[50] Antibiotics should be administered according to AHA guidelines for SBE prophylaxis,[7] and consideration should be given to overnight observation in intensive care settings for all but the most minor of procedures. Procedures with the potential for marked changes in relative pulmonary blood flow should be performed in centers with expertise in acute IV and inhaled pulmonary vasodilators and ready access to extracorporeal membrane oxygenation support, ventricular assist devices, and organ transplantation.

Arrhythmia Management

Adults with CHD are at increased risk for both atrial and ventricular arrhythmias as a result of long-standing volume load, increased afterload, multiple surgical scars, and myopathic ventricles.[51] Issues of arrhythmias associated with atrial septal defects (ASDs) and repaired tetralogy of Fallot are addressed later in this chapter. Various risk-assessment strategies have been suggested to identify CHD patients at risk for acute tachyarrhythmias and sudden death. Programmed ventricular stimulation in a selected group of CHD patients has been used to identify a subgroup with decreased and increased risk of serious arrhythmic events.[52] However, the overall recommendation remains to place the occurrence of arrhythmia into the context of known baseline anatomy, residual anatomy and physiology, past surgeries, ventricular function, and exercise capacity.

Management strategies include antiarrhythmic drugs, transcatheter radiofrequency ablation, surgical maneuvers and pacemaker or implantable telemetry monitoring for development of proarrhythmia, and negative inotropic effects or symptomatic bradycardia that requires pacemaker placement. Radiofrequency catheter ablation has been successfully used for control of arrhythmias with CHD and may provide years of freedom from the use of antiarrhythmic medications in selected patients.[53] Similarly, right- or left-sided Maze procedures have been effective in reducing incidence of atrial tachyarrhythmias if performed at the time of cardiac surgical repair.[54] Indications for prophylactic atrial or ventricular pacing, in single or multiple sites, to diminish arrhythmia and to improve atrial or ventricular function require further study, although such techniques are increasingly used.

Exercise and Athletic Participation

Adult survivors of CHD frequently raise questions about exercise limitations and benefits. A survey of adults at a tertiary referral clinic for CHD demonstrated considerable patient confusion regarding the appropriate level of exercise for existing cardiac lesions.[55] Exercise tolerance, gas exchange parameters, and cardiorespiratory responses to exercise have been studied in several cohorts with similar findings: baseline functional parameters appear markedly reduced compared with age- and gender-matched controls, and they appear to worsen over time and correlate with a decrease in quality of life and survival.[56-59] To date, adults with CHD remain a paradigm for the multitude of comorbidities that combine to engender functional incapacity.[24]

Studies of physical training in patients with severe left ventricular (LV) dysfunction have demonstrated that supervised exercise conditioning can produce increased peak oxygen consumption, improved cardiac output, decreased resting heart rate, increased skeletal muscle blood flow, delayed lactate accumulation during exercise, and improved sense of well-being, although a more recent randomized controlled multimember study has called this into question.[60,61] Extrapolation from such data suggests that adult patients with CHD may benefit from regular aerobic conditioning, which may improve peripheral muscle function and decrease vascular inflammation and thereby decrease myocardial work and increase functional capacity. Postoperative exercise training has been shown to benefit children after surgery for CHD by improving their fitness level.[62,63] However, the safety and utility of exercise rehabilitation programs for adults with CHD remain underexamined.

Recommendations for fitness training and athletic participation for adults with CHD are in constant evolution, with little data to guide decision making. Conservative restrictive guidelines can be extrapolated from the American College of Cardiology (ACC)/AHA guidelines and consensus statement.[7,64] Strenuous exercise is most restricted in adults with illnesses in which experience has suggested catastrophic potential with exertion. These include severe systemic ventricular outflow obstruction, severe pulmonary hypertension (with near-systemic pulmonary artery blood pressure), aortic root dilation of 4.0 to 4.5 cm or greater, single coronary artery or fixed coronary obstruction, sustained or exercise-induced ventricular arrhythmia, systemic or pulmonary ventricular failure, or oxygen saturation at or below 70%. Practically, in all other cases, given marked individual variation, we recommend goals of exercise set for the population at large, with preexercise assessment with reproduction of the desired level of strenuous exercise under physiologic monitoring. This should include measurement of transcutaneous oxygen saturation, VO_2 max, anaerobic threshold, VE/VCO_2, duration of exercise, observation for electrocardiographic (ECG) evidence of arrhythmia or ischemia, and echocardiographic assessment of transvalvular gradient, ventricular function, and pulmonary artery pressure. Risks and goals of athletic participation are then openly discussed with patients and family members.

Transplantation

Unique aspects of transplantation medicine for adults with CHD lie in a combination of anatomically available cannulation access sites, sources of systemic and pulmonary vascular inflow and outflow, past surgical residuae from prior sternotomies and thoracotomies, challenges of immunosuppression in highly sensitized individuals, multiple organ system comorbidities, and posttraumatic stress associated with lifelong medical illness. Indications for consideration for transplantation include balance of quality of life and survival in the young and older adult.[65-67]

Guidelines for Management of Patients with Specific Congenital Cardiac Lesions

Atrial Septal Defects

ASDs are congenital defects that allow communication between the left and right atria (Figure 42-1). They are typically classified as 1) secundum-type (2-ASD), 2) ostium-primum (1-ASD), 3) sinus venosus, and 4) coronary sinus defects. 2-ASDs comprise approximately 10% of all isolated congenital heart malformations and more than 75% of all ASDs.[68,69] Embryologically, the defect appears

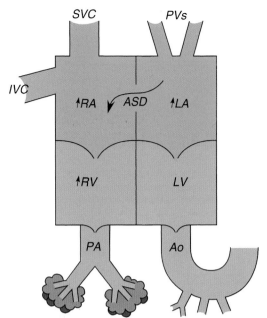

FIGURE 42-1 Atrial septal defect (*ASD*) physiology. Intracardiac shunting is governed by relative resistance to ventricular filling. Unless right ventricular function is compromised, flow is left to right with enlargement of right-sided chambers. Ao, aorta; IVC, inferior vena cava; LA, left atrium; LV, left ventricle; PA, pulmonary artery; PVs, pulmonary veins; RA, right atrium; RV, right ventricle; SVC, superior vena cava.

to stem from abnormal development of the septum primum, resulting in a failure to cover the fossa ovalis. 1-ASDs are a form of endocardial cushion defect almost always associated with abnormality of AV valve formation, in its most benign form, a cleft anterior leaflet of the mitral valve. *Sinus venosus defects* are located at the entrance of the superior vena cava (SVC) to the right atrium and are frequently associated with anomalous right upper pulmonary venous drainage to the SVC–right atrial junction. They comprise 10% of all ASDs, and compared with other ASDs, the sinus venosus type is more commonly associated with elevation of pulmonary vascular resistance if left untreated. The least common type of ASD is the "unroofed" *coronary sinus defect*, which results in a connection between the coronary sinus and left atrium.

Physiologically, the direction and amount of shunting across an ASD depend on the size of the ASD, the respective right- and left-sided chamber compliances, and downstream arterial vessel resistances. Normally, the physiologic parameters are such that shunt flow is from left to right. Over time, left-to-right shunting results in volume overload and, ultimately, in dilation of the right-sided chambers. We rely primarily upon physiologic confirmation of excessive right ventricular (RV) volume loading by echocardiography, rather than primary catheterization-based documentation of significant shunting (pulmonary/systemic flow ≥1.5), as evidence of a hemodynamically significant shunt, although the superiority of this assessment in predicting clinical morbidity is unproven. Routine catheterization of patients with ASD for determination of intracardiac shunting is not indicated, and as such, it is given a class III recommendation (avoidance).[7] TEE and magnetic resonance imaging (MRI) are useful in further defining the location and size of the defect, right-sided chamber sizes, and associated anomalies such as anomalous pulmonary venous drainage.

Large shunts (Qp/Qs >1.5 to 2.0) increase the risk for dyspnea, CHF, atrial arrhythmias, and, less commonly, pulmonary hypertension or paradoxic embolization. Increased shunting may occur with increasing patient age from decreasing LV compliance associated with aging, systemic hypertension, diabetes mellitus, obesity, and ischemic heart disease. All secondary influences on shunting

638

should be medically minimized prior to assessing the importance of any ASD.[70] Endocarditis prophylaxis is not recommended for isolated 2-ASDs, and pregnancy is well tolerated in patients with 2-ASD and even a moderate degree of intracardiac shunting. Discussion might occur concerning the need to close such defects prior to childbirth, theoretically to decrease the rare risk of paradoxical embolization through this defect; we do not recommend ASD closure without hemodynamic indication.

Symptomatic patients with large left-to-right shunts appear to have decreased symptoms and fewer atrial arrhythmias and have improved RV function with ASD closure.[71-75] Although surgical patch or primary suture closure of ASDs, with or without minithoracotomy, remains one of the safest and most effective of adult cardiac surgical procedures, significant morbidity may ensue. Increasing age, medical comorbidities, and the presence of pulmonary hypertension are independent risk factors for increased surgical death. Surgical success is generally uniform, yet it may be accompanied by minor, but persistent, detectable shunting in upward of 7% to 8% of surgically treated patients by echocardiography.[76] The incidence of major or minor neuropsychiatric complications after cardiopulmonary bypass in this population has focused attention on transcatheter closure techniques.

In 1959, Hufnagel and Gillespie[77] were the first to implant a device, a plastic button, on the atrial septum (via thoracotomy) to accomplish ASD closure. The first intracardiac use of a double-umbrella–type device was pioneered by King and Mills in 1974.[78] Device design was refined by Rashkind in 1983 to resemble a barbed single disk and was later modified to become a more flexible double disk.[79] Lock and colleagues[80] altered the wire configuration to allow springed joints on the device arms, forming the first of the modern "clamshell" varieties of closure devices. Subsequent device modifications (e.g., cardioSEAL-STARFlex; NMT Medical, Boston, MA) incorporated changes in device-arm alloys (MP35N) to allow MRI compatibility, adding a second spring to each arm to reduce and displace device-mediated cardiac stress and to lower the device profile, placing nitinol microspring arms in a central interconnecting, arm-to-arm mesh to allow for autoadjustment and maximal defect closure, and creating devices with bioabsorbable potential (e.g., BioSTAR; NMT Medical). However, in the United States, double-umbrella devices have not received Food and Drug Administration (FDA) approval for implantation to close ASDs, and recent results of the randomized controlled trials (RCTs) to assess benefit of patent foramen ovale (PFO) closure with these devices have led to termination of operations for NMT Medical, the manufacturer of these devices.[81] Therefore, double-umbrella devices are typically considered only for small- to moderate-sized (<12 to 14 mm maximal stretch diameter) secundum-type ASDs, in off-label fashion, after specific patient-physician discussion.

Two devices approved by the FDA for catheter closure of 2-ASDs—for all age groups, including pediatrics—include the Amplatzer Septal Occluder (ASO) device (AGA Medical, Plymouth, MN) and the Gore Helex Septal Occluder (W.L. Gore & Associates, Flagstaff, AZ). The ASO device is constructed from a 0.004 to 0.0075 nitinol wire mesh, tightly woven into two flat disks (left atrial [LA] disk larger than the right atrial [RA] disk), with a 3- to 4-mm connecting waist separating the two discs and three Dacron polyester patches sewn into the discs and connecting waist, respectively, to increase thrombogenicity. The wire mesh can be stretched to form a single-wire configuration that allows transport within a guide-catheter delivery system, although the original shape is reformed on deployment because of the memory properties of nitinol. The Helex device is constructed from a curtain of hydrophilic expandable polytetrafluoroethylene (ePTFE) placed over a 0.012-inch nitinol wire frame, wound in a fashion to allow formation of opposing and parallel spiral disks, one on either side of the atrial septum. Similar to the ASO device, the Helex device can be stretched to form a single-wire curtain configuration to allow transport within a narrow catheter delivery system, which obviates the need for a long femoral vein–left atrium sheath; this reconstitutes its opposing spiral shape with a series of push, pinch, and pull

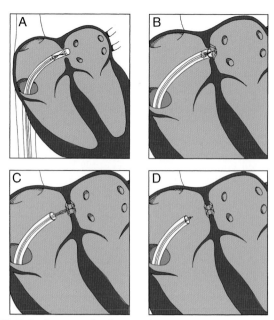

FIGURE 42-2 Prototypical technique of transcatheter deployment of occlusion device for secundum-type atrial septal defect closure.

maneuvers. Both the ASO and Helex devices are fully retrievable with relative ease prior to final deployment and release from their respective delivery systems. Although feasible, post-release retrieval may be extremely difficult, and device embolization often carries substantial patient risk. Under the FDA requirement, operators must be proctored at their own institutions prior to achieving independent implanter status.

For potential closure of 2-ASDs with all approved and investigation closure devices, the atrial septum can be readily crossed from femoral venous access—although on occasion, internal jugular or hepatic venous access may also be used—and the placement of a larger caliber short or longer guiding sheath allows precise extrusion of compacted expandable devices in the desired location (Figure 42-2). The majority of septal closure devices are designed as locked or attachable opposing structures that engage the rim of the tissue surrounding a central hole in the heart wall. Routine use of TEE has been supported by increasing use of intracardiac echocardiography (ICE), and both greatly assist in appropriate device arm placement and success at defect closure.[82]

Clinical experience is greatest with the ASO devices, although in appropriate centers of expertise, results appear similar with various implants, including the Helex Septal Occluder devices and off-label double-umbrella devices.[83-85] Closure rates should typically achieve about 95% complete success for centrally located defects, with a less than 1% to 7% complication rate and 0% mortality rate.[83-85] Patients younger than 40 years have the greatest potential for RV enlargement to return to normal over the 6 months following device implantation, although most patients of all ages with a moderate to large degree of left-to-right intracardiac shunting (Qp/Qs >1.5) and pulmonary vascular resistance below 3 to 5 indexed Wood units (despite potential presence of pulmonary hypertension) demonstrate similar benefit in RV size and function and improvement in sensed and measured functional capacity.[73-75,86,87] Device-related thrombosis and atrial perforations have been recently highlighted but are uncommon.[88,89] A typical postimplantation medical regimen includes aspirin at a dose of 81 mg to 325 mg daily for at least 6 months with or without concomitant clopidogrel at 75 mg daily for 2 to 3 months, although data supporting such recommendations remain theoretic. Antibiotic precautions surrounding dental work or "dirty procedures" are recommended for at least 6 months or until no residual bubble-contrast shunting is recognized on TTE.

CH 42

RECOMMENDATIONS

We recommend closure of ASDs in the presence of echocardiographic evidence of RV volume loading (generally correlating with Qp/Qs ≥1.5) that cannot be explained by concomitant confounding intracardiac pathology, such as pulmonary regurgitation (PR), tricuspid regurgitation, or anomalous pulmonary venous return. We do not routinely measure Qp/Qs as a determinant for ASD closure. Surgical options are among the most successful of modern cardiac surgical procedures, although they still carry associated morbidity. In addition, 2-ASDs less than 36 mm in stretch size (typically <32 mm) are most amenable to transcatheter device closure, although significant diastolic dysfunction and a tendency toward volume retention may remain. The greatest worldwide experience is with the self-centering Amplatzer ASO device for moderate to large 2-ASDs, which has become a standard of care. Nickel allergy, device thrombosis, and device-cardiac interaction, as evidenced by potential for early and late device erosions and as residual diastolic abnormalities, highlight the need for more subtle, compliant, and absorbable devices.

Patent Foramen Ovale

The foramen ovale is a flap-valve communication between the right and left atria. In utero it allows oxygenated blood from the placenta to cross over preferentially to the left side of the heart and perfuse the upper body. Shortly after birth, the pulmonary vascular resistance drops; consequently, the LA pressure rises above the RA pressure and results in functional closure of the foramen ovale. In the majority of patients, this leads to fibrosis and scarring with ultimate closure of the flap-valve communication. However, in up to 25% of the population, permanent closure does not occur, resulting in a PFO. The presence of PFOs has been discussed in association with "idiopathic" stroke and TIA, migraines (particularly with aura), platypnea orthodeoxia, decompression sickness, obstructive sleep apnea, and dementia. Despite highly publicized continued use as treatment for stroke, therapeutic closure of PFOs in patients with stroke and presumed paradoxical embolism (PPE) remains controversial because the causes and natural history of these embolic events are unclear.[90-94] The ability of clinical features (e.g., multiple prior embolic events or silent events by brain scanning, presence of hypercoagulable states, occurrence with Valsalva) or echocardiographic features (e.g., large-volume right-to-left shunting, atrial septal aneurysm or hypermobile atrial septum, and presence of prominent eustachian valve) to identify patients at high risk for recurrence has been suggested but is largely unsubstantiated.[92,93] In an attempt to generate the most meaningful data to guide construction of sufficiently powered RCTs from the disparate and uncontrolled nature and results of series of both medical treatments and percutaneous PFO closure, we performed a systematic review and pooled analysis of uncontrolled studies of transcatheter device closure of PFOs.[95] Results suggested that approximately two thirds of recurrent thromboembolic events could possibly be prevented by percutaneous PFO closure compared with medical therapy, corresponding to a 4% absolute reduction in annual events. These data helped lay a foundation for the establishment of ongoing and completed RCTs to assess the role of PFO closure in addition to short-term medical therapy versus prolonged best medical therapy as treatment for young adults with PPE.

Many factors contributed to the delay and imprecision in construction and completion of adequate trials and assessment of percutaneous PFO closure for relief of neurologic diseases. With intense planning, this milieu radically shifted, setting the stage for randomized controlled comparison of percutaneous PFO closure and other therapies for those affected by cardiac shunting. The largest such trial, the Evaluation of the STARFlex Septal Closure System in Patients with a Stroke or TIA Due to the Possible Passage of a Clot of Unknown Origin Through a Patent Foramen Ovale (CLOSURE-1) study, included more than 1600 patients in an RCT in more than 80 participating centers (neurologist principal investigatorships) to evaluate the cardioSEAL-STARFlex versus tightly controlled best medical therapy; it was sufficiently powered to test superiority of percutaneous PFO closure versus medical therapy in patients with imaging-confirmed index stroke or motor/speech TIA, evaluating similar hard neurologic endpoints as primary outcome. The results of CLOSURE-1 have been released and are insightful. PFO closure in addition to antiplatelet therapy offered no reduction in recurrent stroke (1.5% per year) or TIA (1.5% per year) compared with neurologist-chosen best medical therapy (more than two thirds of patients treated with aspirin alone). Of greatest import was that in the study population of patients defined to have had cryptogenic stroke, nearly all recurrent neurologic events had explainable etiologies. The results of CLOSURE-1 highlight the difficulties of definition of cryptogenic stroke and the need to search for and treat etiologies of stroke in the young other than presence of PFO. Several other percutaneous PFO closure trials remain ongoing.

In light of the above trials, we strongly advocate the following:
- Intensive and reiterative investigation for established etiologies for stroke and TIA and for serologic evidence of procoagulation in all patients with PFO who have stroke or TIA, accompanied by implementation of established therapies designed to reduce these risks
- Patient education regarding inconclusive association of cryptogenic stroke and PFO, with emphasis on available randomized controlled data, as well as individual risk factors for recurrence of symptoms
- Enrollment of willing and eligible patients into further RCTs to evaluate safety and efficacy of treatment arms

PATENT FORAMEN OVALE AND HYPOXEMIA

Pressure overload of the RA may lead to pathologic right-to-left shunting in patients with a PFO. This may accompany chronic alteration of right-sided filling or capacitance—from RV infarction, pulmonary embolism, thoracic surgery, or spinal and ribcage deformity—or transient decrease in RV filling seen with change from a supine to an upright position (orthodeoxia-platypnea syndrome). We and others have closed PFOs in hundreds of such patients with near-uniform short- and intermediate-term improvement (Figure 42-3).[96] However, the long-term benefits of PFO closure in such patients require further study.

PATENT FORAMEN OVALE AND MIGRAINE

Potential for association between migraine syndrome with aura (M+A) and PFO appears to have come full circle over the past few decades. Initial concerns from cardiologists centered around post-implant precipitation of migrainous events that mimic the original neurologic presentation in those who have recently undergone percutaneous PFO closure. True incidence was not catalogued but was sufficient to separately raise suspicions for investigators implanting differing closure devices. Effects from general anesthesia, raised ambient catecholamines, particulate metallic embolization, and embolization of procoagulant microaggregates were all theorized as related to occurrence. Recent assessment of relationship between migraine and PFO failed to demonstrate association in a large case-control analysis.[97]

Although highly publicized and contested in the lay press, the randomized, placebo-controlled (sham procedure) Migraine Intervention with STARFlex Technology (MIST) trial to compare PFO closure with cardioSEAL-STARFlex plus short-term antiplatelet therapy versus best medical antimigraine therapy in patients with resistant migrainous symptoms failed to demonstrate the primary endpoint of migraine elimination. Additional trials remain ongoing, but at present, we do not recommend PFO closure for patients with M+A without cardiac shunting; however, we strongly support further study within the context of RCTs.[98]

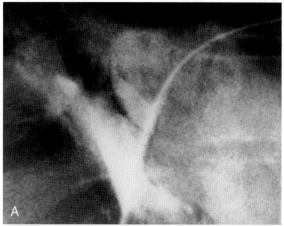

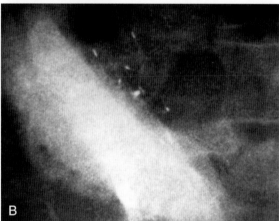

FIGURE 42-3 **A,** Intracardiac passage of contrast across the foramen ovale (orthodeoxia-platypnea) after an injection into the right atrium. A guidewire is anchored in the left upper pulmonary vein. After thoracotomy, the patient was unable to work because of resting aortic oxygen saturation (supine 100%, standing 82%). **B,** Right atrial angiogram demonstrates elimination of shunt flow after implantation of a clamshell occluder on the atrial septum. After patent foramen ovale closure, the patient returned to work with finger oximetry (supine 100%, standing 100%).

RECOMMENDATIONS

The decision to close PFOs associated with PPE is complicated by the high frequency of PFOs in the normal population (25%). An intensive and reiterative search for established etiologies for common syndromes should be carried out, and established therapies for such stroke risks should be used. At present, transcatheter PFO closure is recommended only for PFO associated with orthodeoxia-platypnea or in the presence of right-to-left intracardiac shunting without RV failure.

Bicuspid Aortic Valve

A bicuspid aortic valve is the most common congenital heart defect in the nonpediatric population, found in 1% to 2% of adults older than 18 years, and it may be associated with other left-sided obstructive lesions, such as aortic coarctation, particularly when left-right commissural fusion is present. Progressive pathologic dilation of the aortic root, with or without dissection, may be seen even in the absence of an obstructive gradient or regurgitation. Valvulopathy is more common in bicuspid aortic valves with right noncoronary commissural fusion. Stenosis of the bicuspid valve is associated with, but not dependent on, increasing age and presence of fibrocalcific disease. Aortic insufficiency occurs in younger patients and may represent an isolated hemodynamic lesion as a result of endocarditis or cystic medial necrosis or aortic

root dilation. Endocarditis prophylaxis is recommended for all adults with bicuspid aortic valves.

Although the first and second Natural History of Congenital Heart Defects Studies outlined the course and treatment of bicuspid aortic valve disease, primarily in infants and children, the natural history of bicuspid aortic valve disease and criteria for intervention in the nonpediatric patient population are less well defined.[99] Sudden death in the occasional asymptomatic patient with apparent preserved ventricular function and only moderate obstructive gradient suggests an inability to extrapolate from natural history and intervention studies derived from adults with acquired calcific stenosis.

Surgical aortic valve replacement is the treatment of choice when aortic root surgery is required. The increased complexity of surgical translocation of a pulmonary autograft to the aortic position and subsequent homograft implantation into the pulmonary position (Ross procedure) compared with standard homograft, tissue, or prosthetic valve alternatives are left to the relative expertise and experience of particular surgeons, teams, and centers. Excellent results can be obtained with all the approaches noted above, although each procedure carries its own immediate and long-term complications.

The acceptance of balloon aortic valvuloplasty (BAV) as palliation for children with bicuspid aortic stenosis is in contradistinction to the treatment of elderly patients with calcific aortic stenosis. Two reports have underscored the utility of BAV in selected young and intermediate-aged adults with noncalcified stenotic aortic valves.[100,101] Patients with increased valvular calcification demonstrated a trend toward higher gradients both before and after BAV, and their incident-free survival was lower compared with patients without calcified valves. Balloon-mediated worsening of aortic regurgitation, a rare adverse sequela of BAV, did not preclude the potential for subsequent successful surgical valvuloplasty.

The potential use of transcatheter aortic valve implantation (TAVI) for people with bicuspid aortic valve and aortic stenosis or regurgitation is currently highly investigational and remains unclear, especially when the stenosis and regurgitation are the result of dilation, and in the setting of less calcification and asymmetry. Such patients were excluded from large RCTs, although limited experience in select patients and in experienced hands is encouraging.[102,103]

RECOMMENDATIONS

The above findings support BAV for noncalcified congenital bicuspid aortic stenosis in young and intermediate-aged adults. This procedure can provide effective palliation and can prolong the interval to surgical intervention without significantly increasing cardiac morbidity or serious complications. Immediate recognition of the uncommon complication of balloon-induced avulsion of a valvular cusp during BAV allows effective and timely surgical therapy. Surgical options remain acceptable for the symptomatic patient with calcific disease, noncalcific disease associated with an enlarged aortic root (>4.5 cm), or moderate to severe valvular regurgitation. We recommend an attempt at balloon valvuloplasty for symptomatic adults up to age 40 years with at most a mildly calcified bicuspid aortic valve, a gradient of 60 mm Hg or more with preserved ventricular function, or a gradient less than 60 mm Hg with associated ventricular dysfunction. Despite treatment of valvular disease, vigilant lifelong assessment of the health of the ascending aorta is warranted. Utility and risks of TAVI for bicuspid aortic valvulopathy, stenosis or regurgitation, or regurgitation in other forms of CHD that involve aortic root enlargement require further investigation.

Pulmonary Stenosis

Pulmonary stenosis—most commonly valvular, although branch pulmonary artery and subvalvular obstruction are also possible—occurs in more than 10% of patients with CHD. Adult presentations may range from no symptoms to profound fatigue and dyspnea, depending on the degree of stenosis and RV impairment.

The first and second Natural History of Congenital Heart Disease Studies led to classification of degree of stenosis as *mild*, characterized by RV systolic pressure of 50 mm Hg or less; *moderate*, with RV systolic pressure of 50 to 100 mm Hg; or *severe*, in which RV pressure is over 100 mm Hg.[104] Given the unclear natural history of VPS in adults, the criteria for timing and the nature of the intervention have become dependent in large part on development of symptoms, extrapolation from the natural history in children, and decreasing risk of interventions.

Although open surgical valvotomy was historically the initial therapeutic approach, the current treatment of choice for patients with nondysplastic VPS is balloon pulmonary valvuloplasty (BPV; Figure 42-4). Numerous single-center reports, each with 4 to 53 patients, have demonstrated similar immediate gradient reductions with BPV in adolescents and middle-aged adults aged 13 to 55 years, using standard single, Inoue, or double-balloon techniques to achieve a balloon/annulus ratio between 1.1 and 1.4.[105] The mean follow-up in these series ranged from 0.5 to 6.9 years; when compared with results in pediatrics, it revealed a decreased incidence of periprocedural morbidity and restenosis in the adult. Infundibular spasm leading to hemodynamic compromise or requiring therapy is uncommon and has not been seen either in our experience or in the largest reported series, although individual instances of surgically treated pericardial tamponade, severe infundibular obstruction, periprocedural sepsis, and postprocedural diffuse pulmonary edema have been reported. Brief inflations with rapidly deflating balloons allow avoidance of prolonged reductions in cardiac output in the elderly or in those with low output at baseline. PR after BPV is usually mild, although anecdotal experiences suggest an increasing potential for surgical valve intervention to decrease symptoms of fatigue as a result of decreased RV performance at late (30-year) follow-up.[106]

RECOMMENDATIONS

Given the low attendant morbidity of BPV, we perform this procedure for any adult patient with a gradient above 40 mm Hg and normal RV function—and a lower gradient if cardiac output is reduced, RV systolic function appears subnormal, or RV end-diastolic pressure is 12 mm Hg or more—in the individual either with unoperated VPS or with recurrent VPS after initial surgical treatment. Long-term follow-up for potential effects of PR on RV function is warranted.

Aortic Coarctation

Aortic coarctation (CoA), typically a narrowing of the descending aorta at the site of insertion of the ductus arteriosus distal to the origin of the left subclavian artery, occurs in 5% to 10% of patients with CHD. An accompanying bicuspid aortic valve, most frequently with right-left commissural fusion, is present in 40% to 80% of patients with CoA.

Clinically detectable CoA in the adult, with a resting gradient of 20 mm Hg or more between upper and lower extremities, carries an increasing risk of progressive LV dysfunction, persistent systemic arterial systolic hypertension, and premature cerebrovascular and coronary atherosclerosis, and the potential for dissection or rupture of the aorta or coronary or cerebral vessels, especially during pregnancy, surgery, or catheterization (Figure 42-5). Echocardiography and MRI are the diagnostic modalities used to confirm the diagnosis of CoA and further delineate precise anatomic detail, the presence of cerebral vascular anomalies, and the presence of LV hypertrophy.

As a result of the combination of amplification of the gradient wave and stress on the myocardium and vasculature at all portions of ejection phase in the cardiac cycle (ventricular-arterial coupling), the effects of seemingly mild gradients across CoA may be profound. We consider indications for repair to be 1) the presence of a resting gradient of 20 to 25 mm Hg or more with normal LV function; 2) less gradient with accompanying abnormal LV function, significant ascending aortic enlargement, or significant aortic valve disease; 3) systemic hypertension that requires more than moderate therapy to achieve normotension; or 4) symptoms of abdominal or lower extremity hypoperfusion. Surgical end-to-end or bypass repair has previously been the standard approach, with excellent results and perioperative mortality rates of 2% or less for native CoA repair. Perioperative concerns of low but present risk of spinal cord ischemia or bleeding from collateral vessels are

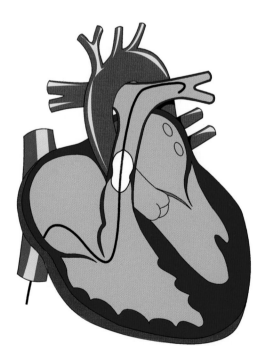

FIGURE 42-4 The technique of balloon pulmonary valvuloplasty.

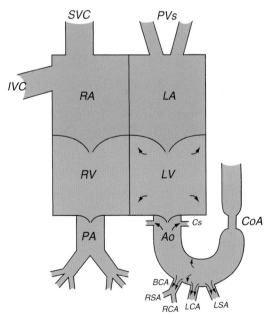

FIGURE 42-5 Aortic coarctation physiology. Narrowing in the descending aorta, just distal to the origin of the left subclavian artery. Wall stress is raised in all proximal chambers and vessels, leading to potential for advanced atherosclerosis, vascular dissection or rupture, and chamber hypertrophy. Ao, aorta; CoA, coarctation; IVC, inferior vena cava; LA, left atrium; LV, left ventricle; PA, pulmonary artery; PVs, pulmonary veins; RA, right atrium; RV, right ventricle; SVC, superior vena cava.

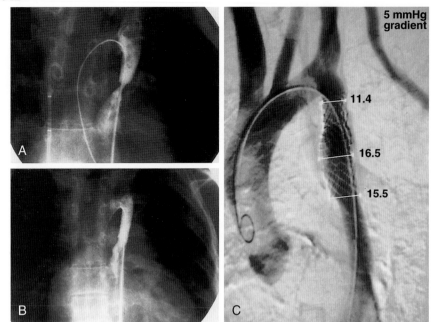

FIGURE 42-6 Unrecognized coarctation of the aorta (80 mm peak systolic gradient) leading to left heart failure and premature atherosclerosis of the coronary and cerebral arterial vasculature (**A**). Initial balloon dilation and stent implantation, with small distal dissection (**B**), later covered with a second stent (**C**). A residual gradient across the entire segment of more than 5 mm Hg was noted.

amplified in the patient with recurrent stenosis after initial repair. Late postoperative complications that include the development of aortic aneurysms and recurrent CoA have been reported in up to 20% of patients who undergo surgical repair, although recent surgical risk of death at reoperation, paraplegia, and late aneurysm formation has been estimated at 2% or less at appropriate centers. A high incidence of late postoperative recurrence of systemic hypertension, inversely correlated with age at repair, has been noted. Patients must be screened on a continuing basis for sequelae of aortic and systemic capacitance vessel noncompliance, aneurysms of the cerebral vasculature,[107] aortic enlargement or dissection, and premature systemic arterial or coronary atherosclerosis. We recommend that patients be examined yearly, with particular emphasis on symptoms suggestive of lower extremity or coronary ischemia or cerebral aneurysm. In addition, we suggest noninvasive imaging with MRI every 3 to 5 years, more frequently if aneurysm or restenosis is present, and exercise testing as suggested by history and examination.

The presence of abnormal vascular elasticity and elevation of mediators of vascular inflammation in patients after apparently successful mechanical relief of aortic CoA and the normalization of these markers with ramipril therapy have led some clinicians to use ACE inhibition or angiotensin receptor blockade to treat those with residual systemic arterial hypertension after repair of aortic CoA.[108] The effects of these agents on long-term outcomes are unstudied.

In children and adults, balloon dilation or stenting of recurrent or persistent CoA following surgical correction is now considered the therapy of choice. Moreover, balloon dilation and stenting are also considered effective alternatives to surgical correction as therapy for native CoA, with up to 15-year follow-up reported at some centers.[109-116] Early studies highlighted a low morbidity rate and high procedural success (>80%), defined in the past either as gradient reduction of 50% or more and an increase in angiographic luminal diameter of 30% or more as a residual gradient of 20 mm Hg or less with near universal reduction in antihypertensive therapy, with balloons chosen to be three to four times the diameter of CoA and not more than 150% of the transverse arch diameter. Estimates of complications included procedure-related death in 0.7%, periprocedural stroke in 0.6%, transmural (0.7%) or intimal (1.6%) dissection with rare need for surgical intervention, and postprocedural aneurysm (7% to 12%). Risk of complication

may be increased with increasing age and in the presence of concomitant bicuspid aortic valvular disease.[117] Balloon-assisted stenting of the aorta (Figure 42-6) without prior maximal balloon dilation permits use of smaller, nonoversized balloons, theoretically with less risk of dissection and rupture of the aortic wall.[118] Predilation of lesions allows for assessment of vessel compliance and for more optimal localization for stent deployment. Care should be taken to avoid extrapolation to the adult population of those results obtained with similar techniques in children, especially given the potential for increased changes in capacitance, compliance, and atherosclerosis in the walls of conduit arterial vessels proximal to the CoA. The relative safety of surgical versus transcatheter balloon and stenting repair of CoA in adults who may wish to become pregnant or sustain significant physical exertion remains to be clarified. Standardization of indication, procedural technique, follow-up, and outcomes assessment remains the major limitation of most studies. Utility of surgery versus endovascular transcatheter therapies when concomitant aortic dilation or aneurysm is present remains undefined. Large, single-center evaluation of adverse outcomes, combined with results from recently formed congenital interventional registries—Improving Pediatric and Adult Congenital Treatment National Cardiovascular Data Registry (IMPACT-NCDR), Congenital Cardiovascular Interventional Study Consortium (CCISC), Congenital Cardiac Catheterization Project on Outcomes (C3PO)—are expected to help standardize indications for the procedure, techniques of intervention, and follow-up and to better assess safety and efficacy of catheter-based and surgical therapies.[119,120]

RECOMMENDATIONS

We recommend balloon-assisted stent implantation, or balloon dilation alone, as an effective alternative therapy for all adults with native or recurrent CoA and a 20 mm Hg or higher gradient or a 20 mm Hg or lower gradient with decreased LV function or symptoms of LV failure, coronary ischemia, or lower extremity claudication. Definition of indications and techniques for catheter-based and surgical intervention based on natural outcomes in a modern era, coupled with standardized long-term follow-up, is eagerly awaited. We consider long-term annual interviews and examinations essential, along with noninvasive imaging at least every 3 to 5 years to assess systemic arterial and LV sequelae after CoA repair.

Optimal management of the patient with aortic CoA with associated aortic dilation remains undefined.

Tetralogy of Fallot

Tetralogy of Fallot (TOF) is the most common cyanotic congenital lesion with patient survival into adulthood, with approximately 2000 affected individuals reaching adulthood with TOF each year in the United States. Based on a modern understanding of TOF, this lesion appears to be more appropriately classified as a monology, a condition caused by a single, unifying abnormality, namely hypoplasia and displacement of the conal, or infundibular, septum. This anterior and superior displacement results in obstruction of the RV outflow tract (pulmonary stenosis) with resultant RV hypertrophy, leaving behind a VSD in the conal septum (Figure 42-7). The aortic annulus is intimately opposed to the conal septum, and displacement of one leads to opposing displacement of the other; in effect, posterior-inferior displacement of the aortic annulus takes a position overriding the ventricular septum.

The degree of hypoplasia and septal malalignment determines the severity of encroachment into the RVOT—although this is always associated with a large conoventricular VSD—with clinical presentations that include 1) minimal RVOT obstruction ("pink" TOF), with predominant left-to-right shunting; 2) moderate RVOT obstruction (most common), with bidirectional shunting and cyanosis; 3) and severe forms of RVOT obstruction (pulmonary atresia), in which cyanosis is obligatory, and pulmonary artery flow arises from persistent, primitive aorta–pulmonary artery collaterals.

In patients with TOF or pulmonary atresia, aorta–pulmonary artery collateral vessels make up many or all of the various subdivisions of the lung vascular tree, ranging from the main or central pulmonary arteries, which may be absent, to individual or multiple proximal branch pulmonary arteries to subsegments of lung vasculature. These collaterals frequently have failed involution, retain stenoses and abnormal vascular walls, and may undersupply or oversupply particular lung segments.

Although TOF is typically diagnosed and repaired in childhood, presentation during adult years can occur in patients who have previously undergone palliative operations and in those who have not. In the past, prior to development of a successful complete repair strategy, patients were managed with systemic–pulmonary arterial shunts (central Waterston, Potts, and classic or modified Blalock-Taussig shunts; see Table 42-1). Residual postoperative shunt complications include pulmonary artery distortion, pulmonary vascular disease, hypertension, and peripheral pulmonary artery stenoses. Complete repair of TOF includes obliteration of any preexisting shunts, elimination of RV outflow obstruction (with or without transpulmonary annular incision and patching), and VSD closure. Additional residual postoperative lesions may include residual VSD, RV outflow obstruction, and PR.

Data regarding long-term follow-up of repaired TOF reveal excellent long-term survival after the initial operative period, with a 32-year survival rate of 86% compared with 96% in a control-matched population. Repaired TOF appears most favorable when the VSD is closed, RVOT obstruction is almost completely relieved, and severe PR and RV dysfunction are not present.[121] More recent multicenter data have suggested a 35-year survival rate greater than 90%.[122] Although the majority of patients have excellent functional capacity, some patients have exercise limitation, RV or LV failure (Table 42-2), RVOT obstruction or aneurysms (<29%), or arrhythmia (<33%) experience sudden death (1% to 3%).[123] Although promising, most recent data on the impact of surgical repair of tetralogy on neonates and young infants are insufficient to assess long-term outcomes.[124,125]

Implicated risk factors for death after TOF repair have most commonly been sought as risks for sudden cardiac death (SCD), with little discrimination between worsened functional status and cardiac muscle dysfunction leading to premature death versus presumed arrhythmic death. These risks have been mostly defined in single-center cohort studies, and the most recent and robust data include multicenter combined assessments.[122,126,127] Of note, most series have not considered immediate surgical risk in such assessments (see below) and have excluded either immediate or first-year nonsurvivors, who frequently comprise a substantial population—up to 10% to 30% in some series.[121,128] Single-center cohorts have continued to suggest older age at repair, prior presence or absence of palliative shunts, radiographic/cardiothoracic ratio, presence of RVOT patch, increased RV systolic pressure, and LV dysfunction as markers for poor outcome in addition to pure electrical markers. Multicenter trials have emphasized older age at repair, presence of PR,[122] older patient age, presence of prior palliative surgery, and increased radiographic/cardiothoracic ratio as independent risk factors for poor outcome[124] in addition to specific additional markers of electrical instability and LV dysfunction.[127]

Increasing time from surgery, in and of itself, has been postulated as changing the risk of death after TOF repair, with recent single-center cohort data that confirm risk of sudden death increasing from 1.2%, 2.2%, 4%, and 6% at 10, 20, 25, and 35 years after operative repair, respectively, with mortality risk of 0.27% per year until 25 years after surgical correction and 0.94% per year thereafter.[128]

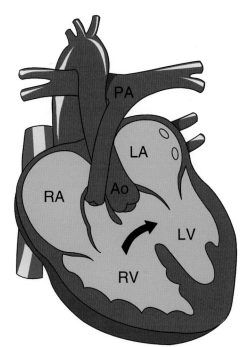

FIGURE 42-7 Tetralogy of Fallot. Ao, aorta; LA, left atrium; LV, left ventricle; PA, pulmonary artery; RA, right atrium; RV, right ventricle.

TABLE 42-2	Causes of Ventricular Failure Following Surgical Repair of Tetralogy of Fallot	
LEFT HEART FAILURE	**RIGHT HEART FAILURE**

• Residual aorta–pulmonary artery
  Shunt
  Collateral
• Residual ventral septal defect
  Patch margin
  Native
• Aortic insufficiency
• Arrhythmias
• Coronary artery
  Anomaly
  Ligation
• Myocardial preservation
	• Right ventricle outflow obstruction
	  Valvular
	  Supravalvular or peripheral PS
	  Pulmonary vascular disease
	• Pulmonary regurgitation
	• Tricuspid regurgitation
	• Atrial septal defect
	• Arrhythmias
	• Left heart failure
	• Myocardial preservation

PS, pulmonary stenosis.

Risks for worsened functional capacity after surgical repair of TOF have been recently studied using NYHA functional status, with its subjective limitations, as a standard of functional ability. RVOT patch repair and transannular patch repair had a similar risk for worsened functional ability and cardiac death in single-center cohort assessment. More recent single-center cohort studies using MRI measures of RV and LV function suggest older age at repair as well as lower LV ejection fraction (LVEF) and RV ejection fraction (RVEF), which correlate with each other, as markers for worsened clinical status by NYHA functional class[129]; this confirms older reports of the import of LV function in patients with TOF.[130-132] Of note, in this single-center study,[133] PR fraction and RV diastolic dimensions did not independently correlate with functional status. Similar recent findings that raised questions regarding the negative predictive potential of PR fraction include additional single-center cohorts and a surgical RCT that emphasized presence of RVOT aneurysm or akinesia, increased RV dimensions and decreased RVEF by MRI, and increased electrocardiographic QRS duration as independent risks for worsened functional ability, decreased RV function at baseline, and lack of RV functional improvement after surgical PV replacement for PR in adults with TOF.[134-140]

Atrial arrhythmias that include sinus node dysfunction, atrial flutter, and atrial fibrillation have been noted in up to 20% to 30% of repaired patients and correlate with the presence of old scar, numbers of prior surgeries, systemic arterial hypertension, atrial enlargement, or hemodynamic abnormalities consistent with ventricular dysfunction.[141] Acute intervention is frequently recommended, especially with associated ventricular or atrial dysfunction. Control of frequently recurring or incessant atrial flutter may be equally effective with radiofrequency ablation compared with the most effective medical therapy, and strategies are frequently combined. Late-onset complete heart block has been diagnosed with an incidence of 4% after a mean follow-up of 20 years. The strongest risk factor for the development of complete heart block is the presence of perioperative complete heart block at the time of surgical repair.

Although pulmonary valve replacement has been proposed as a treatment option for symptomatic patients, several investigators have noted that placing a pulmonary valve in patients with severe RV dilation and dysfunction may not lead to adequate functional recovery of the RV.[139] These observations have led several centers to advocate pulmonary valve replacement before the onset of symptoms in order to preserve RV mechanics; however, uncertainty persists regarding the optimal timing of intervention. Recent investigation suggests that although PR is the primary source of chronic RV volume overload in these patients and correlates closely with RV size, major adverse clinical outcomes in adults with TOF and PR that include death, high-grade ventricular arrhythmia, and heart failure relate primarily to the effects of PR on the RV myocardium: dilation and dysfunction as measured by end-systolic and diastolic volume Z scores and increasing myocardial fibrosis.[137-140,142] Until these predictors are optimally defined, we currently recommend monitoring all patients with TOF and PR with serial MRI to assess for RV forward and regurgitant volumes, ventricular function and scarring, and presence of additional anatomic abnormalities. This should be combined with assessment of functional capacity (cardiopulmonary exercise testing) and ECG and rhythm parameters to assist in the accumulation of sufficient potential predictive data.

Investigational valves, such as the Edwards Sapien transcatheter heart valve (Edwards Lifesciences, Irvine, CA), and FDA-approved percutaneous pulmonary valves, such as the Melody transcatheter pulmonary valve (Medtronic, Minneapolis, MN), have recently been developed. The Melody system uses bioprosthetic valve leaflets (bovine jugular vein) mounted on a balloon-expandable Cheatham platinum-iridium stent delivered via a 22-Fr system using a 22 × 4 cm balloon-in-balloon delivery sheath.[143,144] The Edwards Sapien transcatheter heart valve uses three wire pericardial leaflets sewn inside a 14-mm-long stainless steel stent, with two thirds of the stent covered with a fabric cuff delivered via a 24- to 26-Fr

sheath, available in diameters of 23 to 26 mm and expanded on a 23 × 3 cm or 26 × 3 cm high-pressure balloon.

To date, trials of transcatheter pulmonary valve placement have been most extensive with the Melody valve (Medtronic), demonstrating high rates of procedural success in expert centers with encouraging short-term valve function and improvement in indexes of RV and LV function and patient functional ability. Longer term follow-up is expected to better elucidate risks and benefits of this technique as it becomes more widely applied in CHD. Current humanitarian use approval for Melody valve implantation is limited to placement within regurgitant tube conduits with relatively definable diameters. Compassionate use extrapolation of this technique to larger and less definable outflow positions, as well as to use on the left side of the heart, has been limited but encouraging.

After surgical repair of TOF, patients may have up to a 25% incidence of recurrence or residual obstruction at any level of the RV outflow. In adults, use of balloon dilation and balloon-assisted stent implantation as primary therapy for native and postoperative narrowings in the RVOT, with or without conduit/homograft placement, and in the proximal and distal pulmonary vasculature has success rates similar to those observed in children. Pulmonary artery and RVOT dilations are the most commonly performed interventional procedures in our catheterization laboratory (Figure 42-8). A strategy combining dilations with low- or high-pressure balloons may achieve up to 75% procedural success in relief of obstruction in peripheral pulmonary arteries, defined as an increase of 50% or more in predilation vessel diameter, an increase of more than 20% of flow to the affected lung, or a decrease of more than 20% in systolic RV/aortic pressure ratio.[145] Dilation of

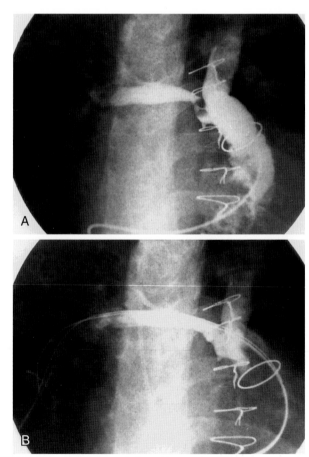

FIGURE 42-8 High-pressure balloon dilation of postoperative proximal right pulmonary artery stenosis (**A**) leads to elimination of gradient, increased angiographic vessel caliber (**B**), and resolution of flow imbalance by nuclear lung scintigraphy.

vessels that exhibit kinking or significant recoil (proximal branch pulmonary arteries) can be improved with placement of intraluminal stents, with a greater than 90% initial procedural success rate.[146] Stent implantation within stenotic valved homografts or conduits must be tempered by the potential for an increase in pulmonary valvular insufficiency. Complications of conduit or vessel rupture, aneurysm formation, or development of high-flow reperfusion edema may occur and have been infrequently correlated (<1% incidence each) with oversizing balloons, especially in calcified conduits or homografts, and postprocedural mean pulmonary artery pressures of 40 mm Hg or more. Balloon dilation or stent implantation remains the procedure of choice for such patients when additional surgery is not required and when obstruction is at the level of the pulmonary trunk or beyond.

We have extended these dilation techniques to adult patients with either isolated peripheral pulmonary artery stenoses or acquired chronic distal thromboembolic pulmonary hypertension (Figure 42-9).[147] Most patients were profoundly debilitated and were referred for evaluation for lung transplantation. The most frequently encountered complication was early development of transient reperfusion pulmonary edema in segments of lung with restored pulmonary blood flow after dilation. After 3 to 4 years of follow-up, survivors show improvement in exercise tolerance.

Embolization coils, vascular occlusion devices, and covered stents have been used in adults with TOF to eliminate residual central aorta shunts or systemic artery–pulmonary artery shunts and duplicate aorta–pulmonary artery collateral vessels.

RECOMMENDATIONS

The adult with repaired TOF faces excellent chances of prolonged survival. Long-term risks include development of 1) RV central or peripheral outflow obstruction; 2) PR; 3) RV dilation and scarring; 4) residual shunting at the septal, aorta–pulmonary shunt, or collateral level; 5) conduction disease with potential heart block; 6) atrial arrhythmias; 7) ventricular arrhythmias; and 8) sudden death. Patients should undergo annual interview and physical examination, pulse oximetry and ECG, and periodic exercise testing with measurement of gas-exchange parameters. We recommend 24-hour ambulatory ECG monitoring every 2 to 3 years and either echocardiography or MRI every 3 to 5 years, and even more frequently if anatomic, arrhythmic, or functional abnormality is documented. Increasing QRS duration, decreasing functional ability, increasing end-systolic and end-diastolic RV volumes, and decreasing RV and LV ejection fractions by MRI and echocardiography all appear to elevate the risk of cardiovascular morbidity and mortality, and they prompt intervention as feasible. We consider balloon dilation or stent implantation to be the procedures of choice for relief of outflow obstruction, and transcatheter embolization is the procedure of choice for elimination of residual shunting and extraneous vessels when additional surgery is not required. The role of percutaneous pulmonary valve implantation, compared with surgical valve replacement and RV remodeling, remains undefined, but results are encouraging and expectations are high in appropriate centers of expertise. Although electrophysiologic study (EPS) may highlight populations at highest risk for SCD, widespread application of EPS to the total adult TOF population remains impractical given the relatively low overall SCD rate. Use of risk scales derived from both clinical experience and multicenter study is suggested to assist in determination of appropriate use of implantable cardioverter-defibrillator (ICD) therapy as primary and secondary prevention in this population.

Patent Ductus Arteriosus

The ductus arteriosus connects the descending aorta and the junction of the main and left pulmonary arteries. It remains patent in approximately 0.07% of live births, which represents 5% to 10% of all cases of CHD. Anatomically, the ductus varies in size and shape and may be calcified or aneurysmal. Difference in relative vascular resistance and physical restriction of the ductus determine the degree and nature of intravascular shunting, but it is typically left-to-right (Figure 42-10). A patent ductus arteriosus in adults usually is asymptomatic, although it may produce symptoms caused by increased volume load on the LV. The diagnosis should be suspected in the setting of a continuous murmur at the left upper sternal-subclavicular border. Intervention to close a patent ductus ateriosus (PDA) is suggested when the shunt is suspected to be substantial and LV enlargement or dysfunction is otherwise unexplained.[7]

Endocarditis remains a constant risk (0.5% to 1.0% per year), although this is debated in the modern antibiotic SBE prophylaxis era. The risk of developing LV dysfunction increases with age, and although operative closure in infancy is both safe and relatively straightforward, surgical repair requires general anesthesia, thoracotomy, and postoperative recuperation. In adults, surgical closure may be more complicated because of anatomic features of the patent ductus that include calcification, friability, and aneurysmal dilation and because of increased incidence of multiple organ system comorbidity.

A transarterial transcatheter device approach to PDA closure was devised by Portsman and colleagues.[148] Today, the most common devices used for transcatheter PDA occlusion are the

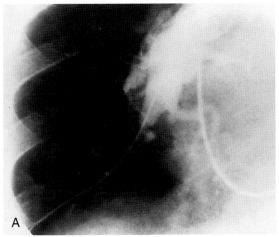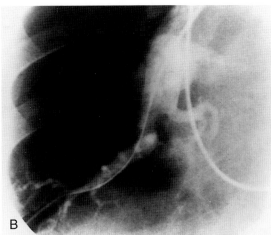

FIGURE 42-9 Right lower lobe segmental vessel before (**A**) and after (**B**) 7 mm balloon dilation. Mean central pulmonary artery pressure fell from 60 mm Hg to 40 mm Hg. Reperfusion pulmonary edema was recognized 15 minutes after dilation.

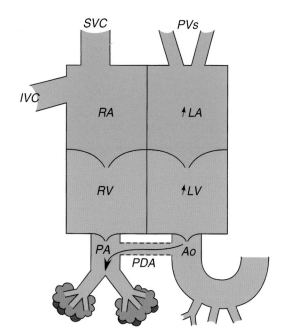

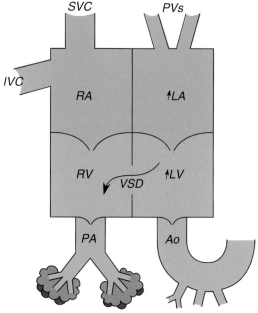

FIGURE 42-10 *Patent ductus arteriosus (PDA) physiology.* Intravascular shunting is governed by relative resistance of pulmonary versus systemic arterial bed. Unless pulmonary vascular disease exists, flow is left to right with enlargement of left-sided chambers. Ao, aorta; IVC, inferior vena cava; LA, left atrium; LV, left ventricle; PA, pulmonary artery; RA, right atrium; RV, right ventricle; SVC, superior vena cava.

FIGURE 42-11 *Ventral septal defect (VSD) physiology.* Intracardiac shunting is governed by relative resistance to ventricular contraction and less so by ventricular filling. Unless right ventricular function is significantly compromised or severe pulmonary hypertension or vascular disease exists, flow is left to right with enlargement of left-sided chambers. Ao, aorta; IVC, inferior vena cava; LA, left atrium; LV, left ventricle; PA, pulmonary artery; RA, right atrium; RV, right ventricle; SVC, superior vena cava.

Amplatzer PDA Occluder device (St. Jude Medical, Plymouth, MN) and embolization coils, with nearly universal success at closure of PDA with one device or another.[149] The low cost and ease and effectiveness of occlusion make the embolization coils the ideal device for closure of PDAs.[150-153] We tend to use coils (single vs. multiple, standard, controlled delivery, or shaped) for PDAs with a minimal diameter less than 2 to 3 mm, and we use Amplatzer PDA Occluders for those with a minimal diameter of 3 mm or more.

In our clinical service, we close audible PDAs with concomitant LV enlargement or dysfunction via a transcatheter approach, and patients do not leave the catheterization laboratory with evidence of residual ductal flow. After device closure, bacterial endocarditis precautions are maintained for 6 months.

RECOMMENDATIONS

Despite unclear risks of bacterial endocarditis in the current antimicrobial era, we recommend transcatheter PDA occlusion with either coil embolization (PDA <3 mm diameter) or Amplatzer PDA Occluders (≥3 mm diameter) for adults with audible PDA associated with LV dysfunction or enlargement.

Ventricular Septal Defects

Isolated VSDs are the most common congenital defect seen in childhood but are much less frequently encountered in adult life as a result of either spontaneous or surgical closure during infancy or childhood. Anatomic classification is based on septal location and includes perimembranous, subpulmonary, AV canal-type, and muscular VSDs. Nature and degree of intracardiac shunting depend on the relative pressure difference, ventricular chamber compliance and capacitance, and anatomic restriction of the VSD (Figure 42-11). VSD closure is recommended for relief of symptoms such as dyspnea and exercise incapacity when accompanied by excessive pulmonary blood flow, typically with pulmonary/systemic blood flow ratio greater than 1.5 to 2.0 and with LV volume loading

in the absence of excessive pulmonary vascular resistance, typically less than 7 to 8 Wood units/m^2 or 280 to 430 dynes/sec/cm^{-5} without reactivity to pulmonary vasodilators. We also consider closing VSDs with a pulmonary/systemic flow ratio below 1.5 to 2 if LV failure is present. Spontaneous closure of tiny to small defects has been reported even into adulthood, and we recommend that adults with persistent nonhemodynamically significant VSDs have an interview and physical examination every 2 years, with echocardiography every 3 years to screen for development of aortic regurgitation, arrhythmia, and potential for SBE. Excessive flow or excessive pressure entering the pulmonary vasculature may contribute as an additional trigger to the development of pulmonary vascular hypertension and potential for shunt reversal, cyanosis, and the sequelae of Eisenmenger disease.

We have applied transcatheter closure techniques for the treatment of congenital, postoperative residual, and acquired VSDs using FDA-approved double-umbrella devices in an attempt to eliminate the need for, or to reduce the risk and complexity of, surgical repair.[81,154,155] To date, the majority of closures have been in patients with muscular VSDs anatomically distant from the aortic valve, rather than the commonly encountered congenital perimembranous VSD, or in those with post–myocardial infarction (MI) ventricular septal rupture.

Transcatheter closure technique requires significant operator experience to reduce procedural morbidity and is one of the most technically demanding of interventional catheter procedures performed in our laboratory (Figure 42-12). A guidewire is typically placed from a transeptal approach into the left atrium and ventricle and across the VSD, and occasionally a retrograde arterial approach is used, especially in patients with TOF with postoperative residual patch margin defects. The left-to-right ventricular approach facilitates subsequent passage of a balloon flotation catheter through the widest portion of the defect; the guidewire is snared and delivered from either the contralateral femoral vein or a jugular vein, depending on the location of the defect. Balloon stretch sizing of the central portion of the defect may

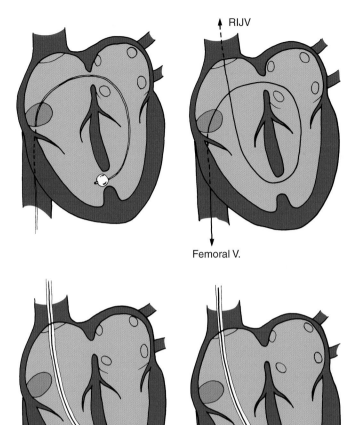

FIGURE 42-12 Transcatheter technique of ventral septal defect closure. RIJV, right internal jugular vein; V., vein.

be compounded by the location of the VSR, the presence of RV or LV dysfunction, multiple organ system failure, medical comorbidities, or prior incomplete surgical attempt at repair. Since February 1990, we have used double-umbrella closure devices—most recently cardioSEAL and cardioSEAL-STARFlex devices, but only the cardioSEAL is approved for limited indications—in attempts to limit VSR after MI. Primary acute VSR typically forms a serpiginous tract with a wide (18 to 21 mm) necrotic "lake" within the septum. More mature defects and postoperative patch margin dehiscence defects ranged from 8 to 25 mm by maximal balloon stretching (Figure 42-13). To date, we have not encountered a defect that was not anatomically or procedurally amenable to device implantation, although success widely varies with technique and devices used. To date, single-center experience with transcatheter closure of post-MI VSR closure remains anecdotal but encouraging. We expect future trials of a more aggressive combined transcatheter-surgical strategy with larger devices and an intense medical-surgical collaboration in an attempt to offer prolonged improvement in patients deemed to be at extreme surgical risk.

Perimembranous Ventral Septal Defect Closure

The use of specifically designed investigational AGA Amplatzer membranous devices in the closure of perimembranous VSDs has been reported in single-center and multicenter studies. Experience is limited, and indications for use are unclear; in addition, adversity is still not fully defined, with particular concern regarding development of complete heart block and semilunar or atrioventricular valve regurgitation. Because of this, further study is required.[157,158]

RECOMMENDATIONS

Transcatheter device closure of native or postoperative residual VSDs anatomically distant from the aortic valve, particularly using double-umbrella cardioSEAL devices, has reduced the need for operation as well as operative morbidity in many patients with complex defects. At present, until larger devices are available, closure of a VSR after MI appears most successful when orchestrated by a combined surgical-medical team using a strategy of expeditious primary surgical repair followed by transcatheter device closure of a residual defect as required. Because of the technical demands of these procedures, transcatheter device closure of VSDs and post-MI VSR remains limited to a few centers.

Postoperative Residual Defects, Collaterals, and Fenestrations

Embolization coils and occlusion devices have been used in adults and children at high or prohibitive surgical risk to successfully eliminate 1) residual central aorta or systemic artery–pulmonary artery shunts or collaterals, 2) systemic venous–pulmonary artery or pulmonary–venous shunts or collaterals, 3) interatrial baffle communications or iatrogenic Fontan fenestrations, 4) left superior or inferior vena caval connections to the left atrium, 5) coronary artery fistulas,[159] 6) systemic and pulmonary arteriovenous malformations, and 7) paravalvular leaks (Figure 42-14).

Increasing recognition of cross-dependency between events and interventions in youth and later in life has led to greater collaboration in management, investigation, and registry of outcomes between caregivers for patients of all ages with CHD. This change in milieu has led to a new and successful age of innovation that couples physiology, pathology, and both medical and mechanical interventions with more extensive application of outcomes and quality assessment. As CHD care for the adult emerges as its own certified and credentialed medical subspecialty, such practice is both necessary and welcomed by all involved in the care of such patients.

facilitate choosing device size. A curved guiding sheath follows the guidewire through the right or left side of the heart across the central channel of the defect, and a device system is delivered in a fashion similar to the technique described for ASD closure. The guiding sheath frequently traverses the intraventricular septum at an acute angle, making fluoroscopic confirmation of arm positioning difficult during deployment. The use of TEE greatly assists in appropriate placement of the arms of the device and aids in successful closure of the defect.

Reviews of procedural, short-, and intermediate-term outcomes of transcatheter muscular VSD closure have been most rigorously reported with double-umbrella devices in 170 highly complex and highest risk patients, with predefined assessment of adversity and outcomes scales.[156] Procedural success was high, with successful implantation in 99% of patients and accompanying marked improvement in clinical severity scale. Potential for device-related adversity was considerable and occurred in 20% of patients, and similar patients and families should be appropriately counseled.

Post–Myocardial Infarction Ventricular Septal Rupture

Although surgical advances have dramatically improved the short- and intermediate-term survival of adults with ventricular septal rupture (VSR) after MI, operative risk remains substantial and may

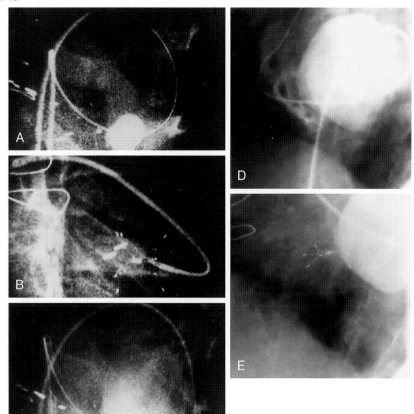

FIGURE 42-13 Balloon stretch sizing (**A**) of the central necrotic portion of a postoperative residual patch margin defect after primary surgical repair of ventricular septal rupture (VSR) after myocardial infarction (MI) in a patient requiring mechanical inotropic support. Transseptal deployment of a clamshell occluder (**B**) leads to modest acute decrease in angiographic shunt (**C**), but patient markedly improves to New York Hospital Association class II symptoms. Shunt flow (**D**) can be totally eliminated (**E**) in some patients with postoperative residual shunting after VSR after MI.

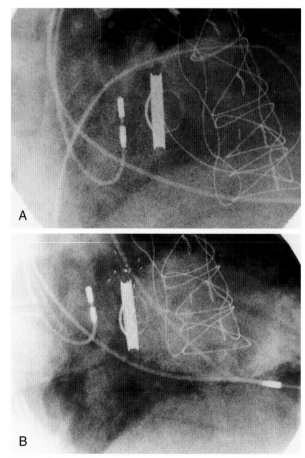

FIGURE 42-14 **A,** Paravalvular mitral regurgitation results in left atrial hypertension and dyspnea. **B,** It is eliminated after placement of an occlusion device, with resolution of symptoms.

REFERENCES

1. Marelli AJ, Mackie AS, Ionescu-Ittu R, Rahme E, Pilote L. Congenital heart disease in the general population: changing prevalence and age distribution. *Circulation* 2007;115:163-172.
2. Warnes CA, Liberthson R, Danielson GK, et al. Task force 1: the changing profile of congenital heart disease in adult life. *J Am Coll Cardiol* 2001;37:1170-1175.
3. Gatzoulis, MA, Hechter, S, Siu SC, et al. Outpatient clinics for adults with congenital heart disease: increasing workload and evolving patterns of referral. *Heart* 1999;81:57.
4. Mackie AS, Ionescu-Ittu R, Pilote L, Rahme E, Marelli AJ. Hospital readmissions in children with congenital heart disease: a population-based study. *Am Heart J* 2008;155:577-584.
5. Gurvitz MZ, Inkelas M, Lee M, et al. Changes in hospitalization patterns among patients with congenital heart disease during the transition from adolescence to adulthood. *J Am Coll Cardiol* 2007;49:875-882.
6. Landzberg MJ, Murphy DJ Jr, Davidson WR, et al. Task force 4: organization of delivery systems of adults with congenital heart disease. *J Am Coll Cardiol* 2001;37:1187-1193.
7. Warnes CA, Williams RG, Bashore TM, et al. ACC/AHA 2008 Guidelines for the Management of Adults with Congenital Heart Disease: a report of the American College of Cardiology/American Heart Association Task Force on Practice Guidelines (writing committee to develop guidelines on the management of adults with congenital heart disease). *Circulation* 2008;118:e714-e833.
8. Morris CD, Reller MD, Menashe VD. Thirty-year incidence of infective endocarditis after surgery for congenital heart defect. *JAMA* 1998;279:599.
9. Durack DT, Lukes AS, Bright DK. New criteria for diagnosis of infective endocarditis: utilization of specific echocardiographic findings. Duke Endocarditis Service. *Am J Med* 1994;96:200.
10. Bayer AS, Bolger AF, Taubert KA, et al. Diagnosis and management of infective endocarditis and its complications. *Circulation* 1998;98:2936.
11. Wilson WR, Karchmer AW, Dajani AS, et al. Antibiotic treatment of adults with infective endocarditis due to streptococci, enterococci, staphylococci and HACEK microorganisms. American Heart Association. *JAMA* 1995;274:1706.
12. Thilen U, Astrom-Olsson K. Does the risk of infective endarteritis justify routine patent ductus arteriosus closure? *Eur Heart J* 1997;18:503.
13. Hoffman JI, Rudolph AM, Heymann MA. Pulmonary vascular disease with congenital heart lesions: pathologic features and causes. *Circulation* 1981;64:878.
14. Wood P. The Eisenmenger syndrome. *Br Med J* 1958;2:701, 755.
15. Pineda CJ, Guerra J, Weisman MH, et al. The skeletal manifestations of clubbing: a study in patients with cyanotic congenital heart disease and hypertrophic osteoarthropathy. *Semin Arth Rheum* 1985;4:263.
16. Rosove MH, Perloff JK, Hocking WG, et al. Chronic hypoxaemia and decompensated erythrocytosis in cyanotic congenital heart disease. *Lancet* 1986;2:313.
17. Lindercamp O, Klose HJ, Betke K, et al. Increased blood viscosity in patients with cyanotic congenital heart disease and iron deficiency. *J Pediatrics* 1979;95:567.
18. Perloff JK, Rosove MH, Child JS, et al. Adults with cyanotic congenital heart disease: hematologic management. *Ann Intern Med* 1988;109:406.
19. Broberg CS, Bax BE, Okonko DO, et al. Blood viscosity and its relationship to iron deficiency, symptoms, and exercise capacity in adults with cyanotic congenital heart disease. *J Am Coll Cardiol* 2006;48:356-365.
20. Tay EL, Peset A, Papaphylactou M, et al. Replacement therapy for iron deficiency improves exercise capacity and quality of life in patients with cyanotic congenital heart disease and/or the Eisenmenger syndrome. *Int J Cardiol* 2011;151:307-312.
21. Flanagan MF, Hourihan M, Keane JF. Incidence of renal dysfunction in adults with cyanotic congenital heart disease. *Am J Cardiol* 1991;68:403.
22. Graham TP. Ventricular performance in adults after operation for congenital heart disease. *Am J Cardiol* 1991;68:403.
23. Driscoll DJ, Staats BA, Heise CT, et al. Functional single ventricle: cardiorespiratory response to exercise. *J Am Coll Cardiol* 1984;4:337.
24. Diller GP, Dimopoulos K, Okonko D, et al. Exercise intolerance in adult congenital heart disase: comparative severity, correlates, and prognostic implication. *Circulation* 2005;112:828-835.
25. Ammash N, Warnes CA. Cerebrovascular events in adult patients with cyanotic congenital heart disease. *J Am Coll Cardiol* 1991;28:768.
26. Aram DM, Ekelman BL, Ben-Shachar G, et al. Intelligence and hypoxemia in children with congenital heart disease: fact or artifact. *J Am Coll Cardiol* 1985;6:889.
27. Galiè N, Beghetti M, Gatzoulis MA, et al.; Bosentan Randomized Trial of Endothelin Antagonist Therapy-5 (BREATHE-5) Investigators. Bosentan therapy in patients with Eisenmenger syndrome: a multicenter, double-blind, randomized, placebo-controlled study. *Circulation* 2006;114(1):48-54.
28. Bowyer JJ, Busst CM, Denison DM, et al. Effect of long term oxygen treatment at home in children with pulmonary vascular disease. *Br Heart J* 1986;55:385.
29. Rosenzweig EB, Kerstein D, Barst RJ. Long-term prostacyclin for pulmonary hypertension with associated congenital heart defects. *Circulation* 1999;99:1858.
30. McLaughlin VV, Genthner De, Panell MM, et al. Compassionate use of continuous prostacyclin in the management of secondary pulmonary hypertension: a case series. *Ann Intern Med* 1999;130:740.
31. Fernandes S, Lang P, Benisty J, et al. Prostacyclin therapy in the adolescent/adult with Eisenmenger syndrome. *Circulation* 1999;100:I-670.
32. Benisty J, Graydon-Baker E, Fernandes S, Pearson D, Landzberg M. Domiciliary inhaled nitric oxide therapy for secondary pulmonary hypertension. *Circulation* 1999;100:I-240-241.
33. Galiè N, Beghetti M, Gatzoulis MA, et al. Bosentan therapy in patients with Eisenmenger syndrome: a multicenter, double-blind, randomized, placebo-controlled study. *Circulation* 2006;114:48-54.
34. Dimopoulos K, Inuzuka R, Goletto S, et al. Improved survival among patients with Eisenmenger syndrome receiving advanced therapy for pulmonary arterial hypertension. *Circulation* 2010;121:20-25.
35. Landzberg MJ, Morrison BJ, Pass RH, et al. Angiotensin converting enzyme inhibition in adults with cyanotic congenital heart disease. *J Am Coll Cardiol* 1995;377A.
36. Harinck E, Hutter PA, Hoorntje TM, et al. Air travel and adults with cyanotic congenital heart disease. *Circulation* 1996;93:272.
37. Broberg CS, Uebing A, Cuomo L, et al. Adult patients with Eisenmenger syndrome report flying safely on commercial airlines. *Heart* 2007;93:1599-1603.
38. Connolly HM, Grogan M, Warnes CA. Pregnancy among women with congenitally corrected transposition of great arteries. *J Am Coll Cardiol* 1999;33:1692.
39. Connolly HM, Warnes CA. Ebstein's anomaly: outcome of pregnancy. *J Am Coll Cardiol* 1994;23:1194.
40. Tobler D, Fernandes SM, Wald RM, et al. Pregnancy outcomes in women with transposition of the great arteries and arterial switch operation. *Am J Cardiol* 2010;106:417-420.
41. Siu SC, Sermer M, Harrison DA, et al. Risk and predictors for pregnancy-related complications in women with heart disease. *Circulation* 1997;96:2789.
42. Khairy P, Ouyang DW, Fernandes SM, et al. Pregnancy outcomes in women with congenital heart disease. *Circulation* 2006;113:517-524.
43. Drenthen W, Boersma E, Balci A, et al. Predictors of pregnancy complications in women with congenital heart disease. *Eur Heart J* 2010;31:2124-2132.
44. Presbitero P, Somerville J, Stone S, et al. Pregnancy in cyanotic congenital heart disease. *Circulation* 1994;89:2673.
45. Bédard E, Dimopoulos K, Gatzoulis MA. Has there been any progress made on pregnancy outcomes among women with pulmonary arterial hypertension? *Eur Heart J* 2009;30:256-265.
46. Lui GK, Silversides CK, Khairy P, et al. Heart rate response during exercise and pregnancy outcome in women with congenital heart disease. *Circulation* 2011;123:242-248.
47. Warner MA, Lunn RJ, O'Leary PW, et al. Outcomes of noncardiac surgical procedures in children and adults with congenital heart disease. Mayo Perioperative Outcomes Group. *Mayo Clin Proc* 1998;73:728.
48. Ammash, NM, Connolly, HM, Abel, MD, et al. Noncardiac surgery in Eisenmenger syndrome. *J Am Coll Cardiol* 1999;33:2222.
49. Laishley RS, Burrows FA, Lerman J, Roy WL. Effect of anesthetic induction regimens on oxygen saturation in cyanotic congenital heart disease. *Anesthesiology* 1986;65:673-677.
50. Baum VC, Perloff JK. Anesthetic implications of adults with congenital heart disease. *Anesth Analg* 1993;76:1342-1358.
51. Walsh EP, Cecchin F. Arrhythmias in adult patients with congenital heart disease. *Circulation* 2007;115:534-545.
52. Alexander ME, Walsh EP, Saul JP, et al. Value of programmed ventricular stimulation in patients with congenital heart disease. *J Cardiovasc Electrophysiol* 1999;10:1033.
53. Triedman JK, Bergau DM, Saul JP, et al. Efficacy of radiofrequency ablation for control of intraatrial reentrant tachycardia in patients with congenital heart disease. *J Am Coll Cardiol* 1997;30:1032.
54. Theodoro DA, Danielson GK, Porter CJ, et al. Right-sided maze procedure for right atrial arrhythmias in congenital heart disease. *Ann Thorac Surg* 1998;65:149.
55. Swan L, Hillis WS. Exercise prescription in adults with congenital heart disease: a long way to go. *Heart* 2000;83:685.
56. Giardini A, Specchia S, Berton E, et al. Strong and independent prognostic value of peak circulatory power in adults with congenital heart disease. *Am Heart J* 2007;154:441-447.
57. Dimopoulos K, Okonko DO, Diller GP, et al. Abnormal ventilatory response to exercise in adults with congenital heart disease relates to cyanosis and predicts survival. *Circulation* 2006;113:2796-2802.
58. Giardini A, Hager A, Pace Napoleone C, Picchio FM. Natural history of exercise capacity after the Fontan operation: a longitudinal study. *Ann Thorac Surg* 2008;85:818-821.
59. Fernandes SM, McElhinney DB, Khairy P, et al. Serial cardiopulmonary exercise testing in patients with previous Fontan surgery. *Pediatr Cardiol* 2010;31:175-180.
60. O'Connor CM, Whellan DJ, Lee KL. Efficacy and safety of exercise training in patients with chronic heart failure: HF-ACTION randomized controlled trial. *JAMA* 2009;301:1439-1450.
61. Dracup K, Baker DW, Dunbar SB, et al. Management of heart failure II: Counseling, education and lifestyle modifications. *JAMA* 272;272:1442.
62. Longmuir PE, Tremblay MS, Goode RC. Postoperative exercise training develops normal levels of physical activity in a group of children following cardiac surgery. *Pediatr Cardiol* 1990;11:126.
63. Ruttenberg HD, Adams TD, Orsmond GS, et al. Effects of exercise training on aerobic fitness in children after open heart surgery. *Pediatr Cardiol* 1983;4:19.
64. Graham TP, Bricker JT, James FW, et al. Task Force 1: congenital heart disease. *J Am Coll Cardiol* 1994;24:845.
65. Davies RR, Russo MJ, Yang J, et al. Listing and transplanting adults with congenital heart disease. *Circulation* 2011;123:759-767.
66. McGlothlin D, De Marco T. Transplantation in adults with congenital heart disease. *Prog Cardiovasc Dis* 2011;53:312-323.
67. Everitt MD, Donaldson AE, Stehlik J, et al. Would access to device therapies improve transplant outcomes for adults with congenital heart disease? Analysis of the United Network for Organ Sharing (UNOS). *J Heart Lung Transplant* 2011;30:395-401.
68. Webb G, Gatzoulis MA. Atrial septal defects in the adult: recent progress and overview. *Circulation* 2006;114:1645-1653.
69. Feltdt RH, Co-Burn JP, Edwards SD, et al. Atrioventricular Septal Defects. In Adams FH, Emmanouilides GC, Reimenschneider TA, editors. *Heart disease in infants, children and adolescents*, 5th ed. Baltimore, 1995, Williams & Wilkins, p 704.
70. Martucci G, Landzberg M. Not just big kids: closing atrial septal defects in adults older than 60 years. *Circ Cardiovasc Interv* 2009;2:83-84.
71. Murphy JG, Gersh BJ, McGoon MD, et al. Long-term outcome after surgical repair of isolated atrial septal defect: follow-up at 27 to 32 years. *N Engl J Med* 1990;323:1645.
72. Konstantinides S, Geibel A, Olschewski M, et al. A comparison of surgical and medical therapy for atrial septal defect in adults. *N Engl J Med* 1995;333:469.
73. Veldtman GR, Razack V, Siu S, et al. Right ventricular form and function after percutaneous atrial septal defect device closure. *J Am Coll Cardiol* 2001;37:2108-2113.

74. Giardini A, Donti A, Formigari R, et al. Determinants of cardiopulmonary functional improvement after transcatheter atrial septal defect closure in asymptomatic adults. *J Am Coll Cardiol* 2004;43:1886-1891.
75. Brochu MC, Baril JF, Dore A, et al. Improvement in exercise capacity in asymptomatic and mildly symptomatic adults after atrial septal defect percutaneous closure. *Circulation* 2002;106:1821-1826.
76. Pastorek JS, Allen HD, Davis JT. Current outcomes of surgical closure of secundum atrial septal defect. *Am J Cardiol* 1994;74:75.
77. Hufnagel C, Gillespie J. Closure of intra-auricular septal defects. *Bull Georgetown Univ Med Center* 1959;4:137.
78. King TD, Thompson SL, Steiner C, et al. Secundum atrial septal defect-nonoperative closure during cardiac catheterization. *JAMA* 1976;235:2506.
79. Rashkind WJ. Interventional cardiac catheterization in congenital heart disease. *Int J Cardiol* 1985;7:1.
80. Lock JE, Rome JJ, Davis R, et al. Transcatheter closure of ventricular septal defects-experimental studies. *Circulation* 1989;779:1091.
81. Furlan AJ, Reisman M, Massaro J, et al. Study design of the CLOSURE I Trial: a prospective, multicenter, randomized, controlled trial to evaluate the safety and efficacy of the STARFlex septal closure system versus best medical therapy in patients with stroke or transient ischemic attack due to presumed paradoxical embolism through a patent foramen ovale. *Stroke* 2010;41:2872-2883.
82. Hellenbrand WE, Fahey JT, McGowan FX, et al. Transesophageal echocardiographic guidance of transcatheter closure of atrial septal defect. *Am J Cardiol* 1990;66:207.
83. Latson LA, Benson LN, Hellenbrand WE, et al. Transcatheter closure of ASD-early results of multicenter trial of the Bard clamshell septal occluder [abstract]. *Circulation* 1991;84:II-544.
84. Du ZD, Hijazi ZM, Kleinman CS, Silverman NH, Larntx K, for the Amplatzer investigators. Comparison between transcatheter and surgical closure of secundum atrial septal defect in children and adults: results of a multi-center non-randomized trial. *J Am Coll Cardiol* 2000;39:1836-1844.
85. Jones TK, Fagan TE, Zahn EM, Jacobson JL, Latson LA, for the HELEX Septal Occluder US Pivotal Study Investigators. US multicenter pivotal study of the HELEX Septal Occluder. *J Am Coll Cardiol* 2005;45:322A.
86. Yong G, Khairy P, De Guise P. Pulmonary arterial hypertension in patients with transcatheter closure of secundum atrial septal defects: a longitudinal study. *Circ Cardiovasc Interv* 2009;2:455-462.
87. Balint OH, Samman A, Haberer K. Outcomes in patients with pulmonary hypertension undergoing percutaneous atrial septal defect closure. *Heart* 2008;94:1189-1193.
88. Krumsdorf U, Ostermayer S, Billinger K, et al. Incidence and clinical course of thrombus formation on atrial septal defect and patent foramen ovale closure devices in 1000 consecutive patients. *J Am Coll Cardiol* 2004;43:302-309.
89. Amin Z, Hijzai ZM, Bass JL, et al. Erosion of Amplatzer septal occlusion device after closure of secundum atrial septal defects: review of registry of complications and recommendations to minimize future risk. *Catheter Cardiovasc Interv* 2004;63:496-502.
90. Mohr JP, Thompson JL, Lazar RM, et al. A comparison of warfarin and aspirin for the prevention of recurrent ischemic stroke. *N Engl J Med* 2001;345:1444-1451.
91. Homma S, Sacco RL, Di tullio MR, et al. Effect of medical treatment in stroke patients with patent foramen ovale: patent foramen ovale in Cryptogenic Stroke Study. *Circulation* 2002;105:2725-2631.
92. Mas JL, Arquizan C, Lamy C, et al. Recurrent cerebral events associated with patent foramen ovale, atrial septal aneurysm, or both. *N Engl J Med* 2001;345:1740-1746.
93. Rigatelli G, Dell'Avvocata F, Giordan M, et al. Embolic implications of combined risk factors in patients with patent foramen ovale (the CARPE criteria): consideration for primary prevention closure? *J Interv Cardiol* 2009;22:398-403.
94. Kizer JR, Devereaux RB. Patent foramen ovale in young patients with unexplained stroke. *N Engl J Med* 2005;353:2361-2372.
95. Khairy P, O'Donnell CP, Landzberg MJ. Transcatheter closure versus medical therapy of patent foramen ovale and presumed paradoxical thromboemboli: a systematic review. *Ann Intern Med* 2003;139:753-760.
96. Landzberg MJ, Sloss LJ, Faherty CE, et al. Orthodeoxia-platypnea due to intracardiac shunting-relief with transcatheter double umbrella closure. *Cathet Cardiovasc Diagn* 1995;36:247.
97. Garg P, Servoss SJ, Wu JC, et al. Lack of association between migraine headache and patent foramen ovale: results of a case-control study. *Circulation* 2010;121(12): 1406-1412.
98. Dowson A, Mullen MJ, Peatfield R, et al. Migraine Intervention With STARFlex Technology (MIST) trial: a prospective, multicenter, double-blind, sham-controlled trial to evaluate the effectiveness of patent foramen ovale closure with STARFlex septal repair implant to resolve refractory migraine headache. *Circulation* 2008;117:1397-1404.
99. Wagner HR, Ellison RC, Keane JF, et al. Clinical course in aortic stenosis. *Circulation* 1977;56(suppl I):I-47.
100. Rosenfeld HM, Landzberg MJ, Perry SB, et al. Balloon aortic valvuloplasty in the young adult with congenital aortic stenosis. *Am J Cardiol* 1994;73:1112.
101. Sandhu SK, Lloyd TR, Crowley DC, et al. Effectiveness of balloon valvuloplasty in the young adult with congenital aortic stenosis. *Cathet Cardiovasc Diagn* 1995;36:122.
102. Leon MB, Smith CR, Mack M, et al. Transcatheter aortic-valve implantation for aortic stenosis in patients who cannot undergo surgery. *N Engl J Med* 2010;363:1597-1607.
103. Wijesinghe N, Ye J, Rodés-Cabau J, et al. Transcatheter aortic valve implantation in patients with bicuspid aortic valve stenosis. *JACC Cardiovasc Interv* 2010;3:1122-1125.
104. Nugent EW, Freedom RM, Nora JJ, et al. Clinical course in pulmonary stenosis. *Circulation* 1977; 56(Suppl I): I-38.
105. Chen CR, Cheng TO, Huang T, et al. Percutaneous balloon valvuloplasty for pulmonic stenosis in adolescents and adults. *N Engl J Med* 1996;335:21.
106. Earing MG, Connolly HM, Dearani JA, et al. Long-term follow-up of patients after surgical treatment for isolated pulmonary valve stenosis. *Mayo Clin Proc* 2005;80:871-876.
107. Connolly HM, Huston J 3rd, Brown RD Jr, et al. Intracranial aneurysms in patients with coarctation of the aorta: a prosepective magnetic resonance angiographic study of 100 patients. *Mayo Clin Proc* 2003;78:1491-1499.
108. Brili S, Tousoulis D, Antoniades C, et al. Effects of ramipril on endothelial function and the expression of proinflammatory cytokines and adhesion molecules in young normotensive subjects with successfully repaired coarctation of aorta: a randomized cross-over study. *J Am Coll Cardiol* 2008;51:742-749.
109. Tyagi S, Arora R, Kaul UP, et al. Balloon angioplasty of native aortic coarctation of the aorta in adolescents and young adults. *Am Heart J* 1992;123:674.
110. Fawzy ME, Dunn B, Galal O, et al. Balloon coarctation and angioplasty in adolescents and adults: early and intermediate results. *Am Heart J* 1992;124:167.
111. McCrindle BW, Jones TK, Morrow WR, et al. Acute results of balloon angioplasty of native coarctation versus recurrent aortic obstruction are equivalent. *J Am Coll Cardiol* 1996;28:1810.
112. de Giovanni JV, Lip GY, Osman K, et al. Percutaneous balloon dilation of aortic coarctation in adults. *Am J Cardiol* 1996;77:435.
113. Fawzy ME, Sivanandam V, Galal O, et al. One- to ten-year follow-up results of balloon angioplasty of native coarctation of the aorta in adolescents and adults. *J Am Coll Cardiol* 1997;30:1534.
114. Shim D, Lloyd TR, Moorehead CP, et al. Comparison of hospital charges for balloon angioplasty and surgical repair in children with native coarctation of the aorta. *J Am Coll Cardiol* 1997;79:1143.
115. Fawzy ME, Awad M, Hassan W, et al. Long-term outcome (up to 15 years) of balloon angioplasty of discrete native coarctation of the aorta in adolescents and adults. *J Am Coll Cardiol* 2004;43:1062-1067.
116. Suarez de Lezo J, Pan M, Romero M, et al. Percutaneous interventions on severe coarctation of the aorta: a 21-year experience. *Pediatr Cardiol* 2005;26:176-189.
117. Oliver JM, Gallego P, Gonzalez A, et al. Risk factors for aortic complications in adults with coarctation of the aorta. *J Am Coll Cardiol* 2004;44:1641-1647.
118. Thanopoulos BV, Triposkiadis F, Margetakis A, Mullins CE. Long segment coarctation of the thoracic aorta: treatment with multiple balloon-expandable stent implantation. *Am Heart J* 1997;133:470.
119. Qureshi AM, McElhinney DB, Lock JE, et al. Acute and intermediate outcomes, and evaluation of injury to the aortic wall, as based on 15 years' experience of implanting stents to treat aortic coarctation. *Cardiol Young* 2007;17:307-318.
120. Holzer R, Qureshi S, Ghasemi A, et al. Stenting of aortic coarctation: acute, intermediate, and long-term results of a prospective multi-institutional registry: Congenital Cardiovascular Interventional Study Consortium (CCISC). *Catheter Cardiovasc Interv* 2010; 76:553-563.
121. Murphy JG, Gersh BJ, Mair DD, et al. Long-term outcome in patients undergoing surgical repair of tetralogy of Fallot. *N Engl J Med* 1993;329:593.
122. Gatzoulis MA, Balaji S, Webber SA, et al. Risk factors for arrhythmia and sudden cardiac death late after repair of tetralogy of Fallot: a multicentre study. *Lancet* 2000;356: 975-981.
123. Rowe SA, Zahka KG, Manolio TA, et al. Lung function and pulmonary regurgitation limit exercise capacity in postoperative tetralogy of Fallot. *J Am Coll Cardiol* 1991;17:461.
124. Hirsch JC, Mosca RS, Bove EL. Complete repair of tetralogy of Fallot in the neonate: results in the modern era. *Ann Surg* 2000;232:508-514.
125. Pigula FA, Khalil PN, Mayer JE, delNido PJ, Jonas RA. Repair of tetralogy of Fallot in neonates and young infants. *Circulation* 1999:100(Suppl II):157-161.
126. Khairy P, Landzberg MJ, Gatzoulis MA, et al. Value of programmed ventricular stimulation after tetralogy of Fallot repair: a multicenter study. *Circulation* 2004;109:1994-2000.
127. Khairy P, Harris L, Landzberg MJ. Implantable cardioverter-defibrillators in tetralogy of Fallot. *Circulation* 2008;117:363-370.
128. Nollert G, Fischlein T, Bouterwek S, et al. Long-term survival in patients with repair of Tetralogy of Fallot: 36 year follow-up of 490 survivors of the first year after surgical repair. *J Am Coll Cardiol* 1997;30:1374-1383.
129. D'Udekem Y, Ovaert C, Frandjean F, et al. Tetralogy of Fallot: transannular and right ventricular patching equally affect late functional status. *Circulation* 2000;102(Suppl III):116-122.
130. Geva T, Sandweiss BM, Gauvreau K, Lock JE, Powell AJ. Factors associated with impaired clinical status in long-term survivors of tetralogy of Fallot repair evaluated by magnetic resonance imaging. *J Am Coll Cardiol* 2004;43:1068-1074.
131. Hausdorf G, Hinrichs C, Nienaber CA, Schark C, Keck EW. Left ventricular contractile state after surgical correction of tetralogy of Fallot: risk factors for late left ventricular dysfunction. *Pediatr Cardiol* 1990;11:61-68.
132. Kondo C, Nakazawa M, Kusakabe K, Momma K. Left ventricular dysfunction on exercise long-term after total repair of tetralogy of Fallot. *Circulation* 1995;92:(Suppl II)250-255.
133. Niezen RA, Helbing WA, van Der Wall, EE et al. Left ventricular function in adults with mild pulmonary insufficiency late after Fallot repair. *Heart* 1999;82:697-703.
134. Davlouros PA, Kilner PJ, Hornung TS, et al. Right ventricular function in adults with repaired tetralogy of Fallot assessed with cardiovascular magnetic resonance imaging: detrimental role of right ventricular outflow aneurysms or akinesia and adverse right-to-left ventricular interaction. *J Am Coll Cardiol* 2002;40:2044-2052.
135. Therrien J, Siu SC, McLaughlin PR, et al. Pulmonary valve replacement in adults late after repair of tetralogy of Fallot: are we operating too late? *J Am Coll Cardiol* 2000;36:1670-1675.
136. Harrild DM, Berul CI, Cecchin F, et al. Pulmonary valve replacement in tetralogy of Fallot: impact on survival and ventricular tachycardia. *Circulation* 2009;119:445-451.
137. Knauth AL, Gauvreau K, Powell AJ, et al. Ventricular size and function assessed by cardiac MRI predict major adverse clinical outcomes late after tetralogy of Fallot repair. *Heart* 2008;94:211-216.
138. Meadows J, Powell AJ, Geva T, et al. Cardiac magnetic resonance imaging correlates of exercise capacity in patients with surgically repaired tetralogy of Fallot. *Am J Cardiol* 2007;100:1446-1450.
139. Geva T, Gauvreau K, Powell AJ, et al. Randomized trial of pulmonary valve replacement with and without right ventricular remodeling surgery. *Circulation* 2010;122: S201-S208.
140. Therrien J, Siu SC, McLaughlin PR, et al. Pulmonary valve replacement in adults late after repair of tetralogy of fallot: are we operating too late? *J Am Coll Cardiol* 2000;36:1670-1675.

141. Khairy P, Aboulhosn J, Gurvitz MZ. Arrhythmia burden in adults with surgically repaired tetralogy of Fallot: a multi-institutional study. *Circulation* 2010;122:868-875.

142. Babu-Narayan SV, Goktekin O, Moon JC, et al. Late gadolinium enhancement cardiovascular magnetic resonance of the systemic right ventricle in adults with previous atrial redirection surgery for transposition of the great arteries. *Circulation* 2005; 111:2091-2098.

143. Bonhoeffer P, Boudjemline Y, Saliba Z, et al. Percutaneous replacement of pulmonary valve in a right ventricle to pulmonary artery prosthetic conduit with valve dysfunction. *Lancet* 2000;356:1403-1405.

144. Bonhoeffer P, Boudjemline Y, Qureshi SA, et al. Percutaneous insertion of the pulmonary valve. *J Am Coll Cardiol* 2002;39:1664-1669.

145. Gentles TL, Lock JE, Perry SB. High pressure balloon angioplasty for branch pulmonary artery stenosis: early experience. *J Am Coll Cardiol* 1993;22:867.

146. O'Laughlin MP, Slack MC, Perry SB, et al. Stent results and follow-up: an improved outlook for pulmonary arterial and systemic venous stenoses [abstract]. *Circulation* 1992;86 (Suppl I):632.

147. Feinstein JA, Goldhaber SZ, Lock JE, Fernandes SM, Landzberg MJ. Balloon pulmonary angioplasty for treatment of chronic thromboembolic pulmonary hypertension. *Circulation* 2001;103:10-13.

148. Verin VE, Saveliev A, Kolody SM, et al. Results of transcatheter closure of the patent ductus arteriosus with the adjustable button device in adults: initial clinic experience [abstract]. *Circulation* 1994;90(Suppl I):387.

149. Pass RH, Hijzai Z, Hsu DT, Lewis V, Hellenbrand WE. Multicenter USA Amplatzer patent ductus arteriosus occlusion device trial: initial and one-year results. *J Am Coll Cardiol* 2004;44:513-519.

150. Cambier PA, Kirby WC, Wortham DC, et al. Percutaneous closure of the small (<2.5 mm) patent ductus arteriosus using coil embolization. *Am J Cardiol* 1992;69:815.

151. Hijzai ZM, Geggel RL. Transcatheter closure of patent ductus arteriosus using coils. *Am J Cardiol* 1997;77:1279.

152. Podnar T, Masura J. Percutaneous closure of patent ductus arteriosus using special screwing detachable coils. *Cathet Cardiovasc Diagn* 1997;41:386.

153. Ing FF, Recto MR, Saidi A, et al. A method providing bidirectional control of coil delivery in occlusions of patent ductus arteriosis with shallow ampulla and Pott's shunts. *Am J Cardiol* 1997;79:1561.

154. Bridges ND, Perry SB, Keane JF, et al. Preoperative transcatheter closure of congenital muscular ventriuclar septal defects. *N Engl J Med* 1991;324:1312.

155. Landzberg MJ, Lock JE. Transcatheter management of ventricular septal rupture after myocardial infarction. *Semin Thorac Cardiovasc Surg* 1998;10:128.

156. Knauth AL, Lock JE, Perry SB, et al. Transcatheter device closure of congenital and post-operative residual ventricular septal defects. *Circulation* 2004;110:501-507.

157. Holzer R, de Giovanni J, Walsh KP, et al. Transcatheter closure of perimembranous ventricular septal defects using the Amplatzer membranous VSD occluder: immediate and midterm results of an international registry. *Catheter Cardiovasc Interv* 2006;68: 620-628.

158. Butera G, Carminati M, Chessa M, et al. Transcatheter closure of perimembranous ventricular septal defects: early and long-term results. *J Am Coll Cardiol* 2007;50: 1189-1195.

159. Valente AM, Lock JE, Gauvreau K, et al. Predictors of long-term adverse outcomes in patients with congenital coronary artery fistulae. *Circ Cardiovasc Interv* 2010;3: 134-139.

CH
42

CARE FOR ADULTS WITH CONGENITAL HEART DISEASE

Prevention and Treatment of Infective Endocarditis

Amy B. Stancoven and Gail E. Peterson

OVERVIEW, 652

DIAGNOSIS, 652

Echocardiography in the Diagnosis and Management of
  Endocarditis, 652

ANTIBIOTIC THERAPY, 654

IDENTIFYING PATIENTS AT RISK OF POOR CLINICAL
OUTCOMES, 657

SURGICAL THERAPY AND COMPLICATED INFECTIVE
ENDOCARDITIS, 658

Heart Failure, 659
Abscess, 660
Embolic Events, 660
Prosthetic Valve Infections, 661
Cardiac Device Infections, 661

LONG-TERM OUTCOMES AND MANAGEMENT, 662

PREVENTION, 662

FUTURE DIRECTIONS, 663

CONCLUSIONS, 663

REFERENCES, 663

Overview

At the time Sir William Osler so eloquently delivered the Gulstonian Lectures in 1885, the understanding of infective endocarditis (IE) was based on clinical observations, autopsy findings, and small case series. Even in modern times, our knowledge of this disease is primarily based on traditional case series with relatively small numbers of patients. The study of endocarditis is hampered by the rarity of the disease, diverse underlying risk factors, a heterogeneous patient population, and a wide array of infecting organisms. A small number of randomized trials for the treatment of endocarditis have been performed, but no randomized trials exist to test strategies for the prevention of infective endocarditis. As a result of these limitations, it is acknowledged that clinical practice guidelines[1-3] are based largely on expert opinion and practice experience rather than evidence-based medicine grounded in large-scale clinical trials.

Diagnosis

Diagnosis of IE has advanced over the last century with the evolution of standardized diagnostic criteria first proposed in 1994 by Durack and colleagues from Duke University.[4] These diagnostic criteria incorporated microbiologic evidence of IE, echocardiographic findings, and a host of other clinical variables, including injection drug use (IDU) as a predisposing condition.[4] The clinical utility, sensitivity, and specificity of the Duke criteria have been independently validated and were found to have superior performance compared with older criteria that excluded echocardiography.[5,6]

As the epidemiology of IE has evolved, and basic understanding of the disease process has improved, modifications have been proposed. These include the modified Duke criteria, which expanded the major criteria to include nosocomial *Staphylococcus aureus* bacteremia and serologic criteria for *Coxiella burnetii*.[7] Although the modified Duke criteria provide a framework for the diagnosis of IE, the criteria were originally developed for research purposes, and clinicians must incorporate clinical judgment in their assessment of patients with suspected IE.

Echocardiography in the Diagnosis and Management of Endocarditis

Echocardiography provides excellent visualization of cardiac anatomy and has contributed to the earlier diagnosis and detection of complications in IE. The hallmark lesion of IE is a vegetation (Figure 43-1, *A*), evident in 67% to 87% of cases of definite IE.[8-11] Vegetations typically occur on the low-pressure side of a high-velocity turbulent jet and are often accompanied by other hemodynamic or anatomic abnormalities. When infection invades contiguous structures, an abscess may result (Figure 43-1, *B*). Abscesses most commonly involve the aortic root and the anterior mitral annulus and may extend into the ventricular or atrial septum, right ventricular (RV) outflow tract, and anterior mitral valve leaflet. A pseudoaneurysm forms when the abscess cavity communicates with the lumen, and it is recognized by color Doppler flow within the perivalvular echo-free space. Periannular extension may result in tissue necrosis and ultimately results in a fistulous communication between areas external to chambers. Periannular invasion that occurs in the setting of a prosthetic valve can lead to valve dehiscence and perivalvular regurgitation (Figure 43-1, *C*). Echocardiographic features identifying patients at high risk for complications are large vegetations (>1 cm), severe left-sided valvular regurgitation, abscess or pseudoaneurysms, valve perforation or dehiscence, premature mitral valve closure in the setting of aortic insufficiency, pulmonary hypertension, and secondary ventricular dysfunction.[12]

Transthoracic echocardiography (TTE) is noninvasive, is easily performed, and does not require conscious sedation; however, in 10% to 15% of adults, sound transmission is compromised by interfering tissue and/or air attenuation, leading to poor spatial resolution. Transesophageal echocardiography (TEE) is more invasive and labor intensive, but it has improved the ability to detect smaller vegetations and complications of endocarditis. The sensitivity and specificity for TTE and TEE are shown in Table 43-1. Technologic advances in harmonic imaging have improved the diagnostic value of TTE, but it remains less sensitive than TEE.[13-16]

During the initial evaluation of patients with suspected IE, echocardiography should be performed promptly, and the appropriate mode depends in part on the probability of disease.[17,18] For example, TEE is an appropriate initial test when the pretest probability of IE is moderate to high.[1,15] Based on a decision-tree analysis and Markov modeling, Heidenreich and colleagues demonstrated that TEE was cost effective for patients with an intermediate pretest probability of IE, such as patients with predisposing conditions and bacteremia with an organism typical for IE, whereas TTE was better only for those patients with a very low pretest probability of IE.[17] Evidence supports that TEE-guided therapy is cost effective in patients with catheter-associated *S. aureus* infections.[18] Clinical findings suggestive of IE are listed in Box 43-1. In patients with a very low probability of IE based on clinical data, echocardiographic findings are unlikely to change patient management.[19] Clinical criteria that suggest a higher likelihood of IE include vasculitic or embolic phenomena, presence of central venous access, presence of a prosthetic valve, recent IDU, and positive blood cultures.

Other clinical situations in which TEE is preferred as an initial study over TTE are shown in Box 43-2 and include those with a high risk for complications, such as perivalvular extension and

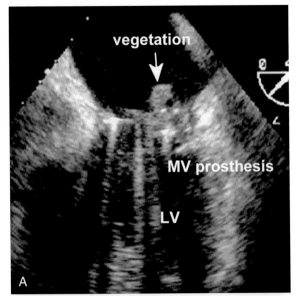

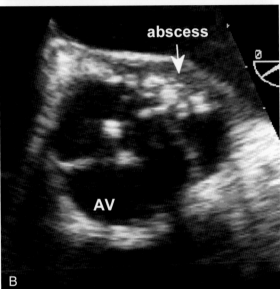

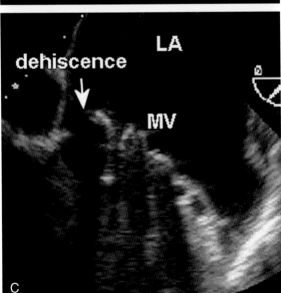

FIGURE 43-1 Echocardiographic findings meeting Duke major criteria for the diagnosis of infective endocarditis. **A,** Vegetation on mitral valve (*MV*) prosthesis. **B,** Periannular aortic abscess. **C,** Prosthetic mitral valve dehiscence. AV, aortic valve; LA, left atrium; LV, left ventricle.

TABLE 43-1	Sensitivity and Specificity of Echocardiography in the Diagnosis of Infective Endocarditis			
	TTE		*TEE*	
	SENSITIVITY (%)	SPECIFICITY (%)	SENSITIVITY (%)	SPECIFICITY (%)
NVE	55-84	62-98	87-94	91-100
PVE	17-45	100	92	97
Abscess	28-36	99	75-87	95

NVE, native valve endocarditis; PVE, prosthetic valve endocarditis; TEE, transesophageal echocardiography; TTE, transthoracic echocardiography.
Data from references 16, 89, and 164-172.

Box 43-1 Clinical Findings that Raise Suspicion for Infective Endocarditis

New murmur or valvular abnormality
Embolism of unknown origin
Sepsis of unknown origin
Fever with any of the following:
- Cardiac device or prosthesis
- History of IE
- Predisposition for IE
  - Valvular or congenital heart disease
  - Intravenous drug use
  - Immunocompromised state
- New conduction disturbance
- Manifestations of heart failure
- Blood cultures growing organisms typical for IE or serology for chronic Q fever
- Evidence of pulmonary infiltrates or embolism
- Abscess of the kidney, spleen, or spine without clear origin

IE, infective endocarditis.
Modified from Habib G, Hoen B, Tornos P, et al. Guidelines on the prevention, diagnosis, and treatment of infective endocarditis (new version, 2009): the Task Force on the Prevention, Diagnosis, and Treatment of Infective Endocarditis of the European Society of Cardiology (ESC). Endorsed by the European Society of Clinical Microbiology and Infectious Diseases (ESCMID) and the International Society of Chemotherapy (ISC) for Infection and Cancer. *Eur Heart J* 2009;30:2369-2413.

Box 43-2 Situations in Which Transesophageal Echocardiography Is Preferable to Transthoracic Echocardiography

With prosthetic heart valves
With intracardiac devices (pacemaker, ICD)
In patients at high risk for complications:
- Those with *Staphylococcus aureus* or fungal infection, prior IE, new heart block, cyanotic congenital heart disease, systemic-pulmonary shunts, poor response to antimicrobials
Intermediate clinical suspicion of IE:
- Unexplained bacteremia with gram-positive cocci, catheter-associated *S. aureus* bacteremia, IDU with fever or bacteremia
Meets modified Duke criteria for possible IE
Inadequate TTE images

ICD, implantable cardioverter-defibrillator; IDU, injection drug use; IE, infective endocarditis, TTE transthoracic echocardiography.
Modified from Baddour LM, Wilson WR, Bayer AS, et al. Infective endocarditis: diagnosis, antimicrobial therapy, and management of complications: a statement for healthcare professionals from the Committee on Rheumatic Fever, Endocarditis, and Kawasaki Disease, Council on Cardiovascular Disease in the Young, and the Councils on Clinical Cardiology, Stroke, and Cardiovascular Surgery and Anesthesia, American Heart Association— executive summary. Endorsed by the Infectious Diseases Society of America. *Circulation* 2005;111:3167-3184; and Douglas PS, Khandheria B, Stainback RF, et al. ACCF/ASE/ ACEP/ASNC/SCAI/SCCT/SCMR 2007 appropriateness criteria for transthoracic and transesophageal echocardiography: a report of the American College of Cardiology Foundation Quality Strategic Directions Committee Appropriateness Criteria Working Group, American Society of Echocardiography, American College of Emergency Physicians, American Society of Nuclear Cardiology, Society for Cardiovascular Angiography and Interventions, Society of Cardiovascular Computed Tomography, and the Society for Cardiovascular Magnetic Resonance. Endorsed by the American College of Chest Physicians and the Society of Critical Care Medicine. *J Am Soc Echocardiogr* 2007;20:787-805.

valve perforation,[1] as well as those with heart failure (HF), new heart block, and persistent fever or bacteremia while receiving appropriate antimicrobial therapy. TEE should also be used as the initial exam in the setting of prosthetic valves and intracardiac devices because of the low sensitivity (~25%) for diagnosing infection with TTE in these conditions.[15] Up to half of patients with prosthetic valves and *S. aureus* bacteremia have endocarditis and should be comprehensively evaluated by TEE.[20] When patients meet the modified Duke criteria for possible IE prior to imaging, TEE usually is the most rational next step for diagnosis. A decision tree to assist in the initial choice of imaging in the setting of suspected IE is shown in Figure 43-2. If the initial TEE findings are negative or nondiagnostic, a follow-up study is recommended 7 to 10 days later if IE is still suspected. Intraoperative TEE is recommended in patients undergoing surgical therapy for IE. After the completion of therapy, TTE should be performed to establish a new baseline for valve function, morphology, ventricular size, and systolic function.[1]

Echocardiographic images should be interpreted only in conjunction with clinical findings because examining echocardiographic images in isolation may lead to both false-positive and false-negative results. False-negative studies may result from vegetations smaller than the limits of imaging resolution, recent loss of a vegetation that has embolized, or acoustic shadowing from a heavily calcified or prosthetic valve. False-positive studies occur in patients with severe myxomatous valvular disease, ruptured chordae, nonbacterial thrombotic (marantic) endocarditis, Libman-Sacks endocarditis, cardiac tumors, or Lambl's excrescences—small tags that occur on 70% to 90% of adult heart valves. Advancements in cardiac imaging modalities, including three-dimensional TEE, computed tomography (CT), and magnetic resonance (MR) are currently being evaluated for their future potential role in the diagnosis and characterization of IE.

Antibiotic Therapy

The cornerstone of antibiotic therapy centers on the isolation of the microorganism and on susceptibility testing, which aids in the appropriate choice and route of antibiotic therapy. Basic principles of antibiotic therapy include the need for bactericidal agents, an adequate duration of treatment, and selection of doses that result in predictable and therapeutic serum levels. Most patients with native valve endocarditis (NVE) are treated with a 4-week course of antibiotics. Patients at higher risk for complications and relapse, such as prosthetic valve endocarditis (PVE), are treated for at least 6 weeks regardless of whether surgery is performed. In patients undergoing surgery, postoperative antibiotic therapy is based on the recommendations for prosthetic valve infections, calculated from the date of surgical intervention, and treatment duration depends on tissue culture results.[1] In selected patients with NVE, such as those with highly sensitive *Streptococcus viridans* infection or uncomplicated right-sided endocarditis as a result of methicillin-sensitive *Staphylococcus aureus* (MSSA), a 2-week course of antibiotic therapy results in high cure rates without substantial recurrence.[21-23] For organisms with sensitivities that are difficult to characterize and that are less responsive to antimicrobials, such as *Abiotrophia defectiva*, *Granulicatella* spp., and *viridans* group streptococci with penicillin mean inhibitory concentration greater than 0.5 μg/mL, the regimen should follow that for enterococcal endocarditis.[3] Details of recommended antibiotic therapy for the most common infecting organisms in IE can be found in Tables 43-2 and 43-3 and in the references.[1,12,21]

Once the diagnosis of IE has been established, treatment with antibiotic therapy should be started immediately. In patients with a high clinical suspicion for IE or those at high risk for complications—such as patients with prosthetic valves with fever and HF or new conduction block or patients with fever, new

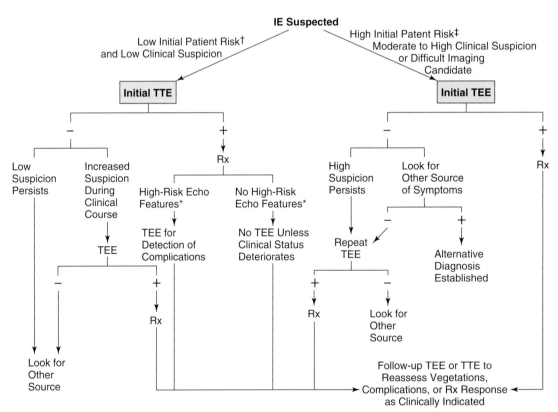

FIGURE 43-2 An approach to the diagnostic use of echocardiography. *High-risk echocardiographic features include large and/or mobile vegetations, valvular insufficiency, suggested perivalvular extension, or secondary ventricular dysfunction. †For example, a patient with fever and a previously known heart murmur and no other signs of IE. ‡For example, patients with risks such as prosthetic heart valves, congenital heart disease, previous endocarditis, new murmur, heart failure, or other signs of endocarditis. IE, infective endocarditis; Rx, antibiotic treatment for endocarditis; TEE, transesophageal echocardiography; TTE, transthoracic echocardiography. *(From Bayer AS, Bolger AF, Taubert KA, et al. Diagnosis and management of infective endocarditis and its complications. Circulation 1998;98:2936-2948.)*

TABLE 43-2 Recommended Antimicrobial Therapy for Common Microorganisms in Infective Endocarditis

MICROORGANISM	NATIVE VALVE	PROSTHETIC VALVE	NOTES
PCN-susceptible *Streptococcus viridans* spp. and *S. bovis*, MIC ≤0.12 μg/mL	PCN G 12 to 18 million U/24 h IV continuously or in 4 to 6 divided doses for 4 wk *or* ceftriaxone 2 g/24 h IV/IM in 1 dose for 4 wk *or* vancomycin 30 mg/kg/24 h IV in 2 divided doses (not to exceed 2 g/24 h) for 4 wk	PCN G 24 million U/24 h IV continuously or in 4 to 6 divided doses for 6 wk *or* ceftriaxone 2 g/24 h IV/IM in 1 dose for 6 wk *with or without* gentamicin 3 mg/kg/24 h IV/IM in 1 dose for 2 wk *or* vancomycin 30 mg/kg/24 h IV in 2 divided doses (not to exceed 2 g/24 h) for 6 wk	2-wk course of PCN G plus gentamicin (3 mg/kg/24 h in 1 dose) *or* ceftriaxone plus gentamicin (3 mg/kg/24 h in 1 dose) as an alternative in uncomplicated cases in patients at low risk for gentamicin toxicity
Relative PCN-resistant *S. viridans* spp. and *S. bovis*, MIC >0.12 μg/mL and <0.5 μg/mL	PCN G 24 million U/24 h IV continuously or in 4 to 6 divided doses for 4 wk *or* ceftriaxone 2 g/24 h IV/IM in 1 dose for 4 wk *plus* gentamicin 3 mg/kg/24 h IV/IM in 1 dose for 2 wk *or* vancomycin 30 mg/kg/24 h IV in 2 divided doses (not to exceed 2 g/24 h) for 4 wk	PCN G 24 million U/24 h IV continuously or in 4 to 6 divided doses for 6 wk *or* ceftriaxone 2 g/24 h IV/IM in 1 dose for 6 wk *plus* gentamicin 3 mg/kg/24 h IV/IM in 1 dose for 6 wk *or* vancomycin 30 mg/kg/24 h IV in 2 divided doses (not to exceed 2 g/24 h) for 6 wk	MIC >0.5 μg/mL, strains treated with regimen recommended for enterococcal endocarditis below Vancomycin should only be used for patients unable to tolerate PCN or ceftriaxone
Oxacillin-susceptible staphylococci	Nafcillin or oxacillin 12 g/24 h IV in 4 to 6 divided doses for 6 wk *with (optional)* gentamicin 3 mg/kg/24 h IV/IM in 2 or 3 divided doses for 3 to 5 days	Nafcillin or oxacillin 12 g/24 h IV in 6 divided doses for at least 6 wk *with* rifampin 900 mg/24 h IV/PO in 3 divided doses for at least 6 wk *with* gentamicin 3 mg/kg/24 h IV/IM in 2 or 3 divided doses for 2 wk	For uncomplicated right-sided IE, 2-wk course of nafcillin or oxacillin *with (optional)* gentamicin 3 mg/kg/24 h in 2 to 3 divided doses If history of nonanaphylactoid hypersensitivity reactions to β-lactams, cefazolin 6 g/24 h IV in 3 divided doses for 6 wk *with (optional)* gentamicin 3 mg/kg/24 h IV/IM in 2 or 3 divided doses for 3 to 5 days If history of anaphylactoid hypersensitivity to β-lactams, vancomycin based on oxacillin-resistant procotol
Oxacillin-resistant staphylococci	Vancomycin 30 mg/kg/24 h IV in 2 divided doses for 6 wk	Vancomycin 30 mg/kg/24 h IV in 2 divided doses for at least 6 wk *with* rifampin 900 mg/24 h IV/PO in 3 divided doses for at least 6 wk *with* gentamicin 3 mg/kg/24 h IV/IM in 2 or 3 divided doses for 2 wk	
HACEK microorganisms (*Haemophilus, Actinobacillus, Cardiobacterium, Eikenella, Kingella*)	Ceftriaxone 2 g/24 h IV/IM in 1 dose for 4 wk *or* ampicillin-sulbactam 12 g/24 h IV in 4 divided doses for 4 wk *or* ciprofloxacin 1000 mg/24 h PO or 800 mg/24 h IV in 2 divided doses for 4 wk	Same protocol as native valve HACEK infection but for 6-wk course	May substitute cefotaxime or another third- or fourth-generation cephalosporin Fluoroquinolone therapy is recommended only for patients intolerant to cephalosporins and ampicillin

Vancomycin dosage should be adjusted to obtain a peak 1 hour after completed infusion of 30 to 45 μg/mL with a trough of 10 to 14 μg/mL. A dosage >2 g/day is acceptable if serum concentrations are inappropriately low.

Gentamicin dosage should be adjusted to obtain a peak of 3 to 4 μg/mL and trough <1 μg/mL when 3 divided doses are used. A nomogram is used for once-daily dosing.

IE, infective endocarditis; IM, intramuscularly; IV, intravenously; MIC, minimum inhibitory concentration; PCN, penicillin; PO, orally.

Modified from references 1, 21, and 173.

pathologic murmur, and HF—empiric therapy should be started. Three sets of blood cultures should be drawn at least 1 hour apart prior to initiation of therapy. The choice of empiric therapy depends on whether the patient has received prior antibiotics, whether a prosthetic valve is present, and whether the surgery was recent, in which case the regimen should include coverage for early PVE. In addition, working knowledge of local epidemiology and antibiotic resistance is helpful.

Outpatient parenteral antibiotic therapy (OPAT) may be safely and effectively used in the modern clinical setting, but it must be used carefully and only in the appropriate patient populations.[24] Within the first 2 weeks of diagnosis, OPAT may be considered in

CH
43

TABLE 43-3   Recommended Antimicrobial Therapy for Enterococcal Infective Endocarditis

MICROORGANISM	NATIVE OR PROSTHETIC VALVE	NOTES
Enterococcus susceptible to PCN, gentamicin, and vancomycin	Ampicillin 12 g/24 h IV in 6 divided doses *or* PCN G 18 to 30 million U/24 h IV continuously or in 6 divided doses for 4 to 6 wk *plus* gentamicin 3 mg/kg/24 h IV/IM in 3 divided doses for 4 to 6 wk *or* vancomycin 30 mg/kg/24 h in 2 divided doses for 6 wk *plus* gentamicin 3 mg/kg/24 h IV/IM in 3 divided doses for 6 wk	Native valve: 4-wk dual therapy if ≤3 months of symptoms; 6-wk dual therapy if >3 months of symptoms Prosthetic valve: minimum 6 wk of dual therapy Vancomycin used only for patients intolerant to penicillin or ampicillin
Enterococcus susceptible to PCN, streptomycin, and vancomycin but resistant to gentamicin	Ampicillin 12 g/24 h IV in 6 divided doses *or* PCN G 24 million U/24 h IV continuously or in 6 divided doses for 4 to 6 wk *plus* streptomycin 15 mg/kg/24 h IV/IM in 2 divided doses for 4 to 6 wk *or* vancomycin 30 mg/kg/24 h in 2 divided doses for 6 wk *plus* streptomycin 15 mg/kg/24 h IV/IM in 2 divided doses for 6 wk	Native valve: 4-wk dual therapy if ≤3 months of symptoms; 6-wk dual therapy if >3 months of symptoms Prosthetic valve: minimum 6 wk of dual therapy Vancomycin is used only for patients intolerant to penicillin or ampicillin
Enterococcus resistant to PCN and susceptible to aminoglycoside and vancomycin	Ampicillin-sulbactam 12 g/24 h IV in 4 divided doses for 6 wk *plus* gentamicin 3 mg/kg/24 h IV/IM in 3 divided doses for 6 wk *or* vancomycin 30 mg/kg/24 h IV in 2 divided doses for 6 wk *plus* gentamicin 3 mg/kg/24 h IV/IM in 3 divided doses for 6 wk	If strain is gentamicin resistant, >6 wk of ampicillin-sulbactam Vancomycin used only for patients intolerant to ampicillin-sulbactam If intrinsic penicillin resistance is present, use vancomycin plus gentamicin dosing; consultation with an infectious disease specialist recommended
Enterococcus resistant to PCN, aminoglycoside, and vancomycin	*E. faecium*: Linezolid 1200 mg/24 h IV/PO in 2 divided doses >8 wk *or* quinupristin-dalfopristin 22.5 mg/kg/24 h IV in 3 divided doses >8 wk *E. faecalis*: Imipenem-cilastatin 2 g/24 h IV in 4 divided doses for at least 8 wk *plus* ampicillin 12 g/24 h IV in 6 divided doses for at least 8 wk *or* ceftriaxone 4 g/24 h IV in 2 divided doses for at least 8 wk *plus* ampicillin 12 g/24 h IV in 6 divided doses for at least 8 wk	Consultation with an infectious disease specialist recommended Cure with antibiotics alone <50%; valve replacement may be needed for cure

Vancomycin dosage should be adjusted to obtain a peak 1 hour after completed infusion of 30 to 45 μg/mL with a trough of 10 to 14 μg/mL. A dosage greater than 2 g/24 h is acceptable if serum concentrations are inappropriately low.
Gentamicin dosage should be adjusted to obtain a peak of 3 to 4 μg/mL and a trough below 1 μg/mL when 3 divided doses are used. A nomogram is used for once-daily dosing.
IM, intramuscularly; IV, intravenously; PCN, penicillin; PO, orally.
Modified from references 1, 21, and 173.

uncomplicated native valve infections with penicillin-susceptible *viridans* group streptococci.[24] Otherwise, patients should be stabilized as an inpatient for a suitable period, usually about 2 weeks, after which OPAT may be considered if the patient is at low risk for complications (e.g., HF and emboli) and is clinically stable without HF, renal impairment, high-risk echocardiographic features, or neurologic symptoms.[3] Appropriate outpatient candidates should also have adequate social support, daily visits by an infusion nurse, and physician visits every 1 to 2 weeks to evaluate for IE complications.[1,3]

A growing concern in the antimicrobial treatment of IE is the emergence of resistant microorganisms, especially multidrug-resistant enterococci and staphylococci. In some cases of resistant organisms, antimicrobial therapy may be required for up to 8 weeks, and surgical intervention may be necessary for a cure.[1] A promising therapy in patients with drug-resistant staphylococci is daptomycin; early studies have demonstrated noninferiority compared with standard therapy in the treatment of *S. aureus* bacteremia with or without right-sided IE.[25] It is hoped that the efficacy of daptomycin, in combination or alone, will extend to

other gram-positive organisms and other types of IE other than right-sided NVE.

In the setting of IDU, the choice of antimicrobial therapy may be tailored based on the type of injected drug. Although *Staphylococcus* species are the most common pathogens in this patient population, patients with IDU are also at risk for less common pathogens and polymicrobial infections. Users of pentazocine are at risk for *Pseudomonas* infections, and those using brown heroin dissolved in lemon juice are at risk for infection with *Candida* species. Patients with IDU who have underlying valvular disease or left-sided IE are also at risk for streptococcal and enterococcal infections.

The most common cause of culture-negative IE is prior antimicrobial therapy. In the setting of concurrent antimicrobial therapy, discontinuing antibiotics and waiting 3 days to draw blood cultures during evaluation for suspected IE is more likely to yield the etiologic pathogen. However, in certain situations—including HF, new conduction abnormalities, and embolism—empiric antibiotic therapy should be started without delay. Recommended antibiotic therapy for culture-negative endocarditis is found in Table 43-4.

TABLE 43-4 **Recommended Antimicrobial Therapy for Culture-Negative Infective Endocarditis, Including *Bartonella***

	NATIVE VALVE	PROSTHETIC VALVE	NOTES
Culture-negative endocarditis	Ampicillin-sulbactam 12 g/24 h IV in 4 divided doses for 4 to 6 wk *plus* gentamicin 3 mg/kg/24 h IV/IM in 3 divided doses for 4 to 6 wk *or* vancomycin 30 mg/kg/24 h IV in 2 divided doses for 4 to 6 wk *plus* gentamicin 3 mg/kg/24 h IV/IM in 3 divided doses for 4 to 6 wk *plus* ciprofloxacin 1000 mg/24 h PO or 800 mg/24 hr IV in 2 divided doses for 4 to 6 wk	*Early (≤1 year):* Vancomycin 30 mg/kg/24 h IV in 2 divided doses for 6 wk *plus* gentamicin 3 mg/kg/24 h IV/IM in 3 divided doses for 2 wk *plus* cefepime 6 g/24 h in 3 divided doses for 6 wk *plus* rifampin 900 mg/24 h PO/IV in 3 divided doses for 6 wk *Late (>1 year):* Same regimen as for culture-negative native valve IE	Consultation with an infectious disease specialist recommended Vancomycin only for patients who cannot tolerate penicillins
Suspected *Bartonella*, culture negative	Ceftriaxone 2 g/24 h IV/IM in 1 dose for 6 wk *plus* gentamicin 3 mg/kg/24 h IV/IM in 3 divided doses for 2 wk *with or without* doxycycline 200 mg/24 h IV/PO in 2 divided doses for 6 wk	Consultation with an infectious disease specialist is recommended	Consultation with an infectious disease specialist recommended
Documented *Bartonella*, culture positive	Doxycycline 200 mg/24 h IV/PO in 2 divided doses for 6 wk *plus* gentamicin 3 mg/kg/24 h IV/IM in 3 divided doses for 2 wk		Consultation with an infectious disease specialist recommended Use rifampin 600 mg/24 h PO/IV in 2 divided doses if gentamicin cannot be given

Vancomycin dosage should be adjusted to obtain a peak 1 hour after completed infusion of 30 to 45 μg/mL with a trough of 10 to 14 μg/mL. A dosage >2 g/24 h is acceptable if serum concentrations are inappropriately low.
Gentamicin dosage should be adjusted to obtain a peak of 3 to 4 μg/mL and a trough <1 μg/mL when 3 divided doses are used. A nomogram is used for once-daily dosing.
Modified from references 1, 21, and 173.

Identifying Patients at Risk of Poor Clinical Outcomes

Despite improved diagnostic methods and advances in medical and surgical therapies, mortality rates from IE have not significantly changed since 1950. Modern case series report an in-hospital mortality rate of 15% to 20%.[9,11,26] The reason for the lack in improvement in outcomes is related in large part to a change in the epidemiology of IE. Paradoxically, advancements in medical technology have led to a shift in IE from a subacute disease to an acute, aggressive disease that increasingly involves the elderly, patients receiving hemodialysis, and those with prosthetic cardiac devices. Injection drug users are at an increased risk of IE, and poor clinical outcomes can be expected in the setting of left-sided IE.[27] Results from an international, multicenter cohort of patients indicate that age, prosthetic valve endocarditis, pulmonary edema, mitral valve vegetations, paravalvular complications, and infection with *S. aureus* or coagulase-negative *Staphylococcus* are associated with in-hospital death.[11]

The U.S. population is aging, and elderly patients constitute a particularly vulnerable group because of the comorbidities associated with medical illness at an advanced age. The incidence of endocarditis in the elderly is four to nine times greater than in the general population, and it has increased in recent years.[9,28,29] Endocarditis in the elderly is associated with a higher mortality rate, ranging from 17% to 28%,[30,31] and with a higher risk of complications, including abscess formation, compared with endocarditis in younger patients.[32] This may be related to a greater incidence of comorbid disease in this population along with more aggressive pathogens. In addition, the elderly more often undergo invasive medical procedures that introduce greater opportunity for bacteremia, which explains the higher rates of health care–associated IE.[32] In at least one observational study, early surgical therapy in elderly patients with IE was independently associated

with a lower in-hospital mortality rate,[31] although data indicate the elderly receive surgery less often compared with younger cohorts.[32]

The incidence of IE in patients receiving hemodialysis has increased over the past decade. Patients on hemodialysis have a fivefold increase in the incidence of valve disease,[33] and the incidence of IE in hemodialysis patients is 50-fold to 70-fold higher than in the general population.[9,34] A trend analysis of the Duke IE database showed that the overall proportion of IE cases that occur in hemodialysis patients increased over a 10-year period and indicated that hemodialysis was strongly associated with *S. aureus* as the infecting microorganism.[26] Because of more aggressive organisms and underlying comorbid disease, the in-hospital and 1-year mortality rates are extremely high in patients receiving hemodialysis (23% to 52% and 38% to 65%, respectively).[35-39] Factors identified with worse outcomes include advanced age, large vegetations, diabetes as a cause for end-stage renal disease (ESRD), fever on admission, elevated white blood cell count (WBC), multivalve IE, mitral annular calcification or severe mitral regurgitation in the setting of mitral valve IE, severe aortic regurgitation in the setting of aortic valve IE, and negative blood cultures.[35,36,38,39]

When treating hemodialysis patients medically, it is tempting to use vancomycin for MSSA because of the ease of administration. However, vancomycin exerts only a slow bactericidal effect, it penetrates vegetations poorly, and it is less active than β-lactams for MSSA.[40] In addition, there is justifiable concern that overuse of this agent will lead to emergence of vancomycin-resistant microorganisms. When a tunneled or other central catheter is in place, every effort should be taken to remove the catheter because cure is unlikely when catheter salvage is attempted.[41]

Prosthetic cardiac devices, which include prosthetic heart valves and implantable cardiac devices, have become increasingly prevalent and are associated with a disproportionate rise in infections.[42] PVE makes up 20% of IE in modern reports, and the majority of infections are caused by *S. aureus*.[43] The in-hospital mortality rate in patients with PVE is higher (23% to 28%) than that associated with NVE (10% to 17%).[11,43] Endocarditis that involves implantable cardiac devices is associated with substantial morbidity and usually requires explantation of the device for cure. Patients with a cardiac device and *S. aureus* bacteremia have a high likelihood of device infection, and a high clinical suspicion for IE is warranted.[20,44]

IDU is an important risk factor for IE, with incidences in this group of 710 per 100,000 person-years[45] compared with 5 to 7.9 per 100,000 person-years in the general population.[46] Patients who use injectible drugs more commonly have right-sided IE, which is associated with a low (<5%) in-hospital mortality rate, provided that vegetations are not large (<20 mm).[27] However, left-sided IE in these patients carries a mortality rate of 20% to 30%,[27] and *S. aureus* infections in this cohort are common.[11] In patients positive for human immunodeficiency virus (HIV), IE is uncommon in the absence of IDU.[47] However, the combination of HIV and IDU is associated with an even greater risk for developing IE.[45,48] The presence of HIV alone is not associated with an adverse prognosis from IE,[49] although more severe HIV infection (CD4 levels <200 cells/μL) is associated with higher mortality rates.[27]

Surgical Therapy and Complicated Infective Endocarditis

The management of complicated IE that includes HF, cardiac abscess, embolic phenomena, and prosthetic valve infection often involves both surgical and medical therapy (Figure 43-3). Goals of surgical therapy are 1) correction of valvular abnormalities,

generally with valvular repair or replacement; 2) control of infection; and 3) prevention of embolic complications. Surgical therapy is performed during the early phase of IE in 20% to 50% of patients and, after the completion of antibiotics, in another 20% to 40%; highest operative rates exist in cases of mitral valve IE.[9,50-54] Published experiences of surgery during active IE show operative mortality rates that range from 5% to 25%, with actuarial 5- and 10-year survival rates of 75% and 61%, respectively.[53,55-60] In comparison, mortality for the same operative procedures is lower when performed for reasons other than IE.[59,61] Both the American Heart Association (AHA) and the European Society of Cardiology (ESC) have published guidelines for performing surgery in IE and largely concur, although their recommendations have subtle differences (Table 43-5).[1,3] The ESC makes further recommendations regarding the timing of surgery in IE.

The decision for surgical therapy should not be based on absolute indications but on serial clinical evaluations, microbiologic results that include surveillance blood cultures on appropriate therapy, and echocardiographic findings. No randomized trials have compared surgical therapy to medical therapy alone. When patients undergoing surgery are carefully matched by propensity scoring, surgery in a diverse group of patients with IE and HF is associated with a 50% reduction in 6-month mortality rate over medical therapy alone.[62] Others have indicated that survivor bias is the basis for favorable results demonstrated with surgery, and caution should be used when interpreting observational data.[63] In a recently published analysis by the International Collaboration on Endocarditis, 619 patients who underwent early surgery were propensity matched to patients receiving medical therapy with

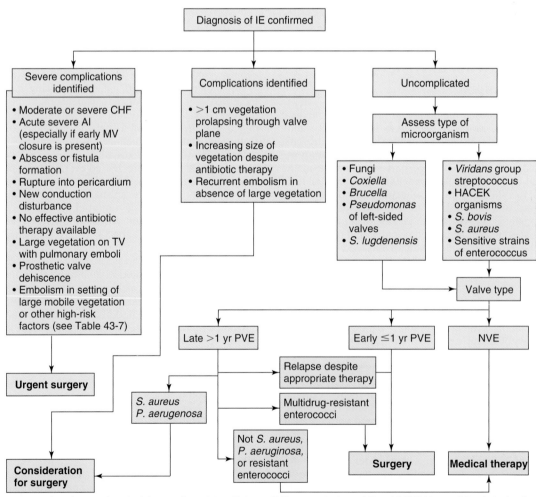

FIGURE 43-3 An approach to the use of surgical therapy. AI, aortic insufficiency; CHF, congestive heart failure; HACEK, *Haemophilus, Actinobacillus, Cardiobacterium, Eikenella, Kingella*; IE, infective endocarditis; MV, mitral valve; NVE, native valve endocarditis; PVE, prosthetic valve endocarditis; TV, tricuspid valve.

TABLE 43-5	American Heart Association and European Society of Cardiology Indications for Surgical Therapy in Infective Endocarditis			
INDICATION		**TIMING***	**CLASS†**	**LOE‡**
Heart Failure				
Acute severe aortic or mitral regurgitation, obstruction, or fistula causing pulmonary edema or shock		*Emergency*	I	B
Acute severe aortic or mitral regurgitation, obstruction, or fistula with persistent HF or echocardiographic evidence of poor hemodynamic tolerance		*Urgent*	I	B
Aortic or mitral valve IE or severe prosthetic dehiscence with severe regurgitation and no HF		*Elective*	IIa	B
Right heart failure as a result of severe TR and poor response to medical therapy		*Urgent/Elective*	*IIa*	*C*
Uncontrolled Infection				
Local (abscess, pseudoaneurysm, fistula, enlarging vegetation, heart block)		*Urgent*	I	B
Persistent fever and positive blood cultures for >7 to 10 days unrelated to extracardiac source		*Urgent*	I	B
Fungal or multidrug-resistant infections		*Urgent/Elective*	I	B
PVE caused by staphylococci or gram-negative rods		*Urgent/Elective*	*IIa*	*C*
Prevention of Embolization				
Aortic, mitral, or prosthetic valve endocarditis with a large vegetation and an embolic event on appropriate therapy		*Urgent*	I/IIa	B/C
Aortic, mitral, or prosthetic valve endocarditis with a large vegetation and other predictors of a complicated course (CHF, persistent infection, embolization)		*Urgent*	I	C
Aortic, mitral, or prosthetic valve endocarditis with isolated, large (>15 mm) mobile vegetation		*Urgent*	IIb	C
Persistent TV vegetation after recurrent pulmonary emboli (>20 mm)		*Urgent/Elective*	*IIa*	*C*

Italics indicate recommendations found only in ESC guidelines.
*Emergency, within 24 hours; urgent, within a few days; elective, after at least 1 to 2 weeks of antimicrobial therapy.
†I, procedure should be performed; IIa, procedure is reasonable; IIb, procedure may be considered.
‡A, multiple population risk strata evaluated with consistent direction and magnitude of treatment effect; B, limited population risk strata evaluated; C, very limited population risk strata evaluated.
CHF, congestive heart failure; HF, heart failure; IE, infective endocarditis; LOE, level of evidence; PVE, prosthetic valve endocarditis; TR, tricuspid regurgitation; TV, tricuspid valve.
From Baddour LM, Wilson WR, Bayer AS, et al. Infective endocarditis: diagnosis, antimicrobial therapy, and management of complications: a statement for healthcare professionals from the committee on rheumatic Fever, Endocarditis, and Kawasaki Disease, Council on Cardiovascular Disease in the Young, and the Councils on Clinical Cardiology, Stroke, and Cardiovascular Surgery and Anesthesia, American Heart Association—executive summary: endorsed by the Infectious Diseases Society of America. *Circulation* 2005; 111:3167-3184; and Habib G, Hoen B, Tornos P, et al. Guidelines on the prevention, diagnosis, and treatment of infective endocarditis (new version 2009): the Task Force on the Prevention, Diagnosis, and Treatment of Infective Endocarditis of the European Society of Cardiology (ESC). Endorsed by the European Society of Clinical Microbiology and Infectious Diseases (ESCMID) and the International Society of Chemotherapy (ISC) for Infection and Cancer.
Eur Heart J 2009;30:2369-2413.

adjustment for survivor bias.[64] In their analysis, *early surgery*, defined as surgery during the initial hospitalization for IE, was associated with a decrease in mortality rate, with an absolute risk reduction of 5.9%.[64] In a subgroup analysis, surgery conferred a survival benefit in patients with stronger indications for surgery, *S. aureus* infection, embolic events, and stroke. The need for a definitive answer about IE and surgery has led to the Early Surgery in Infective Endocarditis Study (ENDOVAL 1), the first ongoing, prospective, randomized trial in IE.[65] A second randomized trial, Early Surgery Versus Conventional Treatment in Infective Endocarditis (EASE), is evaluating the effects on in-hospital death and clinical embolic events of very early surgery (within 48 hours) in patients with NVE, severe left-sided valvular regurgitation, and large vegetations (ClinicalTrials.gov, NCT00750373). Initial results from the EASE trial for the primary endpoint of death plus embolic events within 6 weeks of study randomization demonstrated superior results with early surgery compared with conventional treament (3% vs. 23%; *P* = .014).

In patients chosen for surgical therapy, coronary angiography should be considered preoperatively in men older than 40 years, in postmenopausal women, and in those at high risk for coronary artery disease. Caution should be taken in the setting of large aortic valve vegetations, and coronary CT scan may be considered in this setting for assessment of coronary anatomy, if heart rate allows. All patients with neurologic symptoms should undergo CT of the brain to clarify the nature and extent of disease and to identify hemorrhage before undergoing surgery. At present, results of surgery depend on many factors, including the preoperative condition of the patient, timing of the surgery, surgical techniques, and postoperative management. Preoperative predictors of death include higher New York Hospital Association (NYHA) classification, older age, and the presence of renal failure.[55-58,66,67] Aggressive disease of a shorter duration, as with *S. aureus*, is also associated with increased surgical mortality rate.[29]

Early surgical intervention in the acute phase, particularly in the presence of uncontrolled infection, may seem risky in light of concerns about placing prosthetic material into a highly infected field, with the potential for failure and recurrence of IE. Some investigators have reported that surgical intervention during the acute phase of IE was associated with increased risk for persistent or early recurrent PVE.[61,68] In contrast, others did not find this to be true,[50,69-71] particularly for mitral valve disease.[59,68] With increasing experience and good results, there is a trend for earlier operation in patients with IE. The final surgical outcome appears to have little relation to the duration and intensity of antibiotic therapy before surgery.[71] However, it is important that adequate bactericidal concentrations of antibiotics be present to kill bacteria that enter the circulation during surgical debridement. In general, when surgery is indicated, prognosis is improved if surgery is performed early, before the general condition of the patient has deteriorated.[50,51,64,72]

The choice of surgical technique plays a role in both short- and long-term outcomes. In the setting of mitral valve IE, valve repair should be performed when possible because it is associated with a lower mortality rate (0% to 9%) compared with mitral valve replacement (5% to 25%), and it has low rates of recurrent infection.[72-75] Ten-year survival rates in the setting of mitral valve repair are 80%[76] compared with 61% after mitral valve replacement.[57] For aortic valve IE, homograft replacement may be a better option in terms of reducing recurrent IE,[67] although it may be associated with a greater rate of late valve-related complications.[76] Homografts also offer an advantage in the setting of extensive periannular destruction by infection.[77,78]

Heart Failure

HF is the most common cause of death in IE and usually is the result of infection-related valvular dysfunction such as regurgitation from valvular destruction, valvular perforation, or rupture of infected chordae; but it may also be due to a fistula that results in intracardiac shunting or, rarely, in obstruction from a vegetation. Endocarditis complicated by acute aortic insufficiency is associated with particularly high risk because it is poorly tolerated and results in rapid progression of HF in most cases.[60] The risk of HF is also increased in the presence of virulent pathogens such as *S. aureus;* hemolytic streptococci groups A, B, C, F, and G; and *Streptococcus pneumoniae.*[52] HF may develop at any point during a patient's treatment course, and routine assessment for signs and symptoms of HF should be performed.[79]

Based on observational studies, HF carries a worse prognosis with medical therapy alone and confers a higher surgical risk. Operative mortality rates for IE range from 6% to 11% in the absence of HF compared with 11% to 35% when HF has developed.[12,60,80] In early observational studies, the mortality rates for surgically treated patients with decompensated HF are consistently lower compared with patients treated conservatively.[52,56] In patients with HF that complicates IE, no randomized trials have compared surgical therapy with medical management, and treatment bias likely exists in available observational studies. The most compelling evidence for the benefit of surgical therapy in IE complicated by HF was presented by Vikram and associates,[62] who used propensity analysis to address selection bias and found that patients with left-sided NVE and moderate to severe HF had a significant reduction in mortality rate with surgery compared with conservative therapy (hazard ratio [HR], 0.22; 95% confidence interval [CI], 0.08 to 0.53), whereas patients with mild or no HF derived no benefit from surgery. These results differed from a recent propensity score analysis performed by the International Collaboration on Endocarditis (ICE). Although early surgery was beneficial in the group as a whole, it did not confer a survival benefit in the subgroup of patients with HF when compared with medical therapy.[64] Limits to the ICE propensity analysis include the inability to classify the severity or timing of HF; the inclusion of milder forms of HF may in part explain the lack of benefit with surgical therapy.[64] Despite these limitations, moderate and severe HF are a class I indication for surgical therapy and constitute the primary indication for surgery in most cases of surgically treated IE (22% to 71%).[61,67] When possible, surgery should be performed before the development of intractable HF because postoperative death is related to the severity of hemodynamic impairment at the time of surgery.[57] The mortality benefit is most apparent when surgery is performed early in the course of disease,[56] and no evidence is available to support that delaying surgery to give additional antibiotics improves outcomes. The small (2% to 7%) potential risk of recurrent IE following surgery in the acute phase is far less than the mortality rate from uncontrolled HF.[50,81]

Abscess

Cardiac abscess, or extension of infection beyond the valvular leaflets, occurs in 8% to 40% of patients with NVE,[1,82] most commonly in the aortic annular region, and has been reported in 30% to 100% of patients with PVE.[43,73,82,83] Periannular invasion is more common in bioprosthetic valves during the first postoperative year compared with later infections, whereas invasive disease occurs in mechanical valves regardless of time from implantation.[84]

Significant predictors of abscess include aortic valve involvement, IDU, and new atrioventricular (AV) or bundle branch block from extension of infection into the conduction system.[82,85] The development of new AV or bundle branch block has a positive predictive value of 77% but a relatively low sensitivity (42%) for abscess formation.[82] The presence of intraventricular block (bundle branch or hemiblock) also has prognostic implications, with mortality rates of 31% compared with 15% in patients without block.[86] Periannular extension is more common in patients with *S. aureus* IE,[87] and it should be suspected in patients with NVE with uncontrolled infection or acute hemodynamic deterioration. All patients with PVE that involves the aortic valve are at high risk for abscess and should be carefully evaluated with TEE.

Delivery of antibiotics to extravalvular tissue is difficult; for this reason, mortality rates of medically treated patients with abscess may be 75% or higher.[87,88] As a result, surgical therapy is preferred

in most cases of abscess formation, with operative mortality rates in many,[89,90] but not all, series[57] not significantly different from patients operated on without abscess. If the surgical procedure is radical, resulting in complete resection of the abscess cavity and restoration of near-normal hemodynamics, presurgical abscess is not a predictor of early surgical death or reinfection rate.[58] A very small number of patients with abscesses may be treated medically, provided they are followed up closely by serial TEEs for progression of disease.[91] Contraindications for medical management include heart block, severe or worsening valvular regurgitation, and prosthetic valve dehiscence. If any of these conditions occurs during medical management, prompt surgical intervention should be pursued.[91]

Aortocavitary fistulae are a rare complication of aortic abscess, with an overall prevalence of 1.7%, rising to 5.8% in patients with PVE in the largest series (n = 76) to date.[92] Although every patient did not undergo TEE, it detected 97% of fistulas, whereas TTE detected only 53%.[92] In this series, 87% of patients underwent surgery. The clinical outcome of an aortocavitary fistula is poor; in-hospital mortality rate was 42%, and it was associated with HF and the need for urgent or emergency surgery.[92]

Embolic Events

The incidence of clinically significant embolic events in IE ranges from 40% to 50% in prospective analyses.[11,93] Stroke represents 50% to 65% of these cases and is a major contributor to the morbidity and mortality associated with IE.[94] The majority of strokes are diagnosed before antibiotic treatment begins,[94,95] and most "preventable strokes," defined as those occurring after the initiation of treatment, occur early. In addition, the frequency of embolism dramatically declines after initiation of antimicrobials.[52,96]

Clinical, microbiologic, and echocardiographic factors associated with embolization in IE are summarized in Table 43-6.[97] Echocardiographic risk factors for embolism include vegetation size, morphology, and location.[98] In a meta-analysis of 10 studies that involved a total of 738 patients, 37% of the 323 patients with vegetations more than 10 mm in diameter had an embolism—a risk almost three times greater than that for patients with smaller vegetations.[99] Investigators have also consistently demonstrated that IE secondary to *S. aureus* is associated with increased rates of symptomatic cerebral emboli.[100,101] Evidence also suggests that vegetations on the mitral valve, particularly those on the anterior leaflet, are associated with the highest risk for embolism and stroke (21% to 32% with mitral valve IE vs. 11% to 15% with aortic valve IE).[9,95] The degree of vegetation mobility may also predict embolic risk.[102] When silent emboli, as assessed by cerebral and thoracoabdominal CT scans, and clinically apparent emboli are included together, the composite rate of embolic events is particularly high (83%) when vegetations are both very large (>15 mm) and mobile.[102]

Although current guidelines suggest that surgery be performed after embolic events occur on antimicrobial therapy, many experts advocate earlier, preventative surgical intervention, although evidence to support this position is limited. In a prospective observational study of patients with only embolic-related indications for

TABLE 43-6	Risk Factors for Embolism	
CLINICAL	**MICROBIOLOGIC**	**ECHOCARDIOGRAPHIC**
Prior embolism	*Staphylococcus aureus*	Mitral valve infection
Short symptom duration	*Candida* species	Prosthetic valve infection
Older age	*Abiotrophia* species	Perivalvular extension
Atrial fibrillation	HACEK organisms	Enlarging vegetation on treatment
		Vegetation numbers
		Mobility and size (>10 mm)

HACEK, *Haemophilus, Actinobacillus, Cardiobacterium, Eikenella, Kingella.*

surgery, fewer deaths and fewer embolic complications were reported if surgery was performed within 7 days of diagnosis, although differences in vegetation size and mobility were apparent between the two groups.[103] If a patient has another indication for surgical therapy, such as significant valvular regurgitation or HF, the decision for surgery is easier because it will achieve a twofold objective. Likewise, surgery may be considered after a single embolic episode in patients with a persistent vegetation, when the risk of repeat embolism is believed to be high based on clinical, microbiologic, or echocardiographic parameters.[104,105] It is unclear whether surgery is warranted when a large, mobile vegetation is present without evidence of embolism. However, when the goal is to prevent embolic events, surgery is best performed early because the rate of embolism decreases significantly after the first 1 to 2 weeks of medical treatment.[106]

After a stroke has occurred, the risk of possible further neurologic damage during cardiopulmonary bypass becomes a concern. Patients who have had transient ischemic attacks (TIAs) or asymptomatic stroke appear to be at low risk for further neurologic complications during cardiopulmonary bypass, and these findings should not delay necessary surgery.[107] The optimal timing of surgery following symptomatic ischemic stroke is less clear.[104,105,107,108] Based on more recent data, surgery can be performed 72 hours or later following an ischemic cerebral infarct with only a 3% to 6% risk of neurologic sequelae and a good chance of long-term recovery.[104] Therefore, in the presence of urgent surgical indications that include HF, uncontrolled infection, or high-risk findings for recurrent embolism, it is generally agreed that surgery should not be postponed.[53] In the presence of intracranial hemorrhage, the neurologic prognosis is more guarded, and surgical therapy should be delayed for up to 1 month.[105] Surgical decisions should be made in conjunction with neurologists and, in some cases, neurosurgeons in addition to cardiologists, cardiothoracic surgeons, and infectious disease specialists.

In patients with CT evidence of hemorrhage, cerebral angiography is recommended because 10% to 50% of these patients have a ruptured mycotic aneurysm (MA).[108,109] MAs occur in 1.2% to 5% of IE patients and result from embolization of vegetations to the vasa vasorum.[110,111] The infection then spreads into the intima and through the vessel walls.[110,111] MAs are associated with an increased mortality rate that ranges from 30% for unruptured aneurysms to 80% for ruptured aneurysms.[112] The most common location for an MA is at the branch points of cerebral arteries, but visceral arteries and arteries of the extremities also may be involved. In the absence of signs or symptoms, routine screening for MAs is not indicated. When symptoms are present that suggest an MA, such as a focal neurologic deficit or localized severe headaches, magnetic resonance angiography (MRA) often is performed as the initial step. Conventional angiography is the procedure of choice for diagnosis, especially in the setting of inconclusive non-invasive imaging.[110]

Once the diagnosis of an intracranial MA has been established, monitoring with serial angiograms is recommended. If an MA is enlarging or bleeds, prompt repair should be performed.[108] Endovascular therapy is less invasive and offers a viable alternative to surgical clipping or ligation. It is recommended that cardiac surgery be delayed up to 2 weeks in patients with cerebral MAs that have ruptured or in those that have been repaired, but surgery may be considered earlier when a single MA is present and is adequately repaired, and the risk of bleeding with cardiopulmonary bypass is believed to be low.[113] Intracranial MAs often heal with medical therapy, whereas extracranial MAs usually rupture, so preemptive repair for these MAs is recommended. Symptoms of extracranial MA rupture include massive diarrhea (rupture of an MA into the bowel) or hematuria and increased blood pressure (rupture of a renal MA).

Although aspirin has been shown in some animal models to reduce vegetation size and embolism, a recent randomized clinical trial did not show any benefit related to embolization rate or in patients receiving aspirin therapy. Notably, patients receiving aspirin therapy in this trial had a high rate of bleeding complications[114]; therefore the routine use of aspirin is not recommended for the sole purpose of preventing embolic events, but it may be continued in patients with other clinical indications for aspirin therapy.[1] The risks and benefits of anticoagulation in the setting of IE are discussed in the next section in the context of PVE.

Prosthetic Valve Infections

Prosthetic valve IE can be devastating. The increased frequency of paravalvular invasion, particularly in early PVE, results in a greater incidence of complications such as HF, persistent fever, or new conduction abnormalities compared with NVE. The typical in-hospital mortality rates for PVE range from 13% to 25%, with long-term mortality rates that range from 29% to 48%.[10,69,84,115] Early PVE, defined as occurring within the first postoperative year, is associated with a particularly high mortality rate[10] and is more likely to be associated with paravalvular invasion and hemodynamically significant valvular lesions.

The frequency of PVE is highest during the first 3 months following implantation, remains high through the sixth postoperative month, and gradually declines to a relatively constant rate of 0.3% to 0.8% per year at 12 months and thereafter.[116-118] The infection risk may be higher for mechanical valves during the first year after implantation, but over time the risk of infection for a bioprosthetic valve increases, so that no overall difference is seen in infection rates between the two valve types 5 years postoperatively.[117,118] Patients with prosthetic valves who develop nosocomial bacteremia are at high risk for developing PVE, with an incidence of 11%.[119]

Anticoagulation therapy is controversial, although it is agreed that there is no role for the introduction of anticoagulation in patients who do not otherwise require it. Most experts continue administration of anticoagulation during therapy for mechanical valve IE; however, this approach has been questioned, particularly in patient populations at high risk for embolism, such as those with S. aureus infection, for the first 1 to 2 weeks of therapy.[120] In patients with S. aureus PVE with embolism, discontinuation of anticoagulation for a period of 2 weeks is recommended.[1] When anticoagulation is to be continued, oral anticoagulation should be discontinued during the acute phase and replaced with intravenous unfractionated heparin.

Certain clinical findings help to identify patients with PVE who are at high risk for complications and death when treated with medical therapy alone. Patients who develop pathologic murmurs or moderate to severe HF as a result of valve dysfunction, fever more than 10 days despite appropriate medical therapy, new-onset heart block, or echocardiographic evidence of abscess or valve dehiscence are at high risk for significant complications and death; such patients are unlikely to respond to medical therapy alone.[121,122] The addition of surgery to the treatment plan for high-risk patients results in greater survival rates, fewer relapses, and fewer rehospitalizations for valve surgery.[121,123,124] S. aureus PVE is associated with a particularly grave prognosis, with mortality rates that range from 28% to 82%.[68,69,121,122,125] Surgery appears to improve outcomes in S. aureus PVE regardless of the presence of cardiac complications.[125] Indications for surgical therapy of PVE are not absolute and should be implemented with careful attention to the relative risks and benefits in a given patient. For instance, observational evidence supports medical therapy alone for patients with late-onset PVE caused by viridans streptococci, HACEK group microorganisms (Haemophilus, Actinobacillus, Cardiobacterium, Eikenella, Kingella), or enterococci without evidence of paravalvular invasion or valve dysfunction.[126] If medical therapy alone is pursued, close and consistent follow-up is required.

Cardiac Device Infections

Cardiac device infections (CDIs) are becoming increasingly important and represent a serious cause of morbidity and mortality after device implantation. The published incidence varies from 1% to 5.6% in recent series,[127-130] and 10% to 15% of all CDIs involve an intracardiac lead; this type of infection is classified as *device endocarditis*.[131,132] Reported implantable cardioverter-defibrillator (ICD) infection rates, although not studied systematically, appear to be at least 0.8% to 1.5% in nonthoracotomy devices.[133-135] In the Medicare population, CDIs outpaced the increase in implantations from 1990 to 1999 with an increase from 0.94 to 2.11 infections per 1000 Medicare beneficiaries. This 124% relative increase may represent both an increase in the absolute number of patients with intracardiac devices and an increase in the at-risk years in the cohort.[136] With recent expanded indications for defibrillators and biventricular pacemakers,[137-140] rates of device infections can be expected to increase even further.

The importance of CDIs is further underscored when the cost of standard therapy is considered, which includes removal of the entire device, intravenous antibiotics, and, in most instances, reimplantation.[141] Once device endocarditis or other complicated device infection is confirmed, 4 to 6 weeks of appropriate antibiotic therapy is recommended based on microorganism susceptibilities.[142] The diagnosis of cardiac device endocarditis can be made using the modified Duke criteria for pacemaker leads, which also incorporates pulmonary emboli and local pocket symptoms. In addition, if a patient with an implanted cardiac device has typical signs and symptoms of right- or left-sided IE that include a murmur, recurrent or persistent bacteremia (>4 days on appropriate antibiotics) with a typical organism, or microscopic hematuria, cardiac device endocarditis should be considered high on the differential diagnosis. The initial exam in suspected device endocarditis is TEE because visualization of vegetations on intracardiac leads with TEE is superior to that of TTE. However, negative TEE findings do not exclude the possibility of a CDI in the appropriate clinical setting, particularly if a patient has high-grade bacteremia without an alternate source. Patients found to have bacteremia and a localized, uncomplicated CDI should be treated with 10 to 14 days of antimicrobial therapy after device removal.[142] *Staphylococcus epidermidis* and *S. aureus* are the most common infecting organisms.[128,141,143] Empiric therapy should be initiated accordingly and tailored later based on the identification and susceptibilities of the infecting organism.

Because of the unacceptably high relapse and death rates in patients with incomplete device removal, it is recommended that patients with CDIs undergo complete system removal in addition to antibiotic therapy.[128,141] Removal can be performed using a locking stylet, sheath, or percutaneous laser, with complete extraction success of 95%.[142,144] Historically, it has been recommended that vegetations greater than 1 cm be removed via an open surgical procedure.[145-147] However, percutaneous removal has been described in vegetations up to 7 cm in length without complications.[128,148] Prior to percutaneous removal of an intracardiac lead, an echocardiogram with contrast is recommended to rule out a right-to-left cardiac shunt, particularly when a large vegetation is evident. At the time of device removal, cultures should be performed from the device pocket and from all lead tips and mesh. Surgical removal is required in the setting of epicardial leads or in the presence of a right-to-left shunt, and it may be considered in the setting of a large, mobile vegetation on the lead. In pacemaker-dependent patients, temporary pacing is required, with leads placed on the ipsilateral side of infection proximal to the infected site.[149] Most authors recommend waiting at least 7 to 10 days prior to device replacement on the contralateral side and until serial blood cultures are sterile and signs of infection are absent.

Preventive measures can reduce CDIs. A preimplantation fever, the use of a temporary pacing wire prior to implantation, and early reintervention all increase the risk for infection.[150] Infections often are acquired at the time of device placement or during subsequent manipulation and often are latent. A meta-analysis and a randomized controlled trial of antibiotic prophylaxis prior to pacemaker placement have demonstrated a consistent protective effect, and prophylactic antibiotic use prior to device implantation should be considered the standard of care.[151,152]

Long-Term Outcomes and Management

Patients who survive an initial hospitalization for IE are subject to long-term complications related to the predisposing factors that led to the initial infection, progressive valvular damage, or the prosthetic heart valve placed in response to the initial infection. *Relapse*, defined as resumption of IE within 6 months of treatment with the same microorganism, occurs in approximately 3% of patients.[69,70,153] Recurrence, infection with a different organism or infection more than 6 months after the initial episode, occurs in 2.5% to 12.3% of hospital survivors.[10,69,153,154] It has also been noted that the probability of recurrence-free survival is lower in men and in the elderly.

Between 20% and 47% of patients with IE treated medically eventually require valve replacement, most within the first 2 years of follow-up.[69,70,153] Patients who receive valve replacements during the acute episode of IE or during the follow-up period are at risk for the complications associated with prosthetic heart valves, including valve degeneration, thromboembolic events, bleeding, and recurrent infection.[155] In published series, long-term mortality rates in hospital survivors vary greatly, and 10-year survival rates range from 48% to 80%.[59,61,70] Older age and recurrent endocarditis are significant predictors of death in the follow-up period.[153]

After the patient has completed the antibiotic course, any indwelling lines used for therapy should be promptly removed.[1] Surveillance blood cultures should be performed 5 to 7 days after discontinuation of antibiotics to confirm the effectiveness of therapy. A repeat TTE should be obtained after therapy to document the extent of residual valvular abnormalities and to reestablish baseline hemodynamics following valve repair or replacement surgery, and patients should be educated regarding antibiotic prophylaxis because they represent a high-risk group for recurrent IE. In addition, patients should be referred for dental treatment if necessary and scheduled for regular follow-up to assess for HF symptoms and evaluate for progressive valvular disease.[1]

Prevention

Approximately two thirds (53% to 70%) of patients with endocarditis have preexisting cardiac disease,[9,52,156] but no prospective, randomized, placebo-controlled studies have been done to evaluate IE prevention. Historically, the AHA had based recommendations for endocarditis prophylaxis on in vitro susceptibilities of microorganisms known to cause IE, on animal models of IE, and on the assumption that antimicrobial prophylaxis would prevent it. However, the effectiveness of antibiotic prophylaxis for prevention of IE was controversial and, in 2007, the AHA revised its IE prevention guidelines to reflect the paucity of data. The 2007 AHA guidelines on the prevention of IE concluded that most patients are at a greater risk of IE from bacteremia associated with daily activities, including tooth brushing, than from most dental and medical procedures; only a small number of IE cases were potentially prevented with IE prophylaxis, the risk of antibiotic-associated adverse events likely negated any benefit, and maintenance of optimal oral health was more important than prophylactic antibiotics prior to a dental procedure.[2]

The revised 2007 AHA guidelines on the prevention of IE recommend that only patients at the highest risk for IE-related complications should be considered for antibiotic therapy prior to *dental procedures*, defined as manipulation of gingival or periapical regions of teeth or perforation of the oral mucosa, because those patients are most likely to derive benefit from antibiotic prophylaxis (as defined in Table 43-7).[2] Antimicrobial therapy is primarily directed against *viridans* group streptococci. Prophylactic regimens are also recommended in high-risk patients undergoing invasive respiratory tract procedures and in those with infections that involve the skin or musculoskeletal tissue. IE prophylaxis is no

TABLE 43-7	Cardiac Conditions and Recommended Antibiotic Regimens with the Highest Risk of Adverse Outcomes from Infective Endocarditis in Which Dental Prophylaxis is Reasonable	
CARDIAC CONDITIONS	**ANTIBIOTIC PROPHYLACTIC REGIMEN***	**ANTIBIOTIC PROPHYLACTIC REGIMEN FOR PCN-ALLERGIC PATIENTS***
Prosthetic cardiac valve or prosthetic material used for cardiac valve repair Previous episode of IE Unrepaired cyanotic CHD (includes palliative shunts and conduits) Completely repaired CHD with prosthetic material or device during the first 6 months after the procedure Repaired CHD with residual defects at the site or adjacent to the site of a prosthetic patch or prosthetic device Cardiac transplant recipients with cardiac valvulopathy	*Able to take orally:* amoxicillin 2 g *Unable to take orally:* ampicillin 2 g IM or IV *or* cefazolin or ceftriaxone 1 g IM or IV	*Able to take orally:* cephalexin 2 g *or* other first- or second-generation oral cephalosporin in equivalent dosage *or* clindamycin 600 mg *or* azithromycin or clarithromycin 500 mg *Unable to take orally:* cefazolin or ceftriaxone 1 g IV *or* clindamycin 600 mg IV

*Antibiotics are given as a single dose 30 to 60 min before the procedure.
Avoid cephalosporins in patients with immediate hypersensitivity reactions to penicillins or ampicillin.
Avoid IM administration in patients receiving anticoagulant therapy.
CHD, congestive heart disease; IE, infective endocarditis; IM, intramuscular; IV, intravenous; PCN, penicillin.
From Wilson W, Taubert KA, Gewitz M, et al. Prevention of infective endocarditis: guidelines from the American Heart Association: a guideline from the American Heart Association Rheumatic Fever, Endocarditis, and Kawasaki Disease Committee, Council on Cardiovascular Disease in the Young, and the Council on Clinical Cardiology, Council on Cardiovascular Surgery and Anesthesia, and the Quality of Care and Outcomes Research Interdisciplinary Working Group. *Circulation* 2007;116:1736-1754.

longer recommended in patients who undergo routine gastrointestinal (GI) or genitourinary (GU) procedures.

The changes made in the 2007 AHA guidelines have been met with reluctance from some investigators, and they vary slightly from other published guidelines, including those of the National Institute for Health and Clinical Excellence and the ESC.[3,157] A recent Cochrane Review concluded that no evidence was available to support whether antibiotic prophylaxis was effective in the prevention of IE, but the review only included one case-control study with 349 patients.[158] Some argue that the actual risk of antibiotic use is low and that it is best to err on the side of caution, administering antibiotic prophylaxis until evidence to refute its effectiveness is presented, while also considering the desires of the patient.[159] Prospective randomized studies are needed to define the role of antibiotic prophylaxis in IE once and for all. These trials will be challenging to perform given widely differing predisposing cardiac conditions and the large sample size that would be required to produce meaningful results.

Future Directions

Identifying patients at risk for poor clinical outcomes remains difficult. A few studies have examined the correlation of cardiac biomarkers, including cardiac troponin and brain-type natriuretic peptide, with adverse events in IE patients.[160,161] Results of these pilot studies are promising and warrant further investigation.

Future directions in therapy for IE include possible novel preventive and therapeutic agents. As previously discussed, daptomycin provides promise in an era of multidrug-resistant organisms. Several novel antigens, monoclonal antibodies, and immunoglobulin therapies for *S. aureus* have been investigated in the treatment and prevention of bacteremia and infections, but the clinical benefit has been limited.[162,163] Pagibaximab, a monoclonal antibody directed against lipoteichoic acid, a cell-wall component of gram-positive bacteria, has demonstrated promise and is under continued investigation in low-birth-weight infants in the prevention of *S. aureus* infections (ClinicalTrials.gov, NCT00646399).

A shift in approach is necessary to further the understanding of IE. To develop the quality evidence needed to make therapeutic decisions that improve the outcomes of our patients, we must take advantage of recent advances in technology and information systems. An international effort in this area has led to opportunities to share data and conduct large-scale prospective cohort studies through the creation of the International Collaboration of Endocarditis (ICE) investigation. The first phase of the collaborative effort was to merge all existing databases into a single analysis database from which retrospective, descriptive studies are being performed. The second phase, the ICE Prospective Cohort Study (ICE-PCS), involved the development of a large global database of IE patients whose clinical, echocardiographic, and microbiologic findings have been characterized with standardized, predefined methods. The ICE-PCS enrolled 4794 patients from 64 centers in 28 countries who met the Duke criteria for definite IE. The multinational aspect provides a global view of IE in contrast to the relatively small case series, largely from single centers. Efforts of ICE investigators continue with a project-specific recruitment phase called *ICE-Plus.* Identifying patients at high risk for complications and targeting this population for preventative therapy is one of many potential benefits. It is hoped that the information gained from these efforts will be used to design and conduct randomized, controlled trials of treatment strategies to provide the definitive evidence needed to assist with therapeutic decision making.

Conclusions

Despite an improved understanding of the pathogenesis of IE and better diagnostic and therapeutic methods, the overall mortality rate has changed little over the past 50 years. The use of global databases, such as ICE, can improve knowledge about this heterogeneous disease, identify populations at risk for IE and its complications, and create collaborations among investigators that will lead to new therapeutic and preventative strategies.

We thank Dr. Christopher H. Cabell for his contributions to this chapter in earlier editions.

REFERENCES

1. Baddour LM, Wilson WR, Bayer AS, et al. Infective endocarditis: diagnosis, antimicrobial therapy, and management of complications: a statement for healthcare professionals from the Committee on Rheumatic Fever, Endocarditis, and Kawasaki Disease, Council on Cardiovascular Disease in the Young, and the Councils on Clinical Cardiology, Stroke, and Cardiovascular Surgery and Anesthesia, American Heart Association—executive summary. Endorsed by the Infectious Diseases Society of America. *Circulation* 2005;111:3167-3184.
2. Wilson W, Taubert KA, Gewitz M, et al. Prevention of infective endocarditis: guidelines from the American Heart Association: a guideline from the American Heart Association Rheumatic Fever, Endocarditis, and Kawasaki Disease Committee, Council on Cardiovascular Disease in the Young, and the Council on Clinical Cardiology, Council on Cardiovascular Surgery and Anesthesia, and the Quality of Care and Outcomes Research Interdisciplinary Working Group. *Circulation* 2007;116:1736-1754.
3. Habib G, Hoen B, Tornos P, et al. Guidelines on the prevention, diagnosis, and treatment of infective endocarditis (new version, 2009): the Task Force on the Prevention, Diagnosis, and Treatment of Infective Endocarditis of the European Society of Cardiology (ESC). Endorsed by the European Society of Clinical Microbiology and Infectious Diseases

(ESCMID) and the International Society of Chemotherapy (ISC) for Infection and Cancer. *Eur Heart J* 2009;30:2369-2413.
4. Durack DT, Lukes AS, Bright DK. New criteria for diagnosis of infective endocarditis: utilization of specific echocardiographic findings. Duke Endocarditis Service. *Am J Med* 1994;96:200-209.
5. Habib G, Derumeaux G, Avierinos JF, et al. Value and limitations of the Duke criteria for the diagnosis of infective endocarditis. *J Am Coll Cardiol* 1999;33:2023-2029.
6. Olaison L, Hogevik H. Comparison of the von Reyn and Duke criteria for the diagnosis of infective endocarditis: a critical analysis of 161 episodes. *Scand J Infect Dis* 1996; 28:399-406.
7. Li JS, Sexton DJ, Mick N, et al. Proposed modifications to the Duke criteria for the diagnosis of infective endocarditis. *Clin Infect Dis* 2000;30:633-638.
8. Cabell CH, Peterson GE, Anderson DJ, et al. Echocardiographic findings in 228 patients with endocarditis: the experience of the Duke Endocarditis Service from 1991-2000. *Circulation* 2000;102:II-445.
9. Hoen B, Alla F, Selton-Suty C, et al. Changing profile of infective endocarditis: results of a 1-year survey in France. *JAMA* 2002;288:75-81.
10. Castillo JC, Anguita MP, Ramirez A, et al. Long term outcome of infective endocarditis in patients who were not drug addicts: a 10 year study. *Heart* 2000;83:525-530.
11. Murdoch DR, Corey GR, Hoen B, et al. Clinical presentation, etiology, and outcome of infective endocarditis in the 21st century: the International Collaboration on Endocarditis-Prospective Cohort Study. *Arch Intern Med* 2009;169:463-473.
12. Bayer AS, Bolger AF, Taubert KA, et al. Diagnosis and management of infective endocarditis and its complications. *Circulation* 1998;98:2936-2948.
13. Chirillo F, Pedrocco A, De Leo A, et al. Impact of harmonic imaging on transthoracic echocardiographic identification of infective endocarditis and its complications. *Heart* 2005;91:329-333.
14. Jassal D, Aminbakhsh A, Fang T, et al. Diagnostic value of harmonic transthoracic echocardiography in native valve infective endocarditis: comparison with transesophageal echocardiography. *Cardiovasc Ultrasound* 2007;5:20.
15. Douglas PS, Khandheria B, Stainback RF, et al. ACCF/ASE/ACEP/ASNC/SCAI/SCCT/SCMR 2007 appropriateness criteria for transthoracic and transesophageal echocardiography: a report of the American College of Cardiology Foundation Quality Strategic Directions Committee Appropriateness Criteria Working Group, American Society of Echocardiography, American College of Emergency Physicians, American Society of Nuclear Cardiology, Society for Cardiovascular Angiography and Interventions, Society of Cardiovascular Computed Tomography, and the Society for Cardiovascular Magnetic Resonance. Endorsed by the American College of Chest Physicians and the Society of Critical Care Medicine. *J Am Soc Echocardiogr* 2007;20:787-805.
16. Kini V, Logani S, Ky B, et al. Transthoracic and transesophageal echocardiography for the indication of suspected infective endocarditis: vegetations, blood cultures and imaging. *J Am Soc Echocardiogr* 2010;23:396-402.
17. Heidenreich PA, Masoudi FA, Maini B, et al. Echocardiography in patients with suspected endocarditis: a cost-effectiveness analysis. *Am J Med* 1999;107:198-208.
18. Rosen AB, Fowler VG Jr, Corey GR, et al. Cost-effectiveness of transesophageal echocardiography to determine the duration of therapy for intravascular catheter-associated *Staphylococcus aureus* bacteremia. *Ann Int Med* 1999;130:810-820.
19. Kuruppu JC, Corretti M, Mackowiak P, et al. Overuse of transthoracic echocardiography in the diagnosis of native valve endocarditis. *Arch Int Med* 2002;162:1715-1720.
20. El-Ahdab F, Benjamin DK Jr, Wang A, et al. Risk of endocarditis among patients with prosthetic valves and *Staphylococcus aureus* bacteremia. *Am J Med* 2005;118: 225-229.
21. Wilson WR, Karchmer AW, Dajani AS, et al. Antibiotic treatment of adults with infective endocarditis due to streptococci, enterococci, staphylococci, and HACEK microorganisms. American Heart Association. *JAMA* 1995;274:1706-1713.
22. Torres-Tortosa M, de Cueto M, Vergara A, et al. Prospective evaluation of a two-week course of intravenous antibiotics in intravenous drug addicts with infective endocarditis. Grupo de Estudio de Enfermedades Infecciosas de la Provincia de Cadiz. *Eur J Clin Microbiol Infect Dis* 1994;13:559-564.
23. Chambers HF. Short-course combination and oral therapies of *Staphylococcus aureus* endocarditis. *Infect Dis Clin North Am* 1993;7:69-80.
24. Monteiro CA, Cobbs CG. Outpatient management of infective endocarditis. *Curr Infect Dis Rep* 2001;3:319-327.
25. Fowler VG, Boucher HW, Corey GR, et al. Daptomycin versus standard therapy for bacteremia and endocarditis caused by *Staphylococcus aureus*. *N Engl J Med* 2006; 355:653-665.
26. Cabell CH, Jollis JG, Peterson GE, et al. Changing patient characteristics and the effect on mortality in endocarditis. *Arch Int Med* 2002;162:90-94.
27. Miro JM, del Rio A, Mestres CA. Infective endocarditis in intravenous drug abusers and HIV-1 infected patients. *Infect Dis Clin North Am* 2002;16:273-295, vii-viii.
28. Delahaye F, Ecochard R, de Gevigney G, et al. The long term prognosis of infective endocarditis. *Eur Heart J* 1995;16(Suppl B):48-53.
29. Steckelberg JM, Melton LJ 3rd, Ilstrup DM, et al. Influence of referral bias on the apparent clinical spectrum of infective endocarditis. *Am J Med* 1990;88:582-588.
30. Selton-Suty C, Hoen B, Grentzinger A, et al. Clinical and bacteriological characteristics of infective endocarditis in the elderly. *Heart* 1997;77:260-263.
31. Di Salvo G, Thuny F, Rosenberg V, et al. Endocarditis in the elderly: clinical, echocardiographic, and prognostic features. *Eur Heart J* 2003;24:1576-1583.
32. Durante-Mangoni E, Bradley S, Selton-Suty C, et al. Current features of infective endocarditis in elderly patients: results of the International Collaboration on Endocarditis Prospective Cohort Study. *Arch Intern Med* 2008;168:2095-2103.
33. Abbott KC, Agodoa LY. Hospitalizations for valvular heart disease in chronic dialysis patients in the United States. *Nephron* 2002;92:43-50.
34. Abbott KC, Agodoa LY. Hospitalizations for bacterial endocarditis after initiation of chronic dialysis in the United States. *Nephron* 2002;91:203-209.
35. McCarthy JT, Steckelberg JM. Infective endocarditis in patients receiving long-term hemodialysis. *Mayo Clinic Proceedings* 2000;75:1008-1014.
36. Maraj S, Jacobs LE, Kung SC, et al. Epidemiology and outcome of infective endocarditis in hemodialysis patients. *Am J Med Sci* 2002;324:254-260.
37. Doulton T, Sabharwal N, Cairns HS, et al. Infective endocarditis in dialysis patients: new challenges and old. *Kidney Int* 2003;64:720-727.
38. Spies C, Madison JR, Schatz IJ. Infective endocarditis in patients with end-stage renal disease: clinical presentation and outcome. *Arch Intern Med* 2004;164:71-75.
39. Shroff GR, Herzog CA, Ma JZ, et al. Long-term survival of dialysis patients with bacterial endocarditis in the United States. *Am J Kidney Dis* 2004;44:1077-1082.
40. González C, Rubio M, Romero-Vivas J, et al. Bacteremic pneumonia due to *Staphylococcus aureus:* a comparison of disease caused by methicillin-resistant and methicillin-susceptible organisms. *Clin Infect Dis* 1999;29:1171-1177.
41. Marr KA, Sexton DJ, Conlon PJ, et al. Catheter-related bacteremia and outcome of attempted catheter salvage in patients undergoing hemodialysis. *Ann Intern Med* 1997;127:275-280.
42. Cabell CH, Heidenreich PA, Chu VH, et al. Increasing rates of cardiac device infections among Medicare beneficiaries: 1990-1999. *Am Heart J* 2004;147:582-586.
43. Wang A, Athan E, Pappas PA, et al. Contemporary clinical profile and outcome of prosthetic valve endocarditis. *JAMA* 2007;297:1354-1361.
44. Chamis AL, Peterson GE, Cabell CH, et al. *Staphylococcus aureus* bacteremia in patients with permanent pacemakers or implantable cardioverter-defibrillators. *Circulation* 2001;104:1029-1033.
45. Wilson LE, Thomas DL, Astemborski J, et al. Prospective study of infective endocarditis among injection drug users. *J Infect Dis* 2002;185:1761-1766.
46. Hogevik H, Olaison L, Andersson R, et al. Epidemiologic aspects of infective endocarditis in an urban population: a 5-year prospective study. *Medicine* 1995;74:324-339.
47. Currie PF, Sutherland GR, Jacob AJ, et al. A review of endocarditis in acquired immunodeficiency syndrome and human immunodeficiency virus infection. *Eur Heart J* 1995;16(Suppl B):15-18.
48. Gebo KA, Burkey MD, Lucas GM, et al. Incidence of, risk factors for, clinical presentation, and 1-year outcomes of infective endocarditis in an urban HIV cohort. *J Acquir Immune Defic Syndr* 2006;43:426-432.
49. De Rosa F, Cicalini S, Canta F, et al. Infective endocarditis in intravenous drug users from Italy: the increasing importance in HIV-infected patients. *Infection* 2007;35:154-160.
50. Jault F, Gandjbakhch I, Rama A, et al. Active native valve endocarditis: determinants of operative death and late mortality. *Ann Thorac Surg* 1997;63:1737-1741.
51. Larbalestier RI, Kinchla NM, Aranki SF, et al. Acute bacterial endocarditis: optimizing surgical results. *Circulation* 1992;86:68-74.
52. Alestig K, Hogevik H, Olaison L. Infective endocarditis: a diagnostic and therapeutic challenge for the new millennium. *Scand J Infect Dis* 2000;32:343-356.
53. Prendergast BD, Tornos P. Surgery for infective endocarditis: who and when? *Circulation* 2010;121:1141-1152.
54. Thuny F, Beurtheret S, Mancini J, et al. The timing of surgery influences mortality and morbidity in adults with severe complicated infective endocarditis: a propensity analysis. *Eur Heart J* 2011;32(16):2027-2033. Epub 2009 Mar 26.
55. d'Udekem Y, David TE, Feindel CM, et al. Long-term results of surgery for active infective endocarditis. *Eur J Cardiothorac Surg* 1997;11:46-52.
56. Olaison L, Hogevik H, Myken P, et al. Early surgery in infective endocarditis. *QJM* 1996;89:267-278.
57. Alexiou C, Langley SM, Stafford H, et al. Surgery for active culture-positive endocarditis: determinants of early and late outcome. *Ann Thorac Surg* 2000;69:1448-1454.
58. Bauernschmitt R, Jakob HG, Vahl C-F, et al. Operation for infective endocarditis: results after implantation of mechanical valve. *Ann Thorac Surg* 1998;65:359-364.
59. Aranki SF, Adams DH, Rizzo RJ, et al. Determinants of early mortality and late survival in mitral valve endocarditis. *Circulation* 1995;92(9 Suppl):II143-II149.
60. Moon MR, Stinson EB, Miller DC. Surgical treatment of endocarditis. *Prog Cardiovasc Dis* 1997;40:239-264.
61. Aranki SF, Santini F, Adams DH, et al. Aortic valve endocarditis: determinants of early survival and late morbidity. *Circulation* 1994;90(5 Pt 2):II175-II182.
62. Vikram HR, Buenconsejo J, Hasbun R, et al. Impact of valve surgery on 6-month mortality in adults with complicated, left-sided native valve endocarditis: a propensity analysis. *JAMA* 2003;290:3207-3214.
63. Sy RW, Bannon PG, Bayfield MS, et al. Survivor treatment selection bias and outcomes research: a case study of surgery in infective endocarditis. *Circ Cardiovasc Qual Outcomes* 2009;2:469-474.
64. Lalani T, Cabell CH, Benjamin DK, et al. Analysis of the impact of early surgery on in-hospital mortality of native valve endocarditis: use of propensity score and instrumental variable methods to adjust for treatment-selection bias. *Circulation* 2010;121:1005-1013.
65. San Román JA, López J, Revilla A, et al. Rationale, design, and methods for the early surgery in infective endocarditis study (ENDOVAL 1): a multicenter, prospective, randomized trial comparing the state-of-the-art therapeutic strategy versus early surgery strategy in infective endocarditis. *Am Heart J* 2008;156:431-436.
66. Haydock D, Barratt-Boyes B, Macedo T, et al. Aortic valve replacement for active infectious endocarditis in 108 patients: a comparison of freehand allograft valves with mechanical prostheses and bioprostheses. *J Thorac Cardiovasc Surg* 1992;103:130-139.
67. McGiffin DC, Galbraith AJ, McLachlan GJ, et al. Aortic valve infection: risk factors for death and recurrent endocarditis after aortic valve replacement. *J Thorac Cardiovasc Surg* 1992;104:511-520.
68. Wolff M, Witchitz S, Chastang C, et al. Prosthetic valve endocarditis in the ICU: prognostic factors of overall survival in a series of 122 cases and consequences for treatment decision. *Chest* 1995;108:688-694.
69. Tornos MP, Permanyer-Miralda G, Olona M, et al. Long-term complications of native valve infective endocarditis in non-addicts. A 15-year follow-up study. *Ann Intern Med* 1992;117:567-572.
70. Verheul HA, van den Brink RB, van Vreeland T, et al. Effects of changes in management of active infective endocarditis on outcome in a 25-year period. *Am J Cardiol* 1993; 72:682-687.

71. Mekontso Dessap A, Zahar JR, Voiriot G, et al. Influence of preoperative antibiotherapy on valve culture results and outcome of endocarditis requiring surgery. *J Infect* 2009; 59:42-48.
72. Middlemost S, Wisenbaugh T, Meyerowitz C, et al. A case for early surgery in native left-sided endocarditis complicated by heart failure: results in 203 patients. *J Am Coll Cardiol* 1991;18:663-667.
73. Iung B, Rousseau-Paziaud J, Cormier B, et al. Contemporary results of mitral valve repair for infective endocarditis. *J Am Coll Cardiol* 2004;43:386-392.
74. Sternik L, Zehr KJ, Orszulak TA, et al. The advantage of repair of mitral valve in acute endocarditis. *J Heart Valve Dis* 2002;11:91-97; discussion 97-98.
75. Zegdi R, Debieche M, Latremouille C, et al. Long-term results of mitral valve repair in active endocarditis. *Circulation* 2005;111:2532-2536.
76. Musci M, Weng Y, Hubler M, et al. Homograft aortic root replacement in native or prosthetic active infective endocarditis: twenty-year single-center experience. *J Thorac Cardiovasc Surg* 2010;139:665-673.
77. Glazier JJ, Verwilghen J, Donaldson RM, et al. Treatment of complicated prosthetic aortic valve endocarditis with annular abscess formation by homograft aortic root replacement. *J Am Coll Cardiol* 1991;17:1177-1182.
78. Ross D. Allograft root replacement for prosthetic endocarditis. *J Card Surg* 1990;5:68-72.
79. Sexton DJ, Spelman D. Current best practices and guidelines: assessment and management of complications in infective endocarditis. *Cardiol Clin* 2003;21:273-282, vii-viii.
80. Wilson WR, Danielson GK, Giuliani ER, et al. Cardiac valve replacement in congestive heart failure due to infective endocarditis. *Mayo Clin Proc* 1979;54:223-226.
81. Netzer RO, Altwegg SC, Zollinger E, et al. Infective endocarditis: determinants of long term outcome. *Heart* 2002;88:61-66.
82. Blumberg EA, Karalis DA, Chandrasekaran K, et al. Endocarditis-associated paravalvular abscesses. Do clinical parameters predict the presence of abscess? *Chest* 1995;107: 898-903.
83. Petrou M, Wong K, Albertucci M, et al. Evaluation of unstented aortic homografts for the treatment of prosthetic aortic valve endocarditis. *Circulation* 1994;90:II198-II204.
84. Lytle BW, Priest BP, Taylor PC, et al. Surgical treatment of prosthetic valve endocarditis. *J Thorac Cardiovasc Surg* 1996;111:198-207; discussion 207-210.
85. Omari B, Shapiro S, Ginzton L, et al. Predictive risk factors for periannular extension of native valve endocarditis: clinical and echocardiographic analyses. *Chest* 1989;96: 1273-1279.
86. Meine TJ, Nettles RE, Anderson DJ, et al. Cardiac conduction abnormalities in endocarditis defined by the Duke criteria. *Am Heart J* 2001;142:280-285.
87. Aguado JM, Gonzalez-Vilchez F, Martin-Duran R, et al. Perivalvular abscesses associated with endocarditis: clinical features and diagnostic accuracy of two-dimensional echocardiography. *Chest* 1993;104:88-93.
88. Choussat R, Thomas D, Isnard R, et al. Perivalvular abscesses associated with endocarditis; clinical features and prognostic factors of overall survival in a series of 233 cases. Perivalvular Abscesses French Multicentre Study. *Eur Heart J* 1999;20:232-241.
89. San Roman JA, Vilacosta I, Sarria C, et al. Clinical course, microbiologic profile, and diagnosis of periannular complications in prosthetic valve endocarditis. *Am J Cardiol* 1999;83:1075-1079. .
90. d'Udekem Y, David TE, Feindel CM, et al. Long-term results of operation for paravalvular abscess. *Ann Thorac Surg* 1996;62:48-53.
91. Vlessis AA, Hovaguimian H, Jaggers J, et al. Infective endocarditis: ten-year review of medical and surgical therapy. *Ann Thorac Surg* 1996;61:1217-1222.
92. Anguera I, Miro JM, Evangelista A, et al. Periannular complications in infective endocarditis involving native aortic valves. *Am J Cardiol* 2006;98:1254-1260.
93. Millaire A, Leroy O, Gaday V, et al. Incidence and prognosis of embolic events and metastatic infections in infective endocarditis. *Eur Heart J* 1997;18:677-684.
94. Heiro M, Nikoskelainen J, Engblom E, et al. Neurologic manifestations of infective endocarditis: a 17-year experience in a teaching hospital in Finland. *Arch Intern Med* 2000;160:2781-2787.
95. Cabell CH, Pond KK, Peterson GE, et al. The risk of stroke and death in patients with aortic and mitral valve endocarditis. *Am Heart J* 2001;142:75-80.
96. Dickerman SA, Abrutyn E, Barsic B, et al. The relationship between the initiation of antimicrobial therapy and the incidence of stroke in infective endocarditis: an analysis from the ICE Prospective Cohort Study (ICE-PCS). *Am Heart J* 2007;154:1086-1094.
97. Anavekar NS, Tleyjeh IM, Anavekar NS, et al. Impact of prior antiplatelet therapy on risk of embolism in infective endocarditis. *Clin Infect Dis* 2007;44:1180-1186.
98. Thuny F, Disalvo G, Belliard O, et al. Risk of embolism and death in infective endocarditis: prognostic value of echocardiography: a prospective multicenter study. *Circulation* 2005;112:69-75.
99. Tischler MD, Vaitkus PT. The ability of vegetation size on echocardiography to predict clinical complications: a meta-analysis. *J Am Soc Echocardiogr* 1997;10:562-568.
100. Snygg-Martin U, Gustafsson L, Rosengren L, et al. Cerebrovascular complications in patients with left-sided infective endocarditis are common: a prospective study using magnetic resonance imaging and neurochemical brain damage markers. *Clin Infect Dis* 2008;47:23-30.
101. Hill EE, Herijgers P, Claus P, et al. Clinical and echocardiographic risk factors for embolism and mortality in infective endocarditis. *Eur J Clin Microbiol Infect Dis* 2008;27:1159-1164.
102. Di Salvo G, Habib G, Pergola V, et al. Echocardiography predicts embolic events in infective endocarditis. *J Am Coll Cardiol* 2001;37:1069-1076.
103. Kim D-H, Kang D-H, Lee M-Z, et al. Impact of early surgery on embolic events in patients with infective endocarditis. *Circulation* 2010;122:S17-S22.
104. Ruttmann E, Willeit J, Ulmer H, et al. Neurological outcome of septic cardioembolic stroke after infective endocarditis. *Stroke* 2006;37:2094-2099.
105. Piper C, Wiemer M, Schulte HD, et al. Stroke is not a contraindication for urgent valve replacement in acute infective endocarditis. *J Heart Valve Dis* 2001;10:703-711.
106. Durante Mangoni E, Adinolfi LE, Tripodi MF, et al. Risk factors for "major" embolic events in hospitalized patients with infective endocarditis. *Am Heart J* 2003;146: 311-316.
107. Thuny F, Avierinos JF, Tribouilloy C, et al. Impact of cerebrovascular complications on mortality and neurologic outcome during infective endocarditis: a prospective multicentre study. *Eur Heart J* 2007;28:1155-1161.
108. Gillinov AM, Shah RV, Curtis WE, et al. Valve replacement in patients with endocarditis and acute neurologic deficit. *Ann Thorac Surg* 1996;61:1125-1129, discussion 1130.
109. Hart RG, Kagan-Hallet K, Joerns SE. Mechanisms of intracranial hemorrhage in infective endocarditis. *Stroke* 1987;18:1048-1056.
110. Camarata PJ, Latchaw RE, Rufenacht DA, et al. Intracranial aneurysms. *Invest Radiol* 1993;28:373-382.
111. Clare CE, Barrow DL. Infectious intracranial aneurysms. *Neurosurg Clin N Am* 1992;3:551-566.
112. Bohmfalk GL, Story JL, Wissinger JP, et al. Treatment of mycotic aneurysms. *J Neurosurg* 1981;54:566-567.
113. Chapot R, Houdart E, Saint-Maurice J-P, et al. Endovascular treatment of cerebral mycotic aneurysms. *Radiology* 2002;222:389-396.
114. Chan KL, Dumesnil JG, Cujec B, et al. A randomized trial of aspirin on the risk of embolic events in patients with infective endocarditis. *J Am Coll Cardiol* 2003;42:775-780.
115. Habib G, Tribouilloy C, Thuny F, et al. Prosthetic valve endocarditis: who needs surgery? A multicentre study of 104 cases. *Heart* 2005;91:954-959.
116. Glower DD, Landolfo KP, Cheruvu S, et al. Determinants of 15-year outcome with 1,119 standard Carpentier-Edwards porcine valves. *Ann Thorac Surg* 1998;66:S44-S48.
117. Calderwood SB, Swinski LA, Waternaux CM, et al. Risk factors for the development of prosthetic valve endocarditis. *Circulation* 1985;72:31-37.
118. Grover FL, Cohen DJ, Oprian C, et al. Determinants of the occurrence of and survival from prosthetic valve endocarditis. Experience of the Veterans Affairs Cooperative Study on Valvular Heart Disease. *J Thorac Cardiovasc Surg* 1994;108:207-214.
119. Fang G, Keys TF, Gentry LO, et al. Prosthetic valve endocarditis resulting from nosocomial bacteremia: a prospective, multicenter study. *Ann Int Med* 1993;119:560-567.
120. Tornos P, Almirante B, Mirabet S, et al. Infective endocarditis due to *Staphylococcus aureus:* deleterious effect of anticoagulant therapy. *Arch Intern Med* 1999;159:473-475.
121. Calderwood SB, Swinski LA, Karchmer AW, et al. Prosthetic valve endocarditis: analysis of factors affecting outcome of therapy. *J Thorac Cardiovasc Surg* 1986;92:776-783.
122. Yu VL, Fang GD, Keys TF, et al. Prosthetic valve endocarditis: superiority of surgical valve replacement versus medical therapy only. *Ann Thorac Surg* 1994;58:1073-1077.
123. Koya D, Ryuichi K, Haneda M. Infective endocarditis. *New Engl J Med* 2002;346:782-783.
124. Tornos P, Almirante B, Olona M, et al. Clinical outcome and long-term prognosis of late prosthetic valve endocarditis: a 20-year experience. *Clin Infect Dis* 1997;24: 381-386.
125. John MD, Hibberd PL, Karchmer AW, et al. *Staphylococcus aureus* prosthetic valve endocarditis: optimal management and risk factors for death. *Clin Infect Dis* 1998;26:1302-1309.
126. Akowuah EF, Davies W, Oliver S, et al. Prosthetic valve endocarditis: early and late outcome following medical or surgical treatment. *Heart* 2003;89:269-272.
127. Mela T, McGovern BA, Garan H, et al. Long-term infection rates associated with the pectoral versus abdominal approach to cardioverter-defibrillator implants. *Am J Cardiol* 2001;88:750-753.
128. del Rio A, Anguera I, Miro JM, et al. Surgical treatment of pacemaker and defibrillator lead endocarditis: the impact of electrode lead extraction on outcome. *Chest* 2003;124:1451-1459.
129. Nery PB, Fernandes R, Nair GM, et al. Device-related infection among patients with pacemakers and implantable defibrillators: incidence, risk factors, and consequences. *J Cardiovasc Electrophysiol* 2010;21:786-790.
130. Catanchin A, Murdock CJ, Athan E. Pacemaker infections: a 10-year experience. *Heart Lung Circ* 2007;16:434-439.
131. Baddour LM, Bettmann MA, Bolger AF, et al. Nonvalvular cardiovascular device-related infections. *Circulation* 2003;108:2015-2031.
132. Gandelman G, Frishman WH, Wiese C, et al. Intravascular device infections: epidemiology, diagnosis, and management. *Cardiol Rev* 2007;15:13-23.
133. Gold MR, Peters RW, Johnson JW, et al. Complications associated with pectoral implantation of cardioverter defibrillators. World-Wide Jewel Investigators. *Pacing Clin Electrophysiol* 1997;20:208-211.
134. Smith PN, Vidaillet HJ, Hayes JJ, et al. Infections with nonthoracotomy implantable cardioverter defibrillators: can these be prevented? Endotak Lead Clinical Investigators. *Pacing Clin Electrophysiol* 1998;21:42-55.
135. O'Nunain S, Perez I, Roelke M, et al. The treatment of patients with infected implantable cardioverter-defibrillator systems. *J Thorac Cardiovasc Surg* 1997;113:121-129.
136. Cabell CH, Heidenreich PA, Chu V, et al. Increasing rates of cardiac device infections among Medicare beneficiaries: 1990-1999. *Am Heart J* 2003;147(4)582-586.
137. Moss AJ, Hall WJ, Cannom DS, et al. Improved survival with an implanted defibrillator in patients with coronary disease at high risk for ventricular arrhythmia. Multicenter Automatic Defibrillator Implantation Trial Investigators. *N Engl J Med* 1996;335: 1933-1940.
138. Buxton AE, Lee KL, Fisher JD, et al. A randomized study of the prevention of sudden death in patients with coronary artery disease. Multicenter Unsustained Tachycardia Trial Investigators. *N Engl J Med* 1999;341:1882-1890.
139. Cazeau S, Leclercq C, Lavergne T, et al. Effects of multisite biventricular pacing in patients with heart failure and intraventricular conduction delay. *N Engl J Med* 2001;344:873-880.
140. Gras D, Leclercq C, Tang AS, et al. Cardiac resynchronization therapy in advanced heart failure: the multicenter InSync clinical study. *Eur J Heart Fail* 2002;4:311-320.
141. Chua JD, Wilkoff BL, Lee I, et al. Diagnosis and management of infections involving implantable electrophysiologic cardiac devices. *Ann Intern Med* 2000;133:604-608.
142. Baddour LM, Epstein AE, Erickson CC, et al. Update on cardiovascular implantable electronic device infections and their management: a scientific statement from the American Heart Association. *Circulation* 2010;121:458-477.
143. Cacoub P, Leprince P, Nataf P, et al. Pacemaker infective endocarditis. *Am J Cardiol* 1998;82:480-484.

144. Wilkoff BL, Byrd CL, Love CJ, et al. Pacemaker lead extraction with the laser sheath: results of the pacing lead extraction with the excimer sheath (PLEXES) trial. *J Am Coll Cardiol* 1999;33:1671-1676.

145. Victor F, De Place C, Camus C, et al. Pacemaker lead infection: echocardiographic features, management, and outcome. *Heart* 1999;81:82-87.

146. Meier-Ewert HK, Gray ME, John RM. Endocardial pacemaker or defibrillator leads with infected vegetations: a single-center experience and consequences of transvenous extraction. *Am Heart J* 2003;146:339-344.

147. Grammes JA, Schulze CM, Al-Bataineh M, et al. Percutaneous pacemaker and implantable cardioverter-defibrillator lead extraction in 100 patients with intracardiac vegetations defined by transesophageal echocardiogram. *J Am Coll Cardiol* 2010;55:886-894.

148. Sohail MR. Management of infected pacemakers and implantable cardioverter-defibrillators. *Intern Med J* 2007;37:509-510; author reply 510.

149. Rastan AJ, Doll N, Walther T, et al. Pacemaker dependent patients with device infection: a modified approach. *Eur J Cardiothorac Surg* 2005;27:1116-1118.

150. Klug D, Balde M, Gilles L, et al. Implantable antiarrhythmic systems-related infections: results of a large prospective study on 6319 patients. *Heart Rhythm* 2005;2:S41.

151. de Oliveira JC, Martinelli M, Nishioka SA, et al. Efficacy of antibiotic prophylaxis before the implantation of pacemakers and cardioverter-defibrillators: results of a large, prospective, randomized, double-blinded, placebo-controlled trial. *Circ Arrhythm Electrophysiol* 2009;2:29-34.

152. Da Costa A, Kirkorian G, Cucherat M, et al. Antibiotic prophylaxis for permanent pacemaker implantation: a meta-analysis. *Circulation* 1998;97:1796-1801.

153. Mansur AJ, Dal Bo CM, Fukushima JT, et al. Relapses, recurrences, valve replacements, and mortality during the long-term follow-up after infective endocarditis. *Am Heart J* 2001;141:78-86.

154. Cherubin CE, Neu HC. Infective endocarditis at the Presbyterian Hospital in New York City from 1938-1967. *Am J Med* 1971;51:83-96.

155. Vongpatanasin W, Hillis LD, Lange RA. Prosthetic heart valves. *N Engl J Med* 1996;335:407-416.

156. Werner GS, Schulz R, Fuchs JB, et al. Infective endocarditis in the elderly in the era of transesophageal echocardiography: clinical features and prognosis compared with younger patients. *Am J Med* 1996;100:90-97.

157. Richey R, Wray D, Stokes T. Prophylaxis against infective endocarditis: summary of NICE guidance. *BMJ* 2008;336:770-771.

158. Esposito M, Grusovin MG, Coulthard P, et al. The efficacy of antibiotic prophylaxis at placement of dental implants: a Cochrane systematic review of randomised controlled clinical trials. *Eur J Oral Implantol* 2008;1:95-103.

159. Bach DS. Perspectives on the American College of Cardiology/American Heart Association guidelines for the prevention of infective endocarditis. *J Am Coll Cardiol* 2009; 53:1852-1854.

160. Purcell JB, Patel M, Khera A, et al. Relation of troponin elevation to outcome in patients with infective endocarditis. *Am J Cardiol* 2008;101:1479-1481.

161. Shiue AB, Stancoven AB, Purcell JB, et al. Relation of level of B-type natriuretic peptide with outcomes in patients with infective endocarditis. *Am J Cardiol* 2010; 106:1011-1015.

162. Weems JJ, Jr., Steinberg JP, Filler S, et al. Phase II, randomized, double-blind, multicenter study comparing the safety and pharmacokinetics of tefibazumab to placebo for treatment of *Staphylococcus aureus* bacteremia. *Antimicrob Agents Chemother* 2006; 50:2751-2755.

163. Shah PS, Kaufman DA. Antistaphylococcal immunoglobulins to prevent staphylococcal infection in very low birth weight infants. *Cochrane Database Syst Rev* 2009:CD006449.

164. Casella F, Rana B, Casazza G, et al. The potential impact of contemporary transthoracic echocardiography on the management of patients with native valve endocarditis: a comparison with transesophageal echocardiography. *Echocardiography* 2009;26: 900-906.

165. Jassal DS, Aminbakhsh A, Fang T, et al. Diagnostic value of harmonic transthoracic echocardiography in native valve infective endocarditis: comparison with transesophageal echocardiography. *Cardiovasc Ultrasound* 2007;5:20.

166. Shively BK, Gurule FT, Roldan CA, et al. Diagnostic value of transesophageal compared with transthoracic echocardiography in infective endocarditis. *J Am Coll Cardiol* 1991;18:391-397.

167. Shapiro SM, Young E, De Guzman S, et al. Transesophageal echocardiography in diagnosis of infective endocarditis. *Chest* 1994;105:377-382.

168. Reynolds HR, Jagen MA, Tunick PA, et al. Sensitivity of transthoracic versus transesophageal echocardiography for the detection of native valve vegetations in the modern era. *J Am Soc Echocardiogr* 2003;16:67-70.

169. Morguet AJ, Werner GS, Andreas S, et al. Diagnostic value of transesophageal compared with transthoracic echocardiography in suspected prosthetic valve endocarditis. *Herz* 1995;20:390-398.

170. Vered Z, Mossinson D, Peleg E, et al. Echocardiographic assessment of prosthetic valve endocarditis. *Eur Heart J* 1995;16(Suppl B):63-67.

171. Khandheria BK. Transesophageal echocardiography in the evaluation of prosthetic valves. *Am J Card Imaging* 1995;9:106-114.

172. Daniel WG, Mugge A, Martin RP, et al. Improvement in the diagnosis of abscesses associated with endocarditis by transesophageal echocardiography. *New Engl J Med* 1991;324:795-800.

173. Mylonakis E, Calderwood SB. Infective endocarditis in adults. *New Engl J Med* 2001;345:1318-1330.

CHAPTER 44 Treatment of Pericardial Disease

Brian D. Hoit

ACUTE PERICARDITIS, 667

RECURRENT PERICARDITIS, 668

PERICARDIAL EFFUSION AND TAMPONADE, 669

CONSTRICTIVE PERICARDITIS, 671

TREATMENT OF SPECIFIC CAUSES OF PERICARDITIS, 672

Purulent Pericarditis, 672
Mycobacterial and Fungal Pericarditis, 672

Human Immunodeficiency Virus–Associated Pericarditis, 673
Neoplastic Pericarditis, 673
Pericarditis Complicating Myocardial Infarction and the
    Postpericardial Injury Syndrome, 673
Radiation-Induced Pericardial Disease, 673
Traumatic Pericardial Disease, 674
Chylopericardium, 674
Pericardial Disease in Patients with Renal Failure, 674

Myxedema Pericardial Disease, 674
Connective Tissue Disease–Related Pericardial Disease, 674
Pericardial Disease and Pregnancy, 674
Drug-Induced and Iatrogenic Pericardial Disease, 674
Anticoagulation in Pericarditis, 674

REFERENCES, 675

The treatment of pericardial disease is often simple and rewarding; however, it may offer unexpected challenges and frustrations to both clinician and patient for a number of reasons. First, the presence of pericardial heart disease may elude detection because it often remains clinically silent, apparent only during the evaluation of unrelated symptoms. Moreover, although pericardial disease may be seen as an isolated phenomenon, it may complicate a number of systemic disorders and be overshadowed by extracardiac manifestations. Second, although the European Society of Cardiology (ESC) published guidelines for the diagnosis and management of pericardial diseases,[1] a paucity of randomized, placebo-controlled trials exist (level of evidence: A) from which appropriate therapy may be selected and important clinical decisions made (Table 44-1). Thus the physician often must rely heavily on clinical judgment because most data originate from small, uncontrolled trials and anecdotal experience. Finally, therapeutic options, in most cases, are limited to nonspecific antiinflammatory agents, drainage of pericardial fluid, and pericardiectomy. Although there is general agreement on how these measures should be applied in the patient with either mild or severe disease, there is little consensus on how the large number of cases encountered with clinical manifestations between these two extremes should be managed. Recognizing the subjective nature of many of the therapeutic recommendations, this chapter reviews the options available for treating pericardial heart disease.

Acute Pericarditis

Acute fibrinous, or "dry," pericarditis is a syndrome characterized by typical chest pain, a pathognomonic pericardial friction rub, and specific electrocardiographic (ECG) changes. To determine an etiology and to watch for the development of cardiac tamponade, hospitalization is warranted for most patients who come to medical attention with an initial episode of acute pericarditis, particularly those with moderate or large effusions or those with high-risk features such as elevated temperature, subacute onset, immunosupression, recent trauma, oral anticoagulant therapy, aspirin or nonsterioidal antiinflammatory drug (NSAID) failure, and myopericarditis. Close early follow-up is important in the remainder. Establishing the exact cause of acute pericarditis is an important part of management, but considerable judgment must be exercised when deciding whether and how to investigate the possibility of concomitant systemic disease. For example, an extensive evaluation is generally unnecessary in a young, previously healthy adult who is seen initially with a viral syndrome, typical pericardial chest pain, and a pericardial friction rub. Despite the availability of polymerase chain reaction (PCR) and histochemistry for etiolopathogenetic classification,[2] most cases of viral pericarditis are recognized long after the period of viral activity, making a specific etiologic diagnosis and antiviral chemotherapy unnecessary. Recently, a prospective study of 300 consecutive patients with acute pericarditis addressed this issue. Patients at low risk (n = 254, or 85%) were not hospitalized but were treated empirically with aspirin (800 mg every 6 to 8 hours for 7 to 10 days) without an etiologic search. The strategy was both cost effective and safe; no cases of cardiac tamponade were seen, and the majority of low-risk cases (91%) had a final diagnosis of viral or idiopathic pericarditis after a mean follow-up of 38 months.[3]

Acute pericarditis usually responds to oral NSAIDs, such as acetylsalicylic acid (ASA) 650 mg every 3 to 4 hours or ibuprofen 300 to 800 mg every 6 hours for 7 to 10 days. Indomethacin reduces coronary blood flow and should be avoided. Prophylaxis against gastrointestinal (GI) bleeding with H2 blockers or proton pump inhibitors is warranted, particularly in those at high risk or in those who require longer durations of treatment. Selective cyclooxygenase (COX)-2 inhibitors are NSAIDs with few adverse GI effects, but they have been implicated in adverse cardiovascular events[4]; moreover, COX-2 inhibitors have not been tested in acute pericarditis.

Cumulative anecdotal data, expert consensus, and an open-label clinical trial[5] suggest that addition of colchicine at 1 mg/day for 3 months, with or without a 2-mg loading dose, is effective for the acute episode, is well tolerated, and may prevent recurrences. Accordingly, it has been given a class IIa recommendation in the ESC guidelines.[1] Side effects of colchicine include diarrhea, nausea, and abdominal pain but are usually mild and rarely necessitate withdrawal of the drug. Common side effects (1% to 10%) at higher doses include elevated transaminases and alopecia. Bone marrow suppression, hepatotoxicity, and myotoxicity are less common, and azoospermia is rare. Colchicine is contraindicated in those with severe renal, GI, hepatic, or cardiac disorders and with blood dyscrasias and pregnancy.[5]

Chest pain is alleviated in 1 to 2 days, and the friction rub and ST-segment elevation resolve shortly thereafter. Although most mild cases of idiopathic and viral pericarditis are adequately treated with 1 week of treatment, the optimal duration of treatment is controversial. In the open-label, randomized Colchicine for Acute Pericarditis (COPE) trial, colchicine (0.5 to 1 mg/day for 3 months) as an adjunct to conventional treatment significantly decreased the recurrence rate (10.7% vs. 32.3% at 18 months) and also decreased symptom persistence at 72 hours (11.7% vs. 36.7%) in 120 patients with a first episode of acute pericarditis.[6] The intensity of therapy is dictated by the distress of the patient, and narcotics may be required for severe pain. Some cases necessitate steroid therapy (prednisone 60 to 80 mg/day) for 1 week to control pain, with the dosage tapered carefully on an individual basis thereafter. However, corticosteroids should be avoided unless there are specific indications, such as connective tissue disease and autoreactive or uremic pericarditis, because corticosteroids enhance viral multiplication and may result in recurrences when the dosage is tapered; colchicine may be particularly useful in this situation. Importantly, tuberculous

TABLE 44-1	Summary of the European Society of Cardiology Guidelines on the Diagnosis and Management of Pericardial Heart Disease		
		INDICATION	EVIDENCE
Acute Pericarditis			
Nonsteroidal antiinflammatory drugs		Class I	Level B
Colchicine*		Class IIa	Level B
Systemic corticosteroids†		Class IIa	Level B
Chronic Pericarditis			
Balloon pericardiotomy or pericardiectomy‡		Class IIb	Level B
Recurrent Pericarditis			
Colchicine		Class I	Level B
Systemic corticosteroids§		Class IIa	Level C
Pericardiectomy¶		Class IIa	Level B
Pericardial Effusion			
Pericardiocentesis for cardiac tamponade		Class I	Level B
Pericardiocentesis for smaller effusions		Class IIa	Level B
Analysis of Pericardial Fluid			
Pericardial fluid and blood for bacteria		Class I	Level B
PCR, ADA, IF-γ, lysozyme for tuberculosis		Class I	Level B
PCR, in situ hybridization for virus		Class IIa	Level B
PCR, in situ hybridization for virus		Class IIb	Level B
Pericardial chemistry (specific gravity, protein, LDH, glucose)		Class IIb	Level B
Specific Forms of Pericarditis			
Corticosteroids for tuberculous pericarditis		Class IIb	Level A
Pericardiocentesis for tamponade and large effusions unresponsive to dialysis		Class IIa	Level B
Pericardiocentesis for large neoplastic effusions		Class I	Level B
Diagnostic pericardiocentesis in suspected neoplastic effusion		Class IIa	Level B
Intrapericardial instillation of cytotoxic sclerosing agent for neoplastic pericarditis		Class IIa	Level B
Radiation therapy for control of effusions in patients with radiosensitive tumors		Class IIa	Level B
Percutaneous balloon pericardiotomy for malignant effusions		Class IIa	Level B
Pleuropericardiotomy to drain malignant effusions		Class IIb	Level C
Surgical therapy of chylous effusion resistant to diet and pericardiocentesis		Class I	Level B
Thyroid hormone for effusion secondary to myxedema		Class I	Level B

*For initial attack and prevention of recurrences.
†For connective tissue disease–associated, autoreactive, and uremic effusions.
‡For frequent and symptomatic recurrences.
§For recurrent pericarditis in patients in poor general condition or in frequent crises.
¶For frequent, highly symptomatic recurrences resistant to medical therapy.
ADA, adenosine deaminase; IF-γ, interferon-γ; LDH, lactate dehydrogenase; PCR, polymerase chain reaction.
From Maisch B, Seferovic PM, Ristic AD, et al. Guidelines on the diagnosis and management of pericardial diseases: executive summary. The Task Force on the Diagnosis and Management of Pericardial Diseases of the European Society of Cardiology. *Eur Heart J* 2004;25:587-610.

and pyogenic pericarditis should be excluded before steroid therapy is initiated. Intrapericardial instillation of triamcinolone (300 mg/m^2) avoids systemic side effects and is highly effective.[2] Patients in whom pericarditis represents one manifestation of systemic illness—such as sepsis, uremia, connective tissue disease, or neoplasia—should also receive therapy directed toward the primary disorder in addition to palliative and supportive treatment.

Recurrent Pericarditis

Recurrent or relapsing acute pericarditis is one of the most distressing disorders of the pericardium for both patient and physician. It may occur with or without pericardial effusion and occasionally is associated with pleural effusion or parenchymal pulmonary lesions. Atypical features, such as the absence of physical findings, offer challenges for diagnosis and management and often necessitate close follow-up and rigorous emotional support. Recurrences occur with highly variable frequency over a course of many years. Although they may be spontaneous, recurrences are more commonly associated with either discontinuation or tapering of antiinflammatory drugs.

Painful recurrences of pericarditis may respond to NSAIDs but may require corticosteroids. Increasing evidence suggests that colchicine (0.5 mg orally twice a day for 6 to 12 months with a gradual taper) should be used with NSAIDs before steroid therapy. In the Colchicine for Recurrent Pericarditis (CORE) trial, adjunctive colchicine (0.5 to 1 mg/day for 6 months) significantly decreased symptom persistence at 72 hours (9.5% vs. 31.0%) and also decreased the recurrence rate at 18 months (24.0% vs. 50.6%).[7] A number of ongoing multicenter, double-blind, randomized trials should clarify the role of colchicine in the treatment and prevention of pericarditis.

Once steroids are administered, dependency and the development of steroid-induced abnormalities are potential sequelae. Prednisone is usually begun at a high dose (60 to 80 mg/day) for at least 4 weeks and is slowly tapered over the next 3 months.[8] When necessary, the risks of long-term steroid use should be minimized by using the lowest possible dose, initiating alternate-day therapy, and/or selecting combinations with nonsteroidal drugs or colchicine. In the most difficult cases, relapse occurs every time the dose of prednisone is reduced below 5 to 20 mg/day. When this occurs, the patient should be maintained for several weeks on the lowest suppressive dose before the next taper commences (e.g., 1 to 2.5 mg at intervals of 2 to 6 weeks). During tapering, colchicine should be considered, starting with low doses (0.5 to 0.6 mg). Intrapericardial administration of triamcinolone (300 mg/m^2) has been shown to relieve symptoms in patients with recurrent autoreactive myopericarditis,[9] and azathioprine (50 to 100 mg/day) has also been used to prevent recurrent episodes.[8] Although encouraging results have been reported in a series of patients who underwent pericardiectomy for recurrent pericarditis, pericardiectomy may simply abbreviate, rather than terminate, the painful recurrences. Thus, pericardiectomy should be considered only when repeated attempts at medical treatment have clearly failed.

A recent retrospective, nonrandomized study in 100 patients with recurrences challenges the common practice of using high doses of corticosteroids.[10] Patients were assigned to either a low dose (0.2 to 0.5 mg/kg/day) or high dose (1 mg/kg/day) of prednisone for 4 weeks, followed by a slow taper. Those who received high doses of prednisone, compared with those who received low doses, had a higher rate of severe side effects (23.5% vs. 2%), recurrences (64.7% vs. 32.6%), and disease-related hospitalizations (31.4% vs. 8.2%). Guidelines recommend osteoporosis prevention when corticosteroids are used (calcium 1500 mg/day and vitamin D 800 IU/day) or an activated form of vitamin D, and bisphosphonates are given to prevent bone loss in men and in postmenopausal women; long-term treatment is initiated at a dose greater than 5 mg/day for postmenopausal women.[11]

Pericardial Effusion and Tamponade

In the absence of tamponade or suspected purulent pericarditis, there are few indications for pericardial drainage. Persistent, large, and unexplained effusions, especially when tuberculosis is suspected or present for more than 3 months, may warrant pericardiocentesis. Occasionally, suspected malignancy or systemic disease may necessitate pericardial drainage and biopsy. However, routine drainage of large effusions (20 mm, echo-free space in diastole) has a low diagnostic yield (7%) and no therapeutic benefit.[12] Figure 44-1 presents an approach to the management of moderate and large pericardial effusions.

Remembering that significant tamponade is a clinical diagnosis, and that echocardiographic signs of tamponade are not by themselves an indication for pericardiocentesis, is important. Although the absence of any cardiac chamber collapse has a high negative predictive value (92%), the positive predictive value is low (58%). Also, although positive and negative predictive values were high (82% and 88%, respectively) for abnormal right-sided venous flows (i.e., systolic predominance and expiratory diastolic reversal), they could not be evaluated in more than one third of patients.[13]

Removal of small amounts of tamponading pericardial fluid (approximately 50 mL) produces considerable symptomatic and hemodynamic improvement because of the steep pericardial pressure/volume relation. Unless there is concomitant cardiac disease or coexisting constriction (i.e., effusive-constrictive pericarditis), removal of all of the pericardial fluid normalizes pericardial, atrial, ventricular diastolic, and arterial pressures and cardiac output (see Figure 44-1). Mild or low-pressure tamponade does not require pericardiocentesis—that is, when the venous pressure is less than 10 cm of water, arterial blood pressure is normal, and pulsus paradoxus is absent—particularly when the etiology is idiopathic or viral, or when it is responsive to specific therapy, such as thyroid hormone. At the other extreme, hyperacute tamponade, usually resulting from cardiac trauma, necessitates immediate pericardiocentesis as an initial triage measure. However, most patients fall between these two extremes and require pericardial drainage; this can be accomplished percutaneously, with a needle or balloon catheter, or by surgical means, via a subxiphoid incision, video-assisted thoracoscopy, or thoracotomy.

Unless the situation is immediately life threatening, experienced staff should perform pericardiocentesis in a facility equipped with radiographic, echocardiographic, and hemodynamic monitoring to optimize the success and safety of the procedure. Monitoring the cardiac rhythm and systemic blood pressure is a minimum requirement, and invasive hemodynamics and measurement of pericardial pressures are useful for the diagnosis, particularly in questionable cases. Monitoring the local ECG from the needle tip is not recommended by all authors, and if such monitoring is used, it is essential that the apparatus have equipotential grounding. The advantages of needle pericardiocentesis include the ability to perform careful hemodynamic measurements and the relatively simple logistic and personnel requirements (Table 44-2). The safety of the procedure has been increased by using two-dimensional echo guidance (Figure 44-2) with a 1.2% major complication rate in 1127 cases over 21 years.[14] Injection of agitated saline or small quantities of radiographic contrast with imaging can confirm pericardial puncture with echocardiography or fluoroscopy, respectively (Figure 44-3). Unless there has been massive intrapericardial hemorrhage, bloody fluid originating from the pericardium does not clot.

A 6- to 8-Fr catheter may be placed over a guidewire when pericardial fluid can be freely withdrawn, and the catheter can be left in place for continued drainage using only slight negative pressure. Drainage of the pericardial fluid using a catheter minimizes trauma, allows measurement of pericardial pressure and instillation of drugs into the pericardium, and helps prevent, but does not guarantee, reaccumulation of pericardial fluid.

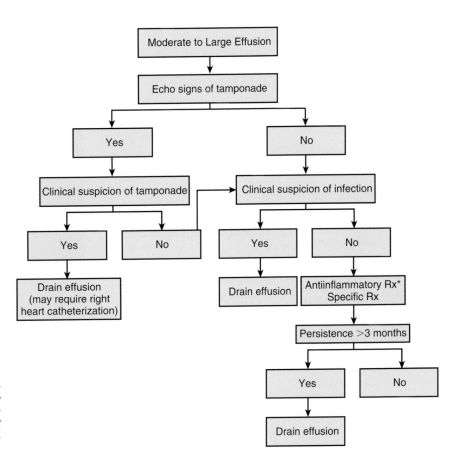

FIGURE 44-1 Algorithm for the management of moderate to large pericardial effusions. *Antiinflammatory treatment if there are signs of pericarditis. Rx, medication. *(Redrawn with permission from Hoit BD. Management of effusive and constrictive pericardial heart disease. Circulation 2002;105:2939-2342.)*

TABLE 44-2	Advantages and Disadvantages of Pericardial Drainage Methods	
METHOD	**ADVANTAGES**	**DISADVANTAGES**
Pericardiocentesis	Acquisition of hemodynamic data	No biopsy material available
	Provides effective relief, particularly if no clots are present	Effusion may recur
	Less postoperative pain than other methods	Drainage may not be adequate, particularly if effusion is loculated
Pericardiotomy (subxiphoid or balloon)	Clots and loculations removed	Evacuation may not be complete
	"Minor" surgical procedure	Frequent pericardial-pleural window closure
Open surgical drainage	Complete drainage	Surgical procedure
	Less reaccumulation, constriction (if total pericardiectomy)	Hemodynamics not readily available
	Access to pericardial tissue	Longer hospitalization, more postoperative pain
	Avoidance of "blind" trauma to pericardium	

Extended catheter drainage over 3 to 5 days is associated with a trend toward lower recurrence rates over a nearly 4-year follow-up.[15] Generally speaking, drainage should continue until the volume of the aspirated fluid is less than 25 mL per day. Although pericardiocentesis is usually well tolerated, pulmonary edema, circulatory collapse, and acute right and left ventricular dysfunction have been reported after drainage. Patients should be monitored for recurrent tamponade, particularly those with hemorrhagic effusions, which may occur despite the presence of an intrapericardial catheter. Dilute heparin or fibrinolytic agents may be instilled in the catheter to prevent clotting, and patients generally should be observed for 24 hours in an intensive care unit.

Major complications of pericardiocentesis include laceration of a coronary vessel or perforation of the myocardium (the thin-walled coronary veins and right heart chambers are particularly prone to brisk bleeding), a lung, or a GI viscus; hypotension that is often reflex in origin; and atrial and ventricular arrhythmia.

Although pericardiocentesis may provide effective relief, percutaneous balloon pericardiotomy, subxiphoid pericardiotomy, or the surgical creation of a pleuropericardial or a peritoneal-pericardial window[16] may be required. In a retrospective review, pericardiocentesis with intrapericardial sclerotherapy was as effective as an open surgical drainage in patients with malignant pericardial effusion.[17] However, the safety and efficacy of subxiphoid pericardiostomy was found to be superior to percutaneous drainage in both benign and malignant effusions.

Open surgical procedures offer several advantages; these include complete drainage, access to pericardial tissue for histopathologic and microbiologic diagnoses, the ability to evacuate

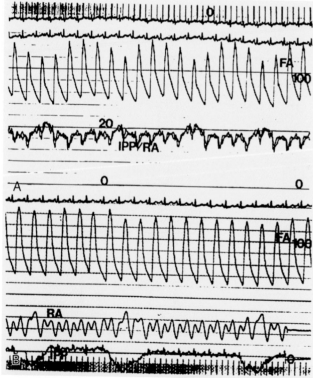

FIGURE 44-2 Hemodynamic record from a patient with cardiac tamponade before (**A**) and after (**B**) pericardiocentesis. **A,** Pulsus paradoxus is evident from the femoral artery (*FA*) pressure tracing. Note the absent Y descent on the right atrial (*RA*) tracing and the equal and elevated RA and pericardial pressures (*IPP*). **B,** After removal of pericardial fluid, pericardial and RA pressures decrease and the pulsus paradoxus disappears. (*Courtesy Noble O. Fowler, MD. From Hoit BD. Pericardial disease and pericardial heart disease. In O'Rourke RA, editor: Steins' internal medicine, 5th ed, St. Louis, Mosby–Year Book, 1998, p 273.*)

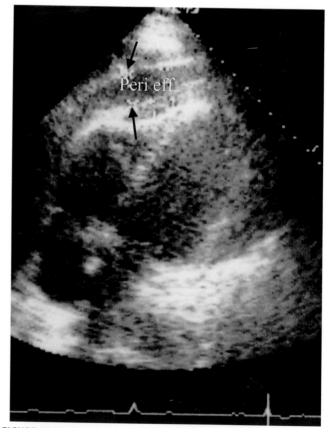

FIGURE 44-3 Two-dimensional echocardiographic image of an acute pericardial effusion (*Peri eff*) complicating percutaneous transluminal myocardial revascularization. Localization of a loculated collection of fluid is used to direct needle pericardiocentesis.

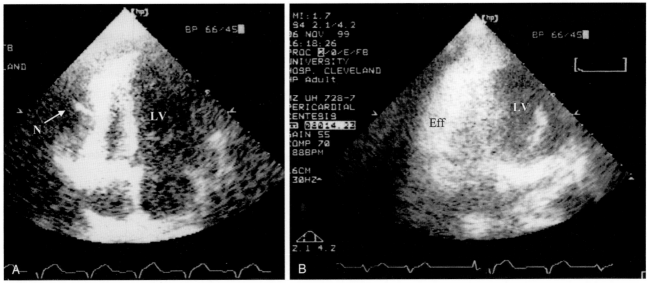

FIGURE 44-4 Echocardiographic imaging can be used to verify the intrapericardial location of the needle (*N*) by either direct imaging (**A**) or by the production of an intrapericardial contrast effect (*Eff*) after injection of agitated saline (**B**). LV, left ventricle.

loculated effusions, and the absence of traumatic injury as a result of blind placement of a needle into the pericardial space. The choice between needle pericardiocentesis and surgical drainage depends on institutional resources, physician experience, the etiology of the effusion, the need for diagnostic tissue samples, and the prognosis of the patient. Needle pericardiocentesis is often the best option when the etiology is known, the diagnosis of tamponade is in question, or both; surgical drainage is optimal when the presence of tamponade is certain, but the etiology is unclear. Pericardiocentesis is ill advised in the presence of loculation, less than 1 cm of effusion, or evidence of fibrin and adhesion (Figure 44-4). It should be recognized that surgical approaches, such as subxiphoid pericardiotomy or thoracoscopic drainage, can be performed using local anesthesia with little attendant morbidity. Irrespective of the method of retrieval, pericardial fluid should be sent for hematocrit and cell count; measurement of glucose levels; Gram, Ziehl-Nielsen, and fungal smears; viral, bacterial, and fungal culture; and cytology. Depending on the clinical circumstances, cytology; assessment of tumor markers and carbohydrate antigens (for suspected malignant disease); analysis of adenosine deaminase, interferon-γ (IF-γ), and pericardial lysozyme; and PCR for suspected tuberculosis should be undertaken.

Volume expansion with agents such as blood, plasma, dextran, or saline may be used, but only as a temporizing measure. The efficacy of volume expansion was evaluated in a study of 49 patients with large pericardial effusions and hemodynamic criteria for cardiac tamponade who were treated with intravenous (IV) administration of 500 mL of normal saline over 10 minutes.[18] Cardiac index increased by more than 10% in 47% of patients, remained unchanged in 22%, and decreased in 31%. Volume expansion significantly increased intrapericardial pressure, right atrial pressure, and left ventricular end-diastolic pressure, and systolic blood pressure below 100 mm Hg was predictive of favorable response to volume expansion. Vagal reflexes complicating tamponade or pericardiocentesis are treated with atropine (1 mg IV); positive-pressure breathing should be avoided because it reduces venous return, right ventricular transmural pressure, and cardiac output.

Recurrent effusions may be treated by either repeat pericardiocentesis, sclerotherapy with tetracycline, surgical creation of a pericardial window, or pericardiectomy. Subtotal pericardiectomy is preferred when the patient is expected to survive more than 1 year. A pleuropericardial window provides a large area for fluid to be reabsorbed and is often performed in patients with malignant effusions. Pericardiectomy may be required for recurrent effusions in dialysis patients, and in critically ill patients, a pericardial window may be created percutaneously with a balloon catheter.

Constrictive Pericarditis

Constrictive pericarditis is a condition in which a thickened, scarred, and often calcified pericardium limits diastolic filling of the ventricles. Although acute pericarditis from most causes may eventuate in constrictive pericarditis, the most common antecedents are idiopathic pericarditis; cardiac trauma and surgery; mediastinal irradiation; infectious diseases such as tuberculosis, which is particularly common in nonindustrialized countries; neoplasms, particularly of the lung and breast; renal failure; and connective tissue diseases. Although it is commonly thought that a normal pericardial thickness excludes the diagnosis of constrictive pericarditis, 28% of 143 surgically confirmed cases revealed normal pericardial thickness on CT scan, and 18% showed normal thickness on histopathologic examination.[19]

Classic chronic constrictive pericarditis is less frequently encountered than in the past, whereas subacute constrictive pericarditis weeks to months after the inciting injury, such as after cardiac surgery, is becoming more common. In this latter group of patients, constriction may be transitory, with a course that may span a matter of weeks to a few months. Not surprisingly, pericardial calcification is uncommon. Doppler-detected constrictive physiology resolved without pericardiectomy in 36 of 212 patients studied retrospectively at the Mayo Clinic after an average of approximately 8 weeks.[20] In asymptomatic patients who may have occult constrictive pericarditis, exercise testing and maximal O_2 consumption, if available, should be quantified, jugular venous pressure should be carefully estimated, and liver function tests should be done. Increasing jugular venous pressure, the need for diuretic therapy, evidence of hepatic insufficiency, and reduced exercise tolerance indicate the need for surgery.

Pericardiectomy is the definitive treatment for constrictive pericarditis but is unwarranted either in early constriction (occult and functional class I) or in severe, advanced disease (functional class IV), when the risk of surgery is excessive (operative mortality rates of 30% to 40% vs. 6% to 19%) and the benefits are diminished.[21] Because some cases of constriction spontaneously resolve before pericardiectomy is recommended, it is prudent that patients with subacute constrictive pericarditis who are hemodynamically stable be given a trial of conservative management for 2 to 3 months until it is clear that the constrictive process is permanent. After pericardiectomy, symptomatic relief and normalization of cardiac pressures may take several months, occurring sooner when the operation is carried out before the disease becomes too chronic. Calcification may correlate with disease chronicity in populations with a low incidence of tuberculous pericarditis[22] and when the pericardiectomy is almost complete. Complete or extensive pericardial resection is desirable. In one study, the long-term outcome was predicted by three variables in a stepwise logistic regression analysis. Specifically, the prognosis was worse with increasing age and with New York Heart Association (NYHA) class and a postirradiation etiology.[21] In another study, age, renal dysfunction, pulmonary hypertension, left ventricular dysfunction, and hyponatremia were independent adverse predictors.[23]

Pericardiectomy is commonly carried out via a median sternotomy, although some surgeons prefer access through a thoracotomy. Despite a decline, the risk of mortality remains approximately 6% to 19% and is increased by heavy calcification and involvement of the visceral pericardium. Left ventricular systolic dysfunction may occur after decortication of a severely constricted heart. Although the left ventricular dysfunction may require treatment for several months, it usually resolves completely. In highly selected patients, orthotopic transplantation may be considered.[21]

Medical therapy of constrictive pericarditis has a small but important role. In some patients constrictive pericarditis resolves either spontaneously or in response to various combinations of NSAIDs, steroids, and antibiotics[20]; in the remaining patients, medical therapy is adjunctive. Specific antibiotic therapy, such as antituberculous medications, should be initiated before surgery and continued afterward. Preoperative diuretics should be used sparingly with the goal of reducing, not eliminating, elevated jugular pressure, edema, and ascites. Postoperatively, diuretics should be given if spontaneous diuresis does not occur. The central venous pressure may take weeks to months to return to normal after pericardiectomy, and the left ventricular ejection fraction may decrease postoperatively, only to return to normal months later. In the interim, digoxin, diuretics, and vasodilators may be useful. In the presence of atrial fibrillation, diuretics and digoxin are useful in patients who are not candidates for pericardiectomy because of their high surgical risk.

Prevention of pericardial constriction consists of appropriate therapy of acute pericarditis and adequate pericardial drainage. Although instillation of fibrinolytics is preventative (urokinase 400,000 U per instillation to 1.6 million U; streptokinase 250,000 IU per instillation to 1 million IU), cortinosteroid instillation is often ineffective.[24]

Treatment of Specific Causes of Pericarditis

Purulent Pericarditis

The incidence and bacterial spectrum of purulent pericarditis have changed because of the increasing frequency of cardiac surgery and instrumentation, selection-induced changes in the flora responsible for hospital-acquired infections, and the prolonged survival of immunocompromised hosts. Bacterial pericarditis is treated with surgical exploration and drainage (pericardiectomy is preferable) and appropriate systemic antibiotics, which should be considered adjuvant. A high index of suspicion is critical; in the appropriate setting, pericardial involvement is often unrecognized when it complicates systemic infection, and the characteristic features of acute pericarditis are frequently absent. The threshold for echocardiography in the septic patient should be low, and whenever purulent pericarditis

is suspected, the pericardial space should be explored. Iodine-containing irrigants may provoke constriction and should be avoided. Fibrinolytics, which were discussed earlier, may be used to lyse fibrous adhesions, liquefy purulent exudate, and prevent constrictive pericarditis.[24]

Mycobacterial and Fungal Pericarditis

Tuberculosis is a major cause of pericarditis in nonindustrialized countries but is an uncommon cause of pericarditis in the United States. Nevertheless, its incidence has increased because of human immunodeficiency virus (HIV) infection.[25] Tuberculous pericarditis results from hematogenous spread of primary tuberculosis or from breakdown of infected mediastinal lymph nodes; therefore, typical symptoms and signs and radiologic evidence of pulmonary tuberculosis are usually absent. Fibrinous pericarditis with caseating necrosis and mononuclear infiltrate gives rise to an effusive phase, which is often voluminous and hemodynamically significant. An adhesive phase follows resolution of the effusion and eventuates in dense, calcific adhesions with clinical constriction in nearly half of patients.

The diagnosis of tuberculous pericarditis is based on histologic identification, culture of *Mycobacterium tuberculosis*, pericarditis with proven extracardiac tuberculosis, or pericardial effusion responsive to antituberculosis therapy.[1-4] PCR-detected *M. tuberculosis* DNA, high adenosine deaminase activity, lysozyme, and interferon-γ concentration in the pericardial fluid are useful indirect diagnostic tools. A "definite" diagnosis of tuberculous pericarditis is made upon demonstration of tubercle bacilli in pericardial fluid (diagnostic sensitivity, 53% to 75%) or pericardial biopsy (diagnostic sensitivity, 10% to 64%). A "probable" diagnosis is made when there is proof of tuberculosis elsewhere in a patient with unexplained pericarditis, a lymphocytic pericardial exudate with high adenosine deaminase activity levels, and/or a good response to antituberculosis therapy.[26] A presumptive diagnosis generally requires a history of contact and/or purified protein derivative conversion, although the latter lacks sensitivity and specificity. Gadolinium-enhanced magnetic resonance imaging and (MRI) may also be useful in early diagnosis.

Fluid should be removed and cultured and antituberculosis therapy begun. Depending on the echocardiographic appearance, subxiphoid drainage may be necessary. Early pericardiectomy has been recommended by some in all cases of tuberculous pericarditis, but the long-term prognosis is excellent for patients without cardiac compression during the acute illness who are treated with medical therapy alone.[26] Multidrug therapy and corticosteroids are effective in tuberculous pericarditis, whereas atypical mycobacterial infections, especially *M. avium-intracellulare*, may be resistant to treatment. Patients with tuberculous pericarditis should receive a regimen of isoniazid (5 mg/kg to a maximum of 300 mg), rifampin (10 mg/kg to a maximum of 600 mg), pyrazinamide (15 to 30 mg/kg/day up to 3 g), and ethambutol (5 to 25 mg/kg to a maximum of 2.5 g) for a minimum of 2 months followed by isoniazid and rifampin for a total of 6 months; this short course of chemotherapy is as effective as 9 months of therapy and is effective in HIV-infected patients.[26] Corticosteroids (prednisone 1 to 2 mg/kg/day) may be useful if pericardial effusion persists or recurs during therapy, and they are beneficial acutely in reducing morbidity and mortality, but definitive data supporting their use to prevent constriction in primary pericardial effusion are lacking.[27] Pericardiectomy may be necessary for recurrent cardiac tamponade.

Patients should be observed for constriction because up to half of them will require pericardiectomy.[28] Failure to improve or worsening over 1 to 2 months, pericardial thickening, or evidence of constriction require urgent pericardiectomy. For patients with hemodynamics consistent with effusive-constrictive pericarditis, plans for visceral and parietal pericardiectomy after a few weeks of chemotherapy should be made. Persistent hypotension may signify tuberculous adrenal insufficiency.

Pericarditis complicating deep fungal infection with *Histoplasma* or *Coccidioides immitis* may be immunologic, may resolve spontaneously, and may not require specific therapy. Amphotericin B (up to 2.5 g total), itraconazole (200 to 400 mg/day), ketoconazole (200 to 400 mg/day), and fluconazole (200 to 400 mg/day) are rarely required. Surgical decompression and specific antifungal or antimicrobial therapy may be necessary for disseminated infection with *Candida*, *Aspergillus*, *Actinomycetes*, and *Nocardia*.

Human Immunodeficiency Virus–Associated Pericarditis

HIV is an important cause of pericardial heart disease. Typically, pericardial effusions are small and asymptomatic in outpatients, but large effusions and tamponade are common in hospitalized patients with late-stage acquired immunodeficiency syndrome (AIDS). Large, symptomatic pericardial effusion in patients with HIV infection should be aggressively investigated, as two thirds of these cases have an identifiable cause.[29] Tamponade in patients with HIV is mycobacterial in origin (*M. tuberculosis* or *M. avium-intracellulare*) in approximately one third of patients.[29]

Neoplastic Pericarditis

Metastatic neoplasia remains the leading cause of pericardial disease in hospitalized patients, most often in those with lung or breast cancer, melanoma, lymphoma, and acute leukemia. Many cases are asymptomatic and are found only incidentally at autopsy, but others cause symptoms and may progress to cardiac tamponade. The pericardium may be thickened and may cause constriction; less commonly, effusive-constrictive pericarditis occurs.

In almost all cases, fluid should be removed if large effusions are refractory or if tamponade ensues.[30] The specific approach depends on the patient's expected longevity and medical condition. Pericardiocentesis is associated with a high recurrence rate and does not provide tissue for biopsy. Sclerosing agents, such as tetracycline (500 to 1000 mg in 20 mL of sterile saline), reduce recurrences, and their use can be considered for patients with a poor prognosis. However, sclerosis is painful, it does not improve prognosis, and it may not be superior to an indwelling catheter alone. Subtotal pericardiectomy is most effective but should only be performed in carefully selected patients. Balloon pericardiotomy avoids the discomfort and risk of surgery and will likely replace surgical subxiphoid pericardiotomy in critically ill patients with predictably limited survival. Radiation therapy and intrapericardial instillation of P32-colloid, a suspension of radioactive phosphorus, are effective strategies to control pericardial effusion but are not without significant practical difficulties and toxicities.[30,31]

Pericarditis Complicating Myocardial Infarction and the Postpericardial Injury Syndrome

Prior to the reperfusion era, pericarditis was common in the first few days after myocardial infarction (MI), occurring in up to 28% to 43% of fatal infarctions, but it was clinically apparent in 7% of cases. Today, pericarditis is much less common, probably as a result of the much lower rate of transmural MI than in the previous era. Pericardial involvement is related to infarct size and is associated with a poor prognosis. An important clinical issue is the extent to which acute pericarditis in MI influences management with anticoagulants. A pericardial friction rub that occurs in the first 2 or 3 days without an associated pericardial effusion should not influence clinical decisions, but pericarditis that occurs later in the course, or pericarditis accompanied by pericardial effusion or tamponade, is a contraindication to anticoagulant therapy.

Cardiac tamponade seldom occurs, except in patients who receive systemic anticoagulants or in those who have cardiac rupture. Fibrinolytic therapy almost invariably precedes the development of pericarditis; therefore, clinical decision making is not usually affected. However, when acute pericarditis is mistaken for acute MI, thrombolytic therapy can have calamitous consequences.

Pericarditis or pericardial effusion that results from earlier injury of the pericardium together constitutes the postpericardial injury syndrome (PPIS), which includes post-MI syndrome or Dressler syndrome and postpericardiotomy syndrome. PPIS is characterized by latency between the inciting pericardial event and pericarditis, tendency to recurrence, and fever or other markers of systemic inflammation. The presentation and clinical course of the postpericardiotomy syndrome are comparable to that of the post-MI syndrome. The most frequent complaint is chest pain occurring a few days to several weeks after a cardiac operation. As with post-MI pericarditis, delayed pericarditis after cardiac surgery is more common in patients who had active pericarditis early after the cardiac operation. Postpericardiotomy syndrome is an important contributing factor in approximately one third of effusions that occur after 7 days in postoperative patients. Treatment of postpericardial syndrome consists of ASA; NSAIDs; colchicine, which may also be preventative; and, if necessary, a short course of steroids, which are not preventative. Therapy with intrapericardial instillation of triamcinolone appears promising but requires further investigation.

Colchicine has been demonstrated to significantly reduce the incidence of PPIS following cardiac surgery.[32] In the largest multicenter study of colchicine in the prevention of postpericardiotomy syndrome, the Colchicine for the Prevention of Post-Pericardiotomy Syndrome (COPPS) study, 360 cardiac surgery patients were randomly assigned on postoperative day 3 to colchicine or placebo administered for 30 days. The primary endpoint was the development of postpericardiotomy syndrome by 12 months.[32] Colchicine significantly reduced the occurrence of the postpericardiotomy syndrome at 12 months compared with placebo (9% vs. 21%). The rate of side effects, primarily related to GI intolerance, was similar in the colchicine and placebo groups.

For patients who develop PPIS, first-line treatment consists of aspirin; if that fails, an NSAID such as ibuprofen may be considered if there are no contraindications, such as those discussed above. In pericarditis associated with an acute MI, aspirin is preferred, and the use of an NSAID other than aspirin should probably be avoided because antiinflammatory therapy may impair scar formation. Aspirin may also be the first choice in patients who require concomitant antiplatelet therapy for any reason. With any aspirin or NSAID regimen, GI protection should be provided.

When the patient does not respond to aspirin, NSAIDs, or colchicine, a short course of steroids is generally effective. Prednisone is typically begun at a dose of 60 mg/day. Once the patient is asymptomatic and objective findings are beginning to improve, the dose is tapered—at first rapidly, such as 5 mg every 3 days until a dose of 20 mg/day is achieved, and then more slowly. If pericarditis recurs, the dose is raised to the lowest dose that suppressed the syndrome, maintained there for several weeks, and then tapered again.

Among patients with recurrent or persistent autoreactive pericarditis with effusion (not limited to PPIS), pericardiocentesis with intrapericardial instillation of triamcinolone (300 mg/m^2) has been proposed as an alternative to systemic therapy to avoid systemic side effects.[33] However, because the data on this are limited, this approach requires further investigation.

Radiation-Induced Pericardial Disease

Acute pericarditis that occurs early during radiation therapy is uncommon and is most likely the result of radiation-induced effects on the tumor rather than a direct toxic effect of radiation on the pericardium. In this instance, therapy should not be disrupted, although a reduction in dose may be necessary. A form of pericardial injury that is delayed—usually less than 1 year, but this is highly variable—may present as acute pericarditis or effusion, often with some degree of cardiac compression. The reaction of the pericardium to radiation is fibrinous inflammation, often with an effusion. Although the acute lesion usually subsides within 2 years without sequelae, constrictive and effusive-constrictive pericarditis may manifest only after many years.

In the effusive stage, the differential diagnosis includes recurrence of the neoplasm; examination of pericardial fluid is then helpful because the fluid frequently shows evidence of malignancy. When the diagnosis remains in doubt, biopsy, particularly epicardial biopsy, may be necessary.[34] Effusion may be due to a radiation therapy–induced hypothyroid state.

Acute radiation-induced pericarditis can be managed symptomatically as acute idiopathic pericarditis. Hemodynamically insignificant pericardial effusion can also be managed conservatively because spontaneous resolution is the rule; however, pericardiectomy should be offered to symptomatic patients with large, recurrent pericardial effusions. Constrictive pericarditis requires pericardiectomy, unless a biopsy obtained to distinguish constriction from restrictive cardiomyopathy secondary to radiation reveals significant endomyocardial fibrosis.

Traumatic Pericardial Disease

Blunt and penetrating trauma are important causes of pericarditis, particularly among young men. Chronic constrictive pericarditis, recurrent pericardial effusion, and recurrent acute pericarditis are well-recognized complications of such trauma. Although traumatic pericarditis is often overshadowed by associated injuries and usually resolves uneventfully, pericardial involvement may be life threatening. Echocardiography used in the trauma unit rapidly and accurately diagnoses hemopericardium in patients with potentially penetrating cardiac wounds. Failure to repair the injury responsible for tamponade is associated with a poor clinical outcome. Constrictive pericarditis occasionally occurs and may be delayed for weeks or years after the injury.

Chylopericardium

Chylous pericardial effusions generally follow traumatic or surgical injury to the thoracic duct but may result from neoplastic obstruction of the thoracic duct (*secondary chylopericardium*); less commonly, they may be idiopathic (*primary chylopericardium*). Failure to respond to a diet rich in medium-chain triglycerides and pericardiocentesis warrants ligation of the thoracic duct and pericardiectomy.[35] In cases deemed inappropriate for aggressive therapy, a valved pericardioperitoneal conduit can be implanted.[35]

Pericardial Disease in Patients with Renal Failure

Pericarditis complicates both uremia and dialytic therapy (hemoperitoneal and peritoneal) and may be clinically silent. The clinical manifestation of nephrogenic pericardial disease may be acute fibrinous pericarditis, pericardial effusion, or cardiac tamponade; classic constrictive pericarditis is rare.

Although intensification of dialysis is an accepted treatment modality for hemodynamically insignificant disease, considerable controversy exists regarding the optimal management of large, persistent, or recurrent pericardial effusion. Tamponade is an indication for pericardial drainage, and large, resistant chronic effusion warrants pericardiocentesis. A conservative approach, such as intensification of dialysis and NSAIDs, may suffice in less

severe cases. The instillation of nonabsorbable steroids (triamcinolone 50 mg every 6 hours for 2 to 3 days) directly into the pericardial space has been advocated,[36] but randomized, controlled data on this form of therapy are absent. If needle drainage is necessary, an indwelling catheter should be left in the pericardial space for at least 2 to 3 days. Dialysis-associated effusive pericarditis usually responds to an intensification of dialysis and regional heparinization or a change to peritoneal dialysis. Pericardiectomy may be necessary for intractable effusions.

Myxedema Pericardial Disease

Pericarditis with effusion, sometimes containing cholesterol, occurs in about one third of patients with myxedema. Effusions develop slowly and may reach prodigious size, and slow resolution usually follows institution of thyroid replacement therapy. Pericardial drainage is generally not indicated because myxedema effusions seldom cause tamponade.

Connective Tissue Disease–Related Pericardial Disease

Pericarditis may accompany virtually any connective tissue disease and manifests as either acute or chronic pericarditis with or without an effusion. Although tamponade, effusive-constrictive disease, and constrictive pericarditis are recognized complications, most cases are subclinical and in many instances are recognized only at autopsy. In the absence of tamponade or secondarily infected effusions, NSAIDs and corticosteroids are useful.

Pericardial Disease and Pregnancy

Small- to moderate-sized effusions occur in the last trimester of approximately 40% of healthy pregnancies, whereas larger accumulations should raise concern of another disorder.[37] Most pericardial diseases in pregnancy are managed the same as for nonpregnant patients. However, colchicine is contraindicated, and high-dose ASA may prematurely close the ductus.[37] Pericardiocentesis should be reserved for large, tamponading effusions and suspected infection; echocardiographic guidance avoids fetal irradiation.

Drug-Induced and Iatrogenic Pericardial Disease

A wide variety of drugs and toxins may cause pericardial heart disease (Table 44-3) by producing either drug-induced lupus, a hypersensitivity or idiosyncratic reaction, pericardial irritation, or hemorrhage. Iatrogenic pericardial disease results from both the calculated complications and the unanticipated misadventures of diagnostic and therapeutic procedures, and specific management depends on the particular procedure. For example, although transseptal punctures may require rescue pericardiocentesis, perforation of a coronary artery by a guidewire may require only withdrawal of the wire and watchful waiting. Coronary artery transections during coronary interventional procedures are treated with either a covered stent or perfusion balloon. Routine echocardiography is recommended after myocardial biopsy and pacemaker lead implantation.[1]

Anticoagulation in Pericarditis

The management of anticoagulation in patients with acute pericarditis and effusion requires analysis of the competing risks and benefits, although few objective data are available for decision making. Acute pericarditis generally responds to NSAIDs within a few days, during which time anticoagulants may be withheld

TABLE 44-3	Drugs and Toxins Implicated as Causes in Pericardial Heart Disease		
DRUG-INDUCED LUPUS	**HYPERSENSITIVITY OR IDIOSYNCRATIC REACTION**	**PERICARDIAL IRRITATION/ HEMORRHAGE**	
Procainamide	Penicillins, sulfa drugs	Anticoagulants	
Tocainide	Cephalosporins	Thrombolytics	
Hydralazine	Streptomycin	Pericardial contact	
Methyldopa	Arabinofuranosyl cytidine	with:	
Phenytoin	(Ara-C)	Tetracycline	
Reserpine	Minoxidil	Talc	
Mesalazine	Practolol	Asbestos	
Isoniazid	Thiazides	Silicones	
Betaxolol	Amiodarone		
	Cyclophosphamide,		
	azathioprine		
	Anthracyclines		
	Psicofuranine		
	5-Fluorouracil		
	Methotrexate		
	Cyclosporine		
	Methysergide, ergoline drugs		
	Cromolyn sodium		
	Carbamazepine		
	Clozapine		
	Streptokinase		
	Phenylbutazone		
	Doxorubicin		
	Polymer fume inhalation		
	Vaccines (smallpox, yellow		
	fever)		
	GM-CSF, cytokines (IL-2, IF-α)		
	Serum sickness, scorpion fish		
	sting		

GM-CSF, granulocyte macrophage colony–stimulating factor; IF-α, interferon-α; IL-2, interleukin 2.
Modified from Spodick DH. *The pericardium: a comprehensive textbook.* 1997, New York, Marcel Dekker, p 412.

in low-risk patients; patients at higher thromboembolic risk can be switched to heparin while awaiting a clinical response. Unexplained effusions should be thoroughly evaluated to exclude hemorrhage.

ACKNOWLEDGMENT

Thanks to Ralph Shabetai for his helpful discussions and encouragement.

REFERENCES

1. Maisch B, Seferovic PM, Ristic AD, et al. Guidelines on the diagnosis and management of pericardial diseases executive summary; The task force on the diagnosis and management of pericardial diseases of the European Society of Cardiology. *Eur Heart J* 2004;25:587-610.
2. Maisch B, Ristic AD, Pankuweit S. Intrapericardial treatment of autoreactive pericardial effusion with triamcinolone: the way to avoid side effects of systemic corticosteroid therapy. *Eur Heart J* 2002;23:1503-1508.
3. Imazio M, Demichelis B, Parrini I, et al. Day-hospital treatment of acute pericarditis: a management program for outpatient therapy. *J Am Coll Cardiol* 2004;43:1042-1046.
4. Topol EJ. Arthritis medicines and cardiovascular events—"house of coxibs." *JAMA* 2005;293:366-368.
5. Imazio M, Brucato A, Trinchero R, et al. Colchicine for pericarditis: hype or hope? *Eur Heart J* 2009;30:532-539.
6. Imazio M, Bobbio M, Cecchi E, et al. Colchicine in addition to conventional therapy for acute pericarditis: results of the Colchicine for acute Pericarditis (COPE) trial. *Circulation* 2005;112:2012-2016.
7. Imazio M, Bobbio M, Cecchi E, et al. Colchicine as first-choice therapy for recurrent pericarditis: results of the CORE (Colchicine for Recurrent Pericarditis) trial. *Arch Intern Med* 2005;165:1987-1991.
8. Marcolongo R, Russo R, Laveder F, et al. Immunosuppressive therapy prevents recurrent pericarditis. *J Am Coll Cardiol* 1995;26:1276-1279.
9. Maisch B, Ristic AD, Pankuweit S. Intrapericardial treatment of autoreactive pericardial effusion with triamcinolone: the way to avoid side effects of systemic corticosteroid therapy. *Eur Heart J* 2002;23:1503-1508.
10. Imazio M, Brucato A, Cumetti D, et al. Corticosteroids for recurrent pericarditis: high versus low doses: a nonrandomized observation. *Circulation* 2008;118:667-671.
11. Imazio M, Spodick DH, Brucato A, Trinchero R, Adler Y. Contemporary issues in the management of pericardial diseases. *Circulation* 2010;121:916-928.
12. Merce J, Sagrista-Sauleda J, Permanyer-Miralda G, et al. Should pericardial drainage be performed routinely in patients who have a large pericardial effusion without tamponade? *Am J Med* 1998;105:106-109.
13. Merce J, Sagrista-Sauleda J, Permanyer-Miralda G, et al. Correlation between clinical and Doppler echocardiographic findings in patients with moderate and large pericardial effusion: implications for the diagnosis of cardiac tamponade. *Am Heart J* 1999;138:759-764.
14. Tsang TS, Enriquez-Sarano M, Freeman WK, et al. Consecutive 1127 therapeutic echocardiographically guided pericardiocentesis: clinical profile, practice patterns, and outcomes spanning 21 years. *Mayo Clin Proc* 2002;77:429-436.
15. Tsang TS, Barnes ME, Gersh BJ, et al. Outcomes of clinically significant idiopathic pericardial effusion requiring intervention. *Am J Cardiol* 2003;91:704-707.
16. Allen KB, Faber LP, Warren WH, et al. Pericardial effusion: subxiphoid pericardiostomy versus percutaneous catheter drainage. *Ann Thorac Surg* 1999;67:437-440.
17. Girardi LN, Ginsberg RJ, Burt ME. Pericardiocentesis and intrapericardial sclerosis: effective therapy for malignant pericardial effusions. *Ann Thorac Surg* 1997;64:1427-1428.
18. Sagristà-Sauleda J, Angel J, Sambola A, Permanyer-Miralda G. Hemodynamic effects of volume expansion in patients with cardiac tamponade. *Circulation* 2008;117:1545.
19. Talreja DR, Edwards WD, Danielson GK, et al. Constrictive pericarditis in 26 patients with histologically normal pericardial thickness. *Circulation* 2003;108:1852-1857.
20. Haley JH, Tajik AJ, Danielson GK, et al. Transient constrictive pericarditis: causes and natural history. *J Am Coll Cardiol* 2004;43:271-275.
21. Ling LH, Oh JK, Schaff HV, et al. Constrictive pericarditis in the modern era: evolving clinical spectrum and impact on outcome after pericardiectomy. *Circulation* 1999;100:1380-1386.
22. Ling L, Oh J, Breen J, et al. Calcific constrictive pericarditis: Is it still with us? *Ann Intern Med* 2000;132:444-450.
23. Bertog SC, Thambidorai SK, Parakh K, et al. Constrictive pericarditis: etiology and cause-specific survival after pericardiectomy. *J Am Coll Cardiol* 2004;43:1445-1452.
24. Ustunsoy H, Celkan MA, Sivrikoz MC, et al. Intrapericardial fibrinolytic therapy in purulent pericarditis. *Eur J Cardiothorac Surg* 2002;22:373-376.
25. Mastroianni A, Coronado O, Chiodo F. Tuberculous pericarditis and AIDS: case reports and review. *Eur J Epidemiol* 1997;13:755-759.
26. Mayosi BM, Burgess LJ, Doubell AF. Tuberculous pericarditis. *Circulation* 2005;112:3608-3616.
27. Ntsekhe M, Wiysonge C, Volmink JA, et al. Adjuvant corticosteroids for tuberculous pericarditis: promising, but not proven. *QJM* 2003;96:593-599.
28. Fowler N. Tuberculous pericarditis. *J Am Med Assn* 1991;266:99-103.
29. Estok L, Wallach F. Cardiac tamponade in a patient with AIDS: a review of pericardial disease in patients with HIV infection. *Mt Sinai J Med* 1998;65:33-39.
30. Tsang TS, Seward JB, Barnes ME, et al. Outcomes of primary and secondary treatment of pericardial effusion in patients with malignancy. *Mayo Clin Proc* 2000;75:248-253.
31. Dempke W, Firusian N. Treatment of malignant pericardial effusion with 32P-colloid. *Br J Cancer* 1999;80:1955-1957.
32. Imazio M, Trinchero R, Brucato A, et al. Colchicine for the Prevention of the Postpericardiotomy Syndrome (COPPS): a multicentre, randomized, double-blind, placebo-controlled trial. *Eur Heart J* 2010;31:2749-2754.
33. Maisch B, Ristić AD, Pankuweit S. Intrapericardial treatment of autoreactive pericardial effusion with triamcinolone: the way to avoid side effects of systemic corticosteroid therapy. *Eur Heart J* 2002;23:1503.
34. Maisch B, Pankuweit S, Brilla C, et al. Intrapericardial treatment of inflammatory and neoplastic pericarditis guided by pericardioscopy and epicardial biopsy—results from a pilot study. *Clin Cardiol* 1999;22:l17-l12.
35. Hoit BD. Chylopericardium and cholesterol pericarditis. LeWinter MM, Downey BC, editors. Available at http://www.uptodate.com.
36. Wood JE, Mahnensmith RL. Pericarditis associated with renal failure: evolution and management. *Semin Dial* 2001;14:61-66.
37. Ristic AD, Seferovic PM, Ljubic A, et al. Pericardial disease in pregnancy. *Herz* 2003;28:209-215.

CHAPTER 45

Optimal Timing of Surgical and Mechanical Intervention in Native Valvular Heart Disease

Melanie S. Sulistio, Edmund A. Bermudez, and William H. Gaasch

OVERVIEW, 676

AORTIC STENOSIS, 676

Assessment of Severity, 676
Timing of Surgical Intervention, 677
Overall Approach, 678

MITRAL STENOSIS, 678

Assessment of Severity, 678
Overall Approach, 680

AORTIC INSUFFICIENCY, 681

Assessment of Severity, 681
Timing of Surgical Intervention, 683
Overall Approach, 683

MITRAL INSUFFICIENCY, 683

Assessment of Severity, 683
Timing of Intervention, 686
Overall Approach, 686

RIGHT-SIDED VALVE DISEASE, 687

Tricuspid Valve Disease, 687
Pulmonary Valve Disease, 687

FUTURE DIRECTIONS, 688

REFERENCES, 688

Overview

The timing of surgical intervention in the management of isolated native valvular dysfunction depends on several elements. The presence of symptoms is important and often reflects the hemodynamic burden that lesions place on ventricular size and function. When lesions are mild in severity, ventricular systolic function remains largely unchanged, and the patient remains asymptomatic. However, as lesions progress in severity, their hemodynamic impact may begin to emerge as ventricular geometry and function change. Cardiovascular symptoms may eventually follow, and, if left untreated, persistent ventricular dysfunction and circulatory compromise may ensue. Native valve heart disease is therefore a triad of lesion severity, ventricular function, and symptoms that largely guides the timing of intervention in an effort to avoid irreversible ventricular dysfunction and cardiovascular morbidity and mortality.[1]

Advances in technology have enabled accurate noninvasive detection and assessment of valvular dysfunction. In particular, echocardiography has become the cornerstone of assessment of valvular lesions. The hemodynamic impact of valvular heart disease can be readily assessed and quantified using multiparametric analyses that include an assessment of ventricular size and function.[2] In some cases, however, the severity of valvular disease may be ambiguous or disparate from other clinical findings, leaving the diagnosis of severity in doubt. In these cases, invasive hemodynamics can be obtained at cardiac catheterization and may be used to help clarify lesion severity. Still, the severity of the lesion alone does not necessarily mandate surgical correction.

Corrective therapy for valvular heart disease is mechanical and absolute. The decision process in arriving at a referral for surgical correction is often complex and requires consideration of the risk of the procedure itself and the risks of prosthetic heart valves in relation to patient-specific conditions. Therefore the type of mechanical intervention—percutaneous or surgical, or repair versus replacement—is a factor in the timing of intervention.

Aortic Stenosis
Assessment of Severity

The severity of aortic stenosis can be assessed noninvasively through echocardiography or invasively during cardiac catheterization.[3] Both methods can provide an accurate assessment of

valve area and transaortic gradients. However, because of its ease and relative accuracy, echocardiography remains the primary modality for the assessment and follow-up of aortic stenosis. In virtually all patients, transthoracic evaluation provides adequate hemodynamic information for the assessment of stenosis severity so that management strategies can be well formulated. Morphologic information, such as pattern and degree of calcification and number of cusps, as well as an assessment of ventricular function and hypertrophy, can readily be obtained.

Lesion severity can usually be categorized by calculation of the aortic valve area (AVA) and measurement of the mean transvalvular pressure gradient.[4] By echocardiography, the continuity equation can be applied to determine valve area with mean gradients measured by Doppler techniques.

$$AVA = \frac{\pi (D/2)^2 \times V_{lvot}}{V_{AV}}$$

In this equation, D is the diameter of the left ventricular outflow tract (LVOT), V_{lvot} is the velocity of blood through the LVOT measured by pulse-wave Doppler, and V_{AV} is the maximum velocity across the aortic valve (AV) measured by continuous-wave Doppler. Accuracy in determining valve area by echocardiography depends on the accuracy of measuring these elements, which can be highly dependent on the sonographer. Direct planimetry of the AV can be performed through transesophageal echocardiography (TEE). However, overestimation of the valve area occurs when planimetry is performed closer to the annulus rather than at the leaflet tips, where coaptation occurs.

If cardiac catheterization is performed, the formula derived by Gorlin and Gorlin[5] is applied to calculate the orifice area.

$$AVA = \frac{CO/SEP(HR)}{44.3\sqrt{MG}}$$

Here, AVA represents aortic valve area (cm^2), CO is cardiac output (mL/min), SEP is systolic ejection period (seconds), HR is ventricular rate (beats/min), and MG is mean transvalvular gradient. An accurate cardiac output calculation will depend on the appropriate use of thermodilution, the Fick calculation, and angiographic technique.[5] Thermodilution is less accurate in low-flow states, significant tricuspid insufficiency, and irregular rhythms. The Fick calculation requires accurate measurement of oxygen consumption. Transducer placement and timing of measurements are important variables in calculating accurate valve areas.

Both techniques to assess valve area depend on flow, so that calculated valve areas may be artifactually small in the presence of low flow (i.e., low cardiac output) and low pressure gradients. During catheterization, calculation of valve resistance may be helpful in these situations.[6] Because resistance may be less sensitive to changes in flow, higher valve resistance (>250 dynes/sec/cm[-5]) is generally seen with truly severe aortic stenosis. The use of dobutamine, either at cardiac catheterization or coupled with echocardiography, may be of benefit in these conditions to help differentiate pseudostenosis from true stenosis.[7] Alternatively, the presence of increased flow, such as in aortic regurgitation, increases the aortic pressure gradient and peak velocity. The dimensionless velocity index (DVI) can be used and is as follows:

$$DVI = \frac{VTI_{lvot}}{VTI_{AV}}$$

In this equation, the velocity-time integral (*VTI*) of both the LVOT and the AV is the sum of the velocities, using the same technique by Doppler as the continuity equation. The increased flow seen in aortic regurgitation affects both the LVOT and the AV proportionally; therefore the DVI remains the same despite the increased flow. A DVI of less than 0.25 is suggestive of severe aortic stenosis. This calculation is also valuable when assessing prosthetic valves and patient-prosthesis mismatch.

Assuming normal cardiac output, severe aortic stenosis is usually present when mean gradients exceed 40 mm Hg. By echocardiography, this usually corresponds to a peak transaortic velocity that exceeds 4.0 to 4.5 m/s.[8] Aortic stenosis is considered severe when these are present or when the calculated valve area is less than 1.0 cm.[2] Definitions of mild, moderate, and severe aortic stenosis are provided in Table 45-1.

Occasionally, noninvasive and invasive measures provide differing results with regard to severity. Aside from the fidelity of technical measurement, the phenomenon of pressure recovery may explain some differences. Distal to the stenosis, some of the blood flow kinetic energy may be recovered in pressure, a phenomenon that is more apparent when the ascending aorta is small. In these cases, echocardiographic velocity may be higher, and the valve area may appear smaller than that determined at cardiac catheterization. Garcia and colleagues[9-11] propose that use of their equation, which takes into account the energy loss across a stenotic AV and can also be indexed for body surface area, would resolve the discrepancy often seen between AVA calculated from transvalvular gradients by Doppler versus catheterization. This calculation, which they refer to as *energy loss coefficient* (ELCo), uses the AVA calculated by Doppler and appears to correlate well with the effective orifice area measured by catheter (EOA_{cath}), particularly when this is significantly different from the effective orifice area measured by Doppler (EOA_{Dop}), although this is secondary to the phenomenon of pressure recovery. Theoretically, this is useful with discrepant noninvasive and invasive measurements, and when the ascending aorta is particularly small (diameter < 3.0 cm). However, the equation has not been applied clinically in large studies to show a significantly improved outcome with application. In addition, it can be argued that when using the current guidelines, and symptoms prompt the need for intervention, the difference in these calculations is merely academic. Further outcome-directed studies are

needed before these calculations are used in the mainstream, but the concept is important to understand differing calculations in AVA.[9-11]

Overall, pressure gradients and valve areas assessed by echocardiography and cardiac catheterization correlate very well with one another, such that in most cases, only echocardiography is needed to define the severity of aortic stenosis. Therefore, unless noninvasive evaluation is ambiguous, cardiac catheterization is used only for the identification of coronary artery disease prior to AV surgery.

Timing of Surgical Intervention

SYMPTOMATIC PATIENTS

The timing of surgical intervention in severe aortic stenosis is clear from its natural history. Once symptoms of heart failure (HF), angina, or syncope develop, the prognosis abruptly changes; the 2-year survival of patients who come to medical attention with HF approaches 50% without surgical correction.[12] No randomized clinical trials are available that compare outcome with medical therapy versus surgical correction in symptomatic patients, but observational data consistently demonstrate that aortic valve replacement (AVR) is associated with a substantial improvement in overall survival and symptomatology.[13-16] Therefore, it is universally recommended that symptomatic patients with severe aortic stenosis undergo surgical correction.

The outcome and risk of surgery is in part related to left ventricular (LV) function.[17] Excessive afterload, also called *afterload mismatch,* is thought to be the prime cause of the dysfunction in many of these patients and is often corrected after valve replacement.[18] In those with severely reduced LV function, complete resolution of symptoms and LV dysfunction may not ensue.[19] Despite this, the operative risk of AVR is acceptable, and the majority of patients demonstrate improved functional status.[20-24] In one study, the presence of coronary artery disease was associated with increased mortality rate after surgery in patients with severely decreased LV ejection fraction (LVEF).[25] Another more recent small study of 86 patients showed that predictors of outcome included not just the presence of LV dysfunction but its severity; those with an LVEF below 40% fared worse. It also found that presence of restrictive filling and a systolic pulmonary artery (PA) pressure of 45 mm Hg or greater were poor prognostic indicators.[26] Therefore, attention to degree of LV dysfunction and its secondary effects, such as pulmonary hypertension (PHTN), need to be considered prior to surgery.

LOW-GRADIENT AORTIC STENOSIS

Patients with severe aortic stenosis (AVA <1.0 cm[2]) may come to medical attention with low transvalvular pressure gradients (mean gradient <30 to 40 mm Hg) in the setting of severe LV dysfunction.[27] This discrepancy occurs in the presence of low transvalvular flow and may be seen in patients with primary contractile dysfunction or excessive afterload or some combination of the two. In those with truly severe stenosis, the use of low-dose dobutamine infusion generally produces an increase in flow and an increase in the transvalvular pressure gradient with little or no change in the valve area. By contrast, a pseudostenosis may be related to the reduced valve-opening force caused by the weakened ventricle. In this situation, dobutamine infusion augments valve opening; an increase in transvalvular flow is seen with little or no change in the pressure gradients, and the calculated effective valve area increases. Dobutamine infusion also provides important information about LV contractile reserve. Patients who lack *contractile reserve,* defined as failure to increase stroke volume by 20% or more during dobutamine infusion, have a poor prognosis, regardless of medical or surgical treatment.[28,29] However, recent literature suggests that for these patients, although the surgical mortality rate is higher than in patients with

TABLE 45-1	Measures of Severity in Aortic Stenosis			
SEVERITY OF AORTIC STENOSIS	MILD	MODERATE	SEVERE	VERY SEVERE
Doppler jet velocity (m/s)	<3.0	3.0-4.0	>4.0	>5.0
Mean gradient (mm Hg)	<25	25-40	>40	>60
Aortic valve area (cm²)	>1.5	1.0-1.5	<1.0	<0.6

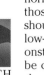

normal LV function, those sent for AVR have better outcomes than those treated with medical management. This implies that surgery should not necessarily be withheld from patients with low-flow/low-gradient aortic stenosis who lack contractile reserve as demonstrated by dobutamine echo.[30-32] Regardless, each patient must be counseled on the risk/benefit ratio of surgery, and decisions should be made on an individual basis.

ELDERLY PATIENTS

Calcific aortic stenosis is the most common valvular lesion seen in elderly patients, but the indications for surgery are the same as for younger patients. Although advanced age has been shown to be a determinant of outcome, it does not preclude surgery because the majority of elderly patients have a good outcome following surgery. For example, in a large retrospective study of 1100 patients aged 80 years or older who underwent AVR, 30-day cardiac and all-cause mortality rates were 4% and 6.6%, respectively.[33] Overall, elderly patients had an improvement in function and quality of life to a degree similar to that of age-matched controls.[34-39]

Elderly patients may come to medical attention with anatomic features that may necessitate further surgical consideration.[34,40] For example, elderly women may have narrow outflow tracts and smaller aortic annular dimensions, which may require annular dilation to allow for a larger prosthesis and may occasionally require a composite graft. In addition, heavy calcification is not uncommon and may require extensive debridement. Comorbidities and the patient's wishes and expectations must also be considered.

ASYMPTOMATIC PATIENTS

AVR in asymptomatic patients with severe stenosis remains controversial. The 2006 American College of Cardiology (ACC)/American Hospital Association (AHA) guidelines provide a class I recommendation for AVR in asymptomatic patients with severe aortic stenosis if they have either LV systolic dysfunction or are undergoing sternotomy for another indication, such as coronary artery bypass grafting (CABG). AVR is given a class IIb recommendation for patients with asymptomatic severe aortic stenosis if there is an abnormal response to exercise, a high likelihood of rapid progression, or the response to exercise is extremely severe (defined as AVA <0.6 cm^2, mean gradient [MG] >60 mm Hg, and pressure velocity [PV] >5.0 m/s), provided the expected operative mortality rate is 1.0% or less.[41] Evidence suggests that exercise testing can be used as a method of risk stratification in patients with severe aortic stenosis but without clear symptomatology.[42,43] Exercise testing should not be performed in those whose symptoms are attributable to aortic stenosis, but with close physician supervision, it can be considered and may uncover exercise-induced symptoms and intolerance. The presence of exercise-induced hypotension portends a poor prognosis. In one study, 66 asymptomatic patients with severe aortic stenosis, but without angiographic coronary artery disease, were followed for a mean of 15 months: four patients died suddenly, and all four had an abnormal stress test.[44,45] Likewise, increased rate of progression has been linked to adverse outcomes, particularly in those who showed an increase in Doppler velocities greater than 0.3 m/sec or a decrease in valve area greater than 0.1 cm^2 per year.[46] Thus, regular monitoring is warranted in asymptomatic patients with severe stenosis.

Since these guidelines were released in 2006, new data have been reported that support surgery in asymptomatic patients with very severe aortic stenosis.[47-49] The favorable risk/benefit ratio of AVR in this population is due both to increased risk of death and adverse events in patients managed conservatively and to improved perioperative mortality rates in isolated AVR, with one study showing a 30-day postoperative mortality rate of 0%, except that one in-hospital death resulted from esophageal perforation

Box 45-1 Recommendations for Aortic Valve Replacement in Patients with Aortic Stenosis

Indications

Patients with severe aortic stenosis and symptoms (angina, syncope, or heart failure)

Patients with severe or moderate aortic stenosis who are undergoing coronary artery bypass graft surgery or surgery on the aorta or other heart valves

Possible Indications

Asymptomatic patients with severe aortic stenosis and at least one of the following*:
- Ejection fraction <50%
- Hemodynamic instability during exercise (e.g., hypotension)
- Ventricular arrhythmia
- High likelihood of progression
- Extremely severe stenosis (AVA <0.6 cm^2, MG >60 mm Hg, PV >5.0 m/s) when operative mortality rate is <1.0%

*Aortic valve replacement is not indicated to prevent sudden death in asymptomatic patients with none of the findings listed.

AVA, aortic valve area; MG, mean transvalvular gradient; PV, pressure velocity.

Modified from Carabello BA. Clinical practice: aortic stenosis. *N Engl J Med* 2002;346:677-682.

(0.5%).[50] However, aside from the risk of surgery, the attendant long-term prosthesis risks must be weighed as well. Implantation of a prosthesis is known to be associated with a significant annual complication rate, which should be taken into account and weighed on a case-by-case basis.[51] Therefore, the best approach is to use symptoms as the primary guide to refer a patient to surgery. In the case of an asymptomatic patient with high-risk features, the physician should at least consider sending the patient for surgery if the institution has excellent surgical outcomes, and if the patient would be compliant with the precautions taken for prosthetic valves.[52,53]

Overall Approach

ROLE OF PERCUTANEOUS INTERVENTION

Percutaneous intervention for aortic stenosis is discussed in Chapter 47. Various techniques will be discussed, but readers should understand how transcatheter aortic valve implantation (TAVI) changes the population of patients who would be considered for intervention.

Surgical correction should be performed in all patients with symptomatic severe aortic stenosis (Box 45-1). AVR has been associated with marked improvements in morbidity and mortality across numerous symptomatic subgroups. In general, patients with only moderate aortic stenosis and symptoms resembling those of aortic stenosis do not require surgical intervention, and other causes for symptoms should be sought. In regard to asymptomatic patients with severe aortic stenosis, the patient should be screened with exercise testing if possible and also for rapid progression of disease. If either of these exist, or if the patient has very severe aortic stenosis in the setting of very good surgical outcomes within the institution to perform the procedure, early referral to surgery should be considered. If referral to surgery is not the best option, then these high-risk patients should be followed closely for progression of disease. Figure 45-1 provides an algorithmic approach that incorporates these recommendations.[27,41]

Mitral Stenosis

Assessment of Severity

Echocardiography is the preferred modality to assess for the presence and severity of mitral stenosis.[54] Classic doming of the

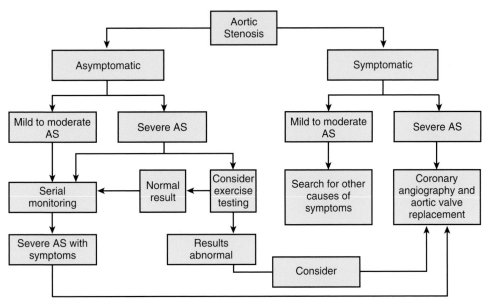

FIGURE 45-1 Algorithm for the timing of surgery in patients with aortic stenosis (*AS*).

anterior leaflet is readily identified from two-dimensional (2D) images, as are other morphologic features important in the assessment of mitral stenosis. Doppler techniques are used to measure the transmitral pressure gradients, with the modified Bernoulli equation, as well as to calculate the mitral valve area (MVA), with the diastolic pressure half-time method or the continuity equation. These measures correlate well with valve areas derived at cardiac catheterization.[55] The pressure half-time method should not be used when significant aortic regurgitation is present or immediately after mitral valvotomy, because abnormalities of atrial or ventricular compliance can affect MVA calculation.[56] Other techniques used to calculate MVA include the proximal isovelocity surface area (PISA) method, and direct planimetry[57] is a good option as long as the image acquisition is adequate and the measurement is taken at the leaflet tips. A measurement closer to the annulus gives a falsely increased valve area. PISA has recently begun to lose favor because of its difficulty in consistent reproducibility, but this has been seen more with regurgitant lesions.[58] Importantly, PA pressures should be determined to aid in the hemodynamic assessment.

Morphologic assessment of the mitral apparatus provides important information that may help guide the type of mechanical intervention (i.e., percutaneous balloon mitral valvuloplasty, surgical commissurotomy, or valve replacement). Echocardiography provides an assessment of leaflet mobility, thickness, calcification, and subvalvular thickening. When leaflets are relatively mobile, noncalcified, and have little subvalvular involvement, percutaneous mitral balloon valvuloplasty (PMBV) is generally successful and provides a safe and effective nonsurgical approach.[59] An echocardiographic scoring system described by Wilkins and colleagues[60] combines these factors into a useful approach to predict procedural success (Box 45-2). The degree of commissural calcification has also been used to help identify the most appropriate candidates for PMBV.[61,62] Higher scores indicate more severe disease and predict a lower likelihood of procedural success of PMBV. A similar scoring system has been described to predict the likelihood of postprocedural severe mitral regurgitation (MR).[63] When patients have significant mitral abnormalities (score >10), the sensitivity and specificity for predicting severe MR is 82% and 91%, respectively. Finally, higher echocardiographic morphologic scores have been related to higher inpatient costs.[64]

Hemodynamic measurements during cardiac catheterization can be performed when noninvasive findings are ambiguous or discordant with clinical findings. Transmitral pressure gradients

can be measured, and the MVA can be calculated using the Gorlin hydraulic formula.[65] Pulmonary pressures and resistance are routinely obtained to assess the hemodynamic effect of the stenosis on the pulmonary circulation. When PA balloon occlusion or wedge pressure is used as a surrogate for left atrial pressure, the transmitral pressure gradient may be overestimated despite adjustment for phase delay. Transseptal puncture is therefore more appropriate in determining the pressure gradient, especially if the accuracy of the wedge pressure is questioned.[66] Left ventriculography is used to assess for the presence of significant mitral insufficiency, and coronary angiography is performed if intervention is contemplated.

The resting MVA and mean pressure gradient are used to categorize the severity of mitral stenosis (Table 45-2). Not

TABLE 45-2   Grades of Mitral Stenosis Severity

SEVERITY	MVA (CM²)	GRADIENT (MM HG)	PAP	SYMPTOMS	ECG SIGNS	THERAPY
Mild	>1.8	2-4	Normal	Usually absent	S_2 to S >120 ms; normal P_2	IE prophylaxis
Moderate	1.2-1.6	4-9	Normal	Class I to II	S_2 to OS 100-120 ms; normal P_2	IE prophylaxis; diuretics
Moderate to severe	1.0-1.2	10-15	Mild pulmonary HTN	Class II to III	S_2 to OS 80-100 ms; P_2 increase	IE prophylaxis; BMV if applicable or surgery
Severe	<1.0	>15	Mild to severe pulmonary HTN	Class II to IV	S_2 to OS <80 ms; P_2 increase; RV lift Sx if right heart fails	IE prophylaxis; BMV or surgery

BMV, balloon mitral valvuloplasty; ECG, electrocardiogram; HTN, hypertension; IE, infective endocarditis; MVA, mitral valve area; OS, opening snap; PAP, pulmonary artery pressure; RV, right ventricular; Sx, symptoms.
Modified from Carabello BA. Modern management of mitral stenosis. *Circulation* 2005;112:432-437.

infrequently, however, the patient's symptoms may be out of proportion to the severity of the stenosis in the basal or resting state. Alternatively, measurements might reflect severe mitral stenosis in a patient without any symptoms. In these cases, assessment of hemodynamics with exercise or dobutamine at catheterization or coupled with echocardiography can help clarify the physiologic burden of mitral stenosis.[43,67] The reasoning behind this "masked" severity is multiple: diastolic filling is highly dependent on heart rate, and when the stenosis appears moderate at rest, a more significant gradient can occur during tachycardia with the increase in heart rate. In addition, some individuals have decreased atrioventricular compliance, which can also contribute. If a significant rise in mean transmitral pressure gradient (>5 mm Hg) or pulmonary capillary wedge pressure (>25 mm Hg) is observed, or if PHTN results (systolic pressure >60 mm Hg), percutaneous intervention should be considered if valve morphology is appropriate.[68] Therefore, an assessment of severity with exercise can help resolve clinical discrepancies in severity and can aid in planning for mechanical intervention.[43]

Overall Approach

PERCUTANEOUS MITRAL BALLOON VALVULOPLASTY

Details of valvuloplasty for mitral stenosis are discussed in Chapter 46. Approach and indications are detailed here.

In asymptomatic patients, percutaneous mechanical intervention is not generally entertained unless hemodynamic abnormalities coexist with at least moderate stenosis (Figure 45-2).[69] Thus if resting PHTN exists (>50 mm Hg) or exercise testing reveals exercise intolerance, induced PHTN (>60 mm Hg), or high PA wedge pressures (>25 mm Hg), PMBV should be considered, although confirmatory data to support this approach are not available.[41]

Symptomatic patients with moderate or severe mitral stenosis (MVA <1.5 cm²) are generally considered for PMBV if valve morphology is favorable and significant mitral insufficiency and left atrial thrombus are excluded (Figures 45-3 and 45-4).[70] If hemodynamically mild mitral stenosis is observed at rest in the presence of symptoms, exercise testing should be used to assess for adverse hemodynamics during stress. If PHTN or high PA wedge pressure is observed, other problems such as LV dysfunction should be considered. If a significant increase in transmitral gradient is observed, PMBV is considered. When patients are severely symptomatic (New York Hospital Association [NYHA] class III to IV) and conditions are not favorable for percutaneous intervention, referral for mitral valve (MV) surgery is recommended. This includes patients with significant mitral insufficiency (3 to 4+) or heavily calcified valves that would predict adverse periprocedural and clinical outcomes.

If left atrial or left atrial appendage thrombus is present, but conditions otherwise favor PMBV, a period of anticoagulation can be advocated to facilitate a later attempt at PMBV.[71] Percutaneous intervention may be feasible after several months of

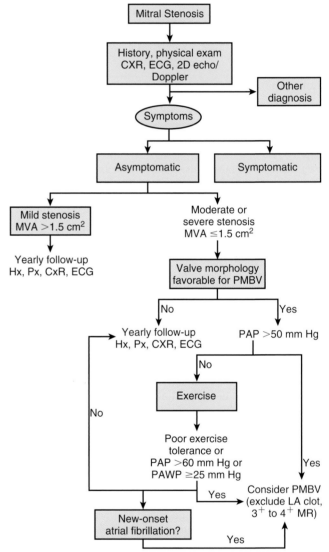

FIGURE 45-2 Management strategy for asymptomatic patients with mitral stenosis. 2D, two dimensional; CxR, chest radiograph; ECG, electrocardiogram; Hx, history; LA, left atrial; MR, mitral regurgitation; MVA, mitral valve area; PAP, pulmonary artery pressure; PAWP, pulmonary artery wedge pressure; PMBV, percutaneous mitral balloon valvuloplasty; Px, physical examination. *(Modified from ACC/AHA guidelines for the management of patients with valvular heart disease: a report of the American College of Cardiology/American Heart Association Task Force on Practice Guidelines [Committee on Management of Patients with Valvular Heart Disease]. J Am Coll Cardiol 2008;52:e1-e142.)*

anticoagulation, as long as thrombus resolution or organization is confirmed by echocardiography.

Surgical approaches to mitral stenosis are used when PMBV is not favorable or is unavailable. MV replacement or open commissurotomy is usually used (Table 45-3). Patients at high risk for surgery can be considered for PMBV, even though they may not be optimal candidates for the percutaneous procedure.[72] Recurrent stenosis can either be managed with repeat PMBV or with MV replacement,[73,74] but the risks of each should be considered given patient comorbidities and valve morphology.

Aortic Insufficiency

Assessment of Severity

The severity of aortic insufficiency can be assessed by Doppler echocardiography. Color flow and spectral Doppler imaging provide the foundation for the determination of the severity of insufficiency. An integrative approach is usually applied that uses all the information from the echocardiography study to arrive at

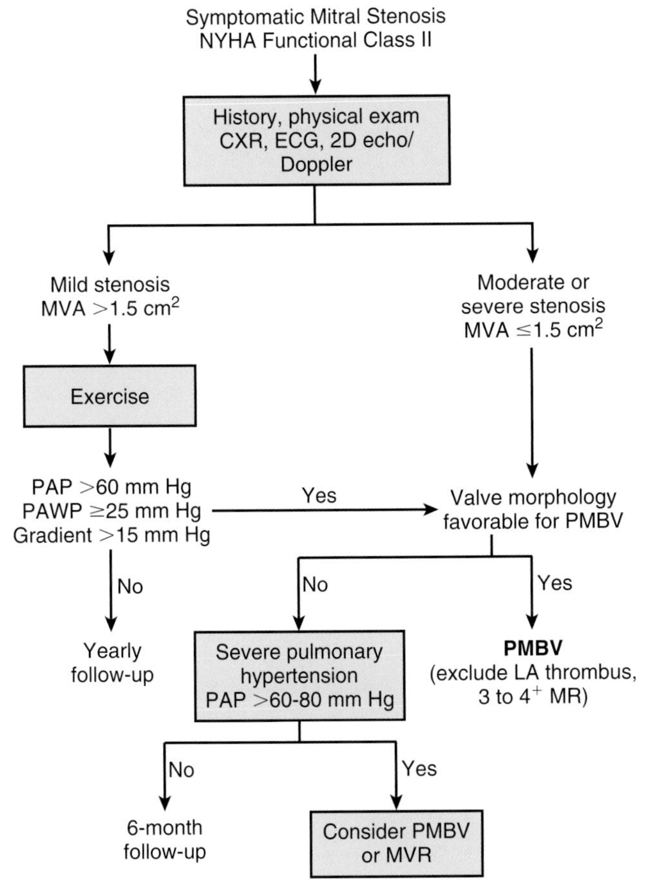

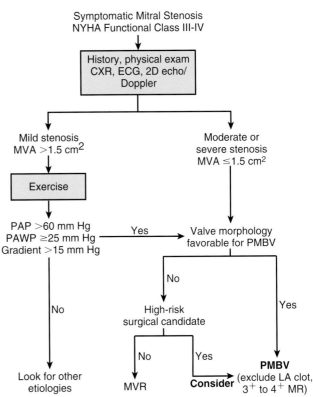

FIGURE 45-3 Management strategy for patients with mitral stenosis and mild symptoms. 2D, two dimensional; CXR, Chest radiograph; ECG, electrocardiogram; LA, left atrial; MR, mitral regurgitation; MVA, mitral valve area; NYHA, New York Hospital Association; PMBV, percutaneous mitral balloon valvuloplasty; PAP, pulmonary artery pressure; PAWP, pulmonary artery wedge pressure. (*Modified from ACC/AHA guidelines for the management of patients with valvular heart disease: a report of the American College of Cardiology/American Heart Association Task Force on Practice Guidelines [Committee on Management of Patients with Valvular Heart Disease].* J Am Coll Cardiol *2008;52:e1-e142.*)

FIGURE 45-4 Management strategy for patients with mitral stenosis and moderate to severe symptoms. CXR, Chest radiograph; LA, left atrial; MR, mitral regurgitation; MVA mitral valve area; NYHA, New York Heart Association; PAP, pulmonary artery pressure; PAWP, pulmonary artery wedge pressure; PMBV, percutaneous mitral balloon valvuloplasty. (*Modified from ACC/AHA guidelines for the management of patients with valvular heart disease: a report of the American College of Cardiology/American Heart Association Task Force on Practice Guidelines [Committee on Management of Patients with Valvular Heart Disease].* J Am Coll Cardiol *2008;52:e1-e142.*)

TABLE 45-3	Mechanical Therapy for Mitral Stenosis			
PROCEDURE	**INDICATIONS**	**CONTRAINDICATIONS**	**ADVANTAGES**	**DISADVANTAGES**
Balloon valvuloplasty	Sx; MVA <1.5 cm^2 with good valve score Pulmonary HTN, MVA <1.5 cm^2 with good valve score Sx or pulmonary HTN + high-risk surgery and any valve score	MVA >1.5 cm^2 LA thrombus, more than moderate MR	Percutaneous	Reduced applicability with poor valve morphology
Open commissurotomy	Sx, MVA <1.5 cm^2; pulmonary HTN with MVA <1.5 cm^2	MVA >1.5 cm^2	Avoids prosthetic valve	Risks of surgery and limited applicability
Mitral valve repair	Sx, MVA <1.5 cm^2 or pulmonary HTN with MVA < 1.5 cm^2	MVA >1.5 cm^2	Applicable when BMV and open commissurotomy fail	All the risks of surgery and of a prosthesis

BMV, balloon mitral valvuloplasty; HTN, hypertension; LA, left atrial; MR, mitral regurgitation; MVA, mitral valve area; Sx, symptoms
Modified from Carabello BA. Modern management of mitral stenosis. Circulation 2005;112:432-437.

TABLE 45-4	Echocardiographic Grading of Aortic Regurgitation				
PARAMETER	**MILD**	**MILD TO MODERATE**	**MODERATE**	**SEVERE**
Specific signs for AR severity	Central jet width <25% of LVOT		Signs of AR more than mild, but no criteria for severe AR	Central jet width ≥65% of LVOT
	Vena contracta <0.3 cm* No or brief early diastolic flow reversal in descending aorta			Vena contracta >0.6 cm*
Supportive signs	Pressure half-time >500 ms Normal LV size†		Intermediate values	Pressure half-time <200 ms Holodiastolic aortic flow reversal in descending aorta Moderate or greater LV enlargement‡
Quantitative Parameters§				
Rvol (mL/beat)¶	<30	30-44	45-59	≥60
RF (%)	<30	30-39	40-49	≥50
EROA (cm²)¶	<0.10	0.10-0.19	0.20-0.29	≥0.30

Caution should be used when interpreting nonnormalized volumes in isolation.
*At a Nyquist limit of 50-60 cm/s.
†LV size applied only to chronic lesions; normal two-dimensional measurements: LV minor axis <2.8 cm/m².
‡In the absence of other etiologies of LV dilation.
§Quantitative parameters can help subclassify the moderate regurgitation group into ranges of mild to moderate and moderate to severe regurgitation, as shown.
¶Consider body size.
AR, aortic regurgitation; EROA, effective regurgitant orifice area; LV, left ventricle; LVOT, left ventricular outflow tract; RF, regurgitant fraction; Rvol, regurgitant volume.
From Zoghbi WA, Enriquez-Sarano M, Foster E, et al. Recommendations for evaluation of the severity of native valvular regurgitation with two-dimensional and Doppler echocardiography. *J Am Soc Echocardiogr* 2003;16:777-802.

a coherent assessment. This should routinely include a 2D assessment of the AV, aorta, and LV chamber size and function.

Color-flow imaging of the regurgitant jet provides important clues to severity. The length alone of the color jet in the LV during diastole is a limited measure of severity; its width and area in the parasternal views are more reliable indicators of regurgitant severity. In addition, the size of the vena contracta provides a useful measure of severity when its size exceeds 6 mm.[75] The vena contracta is the narrowest central flow portion of any color-flow jet. It is essentially the smallest jet size measured at the level of the AV in aortic regurgitation. With these measures, the larger the width or area, the greater the severity of regurgitation. Supportive signs of severe aortic regurgitation include a short pressure half-time of the aortic regurgitant signal, holodiastolic flow reversal in the descending thoracic aorta, and at least moderate LV enlargement.[76] Parameters for the diagnosis of severe aortic regurgitation by echocardiography have been published (Table 45-4).

The aforementioned measures provide a qualitative or semi-quantitative measure of severity. The flow convergence method or proximal isovelocity surface area can be applied, but there is considerably less experience with proximal isovelocity surface area in aortic regurgitation compared with its use in mitral insufficiency.[77] As mentioned earlier in the chapter, this method also seems to be losing favor.[58] However, with this method, the size of the regurgitant orifice can be calculated, and an assessment of regurgitant volumes and severity can be made. A similar volumetric assessment[78] is made by comparing aortic stroke volume (i.e., time-velocity integral of LV outflow) with that of another, uninvolved valve, usually the mitral or pulmonic valve.

Another imaging option is cardiac magnetic resonance imaging (MRI). Advantages of this modality include highly accurate assessments of LV volumes, mass, and ejection fraction. This provides excellent evaluation of regurgitant volume and flow, and imaging of the aorta and aortic root can also be obtained. Disadvantages are the typical limitations of any MRI study: exclusion in the presence of an automatic implantable cardioverter-defibrillator or pacemaker, the length of the study, induced claustrophobia in the patient, and lack of availability or expertise.

Hemodynamic assessment at cardiac catheterization is used when noninvasive techniques fail to provide reliable results.[65] Qualitative assessment of severity is made by evaluating the

TABLE 45-5	Qualitative Grading of Aortic Regurgitation at Cardiac Catheterization
GRADE	**DESCRIPTION**
1+	Incomplete, faint LV opacification that clears with systole
2+	Faint, complete LV opacification not completely cleared with each systole
3+	Progressive opacification such that the LV equals the density of aortic root
4+	LV opacification on the first or second diastole greater than aortic root

LV, left ventricle.

persistence of opacification of the LV during diastole and comparing this with aortic opacification (Table 45-5). Quantitative left ventriculography can be used to calculate regurgitant volumes and regurgitant fraction. Total stroke volume can be obtained by a careful angiographic assessment of end-diastolic and end-systolic volumes. When forward stroke volume obtained from thermodilution or Fick cardiac output techniques is subtracted from total stroke volume, regurgitant volume is derived. Further division by the total stroke volume results in the regurgitant fraction, and a regurgitant fraction that exceeds 50% is consistent with severe aortic insufficiency. Coronary angiography is performed to assess the status of the coronary arteries in those at risk prior to surgical intervention.

Another useful tool in assessing severity of disease is exercise testing and stress echocardiography, which can be useful in many scenarios. Because symptoms often drive the decision to proceed with invasive therapies, exercise testing can demonstrate poor functional status and may induce symptoms in a patient who is relatively sedentary. Moreover, exercise evaluation can provide a baseline for which future studies can be compared to ensure that the function of the patient is stable. High-risk patient groups are also identifiable by this modality and include those who have increased PA pressures with stress (PA systolic pressure >60 mm Hg), those who develop LV dysfunction, and those whose MR worsens with stress. It can also be helpful in elucidating increasing PA pressures or higher degrees of regurgitation during exercise in those patients whose symptoms are out of proportion to the degree of the disease seen at rest.[43,79]

Timing of Surgical Intervention

As with other cardiac valves, recommendations are largely based upon observational data in relatively small populations, because prospective and adequately powered clinical trials have not been performed. Despite this, robust data are available that favor surgical intervention based upon the presence of severe insufficiency, symptoms, and the size and function of the LV. The vast majority of patients with aortic insufficiency undergo valve replacement, although experience with valve repair is accumulating in selected patient populations.

SYMPTOMATIC PATIENTS WITH NORMAL LEFT VENTRICULAR FUNCTION

The prognosis of patients with significant aortic insufficiency has been shown to be related to the presence of HF symptoms. In a study that involved 246 patients followed conservatively with severe or moderately severe insufficiency, NYHA class III or IV patients had an annual mortality rate of 25%, whereas class II patients had an annual mortality rate of 6%.[80] Patients who underwent surgery demonstrated a decreased cardiovascular mortality rate. The presence of significant symptoms of HF or angina in other studies indicates high annual mortality rates (>10%) in those treated conservatively.[81,82]

AV surgery is indicated in patients with normal LV function when NYHA class III or IV symptoms of HF are present.[83] However, when milder symptoms are present, it is often unclear whether symptoms are cardiac in origin, and exercise stress testing may provide helpful information in such patients.[84] When marked LV enlargement is present (>75 mm at end diastole) or when LV ejection fraction (LVEF) is borderline (50% to 55%), the presence of even mild symptoms should prompt a consideration of surgical correction.

The aforementioned applies chiefly to patients with chronic aortic insufficiency. Patients with acute severe insufficiency invariably come to medical attention with advanced symptoms, such as pulmonary edema or cardiogenic shock, and they often have normal LV systolic function and normal LV chamber sizes with tachycardia. In these settings, compensatory mechanisms are often inadequate, and poor outcomes are seen without prompt surgical intervention. Therefore nearly all patients with symptomatic severe aortic insufficiency, whether chronic or acute, should be considered candidates for surgical correction.[85]

SYMPTOMATIC PATIENTS WITH LEFT VENTRICULAR DYSFUNCTION

Surgical correction of symptomatic severe aortic insufficiency usually produces improvement in symptoms irrespective of the state of the LV. In a small study of symptomatic patients with a mean preoperative LVEF of 45%, the majority had a decrease in symptoms and a postoperative increase in LV function (mean postoperative LVEF, 59%).[86] Likewise, symptomatic patients with mild or moderate LV dysfunction also benefit from corrective AV surgery. Patients with severe LV dysfunction or class IV symptoms have previously been shown to have increased mortality rates and less chance of complete functional recovery postoperatively.[87] These patients often present difficult management issues, because irreversible ventricular dysfunction may be present. Although perioperative risk is high in such patients, AV surgery often provides a better alternative than medical therapy alone. In a study from the Mayo Clinic that involved 450 patients who underwent AV surgery for chronic aortic insufficiency, approximately 10% had an LVEF below 35%. In such patients, operative mortality rate was 14%. However, the LVEF increased by 4.9% after surgery, and most patients had prolonged survival

without progression to HF.[88] More recently, the outcomes of AVR at the Cleveland Clinic, specifically in patients with severe LV dysfunction (LVEF <30%), from 1972 to 1999 were described. As expected, mortality rates initially were higher in patients with LV dysfunction compared with matched controls. However, hospital mortality rate in these patients decreased from the initial 50% in 1975 to 0% after 1985. Further survival curves in those patients with LV dysfunction operated on after 1985 matched those of controls with nonsevere LV dysfunction.[89] Thus, even though a randomized controlled trial has not been performed, it can be recommended that such patients should not be denied the potential benefits of surgery.[90] Based on recent data, improved surgical outcomes may have mitigated increased risk in this population, but more data are needed for this to be proven. A period of intense medical treatment to relieve the signs and symptoms of HF is warranted prior to surgical correction.

ASYMPTOMATIC PATIENTS

Some controversy exists regarding surgery for severe aortic regurgitation among asymptomatic individuals, particularly when LV systolic function is normal. LV size by echocardiography at end diastole and end systole has been suggested as a guide for recommending surgical intervention. Severe LV dilation (LV end-diastolic dimension >75 mm) or systolic dysfunction (LV end-systolic dimension >55 mm) appears to represent high-risk patients with an increased incidence of adverse outcomes without intervention.[91,92] Despite the lack of large-scale studies to evaluate patients with asymptomatic severe aortic insufficiency, conventional wisdom indicates that LVEF and end-systolic dimension are important predictors of survival and LV function following surgical correction.[92] Thus, an LVEF below 50% or an end-systolic diameter greater than 55 mm can be considered an indication for AVR in an asymptomatic patient. However, patients with moderately severe dilatation (LV end-diastolic dimension >70 to 75 mm) have been shown to have acceptable outcomes with conservative management.[93] This suggests that end-diastolic size alone is not a strong indication for AVR.

Serial monitoring is required in patients with severe aortic insufficiency who do not yet meet criteria for surgical correction and who remain asymptomatic.[94] Patients with a declining ejection fraction represent a subgroup at higher risk, for whom regular monitoring is mandatory.[95] In addition, some patients who develop systolic dysfunction do so without premonitory symptom development.[96] Therefore in addition to serial follow-up for symptom evaluation, objective evidence by echocardiography is invaluable to identify asymptomatic patients with LV dysfunction, in whom surgical intervention is appropriate.

Overall Approach

An algorithm to guide the timing of surgery in severe chronic aortic insufficiency has been developed (Figure 45-5).[91] In essence, all patients with symptoms (NYHA functional class III or IV), or those with LV dysfunction irrespective of symptoms, should undergo corrective AV surgery. Serial noninvasive monitoring is mandatory for asymptomatic patients without resting ventricular dysfunction and for those who are not yet candidates for correction.

Mitral Insufficiency

Assessment of Severity

An integrative approach is recommended when using echocardiography to assess the severity of MR.[76] The combination of 2D, color-flow, and spectral Doppler measurements, as well as quantitative parameters, aid in identifying severe MR in a more accurate and reproducible fashion. When transthoracic images are inadequate, or when further[8] imaging can assist in planning of

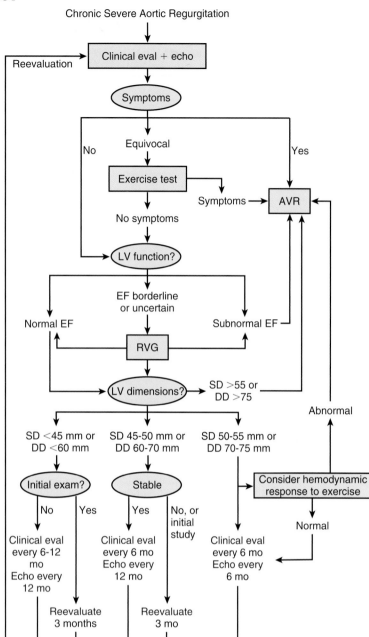

FIGURE 45-5 Timing of surgery for aortic regurgitation. AVR, aortic valve replacement; DD, end-diastolic dimension; EF, ejection fraction; LV, left ventricle; RVG, radionuclide ventriculography; SD, end-systolic dimension. *(Modified from ACC/AHA guidelines for the management of patients with valvular heart disease: a report of the American College of Cardiology/American Heart Association Task Force on Practice Guidelines [Committee on Management of Patients with Valvular Heart Disease].* Circulation *2006;114(5):e84-e231.)*

surgery, transesophageal images may be useful. An application of specific and supportive parameters in MR is shown in Table 45-6, but it should be noted that the degree of MR varies depending on such factors as patient volume status and blood pressure.

Two-dimensional echo imaging gives clues about chronicity and etiology, both of which assist in the assessment of the severity of mitral insufficiency. In acute MR, when compensatory measures have not yet developed, the chamber sizes may be normal. In chronic MR, LV and left atrial enlargement should be present. Two-dimensional imaging also defines whether the MR is due to rheumatic disease or degenerative disease, or is functional, to name some of the more common causes.

Color-flow Doppler parameters can also be helpful in grading severity of mitral insufficiency. Regurgitant jet area lacks accuracy, especially when the jet is eccentric, and it should not be used as a single measure of severity.[97] However, significant MR is likely present when large jets reach the posterior aspect of the left atrium and penetrate the pulmonary veins. Measurement of the vena contracta may provide a more specific sign of severity, especially when measurements exceed 0.6 to 0.8 cm in long-axis views.[98,99] Clinicians should avoid making this measurement in the apical two-chamber view because the vena contracta may be erroneously wide along the coaptation margins. Although measurement of the vena contracta works well with central or eccentric jets, multiple jets create fundamental problems with this technique. Another challenge in using color-flow Doppler is in acute severe MR. Because of the relative lack of difference between the left atrial and LV pressures, the color jet is small and is often mistaken for mild regurgitation. In this circumstance, history, physical exam, and the 2D image—which may elucidate an acute cause, such as flail leaflet—can be crucial.

Spectral Doppler measurements provide important adjunctive information to indicate severe MR. Pulmonary vein systolic flow reversal is a specific sign of hemodynamically severe regurgitation when seen in more than one pulmonary vein.[100] This finding is more reliable in acute or subacute than in chronic mitral insufficiency. The height of the mitral E velocity is greater than the

TABLE 45-6   Echocardiographic Grading of Mitral Regurgitation

	MILD	MILD TO MODERATE	MODERATE	SEVERE
Specific signs of severity	Small central jet <4 cm² or <20% of LA area* Vena contracta width <0.3 cm Minimal or no flow convergence†		Signs of MR more than mild, but no criteria for severe MR	Vena contracta width >7 cm with large central MR jet (area >40% of LA) or with a wall-impinging jet of any size, swirling in LA* Large flow convergence† Systolic reversal in PVs Prominent flail MV leaflet or ruptured papillary muscle
Supportive signs	Systolic dominant flow in pulmonary veins A-wave dominant mitral inflow‡ Soft density, parabolic CW Doppler MR signal Normal LV size¶		Intermediate signs/findings	Dense, triangular CW¶ Doppler MR jet¶ E-wave dominant mitral inflow (>1.2 m/s)‡¶ Enlarged LV and LA size,§ particularly when normal LV function is present
Quantitative Parameters§¶				
Rvol (mL/beat)**	<30	30-44	45-59	≥60
RF (%)	<30	30-39	40-49	≥50
EROA (cm²)**	<0.20	0.20-0.29	0.30-0.39	≥0.4

Caution should be used when interpreting nonnormalized volumes in isolation.

*At a Nyquist limit of 50 to 60 cm/s.

†Minimal and large-flow convergence, defined as a flow convergence radius <0.4 cm and ≤0.9 cm for central jets, respectively, with a baseline shift at a Nyquist limit of 40 cm/s. Cutoffs for eccentric jets are higher and should be angle corrected.

‡Usually >50 years or in conditions of impaired relaxation, in the absence of mitral stenosis, or with other causes of elevated LA pressure.

§In the absence of other etiologies of LV and LA dilation and acute MR.

¶LV size applied only to chronic lesions; normal two-dimensional measurements: LV minor axis of ≤2.8 cm/m², LV end-diastolic volume of ≤82 mL/m², maximal LA anteroposterior diameter of ≤2.8 cm/m², maximal LA volume of ≤36 mL/m².

¶Quantitative parameters can help subclassify the moderate regurgitation group into ranges of mild to moderate and moderate to severe, as shown.

**Consider body surface area.

CW, continuous wave; EROA, effective regurgitant orifice area; LA, left atrium; LV, left ventricle; MR, mitral regurgitation; MV, mitral valve; PVs, pulmonary veins; RF, regurgitant fraction; Rvol, regurgitant volume

Modified from Zoghbi WA, Enriquez-Sarano M, Foster E, et al. Recommendations for evaluation of the severity of native valvular regurgitation with two-dimensional and Doppler echocardiography. *J Am Soc Echocardiogr* 2003;16:777-802.

A-wave velocity in severe MR and is usually greater than 1.2 cm/s. An A-wave dominant pattern virtually excludes severe mitral insufficiency.[101] Another sign supportive of severe insufficiency is a dense, triangular, early peaking mitral insufficient envelope on continuous-wave Doppler sampling.

Quantitative methods can be used to assess the severity of mitral insufficiency. Calculation of stroke volumes in a manner similar to those described above for aortic regurgitation enables the calculation of regurgitant volume, fraction, and orifice area. Studies confirm the validity of this method to assess the severity of mitral insufficiency.[102] The PISA method has been validated previously and allows for regurgitant flow and effective regurgitant area (EROA) to be derived (EROA ≥0.4 cm² is consistent with severe mitral insufficiency). However, the PISA method is decreasing in popularity because of high interobserver variability as described by Biner and colleagues.[58] Also, with the advent of three-dimensional (3D) echo, it has been noted that the assumption of a hemispheric proximal flow convergence, which the PISA method relies on, is not always present. In fact, in functional MR, the flow convergence is more elliptical.[103] As 3D echo becomes more readily available, regurgitant volumes may be more accurately assessed without the prior geometric assumptions.[104]

Hemodynamic evaluation at cardiac catheterization is used when clinical and noninvasive measures are disparate or inconclusive. Semiquantitative and quantitative measures are used to assess for severe insufficiency,[65] and a qualitative scheme is shown in Table 45-7. In a manner similar to that described for aortic insufficiency, regurgitant volumes and regurgitant fraction can be derived, and fractions that exceed 50% signify severe mitral insufficiency.

Another emerging method of evaluating MR is exercise echocardiography. Three different ways to apply exercise echocardiography can be used in this setting. In patients who are

TABLE 45-7   Qualitative Grading of Mitral Regurgitation at Cardiac Catheterization

GRADE	DESCRIPTION
1+	Contrast enters the LA without complete chamber opacification.
2+	Complete opacification of the LA is not as dense as the LV.
3+	Progressive and complete opacification of the LA is equal in density to the LV.
4+	Early opacification is seen, with the LA being denser than the LV, often with opacification of the pulmonary veins.

LA, left atrium; LV, left ventricle.

asymptomatic but relative sedentary, exercise echocardiography may elucidate symptoms previously masked by the patient's lack of activity. Echocardiography with exercise may also reveal high-risk findings that factor into the decision making of whether to refer for surgery. These high-risk findings show either an increase in PA pressure (PA systolic pressure >60 mm Hg) or the development of wall-motion abnormalities and subsequent LV dysfunction. Patients whose symptoms seem to outweigh the severity of MR may also undergo exercise echocardiography to assess whether the regurgitation worsens with exercise, as can be seen in ischemic MR among other scenarios. Findings of increased pulmonary pressures or worsened MR with exercise, as quantified by regurgitant volume, were associated with reduced symptom-free survival in one small study.[79] In general, exercise echocardiography should be considered in the aforementioned scenarios, when patients are capable of performing the test.

Timing of Intervention

As with other valvular lesions, there is a paucity of large-scale randomized trials, and recommendations regarding the optimal time of surgery have been largely based upon observational data regarding predictors of outcome.

The etiology of severe mitral insufficiency appears to impact prognosis. Those patients with primary leaflet abnormalities appear to have a more favorable outcome with surgical intervention, whereas those with secondary insufficiency tend to have a prognosis that primarily depends on the underlying process. The following discussion centers on chronic mitral insufficiency that originates from organic leaflet dysfunction, and the section following it gives special attention to functional ischemic MR.

SYMPTOMATIC PATIENTS

As with many of the other valve diseases, presence of symptoms is a critical factor. Symptomatic patients with severe chronic mitral insufficiency should be considered candidates for surgical intervention.[105] However, because of the dynamic nature of MR, this assessment is often confusing. As mentioned earlier, the degree of regurgitation depends on a patient's status; in the presence of hypertension or hypervolemia, symptoms may be transient. Although no study addresses this particular scenario, given the recent data in support of earlier surgery in asymptomatic patients, it might be deduced that even transient symptoms in the presence of severe MR should prompt consideration for surgery.[106]

ASYMPTOMATIC PATIENTS

Other than etiology and the presence of symptoms, three other factors should be taken into account when determining timing of surgery or intervention: 1) the presence of LV systolic dysfunction, 2) the presence of other high-risk factors, and 3) the type of surgery the patient would be expected to undergo. An LVEF below 60% in a patient without symptoms should be considered an indication for MV surgery. For patients with an LVEF of 60% or more, additional higher-risk findings—such as LV end-systolic dimension below 40 mm, new-onset atrial fibrillation, or the presence of PHTN—should be noted before referral. In addition, the type of surgery and the expertise of the surgical center are other key elements in the decision-making process. MV replacement has lost favor because of the associated problems with the subsequent management of a prosthesis, such as with anticoagulation, and the potential decrease in LV systolic function that results from resection of the MV apparatus. MV repair and preservation of the subvalvular apparatus is now the preferred surgery.[107] When the latter operation is possible, particularly in a surgical center experienced in MV repair, a patient with chronic severe MR might be considered for surgery even in the absence of symptoms, LV dysfunction, and significant high-risk factors, if the predicted outcome of successful repair is greater than 90%.

The feasibility of repair versus replacement can be assessed echocardiographically, either with transthoracic or transesophageal methods.[108] Repair is usually feasible when limited calcification of the leaflets or annulus is present, limited prolapse of only one leaflet exists, or pure annular dilatation or valvular perforation is present. On the other hand, replacement may be required if extensive calcification, severe prolapse, infection, or subvalvular involvement is seen.[109,110]

Debate is ongoing as to the optimal timing of surgery. In 2005, a cohort study described mortality rates that were higher than previously reported in patients with asymptomatic organic MR. In particular, patients with an EROA greater than 40 mm^2 had an increased risk of death from any cause.[111] Shortly thereafter, Rosenhek and colleagues published a study that followed 132 patients with asymptomatic severe MR, which showed comparable mortality rates to Austrian life tables from the Austrian Statistical Office. Rosenhek argued that outcomes are excellent for asymptomatic patients with severe MR when guideline-directed referral for surgery is adhered to and that early referral is not necessary and does not adequately take into account the risks of surgery.[112] Most recently, a study conducted from 1996 to 2005 followed 447 patients with organic, asymptomatic, severe MR who were either sent for early surgery—without yet meeting traditional criteria, such as LV dysfunction, symptoms, or high risk factors—followed with conventional treatment. They demonstrated that the early-surgery group had a significant improvement in 7-year event-free survival compared with the conventional group, arguing that early surgery is beneficial in this subset of patients.[113] Given that consensus of opinion has still not been reached, it appears that a case-by-case evaluation is necessary that takes into particular account the likelihood of repair versus replacement and the current surgical outcomes at each institution.

On the horizon, yet still in clinical studies, is the option of percutaneous MV repair. Mimicking the Alfieri stitch, which was previously used surgically, the percutaneous system aims to provide an edge-to-edge attachment of the anterior and posterior leaflets by means of deployment of a clip with mild residual regurgitation. Based on enrollment in recent trials, patients who might be considered for this procedure include those with moderate to severe MR (3 to 4+), with or without symptoms, and with either functional or degenerative MR, with LVEF below 60% or LV end-systolic diameter greater than 45 mm. The patient should also have the primary regurgitant jet originating from malcoaptation of the A2 and P2 scallops, with presence of any secondary jets being clinically insignificant, and it must be feasible for the patient to undergo transseptal catheterization.[114]

Overall Approach

The decision for surgery is based upon the presence or absence of symptoms, the size and function of the LV, the presence of high-risk factors, and the type of surgery performed. If surgery is performed, valve repair is preferred over replacement, and if replacement is performed, chordal preservation is always preferred. Patients with echocardiographic indicators of LV dysfunction are candidates for surgery irrespective of symptoms. When severe LV dysfunction is present, MV surgery is reasonable when *repair* is feasible, but it can be problematic when valve *replacement* is attempted. When atrial fibrillation or PHTN is present in asymptomatic individuals, early surgery should be considered, especially when repair is likely. Otherwise, close monitoring is usually advocated with noninvasive measures, with possible consideration for early surgery, depending on current surgical outcomes and feasibility of repair (Figure 45-6).

FUNCTIONAL (ISCHEMIC) MITRAL REGURGITATION

Ischemia can cause a variety of MV pathologies that include functional MR (structurally normal leaflets and valve apparatus), papillary muscle rupture, and infarction. Special attention over the past several years has been paid as to what the best course of management is for functional ischemic MR, and for good reason; it has been shown that the presence of ischemic MR predicts a worse mortality, both in comparison with those who have MR from other etiologies and those with ischemia without associated MR.[115-118] Some trials have shown a mortality benefit with surgical intervention for ischemic MR.[119] However, the majority of the evidence shows no clear-cut benefit despite advancing techniques and documentation of improvement in postoperative MR.[120-122] It is also important to note that addition of MV repair or replacement to CABG increases the operative risk above revascularization alone. Ongoing studies are examining the reason behind this lack of significant benefit. Currently the focus is on specific anatomic changes from ischemia, such as papillary muscle tethering from LV remodeling. On the horizon are new annuloplasty rings, undersized rings for the purpose of restrictive

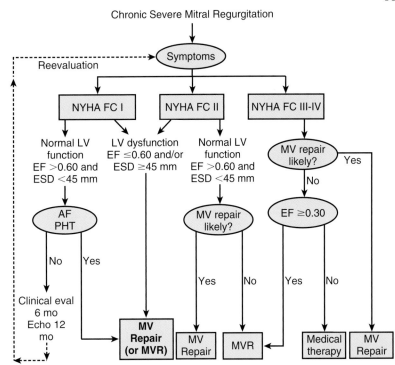

FIGURE 45-6 Management strategy and timing of surgery in patients with mitral regurgitation. AF, atrial fibrillation; EF, ejection fraction; ESD, end-systolic dimension; LV, left ventricle; MV, mitral valve; MVR, mitral valve replacement; NYHA FC, New York Heart Association functional class; PHT, pulmonary hypertension. *(Modified from ACC/AHA guidelines for the management of patients with valvular heart disease: a report of the American College of Cardiology/American Heart Association Task Force on Practice Guidelines [Committee on Management of Patients with Valvular Heart Disease]. J Am Coll Cardiol 1998;32:1486-588.)*

mitral annuloplasty, and chordal cutting; all of these modalities are being examined as potential therapies. Until more studies prove otherwise, MV surgery has not been adequately shown to improve mortality in functional ischemic MR.

Right-Sided Valve Disease

Tricuspid Valve Disease

In adults, severe tricuspid insufficiency can result from a host of primary structural leaflet abnormalities or functional abnormalities (normal leaflets with annular dilation). Primary leaflet abnormalities are divided into *congenital abnormalities*—such as Ebstein anomaly, tricuspid valve (TV) cleft, and double-orifice TV—and *acquired abnormalities* that include endocarditis, carcinoid disease, rheumatic disease, and trauma. Functional abnormalities include right ventricular (RV) dysplasia, primary or secondary PHTN, atrial septal defects, and anomalous pulmonary venous drainage.[123,124] Evaluation is best done with echocardiography, in which a systematic approach allows for determination of severity. In particular, a dense, triangular, early-peaking tricuspid regurgitant envelope seen on spectral Doppler; systolic reversal of hepatic vein flow; a large vena contracta width (>0.7 cm); and dilation of right-sided chambers and the inferior vena cava (IVC) are echocardiographic indicators of severe tricuspid insufficiency.[76,125]

Although it is still standard practice to use 2D echocardiography and Doppler imaging to evaluate valvular lesions, it has become increasingly evident that 3D echocardiography offers several advantages, particularly in regard to the TV. In addition, 2D echocardiography typically only visualizes two of the three TV leaflets, whereas 3D echo demonstrates all three leaflets. The TV annulus is oval and saddle-shaped, which makes it difficult to quantify by a single linear measure, and 3D echo provides a better conceptualization of the annulus and its pathology.[126,127] Therefore, it is not only anticipated that TV pathology will be better defined by this imaging technique, but it is also hoped that therapies for TV pathology will advance with the use of this modality.

Severe tricuspid insufficiency may be a marker for poor outcomes when present alone or in combination with other valve disease.[128] In a retrospective study of more than 5000 predominantly male patients over 4 years, increasing tricuspid regurgitation (TR) severity was associated with worse survival regardless of LVEF or PA pressure. This was notable independent of age, RV size, and IVC dilatation. Mortality rates ranged from a 1-year survival of 91% in patients without TR to 64% in patients with severe TR.[129] When RV failure and tricuspid insufficiency result from reversible left-sided cardiac disease, particularly mitral stenosis, improvement in tricuspid insufficiency may result with surgical or percutaneous correction of the mitral stenosis.[130] However, balloon valvuloplasty for mitral stenosis alone may not completely resolve tricuspid insufficiency[131]; therefore tricuspid annuloplasty at the time of surgical correction for mitral stenosis may be appropriate, particularly if the tricuspid annulus diameter exceeds 3.5 cm.[132-134]

Timing of surgical intervention in severe, isolated tricuspid insufficiency is controversial. However, when symptoms are refractory to medical therapy, surgical intervention is reasonable. When surgical intervention is contemplated, tricuspid annuloplasty is usually performed; when the leaflets are abnormal or severely diseased, however, valve replacement may be necessary.[41]

Significant tricuspid stenosis is a relatively rare entity, but when present, it is usually the result of rheumatic involvement, and both stenosis and regurgitation may be present. The clinical status of the patient usually determines the treatment strategy. Although balloon valvuloplasty has been attempted,[135] significant TR may result; therefore, bioprosthetic valve replacement is often necessary.[136,137]

Pulmonary Valve Disease

Acquired pulmonary valve disease in adults is rare, with the vast majority of lesions originating from congenital malformation of the valve. Pulmonic stenosis in adolescents and young adults is often approached percutaneously and is performed when peak transpulmonic gradients exceed 30 mm Hg in symptomatic patients or 40 mm Hg in asymptomatic patients, or when there is a peak-to-peak RV to PA gradient of 30 to 39 mm Hg.[41,138] Significant pulmonic insufficiency can result following surgical repair of tetralogy of Fallot.[139] On the horizon, and currently being tested, are percutaneous pulmonic valves. Pending further testing and approval of percutaneous pulmonic valves for insufficiency, the timing of pulmonic valve replacement with a bioprosthesis will continue to be debated, although replacement prior to the development of irreversible RV dysfunction is optimal.[140,141]

Future Directions

Increasing clinical data suggest a role for the measurement of circulating biomarkers to help predict adequate timing of intervention for valvular heart disease. Natriuretic peptides have not only been shown to help in the diagnosis of HF,[142] they have also been shown to be independent predictors of outcome.[143] In valvular disease, natriuretic peptides may be a reflection of LV wall stress.[144] Clinically, plasma levels of brain-type natriuretic peptide (BNP) have been shown to parallel the severity of valvular disease and NYHA class among patients with aortic stenosis and mitral insufficiency.[145,146] Additional clinical data suggest that BNP measurement may be helpful in discerning symptom onset[147] or clinical deterioration[148] in aortic stenosis and appear to predict symptom-free survival and postoperative outcome among such patients.[149] Although clinical data are still emerging, measurement of natriuretic peptides may soon complement our current strategies in timing surgical intervention in valvular heart disease.[150]

As our noninvasive imaging techniques continue to improve, new data are available to support that these techniques will further contribute to decision making for the treatment of valvular heart disease. Cardiac MRI, with its ability to assess degree of fibrosis, may be a predictive tool in assessing outcomes of AVR.[151] Likewise, 3D echocardiography is emerging as an exclusive means to allow better assessment of valvular lesions from a geometric standpoint and may provide better quantitative direct measurements. In addition, 3D echocardiography is an excellent imaging modality to use in real time during procedures for rapid assessment of the valve before and after intervention.

REFERENCES

1. Thomas D, Choussat R, Isnard R, et al. Cardiac abscess in infectious endocarditis: a multicenter study apropos of 233 cases. The Working Group on Valvulopathy of the French Society of Cardiology. Arch Mal Coeur Vaiss 1998;91(6):745-752.
2. Cheitlin MD, Armstrong WF, Aurigemma GP, et al. ACC/AHA/ASE 2003 guideline update for the clinical application of echocardiography: summary article. A report of the American College of Cardiology/American Heart Association Task Force on Practice Guidelines (ACC/AHA/ASE Committee to Update the 1997 Guidelines for the Clinical Application of Echocardiography). Circulation 2003;108(9):1146-1162.
3. Weyman AE, Scherrer-Crosbie M. Aortic stenosis: physics and physiology—what do the numbers really mean? Rev Cardiovasc Med 2005;6(1):23-32.
4. Feigenbaum H, Armstrong WF, Ryan T, eds. Feigenbaum's echocardiography, 6th ed. 2005, Philadelphia, Lippincott, Williams & Wilkins, pp 243-244.
5. Gorlin R, Gorlin SG. Hydraulic formula for calculation of the area of the stenotic mitral valve, other cardiac valves, and central circulatory shunts. Am Heart J 1951;41(1):1-29.
6. Cannon JD Jr, Zile MR, Crawford FA Jr, Carabello BA. Aortic valve resistance as an adjunct to the Gorlin formula in assessing the severity of aortic stenosis in symptomatic patients. J Am Coll Cardiol 1992;20(7):1517-1523.
7. Grayburn PA, Eichhorn EJ. Dobutamine challenge for low-gradient aortic stenosis. Circulation 2002;106(7):763-765.
8. Currie PJ, Seward JB, Reeder GS, et al. Continuous-wave Doppler echocardiographic assessment of severity of calcific aortic stenosis: a simultaneous Doppler-catheter correlative study in 100 adult patients. Circulation 1985;71(6):1162-1169.
9. Garcia D, Dumesnil JG, Durand LG, Kadem L, Pibarot P. Discrepancies between catheter and Doppler estimates of valve effective orifice area can be predicted from the pressure recovery phenomenon: practical implications with regard to quantification of aortic stenosis severity. J Am Coll Cardiol 2003;41(3):435-442.
10. Garcia D, Pibarot P, Dumesnil JG, Sakr F, Durand LG. Assessment of aortic valve stenosis severity: a new index based on the energy-loss concept. Circulation 2000;101(7):765-771.
11. Bahlmann E, Cramariuc D, Gerdts E, et al. Impact of pressure recovery on echocardiographic assessment of asymptomatic aortic stenosis: an SEAS substudy. JACC: Cardiovasc Imaging 2010;3(6):555-562.
12. Ross J Jr, Braunwald E. Aortic stenosis. Circulation 1968;38(1 Suppl):61-67.
13. Lund O, Magnussen K, Knudsen M, et al. The potential for normal long-term survival and morbidity rates after valve replacement for aortic stenosis. J Heart Valve Dis 1996;5(3):258-267.
14. Kvidal P, Bergstrom R, Horte LG, Stahle E. Observed and relative survival after aortic valve replacement. J Am Coll Cardiol 2000;35(3):747-756.
15. Schwarz F, Baumann P, Manthey J, et al. The effect of aortic valve replacement on survival. Circulation 1982;66(5):1105-1110.
16. Lindblom D, Lindblom U, Qvist J, Lundstrom H. Long-term relative survival rates after heart valve replacement. J Am Coll Cardiol 1990;15(3):566-573.
17. Lund O, Flo C, Jensen FT, et al. Left ventricular systolic and diastolic function in aortic stenosis: prognostic value after valve replacement and underlying mechanisms. Eur Heart J 1997;18(12):1977-1987.
18. Villari B, Vassalli G, Betocchi S, et al. Normalization of left ventricular nonuniformity late after valve replacement for aortic stenosis. Am J Cardiol 1996;78(1):66-71.
19. Zile MR, Gaasch WH. Heart failure in aortic stenosis: improving diagnosis and treatment. N Engl J Med 2003;348(18):1735-1736.
20. Tarantini G, Buja P, Scognamiglio R, et al. Aortic valve replacement in severe aortic stenosis with left ventricular dysfunction: determinants of cardiac mortality and ventricular function recovery. Eur J Cardiothorac Surg 2003;24(6):879-885.
21. Sharony R, Grossi EA, Saunders PC, et al. Aortic valve replacement in patients with impaired ventricular function. Ann Thorac Surg 2003;75(6):1808-1814.
22. Sharma UC, Barenbrug P, Pokharel S, et al. Systematic review of the outcome of aortic valve replacement in patients with aortic stenosis. Ann Thorac Surg 2004;78(1):90-95.
23. Connolly HM, Oh JK, Schaff HV, et al. Severe aortic stenosis with low transvalvular gradient and severe left ventricular dysfunction: result of aortic valve replacement in 52 patients. Circulation 2000;101(16):1940-1946.
24. Rothenburger M, Drebber K, Tjan TD, et al. Aortic valve replacement for aortic regurgitation and stenosis in patients with severe left ventricular dysfunction. Eur J Cardiothorac Surg 2003;23(5):703-709.
25. Connolly HM, Oh JK, Orszulak TA, et al. Aortic valve replacement for aortic stenosis with severe left ventricular dysfunction: prognostic indicators. Circulation 1997;95(10):2395-2400.
26. Ding WH, Lam YY, Duncan A, et al. Predictors of survival after aortic valve replacement in patients with low-flow and high-gradient aortic stenosis. Eur J Heart Fail 2009;11(9):897-902.
27. Carabello BA. Clinical practice: aortic stenosis. N Engl J Med 2002;346(9):677-682.
28. Monin JL, Monchi M, Gest V, et al. Aortic stenosis with severe left ventricular dysfunction and low transvalvular pressure gradients: risk stratification by low-dose dobutamine echocardiography. J Am Coll Cardiol 2001;37(8):2101-2107.
29. Levy F, Laurent M, Monin JL, et al. Aortic valve replacement for low-flow/low-gradient aortic stenosis: operative risk stratification and long-term outcome: a European multicenter study. J Am Coll Cardiol 2008;51(15):1466-1472.
30. Clavel M-A, Fuchs C, Burwash IG, et al. Predictors of outcomes in low-flow, low-gradient aortic stenosis: results of the multicenter TOPAS study. Circulation 2008;118(14 Suppl 1):S234-S242.
31. Tribouilloy C, Lévy F, Rusinaru D, et al. Outcome after aortic valve replacement for low-flow/low-gradient aortic stenosis without contractile reserve on dobutamine stress echocardiography. J Am Coll Cardiol 2009;53(20):1865-1873.
32. Vaquette B, Corbineau H, Laurent M, et al. Valve replacement in patients with critical aortic stenosis and depressed left ventricular function: predictors of operative risk, left ventricular function recovery, and long-term outcome. Heart 2005;91(10):1324-1329.
33. Asimakopoulos G, Edwards MB, Taylor KM. Aortic valve replacement in patients 80 years of age and older: survival and cause of death based on 1100 cases: collective results from the UK Heart Valve Registry. Circulation 1997;96(10):3403-3408.
34. Bouma BJ, van den Brink RB, Zwinderman K, et al. Which elderly patients with severe aortic stenosis benefit from surgical treatment? An aid to clinical decision making. J Heart Valve Dis 2004;13(3):374-381.
35. Beyerbacht HP, Lamb HJ, van Der Laarse A, et al. Aortic valve replacement in patients with aortic valve stenosis improves myocardial metabolism and diastolic function. Radiology 2001;219(3):637-643.
36. Chiappini B, Camurri N, Loforte A, et al. Outcome after aortic valve replacement in octogenarians. Ann Thorac Surg 2004;78(1):85-89.
37. Gilbert T, Orr W, Banning AP. Surgery for aortic stenosis in severely symptomatic patients older than 80 years: experience in a single UK centre. Heart 1999;82(2):138-142.
38. Levin IL, Olivecrona GK, Thulin LI, Olsson SB. Aortic valve replacement in patients older than 85 years: outcomes and the effect on their quality of life. Coron Artery Dis 1998;9(6):373-380.
39. Langanay T, Verhoye JP, Ocampo G, et al. Current hospital mortality of aortic valve replacement in octogenarians. J Heart Valve Dis 2006;15(5):630-637.
40. Logeais Y, Langanay T, Roussin R, et al. Surgery for aortic stenosis in elderly patients: a study of surgical risk and predictive factors. Circulation 1994;90(6):2891-2898.
41. Bonow RO, Carabello BA, Kanu C, et al. ACC/AHA 2006 guidelines for the management of patients with valvular heart disease: a report of the American College of Cardiology/American Heart Association Task Force on Practice Guidelines (writing committee to revise the 1998 Guidelines for the Management of Patients with Valvular Heart Disease), developed in collaboration with the Society of Cardiovascular Anesthesiologists, endorsed by the Society for Cardiovascular Angiography and Interventions and the Society of Thoracic Surgeons. Circulation 2006;114(5):e84-e231.
42. Alborino D, Hoffmann JL, Fournet PC, Bloch A. Value of exercise testing to evaluate the indication for surgery in asymptomatic patients with valvular aortic stenosis. J Heart Valve Dis 2002;11(2):204-209.
43. Picano E, Pibarot P, Lancellotti P, et al. The emerging role of exercise testing and stress echocardiography in valvular heart disease. J Am Coll Cardiol 2009;54(24):2251-2260.
44. Amato MC, Moffa PJ, Werner KE, Ramires JA. Treatment decision in asymptomatic aortic valve stenosis: role of exercise testing. Heart 2001;86(4):381-386.
45. Chung EH, Gaasch WH. Exercise testing in aortic stenosis. Curr Cardiol Rep 2005;7(2):105-107.
46. Otto CM, Burwash IG, Legget ME, et al. Prospective study of asymptomatic valvular aortic stenosis: clinical, echocardiographic, and exercise predictors of outcome. Circulation 1997;95(9):2262-2270.
47. Pellikka PA, Sarano ME, Nishimura RA, et al. Outcome of 622 adults with asymptomatic, hemodynamically significant aortic stenosis during prolonged follow-up. Circulation 2005;111(24):3290-3295.

48. Rosenhek R, Zilberszac R, Schemper M, et al. Natural history of very severe aortic stenosis. *Circulation* 2010;121(1):151-156.
49. Kang D-H, Park S-J, Rim JH, et al. Early surgery versus conventional treatment in asymptomatic very severe aortic stenosis. *Circulation* 2010;121(13):1502-1509.
50. Malaisrie SC, McCarthy PM, McGee EC, et al. Contemporary perioperative results of isolated aortic valve replacement for aortic stenosis. *Ann Thorac Surg* 2010; 89(3):751-756.
51. Hammermeister K, Sethi GK, Henderson WG, et al. Outcomes 15 years after valve replacement with a mechanical versus a bioprosthetic valve: final report of the Veterans Affairs randomized trial. *J Am Coll Cardiol* 2000;36(4):1152-1158.
52. Iung B. Management of asymptomatic aortic stenosis. *Heart* 2011;97(3):253-259.
53. Vaishnava P, Fuster V, Goldman M, Bonow RO. Surgery for asymptomatic degenerative aortic and mitral valve disease. *Nat Rev Cardiol* 2011;8(3):173-177.
54. Hillis GS, Bloomfield P. Basic transthoracic echocardiography. *Br Med J* 2005; 330(7505):1432-1436.
55. Popovic AD, Stewart WJ. Echocardiographic evaluation of valvular stenosis: the gold standard for the next millennium? *Echocardiography* 2001;18(1):59-63.
56. Pitsavos CE, Stefanadis CI, Stratos CG, et al. Assessment of accuracy of the Doppler pressure half-time method in the estimation of the mitral valve area immediately after balloon mitral valvuloplasty. *Eur Heart J* 1997;18(3):455-463.
57. Oh JK, Seward JB, Tajik AJ. *The echo manual*, 2nd ed. 1999, Lippincott Williams & Wilkins, pp 116-117.
58. Biner S, Rafique A, Rafii F, et al. Reproducibility of proximal isovelocity surface area, vena contracta, and regurgitant jet area for assessment of mitral regurgitation severity. *JACC: Cardiovasc Imaging* 2010;3(3):235-243.
59. Palacios IF, Sanchez PL, Harrell LC, Weyman AE, Block PC. Which patients benefit from percutaneous mitral balloon valvuloplasty? Prevalvuloplasty and postvalvuloplasty variables that predict long-term outcome. *Circulation* 2002;105(12): 1465-1471.
60. Wilkins GT, Weyman AE, Abascal VM, Block PC, Palacios IF. Percutaneous balloon dilatation of the mitral valve: an analysis of echocardiographic variables related to outcome and the mechanism of dilatation. *Br Heart J* 1988;60(4):299-308.
61. Sutaria N, Northridge DB, Shaw TR. Significance of commissural calcification on outcome of mitral balloon valvotomy. *Heart* 2000;84(4):398-402.
62. Cannan CR, Nishimura RA, Reeder GS, et al. Echocardiographic assessment of commissural calcium: a simple predictor of outcome after percutaneous mitral balloon valvotomy. *J Am Coll Cardiol* 1997;29(1):175-180.
63. Padial LR, Abascal VM, Moreno PR, et al. Echocardiography can predict the development of severe mitral regurgitation after percutaneous mitral valvuloplasty by the Inoue technique. *Am J Cardiol* 1999;83(8):1210-1213.
64. Eisenberg MJ, Ballal R, Heidenreich PA, et al. Echocardiographic score as a predictor of in-hospital cost in patients undergoing percutaneous balloon mitral valvuloplasty. *Am J Cardiol* 1996;78(7):790-794.
65. Kern MJ. *The cardiac catheterization handbook*, 4th ed. 2003, Mosby–Year Book. pp 273-274.
66. Nishimura RA, Rihal CS, Tajik AJ, Holmes DR Jr. Accurate measurement of the transmitral gradient in patients with mitral stenosis: a simultaneous catheterization and Doppler echocardiographic study. *J Am Coll Cardiol* 1994;24(1):152-158.
67. Cheriex EC, Pieters FA, Janssen JH, et al. Value of exercise Doppler-echocardiography in patients with mitral stenosis. *Int J Cardiol* 1994;45(3):219-226.
68. Aviles RJ, Nishimura RA, Pellikka PA, Andreen KM, Holmes DR Jr. Utility of stress Doppler echocardiography in patients undergoing percutaneous mitral balloon valvotomy. *J Am Soc Echocardiogr* 2001;14(7):676-681.
69. Carabello BA. Modern management of mitral stenosis. *Circulation* 2005;112(3): 432-437.
70. Rahimtoola SH, Durairaj A, Mehra A, Nuno I. Current evaluation and management of patients with mitral stenosis. *Circulation* 2002;106(10):1183-1188.
71. Silaruks S, Thinkhamrop B, Tantikosum W, et al. A prognostic model for predicting the disappearance of left atrial thrombi among candidates for percutaneous transvenous mitral commissurotomy. *J Am Coll Cardiol* 2002;39(5):886-891.
72. Sutaria N, Elder AT, Shaw TR. Long-term outcome of percutaneous mitral balloon valvotomy in patients aged 70 and over. *Heart* 2000;83(4):433-438.
73. Iung B, Garbarz E, Michaud P, et al. Immediate and mid-term results of repeat percutaneous mitral commissurotomy for restenosis following earlier percutaneous mitral commissurotomy. *Eur Heart J* 2000;21(20):1683-1689.
74. Iung B, Garbarz E, Michaud P, et al. Percutaneous mitral commissurotomy for restenosis after surgical commissurotomy: late efficacy and implications for patient selection. *J Am Coll Cardiol* 2000;35(5):1295-1302.
75. Tribouilloy CM, Enriquez-Sarano M, Bailey KR, Seward JB, Tajik AJ. Assessment of severity of aortic regurgitation using the width of the vena contracta: a clinical color Doppler imaging study. *Circulation* 2000;102(5):558-564.
76. Zoghbi WA, Enriquez-Sarano M, Foster E, et al. Recommendations for evaluation of the severity of native valvular regurgitation with two-dimensional and Doppler echocardiography. *J Am Soc Echocardiogr* 2003;16(7):777-802.
77. Tribouilloy CM, Enriquez-Sarano M, Fett SL, et al. Application of the proximal flow convergence method to calculate the effective regurgitant orifice area in aortic regurgitation. *J Am Coll Cardiol* 1998;32(4):1032-1039.
78. Enriquez-Sarano M, Seward JB, Bailey KR, Tajik AJ. Effective regurgitant orifice area: a noninvasive Doppler development of an old hemodynamic concept. *J Am Coll Cardiol* 1994;23(2):443-451.
79. Magne J, Lancellotti P, Piérard LA. Exercise-induced changes in degenerative mitral regurgitation. *J Am Coll Cardiol* 2010;56(4):300-309.
80. Dujardin KS, Enriquez-Sarano M, Schaff HV, et al. Mortality and morbidity of aortic regurgitation in clinical practice: a long-term follow-up study. *Circulation* 1999;99(14):1851-1857.
81. Aronow WS, Ahn C, Kronzon I, Nanna M. Prognosis of patients with heart failure and unoperated severe aortic valvular regurgitation and relation to ejection fraction. *Am J Cardiol* 1994;74(3):286-288.
82. Ishii K, Hirota Y, Suwa M, et al. Natural history and left ventricular response in chronic aortic regurgitation. *Am J Cardiol* 1996;78(3):357-361.
83. Klodas E, Enriquez-Sarano M, Tajik AJ, et al. Optimizing timing of surgical correction in patients with severe aortic regurgitation: role of symptoms. *J Am Coll Cardiol* 1997;30(3):746-752.
84. Wahi S, Haluska B, Pasquet A, et al. Exercise echocardiography predicts development of left ventricular dysfunction in medically and surgically treated patients with asymptomatic severe aortic regurgitation. *Heart* 2000;84(6):606-614.
85. Nkomo VT. Indications for surgery for aortic regurgitation. *Curr Cardiol Rep* 2003;5(2):105-109.
86. Carabello BA, Usher BW, Hendrix GH, et al. Predictors of outcome for aortic valve replacement in patients with aortic regurgitation and left ventricular dysfunction: a change in the measuring stick. *J Am Coll Cardiol* 1987;10(5):991-997.
87. Carabello BA. Is it ever too late to operate on the patient with valvular heart disease? *J Am Coll Cardiol* 2004;44(2):376-383.
88. Chaliki HP, Mohty D, Avierinos J-F, et al. Outcomes after aortic valve replacement in patients with severe aortic regurgitation and markedly reduced left ventricular function. *Circulation* 2002;106(21):2687-2693.
89. Bhudia SK, McCarthy PM, Kumpati GS, et al. Improved outcomes after aortic valve surgery for chronic aortic regurgitation with severe left ventricular dysfunction. *J Am Coll Cardiol* 2007;49(13):1465-1471.
90. Chaliki HP, Mohty D, Avierinos JF, et al. Outcomes after aortic valve replacement in patients with severe aortic regurgitation and markedly reduced left ventricular function. *Circulation* 2002;106(21):2687-2693.
91. Gruber T, Kohrer C, Lung B, Shcherbakov D, Piendl W. Affinity of ribosomal protein S8 from mesophilic and (hyper)thermophilic archaea and bacteria for 16S rRNA correlates with the growth temperatures of the organisms. *FEBS Lett* 2003;549(1-3): 123-128.
92. Carabello BA, Crawford FA Jr. Valvular heart disease. *N Engl J Med* 1997;337(1):32-41.
93. Tarasoutchi F, Grinberg M, Spina GS, et al. Ten-year clinical laboratory follow-up after application of a symptom-based therapeutic strategy to patients with severe chronic aortic regurgitation of predominant rheumatic etiology. *J Am Coll Cardiol* 2003;41(8):1316-1324.
94. Borer JS, Bonow RO. Contemporary approach to aortic and mitral regurgitation. *Circulation* 2003;108(20):2432-2438.
95. Bonow RO, Lakatos E, Maron BJ, Epstein SE. Serial long-term assessment of the natural history of asymptomatic patients with chronic aortic regurgitation and normal left ventricular systolic function. *Circulation* 1991;84(4):1625-1635.
96. Scognamiglio R, Rahimtoola SH, Fasoli G, Nistri S, Dalla Volta S. Nifedipine in asymptomatic patients with severe aortic regurgitation and normal left ventricular function. *N Engl J Med* 1994;331(11):689-694.
97. Enriquez-Sarano M, Tajik AJ, Bailey KR, Seward JB. Color flow imaging compared with quantitative Doppler assessment of severity of mitral regurgitation: influence of eccentricity of jet and mechanism of regurgitation. *J Am Coll Cardiol* 1993; 21(5):1211-1219.
98. Hall SA, Brickner ME, Willett DL, et al. Assessment of mitral regurgitation severity by Doppler color flow mapping of the vena contracta. *Circulation* 1997;95(3): 636-642.
99. Heinle SK, Hall SA, Brickner ME, Willett DL, Grayburn PA. Comparison of vena contracta width by multiplane transesophageal echocardiography with quantitative Doppler assessment of mitral regurgitation. *Am J Cardiol* 1998;81(2):175-179.
100. Pu M, Griffin BP, Vandervoort PM, et al. The value of assessing pulmonary venous flow velocity for predicting severity of mitral regurgitation: a quantitative assessment integrating left ventricular function. *J Am Soc Echocardiogr* 1999;12(9):736-743.
101. Thomas L, Foster E, Schiller NB. Peak mitral inflow velocity predicts mitral regurgitation severity. *J Am Coll Cardiol* 1998;31(1):174-179.
102. Pu M, Prior DL, Fan X, et al. Calculation of mitral regurgitant orifice area with use of a simplified proximal convergence method: initial clinical application. *J Am Soc Echocardiogr* 2001;14(3):180-185.
103. Matsumura Y, Fukuda S, Tran H, et al. Geometry of the proximal isovelocity surface area in mitral regurgitation by 3-dimensional color Doppler echocardiography: difference between functional mitral regurgitation and prolapse regurgitation. *Am Heart J* 2008;155(2):231-238.
104. Pirat B, Little SH, Igo SR, et al. Direct measurement of proximal isovelocity surface area by real-time three-dimensional color Doppler for quantitation of aortic regurgitant volume: an in vitro validation. *J Am Soc Echocardiogr* 2009;22(3):306-313.
105. Otto CM. Timing of surgery in mitral regurgitation. *Heart* 2003;89(1):100-105.
106. Samad Z, Kaul P, Shaw LK, et al. Impact of early surgery on survival of patients with severe mitral regurgitation. *Heart* 2011;97(3):221-224.
107. Gaasch WH, Meyer TE. Left ventricular response to mitral regurgitation: implications for management. *Circulation* 2008;118(22):2298-2303.
108. Enriquez-Sarano M, Freeman WK, Tribouilloy CM, et al. Functional anatomy of mitral regurgitation: accuracy and outcome implications of transesophageal echocardiography. *J Am Coll Cardiol* 1999;34(4):1129-1136.
109. Hellemans IM, Pieper EG, Ravelli AC, et al. Prediction of surgical strategy in mitral valve regurgitation based on echocardiography. Interuniversity Cardiology Institute of the Netherlands. *Am J Cardiol* 1997;79(3):334-338.
110. Chaudhry FA, Upadya SP, Singh VP, et al. Identifying patients with degenerative mitral regurgitation for mitral valve repair and replacement: a transesophageal echocardiographic study. *J Am Soc Echocardiogr* 2004;17(9):988-994.
111. Enriquez-Sarano M, Avierinos J-F, Messika-Zeitoun D, et al. Quantitative determinants of the outcome of asymptomatic mitral regurgitation. *N Engl J Med* 2005;352(9): 875-883.
112. Rosenhek R, Rader F, Klaar U, et al. Outcome of watchful waiting in asymptomatic severe mitral regurgitation. *Circulation* 2006;113(18):2238-2244.
113. Kang DH, Kim JH, Rim JH, et al. Comparison of early surgery versus conventional treatment in asymptomatic severe mitral regurgitation. *Circulation* 2009;119(6): 797-804.

114. Tamburino C, Ussia GP, Maisano F, et al. Percutaneous mitral valve repair with the MitraClip system: acute results from a real world setting. *Eur Heart J* 2010; 31(11):1382-1389.

115. Akins CW, Hilgenberg AD, Buckley MJ, et al. Mitral valve reconstruction versus replacement for degenerative or ischemic mitral regurgitation. *Ann Thorac Surg* 1994;58(3):668-675; discussion 675-676.

116. Connolly MW, Gelbfish JS, Jacobowitz IJ, et al. Surgical results for mitral regurgitation from coronary artery disease. *J Thorac Cardiovasc Surg* 1986;91(3):379-388.

117. Lamas GA, Mitchell GF, Flaker GC, et al. Clinical significance of mitral regurgitation after acute myocardial infarction. Survival and Ventricular Enlargement Investigators. *Circulation* 1997;96(3):827-833.

118. Hickey MS, Smith LR, Muhlbaier LH, et al. Current prognosis of ischemic mitral regurgitation: implications for future management. *Circulation* 1988;78(3 Pt 2):I51-I59.

119. Schroder JN, Williams ML, Hata JA, et al. Impact of mitral valve regurgitation evaluated by intraoperative transesophageal echocardiography on long-term outcomes after coronary artery bypass grafting. *Circulation* 2005;112(9 Suppl):I293-I298.

120. Badiwala MV, Verma S, Rao V. Surgical management of ischemic mitral regurgitation. *Circulation* 2009;120(13):1287-1293.

121. Kim YH, Czer LS, Soukiasian HJ, et al. Ischemic mitral regurgitation: revascularization alone versus revascularization and mitral valve repair. *Ann Thorac Surg* 2005;79(6): 1895-1901.

122. Mihaljevic T, Lam BK, Rajeswaran J, et al. Impact of mitral valve annuloplasty combined with revascularization in patients with functional ischemic mitral regurgitation. *J Am Coll Cardiol* 2007;49(22):2191-2201.

123. Waller BF, Howard J, Fess S. Pathology of tricuspid valve stenosis and pure tricuspid regurgitation. Part III. *Clin Cardiol* 1995;18(4):225-230.

124. Bruce CJ, Connolly HM. Right-sided valve disease deserves a little more respect. *Circulation* 2009;119(20):2726-2734.

125. Shapira Y, Porter A, Wurzel M, Vaturi M, Sagie A. Evaluation of tricuspid regurgitation severity: echocardiographic and clinical correlation. *J Am Soc Echocardiogr* 1998;11(6):652-659.

126. Muraru D, Badano LP, Sarais C, Solda E, Iliceto S. Evaluation of tricuspid valve morphology and function by transthoracic three-dimensional echocardiography. *Curr Cardiol Rep* 2011;13(3):242-249.

127. Min SY, Song JM, Kim JH, et al. Geometric changes after tricuspid annuloplasty and predictors of residual tricuspid regurgitation: a real-time three-dimensional echocardiography study. *Eur Heart J* 2010;31(23):2871-2880.

128. Sagie A, Schwammenthal E, Newell JB, et al. Significant tricuspid regurgitation is a marker for adverse outcome in patients undergoing percutaneous balloon mitral valvuloplasty. *J Am Coll Cardiol* 1994;24(3):696-702.

129. Nath J, Foster E, Heidenreich PA. Impact of tricuspid regurgitation on long-term survival. *J Am Coll Cardiol* 2004;43(3):405-409.

130. Hannoush H, Fawzy ME, Stefadouros M, et al. Regression of significant tricuspid regurgitation after mitral balloon valvotomy for severe mitral stenosis. *Am Heart J* 2004;148(5):865-870.

131. Song JM, Kang DH, Song JK, et al. Outcome of significant functional tricuspid regurgitation after percutaneous mitral valvuloplasty. *Am Heart J* 2003;145(2):371-376.

132. Duran CM. Tricuspid valve surgery revisited. *J Card Surg* 1994;9(2 Suppl):242-247.

133. Shiran A, Sagie A. Tricuspid regurgitation in mitral valve disease incidence, prognostic implications, mechanism, and management. *J Am Coll Cardiol* 2009;53(5):401-408.

134. Bernal JM, Ponton A, Diaz B, et al. Combined mitral and tricuspid valve repair in rheumatic valve disease: fewer reoperations with prosthetic ring annuloplasty. *Circulation* 2010;121(17):1934-1940.

135. Orbe LC, Sobrino N, Arcas R, et al. Initial outcome of percutaneous balloon valvuloplasty in rheumatic tricuspid valve stenosis. *Am J Cardiol* 1993;71(4):353-354.

136. Porter A, Shapira Y, Wurzel M, et al. Tricuspid regurgitation late after mitral valve replacement: clinical and echocardiographic evaluation. *J Heart Valve Dis* 1999; 8(1):57-62.

137. Scully HE, Armstrong CS. Tricuspid valve replacement: fifteen years of experience with mechanical prostheses and bioprostheses. *J Thorac Cardiovasc Surg* 1995;109(6): 1035-1041.

138. Chen CR, Cheng TO, Huang T, et al. Percutaneous balloon valvuloplasty for pulmonic stenosis in adolescents and adults. *N Engl J Med* 1996;335(1):21-25.

139. Hazekamp MG, Kurvers MM, Schoof PH, et al. Pulmonary valve insertion late after repair of Fallot's tetralogy. *Eur J Cardiothorac Surg* 2001;19(5):667-670.

140. Therrien J, Provost Y, Merchant N, et al. Optimal timing for pulmonary valve replacement in adults after tetralogy of Fallot repair. *Am J Cardiol* 2005;95(6):779-782.

141. Therrien J, Siu SC, McLaughlin PR, et al. Pulmonary valve replacement in adults late after repair of tetralogy of Fallot: are we operating too late? *J Am Coll Cardiol* 2000;36(5):1670-1675.

142. Maisel AS, Krishnaswamy P, Nowak RM, et al. Rapid measurement of B-type natriuretic peptide in the emergency diagnosis of heart failure. *N Engl J Med* 2002;347(3):161-167.

143. Richards AM, Nicholls MG, Espiner EA, et al. B-type natriuretic peptides and ejection fraction for prognosis after myocardial infarction. *Circulation* 2003;107(22):2786-2792.

144. Ikeda T, Matsuda K, Itoh H, et al. Plasma levels of brain and atrial natriuretic peptides elevate in proportion to left ventricular end-systolic wall stress in patients with aortic stenosis. *Am Heart J* 1997;133(3):307-314.

145. Weber M, Arnold R, Rau M, et al. Relation of N-terminal pro-B-type natriuretic peptide to severity of valvular aortic stenosis. *Am J Cardiol* 2004;94(6):740-745.

146. Sutton TM, Stewart RA, Gerber IL, et al. Plasma natriuretic peptide levels increase with symptoms and severity of mitral regurgitation. *J Am Coll Cardiol* 2003;41(12): 2280-2287.

147. Gerber IL, Stewart RA, Legget ME, et al. Increased plasma natriuretic peptide levels reflect symptom onset in aortic stenosis. *Circulation* 2003;107(14):1884-1890.

148. Gerber IL, Legget ME, West TM, Richards AM, Stewart RA. Usefulness of serial measurement of N-terminal pro-brain natriuretic peptide plasma levels in asymptomatic patients with aortic stenosis to predict symptomatic deterioration. *Am J Cardiol* 2005;95(7):898-901.

149. Bergler-Klein J, Klaar U, Heger M, et al. Natriuretic peptides predict symptom-free survival and postoperative outcome in severe aortic stenosis. *Circulation* 2004;109(19): 2302-2308.

150. Pizarro R, Bazzino OO, Oberti PF, et al. Prospective validation of the prognostic usefulness of brain natriuretic peptide in asymptomatic patients with chronic severe mitral regurgitation. *J Am Coll Cardiol* 2009;54(12):1099-1106.

151. Azevedo CF, Nigri M, Higuchi ML, et al. Prognostic significance of myocardial fibrosis quantification by histopathology and magnetic resonance imaging in patients with severe aortic valve disease. *J Am Coll Cardiol* 2010;56(4):278-287.

CHAPTER 46 Surgery for Valvular Heart Disease

Matthias Peltz

OVERVIEW, 691

GENERAL CONSIDERATIONS, 691

Epidemiology, 691
Indications, 691
Preoperative Evaluation and Optimization, 692
Surgical Approaches, 694
Prostheses, 694
Postoperative Care, 699

AORTIC VALVE SURGERY, 699

Overview, 699
Indications, 699

Aortic Valve Replacement, 700
Aortic Valve Repair, 702
Results, 702

MITRAL VALVE SURGERY, 702

Overview, 702
Indications, 704
Mitral Valve Repair, 704
Mitral Valve Replacement, 706
Results, 706

TRICUSPID VALVE SURGERY, 708

Overview, 708

Indications, 708
Surgical Techniques, 708
Results, 708

SPECIAL CONSIDERATIONS, 709

Multiple Valves, 709
Reoperation, 709
Endocarditis, 709
Ischemic Heart Disease, 710
Atrial Fibrillation, 711

REFERENCES, 711

Overview

Although medical therapy can ameliorate symptoms and, in some instances, slow the progression of early-stage valvular heart disease, surgical intervention has been, and remains, the primary and only definitive therapy for nearly all patients with advanced valvular heart disease.

Before the introduction of closed mitral commissurotomy by Elliot Cutler in 1923, the natural history of most forms of valvular heart disease included progressive cardiopulmonary dysfunction and death. Although his subsequent results were poor, Cutler showed for the first time that surgical manipulation of the diseased valve could correct the physiologic dysfunction, alleviate symptoms, and alter the natural history of the disease. Twenty-five years later Dwight Harken, Charles Bailey, and others perfected the technique and demonstrated that surgical correction of valvular heart disease could be routine and durable.

Not until the clinical introduction of the heart-lung machine (John Gibbons, 1953) and the successful deployment of valvular prostheses, first in the descending aorta (Charles Hufnagel, 1952) and then in the heart itself (Nina Braunwald, 1960), could the full spectrum of valvular lesions be approached surgically.[1,2] The modern era of valvular heart surgery began soon after with the introduction of the first widely used and highly successful prosthesis, the Starr-Edwards caged-ball mechanical valve (Albert Starr, 1961).[3]

Other milestones in surgical therapy for valvular heart disease (Table 46-1) include the introduction of xenograft bioprostheses, valved-conduit replacement of the aortic root, development of reproducible techniques for mitral valve (MV) repair by Alain Carpentier,[4,5] introduction of minimally invasive techniques in the late 1990s, and, most recently, development of transcatheter technologies.[6]

Currently, the vast majority of patients with advanced valvular heart disease can be offered surgical therapy with very good short- and long-term results, including those with severe ventricular dysfunction, advanced age, significant pulmonary hypertension, and other comorbidities. Operative mortality rates have declined despite a higher risk patient profile, presumably as a result of refined surgical techniques and technologies, improved myocardial protection, and advances in perioperative care. Recent advances in less-invasive surgical approaches and accelerated postoperative care plans have decreased hospital stays and recovery times. Refined repair techniques and improved prostheses have resulted in better long-term outcomes that include reduced reoperation rates and fewer thromboembolic complications. Finally, the development of transcatheter approaches for both aortic[7] and MV disease may offer treatment options to patients otherwise not considered to be surgical candidates. These technologies are discussed in Chapter 47.

General Considerations

Epidemiology

Approximately 100,000 patients in the United States undergo valvular heart surgery each year, and the overall volume of valvular surgery appears to be growing. As expanding percutaneous interventions erode into isolated coronary surgery volume, most centers are reporting an increasing share of valvular surgery (Figure 46-1, A).[8] The most commonly performed procedure is aortic valve replacement (AVR) with or without concomitant coronary artery bypass grafting (CABG; Figure 46-1, B). MV repair is growing steadily,[9] with a greater appreciation of the importance of correcting tricuspid regurgitation (TR), often concomitant with MV surgery. Pulmonic valve surgery is quite rare in adults and is usually performed in the context of long-standing congenital heart disease or carcinoid heart disease. Pulmonic valve surgery is not discussed in this chapter.

Indications

Timing of valve surgery is discussed in Chapter 45. The specific indications for surgical intervention vary from valve to valve and are discussed separately. In general, however, the indications may be primary or secondary. Traditionally, the primary indication for surgery has been the onset of symptoms, most notably symptoms of left or right heart failure or both, but symptoms also include angina, syncope, and arrhythmias. With wider utilization of echocardiography and improved surgical outcomes, echocardiographic evidence of ventricular strain (dilation or dysfunction) has become the primary indication for surgery in an increasing number of asymptomatic or mildly symptomatic patients. Most recently, the primary indications for MV repair have been broadened to include some asymptomatic patients with normal ventricular function and dimensions.[10]

Many patients who have no primary indication for intervention on a particular valve will undergo valve surgery at the time of another cardiac surgery procedure, such as coronary bypass surgery, other valve surgery, or aortic surgery. The threshold for intervention as a concomitant procedure is usually lower than as a primary procedure, and valve repair or replacement may be indicated for moderate degrees of stenosis or regurgitation. The decision to intervene is based on an understanding of the natural history of these valvular lesions and is primarily aimed at

TABLE 46-1		Historic Highlights
1914	Tuffier	Closed aortic valvulotomy (digital)
1923	Culter	Closed mitral valvulotomy (valvulotome)
1925	Soutter	Closed mitral valvulotomy (digital)
1948	Harken, Bailey	Closed mitral valvulotomy (digital), first large series
1952	Hufnagel	Descending thoracic aortic prosthesis (caged ball), first AR surgery
1953	Gibbons	Heart-lung machine
1956	Murray	Descending thoracic aortic prosthesis (homograft)
1956	Lillehei	Open mitral commissurotomy
1956	Lillehei	Open mitral annuloplasty, first MR surgery
1960	Braunwald	Mechanical prosthetic MVR (polyurethane)
1960	Harken	Mechanical prosthetic AVR (caged ball)
1961	Starr	Mechanical prosthetic MVR with long-term survival (caged ball)
1962	Ross, Barrett-Boyes	Homograft AVR (orthotopic)
1965	Carpentier	Xenograft prosthetic AVR (porcine)
1967	Ross	Autograft AVR
1968	Carpentier	Prosthetic annuloplasty ring
1968	Bentall	Aortic root replacement (valved conduit)
1970s	Carpentier	Functional approach to mitral valve repair
1983	Yacoub	Valve-sparing aortic root replacement (remodeling)
1992	David	Valve-sparing aortic root replacement (inclusion)
1996	Cosgrove, Gundry	Minimally invasive aortic and mitral valve surgery (direct access)
1996	Carpentier, Chitwood	Minimally invasive mitral valve surgery (video assisted)
1998	Carpentier	Minimally invasive mitral valve surgery (robotic)
2002	Cribier	Transcatheter aortic valve implantation

AR, aortic regurgitation; AVR, aortic valve replacement; MR, mitral regurgitation; MVR, mitral valve replacement.

preventing subsequent progression of heart failure symptoms and the need for late reoperation.

Preoperative Evaluation and Optimization

Patients undergoing valvular surgery require thorough preoperative evaluation and optimization to ensure the best possible outcomes.

HISTORY AND PHYSICAL EXAMINATION

A detailed history and physical examination are fundamental. In addition to carefully characterizing the symptom profile of the valve disease, it is important to determine whether there is a history of palpitations or known arrhythmia; risk factors or known coronary artery disease (CAD); stroke or transient ischemic attacks (TIAs); lung, liver, or renal disease; gastrointestinal (GI) bleeding; peripheral vascular disease; bleeding or hypercoagulable conditions; and recent infections. In addition to careful cardiopulmonary auscultation, key elements of the physical

examination include a good dental examination, assessment of jugular venous pressures, carotid bruits and peripheral pulses, hepatomegaly, and availability of venous or arterial conduits for possible concomitant bypass grafting.

Documenting the baseline rhythm, any bundle branch blocks, and baseline ST- and T-wave changes is important for intraoperative and postoperative management. In addition to identifying unsuspected cardiopulmonary pathology, the chest radiograph provides a plethora of useful preoperative information, including chest wall anatomic details that may be helpful for planning less-invasive surgical incisions and for assessing the presence of pathologic calcification of the aorta, valves, or annuli. Each of these elements can have a significant impact on surgical decision making, timing, and choice of prosthesis.

ECHOCARDIOGRAPHY

Nearly all patients referred for surgery will have undergone a transthoracic echocardiogram (TTE) to make the diagnosis, often supplemented by a transesophageal study. Careful characterization of the primary valve lesion is important and can be invaluable for surgical planning and for counseling the patient on the likely intraoperative events. In addition to measuring the degree of stenosis and/or regurgitation, the specific etiology can often be determined. The use of quantitative methods for measuring mitral regurgitation (proximal isovelocity surface area [PISA], effective regurgitant orifice [ERO], and right ventricle [RV]) should be encouraged. The other valves should be carefully interrogated to rule out multivalve disease. Estimation of biventricular function is obviously critical, but so are ventricular dimensions, hypertrophy, any ventricular outflow tract obstruction, and TR jet–derived estimates of pulmonary artery (PA) pressure. Other important findings include atrial dilation, thrombus, patent foramen ovale, and occasional rare anomalies such as a persistent left-sided superior vena cava (SVC). In young patients in whom coronary arteriography may be deferred, echocardiographic identification of the coronary ostia may be important.

Even if the primary valve lesion was well characterized on a series of older echocardiograms, it is advisable to repeat the study within a month or so of surgery to reassess ventricular and other valvular function, which can sometimes progress rather rapidly. In some patients in whom the decision to proceed with surgery is equivocal, such as in cases of low-gradient aortic stenosis (AS) with poor left ventricular (LV) function, stress echocardiography may provide useful information.

CARDIAC CATHETERIZATION

In the majority of patients about to undergo valvular surgery, the complete hemodynamic picture can be obtained with echocardiography alone. Occasionally, however, right and/or left heart catheterization may be indicated to delineate more precisely the hemodynamic picture, especially stenotic gradients and the severity of pulmonary hypertension. Angiographic assessment of valvular regurgitation does not add much to the echocardiogram and can frequently underestimate eccentric jets.

As echocardiography has improved, the primary indication for preoperative catheterization is now coronary angiography, which is indicated in patients with known CAD or significant CAD risk factors. The age threshold for coronary angiography in patients without risk factors is usually 40 years for men and 50 years for women, although some would recommend routine coronary angiography in men as young as 35 years. The likelihood of CAD in preoperative valve patients varies from about 1% in degenerative MV disease to more than 50% in calcific AS.

The specific question of whether a stenotic aortic valve should be crossed to confirm hemodynamics is controversial. Most surgeons are comfortable proceeding on the basis of a good echocardiogram with catheter-based hemodynamic assessment only in equivocal cases. A contemporary study highlighted the real

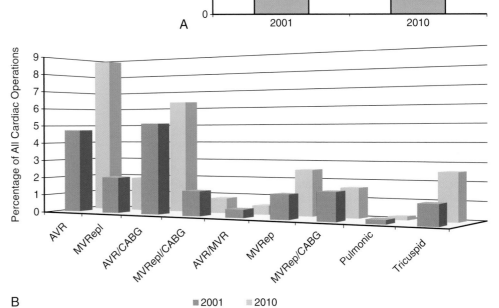

FIGURE 46-1 Valve surgery statistics. **A,** Valve operations as a percentage of all cardiac operations in 2001 vs. 2010. **B,** Specific valve operations as a percentage of all valve operations in 2001 vs. 2010. AVR, aortic valve replacement; CABG, coronary artery bypass graft; MVRep, mitral valve repair; MVRepl, mitral valve replacement; pulmonic, pulmonary valve procedure; tricuspid, tricuspid valve procedure. *(From Society of Thoracic Surgery Database. 2010 Executive Summary. Available at www.sts.org.)*

risk of embolism during attempts to cross a stenotic valve and encouraged a selective approach.[11]

OTHER PREOPERATIVE TESTING

Although echocardiography remains the mainstay of preoperative testing, cardiac magnetic resonance imaging (MRI) provides excellent anatomic and physiologic data in patients with valve disease. The specific indications for its use in this setting, however, have not been established. Other imaging may be indicated in specific clinical scenarios. A computed tomography (CT) scan or MRI of the head may be useful in patients with prior cerebrovascular accident (CVA) or to rule out mycotic aneurysms in patients with endocarditis. Preoperative carotid ultrasound is frequently performed if carotid stenoses are suspected, and a chest CT scan may be useful to determine more precisely the relationship between the heart and chest wall structures to plan minimally invasive surgery.

Holter monitoring may be useful in patients with suspected atrial arrhythmia to determine whether concomitant arrhythmia surgery should be considered. If indicated, formal electrophysiologic testing for ventricular arrhythmias is typically performed postoperatively because the substrate may be altered by surgical intervention.

In patients with dyspnea as a primary symptom, it may be difficult to determine the relative cardiac and pulmonary contributions to their symptoms and the degree to which correcting the cardiac lesion will improve their symptoms. Pulmonary function tests can help clarify this and will allow the physician to provide the patients with realistic expectations from surgery.

MEDICAL THERAPY

Whether a patient comes to medical attention for urgent AVR for acute aortic regurgitation secondary to endocarditis or for purely elective MV repair, the potential for preoperative medical optimization should be considered. Such efforts may significantly assist intraoperative care and may improve postoperative outcomes, especially in high-risk patients. Even in the most urgent settings, such as a patient in shock with acute mitral regurgitation (MR) from papillary muscle rupture, the time waiting for the operating room to be ready can be used to stabilize the hemodynamics with inotropic agents and an intraaortic balloon pump, if these are not contraindicated.

In less urgent settings, every effort should be made to optimize the patient for surgery, remaining careful not to miss the opportunity to intervene by trying to make the patient "perfect." Patients with decompensated heart failure may benefit from aggressive outpatient or inpatient diuresis and titration of other cardiac medications. Elderly or debilitated patients may benefit from preoperative physical therapy or nutritional support. Efforts to improve heart rate control or even cardioversion may be indicated in patients with supraventricular arrhythmias, including atrial fibrillation (AF). Smoking cessation programs or formal pulmonary rehabilitation may be helpful. Patients on hemodialysis are often admitted a few days preoperatively for more aggressive dialysis runs. Patients on warfarin should stop therapy at least 4 to 5 days before surgery, and those with strong indications for anticoagulation are usually admitted for intravenous (IV) heparin or are treated as an outpatient with low-molecular-weight heparin (LMWH). On the other hand, the current practice is to continue aspirin therapy for surgical patients with coronary disease.

Preoperative optimization of high-risk patients undergoing MV surgery may be particularly important, especially for those with significant pulmonary hypertension and ventricular dysfunction. Medical therapy resulting in reduced preoperative PA pressures may improve surgical outcomes.[12]

Surgical Approaches

MEDIAN STERNOTOMY

The median sternotomy remains the primary approach for most patients undergoing valve surgery. Median sternotomy is the only viable approach for those undergoing concomitant bypass grafting; it provides direct access to all important cardiovascular structures, and valve exposure is usually excellent. A full sternotomy can be performed through a fairly limited skin incision (12 to 18 cm) in patients with a favorable body habitus who desire a better cosmetic result. After pericardiotomy, the heart and great vessels are inspected, and increasingly the ascending aorta is scanned with epiaortic ultrasound to rule out significant plaque or atheroma, which might alter cannulation or aortic clamping techniques.

MINIMALLY INVASIVE APPROACHES

Over the past decade, surgeons have explored alternative incisions for accessing heart valves. Such alternatives aim to reduce surgical invasiveness and also yield a better cosmetic result. The primary incisions (Figure 46-2) are typically 5 to 10 cm and include minithoracotomies (anterior, lateral, and axillary) and partial sternotomies (upper and lower). The approaches can be categorized as *direct access, videoscopic,* or *robot assisted.* With direct-access approaches, surgical manipulation is performed under direct vision through the primary incision. Cannulation for cardiopulmonary bypass can be performed centrally through this incision or peripherally. Videoscopic MV surgery is performed through a small working incision and one or more additional endoscopic ports, and cannulation for cardiopulmonary bypass is usually performed peripherally. The valve is viewed on a monitor, and the tissues are manipulated using specialized endoscopic instruments. Robotic MV surgery is similar, but the imaging and instruments are integrated into a robotic surgical device (da Vinci Surgical System; Intuitive Surgical, Sunnyvale, CA) manipulated remotely from a separate console. Some surgeons have used this technology to perform truly endoscopic MV surgery.

The major advantage of minimally invasive approaches is improved cosmesis. Other potential advantages include less pain because of less tissue retraction, shorter length of stay, and less bleeding as a result of less dissection. All minimally invasive approaches leave at least part of the sternum intact, thereby preserving chest wall integrity and possibly resulting in less wound dehiscence and less respiratory morbidity. Minimally invasive approaches are more technically demanding, require more surgical skill, and pose unique surgical challenges owing to reduced tactile feedback, modification of cannulation techniques, difficulties in myocardial protection, and de-airing. A learning curve is involved, and the procedures generally take longer to perform. However, with adequate training and experience, minimally invasive valve surgery can be undertaken with results comparable or superior to those of conventional techniques.

Minimally invasive AVR through a partial upper sternotomy is now widely practiced and has become the standard approach for isolated AVR at many centers. Although published data support the safety and efficacy of this approach, reports are mixed on whether real clinical advantages beyond cosmesis exist.[13-16] Videoscopic and robotic MV surgery are being performed mostly at specialized centers. Again, published data support the safety and efficacy of these approaches, but they have not shown either of these to be superior with regard to hard clinical endpoints.[17,18]

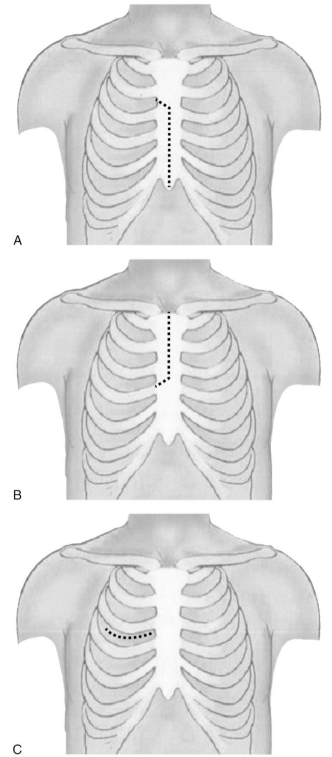

A

B

C

FIGURE 46-2 Minimally invasive valve surgery incisions. **A,** Lower partial sternotomy. **B,** Upper partial sternotomy. **C,** Right minithoracotomy.

Prostheses

Currently available valve prostheses are the product of nearly half a century of engineering, biochemical, and clinical research. Such prostheses are designed to provide maximal hemodynamic performance, durability, and freedom from complications. Nonetheless, the "holy grail" of the perfect valve prosthesis—with no obstruction to flow, no regurgitation, lifelong durability, and no significant complications—may never be reached. In fact, patients and physicians will likely always be faced with the need to balance the pros and cons of each prosthesis. The currently available Food and Drug Administration (FDA)-approved prostheses, and the relative advantages and disadvantages of each class of prostheses, are noted in Tables 46-2 and 46-3. Some of the more commonly used valves are shown in Figure 46-3, and the annuloplasty devices are described later with MV repair.

The primary differentiating characteristics of valve prostheses are their hemodynamic profile and the incidence of valve-related complications. A consensus panel of the Society of Thoracic Surgery (STS) and the American Association of Thoracic Surgery (AATS) published standard definitions and guidelines for reporting valve-related complications in 1996.[2] The panel defined six specific nonfatal valve-related events: 1) structural valve degeneration, 2) nonstructural valve degeneration, 3) valve thrombosis, 4) embolism, 5) bleeding, and 6) operated valvular endocarditis (Box 46-1). Time-related complications are typically reported as linearized rates (thrombosis, embolism, bleeding) or by using actuarial methods (structural valve degeneration, endocarditis).

As more elderly patients underwent valve surgery, it became apparent that actuarial methods can overestimate these rates because they do not censor patients who die from other causes. Reporting actual survival on the basis of Grunkemeier's cumulative incidence method has become more popular because it is more relevant to clinical decision making.[19-21]

MECHANICAL VALVES

Mechanical valves are generally characterized by good hemodynamics, excellent durability, and ease of implantation. These benefits must be balanced against a lifelong need for moderate anticoagulation and sometimes troubling valve noise. Their dominant position has been steadily eroded over the past decade by improved bioprostheses and increasing MV repair.

Mechanical valves are of three types: 1) caged ball, 2) tilting disk, and 3) bileaflet. The Starr-Edwards valve, which consists of a Silastic ball within a titanium cage, remained on the market,

TABLE 46-2 FDA-Approved and U.S.-Marketed Heart Valve Prostheses

TYPE	NAME	MANUFACTURER	APPROVAL YEAR	Size (Range, mm)		MODELS
				AORTIC	MITRAL	
Mechanical Valves						
Caged ball	Starr-Edwards	Edwards Lifesciences	1966	21-31		Discontinued in 2007
Tilting disk	Medtronic Hall	Medtronic	1977	20-31	23-33	Discontinued in 2010
Bileaflet	St. Jude Medical	St. Jude Medical	1977	17-31	17-33	Standard, Masters HP, Regent
	CarboMedics	Sorin Group	1993	16-31	16-33	Standard, Reduced, Optiform, TopHat
	On-X	On-X Life Technologies	2001	19-29	23-33	Standard, Conform-X
	Open Pivot	Medtronic	2000	16-31	16-33	Standard, AP, AP360
Biologic Valves						
Stented porcine	Carpentier-Edwards	Edwards Lifesciences	1975	19-31	25-35	Standard, SAV, Duraflex
	Hancock I	Medtronic	1989	21-29	25-33	Standard, II Ultra
	Hancock II	Medtronic	1999	21-29	25-33	
	Mosaic	Medtronic	2000	19-29	25-33	Standard, Ultra
	Biocor	St. Jude Medical	2005	19-29	25-35	Standard, Supra
	Epic	St. Jude Medical	2007	19-29	27-33	
Stented bovine pericardial	Carpentier-Edwards PERIMOUNT	Edwards Lifesciences	1991 (A) 2000 (M)	19-29	25-33	Standard, Theon, Plus, Magna, Magna Ease
Stentless porcine	Freestyle	Medtronic	1997	19-29	NA	
	Prima Plus	Edwards Lifesciences	2001	21-29	NA	
	Toronto SPV	St. Jude Medical	1997	21-29	NA	
Stentless equine pericardial	3F	Medtronic	2008	21-29	NA	
Aortic homograft		CryoLife, LifeNet	NA	Varies	Varies	
Annuloplasty Devices						
Complete						
Rigid/semirigid	Carpentier-Edwards Classic	Edwards Lifesciences	1968	26-40	26-40	Different mitral and tricuspid models
	Carpentier-Edwards Physio	Edwards Lifesciences	1993	24-40		
	CarboMedics AnnuloFlo	Sorin Group	1997	26-30		
	Seguin	St. Jude Medical	1997	24-40		
	Edwards MC3	Edwards Lifesciences	2002		26-36	Tricuspid only
	Carpentier-McCarthy-Adams IMR ETlogix	Edwards Lifesciences	2003	24-34		
	Geoform	Edwards Lifesciences	2003	26-32		
Flexible	Duran	Medtronic	1989	25-35	*	
	CarboMedics AnnuloFlex	Sorin Group	1999	26-30		
	Tailor	St. Jude Medical	2000	25-35		
Partial						
Rigid/semirigid	Colvin-Galloway Future	Medtronic	2001	26-38		
Flexible	Cosgrove-Edwards	Edwards Lifesciences	1993	26-38	*	Complete ring can be converted to partial band by excising anterior segment.
	Duran	Medtronic	1989	25-35		
	CarboMedics AnnuloFlex	Sorin Group	1999	26-30		
	Tailor	St. Jude Medical	2000	25-35		

A, aortic; FDA, U.S. Food and Drug Administration; M, mitral; NA, not applicable.

CH
46

TABLE 46-3   Valve Prostheses Characteristics

	MECHANICAL	STENTED XENOGRAFT	STENTLESS XENOGRAFT	HOMOGRAFT	AUTOGRAFT
Need for anticoagulation	+	++	+++	+++	+++
Freedom from thromboembolism	+	++	+++?	+++	+++
Durability	+++	++	++?	++	+++
Ease of operation	+++	+++	++	++	+
Hemodynamic performance	++	+	+++	+++	+++
Resistance to infection	+	+	++?	+++	+++
Noise	++	+++	+++	+++	+++

The more plus signs, the greater the relative advantage of a particular valve type. Question marks indicate that the benefit is controversial or uncertain.

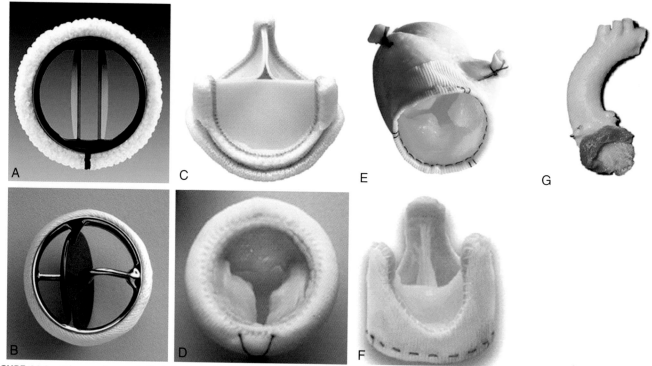

FIGURE 46-3   Valve prostheses. **A,** St. Jude Medical bileaflet mechanical valve. **B,** Medtronic-Hall tilting disk mechanical valve. **C,** Carpentier-Edwards Magna stented bovine pericardial aortic bioprosthesis. **D,** Medtronic Mosaic stented porcine mitral bioprosthesis. **E,** Medtronic Freestyle stentless porcine full-root bioprosthesis. **F,** St. Jude Medical Toronto-SPV stentless porcine subcoronary bioprosthesis. **G,** Aortic homograft.

Box 46-1 Definition of Valve-Related Complications

Structural valve deterioration: Any change in function of an operated valve resulting from an intrinsic abnormality of the valve that causes stenosis or regurgitation exclusive of infection or thrombosis, such as wear, calcification, or leaflet tear.

Nonstructural dysfunction: Any abnormality that results in stenosis or regurgitation at the operated valve that is not intrinsic to the valve itself, exclusive of thrombosis and infection, such as pannus overgrowth, paravalvular leak, inappropriate sizing or positioning, residual leak or obstruction, and clinically important hemolytic anemia.

Valve thrombosis: Any thrombus, in the absence of infection, attached to or near an operated valve that occludes part of the blood flow path or that interferes with valvular function.

Embolism: Any embolic event that occurs in the absence of infection after the immediate perioperative period. A neurologic event includes any

new, temporary, or permanent focal or global neurologic deficit. A peripheral embolic event produces symptoms from complete or partial obstruction of a peripheral artery. Immediate postoperative neurologic deficits and myocardial infarction are generally excluded.

Bleeding event: Any episode of major internal or external bleeding that causes death, hospitalization, or permanent injury or that requires transfusion, regardless of whether anticoagulants or antiplatelet drugs are being taken.

Operated valvular endocarditis: Any infection involving an operated valve, based on customary clinical criteria. Morbidity associated with active infection—such as valve thrombosis, thrombotic embolus, bleeding event, or paravalvular leak—is included under this category and is not included in other categories of morbidity.

essentially unchanged, for nearly 4 decades until its discontinuation in 2007. Despite a remarkable history and excellent durability, recently it was rarely used because it has been surpassed by mechanical valves with superior thromboembolic and hemodynamic profiles. In a tilting-disk valve—such as the Medtronic-Hall valve (Medtronic, Inc., Minneapolis, MN), introduced in 1977 and discontinued in 2010, the ball is replaced by a flat disk that tilts open along retaining guides during systole,

increasing central flow and improving hemodynamics and thromboresistance. The St. Jude mechanical valve (St. Jude Medical, St. Paul, MN), also introduced in 1977, was the first bileaflet valve. With more than 1 million implants, it remains the world's most popular valve prosthesis. It is manufactured from pyrolytic carbon, and each leaflet rotates over a fixed range within pivots in the inner surface of the ring. Several other companies market similar pyrolytic carbon bileaflet valves that purport advantages on the basis of the purity of the carbon (On-X; On-X Life Technologies, Austin, TX), pivot designs (Medtronic Open Pivot, formerly ATS Medical, On-X), and supraannular location of the leaflets and pivots (CarboMedics; Sorin Group, Milan, Italy).

Numerous long-term studies have evaluated the absolute and relative performance of currently available mechanical valves, and several primary findings have been reported. The incidence of structural valve degeneration of the currently marketed mechanical valves is exceedingly low. The annual linearized rates (events per patient-year) of thromboembolism (0.5% to 4%), thrombosis (0% to 0.5%), and major bleeding complications (0.5% to 4%) vary widely from study to study and are greater for valves in the mitral position compared with those in the aortic position. A low but finite incidence of reoperation (5% to 10% at 15 to 20 years) exists for endocarditis, thrombosis, or nonstructural dysfunction such as pannus overgrowth, endocarditis, and perivalvular leak.

Grunkemeier and Wu[21] performed a meta-analysis of complication rates from the two most popular mechanical valves, the St. Jude and CarboMedics valves, and found similar rates of thromboembolism (1.6% aortic, 2% to 2.5% mitral) and bleeding (1.5% aortic, 1.3% to 1.4% mitral). The CarboMedics valve had a lower thrombosis rate in the aortic position (0.02% vs. 0.15%) but was higher in the mitral position (0.33% vs. 0.17%; Table 46-4, Figure 46-4). Several retrospective studies have suggested slightly higher long-term complication rates with the Medtronic-Hall valve compared with the bileaflet valves,[22,23] although a small randomized trial could not detect a difference.[24] The data on the newer valves (On-X) are also comparable, but so far no irrefutable data support their superiority. The recommended target international normalized ratio (INR) for the bileaflet and Medtronic-Hall valves is 2.0 to 3.0 in the aortic position and 2.5 to 3.5 in the mitral position. Low-dose aspirin (75 to 100 mg) is recommended for all patients with mechanical heart valves.[10] More intense anticoagulation and the addition of full-dose aspirin should be considered in patients who are at higher risk for thromboembolism, such as those with AF, prior thromboembolism, hypercoagulable states, or LV dysfunction. Clopidogrel is recommended for patients who cannot take aspirin and those who have had thromboembolic events on higher intensity anticoagulation. Significant interest has been expressed in alternatives to warfarin anticoagulation, such as the new oral, direct thrombin inhibitor dabigatran; emerging factor Xa inhibitors; and dual antiplatelet therapy with aspirin and clopidogrel in AVs. The On-X valve is currently being investigated in a randomized trial to compare standard anticoagulation to lower-intensity anticoagulation for MV replacement (MVR) and high-risk AVR. This trial is also evaluating therapy with aspirin plus clopidogrel in low-risk AVR patients. Data to determine whether these alternatives to full warfarin anticoagulation will be safe and effective are inadequate to date.

STENTED XENOGRAFTS

The first xenograft bioprostheses were developed by Carpentier and Hancock in 1969. They consisted of a rigid or semirigid cloth-covered stent to which porcine aortic valve cusps were attached; cusps created from bovine pericardium were later applied to similar stent structures. The key development was the introduction of glutaraldehyde fixation. By cross-linking collagen fibers and eliminating viable cells, this treatment increases the durability of the xenograft tissue and decreases its antigenicity. It soon became clear, however, that the Achilles heel of glutaraldehyde fixation was subsequent calcification, which is the final common pathway for structural valve degeneration of most bioprostheses. In addition to the loss of cusp mobility, areas of calcification become stress points that can lead to cusp tears. Extensive research over the past 3 decades has led to improved techniques of tissue preservation. Low- or zero-pressure fixation techniques combined with antimineralization treatment have led to significant gains in bioprosthesis durability. This has resulted in a dramatic shift over the past decade away from mechanical prostheses and lowered the age threshold for bioprostheses.

The most commonly used stented xenograft in the United States is the Carpentier-Edwards PERIMOUNT Pericardial Valve (Edwards Lifesciences, Irvine, CA). The most recent design iteration, the Magna valve, purports to maximize hemodynamics through a true supraannular design. Stented porcine valves currently marketed in the United States include versions of the Carpentier-Edwards Porcine valve (Edwards Lifesciences); the Hancock (I, II, and MO) and Mosaic valves (Medtronic); and the recently approved Biocor (St. Jude Medical) and MitroFlow (Sorin Group) valves. Durability data are discussed separately for aortic and mitral valve prostheses.

STENTLESS XENOGRAFTS

Stentless xenograft bioprostheses were developed to mimic the near-native hemodynamics of homografts and autografts while maintaining the ease of use and off-the-shelf convenience of stented bioprostheses. Eliminating the stent permits a larger valve to be inserted but increases the surgical complexity to some degree. Stentless valves can be inserted by one of several techniques. In a subcoronary implantation, the valve is seated

TABLE 46-4 Pooled Event Rates and Hazard Ratios for Comparison of Event Rates

		Pooled Event Rates		Valve Only in Model	
EVENT	VALVE	RATE (%/YEAR)	P VALUE*	HR†	95% CI
Aortic Position					
Thromboembolism	St. Jude	1.58	<.001	1.06	0.68-1.66
	CarboMedics	1.59	<.001		
Valve thrombosis	St. Jude	0.14	.005	0.16	0.05-0.56
	CarboMedics	0.02	.777		
Bleeding	St. Jude	1.32	<.001	1.06	0.66-1.70
	CarboMedics	1.45	<.001		
Mitral Position					
Thromboembolism	St. Jude	2.45	<.001	0.72	0.38-1.38
	CarboMedics	1.95	<.001		
Valve thrombosis	St. Jude	0.17	.111	1.94	0.98-3.84
	CarboMedics	0.33	.03		
Bleeding	St. Jude	1.26	<.001	1.1	0.60-2.00
	CarboMedics	1.41	<.001		

*Heterogeneity assessment among series.
†Valve model effects for CarboMedics valve.
CI, confidence interval; HR, hazard ratio.

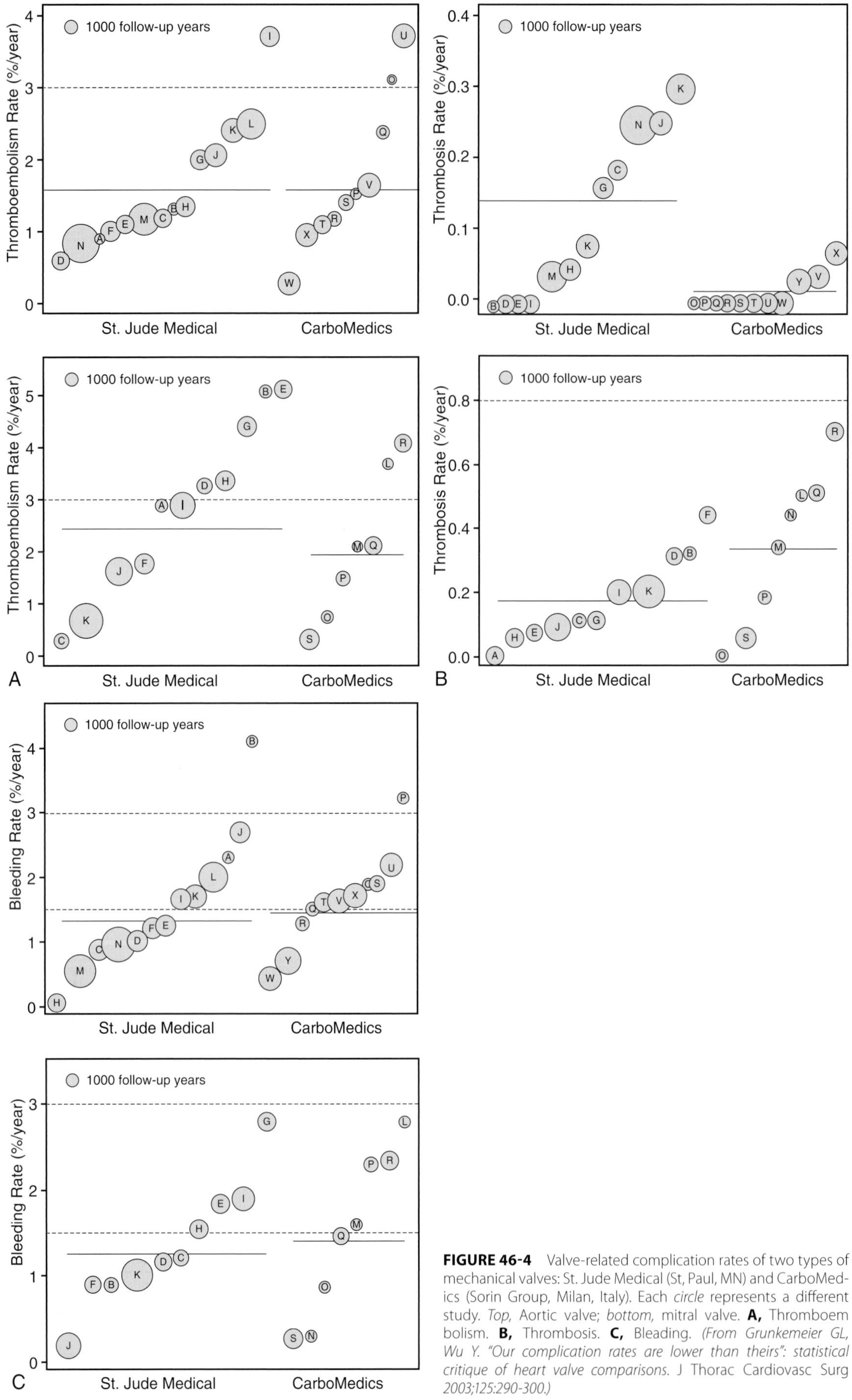

FIGURE 46-4 Valve-related complication rates of two types of mechanical valves: St. Jude Medical (St, Paul, MN) and CarboMedics (Sorin Group, Milan, Italy). Each *circle* represents a different study. *Top,* Aortic valve; *bottom,* mitral valve. **A,** Thromboembolism. **B,** Thrombosis. **C,** Bleeding. *(From Grunkemeier GL, Wu Y. "Our complication rates are lower than theirs": statistical critique of heart valve comparisons.* J Thorac Cardiovasc Surg *2003;125:290-300.)*

within the native aortic root. This typically requires two suture lines: a proximal suture line at the annulus and a distal one to secure the valve and commissures to the sinuses of Valsalva. The hemiroot or full-root techniques involve replacing part of the patient's aortic root with the bioprosthesis. The full-root technique usually requires coronary reimplantation. Whichever technique is used, the implantation of a stentless valve is technically more challenging than that of a stented valve. Once implanted, stentless valves have an excellent hemodynamic profile, and some evidence suggests that they promote greater regression of LV hypertrophy.[25,26] The technical challenge and the lack of data that show an advantage with regard to hard endpoints have limited the adoption of stentless valves since their introduction in the early 1990s. Although some centers have adopted stentless valves as their valve of choice in the aortic position, most limit their use to specific indications, such as a small aortic annulus or diseased root.

Four stentless aortic valves are currently marketed in the United States. The Medtronic Freestyle and the Edwards Prima Plus are both delivered as full porcine aortic roots with the coronaries ligated and a cloth covering the annulus. They can be used for a full-root replacement or can be trimmed for subcoronary implantation. The Toronto Stentless SPV valve (St. Jude Medical) is designed only for subcoronary implantation. The Medtronic 3F valve (formerly ATS Medical) is an equine pericardial valve that only requires suturing of the commissures to the aortic wall, thereby avoiding a second suture line.

HOMOGRAFTS

Homograft valves have been used in the aortic position since the early 1960s, following pioneering work by Ross and Barrett-Boyes. A variety of earlier preservation techniques have been replaced by cryopreservation. Homografts share many of the advantages of stentless valves, including excellent hemodynamics, and they can also be used as full-root or subcoronary implants. They appear to have a greater resistance to infection and are therefore commonly used in the setting of endocarditis. The primary limitations of homografts have been availability and storage requirements. However, utilization of homografts appears to be declining; the most recent data indicate that their durability is not significantly better than that of modern bioprostheses.[27] Homografts tend to calcify as they fail, making reoperation in patients who have received full-root replacements difficult.

Efforts to use MV homografts have not been successful.[28] These efforts have been limited by the complex geometry of the MV and by accelerated degeneration. The increased utilization of valve repair and improvement in bioprostheses have also led to a decline in interest in this approach.

Postoperative Care

The postoperative care of patients undergoing valvular surgery must be tailored to the individual patient's specific condition. The immediate postoperative period is focused on maintaining an adequate cardiac output and monitoring for bleeding. Many, if not most, valve surgery patients are candidates for a fast-track protocol in which the anesthetic management is designed to permit extubation within 1 to 6 hours of arrival in the intensive care unit (ICU) once hemodynamic stability and hemostasis have been achieved.

An increasing proportion of patients have decreased ventricular function, so it is not uncommon that patients will arrive in the ICU on inotropic support. In most patients the support can be weaned over the first 24 hours or so, but this process occasionally can take longer in those with poor function.

When present, pulmonary hypertension must be addressed carefully to protect the RV, which is more difficult to protect and is therefore particularly vulnerable to myocardial stunning. Maneuvers may include avoiding hypoxia or hypercarbia, avoiding α-agonists, and using pulmonary vasodilators such as milrinone or, in severe cases, inhaled nitric oxide.

Patients with severe LV hypertrophy and diastolic dysfunction warrant careful postoperative hemodynamic management. These patients will often need aggressive volume resuscitation and require higher than expected intracardiac filling pressures to maintain an adequate stroke volume. An occasional patient with severe hypertrophy may develop dynamic outflow tract obstruction, the so-called *suicide ventricle*. In addition to maintaining adequate preload, inotropic agents should be avoided, and peripheral vasoconstrictors should be used if necessary to maintain systemic blood pressure. If pacing is necessary, atrioventricular pacing is preferred because the hypertrophied ventricle will usually benefit from atrial contraction.

The next few days in the hospital course are typically focused on diuresis, rhythm management, reinstitution of cardiac and noncardiac medications, pulmonary toilet, mobilization, and anticoagulation. The incidence of postoperative AF is higher in valve patients than in coronary patients.[29,30] Preoperative prophylactic regimens have been proposed but are not widely used. Postoperative AF protocols vary from one institution to another but include β-blockers, amiodarone, calcium channel blockers, and, less commonly, digoxin.[31,32] Transient heart block is not uncommon, so most surgeons will place temporary pacing wires at the time of surgery. Most of the time this will resolve as edema subsides and electrolyte imbalances are corrected. Occasionally, however, a permanent pacemaker is required before discharge. It can be difficult to determine when to proceed with pacemaker implantation, but waiting 5 to 7 days for signs of recovery of the rhythm is reasonable.

All patients with mechanical valves, most MV patients, and those in AF will be anticoagulated in the immediate postoperative period. Warfarin is usually initiated soon after surgery, and some surgeons are reluctant to bridge with IV heparin for fear of bleeding and tamponade. At a minimum, patients with mechanical MVs should be considered at high risk for early thromboembolism and should receive IV heparin, if the INR is not therapeutic within a few days of surgery. Most centers still anticoagulate patients undergoing MV repair, although some high-volume centers have chosen to be selective, using aspirin alone in younger, healthier patients with normal sinus rhythm and good ventricular function. Another area of controversy is whether to anticoagulate patients with aortic bioprostheses.[33-35] A survey indicated that most patients are not being anticoagulated in the absence of other indications.[36]

A baseline postoperative echocardiogram is usually performed before discharge in patients undergoing valve repair or stentless valve replacement. Predischarge education regarding antibiotic prophylaxis and anticoagulant therapy is important.

Aortic Valve Surgery

Overview

AVR is the most commonly performed valve operation. It has been shown to be an effective therapy in all age groups, including the very elderly (age >90 years).[37] The most common etiologies for AS are calcific degeneration, rheumatic disease, and congenital bicuspid valves. The most common causes of pure aortic regurgitation include annuloaortic ectasia and associated dilation of the aortic root, endocarditis, aortic dissection, and rheumatic disease. The indications for surgery depend on the pathophysiology and symptoms. The choice of prosthesis can be difficult and depends on multiple clinical and lifestyle considerations. Early and late outcomes are generally quite good, even in high-risk patients.

Indications

AORTIC STENOSIS/MIXED AORTIC VALVE DISEASE

The indications for aortic valve surgery in pure AS and mixed disease are fairly well established[10] and are described in greater

CH
46

detail in Chapter 45. Current class I indications include severe AS with symptoms or signs of LV dysfunction, as well as other concomitant cardiac surgery. AVR is also recommended (class IIa) in patients with moderate AS undergoing CABG or other valve surgery to decrease the risk of early reoperation for progression of AS. Intervening in mild AS at the time of CABG is more controversial but has been suggested, especially in patients who appear to be at high risk for progression, such as those with significant calcification.[38-40] Other possible but controversial indications for AVR include asymptomatic patients with normal ventricular function and severe AS (valve area <0.6 cm^2), those with severe AS but abnormal response to stress testing (e.g., hypotension), and those with risk factors for more rapid progression.

Patients with poor LV function (ejection fraction <30%) with AS will often come to medical attention with relatively low gradients. Recent data suggest that carefully selected patients in this subgroup benefit from surgery.[41]

AORTIC REGURGITATION

The natural history of AR makes the timing of aortic valve surgery more difficult. Patients can remain relatively asymptomatic until significant ventricular damage has occurred. Class I indications include symptomatic severe AR and asymptomatic severe AR with LV dysfunction. Surgery is also recommended (class IIa) in asymptomatic patients with normal LV function but severe dilation (end-diastolic or end-systolic dimensions >75 mm or >55 mm, respectively). Severe, and probably moderate, AR should be corrected at the time of CABG or other valve surgery.

Aortic Valve Replacement

SURGICAL TECHNIQUE

The steps involved in replacing the aortic valve are fairly well established (Figure 46-5, A). Routine scanning of the aorta is increasingly used before cannulation for cardiopulmonary bypass, usually via the distal aorta and right atrium. The aorta is clamped, and the heart is protected with hyperkalemic cardioplegia solution delivered anterograde in the aortic root or coronary ostia, retrograde via the coronary sinus, or both. This is usually supplemented with mild systemic and/or topical hypothermia. The LV typically is vented through the right superior pulmonary vein. An incision is made in the proximal aorta, and the valve is inspected. Debriding a highly calcified valve and annulus can be a significant challenge; careful attention must be paid to removing all the calcium while maintaining adequate annular tissue and removing all loose debris that can later embolize. The calcium will sometimes continue up the aortic wall, and localized endarterectomies may be required.

Once the annulus is fully debrided, the valve is secured with sutures. The specific suture technique—pledgets versus no pledgets, interrupted versus running, everting versus noneverting, supraannular versus intraannular—can vary from surgeon to surgeon. The suturing technique does not vary significantly between stented xenografts and mechanical valves. Subcoronary implantation of stentless valves, homografts, or even autografts requires a second outflow suture line to secure the valve to the aortic wall. The largest valve that can be comfortably implanted is usually selected. If the annulus is small, the surgeon can enlarge it with a patch to permit a larger prosthesis to be implanted or may opt to use a stentless valve.

The aortotomy is sutured closed, air is evacuated from the heart, and the cross-clamp is removed. The patient is weaned off cardiopulmonary bypass, heparin is reversed with protamine, and the cannulas are removed. Temporary epicardial pacing wires and chest drains are placed before sternal closure.

An aortic root replacement with coronary reimplantation (Bentall procedure) may be performed in the presence of concomitant aortic root disease (dilation, calcification) or if the

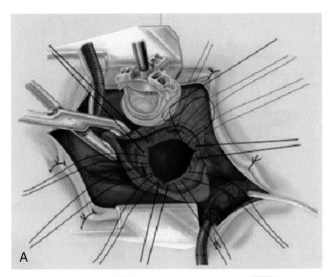

A

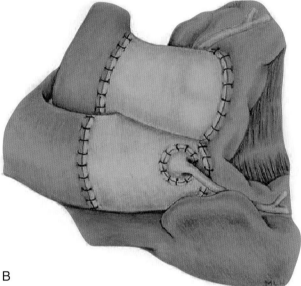

B

FIGURE 46-5 Surgical technique of aortic valve replacement. **A,** Stented xenograft. **B,** The Ross (pulmonary autograft aortic valve replacement) procedure. The patient's pulmonary valve and root are translocated into the aortic position and replaced with a homograft. The figure shows a completed procedure as seen by the surgeon standing to the patient's right. The patient's head is to the left, and the feet are to the right. The confluence of the superior vena cava and right atrial appendage is at the bottom of the figure. Moving up, from the patient's right to left, are the pulmonary autograft with its distal suture line to the ascending aorta and proximal suture line to the aortic annulus—the right coronary artery has been reimplanted as a button, the left coronary button is posterior and not visualized—and the pulmonary homograft with its distal suture line to the confluence of the pulmonary arteries and the proximal arteries and the proximal suture line to the right ventricular outflow tract.

surgeon chooses to implant a stentless prosthesis or homograft as a full root. The aorta is resected from the annulus to the ascending aorta, or further distally if indicated, and the coronary ostia are preserved as buttons. A valved conduit, a mechanical or stented valve attached to a Dacron tube graft, a stentless valve (porcine root), or a homograft is selected and secured proximally and distally to the annulus and aorta, respectively. The coronary buttons are sutured to holes created in the conduit.

The pulmonary autograft or Ross procedure is usually performed as an aortic root replacement using the patient's own pulmonary valve/artery as the prosthesis (Figure 46-5, B). The implant is similar to other root replacements, except that the annulus and sinotubular junction are often reinforced with prosthetic material to prevent late dilation. A pulmonary homograft is usually used to reconstruct the RV outflow tract.

CHOICE OF PROSTHESIS

Selecting the most appropriate prosthesis in a patient undergoing AVR is a complex decision with significant long-term consequences for the patient. As noted in Table 46-3, the available prostheses differ significantly with regard to key parameters, such as the need for anticoagulation, freedom from thromboembolism, durability, ease of operation, hemodynamic performance, and resistance to infection. Although broad age-based guidelines do exist, the final choice should be tailored to the individual patient and should take into consideration multiple factors in addition to age, such as concomitant diseases, especially those affecting life expectancy, general lifestyle and physical activity, surgeon expertise, and, ultimately, overall patient preference.

The primary factor in prosthesis selection is patient age. Elderly patients have lower life expectancies and tend to be less physically active. Younger patients, on the other hand, place a greater demand on the prosthesis with regard to durability and hemodynamic performance. Age has long been recognized as the primary determinant of bioprosthesis calcification and thus durability. Long-term follow-up of the Carpentier-Edwards pericardial valve confirms a strong correlation between age at implant and the likelihood of explant at 15 years (Figure 46-6). The age threshold for a bioprosthesis has traditionally been between 65 and 70 years, and the actual lifetime likelihood of reoperation for structural valve dysfunction in a 65-year-old person is less than 10%. Given the excellent durability of modern bioprostheses, it is uncommon to implant a mechanical valve in an elderly patient. The fact that the patient is already on warfarin for another indication, such as AF, does not necessarily favor the use of a mechanical valve because it converts a relative indication for low-level anticoagulation to an absolute indication for higher levels. It also eliminates the option to discontinue anticoagulation in the event of a major bleeding episode. Even the presence of another mechanical valve does not mandate a second mechanical valve, because risk of thromboembolic and bleeding complications is higher with two mechanical valves than it is with one.

The choice of prosthesis in patients younger than 65 years is more complex and controversial. These patients would traditionally receive a mechanical valve; however, the improvement in bioprosthesis durability and the decrease in the operative risk of replacing a failed prosthesis have led to an increase in the number of patients younger than 65 years who receive bioprostheses, including patients in their 50s and even younger. Women of childbearing age pose a particular dilemma and often choose a bioprosthesis to avoid warfarin, with the understanding that they will face at least one reoperation in their lifetime.

By eliminating the stent and most of the prosthetic material, stentless valves—such as the Toronto SPV, Freestyle, and Prima Plus valves—allow implantation of a larger valve than would be possible with a stented xenograft. The most commonly implanted stentless valve sizes are 25 to 29 mm, whereas most stented valve patients receive a 21- to 25-mm valve. In addition, when matched for size, the hemodynamic profiles of stentless valves are superior to those of stented valves, especially at the smaller sizes.[42] These differences are even greater when measured during exercise or pharmacologic stress.[43] These hemodynamic benefits may justify the use of stentless valves in younger, more active patients in whom a bioprosthesis is being considered. However, whether this hemodynamic benefit translates into real clinical benefit remains controversial. Although the 10-year follow-up with the Freestyle valve is excellent,[44] duration of follow-up is not adequate to show improved durability. Others suggest improved LV mass regression,[45,46] but whether this translates into improved survival is unclear.[47,48] Some data suggest fewer thromboembolic complications.[49] Despite these data, the specific indications for the use of a stentless valve are not well defined, and at this point their use is primarily driven by surgeon preference.

The use of homografts as a primary aortic valve substitute has declined in recent years. Like stentless valves, homografts have excellent hemodynamics and are resistant to thromboembolism and infection. However, recent data suggest that their durability is not significantly better than that of stented xenografts. Without a durability advantage, it is difficult to justify their routine use given their limited availability and the cumbersome storage requirements, although their resistance to infection makes them an excellent choice for patients with endocarditis.

The pulmonary autograft, or Ross procedure, involves replacing the aortic valve with the patient's own pulmonic valve, which in turn is replaced with a homograft or a stentless xenograft. The advantages are near-native hemodynamics and excellent autograft durability; the disadvantages are the high degree of technical complexity and need for reoperation for the homograft. On the basis of the data from the Ross Procedure International Registry, the procedure peaked in popularity in the mid to late 1990s, but procedure volume has declined since then. Several centers continue to report excellent results,[50,51] although it is now primarily a procedure for pediatric patients, in whom the potential for growth is important, and for young adults in their 20s and 30s, when no other good alternatives exist.

PATIENT-PROSTHESIS MISMATCH

The topic of patient-prosthesis mismatch (PPM) remains hotly debated. Strictly speaking, it is defined as a prosthesis that is too small relative to the patient's size and therefore provides residual obstruction to flow despite normal prosthesis function. The most common measure is the indexed effective orifice area (EOA), which is EOA divided by body surface area (BSA). The incidence of PPM depends on the cutoff used. Severe PPM, defined as an EOA index less than 0.65 cm^2/m^2, occurs in up to 10% of patients; *moderate PPM* occurs in up to 70%.[52] Some authors argue that PPM is not clinically relevant and that LV mass regression and early and late cardiac events are not affected.[53-55] Others, led by Pibarot and colleagues, argue vigorously that PPM dramatically affects LV mass regression, operative mortality, late functional status, heart failure, and overall mortality.[52,56]

Because surgeons routinely attempt to implant the largest possible prosthesis, the debate can ultimately be distilled down to the question of whether the surgical technique or valve choice should be modified to avoid PPM.[57] Specific maneuvers include aortic annular enlargement and use of a stentless or a mechanical prosthesis. Opponents of annular enlargement procedures argue that these maneuvers carry additional operative complexity and risk and may therefore not be justified, particularly when surgeons are not familiar with these procedures.[58]

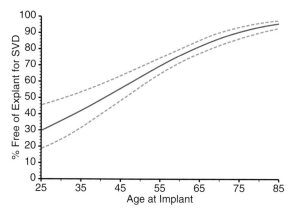

FIGURE 46-6 Age dependence of structural valve degeneration (*SVD*) of Carpentier-Edwards (Edwards Lifesciences, Irvine, CA) pericardial valve in the aortic position. (*From Banbury MK, Cosgrove DM III, White JA, et al. Age and valve size effect on the long-term durability of the Carpentier-Edwards aortic pericardial bioprosthesis. Ann Thorac Surg 2001;72:753-757.*)

Aortic Valve Repair

Selected patients with aortic insufficiency may be candidates for aortic valve repair, although these operations are rarely performed. Patients occasionally come to medical attention with isolated cusp perforation (iatrogenic, healed endocarditis) or cusp prolapse. These valves can be repaired with a pericardial patch over the perforation or plication of the prolapsing segment. Patients with retracted but mobile and noncalcified cusps from rheumatic disease can undergo leaflet extension with pieces of pericardium, and those with noncalcified congenital bicuspid valve disease and AR are offered repair at some centers.[59-61] This typically involves resection of the redundant cusp and commissural plication.

Patients with normal cusps and aortic insufficiency secondary to concomitant aortic root dilation can avoid valve replacement by undergoing one of several valve-sparing aortic root operations. These operations, pioneered by Yacoub[62,63] and David,[64,65] seek to reestablish the three-dimensional support of the native valve to permit adequate coaptation. Although technically difficult, these operations have good results in selected patients when performed at experienced centers.

Results

EARLY

The operative mortality rate for patients who undergo AVR continues to decline. The unadjusted mortality rate is now 3.0% for isolated AVR and 4.5% for AVR with CABG in the STS 2010 Executive Report, despite an older patient population with greater comorbidities. A young, otherwise healthy patient with good ventricular function can be offered the procedure, with a predicted operative mortality rate of 1% (STS Risk Calculator). Elderly patients[37,66,67] and those with decreased ventricular function[41,68,69] do surprisingly well following AVR for AS, presumably because of the immediate benefits of unloading the LV. However, the operative risk does increase in the presence of multiple risk factors that include age, female gender, poor LV function, class IV heart failure, CAD, renal failure, endocarditis, urgent/emergent surgery, and reoperation. The most common causes of operative death are myocardial failure and stroke. Trends in mortality and stroke after AVR were reported by Brown and colleagues over a recent 10-year period (Figure 46-7).[70]

The most common complications following aortic valve surgery are similar to those of other cardiac surgeries and include stroke

(1% to 4%), deep sternal wound infection (1% to 2%), reoperation for bleeding (1% to 3%), and myocardial infarction (MI; 1% to 5%). Transient heart block is not uncommon, presumably as a result of traction or edema of the bundle of His in the vicinity of the right noncoronary commissure. It usually resolves within 5 to 6 days of surgery. The risk of complete heart block requiring pacemaker insertion is 3% to 5%.[71]

LATE

Long-term survival following AVR depends on the patient's characteristics and comorbidity. Estimated 10-year survival can range from 85% in younger, healthier patients to 40% in elderly patients with CAD, class IV congestive heart failure (CHF), and decreased LV function.[72] Low-risk elderly patients undergoing AVR have survival rates similar to those of their peers without aortic valve disease.[73] Approximately 40% of deaths following AVR are valve related, and another 20% are related to nonvalvular cardiac causes. A clinically significant difference in survival is not apparent between mechanical and biologic valves, when age and other risk factors are controlled.

Freedom from reoperation depends on both the prosthesis and patient age. Although they do not degenerate, modern mechanical valves do have a finite reoperation rate of 0.5% to 1% per year from endocarditis, pannus overgrowth, and thrombosis. Actual freedom from reoperation of modern bioprostheses at 15 years approaches 100% in elderly patients older than 70 years, but it can be as low as 50% in patients younger than 50 years.[74,75]

Mitral Valve Surgery

Overview

Although aortic valve surgery remains the most common valve operation (see Figure 46-1, B), the field of MV surgery has been very dynamic, and several important trends and advances have emerged in the past decade.[9] The incidence of rheumatic heart disease has declined, and techniques of percutaneous balloon mitral valvuloplasty have improved; this has led to a decline in the number of patients undergoing surgery for mitral stenosis. In contrast, the number of patients undergoing MV repair, nearly all for MR, has doubled in the past decade (see Figure 46-1, B). A greater understanding of the benefits and techniques of MV repair for degenerative disease has contributed to this trend, and MV repair is now the most common operation for isolated MV disease (Figure 46-8). Other contributing factors include 1) broadening

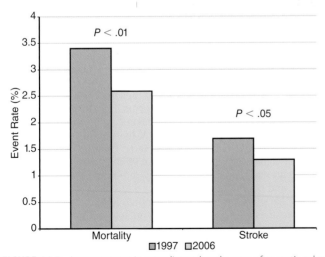

FIGURE 46-7 Improvements in mortality and stroke rates after aortic valve replacement (*AVR*) 1997 compared to 2006. (*Data from Brown JM, O'Brien SM, Wu C, et al. Isolated aortic valve replacement in North America comprising 108,687 patients in 10 years: changes in risks, valve types, and outcomes in the Society of Thoracic Surgeons National Database. J Thorac Cardiovasc Surg 2009;137:82-90.*)

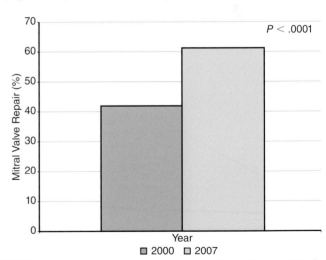

FIGURE 46-8 Trends in mitral valve surgery. By 2007, mitral valve repair had become the most frequent mitral valve operation. (*Data from Gammie JS, Sheng S, Griffith BP, et al. Trends in mitral valve surgery in the United States: results from the Society of Thoracic Surgeons Adult Cardiac Surgery Database. Ann Thorac Surg 2009;87:1431-1439.*)

indications for surgical intervention to include asymptomatic patients with normal ventricles; 2) a greater understanding of the pathophysiology, clinical course, and role of MV surgery in ischemic MR; and 3) a greater acceptance of isolated or concomitant MV repair in patients with poor ventricular function. Repair rates for isolated MR are now approaching 70%.

ANATOMY

The surgical anatomy of the MV is shown in Figure 46-9. The leaflets are divided into eight segments: the posterior leaflet is divided into three segments—P1, P2, and P3—on the basis of anatomically distinct scallops; each anterior leaflet segment—A1, A2, and A3—is defined by its corresponding posterior segment; and the anterolateral commissure (Ac) and posteromedial commissure (Pc) have small but distinct leaflet scallops. The subvalvular apparatus consists of the papillary muscles and chordae tendineae, which are further subdivided into *primary/marginal*, attached to the free margin; *secondary*, attached to the underbelly of the leaflet; and *tertiary/basal*, attached to annulus.

CARPENTIER'S FUNCTIONAL CLASSIFICATION

Although several systems for classifying MV dysfunction have been proposed, Carpentier's functional classification of MR based on the *pathophysiologic triad*—etiology, lesions, and dysfunction—is the most robust (Table 46-5). Each etiology—whether degenerative, rheumatic, ischemic, or related to dilated cardiomyopathy or endocarditis and so on—results in one or more lesions of the annulus, leaflets, or subvalvular apparatus.

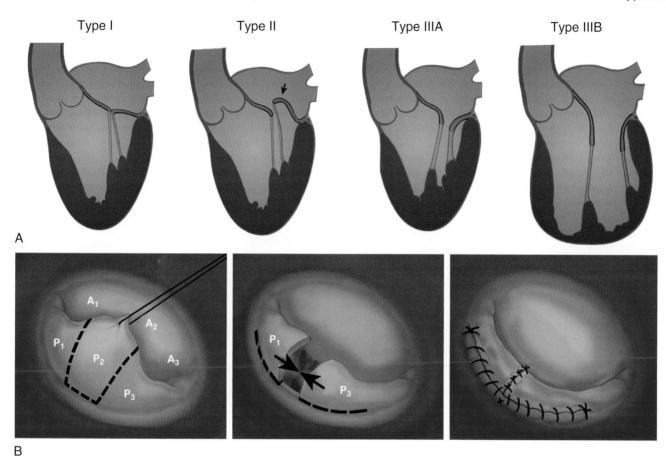

FIGURE 46-9 Principles of mitral valve repair. **A,** Carpentier's functional classification of mitral regurgitation. **B,** Quadrangular resection of the posterior leaflet with sliding valvuloplasty for P2 prolapse. A, anterior leaflet; P, posterior leaflet.

TABLE 46-5	**Carpentier's Functional Classification of Mitral Regurgitation**		
DYSFUNCTION	**LEAFLET MOTION**	**LESIONS**	**COMMON ETIOLOGIES**
Type I	Normal	Annular dilation Leaflet perforation	Dilated cardiomyopathy Ischemic (basal infarction) Endocarditis
Type II	Increased (prolapse)	Chordal elongation Chordal rupture Papillary muscle elongation Papillary muscle rupture	Degenerative Endocarditis Ischemic (PM infarction)
Type III (restricted) A B	 Systole and diastole Systole	Leaflet thickening and retraction Subvalvular thickening and shortening Papillary muscle displacement Annular calcification	Rheumatic Dilated cardiomyopathy Ischemic

PM, papillary muscle.

These lesions result in a specific type of dysfunction on the basis of leaflet motion (see Figure 46-9, *A*). In a normally functioning MV, the leaflets come together within the valve orifice and result in a surface of coaptation. The free margins of the leaflets remain below the plane of the annulus.

In *type I dysfunction,* the leaflets exhibit normal motion. The regurgitation results in annular dilation, which prevents coaptation, or from leaflet perforation. *Type II dysfunction* results from leaflet prolapse, in which the free margins of the involved portions of the leaflets rise above the plane of the annulus into the left atrium, preventing leaflet coaptation. The most common lesions resulting in leaflet prolapse and type II dysfunction include chordal elongation or rupture as a result of degenerative changes. Finally, *type III dysfunction* results from restricted leaflet motion. Here, the free margins of portions of one or both leaflets are pulled below the plane of the annulus into the LV, preventing them from rising up to the plane of the annulus and coapting during systole. The restricted leaflet motion can occur during both systole and diastole, related to valvular or subvalvular pathology (rheumatic fibrosis); this is referred to as *type IIIA dysfunction.* Type III dysfunction more commonly occurs when abnormal ventricular geometry or function leads to papillary muscle displacement, which pulls the otherwise normal leaflets into the ventricle. This is known as *type IIIB dysfunction* and usually results from prior MI (ischemic) or severe ventricular dilation and dysfunction. Frequently, types I and IIIB dysfunction (except leaflet perforation) are referred to as *functional MR* because they occur in the absence of structural abnormalities of the valve.

PREOPERATIVE EVALUATION

A quality echocardiogram is particularly important in the preoperative evaluation of patients with MV disease. Transesophageal echocardiography (TEE) may be necessary to obtain all the important anatomic and physiologic data. The severity of mitral stenosis or MR may have already been established, but more quantitative assessment of MR (PISA, ERO, or RV) may be particularly useful in patients with functional MR (types I and IIIB). The specific type of dysfunction (type I, II, IIIA, or IIIB) should be determined preoperatively by carefully assessing the motion of each segment of each leaflet. The etiology can usually be determined with a combination of history, physical examination, and echocardiography. Distinguishing between specific lesions, such as a ruptured versus elongated chord, is less important because both the likelihood of repair and the surgical technique used are determined by the etiology and type of dysfunction. Extensive mitral annular calcification (MAC) is an important finding because it can significantly increase the complexity of the surgical procedure. Other echocardiographic characteristics, such as atrial and ventricular dimensions, ventricular function, estimated PA pressures, and the status of the other valves, remain critical.

Indications

MITRAL REGURGITATION

The indications for surgical intervention in MR have steadily expanded as the results of MV repair have improved. Class I indications include severe MR in the presence of symptoms or LV dysfunction. On the basis of recent natural history data,[10,76] surgery is also recommended (class IIa) for asymptomatic patients with severe MR and normal LV function, as long as valve repair is deemed likely with a reasonable operative risk. Because the likelihood of repair is lower, surgery is usually deferred in patients with rheumatic disease until the onset of symptoms or LV dysfunction.

Poor LV function and class III to IV heart failure were once considered an absolute contraindication to MV surgery. This was based on data that showed poorer early and late outcomes in these patients, especially when they undergo non–chordal-sparing valve replacement. It was theorized that the MR served as a "pop-off" valve that provided a low-afterload circuit (the left atrium) for the failing ventricle. This concept is now known to be false; it is clear that MR causes volume overload and increases wall stress on the ventricle. Severe ventricular function is no longer an absolute contraindication to MV surgery. Data from Bolling[77] and others have demonstrated that patients with severe LV function can undergo valve repair with a downsized annuloplasty with reasonable early outcomes. Whether valve repair in this setting improves long-term outcomes is unknown; therefore it remains a class IIb indication.[10,78]

MITRAL STENOSIS

The indications for surgery with mitral stenosis are more conservative than for MR for several reasons. First, the etiology is usually rheumatic heart disease, which has a slower, more predictable natural history. A smaller proportion of patients are candidates for MV repair, so the additional risks associated with an MV prosthesis must be taken into consideration in the remaining patients. Finally, patients who are good candidates for percutaneous balloon mitral valvuloplasty (PBMV) can avoid surgery, at least for the medium term. Currently accepted indications for surgery include symptomatic moderate to severe mitral stenosis when PBMV either is unavailable or is contraindicated because of thrombus, significant MR, or unfavorable morphology. Mildly symptomatic patients with severe pulmonary hypertension should also be considered for surgery before the onset of right heart failure.

Mitral Valve Repair

PRINCIPLES

The techniques of MV repair are based on certain fundamental principles developed by Carpentier and others over the past 35 years. They start with the notion that, in theory, any regurgitant valve with adequate, pliable, noncalcified leaflet tissue can be repaired as long as a systematic approach is applied, based on pathophysiologic principles described earlier. The likelihood of a successful repair depends on surgeon experience and on the complexity of the repair, which in turn depends on the etiology, the type of dysfunction, and the distribution of lesions among the various anatomic components of the valve: leaflets, annulus, and subvalvular apparatus. The complexity can range from a simple annuloplasty to a complicated Barlow valve repair that involves interventions to multiple leaflet segments. Although it can vary from patient to patient, generally anterior leaflet pathology is more difficult to repair than posterior leaflet pathology, and rheumatic valves are more challenging than degenerative valves.

The first step in any repair is precise, systematic valve analysis, initially by TEE and then by direct assessment (see Figure 46-9, *B*). The primary goal is to determine the type of dysfunction of each of the eight leaflet segments. This is done by pulling the free margins of the leaflet segment up using a hook and determining whether the leaflet motion is *normal* (type I), *excessive* (type II), or *restricted* (type III). The annulus is assessed separately, noting its size and symmetry and any calcification. Once the valve analysis is complete, the operative plan is established. The specific techniques used depend on the type of dysfunction and are described here.

ANNULOPLASTY

Implantation of a prosthetic annuloplasty ring is an essential part of nearly all MV repairs. The exceptions include the occasional patient with endocarditis that involves only the body of a leaflet.

Nonprosthetic annuloplasty techniques using suture or pericardium do not have a role in modern MV repair because the results with these techniques are much less favorable than those of prosthetic rings.

The primary purpose of annuloplasty is to restore the annular dimensions, bringing the leaflets together and permitting a broad surface of coaptation—a critical element to a durable repair. It also stabilizes the annulus and takes stress off sutures lines. An annuloplasty ring typically is constructed from a core material, either silicone or metal, that determines its rigidity (flexible, semirigid, or rigid); it is sheathed in a cloth material, either Dacron or polyester, through which the sutures are placed. Annuloplasty rings come in numerous sizes, rigidities, and shapes and are sometimes a partial band or complete ring, but they can be broadly categorized as either *remodeling* or *nonremodeling*. A *remodeling annuloplasty* seeks to restore the size and physiologic shape (a "D" or "kidney") of the annulus in contrast to a restrictive *nonremodeling annuloplasty*, which merely decreases the overall circumference of the annulus. Many surgeons, especially those who subscribe to the Carpentierian principles of valve repair, believe that a complete remodeling annuloplasty (e.g., Carpentier-Edwards Physio) should be performed in all repairs to ensure a long-term durable result. Others favor partial or complete flexible rings (e.g., Cosgrove-Edwards Band, Edwards Lifesciences). However, most surgeons now acknowledge that a remodeling annuloplasty is superior in patients with type IIIB MR secondary to ischemic disease or dilated cardiomyopathy. The size of the annuloplasty ring is determined by the height of the anterior leaflet and the intercommissural, or intertrigonal, distance. Patients with degenerative disease and type II dysfunction will typically receive a ring in the 32- to 40-mm range, whereas those with type IIIB dysfunction from ischemic disease or cardiomyopathy will receive much smaller rings, in the 24- to 30-mm range.

MAC is not an infrequent finding in patients undergoing MV surgery, especially elderly patients and those with CAD. MAC poses serious challenges to the surgeon in both MV repair and replacement. It can interfere with seating of the annuloplasty ring and can restrict and distort leaflet tissue; in severe cases, it may extend deep into the subannular ventricular muscle. Ideally, all annular calcification is removed en bloc prior to reconstruction and ring implantation. This is usually straightforward for discrete superficial nodules in the posterior annulus but becomes progressively more challenging if it involves the commissures and is more diffuse and deep. Carpentier has shown that complete en bloc excision of even massive MAC, with subsequent reconstruction of the atrioventricular junction, can be performed safely. However, many surgeons remain wary of this approach for fear it will lead to atrioventricular rupture, a dreaded complication that is usually fatal.

LEAFLET PROLAPSE REPAIR TECHNIQUES (TYPE II)

Leaflet prolapse can be corrected through one of several approaches that involve the leaflets and subvalvular apparatus. The specific technique used depends on the specific prolapsing segment more than the actual lesion (chordal rupture or chordal elongation). The ultimate goal is to leave an adequate amount of mobile, well-supported leaflet to participate in coaptation.

Posterior leaflet prolapse is usually treated by resecting the prolapsing segment and reapproximating the nonprolapsing segments (see Figure 46-9, *B*). This most commonly involves a quadrangular resection of a prolapsed P2 segment. If the resection is relatively small, the annular gap can simply be plicated and the cut edges reapproximated. Usually, however, a sliding valvuloplasty is recommended. Here, the remaining P1 and P3 segments are partially detached from the annulus and then reattached, stretching them across the annular gap, which can be decreased with compression sutures. The sliding valvuloplasty technique has two advantages. First, it avoids the need to plicate a large

annular gap, which can lead to kinking of the circumflex artery. Second, during the process of detaching and reattaching the remaining segments, the surgeon can decrease the height of the posterior leaflet. Left alone, the excessively tall posterior leaflets seen in patients with Barlow disease can lead to a systolic anterior motion (SAM) in which the anterior leaflet is pushed into the LV outflow tract, causing obstruction.

Anterior leaflet prolapse can be corrected by resecting the prolapsing segment or reestablishing its subvalvular support. Triangular resections with direct reapproximation of the cut edges can correct small areas of prolapse, especially when there is redundant tissue, such as in Barlow disease. However, there is a limit to how much anterior leaflet tissue can be resected before the remaining tissue is inadequate for coaptation. If redundant tissue is not present or large areas of prolapse exist, subvalvular support to these areas must be reestablished. Chordal transfer involves detaching normal secondary chords attached to the body of the anterior leaflet and reattaching them to the margin of the prolapsing segments. With chordal transposition the chords are detached, along with some leaflet tissue, from a normal portion of the posterior leaflet; they are then flipped anteriorly and reattached to the prolapsing segment, after which the gap in the posterior leaflet is closed primarily. Finally, if no good chords are available, an artificial chordoplasty can be performed. The new chords are created using GoreTex sutures secured to the papillary muscle and prolapsing leaflet segment. Chordal shortening techniques, in which the length of the elongated chord is decreased by burying the excess into the papillary muscle, were abandoned when retrospective studies showed that they were less durable.

Correcting commissural prolapse can be particularly challenging. Sliding valvuloplasty techniques similar to those used on the posterior leaflet can be applied, but care must be taken to avoid distortion of the valve. Chordal support to the prolapsing commissure can also be established using the same techniques as in the anterior leaflet.

RESTRICTED LEAFLET TECHNIQUES (TYPE III)

In patients with type IIIA dysfunction, usually from rheumatic disease, the restricted leaflet motion results when the fibrotic process leads to thickening and fusion of the subvalvular structures and thickening and retraction of the leaflets, particularly the posterior leaflets. As long as adequate pliable leaflet tissue is available, valve repair can successfully be performed with good long-term results, but this type of repair is not widely practiced outside of major valve-repair centers. Leaflet mobilization is accomplished by resecting secondary chordae and by splitting or fenestrating fused marginal chordae. Leaflet enlargement, typically to the posterior leaflet, can be performed by detaching the leaflet annulus and suturing a patch of autologous glutaraldehyde-fixed pericardium. Patients with rheumatic mitral stenosis, pure or in combination with MR, are treated with open commissurotomy. The fused commissures are split sharply within a few millimeters of the annulus, and the associated fused chords are split down the papillary muscles or are fenestrated.

Patients with type IIIB dysfunction, resulting from ischemic heart disease or dilated cardiomyopathy, have structurally normal leaflets that are restricted as a result of papillary displacement from ventricular dilation and regional wall motion abnormalities. To reestablish an adequate surface of coaptation, the restricted leaflets must be brought toward each other. The final anteroposterior dimension of the valve must be less than its original dimension to overcome the fact that the restricted leaflets cannot rise to their normal systolic position just below the plane of the annulus.

This can be accomplished with a downsized remodeling annuloplasty alone. The intercommissural or intertrigonal distance and the anterior leaflet height are measured, and a ring 2 to 4 mm smaller is selected to achieve proper downsizing. Recently introduced rings specifically designed for type IIIB dysfunction—the asymmetric Carpentier-McCarthy-Adams ET-Logix ring for ischemic MR and the GeoForm ring for cardiomyopathy (both Edwards Lifesciences)—are "predownsized." In other words, they are designed to be more squat with a significantly reduced antero-posterior dimension relative to the intercommissural dimension, allowing good leaflet coaptation while maximizing the overall orifice area.

Although insertion of an annuloplasty ring alone suffices in the vast majority of patients undergoing repair for type IIIB MR, adjunctive techniques may occasionally be useful. Resection of secondary chordae, particularly to the anterior leaflet, can increase leaflet mobility and correct the "hockey stick" deformity seen in patients with severe leaflet restriction. Occasionally, prominent clefts between the posterior leaflet scallops will be splayed out by the leaflet restriction, and closing these clefts can prevent small areas of residual MR. Other techniques, such as papillary muscle relocation and patch extension of the posterior leaflet, have been reported but are not widely used in this condition.

OTHER TECHNIQUES

The edge-to-edge or Alfieri technique involves suturing the free edges of the anterior and posterior leaflets together, usually at A2-P2, creating a double-orifice MV. The technique can correct prolapse in one leaflet by using the other leaflet's chordae. In the process, however, it decreases the MV orifice area. No long-term data are available on the durability of this type of repair,[79] but early data clearly document poor outcomes in the absence of a concomitant annuloplasty[80] and in ischemic MR.[81] The percutaneous application of this technique is the basis of the MitraClip (Abbott Vascular, Abbott Park, IL).[82]

Mitral Valve Replacement

The evidence base supporting valve repair, when feasible, and the increased number of surgeons proficient in these techniques have led to a reduction in the fraction of patients undergoing MV replacement. Even so, the total number of MV replacements has increased, correlating with the increase in the total number of valve surgeries performed. Some valve replacements are being performed in patients with valves that are not repairable, such as those with advanced rheumatic disease with calcification, endocarditis with extensive leaflet destruction, or ruptured papillary muscles following MI. However, even now a number of replaced valves could have been repaired by surgeons experienced in MV repair. In particular, many surgeons are reasonably comfortable repairing valves with isolated posterior leaflet prolapse but proceed with valve replacement when they encounter prolapse of the anterior leaflet. Experienced surgeons, however, can repair more than 90% of degenerative valves, whether the anterior leaflet, posterior leaflet, or both are involved.

CHORDAL-SPARING MITRAL VALVE REPLACEMENT

In the early days of MV replacement, the entire valve, including leaflets and chordae, were resected before implantation of the valve. In the late 1970s and 1980s, however, it became clear that the subvalvular apparatus was an integral component to global ventricular function, and this practice frequently led to decreased LV function following valve replacement. Chordal-sparing techniques were developed and were shown to be superior in terms of preservation of LV function and in terms of early and late outcomes.

The posterior leaflet is now almost always left intact and is plicated within the posterior suture line. The chordal apparatus to the anterior leaflet can also be preserved by resecting an elliptical portion of the body of the leaflet, splitting the remaining rim of leaflet with attached chordae in two and reattaching them to the anterior annulus. Occasionally, in patients with extensive rheumatic fibrosis, calcification, or endocarditic destruction, it may be impossible to preserve the chordal apparatus. In these cases, artificial GoreTex chords can be used to reestablish papillary muscle–annulus continuity.

The actual implantation of the valve is similar to that of a prosthetic AVR and can be performed using a variety of suturing techniques: interrupted versus running, pledgeted versus non-pledgeted, everting versus noninverting. As with AVR, complete debridement of annular calcification is important to prevent perivalvular leaks, although this must be done with great care to avoid atrioventricular disruption, a highly fatal complication.

CHOICE OF PROSTHESIS

The choice of valve prosthesis is somewhat less complicated in the mitral position than in the aortic position. For example, the options are limited to mechanical valves or stented xenografts (porcine or pericardial). In addition, although the durability of mitral bioprostheses has improved significantly, it is not yet good enough to justify routine use in middle-aged adults. Patients younger than 65 years typically receive mechanical valves, and those 65 years and older receive biologic valves. The age threshold can certainly be lowered in selected situations, and recent trends suggest that an increasing number of patients are receiving bioprosthetic valves (Figure 46-10). Patients with CAD, poor LV function, or comorbidities that portend decreased life expectancy may be candidates for biologic valves. Younger patients who cannot or will not take warfarin may also receive a biologic valve, but they need to understand that they almost certainly will face one, if not two, reoperations in their lifetime. Whenever possible, of course, valve repair is preferable in patients of all age groups.

Results

EARLY

The operative risk of MV surgery varies significantly depending on the patient profile and operation. It can be as low as 1% for young, healthy patients undergoing elective MV repair for degenerative disease or more than 50% in an ill elderly patient undergoing emergent surgery for endocarditis. The overall operative mortality rates for isolated MV repair and replacement are 1.4% and 5.9%, respectively.[8] Those rates are significantly higher for

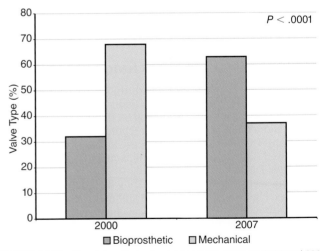

FIGURE 46-10 Trends in mitral valve replacement. Between 2000 and 2007, bioprosthetic mitral valve replacement became the most frequent prosthetic mitral valve choice. (Data from Gammie JS, Sheng S, Griffith BP, et al. Trends in mitral valve surgery in the United States: results from the Society of Thoracic Surgeons Adult Cardiac Surgery Database. Ann Thorac Surg 2009;87:1431-1439.)

patients undergoing concomitant CABG—5.0% for repair and 8.9% for replacement. In a recent study from the Northern New England Cardiovascular Disease Study Group, 10 variables were identified as independent predictors of in-hospital death: female sex, advanced age, diabetes, CAD, prior CVA, elevated creatinine level, New York Heart Association (NYHA) class IV status, CHF, acuity, and valve replacement.[83] Ventricular function, prior cardiac surgery, and pulmonary hypertension have also been found to increase operative risk. Enriquez-Sarano and colleagues[84] have documented improved preservation of ventricular function with MV repair relative to replacement.

The incidence of major morbidity in most MV surgeries remains low, and overall risk of stroke has been reported to be 2% to 3%. Deep sternal wound infections and reoperation for bleeding occur at rates similar to those for other valve surgery, at 2% to 5%. MV surgery is a significant risk factor for postoperative AF, with overall rates of approximately 50%. The incidence of heart block requiring permanent pacemaker insertion is about 3%.[85]

LATE

The late outcomes of MV surgery depend to a large degree on the underlying etiology of the MV disease and whether a valve repair or replacement is performed. Long-term survival in generally healthy patients undergoing MV repair for degenerative valve disease approaches that of an age-matched population. Several studies have documented improved long-term survival with valve repair, at least for degenerative and rheumatic etiologies. Moss and colleagues[86] recently used propensity score methods to show improved late survival (relative risk [RR], 0.52) with MV repair relative to replacement. Late survival is decreased with ischemic compared with nonischemic etiologies. Additional predictors of late survival include ventricular function, NYHA functional status, age, and concomitant CAD. The leading causes of late death include heart failure, thromboembolism, stroke, endocarditis, anticoagulation-related hemorrhage, and MI. Late functional status following MV surgery is good, and most studies report 90% of patients in NYHA class I or II. The durability of MV repair is most directly related to the etiology of the disease, but the long-term results for repair of degenerative valves are excellent (Figure 46-11). Carpentier's group reported their 20-year results,[87] and the overall linearized rate of reoperation was 0.4% per year. Freedom from reoperation was 97% for patients with isolated posterior leaflet prolapse, whereas it was 86% and 83% for those with anterior or bileaflet prolapse, respectively. The results for repair of rheumatic valves, even at experienced centers, are not as good.

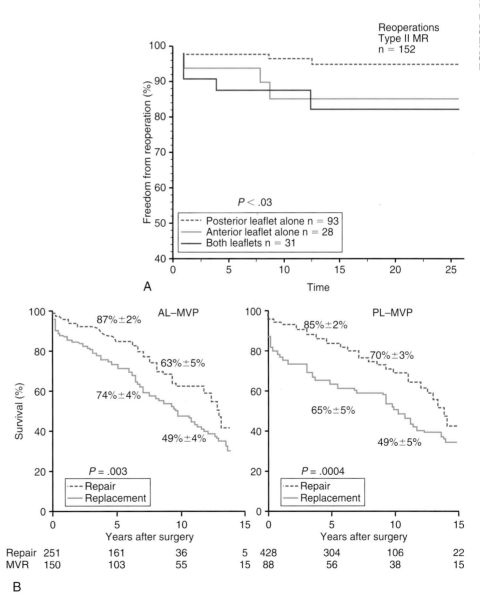

FIGURE 46-11 Long-term outcomes following mitral valve surgery for degenerative disease. **A,** Freedom from reoperation following mitral valve repair for type II mitral regurgitation (*MR*) (Carpentier's experience[87]). **B,** Long-term survival following mitral valve repair or replacement (*MVR*) following mitral valve repair for anterior leaflet (AL) and posterior leaflet (PL) disease (Mayo Clinic experience). MVP, mitral valve prolapse. (*From Mohty D, Orszulak TA, Schaff HV, et al. Very long-term survival and durability of mitral valve repair for mitral valve prolapse. Circulation 2001;104[12 Suppl 1]:I1-I17.*)

Carpentier's group reported linearized rates of reoperation of 1.9% to 2.7% and 20-year freedom of reoperation of 46% to 65%, depending on whether the initial dysfunction was type II, leaflet prolapse, or type III, leaflet restriction.[88]

As with AVR, the long-term freedom from reoperation following MV replacement is a function of the prosthesis type and age. Although structural valve degeneration (SVD) of current-generation mechanical valves is extremely rare, it is important to remember that the reoperation rate is not zero. Linearized rates of reoperation for prosthetic valve endocarditis, pannus overgrowth, and thrombosis are similar to those for atrioventricular mechanical valves—about 1% per year. Durability of bioprostheses was believed to be inferior in the mitral position compared with the aortic position, presumably because mitral bioprostheses are exposed to greater forces during systole.[89,90] More recent data suggest structural deterioration may be similar.[91] Durability remains excellent in elderly patients. Ten-year freedom from SVD for the Carpentier-Edwards pericardial valve was 100% in patients 70 years and older. Performance in patients 60 years and younger is significantly worse, with 60% to 80% rates of freedom from SVD at 8 to 10 years,[89,92] highlighting the importance of achieving high rates of valve repair in these patients. Interestingly, Ruel and colleagues reported that initial valve choice does not seem to influence long-term survival in these patients.[92]

Tricuspid Valve Surgery

Overview

Because most tricuspid valve dysfunction is a result of left heart lesions, isolated tricuspid valve surgery is relatively rare. Causes of isolated tricuspid disease that require surgical correction include congenital anomalies, such as Ebstein anomaly; RV dilation from primary pulmonary hypertension; trauma, such as that following endomyocardial biopsies; and endocarditis. Most tricuspid valve surgery is performed in conjunction with other valve surgery, usually MV repair or replacement. Interest in tricuspid valve surgery has increased in recent years,[93,94] correlating with a greater number of tricuspid valve operations reported in the STS database.

Indications

The indications for tricuspid valve surgery vary depending on whether the disease is primary or secondary. The data supporting these indications are not as well established as they are for aortic and mitral valve disease. Tricuspid stenosis is almost always rheumatic and is rarely isolated, usually presenting with concomitant MV disease. Severe symptomatic TR is considered a class IIA indication for isolated tricuspid valve surgery, and the threshold for correcting it at the time of other valve surgery has fallen in recent years. In the past, even moderate degrees of TR were left alone with the assumption that correction of the left-sided lesions would decrease the PA pressures and the degree of TR. However, recent data suggest that this does not reliably occur, and most patients with moderate TR undergo concomitant tricuspid annuloplasty. A report by Dreyfus and colleagues[94] suggested that annular circumference alone, even in the absence of significant TR, should trigger concomitant annuloplasty. On the other hand, Yilmaz and colleagues recently reported favorable results with observing 3+ or greater functional TR after MV repair in the absence of RV dysfunction.[95]

Surgical Techniques

APPROACH

Tricuspid valve surgery frequently occurs in the context of multivalve surgery and thus is performed through a median sternotomy. Cannulation for cardiopulmonary bypass is usually performed in the ascending aorta and vena cavae, which are occluded below the cannulae to isolate the right atrium before atriotomy. The procedure can be performed under full cardioplegic arrest, under fibrillatory arrest, or on a beating heart under cardiopulmonary bypass, usually during rewarming.

VALVE REPAIR

Most patients with TR will have type I or IIIB dysfunction without leaflet pathology, so-called *functional TR,* and can be successfully treated with annuloplasty alone. Commissuroplasty techniques, such as bicuspidization (obliterating the posterior leaflet), have largely been abandoned. Suture annuloplasty techniques, such as the DeVega annuloplasty, have been popular because they can be rapidly performed. Most data, however, suggest that a formal prosthetic remodeling ring annuloplasty is superior to other techniques and should be the procedure of choice.[93] Many surgeons adapt MV annuloplasty prostheses to tricuspid valve repairs. Devices specifically designed for the tricuspid valve, such as the Edwards MC3, have been developed and are being used with increasing frequency.

Tricuspid valve repair of type II and IIIA dysfunction is rarely performed. Patients with Ebstein anomaly can undergo successful repair with techniques developed by Carpentier and others. Those with degenerative changes or localized damage from trauma or endocarditis can undergo localized leaflet resection and reconstruction using techniques analogous to MV repair.

VALVE REPLACEMENT

Patients undergoing tricuspid valve replacement usually have extensive leaflet damage—such as from rheumatic disease, endocarditis, or biopsy trauma—or have failed prior valve repairs. The trade-offs between tissue and mechanical valves are similar to valves in other positions, but there are fewer data. In the past, surgeons tended to avoid mechanical valves because of reports of high thrombosis rates secondary to low flow velocities; however, more current data with bileaflet valves are significantly better.[96,97] Although the rates of structural valve degeneration for bioprostheses in the tricuspid position appear to be lower than in the mitral position, the incidence of nonstructural degeneration, primarily pannus formation, appears to be higher, presumably as a result of organized thrombotic material. Most patients undergoing tricuspid valve replacement have limited life expectancy as a result of age or underlying disease and therefore receive a bioprosthesis. Mechanical valves are generally reserved for younger, healthier patients and those who have or require another mechanical valve.

The techniques of implantation are similar to those for MV replacement. Sutures along the septal leaflet must be taken superficially to avoid injury to the conduction system in the triangle of Koch. Patients undergoing mechanical valve implantation often have a permanent epicardial pacing lead placed in the operating room.

Results

Operative mortality rates following isolated tricuspid valve surgery are generally high, approximately 10% to 25%,[98,99] because many of these patients have complex medical conditions and advanced right heart disease. Data on the additional risk of concomitant tricuspid valve repair in patients undergoing MV surgery are limited. The operative mortality rate does appear to be higher but is probably due to the fact that the presence of TR is a marker for more advanced cardiopulmonary disease. A major early morbidity risk is complete heart block that requires pacemaker insertion.

Special Considerations

Multiple Valves

Many patients who come in for heart valve surgery have multiple valve dysfunctions. Occasionally, two or more primary valve dysfunctions coexist and are both of sufficient severity to mandate surgery, such as in advanced rheumatic heart disease. More frequently, however, when valve dysfunctions coexist, it is usually possible to identify a primary dysfunction that mandates surgery and secondary dysfunctions that arise from, or coexist with, the primary dysfunction. When the primary dysfunction is of the aortic valve, secondary atrioventricular valve regurgitation may be a direct result of aortic valve disease and could resolve with isolated correction of the aortic lesion. In some patients, however, the secondary process is unrelated or may be so advanced that surgical correction of the aortic lesion alone will not suffice. Atrioventricular valve dysfunction as a primary lesion does not result in secondary aortic valve disease; the aortic valve disease in such cases is treated on its own merit.

MITRAL AND TRICUSPID DISEASE

Tricuspid valve regurgitation often coexists in patients with MV disease who come in for surgery. Traditionally such regurgitation was left uncorrected because it was assumed to be "functional," and correction of MR results in resolution of TR. However, more recent studies have challenged this thinking, and evidence suggests that patients left with uncorrected tricuspid disease fare less well after surgery in terms of long-term symptoms and survival. Patients who initially have absent or mild or moderate TR at the time of MV surgery may also go on to develop worsening TR in the follow-up period.[94,100] Patients who do not have tricuspid repair at the time of surgery have a greater incidence of significant TR and higher incidence of CHF on long-term follow-up,[101,102] although patients without evidence of right heart failure may be an exception to this paradigm.[95] Mortality rates are high for reoperations performed to correct TR—up to 30%.[93]

AORTIC AND MITRAL DISEASE

Patients with primary aortic valve disease sometimes have secondary MV disease. In patients with rheumatic disease, concomitant MV repair or replacement is indicated if there is moderate MR or stenosis. In patients with degenerative AS, secondary MR is not uncommon, presumably as a result of LV dilation and pressure overload. MV repair is certainly indicated if the MR is severe, but most mild to moderate MR is left alone because the data for intervening at this threshold are mixed.[103-105] In the past, some have argued that patients who undergo concomitant aortic and mitral valve surgery should receive a second prosthesis instead of an MV repair. Given the current results of MV repair, this does not appear justified, and every effort should be made to repair the MV in this setting. Gillinov and colleagues[106] have documented improved survival with this approach.

Reoperation

The success and improved long-term outcomes of cardiac surgery in the 1980s and 1990s have resulted in millions of surviving patients worldwide who have had previous cardiac surgery. As these patients age, a proportion will require reoperative valve surgery for valve-related complications or for progression of native valve disease.

Valve surgery in the reoperative setting is more complex compared with first-time surgery because of pericardial adhesions, patent bypass grafts, often advanced cardiac dysfunction with pulmonary hypertension, and technical issues relating to re-replacing heart valves. The mortality risk is higher than for first-time surgery, although this risk has fallen in recent years, with some centers reporting rates less than 5%.

The indications for surgery differ slightly in the reoperative setting because the risk of operative death may outweigh the benefits if conventional indications are applied the same as for first-time surgery. The major consideration in deciding to offer valve reoperation is the relief of symptoms rather than prolongation of life expectancy. In some instances reoperative surgery is undertaken for survival benefit, such as in young patients with SVD, and in those in whom the valve disease would otherwise be fatal, such as patients with endocarditis.

Patients who require reoperation present unique surgical challenges. These patients are often managed medically until the disease is advanced, and surgery is only undertaken when no nonsurgical options are available. Subsequently, many patients have poor LV function, are severely compromised or debilitated with poor functional state, or are elderly with comorbidities. These patients must have a detailed preoperative workup because even small lapses can precipitate a major catastrophe. Cardiac catheterization is performed to delineate coronary anatomy and measure pulmonary pressures. CT is useful in defining the relationship of the cardiac chambers and great vessels to the sternum; sternal reentry may be considered so hazardous that alternative surgical or transcatheter approaches are required. Thorough echocardiographic assessment of all heart valves is necessary because many patients have multiple valve dysfunctions. Details of the prior cardiac operations should be obtained because previous difficulties, observations, or complications may be relevant to the planned procedure. Screening for peripheral vascular disease is necessary in older patients because cannulation of peripheral vessels for cardiopulmonary bypass may be required and is occasionally lifesaving.

Principles of surgical repair or replacement are similar to those for primary valve surgery. When valves are repairable, this remains the treatment of choice. A failed prior valve repair does not mandate a valve replacement if the valve is easily repairable. If valve replacement is required, choice of prosthesis should consider the balance between the risks of anticoagulation and the probability and risks of another future reoperation for biologic valve degeneration. Sometimes the surgeon may choose to re-replace a normally functioning prosthetic valve—that is, to replace a mechanical valve with a bioprosthesis—so the patient can stop anticoagulation or to avert inevitable future structural valve degeneration, such as in a patient with a 10-year-old functioning porcine valve, requiring another cardiac procedure.

Endocarditis

Although medical management remains the cornerstone of therapy for most cases of bacterial endocarditis, surgery has a critical and lifesaving role in the treatment of complicated cases. A detailed discussion of the surgical management of patients with endocarditis is beyond the scope of this chapter.

Diagnosis is usually based on characteristic lesions seen on echocardiography, with or without positive blood cultures (see Chapter 43). TEE is the most sensitive and specific investigation for defining endocarditis lesions, and it is performed in most cases of endocarditis to evaluate for indications for surgery. Surgery is performed urgently for patients who come to medical attention with life-threatening heart failure. The timing of an operation for other indications is less clear, although early surgery is generally favored.[107] One exception is the presence of an embolic stroke, in which case early surgery carries a higher risk of hemorrhagic extension of the stroke.[108] The threshold for surgery tends to be higher for right-sided endocarditis.

The principles of surgical treatment are debridement of all infected tissues, drainage of abscesses, and correction of hemodynamic dysfunction. Following debridement, if the valve annulus is affected, it is reconstructed and the valve is repaired when feasible or is replaced. Abscesses of the aortic root usually necessitate root replacement, and choice of valve prosthesis usually depends on surgeon preference. Allografts and autografts are more resistant to infection, but with thorough debridement and continuation of antibiotic therapy, reinfection of the newly implanted valve is uncommon regardless of the type of prosthesis used.

Ischemic Heart Disease

Ischemic and valvular heart diseases frequently coexist, making surgical decision making and management more complex. Although a patient with advanced disease can certainly come to medical attention with both ischemia and CHF, in most patients, one disease dominates the presentation and the other is more incidental. Management depends on which disease dominates the clinical picture.

INCIDENTAL CORONARY DISEASE IN VALVE SURGERY PATIENTS

Patients with risk factors for CAD, such as advanced age, who require heart valve surgery generally undergo preoperative screening angiography because the presence of concomitant CAD reduces survival after heart valve surgery.[109] Furthermore, the presence of CAD can lead to patchy distribution of cardioplegic solution, which complicates myocardial preservation. The subendocardial region is most vulnerable to poor protection and intraoperative ischemic injury in the presence of coronary disease, particularly in the setting of LV hypertrophy. In patients who have poor ventricular function, incidental CAD may be a contributing factor; MRI is useful in this setting to identify ischemic or infarcted myocardium and to define the potential utility of bypass grafting.

Most surgeons would perform concurrent CABG at the time of heart valve surgery when there are critical coronary lesions (>70% stenosis in a proximal coronary artery or >50% in the left main coronary artery). Surgery classically consists of an internal mammary artery graft to the left anterior descending artery and venous conduits for other vessels. Although concurrent coronary artery bypass surgery is associated with higher perioperative mortality rates compared with isolated valve surgery, no evidence suggests that this is related to the additional surgical procedure per se. Higher mortality rates are probably a reflection of the increased risk of valve surgery in the setting of concurrent ischemic heart disease. If critical coronary lesions are not bypassed, the patient is at greater risk of perioperative MI.

Staged procedures that use percutaneous coronary revascularization followed by valve surgery are an alternative strategy for handling concomitant CAD. Revascularization before surgery allows for an expeditious valve operation with shorter ischemic and cardiopulmonary bypass times. The timing of percutaneous intervention relative to valve surgery and management of antiplatelet therapy are important considerations with this approach.

INCIDENTAL VALVE DISEASE IN CORONARY SURGERY PATIENTS

Widespread use of echocardiography in the workup of cardiovascular disease has led to increased diagnosis of incidental valvular pathology in patients undergoing nonvalvular heart surgery, particularly coronary surgery. If the valve disease is truly incidental, patients are asymptomatic by definition. The indications for valve surgery in any asymptomatic valve patient (see earlier discussion) also apply in the patient having coronary artery bypass surgery. For example, severe AS and severe MR require surgical correction.

Patients undergoing coronary bypass surgery who have valve lesions that do not warrant surgery on their own pose a diagnostic dilemma. These include patients with moderate degrees of valve regurgitation or stenosis. In these patients, a balance must be struck between the risks of concurrent valve surgery and the anticipated rate of disease progression if the valve were left untreated as well as the likelihood and implications of future reoperation. Untreated disease may progress such that the patient requires future reoperation at higher risk. Another important consideration is whether the valve is repairable or if it requires replacement. The threshold for intervention may be lower in patients with repairable valves, but when a valve with moderate dysfunction is irreparable, decisions regarding valve replacement should be taken seriously. A moderately diseased native valve is replaced by a prosthetic valve, which is at risk of prosthesis-related disease. Age also plays a role; younger patients are generally treated more aggressively, and moderate lesions are often ignored in elderly patients.

AORTIC STENOSIS IN CORONARY ARTERY BYPASS GRAFTING PATIENTS

AS is the most frequently diagnosed incidental valve disease. Elderly patients undergoing CABG frequently have coexisting mild to moderate AS. Review of the literature shows that the AS gradient progresses at a rate of 5 to 10 mm Hg/year, and that the valve area decreases by about 0.1 cm²/year.[40] Therefore, young patients and older patients who have a life expectancy of more than 5 years should be offered concurrent AVR for moderate stenosis because future symptomatic AS is likely. Concurrent valve replacement in this setting does not substantially increase mortality rate, but reoperative surgery for AVR in the presence of patent coronary grafts has traditionally carried significant risk. These factors have led to upgrading AVR for moderate AS in patients undergoing CABG to a class I, level of evidence B recommendation in the most recent revascularization guidelines.[110] The presence of significant valve calcification or severely restricted leaflet motion on echocardiography also is an indicator of aggressive disease, and AVR in this setting may be reasonable even in patients with mild AS (gradient <25 mm Hg).[10]

MITRAL REGURGITATION IN CORONARY ARTERY BYPASS GRAFTING PATIENTS

Although unsuspected degenerative or rheumatic MR can occasionally be seen in patients undergoing CABG, in the vast majority of patients with MR at the time of surgery, the underlying etiology is ischemic. Our understanding of ischemic MR has dramatically improved over the past decade. The mechanism is complex but fundamentally results from displacement of the papillary muscles that results in leaflet tethering and restricted leaflet motion (type IIIB dysfunction).

Severe ischemic MR has always been considered a class I indication for concomitant MV surgery.[10] The management of moderate ischemic MR, however, has been more controversial. Data from the early 1990s suggested that moderate ischemic MR could be ignored at the time of CABG,[111] whereas more recent data overwhelmingly support concomitant valve repair for moderate (3+) ischemic MR in most patients. Aklog et al have shown that CABG alone does not reliably correct moderate MR, and 90% of patients are left with 2+ or greater MR (Figure 46-12, A).[112] This and other studies have also documented marked intraoperative downgrading of ischemic MR. The decision to intervene should therefore be based on a preoperative transthoracic echo. Aklog et al have also shown that concomitant mitral annuloplasty can be performed with an operative risk of less than 4%.[113] Patients with 2 to 3+ MR are particularly challenging, especially if they are elderly and have comorbidities that increase the risk of concomitant MV surgery. Considering factors that indicate the ischemic MR is chronic and physiologically significant—such as ventricular dysfunction, AF, and left atrial dilatation—intraoperative provocative testing is important and may be useful in equivocal cases (see Figure 46-12, B).[114] The optimal operation for ischemic MR is unclear.[115] A randomized trial sponsored by the National

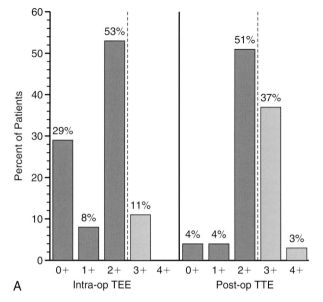

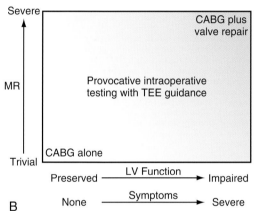

FIGURE 46-12 Ischemic mitral regurgitation (*MR*) at the time of coronary artery bypass graft (*CABG*). **A,** Data showing that CABG alone does not correct moderate ischemic MR, and intraoperative transesophageal echocardiography (*TEE*) downgrades ischemic MR. All patients had 3+ preoperative MR and underwent CABG alone.[112] **B,** Decision making in ischemic MR at the time of CABG.[114] LV, left ventricle; TTE, transthoracic echocardiography.

Institutes of Health (NIH) is currently underway to compare MV repair, usually annuloplasty, with MV replacement for ischemic MR.

Atrial Fibrillation

Surgical treatment of AF is based on the Maze operation, which was developed by Cox in the 1980s.[116] The operation is reported to be effective in curing AF in 80% to 90% of patients; it involves making encircling incisions around the venous atrial inflows to stop the propagation of abnormal atrial impulses, which usually originate around these veins (see Chapter 20). The classic Maze procedure, however, involved making a complex network of atrial incisions, which prolonged the operation and were associated with increased morbidity. For this reason, the Maze operation, despite its effectiveness, was not widely adopted by surgeons.

A recent resurgence of interest in AF surgery has occurred because of the availability of technology that allows surgeons to easily perform ablation around the pulmonary veins without the added complexity and morbidity associated with the original "cut and sew" operation. With several commercially available devices and energy sources—such as radiofrequency, cryotherapy, laser, microwave, and ultrasound—the surgeon can create transmural lesions in the atria without making surgical incisions. These transmural lesions have been shown to be as effective as the original cut-and-sew lesions. Although the focus is primarily on pulmonary vein isolation, the surgeon can also create additional left and right atrial lesions to mimic a complete Maze operation, which may improve the efficacy compared with pulmonary vein isolation alone. Using the commercially available probes and clamps, ablation for AF can be undertaken epicardially, before the surgeon commences cardiopulmonary bypass, or endocardially, with the atrium open for the mitral repair. Modern devices are relatively simple to apply, do not require much specialized surgical skill, and do not unduly prolong the operation. Concurrent AF surgery is now the standard of care for patients undergoing heart valve surgery who have a prior history of AF, and the left atrial appendage is often excised or oversewn at the time of MV surgery.

REFERENCES

1. Gott VL, Alejo DE, Cameron DE. Mechanical heart valves: 50 years of evolution. *Ann Thorac Surg* 2003;76(6):S2230-S2239.
2. Edmunds LH Jr. Evolution of prosthetic heart valves. *Am Heart J* 2001;141(5):849-855.
3. Starr A, Edwards ML. Mitral replacement: clinical experience with a ball-valve prosthesis. *Ann Surg* 1961;154:726-740.
4. Carpentier A. Cardiac valve surgery—the "French correction." *J Thorac Cardiovasc Surg* 1983;86:323-337.
5. Carpentier A, Deloche A, Dauptain J, et al. A new reconstructive operation for correction of mitral and tricuspid insufficiency. *J Thorac Cardiovasc Surg* 1971;61:1-13.
6. Cribier A, Eltchaninoff H, Bash A, et al. Percutaneous transcatheter implantation of an aortic valve prosthesis for calcific aortic stenosis. *Circulation* 2002;106:3006-3008.
7. Leon MB, Smith CR, Mack M, et al. Transcatheter aortic valve implantation for aortic stenosis in patients who cannot undergo surgery. *N Engl J Med* 2010;363:1597-1607.
8. Cardiac Surgery Database Executive Summary: 10 Years. STS report period ending 12/31/2010. Accessed at www.sts.org.
9. Gammie JS, Sheng S, Griffith BP, et al. Trends in mitral valve surgery in the United States: results from the Society of Thoracic Surgeons adult cardiac database. *Ann Thorac Surg* 2009;87:1431-1439.
10. Bonow RO, Carabello BA, Chatterjee K, et al. 2008 Focused update incorporated into the ACC/AHA 2006 guidelines for the management of patients with valvular heart disease: a report of the American College of Cardiology/American Heart Association Task Force on Practice Guidelines. *Circulation* 2008;118:e523-e661.
11. Omran H, Schmidt H, Hackenbroch M, et al. Silent and apparent cerebral embolism after retrograde catheterisation of the aortic valve in valvular stenosis: a prospective, randomised study. *Lancet* 2003;361:1241-1246.
12. Salzberg SP, Filsoufi F, Anyanwu A, et al. High-risk mitral valve surgery: perioperative hemodynamic optimization with nesiritide (BNP). *Ann Thorac Surg* 2005;80:502-506.
13. Aris A, Camara ML, Montiel J, et al. Ministernotomy versus median sternotomy for aortic valve replacement: a prospective, randomized study. *Ann Thorac Surg* 1999;67:1583-1587.
14. Bonacchi M, Prifti E, Giunti G, et al. Does ministernotomy improve postoperative outcome in aortic valve operation? A prospective randomized study. *Ann Thorac Surg* 2002;73:460-465.
15. Dogan S, Dzemali O, Wimmer-Greinecker G, et al. Minimally invasive versus conventional aortic valve replacement: a prospective randomized trial. *J Heart Valve Dis* 2003;12:76-80.
16. Sharony R, Grossi EA, Saunders PC, et al. Propensity score analysis of a six-year experience with minimally invasive isolated aortic valve replacement. *J Heart Valve Dis* 2004;13:887-893.
17. Nifong LW, Chitwood WR, Pappas PS, et al. Robotic mitral valve surgery: a United States multicenter trial. *J Thorac Cardiovasc Surg* 2005;129:1395-1404.
18. Casselman FP, Van Slycke S, Wellens F, et al. Mitral valve surgery can now routinely be performed endoscopically. *Circulation* 2003;108(Suppl 1):II48-II54.
19. Kaempchen S, Guenther T, Toschke M, et al. Assessing the benefit of biological valve prostheses: cumulative incidence (actual) vs. Kaplan-Meier (actuarial) analysis. *Eur J Cardiothorac Surg* 2003;23:710-713; discussion 713-714.
20. Grunkemeier GL, Anderson RP, Miller DC, et al. Time-related analysis of nonfatal heart valve complications: cumulative incidence (actual) versus Kaplan-Meier (actuarial). *Circulation* 1997;96(9 Suppl):II70-II74; discussion II74-II75.
21. Grunkemeier GL, Wu Y. "Our complication rates are lower than theirs": statistical critique of heart valve comparisons. *J Thorac Cardiovasc Surg* 2003;125:290-300.
22. Attila V, Heikkinen J, Biancari F, et al. A retrospective comparative study of aortic valve replacement with St. Jude medical and Medtronic Hall prostheses: a 20-year follow-up study. *Scand Cardiovasc J* 2002;36:53-59.
23. Masters RG, Helou J, Pipe AL, et al. Comparative clinical outcomes with St. Jude Medical, Medtronic Hall and CarboMedics mechanical heart valves. *J Heart Valve Dis* 2001;10:403-409.
24. Fiore AC, Barner HB, Swartz MT, et al. Mitral valve replacement: randomized trial of St. Jude and Medtronic Hall prostheses. *Ann Thorac Surg* 1998;66:707-712; discussion 712-713.
25. Borger MA, Carson SM, Ivanov J, et al. Stentless aortic valves are hemodynamically superior to stented valves during mid-term follow-up: a large retrospective study. *Ann Thorac Surg* 2005;80:2180-2185.

26. Walther T, Falk V, Langebartels G, et al. Regression of left ventricular hypertrophy after stentless versus conventional aortic valve replacement. *Semin Thorac Cardiovasc Surg* 1999;11:18-21.

27. O'Brien MF, Harrocks S, Stafford EG, et al. The homograft aortic valve: a 29-year, 99.3% follow up of 1022 valve replacements. *J Heart Valve Dis* 2001;10:334-344; discussion 335.

28. Ali M, Iung B, Lansac E, et al. Homograft replacement of the mitral valve: eight-year results. *J Thorac Cardiovasc Surg* 2004;128:529-534.

29. McKeown PP, Gutterman D. Executive summary: American College of Chest Physicians guidelines for the prevention and management of postoperative atrial fibrillation after cardiac surgery. *Chest* 2005;128(2 Suppl):1S-5S.

30. Hogue CW Jr, Creswell LL, Gutterman DD, et al. Epidemiology, mechanisms, and risks: American College of Chest Physicians guidelines for the prevention and management of postoperative atrial fibrillation after cardiac surgery. *Chest* 2005;128(2 Suppl): 9S-16S.

31. Podgoreanu MV, Mathew JP. Prophylaxis against postoperative atrial fibrillation: current progress and future directions. *JAMA* 2005;294:3140-3142.

32. Onalan O, Lashevsky I, Crystal E. Prophylaxis and management of postoperative atrial fibrillation. *Curr Cardiol Rep* 2005;7:382-390.

33. Sundt TM, Zehr KJ, Dearani JA, et al. Is early anticoagulation with warfarin necessary after bioprosthetic aortic valve replacement? *J Thorac Cardiovasc Surg* 2005;129: 1024-1031.

34. di Marco F, Meneghetti G, Gerosa G. Early anticoagulation after aortic valve replacement with bioprostheses: time to abandon it? *J Thorac Cardiovasc Surg* 2005;130: 1482-1483.

35. Moinuddeen K, Quin J, Shaw R, et al. Anticoagulation is unnecessary after biological aortic valve replacement. *Circulation* 1998;98(19 Suppl):II95-II98; discussion II98-II99.

36. Gherli T, Colli A, Nicolini F. Incidence of anticoagulation in patients with bioprostheses. *J Heart Valve Dis* 2004;13(Suppl 1):S88-S89.

37. Bridges CR, Edwards FH, Peterson ED, et al. Cardiac surgery in nonagenarians and centenarians. *J Am Coll Surg* 2003;197:347-356.

38. Pereira JJ, Balaban K, Lauer MS, et al. Aortic valve replacement in patients with mild or moderate aortic stenosis and coronary bypass surgery. *Am J Med* 2005;118: 735-742.

39. Smith WT, Ferguson TB Jr, Ryan T, et al. Should coronary artery bypass graft surgery patients with mild or moderate aortic stenosis undergo concomitant aortic valve replacement? A decision analysis approach to the surgical dilemma. *J Am Coll Cardiol* 2004;44:1241-1247.

40. Filsoufi F, Aklog L, Adams DH, et al. Management of mild to moderate aortic stenosis at the time of coronary artery bypass grafting. *J Heart Valve Dis* 2002;11(Suppl 1): S45-S49.

41. Levy F, Laurent M, Monin JL, et al. Aortic valve replacement for low-flow/low-gradient aortic stenosis: operative risk stratification and long-term outcome—a European multicenter study. *J Am Coll Cardiol* 2008;51:1466-1472.

42. Bach DS, Cartier PC, Kon ND, et al. Impact of implant technique following freestyle stentless aortic valve replacement. *Ann Thorac Surg* 2002;74:1107-1113; discussion 1112-1113.

43. Eriksson MJ, Brodin LA, Dellgren GN, et al. Rest and exercise hemodynamics of an extended stentless aortic bioprosthesis. *J Heart Valve Dis* 1997;6:653-660.

44. Bach DS, Kon ND, Dumesnil JG, et al. Ten-year outcome after aortic valve replacement with the freestyle stentless bioprosthesis. *Ann Thorac Surg* 2005;80:480-486; discussion 486-487.

45. Jin XY, Zhang ZM, Gibson DG, et al. Effects of valve substitute on changes in left ventricular function and hypertrophy after aortic valve replacement. *Ann Thorac Surg* 1996;62:683-690.

46. Walther T, Falk V, Langebartels G, et al. Prospectively randomized evaluation of stentless versus conventional biological aortic valves: impact on early regression of left ventricular hypertrophy. *Circulation* 1999;100(19 Suppl):II6-II10.

47. Westaby S, Horton M, Jin XY, et al. Survival advantage of stentless aortic bioprostheses. *Ann Thorac Surg* 2000;70:785-790; discussion 781-790.

48. D'Onofrio A, Cresce GD, Bolgan I, et al. Clinical and hemodynamic outcomes after aortic valve replacement with stented and stentless pericardial xenografts: a propensity-matched analysis. *J Heart Valve Dis* 2011;20:319-326.

49. Dellgren G, Feindel CM, Bos J, et al. Aortic valve replacement with the Toronto SPV: long-term clinical and hemodynamic results. *Eur J Cardiothorac Surg* 2002;21:698-702.

50. Knott-Craig CJ, Elkins RC, Santangelo KL, et al. Aortic valve replacement: comparison of late survival between autografts and homografts. *Ann Thorac Surg* 2000;69: 1327-1332.

51. Stelzer P, Weinrauch S, Tranbaugh RF. Ten years of experience with the modified Ross procedure. *J Thorac Cardiovasc Surg* 1998;115:1091-1100.

52. Pibarot P, Dumesnil JG. Prosthesis-patient mismatch: definition, clinical impact, and prevention. *Heart* 2005;92:1022-1029.

53. Hanayama N, Christakis GT, Mallidi HR, et al. Determinants of incomplete left ventricular mass regression following aortic valve replacement for aortic stenosis. *J Card Surg* 2005;20:307-313.

54. Blackstone EH, Cosgrove DM, Jamieson WR, et al. Prosthesis size and long-term survival after aortic valve replacement. *J Thorac Cardiovasc Surg* 2003;126:783-796.

55. Howell NJ, Keogh B, Ray D, et al. Patient-prosthesis mismatch in patients with aortic stenosis undergoing isolated aortic valve replacement does not affect survival. *Ann Thorac Surg* 2010;89:60-64.

56. Rao V, Jamieson WR, Ivanov J, et al. Prosthesis-patient mismatch affects survival after aortic valve replacement. *Circulation* 2000;102(19 Suppl 3):III5-III9.

57. Garatti A, Mori F, Innocente F, et al. Aortic valve replacement with 17 mm mechanical prostheses: is patient-prosthesis mismatch a relevant phenomenon? *Ann Thorac Surg* 2011;91:71-78.

58. LaPar DJ, Ailawadi G, Bhamidipati CM, et al. Small prosthesis size in aortic valve replacement does not affect mortality. *Ann Thorac Surg* 2011;92:880-888.

59. Minakata K, Schaff HV, Zehr KJ, et al. Is repair of aortic valve regurgitation a safe alternative to valve replacement? *J Thorac Cardiovasc Surg* 2004;127:645-653.

60. Casselman FP, Gillinov AM, Akhrass R, et al. Intermediate-term durability of bicuspid aortic valve repair for prolapsing leaflet. *Eur J Cardiothorac Surg* 1999;15:302-308.

61. Alsoufi B, Borger MA, Armstrong S, et al. Results of valve preservation and repair for bicuspid aortic valve insufficiency. *J Heart Valve Dis* 2005;14:752-758; discussion 758-759.

62. Leyh RG, Schmidtke C, Sievers HH, et al. Opening and closing characteristics of the aortic valve after different types of valve-preserving surgery. *Circulation* 1999; 100:2153-2160.

63. Sarsam MA, Yacoub M. Remodeling of the aortic valve annulus. *J Thorac Cardiovasc Surg* 1993;105:435-438.

64. David TE, Ivanov J, Armstrong S, et al. Aortic valve-sparing operations in patients with aneurysms of the aortic root or ascending aorta. *Ann Thorac Surg* 2002;74:S1758-S1761; discussion S1792-S1799.

65. David TE. Aortic valve-sparing operations for aortic root aneurysm. *Semin Thorac Cardiovasc Surg* 2001;13:291-296.

66. Chiappini B, Camurri N, Loforte A, et al. Outcome after aortic valve replacement in octogenarians. *Ann Thorac Surg* 2004;78:85-89.

67. Sundt TM, Bailey MS, Moon MR, et al. Quality of life after aortic valve replacement at the age of > 80 years. *Circulation* 2000;102(19 Suppl 3):III70-III74.

68. Vaquette B, Corbineau H, Laurent M, et al. Valve replacement in patients with critical aortic stenosis and depressed left ventricular function: predictors of operative risk, left ventricular function recovery, and long-term outcome. *Heart* 2005;91: 1324-1329.

69. Sharony R, Grossi EA, Saunders PC, et al. Aortic valve replacement in patients with impaired ventricular function. *Ann Thorac Surg* 2003;75:1808-1814.

70. Brown JM, O'Brien SM, Wu C, et al. Isolated aortic valve replacement in North America comprising 108,687 patients in 10 years: changes in risks, valve types, and outcomes in the Society of Thoracic Surgeons National Database. *J Thorac Cardiovasc Surg* 2009;137:82-90.

71. Elahi MM, Osman KA, Bhandari M, et al. Does the type of prosthesis influence the incidence of permanent pacemaker implantation following isolated aortic valve replacement? *Heart Surg Forum* 2005;8:E396-E400.

72. Cohen G, David TE, Ivanov J, et al. The impact of age, coronary artery disease, and cardiac comorbidity on late survival after bioprosthetic aortic valve replacement. *J Thorac Cardiovasc Surg* 1999;117:273-284.

73. Ashikkmina EA, Schaff HV, Dearani JA, et al. Aortic valve replacement in the elderly: determinants of late outcome. *Circulation* 2011;124:1070-1078.

74. Banbury MK, Cosgrove DM III, White JA, et al. Age and valve size effect on the long-term durability of the Carpentier-Edwards aortic pericardial bioprosthesis. *Ann Thorac Surg* 2001;72:753-757.

75. McClure RS, Narayanasamy N, Wiegerinck BA, et al. Late outcomes for aortic valve replacement with the Carpentier-Edwards pericardial prosthesis: up to 17-year follow-up in 1,000 patients. *Ann Thorac Surg* 2010;89:1410-1416.

76. Enriquez-Sarano M, Avierinos JF, Messika-Zeitoun D, et al. Quantitative determinants of the outcome of asymptomatic mitral regurgitation. *N Engl J Med* 2005;352: 875-883.

77. Bolling SF. Mitral reconstruction in cardiomyopathy. *J Heart Valve Dis* 2002;11(Suppl 1):S26-S31.

78. Wu AH, Aaronson KD, Bolling SF, et al. Impact of mitral valve annuloplasty on mortality risk in patients with mitral regurgitation and left ventricular systolic dysfunction. *J Am Coll Cardiol* 2005;45:381-387.

79. Alfieri O, Maisano F, De Bonis M, et al. The double-orifice technique in mitral valve repair: a simple solution for complex problems. *J Thorac Cardiovasc Surg* 2001;122: 674-681.

80. Maisano F, Caldarola A, Blasio A, et al. Midterm results of edge-to-edge mitral valve repair without annuloplasty. *J Thorac Cardiovasc Surg* 2003;126:1987-1997.

81. Bhudia SK, McCarthy PM, Smedira NG, et al. Edge-to-edge (Alfieri) mitral repair: results in diverse clinical settings. *Ann Thorac Surg* 2004;77:1598-1606.

82. Franzen O, van der Heyden J, Baldus S et al. MitraClip therapy in patients with end-stage systolic heart failure. *Eur J Heart Fail* 2011;13:569-576.

83. Nowicki ER, Birkmeyer NJ, Weintraub RW, et al. Multivariable prediction of in-hospital mortality associated with aortic and mitral valve surgery in Northern New England. *Ann Thorac Surg* 2004;77:1966-1977.

84. Enriquez-Sarano M, Schaff HV, Orszulak TA, et al. Valve repair improves the outcome of surgery for mitral regurgitation: a multivariate analysis. *Circulation* 1995;91: 1022-1028.

85. Meimoun P, Zeghdi R, D'Attelis N, et al. Frequency, predictors, and consequences of atrioventricular block after mitral valve repair. *Am J Cardiol* 2002;89:1062-1066.

86. Moss RR, Humphries KH, Gao M, et al. Outcome of mitral valve repair or replacement: a comparison by propensity score analysis. *Circulation* 2003;108(Suppl 1): II90-II97.

87. Braunberger E, Deloche A, Berrebi A, et al. Very long-term results (more than 20 years) of valve repair with Carpentier's techniques in nonrheumatic mitral valve insufficiency. *Circulation* 2001;104(Suppl 1):I8-I11.

88. Chauvaud S, Fuzellier JF, Berrebi A, et al. Long-term (29 years) results of reconstructive surgery in rheumatic mitral valve insufficiency. *Circulation* 2001;104(12 Suppl 1): I12-I15.

89. Marchand MA, Aupart MR, Norton R, et al. Fifteen-year experience with the mitral Carpentier-Edwards PERIMOUNT pericardial bioprosthesis. *Ann Thorac Surg* 2001;71(5 Suppl):S236-S239.

90. Eric Jamieson WR, Marchand MA, Pelletier CL, et al. Structural valve deterioration in mitral replacement surgery: comparison of Carpentier-Edwards supra-annular porcine and perimount pericardial bioprostheses. *J Thorac Cardiovasc Surg* 1999;118: 297-304.

91. Jamieson WR, Riess FC, Raudkivi PJ, et al. Medtronic mosaic porcine bioprosthesis: assessment of 12-year performance. *J Thorac Cardiovasc Surg* 2011;142:302-307.

92. Ruel M, Chan V, Bédard P et al. Very long-term survival implications of heart valve replacement with tissue versus mechanical prosthesis in adults < 60 years of age. *Circulation* 2007;116(11 Suppl):I294-I300.

93. McCarthy PM, Bhudia SK, Rajeswaran J, et al. Tricuspid valve repair: durability and risk factors for failure. *J Thorac Cardiovasc Surg* 2004;127:674-685.

94. Dreyfus GD, Corbi PJ, Chan KM, et al. Secondary tricuspid regurgitation or dilatation: which should be the criteria for surgical repair? *Ann Thorac Surg* 2005;79:127-132.

95. Yilmaz O, Suri RM, Dearani JA, et al. Functional tricuspid regurgitation at the time of mitral valve repair for degenerative leaflet prolapse: the case for a selective approach. *J Thorac Cardiovasc Surg* 2011;142:608-613.

96. Rizzoli G, Vendramin I, Nesseris G, et al. Biological or mechanical prostheses in tricuspid position? A meta-analysis of intra-institutional results. *Ann Thorac Surg* 2004;77:1607-1614.

97. Kaplan M, Kut MS, Demirtas MM, et al. Prosthetic replacement of tricuspid valve: bioprosthetic or mechanical. *Ann Thorac Surg* 2002;73:467-473.

98. Filsoufi F, Anyanwu AC, Salzberg S, et al. Long-term outcomes of tricuspid valve replacement in the current era. *Ann Thorac Surg* 2005;80:845-850.

99. Moraca RJ, Moon MR, Lawton JS, et al. Outcomes of tricuspid valve repair and replacement: a propensity analysis. *Ann Thorac Surg* 2009;87:83-89.

100. Gold JP. When should tricuspid valve replacement/repair accompany mitral valve surgery? *Adv Cardiol* 2004;41:133-139.

101. Matsunaga A, Duran CM. Progression of tricuspid regurgitation after repaired functional ischemic mitral regurgitation. *Circulation* 2005;112(9 Suppl):I453-I457.

102. Kirali K, Omeroglu SN, Uzun K, et al. Evolution of repaired and non-repaired tricuspid regurgitation in rheumatic mitral valve surgery without severe pulmonary hypertension. *Asian Cardiovasc Thorac Ann* 2004;12:239-245.

103. Absil B, Dagenais F, Mathieu P, et al. Does moderate mitral regurgitation impact early or mid-term clinical outcome in patients undergoing isolated aortic valve replacement for aortic stenosis? *Eur J Cardiothorac Surg* 2003;24:217-222; discussion 222.

104. Barreiro CJ, Patel ND, Fitton TP, et al. Aortic valve replacement and concomitant mitral valve regurgitation in the elderly: impact on survival and functional outcome. *Circulation* 2005;112(9 Suppl):I443-I447.

105. Tassan-Mangina S, Metz D, Nazeyllas P, et al. Factors determining early improvement in mitral regurgitation after aortic valve replacement for aortic valve stenosis: a transthoracic and transesophageal prospective study. *Clin Cardiol* 2003;26:127-131.

106. Gillinov AM, Blackstone EH, Cosgrove DM III, et al. Mitral valve repair with aortic valve replacement is superior to double valve replacement. *J Thorac Cardiovasc Surg* 2003;125:1372-1387.

107. Habib G, Avierinos JF, Thuny F. Aortic valve endocarditis: is there an optimal surgical timing? *Curr Opin Cardiol* 2007;22:77-83.

108. Byrne JG, Rezai K, Sanchez JA, et al. Surgical management of endocarditis: the Society of Thoracic Surgeons clinical practice guideline. *Ann Thorac Surg* 2011;91:2012-2019.

109. Jones EL, Weintraub WS, Craver JM, et al. Interaction of age and coronary disease after valve replacement: implications for valve selection. *Ann Thorac Surg* 1994;58:378-384; discussion 384-385.

110. Hillis LD, Smith PK, Anderson JL, et al. 2011 ACCF/AHA guideline for coronary artery bypass graft surgery: executive summary. A report of the American College of Cardiology Foundation/American Heart Association Task Force on Practice Guidelines. *Circulation* 2011;124:2610-2642.

111. Duarte IG, Shen Y, MacDonald MJ, et al. Treatment of moderate mitral regurgitation and coronary disease by coronary bypass alone: late results. *Ann Thorac Surg* 1999;68:426-430.

112. Aklog L, Filsoufi F, Flores KQ, et al. Does coronary artery bypass grafting alone correct moderate ischemic mitral regurgitation? *Circulation* 2001;104(12 Suppl 1):I68-I75.

113. Filsoufi F, Aklog L, Byrne JG, et al. Current results of combined coronary artery bypass grafting and mitral annuloplasty in patients with moderate ischemic mitral regurgitation. *J Heart Valve Dis* 2004;13:747-753.

114. Byrne JG, Aklog L, Adams DH. Assessment and management of functional or ischaemic mitral regurgitation. *Lancet* 2000;355:1743-1744.

115. Magne J, Girerd N, Sénéchal M, et al. Mitral repair versus replacement for ischemic mitral regurgitation: comparison of short-term and long-term survival. *Circulation* 2009;120(Suppl 1):S104-S111.

116. Cox JL, Schuessler RB, Cain ME, et al. Surgery for atrial fibrillation. *Semin Thorac Cardiovasc Surg* 1989;1:67-73.

CH
46

SURGERY FOR VALVULAR HEART DISEASE

Percutaneous Treatment for Valvular Heart Disease

Steven R. Bailey

OVERVIEW, 714

PERCUTANEOUS AORTIC VALVE IMPLANTATION, 714

CURRENT PERCUTANEOUS AORTIC VALVES, 714

Edwards Sapien Valve, 714
Medtronic CoreValve Revalving System, 715

PATIENT EVALUATION AND IMAGING PRIOR TO
TRANSCATHETER AORTIC VALVE
IMPLANTATION, 715
Access Site Evaluation, 716
Measurement of Aortic Valve Annulus, 716

TRANSCATHETER AORTIC VALVE IMPLANTATION
PROCEDURE, 717

Patient Outcomes, 717
New Access Approaches, 719
New Applications, 719
Potential Complications, 719
Next-Generation Aortic Valve Therapy, 720

PERCUTANEOUS MITRAL VALVE THERAPY, 721

Approach to Leaflet Repair, 722
Chamber Remodeling, 724

Direct Annuloplasty, 724
Ventricular Remodeling, 725
Chordal Implantation, 725
Mitral Valve Replacement, 725

SUMMARY, 726

REFERENCES, 726

Overview

Every year, tens of thousands of patients come to medical attention with either symptomatic valvular heart disease or evidence of progressive myocardial dysfunction related to underlying valvular dysfunction.[1] Aortic stenosis is the most common valve pathology in the elderly and is present in 1% to 2% of individuals older than 65 years and more than 4% in those older than 85 years.[2] Patients today with aortic stenosis are typically not referred for surgical valve replacement until symptoms of angina, heart failure (HF), or syncope develop.[3] These symptoms, although long-trusted over time, often present late in the disease process, and all too often they occur in elderly patients with multiple comorbid medical conditions. Percutaneous aortic balloon valvuloplasty (PABV) was introduced in 1986 by Cribier and colleagues[4] as the initial percutaneous therapeutic option for high-risk or nonsurgical patients with multiple comorbidities.

Mitral valve (MV) disease, which used to commonly manifest as rheumatic mitral stenosis, is now more commonly the result of either degenerative valve disorders, such as myxomatous valves, or functional mitral regurgitation (MR) as a result of myocardial ischemia or myocardial dilation.[5] New percutaneous therapies have been developed that focus on direct treatments of the leaflet pathology, mitral annular reduction, or percutaneous valve replacement.

This chapter focuses on the new percutaneous technologies that have been developed to treat aortic and mitral valve disease in adults. Current results are assessed to determine the likely clinical role of percutaneous devices.

Percutaneous Aortic Valve Implantation

In the elderly, surgical aortic valve replacement (AVR) represents 60% to 70% of all valve surgery performed and as such is the most common heart valve operation performed in adults. Surgical AVR is associated with a perioperative mortality risk of approximately 3% to 4%, increasing to 5.5% to 6.8% when combined with coronary artery bypass grafting (CABG).[6-7] Unfortunately, a significant number of patients who might potentially benefit from AVR either are not referred or do not receive the procedure. One survey of 92 European heart centers found that 31.8% of patients with severe, symptomatic single-valve disease did not undergo intervention, most frequently because of comorbid conditions that placed the patient at high surgical risk.[8]

Although surgical AVR for aortic stenosis is the only procedure demonstrated to improve mortality rate, use of PABV has been demonstrated to improve short-term symptoms and to decrease morbidity. The risk of stroke is less than 0.5%, and moderate to severe aortic insufficiency is reported in less than 1% of patients undergoing PABV. The duration of benefits is unpredictable but is typically less than 1 year, and the need for repeat procedures has limited the number of patients who are candidates for this procedure. Based on these considerations, the American College of Cardiology (ACC)/American Heart Association (AHA) guidelines have rated this a class IIb indication.[9]

The introduction of coronary and endovascular stent technology sparked new interest in endovascular therapies with the demonstration that stents with sufficiently large final expanded diameters to treat the aorta could be delivered percutaneously. Andersen and colleagues[10] published their experience with a transluminal valve. These results gave rise to the emerging field of percutaneous heart valve replacement (PHVR) using catheter-based technology, with early work reported by Paniagua and colleagues[11] that allows for implantation of a prosthetic valve from transvascular (transfemoral or transaxillary) and transapical approaches.[12] Designed primarily to treat stenotic aortic valves, these technologies permit the implantation of a prosthetic heart valve, known as a *transcatheter aortic valve implant* (TAVI), within the diseased native aortic valve without the need for open heart surgery or cardiopulmonary bypass.[13]

Current Percutaneous Aortic Valves

Edwards Sapien Valve

The Edwards Sapien transcatheter heart valve (Edwards Lifesciences, Irvine, CA) was the first percutaneous valve system systematically implanted in a trial in humans.[14] It is a balloon-expandable system with a balloon-mounted bovine pericardial valve within a stainless steel stent (Figure 47-1) that is mechanically compressed onto the delivery balloon in the procedural suite. It is currently available in two valve diameters, 23 and 26 mm, delivered initially on catheters with diameters of 22 and 24 Fr, respectively. These valve diameters are suitable for implantation in aortic annulus diameters of 18 to 25 mm. Given their large diameter, these catheters currently require minimal vessel diameters of 7 and 8 mm, respectively, for the transfemoral approach. Recent modifications to the device with the introduction of a cobalt-chrome frame, which allows thinner struts, have reduced the delivery profile to 18 Fr. Modifications to the delivery system have also included a longer intravascular sheath to facilitate delivery of the device to the descending aorta; improved maneuverability in the ascending aorta;

and availability of larger valve diameters. This is expected to broaden the population of patients who can receive this therapy while improving the short-term outcomes and reducing complications.

Medtronic CoreValve Revalving System

The CoreValve (Medtronic, Minneapolis, MN) is a self-expanding nitinol frame containing a porcine pericardial valve that is sewn into the frame (Figure 47-2). The delivery catheter diameter has been reduced from the original diameter of 25 Fr to the current 18 Fr.[15] It is currently available in valve diameters of 26 and 29 mm to allow implantation in aortic valve annulus diameters of 20 to 24 mm and 24 to 27 mm, respectively. The smaller diameter of the delivery sheath allows transfemoral implantation in patients with an iliac artery diameter of 6 mm or more, allowing broader application in women. As operator experience has increased, the newer generation CoreValve PHV has demonstrated a lower rate of major adverse cardiac and cerebrovascular events and a higher rate of primary procedural success compared with earlier versions of the CoreValve.[16]

Patient Evaluation and Imaging Prior to Transcatheter Aortic Valve Implantation

TAVI is currently intended for implantation in patients with symptomatic severe calcific aortic stenosis that requires AVR who are at high risk for open chest surgery as a result of comorbid conditions and in those who are considered inoperable.

A new change in clinical practice is the development of multi-specialty teams to evaluate patients prior to TAVI procedures. This team typically includes a cardiologist, cardiothoracic and vascular surgeons, an imaging specialist, anesthesiologists, geriatricians, and physical therapy specialists. Figure 47-3 is a suggested algorithm for evaluation of patients being considered for TAVI.

In symptomatic patients, quantification of the severity of aortic stenosis still rests on echocardiographic Doppler techniques with

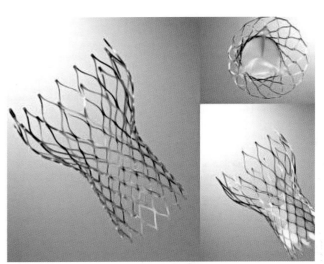

FIGURE 47-2 Medtronic (Minneapolis, MN) CoreValve Revalving System aortic bioprosthesis.

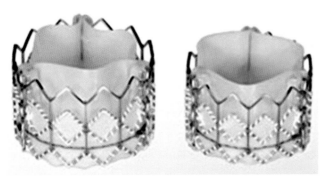

FIGURE 47-1 Edwards Sapien Percutaneous Heart Valve and Edwards Sapien Transcatheter Heart Valve (Edwards Lifesciences, Irvine, CA). This balloon-expandable cobalt-chrome frame contains a valve and is currently available in 23- and 26-mm sizes.

PERCUTANEOUS TREATMENT FOR VALVULAR HEART DISEASE

CH 47

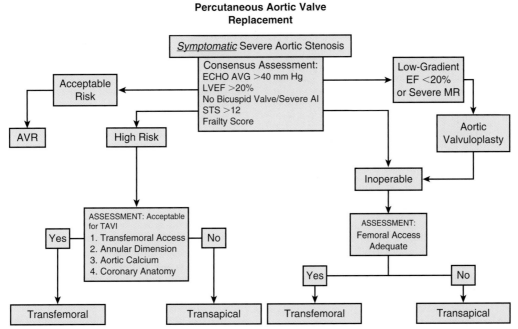

FIGURE 47-3 Evaluation of the patient with symptomatic aortic stenosis for transcatheter aortic valve insertion. AVG, aortic valve gradient; AVR, aortic valve replacement; ECHO, echocardiography; EF, ejection fraction; LVEF, left ventricular ejection fraction; MR, mitral regurgitation; STS, ST segment; TAVI, transcatheter aortic valve implementation.

the standard definitions of an aortic valve area (AVA) less than 1 cm^2 (<0.6 cm^2/m^2) or a mean gradient greater than 40 mm Hg. For TAVI, current studies[17-18] have required an AVA of less than 0.8 cm^2. The echocardiogram is also critically important for assessing the anatomy and morphology of the aortic valve. As an example, a bicuspid valve as assessed by echo is considered a contraindication for TAVI because of the possibility of more severe aortic insufficiency during the preparatory PABV and a higher probability of asymmetric prosthesis deployment.

Evaluation of left ventricular (LV) dimensions and function is a critical step in the preprocedural screening of candidates for TAVI. Intracardiac thrombus is a strong contraindication for a TAVI procedure. Apical myocardial infarction with apical wall thinning may contraindicate the transapical approach because it predisposes to LV tearing and pseudoaneurysm formation. Severe primary MR is also an exclusion criterion for TAVI. If there is concern regarding the contribution of critical aortic stenosis to the MR, the interventionist could perform aortic valvuloplasty and may subsequently reevaluate the severity of MR. In many patients, LV function may improve with diminished MR after valvuloplasty, and the patient may then be a candidate for TAVI. In addition, the strategy of TAVI alone may be appropriate in many patients in whom the risk of double-valve surgery may be prohibitive.[19]

Evaluation of a patient's surgical risk remains clinically challenging. Currently, a Society of Thoracic Surgeons (STS) risk score greater than 10 and a logistic EuroSCORE greater than 20[20-26] are most often used to define high risk. Unfortunately, these scores do not include important variables present in many patients being considered for TAVI that increase the risk of complications, such as small vessels,[27] plaque at the coronary ostia,[28] a porcelain aorta, cirrhosis, previous mediastinal radiation, prior sternotomies, history of mediastinitis, chest wall deformities, severely compromised respiratory function, and frailty.

The STS score has been shown to underestimate appreciably the true mortality rate after cardiac surgery, but it more closely reflects the operative and 30-day mortality rates for the highest risk patients undergoing AVR. The EuroSCORE overestimates the mortality risk of AVR,[20] with the greatest overestimation in high-risk patients.[21] Therefore, it is recommended that high-risk patients not be selected for TAVI based on the EuroSCORE alone because it has been shown to have insufficient discrimination and calibration.[22] It is likely that new scores specific to high-risk patients will be developed to better define patient outcomes from TAVI.

Clinical judgment remains the key in the patient selection process. TAVI is currently designed for high-risk patients in whom comorbidities would not interfere with recovery after the procedure. Patients who have decompensated HF and severely depressed LV function, have concomitant severe valvular lesions, and are bedridden or have an abbreviated life expectancy of less than 1 year should not undergo this procedure. Patients undergoing TAVI must be in stable condition before the procedure.

For patients whose clinical condition might be improved or stabilized, medical optimization, and possibly balloon valvuloplasty, should be undertaken to allow for improvement of their clinical status and ventricular function prior to consideration for TAVI. In addition, the coronary arterial anatomy should be evaluated by coronary angiography because the presence of significant coronary artery disease not amenable to percutaneous intervention may be a relative contraindication for TAVI.[28]

The hemodynamic results obtained with TAVI have been demonstrated to be comparable or better than those seen with surgical aortic valve implantation.[29]

Access Site Evaluation

Vascular access anatomy is one of the most important determinants of procedural success and potential complications. The larger 24-Fr sheaths used require minimum vessel diameters of 7 and 8 mm and even smaller, and 18-Fr sheaths require minimum vessel diameters of 6 mm. These vascular access concerns are modified by the presence of extensive calcification, bulky atheroma, and severe tortuosity, all of which can prevent the large sheath from advancing to the abdominal aorta.[30,31]

Several imaging modalities are currently used for specific evaluation of the access vessels and aorta: angiography, contrast-enhanced computed tomography (CT), and intravascular ultrasound (IVUS). Conventional abdominal aortography has been clinically useful for evaluation of the aorta and its branches and produces excellent images, but it often requires up to 150 mL (2 to 2.5 mL/kg) of contrast media.[32] Utilization of digital subtraction angiography often produces better images and requires a smaller amount of contrast (20 to 40 mL). Vessel diameters should be measured by quantitative coronary angiography and a reference marker such as a pigtail catheter.

A detailed CT analysis is very important because it can potentially indicate access problems that result from calcification or tortuosity. Calcification is often not well appreciated by angiography. The CT images are typically evaluated in axial, longitudinal, and three-dimensional views.[33,34] The noncontrast CT is often critical for quantifying the amount of calcification present and is typically best visualized in the longitudinal and axial views. Significant calcification, especially in long segments, does not allow the straightening of the arteries required for successful device delivery. Severe calcification in the distal aorta at the bifurcation of the internal and external iliac arteries is notable because it will not allow expansion or displacement. The presence on CT of severe calcification may result in a patient being rejected for transfemoral access; this is one of the most frequent reasons for selection of alternative access routes (axillary or transapical). CT images of the chest are also helpful to plan the transapical procedure, allowing for visualization of the relationship of the apex to the chest wall and for evaluating the angle of approach to the LV outflow tract.

When a discrepancy is present in the assessment by angiography and CT, IVUS is an excellent way to measure vessel lumen diameter. Unfortunately, this technology is poor for the definition and analysis of the extent of calcification.

Patients with extensive atherosclerosis of the aorta and those with porcelain aortas or large, mobile, protruding aortic atheromas are at high risk for a neurologic event during the procedure. Atherosclerotic debris can also be dislodged from the calcific aortic valve itself or from the peripheral vessels and is embolized to the brain, resulting in ischemic stroke.[35] Surveillance monitoring after TAVI has shown that the incidence of clinically silent periinterventional cerebral embolic lesions after TAVI is very high (up to 85%), but clinical significance is much lower, at approximately 3%.[36] Because of the risk of embolic lesions and events, embolic protection devices are currently under development, but whether they will lower the risk of stroke remains to be determined. Aortic aneurysms, if present, may not be problematic when advancing the delivery system, but their presence increases the risk of plaque or thrombus dislodgment and may therefore lead to procedural complications.

Measurement of Aortic Valve Annulus

The shape of the aortic valve annulus is oval rather than circular, with the coronal diameter larger than the sagittal diameter. Two-dimensional echocardiography is not the best approach because only one dimension of the aortic valve annulus can be measured, and it underestimates the annular size.[31] Because transesophageal echocardiography (TEE) underestimates the aortic valve annulus, magnetic resonance imaging (MRI) and CT have been shown to be more accurate than TEE to measure the aortic valve annulus, using perioperative measurements as the reference.[32] A recent study evaluated the aortic annulus with transthoracic echocardiography (TTE), TEE, and CT in 187 patients referred for

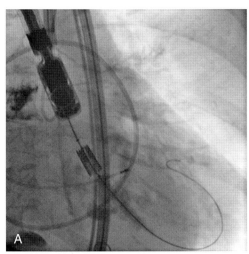
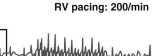
RV pacing: 200/min
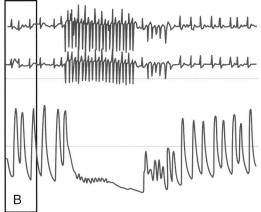

FIGURE 47-4 **A,** Demonstrated placement of an Edwards Sapien transcatheter aortic valve (Edwards Lifesciences, Irvine, CA) at the level of the aortic annulus. **B,** Rapid ventricular (*RV*) pacing.

TAVI, and strong correlation was found among the measurement techniques; however, differences up to 3 mm appeared in all measurement methods. Interobserver and intraobserver variability was better for TEE than for CT, and the TEE annulus measurement as a decisive parameter for TAVI was safe, with a low complication rate.[39]

Transcatheter Aortic Valve Implantation Procedure

The original Edwards Sapien TAVI implants with the percutaneous valve technology system were placed in an antegrade fashion that required transseptal puncture with passage of the Edwards Sapien Percutaneous Valve across the MV and the LV and implanting the prosthesis at the level of the annulus of the native the aortic valve.[40] Although effective, this technique led to complications that included acute MV regurgitation and ventricular perforation. Currently, seven delivery or implantation approaches have been used for TAVI implantation: 1) femoral vein, 2) femoral artery, 3) subclavian artery, 4) axillary artery, 5) common carotid artery, 6) ascending aorta, and 7) directly through the apex of the heart by thoracotomy incision (transapical).

The development of a simplified retrograde transaortic technique has been critical in the broader application of the TAVI systems and is the most frequently used technique.[41] With standard techniques for arterial cannulation and after baseline aortography, a 14-Fr access sheath placement and the use of preclosure techniques have contributed to a wider dissemination of this procedure. Crossing of the valve uses a 0.035-inch guidewire placed by a catheter used to cross the aortic valve, and baseline gradients are obtained. A 0.035-inch, 270-cm extra-stiff guidewire with an exaggerated loop at the distal tip is then advanced through the catheter in the LV. The exaggerated loop minimizes the risk of LV trauma or arrhythmia. With this very stiff wire, the aortic valve is predilated, typically with a 23-mm balloon; currently, rapid cardiac pacing is performed to prevent ejection of the balloon during inflation. After successful balloon valvuloplasty, the 14-Fr sheath is exchanged by using sequential dilation for the appropriate-sized sheath (18 to 24 Fr) to allow the valve delivery system to be advanced. With fluoroscopic landmarks and echo imaging, the valve is positioned across the aortic annulus. By using rapid right ventricular pacing, the valve is expanded with the balloon, or the constraining sheath is withdrawn (self-expanding) and adequate expansion is confirmed. Implantation of a Sapien valve and rapid ventricular pacing are illustrated in Figure 47-4. Repeat hemodynamic assessment is performed, and

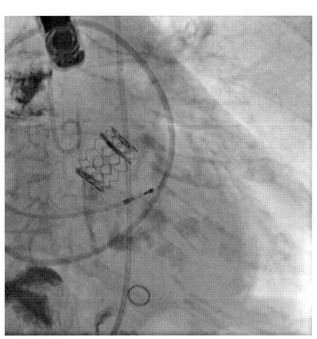

FIGURE 47-5 After implantation of a Sapien aortic valve (Edwards Lifesciences, Irvine, CA).

the aortogram is repeated to confirm adequate placement, image the coronary arteries, and grade the severity of any perivalvular leak. Figure 47-5 demonstrates an expanded Sapien valve in the aortic position. The CoreValve may be slightly repositioned prior to release if the placement is inadequate.

Patient Outcomes

If defined as technical success implanting the valve, procedural success rates have increased steadily, from 82% in the initial transvenous experience to more than 95% in more contemporary series. It appears that when patients are appropriately selected, TAVI is a procedure that can be reproducibly and reliably performed.[42] As previously cited, in a recent review of 2356 patients from more than 80 published reports of patients receiving the Edwards Lifesciences and Medtronic transthoracic heart valves (THVs),[12] survival at 30 days was reported to be 89% and was similar for both valves. As might be expected, survival continues

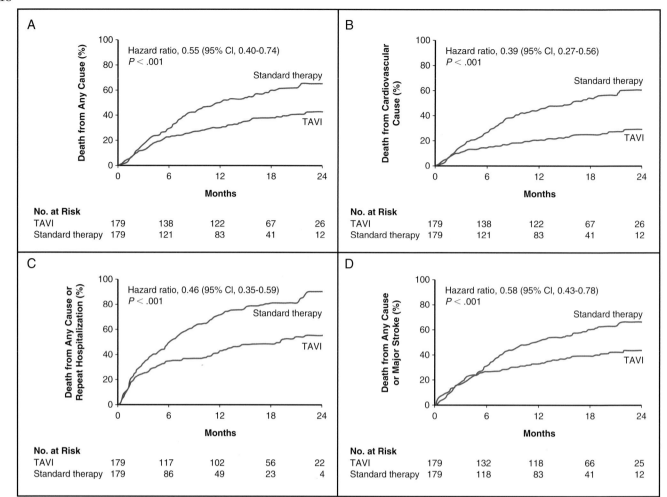

FIGURE 47-6 Time-to-event curves for the primary endpoint and other selected endpoints. Placement of Aortic Transcatheter Valves (PARTNER) Cohort B trial. CI, confidence interval; TAVI, transcatheter aortic valve implantation. *(From Leon MB, Smith CR, Mack M, et al. Transcatheter aortic-valve implantation for aortic stenosis in patients who cannot undergo surgery.* N Engl J Med *2010;363:1597-1607.)*

to improve, with contemporary reports documenting 30-day survival rates of 93% to 95%.[36] To date, the literature has consisted primarily of registries, with varying entry criteria, endpoints, and lengths of follow-up. Registries provide the opportunity to evaluate evolutions in technology and to generate hypotheses, but they lack the rigor of randomized trials to provide comparative outcomes.

We are now able to better understand patient outcomes after TAVI compared with medical management alone from the results of the Placement of Aortic Transcatheter Valves (PARTNER) Cohort B trial (Figure 47-6).[44] Patients were only randomized if they were declined as surgical candidates because of prohibitive risk based on a common set of criteria that required a consensus of more than two senior surgeons at multiple clinical sites. This investigation occurred at a time when large first-generation devices were used, and most operators were early in their experience with TAVI. Despite these disadvantages, the procedural teams achieved a very low 30-day mortality rate of 6.4%.

In the PARTNER 1B trial, the nonoperative patients (those who did not undergo TAVI) had a poor outlook, and only 50% survived 1 year. The most important finding in this trial was the remarkable 20% absolute improvement in survival at 1 year in the patients who underwent percutaneous TAVI with the Sapien valve. Notably, the survival curves continue to diverge at 1 year, which suggests a sustained benefit in the TAVI group.

A randomized evaluation of high-risk *operable* patients was recently published that compared conventional AVR surgery with

TAVI using the Sapien valve (Figure 47-7).[42] In this prospective trial at 25 centers, 699 high-risk patients (median age, 84.1 years) with critical aortic stenosis and a mean STS score of 11.8 (logistic EuroSCORE of 29.3; Table 47-1) were randomized to surgical AVR or TAVI with the Sapien valve. The patients were all greater than New York Hospital Association (NYHA) class II. The predicted operative mortality rate was independently determined by site surgeons and cardiologists, and patients included in the study had an estimated STS score of 10 or higher. In addition, the LV ejection fraction (LVEF) had to be greater than 20% without a bicuspid aortic valve or severe aortic insufficiency. At the end of 1 year, both groups had similar mortality rates (surgical AVR, 26.8% vs. TAVI, 24.2%). A second group of patients received transapical implantations; these patients demonstrated a trend toward worse outcomes, compared with surgical AVR, at 30 days and 1 year, which does raise some concern over procedural events with transapical implantation. One of the greatest concerns has been the rate of procedural, as well as late, stroke. This may represent either procedural or technical issues, or it may reflect the complex patient population. Randomized evaluations in lower risk operable patients with the CoreValve and Sapien XT devices began enrollments in the United States in 2011.

Late survival rates in the high-risk patient populations at 1 year have been reported to range from 69% to 85%, which likely primarily reflects the underlying comorbidities in the very ill patients undergoing TAVI rather than aortic valve performance. Investigations of multiple factors have demonstrated that the logistic

EuroSCORE, STS score, age, liver disease, severe MR, anemia, prior stroke, pulmonary disease, and renal failure are all predictors of late death following TAVI.

In this ill population, improvement in functional class, rather than decreased mortality rate, may be a more important clinical endpoint. Decreased symptoms and sustained improvements in exercise tolerance have been reported in most published series. Typically, NYHA class improves from class III to IV at baseline to class I to II late after TAVI.[46] It remains unclear which elderly patients with comorbidities will derive significant symptomatic and clinical benefit from TAVI. As noted in the section on patient selection, these critical issues require multidisciplinary assessment of these complex patients.

New Access Approaches

The transapical approach still plays an important role in this patient population. The patients who undergo transapical TAVI typically have more comorbidities, more difficult vascular access, and smaller aortic annular dimensions.[47] This approach may have unique complications, including aneurysm formation at the site of the apical access, device embolization, and paravalvular leak.[48]

New Applications

Early experience is now accumulating with valve-in-valve implantation, or a percutaneous valve within a degenerated surgical bioprosthesis, with both the Sapien and CoreValve devices. In contrast to degenerative native aortic stenosis, the surgical valve facilitates positioning and paravalvular sealing and may protect the atrioventricular conduction system and the left main ostium.[49] Unfortunately, not all surgical valves are appropriate for valve-in-valve implantation. They may compromise coronary ostia,[50,51] be difficult to image, or simply be too small for a valve-in-valve implant. For instance, one widely used 21-mm surgical tissue valve has an internal diameter of 17 mm, meaning that even the smallest THV currently available will be underexpanded, resulting in moderate stenosis.

Hypothetically, an inadequate TAVI, like a percutaneous coronary stent, may allow repeat valve-in-valve implantation. Although repeat implantation has been demonstrated acutely, significant experience is lacking with repetitive TAVI implantation.

Potential Complications

Concern over the incidence of embolic stroke has risen as TAVI has expanded into clinical practice. When comparing the first generation of Sapien TAVI systems, the Sapien Aortic Bioprosthesis European Outcome (SOURCE) registry (with self-reported and nonadjudicated events) reported a stroke rate of 2.4%, whereas the more rigorously monitored PARTNER B trial reported a major stroke rate of 5.0%. Stroke rates in the literature have varied widely, and the reported incidence has been 0% to 10% with TAVI. Procedural stroke is often due to embolization of the friable material found in the diseased aorta or aortic valve, as demonstrated by transcranial Doppler. New cerebral lesions, as assessed by diffusion-weighted MRI, have been reported in 58% to 91% of patients undergoing TAVI, although these findings do not appear to correlate with clinical neurologic deficits. Experimental approaches to mitigation include catheters and filters. The risk of procedural stroke seems to be falling with smaller and less traumatic catheters, improved technique, and lower risk patients. However, not all strokes are atheroembolic. Possible additional factors include valve thrombosis, atrial fibrillation, institution of anticoagulation that leads to hemorrhagic stroke, or discontinuation of anticoagulation. In the absence of data, the standard approach to prevention of valve thromboembolism has been long-term aspirin and 1 to 3 months of clopidogrel or, in the presence of additional risk factors such as atrial fibrillation, warfarin or dabigatran.

Placing the open cells of a THV over a coronary ostium appears to be generally well tolerated, at least acutely. However, coronary obstruction may rarely occur as a consequence of THV displacement of the native valve leaflet over the left main ostium. Successful management may require temporary cardiopulmonary support and percutaneous or surgical revascularization. Risk factors for left main occlusion include a low origin of the coronary ostium, a shallow sinus of Valsalva, a bulky native valve, and design characteristics of the prosthesis.[52] Concomitant coronary artery disease is common and negatively impacts both procedural

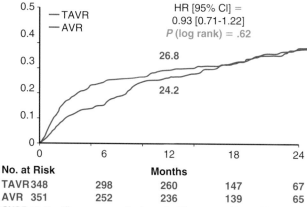

Primary Endpoint:
All-Cause Mortality at 1 Year

HR [95% CI] = 0.93 [0.71-1.22]
P (log rank) = .62

26.8
24.2

No. at Risk				
		Months		
TAVR 348	298	260	147	67
AVR 351	252	236	139	65

FIGURE 47-7 All-cause mortality from the Placement of Aortic Transcatheter Valves (PARTNER) Cohort A trial. AVR, aortic valve replacement; CI, confidence interval; HR, hazard ratio; TAVR, transcatheter aortic valve replacement. *(From Smith CR, Leon MB, Mack MJ, et al. Transcatheter versus surgical aortic valve replacement in high risk patients. N Engl J Med 2011;364:2187-2198.)*

TABLE 47-1	**Neurologic Events at 30 Days and 1 Year (N = 699)**					
	30 Days			*1 Year*		
OUTCOME (N [%])	**TAVR (N = 348)**	**AVR (N = 351)**	**P VALUE**	**TAVR (N = 348)**	**AVR (N = 351)**	**P VALUE**
All stroke or TIA	19 (5.5)	8 (2.4)	.04	27 (8.3)	13 (4.3)	.04
TIA	3 (0.9)	1 (0.3)	.33	7 (2.3)	4 (1.5)	.47
All stroke	16 (4.6)	8 (2.4)	.12	20 (6.0)	10 (3.2)	.08
Major stroke	13 (3.8)	7 (2.1)	.20	17 (5.1)	8 (2.4)	.07
Minor stroke	3 (0.9)	1 (0.3)	.34	3 (0.9)	2 (0.7)	.84
Death/major stroke	24 (6.9)	28 (8.2)	.52	92 (26.5)	93 (28.0)	.68

TIA, transient ischemic attack.
From Smith CR, Leon MB, Mack MJ, et al. Transcatheter versus surgical aortic valve replacement in high risk patients. *N Engl J Med* 2011;364:2187-2198.

outcomes and late survival following TAVI. Clinical experience to date suggests that the majority of coronary disease in patients undergoing TAVI can be managed conservatively.

Injury to the atrioventricular conduction system as it courses through the interventricular septum below the aortic valve may be associated with new left bundle block or complete heart block. Surgical AVR is associated with a need for permanent pacing in 3% to 18%. TAVI is reportedly associated with new pacemaker implantation in 3% to 36% of patients; however, comparisons are difficult because current TAVI patients represent a particularly high-risk group, and local practice varies widely in terms of the threshold for pacemaker implantation. In the PARTNER trials, no difference was reported in the need for permanent pacemaker insertion in the TAVI group compared with the surgical group at 30 days (3.8% vs. 3.6%; at 1 year, 5.7% vs. 5.0%). We are faced with reports that the 9% to 36% rate of new pacemaker implantation with the CoreValve device is clearly higher than the 3% to 12% rate reported with the Edwards Lifesciences device, presumably because this device often extends further into the LV outflow tract. Additional risk factors for new heart block may include advanced age, preexisting right bundle branch block, or atrioventricular delay and oversizing.

Next-Generation Aortic Valve Therapy

With the success of the first-generation valves, it has become increasingly clear that we still need improvement in percutaneous heart valve designs. The next generation of TAVI will demonstrate diameters smaller than 18 Fr, improved access, enhanced ease of passage through the stenotic native aortic valve, coaxial alignment, repositionable valves, and the opportunity to recapture and remove the valve, if necessary, even after initial deployment. Some next-generation valves that fit these criteria are in early evaluation and are reviewed in this section. Table 47-2 lists valves that have been implanted in humans to date.

The Direct Flow Valve (Direct Flow Medical, Santa Rosa, CA) differs from other percutaneous valves in that it has no metallic components. This percutaneous valve (Figure 47-8) includes two expandable tubular cuffs, buttressed with polyester, that contain a bovine pericardial valve (see Figure 47-8).[53] The valve is designed to be positioned below the aortic annulus and anchored distally above the tips of the native valve leaflets. Expanded with saline, the first cuff within the LV outflow tract frees the valve, which immediately functions and allows hemodynamic stability throughout deployment, so rapid pacing is not required. After deployment, valve function, paravalvular leak,

TABLE 47-2	Current Studies of Percutaneous Aortic Valve Therapies Used for Human Implants		
COMPANY	VALVE NAME	VALVE POSITION	VALVE TYPE
Medtronic	CoreValve ReValving System	Aortic	Porcine
Direct Flow Medical	Direct Flow Medical Valve	Aortic	Equine
Edwards Lifesciences	Edwards Sapien, Sapien XT, Cribier Edwards, and Percutaneous Heart Valve Technologies	Aortic	Equine
Medtronic	Melody Valve	Aortic	Bovine
Sadra	Lotus Valve	Aortic	Bovine
Unknown	Paniagua Heart Valve	Aortic	Unknown

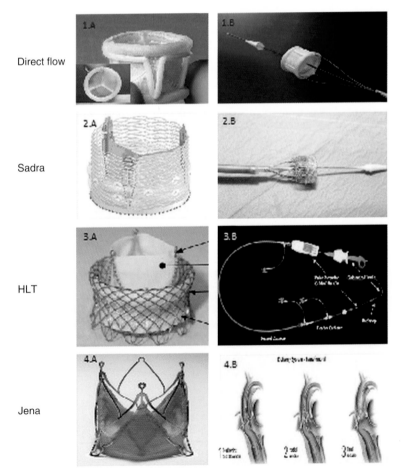

Direct flow

Sadra

HLT

Jena

FIGURE 47-8 Next-generation percutaneous aortic valves for transcatheter implantation. Direct flow, Direct Flow Valve (Santa Rosa, CA); HLT, Heart Leaflet Technologies (Maple Grove, MN); Jena, JenaValve (Munich, Germany); Sadra, Lotus Valve (Sadra/Boston Scientific, Boston, MA).

Medtronic Engager Transapical Valve

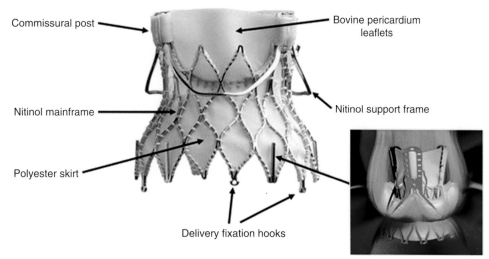

Commissural post

Bovine pericardium leaflets

Nitinol mainframe

Nitinol support frame

Polyester skirt

Delivery fixation hooks

FIGURE 47-9 The Medtronic (Minneapolis, MN) Engager transapical valve.

and positioning are then reevaluated by echocardiography. If the valve is not ideally positioned or if paravalvular leakage is present, the valve can be collapsed, repositioned, or withdrawn, and the procedure can be repeated. If the valve is positioned well, and hemodynamic function is acceptable, the saline is replaced with a water-soluble epoxy inflation medium that rapidly cures in situ to allow rapid detachment. The current status of in vivo implants consists of 31 patients at two centers in Europe. Out of those, only 22 patients underwent implantation in this feasibility study. Because of technical issues, 9 patients did not have the valve implanted, 2 patients died after implantation (1 from myocardial infarction and 1 from HF), and 18 patients were implanted and discharged from the hospital. Aortic gradients were approximately 20 mm Hg with an effective valve area by transthoracic echocardiography of 1.5 cm^2. During the 6-month follow-up, 2 patients died: 1 from respiratory problems and 1 of unknown causes. The remaining 16 patients (72%) were reported to be stable for more than 24 months, in NYHA class I or II, with a paravalvular leak of grade 1 or less.[54] A European trial using the 18-Fr system is scheduled to begin in the near future, and a 16-Fr device is under development.

The Lotus Valve (Sadra/Boston Scientific, Boston, MA) is a percutaneous system that comprises a nitinol self-expanding ring that holds a bovine pericardial valve and has a delivery system for guidance and placement (see Figure 47-8). This second-generation valve is deployed without the need for rapid pacing. Paravalvular leakage is minimized by the use of an outer-diameter seal. Despite its initial flexibility, final expansion results in a rigid cage, but the valve can be retracted into the delivery sheath at any time before final separation of the delivery device. The first clinical deployment of the Lotus Valve was performed in July 2007 in Germany.[55] A feasibility trial of 10 patients was conducted to evaluate this device. Four patients continue to be followed with the longest follow-up greater than 24 months. The Lotus Valve demonstrates valve areas exceeding 1.5 cm^2 and pressure gradients of less than 20 mm Hg. Plans for a larger clinical experience are being developed.

The Heart Leaflet Technologies valve (Heart Leaflet Technologies, Maple Grove, MN) is composed of a super-elastic nitinol wire form that supports the glutaraldehyde cross-linked, trileaflet, porcine pericardial tissue valve (see Figure 47-8). In addition, a braided polyester liner minimizes the regurgitant flow around the valve; it uses a proprietary configuration that allows antegrade blood flow, decreasing the need for rapid ventricular pacing for implantation.

The JenaValve technology platform (JenaValve, Munich, Germany) is developing transapical and transfemoral prosthesis platforms that use a self-expanding nitinol stent with a bovine pericardial valve (see Figure 47-8).[56] One aspect unique to the JenaClip design is integrated feelers that capture, or clip, the leaflets to avoid potential coronary flow obstruction. This valve has a full range of sizes, from 19 to 27 mm, and is 30 mm in height. A transapical approach system is also in development, and both systems can deploy the prosthesis with the heart beating, without the use of cardiopulmonary bypass or rapid pacing. As of this writing, JenaValve's transapical device was in the implementation process of a first-in-human trial.

TRANSAPICAL VALVES

The Engager (formerly Embracer Valve, Medtronic) is dedicated to apical delivery (Figure 47-9). The system utilizes a self-expanding nitinol frame, a second support frame with three commissural posts, valve leaflets of bovine pericardium attached to the self-expanding nitinol frame, and fixation hooks with barbs at the LV outflow tract side of the device. A polyester skirt is contiguous with the bovine pericardial leaflets. First-in-human trials have been done in 20 patients, and more extensive human trials are pending (www.ClinicalTrials.gov identifier NCT00677638).

Percutaneous Mitral Valve Therapy

The pandemic of rheumatic mitral stenosis has presented therapeutic challenges in providing surgical therapy to individuals suffering from this debilitating disease. Both closed and open surgical commissurotomy were utilized prior to valve replacement in an effort to decrease the severity of stenosis. The introduction of balloon mitral valvuloplasty as a therapy for rheumatic mitral stenosis more than 25 years ago arose from attempts to simulate the surgical procedure using endovascular techniques. Such percutaneous balloon therapies provided the initial step in a journey of developing percutaneous treatments for MV disorders.[56] In the recent past, using devices adapted from atrial septal defect and patent foramen oval (PFO) closures, percutaneous device closure of paravalvular leaks after surgical valve implantation was shown to have a potential, albeit limited, role.[57-60] MR, as a result of either degenerative valve disease or functional etiologies, has required surgical valve repair or replacement. Advances in surgical valve techniques that allow patients to benefit from less invasive surgical procedures, without the need

TABLE 47-3   **Current Studies of Percutaneous Mitral Repair Approaches: Compendium of Targeted Therapy and Devices**

SITE OF THERAPY	TREATMENT APPROACH	DEVICE	STATUS
Leaflets	Edge-to-edge (leaflet plication)	MitraClip	Randomized trial data presented
		MitraFlex	Preclinical development
	Space occupier (leaflet coaptation)	Percu-Pro System	Phase 1 trial
	Leaflet ablation	ThermoCool	Animal models
Annulus	Indirect annuloplasty	—	—
	Coronary sinus approach, with sinus reshaping	Monarc	FIH results; feasibility study ongoing
		Carillon	FIH results; feasibility study complete
		Viacor	FIH results; feasibility study ongoing
	Asymmetrical approach	St. Jude	Animal models
		NIH-Cerclage technology	Animal models
Direct annuloplasty	Percutaneous mechanical cinching	Mitralign	FIH results
		Accucinch GDS	FIH results
		Millipede ring system	Preclinical development
	Percutaneous energy-mediated cinching	QuantumCor	Animal models
		ReCor	Preclinical development
	Hybrid	Mitral solutions	Preclinical development
		MiCardia	Preclinical development
Chordal implants	Transapical	—	—
	Artificial chord	NeoChord, MitraFlex	Preclinical development
	Transapical-transseptal	—	—
	Artificial chord	Babic	Preclinical development
LV	LV (and MA) remodeling	Mardil-BACE	Temporary human implant
Valve implants	Right minithoracotomy	EndoValve-Hermann prosthesis	Animal models
	Transapical	Lutter prosthesis	Animal models
	Transseptal	CardiaQ prosthesis	Preclinical development

FIH, first in human; LV, left ventricle; MA, mitral annulus; NIH, National Institutes of Health.

for thoracotomy or cardiopulmonary bypass, have been met with enthusiasm.

Adaptation of these surgical strategies to new percutaneous approaches has resulted in a large number of new technologies. These percutaneous devices for mitral repair can be categorized by procedures that approach the various components of the MV and its apparatus. It is important to recall that the MV consists of multiple components: anterior and posterior leaflets, a subvalvular apparatus (chordae tendineae and papillary muscles), the annulus, and the left atrial and LV chamber.[61] Individually, each of these components may be a potential treatment target to reduce MR. An abbreviated review of the current percutaneous therapies being developed and evaluated for the management of MR is presented in Table 47-3.

Approach to Leaflet Repair

Surgery can achieve complex valve leaflet and chordal repair, but such things are currently beyond the reach of percutaneous approaches, which have been designed to treat a single pathologic component. Currently, a percutaneous leaflet-to-leaflet technique has been developed that simulates the double-orifice surgical repair initially described by Maisano and coworkers.[62] During the surgery, the free edges of the mitral leaflets are sutured together in the midportion (A2-P2 segment) to create two separate, smaller orifices. During surgery an annuloplasty ring can be implanted, which seems to decrease the need for reoperation in patients with more severe MR.[63-65]

The MitraClip device (Evalve, Abbot Vascular) was proven safe and effective in animal models[66] and has been used in the treatment of carefully selected patients.[67] The procedure is accomplished under TEE guidance, using a unique transseptal catheter delivery system that allows a metallic clip to grasp and approximate the free edges of the two MV leaflets (Figure 47-10). TEE guidance is used to position the implant and assess the effect. If the initial placement is unsatisfactory, the clip can be removed or repositioned. In addition, to achieve optimal reduction in the severity of MR, one additional clip can be implanted adjacent

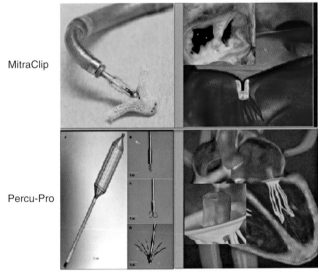

MitraClip

Percu-Pro

FIGURE 47-10 Approaches for leaflet-to-leaflet transcatheter mitral valve therapies. MitraClip, Abbott Vascular (Abbott Park, IL); Percu-Pro, Cardiosolutions (Stoughton, MA).

to the first clip.[68] Clinically significant mitral stenosis has not been observed after this procedure, and a minimal increase has been noted in transmitral gradient, from 1.7 ± 0.9 mm Hg to only 4.1 ± 2.2 mm Hg ($P < .001$).[69] Great care has been taken to assess the transmitral gradient prior to implantation of more than one clip because of the concern of creating mitral stenosis.[70]

In the randomized Endovascular Valve Edge-to-Edge Repair Study (EVEREST II), experience was limited with functional MR.[70] In an echocardiographic substudy of the EVEREST registry, 8 of the 37 patients had functional MR with normal leaflet morphology, and they experienced reductions in MR similar to the degenerative group with similar favorable LV remodeling.[71]

The pivotal EVEREST II study[72] randomized 279 patients with a core lab-assessed MR of grade 3 or higher, irrespective of symptomatic status, in a 2:1 fashion to MitraClip implantation or surgical MV repair or replacement. The primary efficacy endpoint was freedom from death, freedom from surgery for valvular dysfunction, or MR of grade 3 or higher at 1 year, which occurred in 55.2% in the percutaneous arm and 73.0% in the surgical arm ($P < .001$); at 2 years, it was 51.7% in the percutaneous arm and 66.3% in the surgical arm ($P < .001$). In the per-treatment protocol, in which patients (n = 20) not receiving clip implantation were excluded, efficacy at 1 year was 67.4% in the percutaneous arm and 73.0% in the surgical arm ($P < .67$); at 2 years, efficacy was 62.7% in the percutaneous arm and 66.3% in the surgical arm ($P < .67$). This finding demonstrates that if the clip procedure can be performed successfully, it has similar results to MV surgery for these composite endpoints. Device failure, if it occurred, was seen early, with rare late clip failures requiring surgery (Figure 47-11). A high-risk registry for patients with elevated surgical risk (estimated 30-day mortality rate >12% using the STS risk-assessment tool) was also completed and is in the long-term follow-up phase.

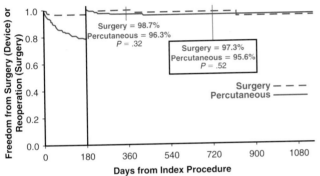

FIGURE 47-11 Landmark analysis of the Endovascular Valve Edge-to-Edge Repair Study (EVEREST II).

Unresolved questions regarding the MitraClip percutaneous edge-to-edge procedure remain. Although durability out to 2 years has been established, comparative long-term durability data are not available. Concerns regarding the potential for the late presentation of chronic leaflet injury that requires eventual surgical repair remain. Nevertheless, these data have been sufficiently compelling for commercial release of the MitraClip in Europe with an expectation for submission to the U.S. Food and Drug Administration (FDA) panel in the near future.

Mitral annuloplasty using an undersized ring is often a routine component of surgical MV repair.[73] A number of percutaneous devices have attempted to reproduce the beneficial effects of surgical annuloplasty by taking advantage of the proximity of the coronary sinus to the mitral annulus. The coronary sinus and its major tributary, the great cardiac vein, somewhat parallel the annulus of the MV along its posterior and lateral aspects. The epicardial coronary venous system is most easily accessible from the internal jugular vein, as the confluence of the coronary sinus drains directly into the right atrium. Percutaneous approaches have generally used the internal jugular or subclavian access to the right atrium to allow intubation of the coronary sinus. Various remodeling devices (Figure 47-12) can be introduced into the coronary sinus, with the objective being to displace the adjacent posterior mitral annulus toward the anterior aspect of the annulus and thereby improve coaptation of the mitral leaflets.

The coronary sinus approach is appealing for its simplicity, with transvenous access using fluoroscopic guidance. Unfortunately, there are many potentially significant limitations. First, the anatomic relationship of the coronary sinus to the mitral annulus is highly variable.[74] Somewhat surprisingly, very early data suggest that benefit from coronary sinus annuloplasty cannot be predicted by preprocedural imaging assessment.[75] A second concern is that the circumflex artery travels beneath the great cardiac vein in more than 50% of patients. Coronary artery compression resulting in ischemia and infarction have occurred. The use of the coronary sinus to place biventricular pacing leads, often in patients with decreased ventricular function and functional MR, may present issues regarding this approach as well.[76,77]

Monarc

Carillon XE Device

Viacor

St. Jude

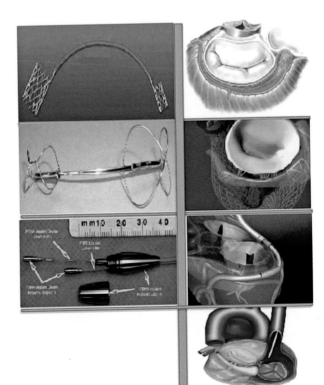

FIGURE 47-12 Percutaneous approaches to mitral annuloplasty. Carillon, Cardiac Dimensions (Kirkland, WA); St. Jude, St. Jude Medical (St. Paul, MN); Monarc, Edwards Lifesciences (Irvine, CA); VIACOR, Viacor, Inc. (Wilmington, MA).

The Edwards Lifesciences Monarc transvenous annuloplasty device is formed from a stent-like anchor placed in the great cardiac vein, connected by a bridge segment with biodegradable spacers that connect to a second anchor located proximally at the coronary sinus ostium. The self-expanding cage is compressed into a delivery sheath placed from the jugular vein. Once positioned, the sheath is withdrawn to allow the nitinol alloy anchors to expand, fixing the device. Tension on the device allows the system to acutely decrease the coronary sinus dimension. Over a few weeks, the spacers dissolve, shortening the bridge and drawing the anchors closer together, potentially shortening the coronary sinus. The Monarc coronary sinus device is anchored into the anterior interventricular vein and exerts a slight effect on the LV.

The Carillon Mitral Contour System (Cardiac Dimensions, Kirkland, WA), also an indirect annuloplasty device, uses two self-expanding nitinol anchors connected by a manual tensioning wire that immediately shortens the coronary sinus. Using echocardiographic or angiographic imaging, the tension can be adjusted prior to final deployment. Initial feasibility studies showed a reduction in annular dimension and MR severity limited by anchor slippage.[78] The Carillon XE is a device modification used in the multicenter Evaluating the Use of SR34006 Compared to Warfarin or Acenocoumarol in Patients with Atrial Fibrillation (AMADEUS) trial. It was permanently deployed in 30 of 43 patients, and the failure modes were inadequate MR reduction or arterial compression. New modifications (Carillon XE2) resulted in the 36-patient Transcatheter Implantation of the Carillon Mitral Annuloplasty (TITAN) trial,[79] which resumed enrollment in 2011.

The Viacor (Wilmington, MA) percutaneous transvenous mitral annuloplasty device[80] represents the third indirect approach to coronary sinus mitral annuloplasty (see Figure 47-12). Using a delivery catheter, deflecting metallic rods are implanted in the coronary sinus using a subclavian cutdown; the rods deflect the posterior annulus anteriorly. Rod exchange may require surgical reaccess, but proof-of-concept temporary implants have suggested efficacy,[81] and the subsequent Safety and Efficacy of the Percutaneous Transvenous Mitral Annuloplasty Device to Reduce Mitral Regurgitation (PTOLEMY) feasibility trial temporarily reduced MR by at least one grade in 13 of 19 patients, but permanent implantation was achieved in only 9 of 27 patients.[82]

Chamber Remodeling

As discussed above, the variable relationship of the coronary sinus and great cardiac vein to the mitral annulus creates significant challenges. Anchors, in either the atrium or ventricle, have been developed to directly remodel these chambers to decrease chamber diameters and to decrease the diameter of the mitral annulus (Figure 47-13). The opportunity to use an anchor in the coronary sinus, combined with a second anchor system in the right atrium, has been evaluated as a means of applying more traction on the mitral annulus.

The St. Jude Medical (Minneapolis, MN) system is composed of four helical anchors, two loading spacers, a tether rope, and a locking mechanism. The distal pair of anchors is delivered via the coronary sinus into the LV myocardium near the posterior leaflet scallop; the proximal pair of anchors is delivered via the right atrium into the posteromedial trigone. The double anchors are connected by a cable to enable reduction of the posteromedial MA and are locked via a self-retracting nitinol structure. Proof of concept has been demonstrated in animal models.[83]

Direct Annuloplasty

Direct modification of the mitral annulus is an appealing method of mimicking the effects of surgical annuloplasty. Attempts to develop systems that allow annuloplasty rings to be introduced through a catheter have been frustrating, as positioning and fixation have proven unreliable (Figure 47-14).

Surgical suture plication of the posterior portion of the annulus has been reported to offer benefit even without implantation of a ring.[84] Application of radiofrequency to the annulus via a catheter to shrink the annulus via collagen contraction has been proposed (QuantumCor, Lake Forest, CA).[85,86] A system that also uses energy to remodel the annulus is the ReCor device (ReCor, Paris, France), which delivers high-intensity focused ultrasound circumferentially and perpendicularly to the shaft of a delivery catheter, resulting in tissue heating and collagen shrinkage of the mitral annulus. The limitations of both energy delivery systems stem from the lack of precision in energy delivery and include possible development of annular stenosis of the MV and perforation or other damage of adjacent structures, although these seem

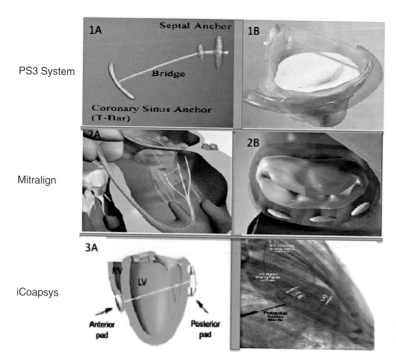

FIGURE 47-13 Percutaneous mitral transvenous annuloplasty devices. iCoapsys, Myocor (Maple Grove, MN); Mitralign (Tewksbury, MA); PS3, Ample Medical (Foster City, CA).

more theoretical, as they have not been reported in the animal model evaluations.

The Mitralign Percutaneous Annuloplasty System (Mitralign, Tewksbury, MA) uses a guide catheter passed between the two papillary muscles (see Figure 47-13) to access this subvalvular space in the region of the mitral P2 scallop. The Accucinch system (Guided Delivery Systems, Santa Clara, CA) uses a transventricular approach for anchor placement, entering medial or lateral to the papillary muscles. The posterior annulus is cinched circumferentially from trigone to trigone (see Figure 47-14), and improvement in MR has been reported; this device does have reported but unpublished first-in-human results. The Millipede system (Millipede, Ann Arbor, MI) places a novel repositionable and retrievable annular ring (see Figure 47-14) with a unique attachment system via a transseptal approach or using a minimally invasive technique.

Ventricular Remodeling

The iCoapsys device[87] (Myocor, Maple Grove, MN) is designed to produce a reduction in MR by remodeling the LV (see Figure 47-13). This percutaneous device is implanted with a subxiphoid

pericardial access sheath. Using a sophisticated positioning system, two fixation pads are placed on the surface of the LV, one anterior and one posterior. LV puncture allows a cable to connect the two pads, and tensioning the cable draws the pads together. As the anteroposterior diameter of the LV is reduced, the anteroposterior dimension of the mitral annulus also shrinks, with the aim of resulting in improved leaflet coaptation, reduced chordal tethering, and improved LV function.[88,89]

The BACE system (Mardil, Morrisville, NC) requires a minithoracotomy but is implanted on a beating heart. A silicone band is placed around the atrioventricular groove with built-in inflatable chambers placed on the mitral annulus (MA). This reshapes the MA for better leaflet coaptation, and it can be remotely adjusted after implantation. No coronary artery compromise was shown in animal models, and proof of concept was demonstrated in 15 patients (unpublished data).

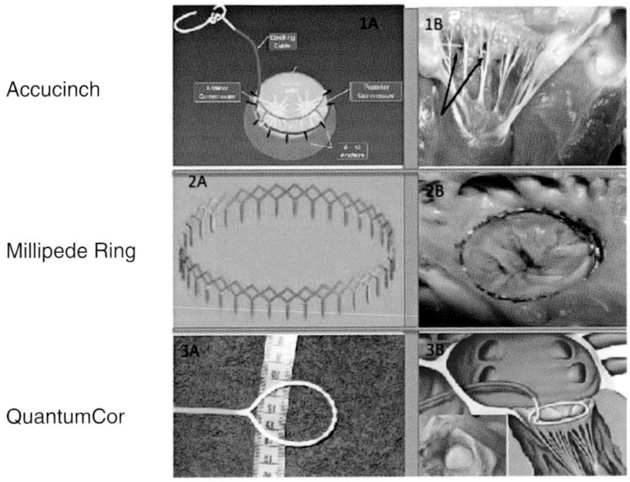

Chordal Implantation

Transcatheter and percutaneous chordal procedures are currently under development that include chordal cutting and chordal implantation.[90] Three devices are currently in development: the transapically delivered MitraFlex (TransCardiac Therapeutics, Atlanta, GA) and Neochord devices (Neochord, Minnetonka, MN; Figure 47-15) and the transapical-transseptal Babic (Belgrade, Serbia) device. The MitraFlex and Neochord devices place an anchor in the inner LV myocardium and another on the leaflet via a transapical approach, and they connect the two with a synthetic "chord." In the Babic device,[91] two continuous suture tracks are created from the LV puncture site through the puncture of the target leaflet and are exteriorized via the transseptal route. A pledget is apposed onto the exteriorized venous sutures and is anchored onto the atrial side of the leaflet by retracting the guiding sutures from the epicardial end. A polymer tube is then interposed between the leaflet and free myocardial wall and is secured at the epicardial surface by an adjustable knob.

Mitral Valve Replacement

The goal of percutaneous approaches is to provide results comparable to those of surgery. As surgical MV repair is often not feasible, and MV replacement is required, percutaneous MV replacement may have a role as well (Figure 47-16). To accomplish delivery of a percutaneous MV, several formidable obstacles

Accucinch

Millipede Ring

QuantumCor

FIGURE 47-14 Direct annuloplasty using percutaneous therapy. Accucinch, Guided Delivery Systems (Santa Clara, CA); Millipede (Ann Arbor, MI); Quantum-Cor (Lake Forest, CA).

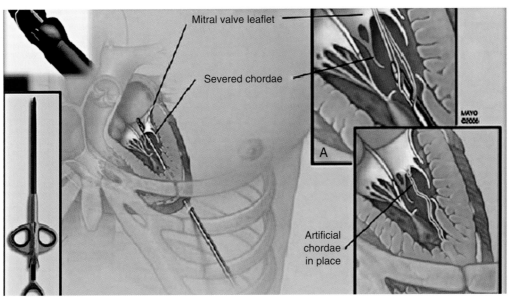

FIGURE 47-15 Minimally invasive percutaneous mitral chord reconstruction.

726

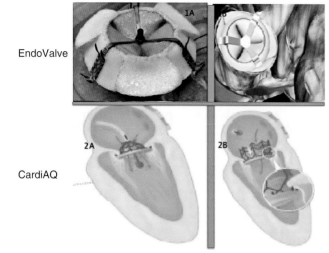

EndoValve

CardiAQ

FIGURE 47-16 Percutaneous mitral valve replacement. CardiAQ, CardiAQ Valve Technologies (Winchester, MA); EndoValve (Princeton, NJ).

must be overcome. First, the asymmetrical shape of the annulus presents great difficulty in fabrication of device rings. Second, a family of anchoring designs might be required to treat differing etiologies of MR. Third, LV outflow obstruction might occur as a result of retained native valve tissue. Fourth, paravalvular leaks that occur in surgically implanted valves may continue to be a significant issue.

Three devices are currently in various stages of development. The EndoValve-Herrmann prosthesis (EndoValve, Princeton, NJ) is currently designed to be implanted through the left atrium via a right minithoracotomy on a beating heart. This foldable, valve-sparing nitinol structure attaches to the native valve with specially designed grippers that allow repositioning before release. Feasibility has been demonstrated in animal models of MR, and fully percutaneous versions are in development. A nitinol stent-valve, the Lutter prosthesis (Bonn, Germany), has been implanted trans-apically in porcine models, and the CardiAQ transseptal prosthesis (CardiAQ Valve Technologies, Winchester, MA) is also in preclinical development. Given the myriad complexities with these systems, we should anticipate the need for further refinements prior to any clinical studies.

Summary

The clinical evaluation of percutaneous approaches to AVR and MV repair remains limited to relatively small case experiences and one pivotal randomized trial in each arena. Currently, the clinical role for transcatheter AVR in inoperable patients has been established. The most recent data suggest that TAVI will likely be a clinical choice for high-risk surgical patients as well.

Percutaneous edge-to-edge repair is promising based upon its initial data and early clinical use, although application of this technology in the general population of patients remains to be determined. The opportunity is certainly promising for new percutaneous repair and replacement technologies, as more devices are evaluated in human trials.

REFERENCES

1. Nkomo, VT, Gardin JM, Skelton TH, et al. Burden of valvular heart diseases: a population-based study. *Lancet* 2006;368:1005-1011.
2. Lindroos M, Kupari M, Heikkila J, et al. Prevalence of aortic valve abnormalities in the elderly: an echocardiographic study of a random population sample. *J Am Coll Cardiol* 1993;21(5):1220-1225.
3. Ross J Jr, Braunwald E. Aortic stenosis. *Circulation* 1968;38:61-67.
4. Cribier A, Savin T, Saoudi N, et al. Percutaneous transluminal valvuloplasty of acquired aortic valve stenosis in elderly patients: an alternative to valve replacement. *Lancet* 1986;1:63-67.
5. Perloff JK, Rogers WC. The mitral apparatus: functional anatomy of mitral regurgitation. *Circulation* 1972;46:227-239.
6. Murphy ES, Lawson RM, Starr A, Rahimtoola SH. Severe aortic stenosis in patients 60 years of age or older: left ventricular function and 10-year survival after valve replacement. *Circulation* 1981;64:II184-II188.
7. O'Brien SM, Shahian DM, Filardo G, et al. The Society of Thoracic Surgeons 2008 cardiac surgery risk models: part 2—isolated valve surgery. *Ann Thorac Surg* 2009;88(1 Suppl):S23-S42.
8. Iung B, Cachier A, Baron G, et al. Decision-making in elderly patients with severe aortic stenosis: why are so many denied surgery? *Eur Heart J* 2005;26:2714-2720.
9. Bonow RO, Carabello BA, Kanu C, et al. ACC/AHA 2006 guidelines for the management of patients with valvular heart disease: a report of the American College of Cardiology/American Heart Association Task Force on Practice Guidelines. *Circulation* 2006;114:e84-e231.
10. Andersen HR, Knudsen LL, Hasemakam JM. Transluminal implantation of artificial heart valves: description of a new expandable aortic valve and initial results with implantation by catheter techniques in closed chest pigs. *Eur Heart J* 1992;13:704-708.
11. Paniagua D, Condado JA, Besso J, et al. First human case of retrograde transcatheter implantation of an aortic valve prosthesis. *Tex Heart Inst J* 2005;32:393-398.
12. Percutaneous Heart Valve Replacement. Technical Brief No. 2. Prepared by Duke Evidence-based Practice Center under Contract No. 290-02-0025. 2010, Rockville, MD, Agency for Healthcare Research and Quality. Accessed 2010 July 28 at www.effectivehealthcare.ahrq.gov/reports/final.cfm.
13. Cribier A, Eltchaninoff H, Bash A, et al. Percutaneous transcatheter implantation of an aortic valve prosthesis for calcific aortic stenosis: first human case description. *Circulation* 2002;106:3006-3008.
14. Buellesfeld L, Gerckens U, Grube E. Percutaneous implantation of the first repositionable aortic valve prosthesis in a patient with severe aortic stenosis. *Catheter Cardiovasc Interv* 2008;71:579-584.
15. Piazza N, Grube E, Gerckens U, et al. Procedural and 30-day outcomes following transcatheter aortic valve implantation using the third generation (18 Fr) CoreValve revalving system: results from the multicentre, expanded evaluation registry 1-year following CE mark approval. *EuroIntervention* 2008;4:242-249.
16. Rodés-Cabau J, Dumont E, De LaRochellière R, et al. Feasibility and initial results of percutaneous aortic valve implantation including selection of the transfemoral or transapical approach in patients with severe aortic stenosis. *Am J Cardiol* 2008;102:1240-1246.
17. Coeytaux RR, Williams JW Jr, Gray RN, Wang A. Percutaneous heart valve replacement for aortic stenosis: state of the evidence. *Ann Intern Med* 2010;153:314-324.
18. Piazza N, Serruys PW, de Jaegere P. Feasibility of complex coronary intervention in combination with percutaneous aortic valve implantation in patients with aortic stenosis using percutaneous left ventricular assist device (TandemHeart). *Catheter Cardiovasc Interv* 2009;73:161-166.
19. Nashef SA, Roques F, Michel P, et al. European system for cardiac operative risk evaluation (EuroSCORE). *Eur J Cardiothorac Surg* 1999;16:9-13.
20. Nashef SA, Roques F, Hammill BG, et al.; EuroSCORE Project Group. Validation of European System for Cardiac Operative Risk Evaluation (EuroSCORE) in North American cardiac surgery. *Eur J Cardiothorac Surg* 2002;22:101-105.
21. Shroyer AL, Coombs LP, Peterson ED, et al.; Society of Thoracic Surgeons. The Society of Thoracic Surgeons: 30-day operative mortality and morbidity risk models. *Ann Thorac Surg* 2003;75:1856-1864; discussion 1864-1865.
22. Dewey TM, Brown D, Ryan WH, et al. Reliability of risk algorithms in predicting early and late operative outcomes in high-risk patients undergoing aortic valve replacement. *J Thorac Cardiovasc Surg* 2008;135:180-187.
23. Osswald BR, Gegouskov V, Badowski-Zyla D, et al. Overestimation of aortic valve replacement risk by Euro SCORE: implications for percutaneous valve replacement. *Eur Heart J* 2009;30:74-80.
24. Brown ML, Schaff HV, Sarano ME, et al. Is the European System for Cardiac Operative Risk Evaluation model valid for estimating the operative risk of patients considered for percutaneous aortic valve replacement? *J Thorac Cardiovasc Surg* 2008;136:566-571.
25. Schenk S, Fritzsche D, Atoui R, et al. EuroSCORE-predicted mortality and surgical judgment for aortic valve replacement. *J Heart Valve Dis* 2010;19:5-15.
26. Berry C, Cartier R, Bonan R. Fatal ischemic stroke related to nonpermissive peripheral artery access for percutaneous aortic valve replacement. *Catheter Cardiovasc Interv* 2007;69:56-63.
27. Bagur R, Dumont E, Doyle D, et al. Coronary ostia stenosis after transcatheter aortic valve implantation. *JACC Cardiovasc Interv* 2010;3:253-255.
28. Clavel MA, Webb JG, Pibarot P, et al. Comparison of the hemodynamic performance of percutaneous and surgical bioprostheses for the treatment of severe aortic stenosis. *J Am Coll Cardiol* 2009;53:1883-1891.
29. Eltchaninoff H, Tron C, Cribier A. Percutaneous implantation of aortic valve prosthesis in patients with calcific aortic stenosis: technical aspects. *J Interv Cardiol* 2003;16:515-521.
30. Ghanem A, Müller A, Nähle CP, et al. Risk and fate of cerebral embolism after transfemoral aortic valve implantation: a prospective pilot study with diffusion-weighted magnetic resonance imaging. *J Am Coll Cardiol* 2010;55:1427-1432.
31. Smíd M, Ferda J, Baxa J, et al. Aortic annulus and ascending aorta: comparison of preoperative and perioperative measurement in patients with aortic stenosis. *Eur J Radiol* 2010;74:152.
32. Ng AC, Delgado V, van der Kley F, et al. Comparison of aortic root dimensions and geometries before and after transcatheter aortic valve implantation by 2- and 3-dimensional transesophageal echocardiography and multislice computed tomography. *Circ Cardiovasc Imaging* 2010;3:94-102.
33. Messika-Zeitoun D, Serfaty JM, Brochet E, et al. Multimodal assessment of the aortic annulus diameter: implications for transcatheter aortic valve implantation. *J Am Coll Cardiol* 2010;55:186-194.

34. Thomas M, Schymik G, Walther T, et al. Thirty-day results of the SAPIEN Aortic Bioprosthesis European Outcome (SOURCE) Registry: a European registry of transcatheter aortic valve implantation using the Edwards SAPIEN valve. *Circulation* 2010;122:62-69.

35. Kahlert P, Knipp SC, Schlamann M, et al. Silent and apparent cerebral ischemia after percutaneous transfemoral aortic valve implantation: a diffusion-weighted magnetic resonance imaging study. *Circulation* 2010;121:870-878.

36. Cribier A, Eltchaninoff H, Tron C, et al. Treatment of calcific aortic stenosis with the percutaneous heart valve: mid-term follow-up from the initial feasibility studies—the French experience. *J Am Coll Cardiol* 2006;47:1214-1223.

37. Reference deleted in proofs.

38. Reference deleted in proofs.

39. Messika-Zeitoun D, Serfaty JM, Brochet E, et al. Multimodal assessment of the aortic annulus diameter: implications for transcatheter aortic valve implantation. *J Am Coll Cardiol* 2010;55:186-194.

40. Cribier A, Eltchaninoff H, Tron C, et al. Early experience with percutaneous transcatheter implantation of heart valve prosthesis for the treatment of end-stage inoperable patients with calcific aortic stenosis. *J Am Coll Cardiol* 2004;43:698-703.

41. Webb JG, Chandavimol M, Thompson CR, et al. Percutaneous aortic valve implantation retrograde from the femoral artery. *Circulation* 2006;113:842-850.

42. Smith CR, Leon MB, Mack MJ, et al. Transcatheter versus surgical aortic-valve replacement in high-risk patients. *N Engl J Med* 2011;364:2187-2198.

43. Reference deleted in proofs.

44. Leon MB, Smith CR, Mack M, et al.; PARTNER Trial Investigators. Transcatheter aortic-valve implantation for aortic stenosis in patients who cannot undergo surgery. *N Engl J Med* 2010;363:1597-1607.

45. Reference deleted in proofs.

46. Rodés-Cabau J, Houde C, Perron J, Benson LN, Pibarot P. Delayed improvement in valve hemodynamic performance after percutaneous pulmonary valve implantation. *Ann Thorac Surg* 2008;85:1787-1788.

47. Falk V, Schwammenthal EE, Kempfert J, et al. New anatomically oriented transapical aortic valve implantation. *Ann Thorac Surg* 2009;87:925-926.

48. Webb JG, Altwegg L, Masson JB, et al. A new transcatheter aortic valve and percutaneous valve delivery system. *J Am Coll Cardiol* 2009;53:1855-1858.

49. Ye J, Webb JG, Cheung A, et al. Transcatheter valve-in-valve aortic valve implantation: 16-month follow-up. *Ann Thorac Surg* 2009;88:1322-1324.

50. Ng AC, van der Kley F, Delgado V, et al. Percutaneous valve-in-valve procedure for severe paravalvular regurgitation in aortic bioprosthesis [Letter]. *JACC Cardiovasc Imaging* 2009;2:522-523.

51. Rodés-Cabau J, Dumont E, Doyle D. "Valve-in-valve" for the treatment of paravalvular leaks following transcatheter aortic valve implantation. *Catheter Cardiovasc Interv* 2009;74:1116-1119.

52. Bartorelli AL, Andreini D, Sisillo E, et al. Left main coronary artery occlusion after percutaneous aortic valve implantation. *Ann Thorac Surg* 2010;89:953-955.

53. Schofer J, Schlater M, Treedeet H, et al. Retrograde transarterial implantation of a nonmetallic aortic valve prosthesis in high-surgical-risk patients with severe aortic stenosis: a first-in-man feasibility and safety study. *Circ Cardiovasc Interv* 2008;1:126-133.

54. Bijulic K, Tuebler T, Reichenspurner H, et al. Midterm stability and hemodynamic performance of transfemorally implantable nonmetallic, retrievable and repositionable aortic valve in patients with severe aortic stenosis. Up to 2-year follow-up of the direct-flow medical valve: a pilot study. *Circ Cardiovasc Interv* 2011;4:595-601.

55. Buellesfeld L, Gerckens U, Grube E. Percutaneous implantation of the first repositionable aortic valve prosthesis in a patient with severe aortic stenosis. *Catheter Cardiovasc Interv* 2008;71:579-584.

56. Figulla HR, Ferrari M. Percutaneously implantable aortic valve: the JenaValve concept evolution. *Herz* 2006;31:685-687.

57. Inoue K, Owaki T, Nakamura T, Kitamura F, Miyamoto N. Clinical application of transvenous mitral commissurotomy by a new balloon catheter. *J Thorac Cardiovasc Surg* 1984;87:394-402.

58. Pate GE, Al Zubaidi A, Chandavimol M, et al. Percutaneous closure of prosthetic paravalvular leaks: case series and review. *Catheter Cardiovasc Interv* 2006;68:528-533.

59. Pate GE, Thompson CR, Munt BI, Webb JG. Techniques for percutaneous closure of prosthetic paravalvular leaks. *Catheter Cardiovasc Interv* 2006;67:158-166.

60. Hein R, Wunderlich N, Wilson N, Sievert H. New concepts in transcatheter closure of paravalvular leaks. *Future Cardiol* 2008;4:373-378.

61. Perloff JK, Rogers WC. The mitral apparatus: functional anatomy of mitral regurgitation. *Circulation* 1972;46:227-239.

62. Maisano F, Torracca L, Oppizzi M, et al. The edge-to-edge technique: a simplified method to correct mitral insufficiency. *Eur J Cardiothorac Surg* 1998;13:240-246.

63. Bhudia SK, McCarthy P, Smedira NG, et al. Edge-to-edge (Alfieri) mitral repair results in diverse clinical settings. *Ann Thorac Surg* 2004;77:1598-1606.

64. Alfieri OMF, De Bonis M, Stefano PL, et al. The double-orifice technique in mitral valve repair: a simple solution for complex problems. *J Thorac Cardiovasc Surg* 2001;122:674-681.

65. Bach DS, Bolling SF. Improvement following correction of secondary mitral regurgitation in end-stage cardiomyopathy with mitral annuloplasty. *Am J Cardiol* 1996;78:966-969.

66. Naqvi TZ, Buchbinder M, Zarbatany D, et al. Edge-to-edge repair utilizing a percutaneous suture device in an animal model. *Cathet Cardiovasc Interv* 2007;69:525-531.

67. Silvestry FE, Rodriguez LL, Herrmann HC, et al. Echocardiographic guidance and assessment of percutaneous repair for mitral regurgitation with the Evalve MitraClip: lessons learned from EVEREST I. *J Am Soc Echocardiogr* 2007;20:1131-1140.

68. Foster E, Wasserman HS, Gray W, et al. Quantitative assessment of severity of mitral regurgitation by serial echocardiography in a multicenter clinical trial of percutaneous mitral valve repair. *Am J Cardiol* 2007;100:1577-1583.

69. Feldman T. EVEREST Registry (Endovascular Valve Edge-to-edge REpair Studies): reduction in mitral regurgitation 12 months following percutaneous mitral valve repair. *Clin Cardiol* 2007;30:416-417.

70. Herrmann HC, Kar S, Siegel R, et al. Effect of percutaneous mitral valve repair with the MitralClip on mitral valve area and gradient. *EuroIntervention* 2009;4:437-442.

71. Feldman T, Glower D. Patient selection for percutaneous mitral valve repair: insight from early clinical trial applications. *Nat Clin Pract Cardiovasc Med* 2008;5:84-90.

72. Feldman T, Foster E, Glower DG, et al, for the EVEREST II Investigators. Percutaneous repair or surgery for mitral regurgitation. *N Engl J Med* 2011;364:1395-1406.

73. Savage EB, Ferguson B Jr, DiSesa VJ. Use of mitral valve repair: analysis of contemporary United States experience reported to the Society of Thoracic Surgeons National Cardiac Database. *Ann Thorac Surg* 2003;75:820-825.

74. Webb JG, Harnek J, Munt BI, et al. Percutaneous transvenous mitral annuloplasty: initial human experience with device implantation in the coronary sinus. *Circulation* 2006;113:851-855.

75. Maselli D, Guarracino F, Chiaramonti F, et al. Percutaneous mitral annuloplasty: an anatomic study of human coronary sinus and its relation with mitral valve annulus and coronary arteries. *Circulation* 2006;114:377-380.

76. Goldberg SL, Van Bibber R, Schofer J, et al. The frequency of coronary artery compression and management using a removable mitral annuloplasty device in the coronary sinus. *J Am Coll Cardiol* 2008;51(10 Suppl B):28.

77. Bax JJ, Poldermans D. Mitral regurgitation and left ventricular dyssynchrony: implications for treatment. *Heart* 2006;92:1363-1364.

78. Kuck HK, Webb JG, Harnek J, et al. Percutaneous treatment of functional mitral regurgitation: interim EVOLUTION study results with the MONARC system. *Am J Cardiol* 2007;100(8 Suppl 1):58L.

79. Maniu CV, Patel JB, Reuter DG, et al. Acute and chronic reduction of functional mitral regurgitation in experimental heart failure by percutaneous mitral annuloplasty. *J Am Coll Cardiol* 2004;44:1652-1661.

80. Duffy SJ, Federman J, Farrington C, et al. Feasibility and short-term efficacy of percutaneous mitral annular reduction for the therapy of functional mitral regurgitation in patients with heart failure. *Catheter Cardiovasc Interv* 2006;68:205-210.

81. Siminiak T, Jerzykowska O, Kalmucki P, et al. Percutaneous trans-coronary-venous repair of functional mitral regurgitation: single-center experience with CARILLON mitral contour system. *Eur Heart J* 2008;29(abstract supplement):60.

82. Siminiak T, Hoppe UC, Schofer J, et al. Functional mitral regurgitation: percutaneous trans-coronary-venous repair mitral contour system: acute results from AMADEUS trial. *Eur Heart J* 2008;29(abstract supplement):780.

83. Sorajja PNR, Thompson J, Zehr K. A novel method of percutaneous mitral valve repair for ischemic mitral regurgitation. *JACC Cardiovasc Interv* 2008;1:663-672.

84. Burr LH, Krayenbuhl C, Sutton MS. The mitral plication suture: a new method of mitral valve repair. *J Thorac Cardiovasc Surg* 1977;73:589-595.

85. Barlow CW, Ali ZA, Lim E, Barlow JB, Wells FC. Modified technique for mitral repair without ring annuloplasty. *Ann Thorac Surg* 2003;75:298-300.

86. Heuser RR, Witzel T, Dickens D, Takeda PA. Percutaneous treatment for mitral regurgitation: the QuantumCor system. *J Interv Cardiol* 2008;21:178-182.

87. Grossi EA, Saunders PC, Woo YJ, et al. Intraoperative effects of the Coapsys annuloplasty system in a randomized evaluation (RESTOR-MV) of functional ischemic mitral regurgitation. *Ann Thorac Surg* 2005;80:1706-1711.

88. Mishra YK, Mittal S, Jaguri P, Trehan N. Coapsys mitral annuloplasty for chronic functional ischemic mitral regurgitation: 1-year results. *Ann Thorac Surg* 2006;81:42-46.

89. Pedersen WR, Block P, Leon M, et al. iCoapsys mitral valve repair system: percutaneous implantation in an animal model. *Catheter Cardiovasc Interv* 2008;72:125-131.

90. Messas E, Guerrero JL, Handschumacher MD, et al. Chordal cutting: a new therapeutic approach for ischemic mitral regurgitation. *Circulation* 2001;104:1958-1963.

91. Maisano F, Michev I, Vigano G, Alfieri O, Colombo A. Transapical mitral valve repair: chordal implantation with a suction and suture device. *Am J Cardiol* 2008;102(abstract suppl):8i.

Manifestations, Mechanisms, and Treatment of HIV-Associated Cardiovascular Disease

David C. Lange, Eric A. Secemsky, Jennifer E. Ho, and Priscilla Y. Hsue

OVERVIEW, 728

ANTIRETROVIRAL THERAPY, 728

Protease Inhibitors, 728
Nucleoside/Nucleotide Reverse Transcriptase Inhibitors, 729
Nonnucleoside Reverse Transcriptase Inhibitors, 729
Fusion Inhibitors, 729
Integrase Inhibitors, 729
Combination Medications, 729

METABOLIC EFFECTS OF HIV INFECTION AND
ANTIRETROVIRAL THERAPY, 730

Hypertension, 730
Lipodystrophy and the Metabolic Syndrome, 731

SCREENING FOR CARDIOVASCULAR DISEASE IN
HIV-POSITIVE PATIENTS, 731

HIV INFECTION AND MYOCARDIAL INFARCTION, 731

CLINICAL FEATURES OF CORONARY DISEASE IN HIV
PATIENTS, 732

Pathogenesis of Coronary Heart Disease in HIV
Infection, 732

TREATMENT OF CORONARY RISK FACTORS IN HIV
PATIENTS, 733

Myocardial Involvement in HIV, 734
Pericardial Disease in Patients with HIV Infection, 734

HIV-RELATED PULMONARY HYPERTENSION, 734

Cerebrovascular Disease, 735
Endocarditis and Other Cardiac Disease, 735

SUMMARY, 735

REFERENCES, 735

Overview

In 2008, an estimated 33 million people were living with human immunodeficiency virus (HIV) worldwide, including approximately 1.4 million people in North America.[1] The introduction of highly active antiretroviral therapy (HAART) in the mid to late 1990s led to a dramatic decrease in the rates of HIV-associated morbidity and mortality.[2] In one HIV outpatient study, the mortality rate among 1255 patients in the United States with at least one CD4+ count below 100 cells/μL declined from 29.4 to 8.8 per 100 patient-years from 1995 to the second quarter of 1997.[2] This period coincides with the initiation of protease inhibitors. Similarly, in a European cohort study of 4270 patients who had a CD4+ count below 500 cells/μL, the mortality rate fell from 23.3 to 4.1 per 100 patient-years during mid 1995 and late 1997 to early 1998.[3] These studies not only demonstrated a decrease in mortality rates among HIV patients but also showed a decline in the incidence of opportunistic infections,[2] which correlated with the intensity of the antiretroviral therapy.[3] More recent studies have continued to demonstrate improved mortality rates in the HAART era.[4-8]

With these advances in HIV treatment and subsequent improvement in life expectancy, new health concerns have arisen for HIV-infected individuals. Emerging evidence suggests that HIV-infected individuals who are successfully treated with long-term antiretroviral medications, with restoration of normal CD4+ counts and undetectable HIV viral loads, still have a shorter lifespan compared with uninfected individuals.[9,10] Of note, for HIV-positive patients with a CD4+ count above 200 cells/μL, risk for death unrelated to acquired immunodeficiency syndrome (AIDS) is greater than AIDS-related death.[11] In particular, premature cardiovascular disease has become a prominent issue in HIV patients because HIV-positive patients have increased rates of coronary atherosclerotic events and cardiovascular mortality compared with noninfected controls.[12-14] In addition, metabolic abnormalities such as hyperlipidemia, hypertension, and hyperglycemia are more common in HIV-positive individuals than in the general population. Multiple etiologies are likely to contribute to premature cardiovascular disease in the setting of HIV infection. Altered immune responses and a chronic inflammatory state resulting from HIV infection and off-target effects from antiretroviral medications have been implicated in accelerating cardiovascular disease.

Antiretroviral Therapy

Uncontrolled HIV replication leads to both increased cardiovascular risk and other non-AIDS complications.[11,15,16] HAART generally consists of a multidrug regimen that includes either a protease inhibitor, a nonnucleoside reverse transcriptase inhibitor, or a combination of the two,[5] and it represents the most common treatment regimen for suppressing HIV replication. The International AIDS Society USA Panel Guidelines recommend the initiation of HAART for all asymptomatic individuals with CD4+ counts below 350 cells/μL and "individualized" therapy for selected patients with CD4+ counts above 350 cells/μL.[17] Patients for whom early HAART should be considered include those with high cardiovascular risk, high viral loads (>100,000 copies/mL), a rapidly declining CD4+ count (>100/μL decrease per year), active hepatitis B or C infections, or the presence of HIV-associated nephropathy.[17] Whether earlier initiation of HAART at higher CD4+ counts will improve cardiovascular risk in high-risk HIV-infected individuals is not yet known.

The initial choice of HAART regimen is primarily determined by HIV genotype and drug-resistance patterns; however, drug-drug interactions and metabolic side effects should be considered in patients at high cardiovascular risk. Novel antiretroviral agents, such as integrase inhibitors and viral entry inhibitors, may have more favorable cardiovascular side-effect profiles compared with traditional HAART medications and can be considered in patients at increased cardiovascular risk.[18]

Protease Inhibitors

Protease inhibitors (PIs) are the most widely used class of antiretroviral agents used to treat HIV and are listed in Table 48-1 along with important drug-drug interactions and side effects.[19] PIs bind to the site of the HIV-1 protease enzyme and inhibit cleavage of viral polyprotein precursors into the functional proteins required for infectious HIV. This results in the formation of immature, noninfectious viral particles. PIs are associated with a wide range of side effects that include disorders of glucose and lipid metabolism, hepatotoxicity, gastrointestinal complaints, sexual dysfunction, and an increased risk of bleeding.[20] These adverse effects are frequently severe enough to cause discontinuation of therapy.[21]

TABLE 48-1 Protease Inhibitors

GENERIC NAME	CARDIAC/METABOLIC EFFECTS	COMMON ADVERSE EVENTS	IMPORTANT DRUG INTERACTIONS*
Amprenavir	Hyperglycemia, ↑TG, ↑QTc interval	Lactic acidosis, periorbital and peripheral numbness, rash, nausea, diarrhea	Lovastatin, simvastatin, bepridil
Atazanavir	↑PR interval	Lactic acidosis, hyperbilirubinemia	Proton pump inhibitors, bepridil
Darunavir/ritonavir	↑LDL, ↑TG, hyperglycemia, ↓HR, MI, fat redistribution	GI side effects, neutropenia, ↑ALT/AST	Lovastatin, simvastatin, midazolam, rifampin, sildenafil (if dosed for pulmonary HTN)
Fosamprenavir	↑Blood glucose, ↑TG	Same as with amprenavir	Flecainide, propafenone, lovastatin, simvastatin
Indinavir	Hyperglycemia, fat redistribution, MI, ↑TG, ↑QTc interval	Dry eyes, mouth, and skin; nephrolithiasis, hyperbilirubinemia, neutropenia, paronychia, vasculitis	
Lopinavir/ritonavir	↑LDL, ↑TG, hyperglycemia, weight loss, atrial fibrillation, ↑PR interval, fat redistribution, ↓HR, MI, ↑QTc interval	Pancreatitis, GI side effects common but mild	See ritonavir
Nelfinavir	Fat redistribution, hyperglycemia/hypoglycemia, ↑LDL, ↑QTc interval	Nephrolithiasis, more diarrhea than other PIs	Amiodarone quinidine, lovastatin, simvastatin, atorvastatin
Ritonavir	↑LDL, ↑TG, syncope, ↑PR interval, ↓HR, MI, ↑QTc interval	Pancreatitis, altered taste sensation	Same as for nelfinavir; bepridil, clozapine, estradiol, flecainide, methadone, propafenone
Saquinavir	Fat redistribution, hyperglycemia	Altered sense of taste	
Tipranavir/ritonavir	↑LDL, ↑TG, hyperglycemia	Rash, GI side effects, ↑ALT/AST, myalgias	Lovastatin, simvastatin, sildenafil (if dosed for pulmonary HTN)

*All PIs interact with antiarrhythmic drugs, ergots, triazolobenzodiazepines (alprazolam [Xanax], midazolam [Versed], and triazolam [Halcion]), and pan inducers of the cytochrome P450 enzymes (barbiturates, carbamazepine, ethanol, phenytoin, and rifamycins). These drugs should not be used with PIs.
ALT, alanine transaminase; AST, aspartate aminotransferase; GI, gastrointestinal; HR, heart rate; HTN, hypertension; LDL, low-density lipoprotein; MI, myocardial infarction; PI, protease inhibitor; TG, triglycerides.

In addition, because all PIs inhibit metabolism of the cytochrome (CY) P450 3A4 enzyme, they interact with many cardiac medications, as shown in Table 48-1. Rhabdomyolysis has been reported with the combination of a PI and a statin metabolized by the cytochrome P450 3A liver enzymes, such as simvastatin.[22,23]

Nucleoside/Nucleotide Reverse Transcriptase Inhibitors

Nucleoside/nucleotide reverse transcriptase inhibitors (NRTIs) are structurally defective analogues of viral nucleotides. After being incorporated into viral DNA, they prematurely terminate viral strand synthesis and inhibit viral replication. Unlike PIs, NRTIs are generally well tolerated and do not interfere with the CYP450 system. However, they do cause mitochondrial toxicity, which is expressed clinically as peripheral neuropathy, myopathy, lactic acidosis, hepatic steatosis, pancreatitis, and lipodystrophy.[24] Table 48-2 demonstrates several NRTIs, their doses, and common side effects.

Nonnucleoside Reverse Transcriptase Inhibitors

Nonnucleoside reverse transcriptase inhibitors (NNRTIs) block DNA elongation by directly binding to the reverse transcriptase enzyme.[24,25] The antiviral potency and good tolerability of NNRTIs make them a favored component of HAART regimens, particularly because toxicity and viral cross-resistance do not overlap with NRTIs. Their most frequently reported side effects are rash, elevation of liver enzymes, and fat redistribution.[24,25] Table 48-2 demonstrates several NNRTIs, their doses, and common side effects.

Fusion Inhibitors

Enfuvirtide is one of the newer classes of antiretroviral drugs known as *fusion inhibitors*,[26] and it prevents the conformational changes necessary for the fusion of virions to host cells. Because this drug is costly and requires administration by injection, enfuvirtide is generally reserved for patients who have failed other antiretroviral regimens. Maraviroc, another fusion inhibitor, blocks the CCR5 receptor of host CD4+ cells; it is dosed orally. Although short-term studies of maraviroc have shown good safety and efficacy and a generally favorable cardiovascular profile, the long-term effects of blocking the host CCR5 receptor are not known.[27]

Integrase Inhibitors

Another new class of antiretroviral medications are integrase inhibitors, such as raltegravir, which inhibits HIV-1 integrase, an important enzyme that allows for the insertion of HIV-1 viral DNA into the host cellular genome. Raltegravir has been demonstrated to be both safe and effective, although drug resistance develops relatively quickly.[28] The most common side effects of raltegravir use include headache, fatigue, and nausea, but no consistent treatment-related cardiac or metabolic changes have been reported.[28]

Combination Medications

In an effort to reduce the high pill burdens associated with several of the HAART regimens, several combination pills are now available. These combination pills include atripla (efavirenz/emtricitabine/tenofovir), combivir (zidovudine/lamivudine), epzicom (abacavir/lamivudine), trizivir (abacavir/lamivudine/zidovudine), and truvada (emtricitabine/tenofovir). The side-effect

TABLE 48-2 Nucleoside/Nucleotide Reverse Transcriptase Inhibitors and Nonnucleoside Reverse Transcriptase Inhibitors

GENERIC NAME	CARDIAC/METABOLIC EFFECTS	COMMON ADVERSE EVENTS
NRTIs		
Abacavir (ABC)	↑TG, MI, fat redistribution	Hypersensitivity reaction in about 4%
Didanosine (ddI)	Hyperglycemia	Peripheral neuropathy in 15%, optic neuritis, rare pancreatitis
Emtricitabine	↑TG, hyperglycemia	Stopping may exacerbate hepatitis B
Entecavir	Hyperglycemia, peripheral edema	↑ALT/AST, headache, fatigue, dizziness, GI upset, hematuria
Lamivudine (3TC)	Fat redistribution	Generally well tolerated
Stavudine (d4T)	None	Peripheral neuropathy; higher risk in patients with CD4+ counts <50 cells/μL
Tenofovir	↑TG, hyperglycemia	Nausea; generally well tolerated
Zalcitabine (ddC)	None	High rate of peripheral neuropathy, oral ulcers; rarely used because of toxicity
Ziduvidine (AZT)	None	Nausea, headache, fatigue, anemia, neutropenia, neuropathy, myopathy
Combination NRTIs		
ABC/3TC	Same as ABC	Same as ABC
AZT/3TC	None	Same as AZT
AZT/3TC/ABC	Same as AZT and ABC	Same as AZT and ABC
Efavirenz/emtricitabine/tenofovir	Same as efavirenz, emtricitabine, and tenofovir	Same as efavirenz, emtricitabine, and tenofovir singly
Emtricitabine/tenofovir	Same as emtricitabine and tenofovir	Same as emtricitabine and tenofovir
NNRTIs		
Delavirdine	Fat redistribution	Rash, ↑ALT/AST
Efavirenz	↑TG, hyperglycemia	Rash, CNS symptoms (insomnia)
Etravirine	Hyperglycemia, ↑LDL, ↑TG, HTN	Rash, nausea, ↑ALT/AST, neuropathy
Nevirapine	None	Rash, hepatitis

ALT, alanine transaminase; AST, aspartate aminotransferase; CNS, central nervous system; GI, gastrointestinal; HTN, hypertension; LDL, low-density lipoprotein; MI, myocardial infarction; NNRTI, nonnucleoside reverse transcriptase inhibitors; NRTIs, nucleoside/nucleotide reverse transcriptase inhibitors; TG, triglycerides.

profiles of these medications generally follow those of the individual components. Retrospective studies have shown increased durability of HAART regimens that contain combination pills, presumably because of decreased pill burden, improved side-effect profiles, and increased medication compliance.[29]

Metabolic Effects of HIV Infection and Antiretroviral Therapy

HIV disease and antiretroviral therapy have been associated with many different metabolic effects that include hyperlipidemia, insulin resistance, and hypertension. However, the relationships among HIV infection, antiretroviral therapy, and cardiac risk factors are complex and remain poorly understood. In untreated HIV patients, lower CD4+ counts are associated with lower total blood cholesterol, lower high-density lipoprotein (HDL) cholesterol, and higher triglyceride levels.[30] Independent of changes in body composition, PIs induce hyperlipidemia and insulin resistance in HIV patients.[31] Different PIs appear to have differing effects on lipid metabolism. For example, ritonavir raises triglycerides and slightly lowers HDL cholesterol, but it has no effect on low-density lipoprotein (LDL) cholesterol.[32,33] Indinavir has no effect on lipoproteins but induces insulin resistance.[34] Lopinavir/ritonavir increases triglycerides but has no effect on LDL or HDL cholesterol, nor does it affect insulin resistance.[35] It should be noted that these studies were intended to isolate the side effects of the drugs; they were relatively short in duration and involved HIV-negative subjects. Atazanavir most likely has the least effect on triglyceride levels.[36] The newer classes of antiretroviral medications, namely integrase inhibitors and CCR5 inhibitors, do not appear to be associated with significant dyslipidemia.

In 2003, a multicenter AIDS cohort study included HIV-infected patients treated for longer periods; the results of this study help to provide a clearer picture of lipid changes associated with HIV disease and treatment.[37] In this study, 50 HIV patients had blood samples available from before they became HIV positive, before HAART was initiated, at a mean of 7.8 years later, and at four follow-up visits during treatment. As shown in Figure 48-1, total and LDL cholesterol decreased after the onset of HIV disease but returned to preinfection levels or higher with HAART. However, HDL cholesterol levels decreased markedly after the onset of HIV and did not recover. Triglycerides were measured once during treatment and were elevated.

Another study of the effects of PIs on lipids in HIV patients showed that these drugs increase total and LDL cholesterol by 20% to 60% and may more than double triglyceride levels.[38] Replacement of a PI with an alternative class of medication—including an NNRTI such as nevirapine or efavirenz or an NRTI such as abacavir—has been shown to reduce LDL cholesterol and triglyceride levels and to increase HDL cholesterol.[39]

Hypertension

Hypertension has been reported in up to one third of HIV patients.[40,41] Some studies link NNRTIs and PIs to hypertension,[42,43] whereas other studies show no association.[40] In general, hypertension associated with HIV appears to be linked to insulin resistance and the metabolic syndrome.[41] Unfortunately, studies that examine long-term effects of HIV- or HAART-associated hypertension are lacking. Thus, most guidelines recommend aggressive management of traditional cardiovascular risk factors, including hypertension; however, hypertension is not currently mentioned as a treatment consideration prior to initiating, nor

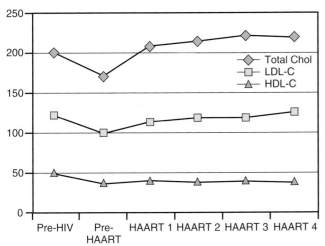

FIGURE 48-1 This figure shows lipid levels in HIV-infected men before HIV seroconversion (*pre-HIV*), before starting highly active antiretroviral therapy (*Pre-HAART*), first visit after starting HAART (*HAART 1*), second visit after HAART (*HAART 2*), third visit after HAART (*HAART 3*), and fourth visit after HAART (*HAART 4*). The mean interval between the pre-HIV measurement and the pre-HAART measurement was 7.8 years. Between pre-HAART and the first post-HAART measurement, the interval was 1.3 years; the subsequent mean intervals between measurements were 0.5, 2.1, and 0.6 years. Total and low-density lipoprotein cholesterol (*LDL-C*) levels increased during HAART but were depressed before treatment compared with the values before HIV infection. HDL-C, high-density lipoprotein cholesterol; Total Chol, total cholesterol. (*Data from Riddler SA, Smit E, Cole SR, et al. Impact of HIV infection and HAART on serum lipids in men. JAMA 2003;289:2978-2982.*)

as an indication for changing, a HAART regimen for a given patient.

Lipodystrophy and the Metabolic Syndrome

HIV-associated fat redistribution, also called *lipodystrophy* or *lipoatrophy*, is characterized by a selective loss of fat from the face and extremities with or without an accumulation of fat in the neck, dorsocervical region, abdomen, and trunk.[39,44] Lipodystrophy in HIV patients is associated with metabolic abnormalities such as insulin resistance, impaired glucose tolerance, elevated triglycerides, low HDL cholesterol, and hypertension.[45,46]

Lipodystrophy becomes clinically evident in 20% to 35% of patients after 1 to 2 years of combination HAART.[47] The type and duration of antiretroviral therapy are strongly associated with the development and severity of lipodystrophy. Combination therapy with a PI and two NRTIs, particularly stavudine with didanosine, is most likely to induce severe lipodystrophy.[39] Exercise training, either alone[48] or in combination with metformin,[49] has been reported to improve body composition in patients with lipodystrophy. Injection of synthetic fillers has been reported to improve cosmetic appearances in HIV patients,[50] but it does not ameliorate the metabolic effects. The use of stavudine and lopinavir/ritonavir was associated with metabolic syndrome in a cross-sectional study of HIV-infected individuals.[51] Another study showed that initiation of HAART in treatment-naive HIV patients was associated with development of metabolic syndrome, thereby increasing cardiovascular risk.[52]

Screening for Cardiovascular Disease in HIV-Positive Patients

Although several multivariate models have been developed to estimate the probability of coronary heart disease (CHD) in the general population, these models have not been validated in patients with HIV infection. The most widely used model, the Framingham risk score, appears to underestimate CHD risk in HIV patients who are smokers.[53] Developing a unique model for HIV-positive patients is difficult, because it is not clear which HIV-specific risk factors or exposures are relevant to the development of CHD. One HIV-specific CHD risk prediction model from the Data Collection on Adverse Events of Anti-HIV Drugs (DAD) study group incorporated PI exposure with traditional CHD risk factors. This model appeared to be reasonably accurate in preliminary studies. For example, among the 33,594 person-years observed in this study, 157 CHD events occurred; the DAD equation predicted 153 events, and the area under the receiver-operating characteristics curve was 0.78 (95% confidence interval [CI], 0.75 to 0.82).[53] The Infectious Diseases Society of America/HIV Medicine Association recommends checking fasting lipid panels and fasting glucose levels before and within 4 to 6 weeks after starting HAART; it also recommends routine measurements of body weight and changes in body shape.[54]

As is the case with multivariate CHD risk-prediction models, the sensitivity and specificity of exercise and pharmacologic stress testing are not well established in the HIV-positive patient population. In general, use of this risk-stratification tool currently follows guidelines for the general population. Similarly, further work is needed to clarify the role of surrogate markers of CHD such as carotid artery intima-media thickness (carotid IMT), inflammatory biomarkers such as high-sensitivity C-reactive protein (hs-CRP), and apolipoprotein B100, as these tests have not been validated in the early detection of CHD in HIV patients.[55] One study that evaluated HIV-infected individuals found that both elevated CRP and HIV were independently associated with increased risk of myocardial infarction (MI).[56]

HIV Infection and Myocardial Infarction

The first cases of coronary disease in two young HIV-infected men who received PIs were reported in 1998.[57,58] Whether the rate of coronary events is actually increased in HIV patients and whether this increase is mediated by HAART are areas of present controversy.

A retrospective study of 36,766 HIV patients treated at Veterans Affairs facilities between 1993 and 2001 found no increase in cardiovascular or cerebrovascular events in patients who received HAART during a mean follow-up period of 40 months.[59] Similarly, in a meta-analysis of 30 randomized clinical trials, the incidence of MI was not higher in patients receiving PIs compared with NRTIs; however, the duration of treatment was only 1 year, and the number of events was small.[60]

However, in the HIV Outpatient Study (HOPS), the frequency of MI increased after the introduction of PIs, and MI occurred in 19 of 3247 patients taking PIs but in only 2 of 2425 not taking PIs.[61] The DAD study group prospectively followed 23,468 HIV patients for a mean duration of 1.6 years, with an average exposure to antiretroviral therapy of 1.9 years, and showed that the risk of MI increased with longer exposure to combination antiretroviral therapy.[62] In particular, exposure to protease inhibitors for greater than 6 years was associated with an increased risk of MI, a finding which was only partially attenuated after accounting for dyslipidemia.[63] Additional data from the DAD study showed that specific agents, such as the protease inhibitors indinavir and lopinavir/ritonavir, and NRTIs, including didanosine and abacavir, were associated with a higher risk of MI in their cohort.[64]

In the French Hospital Database on HIV, MI was diagnosed in 60 of 34,976 patients during a median follow-up of 33 months.[65] In this study, patients taking PIs had a significantly higher risk of MI compared with patients not taking PIs, with a relative risk of 2.56; the relative risk for those taking PIs for 30 months or more compared with those taking PIs for less than 18 months was 3.6. In the Kaiser Permanente Medical Care Program of Northern California database, 72 coronary events, including 47 MI events, were documented in 4159 HIV patients during a median follow-up of 4.1 years.[66] Median exposure time to PIs was 2.8 years. The coronary event rate was similar in patients taking and not taking PIs; however, HIV-infected patients had a rate of 6.5, compared with 3.8 events per 1000 patient-years in non–HIV-infected controls. Abacavir-related cardiovascular toxicity has been the source of recent controversy. Abacavir appeared to increase the risk of MI in some observational studies but not in others.[67,68] The discrepancies in study findings are most likely due to differences in study design, short follow-up times, lack of control groups, and limited data on HAART.[69]

By contrast, the Strategies for Management of Anti-Retroviral Therapy (SMART) study, which involved 5472 HIV-infected patients randomized to a viral suppression strategy (continuous HAART) versus a drug-conservation strategy (intermittent HAART), demonstrated that patients assigned to continuous HAART had a decreased risk of fatal or nonfatal cardiovascular disease compared with those on intermittent HAART.[16] In addition, the initiation of HAART in treatment-naive patients resulted in a dramatic improvement in endothelial function, suggesting that in the short term, HAART therapy may actually decrease cardiovascular risk.[71]

In aggregate, these studies suggest possible short-term beneficial effects from HAART related to suppression of viral replication, and these are counterbalanced by long-term detrimental cardiovascular effects related to insulin resistance and dyslipidemia. These data provide additional support for the hypothesis that HIV itself is mechanistically associated with increased CHD risk. These studies suggest that the rate of MI is higher in HIV patients who take PIs and that the risk increases as the duration of treatment lengthens. Although the coronary event rates in these studies are relatively low, risk may prove to be higher as the HIV population ages. Additional studies are needed with longer-term follow-up to further define the mechanism underlying HIV medications and CV risk.

Clinical Features of Coronary Disease in HIV Patients

The clinical features of 334 patients, 225 (67%) of whom presented with acute MI, were analyzed from seven different reports and are shown in Table 48-3.[21,72-78] Only 31 (9%) of these patients were women. The average age of the patients with HIV and MI was approximately 8 to 11 years younger than in HIV-negative patients with MI, evidence that further supports the role of HIV or its treatment in the pathogenesis of MI. The proportion of patients receiving PIs ranged from 49% to 71%. In each of these studies, more than half of the patients smoked cigarettes at the time of their coronary event.

When they were reported, mean HDL cholesterol levels were very low in each of the three studies, ranging from 28 to 35 mg/dL.[73,74,78] These levels were significantly lower than those of HIV-positive patients without coronary disease[74] and lower

than non-HIV controls with coronary disease.[73,78] Mean LDL cholesterol levels were lower in HIV-positive coronary patients than in non–HIV-positive coronary controls in one study[73] but not in another.[78] In the French cohort, LDL cholesterol levels were much higher in the HIV patients with coronary disease than in those without.[74]

As might be expected in a younger population, single-vessel disease is common,[73-76,78] and the Thrombolysis in Myocardial Infarction (TIMI) risk score[79] is low if an acute coronary syndrome is present.[78] Thus, HIV-infected patients tend to have good outcomes after coronary events. Only nine in-hospital deaths (4.8%) occurred among 189 patients in the studies included in Table 48-3 that reported follow-up.[73,74,76-78]

Coronary angioplasty or stenting has often been performed in these patients, and the immediate results have been excellent; however, the restenosis rate appears to be higher than that in patients without HIV infection.[73,78] This may be related to differences in pathologic features of atherosclerosis in HIV-positive patients, as will be discussed below. In one study, restenosis developed in 15 of 29 HIV-positive patients compared with 3 of 21 non–HIV-positive controls (52% vs. 14%) undergoing percutaneous coronary intervention in the era before the drug-eluting stent (DES).[78] Similarly, in another study, 6 of 14 HIV patients had restenosis that required target vessel revascularization, compared with 4 of 38 uninfected controls (43% vs. 11%).[73] Restenosis rates are higher after both balloon angioplasty and stenting, and HIV-positive patients should be considered for DES, given lower rates of in-stent restenosis with DES compared with bare-metal stents in HIV-positive patients.[80] Compared with controls at 1 year of follow-up, recurrent acute coronary syndromes were more frequent among HIV-infected individuals.[81]

Few data are available describing outcomes following coronary artery bypass surgery (CABG) in HIV-positive patients. In one small series of 37 HIV patients who were followed after coronary bypass surgery, event-free survival was 81% at 3 years.[82] Of note, the median age of the bypass patients in this study was only 44 years. In another study to evaluate individuals treated in the Kaiser health system, HIV patients undergoing cardiothoracic surgery had fewer complications than uninfected controls (5.3% vs. 26.3%).[83] There have been no large-scale studies of HIV patients who were referred for a bypass grafting study with long-term follow-up, and no studies have reported graft patency rates after coronary bypass in HIV patients.

Pathogenesis of Coronary Heart Disease in HIV Infection

Compared with the general population, atherosclerosis in HIV patients seems to represent a pathologically distinct entity, although autopsy results vary. One autopsy study demonstrated accelerated atherosclerosis in young HIV-1 infected patients with

TABLE 48-3	Clinical Features of Coronary Heart Disease in HIV Patients						
STUDY	PATIENTS (N)	AGE (YEARS)	CURRENT SMOKING	CD4+ COUNT (CELLS/μL)	PI USE	MI ON PRESENTATION	SINGLE-VESSEL DISEASE
David et al[72]	16	43*	81%	234 (74 to 731)*	69%	8/16 (50%)	NR
Matetzky et al[73]	24	47 ± 9	58%	318 ± 210	71%	All MI	5/21 (24%)
Escaut et al[74]	17	46 ± 6	71%	272 ± 185	65%	11/17 (65%)	9/17 (53%)
Mehta et al[75]	129†	42 ± 10	NR	313 ± 209	NR	109/129 (77%)	26/76 (34%)
Ambrose et al[76]	51	48 ± 9	55%	426 ± 290	59%	34/51 (67%)	21/45 (47%)
Varriale et al[77]	29	46 ± 10	55%	>500 in 18/29	66%	All MI	NR
Hsue et al[78]	68	50 ± 8	68%	341 (3 to 4360)*	49%	37/68 (54%)	20/56 (36%)

*Median value; all other values are means.
†Patients were drawn from 25 previous reports.
HIV, human immunodeficiency virus; MI, myocardial infarction; NR, not reported; PI, protease inhibitor.

lesions indicative of both "typical" atherosclerotic CHD and a vasculopathy similar to that seen in patients after cardiac transplant.[84] Another autopsy study revealed that HIV-associated atherosclerosis was characterized by unusual proliferation of smooth muscle cells and elastic fibers that formed endoluminal protrusions in a diffuse circumferential pattern.[75] This may contribute to the higher rates of restenosis seen in HIV-positive patients.

The underlying mechanism of early atherosclerosis in HIV disease is likely multifactorial; direct viral effects, CD4+ suppression,[14,86] the use of HAART and associated metabolic changes,[59-62,65-67] and host immune responses all potentially play a role.[87-89]

Treatment of Coronary Risk Factors in HIV Patients

Currently, there is no direct evidence that treating risk factors for CHD in HIV-positive patients improves outcomes, although it appears reasonable to extrapolate from observations on the treatment of traditional risk factors in non–HIV-positive patients.

Cigarette smoking is one of the most common and modifiable risk factors in patients with HIV infection; the prevalence of cigarette smoking in HIV-positive patients has been reported to be as high as 70% to 80% in some areas,[90] and compared with other smokers, HIV-positive patients are less likely to have contemplated quitting.[90] Different treatments that have been tested in pilot studies of HIV-infected smokers include interventions led by nurses[91] and the provision of cellular telephones to low-income, HIV-infected smokers to facilitate counseling.[92] Cigarette smoking is implicated in many complications of HIV,[90] including atherosclerosis and pulmonary disease, and it should be a major focus of attention by physicians who treat HIV patients.

Regarding the evaluation and management of HAART-related hyperlipidemia, the Infectious Diseases Society of America (IDSA) and the Adult AIDS Clinical Trials Group (AACTG) have developed specific guidelines[93] based largely on the National Cholesterol Education Program Adult Treatment Panel III (NCEP ATP III) guidelines. These guidelines call for individualized cholesterol targets based on the patient's Framingham 10-year risk assessment.[94] A general algorithm for the treatment of hyperlipidemia in HIV patients is shown in Figure 48-2.

It is important to keep specific drug-drug interactions in mind when initiating lipid-lowering therapy in HIV-positive patients. This is especially true in patients on PIs and NNRTIs, because both can interact with the CYP450 pathway. In general, all PIs inhibit CYP3A4, as does the NNRTI delavirdine. However, other NNRTIs, including nevirapine and efavirenz, induce the CYP3A4 enzyme. Because pravastatin is not metabolized by CYP3A4, it is a first-line agent for LDL lowering in HIV patients, including those on HAART. Conversely, both simvastatin and lovastatin are contraindicated in the setting of PI use, because their serum levels increase dramatically in this setting, and cases of rhabdomyolysis and death have been reported.[95] Acceptable first-line alternatives to pravastatin include atorvastatin and rosuvastatin, which may be used at lower doses in HIV patients, because serum levels appear to be increased to a lesser degree than those of simvastatin or lovastatin.[96,97] Fluvastatin is metabolized by CYP2C9 and can be used as a second-line agent.[93]

Fibrates, such as gemfibrozil or micronized fenofibrate, are the treatment of choice for hypertriglyceridemia in HIV-positive patients. Dosing for gemfibrozil is typically 600 mg twice daily, and micronized fenofibrate is given at doses of 54 to 160 mg daily. Treatment is recommended for triglyceride levels that exceed 500 mg/dL.[93] Niacin is not recommended in patients with concurrent PI use or in the presence of lipodystrophy, because it can cause or worsen insulin resistance.[93] Bile-sequestering resins are not recommended for use in HIV-positive patients.[93] Ezetimibe is effective as second-line therapy when added to maximally tolerated doses of lipid-lowering theapy.[98] When used as a single agent, ezetimibe has modest lipid-lowering activity.[99] Omega-3 fatty acid supplementation has been shown to be both safe and effective in lowering triglycerides in HIV-positive patients on HAART[100,101]; however, some studies have shown an increase in LDL cholesterol.[100] It is unclear whether this increased LDL attenuates any cardiovascular benefit that would otherwise be derived from these supplements.[100] An algorithm for management of elevated triglycerides is shown in Figure 48-2.

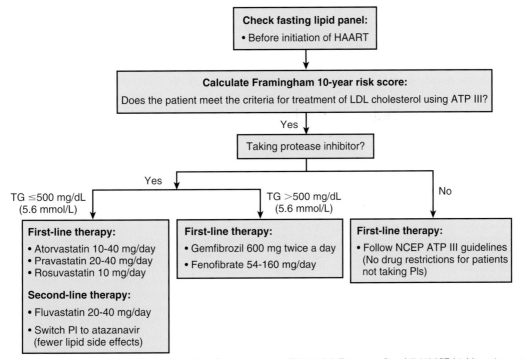

FIGURE 48-2 Algorithm for management of dyslipidemia in HIV-infected patients. ATP III, Adult Treatment Panel III; HAART, highly active antiretroviral therapy; LDL, low-density lipoprotein; NCEP, National Cholesterol Education Program; PI, protease inhibitor; TG, triglyceride.

Hypertriglyceridemia is often accompanied by the other components of the metabolic syndrome: low HDL cholesterol, increased remnant lipoproteins, small LDL particle size, abdominal obesity, hypertension, insulin resistance, and glucose intolerance (a proinflammatory state and a prothrombotic state).[102] The primary treatment target for the metabolic syndrome is obesity, and the recommended measures include diet and exercise.[103] Even modest reductions in body weight improve dyslipidemia, hypertension, glucose intolerance, and levels of inflammatory and thrombotic markers[103]; thus weight loss is likely to be beneficial in reducing cardiovascular risk among HIV-infected individuals who are obese.

As mentioned above, hypertension is common among patients receiving HAART. Commonly used antihypertensive agents—angiotensin-converting enzyme (ACE) inhibitors, aldosterone receptor blockers (ARBs), β-blockers, and thiazide diuretics—can all be safely used with most HAART regimens. However, many of the dihydropyridine and nondihydropyridine calcium channel blockers (CCBs) are metabolized by the CYP450 system; thus these medications should be used with caution in patients on PIs.[1] Finally, as with HIV-negative patients, primary prevention of coronary disease using aspirin therapy in patients deemed appropriate according to American Heart Association (AHA) guidelines can be considered.

Myocardial Involvement in HIV

The HIV virus has been recognized as an important cause of dilated cardiomyopathy (DCM). The diagnosis of HIV-related DCM carries a very poor prognosis, with a mortality hazard ratio of 4.0 compared with uninfected controls with idiopathic DCM.[104] Myocarditis and HIV-1 infection are the most-studied causes of DCM in HIV disease,[105] but nutritional deficiencies, autoimmune factors, immune activation, HAART toxicity, and coinfection with other viruses, including coxsackievirus B3 and cytomegalovirus (CMV), also seem to play a role.[106]

Before the advent of antiretroviral therapy, global left ventricular (LV) dysfunction was detected by echocardiography in 15% of HIV patients who were selected randomly in one study.[107] In almost all cases, myocardial biopsy revealed myocarditis with cardiotropic viral infection.[108] In autopsy studies of patients with HIV, myocarditis was identified in over 50% of the 71 patients evaluated, and biventricular dilation was present in 10% of cases.[109]

Zidovudine—or azidothymidine, better known as AZT—may cause mitochondrial myopathy in skeletal muscles, providing a possible link to involvement of myocardial muscle.[110] Studies performed on transgenic mice suggest that AZT is associated with diffuse destruction of cardiac mitochondrial ultrastructures and also with inhibition of cardiac mitochondrial DNA replication.[111] Clinical studies on AZT have been mixed and show both association[112] and no association with LV dysfunction.[113,114]

Many organisms—such as herpes simplex virus,[115] CMV, *Mycobacterium tuberculosis, Mycobacterium avium intracellulare,*[116] *Cryptococcus neoformans,*[117] *Toxoplasma gondii,*[118] and *Histoplasma capsulatum*—may cause pericarditis and myocarditis in HIV-infected individuals. In one autopsy series, cardiac toxoplasmosis was diagnosed at autopsy in 21 (12%) of 182 of HIV-infected patients.[119] In another autopsy series performed before the introduction of HAART, myocarditis was documented in 40% to 52% of patients who died of AIDS.[120] In more than 80% of these patients, no specific etiologic factor was found, whereas the remaining cases were attributable to the above-mentioned infectious agents.[120]

The introduction of HAART seems to influence the course of HIV-associated DCM, with a decreasing rate of mortality from heart failure. In a study performed in 1999 that involved 105 ambulatory HIV patients, the prevalence of myocardial systolic dysfunction was low (3%), and none of the patients developed end-stage DCM.[119] A decrease in the prevalence of global cardiac involvement has been shown in a retrospective study that compared HIV-positive patients treated with HAART with those treated with NRTIs.[121] An echocardiographic study of contemporary asymptomatic HIV-infected individuals showed that diastolic dysfunction and LV mass index were independently associated with HIV infection.[122] In another echocardiographic study of HIV-infected individuals, a high prevalence of systolic and diastolic dysfunction and pulmonary hypertension as noted.[123]

Treatment of DCM in HIV patients has not been specifically studied; however, this is an area of active research in the ongoing HIV-HEART study.[124] By extrapolation of studies from HIV-negative patients, diuresis, afterload reduction with ACE inhibitors or ARBs for patients who are ACE-inhibitor intolerant, β-blocker therapy, aldosterone antagonists, hydralazine and nitrates for select patients, and implantable cardioverter-defibrillator therapy and/or cardiac resynchronization therapy would appear to be beneficial, although these interventions have not been studied specifically in the HIV-infected patient population. Discontinuation of possible contributing substances—such as alcohol, cocaine, methamphetamines, and NRTI medication, as mentioned above—should be considered. Only a few cases of DCM have been reported in the literature related to the use of LV-assist devices[125] or heart transplant in HIV-infected individuals.[126]

Pericardial Disease in Patients with HIV Infection

Pericarditis in HIV-infected patients may occur with large effusions and not infrequently with cardiac tamponade.[127-129] The incidence of pericardial effusion in patients with asymptomatic AIDS (defined as patients with CD4+ <200 cells/μL) was 11% per year before the introduction of HAART.[129] The survival of AIDS patients with effusion was significantly shorter than the survival of those without effusion. In contrast, contemporary studies of HIV patients show that the prevalence of pericardial effusion is much lower.[130] The pathogenesis of pericardial effusion in HIV-positive patients is unclear. Case reports have described various neoplastic and infectious comorbidities that include Kaposi sarcoma,[127] bacterial pericarditis,[128] lymphoma,[131] mycobacteria,[132-134] and CMV.[135] However, the patients studied in these case reports were generally inpatients hospitalized for acute illness and may not represent the majority of HIV-positive patients with pericardial effusions, many of whom are asymptomatic.

In HIV patients, culture of pericardial fluid is often unrevealing. Case reports of pathogens such as *Mycobacterium tuberculosis,*[132-134] *Staphylococcus,*[136,137] *Cryptococcus neoformans,*[138] and herpes simplex[139] as causes of pericarditis are isolated. Treatment and evaluation of effusion in the HIV-positive patient are similar to those of noninfected subjects and involve echocardiography and pericardiocentesis, if indicated.

HIV-Related Pulmonary Hypertension

The incidence of HIV-associated symptomatic pulmonary hypertension before the advent of HAART was 1% to 2%.[140] However, the prevalence of asymptomatic elevations in pulmonary arterial systolic pressures (PASPs), as assessed by echocardiography, may in fact be much higher. A recent study found PASPs greater than 30 mm Hg in roughly 35% of HIV-positive patients, compared with 7.7% in noninfected controls.[141] HIV was the sole risk factor for pulmonary arterial hypertension (PAH) in 82% of HIV-infected patients, indicating that this association may be largely independent of other secondary causes of PAH.[142] Additionally, HIV-associated PAH carries higher mortality rates and follows a more rapidly progressive disease course (median survival rate approximately 6 months) when compared with PAH in those without HIV.[143]

The pathogenesis of HIV-associated pulmonary hypertension remains unclear and is likely multifactorial. Contributing factors probably include elevated levels of endothelin-1, a potent vasoconstrictor—which may be mediated by HIV proteins, including glycoprotein 120[144]—increased circulation of inflammatory markers,[145] and autoimmunity.[146]

Treatment of HIV-associated PAH, including the role of HAART, remains unclear. The role of pulmonary vasodilators has not been well studied, although one uncontrolled study showed improvement in clinical measures of heart failure and hemodynamics in HIV-positive patients on bosentan.[147] The recommended dosage of bosentan, if used in patients on a PI, is 62.5 mg daily or every other day, rather than the usual dosing of 125 mg twice daily. To date, there have been no studies describing the use of selective endothelin receptor antagonists (ambrisentan or sitaxsentan) in the setting of HIV, and there have been no controlled trials of sildenafil in HIV-associated PAH. Small prospective studies have shown hemodynamic improvement with the use of prostacyclin analogs in HIV-associated PAH.[148] Finally, treatment of HIV-associated PAH with HAART was not associated with an improvement in hemodynamic parameters in a retrospective analysis of 77 consecutive patients.[149]

Cerebrovascular Disease

The prevalence of ischemic stroke and intracranial hemorrhage is relatively low in HIV-positive patients, in spite of the fact that up to 40% of AIDS patients appear to have some neurologic complications.[150] One cohort study estimated the prevalence of cerebrovascular disease to be 1.9%, with an annual incidence of 216 per 100,000 person-years. Cerebrovascular disease appears to be more common in later stages of infection and in poorer immunologic states.[151] The DAD study results showed an incidence rate of 5.7 per 1000 person-years for the combined endpoint of cardiovascular and cerebrovascular disease events, with an increased risk with longer HAART exposure, although HAART did not change the risk of cerebrovascular disease in another study.[152,153]

Endocarditis and Other Cardiac Disease

HIV does not appear to modify the risk of bacterial endocarditis, and rates in HIV-infected patients are similar to those in cohorts with similar risk profiles. The diagnosis and management of bacterial endocarditis in HIV patients do not differ from that of uninfected patients.[154] Cardiac malignancies, including Kaposi sarcoma and malignant lymphoma, are quite rare in HIV patients.[106] Finally, it has been reported that many HIV-positive patients have prolonged QTc intervals, a finding that may be associated with myocarditis, cardiomyopathy, autonomic neuropathy, and use of PIs.[106]

Summary

As the number of HIV-infected adults increases, and as their life expectancy continues to increase, cardiovascular complications specific to HIV-infected individuals will represent an increasingly important health issue. Although studies on these issues are ongoing, physicians should remain aware of the possibility of HIV-associated cardiovascular complications in their patients with HIV infection, especially atherosclerosis, and physicians should treat all risk factors aggressively.

REFERENCES

1. UNAids Global Facts and Figures. Available at www.unaids.org/en/media/unaids/contentassets/dataimport/pub/factsheet/2009/20091124_fs_global_en.pdf. Accessed June 3, 2012.
2. Palella FJ Jr, Delaney KM, Moorman AC, et al. Declining morbidity and mortality among patients with advanced human immunodeficiency virus infection. N Engl J Med 1998;338:853-860.
3. Mocroft A, Vella S, Benfield TL, et al. Changing patterns of mortality across Europe in patients infected with HIV-1. Lancet 1998;352:1725-1730.
4. Mocroft A, Ledergerber B, Katlama C, et al. Decline in the AIDS and death rates in the EuroSIDA study: an observational study. Lancet 2003;362:22-29.
5. Palella FJ Jr, Baker RK, Moorman AC, et al. Mortality in the highly active antiretroviral therapy era: changing causes of death and disease in the HIV outpatient study. J Acquir Immune Defic Syndr 2006;43:27-34.
6. Aldaz P, Castilla J, Moreno-Iribas C, et al. Trends in mortality and causes of death among persons with HIV infection 1985-2004 [in Spanish]. Enferm Infecc Microbiol Clin 2007;25:5-10.
7. Jensen-Fangel S, Pedersen L, Pedersen C, et al. Low mortality in HIV-infected patients starting highly active antiretroviral therapy: a comparison with the general population. AIDS 2004;18:89-97.
8. The Antiretroviral Therapy Cohort Collaboration. Mortality of HIV-infected patients starting potent antiretroviral therapy: comparison with the general population in nine industrialized countries. Int J Epidemiol 2009;38:1624-1633.
9. The Antiretroviral Therapy Cohort Collaboration. Life expectancy of individuals on combination antiretroviral therapy in high-income countries: a collaborative analysis of 14 cohort studies. Lancet 2008;372:293-299.
10. Bhaskaran K, Hamouda O, Sannes M, et al. CASCADE Collaboration. Changes in the risk of death after HIV seroconversion compared with mortality in the general population. JAMA 2008;300:51-59.
11. Lau B, Gange SJ, Moore RD. Risk of non–AIDS-related mortality may exceed risk of AIDS-related mortality among individuals enrolling into care with CD4+ counts greater than 200 cells/mm³. J Acquir Immune Defic Syndr 2007;44:179-187.
12. Holmberg SD, Moorman AC, Williamson JM, et al. Protease inhibitors and cardiovascular outcomes in patients with HIV-1. Lancet 2002;360:1747-1748.
13. Friis-Møller N, Sabin CA, Weber R, et al. Combination antiretroviral therapy and the risk of myocardial infarction. N Engl J Med 2003;349:1993-2003.
14. Hsue PY, Lo JC, Franklin A, et al. Progression of atherosclerosis as assessed by carotid intima-media thickness in patients with HIV infection. Circulation 2004;109:1603-1608.
15. Baker JV, Peng G, Rapkin J, et al. CD4+ count and risk of non-AIDS diseases following initial treatment for HIV infection. AIDS 2008;22:841-848.
16. El-Sadr WM, Lundgren JD, Neaton JD, et al. Strategies for Management of Antiretroviral Therapy (SMART) Study Group. CD4+ count–guided interruption of antiretroviral treatment. N Engl J Med 2006;355:2283-2296.
17. Hammer SM, Eron JJ, Reiss P, et al. Antiretroviral treatment of adult HIV infection: 2008 recommendations of the International AIDS Society–USA panel. JAMA 2008;300:555-570.
18. Stein JH, Hadigan CM, Brown TT, et al. Prevention strategies for cardiovascular disease in HIV-infected patients. Circulation 2008;118:e54-e60.
19. Hsue PY, Waters DD. What a cardiologist needs to know about patients with HIV infection. Circulation 2005;112:3947-3957.
20. Wynn GH, Zapor MJ, Smith BH, et al. Med-psych drug-drug interactions update: antiretrovirals. Part 1: overview, history, and focus on protease inhibitors. Psychosomatics 2004;45:262-270.
21. d'Arminio Monforte A, Lepri AC, Rezza G, et al. Insights into the reasons for discontinuation of the first highly active antiretroviral therapy (HAART) regimen in a cohort of antiretroviral-naïve patients. I.CO.N.A. Study Group. Italian Cohort of Antiretroviral-Naïve Patients. AIDS 2000;14:499-507.
22. Fichtenbaum CJ, Gerber JG, Rosenkranz SL. Pharmacokinetic interactions between protease inhibitors and statins in HIV seronegative volunteers: ACTG Study A5047. AIDS 2002;16:569-577.
23. Hare CB, Vu MP, Grunfeld C. Simvastatin-nelfinavir interaction implicated in rhabdomyolysis and death. Clin Infect Dis 2002;35:E111-E112.
24. Zapor MJ, Cozza KL, Wynn GH, et al. Med-psych drug-drug interactions update: antiretrovirals, part 2: focus on non-protease inhibitor antiretrovirals (NRTIs, NNRTIs and fusion inhibitors). Psychosomatics 2004;45:524-535.
25. Balzarini J. Current status of the non-nucleoside reverse transcriptase inhibitors of human immunodeficiency virus type 1. Curr Top Med Chem 2004;4:921-944.
26. Hardy H, Skolnick PR. Enfuvirtide, a new fusion inhibitor for therapy of human immunodeficiency virus type 1. Pharmacotherapy 2004;24:198-211.
27. Stephenson J. Researchers buoyed by novel HIV drugs: will expand drug arsenal against resistant virus. JAMA 2007;297(4):1535-1536.
28. Hicks C, Gulick R. Raltegravir: the first HIV type 1 integrase inhibitor. Clin Infect Dis 2009;48(7):931-939.
29. Willig J, Abroms S, Westfall AO, et al. Increased durability in the era of once-daily fixed-dose combination antiretroviral therapy. AIDS 2008;22(15):1951-1960.
30. Grunfeld C, Pang M, Coerrier W, et al. Lipids, lipoproteins, triglyceride clearance, and cytokines in HIV infection and the acquired immunodeficiency syndrome. J Clin Endocrinol Metab 1992;74:1045-1052.
31. Mulligan K, Grunfeld C, Tai VW, et al. Hyperlipidemia and insulin resistance are induced by protease inhibitors independent of changes in body composition in patients with HIV infection. J Acquired Immune Defic Syndr 2000;23:35-43.
32. Purnell JQ, Zambon A, Knopp RH, et al. Effect of ritonavir on lipids and post-heparin lipase activities in normal subjects. AIDS 2000;14:51-57.
33. Sadler BM, Piliero PJ, Preston SL, et al. Pharmacokinetics and safety of amprenavir and ritonavir following multiple-dose, co-administration to healthy volunteers. AIDS 2001;15:1009-1018.
34. Noor MA, Lo JC, Mulligan K, et al. Metabolic effects of indinavir in healthy HIV-seronegative men. AIDS 2001;15:F11-F18.
35. Lee GA, Seneviratne T, Noor MA, et al. The metabolic effects of lopinavir/ritonavir in HIV-negative men. AIDS 2004;18:641-649.
36. Sanne I, Piliero P, Squires K, et al. Results of a phase 2 clinical trial at 48 weeks (AI424-007): a dose-ranging, safety, and efficacy comparative trial of atazanavir at three doses in combination with didanosine and stavudine in antiretroviral-naïve subjects. J Acquir Immune Defic Syndr 2003;32:18-29.

MANIFESTATIONS, MECHANISMS, AND TREATMENT OF HIV-ASSOCIATED CARDIOVASCULAR DISEASE

37. Riddler SA, Smit E, Cole SR, et al. Impact of HIV infection and HAART on serum lipids in men. *JAMA* 2003;289:2978-2982.
38. Kannel WB, Giordano M. Long-term cardiovascular risk with protease inhibitors and management of the dyslipidemia. *Am J Cardiol* 2004;94:901-906.
39. Grinspoon S, Carr A. Cardiovascular risk and body-fat abnormalities in HIV-infected adults. *N Engl J Med* 2005;352:48-62.
40. Jung O, Bickel M, Ditting T, et al. Hypertension in HIV-1 infected patients and its impact on renal and cardiovascular integrity. *Nephrol Dial Transplant* 2004;19:2250-2258.
41. Gazzaruso C, Bruno R, Garzaniti A, et al. Hypertension among HIV patients: prevalence and relationships to insulin resistance and metabolic syndrome. *J Hypertens* 2003;21:1377-1382.
42. Chow DC, Souza SA, Chen R, et al. Elevated blood pressure in HIV-infected individuals receiving highly active antiretroviral therapy. *HIV Clin Trials* 2003;4:411-416.
43. Cattelan AM, Trevenzoli M, Sasset L, et al. Indinavir and systemic hypertension. *AIDS* 2001;15:805-807.
44. Lo JC, Mulligan K, Tai VW, Algren H, Schambelan M. "Buffalo hump" in men with HIV-1 infection. *Lancet* 1998;351:871-875.
45. Sattler F, Qian D, Louie S, et al. Elevated blood pressure in subjects with lipodystrophy. *AIDS* 2001;15:2001-2010.
46. Walli R, Herfort O, Michl GM, et al. Treatment with protease inhibitors associated with peripheral insulin resistance and impaired oral glucose tolerance in HIV-1 infected patients. *AIDS* 1998;12:F167-F173.
47. Martinez E, Mocroft A, Carcia-Viejo MA, et al. Risk of lipodystrophy in HIV-1–infected patients treated with protease inhibitors: a prospective cohort study. *Lancet* 2001;357:592-598.
48. Jones SP, Doran DA, Leatt PB, Maher B, Primohamed M. Short-term exercise training improves body composition and hyperlipidaemia in HIV-positive individuals with lipodystrophy. *AIDS* 2001;15:2049-2051.
49. Driscoll SD, Meininger GE, Lareau MT, et al. Effects of exercise training and metformin on body composition and cardiovascular indices in HIV-infected patients. *AIDS* 2004;18:465-473.
50. Moyle GJ. Plastic surgical approaches for HIV-associated lipodystrophy. *Curr HIV/AIDS Rep* 2005;3:127-131.
51. Jerico C, Knobel H, Montero M, et al. Metabolic syndrome among HIV-infected patients: prevalence, characteristics and related factors. *Diabetes Care* 2005;28:132-137.
52. Wand H, Calmy A, Carey DL, et al. Metabolic syndrome, cardiovascular disease and type 2 diabetes mellitus after initiation of antiretroviral therapy in HIV infection. *AIDS* 2007;21(18):2445-2453.
53. Schambelan M, Wilson PW, Yarasheski KE, et al. Development of appropriate coronary heart disease risk prediction models in HIV-infected patients. *Circulation* 2008;118:e48-e53.
54. Aberg JA, Gallant JE, Anderson J, et al. Primary care guidelines for the management of persons infected with human immunodeficiency virus: recommendations of the HIV Medicine Association of the Infectious Diseases Society of America. *Clin Infect Dis* 2004;39:609-629.
55. Hsue PY, Squires K, Bolger AF, et al. Screening and assessment of coronary heart disease in HIV-infected patients. *Circulation* 2008;118:e41-e47.
56. Triant VA, Meigs JB, Grinspoon SK. Association of C-reactive protein and HIV infection with acute myocardial infarction. *J Acquir Immune Defic Syndr* 2009;51:268-273.
57. Henry K, Melroe H, Heubsch J, et al. Severe premature coronary artery disease with protease inhibitors. *Lancet* 1998;351:1328.
58. Vittecoq D, Escaut L, Monsuez JJ. Vascular complications associated with use of HIV protease inhibitors. *Lancet* 1998;351:1959.
59. Bozzette SA, Ake CF, Tam HK, Chang SW, Louis TA. Cardiovascular and cerebrovascular events in patients treated for human immunodeficiency virus infection. *N Engl J Med* 2003;348:702-710.
60. Coplan PM, Nikas A, Japour A, et al. Incidence of myocardial infarction in randomized clinical trials of protease inhibitor–based antiretroviral therapy: an analysis of four different protease inhibitors. *AIDS Res Hum Retroviruses* 2003;19:449-455.
61. Holmberg SD, Moorman AC, Williamson JM, et al. Protease inhibitors and cardiovascular outcomes in patients with HIV-1. *Lancet* 2002;360:1747-1748.
62. Friis-Møller N, Sabin CA, Weber R, et al.; Data Collection on Adverse Events of Anti-HIV Drugs (DAD) Study Group. Combination antiretroviral therapy and risk of myocardial infarction. *N Engl J Med* 2003;349:1993-2003.
63. Friis-Møller N, Reiss P, Sabin CA, et al.; DAD Study Group. Class of antiretroviral drugs and the risk of myocardial infarction. *N Engl J Med* 2007;356:1723-1735.
64. Worm SW, Sabin C, Weber R, et al. Risk of myocardial infarction in patients with HIV infection exposed to specific individual antiretroviral drugs from the 3 major drug classes: the data collection on adverse events of anti-HIV drugs (D:A:D) study. *J Infect Dis* 2010;201:318-330.
65. Mary-Krause M, Cotte L, Simon A, et al. Increased risk of myocardial infarction with duration of protease inhibitor therapy in HIV-infected men. *AIDS* 2003;17:2479-2486.
66. Klein D, Hurley LB, Quesenberry CP Jr, et al. Do protease inhibitors increase the risk for coronary heart disease in patients with HIV-1 infection? *J Acquir Immune Defic Syndr* 2002;30:471-477.
67. Sabin CA, Worm SW, Weber R, et al.; D:A:D Study Group. Use of nucleoside reverse transcriptase inhibitors and risk of myocardial infarction in HIV-infected patients enrolled in the D:A:D study: a multi-cohort collaboration. *Lancet* 2008;371:1417-1426.
68. Brothers CH, Hernandez JE, Cutrell AG, et al. Risk of myocardial infarction and abacavir therapy: no increased risk across 52 GlaxoSmithKline-sponsored clinical trials in subjects. *J Acquir Immune Defic Syndr* 2009;51:20-28.
69. Murphy R, Costagliola D. Increased cardiovascular risk in HIV infection: drug, virus and immunity. *AIDS* 2008;22:1625-1627.
70. Reference deleted in proofs.
71. Torriani FJ, Komarow L, Parker RA, et al. Endothelial function in human immunodeficiency virus-infected antiretroviral-naïve subjects before and after starting potent

antiretroviral therapy: the ACTG (AIDS Clinical Trials Group) Study 5152s. *J Am Coll Cardiol* 2008;52:569-576.
72. David MH, Hornung R, Fichtenbaum CJ. Ischemic cardiovascular disease in persons with human immunodeficiency virus infection. *HIV/AIDS* 2002;34:98-102.
73. Matetzky S, Domingo M, Kar S, et al. Acute myocardial infarction in human immunodeficiency virus-infected patients. *Arch Int Med* 2003;163:457-460.
74. Escaut L, Monsuez JJ, Chioni G, et al. Coronary artery disease in HIV infected patients. *Intensive Care Med* 2003;29:969-973.
75. Mehta NJ, Khan IA. HIV-associated coronary artery disease. *Angiology* 2003;54:269-275.
76. Ambrose JA, Gould RB, Kurian DC, et al. Frequency of and outcome of acute coronary syndromes in patients with human immunodeficiency virus infection. *Am J Cardiol* 2003;92:301-303.
77. Varriale P, Saravi G, Hernandez E, Carbon F. Acute myocardial infarction in patients infected with human immunodeficiency virus. *Am Heart J* 2004;147:55-59.
78. Hsue PY, Giri K, Erickson S, et al. Clinical features of acute coronary syndromes in patients with human immunodeficiency virus infection. *Circulation* 2004;109:316-319.
79. Antman EM, Cohen M, Bernink PJ, et al. The TIMI risk score for unstable angina/non–ST-elevation MI: a method for prognostication and therapeutic decision making. *JAMA* 2000;284:835-842.
80. Ren X, Trilesskaya M, Kwan DM, et al. Comparison of outcomes using bare metal versus drug-eluting stents in coronary artery disease patients with and without human immunodeficiency virus infection. *Am J Cardiol* 2009;104:216-222.
81. Boccara F, Mary-Krause M, Teiger E, et al. Acute coronary syndrome in human immunodeficiency virus-infected patients: characteristics and 1 year prognosis. *Eur Heart J* 2011;32(1):41-50.
82. Trachiotis GD, Alexander EP, Benator D, Gharagozloo F. Cardiac surgery in patients infected with the human immunodeficiency virus. *Ann Thorac Surg* 2003;76:1114-1118.
83. Horberg MA, Hurley LB, Klein DB, et al. Surgical outcomes in human immunodeficiency virus–infected patients in the era of highly active antiretroviral therapy. *Arch Surg* 2006;141:1238-1245.
84. Tabib A, Leroux C, Mornex JF, et al. Accelerated coronary atherosclerosis and arteriosclerosis in young human-immunodeficiency-virus–positive patients. *Coron Artery Dis* 2000;11:41-46.
85. Reference deleted in proofs.
86. Kaplan RC, Kingsley LA, Grange SJ, et al. Low CD4+ count as a major atherosclerosis risk factor in HIV-infected women and men. *AIDS* 2008;22:1615-1624.
87. Hsue PY, Hunt PW, Sinclair E, et al. Increased carotid intima-media thickness in HIV patients is associated with increased cytomegalovirus-specific T-cell responses. *AIDS* 2006;20:2275-2283.
88. Melendez MM, McNurlan MA, Mynarcik DC, et al. Endothelial adhesion molecules are associated with inflammation in subjects with HIV disease. *Clin Infect Dis* 2008;46:775-780.
89. Kuller LH, Tracy R, Belloso W, et al. Inflammatory and coagulation biomarkers and mortality in patients with HIV infection. *PloS Med* 2008;5:e203.
90. Niaura R, Shadel WG, Morrow K, et al. Human immunodeficiency virus infection, AIDS, and smoking cessation: the time is now. *Clin Infect Dis* 2000;31:808-812.
91. Wewers ME, Neidig JL, Kihm KE. The feasibility of a nurse-managed, peer-led tobacco cessation intervention among HIV-positive smokers. *J Assoc Nurses AIDS Care* 2000;11:37-44.
92. Lazev A, Vidrine D, Arduino R, et al. Increasing access to smoking cessation treatment in low-income, HIV-positive population: the feasibility of using cellular telephones. *Nicotine Tob Res* 2004;6:281-286.
93. Dube MP, Stein JH, Aberg JA, et al. Guidelines for the evaluation and management of dyslipidemia in human immunodeficiency virus (HIV)-infected adults receiving antiretroviral therapy: recommendations of the HIV Medical Association of the Infectious Diseases Society of America and the Adult AIDS Clinical Trials Group. *Clin Infect Dis* 2003;37:613-627.
94. Executive Summary of the Third Report of The National Cholesterol Education Program (NCEP) Expert Panel on Detection, Evaluation, and Treatment of High Blood Cholesterol in Adults (Adult Treatment Panel III). *JAMA* 2001;285:2486-2497.
95. Hare CB, Vu MP, Grunfeld C, et al. Simvastatin-nelfinavir interaction implicated in rhabdomyolysis and death. *Clin Infect Dis* 2002;35:e111-e112.
96. van der Lee M, Sankatsing R, Schippers E, et al. Pharmacokinetics and pharmacodynamics of combined use of lopinavir/ritonavir and rosuvastatin in HIV-infected patients. *Antivir Ther (Lond)* 2007;12:1127-1132.
97. Busti AJ, Bain AM, Hall RG, et al. Effects of atazanavir/ritonavir or fosamprenavir/ritonavir on the pharmacokinetics of rosuvastatin. *J Cardiovasc Pharmacol* 2008;51:605-610.
98. Bennett MT, Johns KW, Bondy GP. Ezetimibe is effective when added to maximally tolerated lipid lowering therapy in patients with HIV. *Lipids Health Dis* 2007;6:15.
99. Wohl DA, Waters D, Simpson RJ Jr, et al. Ezetimibe alone reduces low-density lipoprotein cholesterol in HIV-infected patients receiving combination antiretroviral therapy. *Clin Infect Dis* 2008;47:1105-1108.
100. Wohl DA, Tien HC, Busby M, et al. Randomized study of the safety and efficacy of fish oil (omega-3 fatty acid) supplementation with dietary and exercise counseling for the treatment of antiretroviral therapy-associated hypertriglyceridemia. *Clin Infect Dis* 2005;41:1498-1504.
101. DeTruchis P, Kirstetter M, Perier A, et al. Reduction in triglyceride level with N-3 polyunsaturated fatty acids in HIV-infected patients taking potent antiretroviral therapy: a randomized prospective study. *J Acquir Immune Defic Syndr* 2007;44:278-285.
102. Grundy SM, Brewer HB Jr, Cleeman JI, et al. Definition of metabolic syndrome. Report of the National Heart, Lung and Blood Institue/American Heart Association conference on scientific issues related to definition. *Circulation* 2004;109:433-438.
103. Grundy SM, Hansen B, Smith SC, et al. Clinical management of metabolic syndrome. Report of the National Heart, Lung and Blood Institute/American Diabetes Association conference on scientific issues related to management. *Circulation* 2004;109:551-556.

104. Pendergast BD. HIV and cardiovascular medicine. *Heart* 2003;89:793-800.

105. Rerkpattanapipat P, Wongpraparut N, Jacobs LE, et al. Cardiac manifestations of acquired immunodeficiency syndrome. *Arch Intern Med* 2000;160:602-608.

106. Khunnawat C, Mukerji S, Havlichek D, et al. Cardiovascular manifestations in human immunodeficiency virus–infected patients. *Am J Cardiol* 2008;102:635-642.

107. Herskowitz A, Vlahov D, Willoughby S, et al. Prevalence and incidence of left ventricular dysfunction in patients with human immunodeficiency virus infection. *Am J Cardiol* 1993;71:955-958.

108. Herskowitz A, Wu TC, Willoughby SB, et al. Myocarditis and cardiotropic viral infection associated with severe left ventricular dysfunction in late-stage infection with human immunodeficiency virus. *J Am Coll Cardiol* 1994;24:1025-1032.

109. Anderson DW, Virmani R, Reilly JM, et al. Prevalent myocarditis at necropsy in the acquired immunodeficiency syndrome. *J Am Coll Cardiol* 1988;11:792-799.

110. Dalakas MC, Illa I, Pezeshkpour GH, et al. Mitochondrial myopathy caused by long-term zidovudine therapy. *N Engl J Med* 1990;332:1098-1105.

111. Lewis W, Grupp IL, Grupp G, et al. Cardiac dysfunction in the HIV-1 transgenic mouse treated with zidovudine. *Lab Invest* 2000;80:187-197.

112. Herskowitz A, Willoughby SB, Baughman KL, et al. Cardiomyopathy associated with antiretroviral therapy in patients with HIV infection: a report of six cases. *Ann Intern Med* 1992;116:311-313.

113. Cardoso JS, Moura B, Martins L, et al. Left ventricular dysfunction in HIV-infected patients. *Int J Cardiol* 1998;63:37-45.

114. Cardoso JS, Moura B, Mota-Miranda A, Rocha-Concalves F, Lecour H. Zidovudine therapy and left ventricular function and mass in HIV-infected patients. *Cardiology* 1997;88:26-28.

115. Freedberg RS, Gindea AJ, Dieterich DT, et al. Herpes simplex pericarditis in AIDS. *NY State J Med* 1987;87:304-306.

116. Barbaro G. Cardiovascular manifestation of HIV infection. *J R Soc Med* 2001;94:384-390.

117. Schuster M, Valentine F, Holzman R. Cryptococcal pericarditis in an intravenous drug abuser. *J Infect Dis* 1985;152:842.

118. Hofman P, Drici MD, Gibelin P, et al. Prevalence of *Toxoplasma* myocarditis in patients with the acquired immunodeficiency syndrome. *Br Heart J* 1993;70:376-381.

119. Bijl M, Dieleman JP, Simoons M, van der Ende M. Low prevalence of cardiac abnormalities in an HIV-seropositive population on antiretroviral combination therapy. *J Acquir Immune Defic Syndr* 2001;27:318-320.

120. Barbaro G, DiLorenzo G, Grisorio B, Barbarini G. Cardiac involvement in the acquired immunodeficiency syndrome: a multicenter clinical-pathological study. Gruppo Italiano per lo Studio Cardiologico dei pazienti affetti da AIDS investigators *AIDS Res Hum Retroviruses* 1998;14:1071-1077.

121. Pugliese A, Isnardi D, Saini A, et al. Impact of highly active antiretroviral therapy in HIV positive patients with cardiac involvement. *J Infect* 2000;40:282-284.

122. Hsue PY, Hunt PW, Ho JE, et al. Impact of HIV infection on diastolic function and left ventricular mass. *Circ Heart Failure* 2010;3:132-139.

123. Mondy KE, Gottdiener J, Overton ET, et al. High prevalence of echocardiographic abnormalities among HIV-infected persons in the era of highly active antiretroviral therapy. *Clin Infect Dis* 2011;52(3):378-386.

124. Neumann T, Esser S, Potthoff A, et al. Prevalence and natural history of heart failure in outpatient HIV-infected subjects: rationale and design of the HIV-HEART study. *Eur J Med Res* 2007;12:243-248.

125. Brucato A, Colombo T, Concacina E, et al. Fulminant myocarditis during HIV seroconversion: recovery with temporary left ventricular mechanical assistance. *Ital Heart J* 2004;5:228-231.

126. Calabrese LH, Albricht M, Young J, et al. Successful cardiac transplantation in an HIV-1 infected patient with advanced disease. *N Engl J Med* 2003;348:2323-2328.

127. Stotka JC, Good CB, Downer WR, et al. Pericardial effusion and tamponade due to Kaposi's sarcoma in acquired immunodeficiency syndrome. *Chest* 1989;95:1359-1361.

128. Karve MM, Murali MR, Shah HM, et al. Rapid evolution of cardiac tamponade due to bacterial pericarditis in two patients with HIV-1 infection. *Chest* 1992;101:1461-1463.

129. Heidenreich PA, Eisenberg MJ, Kee LL, et al. Pericardial effusion in AIDS: incidence and survival. *Circulation* 1995;92:3229-3234.

130. Hsue PY, Hunt PW, Ho JE, et al. Impact of HIV infection on diastolic function and left ventricular mass. *Circ Heart Fail* 2010;3:132-139.

131. Kelsey RC, Saker A, Morgan M. Cardiac lymphoma in a patient with AIDS. *Ann Intern Med* 1991;115:370-371.

132. D'Cruz IA, Sengupta EE, Abrahams C, et al. Cardiac involvement, including tuberculous pericardial effusion, complicating acquired immune deficiency syndrome. *Am Heart J* 1986;112:1100-1102.

133. Dalli E, Quesada A, Juan G, et al. Tuberculous pericarditis as the first manifestation of acquired immunodeficiency syndrome. *Am Heart J* 1987;114:905-906.

134. de Miguel J, Pedreira JD, Campos V, et al. Tuberculous pericarditis and AIDS. *Chest* 1990;97:1273.

135. Nathan PE, Arsura EL, Zappi M. Pericarditis with tamponade due to cytomegalovirus in the acquired immunodeficiency syndrome. *Chest* 1991;99:765-766.

136. Stechel RO, Cooper DJ, Greenspan J, et al. Staphylococcal pericarditis in a homosexual patient with AIDS-related complex. *NY State J Med* 1986;86:592-593.

137. Decker CF, Tuazon CU. *Staphylococcus aureus* pericarditis in HIV-infected patients. *Chest* 1994;105:615-616.

138. Schuster M, Valentine F, Holzman R. Cryptococcal pericarditis in an intravenous drug abuser. *J Infect Dis* 1985;152:842.

139. Freedberg RS, Gindea AJ, Dieterich DT, et al. Herpes simplex pericarditis in AIDS. *NY State J Med* 1987;304-306.

140. Speich R, Jenni R, Opravil M, et al. Primary pulmonary hypertension in HIV infection. *Chest* 1991;100:1268-1271.

141. Hsue PY, Deeks SG, Farah HH, et al. Role of HIV and human herpesvirus-8 infection in pulmonary arterial hypertension. *AIDS* 2008;22:825-833.

142. Grubb JR, Moorman AC, Baker RK, et al. The changing spectrum of pulmonary disease in patients with HIV infection on antiretroviral therapy. *AIDS* 2006;20:1095-1107.

143. Mehta NJ, Khan IA, Mehta RN, et al. HIV-related pulmonary hypertension: analytic review of 131 cases. *Chest* 2000;118:1133-1141.

144. Ehrenreich H, Rieckmann P, Sinowatz F, et al. Potent stimulation of monocytic endothelin-1 production by HIV-1 glycoprotein 120. *J Immunol* 1993;150:4601-4609.

145. Pellicelli AM, Palmieri F, Cicalini S, et al. Pathogenesis of HIV-related pulmonary hypertension. *Ann N Y Acad Sci* 2001;946:82-94.

146. Opravil M, Pechère M, Speich R, et al. HIV-associated primary pulmonary hypertension: a case control study. Swiss HIV Cohort Study. *Am J Respir Crit Care Med* 1997;155:990-995.

147. Sitbon O, Gressin V, Speich R, et al. Bosentan for the treatment of human immunodeficiency virus-associated pulmonary arterial hypertension. *Am J Resp Crit Care Med* 2004;170:1212-1217.

148. Nunes H, Humbert M, Sitbon O, et al. Prognostic factors for survival in human immunodeficiency virus–associated pulmonary arterial hypertension. *Am J Respir Crit Care Med* 2003;167:1433-1439.

149. Degano B, Guillaume M, Savale L, et al. HIV-associated pulmonary arterial hypertension: survival and prognostic factors in the modern therapeutic era. *AIDS* 2010;24:67-75.

150. Levy RM, Bredesen DE. Central nervous system dysfunction in acquired immunodeficiency syndrome. *J Acquir Immune Defic Syndr* 1988;1:41-64.

151. Bozzette SA, Ake CF, Tam HK, et al. Cardiovascular and cerebrovascular events in patients treated for human immunodeficiency virus infection. *N Engl J Med* 2003;348:702-710.

152. Evers S, Nabavi D, Rahmann A, et al. Ischaemic cerebrovascular events in HIV infection: a cohort study. *Cerebrovasc Dis* 2003;15:199-205.

153. d'Arminio A, Sabin CA, Philliips AN, et al. Cardio- and cerebrovascular events in HIV-infected persons. *AIDS* 2004;18:1811-1817.

154. Dubé MP, Lipshultz SE, Fichtenbaum CJ, et al. Effects of HIV infection and antiretroviral therapy on the heart and vasculature. *Circulation* 2008;118:e36-e40.

CH
48

MANIFESTATIONS, MECHANISMS, AND TREATMENT OF HIV-ASSOCIATED CARDIOVASCULAR DISEASE

CHAPTER 49 Rehabilitation of the Patient with Cardiovascular Disease

Jonathan N. Myers and Victor F. Froelicher

PHYSIOLOGIC EFFECTS OF IMMOBILITY, 738

PHYSICAL TRAINING, 738

Newer Concepts Regarding Physiologic Benefits of
Exercise Training, 739

CARDIAC REHABILITATION AFTER MYOCARDIAL
INFARCTION, 739

Disability from Myocardial Infarction, 739
In-Hospital Exercise After a Coronary Event, 740
Outpatient Cardiac Rehabilitation, 740
Exercise Prescription for Outpatient Rehabilitation, 742
Contraindications to Exercise Training, 743
Rehabilitation in Patients with Chronic Heart
Failure, 744

Meta-Analyses of Survival After Cardiac
Rehabilitation, 744
Evolving Landscape for Cardiac Rehabilitation, 745

SUMMARY, 745

REFERENCES, 745

Before the 1970s, patients were completely immobilized after a myocardial infarction (MI) for 6 weeks or longer; the prevailing view was that this period was necessary for complete healing of the myocardium to occur. The post-MI patient was generally not expected to ever return to normal occupational or recreational activities. The process known as *cardiac rehabilitation* evolved in an effort to restore the patient to optimal physical, psychologic, and social function.

A significant body of data over the last four decades has documented both the benefits of early ambulation and the numerous detrimental effects of strict bed rest; the act of merely sitting in an upright position has been shown to reduce the detrimental effects of remaining supine.[1] As a result, both the indications for and the scope of cardiac rehabilitation services have broadened. Advances in the treatment of cardiovascular (CV) diseases and data supporting the value of secondary prevention have greatly increased the spectrum of patients who may benefit from cardiac rehabilitation to include not only post-MI patients (both ST-segment elevation and non–ST-segment elevation) but also those who have undergone cardiac transplantation; percutaneous coronary interventions (PCI), including stenting and angioplasty; and those with chronic heart failure (CHF), implantable cardioversion devices (ICDs), and pacemakers.

In addition, it is now widely recognized that exercise is only one component of cardiac rehabilitation: objectives for patients include not only preventing the effects of deconditioning but also improving functional capacity, relieving symptoms, and providing education, risk-factor reduction, assistance in returning to normal activities, and psychosocial support. Societal objectives include decreasing health care costs by reductions in treatment time, reductions in medication, and the prevention of premature disability, thus maintaining individual productivity and lessening the need for societal support. It is noteworthy in this context that randomized exercise trials, when combined, have shown that the rate of mortality from CV causes, defined as fatal reinfarction or sudden cardiac death, is reduced 20% to 25% among patients who participate in rehabilitation. Even with major advances in the treatment of acute MI, such as thrombolytic therapy, updates of the meta-analyses of trials performed from the 1970s through the 1990s have shown 25% to 30% reductions in mortality with rehabilitation.[2-4]

Physiologic Effects of Immobility

Data published since the late 1960s on the deleterious physiologic effects of bed rest have been an important stimulus for the growth of cardiac rehabilitation and an appreciation of its benefits. It is now widely recognized that the negative effects of bed rest include not only reductions in functional capacity but also reductions in adverse hemodynamic changes, orthostatic intolerance, risk of thrombus formation, and alterations in cardiac size and function. Patients hospitalized for cardiac events today are encouraged to begin physical activities as soon as possible. Simply exposing the patient to orthostatic stress and early ambulation counteracts the negative physiologic effects of prolonged bed rest[1,5] and also provides the patient with tangible affirmation of improvement and increases self-confidence.

Physical Training

Regular exercise increases work capacity, and hundreds of studies have documented greater exercise capacity among people who are active compared with sedentary individuals. In general, patients with CV disease are equally able to benefit from exercise training. Although some notable differences do exist, the mechanisms underlying the response to training are similar among those with and those without CV disease. The magnitude of the improvement in exercise capacity with training varies widely but generally ranges from 5% to 25%, although increases as great as 50% have been reported. The best metric to quantify the training response is a change in peak VO_2, and the degree of change depends largely on the patient's initial state of fitness, but it is also affected by age and the type, frequency, and intensity of training.

The physiologic benefits of a training program can be classified as *morphologic, hemodynamic,* and *metabolic* (Box 49-1). Many animal studies have demonstrated significant morphologic changes with training, including myocardial hypertrophy with improved myocardial function, increases in coronary artery size, and increases in the myocardial capillary/fiber ratio. However, such changes have been difficult to demonstrate in humans.[6,7] The major morphologic outcome of a training program in humans is probably an increase in cardiac size. However, although this adaptation has been demonstrated by many investigators among young, healthy individuals, it is unlikely to occur among older subjects (>40 years) or in patients with CV disease. Hemodynamic changes after training include reductions in heart rate at rest and at any matched submaximal workload. For the patient with coronary artery disease (CAD), this is beneficial in that it results in a reduction in myocardial demand during activities of daily living. Other hemodynamic changes that have been demonstrated after training include reductions in blood pressure, increases in blood volume, and increases in maximal cardiac output; the latter underlies an increase in peak VO_2.

In patients with heart disease, the major physiologic effects of training occur in the skeletal muscle. The metabolic capacity of the skeletal muscle is enhanced through increases in mitochondrial volume and number, capillary density, and oxidative

> ### Box 49-1 Physiologic Adaptations to Physical Training in Humans
>
> **Morphologic Adaptations**
> Myocardial hypertrophy (generally only in younger, healthy subjects)
>
> **Hemodynamic Adaptations**
> Increased blood volume
> Increased end-diastolic volume
> Increased stroke volume
> Increased cardiac output
> Decreased heart rate for any submaximal workload
>
> **Metabolic Adaptations**
> Increased mitochondrial volume and number
> Greater muscle glycogen stores
> Enhanced fat utilization
> Enhanced lactate removal
> Increased enzymes for aerobic metabolism
> Increased maximal oxygen uptake

now well established that the luminal diameter of epicardial vessels changes rapidly in response to mechanical (flow related) and endogenous or pharmacologic stimuli. Hambrecht and colleagues[14] studied the effects of exercise training in patients with reduced ventricular function and reported that leg blood flow during acetylcholine infusion was enhanced compared with controls. The improvement after training was attributed to an increase in endothelium-dependent vasodilation with an increase in basal nitric oxide formation. In subsequent studies, these investigators have demonstrated improvements in endothelium-dependent vasodilation in epicardial vessels and resistance vessels in patients with CAD.[11-13] After 4 weeks of exercise training, a 29% increase was reported in coronary artery flow reserve in comparison with the nonexercise control group.[11]

These findings have been confirmed by other groups[12,15-18] and suggest that exercise training may have a profound effect on the vasodilatory properties of the vascular endothelium. Further exploration into the effects of exercise training on the dynamic behavior of the endothelium is an important target area for future research in individuals both with and without existing CV disease.

Cardiac Rehabilitation After Myocardial Infarction

Changes in health care economics have drastically altered how cardiac rehabilitation is implemented. Hospital stays are shorter, progression through the program is more rapid, and much of the "cardiac rehabilitation" as it was traditionally known has changed. Reimbursement patterns differ considerably from one state to another and from one program to another. With less time for clinicians to interact with and monitor patients and to cover educational materials adequately, the need for structured outpatient programs in the home or community has increased. Traditionally, typical phases have been included in rehabilitation: *phase I* includes the coronary care unit and inpatient care during the first few days after the event; *phase II* involves convalescence, an outpatient program, or a home program; and *phase III* usually involves a longer-term community-based or home program. The precise course of each program naturally depends on the individual's needs and clinical status.

Disability from Myocardial Infarction

CV diseases are the leading cause of activity limitation and disabled worker benefits in the United States. In fact, CAD alone is responsible for almost one out of five disability allowances paid by the Social Security Administration. However, the total economic impact results from the combination of Social Security benefits, welfare support, disability insurance income, unemployment compensation, loss of taxable revenue, and reduced worker productivity related to CV diseases. From a purely economic standpoint, it is essential that patients with CAD be rehabilitated as quickly and efficiently as possible to enable their return to remunerative employment. Just as important, however, is amelioration of the psychosocial impact of heart disease that includes a lessening of depression and an expedient return to the social roles the patient had in the family and community prior to the illness.

Historically, the patient's return to work, ability to drive, and sexual activity have been based on clinical judgments rather than on physiologic assessments. These decisions should be based on the consequences of the coronary event—such as ischemia, symptoms of CHF, or dysrhythmias—the nature of the patient's occupational or recreational activities, and the response to the predischarge exercise test. In general, if the patient does not exhibit any untoward responses to submaximal exercise testing and achieves five or more metabolic equivalents (METs), it is unlikely that he or she will encounter difficulties during activities

enzyme content. These adaptations enhance perfusion and the efficiency of oxygen extraction.[6,7] Importantly, exercise training has a favorable impact on virtually all the risk factors for CV disease, including blood pressure, obesity, insulin resistance, inflammation, low fitness, and lipid abnormalities. Although the effect of a rehabilitation program on any single factor is likely to be modest, the combined effects of training on overall risk can be significant.

Newer Concepts Regarding Physiologic Benefits of Exercise Training

The effects of exercise training on the coronary vasculature have long been of interest. Although the hypothesis that training might reverse the effects of atherosclerosis in humans had generally been abandoned, studies performed in the last two decades in patients with CAD indicate that exercise training, when combined with multidisciplinary risk management, can improve myocardial perfusion.[8-13] This has been demonstrated indirectly using nuclear imaging[8] and directly by angiography.[9-13] Because most of these studies involved multifactorial risk reduction—improved diet, smoking cessation, stress management, and pharmacologic management of risk factors—in addition to exercise, it is not possible to determine the independent effects of exercise training.

Debate continues regarding the mechanism by which the apparent improvement in myocardial perfusion might occur following training. It is generally considered unlikely that changes in coronary blood flow observed in animals during exercise would apply to humans. Three mechanisms could potentially explain an improvement in perfusion after training: 1) direct regression of atherosclerotic lesions; 2) formation of collateral vessels; or 3) a change in the dynamics of epicardial flow via flow-mediated or endogenous stimuli of the vessel. Evidence of small but significant improvements in lumen diameter has been seen after intensive exercise and risk-reduction programs in patients with CAD, but little evidence exists that collateral vessel formation occurs after training in humans. Interestingly, although changes in lumen diameter after these intervention programs are quite small, they are associated with considerable reductions in hospital admissions for cardiac reasons.[9,13] This suggests that patients in the intervention groups may achieve greater plaque stability without large changes in the coronary artery lumen.

A significant amount of research has demonstrated that training improves endothelial function, thus permitting enhanced peripheral and coronary blood flow in response to exercise. This represents a paradigm shift in the pathophysiology of CAD. It is of daily living. More strenuous jobs or recreational requirements should not be initiated until a symptom-limited exercise test can be performed, and exercise capacity can be determined and related to the desired physical activities of the patient.

Factors that influence a patient's return to work include age, work history, severity of cardiac damage, financial compensation for illness, the employer's ignorance about the patient's abilities, termination of employment, and, most importantly, the patient's perception of his or her clinical status. Efforts of the rehabilitation team to develop a positive attitude and a sense of well-being for the patient may facilitate appropriate vocational adjustments. The physician's attitude also greatly affects the patient's return to work, and encouragement can be very beneficial.

In-Hospital Exercise After a Coronary Event

The purpose of beginning cardiac rehabilitation immediately after an event is to counteract the negative effects of deconditioning rather than to promote training adaptations. It also provides an ideal time to begin education and psychologic support. The first 3 to 5 days after an MI or bypass surgery are critical for beginning these processes, and the literature is replete with studies that document the efficacy and safety of beginning activities, as well as education, in stable patients soon after a coronary event.[19] Appropriate activities initially include sitting at the bedside, active range-of-motion exercises, and self-care with progression to ambulation around the hospital unit under supervision and later to climbing a flight of stairs.

PATIENT EDUCATION

Education should be initiated before physical activities are begun, and the patient may lack self-confidence and may need affirmation that the activities are safe. Patient education during the acute phase usually consists of an explanation of the coronary care or telemetry unit, the cardiac rehabilitation program, cardiac-related symptoms, and the delivery of routine diagnostic and therapeutic modalities. The patient should be educated in terms of the limitations imposed by the disease, potential for improvement, and precautions to be observed; in addition, the program must be individualized for the patient, depending on his or her psychosocial status. Clinical status is determined largely by the severity of the MI, but the medical history must also be considered.

EXERCISE TESTING BEFORE HOSPITAL DISCHARGE

In current clinical practice, most patients undergo an angiogram prior to hospital discharge. When an invasive strategy is not pursued, performing an exercise test prior to hospital discharge provides a great deal of useful information that includes clarification of the response to exercise, development of an exercise prescription, and recognition of the need for medications or interventions. It can also have a beneficial psychologic impact on recovery and begins the rehabilitation process. The test is considered the first step in the outpatient cardiac rehabilitation exercise program; otherwise, the exercise test could be performed at a later date after recovery from PCI or surgery.

Whether the predischarge test should be performed to a maximal level and whether it should be performed in patients with ST-segment elevation MIs (STEMIs) have been debated. Available data indicate that it is safe to perform maximal or near-maximal testing in most post-MI patients, although a distinction has not been made for the presence or absence of STEMIs. The predischarge test has generally been submaximal, but the appropriate "submaximal" endpoint has varied. Traditionally, the test is stopped at a level not exceeding 5 METs or a Borg perceived exertion level of 16. A submaximal target heart rate has also been used, such as 110 beats/min for patients taking β-blockers. The protocol should be modified to accommodate the reduced exercise tolerance of most patients recovering from an MI, and

individualized ramp or Naughton protocols are preferable.[20] Later, when a return to full activities is intended, the test can be symptom- and sign-limited.

The prognostic value of the predischarge test has been widely studied. A meta-analysis[21] and recent results from the Danish Trial in Acute Myocardial Infarction (DANAMI-2)[22] have shown that exercise capacity is a better predictor of risk than is ST-segment depression or other exercise test responses. However, ST-segment depression probably indicates increased risk in men who do not take digoxin and in whom resting electrocardiograms (ECGs) do not show extensive damage. The criterion of 2.0 mm or more of ST-segment depression along with symptoms or abnormal hemodynamic responses appears to be useful for identifying higher-risk patients who should be considered for cardiac catheterization and possibly revascularization.

Outpatient Cardiac Rehabilitation

Multiple approaches to outpatient rehabilitation have been taken. Usually the rehabilitation phase begins 1 to 2 weeks after discharge from the hospital, and it may last from 1 to 4 months. Most commonly, patients attend group exercise sessions three times per week; however, frequency of exercise is often modified by the individual patient's overall goals, functional capabilities, insurance reimbursement, proximity to the hospital or clinic, and personal commitment. The first few exercise sessions usually emphasize warm-up and cool-down activities with only a modest aerobic component. A symptom-limited maximal exercise test is often recommended approximately 6 weeks after hospital discharge to determine appropriate activity limitations.

Changes in reimbursement patterns have changed outpatient programs more than other components of cardiac rehabilitation. In many instances, only a few exercise or educational sessions are reimbursed. The transition from an outpatient to a home-based maintenance program now occurs more rapidly. Randomized trials have demonstrated that patients can return to work quickly and safely during rehabilitation and that participation in rehabilitation facilitates this process. DeBusk and colleagues pioneered the application of home rehabilitation programs in the 1980s; these programs either use unmonitored or include monitored surveillance via telephone or microprocessor.[23] Home programs are now widely used, and the safety and efficacy of these programs have been shown to be similar to those of more conventional programs.[24]

OTHER COMPONENTS OF OUTPATIENT REHABILITATION

In recent years, cardiac rehabilitation programs have undergone a transformation into broader *secondary* prevention centers, beyond exercise-based rehabilitation.[19,25] Changes in reimbursement patterns, the demonstration that clinical outcomes can be improved by *multidisciplinary* risk-factor intervention, and recent observations that a wider spectrum of patients benefit from cardiac rehabilitation—such as the elderly, patients with CHF or peripheral vascular disease, and those who have had valvular surgery, transplants, or cardiac resynchronization therapy—have contributed to the development of new models for cardiac rehabilitation. This change has also occurred because physicians have not been particularly effective in assisting patients in achieving defined risk-factor goals,[25,26] and multidisciplinary secondary prevention approaches have been demonstrated to facilitate a greater proportion of patients meeting evidence-based treatment guidelines. In addition, the typical patient referred to cardiac rehabilitation today has multiple subclinical and clinical diagnoses, and programs have been restructured to include patients with multiple diagnoses. The latter approach—termed the *inclusive chronic disease model*[27] or simply *chronic disease management*[28]—has been shown to be cost-effective and to reduce personnel, program, and facility redundancy.

The concept that cardiac rehabilitation should be the primary medium to implement comprehensive CV risk reduction—and the fact that secondary prevention has been embraced by the American Heart Association (AHA),[29] the Agency for Health Care Policy and Research Clinical Practice Guidelines,[30] and the American Association for Cardiovascular and Pulmonary Rehabilitation[31]—is important. The recent AHA consensus statement on core components of rehabilitation and secondary prevention programs[32] defines specific evidence-based risk-factor goals for management of lipids, blood pressure, weight, smoking cessation, diabetes management, and physical activity (Box 49-2). This model provides an integrated system that includes appropriate triage, education, counseling on lifestyle interventions, and long-term follow-up.

Safety of Cardiac Rehabilitation

The safety of outpatient cardiac rehabilitation has been well documented. Van Camp and Peterson[33] gathered data from 167 randomly selected cardiac rehabilitation centers on more than 51,000 patients who exercised for more than 2 million hours. Over a 4-year period, there were only 21 cardiac resuscitations, 3 of which failed, and 8 MIs. This amounts to 8.9 cardiac arrests, 3.4 infarctions, and 1.3 fatalities per million hours of patient exercise. Surprisingly, ECG monitoring had little influence on complications, which suggests that the additional expense of telemetry may not be necessary. In a 16-year follow-up from William Beaumont Hospital in Michigan, 292,254 patient exercise hours were recorded in phase II and III programs.[34] During this period, only five major CV complications occurred, representing a rate of one per 58,451 patient exercise hours. This event rate is similar to that described in a summary of studies from the AHA, in which an average of one event was reported for every 62,000 hours of exercise in rehabilitation programs.[27] Despite the low incidence of these events, appropriate medical personnel trained in the use of automated external defibrillators must be available to respond when events do occur.

Monitoring in Outpatient Rehabilitation

It is now recognized that only a small percentage of patients require continuous ECG monitoring during exercise. Efforts to reduce the cost of rehabilitation, in addition to the recognition that most patients can exercise safely without continuous telemetry, have brought about this change. Moreover, no predictors have been established for identifying patients in whom monitoring may reduce risk.[35] ECG monitoring can be useful to track compliance with the exercise prescription and to increase the patient's self-confidence for independent activity. ECG monitoring may also be used intermittently in appropriate patients based on clinical judgment. Although no current guidelines have been established specific to this issue, Box 49-3 lists instances in which ECG monitoring may be appropriate during rehabilitation sessions.[35,36]

Maintenance Program

Progression to an out-of-hospital maintenance program is desirable to maintain training adaptations and to help prevent recurrence of events or symptoms. The time required before patients move from a supervised program to a maintenance program can vary considerably, depending on reimbursement, patient stability, exercise capacity, and individual patient needs, but it rarely exceeds 12 weeks. It is important for the patient to understand how to monitor his or her own exercise intensity and recognize symptoms, and the patient must gain a basic knowledge of his or her particular disease and the necessity of any

---

Box 49-2 Core Components for Cardiac Rehabilitation and Secondary Prevention Programs

Lipid Management
- Short-term: Assessment and modification of interventions should continue until LDL is <100 mg/dL.
- Long-term: LDL should be <100 mg/dL. Secondary goals include HDL >40 mg/dL and triglycerides <200 mg/dL.

Hypertension Management
- Short-term: Assessment and modification of interventions should continue until BP is <140 mm Hg systolic and <90 mm Hg diastolic; in patients with heart failure, diabetes, and renal failure, BP should be <130 mm Hg systolic and <85 mm Hg diastolic.
- Long-term: BP <140 mm Hg systolic and <90 mm Hg diastolic is the goal; in patients with heart failure, diabetes, and renal failure, BP should be <130 mm Hg systolic and <85 mm Hg diastolic.

Smoking Cessation
- Short-term: The patient will demonstrate readiness to change by initially expressing a decision to quit (*contemplation*) and selecting a quit date (*preparation*). Subsequently the patient will quit smoking and cease use of all tobacco products (*action*); the patient will adhere to any prescribed pharmacotherapy, will practice strategies as recommended, and will resume a cessation plan as quickly as possible if relapse occurs.
- Long-term: The patient will report complete abstinence from smoking and use of all tobacco products at 12 months from the quit date.

Weight Management
- In patients with a BMI >25 kg/m² and/or a waist circumference >40 inches (102 cm) in men and 35 inches (89 cm) in women, weight loss should be advised.
- Establish reasonable short-term and long-term weight goals individualized to the patient, with consideration given to associated risk factors (e.g., the patient should reduce body weight by at least 10% at a rate of 1 to 2 lb/week over ≤6 months).

- Short-term: Assessment and modification of interventions should continue until progressive weight loss is achieved. Have the patient participate in an on-site weight-loss program, or provide referral to specialized nutrition weight-loss programs such that weight goals are achieved.
- Long-term: Patient should adhere to a diet and exercise program aimed toward attainment of an established weight goal.

Diabetes Management
- Short-term: Develop a regimen of dietary adherence and weight control that includes exercise, oral hypoglycemic agents, insulin therapy, and optimal control of other risk factors. Drug therapy should be provided and/or monitored in concert with the patient's primary health care provider.
- Long-term: The goal should be normalization of fasting plasma glucose (80 to 110 mg/dL or HbA1c <7.0), minimization of diabetic complications, and control of associated obesity, hypertension (<130/85 mm Hg), and hyperlipidemia.
- Refer patients whose fasting glucose is >110 mg/dL without known diabetes to their primary health care provider for further evaluation and treatment.

Physical Activity Counseling
- Increased physical activity includes 20 to 30 min/day of moderate physical activity ≥5 days/week and increased activity in usual routines, such as parking farther away from entrances, walking two or more flights of stairs instead of taking the elevator, and walking 15 minutes during a break from work.
- Patients should increase participation in domestic, occupational, and recreational activities.
- Improved psychosocial well-being, reduction in stress, facilitation of functional independence, prevention of disability, and enhancement of opportunities for independent self-care are important to achieve recommended goals.

BMI, body mass index; BP, blood pressure; HbA1c, glycosylated hemoglobin; HDL, high-density lipoprotein; LDL, low-density lipoprotein.
From Balady GJ, Williams MA, Ades PA, et al. Core components of cardiac rehabilitation secondary prevention programs: 2007 update. *J Cardiopulm Rehabil* 2007;115: 2675-2682.

prescribed medications. When making occupational activity recommendations for patients, it can be helpful to know the estimated energy requirements of various activities (Table 49-1). This way, appropriate recommendations can balance the patient's functional limitations with the need to return to work, the desire to continue recreational activities, or both.

It is useful to perform an exercise test prior to the maintenance program in order to provide an outgoing exercise prescription, confirm the safety of exercise for a given patient, and assess risk for future cardiac events. Funding for this phase must often be borne by the patient, because most types of health insurance do not cover it.

Exercise Prescription for Outpatient Rehabilitation

Exercise prescription has been defined as the process whereby a person's recommended regimen of physical activity is designed in a systematic and individualized manner. An "individualized manner" implies the establishment of specific individualized strategies to optimize return to work or to activities of daily living, to reduce risk factors for future cardiac events, and to maximize the

> ### Box 49-3 Appropriate Circumstances for Electrocardiographic Monitoring During Rehabilitation Sessions
>
> 1. Patient lacks confidence to exercise independently.
> 2. Left ventricular function is severely depressed (ejection fraction <30%).
> 3. Complex ventricular arrhythmias occur at rest.
> 4. Ventricular arrhythmias appear or increase with exercise.
> 5. Patient exhibits a decrease in systolic blood pressure with exercise.
> 6. Patient is a survivor of sudden cardiac death.
> 7. Patient has had a myocardial infarction complicated by congestive heart failure, cardiogenic shock, and/or serious ventricular arrhythmias.
> 8. Patient has severe coronary artery disease and marked exercise-induced ischemia.
> 9. Patient is unable to self-monitor exercise intensity because of a physical or intellectual impairment.

patient's capacity to maintain an active lifestyle. The development of an appropriate exercise prescription to meet the individual patient's needs has a sound scientific foundation,[37,38] but there is also an art to effective exercise programming. No single program is best for all patients or even for one patient over time; capabilities, vocational needs, and expectations differ among patients and can change with the passage of time. Thus, the art of exercise prescription relies on the physician's or exercise physiologist's abilities to synthesize pathophysiologic, psychosocial, and vocational factors and to tailor the exercise prescription to the patient's needs and realistic goals. A final but important consideration is the selection of activities that the individual enjoys, and thus will be more likely to continue to perform, after the formal rehabilitation program ends.

PRINCIPLES OF EXERCISE PRESCRIPTION

Training implies chronic adaptations of the body to the demands placed on it. A *training effect* is best measured as an increase in peak VO$_2$, but not all institutions have gas-exchange equipment, and functional outcomes of rehabilitation can be quantified in many ways. For example, some patients may be better suited after rehabilitation to carry out submaximal levels of activity for longer periods, to remain independent, to continue working, or to rejoin their friends on the golf course. All of these can be important goals for a given patient and may occur even with a minimal change in peak VO$_2$.

The major components of the exercise prescription are the *frequency, intensity, duration, mode,* and *rate of progression.* In general, these principles apply for both the patient with heart disease and the healthy adult; however, the ways in which they are applied differ. It is generally accepted that increases in peak VO$_2$ are achieved if a person exercises dynamically for a period ranging from 15 to 60 minutes, 3 to 5 times per week, at an intensity equivalent to 50% to 80% of his or her maximum capacity. Dynamic exercises are those that use large muscle groups in a rhythmic manner, such as treadmill walking, cycle ergometry, rowing, stepping, and arm ergometry. Short warm-up and cool-down periods are strongly encouraged for participants in cardiac rehabilitation programs.

Much of the art of exercise prescription involves individualizing exercise intensity. Typically, exercise intensity is expressed as a

TABLE 49-1	Energy Cost of Various Occupational and Recreational Activities	
	OCCUPATIONAL	**RECREATIONAL**
1-2 METs	Desk work, auto driving, typing	Standing, walking (1 mph), playing cards, sewing, knitting
2-3 METs	Auto repair, light janitorial work, bartending	Level walking (2 mph), level bicycling (5 mph), operating a riding lawn mower, billiards, bowling, shuffleboard, woodworking (light), powerboat driving, golfing (power cart), canoeing (2.5 mph), horseback riding (at a walk), playing piano and other musical instruments
3-4 METs	Bricklaying, plastering, using a wheelbarrow (light load), machine assembly, welding (moderate load), cleaning windows	Walking (3-3.5 mph), cycling (8 mph), table tennis, golfing (carrying clubs), dancing, badminton (singles), tennis (doubles), raking leaves, hoeing, many calisthenics
4-5 METs	Digging or shoveling light earth	Walking briskly (4 mph), cycling (10 mph), canoeing (4 mph), horseback riding, stream fishing, ice or roller skating (9 mph)
6-7 METs	Shoveling (10 lb), carrying 50- to 75-lb objects, using heavy power tools	Walking quickly (5 mph), cycling (11 mph), playing badminton (competitive) and tennis (singles), splitting wood, shoveling snow, lawn mowing, folk dancing, light downhill skiing, ski touring (2.5 mph), water skiing
7-8 METs	Digging ditches, carrying 80 lb, sawing hardwood	Jogging (5 mph), cycling (12 mph), horseback riding (at a gallop), vigorous downhill skiing, basketball, mountain climbing, ice hockey, canoeing (5 mph), touch football, paddleball
8-9 METs	Moving or pushing objects >75 lb	Running (5.5 mph), cycling (13 mph), ski touring (4 mph), shoveling (14 lb), baling hay, squash (social), handball (social), fencing, basketball (vigorous)
10+ METs	Shoveling >16 lb loads, climbing a ladder in full firefighting gear	Running: 6 mph = 10 METs; 7 mph = 11.5 METs; 8 mph =13.5 METs; 9 mph = 15 METs; 10 mph = 16 METs; ski touring (5+ mph), handball (competitive), racquetball (competitive)

METs, metabolic equivalents.
From Ainsworth BE, Haskell WL, Leon AS, et al. Compendium of physical activities: classification of energy costs of human physical activities. *Med Sci Sports Exerc* 1993;25[1]:71-80.

percentage of maximal capacity, either in absolute terms, such as workload or watts, or in relation to the maximal heart rate, maximal oxygen uptake, or perceived effort. Training benefits have been shown to occur with the use of exercise intensities ranging from 40% to 85% of maximal oxygen uptake, which are generally equivalent to 50% to 90% of maximal heart rate. However, the intensity that a given individual can maintain for a specified period varies widely. In general, the most appropriate intensity for most patients in rehabilitation programs is 50% to 70% of maximal capacity. The actual prescribed exercise intensity for a specific patient should naturally depend on goals, health status, length of time since infarction or surgery, symptoms, and initial state of fitness.

Training is a general phenomenon, and no true threshold exists beyond which patients achieve benefits. Thus as long as patients exercise safely, setting the exercise intensity is a less rigid practice than it was years ago. In addition, the patient's ability to tolerate activities can change daily. Other factors—such as time of day, environment, and time since medications were taken—can influence the patient's response to exercise, and the exercise prescription must be adjusted accordingly. It is also useful to employ a window of intensity that ranges from about 10% above to 10% below the desired level.

The graded exercise test is the foundation on which a safe and effective exercise prescription is based. To achieve a desired training intensity, oxygen uptake or some estimation of it must be quantified during a maximal or symptom-limited exercise test. Because heart rate is easily measured and is linearly related to oxygen uptake, it has become a standard by which training intensity is estimated during exercise sessions. The most useful method is known as the *heart rate reserve*. This method uses a percentage of the difference between maximal heart rate and resting heart rate and adds this value to the resting heart rate. An example of a typical patient given an exercise prescription at 60% of the heart rate reserve is illustrated in Figure 49-1. This is also referred to as the *Karvonen formula,* and it is reliable in patients with normal sinus rhythm whose measurements of resting and maximal heart rates are accurate. An estimated target heart rate for exercise should be supplemented by considering the patient's MET level relative to his or her maximum, the perceived exertion, and symptoms.

RESISTANCE EXERCISE

Once thought to be contraindicated in patients with CV disease, resistance exercise is now widely recommended as a component of rehabilitation programs.[39] Supervised resistance exercise has been shown to improve muscular strength, endurance, functional capacity, and independence while reducing disability.[39,40] In a review of resistance-exercise studies as part of cardiac rehabilitation programs by the Agency for Health Care Policy and Research,[30] all studies reported increases in muscular strength and endurance. The absence of reported symptoms, hemodynamic abnormalities, rhythm disturbances, and CV complications indicates that resistance training is safe for clinically stable patients participating in rehabilitation programs.

In general, recommendations for resistance training in the context of cardiac rehabilitation entail a high-repetition, low-resistance regimen. Typically, this involves one set of 10 to 15 repetitions, using 8 to 10 different stations or exercises that include a broad range of upper- and lower-body muscle groups. As a guide, patients should begin using weights in the range of 40% to 50% of the one-repetition maximum (1-RM), and they should gradually progress to 50% to 70% of their 1-RM. Resistance training should be performed at a moderate to slow speed and should be rhythmic, and the breathing pattern should be normal throughout the movement. Resistance training should be performed 2 to 3 days per week and should include stretching the major muscle groups prior to engaging in the resistance exercise.[39] Most commonly, the resistance portion is performed following the aerobic component, which ensures an adequate warm-up period.

Contraindications to Exercise Training

Appropriate indications and contraindications to exercise training should be considered before initiating an exercise program (Box 49-4). Absolute contraindications to training include

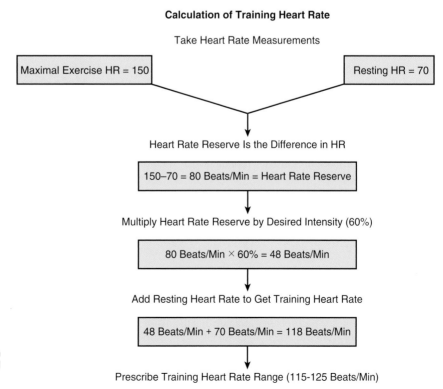

Calculation of Training Heart Rate

Take Heart Rate Measurements

| Maximal Exercise HR = 150 | | Resting HR = 70 |

Heart Rate Reserve Is the Difference in HR

150–70 = 80 Beats/Min = Heart Rate Reserve

Multiply Heart Rate Reserve by Desired Intensity (60%)

80 Beats/Min × 60% = 48 Beats/Min

Add Resting Heart Rate to Get Training Heart Rate

48 Beats/Min + 70 Beats/Min = 118 Beats/Min

Prescribe Training Heart Rate Range (115-125 Beats/Min)

FIGURE 49-1 Flow diagram for development of an exercise prescription using heart rate (*HR*) in a typical patient starting a rehabilitation program.

Box 49-4 Clinical Indications and Contraindications for Inpatient and Outpatient Cardiac Rehabilitation

Indications

- Medically stable after myocardial infarction
- Stable angina
- Coronary artery bypass graft surgery
- Percutaneous transluminal coronary angioplasty or other transcatheter procedure
- Compensated congestive heart failure
- Cardiomyopathy
- Heart or other organ transplantation
- Other cardiac surgery, including valvular and pacemaker insertion or implanted cardioverter defibrillator
- Peripheral vascular disease
- High-risk cardiovascular disease ineligible for surgical intervention
- Sudden cardiac death syndrome
- End-stage renal disease
- At risk for coronary artery disease, with diagnoses of diabetes mellitus, dyslipidemia, hypertension, obesity, or other conditions
- Other patients who may benefit from structured exercise and/or patient education based on physician referral and consensus of the rehabilitation team

Contraindications

- Unstable angina
- Resting systolic blood pressure >200 mm Hg or diastolic BP >110 mm Hg
- Orthostatic blood pressure drop of >20 mm Hg with symptoms
- Moderate to severe aortic stenosis
- Acute systemic illness or fever
- Uncontrolled atrial or ventricular arrhythmias
- Uncontrolled tachycardia (>120 beats/min)
- Uncompensated congestive heart failure
- Third-degree heart block (without pacemaker)
- Active pericarditis or myocarditis
- Recent embolism
- Thrombophlebitis
- Resting ST displacement (>2 mm)
- Uncontrolled diabetes
- Orthopedic problems that prohibit exercise
- Other metabolic conditions such as thyroiditis, hypokalemia, hyperkalemia, or hypovolemia

From the American College of Sports Medicine. *Guidelines for exercise testing and prescription*, 8th ed. 2010, Baltimore, Lippincott, Williams & Wilkins.

unstable angina pectoris, aortic dissection, complete heart block, uncontrolled hypertension, decompensated heart failure, uncontrolled dysrhythmias, thrombophlebitis, and other complicating illnesses that prevent exercise. Relative contraindications include frequent premature ventricular contractions, controlled dysrhythmias, intermittent claudication, metabolic disorders, and moderate anemia or pulmonary disease. Studies show that if these contraindications are considered, the incidence of exertion-related complications in cardiac rehabilitation programs is extremely low and, because of the availability of rapid defibrillation, serious events rarely occur.

Rehabilitation in Patients with Chronic Heart Failure

Until the late 1980s, stable CHF was considered by many authorities to be a contraindication to participation in an exercise program. Today it is known that patients with CHF derive considerable benefits from cardiac rehabilitation. Randomized trials performed over the last two decades indicate that the major physiologic adaptations from training in CHF largely occur in the skeletal muscle rather than in the heart itself.[41]

The clinical approach to the patient with CHF who is considered for a rehabilitation program is similar to that for the post-MI patient described earlier, although several important differences are worth noting. Patients must be stable, and those who exhibit significant dyspnea with exertion, peripheral edema, or other signs indicative of right-sided heart failure should be deferred until the absence of these signs is ensured. The potential for complications during exercise may be higher in patients with CHF compared with patients who have normal left ventricular function. A greater number of medications are to be considered that can influence exercise responses; these include vasoactive, antiarrhythmic, inotropic, and β-blocking agents. Exercise capacity tends to be significantly lower in patients with CHF compared with that in the typical patient with coronary disease. Numerous hemodynamic abnormalities underlie the reduced exercise capacity in CHF and include impaired heart rate responses, inability to distribute cardiac output normally, abnormal arterial vasodilatory capacity, abnormal cellular metabolism in skeletal muscle, elevated systemic and pulmonary vascular resistance, and ventilatory abnormalities that increase the work of breathing and cause exertional dyspnea.[41,42] Studies suggest that many of these abnormalities can be improved by exercise training.[42,43]

Most patients with reduced left ventricular function who are clinically stable and have reduced exercise tolerance are candidates for exercise programs. It is often necessary to exclude patients with signs and symptoms of right-sided heart failure or to treat them judiciously before entry into a program. An exercise test is particularly important before initiating the program to ensure safety of participation. Rhythm abnormalities, exertional hypotension, or other signs of instability should be ruled out. Expired gas-exchange measurements are particularly informative in this group, because they permit an assessment of ventilatory abnormalities that are common in this condition.[44,45] ECG monitoring during exercise is more often indicated in this group than in participants with CAD, given the higher risk for malignant arrhythmias. Attention should be given to daily changes in body weight, rhythm status, and symptoms.

Increasing numbers of patients have undergone cardiac transplantation for end-stage heart failure, and today approximately three-quarters of these patients remain alive after 5 years. Recent reports have addressed the effects of training after cardiac transplantation. These studies have demonstrated increases in peak VO_2, reductions in resting and submaximal heart rates, and improved ventilatory responses to exercise.[46-48] The combination of improved cardiac function, changes in skeletal muscle metabolism, and improvements in strength contributes to improved exercise tolerance with training in these patients.

Meta-Analyses of Survival After Cardiac Rehabilitation

The overall benefits of cardiac rehabilitation are now widely accepted, and comprehensive reviews are available that confirm these benefits.[4,12,19,30,42,43] Because none of the single-center studies alone has been sufficiently powered to adequately document changes in mortality, a series of meta-analyses has been performed to evaluate the impact of cardiac rehabilitation on fatal and nonfatal events. O'Connor and colleagues[49] performed a meta-analysis of 22 randomized trials of cardiac rehabilitation that involved 4554 patients. They found a 20% reduction of risk for total mortality, a 22% reduction for CV mortality, and a 25% reduction in the risk for fatal reinfarction. Oldridge and colleagues[50] performed a similar meta-analysis with 10 randomized trials that included 4347 patients and found a similar reduction for all-cause and CV mortality in the patients undergoing cardiac rehabilitation. The pooled odds ratios for the combined studies suggest 24% and 25% reductions in all-cause and CV deaths, respectively, among the exercise groups. Criticisms of these analyses are that each of the pooled studies was not uniform in its treatment of patients, and a nonexercise intervention done in the different trials may have biased the results. Nevertheless, these two meta-analyses have been widely cited and have been highly influential in support of cardiac rehabilitation.

Taylor and colleagues[2] performed an updated meta-analysis of rehabilitation trials among patients with coronary heart disease that focused on studies performed during the 1970s and 1980s, but another analysis included trials up to 2003. A total of 48 trials that involved 8940 patients met the inclusion criteria. Compared with usual care, cardiac rehabilitation was associated with reduced all-cause mortality (odds ratio, 0.80) and cardiac mortality (odds ratio, 0.74). In addition, participation in cardiac rehabilitation was associated with greater reductions in cholesterol, triglycerides, and systolic blood pressure, although no differences were reported between rehabilitation patients and usual care groups in nonfatal reinfarctions or revascularization rates. Importantly, the effect of rehabilitation on mortality was independent of CHF diagnosis, type of rehabilitation, dosage of exercise intervention, length of follow-up, trial quality, or trial publication date.

Although the mortality effects of exercise-based rehabilitation on outcomes in post-MI patients have been known since the 1980s, meta-analyses among patients with CHF have only recently been performed. Until the late 1980s, activity was generally restricted in patients with CHF, largely because of concerns over safety and unknown effects of training on the myocardial remodeling process. During the 1990s, numerous trials demonstrated that exercise training is safe for these patients, and several landmark trials were published that used advanced imaging techniques to allay concerns over the effects of training on left ventricular remodeling.

A collaborative study of European centers (the ExTraMATCH study) that performed exercise training trials in patients with CHF during the 1990s was undertaken.[3] This meta-analysis included controlled exercise trials and was designed to provide estimates of treatment benefits on mortality and hospital admission. Nine trials met the study inclusion criteria and comprised a total of 395 exercise-intervention patients and 406 controls. After a mean follow-up period of 705 days, it was found that exercise training reduced mortality rate by 35% and reduced the composite outcome of death or hospital admission by 28%. Moreover, no evidence was found that any subgroup—elderly patients, those with severely reduced exercise capacity or ventricular function, patients with a specific type of CHF, those with a specific duration of training, or either gender—was less likely to benefit from training. A more recent meta-analysis of controlled trials that included 3647 patients with CHF demonstrated no differences in mortality between exercise and usual care groups, but a 28% reduction in CHF-related hospital admissions was demonstrated among those in the exercise groups.[51]

Evolving Landscape for Cardiac Rehabilitation

Early and progressive ambulation of patients after an MI is now considered routine care. Despite many new therapies in CV medicine, cardiac rehabilitation maintains an important place in reducing morbidity and mortality rates.[2-4,19,30,49-51] When combined, the controlled trials demonstrate that the efficacy of rehabilitation in reducing mortality is similar to the best medical interventions.[30] Moreover, cardiac rehabilitation has redirected interest to humanistic concerns, providing a balance to the emphasis on complex technology. It also provides an ideal environment for patient supervision and for ensuring stability after an interventional procedure. Cardiac rehabilitation and secondary prevention programs have become the cornerstone of a multifactorial approach to secondary prevention of CV disease,[19,25,52] and available data suggest that cardiac rehabilitation is economically sound.[13,53,54]

Summary

Medicine has experienced an evolution toward assessments of technologic efficacy and outcomes assessment. Health economists and legislators are reexamining the value placed on all forms of medical care. Although this movement has changed the way that cardiac rehabilitation is implemented, studies have confirmed its value. Some of the ways in which the current economic environment has changed cardiac rehabilitation include a lessening of direct ECG monitoring, shorter hospital stays, and a more rapid progression to home programs; advances in therapy for MI and other cardiac events have lessened associated morbidity. Data on efficacy, safety, and technologic advances in the treatment of CV disease have shown that cardiac rehabilitation has changed in such a way that a wider range of patients can benefit from these services than in the past. For example, patients with stable CHF, once excluded from cardiac rehabilitation programs, are now thought to be among those who benefit the most. Pacemaker, post-transplantation, post-PCI, post-bypass, post–valvular surgery, and claudicant patients now make up a significant fraction of the patients in many programs. Despite the many benefits of cardiac rehabilitation, most eligible patients, as many as 80% to 90%, fail to receive these services. This is due in part to the fact that cardiac rehabilitation continues to be perceived as less important than invasive coronary interventions in mainstream cardiology and also to the fact that it is less vigorously promoted. Directing rehabilitation services to a larger proportion of patients who may benefit from them remains one of the important challenges for the field.

Lastly, there has been a change in the public health care message toward physical "activity" as inherently beneficial regardless of the objective measurement of "fitness." This has caused a shift in focus from morbidity, mortality, and exercise capacity to issues related to maintaining an active lifestyle and optimizing the patient's capacity to meet the physical challenges offered by occupational or recreational activities. An important but underappreciated role of the health professional is to motivate patients to include physical activity as a routine part of their lifestyle.[55,56] The cardiac rehabilitation environment provides a unique opportunity for health professionals to counsel patients on health behaviors vitally related to both prognosis and overall health.

REFERENCES

1. Convertino VA. Value of orthostatic stress in maintaining functional status soon after myocardial infarction or cardiac artery bypass grafting. *J Cardiovasc Nurs* 2003;18:124-130.
2. Taylor RS, Brown A, Ebrahim S, et al. Exercise-based rehabilitation for patients with coronary heart disease: systematic review and meta-analysis of randomized controlled trials. *Am J Med* 2004;16:682-692.
3. Piepoli MF, Davos C, Francis DP, Coats AJ. Exercise training meta-analysis of trials in patients with chronic heart failure (ExTraMATCH). *Br Med J* 2004;328:189.
4. Smart N, Marwick TH. Exercise training for heart failure patients: a systematic review of factors that improve patient mortality and morbidity. *Am J Med* 2004;116:693-706.
5. Glasziou AC, Del Mar C. Bed rest: a potentially harmful treatment needing more careful evaluation. *Lancet* 1999;354:1229-1233.
6. Froelicher VF, Myers J. *Exercise and the heart*, 5th ed. Philadelphia, 2006, WB Saunders, pp 419-461.
7. Rowell LB, O'Leary DS, Kellog DL. Integration of cardiovascular control systems during exercise. In Rowell LB, Shepherd JT, editors: *Exercise regulation and integration of multiple systems: handbook of physiology*. New York, 1996, Oxford University Press, pp 770-840.
8. Schuler G, Hambrecht R, Schlierf G, et al. Myocardial perfusion and regression of coronary artery disease in patients on a regimen of intensive physical exercise and low fat diet. *J Am Coll Cardiol* 1992;19:34-42.
9. Hambrecht R, Niebauer J, Marburger C, et al. Various intensities of leisure time physical activity in patients with coronary artery disease: effects on cardiorespiratory fitness and progression of coronary atherosclerotic lesions. *J Am Coll Cardiol* 1993;22:468-477.
10. Haskell WL, Alderman EL, Fair JM, et al. Effects of intensive multiple risk factor reduction on coronary atherosclerosis and clinical cardiac events in men and women with coronary artery disease: the Stanford Coronary Risk Intervention Project (SCRIP). *Circulation* 1994;89:975-990.
11. Hambrecht R, Wolf A, Gielen S, et al. Effect of exercise on coronary endothelial function in patients with coronary artery disease. *N Engl J Med* 2000;342:454-460.
12. Linke A, Erbs S, Hambrecht R. Exercise and the coronary circulation—alterations and adaptations in coronary artery disease. *Prog Cardiovasc Dis* 2006;48:270-284.
13. Hambrecht R, Walther C, Mobius-Winkler S, et al. Percutaneous coronary angioplasty compared with exercise training in patients with stable coronary artery disease: a randomized trial. *Circulation* 2004;109:1371-1378.
14. Hambrecht R, Fiehen E, Weigl C, et al. Regular physical exercise corrects endothelial dysfunction and improves exercise capacity in patients with chronic heart failure. *Circulation* 1998;98:2709-2715.

15. Edwards DG, Schofield RS, Lennon SL, et al. Effect of exercise training on endothelial function in men with coronary artery disease. *Am J Cardiol* 2004;93:617-620.

16. Gokce N, Vita JA, Bader DS, et al. Effect of exercise on upper and lower extremity endothelial function in patients with coronary artery disease. *Am J Cardiol* 2002; 90:124-127.

17. Moyna NM, Thompson PD. The effect of physical activity on endothelial function in man. *Acta Physiol Scand* 2004;180:113-123.

18. Linke A, Erbs S, Hambrecht R. Effects of exercise training upon endothelial function in patients with cardiovascular disease. *Front Biosci* 2008;13:424-432.

19. Ades PA. Cardiac rehabilitation and secondary prevention of coronary heart disease. *N Engl J Med* 2001;345:892-902.

20. Myers J. Optimizing the clinical exercise test: a commentary on the exercise protocol. *Heart Fail Monit* 2004;4:82-89.

21. Shaw LJ, Peterson ED, Kesler K, Hasselblad V, Califf RM. A meta-analysis of predischarge risk stratification after acute myocardial infarction with stress electrocardiographic, myocardial perfusion, and ventricular function imaging. *Am J Cardiol* 1996;78:1327-1337.

22. Valeur N, Clemmensen P, Grande P, Wachtell K, Saunamaki K. Pre-discharge exercise test for evaluation of patients with complete or incomplete revascularization following primary percutaneous coronary intervention: a DANAMI-2 sub-study. *Cardiology* 2008;109:163-171.

23. DeBusk RF, Haskell WL, Miller NH, et al. Medically directed at-home rehabilitation soon after clinically uncomplicated acute myocardial infarction: a new model for patient care. *Am J Cardiol* 1985;55:251.

24. Taylor RS, Dalal H, Jolly K, Moxham T, Zawada A. Home-based versus centre-based cardiac rehabilitation. *Cochrane Database Syst Rev* 2010(20):CD007130.

25. Ades PA, Balady GJ, Berra K. Transforming exercise-based cardiac rehabilitation programs into secondary prevention centers: a national imperative. *J Cardiopulm Rehabil* 2001;21:263-273.

26. Erhardt LR. Managing cardiovascular risk: reality vs. perception. *Eur Heart J* 2005;(Suppl L):L11-L15.

27. Ribisl PM. The inclusive chronic disease model: reaching beyond cardiopulmonary patients. In Jobin J, Maltais F, Poirier P, LeBlanc P, Simard C, editors: *Advancing the frontiers of cardiopulmonary rehabilitation.* Champaign, 2002, IL, Human Kinetics, pp 28-36.

28. Dorland J, McColl MA, editors. *Emerging approaches to chronic disease management in primary health care.* 2007, McGill Queens University Press.

29. Leon AS, Frankin BA, Costa F, et al. Cardiac rehabilitation and secondary prevention of coronary heart disease: an AHA scientific statement from the Council on Clinical Cardiology (Subcommittee on Exercise, Cardiac Rehabilitation, and Prevention) and the Council on Nutrition, Physical Activity, and Metabolism (Subcommittee on Physical Activity), in collaboration with the AACVPR. *Circulation* 2005;111:369-376.

30. Agency for Health Care Policy and Research Clinical Practice Guidelines. *Cardiac Rehabilitation.* Washington, DC, 1995, US Department of Health and Human Services.

31. American Association of Cardiovascular and Pulmonary Rehabilitation. *Guidelines for cardiac rehabilitation and secondary prevention*, 4th ed. 2004, Champaign, Human Kinetics.

32. Balady GJ, Williams MA, Ades PA, et al. Core components of cardiac rehabilitation/secondary prevention programs: 2007 update. *J Cardiopulm Rehabil* 2007;115:2675-2682.

33. Van Camp SP, Peterson RA. Cardiovascular complications of outpatient cardiac rehabilitation programs. *JAMA* 1986;256:1160-1163.

34. Franklin BA, Bonzheim K, Gordon S, Timmis GC. Safety of medically supervised outpatient cardiac rehabilitation exercise therapy: a 16 year follow-up. *Chest* 1998, 114:902-906.

35. Fletcher GF, Balady GJ, Amsterdam EA, et al. Exercise standards: a statement for healthcare professionals from the American Heart Association. *Circulation* 2001;104: 1694-1740.

36. Verril D, Ashley R, Forkner T. Recommended guidelines for monitoring and supervision of North Carolina phase II/III cardiac rehabilitation programs: a position paper by the North Carolina Cardiopulmonary Rehabilitation Association. *J Cardiopulm Rehabil* 1996;16:9-24.

37. American College of Sports Medicine. *Guidelines for exercise testing and exercise prescription*, 8th ed. Baltimore, 2010, Lippincott, Williams & Wilkins.

38. American College of Sports Medicine Position Stand. The recommended quantity and quality of exercise for developing and maintaining cardiorespiratory and muscular fitness and flexibility in healthy adults. *Med Sci Sports Exerc* 1998;30:975-991.

39. Williams MA, Haskell WL, Ades PA, et al. Resistance exercise in individuals with and without cardiovascular disease: 2007 update. A scientific statement from the American Heart Association Council on Clinical Cardiology and Council on Nutrition, Physical Activity, and Metabolism. *Circulation* 2007;116:572-584.

40. Meka N, Katragadda S, Cherian B, Arora RR. Endurance exercise and resistance training in cardiovascular disease. *Ther Adv Cardiovasc Dis* 2008;2:115-121.

41. Duscha BD, Schulze C, Robbins JL, Forman DE. Implications of chronic heart failure on peripheral vasculature and skeletal muscle before and after exercise training. *Heart Fail Rev* 2008;13:13-21.

42. Pina IL, Apstein CS, Balady GJ, et al. Exercise and heart failure: a statement from the American Heart Association Committee on Exercise, Rehabilitation, and Prevention. *Circulation* 2003;107:1210-1225.

43. Keteyian SJ, Piña IL, Hibner BA, Fleg JL. Clinical role of exercise training in the management of patients with chronic heart failure. *J Cardiopulm Rehabil Prev* 2010;30:67-76.

44. Myers, J. Effects of exercise training on abnormal ventilatory responses to exercise in patients with chronic heart failure. *Congest Heart Fail* 2000;6:243-249.

45. Arena R, Myers J, Guazzi M. The clinical and research applications of aerobic capacity and ventilatory efficiency in heart failure: an evidence-based review. *Heart Fail Rev* 2008;13:245-269.

46. Haykowsky M, Eves N, Figgures L, et al. Effect of exercise training on VO₂ peak and left ventricular systolic function in recent cardiac transplant recipients. *Am J Cardiol* 2005;95:1002-1004.

47. Williams MA, Ades PA, Hamm LF, et al. Clinical evidence for a health benefit from cardiac rehabilitation: an update. *Am Heart J* 2006;152:835-841.

48. Kavanagh T. Exercise rehabilitation in cardiac transplant patients: a comprehensive review. *Eura Medicophys* 2005;41:67-74.

49. O'Connor GT, Buring JE, Yusuf S, et al. An overview of randomized trials of rehabilitation with exercise after myocardial infarction. *Circulation* 1989;80:234-244.

50. Oldridge NB, Guyatt GH, Fischer ME, Rimm AA. Cardiac rehabilitation after myocardial infarction: combined experience of randomized clinical trials. *JAMA* 1988;260: 945-950.

51. Davies EJ, Moxham T, Rees K, Singh S, et al. Exercise training for systolic heart failure: Cochrane systematic review and meta-analysis. *Eur J Heart Fail* 2010;12:706-715.

52. Lavie CJ, Thomas RJ, Squires RW, Allison TG, Milani RV. Exercise training and secondary prevention in primary and secondary coronary prevention. *Mayo Clin Proc* 2009;84:373-383.

53. Yu CM, Lau CP, Chau J, et al. A short course of cardiac rehabilitation program is highly cost effective in improving long-term quality of life in patients with recent myocardial infarction or percutaneous coronary intervention. *Arch Phys Med Rehabil* 2004;85:1915-1922.

54. Lee AJ, Strickler GK, Shepard DS. The economics of cardiac rehabilitation and lifestyle modification: a review of the literature. *J Cardiopulm Rehabil Prev* 2007;27(3):135-142.

55. Myers J. Physical activity: the missing prescription. *Eur J Cardiovasc Prev Rehabil* 2005;12:85-86.

56. Peterson JA. Get moving: physical activity counseling in primary care. *J Am Acad Nurse Pract* 2007;19:349-357.

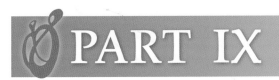

Cardiovascular Devices

Daniel B. Kramer

Treatment of cardiovascular disease increasingly uses a wide variety of devices to support cardiac mechanical or electrical function and to provide critical diagnostic data. Each of the devices described here is routinely used to care for patients with cardiovascular problems. Because of important risks in their use, each device demands specific training, knowledge, and expertise. In experienced hands, these devices may be livesaving for well-selected patients.

Pulmonary Artery Catheters

Pulmonary artery catheters (PACs) allow direct hemodynamic assessment and oximetry of right-sided chambers as well as indirect or calculated measures of left-sided pressure, cardiac output, and resistance of the pulmonary and systemic vasculature.

Indications

Routine use of PACs in the care of critically ill patients remains controversial, and the results of several large studies evaluating their use have not definitely shown improved outcomes.[1,2] In practice, PACs are used most often for diagnosis and management of undifferentiated shock or pulmonary edema and for titration of fluid resuscitation, vasopressors, or inotropes. Common uses for PACs are listed in Table A-1. As with any test, particularly an invasive and potentially hazardous one, insertion of a PAC should only be performed after a clinical decision has been made that the data gathered will either refine the diagnosis or influence therapy in a meaningful way.

Design

A typical PAC is shown in Figure A-1. Catheters used for single measurements during cardiac catheterization have only a single port and are not preformed. These catheters are placed and steered into position under fluoroscopy. Catheters intended to be placed without fluoroscopy are preformed with a curve that facilitates advancement from either the right internal jugular vein or left subclavian vein into the right atrium, right ventricle, through the right ventricular outflow tract, and into either the left or (more commonly) right main pulmonary artery. Some models include an additional port for real-time measurement of mixed venous saturation or temperature.

Technical Aspects of Placement

PACs are inserted through a short introducer sheath placed in either the internal jugular, femoral, or subclavian vein. Some operators are able to place a smaller PAC (5 Fr) through initial access in peripheral veins. For PACs that are expected to remain in place, the catheter should be placed through a sterile covering that will cover the exposed catheter tubing and connect to the introducer hub.

After insertion beyond the sheath (10 to 15 cm), the balloon is inflated with 1 to 1.5 mL of air from a provided syringe that locks into the appropriate port. Balloon inflation allows the catheter to "float" along with right-sided flow into either the left or right pulmonary artery until the wedge position is reached. Accurate pressure calibration should be confirmed with the baseline at 0 mm Hg with the transducer open to atmosphere. Pressure is transduced on inflation of the balloon to allow accurate recordings in each cardiac chamber and confirmation of balloon-tip placement. While under fluoroscopic guidance, a combination of the anatomic landmarks and, more importantly, the catheter waveform is used to identify the position of the distal port. Without fluoroscopy, correct interpretation of the waveform is essential. When a satisfactory position has been reached, the amount of PAC inserted (using the centimeter markers on the catheter) should be noted at the entrance to the sheath; this is important when troubleshooting a malfunctioning catheter. When the catheter is being advanced beyond the sheath, the balloon must always be inflated; the balloon must be deflated whenever the catheter is being withdrawn to avoid vascular or valvular injury.

Placement into the PA is achievable without fluoroscopy in most patients. However, patients with substantial pulmonary hypertension and/or tricuspid regurgitation may prove more challenging; several additional relative contraindications to placement without fluoroscopy are noted in Box A-1. The usual contraindications to central line placement (regardless of PAC insertion) also apply and include significant coagulopathy, known venous occlusion, and contralateral pulmonary compromise. A typical radiographic appearance of PAC placement is shown in Figure A-2.

Interpretation of Waveforms

Characteristic waveforms, normal values, and typical distance from the insertion site in the right internal jugular vein or left subclavian vein in a normal right atrium, right ventricle, pulmonary artery, and pulmonary wedge position are shown in Figure A-3. Tracings at the bedside may not be as easily recognized, however; in these cases, correlation of the waveforms with the electrocardiogram may help define A, C, and V waves and X and Y descents (Figure A-4).

Troubleshooting and Complications

Failure to obtain satisfactory waveforms is common and may be related to air or small clots anywhere in the system from catheter tip through transducer. The catheter should be thoroughly flushed before and after oximetry measurements and whenever waveforms no longer appear to be normal. Failure of transduction may also manifest if the relevant port abuts the wall of a chamber, in

TABLE A-1	Selected Clinical Situations in Which Pulmonary Artery Catheters May Assist Diagnosis or Treatment
CLINICAL SCENARIO	**UTILITY OF PULMONARY ARTERY CATHETER**
Undifferentiated shock	Characterize filling pressures, cardiac output, and vascular resistances to differentiate hypovolemia, cardiogenic shock, sepsis, or mixed physiology Oximetry may provide rapid diagnosis of ventricular septal defect in setting of acute myocardial infarction
Acute decompensated heart failure	Characterize filling pressures, cardiac output, and systemic vascular resistance in response to tailored therapy Establish candidacy and status for cardiac/cardiopulmonary transplantation
Pulmonary edema	Characterize filling pressures to distinguish between cardiogenic and noncardiogenic etiologies
Suspected pericardial tamponade	Determine filling pressures (± equalization) and contours of X and Y descents to establish diagnosis and monitor response to treatment
Pulmonary hypertension	Provide reproducible, real-time measurement of pulmonary pressures and calculated pulmonary vascular resistance at baseline and in response to inhaled oxygen and vasodilatory therapies May be indicated to establish candidacy for surgical procedures or medical therapies (e.g., liver transplantation, selective pulmonary vasodilators)
Valvular heart disease, suspected shunt, or constriction/restriction assessment	Combine with left heart catheterization for precise quanitification of aortic or mitral valvular stenosis, location and degree of shunting, and diagnosis of constriction/restriction

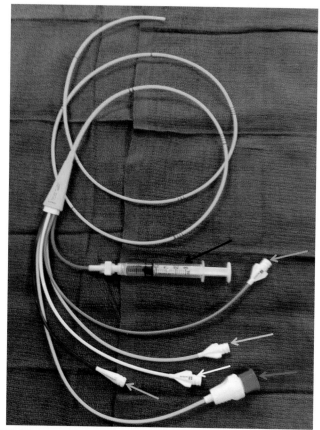

FIGURE A-1 A thermodilution-capable pulmonary artery catheter is shown. The available ports are designed for proximal infusion (*orange arrow*) and positioning in the right atrium (*white arrow*), right ventricle (*gray arrow*), and pulmonary artery (*yellow arrow*). Additionally, there is a connector for temperature measurements (*red arrow*) and inflation of the balloon (*black arrow*).

Box A-1 Relative Contraindications to Pulmonary Artery Catheter Placement Without Fluoroscopic Guidance

Pacemaker or implantable cardioverter-defibrillator
Other intracardiac devices such as patent foramen ovale/atrial septal defect occlusion device
Tricuspid or pulmonary valve prostheses
Left bundle branch block
Right-sided endocarditis
Known or suspected pulmonary embolism
Known unrepaired ventricular septal defect

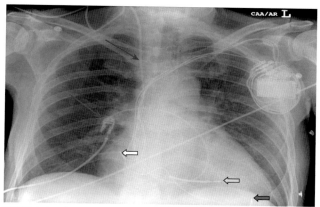

FIGURE A-2 The typical radiographic appearance of a pulmonary artery catheter (PAC) via the right internal jugular vein in a patient with a biventricular implantable cardioverter-defibrillator (ICD) is shown. The *red arrow* indicates the proximal portion of the PAC and the *blue arrow* indicates its tip in the right main pulmonary artery. The ICD system includes a right atrial pacing lead (*white arrow*), right ventricular ICD lead (*yellow arrow*), and left ventricular pacing lead (*green arrow*).

which case gentle advancement (with the balloon up) or retraction (with the balloon down) may improve the tracing. Inability to reproduce a wedge tracing may reflect migration of the catheter, in which case a chest radiograph and confirmation of the insertion distance may be helpful.

Complications of PAC placement include vascular injury, pneumothorax, infection, and arrhythmias. The most serious complication of either acute or indwelling use of a PAC is rupture of a pulmonary artery or branch vessel, which may cause rapid deterioration and death if not quickly identified and managed. Any patient with a PAC inserted who develops new hemoptysis, ipsilateral pleural effusion, or sudden decompensation should be presumed to have a pulmonary artery rupture until proven otherwise. Acute management of suspected pulmonary artery rupture includes turning the patient on his or her side toward the site of last known PAC placement; preparations for intubation with a dual-lumen endotracheal tube; emergency portable chest radiograph; reversal of coagulopathy if appropriate; and evaluation for

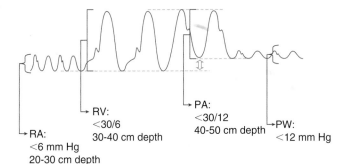

FIGURE A-3 Typical waveforms for the right atrium (*RA*), right ventricle (*RV*), pulmonary artery (*PA*), and pulmonary wedge (*PW*) positions are shown. Note that the depth in centimeters refers to distance from a standard insertion from the right internal jugular vein. *(Courtesy Peter A. Noseworthy, MD.)*

> ### Box A-2 Indications for IABP Placement Categorized by Physiology
>
> Afterload reduction
> - Acute mitral regurgitation
> - Ventricular septal defect/rupture
> - Severe systolic heart failure
> - Cardiogenic shock
> - Bridge to or from cardiopulmonary bypass
>
> Increased coronary perfusion
> - Refractory angina
> - Bridge through high-risk PCI or while awaiting CABG

CABG, coronary artery bypass grafting; IABP, intraaortic balloon pump; PCI, percutaneous coronary intervention.

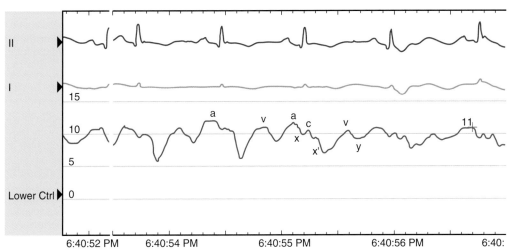

FIGURE A-4 The a, c, and v waves are shown along with the x and y descents relative to the surface electrocardiogram. Note that the A wave is the first positive deflection to follow the p wave, and the V wave is on or shortly after the t wave.

surgical or endovascular stabilization and repair. Until further diagnostics have been performed, the PA catheter should not be removed because this may worsen the hemorrhage. In the case of actual rupture where the patient remains stable, the catheter may need to be removed in the operating room.

Intraaortic Balloon Pump Counterpulsation

Percutaneous placement of an intraaortic balloon pump (IABP) provides hemodynamic support and augments coronary perfusion. Despite their effectiveness, IABPs are associated with morbidity. Approximately 10% of patients have complications, 2% to 3% of which are serious.[3,4] Thus, the risks and benefits of therapy must be weighed at initial insertion, and the need for continued treatment and criteria for discontinuation should be continuously reevaluated to minimize indwelling time and reduce the risk of complications.

Indications

The indications for IABP placement may be organized according to its physiologic effects (Box A-2). IABPs provide systolic unloading and diastolic augmentation of arterial blood pressure. Increased diastolic pressure improves coronary blood flow and provides effective and immediate relief of refractory angina, provides support throughout high-risk percutaneous coronary

interventions, and may temporarily relieve refractory arrhythmias related to ischemia.[5]

Design

IABPs are catheter-based devices with an inflatable balloon mounted on the distal portion of a stiff shaft that facilitates insertion retrograde from the femoral artery into the descending aorta. The inflation port is connected to the drive console, which inflates the balloon with helium. By using gating based on either electrocardiographic gating to the R wave of the QRS complex, the pressure waveform, or a fiberoptic trigger, the balloon inflates during diastole and deflates during systole. A radiopaque marker at the distal end of the catheter allows fluoroscopic localization during placement and position confirmation. The central lumen of the catheter facilitates initial insertion over a wire. After insertion, this lumen allows for monitoring of aortic pressure and facilitates timing of the device.

Technical Aspects of Placement

The IABP is usually placed via percutaneous access in the common femoral artery. A careful vascular exam of both lower extremities and the left arm should be performed before insertion. The catheters can be placed without a sheath or through an introducer sheath. Preinsertion angiography can be performed to determine whether the iliofemoral arteries are large enough to accommodate the catheter and/or sheath. Severe atherosclerotic disease or tortuousity in the common femoral artery, iliac arteries, or aorta may preclude placement of the device. After the appropriate size balloon is chosen based on patient size and the device is prepared, the distal end of the IABP is positioned in the proximal portion of the descending aorta over a guidewire. Placement is confirmed fluoroscopically, with the tip of the IABP roughly at the level of the carina and clearly below the aortic arch (to avoid compromise of the left subclavian artery). The wire is removed, the balloon inflation port is connected to the IABP console, and the central lumen is connected to a pressure transducer on the console.

Timing and Waveforms

Inspection of the arterial waveform with the IABP set to inflate with alternate heartbeats (1:2 counterpulsation) allows assessment of its impact on systolic unloading and diastolic augmentation (Figure A-5). In addition, problems with timing may be identified and adjustments made as needed (Figures A-6 and A-7).

Complications

Complications of IABPs include vascular dissection or laceration, limb ischemia, thrombotic or cholesterol embolization, visceral or renal ischemia, infection, or mechanical failure requiring surgical removal of the device. A contemporary large registry experience with IABPs identified an in-hospital mortality rate of 22% for recipients and a complication rate of 10.3%. Complications are more likely in patients with significant preexisting peripheral vascular disease as well as in female and older patients.[3]

Pericardiocentesis

Indications

Percutaneous access into the pericardial space treats pericardial tamponade, provides diagnostic data in the evaluation of effusions, and allows access to the epicardium for electrophysiologic mapping and ablation.

Technical Aspects

In cases of suspected cardiac tamponade in which the patient is not in danger of imminent arrest, a PAC is used before drainage to obtain baseline measurements to confirm both the diagnosis and response to fluid removal. Arterial pressure monitoring can also be helpful to quantify accurately the pulsus paradoxus and the response to drainage. Pericardiocentesis may be performed with electrocardiographic, echocardiographic, and/or pressure monitoring guidance. Coagulopathy is a relative contraindication to the procedure, although it can be performed despite therapeutic anticoagulation when necessary.

Patients are prepped and draped in a sterile fashion and given local anesthesia; they are ideally positioned with a wedge cushion providing a 45-degree incline to the thorax to direct the effusion anteriorly. Needles should have a short bevel to reduce the likelihood of right ventricular injury and, if clinical stability permits, should be connected to ports for pressure transduction of pericardial pressure as well as evacuation of fluid into a collection container and/or analysis tubes.

Access is most usually achieved via the subxyphoid approach under fluoroscopic or echocardiographic guidance. In either case

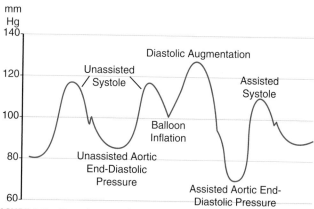

FIGURE A-5 Normal timing of an intraaortic balloon pump (IABP) evaluated at 1:2 counterpulsations is shown. With the first beat, aortic systolic and end-diastolic pressures are shown without IABP support and are therefore unassisted. With the second beat, the balloon inflates with the appearance of the dicrotic notch, and peak-augmented diastolic pressure is inscribed. With balloon deflation, assisted end-diastolic pressure and assisted systolic pressure are observed. To confirm that IABP is producing maximal hemodynamic benefit, the peak diastolic augmentation should be greater than the unassisted systolic pressure, and the two assisted pressures should be less than the unassisted values. *(From Trost JC, Hillis LD. Intra-aortic balloon counterpulsation. Am J Cardiol 2006;97[9]:1391-1398.)*

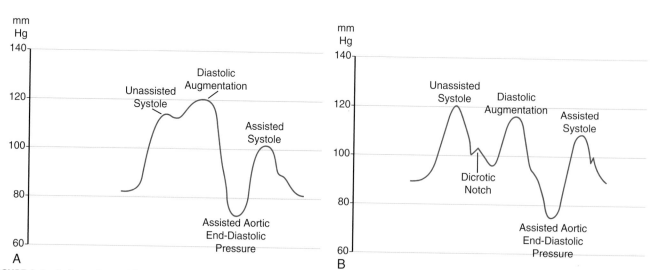

FIGURE A-6 **A,** Systemic arterial pressure waveform from a subject in whom balloon inflation occurs too early, before aortic valve closure. Consequently, the left ventricle is forced to empty against an inflated balloon; the corresponding increase in afterload may increase myocardial oxygen demands and worsen systolic function. **B,** Systemic arterial pressure waveform from a patient in whom balloon inflation occurs too late, well after the beginning of diastole, thereby minimizing diastolic pressure augmentation. *(From Trost JC, Hillis LD. Intra-aortic balloon counterpulsation. Am J Cardiol 2006;97[9]:1391-1398.)*

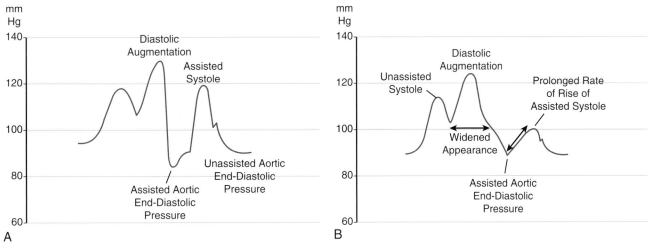

A

B

FIGURE A-7 **A,** Systemic arterial pressure waveform from a patient in whom balloon deflation occurs too early, before the end of diastole. This may shorten the period of diastolic pressure augmentation. A corresponding transient decrease in aortic pressure may promote retrograde arterial flow from the carotid or coronary arteries, possibly inducing cerebral or myocardial ischemia. **B,** Systemic arterial pressure waveform from a subject in whom balloon deflation occurs too late, after the end of diastole, thereby producing the same deleterious consequences as early balloon inflation (increased left ventricular afterload, with a resultant increase in myocardial oxygen demands and a worsening of systolic function). *(From Trost JC, Hillis LD. Intra-aortic balloon counterpulsation. Am J Cardiol 2006;97[9]:1391-1398.)*

the needle is attached to a syringe, and both are directed at a shallow angle toward the left shoulder with continuous aspiration to detect entry into the pericardium (which may be subtle). For effusions deemed to be most accessible from the apex, the needle should be aimed along the main axis of the left ventricle and the left ventricular outflow tract. The needle is advanced to the pericardium under negative pressure. When fluid is aspirated, pressure is immediately transduced to confirm that the end of the needle is in the pericardial space and not in a cardiac chamber and to confirm its relation to right atrial pressure. If an electrocardiographic (ECG) lead has been attached, a current of injury on ECG monitoring may be detected. In some cases, such as with hemorrhagic effusions or when the pressure waveform is atypical, gentle injection of contrast (radiopaque if under fluoroscopy; agitated saline if under echocardiographic guidance) may be helpful to confirm position. A guidewire is then advanced and should be observed coursing laterally and posteriorly toward the left atrium, after which a soft catheter may be placed over the wire and left in place for continued drainage.

Electrical Cardioversion and Defibrillation

External electrical cardioversion is highly successful in terminating atrial and ventricular arrhythmias in acute and elective settings.

Equipment

Several models of defibrillators are available, and most models currently in use have both automatic and manual operating modes. Modern defibrillators use *biphasic* energy waveforms, which terminate atrial and ventricular arrhythmias more successfully and with less energy than *monophasic* waveforms.[6-8] A typical defibrillator for hospital use is pictured in Figure A-8. Key controls common to different models include options for synchronization, ECG lead selection and gain, shock energy, and parameters for transcutaneous pacing.

Setup and Patient Preparation

Specialized adhesive pads with defibrillation electrodes or handheld paddles are positioned to direct the defibrillation waveform. In elective cases, the patient's chest should be shaved and dry;

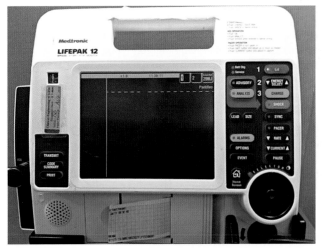

FIGURE A-8 A typical external defibrillator for in-hospital use is shown. Different models vary slightly, but essential features (seen here) include controls for energy selection, synchronization, charge, and discharge, and pacing functions.

note should be made of any preexisting skin wounds or rashes prior to application of conducting gel. Pad placement is done with either an apical-posterior or anterior-lateral alignment (Figure A-9). An anterior-posterior alignment may be more effective for conversion of atrial arrhythmias because the atria are more likely to be captured by the defibrillation waveform.[9,10] If pads are used, additional pressure applied with the paddles (or removing the pads and using paddles alone) may make defibrillation more effective.[11] Stable or conscious patients should be well sedated prior to cardioversion, and equipment for airway management or any unexpected proarrhythmia should be immediately available.

Technical Considerations

Once the patient has been prepared, the device should be synchronized to the R wave for cardioversion; for defibrillation, the device should be left in asynchronous mode. The defibrillator may then be charged to the selected energy while the primary operator ensures that personnel are not directly touching the patient. Biphasic defibrillation protocols for ventricular

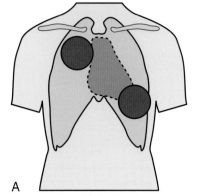 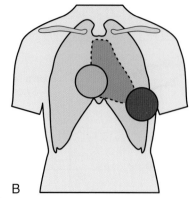 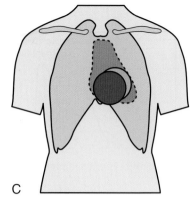

A   B   C

FIGURE A-9   External defibrillator placement. Anterior-lateral (**A**), apical-posterior (**B**), and anterior-posterior (**C**) external defibrillator pad or paddle placement is shown. *(Modified from Kerber RE; Electrical treatment of cardiac arrhythmias: defibrillation and cardioversion. Ann Emerg Med 1993;22:296-301.)*

arrhythmias start at 150 J and may increase to 200 J, 300 J, or 360 J if the initial defibrillation is not successful.[12] However, lower energy defibrillations (50 to 100 J) may be effective in more organized arrhythmias such as atrial flutter or monomorphic ventricular tachycardia.

Permanent Pacemakers

Pacemaker (PM) and implantable cardioverter-defibrillator (ICD) systems consist of a pulse generator and electrodes (leads). Devices may be single chamber, dual chamber, or biventricular. Chest radiograph appearance of typical PM and ICD systems is shown in Figure A-10.

Leads

A variety of pacing leads are commercially available and vary with respect to fixation mechanism (active or passive), insulation type, configuration (unipolar versus bipolar), and connector type (Table A-2). *Lead impedance* may be used as a measure of lead integrity. Low lead impedance may be due to an insulation defect, whereas high lead impedances may indicate a lead fracture.

Basic Pacing Concepts

Stimulation threshold is the minimal electrical stimulus necessary to capture consistently the heart outside its refractory period. The threshold can be described by the strength-duration curve (Figure A-11), which plots amplitude (measured in volts) against pulse width (measured in milliseconds). Values on or above the curve result in capture. Pacing at an output below threshold results in *failure to capture* (Figure A-12). Failure to capture should be distinguished from *no output* conditions (such as those due to a depleted pulse generator battery), in which no pacing artifact is present.

    Sensing is the ability of the PM to detect the heart's intrinsic rhythm. *Intrinsic amplitude* refers to the size (measured in millivolts) of the detected electrical signal from the atrium or ventricle. *Sensitivity* is a programmable setting above which electrical signals will be interpreted as cardiac in origin and below which electrical signals will be ignored. *Undersensing* is the failure of the PM to detect the intrinsic cardiac electrical signal (Figure A-13, *A*). *Oversensing* is the sensing of an inappropriate signal (either physiologic or nonphysiologic) (see Figure A-13, *B*). Box A-3 lists some potential sources of electromagnetic interference that can cause oversensing. A magnet placed over a pacemaker disables the PM's ability to sense and converts the pacing mode to DOO or VOO, resulting in continuous asynchronous pacing. Magnets placed over ICDs, however, do not ordinarily affect *pacing* functions.

Pacemaker Programming Considerations

MODE

The programmable pacing mode determines in which chambers the PM paces and senses and how it responds to sensed signals (Table A-3).[13] Examples of the potential ECG appearance of proper dual-chamber pacing are shown in Figure A-14. Cardiac resynchronization therapy has a characteristic ECG appearance that may be distinguished from right ventricle (RV)-apical or left ventricle (LV)-only pacing, a characterization that may be useful in troubleshooting suspected lead migration or loss of pacing output (Figure A-15).

RATE-RESPONSIVE PACING

Rate-responsive pacing is designed to result in an increase in heart rate proportional to an increase in metabolic demand and helps patients achieve more physiologic heart rates. A variety of sensors is available for detecting increases in metabolic demand (Table A-4).

Pseudo Pacemaker Malfunction

A number of programming features may result in the appearance of PM malfunction, such as failure to capture or failing to pace at the programmed rate (Table A-5).

Temporary Pacemakers

Temporary transvenous or transcutaneous pacing provides definitive management of symptomatic bradycardia and may also be indicated for patients at high risk for heart block (e.g., those undergoing high-risk procedures such as alcohol septal ablation or percutaneous aortic valve implantation).

Indications

Observational studies and clinical experience provide data for current guidelines for the use of temporary pacing in the setting of acute coronary syndromes (Figure A-16). These include patients with unstable bradycardia not responsive to atropine or positive chronotropes, patients with high-grade or complete atrioventricular block, and select patients with intraventricular conduction defects. The risks of placement of a temporary transvenous wire in these settings must be balanced against the risks of vascular access in patients typically receiving multiple antiplatelet and anticoagulant medications. Transcutaneous pacing is an emergency therapy that should be viewed as a bridge to more definitive management.

Text continued on page 758

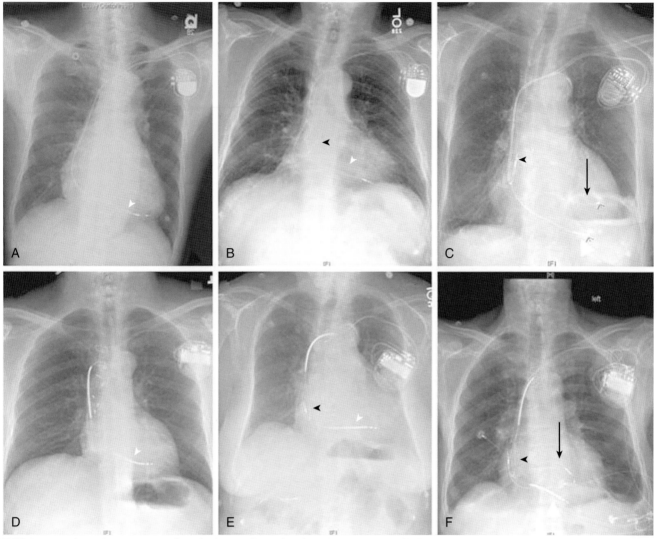

FIGURE A-10 Radiographic appearance of standard pacemaker and implantable cardioverter-defibrillator (ICD) systems is shown. **A,** Single-chamber pacemaker. **B,** Dual-chamber pacemaker. **C,** Biventricular pacemaker. **D,** Single-chamber ICD. **E,** Dual-chamber ICD. **F,** Biventricular ICD. Single-chamber systems consist of a right ventricular electrode (*white arrowhead*). Dual-chamber systems have a right atrial (*black arrowhead*) and right ventricular electrode, whereas biventricular systems have a third lead positioned in the coronary sinus (*black arrow*).

TABLE A-2	Pacing Electrode Features
FEATURE	**COMMENT**
Fixation Mechanism	
Transvenous, passive fixation	Tines become lodged in trabeculations; lower pacing threshold, higher dislodgement rate
Transvenous, active fixation	Helix or screw extends into endocardial tissue to secure lead; higher pacing thresholds, lower dislodgement rate
Epicardial	Surgically implanted on outer surface of heart. Typically higher pacing thresholds. May be used for patients with mechanical tricuspid valve, those with difficult coronary sinus access requiring left ventricular pacing, or those requiring pacemaker undergoing concurrent cardiac surgery
Insulation	
Polyurethane	Easier to pass, more rigid, less durable, thinner
Silicone	Higher coefficient of friction, therefore less "slippery," less rigid, more durable, thicker
Configuration	
Unipolar	Sensing and pacing between the lead tip (distal electrode) and the pacemaker pulse generator; bigger "antenna," therefore more prone to oversensing
Bipolar	Sensing and pacing between two electrodes separated by several millimeters (proximal and distal) located on a single lead; smaller "antenna," therefore less prone to oversensing

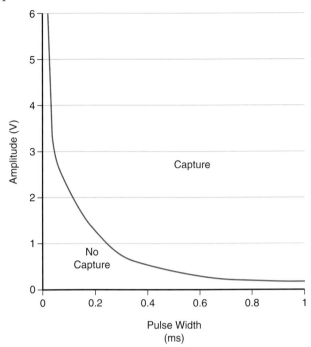

FIGURE A-11 A strength-duration curve describes the relationship between the amplitude and the pulse width. Values on or above the curve result in capture. Values below the curve result in failure to capture.

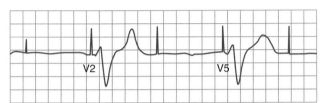

FIGURE A-12 An example of intermittent failure to capture is shown. Pacing spikes can be seen marching steadily through the tracing, but every other beat fails to elicit ventricular depolarization. This can be attributed to elevated pacing thresholds, a low programmed pacemaker output, a depleted pulse generator battery, lead abnormality, or a prolonged refractory period.

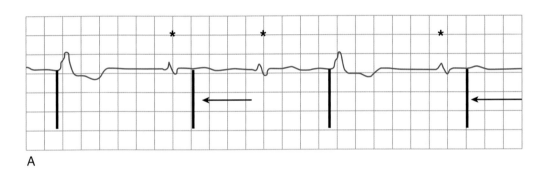

A

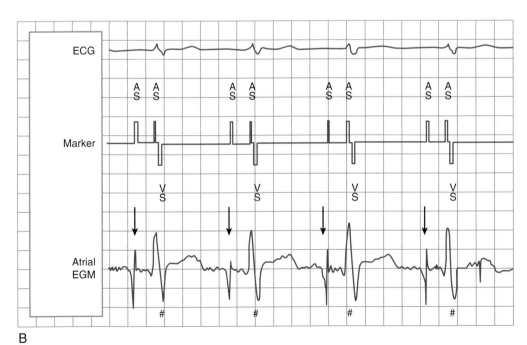

B

FIGURE A-13 A, Undersensing of the QRS complex is demonstrated. The first and fourth QRS complexes are ventricular paced beats. Native QRS complexes (*asterisks*), however, are not appropriately sensed, resulting in a failure to inhibit pacing. As a result, inappropriate ventricular pacing spikes are present (*left arrows*). Because they occur in the ventricular refractory period, they result in failure to capture. Reprogramming the pacemaker to a more sensitive setting overcame this problem. The pacing threshold was not elevated. **B,** Atrial oversensing is present. The atrial electrogram (*EGM*) obtained during routine pacemaker interrogation demonstrates sensing of the intrinsic atrial signal (*down arrows*) and far-field oversensing of the ventricular signal (*pound symbols*). This is confirmed by the marker channel. AS, atrial sensed event; ECG, electrocardiogram; VS, ventricular sensed event.

TABLE A-3	Revised NASPE/BPEG Generic Code for Antibradycardia, Adaptive-Rate, and Multisite Pacing*			
POSITION I CHAMBER PACED	**POSITION II** CHAMBER SENSED	**POSITION III** CHAMBER SENSED	**POSITION IV** RATE MODULATION	**POSITION V** MULTISITE PACING
0 = None	0 = None	0 = None	0 = None	0 = None
A = Atrium	A = Atrium	A = Atrium	A = Atrium	A = Atrium
V = Ventricle	V = Ventricle	V = Ventricle	V = Ventricle	V = Ventricle
D = Dual (A + V)	D = Dual (A + V)	D = Dual (A + V)	D = Dual (A + V)	D = Dual (A + V)
S = Single (A or V)	S = Single (A or V)	S = Single (A or V)	S = Single (A or V)	S = Single (A or V)

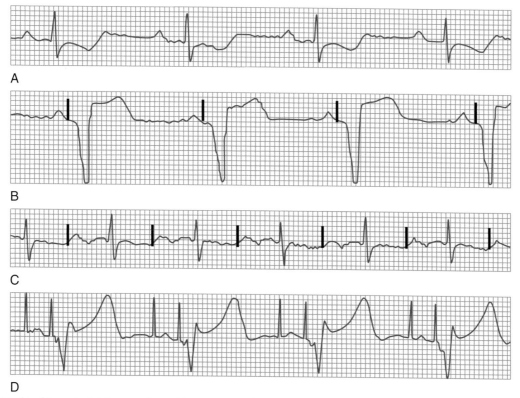

FIGURE A-14 Examples of the potential electrocardiographic appearance of proper dual-chamber pacing are shown. **A,** Sinus rhythm without pacing. **B,** Sinus rhythm with ventricular pacing. **C,** Atrial pacing with intact atrioventricular conduction. **D,** Dual-chamber pacing.

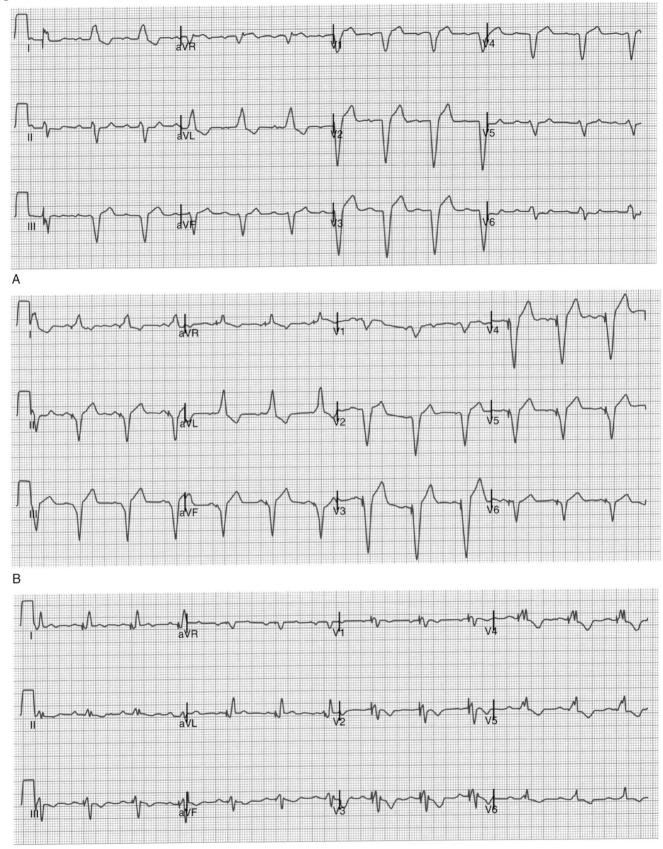

A

B

C

FIGURE A-15   The electrocardiographic appearance of intrinsic left bundle branch block (**A**), right ventricular apical pacing (**B**), left ventricular pacing (**C**), and biventricular pacing (**D**) is shown.

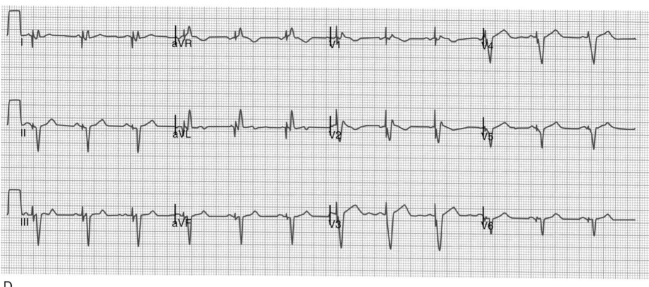

D

FIGURE A-15, cont'd Note that biventricular pacing narrows the QRS considerably with a pseudo-right bundle branch block pattern and initial negative deflections in lead I and aVL, both of which are more prominent in left ventricle–only pacing. The frontal plane axis shifts from left axis deviation at baseline and with right ventricular apical pacing to a rightward axis with left ventricular pacing, and a northwest axis with biventricular pacing (monophasic R wave in aVR compared with a QS in aVR for left ventricular pacing).

TABLE A-4 Sensors for Rate Responsive Pacing

TYPE OF SENSOR	DESCRIPTION	COMMENTS
Motion/activity sensor Example: piezoelectric crystal	Detects physical movement; sensor increases rate according to level of activity Mechanical force causes change in crystal	Brisk response to exercise but does not respond well to other physiologic stresses, such as emotional stress Can be activated by nonphysiologic stimuli structure that generates voltage (e.g., vibration while riding in a car)
Accelerometer	Converts change in velocity in anterior-posterior direction into electrical signal	May not provide adequate response to activities without movement in anterior-posterior direction (e.g., weight lifting)
Minute ventilation	Measures changes in electrical impedance across chest as surrogate marker for respiratory rate	Good correlation with metabolic workload; does not respond as quickly as motion/activity sensors to onset of exercise
Physiologic sensors Example: QT duration	Assess true physiologic measure Measured from onset of QRS to end of the T wave	Rarely stand-alone sensor for rate-responsive pacing; accuracy varies Interval affected by autonomic tone and heart rate; good rate-adaptive measure; does not respond well to non–exercise-related stress

TABLE A-5 Causes of Pseudo-Pacemaker Malfunction

FEATURE	DESCRIPTION
Mode switch	Device switches from tracking mode (such as DDD) to nontracking mode (such as DDI) in response to sustained atrial arrhythmia. Mode switch pacing rate may be separately programmable or may be the lower rate limit of the pacemaker.
Hysteresis	Allows the rate to fall below the programmed lower rate of the pacemaker following an intrinsic beat.
Rate drop response	Delivers pacing at a programmed high rate (e.g., 100 beats/min) for a limited time in response to a drop in heart rate. Used for patients with neurocardiogenic syncope.
Rate-responsive pacing	Increases heart rate in response to activity.
Sleep mode	Allows programming of different lower rate for bedtime hours to minimize pacing and conserve the battery.
Threshold testing	Automated feature to test threshold, typically during sleep. May appear similar to failure to capture.

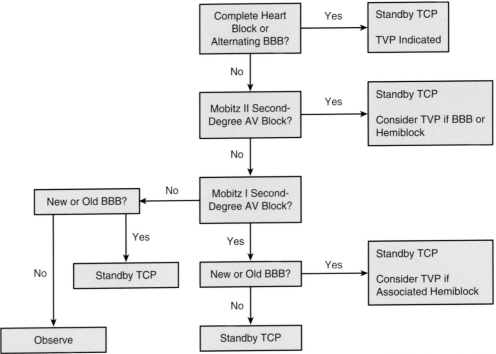

FIGURE A-16 An algorithm is shown for considering either transcutaneous pacing (*TCP*) or transvenous pacing (*TVP*) in the setting of different atrioventricular (*AV*) conduction defects or bundle branch block (*BBB*). *(Modified from Antman EM, Anbe DT, Armstrong PW, et al. ACC/AHA guidelines for the management of patients with ST-elevation myocardial infarction: a report of the American College of Cardiology/American Heart Association Task Force on Practice Guidelines [Committee to Revise the 1999 Guidelines for the Management of Patients with Acute Myocardial Infarction]. Circulation 2004;110[9]:e82-e292.)*

Indications outside acute ischemic syndromes include any symptomatic nonreversible bradycardia; overdrive pacing of ventricular arrhythmias, particularly torsades de pointes; and support through procedures with high rates of acquired complete heart block.

Placement

Placement of a transvenous temporary wire with a balloon tip is similar to PAC placement and may be performed without fluoroscopy in patients who do not have the relevant contraindications noted in Box A-1. The inducer sheath ideally should contain a locking mechanism at the hub to prevent migration of the temporary wire after it has been placed and should include a sterile sleeve to cover the exposed wire. Once the temporary wire has been advanced through the sheath, the balloon is inflated and the pacing function of the wire is activated. In this way, progress through the right atrium and into the RV can be identified by successful capture and by the vector of the paced QRS complex, which ideally will reflect stable placement in the right ventricular apex (with a left bundle branch block [LBBB], superior axis) or outflow tract (LBBB, inferior axis). Temporary PM units include either digital or analog controls to modulate output, pacing mode, rate, and sensitivity.

When a location with a satisfactory paced complex is identified, the pacing output is diminished until the threshold is identified. A safe pacing threshold should be much less than 5 mA, recognizing that the threshold may be affected by metabolic disarray and other features of critical illness. Sensitivity testing may be possible depending on the patient's underlying rhythm and may further confirm stable initial placement. A chest radiograph should be obtained to confirm the absence of any complication related to vascular access or lead position.

Transvenous temporary wire placement can also be quickly done under fluoroscopy with either a balloon-tipped catheter or a electrophysiology multipolar pacing catheter, which may provide a more stable pacing position or placement in the coronary sinus.

Transcutaneous pacing is performed through an external defibrillator as described above. The programmable features include the pacing rate and the output (measured in milliamperes). Electrical capture (on telemetry or ECG) should be confirmed by palpation of the pulse because adequate myocardial capture may be difficult, particularly in unstable patients or those with electrolyte or pH pertubations. Transcutaneous pacing is painful, and conscious patients should be heavily sedated.

Complications and Troubleshooting

Temporary pacing (either transcutaneous or transvenous) may suppress a patient's underlying escape rhythm. Thus, after commitment to pacing, it is imperative to recognize and address promptly any suspected malfunction. Apart from complications related to vascular access and trauma from the pacing wire itself, problems with temporary PMs include failure to pace (no pacing spikes seen on telemetry), failure to capture (pacing spikes seen without a QRS complex), or failure to sense (pacing spikes on or around native QRS complexes). Failure to pace should prompt confirmation that the connections and battery unit are intact and may require empiric replacement of the latter. Lack of capture should prompt formal threshold testing and a chest radiograph to exclude lead migration, including possible cardiac perforation, which may be clinically subtle. Undersensing or oversensing can often be overcome by adjusting the PM sensitivity settings.

Implantable Cardioverter-Defibrillators

Like PMs, ICDs can be single chamber, dual chamber, or biventricular. An ICD system can be radiographically distinguished from a PM system by the presence of one or two shocking coils (Figure A-10). ICD generators consist of a battery, a capacitor, circuitry, and the device housing, or "can."

Programmed Therapies for Ventricular Arrhythmias

ICDs continuously monitor the patient's heart rate. When pre-specified programmable detection criteria are met, the device delivers therapy to restore the patient's rhythm back to normal. Therapies are programmed according to heart rate, or "zones." Each zone is programmable and specifies the heart rate range and duration of arrhythmia required before declaring an arrhythmia present and initiating delivery of therapy.

ICDs can deliver two types of therapies to terminate ventricular arrhythmias: high-voltage therapies (i.e., shocks) or antitachycardia pacing (ATP). High-voltage shocks (typically 30 to 40 J maximum) are usually delivered from the ICD and superior vena cava coil to the RV coil, although alternate shocking configurations may be used (see Figure A-17). As is the case with modern external defibrillators, current implantable defibrillators deliver biphasic shocks (energy flow reverses direction during delivery), which are more energy efficient than older devices that delivered monophasic shocks. Some devices also allow programming of the tilt (the drop in voltage during discharge), with 50% and 65% being the values most frequently used. ATP may be used to terminate ventricular tachycardia painlessly, typically by delivering 6 to 10 paced beats at a rate slightly faster than the tachycardia. ATP is successful at terminating even rapid ventricular tachycardia up to 80% of the time.[14] A typical example of ICD programmed zones and therapy is given in Table A-6.

The defibrillation threshold (DFT) or upper limit of vulnerability (ULV) is typically tested in patients with ICDs at implant and in select patients during follow-up. This value is the amount of energy required to terminate ventricular fibrillation and restore sinus rhythm. The maximum device output should be 7 to 10 J above the DFT or ULV to allow reliable defibrillation under clinical conditions.[15] A number of medications can affect the DFT, most notably antiarrhythmia drugs (Table A-7).

Magnet Operation

All modern ICDs are also PMs; as such, they have the ability to treat tachyarrhythmias as well as bradyarrhythmias. ICDs differ from PMs, however, in their response to magnet application. Although PMs revert to asynchronous pacing in the presence of a magnet, ICDs do not. For most ICDs, magnets deactivate tachyarrhythmia detection (sensing) while the magnet is directly over the device. Removal of the magnet restores device function to normal operation.

Inappropriate Shocks

An inappropriate shock is the delivery of a shock to the patient for a reason other than a sustained ventricular arrhythmia. Rapid heart rates of nonventricular origin (sinus tachycardia or atrial

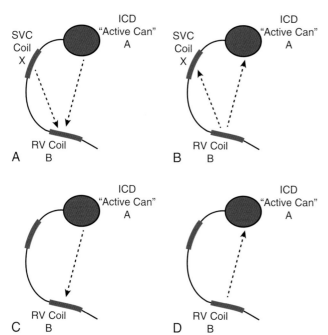

FIGURE A-17 A variety of shocking circuit configurations are shown. Transvenous implantable cardioverter-defibrillator (*ICD*) leads may be dual coil (6A and 6B) or single coil (6C and 6D). For dual-coil leads, energy is delivered from (**A**) the ICD ("*Active Can*") and superior vena cava (*SVC*) coil to the right ventricular (*RV*) coil ("initial" polarity, or "AX to B") or (**B**) from the RV coil to the SVC coil and ICD ("reversed" polarity, or "B to AX"). For single-coil leads, energy delivery is from the (**C**) ICD to the RV coil ("initial" polarity, or "A to B") or (**D**) RV coil to ICD ("reversed" polarity, or "B to A"). Dual-coil systems have defibrillation thresholds (DFTs) of 5 to 7 J lower, on average, than single-coil systems. Mean DFT is approximately equal with standard or reversed polarity, although DFT can vary by 5 to 7 J with different polarity in individual patients. On occasion, an epicardial system may be encountered, in which energy delivery is between two surgically placed epicardial patches or between an epicardial patch and active can (not shown).

TABLE A-6	Typical Implantable Cardioverter-Defibrillator Programming	
	VT ZONE	**VF ZONE**
Heart rate	170-200 beats/min	>200 beats/min
Cycle length	300-350 ms	<300 ms
Detection duration	16 intervals	2 sec
Therapy 1	Burst pacing	24 J
Therapy 2	24 J	35 J
Therapy 3	35 J	35 J
Therapy 4	35 J	35 J
Therapy 5	35 J	35 J

An example of typical implantable cardioverter-defibrillator programming for tachyarrhythmia detection and treatment is shown. The VT zone is programmed to respond to arrhythmias in the 170-200 beats/min range (cycle length, 300 to 350 ms). In this case, if 16 intervals are within the programmed VT range, the device begins to deliver therapy. Antitachycardia pacing will be attempted first. If the arrhythmia persists, a series of shocks is delivered, with the device automatically withholding additional therapy if the rhythm falls below the rate cutoff. If the heart rate is >200 beats/min for 2 seconds, VF therapies will apply. The first programmed shock is typically 10 J above the defibrillation threshold, with the remainder of the therapies programmed to maximal output.

VF, ventricular fibrillation; VT, ventricular tachycardia.

TABLE A-7	Medications that Can Affect the Defibrillation Threshold
MEDICATION	**EFFECT ON DFT**
Amiodarone	Increase
Disopyramide	Increase
Flecainide	Increase
Lidocaine	Increase
Mexilitine	Increase
NAPA	Decrease
Procainamide	Varies
Propafenone	Varies
Sotalol	Decrease
Verapamil	Increase

NAPA, N-acetyl procainamide.

TABLE A-8	Arrhythmia Discriminators	
DISCRIMINATOR	**MECHANISM**	**CLINICAL IMPLICATIONS**
Stability	Measures beat-to-beat variation in arrhythmia cycle length. Withholds therapy for irregular rhythms.	Effective at discriminating between ventricular tachycardia (usually very regular) and rapid atrial fibrillation (usually irregular).
Onset	Measures how sudden the arrhythmia onset was. Withholds therapy unless the arrhythmia begins suddenly.	Effective at discriminating sinus tachycardia from ventricular tachycardia. Ventricular tachycardia is usually sudden in onset, whereas the heart rate increases more gradually for patients with sinus tachycardia.
Morphology	Compares the QRS configuration during arrhythmia with the baseline QRS configuration. Withholds therapy if the arrhythmia QRS is similar to the baseline QRS.	Can help avoid inappropriate shocks for supraventricular arrhythmias.

fibrillation with a rapid ventricular response rate) resulting in ICD shocks occur in 12% of ICD patients. Environmental noise or "noise" due to a lead abnormality (insulation breech or lead fracture) may also lead to inappropriate shocks. Most ICDs have programmable features that may reduce the chances of a patient receiving an inappropriate shock (Table A-8).

Routine Follow-up

ICD patients require routine outpatient follow-up every 3 to 6 months. At each visit, device interrogation is performed to determine if any significant arrhythmias have occurred in the interval since the patient was last seen. Other parameters that are also routinely checked are battery voltage, full energy charge time (6 to 10 seconds in a new device, 12 to 18 seconds in a device near elective replacement), pacing threshold, intrinsic amplitude, and lead impedance. Patients also routinely send in scheduled transmissions from home through a device that relays basic PM or ICD data to the manufacturer. This generates reports that can be downloaded by caregivers. These transmissions typically are staggered with office appointments but can also be done on demand if a patient has symptoms suggestive of a device problem.

REFERENCES

1. Shah MR, Hasselblad V, Stevenson LW, et al. Impact of the pulmonary artery catheter in critically ill patients: meta-analysis of randomized clinical trials. *JAMA* 2005;294:1664-1670.
2. Harvey S, Harrison DA, Singer M, et al. Assessment of the clinical effectiveness of pulmonary artery catheters in management of patients in intensive care (PAC-Man): a randomised controlled trial. *Lancet* 2005;366:472-477.
3. Ferguson JJ 3rd, Cohen M, Freedman RJ Jr, et al. The current practice of intra-aortic balloon counterpulsation: results from the benchmark registry. *J Am Coll Cardiol* 2001;38:1456-1462.
4. Lewis PA, Mullany DV, Townsend S, et al. Trends in intra-aortic balloon counterpulsation: comparison of a 669 record Australian dataset with the multinational Benchmark Counterpulsation Outcomes Registry. *Anaesth Intensive Care* 2007;35:13-19.
5. Antman EM, Hand M, Armstrong PW, et al. 2007 focused update of the ACC/AHA 2004 Guidelines for the Management of Patients with ST-Elevation Myocardial Infarction: a report of the American College of Cardiology/American Heart Association Task Force on Practice Guidelines. *Circulation* 2008;117:296-329.
6. Schneider T, Martens PR, Paschen H, et al. Multicenter, randomized, controlled trial of 150-J biphasic shocks compared with 200- to 360-J monophasic shocks in the resuscitation of out-of-hospital cardiac arrest victims. Optimized Response to Cardiac Arrest (ORCA) investigators. *Circulation* 2000;102:1780-1787.
7. Mittal S, Ayati S, Stein KM, et al. Transthoracic cardioversion of atrial fibrillation: comparison of rectilinear biphasic versus damped sine wave monophasic shocks. *Circulation* 2000;101:1282-1287.
8. Niebauer MJ, Brewer JE, Chung MK, Tchou PJ. Comparison of the rectilinear biphasic waveform with the monophasic damped sine waveform for external cardioversion of atrial fibrillation and flutter. *Am J Cardiol* 2004;93:1495-1499.
9. Botto GL, Politi A, Bonini W, et al. External cardioversion of atrial fibrillation: role of paddle position on technical efficacy and energy requirements. *Heart* 1999;82:726-730.
10. Kirchhof P, Eckardt L, Loh P, et al. Anterior-posterior versus anterior-lateral electrode positions for external cardioversion of atrial fibrillation: a randomised trial. *Lancet* 2002;360:1275-1279.
11. Kirchhof P, Monnig G, Wasmer K, et al. A trial of self-adhesive patch electrodes and hand-held paddle electrodes for external cardioversion of atrial fibrillation (MOBIPAPA). *Eur Heart J* 2005;26:1292-1297.
12. Stiell IG, Walker RG, Nesbitt LP, et al. Biphasic trial: a randomized comparison of fixed lower versus escalating higher energy levels for defibrillation in out-of-hospital cardiac arrest. *Circulation* 2007;115:1511-1517.
13. Bernstein AD, Daubert JC, Fletcher RD, et al. The revised NASPE/BPEG generic code for antibradycardia, adaptive-rate, and multisite pacing. North American Society of Pacing and Electrophysiology/British Pacing and Electrophysiology Group. *Pacing Clin Electrophysiol* 2002;25:260-264.
14. Wathen MS, DeGroot PJ, Sweeney MO, et al. Prospective randomized multicenter trial of empirical antitachycardia pacing versus shocks for spontaneous rapid ventricular tachycardia in patients with implantable cardioverter-defibrillators: Pacing Fast Ventricular Tachycardia Reduces Shock Therapies (PainFREE Rx II) trial results. *Circulation* 2004;110:2591-2596.
15. Russo AM, Sauer W, Gerstenfeld EP, et al. Defibrillation threshold testing: is it really necessary at the time of implantable cardioverter-defibrillator insertion? *Heart Rhythm* 2005;2:456-461.

INDEX

Page numbers followed by "f" indicate figures, "t" indicate tables, and "b" indicate boxes.

A

AAA(s) (abdominal aortic aneurysms), 606-608
  medical management of, 607-608
  surgical management of, 606-607, 607f
AAA trial, 539-540
Abacavir, for HIV infection, 730t
Abacavir/lamivudine, for HIV infection, 729-730, 730t
Abacavir/lamivudine/zidovudine, for HIV infection, 729-730, 730t
Abbreviated New Drug Application (ANDA), 39
ABCB1 gene, in pharmacogenetics of clopidogrel, 55t, 56
  therapeutic implications of, 56-57
ABCD (Alternans Before Cardioverter Defibrillator) trial, 400
ABCD (Appropriate Blood Pressure Control in Diabetes) trial, 542
ABCDE approach, for NSTE-ACS, 165, 166b
Abciximab
  dosage of, 114
  indications for, 114
  mechanism of action of, 114
  for NSTE-ACS, 158
  side effects and contraindications to, 115
  for STEMI
    in acute phase, 182
    with PCI, 189t
Abdominal aortic aneurysms (AAAs), 606-608
  medical management of, 607-608
  surgical management of, 606-607, 607f
Abdominal fat content, 446-448
Abiotrophia defectiva, endocarditis due to, 654
ABPM (ambulatory blood pressure monitoring), 466, 485
  for resistant hypertension, 501-502
Abscess, in infective endocarditis, 652, 653f, 660
Absolute risk difference (ARD), 12-13
Academic research organizations (AROs), 37
ACAS study, 560-561, 561t, 565
ACB study, 557
ACC (American College of Cardiology)
  Door-to-Balloon Alliance of, 71
  on systems of care for STEMI, 179
Accessory pathway(s), 383
Accessory pathway–mediated tachycardias, catheter ablation for, 383-385, 384f
ACCF (American College of Cardiology Foundation), on systems of care for STEMI, 179
ACCOMPLISH trial, 95, 96f, 484
ACCORD trial, 94, 436, 557
Accucinch Guided Delivery System, 722t, 725, 725f
Acculink stent, 563
Accunet filter distal embolic protection device, 563
Accupril (quinapril)
  for heart failure, 246t
  for hypertension, 478t
    in children, 536t
Accuretic (quinapril/hydrochlorothiazide), for hypertension, 485t
ACD (acid citrate dextrose), for LDL apheresis, 455

ACE inhibitors. *See* Angiotensin-converting enzyme (ACE) inhibitors.
Acebutolol (Sectral)
  drug interactions with, 105t
  for hypertension, 481t
  pharmacodynamic properties and cardiac effects of, 98t
  properties of, 102t
Acecainide. *See* *N*-acetylprocainamide (acecainide, NAPA).
Aceon (perindopril)
  for carotid artery stenosis, 555
  for heart failure, 259
  for hypertension, 478t
Acetylsalicylic acid (ASA), for acute pericarditis, 667
ACHD. *See* Adult congenital heart disease (ACHD).
Acid citrate dextrose (ACD), for LDL apheresis, 455
ACLS (Advanced Cardiac Life Support), for cardiac arrest, 415-417, 416f
ACME trial, 141-142
Acquired immunodeficiency syndrome (AIDS). *See* Human immunodeficiency virus (HIV).
Acromegaly, 499-500
  presentation and diagnosis of, 499-500
  principles of treatment of, 500
ACS. *See* Acute coronary syndrome (ACS).
ACSRS study, 566
ACST study, 560-561, 561t, 565
ACTH-dependent Cushing syndrome, 498
ACTH-independent Cushing syndrome, 498
Actinobacillus spp, endocarditis due to, 655t
ACTION (Acute Coronary Treatment and Intervention Outcomes Network), 71-72, 167
Acute coronary syndrome (ACS)
  global cardiovascular therapy for, 75-76, 76f
  hypertensive emergencies with, 513
  non–ST-elevation. *See* Non–ST-elevation acute coronary syndrome (NSTE-ACS).
Acute Coronary Treatment and Intervention Outcomes Network (ACTION), 71-72, 167
Acute Coronary Treatment and Intervention Outcomes Network Registry–Get with the Guidelines (ACTION-GWTG, AR-G), 71-72, 178-179
Acute Decompensated Heart Failure (ADHERE) national registry, 283, 285-286, 291
Acute myocardial infarction (AMI)
  β-adrenergic blockers for survivors of, 99
  bone marrow cells for, 324
  mesenchymal stromal cells for, 326
Adalat. *See* Nifedipine (Adalat, Nifedical, Procardia).
ADAM Veterans Affairs Cooperative Study, 606
Added costs, 24
Adenoma, aldosterone-producing, 494-496
  surgical treatment of, 496-497
Adenosine, 357
  adverse reactions to, 357
  atrial fibrillation induced by, 368, 368f, 369t

Adenosine *(Continued)*
  clinical applications of, 357
  clinical pharmacology of, 357
  dosage and administration of, 357
    modification in disease states of, 357
  drug interactions with, 357
  mechanism of action of, 357
  for paroxysmal supraventricular tachycardia, 368, 368f
  in pregnancy and lactation, 622t-623t
ADHERE national registry, 283, 285-286, 291
Adjudication, of clinical endpoints, 38
ADONIS trial, 358-359
ADOPT trial, 593
Adrenal hyperplasia
  congenital, hypertension due to, 497-498
  primary, 494-496
  surgical treatment of, 496-497
Adrenalectomy, laparoscopic, for primary aldosteronism, 496-497
Adrenocorticotropic hormone (ACTH)-dependent Cushing syndrome, 498
Adrenocorticotropic hormone (ACTH)-independent Cushing syndrome, 498
ADSORB trial, 615-616
Adult congenital heart disease (ACHD), 632-651
  aortic coarctation as, 641-643, 641f-642f
    recommendations for, 642-643
  arrhythmias in, 636-637
  atrial septal defects as, 637-639, 637f-638f
    recommendations for, 639
  bicuspid aortic valve as, 640
    recommendations for, 640
  cyanosis in, 633-635
    cardiopulmonary exercise with, 634
    major organ complications of, 634
    neurologic effects of, 634-635
    recommendations for management of, 635
  endocarditis in, 632
  exercise and athletic participation with, 636-637
  left-to-right shunting in, 632-633
  noncardiac surgery with, 636
    recommendations for, 636
  palliative surgical procedures and surgical repairs for, 632, 633t
  patent ductus arteriosus as, 645-646, 646f
    recommendations for, 646
  patent foramen ovale as, 639-640
    and hypoxemia, 639, 640f
    and migraine, 639
    recommendations for, 640
  postoperative residual defects, collaterals, and fenestrations in, 647, 648f
  and pregnancy, 635-636
    recommendations for, 636
  pulmonary stenosis as, 640-641, 641f
    recommendations for, 641
  tetralogy of Fallot as, 643-645, 643f
    recommendations for, 645
    right ventricular outflow tract obstruction after repair of, 644-645, 644f-645f
    ventricular failure after surgical repair of, 643, 643t
  transplantation for, 637
  ventricular septal defects as, 646-647, 646f-647f

Adult congenital heart disease (ACHD)
  (Continued)
    closure of perimembranous, 647
    post–myocardial infarction ventricular
      septal rupture with, 647, 648f
    recommendations for, 647
Adult Treatment Panel III Therapeutic Lifestyle
  Changes diet, 192
ADVANCE study, 475
Advanced Cardiac Life Support (ACLS), for
  cardiac arrest, 415-417, 416f
Adverse events, in clinical trials, 38
Adverse Events Reporting System (AERS),
  35-36
Advisory panels
  for evaluating IND applications, 35
  for medical device approval, 51
AED (automatic external defibrillator)
  for cardiac arrest, 408
  for STEMI, 179
AERS (Adverse Events Reporting System), 35-36
AF. *See* Atrial fibrillation (AF).
AFCAPS/TEXCAPS study, 425t
AF-CHF trial, 372-373
AFFIRM study, 352, 372-374
Affordability, of cardiovascular drugs in
  low- and middle-income countries, 77-78,
  78f
African-American patients, hypertension in,
  487
Afterload mismatch, in aortic stenosis, 677
AGA Amplatzer membranous devices, 647
Age
  and heart failure risk stratification, 286t
  and human cardiac stem cell function,
    327-330
Age-dependent penetrance, 332
Agonists, 96
AHA (American Heart Association)
  Get with the Guidelines–Coronary Artery
    Disease program of, 71
  on systems of care for STEMI, 179
AHEAD trial, 446
A-HeFT trial, 87, 255
AHI (apnea-hypopnea index), 502
AIDS. *See* Human immunodeficiency virus
  (HIV).
AIM-HIGH trial, 428, 437, 557
AIR study, 600, 600f
AIRE trial, 247t
Airline travel
  by adults with cyanotic congenital heart
    disease, 635
  with pulmonary arterial hypertension, 604
  and venous thromboembolism, 580
ALA (α-linolenic acid), for hyperlipidemia,
  444
Alcohol consumption, with hypertension, 469t
Alcohol septal ablation (ASA), for LVOT
  obstruction, 333-334, 334t
Aldactone. *See* Spironolactone (Aldactone).
Aldomet (methyldopa), for hypertension, 483,
  483t
  in pregnancy, 524t
Aldosterone, plasma concentration of, 495
Aldosterone escape, 253
Aldosterone receptor antagonists (ARAs)
  for heart failure, 253-254
    adverse effects of, 248t
    clinical efficacy of, 253-254
    endpoints with, 242t
    pathophysiologic mechanisms and, 253,
      253t
    practical considerations with, 254
  for hypertension, 477t, 482, 482t
    in children, 536t
    monitoring and adverse effects of, 485t
    resistant, 505-507, 506f-507f

Aldosterone receptor antagonists (ARAs)
  (Continued)
  for STEMI
    during convalescence, 193
    in long-term management, 206
    with pulmonary congestion, 194
Aldosterone-producing adenoma (APA),
  494-496
  surgical treatment of, 496-497
Aldosteronism
  glucocorticoid-remediable, 494-495
    pharmacologic treatment of, 497
  primary, 494-497
    diagnosis of, 495-496, 495f-496f
    pharmacologic treatment of, 497
    principles of treatment of, 496-497
    and resistant hypertension, 503t,
      504-508
    subtypes of, 494-495, 495b, 496f
    surgical treatment of, 496-497
Alemtuzumab, with cardiac transplantation,
  311t
Alfieri technique, for mitral valve repair, 706
Aliskiren (Tekturna)
  for heart failure, 263-264
  for hypertension, 483-484, 483t
Aliskiren/amlodipine (Tekamlo), for
  hypertension, 485t
Aliskiren/hydrochlorothiazide (Tekturna HCT),
  for hypertension, 485t
Aliskiren/valsartan (Valturna), for
  hypertension, 485t
ALLHAT Dissemination Committee, 470
ALLHAT trial, 94, 257, 481-482, 505
ALLHAT-LLA trial, 425t
Allocation ratio, 6
Allopurinol
  for gout in adults with cyanotic congenital
    heart disease, 634
  for heart failure, 264
  for refractory angina, 261
α value, 1-2, 2f, 9-11
α-adrenergic activity, of β-adrenergic blockers,
  101-103
α-adrenergic blockers
  for hypertension, 482, 483t
    due to pheochromocytoma, 491-493, 492t
    for hypertensive emergencies, 514t-515t
α-agonists, for hypertension, 483, 483t
  in children, 536t
α-linolenic acid (ALA), for hyperlipidemia, 444
ALPHABET trial, 600
α-/β-adrenergic blockers, for hypertension,
  481-482, 481t
  in children, 536t
  due to pheochromocytoma, 492t, 493
Altace. *See* Ramipril (Altace).
ALT-CAB (anterolateral thoracotomy–coronary
  artery bypass), 228
Alteplase
  in pregnancy and lactation, 622t-623t
  for STEMI, 186, 188t
Alternans Before Cardioverter Defibrillator
  (ABCD) trial, 400
Alternative hypothesis, 9
AMADEUS trial, 724
Ambrisentan, for pulmonary arterial
  hypertension, 601
  HIV-related, 735
Ambulatory blood pressure monitoring
  (ABPM), 466, 485
  for resistant hypertension, 501-502
AME (apparent mineralocorticoid excess)
  syndromes, hypertension due to, 498-499
American College of Cardiology (ACC)
  Foundation
  Door-to-Balloon Alliance of, 71
  on systems of care for STEMI, 179

American Heart Association (AHA)
  Get with the Guidelines–Coronary Artery
    Disease program of, 71
  on systems of care for STEMI, 179
AMI (acute myocardial infarction)
  β-adrenergic blockers for survivors of, 99
  bone marrow cells for, 324
  mesenchymal stromal cells for, 326
Amiloride (Midamor)
  for heart failure, 243t
  for hypertension, 480t
    in children, 536t
    resistant, 507
Amiodarone, 353-355
  adverse reactions to, 355, 375t
  for atrial fibrillation, 374t, 375
  clinical applications of, 353-354
  clinical pharmacology of, 354
  dosage and administration of, 354-355,
    375t
  modification in disease states of, 355
  drug interactions with, 355
  for heart failure, 258-259
  initiation and monitoring of, 377
  for maintenance of sinus rhythm, 375
  mechanism of action of, 354
  for paroxysmal supraventricular tachycardia,
    369
  in pregnancy and lactation, 622t-623t,
    628-629
  and statins, 60-61
  for sustained monomorphic ventricular
    tachycardia, 411-413
    algorithm for, 412f
    clinical trials of, 411-412, 411f
    recommended dose of, 410t
Amlodipine (Norvasc), 93-94
  for heart failure, 257
  for hypertension, 479t
    in children, 536t
  pharmacodynamic effects of, 91t
Amlodipine besylate/benazepril hydrochloride
  (Lotrel), for hypertension, 485t
Amlodipine/olmesartan medoxomil (Azor), for
  hypertension, 485t
Amlodipine/valsartan/hydrochlorothiazide
  (Exforge HCT), for hypertension, 485t
Amoxicillin, for endocarditis prophylaxis
  during delivery, 630
Amphetamines, hypertensive emergencies due
  to, 518
Ampicillin
  for endocarditis prophylaxis during delivery,
    630
  for infective endocarditis, 656t
Ampicillin-sulbactam, for infective
  endocarditis, 655t-657t
Amplatzer PDA Occluder device, 645-646
Amplatzer Septal Occluder (ASO) device, 638
Amprenavir, for HIV infection, 729t
AMR101, for mixed dyslipidemia, 438
Amyloidosis, cardiac, 336-337
Anacetrapib
  for chronic stable angina, 149
  for low HDL cholesterol, 439
Analgesia, for STEMI in acute phase, 181-182
ANDA (Abbreviated New Drug Application),
  39
ANDROMEDA trial, 358
Anemia
  in heart failure, 264
    acute decompensated, 298
  of pregnancy, 621
Angina pectoris
  β-adrenergic blockers in
    combined with other antianginal
      therapies, 99
    effects of, 97, 97b, 98t

Angina pectoris (Continued)
vs. other antianginal therapies, 97
for unstable angina, 97
calcium channel blockers for, 92
causes of, 131, 132t
chronic stable, 131-152
antiplatelet therapy for
with novel agents, 149
with percutaneous coronary
intervention, 144
for prevention of coronary events,
144-146, 146f
cardiac rehabilitation for, 140
for prevention of coronary events, 144
classification of, 132b
clinical assessment of, 131, 132b
coronary artery bypass graft for, 144
arterial conduits in, 144
complications of, 144, 145f
vs. percutaneous coronary intervention,
142-143
percutaneous coronary intervention
after, 143
results of, 142f
in secondary prevention, 147-149
coronary revascularization for, 141-144
in secondary prevention, 147-149
epidemiology of, 131
invasive evaluation of, 136-137, 137b
lifestyle and risk factor modifications for,
137-140
for diabetes mellitus, 140
dietary intervention as, 138-140
for obesity, 140
smoking in, 137-138
and myocardial infarction, 131, 132f-133f
natural history of, 131, 132f-133f
newer options for treatment of, 104-106
ivabradine as, 104-105
nicorandil as, 104, 105f
ranolazine as, 105-106, 106f
trimetazidine as, 106
noninvasive evaluation of, 131-136
cardiac MRI for, 134
computed tomography for, 135-136
coronary calcium score for, 135
CT coronary angiography for, 135-136,
136f
echocardiography for, 133-134
electrocardiogram for, 131-133, 133b,
134f-135f
myocardial perfusion scintigraphy for,
134-135, 135b
selection and frequency of stress testing
for, 136, 137t, 138f
overall assessment of risk for, 137, 138f
percutaneous coronary intervention for,
141-144
antiplatelet therapy with, 144
complications of, 144
vs. coronary artery bypass graft, 142-143
after coronary artery bypass grafting,
143
culprit lesions, 143
indications for, 142
vs. medical treatment, 142
pharmacologic therapy for, 140-141
with ACE inhibitors, 147
with β-blockers, 140-141, 147
with calcium channel blockers, 141
with cholesteryl ester transfer protein
inhibitors, 149
with ivabradine, 141
with lipid-lowering agents, 146-147, 148f
with nitrates, 141
vs. percutaneous coronary intervention,
142
with potassium channel agonists, 141

Angina pectoris (Continued)
risk stratification for, 131-137, 132b, 133f
secondary prevention of, 139f, 144-149
ACE inhibitors in, 147
antiplatelet therapy in, 144-146, 146f
β-blockers in, 147
cardiac rehabilitation in, 144
coronary artery bypass graft in, 147-149
coronary revascularization in, 147-149
lipid-lowering therapy in, 146-147, 148f
stents for, 142f, 143-144
symptomatic medical management of,
139f, 140-144
therapeutic interventions for, 137-149, 138f
in pregnancy, 626-627
refractory, 325-326
at rest, 97
unstable. See Non–ST-elevation acute
coronary syndrome (NSTE-ACS).
vasospastic, 97
Angiogenesis, therapeutic, for peripheral artery
disease, 549
Angiographic trials, of statins, 423
Angioguard distal embolic protection device,
563
Angiotensin receptor blockers (ARBs)
for abdominal aortic aneurysms, 607-608
for acute myocardial infarction, 76
for carotid artery stenosis, 556
for heart failure, 245-250
acute decompensated, 296-297
clinical efficacy of, 246-248, 247t
dosage of, 246t
endpoints with, 242t
pathophysiologic mechanisms and,
245-246, 245f
practical considerations with, 248t,
249-250
with preserved ejection fraction, 259, 260t
for hypertension, 477t, 478-479, 479t
in children, 535, 536t
in combination products, 485t
monitoring and adverse effects of, 485t
for maintenance of sinus rhythm, 377
for NSTE-ACS, postdischarge, 166-167
for peripheral artery disease, 542
for renal artery stenosis, 574
for STEMI
during convalescence, 193
in long-term management, 206
for valvular heart disease in pregnancy,
623-624
Angiotensin-converting enzyme (ACE)
inhibitors
for abdominal aortic aneurysms, 607-608
for acute coronary syndrome in global
community, 76
for acute myocardial infarction, 76
for carotid artery stenosis, 555
for heart failure, 245-250
acute decompensated, 296
clinical efficacy of, 246, 247t
dosage of, 246t
endpoints with, 242t
pathophysiologic mechanisms and,
245-246, 245f
practical considerations with, 248-249,
248t
with preserved ejection fraction, 259,
260t
for hypertension, 477t-478t, 478
in children, 535, 536t
in combination products, 485t
monitoring and adverse effects of,
485t
for hypertensive emergencies, 514t-515t
after NSTE-ACS, 166-167
for peripheral artery disease, 542

Angiotensin-converting enzyme (ACE)
inhibitors (Continued)
for renal artery stenosis, 574
for secondary prevention of coronary events,
147
for STEMI
during convalescence, 192
in long-term management, 206
with pulmonary congestion, 194
for valvular heart disease in pregnancy,
623-624
AnnuloFlex prosthesis, 695t
AnnuloFlo prosthesis, 695t
Annuloplasty devices, 695t
Annuloplasty ring, in mitral valve repair,
705-706
percutaneous
with direct approach, 722t, 724-725, 725f
with indirect approach, 722t, 723
ANP (atrial natriuretic peptide), in resistant
hypertension, 505f
Antagonists, 96
Anterior leaflet prolapse, 702
Anterolateral thoracotomy–coronary artery
bypass (ALT-CAB), 228
Anteroseptal space, 383-384
Antiarrhythmic drug(s), 343-364
adenosine as, 357
amiodarone as, 353-355
β-adrenergic blockers as, 99
classification of, 344, 345f
disopyramide as, 349-350
dofetilide as, 356-357
dosages and toxicities of, 375-376, 375t
dronedarone as, 358-359
elimination of, 359
flecainide as, 352
for heart failure, 258-259
history of, 343
ibutilide as, 355-356
lidocaine as, 344-347
mexiletine as, 347-348
procainamide as, 348-349
propafenone as, 351-352
quinidine as, 350-351
ranolazine as, 106
sotalol as, 352-353
Antibiotic prophylaxis
for dental procedures, 662-663, 663t
in pregnancy, 630
Antibiotic therapy, for infective endocarditis,
654-656
with common microorganisms, 655t
with enterococcal microorganisms, 656t
with IV drug use, 656
outpatient parenteral, 655-656
with resistant microorganisms, 656
Anticoagulant therapy, 115-120
for acute decompensated heart failure, 298
for cardiac amyloidosis, 337
with cardioversion, 379, 379f
direct thrombin inhibitors as, 118, 119f
argatroban as, 120
bivalirudin (hirulog) as, 120
hirudin (lepirudin) as, 118-120
for heart failure, 258
low-molecular-weight heparin as, 117-118
dosages of, 118
indications for, 118
mechanisms of action of, 117-118
side effects and contraindications to, 118
for NSTE-ACS, 159-163, 159f, 160t
direct thrombin inhibitors as, 161-162,
162f
factor Xa inhibitors as, 162-163, 163f
other, 163
postdischarge, 166
recommendations on, 163, 169b

Anticoagulant therapy (Continued)
　　unfractionated heparin and low-molecular-
　　　　weight heparin as, 159-161, 160t-161t,
　　　　161f
　　oral, 121-123
　　　　novel agents for, 122, 122f
　　　　warfarin for, 121-122
　　for pericarditis, 674-675
　　for peripheral artery disease, 541
　　for STEMI
　　　　in acute phase, 182-183
　　　　with PCI, 189, 190t
　　unfractionated heparin as, 115-117
　　　　dosages of, 117
　　　　indications for, 117
　　　　mechanisms of action of, 115-117, 116f
　　　　side effects and contraindications to, 117
　　for venous thromboembolism, 587-589,
　　　　587b
　　　　direct factor XA and factor IIA inhibitors
　　　　　　for, 589
　　　　duration of, 590, 590f
　　　　with fondaparinux, 588
　　　　and heparin-induced thrombocytopenia,
　　　　　　587, 588f
　　　　with low-molecular-weight heparin, 588
　　　　in pregnancy, 624-625
　　　　with unfractionated heparin, 587
　　　　with warfarin, 588-589, 588b
Antihypertensive medications, 474-489
　　adherence to, 468, 468b
　　for carotid artery disease, 555-556
　　for children, 534-536, 535f, 536t
　　classes of, 476-484, 477t
　　　　ACE inhibitors as, 477t-478t, 478
　　　　　　in combination products, 485t
　　　　　　monitoring and adverse effects of, 485t
　　　　aldosterone antagonists as, 477t, 482, 482t
　　　　　　monitoring and adverse effects of, 485t
　　　　α-blockers as, 482, 483t
　　　　angiotensin receptor blockers as, 477t,
　　　　　　478-479, 479t
　　　　　　in combination products, 485t
　　　　　　monitoring and adverse effects of, 485t
　　　　arterial vasodilators as, 483, 483t
　　　　β-blockers as, 99, 477t, 481-482, 481t
　　　　　　in combination products, 485t
　　　　　　monitoring and adverse effects of, 485t
　　　　calcium channel blockers as, 92, 92t, 477t,
　　　　　　479-480, 479t
　　　　　　in combination products, 485t
　　　　　　dihydropyridine, 477t, 479-480, 479t
　　　　　　monitoring and adverse effects of, 485t
　　　　　　nondihydropyridine, 477t, 479-480,
　　　　　　　　479t
　　　　central α-agonists as, 483, 483t
　　　　direct renin inhibitor as, 483-484, 483t
　　　　　　in combination products, 485t
　　　　other agents as, 482-484, 483t
　　　　rauwolfia alkaloids as, 483t, 484
　　　　thiazide diuretics as, 477t, 480-481, 480t
　　　　　　in combination products, 485t
　　　　　　monitoring and adverse effects of, 485t
　　HIV infection and, 734
　　for hypertensive emergencies, 513-519,
　　　　514t-515t
　　hypertensive emergencies due to acute
　　　　withdrawal of, 517
　　implementation of, 484-486
　　　　adherence in, 468, 468b, 486
　　　　monitoring in, 484-486, 485t
　　　　monotherapy vs. combination therapy in,
　　　　　　484, 485t
　　　　need for 24-hour coverage in, 484
　　　　step-down therapy in, 486
　　labeling of, 35b
　　overview of, 474

Antihypertensive medications (Continued)
　　for peripheral artery disease, 542
　　in pregnancy, 524-525, 524t
　　principles of treatment with, 474
　　　　blood pressure goals in, 474
　　　　evidence-based treatment in, 474
　　selection of, 474-476
　　　　algorithm for, 475f
　　　　with chronic kidney disease, 476
　　　　with compelling indications, 475-476
　　　　with coronary artery disease, 476
　　　　with diabetes, 475-476
　　　　with left ventricular dysfunction, 476
　　　　with previous ischemic stroke, 476
　　　　for uncomplicated hypertension, 475
　　in special populations, 486-487
　　　　African-Americans as, 487
　　　　elderly as, 486-487
Antiischemic medications
　　β-adrenergic blockers as, 96-104
　　calcium channel blockers as, 89-96
　　for chronic stable angina, 140-141
　　　　ACE inhibitors as, 147
　　　　β-blockers as, 140-141, 147
　　　　calcium channel blockers as, 141
　　　　cholesteryl ester transfer protein inhibitors
　　　　　　as, 149
　　　　ivabradine as, 141
　　　　nitrates as, 141
　　　　vs. percutaneous coronary intervention, 142
　　　　potassium channel agonists as, 141
　　newer options for, 104-106
　　　　ivabradine as, 104-105
　　　　nicorandil as, 104, 105f
　　　　ranolazine as, 105-106, 106f
　　　　trimetazidine as, 106
　　for NSTE-ACS, 153-155
　　　　β-adrenergic receptor blockers as, 154
　　　　calcium channel antagonists as, 154-155
　　　　nitrates as, 153-154, 154f
　　　　ranolazine as, 155
　　organic nitrates as, 83-89
Antiplatelet therapy, 107-115
　　aspirin as, 107-109
　　　　dosages of, 109
　　　　indication for, 108-109
　　　　mechanism of action of, 107-108, 108f
　　　　side effects and contraindications to, 109
　　for carotid artery disease, 557-558, 558t
　　for chronic stable angina
　　　　with novel agents, 149
　　　　with percutaneous coronary intervention,
　　　　　　144
　　　　for prevention of coronary events, 144-146,
　　　　　　146f
　　glycoprotein IIB/IIIA receptor antagonists as,
　　　　114-115
　　　　dosages of, 114-115
　　　　indications for, 114
　　　　mechanisms of action of, 114
　　　　side effects and contraindications to, 115
　　for noncardiac vascular surgery, 544
　　novel agents in, 115, 116f
　　for NSTE-ACS, 155-157, 155b
　　　　aspirin as, 155-156, 155f
　　　　clopidogrel as, 156, 156f
　　　　duration of, 157
　　　　intravenous, 158-159, 158f, 159b
　　　　P2Y$_{12}$ antagonists as, 156
　　　　platelet function testing and genetics for,
　　　　　　157-159
　　　　postdischarge, 166
　　　　prasugrel as, 156-157
　　　　ticagrelor as, 157
　　P2Y$_{12}$ receptor antagonists as, 109-114
　　　　dosages of, 112-113
　　　　indication for, 111-112, 112t

Antiplatelet therapy (Continued)
　　mechanism of action of, 109-111, 110f, 110t
　　side effects and contraindications to,
　　　　113-114
　　for peripheral artery disease, 539-541
　　for STEMI
　　　　in acute phase, 182
　　　　in long-term management, 206
　　　　with PCI, 189, 189t
　　　　after stent placement, 218, 219t
Antiretroviral therapy, for HIV infection,
　　728-730
　　combination medications in, 729-730
　　fusion inhibitors in, 729
　　integrase inhibitors in, 729
　　and lipid-lowering therapy, 733, 733f
　　metabolic effects of, 730-731
　　nonnucleoside reverse transcriptase
　　　　inhibitors in, 729, 730t
　　nucleoside/nucleotide reverse transcriptase
　　　　inhibitors in, 729, 730t
　　protease inhibitors in, 728-729, 729t
Antitachycardia pacing (ATP), 759
　　for sustained monomorphic ventricular
　　　　tachycardia, 413, 413f
Antithrombotic therapy
　　for heart failure, 258
　　for STEMI
　　　　in acute phase, 182-183, 183f
　　　　during convalescence, 192
　　for thromboembolism in pregnancy, 625
Antithrombotic Trialists' Collaboration
　　meta-analysis, 109, 144-146, 146f, 540-541
Antithymocyte globulin, with cardiac
　　transplantation, 311t
Anxiety, after NSTE-ACS, 166t
Aorta, balloon-assisted stenting of, 642f, 643
Aortic abscess, in infective endocarditis, 652,
　　653f, 660
Aortic aneurysms
　　abdominal, 606-608
　　　　medical management of, 607-608
　　　　surgical management of, 606-607, 607f
　　thoracic, 608-613
　　　　etiology of, 608
　　　　in Marfan syndrome, 608, 613
　　　　medical management of, 613
　　　　natural history of, 608
　　　　surgical management of, 608-613
　　　　　　of aortic arch, 609-611, 611f
　　　　　　of aortic root, 609, 610f
　　　　　　of ascending aorta, 609, 609f
　　　　　　Bentall procedure for, 609
　　　　　　cerebral protection with, 611
　　　　　　complications of, 612
　　　　　　composite aortic graft for, 609, 610f
　　　　　　David-I technique for, 609
　　　　　　David-V technique for, 609
　　　　　　of descending aorta, 609, 612-613
　　　　　　in Ehlers-Danlos syndrome, 608
　　　　　　elephant trunk technique for, 612, 612f
　　　　　　hemiarch repair for, 609, 611f
　　　　　　hybrid procedure for, 611-612, 612f
　　　　　　interposition prosthetic Dacron graft for,
　　　　　　　　609, 609f
　　　　　　in Loeys-Dietz syndrome, 608
　　　　　　in Marfan syndrome, 608
　　　　　　Ross procedure for, 609
　　　　　　timing of, 608
　　　　　　total aortic arch repair for, 609-611,
　　　　　　　　611f
　　　　　　transluminally placed endovascular
　　　　　　　　stent-graft for, 612-613
　　　　　　valve-sparing root repair for, 609, 610f
Aortic arch endarterectomy, for thoracic aortic
　　atheroembolism, 618
Aortic atheroembolism, thoracic, 617-618

Aortic balloon valvuloplasty, percutaneous, 714
  access site evaluation for, 716
  currently available devices for, 714-715, 715f
  measurement of aortic valve annulus for, 716-717
  new access approaches for, 719
  new applications of, 719
  next generation of, 720-721, 720f, 720t
  patient evaluation and imaging prior to, 715-717, 715f
  patient outcomes with, 717-719, 718f-719f, 719t
  potential complications of, 719-720
  transapical valves in, 721, 721f
  transcatheter implantation procedure for, 717-721, 717f
Aortic coarctation, 641-643, 641f-642f
  hypertension due to, 503t
  recommendations for, 642-643
Aortic disease, 606-619
  aortic aneurysms as. See Aortic aneurysms.
  aortic dissection as. See Aortic dissection.
  intramural hematoma as, 617
  penetrating atherosclerotic ulcer as, 617
  thoracic aortic atheroembolism as, 617-618
Aortic dissection, 613-617
  with aortic regurgitation, 614
  β-adrenergic blockers for, 100
  definitive therapy for, 614-616, 615f-616f
  hypertensive emergencies with, 513-515, 515f
  long-term therapy and late follow-up for, 616-617
  malperfusion in, 614-615, 615f
  type A, 614
  type B, 614-615, 615f
    complicated, 615, 615f-616f
    uncomplicated, 616
Aortic homograft, 695t, 696f, 701
Aortic insufficiency, 681-683
  aortic dissection with, 614
  assessment of severity of, 681-683, 682t
  and mechanical circulatory support, 318
  in pregnancy, 623-624
  timing of surgical intervention for, 683
    in asymptomatic patients, 683
    overall approach to, 683, 684f
    in symptomatic patients with LV dysfunction, 683
    in symptomatic patients with normal LV function, 683
Aortic regurgitation, 681-683
  aortic dissection with, 614
  assessment of severity of, 681-683, 682t
  and mechanical circulatory support, 318
  in pregnancy, 623-624
  timing of surgical intervention for, 683
    in asymptomatic patients, 683
    overall approach to, 683, 684f
    in symptomatic patients with LV dysfunction, 683
    in symptomatic patients with normal LV function, 683
Aortic stenosis (AS), 676-678
  assessment of severity of, 676-677, 677t
  in CABG patients, 710
  in pregnancy, 624
  timing of surgical intervention for, 676-678
    in asymptomatic patients, 678
    in elderly patients, 678
    indications for, 678, 678b, 699-700
    in low-grade stenosis, 677-678
    overall approach to, 678, 678b, 679f
    in symptomatic patients, 677
Aortic valve, bicuspid, 640
  recommendations for, 640
Aortic valve annulus, measurement of, 716-717
Aortic valve area (AVA), 676

Aortic valve disease
  with mitral valve disease, 709
  mixed, 699-700
  percutaneous treatment for, 714
    access site evaluation for, 716
    currently available, 714-715, 715f
    measurement of aortic valve annulus for, 716-717
    new access approaches for, 719
    new applications of, 719
    next generation of, 720-721, 720f, 720t
    patient evaluation and imaging prior to, 715-717, 715f
    patient outcomes with, 717-719, 718f-719f, 719t
    potential complications of, 719-720
    transapical valves in, 721, 721f
    transcatheter implantation procedure for, 717-721, 717f
  surgical treatment for. See Aortic valve surgery.
Aortic valve repair, 702
Aortic valve replacement (AVR)
  in asymptomatic patients, 678
  choice of prosthesis for, 701, 701f
  in elderly patients, 678
  indications for, 678, 678b, 699-700
  in low-grade stenosis, 677-678
  overall approach to, 678, 679f
  patient-prosthesis mismatch in, 701
  results of, 702
    early, 702, 702f
    late, 702
  surgical technique for, 700, 700f
  in symptomatic patients, 677
Aortic valve surgery, 699-702
  for aortic insufficiency/regurgitation, 683, 700
    in asymptomatic patients, 683
    overall approach to, 683, 684f
    in symptomatic patients with LV dysfunction, 683
    in symptomatic patients with normal LV function, 683
  for aortic stenosis, 676-678
    in asymptomatic patients, 678
    in elderly patients, 678
    indications for, 678, 678b, 699-700
    in low-grade stenosis, 677-678
    overall approach to, 678, 678b, 679f
    in symptomatic patients, 677
  aortic valve repair as, 702
  aortic valve replacement as, 700-701
    choice of prosthesis for, 701, 701f
    indications for, 678, 678b
    patient-prosthesis mismatch in, 701
    surgical technique for, 700, 700f
  indications for, 699-700
  for mixed aortic valve disease, 699-700
  overview of, 699-700
  results of, 702
    late, 702
Aortocavitary fistulae, in infective endocarditis, 652, 660
Aortoiliac bifurcation disease, 546-547, 547f
Aortoiliac disease, 545f-547f, 546-547
APA (aldosterone-producing adenoma), 494-496
  surgical treatment of, 496-497
APCSC (Asia Pacific Cohort Studies Collaboration), 556
Apixaban (Eliquis), 122, 160t
  for NSTE-ACS, 163
  for thromboprophylaxis, 592-593
Apnea-hypopnea index (AHI), 502
APOC1 gene, in genome-wide association studies of statins, 62t, 63

APOE gene, in pharmacogenetics of statins, 61, 62t
Apoptosis, 100
Apparent mineralocorticoid excess (AME) syndromes, hypertension due to, 498-499
APPRAISE trial, 122
APPRAISE-2 trial, 163
Appropriate Blood Pressure Control in Diabetes (ABCD) trial, 542
Apresoline. See Hydralazine (Apresoline).
APRICOT study, 207
ARAS. See Atherosclerotic renal artery stenosis (ARAS).
ARAs. See Aldosterone receptor antagonists (ARAs).
ARBITER 2 trial, 437
ARBITER 6-HALTS trial, 437
ARBs. See Angiotensin receptor blockers (ARBs).
ARCH trial, 618
ARD (absolute risk difference), 12-13
Argatroban, 120
  dosages of, 120
  indications for, 120
  mechanisms of action of, 120
  for NSTE-ACS, 161-162
  in pregnancy and lactation, 622t-623t
  side effects and contraindications to, 120
L-Arginine, for prevention of hypertension during pregnancy, 524
ARIC study, 79, 555-556
ARIES-1 and ARIES-2 studies, 601
ARMYDA-2 study, 156
AROs (academic research organizations), 37
Arrhythmias. See also specific arrhythmias, e.g., Atrial flutter.
  in adults with congenital heart disease, 636-637
  antiarrhythmic drugs for. See Antiarrhythmic drug(s).
  in heart failure, 284
  and mechanical circulatory support, 318
  due to pheochromocytoma, 493t
  in pregnancy, 628-629
  after STEMI, 194f, 198-199
Arterial conduits, for coronary artery bypass graft, 144
  non–left descending, 230-232, 231t
    gastroepiploic artery for, 231t, 232
    inferior epigastric artery for, 230, 231t
    left internal mammary artery for, 228, 231t
    radial artery for, 231t, 232
    right internal mammary artery for, 230-232, 231t
Arterial switch operation, 633t
Arterial vasodilators
  for hypertension, 483, 483t
    in children, 536t
  for hypertensive emergencies, 514t-515t
ARTS study, 143
AS. See Aortic stenosis (AS).
ASA (acetylsalicylic acid), for acute pericarditis, 667
ASA (alcohol septal ablation), for LVOT obstruction, 333-334, 334t
ASCEND-HF trial, 292, 293f, 301-302
ASCOT-BPLA trial, 94-95
ASCOT-LLA trial, 425t
ASDs. See Atrial septal defects (ASDs).
Asia Pacific Cohort Studies Collaboration (APCSC), 556
ASO (Amplatzer Septal Occluder) device, 638
Aspiration thrombectomy, for STEMI, 190
ASPIRE-2 study, 575, 576t
Aspirin
  as antiplatelet agent, 107-109
  dosages of, 109

Aspirin *(Continued)*
    indication for, 108-109
    mechanism of action of, 107-108, 108f
    side effects and contraindications to, 109
  for carotid artery disease, 557-558, 558t
  for chronic stable angina, 144-146, 146f
  for NSTE-ACS, 155-156, 155f
    postdischarge, 166
  for peripheral artery disease, 539-541
  for postpericardial injury syndrome, 673
  in pregnancy and lactation, 622t-623t, 627
  for prevention of preeclampsia, 524
  for renal artery stenosis, 574
  for STEMI
    in acute phase, 182
    during convalescence, 192
    in long-term management, 206
    with PCI, 189t
    with pericarditis, 200
    prehospital, 179
  after stent placement, 219t
  for thoracic aortic atheroembolism, 618
  for thromboprophylaxis, 592
    with atrial fibrillation, 378, 378t
Aspirin sensitivity, 109
ASTAMI trial, 324
ASTRAL trial, 576-577, 576t
Atacand. *See* Candesartan cilexetil (Atacand).
Atazanavir, for HIV infection, 729t
Atenolol (Tenormin)
  for hypertension, 481t
    in children, 536t
  indications for, 101
  pharmacodynamic properties and cardiac
    effects of, 98t
  pharmacokinetics of, 103
  in pregnancy and lactation, 622t-623t
  properties of, 102t
Atenolol/chlorthalidone (Tenoretic), for
    hypertension, 485t
ATHENA trial, 358-359
Atheroembolism, thoracic aortic, 617-618
Atherosclerotic carotid artery disease. *See*
    Carotid artery disease.
Atherosclerotic renal artery stenosis (ARAS),
    571-579
  clinical manifestations of, 571, 572b
  diagnostic imaging of, 571-574
    captopril renal scintigraphy for, 572
    catheter-based angiography for, 573f
    choice of correct, 573-574, 573f
    CTA and MRA for, 572
    renal artery duplex ultrasonography for,
      571, 572f, 572t
  vs. fibromuscular dysplasia, 573-574, 573f,
    577
  hypertension due to, 503t, 571-572
  natural history of, 571
  overview of, 571
  treatment of, 574-578
    catheter-based intervention for, 575-577,
      576t
    catheter-based renal artery sympathetic
      denervation for, 578
    medical, 574
    patient selection for revascularization for,
      574-575
    surveillance for, 577-578
Atherosclerotic ulcer, penetrating, of aorta,
    617
Athletic participation, by adults with
    congenital heart disease, 636-637
Atkins diet, for obesity, 446
ATMOSPHERE trial, 263-264
Atopaxar, 115
Atorvastatin
  for carotid artery disease, 556
  for chronic stable angina, 146-147

Atorvastatin *(Continued)*
  clinical trials of, 423, 424f
  dosage of, 422t
  with HIV infection and HAART, 733f
  pharmacodynamics and pharmacokinetics
    of, 60t
  pharmacokinetics of, 422t
  in pregnancy and lactation, 622t-623t, 627
ATP (antitachycardia pacing), 759
  for sustained monomorphic ventricular
    tachycardia, 413, 413f
Atrial arrhythmias, after tetralogy of Fallot
    repair, 644
Atrial fibrillation (AF), 372-382, 386-390
  adenosine-induced, 368, 368f
  cardiac resynchronization therapy in, 276
  after cardiac surgery, 379-380
  catheter ablation for, 386-390
    trigger-based strategies for, 386-387,
      387f-388f
  classification of, 372
  in heart failure, 284
  in hypertrophic cardiomyopathy, 335-336
  immediate (early) recurrence of, 375
  left atrial appendage closure devices for,
    388, 389f
  long-standing, 372
  maintenance of sinus rhythm with, 375-379
    adjunctive therapy for, 377
    nonpharmacologic approaches to, 377
    pacing for, 378
    pharmacologic approaches to, 375-377, 375t
      choice of drug in, 376, 376f
      initiation and monitoring of, 376-377
  new-onset, 372
  paroxysmal, 372
  pericardioversion anticoagulation for, 379,
    379f
  permanent, 372
  persistent, 372, 387-388
  in pregnancy, 628
  rate control for, 373-374
    atrioventricular junction ablation for,
      390-392
    nonpharmacologic approach to, 374
    pharmacologic approach to, 373-374, 373t
    rhythm vs., 372-375
  rhythm control for, 374-375
    electrical cardioversion for, 375
    pharmacologic cardioversion for, 374-375,
      374t
    rate vs., 372-375
  after STEMI, 199
  surgical techniques for, 389-390, 389f,
    711
  thromboembolic prophylaxis for, 378, 378b,
    378t
Atrial flutter, 369-371, 386
  atypical, 369, 386
  catheter ablation of, 369, 370f, 386, 386f
  isthmus-dependent, 386, 386f
  multifocal, 370
  pharmacologic management of
    long-term, 370
    short-term, 370
  in pregnancy, 628
Atrial natriuretic peptide (ANP), in resistant
    hypertension, 505f
Atrial premature contractions, in pregnancy,
    628
Atrial septal defects (ASDs), 637-639
  classification of, 637
  clinical manifestations of, 637-638
  devices for closure of, 638, 638f
  physiology of, 637-639, 637f
  recommendations for, 639
Atrial septostomy, for pulmonary arterial
    hypertension, 602

Atrial tachycardia
  catheter ablation for, 385-386
  focal, 385
  macroreentrant, 385
  mechanisms of, 366f, 367
  pharmacologic treatment of, 369
Atrial-synchronized biventricular pacing. *See*
    Cardiac resynchronization therapy (CRT).
Atrioventricular (AV) conduction disturbances,
    after STEMI, 198-199, 198t
Atrioventricular (AV) junction ablation, for
    atrial fibrillation, 390-392
Atrioventricular nodal reentrant tachycardia
    (AVNRT), 366
  catheter ablation for, 385, 385f
  mechanisms of, 366, 366f, 384f
Atrioventricular reentrant tachycardia (AVRT),
    366
  antidromic, 366-367
  mechanisms of, 366-367, 366f
  orthodromic, 366-367, 367f
Atripla (efavirenz/emtricitabine/tenofovir), for
    HIV infection, 729-730, 730t
ATS prosthetic valve, 695-697
ATTRACT study, 589-590
Autografts, as valve prostheses, 696t
Automatic external defibrillator (AED)
  for cardiac arrest, 408
  for STEMI, 179
Autonomic dysfunction, hypertensive
    emergencies due to, 518
Autonomic function, and risk of sudden
    cardiac death, 398, 400t
AV (atrioventricular) conduction disturbances,
    after STEMI, 198-199, 198t
AV (atrioventricular) junction ablation, for
    atrial fibrillation, 390-392
AVA (aortic valve area), 676
Availability, of cardiovascular drugs in
    low- and middle-income countries, 77-78
Avalide (irbesartan/hydrochlorothiazide), for
    hypertension, 485t
Avapro (irbesartan)
  for heart failure, 259-260
  for hypertension, 479t
AVERT study, 146-147
AVID trial, 353-354, 396, 398t, 409f
AVNRT (atrioventricular nodal reentrant
    tachycardia), 366
  catheter ablation for, 385, 385f
  mechanisms of, 366, 366f, 384f
AVR. *See* Aortic valve replacement (AVR).
AVRT (atrioventricular reentrant tachycardia),
    366
  antidromic, 366-367
  mechanisms of, 366-367, 366f
  orthodromic, 366-367, 367f
AXD6140, 110t
Azathioprine
  with cardiac transplantation, 311t
  for myocarditis, 263
  for recurrent pericarditis, 668
Azidothymidine (AZT), for HIV infection,
    730t
  myocardial effects of, 734
Azilsartan medoxomil (Edarbi), for
    hypertension, 479t
Azor (amlodipine/olmesartan medoxomil), for
    hypertension, 485t

B

Babic device, 722t, 725
BACE system, 722t, 725
Bacterial endocarditis. *See* Infective
    endocarditis (IE).
Bailey, Charles, 691

Bailout stent implantation, 143
BALANCE study, 324-325
Balloon angioplasty, 214
    for femoral-popliteal disease, 548, 549f
    for infrapopliteal disease, 549, 550f
    for STEMI, 189t
Balloon aortic valvuloplasty (BAV), for
    bicuspid aortic valve, 640
Balloon pulmonary valvuloplasty (BPV), for
    pulmonary stenosis, 641, 641f
Balloon valvuloplasty
    for bicuspid aortic valve, 640
    for mitral stenosis, 681t
    for pulmonary stenosis, 641, 641f
Balloon-assisted stenting, of aorta, 642f, 643
Balloon-expandable stents, for aortoiliac
    disease, 546-547, 547f
Bare-metal stent (BMS), 214-215
    for STEMI, 189t, 190
BARI trial, 143
Baroreceptor sensitivity, after STEMI, 204
Baroreflex activation therapy, for resistant
    hypertension, 508
Baroreflex slope, and risk of sudden cardiac
    death, 398, 400t
Bartonella spp, endocarditis due to, 657t
BAS(s). See Bile acid sequestrants (BASs).
Basal metabolic rate (BMR), 448
Base case analysis, 26
Basic life support (BLS) algorithm, for cardiac
    arrest, 415, 415f
BASIC (Brain Attack Surveillance in Corpus
    Christi) Project, 553
BASIL trial, 545
Basiliximab, with cardiac transplantation,
    311t
BAV (balloon aortic valvuloplasty), for
    bicuspid aortic valve, 640
Bayes' rule, 2
Bayesian approach
    for clinical trials, 11
    for meta-analysis, 16-17, 18f-19f
BCIS study, 224
Beating-heart totally endoscopic coronary
    bypass (BH-TECAB), 230
BEAUTIFUL trial, 104-105
Benazepril (Lotensin), for hypertension, 478t
    in children, 536t
Benazepril/hydrochlorothiazide (Lotensin
    HCT), for hypertension, 485t
Benefits
    balancing risks and, 22-23
    incremental, 24
BENESTENT trial, 143, 214
Benicar (olmesartan medoxomil), for
    hypertension, 479t
    in children, 536t
Benicar HCT (olmesartan medoxomil/
    hydrochlorothiazide), for hypertension,
    485t
Bentall procedure, for thoracic aortic
    aneurysms, 609
Benzothiazepine-binding site, 90
Beraprost, for pulmonary arterial hypertension,
    600
BEST trial, 251, 251t
β1 selectivity, 101
β value, 1-2, 2f, 9-11
β-adrenergic blockers, 96-104
    adverse effects of, 103-104
    α-adrenergic activity of, 101-103, 481-482,
        481t
    for angina pectoris, 97, 97b, 98t
        chronic stable angina, 140-141, 147
        at rest and vasospastic, 97
    for aortic aneurysms
        abdominal, 607
        thoracic, 613

β-adrenergic blockers (Continued)
    for aortic dissection, 613-614
    for arrhythmias, 99
    for atrial fibrillation, 373t
    β1 selectivity of, 101
    β-adrenergic receptors and, 96-97
    cardioselective, 102t, 481-482, 481t
    for carotid artery stenosis, 555
    classes of, 250
    for congestive cardiomyopathy, 100
    contraindications to, 104
    for dissecting aneurysms, 100
    drug interactions with, 94, 104, 105t
    for Ehlers-Danlos syndrome, 100
    first-generation, 250
    for heart failure, 250-253
        acute decompensated, 297
        choice of, 253
        clinical efficacy of, 250-252, 251t
        dosage of, 246t
        endpoints with, 242t
        pathophysiologic rationale for, 250
        pharmacology of, 250
        practical considerations with, 252-253
    for hypertension, 99, 477t, 481-482, 481t
        in children, 535, 536t
        in combination products, 485t
        monitoring and adverse effects of,
            485t
        due to pheochromocytoma, 493
    for hypertensive emergencies, 514t-515t
    for hypertrophic cardiomyopathy, 100
    with intrinsic sympathomimetic (partial
        agonist) activity, 101, 481-482, 481t
    for mitral stenosis in pregnancy, 624
    for mitral valve prolapse, 100
    nitric oxide potentiating effect of,
        103
    for noncardiac vascular surgery,
        544
    noncardioselective, 102t, 481-482, 481t
    for NSTE-ACS, 154
        postdischarge, 167
    vs. other antianginal therapies, 97
    with other antianginal therapies, 99
    overdosage with, 104
    for perioperative therapy in high-risk
        patients, 100-101
    for peripheral artery disease, 542
    pharmacodynamic properties of, 98t
    pharmacokinetics of, 103
    pharmacologic differences among, 101-103,
        102t
    potency of, 101
    in pregnancy, 626-627
        for mitral stenosis, 624
    for secondary prevention of coronary events,
        147
    second-generation, 250
    for "silent" myocardial ischemia, 99-100
    for STEMI
        in acute phase, 183-184
        during convalescence, 192
        in long-term management, 206
        with pulmonary congestion, 194
    for survivors of acute myocardial infarction,
        99
    for syndrome X, 100
    third-generation, 250
    vasodilatory, 102t
    withdrawal from, 104
β-adrenergic receptor(s), 96-97
β-adrenergic receptor downregulation, 250
β-blockers. See β-adrenergic blockers.
Betapace. See Sotalol (Betapace).
Betaxolol (Kerlone)
    for hypertension, 481t
    indications for, 101

Betaxolol (Kerlone) (Continued)
    pharmacodynamic properties and cardiac
        effects of, 98t
    properties of, 102t
Betrixaban, 160t
Between-trial variability, 16
BH-TECAB (beating-heart totally endoscopic
    coronary bypass), 230
Bicuspid aortic valve, 640
    recommendations for, 640
Bidirectional Glenn anastomosis, 633t
Bifurcation lesions, 223, 223f
Bile acid sequestrants (BASs)
    for lowering LDL cholesterol, 428-430,
        429t
        clinical efficacy of, 429, 429t
        effects on lipids and lipoproteins of,
            429
        safety/compliance issues for, 429-430
    for peripheral artery disease, 541-542
    in pregnancy, 627
Bileaflet prosthesis, 695-697, 695t, 696f
Biocor prosthesis, 695t, 697
Biodegradable polymers, stents with,
    221
Biodegradable stents, 220
Biolimus-based stents, 220-221
Biologic products, regulation of, 34, 36
Biomarkers
    for STEMI, 181
    as surrogate endpoints of trial, 9, 10f
Biomaterial(s), mechanical failure of, 48
Biomatrix stent, 221
Bioresorbable vascular scaffold (BVS)
    everolimus stent, 220
Biosimilar drugs, 39
BioSTAR device, 638
Biotransformation hypothesis, of nitrate
    tolerance, 87-88
BIP study, 436, 557
Bisoprolol (Zebeta)
    for congestive cardiomyopathy,
        100
    for heart failure, 246t, 250, 252-253
    for hypertension, 481t
    indications for, 101
    properties of, 102t
Bisoprolol/hydrochlorothiazide (Ziac), for
    hypertension, 485t
    in children, 536t
Bitter orange, hypertensive emergency due to,
    511
BiVAD (biventricular assist device), 315
Bivalirudin, 120
    indications and dosage for, 120
    mechanisms of action of, 120
    for NSTE-ACS, 161-162, 162f, 163t
    for STEMI
        in acute phase, 183
        with PCI, 190t
Biventricular assist device (BiVAD), 315
Biventricular pacing. See Cardiac
    resynchronization therapy (CRT).
Blalock-Taussig shunt, 633t
Bleeding event, with valve surgery, 696b
Bleeding risk, with fibrinolytic therapy, 185
Blinded trials, 6
    of cardiovascular devices, 46
Blocadren. See Timolol (Blocadren).
Block size, 6
Blood pressure (BP)
    in acute decompensated heart failure,
        287
    and global cardiovascular disease, 80-81
    in pregnancy, 621
Blood pressure (BP) control
    after NSTE-ACS, 166t, 167
    after STEMI, 205t, 206

Blood pressure (BP) goals, for hypertension, 474
  in elderly patients, 486
Blood pressure (BP) levels, in children, 529
  for boys, 530t-531t
  for girls, 531t-532t
Blood pressure (BP) measurement, 466, 466b
  for hypertensive emergencies, 511-512
Blood pressure (BP) monitoring, for hypertension, 484-486, 485t
  ambulatory, 466, 485, 501-502
  resistant, 501-502
Blood pressure (BP) reduction
  antihypertensive medications for. See Antihypertensive medications.
  high-carbohydrate, low-fat diets for, 442, 443f
Blood urea nitrogen (BUN)
  in acute decompensated heart failure, 287
  and heart failure risk stratification, 285, 285t
Blood volume, in pregnancy, 621
BLS (basic life support) algorithm, for cardiac arrest, 415, 415f
BMCs (bone marrow cells), 322
  and clinical studies, 324-326
  transdifferentiation of, 323
BMI (body mass index), 446, 447t
BMPR2, in pulmonary arterial hypertension, 604
BMR (basal metabolic rate), 448
BMS (bare-metal stent), 214-215
  for STEMI, 189t, 190
BNP (brain natriuretic peptide)
  in acute decompensated heart failure, 287-288, 288f, 288t
  in resistant hypertension, 505f
Body mass index (BMI), 446, 447t
Bone marrow cells (BMCs), 322
  and clinical studies, 324-326
  transdifferentiation of, 323
Bosentan
  in pregnancy and lactation, 622t-623t
  for pulmonary arterial hypertension, 601, 601f
    with HIV infection, 735
BP. See Blood pressure (BP).
BPV (balloon pulmonary valvuloplasty), for pulmonary stenosis, 641, 641f
Bradyarrhythmias, after STEMI, 198-199, 198t
Brain Attack Surveillance in Corpus Christi (BASIC) Project, 553
Brain natriuretic peptide (BNP)
  in acute decompensated heart failure, 287-288, 288f, 288t
  in resistant hypertension, 505f
Braunwald, Nina, 691
Brazil, regulation of new drugs in, 37
Breastfeeding, cardiac drugs during, 622t-623t
BREATHE trial, 601, 601f
Bucindolol
  for heart failure, 251
  pharmacology of, 250
Bumetanide (Bumex)
  for heart failure, 243t
  for hypertension, 480t
BUN (blood urea nitrogen)
  in acute decompensated heart failure, 287
  and heart failure risk stratification, 285, 285t
Bupropion hydrochloride (Zyban), for smoking cessation in peripheral artery disease, 542-543, 543f
BVS (bioresorbable vascular scaffold) everolimus stent, 220
Bystolic. See Nebivolol (Bystolic).

C

CABACS trial, 568
CABG. See Coronary artery bypass graft (CABG).
CABG-Patch trial, 270-271, 399t
CAD. See Coronary artery disease (CAD).
CADUCEUS trial, 326
CAFÉ (complex atrial fractionated electrograms), 387
Caged ball prosthesis, 695-697, 695t
CAH (congenital adrenal hyperplasia), hypertension due to, 497-498
Calcification
  in chronic stable angina, 135
  of prosthetic heart valve, 49f
Calcium antagonists. See Calcium channel blockers (CCBs).
Calcium channel(s)
  L and T types of, 90
  molecular structure of, 90
  as site of action of calcium channel blockers, 89-90, 90f
Calcium channel blockers (CCBs), 89-96
  for aortic dissection, 614
  for atrial fibrillation, 373t
  with β-adrenergic blockers, 99
  calcium channel as site of action of, 89-90, 90f
  for carotid artery stenosis, 555
  for chronic stable angina, 141
  classification of, 91
  dihydropyridines as, 93
  diltiazem as, 93
  drug binding sites for, 90
  drug interactions with, 94
  fundamental mechanisms of, 89-90, 90f
  for heart failure, 257
    with preserved ejection fraction, 259
  for hypertension, 92, 92t, 477t, 479-480, 479t
    in children, 535, 536t
    in combination products, 485t
    monitoring and adverse effects of, 485t
    due to pheochromocytoma, 492t, 493
    pulmonary arterial, 599
    systemic, 92, 92t
  for hypertensive emergencies, 514t-515t
  with L and T type calcium channels, 90
  for maintenance of sinus rhythm, 377
  major cardiovascular actions of, 91
  major indications for, 92
  molecular structure of, 90
  noncardiovascular effects of, 91
  for NSTE-ACS, 154-155
  for paroxysmal supraventricular tachycardia, 368, 369t
  pharmacodynamic effects of, 90-91, 91t
  pharmacokinetics of, 91
  for postinfarct protection, 92
  in pregnancy, 627
  "safety" controversy over, 94-96, 95f-96f
  after STEMI, 193
  for supraventricular tachycardia, 92
  vascular selectivity of, 91
  verapamil as, 92-93
Calibration, 3
Call to Action to Prevent Deep Vein Thrombosis and Pulmonary Embolism, 580
Calorie levels, for weight loss, 448
CAMELOT trial, 94, 542
CAMIAT trial, 353-354
Campestanol, 430
Campesterol, 430
Cancer
  after cardiac transplantation, 313-314
  prevention of venous thromboembolism in patients with, 591-592

Candesartan cilexetil (Atacand)
  for heart failure
    as alternative to ACE inhibitors, 248
    dosage of, 246t, 250
    pathophysiologic mechanisms of, 245-246
    with preserved ejection fraction, 259-260
    in triple therapy, 246-248
  for hypertension, 479t
    in children, 536t
  for STEMI
    during convalescence, 192-193
    in long-term management, 206
Candesartan cilexetil/hydrochlorothiazide (Atacand HCT), for hypertension, 485t
Cangrelor, 110t, 115
  for NSTE-ACS, 158-159
Canola oil (rapeseed oil), for hyperlipidemia, 444
CAP study, 63
Capozide (captopril/hydrochlorothiazide), for hypertension, 485t
CAPRICORN trial, 251t, 252
CAPRIE trial
  for cerebrovascular disease, 557, 558t
  indications in, 111, 112t
  for peripheral artery disease, 540-541
  preventive benefits in, 146
  side effects in, 113
CAPS study, 343
CAPTIM trial, 185
Captopril (Capoten)
  for heart failure, 246t
    acute decompensated, 296
  for hypertension, 478t
    in children, 536t
  in pregnancy and lactation, 622t-623t
  for STEMI
    during convalescence, 192
    with pulmonary congestion, 194
Captopril renal scintigraphy, 572
Captopril-Digoxin Multicenter Research Group, 256
Captopril/hydrochlorothiazide (Capozide), for hypertension, 485t
CAPTURE-1 trial, 563
CAPTURE-2 trial, 563-564
Carbohydrates, glycemic index of, 445
CarboMedics AnnuloFlex prosthesis, 695t
CarboMedics AnnuloFlo prosthesis, 695t
CarboMedics mechanical valve, 695-697, 695t
  complication rates with, 697, 697t, 698f
Cardene. See Nicardipine (Cardene).
Cardiac abscess, in infective endocarditis, 652, 653f, 660
Cardiac allograft vasculopathy (CAV), 313
Cardiac amyloidosis, 336-337
Cardiac arrest
  care after, 417-418
    algorithm for, 417, 418f
    critical care support in, 417
    general approach to, 417
    neurologic prognostication in, 417-418
    therapeutic hypothermia in, 417
  defined, 414
  epidemiology of, 414
  etiology of, 408
  management of, 414-418
    ACLS for, 415-417, 416f
    automatic external defibrillator for, 408
    chain of survival paradigm for, 414, 415f
    CPR for, 414-417
      chest compressions in, 414-415
      defibrillation in, 415, 415f
      rescue breathing in, 415
    general principles for, 414, 415f

Cardiac arrest (Continued)
  out-of-hospital
    quality improvement for, 72
    systems of care for, 70
      need for, 67-68
Cardiac arrhythmias. See Arrhythmias.
Cardiac biology, 322
Cardiac biomarkers, for STEMI, 181
Cardiac catheterization, 223-225
  intravascular assessment of lesion severity
    in, 224-225
  mechanical support for high-risk
    percutaneous coronary intervention in,
    224
  for NSTE-ACS, invasive vs. conservative
    strategy of, 163-165, 164f
  transradial access in, 223-224
  prior to valve surgery, 692-693
Cardiac contractility modulation (CCM), 278
Cardiac device infections (CDIs), infective
  endocarditis with, 661-662
Cardiac filling pressures, in acute
  decompensated heart failure, 285-286,
  290
Cardiac hemochromatosis, 338-339
  treatment of, 338-339
Cardiac index, in acute decompensated heart
  failure, 290
Cardiac magnetic resonance imaging, for
  chronic stable angina, 134
Cardiac magnetic resonance perfusion
  imaging, for chronic stable angina, 134,
  137t
Cardiac malignancies, in HIV-positive patients,
  735
Cardiac niches, 327, 328f-329f
Cardiac output
  in acute decompensated heart failure, 290
  in pregnancy, 621
  procainamide with low, 348-349
Cardiac progenitors, endogenous, 326-327,
  327f-330f
Cardiac rehabilitation, 739-745
  in chronic heart failure, 744
  for chronic stable angina, 140
  contraindications to, 743-744, 744b
  disability from myocardial infarction and,
    739-740
  evolving landscape for, 745
  inpatient
    exercise testing before discharge and, 740
    in-hospital exercise in, 740
    patient education on, 740
  meta-analysis for survival after, 744-745
  outpatient, 740-742
    core components for, 740-742, 741b
    exercise prescription for, 742-743, 743f
    maintenance program for, 741-742, 742t
    monitoring in, 741, 742b
    resistance exercise in, 743
    safety of, 741
  for secondary prevention of coronary events,
    144
Cardiac resynchronization therapy (CRT), 273
  in atrial fibrillation, 276
  ECG appearance of, 756f-757f
  future directions of, 276
  in heart failure
    indications for, 276
    mild, 275-276
    monitoring via, 276-277
  history of, 273
  landmark trials of, 273-275, 274f
  in long-term right ventricle pacing, 276
  for prevention of sudden cardiac death, 401,
    402t, 403f
Cardiac sarcoidosis, 337-338
  treatment of, 338

Cardiac stem cells (CSCs)
  age, cardiac disease and, 327-330
  endogenous, 326-327, 327f-330f
  hematopoietic stem cell transdifferentiation
    to, 323
  in myocardial repair, 322, 324f
Cardiac surgery, atrial fibrillation after,
  379-380
Cardiac syndrome X, 168-169, 169b, 170f
  β-adrenergic blockers for, 100
Cardiac tamponade, 669-671, 670f
Cardiac transplantation, 307-314
  for adults with congenital heart disease,
    637
  for cardiac amyloidosis, 337
  for cardiac hemochromatosis, 339
  for cardiac sarcoidosis, 338
  complications after, 310-314
    cardiac allograft vasculopathy as, 313
    diabetes as, 313
    dyslipidemia as, 313
    hypertension as, 313
    infections as, 312
    malignancy as, 313-314
    renal insufficiency as, 313
  future directions for, 314
  immunosuppressive therapy with, 310, 311t
    drug interactions with, 310, 312b
  listing for, 309, 309t
  for nonobstructive hypertrophic
    cardiomyopathy, 335
  patient management after, 309-310, 310t
  patient management prior to, 309
  patient selection for, 307-309, 308b
    age in, 308
    assessment of cardiac disease severity in,
      307-308
    assessment of pulmonary vasculature in,
      308
    comorbidities in, 308
    immunologic sensitization in, 308-309
  rejection of
    causes of, 309
    diagnosis of, 309-310, 310t
    prevention and treatment of, 310, 311t
  surgical technique for, 309
  total orthotopic, 309
Cardiac troponins
  in heart failure, 284, 284f
  for STEMI, 181
CardiAQ prosthesis, 722t, 726, 726f
Cardiobacterium spp, endocarditis due to, 655t
Cardiogenic shock, after STEMI, 195, 195f
CardioMEMS device, 277, 278f-279f
Cardiomyocyte(s), 322
  death and regeneration of, 322, 323f
  in aging heart, 330
  structural and functional integration of
    newly formed, 327, 330f
Cardiomyopathy
  congestive, β-adrenergic blockers for, 100
  dilated
    bone marrow cells for, 325
    catheter ablation for ventricular
      tachycardia in, 391-392
    with HIV infection, 734
  hypertrophic, 332-336
    atrial fibrillation in, 335-336
    β-adrenergic blockers for, 100
    defined, 332
    LVOT obstruction in, 332-335
      alcohol septal ablation for, 333-334, 334t
      pharmacologic treatment of, 332
      surgical myectomy for, 332, 333f, 334t
      ventricular pacing for, 334-335
    nonobstructive, 335
    screening at-risk family members for, 336
    sudden cardiac death in, 335, 335f

Cardiomyopathy (Continued)
  peripartum, 627-628
  restrictive, 336-340
    due to cardiac amyloidosis, 336-337
    due to cardiac hemochromatosis, 338-339
      treatment of, 338-339
    due to cardiac sarcoidosis, 337-338
      treatment of, 338
    due to endomyocardial fibrosis, 339
    etiology of, 336, 336b
    due to Fabry's disease, 339
    idiopathic, 336
    due to Löffler hypereosinophilic
      syndrome, 339-340
    with mutations in LAMP2 (Danon disease),
      PRKAG2, or mitochondrial genes, 339
    due to storage diseases of myocardium,
      339
Cardiopulmonary bypass (CPB), minimally
  invasive surgical coronary
  revascularization without, 225-227, 226f
Cardiopulmonary resuscitation (CPR)
  for cardiac arrest, 414-417
    chest compressions in, 414-415
    defibrillation in, 415, 415f
    rescue breathing in, 415
  in pregnancy, 629
  for STEMI, 179
  system of care for, 70
Cardiorenal syndrome, 245, 287, 287b
cardioSEAL device, 647
cardioSEAL-STARFlex device
  for atrial septal defects, 638
  for patent foramen ovale, 639
  for ventricular septal rupture, 647
Cardiosphere(s), 326, 327f
Cardiosphere-derived cells (CDCs), 326-327
Cardiovascular and Renal Drugs Advisory
  Committee (CRAC), 35
Cardiovascular (CV) devices. See also Medical
  device(s).
  for electrical cardioversion and
    defibrillation, 751-752
    equipment for, 751, 751f
    set-up and patient preparation for, 751,
      752f
    technical considerations with, 751-752
  implantable cardioverter-defibrillators as,
    758-760
    inappropriate shocks with, 759-760, 760t
    magnet operation with, 759
    programmed therapies for ventricular
      arrhythmias with, 759, 759f, 759t
    routine follow-up with, 760
  intra-aortic balloon pump as, 749-750
    complications of, 750
    design of, 749
    indications for, 749, 749b
    technical aspects of placement of, 749-750
    timing and waveforms with, 750, 750f-751f
  pacemakers as
    permanent, 752
      basic pacing concepts with, 752, 754b,
        754f
      leads for, 752, 753t
      programmable mode for, 752, 755f-757f,
        755t
      pseudo-malfunction of, 752, 757t
      radiographic appearance of, 752, 753f
      rate-responsive pacing with, 752, 757t
    temporary, 752-758
      complications and troubleshooting with,
        758
      indications for, 752-758, 758f
      placement of, 758
  for pericardiocentesis, 750-751
    indications for, 750
    technical aspects of, 750-751

Cardiovascular (CV) devices (Continued)
  pulmonary artery catheters as, 747-749
    design of, 747, 748f
    indications for, 747, 748t
    interpretation of waveforms from, 747, 749f
    technical aspects of placement of, 747,
      748b, 748f
    troubleshooting and complications with,
      747-749
Cardiovascular disease (CVD)
  costs of, 1
  epidemiology of, 1
  global
    burden of, 75, 76f
    economic impact of, 75
    epidemiology of, 75
  lifestyle modification for. See Lifestyle
    modification.
Cardiovascular Health Study, 553-555, 571
Cardiovascular (CV) presentations,
    hypertensive emergencies with, 513-515
  acute coronary syndromes as, 513
  aortic dissection as, 513-515, 515f
  left ventricular failure and acute pulmonary
    edema as, 513
Cardiovascular (CV) risk
  peripheral artery disease and, 539, 540f
  resistant hypertension and, 502
Cardiovascular risk (CV) reduction, for
    peripheral artery disease, 539-543
  ACE inhibitor therapy as, 542
  anticoagulant therapy as, 541
  antihypertensive therapy as, 542
  antiplatelet therapy as, 539-541
  β-blocker therapy as, 542
  lipid-lowering drugs as, 541-542
  smoking cessation as, 542-543, 543b, 543f
Cardioversion, 751-752
  for atrial fibrillation, 375
    anticoagulation with, 379, 379f
    electrical, 375
    pharmacologic, 374-375, 374t
  equipment for, 751, 751f
  set-up and patient preparation for,
    751, 752f
  for sustained monomorphic ventricular
    tachycardia, 413
  technical considerations with, 751-752
Cardioverter
  external, 751, 751f
  implantable. See Implantable cardioverter-
    defibrillators (ICDs).
Cardizem. See Diltiazem.
CARDS study, 425t
Cardura (doxazosin), for hypertension, 482,
    483t
  due to pheochromocytoma, 491-493, 492t
  resistant, 507
CARE study, 146, 425t
CARE-HF trial, 275, 275f
CARESS study, 557
Carillon Mitral Contour System, 722t, 724
Carillon XE device, 723f, 724
CARISA trial, 106, 106f
Carney triad, and pheochromocytomas, 490
Carotid artery disease, 553-570
  clinically significant, 555
  and coronary artery bypass graft surgery,
    566-568
  imaging of, 554f
  medical therapy of, 555-558
    antihypertensive therapy in, 555-556
    antiplatelet therapy in, 557-558, 558t
    lipid-lowering therapy in, 556-557
    smoking cessation in, 555
  prevalence of, 553-555
  revascularization for, 558-568

Carotid artery disease (Continued)
  changing attitude toward, 565-566
  endovascular (carotid artery stenting),
    562-565
    indications for, 562, 562f
    in normal-risk symptomatic patients,
      563-565, 565f
    serial steps during, 559f
    in symptomatic and asymptomatic
      patients at high surgical risk, 563
  surgical (carotid endarterectomy), 559-562
    for asymptomatic carotid artery
      stenosis, 560-562, 561t
    carotid artery bifurcation exposed
      during, 559f
    for symptomatic carotid artery stenosis,
      559-560, 560f, 561t
  and risk of stroke, 553
Carotid artery stenosis. See Carotid artery
    disease.
Carotid artery stenting (CAS), 562-565
  indications for, 562, 562f
  in normal-risk symptomatic patients,
    563-565, 565f
  serial steps during, 559f
  in symptomatic and asymptomatic patients
    at high surgical risk, 563
Carotid endarterectomy (CEA), 559-562
  for asymptomatic carotid artery stenosis,
    560-562, 561t
  carotid artery bifurcation exposed during, 559f
  and coronary artery bypass graft, 566-568
  for symptomatic carotid artery stenosis,
    559-560, 560f, 561t
Carpentier-Edwards Classic prosthesis, 695t
Carpentier-Edwards Magna stented bovine
    pericardial aortic bioprosthesis, 696f, 697
Carpentier-Edwards mechanical valve, 695t
Carpentier-Edwards Perimount Pericardial
    Valve, 695t, 697
  age dependence of structural degeneration
    of, 701, 701f
Carpentier-Edwards Physio prosthesis, 695t
Carpentier-Edwards Porcine valve, 697
Carpentier-McCarthy-Adams ET-Logix ring,
    695t, 705-706
Carpentier's functional classification, of mitral
    regurgitation, 703-704, 703f, 703t
CARPREG, 635-636
CARRESS trial, 292
CART (classification and regression tree)
    analysis, for heart failure, 285
Carteolol (Cartrol)
  indications for, 101
  pharmacodynamic properties and cardiac
    effects of, 98t
  properties of, 102t
Cartia. See Diltiazem.
Carvedilol (Coreg)
  for congestive cardiomyopathy, 100
  drug interactions with, 105t
  for heart failure
    choice of, 253
    clinical trials of, 250-252
    dosage of, 246t
    practical considerations with, 252
  for hypertension, 481t
    in children, 536t
  indications for, 101
  pharmacodynamic properties and cardiac
    effects of, 98t
  pharmacology of, 250
  in pregnancy and lactation, 622t-623t
  properties of, 102t
  after STEMI, 192
  for survivors of acute myocardial infarction, 99
CAS. See Carotid artery stenting (CAS).

CASANOVA trial, 560, 561t
Case(s), 6
Case-control studies, 6
CASH trial, 396, 398t, 409f
CASPAR study, 168
CASS study, 144
CAST trial, 4, 343, 353-354, 356, 628-629
CAT trial, 397-398, 399t
Catapres (clonidine)
  for hypertension, 483, 483t
    in children, 536t
  hypertensive emergencies due to acute
    withdrawal of, 517
Catecholamine synthesis inhibitor, for
    hypertension due to pheochromocytoma,
    492t, 493
Catecholaminergic presentations, hypertensive
    emergencies with, 517-518
  due to acute withdrawal of antihypertensive
    therapy, 517
  due to autonomic dysfunction, 518
  due to pheochromocytoma, 517-518
  due to sympathomimetic drugs, 518
Catecholamine-secreting paragangliomas, 490
Catheter ablation, for tachyarrhythmias, 383-395
  indications for, 383, 384b
  practical considerations with, 383, 384f
  results of, 383, 384t
  supraventricular, 383-386
    accessory pathway–mediated tachycardias
      as, 383-385, 384f
    atrial fibrillation as, 386-390, 387f-388f
    atrial flutter as, 386, 386f
    atrial tachycardia as, 385-386
    atrioventricular node reentry tachycardia
      as, 385, 385f
  ventricular, 390-392
    idiopathic ventricular tachycardia as,
      390-391
    ventricular fibrillation and polymorphic
      ventricular tachycardia as, 392
    ventricular tachycardia in patients with
      structural heart disease as, 391-392,
      391f
Catheter-assisted embolectomy, for pulmonary
    embolism, 590
Catheterization laboratory activation, for
    STEMI, 68-69
CAV (cardiac allograft vasculopathy), 313
CBER (Center for Biologics Evaluation and
    Research), 34, 36
CCISC (Congenital Cardiovascular
    Interventional Study Consortium), 642
CCM (cardiac contractility modulation), 278
CCU (coronary care unit), for STEMI, 190-192
CD34 antibody–eluting stent, 220-221
CDCs (cardiosphere-derived cells), 326-327
CDER (Center for Drug Evaluation and
    Research), 34, 36
CDIs (cardiac device infections), infective
    endocarditis with, 661-662
CDRH (Center for Devices and Radiological
    Health), 34
  interactions with external stakeholders and
    government partners of, 51
  product recall by, 50
CEA. See Carotid endarterectomy (CEA).
Ceftriaxone, for infective endocarditis,
    655t-657t
Cenderitide, for heart failure, 264
Center for Biologics Evaluation and Research
    (CBER), 34, 36
Center for Devices and Radiological Health
    (CDRH), 34
  interactions with external stakeholders and
    government partners of, 51
  product recall by, 50

Center for Drug Evaluation and Research (CDER), 34, 36
Centers for Medicare and Medicaid Services (CMS), on reimbursement for medical device development, 51
Central α-agonists, for hypertension, 483, 483t
    in children, 536t
CER. See Comparative effectiveness research (CER).
CER (control event rate), 15, 16f
Cerebral protection, for aortic arch surgery, 611
Cerebrovascular accidents (CVAs). See Stroke.
Cerebrovascular disease
    due to atherosclerotic carotid artery disease. See Carotid artery disease.
    in HIV-positive patients, 735
Cerebrovascular event, 553
Cerebrovascular syndromes, hypertensive emergencies with
    hemorrhagic, 516
    ischemic, 515-516
CETP gene, in pharmacogenetics of statins, 61-62
CETP (cholesteryl ester transfer protein) inhibition
    for chronic stable angina, 149
    for low HDL cholesterol, 438-439, 438f
CFR (Code of Federal Regulations), 34
CHADS₂ Scoring System, for stroke risk, 378, 378t
Chain of survival
    for cardiac arrest, 414, 415f
    for STEMI, 178-179
Chamber remodeling, in percutaneous mitral valve repair, 722t, 724, 724f
CHAMPION PLATFORM trial, 158-159
CHAMPION-PCI trial, 158-159
CHAMPION-PHOENIX trial, 158-159
Chantix (varenicline), for smoking cessation in peripheral artery disease, 542-543, 543f
Charges, in cost-effectiveness analysis, 24
CHARISMA trial
    for cerebrovascular disease, 557, 558t
    duration of therapy in, 157
    indications in, 111, 112t
    for peripheral artery disease, 540-541
    pharmacogenetics in, 54-56
    preventive benefits in, 146
CHARM-Added study, 246-250, 247t
CHARM-Alternative study, 247t, 248
CHARM-Preserved study, 259-260, 260t
CHD. See Coronary heart disease (CHD).
CHD (congenital heart disease), adult. See Adult congenital heart disease (ACHD).
Chemotherapy-associated venous thromboembolism, 580, 581t
Chest compressions, for cardiac arrest, 414-415
Chest pain, recurrent, after STEMI, 199-200
Chest radiography
    in acute decompensated heart failure, 286
    for pulmonary embolism, 583
CHF (congestive heart failure). See Heart failure (HF).
CHF-STAT trial, 258, 353-354
Children
    hypertension in, 529-537
        classification of, 529, 533t
        confirmation of, 529
        definitions of, 529
            levels for boys in, 530t-531t
            levels for girls in, 531t-532t

Children (Continued)
        evaluation of, 529, 533t
            algorithm for, 532f
            due to medications or illicit drugs, 529, 533t
            overview of, 529
            primary vs. secondary, 529-536
            target organ damage due to, 533-534
            treatment of, 534-536
                algorithm for, 532f
                antihypertensive medications for, 534-536, 535f, 536t
                nonpharmacologic, 534
    hypertensive emergencies in, 518
China
    regulation of new drugs in, 37
    secondary prevention of coronary artery disease in, 77
Chlorothiazide, for heart failure, 243t
Chlorthalidone (Hygroton, Thalitone)
    for heart failure, 243t
    for hypertension, 480t, 481
        in children, 536t
        resistant, 505, 506f
Cholesterol
    and global cardiovascular disease, 81
    high-density lipoprotein. See High-density lipoprotein (HDL) cholesterol.
    HIV infection and, 730, 731f
    low-density lipoprotein. See Low-density lipoprotein (LDL) cholesterol.
    after STEMI, 205t, 206
Cholesterol absorption inhibitors, 430
    effect on lipids and lipoproteins of, 430
    efficacy of, 430
    safety of, 430
Cholesterol management, for NSTE-ACS, postdischarge, 166t, 167-168, 167f-168f
Cholesterol Treatment Trialists' (CTT) collaboration, 424, 426f
Cholesteryl ester transfer protein (CETP) inhibition
    for chronic stable angina, 149
    for low HDL cholesterol, 438-439, 438f
Cholestyramine resin
    for lowering LDL cholesterol
        clinical efficacy of, 429, 429t
        dosage of, 429t
        effects on lipids and lipoproteins of, 429
    in pregnancy, 627
Chordal implantation, in percutaneous mitral valve repair, 722t, 725, 725f
Chordal transfer, for anterior leaflet prolapse, 705
Chordal-sparing mitral valve replacement, 706
Chronic disease management, 740
Chronic kidney disease (CKD)
    in atherosclerotic renal artery stenosis, 571
    hypertension with, 476
    NSTE-ACS with, 172
Chronic total occlusions (CTOs), 222-223
Chylopericardium, 674
CI(s) (confidence intervals), 8
CIBIS I and II studies, 250, 251t
CIDS trial, 396, 398t, 409f
Cigarette smoking
    and chronic stable angina, 137-138
    and global cardiovascular disease, 80
    with HIV infection, 733
    quitting. See Smoking cessation.
Cilostazol
    for carotid artery disease, 558
    for intermittent claudication, 543-544
Ciprofloxacin, for infective endocarditis, 655t, 657t
Circus movement tachycardia, 383

Citrus aurantium, hypertensive emergency due to, 511
CK (creatine kinase) levels, statins and, 427
CKD (chronic kidney disease)
    in atherosclerotic renal artery stenosis, 571
    hypertension with, 476
    NSTE-ACS with, 172
CK-MB (MB fraction of creatine kinase), for STEMI, 181
CLAIR study, 557
CLARITY trial, 111, 112t, 113
CLARITY-TIMI 28 trial, 182
CLAS study, 429t
CLASP study, 627
Class I devices, 42-43
Class II devices, 43
Class III devices, 43
Class labeling, of new drugs, 35
Classic approach, for clinical trials, 11
Classic Glenn anastomosis, 633t
CLASSICS study, 113
Classification and regression tree (CART) analysis, for heart failure, 285
Clevidipine, for hypertensive emergencies, 514t-515t
CLI. See Critical limb ischemia (CLI).
Clinical and Translational Science Awards (CTSA), 39
Clinical event adjudication, for clinical trial, 38
Clinical therapeutic development, cycle of, 33, 34f
Clinical trial(s), 3-11
    anatomy of, 37-38
        clinical events adjudication in, 38
        data management in, 38
        protocol development in, 37-38
        safety surveillance in, 38
        site management in, 38
        statistics in, 38
    checklist of information to include when reporting on, 14t
    design of, 4-11
        Bayesian methodology for, 11
        classic or frequentist, 11
        control group and test treatments in, 5-6, 5b
        crossover, 7
        endpoints in
            adjudication of, 38
            composite, 6-7, 9
            selection of, 9, 10f
            surrogate, 9, 10f
        factorial, 7-8
        false-positive and false-negative error rates in, 9-11
        fixed sample size, 6
        with historical controls, 7
        nonrandomized concurrent control, 7
        open or closed sequential, 6
        randomized controlled, 5-7
        sample size estimations in, 9
        sequential stopping boundaries in, 9-10, 11f
        to test equivalence of therapies, 8-9, 8f
        withdrawal studies as, 7
    international, 36-37
    learning curve in, 5
    need for, 3-4
    phases of, 3-4, 4t
        in new drug development, 33, 34f
    postmarketing, 5
    power of, 8f, 9-11
    reading and interpretation of, 11-15, 12f
        detection of treatment effects in, 13-15, 15f-16f

Clinical trial(s) *(Continued)*
  errors that can affect, 5f
  measures of treatment effect in, 12-13, 14t
  missing data in, 12, 13t
  questions to ask in, 11, 11b
  six-step process for, 5f
  and spectrum of clinical/translational science, 3-4, 3f
  stages of, 3-5, 4t
Clinical/translational science, spectrum of, 3-4, 3f
CLMN gene, in genome-wide association studies of statins, 62t, 63
Clonidine (Catapres)
  for hypertension, 483, 483t
    in children, 536t
  hypertensive emergencies due to acute withdrawal of, 517
Clopidogrel, 53-57, 110t
  absorption, metabolism, and action pathway of, 55f
  for carotid artery disease, 557-558, 558f
  for chronic stable angina, 144, 146
  dosage of, 111-112
  drug interactions with, 53, 54f
  indications for, 53, 111, 112t
  mechanism of action of, 53, 110f, 111
  for NSTE-ACS, 156, 156f
  for peripheral artery disease, 540-541
  pharmacogenetics of, 53-56
    future directions for, 57
    genetic polymorphism in, 54t-55t
    key genes in, 54t
      ABCB1 as, 55t, 56
      CYP2C19 as, 54-56, 55t
      PON1 as, 56
    testing for, 56
      cost effectiveness of, 57
    therapeutic implications of, 56-57
  pharmacology of, 53
  in pregnancy and lactation, 622t-623t
  side effects and contraindications to, 113
  for STEMI
    in acute phase, 182, 182f
    in long-term management, 206
    with PCI, 189t
  for thoracic aortic atheroembolism, 618
Closed sequential design, 6
Closed-cell stents, 214
CLOSURE-1 study, 639
Clubbing, in adults with cyanotic congenital heart disease, 634
CMS (Centers for Medicare and Medicaid Services), on reimbursement for medical device development, 51
CMV (cytomegalovirus), after cardiac transplantation, 312
COAG trial, 60, 589
Coagulation cascade, in acute coronary syndromes, 159, 159f
Coarctation of aorta (CoA), 641-643, 641f-642f
  hypertension due to, 503t
  recommendations for, 642-643
Cocaine
  hypertensive emergencies due to, 518
  NSTE-ACS due to, 169-170, 170b
Coccidioides immitis, pericarditis due to, 673
Code of Federal Regulations (CFR), 34
COGENT trial, 53
Colchicine
  for gout in adults with cyanotic congenital heart disease, 634
  for pericarditis
    acute, 667-668

Colchicine *(Continued)*
    recurrent, 668
    with STEMI, 200
  for postpericardial injury syndrome, 673
Colesevelam
  in diabetes, 429
  dosage of, 429t
  effects on lipids and lipoproteins of, 429
Colestipol resin
  clinical efficacy of, 429, 429t
  dosage of, 429t
  effects on lipids and lipoproteins of, 429
  in pregnancy, 627
  safety/compliance issues with, 429-430
Collaterals, after repair of congenital heart defects, 647
Colvin-Galloway Future prosthesis, 695t
Combination products, 50-51
Combined patient interventions, for antihypertensive medications, 468
Combivir (zidovudine/lamuvidine), for HIV infection, 729-730, 730t
COMET trial, 251-252, 251t
Commissural prolapse, 702
COMMIT trial, 111, 112t, 113, 154
COMMIT/CCS-2 trial, 182-184
Common Market of the South (MERCOSUR), 37
COMPANION trial, 274-275, 401, 402t, 403f
Comparative effectiveness research (CER), 19-23
  balancing risks and benefits in, 22-23
  defined, 19-20
  methods for, 20-22, 22t
  scope of, 19-20, 22t
COMPARE study, 217t
COMPASS-HF study, 277
Compensated erythrocytosis, in adults with cyanotic congenital heart disease, 634
Compensatory mechanisms, in heart failure, 283, 283f
Complex atrial fractionated electrograms (CAFÉ), 387
Complex patient interventions, for antihypertensive medications, 468
Composite endpoints
  for cardiovascular device trials, 45
  for clinical trials, 6-7, 9
Composition of matter patent, 39
Compression stockings
  for deep vein thrombosis, 587
  for peripheral edema in pregnancy, 623
  for thromboprophylaxis, 592
Computed tomography (CT)
  for chronic stable angina, 135-136
  for pulmonary embolism, 584, 584f-585f
Computed tomography (CT) coronary angiography, for chronic stable angina, 135-136, 136f
Concealed pathway, in atrioventricular reentrant tachycardia, 366-367
Conduction abnormalities
  antiarrhythmic drugs for. *See* Antiarrhythmic drugs.
  in heart failure, 273
Confidence intervals (CIs), 8
Confounding by indication, 21-22
Congenital adrenal hyperplasia (CAH), hypertension due to, 497-498
Congenital heart disease (CHD), adult. *See* Adult congenital heart disease (ACHD).
Congestive cardiomyopathy, β-adrenergic blockers for, 100
Congestive heart failure (CHF). *See* Heart failure (HF).
Connective tissue disease–related pericardial disease, 674

CONSENSUS II trial, 247t, 248
CONSENSUS trial, 246, 247t, 248
CONSORT (Consolidated Standards of Reporting Trials) Group, 9, 14t
Constrictive pericarditis, 671-672
CONTAK CD trial, 274
Continuous positive airway pressure (CPAP), for obstructive sleep apnea, 503
Contraception, with pulmonary arterial hypertension, 604
Contract research organizations (CROs), 37
Contractile reserve, in aortic stenosis, 677-678
Control(s), historic, 7
Control event rate (CER), 15, 16f
Control group, 5-6, 5b
Cooperative Cardiovascular Project, 71
COPE trial, 667-668
COPERNICUS trial, 251-253, 251t, 262
COPPS study, 673
CORAL trial, 577
Coreg. *See* Carvedilol (Coreg).
CoreValve Revalving System, 715, 715f, 720t
Corgard. *See* Nadolol (Corgard).
Coronary angiography
  for assessment of lesion severity, 224
  for chronic stable angina, 137, 137b
  after STEMI, 204
Coronary angioplasty, in HIV-positive patients, 732
Coronary artery bypass graft (CABG), 225-234
  carotid artery disease and, 566-568
  for chronic stable angina, 144
    arterial conduits in, 144
    complications of, 144, 145f
    vs. percutaneous coronary intervention, 142-143
    percutaneous coronary intervention after, 143
    results of, 142f
  in secondary prevention, 147-149
  global use of, 76, 76f
  in HIV-positive patients, 732
  hypertensive emergencies after, 519
  minimally invasive, 225-230
    anterolateral thoracotomy, 228
    direct, 227-228, 228f
    endoscopic atraumatic, 228
    multivessel, 228-229, 229f
    off-pump, 225-227, 226f
    robotically assisted, 229-230, 230f
    small-access, 227-230, 227t
    thoracoscopic direct, 228
    totally endoscopic, 229, 230f
  non–left descending arterial conduits in, 230-232, 231t
    gastroepiploic artery for, 231t, 232
    inferior epigastric artery for, 230, 231t
    left internal mammary artery for, 228, 231t
    radial artery for, 231t, 232
    right internal mammary artery for, 230-232, 231t
  after STEMI, 202
  with valvular heart disease
    aortic stenosis as, 710
    incidental, 710
    mitral regurgitation as, 710-711, 711f
Coronary artery disease (CAD)
  hypertension with, 476
  LDL cholesterol concentrations of more than 200 mg/dL and, 455
  multivessel, with STEMI, 204
  in valve surgery patients, 710
Coronary calcium score, for chronic stable angina, 135
Coronary care unit (CCU), for STEMI, 190-192

Coronary Drug Project, 436-437
Coronary heart disease (CHD)
  dietary fat and, 443-444
  epidemiology of, 131
  fish oil to prevent, 445-446
  with HIV infection
    clinical features of, 732-733, 732t
    pathogenesis of, 732-733
    risk factors for, 730-731, 731f
      treatment of, 733-734, 733f
    screening for, 731
Coronary revascularization, 214-239
  for bifurcation lesions, 223, 223f
  catheterization techniques for, 223-225
    intravascular assessment of lesion severity
      in, 224-225
    mechanical support for high-risk
      percutaneous coronary intervention
      in, 224
    transradial access in, 223-224
  for chronic stable angina, 141-144, 147-149
  for chronic total occlusions, 222-223
  drug-coated balloons for, 221-222
  future directions for, 233-234
  global use of, 75
  hybrid, 232-233
    current state of, 233
    defined, 232
    one-stop, 233
    rationale and background of, 232
    technical and timing issues with, 233
    two-staged, 233
  overview of, 214
  saphenous vein grafts for, 222
  stents for, 214-222
    bare-metal, 214-215
    drug-eluting, 215-222
      with changes to drug coatings, 220-221,
        220f
      with changes to polymer structure, 221
      with changes to stent platform, 219-220
      development of, 215
      efficacy of, 218
      indications for, 218-219
      new, 219-222
      paclitaxel, 215-217, 216t
      safety of, 218, 219t
      sirolimus, 215, 216t
      zotarolimus and everolimus, 217-218,
        217t
    pre-stent era and, 214
  surgical, 225-234
    minimally invasive, 225-230
      direct, 227-228, 228f
      multivessel, 228-229, 229f
      off-pump, 225-227, 226f
      robotically assisted, 229-230, 230f
      small-access, 227-230, 227t
      thoracoscopic direct, 228
    non–left descending arterial conduits in,
      230-232, 231t
      gastroepiploic artery for, 231t, 232
      inferior epigastric artery for, 230, 231t
      left internal mammary artery for, 228,
        231t
      radial artery for, 231t, 232
      right internal mammary artery for,
        230-232, 231t
Coronary sinus approach, to mitral
  annuloplasty, 722t, 723, 723f
Coronary sinus defect, 637
Coronary stent(s), 214-222
  antiplatelet therapy after placement of, 218,
    219t
  bare-metal, 214-215
  biodegradable, 220
  with biodegradable polymers, 221
  for chronic stable angina, 142f, 143-144

Coronary stent(s) (Continued)
  drug-eluting, 215-222
    with changes to drug coatings, 220-221,
      220f
    with changes to polymer structure,
      221
    with changes to stent platform,
      219-220
    for chronic stable angina, 143-144
    development of, 215
    efficacy of, 218
    indications for, 218-219
    new, 219-222
    paclitaxel, 215-217, 216t
    safety of, 218, 219t
    sirolimus, 215, 216t
    for STEMI, 189t, 190
    zotarolimus and everolimus, 217-218,
      217t
  with durable polymers, 221
  in HIV-positive patients, 732
  open-cell vs. closed-cell, 214
  polymer-free, 221
  pre-stent era and, 214
  for STEMI, 189t, 190
Corticosteroids
  for cardiac sarcoidosis, 338
  for gout in adults with cyanotic congenital
    heart disease, 634
  for pericarditis
    recurrent, 668
    tuberculous, 672
  for postpericardial injury syndrome, 673
Cortisol resistance, hypertension due to
  primary, 498
Corzide (nadolol/bendroflumethiazide), for
  hypertension, 485t
Cosgrove-Edwards prosthesis, 695t
Cost(s)
  incremental (added), 24
  present vs. future, 27-28
Cost-benefit analysis, 23, 23t
Cost-effectiveness analysis, 23-30
  methods for performing, 24-26
    hybrid approaches as, 26, 26f
    modeling approaches as, 25-26, 25f
    trial-based, 3-4
  objective of, 23-24, 23t
  other methodologic considerations in,
    26-29
    defining when therapy is cost effective as,
      29-30, 30t
    discounting as, 27-28
    perspective as, 27
    sensitivity analysis as, 26-27
      one-way, 26, 26f-27f
      probabilistic, 27, 29f
      two-way, 26-27, 28f
    time horizon as, 28-29, 29f
  and other types of economic evaluation,
    23-24, 23t-24t
  reading and interpretation of, 30, 30b
  relevant costs in, 24
Cost-effectiveness threshold, 29-30
Cost-minimization analysis, 23, 23t
Cost-to-charge ratios, 24
Cost-utility analysis, 23-24, 23t-24t
Coumarin, in pregnancy, 625
COURAGE trial, 142
Covera. See Verapamil (Covera, Verelan).
COX (cyclooxygenase), aspirin inhibition of,
  107-108, 108f
Cox Maze procedure, for atrial fibrillation,
  389-390, 389f
Cozaar. See Losartan potassium (Cozaar).
CPACS trial, 77
CPAP (continuous positive airway pressure),
  for obstructive sleep apnea, 503

CPB (cardiopulmonary bypass), minimally
  invasive surgical coronary
  revascularization without, 225-227, 226f
C3PO, 642
CPR. See Cardiopulmonary resuscitation (CPR).
CPTPs (cyclopentyltriazolopyrimidines), 111
  for NSTE-ACS, 157
CRAC (Cardiovascular and Renal Drugs
  Advisory Committee), 35
Creatine kinase (CK) levels, statins and, 427
Creatinine, serum
  in acute decompensated heart failure, 287
  and heart failure risk stratification, 285,
    285t-286t
CREDO trial, 111, 112t, 113, 156
CREST syndrome, and pulmonary arterial
  hypertension, 596
CREST trial, 564-565
Cribler Edwards valve, 720t
CRISP trial, 546-547
CRISP-AMI trial, 224
Crista terminalis, 369
Critical care support, after cardiac arrest, 417
Critical limb ischemia (CLI)
  indications for revascularization for, 545
  overview of, 539
  smoking cessation for, 542
  therapeutic angiogenesis for, 549
CRO(s) (contract research organizations), 37
Crossover design, 7
  factorial, 7-8
  in withdrawal studies, 7
CRT. See Cardiac resynchronization therapy
  (CRT).
CRUSADE initiative, 71, 167
Crush stenting, for bifurcation lesion, 223,
  223f
CSCs. See Cardiac stem cells (CSCs).
CSPS-2 trial, 558
CT (computed tomography)
  for chronic stable angina, 135-136
  for pulmonary embolism, 584, 584f-585f
CT (computed tomography) coronary
  angiography, for chronic stable angina,
  135-136, 136f
CTAF trial, 352
CTOs (chronic total occlusions), 222-223
CTSA (Clinical and Translational Science
  Awards), 39
CTT collaboration, 424, 426f
Culotte stenting, for bifurcation lesion, 223, 223f
Culprit lesion percutaneous coronary
  intervention, 143
Culture-negative endocarditis, 656, 657t
Cumulative meta-analysis, 16-17, 18f-19f
CURE trial
  dosages in, 109
  indications in, 111, 112t
  for NSTE-ACS, 156
  pharmacogenetics in, 54-56
  side effects in, 113
CURRENT-OASIS-7 trial, 109, 111, 112t, 155-156
Cushing syndrome, 498-499, 503t
  ACTH-dependent, 498
  ACTH-independent, 498
  diagnosis of, 498-499
  presentation of, 498
  principles of treatment of, 499
Cutler, Elliot, 691
CV. See Cardiovascular (CV).
CVAs (cerebrovascular accidents). See Stroke.
CVD. See Cardiovascular disease (CVD).
Cyanotic congenital heart disease, in adults,
  633-635
  cardiopulmonary exercise with, 634
  major organ complications of, 634
  neurologic effects of, 634-635
  recommendations for management of, 635

Cyclooxygenase (COX), aspirin inhibition of, 107-108, 108f
Cyclopentyltriazolopyrimidines (CPTPs), 111
  for NSTE-ACS, 157
Cyclosporine
  with cardiac transplantation, 311t
  and statins, 60-61
CYP2C9 gene
  in pharmacogenetics of warfarin, 58t, 59
    testing for, 59
    therapeutic implications of, 59-60
    and therapeutic modifications, 59-60
    and warfarin dose-response, 589
CYP2C19 gene, in pharmacogenetics of clopidogrel, 54-56, 55t
  testing for, 56
  therapeutic implications of, 56-57
CYP4F2 gene, in pharmacogenetics of warfarin, 58t, 59
  therapeutic implications of, 59-60
Cypher, 215
Cytokinesis, 322
Cytomegalovirus (CMV), after cardiac transplantation, 312

D

da Vinci S robot, 229
Dabigatran (Pradaxa), 122, 160t
  in pregnancy and lactation, 622t-623t
  for thromboembolic prophylaxis with atrial fibrillation, 378
  for venous thromboembolism, 589
DAD study group, 731
Dalcetrapib, for low HDL cholesterol, 436, 439
DALI System, 456-457, 457f, 457t
dal-OUTCOMES trial, 439
dal-PLAQUE trial, 436
Dalteparin
  for NSTE-ACS, 159-161
  in pregnancy, 625-626
dal-VESSEL trial, 436
DALYs (disability-adjusted life years), 23
  global cardiovascular disease and, 75
Damus-Kaye-Stansel operation, 633t
DANAMI 2 trial, 740
Danaparoid, in pregnancy and lactation, 622t-623t
Danon disease, cardiomyopathy associated with, 339
Darbepoetin Alfa, for heart failure, 264
DART trial, 445
Darunavir, for HIV infection, 729t
DASH diet
  for hyperlipidemia, 442-443, 443f
  for hypertension, 471
    in children, 534
  for obesity, 448, 449t
DAD study group, 731
Data management, for clinical trial, 38
Data pooling. See Meta-analysis.
Data Safety Monitoring Boards (DSMBs), 6
  for cardiovascular device trials, 46
Data safety monitoring committee (DSMC), 6
David, Tirone, 609
David-I technique, for thoracic aortic aneurysms, 609
David-V technique, for thoracic aortic aneurysms, 609
DAVIT II trial, 141
D2B (Door-to-Balloon) program, 179
D2B (door-to-balloon) times, for STEMI, 68-69, 185
D-binding site, of calcium channel blockers, 90

DCM (dilated cardiomyopathy)
  bone marrow cells for, 325
  catheter ablation for ventricular tachycardia in, 391-392
  with HIV infection, 734
ddC (zalcitabine), for HIV infection, 730t
ddI (didanosine), for HIV infection, 730t
D-dimer
  in deep vein thrombosis, 582-583
  in pulmonary embolism, 583
Decision tree, 25
Decompensated erythrocytosis, in adults with cyanotic congenital heart disease, 634
Deep vein thrombosis (DVT), 580-595
  diagnosis of, 582-583
    algorithm for, 583, 583f
    clinical likelihood assessment in, 582
    clinical presentation in, 582-583
    imaging in, 583, 583f
    laboratory testing in, 582-583
  epidemiology and risk factors for, 580-581, 581t-582t
  management of, 586-591
    advanced therapy in, 589-591
    anticoagulation in, 587-589, 587b
      direct factor XA and factor IIA inhibitors for, 589
      duration of, 590, 590f
      with fondaparinux, 588
      and heparin-induced thrombocytopenia, 587, 588f
      with low-molecular-weight heparin, 588
      with unfractionated heparin, 587
      with warfarin, 588-589, 588b
    inferior vena cava filters for, 591
    spectrum of disease and, 586-587
  pathophysiology and natural history of, 582
  in pregnancy, 624-626
  prevention of, 591-593
    duration of prophylaxis and extension after discharge in, 593, 593t
    with hip replacement, knee replacement, and hip fracture, 592, 592b
    in-hospital prophylaxis for, 592
    mechanical prophylaxis for, 592-593
    in patients with cancer, 591-592
    unconventional prophylaxis for, 592-593
      with statins, 593
      with vitamin E, 592-593
  after STEMI, 201
Deferasirox, for cardiac hemochromatosis, 338-339
Deferiprone, for cardiac hemochromatosis, 338-339
Deferoxamine, for cardiac hemochromatosis, 338-339
Defibrillation, 751-752
  for cardiac arrest, 415, 415f
  equipment for, 751, 751f
  set-up and patient preparation for, 751, 752f
  technical considerations with, 751-752
Defibrillation threshold (DFT), 759, 759t
Defibrillator
  external, 751, 751f
  automatic
    for cardiac arrest, 408
    for STEMI, 179
  implantable. See Implantable cardioverter-defibrillators (ICDs).
DEFINE trial, 436, 439
DEFINITE trial, 270-271
Delavirdine, for HIV infection, 730t
Delone. See Furosemide.
Demadex (torsemide)
  for heart failure, 243t
  for hypertension, 480t
  in pregnancy and lactation, 622t-623t

Deming, W.E., 70
Dental procedures, endocarditis prophylaxis for, 662-663, 663t
Deoxycorticosterone-producing tumor, hypertension due to, 498
DEP (distal embolic protection) devices
  for carotid artery stenosis, 563
  for renal artery stenosis, 575-576
Department of Health and Human Services (HHS), in device development, 51
Depression
  after NSTE-ACS, 166t
  after STEMI, 207
DES. See Drug-eluting stent (DES).
DESSERT trial, 216t
Destination protocols, for STEMI, 179, 180f
Destination Therapy Risk Score (DTRS), 316-317
Developing countries, ethics of drug development in, 37
Device(s). See Cardiovascular (CV) devices; Medical device(s).
Device endocarditis, 661-662
Dexamethasone, for glucocorticoid-remediable aldosteronism, 497
Dextran sulfate cellulose columns, LDL apheresis using, 456, 456f
DFT (defibrillation threshold), 759, 759t
DHA (docosahexaenoic acid)
  for mixed dyslipidemia, 437-438
  to prevent coronary heart disease, 445-446
DHPs. See Dihydropyridine(s) (DHPs).
Diabetes
  after cardiac transplantation, 313
  and chronic stable angina, 140
  heart failure with, 262
  hypertension with, 475-476
  and peripheral artery disease, 543
    antihypertensive therapy for, 542
  statins and, 428
Diabetes management
  cardiac rehabilitation and, 741b
  after NSTE-ACS, 166t, 168, 170-171, 171b
  after STEMI, 205t, 206
DIABETES trial, 216t
Diagnostic cutoffs, 2-3, 2f
Diagnostic tests
  interpretation of, 1-3, 2f
  tools for assessment of, 1-32
    clinical trials as, 3-11
    comparative effectiveness research as, 19-23
    cost-effectiveness analysis as, 23-30
    meta-analysis as, 15-19
DIAMOND study, 259, 356
Diastolic blood pressure levels
  for boys, 530t-531t
  for girls, 531t-532t
Diazoxide, for hypertensive emergencies, 514t-515t
Didanosine (ddI), for HIV infection, 730t
Diet
  for chronic stable angina, 138-140
  for heart failure, 243, 243t
  for hypertension, 468-469, 469t
    in children, 534
    tips for success in adopting healthier, 471, 471t
  after NSTE-ACS, 166t
  after STEMI, 205t, 206
Dietary Approaches to Stop Hypertension (DASH) diet
  for hyperlipidemia, 442-443, 443f
  for hypertension, 471
    in children, 534
  for obesity, 448, 449t
Dietary Guidelines, 448
Digitalis, in pregnancy and lactation, 622t-623t

Digoxin
for atrial fibrillation, 373t
drug interactions with, 94
for heart failure, 254, 256-257
acute decompensated, 296
endpoints with, 242t
pharmacologic and clinical effects of, 256
practical considerations with, 256-257
for hypertension, pulmonary arterial, 599
for mitral stenosis, in pregnancy, 624
for peripartum cardiomyopathy, 627
Dihydropyridine(s) (DHPs), 93
with β-adrenergic blockers, 99
classification of, 91
contraindications and cautions with, 93
drug interactions with, 94
first-generation, 93
for hypertension, 477t, 479-480, 479t
monitoring and adverse effects of, 485t
for NSTE-ACS, 154-155
second-generation, 93-94
side effects of, 93
Dihydropyridine (DHP)-binding site, 90
Dilacor. See Diltiazem.
Dilated cardiomyopathy (DCM)
bone marrow cells for, 325
catheter ablation for ventricular tachycardia in, 391-392
with HIV infection, 734
Diltia. See Diltiazem.
Diltiazem (Cardizem, Cartia, Dilacor, Diltia, Tiazac, Taztia), 93
for atrial fibrillation, 373t
with β-adrenergic blockers, 99
contraindications to, 93
dose of, 93
drug interactions with, 94
for hypertension, 479t
for maintenance of sinus rhythm, 377
for paroxysmal supraventricular tachycardia, 368, 369t
pharmacodynamic effects of, 91t
pharmacokinetics of, 93
in pregnancy, 93, 622t-623t
for mitral stenosis, 624
side effects of, 93
after STEMI, 193
Dimensionless velocity index (DVI), 677
DINAMIT trial, 272, 397-398, 399t
DIONYSOS trial, 358
Diovan. See Valsartan (Diovan).
Diovan HCT (valsartan/hydrochlorothiazide), for hypertension, 485t
Dipping pattern, in ambulatory blood pressure monitoring, 501-502
Dipyridamole, for carotid artery disease, 557-558, 558t
Direct Flow Valve, 720-721, 720f, 720t
Direct renin inhibitor
for heart failure, 263-264
for hypertension, 483-484, 483t
in combination products, 485t
Direct thrombin inhibitors (DTIs), 118, 119f
argatroban as, 120
bivalirudin (hirulog) as, 120
hirudin (lepirudin) as, 118-120
for NSTE-ACS, 161-162, 162f
in pregnancy, 625
for STEMI, 183
for thromboprophylaxis with atrial fibrillation, 378
Direct-access approaches, for valve surgery, 694
Disability
from myocardial infarction, 739-740
after STEMI, 207

Disability-adjusted life years (DALYs), 23
global cardiovascular disease and, 75
Discounting, 27-28
Discrimination, 3
Disopyramide, 349-350
adverse reactions to, 349-350, 375t
clinical applications of, 349
clinical pharmacology of, 349
dosage and administration of, 349
modification in disease states of, 349
drug interactions with, 350
for LVOT obstruction, 332
mechanisms of action of, 349
Dissecting aneurysms, β-adrenergic blockers for, 100
Dissemination, 67
Distal embolic filter devices, 222
Distal embolic protection (DEP) devices
for carotid artery stenosis, 563
for renal artery stenosis, 575-576
Distal occlusion devices, 222
Diuretic(s)
for carotid artery stenosis, 555
for heart failure, 243-245
acute decompensated
oral, 297
parenteral, 290-291, 291f
adverse effects of, 244
dosage of, 243t
endpoints with, 242t
mechanism of action of, 243-244, 283, 283f
pathophysiologic mechanisms and, 242-243
practical considerations with, 244-245
for hypertension, 477t, 480-481, 480t
in children, 536t
in combination products, 485t
monitoring and adverse effects of, 485t
resistant, 505, 505f-506f
for peripheral edema in pregnancy, 623
for primary aldosteronism, 497
Diuretic resistance, 244-245
Diuretic synergism, 245
Dobutamine
for acute pulmonary edema, 300
for heart failure, 257
acute decompensated, 293-294, 294f, 295t
Docosahexaenoic acid (DHA)
for mixed dyslipidemia, 437-438
to prevent coronary heart disease, 445-446
Dofetilide, 356-357
adverse reactions to, 357, 375t
for atrial fibrillation, 374t
clinical applications of, 356
clinical pharmacology of, 356
dosage and administration of, 356, 375t
modification in disease states of, 356-357
drug interactions with, 357
mechanism of action of, 356
in pregnancy and lactation, 622t-623t
Dominant strategy, 29
Door-to-Balloon Alliance, 71
Door-to-Balloon (D2B) program, 179
Door-to-balloon (D2B) times, for STEMI, 68-69, 185
Dopamine
for acute decompensated heart failure, 295-296, 295f
for acute pulmonary edema, 300, 300f
for cardiac amyloidosis, 337
Dopamine antagonist, for hypertensive emergencies, 514t-515t
DOSE-AHF study, 291, 291f
Double-blind trials, 6
Double-umbrella devices, 638

Doxazosin (Cardura), for hypertension, 482, 483t
due to pheochromocytoma, 491-493, 492t
resistant, 507
Doxycycline, for infective endocarditis, 657t
DRASTIC trial, 576, 576t
DREAM trial, 607
Dressler syndrome, 673
Dronedarone, 358-359
adverse reactions to, 359, 375t
clinical applications of, 358
clinical pharmacology of, 358
dosage of, 375t
individualization of, 358
modification in disease states of, 359
drug interactions with, 359
for heart failure, 259
initiation and monitoring of, 376-377
mechanism of action of, 358
postmarketing surveillance of, 36b
in pregnancy and lactation, 622t-623t
Drug(s), defined, 42
Drug affordability, in low- and middle-income countries, 77-78, 78f
Drug availability, in low- and middle-income countries, 77-78
Drug development, 33-40
anatomy of clinical trials in, 37-38
clinical events adjudication in, 38
data management in, 38
protocol development in, 37-38
safety surveillance in, 38
site management in, 38
statistics in, 38
economics of, 38-39
cost in, 37
funding in, 33
National Institutes of Health Roadmap program in, 39
patent considerations in, 39
Prescription Drug User Fee Act in, 38-39
medical device vs., 42, 43t
overview of, 33-36
cycle of clinical therapeutic development in, 33, 34f
international, 36-37
in developing countries, 37
Investigational New Drug Application in, 34
advisory panels for, 35
data necessary to support, 34-35
emergency use, 35
exemptions from, 36
investigator-initiated, 35-36
treatment, 35
types of, 35
labeling in, 35
phase I to IV paradigm in, 33, 34f
postmarketing surveillance in, 35-36
regulation of new drugs in, 34-35
CDER vs. CBER in, 34, 36
pipeline of, 34f
Drug Price Competition and Patent Term Restoration Act, 39
Drug-coated balloons, 221-222
Drug-eluting stent (DES), 215-222
with changes to drug coatings, 220-221, 220f
with changes to polymer structure, 221
with changes to stent platform, 219-220
for chronic stable angina, 143-144
development of, 215
efficacy of, 218
for femoral-popliteal disease, 548-549
indications for, 218-219
new, 219-222
paclitaxel, 215-217, 216t

Drug-eluting stent (DES) (Continued)
  safety of, 218, 219t
  sirolimus, 215, 216t
  for STEMI, 189t, 190
  zotarolimus and everolimus, 217-218, 217t
Drug-induced pericardial disease, 674, 675t
DSMBs (Data Safety Monitoring Boards), 6
  for cardiovascular device trials, 46
DSMC (data safety monitoring committee), 6
d4T (stavudine), for HIV infection, 730t
DTIs. See Direct thrombin inhibitors (DTIs).
DTRS (Destination Therapy Risk Score), 316-317
Dual-chamber pacing, 752, 755f
Ductus arteriosus, 645
  patent, 645-646, 646f
  recommendations for, 646
Duke criteria, for infective endocarditis, 652, 653f
Durable polymers, stents with, 221
Duran prosthesis, 695t
DVI (dimensionless velocity index), 677
DVT. See Deep vein thrombosis (DVT).
Dynacirc (isradipine), for hypertension, 479t
  in children, 536t
Dyrenium (triamterene)
  for acute decompensated heart failure, 291
  for heart failure, 243t
  for hypertension, 480t
Dyslipidemia
  after cardiac transplantation, 313
  with HIV infection, 733, 733f
  mixed, 434-441
    cholesteryl ester transfer protein inhibition as, 438-439, 438f
    combination therapy for
      non–HDL-c reduction in, 435, 435t
      rationale for, 434-435, 435f
      statin-fibrate, 436
      statin-niacin, 436-437
      statin–omega 3 fatty acids, 437-438
      therapy to modify HDL in, 435-436

E
E5555, 115
Early recurrence of atrial fibrillation (ERAF), 375
ECG. See Electrocardiogram (ECG).
Echocardiography
  of chronic stable angina, 133-134, 137t
  of infective endocarditis, 652-654, 653f
    decision tree for use of, 652-654, 654f
    sensitivity and specificity of, 652, 653t
    transthoracic vs. transesophageal, 652, 653b, 653t
  of pulmonary embolism, 584, 585f
  after STEMI, 202-203
  prior to valve surgery, 692
Eclampsia, 518, 523, 525
ECLIPSE study, 438
ECM (extracellular matrix) production, in pulmonary arterial hypertension, 604
Economic evaluation
  how to use, 30, 30b
  types of, 23-24, 23t-24t
Economics, of drug development, 38-39
  cost in, 37
  funding in, 33
    National Institutes of Health Roadmap program in, 39
    patent considerations in, 39
    Prescription Drug User Fee Act in, 38-39
ECSS study, 144
ECST trial, 560, 561t

ED management. See Emergency department (ED) management.
Edarbi (azilsartan medoxomil), for hypertension, 479t
Edema
  in pregnancy, 623
  pulmonary. See Pulmonary edema.
Edge-to-edge technique, for mitral valve repair, 706, 722-723, 722f-723f
Edoxaban (Lixiana), 160t
Edwards MC3 prosthesis, 695t
Edwards Prima Plus prosthesis, 695t, 699
Edwards Sapien percutaneous heart valve, 714-715, 715f, 720t
Edwards Sapien transcatheter heart valve, 714-715, 715f
  implantation procedure for, 717-721, 717f
  patient outcomes with, 717-719, 718f-719f, 719t
  for tetralogy of Fallot, 644
EECP (enhanced external counterpulsation), for ischemic heart disease with heart failure, 261-262
EF (ejection fraction), left ventricular. See Left ventricular ejection fraction (LVEF).
Efavirenz, for HIV infection, 730t
Efavirenz/emtricitabine/tenofovir (Atripla), for HIV infection, 729-730, 730t
EFFECT study, 71
Effective orifice area (EOA), 701
Effective regurgitant orifice area (EROA), 685-686
Effectiveness, 20
Efficacy, 20
Ehlers-Danlos syndrome
  β-adrenergic blockers for, 100
  thoracic aortic aneurysms in, 608
Eicosapentaenoic acid (EPA)
  for mixed dyslipidemia, 437-438
  to prevent coronary heart disease, 445-446
Eikenella spp, endocarditis due to, 655t
Einstein, Albert, 67
Einstein-DVT study, 589
Eisenmenger syndrome, pregnancy with, 629
Ejection fraction (EF), left ventricular. See Left ventricular ejection fraction (LVEF).
ELCo (energy loss coefficient), 677
Elderly patients
  aortic stenosis in, 678
  hypertension in, 486-487
    blood pressure goals for, 486
    isolated systolic, 486
    and orthostatic hypotension, 486-487
    selecting drug therapy for, 487
  infective endocarditis in, 657
  NSTE-ACS in, 171
Electrical cardioversion and defibrillation, 751-752
  for atrial fibrillation, 375
  equipment for, 751, 751f
  set-up and patient preparation for, 751, 752f
  technical considerations with, 751-752
Electrical substrate assessment, after STEMI, 204
Electrocardiogram (ECG)
  for chronic stable angina, 131-133, 133b, 134f-135f, 137t
  for pulmonary embolism, 583
  signal-averaged, for risk of sudden cardiac death, 398, 400t
  for STEMI, 181
Electrocardiographic (ECG) monitoring, during cardiac rehabilitation, 741, 742b
Electrophysiologic studies, for risk of sudden cardiac death, 398, 400t
Element stent, 219-220

Elephant trunk technique, for thoracic aortic aneurysms, 612, 612f
Elinogrel, 110t
  for NSTE-ACS, 159
Eliquis (apixaban), 122, 160t
  for NSTE-ACS, 163
  for thromboprophylaxis, 592-593
ELITE I study, 246
ELITE II study, 246, 247t
EMA (European Medicines Agency), 37
Embolic events
  infective endocarditis with, 659t-660t, 660-661
  with valve surgery, 696b
Embolic protection devices, 222
  for carotid artery stenosis, 563
  for renal artery stenosis, 575-576
Embolism, pulmonary. See Pulmonary embolism (PE).
Emboshield distal embolic protection device, 563
Emergency department (ED) management, of STEMI, 179-181
  early risk assessment in, 181-190
  medications used in, 181-184
    analgesia as, 181-182
    anticoagulant agents as, 182-183, 183f-184f
    antiplatelet agents as, 182, 182f
    β-blockers as, 183-184
    nitroglycerin as, 181
    oxygen as, 181
  patient evaluation in, 180-181
  patient triage in, 179-180
  reperfusion therapy in, 184-190
    fibrinolytic, 185-186, 187b, 188f, 188t
    general concepts of, 184-185
    in hospitals without on-site cardiac surgery, 190, 191b
    percutaneous coronary intervention as, 186-190, 189f, 189t-190t
    pharmacoinvasive management as, 190
    predicted transfer and door-to-balloon time for, 185, 187f
    risk of bleeding and, 185
    risk stratification and, 185, 186f
    stents in, 190
    thrombus aspiration in, 190
    time from symptom onset to, 185
Emergency medical services (EMS)
  for cardiac arrest, 70
  for STEMI, 68-69, 179
Emergency use IND, 35
EMF (endomyocardial fibrosis), 339
  hypereosinophilic, 339-340
EMIAT trial, 353-354
EMIP-FR trial, 106
EMPHASIS-HF trial, 253-254, 253t
Emtricitabine, for HIV infection, 730t
Emtricitabine/tenofovir (Truvada), for HIV infection, 729-730, 730t
Enalapril (Renitec, Vasotec)
  for heart failure, 246, 246t
  for hypertension, 478t
    in children, 536t
  for peripheral artery disease, 542
  in pregnancy and lactation, 622t-623t
Enalapril maleate/felodipine (Lexxel), for hypertension, 485t
Enalaprilat, for hypertensive emergencies, 514t-515t
Enalapril/hydrochlorothiazide (Vaseretic), for hypertension, 485t
Encephalopathy, hypertensive, 516, 517f
Encephalopathy, hypertensive, 516, 517f
Endeavor stent, 221
ENDEAVOR-I study, 217t
ENDEAVOR-II study, 217, 217t
ENDEAVOR-III study, 217t
ENDEAVOR-IV study, 217t

Endo-ACAB (endoscopic atraumatic coronary artery bypass), 228
Endocarditis
  infective. *See* Infective endocarditis (IE).
  operated valvular, 696b
Endocrine causes, of hypertension, 490-500, 491b
  other forms of mineralocorticoid excess as, 497-499
    apparent mineralocorticoid excess syndromes as, 498-499
    hyperdeoxycorticosteronism as, 497-498
  pheochromocytoma as, 490-494, 503t
    acute hypertensive crises in, 493, 493t
    anesthesia and surgery for, 493-494
    diagnosis of, 490, 492f
    long-term postoperative follow-up for, 494
    malignant, 494
    in pregnancy, 494
    preoperative management of, 490-493, 492t
    presentation of, 490, 491b
    principles of treatment of, 490-494
    syndromic, 490, 491t
  primary aldosteronism as, 494-497, 503t, 504-508
    diagnosis of, 495-496, 495f-496f
    pharmacologic treatment of, 497
    principles of treatment of, 496-497
    subtypes of, 494-495, 495b, 496f
    surgical treatment of, 496-497
  due to thyroid and parathyroid disease, 499-500
    acromegaly as, 499-500
    primary hyperparathyroidism as, 499, 503t
    thyroid dysfunction as, 499
Endogenous cardiac progenitors, 326-327, 327f-330f
Endomyocardial disorders, 339-340
Endomyocardial fibrosis (EMF), 339
  hypereosinophilic, 339-340
ENDORSE study, 591
Endoscopic atraumatic coronary artery bypass (endo-ACAB), 228
Endothelial progenitor cells (EPCs), 322-323
Endothelin receptor antagonism, for pulmonary arterial hypertension, 601, 601f
  HIV-related, 735
Endothelin type A (ETA) receptor antagonists, for pulmonary arterial hypertension, 601
Endothelin type B (ETB) receptor antagonists, for pulmonary arterial hypertension, 601, 601f
ENDOVAL study, 658-659
EndoValve-Hermann prosthesis, 722t, 726, 726f
Endovascular renal artery stent revascularization (ERASR), 574-577
  surveillance following, 577
Endpoints
  adjudication of, 38
  for cardiovascular device trials, 45-46
    composite, 45
    surrogate, 45
  composite, 6-7, 9
    for cardiovascular device trials, 45
  selection of, 9, 10f
  surrogate, 9, 10f
    for cardiovascular device trials, 45
End-stage renal disease (ESRD), in atherosclerotic renal artery stenosis, 571
Energy costs, of occupational and recreational activities, 741-742, 742t
Energy loss coefficient (ELCo), 677
Enfuvirtide, for HIV infection, 729
Engager transapical valve, 721, 721f
Enhanced external counterpulsation (EECP), for ischemic heart disease with heart failure, 261-262

Enoxaparin
  dosages of, 118
  mechanisms of action of, 117-118
  for NSTE-ACS, 159-161, 161f, 163t
  in pregnancy and lactation, 622t-623t, 625-626
  safety and efficacy of, 118
  side effects and contraindications to, 118
  for STEMI
    in acute phase, 183, 184f
    with PCI, 190t
  for thromboprophylaxis, 591, 593
Entecavir, for HIV infection, 730t
Enterococcal endocarditis, 654, 656t
Enterococcus faecalis, endocarditis due to, 656t
Enterococcus faecium, endocarditis due to, 656t
EOA (effective orifice area), 701
EPA (eicosapentaenoic acid)
  for mixed dyslipidemia, 437-438
  to prevent coronary heart disease, 445-446
EPCs (endothelial progenitor cells), 322-323
Ephedra sinica, hypertensive emergency due to, 511
EPHESUS study, 193, 253, 253t
Epinephrine, for acute decompensated heart failure, 296
Eplerenone (Inspra)
  for heart failure
    clinical efficacy of, 253
    pathophysiology and, 253
    practical considerations with, 254
    randomized controlled trials of, 253t
  for hypertension, 482, 482t
    in children, 536t
  in pregnancy and lactation, 622t-623t
  for primary aldosteronism, 497
  for STEMI
    during convalescence, 193
    with pulmonary congestion, 194
Epoprostenol, for pulmonary arterial hypertension, 599, 600f
  in pregnancy and lactation, 622t-623t, 629
Eprosartan mesylate (Teveten), for hypertension, 479t
Eprosartan mesylate/hydrochlorothiazide (Teveten HCT), for hypertension, 485t
Eptifibatide
  dosage of, 114
  indications for, 114
  mechanism of action of, 114
  for NSTE-ACS, 158
  with PCI for STEMI, 189t
Epzicom (abacavir/lamivudine), for HIV infection, 729-730, 730t
Equivalence margin, 8
Equivalence trials, 8-9, 8f
ERAF (early recurrence of atrial fibrillation), 375
ERASR (endovascular renal artery stent revascularization), 574-577
  surveillance following, 577
ERICA study, 106
EROA (effective regurgitant orifice area), 685-686
Erythrityl tetranitrate, side effects of, 87t
Erythrocytosis, compensated vs. decompensated, in adults with cyanotic congenital heart disease, 634
Erythropoiesis-stimulating agents (ESAs), for heart failure, 264
  acute decompensated, 298
Escape phenomenon, with ACE inhibitors, 245-246
ESCAPE study, 287, 289, 289t
Esidrix. *See* Hydrochlorothiazide.

Esmolol
  for aortic dissection, 614
  for atrial fibrillation, 373t
  for cardiac arrhythmias due to pheochromocytoma, 493t
  for hypertensive emergencies, 514t-515t
  indications for, 101
  pharmacodynamic properties and cardiac effects of, 98t
ESPRIT trial, 557-558, 558t
ESPS-2 study, 557-558, 558t
ESRD (end-stage renal disease), in atherosclerotic renal artery stenosis, 571
Essential Drug List, 78
ETA (endothelin type A) receptor antagonists, for pulmonary arterial hypertension, 601
ETB (endothelin type B) receptor antagonists, for pulmonary arterial hypertension, 601, 601f
Ethacrynic acid, for heart failure, 243t
Ethambutol, for tuberculous pericarditis, 672
Ethics, of drug development in developing countries, 37
Etravirine, for HIV infection, 730t
EURIDIS trial, 358-359
EUROASPIRE II study, 76-77
EUROPA study, 147, 248
Europe, regulation of new drugs in, 37
European Medicines Agency (EMA), 37
European Society of Cardiology prognostic model, for pulmonary embolism, 586, 587t
European Stroke Initiative, 565
EuroSCORE, for transcatheter aortic valve implant, 716
EVA-3S trial, 563-564
EVAR trial, 607
EVAR-2 trial, 607
EVEREST II study, 722-723, 723f
EVEREST study, 302
Everolimus
  with cardiac transplantation, 311t
  molecular structure and mechanism of action of, 220f
Everolimus-eluting stents, 217-218, 217t
  with biodegradable polymers, 221
Evidence-based treatment, of hypertension, 474
EVOLVE trial, 221
EXACT trial, 563
EXACT-HF study, 261, 264
Excel stent, 221
EXCLAIM trial, 593
Exercise
  in adults with congenital heart disease, 636-637
    cyanotic, 634
  for chronic stable angina, 140
  for hypertension, 468-469, 469t
    in children, 534
    tips for success in increasing, 471
  after NSTE-ACS, 166t, 168
  for obesity, 448, 450, 452t
  after STEMI, 205t, 207
Exercise prescription, for outpatient cardiac rehabilitation, 742-743
  principles of, 742-743, 743f
Exercise testing
  for chronic stable angina, 132, 133b, 134f-135f, 137t
  after myocardial infarction, 740
  after STEMI, 202
Exercise training, in rehabilitation, 738-739
  contraindications to, 743-744, 744b
  physiologic benefits of, 738, 739b
  newer concepts regarding, 739
  resistance exercise in, 743
Exforge (valsartan/amlodipine), for hypertension, 485t

Exforge HCT (amlodipine/valsartan/ hydrochlorothiazide), for hypertension, 485t
External defibrillation, 751-752
    for cardiac arrest, 415, 415f
    equipment for, 751, 751f
    set-up and patient preparation for, 751, 752f
    technical considerations with, 751-752
Extracellular matrix (ECM) production, in pulmonary arterial hypertension, 604
ExTRACT TIMI 25 trial, 123
ExTraMATCH study, 745
Ezetimibe, 430
    effect on lipids and lipoproteins of, 430
    efficacy of, 430
    for peripheral artery disease, 541-542
    in pregnancy, 627
    safety of, 430

F

Fabry's disease, 339
Factor IIa inhibitors
    oral, 122
    for venous thromboembolism, 589
Factor Xa inhibitors, 121
    indications and dosing for, 121
    mechanisms of action of, 121
    for NSTE-ACS, 162-163, 163f
    oral, 122
    for STEMI
        in acute phase, 183
    for thromboprophylaxis, 592
    for venous thromboembolism, 589
Factorial design, 7-8
Failure mode analysis, 47
Failure to capture, 752, 754f
False-negative rate (FNR), 1-2, 2f, 9-11
False-positive rate (FPR), 1-2, 2f, 9-11
FAME trial, 225
Familial Atherosclerosis Treatment Study (FATS), 429, 429t
Familial hyperaldosteronism (FH), 494-495
Familial hypercholesterolemia (FH), 454-455
Familial paragangliomas, 490, 491t
FASTER study, 557, 558t
FAST-MI registry, 53
Fat(s), dietary
    and coronary heart disease, 443-444
    label language for, 471, 471t
"Fat free," 471t
Fatigue, in acute decompensated heart failure, 287
FATS study, 429, 429t
FCTC (Framework Convention in Tobacco Control), 80
FDA (Food and Drug Administration)
    regulation of new drugs by, 34, 36
    regulation of new medical devices by, 42-44
Feigenbaum, Armand, 70
Felodipine (Plendil), for hypertension, 479t
    in children, 536t
FemPac trial, 548-549
Femoral-popliteal disease, 545f, 547-549, 548f-549f
Fenestrations, after repair of congenital heart defects, 647
Fenofibrate
    additive effects of, 435t
    for carotid artery disease, 557
    for hypertriglyceridemia with HIV infection, 733
    for lowing of LDL cholesterol, 428
    in pregnancy, 627

Fenofibric acid
    additive effects of, 435t
    for mixed dyslipidemia, 436
Fenoldopam, for hypertensive emergencies, 514t-515t
Fetus, risk of cardiac drugs to, 621, 622t-623t
FFR (fractional flow reserve), for assessment of coronary lesion severity, 225
FH (familial hyperaldosteronism), 494-495
FH (familial hypercholesterolemia), 454-455
FH-SCOR, 429t
Fibrates
    for hypertriglyceridemia with HIV infection, 733
    for lowing of LDL cholesterol, 428
    for mixed dyslipidemia, 436
    for peripheral artery disease, 541-542
Fibrinoid necrosis, 510-511
Fibrinolysis, 122-123
    for deep vein thrombosis, 589-590
    dosages of, 123
    global use of, 75
    indications for, 123, 123t
    mechanisms of action of, 122
    in pregnancy, 626
    properties of, 123t
    for pulmonary embolism, 590
    side effects and contraindications to, 123, 124b
    for STEMI, 185-186
        comparison of agents for, 186, 188t
        complications of, 185-186, 188f
        effect on LV function of, 185
        indications and contraindications for, 185, 187b
        mortality benefit of, 185
        PCI vs., 187f
        prehospital, 179, 180f
        risk of bleeding with, 185
Fibromuscular dysplasia (FMD), renal artery stenosis due to, 573-574, 573f, 577
Fick outputs, in acute decompensated heart failure, 290
FIELD study, 436, 557
FilterWire, 222
First messenger, 96
Fish oil, to prevent coronary heart disease, 445-446
Five A Strategy, for smoking cessation, 168
501(k) premarket notification, 41-43
Fixed effects model, 16, 18f
Fixed randomization schemes, 6
Fixed sample size design, 6
Flecainide, 352
    adverse reactions to, 352, 375t
    for atrial fibrillation, 374t
    clinical applications of, 352
    clinical pharmacology of, 352
    dosage and administration of, 352, 375t
        modification in disease states of, 352
    drug interactions with, 352
    initiation and monitoring of, 376
    mechanism of action of, 352
    for paroxysmal supraventricular tachycardia, 368-369
    in pregnancy, 628-629
Floating spheres, 326, 327f
Fluency stent, for femoral-popliteal disease, 548
Fluid management, for acute decompensated heart failure, 290-292, 291f
Fluid restriction, for acute decompensated heart failure, 297
Fluvastatin
    dosage of, 422t
    with HIV infection and HAART, 733f
    pharmacodynamics and pharmacokinetics of, 60t, 422t
    in pregnancy, 627

FMD (fibromuscular dysplasia), renal artery stenosis due to, 573-574, 573f, 577
FNR (false-negative rate), 1-2, 2f, 9-11
Follow-up visit, after STEMI, 207
Fondaparinux, 121
    indications and dosing for, 121
    mechanisms of action of, 121
    for NSTE-ACS, 162, 163t
    in pregnancy and lactation, 622t-623t
    for STEMI
        in acute phase, 183
        with PCI, 190t
    for superficial venous thrombosis, 586-587
    for thromboprophylaxis, 592
    for venous thromboembolism, 588
Fontan procedure, 633t
Food and Drug Administration (FDA)
    regulation of new drugs by, 34, 36
    regulation of new medical devices by, 42-44
Foramen ovale, 639
    patent, 639-640
        and hypoxemia, 639, 640f
        and migraine, 639
        recommendations for, 640
Foreign data, used for U.S. product approval, 46
Fosamprenavir, for HIV infection, 729t
Fosinopril (Monopril)
    for heart failure, 246t
    for hypertension, 478t
        in children, 536t
FPR (false-positive rate), 1-2, 2f, 9-11
Fractional flow reserve (FFR), for assessment of coronary lesion severity, 225
Framingham Heart Study, 553-556
Framingham Heart Study Risk Score, 463-464
    in global therapy, 79
    in HIV-positive patients, 731
Framingham Offspring Study, 79
Fraxiparin, for NSTE-ACS, 160-161
FRAX.I.S trial, 160-161
Free radical hypothesis, of nitrate tolerance, 88
Freestyle stentless porcine full-root bioprosthesis, 695t, 696f, 699
French Hospital Database on HIV, 731-732
Frequency dependence, of antiarrhythmic drugs, 344
Frequentist approach, for clinical trials, 11
FRIC trial, 160-161
FRISC II trial, 164, 164f, 170-171
FRISC trial, 160
Functional status, after STEMI, 207
Fungal pericarditis, 672-673
Furosemide (Lasix, Delone, Furocot, Lo-Aqua)
    for acute decompensated heart failure, 290-291
    for heart failure, 243t, 244
    for hypertension, 480t
        in children, 536t
    in pregnancy and lactation, 622t-623t, 623
Fusion inhibitors, for HIV infection, 729
Futility index, 9-10
FUTURA-OASIS 8 trial, 162
Future prosthesis, 695t

G

Ganciclovir, after cardiac transplantation, 312
Ganglionic blocker, for hypertensive emergencies, 514t-515t
GAP (Guidelines Applied in Practice), 71
Gastroepiploic artery (GEA) graft, for coronary artery bypass, 231t, 232
GCP (Good Clinical Practices), 37

GCS (graduated compression stockings)
  for deep vein thrombosis, 587
  for peripheral edema in pregnancy, 623
  for thromboprophylaxis, 592
Gemfibrozil
  for chronic stable angina, 147
  for hypertriglyceridemia with HIV infection,
    733
  in pregnancy, 627
GEMINI trial, 476
Gene therapy, for severe hypercholesterolemia,
  460-461
Gene transfer, for severe hypercholesterolemia,
  460-461
Generic drugs, development of, 39
Genetic testing, for risk of sudden cardiac
  death, 400
Geneva score, for pulmonary embolism, 583,
  584t
Gentamicin
  for endocarditis prophylaxis during delivery,
    630
  for infective endocarditis, 655t-657t
Geoform ring, 695t, 705-706
German and Austrian Xamoterol Study Group,
  256
German Multicenter Apheresis Trial, 457-458
Gestational hypertension, 521, 523
GFR (glomerular filtration rate), in adults with
  cyanotic congenital heart disease, 634
Gibbons, John, 691
GIFT trial, 589
GISSI trial, 445
GISSI-AF trial, 377
Glenn anastomosis
  bidirectional, 633t
  classic, 633t
Global cardiovascular therapy, 75-82
  for acute coronary syndrome, 75-76, 76f
  burden of cardiovascular disease and, 75,
    76f
  current trends and challenges of, 75-80
  drug availability and affordability for, 77-78,
    78f
  human resource shortages and, 78, 79f
  polypill in, 79-80
  for primary prevention, 75, 79
  for primordial prevention, 75, 80-81
  risk factors and, 80-81
    blood pressure as, 80-81
    lipids as, 81
    obesity as, 81
    tobacco as, 80
  for secondary prevention, 75-77, 77f
  WHO essential drug list and, 78
Glomerular filtration rate (GFR), in adults
  with cyanotic congenital heart disease,
  634
Glucocorticoid-remediable aldosteronism
  (GRA), 494-495
  pharmacologic treatment of, 497
Glycemic control, after STEMI, 193
Glycemic index, of carbohydrates, 445
Glyceryl trinitrate (GTN)
  history of, 83
  mechanisms of action of, 83-84
  nonhemodynamic effects of, 88-89
  pharmacodynamic effects of, 84, 86f
  pharmacokinetics of, 84, 87t
  side effects of, 84-85, 87t
  sublingual, 85, 86t-87t
Glycoprotein (GP) IIB/IIIA receptor, 114
Glycoprotein (GP) IIB/IiIA receptor antagonists,
  114-115
  dosages of, 114-115
  indications for, 114
  mechanisms of action of, 114
  for NSTE-ACS, 158-159, 158f, 159b

Glycoprotein (GP) IIB/IIIA receptor antagonists
    (Continued)
  side effects and contraindications to, 115
  for STEMI
    in acute phase, 182
    with PCI, 189t
GMP (Good Manufacturing Practices), 37
Go-DARTS diabetic cohort, 61
Good Clinical Practices (GCP), 37
Good Manufacturing Practices (GMP), 37
Gore Helix Septal Occluder, 638
Gore Tag thoracic aortic endoprosthesis,
  612-613
Gout, in adults with cyanotic congenital heart
  disease, 634
GP. See Glycoprotein (GP).
GRA (glucocorticoid-remediable
  aldosteronism), 494-495
  pharmacologic treatment of, 497
GRACE registry, 75, 170
GRACE score, 153, 154t, 186f
Graded exercise test, 743, 743f
Graduated compression stockings (GCS)
  for deep vein thrombosis, 587
  for peripheral edema in pregnancy, 623
  for thromboprophylaxis, 592
Granulicatella spp, endocarditis due to, 654
GRAVITAS study, 56, 157
Gray-scale median (GSM) score, 566
GSM (gray-scale median) score, 566
GTN. See Glyceryl trinitrate (GTN).
GUARD trial, 95-96
GuardWire distal occlusion device, 222
Guidant Tetra-D stent, 215
Guidelines Applied in Practice (GAP), 71
GUSTO I trial, 26, 26f, 197
GUSTO II trial, 119, 194
GWTG-CAD (Get with the Guidelines–Coronary
  Artery Disease), 71

H

HAART. See Highly active antiretroviral
  therapy (HAART).
HACEK microorganisms, endocarditis due to,
  655t
Haemophilus spp, endocarditis due to,
  655t
Hancock prosthesis, 695t, 697
Harken, Dwight, 691
Hatch-Waxman Act, 39
HATS study, 437
HCM. See Hypertrophic cardiomyopathy
  (HCM).
HCR. See Hybrid coronary revascularization
  (HCR).
hCSCs (human cardiac stem cells)
  age, cardiac disease and, 327-330
  endogenous, 326-327, 327f-330f
  hematopoietic stem cell transdifferentiation
    to, 323
  in myocardial repair, 322, 324f
HCTZ. See Hydrochlorothiazide.
HDE (Humanitarian Device Exemption),
  44
HDL cholesterol. See High-density lipoprotein
  (HDL) cholesterol.
Health care systems, vs. systems of care,
  67
Heart block, after STEMI, 198-199, 198t
Heart failure (HF)
  acute, 299-301
    defined, 281
    dobutamine for, 300
    dopamine vs. norepinephrine for, 300,
      300f
    LVEF in, 299-300, 300f

Heart failure (HF) (Continued)
    nitroglycerin for, 300
    nitroprusside for, 300, 301f
    noninvasive positive-pressure ventilation
      for, 300, 301f
    parenteral diuretics for, 291
    syndromes of, 281
  acute decompensated, 281-306
    adjustment of oral medications for, 296-297
      for β-blockers, 297
      for nitrates and hydralazine, 297
      for oral diuretics, 297
      for renin-angiotensin-aldosterone system
        inhibitors, 296-297
    comorbidities with, 281, 282t, 298
    epidemiology of, 281-282, 282f, 282t
    future directions for, 301-303, 302f
    general management of, 285-290
      clinical assessment of intracardiac
        filling pressures in, 285-286
      clinical assessment of systemic
        perfusion in, 287
      fluid management in, 290-292, 291f
      hemodynamic goals of therapy in, 290
      hemodynamic profiles in, 289-290
      initial patient evaluation in, 285
      laboratory assessment in, 287-288, 287b,
        288f, 288t
      noninvasive vs. invasive, 288-289, 289t,
        292t
      risk stratification in, 285, 285t-286t, 286f
    goals in treatment of
      general, 288-289, 289t
      hemodynamic, 290
    other management issues in, 297-299
      anticoagulation as, 298
      comorbidities as, 298
      discharge planning and immediate
        postdischarge care as, 298-299,
        298t, 299b
      oxygen supplementation as, 297-298
      sodium and fluid restriction as, 297
      ventricular arrhythmias as, 298
    pathophysiology of, 282-285
    pulmonary artery catheter for, 289, 289t,
      748t
    special considerations with, 299-301
      acute pulmonary edema as, 291,
        299-301, 300f-301f
      mechanical circulatory support as, 299
      preserved ejection fraction as, 301
    terminology for, 281, 282f
    vasoactive therapy for, 292-296
      digoxin as, 296
      dobutamine as, 293-294, 294f, 295t
      dopamine as, 295-296, 295f
      epinephrine and norepinephrine as, 296
      milrinone as, 294-295, 294f
      nesiritide as, 292-293, 293f
      nitroglycerin as, 292, 292t
      nitroprusside as, 293, 294f-295f
  advanced, 307-321
    approach to patient with, 307, 308f
    cardiac transplantation for, 307-314
      drug interactions with, 310, 312b
      future directions for, 314
      listing for, 309, 309t
      patient management after, 309-310, 310t
      patient management prior to, 309
      patient selection for, 307-309, 308b
      prevention and treatment of
        complications after, 310-314
      prevention and treatment of rejection
        of, 310, 311t
      surgical technique for, 309
    mechanical circulatory support for, 314-319
      adverse events with, 319, 319t
      benefits of, 314

Heart failure (HF) (Continued)
cardiac considerations with, 317-318
configuration of, 314-315, 315f
indications for, 315
noncardiac considerations with, 318
other considerations with, 318-319
surgical considerations with, 318
timing of, 315-317, 316f-317f, 317t
overview of, 307
comorbidities with, 264, 281, 282t, 285
conduction abnormalities in, 273
with diabetes, 262
diastolic, 283
epidemiology of, 281-282, 282f
gender, rate, and ethnic considerations with, 262
hemodynamic profiles for, 289-290
implantable devices for, 270-280
for cardiac resynchronization therapy, 273
in atrial fibrillation, 276
future directions of, 276
indications for, 276
landmark trials of, 273-275, 274f
in long-term right ventricle pacing, 276
with mild heart failure, 275-276
future directions for, 278
implantable cardioverter-defibrillators as, 270-272, 271f
early after myocardial infarction, 272
indications for prophylactic, 272
practical considerations for, 272-273
monitoring heart failure through, 276-277, 277f-279f
infective endocarditis with, 659-660, 659t
with ischemic heart disease, 261-262, 261t
with myocarditis, 262-263
nitrates with, 87
pathophysiology of, 241-263, 242f, 282-285
acute compensatory mechanisms in, 283, 283f
common precipitating factors in, 284-285, 284b
myocardial injury in, 284, 284f
with reduced vs. preserved ejection fraction, 282-283
pharmacologic management of, 241-269
aldosterone antagonists for, 253-254
adverse effects of, 248t
clinical efficacy of, 253-254
endpoints with, 242t
pathophysiologic mechanisms and, 253, 253t
practical considerations with, 254
antiarrhythmic therapy for, 258-259
antithrombotic therapy for, 258
β-blockers for, 250-253
choice of, 253
clinical efficacy of, 250-252, 251t
dosage of, 246t
endpoints with, 242t
pathophysiologic rationale for, 250
pharmacology of, 250
practical considerations with, 252-253
calcium channel blockers for, 257
with preserved ejection fraction, 259
with comorbidities, 264
with diabetes, 262
digoxin for, 254, 256-257
endpoints with, 242t
pharmacologic and clinical effects of, 256
practical considerations with, 256-257
diuretics for, 243-245
adverse effects of, 244
dosage of, 243t
endpoints with, 242t
mechanism of action of, 243-244

Heart failure (HF) (Continued)
pathophysiologic mechanisms and, 242-243
practical considerations with, 244-245
endpoints with, 242, 242t
future directions in, 263-264
gender, race, and ethnic considerations for, 262
hydralazine and isosorbide dinitrate for, 254-256, 255f
practical considerations with, 255-256
with ischemic heart disease, 261-262, 261t
with myocarditis, 262-263
pathophysiology and, 241-263, 242f
for patients who remain symptomatic despite standard therapy, 254, 254t
positive inotropic agents for, 257-258
as bridge to end of life, 257-258
as bridge to transplant, 257
intravenous, 257-258
oral, 257
with preserved ejection fraction, 259-261
clinical efficacy of, 259-260
clinical trials of, 259, 260t
mortality and, 259, 259t
practical considerations with, 260-261
recommendations on, 259, 260t
vs. reduced, 282-283
renin-angiotensin system inhibitors (ACE inhibitors and ARBs) for, 245-250
clinical efficacy of, 246-248, 247t
dosage of, 246t
endpoints with, 242t
pathophysiologic mechanisms and, 245-246, 245f
practical considerations with, 248-250, 248t
with preserved ejection fraction, 259, 260t
staging system and, 241-263, 242f, 243t
targets of, 241-263, 242t
with valvular heart disease, 262
in pregnancy, 627-628
with preserved ejection fraction, 259-261, 301
mortality in, 259, 259t
pharmacologic management of, 259-261
clinical efficacy of, 259-260
practical considerations with, 260-261
randomized trials of, 259, 260t
recommendations on, 259, 260t
procainamide with, 348-349
quality improvement for, 72
regenerative therapy for, 322-331
age, cardiac disease, and human cardiac stem cell function in, 327-330
bone marrow cells and clinical studies on, 324-326
cardiomyocyte death and regeneration and, 322, 323f
circulating progenitor cells and myocardial regeneration in, 322-323, 323f-324f
endogenous cardiac progenitors in, 326-327, 327f-330f
hematopoietic stem cell transdifferentiation and, 323-324, 325f
rehabilitation for, 744
risk stratification for, 285, 285t-286t, 286f
sodium restriction for, 243, 243t
pathophysiologic mechanisms and, 242-243
Stage D, 281
staging system for, 241-263, 242f, 243t
systems of care for, 69-70
systolic, 283
time course of, 282f
with valvular heart disease, 262

Heart Leaflet Technologies valve, 720f, 721
Heart rate
and heart failure risk stratification, 286t
training, 743, 743f
Heart rate reserve, 743, 743f
Heart rate variability (HRV)
monitoring of, 276
after STEMI, 204
Heart transplantation. See Cardiac transplantation.
Heart valve(s). See under Valve.
HELLP syndrome
diagnosis of, 523-524, 523b
pathophysiology of, 521-522, 522f
HELP (heparin-induced extracorporeal LDL precipitation), LDL apheresis using, 456, 457f, 457t
HELP-LDL Apheresis Multicenter Study, 457-458
Helsinki Heart Study (HHS), 436
Hematologic changes, due to cyanosis, 634
Hematoma, aortic intramural, 617
Hematopoietic progenitor cells (HPCs), in myocardial repair, 322, 324f
Hematopoietic stem cells (HSCs), 322
in myocardial repair, 322, 324f
transdifferentiation of, 323-324, 325f
Hematuria, hypertensive emergencies with, 517
Hemiarch repair, for thoracic aortic aneurysms, 609, 611f
Hemochromatosis, cardiac, 338-339
treatment of, 338-339
Hemodialysis, infective endocarditis with, 657
Hemodynamic assessment, after STEMI, 193
Hemodynamic benefits, of physical training, 738, 739b
Hemodynamic disturbances, after STEMI, 193-196, 194f
Hemodynamic monitoring
for heart failure, 289, 289t
implantable devices for, 276-277, 277f-279f
Hemodynamic profiles, for heart failure, 289-290
Hemoglobin A1c reduction, ranolazine for, 106
Hemolysis, elevated liver enzymes, low platelets (HELLP) syndrome
diagnosis of, 523-524, 523b
pathophysiology of, 521-522, 522f
Hemorrhage, hypertensive emergencies with, 518-519
intracerebral, 516, 516f
subarachnoid, 516
Hemorrhagic cerebrovascular syndromes, hypertensive emergencies with, 516
Hemorrhagic complications, after STEMI, 201-202, 202b
Heparin
for LDL apheresis, 455
low-molecular-weight, 117-118
dosages of, 118
indications for, 118
mechanisms of action of, 117-118
for NSTE-ACS, 159-161, 160t, 161f
in pregnancy and lactation, 622t-623t, 625
side effects and contraindications to, 118
for STEMI, 182-183, 184f
for thromboprophylaxis, 591-592
for venous thromboembolism, 588
unfractionated, 115-117
dosages of, 117
indications for, 117
mechanisms of action of, 115-117, 116f
for NSTE-ACS, 159-161, 160t-161t, 161f, 163t
in pregnancy and lactation, 622t-623t, 625
side effects and contraindications to, 117
for STEMI

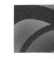

Heparin *(Continued)*
    in acute phase, 182-183, 183f-184f
    during convalescence, 192
    with PCI, 190t
  for thromboprophylaxis, 591
  for venous thromboembolism, 587
Heparin rebound, 117
Heparin resistance, 117
Heparin-coated stents, for chronic stable
    angina, 143-144
Heparin-induced extracorporeal LDL
    precipitation (HELP), LDL apheresis using,
    456, 457f, 457t
Heparin-induced thrombocytopenia (HIT), 117,
    587, 588f
Hepatic dysfunction, and mechanical
    circulatory support, 318
Hepatotoxicity, of statins, 424-426, 427f, 428b
HERCULES study, 575
Herculink Elite Renal Stent, 575
HF. *See* Heart failure (HF).
HHS (Department of Health and Human
    Services), in device development, 51
HHS (Helsinki Heart Study), 436
Hibernating myocardium, 261
High-carbohydrate, low-fat diets, 442, 443f
High-density lipoprotein (HDL) cholesterol
  HIV infection and, 730, 731f
  therapy to manage low, 434-441
    cholesteryl ester transfer protein inhibition
      as, 438-439, 438f
    combination therapy for
      non–HDL-c reduction in, 435, 435t
      rationale for, 434-435, 435f
      statin-fibrate, 436
      statin-niacin, 436-437
      statin–omega 3 fatty acids, 437-438
      therapy to modify HDL in, 435-436
    therapy to modify, 435-436
High-density lipoprotein (HDL) hypothesis,
    436
Highly active antiretroviral therapy (HAART),
    728-730
  combination medications in, 729-730
  fusion inhibitors in, 729
  integrase inhibitors in, 729
  and lipid-lowering therapy, 733, 733f
  metabolic effects of, 730-731
  nonnucleoside reverse transcriptase
    inhibitors in, 729, 730t
  nucleoside/nucleotide reverse transcriptase
    inhibitors in, 729, 730t
  protease inhibitors in, 728-729, 729t
High-voltage shocks, with implantable
    cardioverter-defibrillators, 759, 759f
  inappropriate, 759-760, 760t
Hip fracture, thromboprophylaxis with, 592,
    592b
Hip replacement, thromboprophylaxis with,
    592, 592b
Hirudin, 118-120
  indications and dosages for, 119
  mechanisms of action of, 118
  for NSTE-ACS, 161-162
  side effects and contraindications to, 120
Hirulog, 120
  indications and dosage for, 120
  mechanisms of action of, 120
Histoplasma spp, pericarditis due to, 673
Historic controls, 7
HIT (heparin-induced thrombocytopenia), 117,
    587, 588f
HIV. *See* Human immunodeficiency virus
    (HIV).
HIV Outpatient Study (HOPS), 731
HMG-CoA reductase inhibitors. *See* Statin(s).
HMGCR gene, in pharmacogenetics of statins,
    61

HOBIPACE trial, 276
Homograft valves, 699
  aortic, 696f, 701
  characteristics of, 696t
  currently available, 695t, 696f
HOPE study, 147, 248, 542
HOPS study, 731
HORIZONS-AMI trial, 120, 183, 216t
Hormone replacement therapy, after STEMI,
    207
HPCs (hematopoietic progenitor cells), in
    myocardial repair, 322, 324f
HPS study
  adverse effects in, 428
  drug efficacy in, 423-424, 425t
  ischemic heart disease in, 147
  peripheral artery disease in, 541
  STEMI in, 206
HRV (heart rate variability)
  monitoring of, 276
  after STEMI, 204
HSCs (hematopoietic stem cells), 322
  in myocardial repair, 322, 324f
  transdifferentiation of, 323-324, 325f
HSP (human subject protection), 37
Hufnagel, Charles, 691
Human capital approach, 23
Human cardiac stem cells (hCSCs)
  age, cardiac disease and, 327-330
  endogenous, 326-327, 327f-330f
  hematopoietic stem cell transdifferentiation
    to, 323
  in myocardial repair, 322, 324f
Human immunodeficiency virus (HIV), 728-737
  antiretroviral therapy for, 728-730
    combination medications in, 729-730
    fusion inhibitors in, 729
    integrase inhibitors in, 729
    and lipid-lowering therapy, 733, 733f
    metabolic effects of, 730-731
    nonnucleoside reverse transcriptase
      inhibitors in, 729, 730t
    nucleoside/nucleotide reverse
      transcriptase inhibitors in, 729, 730t
    protease inhibitors in, 728-729, 729t
  and cardiac malignancies, 735
  and cerebrovascular disease, 735
  coronary heart disease with
    clinical features of, 732-733, 732t
    pathogenesis of, 732-733
    risk factors for, 730-731, 731f
      treatment of, 733-734, 733f
    screening for, 731
  and endocarditis, 735
  epidemiology of, 728
  and hypertension, 730-731
    pulmonary, 734-735
    treatment of, 734
  and lipodystrophy, 731
  metabolic effects of, 730-731
  and metabolic syndrome, 731
  and myocardial infarction, 731-732
  myocardial involvement in, 734
  overview of, 728
  pericardial disease with, 673, 734
  screening for cardiovascular disease with, 731
Human resources shortages, for global
    cardiovascular therapy, 78, 79f
Human subject protection (HSP), 37
Humanitarian Device Exemption (HDE), 44
Hybrid approaches, for cost-effectiveness
    analysis, 26, 26f
Hybrid coronary revascularization (HCR),
    232-233
  current state of, 233
  defined, 232
  one-stop, 233
  rationale and background of, 232

Hybrid coronary revascularization (HCR)
    (Continued)
  technical and timing issues with, 233
  two-staged, 233
Hybrid therapy, for maintenance of sinus
    rhythm, 377
Hydralazine (Apresoline)
  for hypertension, 483, 483t
    in children, 536t
    in pregnancy, 524t
  for hypertensive emergencies, 514t-515t
  in pregnancy and lactation, 622t-623t, 627
Hydralazine and isosorbide dinitrate, for heart
    failure, 254-256, 255f
  acute decompensated, 297
  practical considerations with, 255-256
Hydrochlorothiazide (HCTZ, Esidrix,
    HydroDIURIL, Microzide, Oretic)
  for heart failure, 243t
  for hypertension, 480t, 481
    in children, 536t
    resistant, 505, 506f
  in pregnancy and lactation, 622t-623t
  for primary aldosteronism, 497
Hydrocortisone, for glucocorticoid-remediable
    aldosteronism, 497
β-Hydroxy-β-methylglutaryl coenzyme A
    (HMG-CoA) reductase inhibitors. *See*
    Statin(s).
11-β-Hydroxylase deficiency, hypertension due
    to, 498
17-α-Hydroxylase deficiency, hypertension due
    to, 498
Hygroton. *See* Chlorthalidone (Hygroton,
    Thalitone).
Hyperaldosteronism
  familial, 494-495
  idiopathic, 494-495
  pharmacologic treatment of, 497
Hypercholesterolemia
  familial, 454-455
  severe, 454-462
    definition of target population with, 454
    description of patient population with,
      454-455
      homozygous familial, 454-455
      with LDL cholesterol concentrations of
        more than 200 mg/dL and coronary
        artery disease, 455
      with LDL cholesterol concentrations of
        more than 300 mg/dL without
        coronary artery disease, 455
    gene therapy for, 460-461
    LDL apheresis for, 454-458
      benefits of, 457-458
      comparison of methods of, 457t
      failure to treat individuals who may
        benefit from, 458
      risks of, 457
      technical aspects of, 455-457, 456f
      using dextran sulfate cellulose columns,
        456, 456f
      using heparin-induced extracorporeal
        LDL precipitation, 456, 457f, 457t
      using immunoadsorption columns, 456,
        456f, 457t
      using whole blood–compatible systems,
        456-457, 457f, 457t
    options for treatment of, 454
    recommendations for, 461
    surgical procedures for, 454,
      458-461
      liver transplantation as, 459-460, 459t
      partial ileal bypass as, 460
      portacaval shunt as, 458-459, 458f,
        459t
Hyperdeoxycorticosteronism, hypertension
    due to, 497-498

Hypereosinophilic endomyocardial fibrosis, 339-340
Hyperlipidemia
  diet for, 442-446
    clinical trials of low-fat and low saturated fat, 443-444
    DASH, 442-443, 443f
    fish oil in, 445-446
    high-carbohydrate, low-fat, 442, 443f
    moderate unsaturated fat, 444-445, 444t
    reduced-carbohydrate, higher unsaturated fat, and protein, 445, 445t
    type of carbohydrate in, 445
  with HIV infection, 730, 731f
    treatment of, 733, 733f
  with LDL concentrations of more than 200 mg/dL and coronary artery disease, 455
  with LDL concentrations of more than 300 mg/dL without coronary artery disease, 455
  pharmacologic treatment of
    bile acid sequestrants for, 428-430, 429t
      clinical efficacy of, 429, 429t
      effects on lipids and lipoproteins of, 429
      safety/compliance issues for, 429-430
    combination therapy for
      non–HDL-c reduction in, 435, 435t
      rationale for, 434-435, 435f
      statin-fibrate, 436
      statin-niacin, 436-437
      statin–omega 3 fatty acids, 437-438
      therapy to modify HDL in, 435-436
    ezetimibe and cholesterol absorption inhibitors for, 430
      effect on lipids and lipoproteins of, 430
      efficacy of, 430
      safety of, 430
    fibrates and nicotinic acid for, 428
    plant stanol esters for, 430-431
      effects on lipids and lipoproteins of, 430-431
      efficacy against coronary heart disease of, 430-431
      safety of, 431
    statins for. See Statin(s).
Hyperparathyroidism, primary, 499, 503t
  presentation and diagnosis of, 499
  principles of treatment of, 499
Hyperperfusion syndrome, 519
Hypertension
  accelerated, 510
  antihypertensive medications for. See Antihypertensive medications.
  after cardiac transplantation, 313
  in children, 529-537
    classification of, 529, 533t
    confirmation of, 529
    definitions of, 529
      diastolic BP levels for boys in, 531t-532t
      systolic BP levels for boys in, 530t-531t
    evaluation of, 529, 533t
      algorithm for, 532f
    due to medications or illicit drugs, 529, 533t
    overview of, 529
    primary vs. secondary, 529-536
    target-organ damage due to, 533-534
    treatment of, 534-536
      algorithm for, 532f
      antihypertensive medications for, 534-536, 535f, 536t
      nonpharmacologic, 534
  with chronic kidney disease, 476
  classification of, 463, 464t
  with coronary artery disease, 476

Hypertension (Continued)
  defined, 463
  with diabetes, 475-476
  in elderly patients, 486-487
    blood pressure goals for, 486
    isolated systolic, 486
    and orthostatic hypotension, 486-487
    selecting drug therapy for, 487
  endocrine causes of, 490-500, 491b
    other forms of mineralocorticoid excess as, 497-499
      apparent mineralocorticoid excess syndromes as, 498-499
      hyperdeoxycorticosteronism as, 497-498
    pheochromocytoma as, 490-494, 503t
      acute hypertensive crises in, 493, 493t
      anesthesia and surgery for, 493-494
      diagnosis of, 490, 492f
      long-term postoperative follow-up for, 494
      malignant, 494
      in pregnancy, 494
      preoperative management of, 490-493, 492t
      presentation of, 490, 491b
      principles of treatment of, 490-494
      syndromic, 490, 491t
    primary aldosteronism as, 494-497, 503t, 504-508
      diagnosis of, 495-496, 495f-496f
      pharmacologic treatment of, 497
      principles of treatment of, 496-497
      subtypes of, 494-495, 495b, 496f
      surgical treatment of, 496-497
    due to thyroid and parathyroid disease, 499-500
      acromegaly as, 499-500
      primary hyperparathyroidism as, 499, 503t
      thyroid dysfunction as, 499
  epidemiology of, 463, 510
  HIV infection and, 730-731
    pulmonary, 734-735
    treatment of, 734
  with left ventricular dysfunction, 476
  lifestyle modifications for, 468-472, 469t
    approaches to increasing adoption of, 469-471
    barriers to, 469
    DASH diet as, 442-443, 443f
    general tips for adopting healthier lifestyles in, 471-472
    practical approaches to encouraging, 469-472, 470f
    readiness for change and, 470-471, 470f
    tips for success in adopting healthier dietary practices as, 471, 471t
    tips for success in increasing physical activity as, 471
  malignant, 510
  obesity and, 471
  obstructive sleep apnea and, 465, 502-504, 503t
  overview of, 463
    of treatment, 467, 467f
  patient evaluation for, 463-467, 464f
    blood pressure measurement in, 466, 466b
    history in, 463-464
      family, 465
      past medical, 465
      personal, 465, 465b
      of present illness, 464-465
      social, 465
    laboratory evaluation in, 466-467, 466b
    physical examination in, 465-466
    review of symptoms in, 465
  in pregnancy, 521-528
    acute management of severe, 525
    chronic, 521, 523

Hypertension (Continued)
    diagnosis of, 523-524, 523b
    eclampsia as, 525
    epidemiology and risk factors for, 521, 522t
    gestational, 521, 523
    implications for later cardiovascular disease of, 525-526
    overview of, 521
    pathophysiology of, 521-523
    preeclampsia as
      defined, 521
      pathophysiology of, 521-523, 522f
      risk factors for, 521, 522t
    prevention of, 524
    treatment of, 524-525, 524t
  with previous ischemic stroke, 476
  pseudo-, with aortic dissection, 614
  pulmonary, 596, 597t
    HIV-related, 734-735
    in pregnancy, 629-630
    pulmonary artery catheters for, 748t
  pulmonary arterial, 596-605
    chronic thromboembolic, 582
    classification of, 596, 598, 599b
    diagnosis of
      current state of, 596, 597t
      and risk stratification, 596-598, 599b
    epidemiologic associations with, 596, 597b, 597f
    with heart failure, 264
    HIV-related, 734-735
    idiopathic, 596
      epidemiologic associations with, 596
      pathophysiologic paradigm of, 596, 598f
      transplantation for, 602
    pathobiologic paradigm of
      current, 596, 598f
      new, 604
    pregnancy and contraception with, 604
    therapy for
      algorithms for, 602-604, 603f
      atrial septostomy in, 602
      combination, 602, 603f
      conventional, 599
      current state of, 599-602
      endothelin receptor antagonism in, 601, 601f
      new paradigm of, 604
      phosphodiesterase inhibition in, 601-602
      prostanoids in, 599-601, 600f
      transplantation in, 602
  due to renal artery stenosis, 503t
  due to renal parenchymal disease, 503t
  resistant, 467, 501-509
    due to aortic dissection, 614
    baroreflex activation therapy for, 508
    and cardiovascular risk, 502
    causes of, 468b, 502, 502b, 503t
    defined, 501, 502b
    diagnosis of, 464-465
      ambulatory blood pressure monitoring for, 501-502
    epidemiology of, 501
    interfering substances in, 504, 504b
      dietary sodium as, 504
    obstructive sleep apnea and, 502-504, 503t
    pharmacologic treatment of, 504-508
      diuretics for, 505, 505f-506f
      mineralocorticoid receptor antagonists for, 505-507, 506f-507f
      other antihypertensive agents for, 507
    primary aldosteronism and, 503t, 504-508
    pseudo-, 501, 502b
    due to renal artery stenosis, 571

Hypertension (Continued)
   renal sympathetic denervation for, 507-508
   role of hypertension specialist for, 508
   secondary, 465b, 502, 502b, 503t
      in children, 529-536
   uncontrolled, 501
Hypertension management, cardiac rehabilitation and, 741b
Hypertension specialist, for resistant hypertension, 508
Hypertensive crisis, 510-520
   definitions for, 510, 511b
   epidemiology and etiology of, 510
   overview of, 510
   pathophysiology of, 510-513, 511f
   patient evaluation for, 511-513, 512b, 512t
   due to pheochromocytoma, 493, 493t
Hypertensive emergency
   with cardiovascular presentations, 513-515
      acute coronary syndromes as, 513
      aortic dissection as, 513-515, 515f
      left ventricular failure and acute pulmonary edema as, 513
   with catecholaminergic presentations, 517-518
      due to acute withdrawal of antihypertensive therapy, 517
      due to autonomic dysfunction, 518
      due to pheochromocytoma, 517-518
      due to sympathomimetic drugs, 518
   caveats to therapy in, 519
   defined, 510
   epidemiology and etiology of, 510
   follow-up and prognosis for, 519
   with hemorrhagic presentation, 518-519
   management of, 513-519, 514t-515t
   with neurologic presentations, 515-516, 516f
      hemorrhagic cerebrovascular syndromes as, 516
      hypertensive encephalopathy as, 516, 517f
      intracerebral hemorrhage as, 516, 516f
      ischemic cerebrovascular syndromes as, 515-516
      subarachnoid hemorrhage as, 516
   pathophysiology of, 510-513, 511f
   patient evaluation for, 511-513
      ancillary testing in, 512-513, 512t
      history in, 511, 512b
      physical examination in, 511-512, 512b
   pediatric, 518
   during pregnancy, 518
   with renal presentations, 517
   after vascular surgery, 518-519
Hypertensive encephalopathy, 516, 517f
Hypertensive urgency, 510
Hyperthyroidism, hypertension due to, 499
Hypertriglyceridemia
   HIV infection and, 730, 733
   therapy to manage, 434-441
      non–HDL-c reduction in, 435, 435t
      rationale for, 434-435, 435f
      statin-fibrate, 436
      statin-niacin, 436-437
      statin–omega 3 fatty acids, 437-438
      therapy to modify HDL in, 435-436
Hypertrophic cardiomyopathy (HCM), 332-336
   atrial fibrillation in, 335-336
   β-adrenergic blockers for, 100
   defined, 332
   LVOT obstruction in, 332-335
      alcohol septal ablation for, 333-334, 334t
      pharmacologic treatment of, 332
      surgical myectomy for, 332, 333f, 334t
      ventricular pacing for, 334-335
   nonobstructive, 335
   screening at-risk family members for, 336
   sudden cardiac death in, 335, 335f

Hyperviscosity syndromes, in adults with cyanotic congenital heart disease, 634
Hypoalbuminemia, in acute decompensated heart failure, 287
Hypokalemia, in acute decompensated heart failure, 287, 291
Hypomagnesemia, in acute decompensated heart failure, 287
Hyponatremia, in acute decompensated heart failure, 287
Hypotension, after STEMI, 193, 194f
Hypothermia, therapeutic, after cardiac arrest, 417
Hypothesis
   alternative, 9
   null, 8f, 9
Hypothyroidism, hypertension due to, 499
Hypovolemia, after STEMI, 193, 194f
Hypoxemia, patent foramen ovale and, 639, 640f
Hytrin (terazosin), for hypertension, 483t
   due to pheochromocytoma, 491-493, 492t
Hyzaar (losartan potassium/hydrochlorothiazide), for hypertension, 485t

I

IABP. See Intra-aortic balloon pump (IABP).
Iatrogenic pericardial disease, 674, 675t
Ibuprofen
   for acute pericarditis, 667
   for postpericardial injury syndrome, 673
Ibutilide, 355-356
   adverse reactions to, 356
   for atrial fibrillation, 374t
   for atrial flutter, 370
   clinical applications of, 355
   clinical pharmacology of, 355-356
   dosage and administration of, 356
      modification in disease states of, 356
   drug interactions with, 356
   mechanism of action of, 355
iCast Atrium Registry Ultrasound Study (ICARUS), 546-547
ICDs. See Implantable cardioverter-defibrillators (ICDs).
ICE, 660, 663
ICE Plus, 663
ICE-PCS study, 663
ICER (incremental cost-effectiveness ratio), 24
ICH (International Conference on Harmonisation of Technical Requirements for Registration of Pharmaceuticals for Human Use), 37
ICH (intracranial hemorrhage), due to fibrinolytic therapy, 185-186, 188f
iCoapsys device, 724f, 725
ICSS study, 564
ICTUS trial, 164-165
ICUR (incremental cost-utility ratio), 24
IDE (Investigational Device Exemption), 41-44
IDEAL trial, 147, 425t
Idiopathic hyperaldosteronism (IHA), 494-495
   pharmacologic treatment of, 497
Idiopathic pulmonary arterial hypertension (iPAH), 596
   epidemiologic associations with, 596
   pathophysiologic paradigm of, 596, 598f
   transplantation for, 602
IDU (intravenous drug use), infective endocarditis with, 656, 658
IE. See Infective endocarditis (IE).
IEA (inferior epigastric artery) graft, for coronary artery bypass, 230, 231t

Ileal bypass, partial, for severe hypercholesterolemia, 460
   cholesterol lowering via, 459-460
   risks and benefits of, 460
   technique of, 459
ILLUMINATE trial, 149, 439
ILLUSTRATE trial, 439
Iloprost, for pulmonary arterial hypertension, 600, 600f
   in pregnancy and lactation, 622t-623t, 629-630
Imipenem-cilastatin, for enterococcal endocarditis, 656t
Immediate recurrence of atrial fibrillation (IRAF), 375
Immobility, physiologic effects of, 738
Immunoadsorption columns, LDL apheresis using, 454, 456, 457t
Immunosuppressive therapy, with cardiac transplantation, 310, 311t
   drug interactions with, 310, 312b
IMPACT-HF trial, 252
IMPACT-NCDR study, 642
Impella LP2.5 device, 224
Implant retrieval and evaluation, 47-48
Implantable cardioverter-defibrillators (ICDs), 758-760
   for cardiac sarcoidosis, 338
   early after myocardial infarction, 272
   for heart failure, 270-272, 271f
      indications for prophylactic, 272
      monitoring via, 276-277
   for hypertrophic cardiomyopathy, 335
   inappropriate shocks with, 759-760, 760t
   magnet operation with, 759
   practical considerations for, 272-273
   for prevention of sudden cardiac death, 396-407
      cardiac resynchronization, 401, 403f
      indications for, 401-404, 403b, 403f
      primary, 397-398
         age and, 401
         clinical trials of, 397-398, 399t, 400f
         with comorbidities, 400-401, 402f
         with heart failure, 401
         with kidney disease, 401
         risk stratification for, 398-400, 400t
      secondary, 396, 398t
      systems and technology for, 396-406, 397f
   radiographic appearance of, 753f, 758
   routine follow-up with, 760
   after STEMI, 199, 200f
   for ventricular arrhythmias, 759, 759f, 759t
Implantable devices, for heart failure, 270-280
   for cardiac resynchronization therapy, 273
      in atrial fibrillation, 276
      future directions of, 276
      indications for, 276
      landmark trials of, 273-275, 274f
      in long-term right ventricle pacing, 276
      with mild heart failure, 275-276
   future directions for, 278
   implantable cardioverter-defibrillators as, 270-272, 271f
      early after myocardial infarction, 272
      indications for prophylactic, 272
      practical considerations for, 272-273
      monitoring heart failure through, 276-277, 277f-279f
IMPROVE registry, 593
Inappropriate sinus tachycardia, 367
   catheter ablation for, 386
   pharmacologic treatment of, 371
   in pregnancy, 628
Incident investigation, for medical device failures, 48
Inclusive chronic disease model, 740

Incremental benefits, 24
Incremental cost(s), 24
Incremental cost-effectiveness ratio (ICER), 24
Incremental cost-utility ratio (ICUR), 24
IND (Investigational New Drug Application), 34
Indapamide (Lozol)
  for heart failure, 243t
  for hypertension, 480t
Inderal. See Propranolol (Inderal, Innopran).
Inderide (propranolol hydrochloride/
    hydrochlorothiazide), for hypertension, 485t
India
  regulation of new drugs in, 37
  secondary prevention of coronary artery
    disease in, 77
Indinavir, for HIV infection, 729t
Indomethacin, for acute pericarditis, 667
Infection(s)
  after cardiac transplantation, 312
  and mechanical circulatory support, 318
  with prosthetic heart valve, 42f, 49f
Infective endocarditis (IE), 652-666
  in adults with congenital heart disease, 632
  antibiotic therapy for, 654-656
    for common microorganisms, 655t
    for enterococcal microorganisms, 656t
    with IV drug use, 656
    outpatient parenteral, 655-656
    for resistant microorganisms, 656
  diagnosis of, 652-654
    clinical findings in, 652, 653b
    Duke criteria for, 652, 653f
    echocardiography in, 652-654, 653f
      decision tree for use of, 652-654, 654f
      sensitivity and specificity of, 652, 653t
      transthoracic vs. transesophageal, 652,
        653b, 653t
  in elderly, 657
  future directions with, 663
  with hemodialysis, 657
  in HIV-positive patients, 735
  with IV drug use, 656, 658
  long-term outcomes and management of,
    662
  overview of, 652
  with patent ductus arteriosus, 645
  prevention of, 662-663, 663t
  prophylaxis for, 662-663, 663t
    during delivery, 630
  with prosthetic cardiac devices, 657-658
  risk of poor clinical outcomes with, 657-658
  surgical therapy for complicated, 658-662,
    709-710
    with abscess, 652, 653f, 660
    approach to, 658, 658f
    with cardiac device infections, 661-662
    with embolic events, 659t-660t, 660-661
    with heart failure, 659-660, 659t
    indications for, 658, 659t
    with prosthetic valve infections, 661
    with uncontrolled infection, 659t
Inferior epigastric artery (IEA) graft, for
    coronary artery bypass, 230, 231t
Inferior vena cava (IVC) filters, for
    thromboembolic disease, 591
Infinnium stent, 221
In-flow disease, 546
Influenza vaccine, after NSTE-ACS, 168
Infrapopliteal disease, 549, 550f
Innopran. See Propranolol (Inderal, Innopran).
INR (International Normalized Ratio), for
    warfarin, 57, 121, 588
Inspra. See Eplerenone (Inspra).
INSTEAD trial, 615-616
Insulin Resistance Intervention After Stroke
    (IRIS) trial, 397-398, 399t

Integrase inhibitors, for HIV infection, 729
Integrated with classification improvement, 3
Intensification, 13
Interceptor PLUS, 222
INTERMACS registry, 317, 317f, 317t
Intermittent claudication, 543-544, 544f
  cilostazol for, 543-544
  pentoxifylline for, 543
Intermittent pneumatic compression devices,
    for thromboprophylaxis, 592
International Conference on Harmonisation of
    Technical Requirements for Registration of
    Pharmaceuticals for Human Use (ICH), 37
International drug development, 36-37
International Normalized Ratio (INR), for
    warfarin, 57, 121, 588
International Sensitivity Index (ISI), for
    warfarin, 121
Intra-aortic balloon pump (IABP), 224, 749-750
  for acute decompensated heart failure, 299
  complications of, 750
  design of, 749
  indications for, 749, 749b
  after STEMI, 198
  technical aspects of placement of, 749-750
  timing and waveforms with, 750, 750f-751f
Intracardiac filling pressures, in acute
    decompensated heart failure, 285-286
Intracerebral hemorrhage, hypertensive
    emergencies with, 516, 516f
Intracoronary stent(s), for chronic stable
    angina, 142f, 143-144
Intracranial tumor, hypertension due to, 503t
Intrafascicular verapamil-sensitive reentrant
    tachycardia, catheter ablation for, 390-391
Intramural hematoma, aortic, 617
Intrasaccular approach of Creech, for
    abdominal aortic aneurysms, 606
Intrathoracic impedance monitoring, 277, 277f
Intravascular assessment, of coronary lesion
    severity, 224-225
Intravascular ultrasound (IVUS), for
    assessment of coronary lesion severity,
    224-225
Intravenous drug use (IDU), infective
    endocarditis with, 656, 658
Intravenous immune globulin (IVIG), for
    myocarditis, 263
Intrinsic amplitude, 752
INVEST study, 94-95
INVEST trial, 96
Investigational Device Exemption (IDE), 41-44
Investigational New Drug Application (IND), 34
  advisory panels for, 35
  data necessary to support, 34-35
  emergency use, 35
  exemptions from, 36
  investigator-initiated, 35-36
  treatment, 35
  types of, 35
IONA trial, 104, 105f, 141
iPAH. See Idiopathic pulmonary arterial
    hypertension (iPAH).
I-PRESERVE study, 259-260, 260t
IRAF (immediate recurrence of atrial
    fibrillation), 375
Irbesartan (Avapro)
  for heart failure, 259-260
  for hypertension, 479t
Irbesartan/hydrochlorothiazide (Avalide), for
    hypertension, 485t
IRIS trial, 272, 397-398, 399t
Iron chelation therapy, for cardiac
    hemochromatosis, 338-339
ISAR-REACT 3 trial, 162
ISAR-REACT 3A trial, 159
ISAR-REACT 4 trial, 162
ISAR-REACT trial, 144, 158

ISAR-SHOCK trial, 224
Ischemic cerebrovascular syndromes,
    hypertensive emergencies with, 515-516
Ischemic heart disease
  global cardiovascular therapy for, 76-77, 77f
  and heart failure, 261-262, 261t, 284-285
  pharmacologic options for, 83-130
    β-adrenergic blockers as, 96-104
    calcium channel blockers as, 89-96
    newer options for, 104-106
      ivabradine as, 104-105
      nicorandil as, 104, 105f
      ranolazine as, 105-106, 106f
      trimetazidine as, 106
    organic nitrates as, 83-89
    due to thrombosis, 107-123, 107f
      anticoagulant therapy for, 115-120
      antiplatelet therapy for, 107-115
      factor Xa inhibitors as, 121
      oral anticoagulants as, 121-123
  in pregnancy, 626-627
  "silent," β-adrenergic blockers for, 99-100
  stable, 131-152
    antiplatelet therapy for
      with novel agents, 149
      with percutaneous coronary
        intervention, 144
      for prevention of coronary events,
        144-146, 146f
    cardiac rehabilitation for, 140
      for prevention of coronary events, 144
    clinical assessment of, 131, 132b
    coronary artery bypass graft for, 144
      arterial conduits in, 144
      complications of, 144, 145f
      vs. percutaneous coronary intervention,
        142-143
      percutaneous coronary intervention
        after, 143
      results of, 142f
      in secondary prevention, 147-149
    coronary revascularization for, 141-144
      in secondary prevention, 147-149
    epidemiology of, 131
    invasive evaluation of, 136-137, 137b
    lifestyle and risk factor modifications for,
      137-140
      for diabetes mellitus, 140
      dietary intervention as, 138-140
      for obesity, 140
      smoking in, 137-138
    natural history of, 131, 132f-133f
    noninvasive evaluation of, 131-136
      cardiac MRI for, 134
      computed tomography for, 135-136
      coronary calcium score for, 135
      CT coronary angiography for, 135-136,
        136f
      echocardiography for, 133-134
      electrocardiogram for, 131-133, 133b,
        134f-135f
      myocardial perfusion scintigraphy for,
        134-135, 135b
      selection and frequency of stress testing
        for, 136, 137t, 138f
    overall assessment of risk for, 137, 138f
    percutaneous coronary intervention for,
      141-144
      antiplatelet therapy with, 144
      complications of, 144
      vs. coronary artery bypass graft, 142-143
      after coronary artery bypass grafting,
        143
      culprit lesions, 143
      indications for, 142
      vs. medical treatment, 142
    pharmacologic therapy for, 140-141
      with ACE inhibitors, 147

Ischemic heart disease *(Continued)*
  with β-blockers, 140-141, 147
  with calcium channel blockers, 141
  with cholesteryl ester transfer protein
      inhibitors, 149
  with ivabradine, 141
  with lipid-lowering agents, 146-147, 148f
  with nitrates, 141
  vs. percutaneous coronary intervention,
      142
  with potassium channel agonists, 141
  risk stratification for, 131-137, 132b, 133f
  secondary prevention of, 139f, 144-149
    ACE inhibitors in, 147
    antiplatelet therapy in, 144-146, 146f
    β-blockers in, 147
    cardiac rehabilitation in, 144
    coronary artery bypass graft in, 147-149
    coronary revascularization in, 147-149
    lipid-lowering therapy in, 146-147, 148f
  stents for, 142f, 143-144
  symptomatic medical management of,
      139f, 140-144
  therapeutic interventions for, 137-149, 138f
  and valvular heart disease, 710-711
    aortic stenosis in CABG patients as, 710
    incidental coronary disease in valve
        surgery patients as, 710
    incidental valve disease in coronary
        surgery patients as, 710
    mitral regurgitation in CABG patients as,
        710-711, 711f
Ischemic stroke
  hypertension with previous, 476
  after STEMI, 200-201, 201f
ISH (isolated systolic hypertension), in elderly
    patients, 486
ISHIB, 487
ISI (International Sensitivity Index), for
    warfarin, 121
ISIS-2 study, 182
ISIS-4 study, 247t
Isolated systolic hypertension (ISH), in elderly
    patients, 486
Isomer-d-propranolol, pharmacodynamic
    properties and cardiac effects of, 98t
Isoniazid, for tuberculous pericarditis, 672
Isoproterenol
  in pregnancy and lactation, 622t-623t
  for STEMI, 183-184
Isosorbide dinitrate
  for heart failure, 254-256, 255f
    acute decompensated, 297
    practical considerations with, 255-256
  pharmacokinetics of, 87t
  side effects of, 87t
Isosorbide-5-mononitrate, 85-87
  pharmacokinetics of, 87t
  side effects of, 87t
Isradipine (Dynacirc), for hypertension, 479t
  in children, 536t
Ivabradine
  for chronic stable angina, 104-105, 141
  for heart failure, 264
IVC (inferior vena cava) filters, for
    thromboembolic disease, 591
IVIG (intravenous immune globulin), for
    myocarditis, 263
IVUS (intravascular ultrasound), for
    assessment of coronary lesion severity,
    224-225

J

Jactax stent, 221
JenaValve, 720f, 721
Junctional ectopic tachycardia, 371

K

Karvonen formula, 743, 743f
Karyokinesis, 322
KCNJ5 gene, in primary aldosteronism, 494-495
Kerlone. *See* Betaxolol (Kerlone).
KIF6 gene, in pharmacogenetics of statins,
    62-63, 62t
Kingella spp, endocarditis due to, 655t
Kissing stents, for bifurcation lesion, 223, 223f
Knee replacement, thromboprophylaxis with,
    592, 592b
Konno operation, 633t

L

LAA (left atrial appendage) closure devices,
    388, 389f
LAA (left atrial appendage) thrombus, mitral
    stenosis with, 680-681
LAARS study, 458
Labeling
  of cardiovascular devices, 46-47
  of new drugs, 35
Labetalol (Trandate, Normodyne)
  for aortic dissection, 614
  drug interactions with, 105t
  for hypertension, 481t
    in children, 536t
    due to pheochromocytoma, 492t, 493
    in pregnancy, 524t
  for hypertensive emergencies, 514t-515t
  indications for, 101
  pharmacodynamic properties and cardiac
      effects of, 98t
  in pregnancy and lactation, 622t-623t
  properties of, 102t
LACMART trial, 458
Lactation, cardiac drugs in, 622t-623t
Lamivudine (3TC), for HIV infection, 730t
LAMP2 mutations, cardiomyopathy associated
    with, 339
Lanoteplase (nPA), 123t
Laparoscopic adrenalectomy, for primary
    aldosteronism, 496-497
LAPTOP system, 277, 278f-279f
LAPTOP-HF study, 277
LARS study, 457-458
Lasix. *See* Furosemide.
Latent conditions, in medical device failures,
    47-48
Latin America, regulation of new drugs in, 37
LBBB (left bundle branch block)
  in heart failure, 273
  with STEMI, 181
LDL cholesterol. *See* Low-density lipoprotein
    (LDL) cholesterol.
LDLA. *See* Low-density lipoprotein apheresis
    (LDLA).
LDLR gene, in pharmacogenetics of statins, 62
Lead(s), for permanent pacemakers, 752, 753t
Lead impedance, 752
LEADERS trial, 221
Leaflet ablation, 722t
Leaflet coaptation, 722t
Leaflet plication, 722-723, 722f-723f
Leaflet prolapse, 705
Leaflet repair, in percutaneous mitral valve
    therapy, 722-724, 722f-723f, 722t

Leaflet-to-leaflet transcatheter mitral valve
    therapies, 722-723, 722f-723f
Learning curve, in clinical trials, 5
Left atrial appendage (LAA) closure devices,
    388, 389f
Left atrial appendage (LAA) thrombus, mitral
    stenosis with, 680-681
Left atrial thrombus, mitral stenosis with,
    680-681
Left bundle branch block (LBBB)
  in heart failure, 273
  with STEMI, 181
Left internal mammary artery (LIMA) graft, for
    coronary artery bypass, 228, 231t
Left ventricular (LV) aneurysm, after STEMI,
    197-198
Left ventricular assist device (LVAD), 315
  after STEMI, 198
Left ventricular (LV) dysfunction, hypertension
    with, 476
Left ventricular ejection fraction (LVEF)
  in acute pulmonary edema, 299-300, 300f
  heart failure with preserved, 259-261
    mortality in, 259, 259t
    pharmacologic management of, 259-261
      clinical efficacy of, 259-260
      practical considerations with, 260-261
      randomized trials of, 259, 260t
      recommendations on, 259, 260t
    vs. reduced, 282-283
  and risk of sudden cardiac death, 398, 400t
  after STEMI, 204
Left ventricular (LV) failure, hypertensive
    emergencies with, 513
Left ventricular (LV) filling pressure, in acute
    decompensated heart failure, 286
Left ventricular (LV) free wall rupture, after
    STEMI, 197, 197t
Left ventricular (LV) function, after STEMI,
    203-204
Left ventricular hypertrophy (LVH), and
    hypertension in children, 533
Left ventricular outflow tract obstruction
    (LVOTO), 332-335
  alcohol septal ablation for, 333-334, 334t
  etiology of, 332
  pharmacologic treatment of, 332
  surgical myectomy for, 332, 333f, 334t
  ventricular pacing for, 334-335
Left ventricular (LV) pacing, 756f-757f
Left ventricular (LV) scar burden, and risk of
    sudden cardiac death, 398-400, 400t
Left ventricular (LV) systolic dysfunction, and
    heart failure risk stratification, 286t
Left ventricular (LV) thrombus, after STEMI,
    197-198
Left-to-right shunting, in adults with congenital
    heart disease, 632-633
Lepirudin, 118-120
  indications and dosages for, 119
  mechanisms of action of, 118
  side effects and contraindications to, 120
"Less sodium," 471t
Levatrol. *See* Penbutolol (Levatrol).
Levosimendan, for acute decompensated heart
    failure, 302
Levothyroxine, for hypothyroidism, 499
Lexxel (enalapril maleate/felodipinel), for
    hypertension, 485t
Licorice, hypertensive emergency due to, 511
Lidocaine, 344-347
  adverse reactions to, 347
  for cardiac arrhythmias due to
      pheochromocytoma, 493t
  clinical applications of, 344-345
  clinical pharmacology of, 345-346
  dosage and administration of, 346
  modification in disease states of, 346-347

Lidocaine *(Continued)*
  drug interactions with, 347
  mechanism of action of, 345
  in pregnancy and lactation, 622t-623t, 629
  for sustained monomorphic ventricular
    tachycardia, 409-410, 410t
Lietz-Miller risk score, 316-317
Life cycle, of product, 47, 47f
LIFENOX study, 591
Lifestyle modifications, 442-453
  for chronic stable angina, 137-140
  for dietary fats and lipids, 442-446
    DASH diet in, 442-443, 443f
    fish oil in, 445-446
    high-carbohydrate, low-fat diets in, 442,
      443f
    low-fat diets and low saturated fat in,
      443-444
    moderate unsaturated fat diets in, 444-445,
      444t
    reduced-carbohydrate, higher unsaturated
      fat, and protein diets in, 445, 445t
    type of carbohydrate in, 445
  for hypertension, 468-472, 469t
    approaches to increasing adoption of,
      469-471
    barriers to, 469
    in children, 534-536
    general tips for adopting healthier
      lifestyles in, 471-472
    practical approaches to encouraging,
      469-472, 470f
    readiness for change and, 470-471, 470f
    tips for success in adopting healthier
      dietary practices as, 471, 471t
    tips for success in increasing physical
      activity as, 471
  after NSTE-ACS, 165, 166t
  for obesity, 446-450, 446f
    clinical assessment of, 446-448, 447t
    DASH diet in, 448-450, 449t
    determination of calorie levels for weight
      loss in, 448
    goals for weight loss and management in,
      448
    Mediterranean diet in, 448-450, 450f, 451t
    physical activity in, 450, 452t
    2010 Dietary Guidelines in, 448
    overall effect of, 450, 451b
Lifetime time horizon, of cost-effectiveness
    analysis, 28-29
"Light in fat," 471t
"Light sodium," 471t
Likelihood ratio (LR), 2, 2f
LIMA (left internal mammary artery) graft, for
    coronary artery bypass, 228, 231t
Linezolid, for enterococcal endocarditis, 656t
Lipid(s), and global cardiovascular disease, 81
Lipid disorders
  after cardiac transplantation, 313
  diet for, 442-446
    DASH, 442-443, 443f
    fish oil in, 445-446
    high-carbohydrate, low-fat, 442, 443f
    low-fat and low saturated fat, 443-444
    moderate unsaturated fat, 444-445, 444t
    reduced-carbohydrate, higher unsaturated
      fat, and protein, 445, 445t
    type of carbohydrate in, 445
  elevated LDL cholesterol as
    bile acid sequestrants for, 428-430, 429t
      clinical efficacy of, 429, 429t
      effects on lipids and lipoproteins of,
        429
      safety/compliance issues for, 429-430
    combination therapy for
      non–HDL-c reduction in, 435, 435t
      rationale for, 434-435, 435f

Lipid disorders *(Continued)*
    statin-fibrate, 436
    statin-niacin, 436-437
    statin–omega 3 fatty acids, 437-438
    therapy to modify HDL in, 435-436
  with concentrations of more than
    200 mg/dL and coronary artery
    disease, 455
  with concentrations of more than
    300 mg/dL without coronary artery
    disease, 455
  ezetimibe and cholesterol absorption
    inhibitors for, 430
    effect on lipids and lipoproteins of, 430
    efficacy of, 430
    safety of, 430
  fibrates and nicotinic acid for, 428
  high-carbohydrate, low-fat diets for, 442,
    443f
  plant stanol esters for, 430-431
    effects on lipids and lipoproteins of,
      430-431
    efficacy against coronary heart disease
      of, 430-431
    safety of, 431
  statins for. *See* Statin(s).
  mixed, 434-441
    cholesteryl ester transfer protein inhibition
      as, 438-439, 438f
    combination therapy for
      non–HDL-c reduction in, 435, 435t
      rationale for, 434-435, 435f
      statin-fibrate, 436
      statin-niacin, 436-437
      statin–omega 3 fatty acids, 437-438
      therapy to modify HDL in, 435-436
  in pregnancy, 627
Lipid management
  cardiac rehabilitation and, 741b
  after STEMI, 205t, 206
LIPID study, 425
Lipid-lowering therapy
  bile acid sequestrants in, 428-430, 429t
    clinical efficacy of, 429, 429t
    effects on lipids and lipoproteins of, 429
    safety/compliance issues for, 429-430
  for carotid artery disease, 556-557
  combination therapy as
    non–HDL-c reduction in, 435, 435t
    rationale for, 434-435, 435f
    statin-fibrate, 436
    statin-niacin, 436-437
    statin–omega 3 fatty acids, 437-438
    therapy to modify HDL in, 435-436
  ezetimibe and cholesterol absorption
    inhibitors in, 430
    effect on lipids and lipoproteins of, 430
    efficacy of, 430
    safety of, 430
  fibrates and nicotinic acid in, 428
  high-carbohydrate, low-fat diets in, 442,
    443f
  with HIV infection, 733, 733f
  for peripheral artery disease, 541-542
  plant stanol esters in, 430-431
    effects on lipids and lipoproteins of,
      430-431
    efficacy against coronary heart disease of,
      430-431
    safety of, 431
  in pregnancy, 627
  for secondary prevention of coronary events,
    146-147, 148f
  statins in. *See* Statin(s).
Lipodystrophy, HIV infection and, 731
Liposorber-D, 456-457, 457f, 457t
Lisinopril (Prinivil, Zestril)
  for heart failure, 246, 246t

Lisinopril (Prinivil, Zestril) *(Continued)*
  for hypertension, 478t
    in children, 536t
    after STEMI, 192
Lisinopril/hydrochlorothiazide (Prinzide,
    Zestoretic), for hypertension, 485t
Listeria, after cardiac transplantation, 312
LITE study, 580
Literature synthesis. *See* Meta-analysis.
Liver toxicity, of statins, 424-426, 427f, 428b
Liver transplantation, for severe
    hypercholesterolemia, 459-460, 459t
  cholesterol lowering via, 460
  risks and benefits of, 460
  treatment guidelines for, 460
Lixiana (edoxaban), 160t
LMWH. *See* Low-molecular-weight heparin
    (LMWH).
Lo-Aqua. *See* Furosemide.
Loeys-Dietz syndrome, thoracic aortic
    aneurysms in, 608
Löffler hypereosinophilic syndrome, 339-340
Löffler syndrome, 339-340
Loniten (minoxidil), for hypertension, 483,
    483t
  in children, 536t
Look AHEAD trial, 446
Loop diuretics
  for heart failure, 243-244, 243t
  for hypertension, 480t, 481
  for peripheral edema in pregnancy, 623
Lopinavir, for HIV infection, 729t
Lopressor. *See* Metoprolol (Lopressor, Toprol).
Lopressor HCT (metoprolol tartrate/
    hydrochlorothiazide), for hypertension,
    485t
Losartan potassium (Cozaar)
  for heart failure, 246-248, 246t, 250
  for hypertension, 479t
    in children, 536t
  for maintenance of sinus rhythm, 377
  in pregnancy and lactation, 622t-623t
Losartan potassium/hydrochlorothiazide
    (Hyzaar), for hypertension, 485t
Lotensin (benazepril), for hypertension,
    478t
  in children, 536t
Lotensin HCT (benazepril/
    hydrochlorothiazide), for hypertension,
    485t
Lotrel (amlodipine besylate/benazepril
    hydrochloride), for hypertension, 485t
Lotus Valve, 720f, 720t, 721
Lovastatin
  clinical trials of, 423
  dosage of, 422t
  pharmacodynamics and pharmacokinetics
    of, 60t, 422t
  in pregnancy, 627
"Low fat," 471t
"Low saturated fat," 471t
"Low sodium," 471t
Low-density lipoprotein apheresis (LDLA),
    454-458
  benefits of, 457-458
  comparison of methods of, 457t
  failure to treat individuals who may benefit
    from, 458
  risks of, 457
  technical aspects of, 455-457, 456f
  using dextran sulfate cellulose columns, 456,
    456f
  using heparin-induced extracorporeal LDL
    precipitation, 456, 457f, 457t
  using immunoadsorption columns, 456, 456f,
    457t
  using whole blood–compatible systems,
    456-457, 457f, 457t

Low-density lipoprotein (LDL) cholesterol
elevated
bile acid sequestrants for, 428-430, 429t
clinical efficacy of, 429, 429t
effects on lipids and lipoproteins of, 429
safety/compliance issues for, 429-430
combination therapy for
non–HDL-c reduction in, 435, 435t
rationale for, 434-435, 435f
statin-fibrate, 436
statin-niacin, 436-437
statin–omega 3 fatty acids, 437-438
therapy to modify HDL in, 435-436
with concentrations of more than 200 mg/
dL and coronary artery disease, 455
with concentrations of more than 300 mg/
dL without coronary artery disease,
455
ezetimibe and cholesterol absorption
inhibitors for, 430
effect on lipids and lipoproteins of, 430
efficacy of, 430
safety of, 430
fibrates and nicotinic acid for, 428
high-carbohydrate, low-fat diets for, 442,
443f
plant stanol esters for, 430-431
effects on lipids and lipoproteins of,
430-431
efficacy against coronary heart disease
of, 430-431
safety of, 431
statins for. See Statin(s).
HIV infection and, 730, 731f
Low-fat diets, for hyperlipidemia, 443-444
Low–glycemic index diet, 445
Low-molecular-weight heparin (LMWH),
117-118
dosages of, 118
indications for, 118
mechanisms of action of, 117-118
for NSTE-ACS, 159-161, 160t, 161f
in pregnancy and lactation, 622t-623t, 625
side effects and contraindications to, 118
for STEMI, 182-183, 184f
for thromboprophylaxis, 591-592
for venous thromboembolism, 588
Low-output state, after STEMI, 193, 194f-195f
Lozol (indapamide)
for heart failure, 243t
for hypertension, 480t
LR (likelihood ratio), 2, 2f
LRC CPPT trial, 429, 429t
LSD (lysergic acid diethylamide), hypertensive
emergencies due to, 518
L-type calcium channels, 90
Lung scanning, for pulmonary embolism, 584
Lung transplantation, pulmonary arterial
hypertension, 602
Lutter prosthesis, 722t, 726
LV. See Left ventricular (LV).
LVAD (left ventricular assist device), 315
after STEMI, 198
LVEF. See Left ventricular ejection fraction
(LVEF).
LVH (left ventricular hypertrophy), and
hypertension in children, 533
LVOTO. See Left ventricular outflow tract
obstruction (LVOTO).
Lyon Heart Study, 444
Lysergic acid diethylamide (LSD), hypertensive
emergencies due to, 518

M

MA (mycotic aneurysm), infective endocarditis
with rupture of, 661

Ma huang, hypertensive emergency due to, 511
MAC (mitral annular calcification), 704-705
MACE trial, 560
MADIT II trial, 270-271, 271f, 401, 409f
MADIT trial, 270, 399t, 409f
MADIT-CRT trial, 275, 401, 402t
Magnesium, for ventricular tachycardia
polymorphic, 413-414
sustained monomorphic, 413
Magnesium sulfate
for hypertensive emergencies, 514t-515t
for preeclampsia and eclampsia, 525
Magnet operation, in implantable cardioverter-
defibrillators, 759
Magnetic resonance (MR) coronary
angiography, for chronic stable angina,
134
Magnetic resonance imaging (MRI)
for chronic stable angina, 134
for pulmonary embolism, 585
MAINTAIN registry, 167
Malignancy
cardiac, in HIV-positive patients, 735
after cardiac transplantation, 313-314
prevention of venous thromboembolism in
patients with, 591-592
MAO (monoamine oxidase) inhibitors, and
tyramine, hypertensive emergencies due
to, 518
Maraviroc, for HIV infection, 729
Mardil-BACE system, 722t, 725
Marfan syndrome
in pregnancy, 629
thoracic aortic aneurysms in, 608, 613
MARINE trial, 438
MARISA trial, 106
Markov models, 25
MATCH trial, 557, 558t
Matched controls, 6
Matrix metalloproteinase-9 (MMP-9), and
abdominal aortic aneurysms, 608
Mavik (trandolapril)
for heart failure, 246t
for hypertension, 478t
Maze procedure
for atrial fibrillation, 711
for maintenance of sinus rhythm, 377
minimally invasive, 377
MB fraction of creatine kinase (CK-MB), for
STEMI, 181
MDR1 gene, in pharmacogenetics of
clopidogrel, 55t, 56
therapeutic implications of, 56-57
MDUFMA (Medical Device User Fee and
Modernization Act), 50-51
Mechanical circulatory support (MCS),
314-319
for acute decompensated heart failure,
299
adverse events with, 319, 319t
benefits of, 314
biologic, 314
hemodynamic, 314
configuration of, 314-315
cannulation in, 315
continuous flow in, 314-315, 315f
pulsatile flow in, 314, 315f
considerations prior to, 317-319
cardiac, 317-318
noncardiac, 318
other, 318-319
surgical, 318
indications for, 315
timing of, 315-317
as bridge to transplant, 316, 316f
elective, 316
emergent, 315-316

Mechanical circulatory support (MCS)
(Continued)
INTERMACS profile in, 317, 317f, 317t
risk models in, 316-317
univentricular vs. biventricular, 315
Mechanical complications, of STEMI,
196-198
Mechanical failure, of biomaterials, 42f, 48,
49f
Mechanical support, for high-risk percutaneous
coronary intervention, 224
Mechanical support devices, after STEMI,
198
Mechanical valves, 695-697
characteristics of, 696t
currently available, 695t, 696f
pregnancy with, 626
valve-related complications with, 697, 697t,
698f
Mechanical ventilation, for STEMI with
pulmonary congestion, 194
Median sternotomy, for valve surgery, 694
Medical device(s). See also Cardiovascular
(CV) devices.
classification of, 42-43
development of, 41-52
overview of, 41-42, 42f
reimbursement for, 51
trials in
endpoints and surrogate endpoints for,
45-46
foreign, 46
independent oversight of, 46
randomized vs. nonrandomized, 44-45
study blinding for, 46
ensuring safety of, 48-50
cardiologist's role in, 50
device safety and failure concepts for,
47-48, 49f
postmarket assessment tools for, 48-50,
48b
product recall and Center for Devices and
Radiological Health for, 50
reasonable vs. absolute assurance for, 47
risk and benefit in, 47-48
total product life cycle approach to, 47,
47f
failure of, 42f, 47-48, 49f
labeling and off-label use of, 46-47
overview of, 41, 42f
vs. drugs, 42, 43t
preamendment, 43
predicate, 43
regulation of
CDRH interactions with external
stakeholders and government
partners in, 51
for combination products, 50-51
contemporary issues in, 44-47
fundamentals of, 42-44
history of, 42-43
other key topics in, 50-51
pathway for, 43-44, 44f
501(K) premarket notification in, 41-43
Humanitarian Device Exemption in, 44
Investigational Device Exemption in,
41-44
premarket approval application in, 41-43
role of advisory panel in, 51
violative, 50
Medical Device Amendments, 43
Medical device errors, 42f, 47-48, 49f
Medical Device User Fee and Modernization
Act (MDUFMA), 50-51
Medical Dictionary for Regulatory Activities
(MedDRA), 38
Mediterranean diet, 446, 448-450, 450f, 451t
Medtronic ATS prosthetic valve, 695-697

Medtronic CoreValve Revalving System, 715, 715f, 720t
Medtronic Engager transapical valve, 721, 721f
Medtronic Freestyle stentless porcine full-root bioprosthesis, 695t, 696f, 699
Medtronic Melody transcatheter pulmonary valve, 720t
  for tetralogy of Fallot, 644
Medtronic Mosaic stented porcine mitral bioprosthesis, 695t, 696f, 697
Medtronic 3F valve, 699
Medtronic Ventor transapical valve, 721, 721f
Medtronic-Hall tilting disc mechanical valve, 695-697, 695t, 696f
Megatrials, 6-7
MELODIE trial, 546
Melody transcatheter pulmonary valve, 720t
  for tetralogy of Fallot, 644
Melphalan, for cardiac amyloidosis, 337
MEN (multiple endocrine neoplasia) type 2A, pheochromocytomas in, 490, 491t
MEN (multiple endocrine neoplasia) type 2B, pheochromocytomas in, 490, 491t
MERCOSUR (Common Market of the South), 37
MERIT-HF trial
  choice of β-blocker in, 253
  clinical efficacy in, 251t
  congestive heart failure in, 251
  and implantable cardioverter-defibrillators, 270
  practical considerations in, 252-253
  race-stratified data in, 262
MERLIN-TIMI 36 trial, 106, 155, 261
MES (microembolic signals), in carotid artery disease, 557, 566
Mesenchymal stromal cells (MSCs), 323-324
  and clinical studies, 326
Meta-analysis, 15-19, 17f
  in comparative effectiveness research, 20-21, 22t
  complexity of, 15-16, 17f
  cumulative, 16-17, 18f-19f
  defined, 15
  fundamental principle of, 15
  future trends in, 18, 20f-21f
  history of, 15
  indirect, 20-21
  meta-regression in, 17-18
  pooling of data in, 15-16, 17f
  reading and interpretation of, 18-19, 21b
  weighted average in, 15
Metabolic benefits, of physical training, 739, 739b
Metabolic effects, of HIV infection and HAART, 730-731
Metabolic syndrome, 204
  and chronic stable angina, 140
  HIV infection and, 731
Metabolic syndrome X, 168
Meta-regression, 17-18
Metformin, with heart failure, 262
Methamphetamines, NSTE-ACS due to, 169-170, 170b
Methicillin-sensitive Staphylococcus aureus (MSSA), endocarditis due to, 654
Methyldopa (Aldomet), for hypertension, 483, 483t
  in pregnancy, 524t
α-Methyl-L-tyrosine (metyrosine), for hypertension, due to pheochromocytoma, 492t, 493
Metolazone (Mykrox, Zaroxolyn)
  for heart failure, 243t, 245
  for hypertension, 480t
Metoprolol (Lopressor, Toprol)
  for atrial fibrillation, 373t
  for congestive cardiomyopathy, 100

Metoprolol (Lopressor, Toprol) (Continued)
  drug interactions with, 105t
  for heart failure, 246t, 251-253
  for hypertension, 481t
    in children, 536t
    in pregnancy, 524t
  indications for, 101
  long-acting sustained-release, 103
  pharmacodynamic properties and cardiac effects of, 98t
  pharmacokinetics of, 103
  pharmacology of, 250
  in pregnancy and lactation, 622t-623t
  properties of, 102t
  for STEMI
    in acute phase, 183-184
    during convalescence, 192
    choice of β-blocker in, 253
    clinical efficacy in, 251t
    congestive heart failure in, 251
    and implantable cardioverter-defibrillators, 270
    practical considerations in, 252-253
    race-stratified data in, 262
Metoprolol tartrate/hydrochlorothiazide (Lopressor HCT), for hypertension, 485t
Metyrosine, for hypertension due to pheochromocytoma, 492t, 493
Mexico, regulation of new drugs in, 37
Mexiletine, 347-348
  adverse reactions to, 347
  clinical applications of, 347
  clinical pharmacology of, 347
  dosage and administration of, 347
    modification in disease states of, 347
  drug interactions with, 348
  mechanism of action of, 347
  in pregnancy and lactation, 622t-623t
MI. See Myocardial infarction (MI).
MiCardia device, 722t
Micardis (telmisartan), for hypertension, 479t
Micardis HCT (telmisartan/hydrochlorothiazide), for hypertension, 485t
Microembolic signals (MES), in carotid artery disease, 557, 566
Microzide. See Hydrochlorothiazide.
MICS CABG (minimally invasive coronary artery bypass grafting), 228, 228f
Midamor. See Amiloride (Midamor).
MIDCAB (minimally invasive direct coronary artery bypass), 227-228, 228f
  thoracoscopic, 228
MI-FREE trial, 165
Migraine, patent foramen ovale and, 639
Mild Carvedilol Heart Failure study, 250
Millipede ring system, 722t, 725, 725f
Milrinone, for heart failure, 257
  acute decompensated, 294-295, 294f
Mineralocorticoid excess, hypertension due to, 497-499
Mineralocorticoid excess syndromes, apparent, hypertension due to, 498-499
Mineralocorticoid receptor antagonists. See Aldosterone receptor antagonists (ARAs).
Minimally invasive coronary artery bypass grafting (MICS CABG), 228, 228f
Minimally invasive direct coronary artery bypass (MIDCAB), 227-228, 228f
  thoracoscopic, 228
Minimally invasive surgical (MIS) approach
  for atrial fibrillation, 390
  for valve surgery, 694, 694f
Minimally invasive surgical (MIS) coronary revascularization, 225-230
  direct, 227-228, 228f

Minimally invasive surgical (MIS) coronary revascularization (Continued)
  multivessel, 228-229, 229f
  off-pump, 225-227, 226f
  robotically assisted, 229-230, 230f
  small-access, 227-230, 227t
  thoracoscopic direct, 228
Minipress (prazosin), for hypertension, 483t
  due to pheochromocytoma, 491-493, 492t
Minitrials, 6-7
Minoxidil (Loniten), for hypertension, 483, 483t
  in children, 536t
MIRACLE trial, 273-274, 274f
MIRACLE-ICD trial, 274
MIS (minimally invasive surgical) approach. See Minimally invasive surgical (MIS) approach.
Missing data, in clinical trials, 12, 13t
Mission: Lifeline program, 69, 179
MIST trial, 639
Mitochondrial gene mutations, cardiomyopathy associated with, 339
MitraClip device, 722, 722f-723f, 722t
MitraFlex device, 722t, 725
Mitral annular calcification (MAC), 704-705
Mitral annuloplasty, percutaneous approaches to, 722t, 723
  direct, 722t, 724-725, 725f
  indirect, 722t, 723
    with asymmetrical approach, 722t
    with coronary sinus approach, 722t, 723, 723f
Mitral insufficiency, 683-687
  assessment of severity of, 683-685, 685t
    overall approach to, 686-687, 687f
  functional (ischemic), 686-687
  timing of intervention for, 686
    in asymptomatic patients, 686
    in symptomatic patients, 686
Mitral leaflet prolapse repair, 705
Mitral regurgitation (MR), 683-687
  assessment of severity of, 683-685, 685t
    overall approach to, 686-687, 687f
  in CABG patients, 710-711, 711f
  Carpentier's functional classification of, 703-704, 703f, 703t
  functional (ischemic), 686-687
  indications for surgical intervention in, 704
  due to LVOT obstruction, 333, 333f
  in pregnancy, 623-624
  after repair of congenital heart defects, 648f
  after STEMI, 196-197, 197t
  timing of intervention for, 686
    in asymptomatic patients, 686
    in symptomatic patients, 686
Mitral solutions device, 722t
Mitral stenosis, 678-681
  assessment of severity of, 678-680, 679b, 680t
  indications for surgical intervention in, 704
  in pregnancy, 624
  surgical approaches to, 681, 681t
  timing of intervention for, 680-681
    in asymptomatic patients, 680, 680f
    with left atrial or left atrial appendage thrombosis, 680-681
    with mild symptoms, 680, 681f
    with moderate to severe symptoms, 680, 681f
  overall approach to, 680-681
Mitral valve (MV)
  surgical anatomy of, 703, 703f
  systolic anterior motion of, 332-333
Mitral valve area (MVA), 678-680, 680t
Mitral valve (MV) disease
  aortic valve disease with, 709
  percutaneous treatment for, 721-726, 722t

Mitral valve (MV) disease (Continued)
　　chamber remodeling in, 722t, 724, 724f
　　chordal implantation in, 722t, 725, 725f
　　direct annuloplasty in, 722t, 724-725, 725f
　　leaflet repair in, 722-724, 722f-723f, 722t
　　mitral valve replacement in, 725-726, 726f
　　ventricular remodeling in, 722t, 725
　　surgical treatment for. See Mitral valve (MV)
　　　surgery.
　　tricuspid regurgitation with, 709
Mitral valve (MV) prolapse
　　β-adrenergic blockers for, 100
　　surgical repair of, 705
Mitral valve (MV) repair, 704-706
　　annuloplasty in, 704-705
　　leaflet prolapse repair techniques in, 705
　　other techniques in, 706
　　percutaneous, 721-726, 722t
　　　chamber remodeling in, 722t, 724, 724f
　　　chordal implantation in, 722t, 725, 725f
　　　direct annuloplasty in, 722t, 724-725, 725f
　　　leaflet repair in, 722-724, 722f-723f, 722t
　　　ventricular remodeling in, 722t, 725
　　principles of, 703f, 704
　　restricted leaflet techniques in, 705-706
　　timing of, 681t
Mitral valve (MV) replacement, 706
　　choice of prosthesis for, 706, 706f
　　chordal-sparing, 706
　　percutaneous, 725-726, 726f
Mitral valve (MV) surgery, 702-708
　　Carpentier's functional classification and,
　　　703-704, 703f, 703t
　　indications for, 704
　　for mitral insufficiency/regurgitation, 686,
　　　704
　　　in asymptomatic patients, 686
　　　in symptomatic patients, 686
　　for mitral stenosis, 680-681, 704
　　　in asymptomatic patients, 680, 680f
　　　with left atrial or left atrial appendage
　　　　thrombosis, 680-681
　　　overall approach to, 680-681
　　　in patients with mild symptoms, 680, 681f
　　　in patients with moderate to severe
　　　　symptoms, 680, 681f
　　mitral valve repair as, 704-706
　　　annuloplasty in, 704-705
　　　leaflet prolapse repair techniques in, 705
　　　other techniques in, 706
　　　principles of, 703f, 704
　　　restricted leaflet techniques in, 705-706
　　　timing of, 681t
　　mitral valve replacement as, 706
　　　choice of prosthesis for, 706, 706f
　　　chordal-sparing, 706
　　overview of, 702-704, 702f
　　preoperative evaluation for, 704
　　results of, 706-708
　　　early, 706-707
　　　late, 707-708, 707f
　　surgical anatomy for, 703, 703f
Mitralign device, 722t, 724f
Mitralign Percutaneous Annuloplasty System,
　　725
MitroFLow valve, 697
Mixed α-/β-adrenergic blockers, for
　　hypertension, 481-482, 481t
　　due to pheochromocytoma, 492t, 493
Mixed aortic valve disease, 699-700
Mixed dyslipidemia, 434-441
　　cholesteryl ester transfer protein inhibition
　　　as, 438-439, 438f
　　combination therapy for
　　　non–HDL-c reduction in, 435, 435t
　　　rationale for, 434-435, 435f
　　　statin-fibrate, 436

Mixed dyslipidemia (Continued)
　　statin-niacin, 436-437
　　statin–omega 3 fatty acids, 437-438
　　therapy to modify HDL in, 435-436
MMF (mycophenolate mofetil), with cardiac
　　transplantation, 311t
MMP-9 (matrix metalloproteinase-9), and
　　abdominal aortic aneurysms, 608
MOCHA study, 250, 252-253
Modeling approaches, for cost-effectiveness
　　analysis, 25-26, 25f
Moderate unsaturated fat diets, for
　　hyperlipidemia, 444-445, 444t
Moexipril (Univasc), for hypertension, 478t
Moexipril/hydrochlorothiazide (Uniretic), for
　　hypertension, 485t
Monarc transvenous annuloplasty device, 722t,
　　723f, 724
Monoamine oxidase (MAO) inhibitors, and
　　tyramine, hypertensive emergencies due
　　to, 518
Monoclonal antibodies, with cardiac
　　transplantation, 311t
Monopril (fosinopril)
　　for heart failure, 246t
　　for hypertension, 478t
　　　in children, 536t
Monounsaturated fat diets, for hyperlipidemia,
　　444-445
Monte Carlo simulations, 27, 29f
MOOSE study, 15
Morphine sulfate, for STEMI, 181-182
Morphologic benefits, of physical training, 738,
　　739b
Mosaic stented porcine mitral bioprosthesis,
　　695t, 696f, 697
MOSES study, 476, 556
M-PATHY study, 334-335
MR. See Mitral regurgitation (MR).
MR (magnetic resonance) coronary
　　angiography, for chronic stable angina,
　　134
MRFIT trial, 556
MRI (magnetic resonance imaging)
　　for chronic stable angina, 134
　　for pulmonary embolism, 585
MSCs (mesenchymal stromal cells), 323-324
　　and clinical studies, 326
MSSA (methicillin-sensitive Staphylococcus
　　aureus), endocarditis due to, 654
Multicentre Thermocool Ventricular
　　Tachycardia Ablation Trial, 391
Multidisciplinary risk-factor intervention, 740
Multiple endocrine neoplasia (MEN) type 2A,
　　pheochromocytomas in, 490, 491t
Multiple endocrine neoplasia (MEN) type 2B,
　　pheochromocytomas in, 490, 491t
Multivessel small thoracotomy (MVST), 228,
　　228f
Muscle toxicity, of statins, 427-428, 428b
Musculoskeletal changes, due to cyanosis, 634
Mustard procedure, 633t
MUSTIC trials, 273
MUSTT trial, 270-271, 399t, 409f
MV. See Mitral valve (MV).
MVA (mitral valve area), 678-680, 680t
MVST (multivessel small thoracotomy), 228,
　　228f
Mycobacterial pericarditis, 672-673
Mycobacterium avium-intracellulare, pericarditis
　　due to, 672
Mycobacterium tuberculosis, pericarditis due to,
　　672-673
Mycophenolate mofetil (MMF), with cardiac
　　transplantation, 311t
Mycophenolic acid, with cardiac
　　transplantation, 311t

Mycotic aneurysm (MA), infective endocarditis
　　with rupture of, 661
Myectomy, surgical, for LVOT obstruction, 332,
　　333f, 334t
Mykrox (metolazone)
　　for heart failure, 243t, 245
　　for hypertension, 480t
Myocardial infarction (MI)
　　acute
　　　β-adrenergic blockers for survivors of, 99
　　　bone marrow cells for, 324
　　　mesenchymal stromal cells for, 326
　　angina and, 131, 132f-133f
　　cardiac rehabilitation after, 739-745
　　　contraindications to, 743-744, 744b
　　　disability and, 739-740
　　　evolving landscape for, 745
　　　inpatient
　　　　exercise testing before discharge and,
　　　　　740
　　　　in-hospital exercise in, 740
　　　　patient education on, 740
　　　meta-analysis for survival after, 744-745
　　　outpatient, 740-742
　　　　core components for, 740-742, 741b
　　　　exercise prescription for, 742-743, 743f
　　　　maintenance program for, 741-742, 742t
　　　　monitoring in, 741, 742b
　　　　resistance exercise in, 743
　　　　safety of, 741
　　catheter ablation for ventricular tachycardia
　　　with healed, 391-392, 391f
　　disability from, 739-740
　　and heart failure, 284-285
　　HIV infection and, 731-732
　　implantable cardioverter-defibrillators after,
　　　272
　　pericarditis after, 673
　　in pregnancy, 626
　　ST-segment elevation. See ST-segment
　　　elevation myocardial infarction
　　　(STEMI).
　　ventricular septal rupture after, 647, 648f
Myocardial injury, in heart failure, 284, 284f
Myocardial involvement, in HIV infection, 734
Myocardial ischemia, "silent," β-adrenergic
　　blockers for, 99-100
Myocardial niches, 327, 328f-329f
Myocardial perfusion, exercise training and,
　　739
Myocardial perfusion imaging, after STEMI, 203
Myocardial perfusion scintigraphy, for chronic
　　stable angina, 134-135, 135b, 137t
Myocardial regeneration, circulating progenitor
　　cells and, 322-323, 323f-324f
Myocardial repair, by exogenous and
　　endogenous progenitor cells, 322, 324f
Myocardial viability, after STEMI, 204
Myocarditis, heart failure with, 262-263,
　　300-301
Myocarditis Treatment Trial, 263
Myocardium
　　hibernating, 261
　　storage diseases of, 339
　　"stunned", 133-134
Myocyte(s), 322
　　death and regeneration of, 322, 323f
　　in aging heart, 330
Myolimus-based stents, 220-221
Myopathy, statin-associated, 427-428, 428b
Myxedema pericardial disease, 674

N

N-acetylprocainamide (acecainide, NAPA)
　　adverse reactions to, 349

N-acetylprocainamide (acecainide, NAPA) (Continued)
  clinical applications of, 348
  clinical pharmacology of, 348
  dosage and administration of, 348
    modification in disease states of, 348-349
  drug interactions with, 349
  mechanism of action of, 348
  for sustained monomorphic ventricular tachycardia, 410
Nadolol (Corgard)
  for hypertension, 481t
  indications for, 101
  pharmacodynamic properties and cardiac effects of, 98t
  pharmacokinetics of, 103
  properties of, 102t
Nadolol/bendroflumethiazide (Corzide), for hypertension, 485t
Nadroparin, for thromboprophylaxis, 591-592
Nafcillin, for infective endocarditis, 655t
NAPA. See N-acetylprocainamide (acecainide, NAPA).
NASCET trial, 560, 560f, 561t
National Cardiovascular Data Registry, 179
National Cholesterol Education Program Adult Treatment Panel III (NCEP ATP III)
  non–HDL-c goal of, 434
  Therapeutic Lifestyle Changes diet of, 192
National Heart, Lung and Blood Institute (NHLBI) Type II Intervention Study, 429, 429t
National Institutes of Health (NIH), Roadmap for Medical Research of, 39
National Lipid Association Statin Safety Assessment Task Force, 424-426
Native valve endocarditis (NVE), antibiotics for, 654
Natural History of Congenital Heart Defects Studies, 640-641
N-binding site, of calcium channel blockers, 90
NCEP ATP III (National Cholesterol Education Program Adult Treatment Panel III)
  non–HDL-c goal of, 434
  Therapeutic Lifestyle Changes diet of, 192
NDA (new drug application) fees, 38-39
NDHPs. See Nondihydropyridines (NDHPs).
Nebivolol (Bystolic)
  for heart failure, 252-253
  for hypertension, 481t
  indications for, 101
  for peripheral artery disease, 542
  pharmacodynamic properties and cardiac effects of, 98t
  properties of, 102t
Negative predictive value (NPV), 1-2, 2f
NeoChord device, 722t, 725
Neoplastic pericarditis, 673
Nesiritide, for acute decompensated heart failure, 292-293, 293f
Net clinical benefit, 13
Net reclassification improvement, 3
Neurofibromatosis type 1, pheochromocytomas in, 490, 491t
Neurohormonal hypothesis, of nitrate tolerance, 88
Neurologic effects, of cyanotic congenital heart disease, 634-635
Neurologic presentations, hypertensive emergencies with, 515-516, 516f
  hemorrhagic cerebrovascular syndromes as, 516
  hypertensive encephalopathy as, 516, 517f
  intracerebral hemorrhage as, 516, 516f
  ischemic cerebrovascular syndromes as, 515-516
  subarachnoid hemorrhage as, 516

Neurologic prognostication, after cardiac arrest, 417-418
Nevirapine, for HIV infection, 730t
Nevo stent, 221
New drug application (NDA) fees, 38-39
New drug development. See Drug development.
Newborn, risk of cardiac drugs to, 621, 622t-623t
NHLBI (National Heart, Lung and Blood Institute) Type II Intervention Study, 429, 429t
Niacin
  additive effects of, 435t
  for mixed dyslipidemia, 436-437
  for peripheral artery disease, 541-542
  in pregnancy, 627
Nicardipine (Cardene)
  for acute hypertensive crisis due to pheochromocytoma, 493, 493t
  for hypertension, 479t
    due to pheochromocytoma, 492t, 493
  for hypertensive emergencies, 514t-515t
Nicorandil, for chronic stable angina, 104, 105f, 141
Nicotinic acid, for lowing of LDL cholesterol, 428
Nifedipine (Adalat, Nifedical, Procardia), 93
  with β-adrenergic blockers, 99
  for hypertension, 479t
    in children, 536t
  pharmacodynamic effects of, 91t
  in pregnancy and lactation, 622t-623t
NIH (National Institutes of Health), Roadmap for Medical Research of, 39
NIH-Cerclage technology, 722t
NIPPV (noninvasive positive-pressure ventilation), for acute pulmonary edema, 300, 301f
Nisoldipine (Sular), for hypertension, 479t
Nitinol self-expanding stent, for carotid artery stenosis, 563
Nitrates, organic. See Organic nitrates.
Nitric oxide (NO), for pulmonary arterial hypertension, 604
Nitric oxide (NO) potentiating effect, of β-adrenergic blockers, 103
Nitroglycerin
  for acute decompensated heart failure, 292, 292t
  for acute pulmonary edema, 300
  history of, 83
  for hypertensive emergencies, 514t-515t
  mechanisms of action of, 83-84
  nonhemodynamic effects of, 88-89
  for NSTE-ACS, 153-154, 154f
  pharmacodynamic effects of, 84, 86f
  pharmacokinetics of, 84, 87t
  in pregnancy and lactation, 622t-623t, 626-627
  side effects of, 84-85, 87t
  for STEMI
    in acute phase, 181
    during convalescence, 192
    with pulmonary congestion, 193
  sublingual, 85, 86t-87t
Nitroprusside
  for acute decompensated heart failure, 293, 294f-295f
  for acute hypertensive crisis due to pheochromocytoma, 493, 493t
  for acute pulmonary edema, 300, 301f
  for aortic dissection, 613
  for hypertensive emergencies, 514t-515t
  in pregnancy and lactation, 622t-623t
NNH (number needed to harm), 13
  in balancing risks and benefits, 22-23
  in detection of treatment effects, 15

NNRTIs (nonnucleoside reverse transcriptase inhibitors), for HIV infection, 729, 730t
NNT (number needed to treat), 13
  in balancing risks and benefits, 22-23
NO (nitric oxide), for pulmonary arterial hypertension, 604
No output condition, 752
NO (nitric oxide) potentiating effect, of β-adrenergic blockers, 103
"No salt added", 471t
Nobori stent, 221
NOMASS study, 553, 555
Noncardiac surgery, in adults with congenital heart disease, 636
  recommendations for, 636
Nondihydropyridines (NDHPs), 89
  with β-adrenergic blockers, 99
  classification of, 91
  for hypertension, 477t, 479-480, 479t
    monitoring and adverse effects of, 485t
  for NSTE-ACS, 154-155
  for paroxysmal supraventricular tachycardia, 368, 369t
Nondipping pattern, in ambulatory blood pressure monitoring, 501-502
Non–high-density lipoprotein cholesterol (non–HDL-c)
  goals for
    lack of achievement of, 434
    of NCEP, 434
  reduction of, 435, 435t
Noninferiority margin, 8
Noninferiority trials, 8
Noninvasive positive-pressure ventilation (NIPPV), for acute pulmonary edema, 300, 301f
Nonnucleoside reverse transcriptase inhibitors (NNRTIs), for HIV infection, 729, 730t
Nonrandomized concurrent control studies, 7
Nonrandomized studies, of medical devices, 44-45
Nonremodeling annuloplasty, in mitral valve repair, 705
Non–ST-elevation acute coronary syndrome (NSTE-ACS), 153-177
  anticoagulants for, 159-163, 159f, 160t
    direct thrombin inhibitors as, 161-162, 162f
    factor Xa inhibitors as, 162-163, 163f
    other, 163
    recommendations on, 163, 169b
    unfractionated heparin and low-molecular-weight heparin as, 159-161, 160t-161t, 161f
  antiischemic medications for, 153-155
    β-adrenergic receptor blockers as, 154
    calcium channel antagonists as, 154-155
    nitrates as, 153-154, 154f
    ranolazine as, 155
  antiplatelet agents for, 155-157, 155b
    aspirin as, 155-156, 155f
    clopidogrel as, 156, 156f
    duration of, 157
    intravenous platelet inhibitors as, 158-159, 158f, 159b
    P2Y$_{12}$ antagonists as, 156
    platelet function testing and genetics for, 157-159
    prasugrel as, 156-157
    ticagrelor as, 157
  clinical risk score for, 153, 154t
  hospital discharge and postdischarge care for, 165-172
    for cardiac syndrome X, 168-169, 169b, 170f
    cholesterol treatment in, 167-168, 167f-168f
    with chronic kidney disease, 172
    with cocaine and methamphetamine use, 169-170, 170b

Non–ST-elevation acute coronary syndrome
(NSTE-ACS) (Continued)
with diabetes, 168, 170-171, 171b
diet in, 168
for elderly, 171
exercise in, 168
influenza vaccine in, 168
lifestyle modifications in, 165, 166t
medications in, 165, 166b
ACE inhibitors and ARBs as, 166-167
anticoagulants as, 166
antiplatelet agents as, 166
barriers to compliance with, 165, 165f
β-blockers as, 167
multidisciplinary approach to, 165, 166b
smoking cessation in, 167-168
for women, 171-172
invasive vs. conservative strategy for cardiac
catheterization for, 163-165, 164f
Non–ST-elevation myocardial infarction
(NSTEMI). See Non–ST-elevation acute
coronary syndrome (NSTE-ACS).
Nonsteroidal anti-inflammatory drugs (NSAIDs)
for pericarditis
acute, 667
recurrent, 668
for postpericardial injury syndrome, 673
Norepinephrine
for acute decompensated heart failure, 296
for acute pulmonary edema, 300, 300f
Normodyne. See Labetalol (Trandate,
Normodyne).
Northern New England Cardiovascular Disease
Study Group, 706-707
Norvasc. See Amlodipine (Norvasc).
Novolimus-based stents, 220-221
nPA (lanoteplase), 123t
NPV (negative predictive value), 1-2, 2f
NRTIs (nucleoside/nucleotide reverse
transcriptase inhibitors), for HIV infection,
729, 730t
NSAIDs (nonsteroidal anti-inflammatory drugs)
for pericarditis
acute, 667
recurrent, 668
for postpericardial injury syndrome, 673
NSTE-ACS. See Non–ST-elevation acute
coronary syndrome (NSTE-ACS).
NSTEMI (non–ST-elevation myocardial
infarction). See Non–ST-elevation acute
coronary syndrome (NSTE-ACS).
Nucleoside/nucleotide reverse transcriptase
inhibitors (NRTIs), for HIV infection, 729,
730t
Null hypothesis, 8f, 9
Number needed to harm (NNH), 13
in balancing risks and benefits, 22-23
in detection of treatment effects,
15
Number needed to treat (NNT), 13
in balancing risks and benefits, 22-23
Nutritional impairment, and mechanical
circulatory support, 318
NVE (native valve endocarditis), antibiotics for,
654

O

OASIS-2 trial, 119
OASIS-5 trial, 162
OASIS-6 trial, 121
OAT trial, 190
Obesity, 446-450
Atkins diet for, 446
and chronic stable angina, 140
clinical assessment of, 446-448, 447t
DASH diet for, 448-450, 449t

Obesity (Continued)
determination of calorie levels for weight
loss for, 448
diet composition for, 446, 446f
epidemiology of, 446
and global cardiovascular disease, 81
goals for weight loss and management for,
448
health consequences of, 446
and hypertension, 471
Mediterranean diet for, 446, 448-450, 450f,
451t
physical activity for, 448, 450, 452t
2010 Dietary Guidelines for, 448
Objective Performance Criteria (OPC), 45
Observation studies, 7
in comparative effectiveness research, 21-22,
22t
Obstructive sleep apnea (OSA), and
hypertension, 465, 502-504, 503t
Occupational activities, energy costs of,
741-742, 742t
OCP (Office of Combination Products),
50-51
OCT (optical coherence tomography), for
assessment of coronary lesion severity,
224-225
Odds ratio (OR), 12
Office of Combination Products (OCP), 50-51
Off-label use, 36
of cardiovascular devices, 46
Off-pump coronary artery bypass (OPCAB),
225-227, 226f
OHCA (out-of-hospital cardiac arrest)
quality improvement for, 72
systems of care for, 70
need for, 67-68
Olmesartan medoxomil (Benicar), for
hypertension, 479t
in children, 536t
Olmesartan medoxomil/amlodipine/
hydrochlorothiazide (Tribenzor), for
hypertension, 485t
Olmesartan medoxomil/hydrochlorothiazide
(Benicar HCT), for hypertension, 485t
Omecantiv mecarbil, for acute decompensated
heart failure, 302-303
Omega-3 fatty acids
additive effects of, 435t
for mixed dyslipidemia, 437-438
to prevent coronary heart disease, 445-446
OMNI Heart Study, 445, 445t
One-way sensitivity analysis, 26, 26f-27f
On-pump coronary artery bypass (ONCAB),
225, 226f
ONSET/OFFFSET trial, 57
ONTARGET trial, 478-479
On-X mechanical valve, 695-697, 695t
OPAT (outpatient parenteral antibiotic
therapy), for infective endocarditis,
655-656
OPC (objective performance criteria), 45
OPCAB (off-pump coronary artery bypass),
225-227, 226f
Open commissurotomy, for mitral stenosis, 681t
Open Pivot prosthesis, 695t
Open sequential design, 6
Open-cell stents, 214
OPO (Organ Procurement Organization), 309
OPTIC study, 258-259
Optical coherence tomography (OCT), for
assessment of coronary lesion severity,
224-225
OPTIMIZE-HF program, 283-286
OR (odds ratio), 12
Oral anticoagulants, 121-123
novel agents as, 122, 122f
warfarin as, 121-122

Oral hypoglycemic agents, labeling of, 35b
Oretic. See Hydrochlorothiazide.
Organ Procurement Organization (OPO), 309
Organic nitrates, 83-89
for acute relief of angina, 141
with β-adrenergic blockers, 99
for chronic stable angina, 141
clinical efficacy of, 85-87
current perspective on, 89
for heart failure, 87
acute decompensated, 297
isosorbide dinitrate as, 297
nitroglycerin as, 292, 292t
nitroprusside as, 293, 294f-295f
in pregnancy, 627
long-acting, 85-87
mechanism of action of, 83-84, 84f-85f
nonhemodynamic effects of, 88-89
for NSTE-ACS, 153-154, 154f
other indications for, 87
overview of, 83
pharmacodynamic effects of, 84, 86f
pharmacokinetics of, 84, 86t
for prevention of anginal episodes, 141
prophylactic use of, 141
side effects of, 84-85, 87t
for STEMI
in acute phase, 181
during convalescence, 192
sublingual, 85, 86t-87t
tolerance to, 83-84, 85f, 87-88
biotransformation hypothesis of, 87-88
free radical hypothesis of, 88
neurohormonal hypothesis of, 88
Ornish diet, for hyperlipidemia, 443-444
Orthostatic hypotension, in elderly patients,
486-487
OSA (obstructive sleep apnea), and
hypertension, 465, 502-504, 503t
Osler, William, 652
Otamixaban, for NSTE-ACS, 163
Outcome measure, selection of, 9, 10f
Out-of-hospital cardiac arrest (OHCA)
quality improvement for, 72
systems of care for, 70
need for, 67-68
Outpatient parenteral antibiotic therapy
(OPAT), for infective endocarditis,
655-656
Overdrive ventricular pacing, for sustained
monomorphic ventricular tachycardia,
413, 413f
Oversensing, 752, 754f
Overview. See Meta-analysis.
Oxacillin, for infective endocarditis, 655t
Oxacillin-resistant staphylococci, endocarditis
due to, 655t
Oxacillin-susceptible staphylococci,
endocarditis due to, 655t
Oxford Community Stroke Project, 555
Oxprenolol, pharmacodynamic properties and
cardiac effects of, 98t
Oxygen
for acute decompensated heart failure,
297-298
for STEMI
in acute phase, 181
with pulmonary congestion, 193
Oxygen consumption, in acute decompensated
heart failure, 290

P

p³ System, 724f
PA. See Primary aldosteronism (PA).
PABV. See Percutaneous aortic balloon
valvuloplasty (PABV).

PAC(s) (pulmonary artery catheters). *See* Pulmonary artery catheters (PACs).
PAC (plasma aldosterone concentration), 495, 495f
PAC-COCATH ISR 1 study, 221-222
Pacemaker (PM)
  permanent, 752
    basic pacing concepts with, 752
      failure to capture as, 752, 754f
      sensing as, 752, 754b, 754f
      stimulation threshold as, 752, 754f
    leads for, 752, 753t
    programming considerations with, 752
      mode as, 752, 755f-757f, 755t
      rate-responsive pacing with, 752, 757t
    pseudo-malfunction of, 752, 757t
    radiographic appearance of, 752, 753f
  temporary, 752-758
    complications and troubleshooting with, 758
    indications for, 752-758, 758f
    placement of, 758
Pacing
  antitachycardia, 759
  biventricular. *See* Cardiac resynchronization therapy (CRT).
  dual-chamber, 752, 755f
  left ventricular, 756f-757f
  for maintenance of sinus rhythm, 378
  rate-responsive, 752, 757t
  right ventricular apical, 756f-757f
Pacing electrodes, for permanent pacemakers, 752, 753t
Pacing mode, programmable, 752, 755f-757f, 755t
Paclitaxel, molecular structure and mechanism of action of, 220f
Paclitaxel-eluting stent(s), 215-217, 216t
  with biodegradable polymers, 221
  for chronic stable angina, 143-144
  for femoral-popliteal disease, 548-549
PAC/PRA (plasma aldosterone concentration/plasma renin activity) ratio, 495, 495f
PAD. *See* Peripheral artery disease (PAD).
PAD trial, 179
PADI trial, 549
PAH. *See* Pulmonary artery hypertension (PAH).
PAH (primary adrenal hyperplasia), 494-496
  surgical treatment of, 496-497
PAINT trial, 221
PALLAS trial, 376-377
Palmaz-Schatz stent, 214
Paniagua Heart Valve, 720t
Papillary muscle rupture, after STEMI, 197t
PAR-1 (protease activated receptor 1)
  antagonists, 115
  for chronic stable angina, 149
Paragangliomas
  catecholamine-secreting, 490
  familial, 490, 491t
Paravalvular leaks, after repair of congenital heart defects, 647, 648f
Paroxysmal supraventricular tachycardias (PSVTs), 366
  defined, 366
  long-term therapy of, 369, 369f
  management of acute episodes of, 367-369, 368f, 369f
  mechanism of, 366-369, 366f-367f
Partial ileal bypass (PIB), 460
  cholesterol lowering via, 459-460
  risks and benefits of, 460
  technique of, 459
PARTNER 1B trial, 718
PARTNER Cohort A trial, 718, 719f, 719t
PARTNER Cohort B trial, 714, 718, 718f
PASEO trial, 216t
PASSION trial, 216t
Patent(s), for new drugs, 39

Patent ductus arteriosus (PDA), 645-646, 646f
  recommendations for, 646
Patent foramen ovale (PFO), 639-640
  and hypoxemia, 639, 640f
  and migraine, 639
  recommendations for, 640
Patient behavioral interventions, for antihypertensive medications, 468
Patient education
  for antihypertensive medications, 468
  after myocardial infarction, 740
Patient triage, for STEMI, 179-180
Patient-prosthesis mismatch (PPM), 701
Patient-specific barriers, to lifestyle modifications for hypertension, 469
PCI. *See* Percutaneous coronary intervention (PCI).
PCI-CURE trial, 111, 112t, 156
PCN (penicillin), for infective endocarditis, 655t-656t
PCP (phencyclidine hydrochloride), hypertensive emergencies due to, 518
PCSK9 as, 61, 62t
PCWP (pulmonary capillary wedge pressure), in acute decompensated heart failure, 285-286, 290
PDA (patent ductus arteriosus), 645-646, 646f
  recommendations for, 646
PDE (phosphodiesterase) inhibitors
  for heart failure, 257
  for pulmonary arterial hypertension, 601-602
PDE-5 (phosphodiesterase 5) inhibitors, for heart failure, 264
PDUFA (Prescription Drug User Fee Act), 38-39
PE. *See* Pulmonary embolism (PE).
PEACE trial, 147
PEITHO study, 590
Penbutolol (Levatrol)
  for hypertension, 481t
  indications for, 101
  pharmacodynamic properties and cardiac effects of, 98t
  properties of, 102t
Penetrance, age-dependent, 332
Penetrating atherosclerotic ulcer, of aorta, 617
Penicillin (PCN), for infective endocarditis, 655t-656t
Pentaerythritol tetranitrate, 85-87
  side effects of, 87t
Pentoxifylline, for intermittent claudication, 543
PEP trial, 592
PEPCAD III study, 222
PEP-CHF study, 259, 260t
Percu-Pro System, 722t
Percutaneous aortic balloon valvuloplasty (PABV), 714
  access site evaluation for, 716
  currently available, 714-715, 715f
  measurement of aortic valve annulus for, 716-717
  new access approaches for, 719
  new applications of, 719
  next generation of, 720-721, 720f, 720t
  patient evaluation and imaging prior to, 715-717, 715f
  patient outcomes with, 717-719, 718f-719f, 719t
  potential complications of, 719-720
  transapical valves in, 721, 721f
  transcatheter implantation procedure for, 717-721, 717f
Percutaneous coronary intervention (PCI)
  for chronic stable angina, 141-144
    antiplatelet therapy with, 144
    complications of, 144
    vs. coronary artery bypass graft, 142-143
    after coronary artery bypass grafting, 143
    culprit lesions, 143

Percutaneous coronary intervention (PCI) *(Continued)*
    indications for, 142
    vs. medical treatment, 142
  global use of, 75, 76f
  mechanical support for high-risk, 224
  simultaneous surgical and, 233
  for STEMI, 186-190
    anticoagulant therapy with, 189, 190t
    antiplatelet therapy with, 189, 189t
    vs. fibrinolysis, 187f
    at hospitals without on-site cardiac surgery, 190, 191b
    primary, 179, 186-189
    symptom-to-balloon time in, 189, 189f
  before surgical intervention, 233
  surgical intervention before, 233
  systems of care for, 68-69
  transradial access for, 223-224
Percutaneous fenestration, of dissection flap for aortic dissection, 615, 615f
Percutaneous heart valve replacement (PHVR), 714-727
  aortic, 714
    access site evaluation for, 716
    currently available, 714-715, 715f
    measurement of aortic valve annulus for, 716-717
    new access approaches for, 719
    new applications of, 719
    next generation of, 720-721, 720f, 720t
    patient evaluation and imaging prior to, 715-717, 715f
    patient outcomes with, 717-719, 718f-719f, 719t
    potential complications of, 719-720
    transapical valves in, 721, 721f
    transcatheter implantation procedure for, 717-721, 717f
  mitral, 725-726, 726f
  overview of, 714
Percutaneous Heart Valve Technologies, 720t
Percutaneous left atrial ablation, for maintenance of sinus rhythm, 377
Percutaneous mitral balloon valvuloplasty (PMBV), 679
  indications for, 680-681
Percutaneous transluminal renal angioplasty (PTRA), 572-573, 575-577
Percutaneous treatment, for valvular heart disease, 714-727
  aortic, 714
    access site evaluation for, 716
    currently available, 714-715, 715f
    measurement of aortic valve annulus for, 716-717
    new access approaches for, 719
    new applications of, 719
    next generation of, 720-721, 720f, 720t
    patient evaluation and imaging prior to, 715-717, 715f
    patient outcomes with, 717-719, 718f-719f, 719t
    potential complications of, 719-720
    transapical valves in, 721, 721f
    transcatheter implantation procedure for, 717-721, 717f
  mitral, 721-726, 722t
    chamber remodeling in, 722t, 724, 724f
    chordal implantation in, 722t, 725, 725f
    direct annuloplasty in, 722t, 724-725, 725f
    leaflet repair in, 722-724, 722f-723f, 722t
    mitral valve replacement in, 725-726, 726f
    ventricular remodeling in, 722t, 725
  overview of, 714
Percutaneous valvuloplasty, for mitral stenosis in pregnancy, 624

Percutaneously implanted expanding endovascular stent-grafts, for abdominal aortic aneurysms, 606-607, 607f
Perhexiline, for nonobstructive hypertrophic cardiomyopathy, 335
Pericardial disease, 667-675
  chylopericardium as, 674
  connective tissue disease–related, 674
  drug-induced and iatrogenic, 674, 675t
  guidelines to diagnosis and management of, 667, 668t
  HIV-associated, 673, 734
  myxedema, 674
  pericardial effusion as. See Pericardial effusion.
  pericarditis as. See Pericarditis.
  and pregnancy, 674
  radiation-induced, 673-674
  with renal failure, 674
  traumatic, 674
Pericardial effusion, 668t, 669-671
  algorithm for management of, 669, 669f
  pericardial drainage for, 669
    complications of, 670
    hemodynamic improvement with, 669, 670f
    imaging during, 669, 670f-671f
    with loculation, 670-671, 670f
    methods of, 669, 670t
  surgical management of, 670-671, 670f
Pericardial fluid analysis, 668t
Pericardial friction rub, after myocardial infarction, 673
Pericardial tamponade, pulmonary artery catheters for, 748t
Pericardiectomy, for constrictive pericarditis, 671-672
Pericardiocentesis, 750-751
  advantages and disadvantages of, 669, 670t
  alternatives to, 670, 670t
  with catheter drainage, 669-670
  complications of, 670
  hemodynamic improvement with, 669, 670f
  imaging guidance of, 669, 670f-671f
  indications for, 750
  with loculation, 670-671, 670f
  for postpericardial injury syndrome, 673
  technical aspects of, 750-751
Pericardiotomy, 670t
Pericarditis
  acute, 667-668, 668t
  anticoagulation in, 674-675
  chronic, 668t
  connective tissue disease–related, 674
  constrictive, 671-672
  guidelines to diagnosis and management of, 667, 668t
  HIV-associated, 673, 734
  mycobacterial and fungal, 672-673
  after myocardial infarction, 673
  myxedema, 674
  neoplastic, 673
  purulent, 672
  radiation-induced, 673-674
  recurrent, 668, 668t
  with renal failure, 674
  after STEMI, 200
  traumatic, 674
Perindopril (Aceon)
  for carotid artery stenosis, 555
  for heart failure, 259
  for hypertension, 478t
Perioperative bleeding, in adults with cyanotic congenital heart disease, 634
Peripartum cardiomyopathy (PPCM), 627-628
Peripheral artery disease (PAD), 539-552
  and cardiovascular risk, 539, 540f
  defined, 539
  epidemiology of, 539

Peripheral artery disease (PAD) (Continued)
  interventional management of, 544-546
    for aortoiliac disease, 545f-547f, 546-547
    for femoral-popliteal disease, 545f, 547-549, 548f-549f
    indications for, 545, 545f
    for infrapopliteal disease, 549, 550f
    procedural considerations for, 546
  medical therapy of, 539, 540f
    for cardiovascular risk reduction, 539-543
      ACE inhibitor therapy as, 542
      anticoagulant therapy as, 541
      antihypertensive therapy as, 542
      antiplatelet therapy as, 539-541
      β-blocker therapy as, 542
      lipid-lowering drugs as, 541-542
      smoking cessation as, 542-543, 543b, 543f
    with diabetes, 543
    for intermittent claudication, 543-544, 544f
      cilostazol as, 543-544
      pentoxifylline as, 543
    potential benefits of, 541t
  natural history of, 539, 540f
  overview of, 539
  risk factors for, 539
  therapeutic angiogenesis for, 549
Peripheral edema, in pregnancy, 623
Permanent pacemakers, 752
  basic pacing concepts with, 752
    failure to capture as, 752, 754f
    sensing as, 752, 754b, 754f
    stimulation threshold as, 752, 754f
  leads for, 752, 753t
  programming considerations with, 752
    mode as, 752, 755f-757f, 755t
    rate-responsive pacing with, 752, 757t
  pseudo-malfunction of, 752, 757t
  radiographic appearance of, 752, 753f
PERSEUS trial, 219-220
Perspective, of cost-effectiveness analysis, 27
PETTICOAT technique, for aortic dissection, 615
PFO. See Patent foramen ovale (PFO).
PH. See Pulmonary hypertension (PH).
Pharmaceuticals and Medical Devices Agency (PMDA), 37
Pharmacogenetics, 53-66
  of clopidogrel, 53-56
    future directions for, 57
    genetic polymorphism in, 54t
    key genes in, 54t
      ABCB1 as, 55t, 56
      CYP2C19 as, 54-56, 55t
      PON1 as, 56
    testing for, 56
      cost effectiveness of, 57
    therapeutic implications of, 56-57
  defined, 53
  genetic polymorphism in, 54t
  indications for, 53
  key genes in, 54t
  of statins, 61-63
    future directions for, 63
    genetic polymorphism in, 54t, 62t
      and adverse effects, 63
      of SLCO1B1, 62t, 63
    genome-wide association studies in, 63
      APOC1 gene in, 62t, 63
      CLMN gene in, 62t, 63
    key genes in, 54t, 61t
      APOE as, 61, 62t
      CETP as, 61-62
      HMGCR as, 61
      KIF6 as, 62-63, 62t
      LDLR as, 62
      PCSK9 as, 61, 62t

Pharmacogenetics (Continued)
  therapeutic implications of, 63
  of warfarin, 57-59, 58f
    future directions for, 60
    genetic polymorphism in, 54t, 58t
    key genes in, 54t
      CYP2C9 as, 54t, 59
      CYP4F2 as, 54t, 59
      VKORC1 as, 57-59, 58t
    testing for, 59
      cost effectiveness of, 59
    therapeutic implications of, 59-60
    therapeutic modifications as, 59-60
Pharmacoinvasive management, of STEMI, 190
Pharmacokinetics, in pregnancy, 621, 622t
Pharmacomechanical therapy, for pulmonary embolism, 590
Phase I trials, 33, 34f
Phase II trials, 33, 34f
Phase III trials, 33, 34f
Phase IV trials, 33, 34f
Phencyclidine hydrochloride (PCP), hypertensive emergencies due to, 518
Phenoxybenzamine, for hypertension due to pheochromocytoma, 491-493, 492t
Phentolamine
  for acute hypertensive crisis due to pheochromocytoma, 493, 493t
  for hypertensive emergencies, 514t-515t
Phenylalkylamine-binding site, 90
Pheochromocytoma, 490-494, 503t
  acute hypertensive crises in, 493, 493t
  anesthesia and surgery for, 493-494
  defined, 490
  diagnosis of, 490, 492f
  extraadrenal, 490
  hypertensive emergencies due to, 517-518
  long-term postoperative follow-up for, 494
  malignant, 494
  in pregnancy, 494
  preoperative management of, 490-493, 492t
  presentation of, 490, 491b
  principles of treatment of, 490-494
  syndromic, 490, 491t
PHIRST study, 602
Phlebotomy, for cardiac hemochromatosis, 338
Phlegmasia cerulea dolens, 587
Phosphodiesterase 5 (PDE-5) inhibitors, for heart failure, 264
Phosphodiesterase (PDE) inhibitors
  for heart failure, 257
  for pulmonary arterial hypertension, 601-602
PHVR. See Percutaneous heart valve replacement (PHVR).
Physical activity
  for hypertension, 468-469, 469t
    in children, 534
    tips for success in increasing, 471
  for obesity, 448, 450, 452t
  after STEMI, 205t, 207
Physical activity counseling, cardiac rehabilitation and, 741b
Physical training, in rehabilitation, 738-739
  contraindications to, 743-744, 744b
  physiologic benefits of, 738, 739b
    newer concepts regarding, 739
  resistance exercise in, 743
PI(s) (protease inhibitors)
  for HIV infection, 728-729, 729t
  and statins, 423
PIB. See Partial ileal bypass (PIB).
PICCOLETO study, 222
Pindolol (Visken)
  for hypertension, 481t
  indications for, 101

Pindolol (Visken) *(Continued)*
  pharmacodynamic properties and cardiac
    effects of, 98t
  properties of, 102t
Pioglitazone, after STEMI, 206
PIOPED III investigation, 585
PISA (proximal isovolumetric surface area)
    method, for mitral stenosis, 678-679
Pitavastatin
  dosage of, 422t
  pharmacokinetics of, 422t
PLAATO trial, 388
Plant stanol esters, for lowering LDL
    cholesterol, 430-431
  effects on lipids and lipoproteins of, 430-431
  efficacy against coronary heart disease of,
    430-431
  safety of, 431
Plaque vulnerability, markers of, 566
Plasma aldosterone concentration (PAC), 495,
    495f
Plasma aldosterone concentration/plasma
    renin activity (PAC/PRA) ratio, 495, 495f
Plasma exchange, for severe
    hypercholesterolemia, 455
Plasma renin activity (PRA), in primary
    aldosteronism, 494-495, 495f
Plasmapheresis, for severe
    hypercholesterolemia, 455
Platelet aggregation, in acute coronary
    syndromes, 159, 159f
Platelet function testing, 157-159
PLATO trial
  indications in, 112
  NSTE-ACS in, 157
  pharmacogenetics in, 56-57
  STEMI in, 182
Platelet inhibitors. *See* Antiplatelet therapy.
Platelet-mediated thrombosis, 107, 107f
PLATINUM trial, 219-220
Plendil (felodipine), for hypertension, 479t
  in children, 536t
Plexiform lesion, in pulmonary arterial
    hypertension, 604
PM. *See* Pacemaker (PM).
PMA (premarket approval) application, 41-43
PMBV (percutaneous mitral balloon
    valvuloplasty), 679
  indications for, 680-681
PMDA (Pharmaceuticals and Medical Devices
    Agency), 37
PMVT (polymorphic ventricular tachycardia),
    catheter ablation for, 392
Pneumocystis carinii pneumonia, after cardiac
    transplantation, 312
Polyclonal antibodies, with cardiac
    transplantation, 311t
Polymer-free stents, 221
Polymorphic ventricular tachycardia (PMVT),
    catheter ablation for, 392
Polypill, for global cardiovascular therapy,
    79-80
Polytetrafluoroethylene (PTFE)-covered stents
  for aortoiliac disease, 546-547
  for femoral-popliteal disease, 548
Polyunsaturated fatty acids (PUFAs)
  for mixed dyslipidemia, 437-438
  to prevent coronary heart disease, 445-446
Polyunsaturated vegetable oils, for
    hyperlipidemia, 444-445, 444t
P-OM3 (prescription omega-3 ethyl esters)
    therapy, for mixed dyslipidemia, 438
PON1 gene, in pharmacogenetics of
    clopidogrel, 56
Pooled analyses, in comparative effectiveness
    research, 20-21, 22t
Pooling studies, in meta-analysis, 15-16, 17f
POPADAD trial, 539-540

Population strategies, for global cardiovascular
    disease, 75, 80-81
Portacaval shunt, 458-459
  cholesterol lowering via, 454, 459t
  risks and benefits of, 459
  technique of, 458, 458f
  treatment guidelines for, 459
POSCH, 460
Positive inotropic agents, 257-258
  as bridge to end of life, 257-258
  as bridge to transplant, 257
  intravenous, 257-258
  oral, 257
Positive predictive value (PPV), 1-2, 2f
Post CABG trial, 423
Postapproval surveillance, for medical devices,
    48-50, 48b
Posterior leaflet prolapse, 705
Postinfarct protection, calcium channel
    blockers for, 92
Postmarket surveillance
  for medical devices, 48-50, 48b
  for new drugs, 35-36
Postmarketing trials, 5
Post–myocardial infarction syndrome, 673
Postpericardial injury syndrome (PPIS), 673
Postpericardiotomy syndrome, 673
Postthrombotic syndrome, 582, 587
Posttransplant lymphoproliferative disease
    (PTLD), 313-314
Potassium channel agonists, for chronic stable
    angina, 141
Potassium intake, for hypertension, 468-469, 469t
Potassium-sparing diuretics
  for heart failure, 243-244, 243t
    acute decompensated, 291
  for hypertension, 480t
  in pregnancy, 623
Potts shunt, 633t
Power, of clinical trial, 8f, 9-11
P-PCI (primary percutaneous coronary
    intervention), for STEMI, 179, 186-189
PPCM (peripartum cardiomyopathy), 627-628
PPH (primary pulmonary hypertension), 596
PPIs (proton pump inhibitors), and clopidogrel,
    53
PPIS (postpericardial injury syndrome), 673
PPM (patient-prosthesis mismatch), 701
PPV (positive predictive value), 1-2, 2f
PRA (plasma renin activity), in primary
    aldosteronism, 494-495, 495f
Pradaxa. *See* Dabigatran (Pradaxa).
PRAGUE-2 trial, 185
PRAISE study, 93-94, 257
Prasugrel, 110t
  dosage of, 113
  indication for, 111-112
  mechanism of action of, 111
  for NSTE-ACS, 156-157
  in pregnancy and lactation, 622t-623t
  side effects and contraindications to,
    113
  for STEMI
    in acute phase, 182
    with PCI, 189t
Pravastatin
  for cardiac syndrome X, 169
  for chronic stable angina, 147
  dosage of, 422t
  with HIV infection and HAART, 733f
  pharmacodynamics and pharmacokinetics
    of, 60t
  pharmacokinetics of, 422t
  cardiovascular benefits in, 425t
  combination therapy in, 434
  effect on lipids and lipoproteins in, 422
  effect on liver in, 424
  NSTE-ACS in, 167, 167f

Pravastatin *(Continued)*
  pharmacogenetics in, 61
  STEMI in, 206
Prazosin (Minipress), for hypertension,
    483t
  due to pheochromocytoma, 491-493,
    492t
Preamendment device, 43
Precise stent, for carotid artery stenosis, 563
PRECISE trial, 250
Predicate devices, 43
Prednisone
  for cardiac amyloidosis, 337
  for cardiac sarcoidosis, 338
  with cardiac transplantation, 311t
  for glucocorticoid-remediable aldosteronism,
    497
  for myocarditis, 263
  for pericarditis
    recurrent, 668
    tuberculous, 672
  for postpericardial injury syndrome, 673
Preeclampsia, 518
  atypical, 523-524
  complications of, 523
  death from, 521
  defined, 521
  diagnosis of, 523-524, 523b
  epidemiology of, 521
  implications for cardiovascular disease after,
    525-526
  pathophysiology of, 521-523, 522f
  prevention of, 524
  risk factors for, 521, 522t
  treatment of, 524-525, 524t
Pregnancy, 621-631
  altered pharmacokinetics in, 621, 622t
  anemia of, 621
  antibiotic prophylaxis in, 630
  blood volume in, 621
  cardiac arrhythmias in, 628-629
  cardiovascular changes in, 621
  with congenital heart disease, 635-636
    recommendations for, 636
  edema in, 623
  fibrinolysis in, 626
  heart failure in, 627-628
  hypertension in, 521-528
    acute management of severe, 525
    chronic, 521, 523
    diagnosis of, 523-524, 523b
    eclampsia as, 525
    epidemiology and risk factors for, 521, 522t
    gestational, 521, 523
    implications for later cardiovascular
      disease of, 525-526
    overview of, 521
    pathophysiology of, 521-523
    preeclampsia as
      defined, 521
      pathophysiology of, 521-523, 522f
      risk factors for, 521, 522t
    prevention of, 524
    pulmonary, 629-630
    treatment of, 524-525, 524t
  hypertensive emergencies in, 518
  ischemic heart disease in, 626-627
  lipid disorders in, 627
  Marfan syndrome in, 629
  with mechanical heart valve, 626
  pericardial disease and, 674
  pheochromocytoma in, 494
  with pulmonary arterial hypertension, 604
  RBC mass in, 621
  risk of cardiac drugs to fetus and newborn
    in, 621, 622t-623t
  thromboembolic disease in, 624-626
  valvular heart disease in, 623-624

Prehospital diagnosis, of STEMI, 68-69
Prehypertension
  in children, 529
  DASH diet for, 442-443, 443f
  defined, 464t
Preload, in heart failure, 283, 283f
Premarket approval (PMA) application, 41-43
Premarket notification, 41-43
PREMISE study, 76-77
Prescription Drug User Fee Act (PDUFA), 38-39
Prescription omega-3 ethyl esters (P-OM3)
    therapy, for mixed dyslipidemia, 438
Prevention
  of coronary events with ischemic heart
      disease, 139f, 144-149
    ACE inhibitors in, 147
    antiplatelet therapy in, 144-146, 146f
    β-blockers in, 147
    cardiac rehabilitation in, 144
    coronary artery bypass graft in, 147-149
    coronary revascularization in, 147-149
    lipid-lowering therapy in, 146-147, 148f
  of global cardiovascular disease
    primary, 75, 79
    primordial, 75, 80-81
    secondary, 75-77, 77f
  of hypertension in pregnancy, 524
  implantable cardioverter-defibrillators for,
      396-407
    cardiac resynchronization, 401, 403f
    indications for, 401-404, 403b, 403f
    primary, 397-398
      clinical trials of, 397-398, 399t, 400f
      with comorbidities, 400-401, 402f
      risk stratification for, 398-400, 400t
    secondary, 396, 398t
    systems and technology for, 396-406, 397f
  of venous thromboembolism, 591-593
    duration of prophylaxis and extension
        after discharge in, 593, 593t
    with hip replacement, knee replacement,
        and hip fracture, 592, 592b
    in-hospital prophylaxis for, 592
    mechanical prophylaxis for, 592-593
    in patients with cancer, 591-592
    unconventional prophylaxis for, 592-593
      with statins, 593
      with vitamin E, 592-593
Primary adrenal hyperplasia (PAH), 494-496
  surgical treatment of, 496-497
Primary aldosteronism (PA), 494-497
  diagnosis of, 495-496, 495f-496f
  pharmacologic treatment of, 497
  principles of treatment of, 496-497
  and resistant hypertension, 503t, 504-508
  subtypes of, 494-495, 495b, 496f
  surgical treatment of, 496-497
Primary cortisol resistance, hypertension due
    to, 498
Primary PCI centers, transport to, 68-69
Primary percutaneous coronary intervention
    (P-PCI), for STEMI, 179, 186-189
Primary prevention
  of global cardiovascular disease, 75, 79
  implantable cardioverter-defibrillators for,
      397-398
    clinical trials of, 397-398, 399t, 400f
    with comorbidities, 400-401, 402f
    risk stratification for, 398-400, 400t
Primary pulmonary hypertension (PPH), 596
Primordial prevention, of global cardiovascular
    disease, 75, 80-81
PRINCE (Pravastatin Inflammation/CRP
    Evaluation), 63
PRINCIPLE-TIMI 44 trial, 53
Prinivil. See Lisinopril (Prinivil, Zestril).
Prinzide (lisinopril/hydrochlorothiazide), for
    hypertension, 485t

PRISMA, 15
PRISON II study, 223
PRKAG2 mutations, cardiomyopathy
    associated with, 339
Probabilistic sensitivity analysis, 27, 29f
PROBE (prospective, randomized, open-label
    blinded endpoint) design, 6
Procainamide, 348-349
  adverse reactions to, 349, 375t
  clinical applications of, 348
  clinical pharmacology of, 348
  dosage and administration of, 348, 375t
    modification in disease states of, 348-349
  drug interactions with, 349
  mechanism of action of, 348
  in pregnancy and lactation, 622t-623t, 628-629
  for sustained monomorphic ventricular
      tachycardia, 410-411, 410t
Procardia. See Nifedipine (Adalat, Nifedical,
    Procardia).
Processed foods, and hypertension, 471
Product label, for cardiovascular devices, 46-47
Product life cycle, 47, 47f
Product recall, 50
PROFESS trial, 476, 556, 558, 558t
Progenitor cells
  circulating, and myocardial regeneration,
      322-323, 323f-324f
  endogenous cardiac, 326-327, 327f-330f
  endothelial, 322-323
  hematopoietic, in myocardial repair, 322,
      324f
Programmable pacing mode, 752, 755f-757f,
    755t
PROGRESS study, 476, 556
PROMISE trial, 257
Promus Element stent, 219-220
Propafenone, 351-352
  for atrial fibrillation, 374t
  clinical applications of, 351
  clinical pharmacology of, 351
  dosage and administration of, 351, 375t
    modification in disease states of, 351
  drug interactions with, 351-352
  initiation and monitoring of, 376
  for paroxysmal supraventricular tachycardia,
      369
  toxicities of, 375t
Prophylaxis
  endocarditis, 662-663, 663t
    during delivery, 630
  thrombo-, 591-593
    duration of and extension after discharge
        of, 593, 593t
    with hip replacement, knee replacement,
        and hip fracture, 592, 592b
    in-hospital, 592
    mechanical, 592-593
    in patients with cancer, 591-592
    in pregnancy, 624-626
    unconventional agents for, 592-593
      with statins, 593
      with vitamin E, 592-593
Propranolol (Inderal, Innopran)
  for abdominal aortic aneurysms, 607
  adverse effects of, 103
  in angina pectoris, 97
  for aortic dissection, 613-614
  for atrial fibrillation, 373t
  drug interactions with, 105t
  for hypertension, 481t
    in children, 536t
  for hypertrophic cardiomyopathy, 100
  indications for, 101
  long-acting sustained-release, 103
  for paroxysmal supraventricular tachycardia,
      368
  for peripheral artery disease, 542

Propranolol (Inderal, Innopran) (Continued)
  pharmacodynamic properties and cardiac
      effects of, 98t
  pharmacokinetics of, 103
  pharmacology of, 250
  in pregnancy and lactation, 622t-623t
  properties of, 102t
  for survivors of acute myocardial infarction,
      99
Propranolol hydrochloride/
    hydrochlorothiazide (Inderide), for
    hypertension, 485t
Prostacyclin, for pulmonary arterial
    hypertension, 599, 600f
  in pregnancy, 629
Prostanoids, for pulmonary arterial
    hypertension, 599-601, 600f
Prosthetic cardiac devices, infective
    endocarditis with, 657-658
Prosthetic heart valves, 694-699
  annuloplasty devices as, 695t
  autografts as, 696t
  characteristics of, 694-695, 696t
  currently available, 694-695, 695t, 696f
  homografts as, 699
    characteristics of, 696t
    currently available, 695t, 696f
  mechanical, 695-697
    characteristics of, 696t
    currently available, 695t, 696f
    valve-related complications with, 697, 697t,
        698f
  pregnancy with, 626
  valve-related complications of, 695, 696b
  xenografts as
    stented, 697
      characteristics of, 696t
      currently available, 695t, 696f
    stentless, 697-699
      characteristics of, 696t
      currently available, 695t, 696f
Prosthetic valve endocarditis (PVE)
  antibiotics for, 654
  surgical management of, 661
Protease activated receptor 1 (PAR-1)
    antagonists, 115
  for chronic stable angina, 149
Protease inhibitors (PIs)
  for HIV infection, 728-729, 729t
  and statins, 423
PROTECHT study, 591-592
PROTECT II trial, 224
PROTECT-AF study, 388
Proteinuria, 523
Protocol development, for clinical trial, 37-38
Proton pump inhibitors (PPIs), and clopidogrel,
    53
PROVE IT-TIMI 22 trial
  cardiovascular benefits in, 425t
  combination therapy in, 434
  effect on lipids and lipoproteins in, 422
  effect on liver in, 424
  NSTE-ACS in, 167, 167f
  pharmacogenetics in, 61
  STEMI in, 206
PROVE-IT trial, 147
Provider interventions, for antihypertensive
    medications, 468
Provision approach, for bifurcation lesion, 223
Proximal isovolumetric surface area (PISA)
    method, for mitral stenosis, 678-679
Proximally placed occlusion devices, 222
Proxis proximal occlusion device, 222
PRT054021, 160t
PRT060128, 110t
PS (pulmonic stenosis), 640-641, 641f, 687-688
  in pregnancy, 624
  recommendations for, 641

Pseudo pacemaker malfunction, 752, 757t
Pseudoaneurysm, in infective endocarditis, 652
Pseudohypertension, with aortic dissection, 614
Pseudoresistance, vs. resistant hypertension, 501, 502b
PSVTs. See Paroxysmal supraventricular tachycardias (PSVTs).
Psychosocial impact, of STEMI, 207
PTFE (polytetrafluoroethylene)-covered stents
    for aortoiliac disease, 546-547
    for femoral-popliteal disease, 548
PTLD (posttransplant lymphoproliferative disease), 313-314
PTOLEMY feasibility trial, 724
PTRA (percutaneous transluminal renal angioplasty), 572-573, 575-577
PUFAs (polyunsaturated fatty acids)
    for mixed dyslipidemia, 437-438
    to prevent coronary heart disease, 445-446
Pulmonary arterial hypertension (PAH), 596-605
    chronic thromboembolic, 582
    classification of, 596, 598, 599b
    diagnosis of
        current state of, 596, 597t
        and risk stratification, 596-598, 599b
        epidemiologic associations with, 596, 597b, 597f
    with heart failure, 264
    HIV-related, 734-735
    idiopathic, 596
        epidemiologic associations with, 596
        pathophysiologic paradigm of, 596, 598f
        transplantation for, 602
    pathobiologic paradigm of
        current, 596, 598f
        new, 604
    pregnancy and contraception with, 604
    therapy for
        algorithms for, 602-604, 603f
        atrial septostomy in, 602
        combination, 602, 603f
        conventional, 599
        current state of, 599-602
        endothelin receptor antagonism in, 601, 601f
        new paradigm of, 604
        phosphodiesterase inhibition in, 601-602
        prostanoids in, 599-601, 600f
        transplantation in, 602
Pulmonary artery catheters (PACs), 747-749
    for acute decompensated heart failure, 289, 289t
    design of, 747, 748f
    indications for, 747, 748t
    interpretation of waveforms from, 747, 749f
    after STEMI, 193
    technical aspects of placement of, 747, 748b, 748f
    troubleshooting and complications with, 747-749
Pulmonary artery stenosis, after tetralogy of Fallot repair, 644-645, 644f-645f
Pulmonary autograft, 701
Pulmonary capillary wedge pressure (PCWP), in acute decompensated heart failure, 285-286, 290
Pulmonary congestion, after STEMI, 193-194, 194f
Pulmonary disease, and mechanical circulatory support, 318
Pulmonary edema
    acute, 299-301
        defined, 281
        dobutamine for, 300
        dopamine vs. norepinephrine for, 300, 300f

Pulmonary edema (Continued)
    hypertensive emergencies with, 513
    LVEF in, 299-300, 300f
    nitroglycerin for, 300
    nitroprusside for, 300, 301f
    noninvasive positive-pressure ventilation for, 300, 301f
    parenteral diuretics for, 291
    pulmonary artery catheters for, 748t
    after STEMI, 193-194, 194f
Pulmonary embolism (PE), 580-595
    diagnosis of, 583-586
        algorithm for, 585-586, 586f
        chest CT in, 584, 584f-585f
        chest radiography in, 583
        clinical presentation in, 583-586, 584t
        ECG in, 583
        echocardiography in, 584, 585f
        laboratory testing in, 583
        lung scanning in, 584
        MRI in, 585
    epidemiology and risk factors for, 580-581, 581t-582t
    management of, 586-591
        advanced therapy in, 583, 589-591
        anticoagulation in, 587-589, 587b
            direct factor XA and factor IIA inhibitors for, 589
            duration of, 590, 590f
            with fondaparinux, 588
            and heparin-induced thrombocytopenia, 587, 588f
            with low-molecular-weight heparin, 588
            with unfractionated heparin, 587
            with warfarin, 588-589, 588b
        inferior vena cava filters for, 591
        spectrum of disease and, 586-587
    massive, 586-587
    pathophysiology and natural history of, 582, 582f
    in pregnancy, 624-626
    prevention of, 591-593
        duration of prophylaxis and extension after discharge in, 593, 593t
        with hip replacement, knee replacement, and hip fracture, 592, 592b
        in-hospital prophylaxis for, 592
        mechanical prophylaxis for, 592-593
        in patients with cancer, 591-592
        unconventional prophylaxis for, 592-593
            with statins, 593
            with vitamin E, 592-593
    after STEMI, 201
    submassive, 586
Pulmonary hypertension (PH), 596, 597t
    arterial. See Pulmonary arterial hypertension (PAH).
    HIV-related, 734-735
    in pregnancy, 629-630
    primary, 596
    pulmonary artery catheters for, 748t
Pulmonary infarction syndrome, 587
Pulmonary stenosis, 640-641, 641f, 687-688
    in pregnancy, 624
    recommendations for, 641
Pulmonary valve disease, 687-688
Pulmonary valve replacement, for tetralogy of Fallot, 644
Pulmonary vein isolation (PVI), for maintenance of sinus rhythm, 377
Pulmonic stenosis (PS), 640-641, 641f, 687-688
    in pregnancy, 624
    recommendations for, 641
Pulsus alternans, in acute decompensated heart failure, 287
Pulsus paradoxus, 670f
PURE study, 77, 77f
PURSUIT score, 153, 154t

Purulent pericarditis, 672
PVE (prosthetic valve endocarditis)
    antibiotics for, 654
    surgical management of, 661
PVI (pulmonary vein isolation), for maintenance of sinus rhythm, 377
P2Y12 receptor antagonists, 109-115
    dosages of, 112-113
    indication for, 111-112, 112t
    mechanism of action of, 109-111, 110f, 110t
    for NSTE-ACS, 156
    with PCI for STEMI, 189t
    side effects and contraindications to, 113-114
    after stent placement, 219t
Pyrazinamide, for tuberculous pericarditis, 672

Q
QALY (quality-adjusted life-year), 23
QThrombosis algorithm, 580, 581t
Quality improvement
    experience to date with, 71-72
        for heart failure, 72
        for out-of-hospital cardiac arrest, 72
        for STEMI, 71-72
    theory of, 70-71
Quality-adjusted life-year (QALY), 23
Quanam stent, 215
Quantitative review. See Meta-analysis.
QuantumCor device, 722t, 724-725, 725f
Quinapril (Accupril)
    for heart failure, 246t
    for hypertension, 478t
        in children, 536t
Quinapril/hydrochlorothiazide (Accuretic), for hypertension, 485t
Quinidine, 350-351
    adverse reactions to, 351, 375t
    for atrial fibrillation, 374, 374t
    clinical applications of, 350
    clinical pharmacology of, 350
    dosage and administration of, 350, 375t
        modification in disease states of, 350-351
    drug interactions with, 351
    initiation and monitoring of, 376
    mechanism of action of, 350
    in pregnancy and lactation, 622t-623t, 628
Quinupristin-dalfopristin, for enterococcal endocarditis, 656t

R
RAAS. See Renin-angiotensin-aldosterone system (RAAS).
RACE (Reperfusion of Acute MI in Carolina Emergency Departments) program, 69
RACE trial, 372
RADAR trial, 577
Radial artery (RA) graft, for coronary artery bypass, 231t, 232
RADIANCE 1 and 2 trials, 439
RADIANCE study, 7
Radiation-induced pericardial disease, 673-674
Radiofrequency ablation (RFA). See Catheter ablation.
Radiofrequency lesions, histology of, 383, 384f
RADUS (renal artery duplex ultrasonography)
    diagnostic, 571, 572f, 572t
    for surveillance, 577-578
RAFT trial, 275-276, 401, 402t
Rales, in acute decompensated heart failure, 286
RALES study, 193, 253-254, 253t
Raltegravir, for HIV infection, 729
Ramipril (Altace)
    for heart failure, 246t

Ramipril (Altace) (Continued)
  for hypertension, 478t
  for peripheral artery disease, 542
  for STEMI
    during convalescence, 192
    with pulmonary congestion, 194
Random effects model, 16
Ranolazine
  with β-adrenergic blockers, 99
  for chronic stable angina, 105-106, 106f, 141
    with heart failure, 261
  mechanism of action of, 105-106, 106f
  for NSTE-ACS, 155
  other potential uses of, 106
RAPCO trial, 231-232
Rapeseed oil (Canola), for hyperlipidemia, 444
RAR (renal/aortic ratio), 571, 572t
RAS. See Renal artery stenosis (RAS).
Rastelli operation, 633t
Rate control, for atrial fibrillation, 373-374
  atrioventricular junction ablation in, 390-392
  nonpharmacologic approach to, 374
  pharmacologic approach to, 373-374, 373t
  rhythm vs., 372-375
Rate-responsive pacing, 752, 757t
Rauwolfia alkaloids, for hypertension, 483t, 484
RAVEL trial, 215, 216t
RBC (red blood cell) mass, in pregnancy, 621
RCM. See Restrictive cardiomyopathy (RCM).
RCT (reverse cholesterol transport), 436
RCTs (randomized controlled trials), 5-7
  in comparative effectiveness research, 20, 22t
  of medical devices, 44-45
REACT trial, 190
Readiness for change, for hypertension, 470-471, 470f
Receiver operating characteristic (ROC) curve, 2-3, 2f
Receptors, 96
Reclassification, 3
Recombinant tissue plasminogen activator, for pulmonary embolism, 590
ReCor device, 722t, 724-725
RE-COVER trial, 589
Recreational activities, energy costs of, 741-742, 742t
Red blood cell (RBC) mass, in pregnancy, 621
RED-HF trial, 264
"Reduced fat," 471t
"Reduced sodium," 471t
Reduced-carbohydrate diets, for hyperlipidemia, 445, 445t
Reentrant paroxysmal supraventricular tachycardia, after STEMI, 199
Regeneration
  of cardiomyocytes, 322, 323f
  circulating progenitor cells and myocardial, 322-323, 323f-324f
Regenerative therapy, for heart failure, 322-331
  age, cardiac disease, and human cardiac stem cell function in, 327-330
  bone marrow cells and clinical studies on, 324-326
  cardiomyocyte death and regeneration and, 322, 323f
  circulating progenitor cells and myocardial regeneration in, 322-323, 323f-324f
  endogenous cardiac progenitors in, 326-327, 327f-330f
  hematopoietic stem cell transdifferentiation and, 323-324, 325f
Regional transfer protocols, for STEMI, 69
Regulation
  of medical devices

Regulation (Continued)
  CDRH interactions with external stakeholders and government partners in, 51
  for combination products, 50-51
  contemporary issues in, 44-47
  fundamentals of, 42-44
  history of, 42-43
  other key topics in, 50-51
  pathway for, 43-44, 44f
    501(k) premarket notification in, 41-43
    Humanitarian Device Exemption in, 44
    Investigational Device Exemption in, 41-44
    premarket approval application in, 41-43
  role of advisory panel in, 51
  of new drugs, 34-35
    CDER vs. CBER in, 34, 36
Rehabilitation, 738-746
  cardiac, 739-745
    in chronic heart failure, 744
    contraindications to, 743-744, 744b
    disability from myocardial infarction and, 739-740
    evolving landscape for, 745
    inpatient
      exercise testing before discharge and, 740
      in-hospital exercise in, 740
      patient education on, 740
    meta-analysis for survival after, 744-745
    outpatient, 740-742
      core components for, 740-742, 741b
      exercise prescription for, 742-743, 743f
      maintenance program for, 741-742, 742t
      monitoring in, 741, 742b
      resistance exercise in, 743
      safety of, 741
    physical training for, 738-739
      physiologic benefits of, 738, 739b
      newer concepts regarding, 739
    physiologic effects of immobility and, 738
Relative risk (RR), 12-13
  and control event rate, 15, 16f
RELAX-AHF study, 302
Relaxin, for acute decompensated heart failure, 302, 302f
RE-LY trial, 122
REMATCH trial, 46
Remodeling annuloplasty, in mitral valve repair, 705
Remodulin (treprostinil), for pulmonary arterial hypertension, 599-601
Renal angioplasty, percutaneous transluminal, 572-573, 575-577
Renal artery duplex ultrasonography (RADUS)
  diagnostic, 571, 572f, 572t
  for surveillance, 577-578
Renal artery stenosis (RAS), 571-579
  clinical manifestations of, 571, 572b
  diagnostic imaging of, 571-574
    captopril renal scintigraphy for, 572
    catheter-based angiography for, 573f
    choice of correct, 573-574, 573f
    CTA and MRA for, 572
    renal artery duplex ultrasonography for, 571, 572f, 572t
  etiology of, 571
  due to fibromuscular dysplasia, 573-574, 573f, 577
  hypertension due to, 503t, 571-572
  natural history of, 571
  overview of, 571
  treatment of, 574-578
    catheter-based intervention for, 575-577, 576t

Renal artery stenosis (RAS) (Continued)
    catheter-based renal artery sympathetic denervation for, 578
    medical, 574
    patient selection for revascularization for, 574-575
    surveillance for, 577-578
Renal artery stenting, 574-577
Renal artery sympathetic denervation, for resistant hypertension, 507-508, 578
Renal changes, due to cyanosis, 634
Renal failure, pericardial disease with, 674
Renal insufficiency, after cardiac transplantation, 313
Renal parenchymal disease, hypertension due to, 503t
Renal presentations, hypertensive emergencies with, 517
Renal resistive index (RRI), 575
Renal sympathetic denervation, for resistant hypertension, 507-508, 578
Renal/aortic ratio (RAR), 571, 572t
Renin-angiotensin system, and abdominal aortic aneurysms, 607-608
Renin-angiotensin-aldosterone system (RAAS),
  in heart failure, 283
  in preeclampsia, 522
  inhibitors of
    for heart failure, 245-250
      acute decompensated, 296-297
      clinical efficacy of, 246-248, 247t
      dosage of, 246t
      endpoints with, 242t
      pathophysiologic mechanisms and, 245-246, 245f
      practical considerations with, 248-250, 248t
      with preserved ejection fraction, 259, 260t
    for STEMI
      during convalescence, 192-193
      in long-term management, 206
Renitec. See Enalapril (Renitec, Vasotec).
Renovascular disease. See Renal artery stenosis (RAS).
REPAIR-AMI study, 324
Reperfusion of Acute MI in Carolina Emergency Departments (RACE) program, 69
Reperfusion therapy, 184-190
  fibrinolytic therapy in, 185-186
    comparison of agents for, 186, 188t
    complications of, 185-186, 188f
    effect on LV function of, 185
    indications and contraindications for, 185, 187b
    mortality benefit of, 185
    risk of bleeding with, 185
  general concepts of, 184-185
  in hospitals without on-site cardiac surgery, 190, 191b
  percutaneous coronary intervention in, 186-190
    anticoagulant therapy with, 189, 190t
    antiplatelet therapy with, 189, 189t
    vs. fibrinolysis, 187f
    at hospitals without on-site cardiac surgery, 190, 191b
    primary, 179, 186-189
    symptom-to-balloon time in, 189, 189f
  pharmacoinvasive management in, 190
  predicted transfer and door-to-balloon time for, 185, 187f
  risk of bleeding and, 185
  risk stratification and, 185, 186f
  stents in, 190
  thrombus aspiration in, 190
  time from symptom onset to, 185

REPLACE-2 trial, 120, 161-162
Request for Designation process, 51
Rescue breathing, for cardiac arrest, 415
Research synthesis. *See* Meta-analysis.
Reserpine, for hypertension, 483t, 484
RESIST study, 575-576
Resistance exercise, in cardiac rehabilitation, 743
Resistant hypertension (RHTN), 467, 501-509
  due to aortic dissection, 614
  baroreflex activation therapy for, 508
  and cardiovascular risk, 502
  causes of, 468b, 502, 502b, 503t
  defined, 501, 502b
  diagnosis of, 464-465
    ambulatory blood pressure monitoring for, 501-502
  epidemiology of, 501
  interfering substances in, 504, 504b
    dietary sodium as, 504
  obstructive sleep apnea and, 502-504, 503t
  pharmacologic treatment of, 504-508
    diuretics for, 505, 505f-506f
    mineralocorticoid receptor antagonists for, 505-507, 506f-507f
    other antihypertensive agents for, 507
  primary aldosteronism and, 503t, 504-508
  pseudo-, 501, 502b
  due to renal artery stenosis, 571
  renal sympathetic denervation for, 507-508
  role of hypertension specialist for, 508
RESOLUTE All-Comers Trial, 221
Resolute stent, 221
RESOLUTE study, 217t
RESOLUTE US study, 217t
RESOLVED pilot study, 284
Restrictive cardiomyopathy (RCM), 336-340
  associated with mutations in *LAMP2* (Danon disease), *PRKAG2*, or mitochondrial genes, 339
  due to cardiac amyloidosis, 336-337
  due to cardiac hemochromatosis, 338-339
    treatment of, 338-339
  due to cardiac sarcoidosis, 337-338
    treatment of, 338
  due to endomyocardial fibrosis, 339
  etiology of, 336, 336b
  due to Fabry's disease, 339
  idiopathic, 336
  due to Löffler hypereosinophilic syndrome, 339-340
  due to storage diseases of myocardium, 339
Reteplase (rPA), 123, 123t
  for STEMI, 186, 188t
Return to work, after STEMI, 207
Revascularization
  for carotid artery disease, 558-568
    changing attitude toward, 565-566
    endovascular (carotid artery stenting), 562-565
      indications for, 562, 562f
      in normal-risk symptomatic patients, 563-565, 565f
      serial steps during, 559f
    in symptomatic and asymptomatic patients at high surgical risk, 563
    surgical (carotid endarterectomy), 559-562
      for asymptomatic carotid artery stenosis, 560-562, 561t
      carotid artery bifurcation exposed during, 559f
      for symptomatic carotid artery stenosis, 559-560, 560f, 561t
  coronary. *See* Coronary revascularization.
  for peripheral artery disease, 544-546
    aortoiliac, 545f-547f, 546-547

Revascularization (*Continued*)
    femoral-popliteal, 545f, 547-549, 548f-549f
    indications for, 545, 545f
    infrapopliteal, 549, 550f
    procedural considerations for, 546
  for renal artery stenosis, 574-577
REVEAL HPS-3 TIMI-55 trial, 439
Reverse cholesterol transport (RCT), 436
REVERSE study, 275
Reverse-T stenting, for bifurcation lesion, 223f
Reynolds Risk Score, 79
RFA (radiofrequency ablation). *See* Catheter ablation.
Rheumatic mitral stenosis, in pregnancy, 624
RHTN. *See* Resistant hypertension (RHTN).
Rhythm control, for atrial fibrillation, 374-375
  electrical cardioversion in, 375
  pharmacologic cardioversion in, 374-375, 374t
  rate vs., 372-375
RIETE Registry, 580
Rifampin, for tuberculous pericarditis, 672
Right atrial pressure, in acute decompensated heart failure, 290
Right internal mammary artery (RIMA) graft, for coronary artery bypass, 230-232, 231t
Right ventricular (RV) apical pacing, 756f-757f
Right ventricular (RV) dysfunction, due to pulmonary embolism, 582, 582f
Right ventricular (RV) enlargement, in pulmonary embolism, 584, 585f
Right ventricular (RV) function, and mechanical circulatory support, 317-318
Right ventricular (RV) infarction, with STEMI, 181, 196, 196f
Right ventricular outflow tract (RVOT) obstruction, in tetralogy of Fallot, 643
  after repair, 644-645, 644f-645f
Right ventricular (RV) pacing, long-term, cardiac resynchronization therapy in, 276
Right-sided valvular heart disease, 687-688
  pulmonary, 687-688
  tricuspid, 687
RIMA (right internal mammary artery) graft, for coronary artery bypass, 230-232, 231t
Risk(s)
  balancing benefits and, 22-23
  cardiovascular
    peripheral artery disease and, 539, 540f
    resistant hypertension and, 502
  relative, 12-13
    and control event rate, 15, 16f
  of stroke, 553
Risk assessment, for STEMI, 181-190
Risk difference, absolute, 12-13
Risk factor(s)
  for global cardiovascular disease, 80-81
  for peripheral artery disease, 539
  for preeclampsia, 521, 522t
  for venous thromboembolism, 580-581, 581t-582t
Risk factor control, after STEMI, 204-206, 205t
  blood pressure control in, 205t, 206
  diabetes management in, 205t, 206
  lipid management in, 205t, 206
  smoking cessation in, 205t, 206
  weight management in, 204, 205t
Risk factor modification, for chronic stable angina, 137-140
  for diabetes mellitus, 140
  dietary intervention as, 138-140
  for obesity, 140
  smoking in, 137-138

Risk reduction, for peripheral artery disease, 539-543
  ACE inhibitor therapy as, 542
  anticoagulant therapy as, 541
  antihypertensive therapy as, 542
  antiplatelet therapy as, 539-541
  β-blocker therapy as, 542
  lipid-lowering drugs as, 541-542
  smoking cessation as, 542-543, 543b, 543f
Risk scores, 3
Risk stratification
  for heart failure, 285, 285t-286t, 286f
  for STEMI, 202-204, 203f
    assessment of electrical substrate in, 204
    echocardiography in, 202-203
    in emergency department, 185, 186f
    exercise testing in, 202
    invasive evaluation for, 204
    left ventricular function in, 203-204
    myocardial perfusion imaging in, 203
    myocardial viability in, 204
    recurrent, 202-204, 203f
  for sudden cardiac death, 398-400, 400t
    autonomic function (baroreflex slope) in, 398, 400t
    ejection fraction in, 398, 400t
    electrophysiologic studies in, 398, 400t
    genetic testing in, 400
    left ventricular scar burden in, 398-400, 400t
    nonsustained ventricular arrhythmias in, 398, 400t
    signal-averaged ECG in, 398, 400t
    T-wave alternans in, 398, 400t
  for venous thromboembolism
    chest CT for, 584, 584f-585f
    echocardiography for, 584, 585f
    overall, 586, 586f, 586t-587t
RITA-2 trial, 142
Ritonavir, for HIV infection, 729t
Rituximab, with cardiac transplantation, 311t
RIVAL trial, 224
Rivaroxaban (Xarelto), 122, 160t
  for NSTE-ACS, 163, 163t
  for thromboprophylaxis, 592-593
  for venous thromboembolism, 589
Roadmap for Medical Research, 39
Robotic valve surgery, 694
Robotically assisted revascularization, 229-230, 230f
ROC (receiver operating characteristic) curve, 2-3, 2f
ROOBY trial, 226-227
Root cause, of medical device failure, 48
ROSE-AHF study, 296
Ross procedure
  in adults, 633t
  for aortic valve replacement, 701
  for bicuspid aortic valve, 640
  for thoracic aortic aneurysms, 609
Ross Procedure International Registry, 701
Rosuvastatin
  dosage of, 422t
  with HIV infection and HAART, 733f
  pharmacodynamics and pharmacokinetics of, 60t, 422t
  for thromboprophylaxis, 593
rPA (reteplase), 123, 123t
  for STEMI, 186, 188t
RR (relative risk), 12-13
  and control event rate, 15, 16f
RRI (renal resistive index), 575
RRISC study, 222
RV. *See* Right ventricular (RV).
RVOT (right ventricular outflow tract) obstruction, in tetralogy of Fallot, 643
  after repair, 644-645, 644f-645f

S

4S trial, 146, 541
SAFER trial, 222
SAFE-T trial, 352
Safety surveillance, for clinical trial, 38
SAH (subarachnoid hemorrhage), hypertensive emergencies with, 516
SAM (systolic anterior motion), of mitral valve, 332-333
Sample size, 6-7
    estimation of, 9
    fixed, 6
Saphenous vein graft(s) (SVGs), 222, 231t
    alternatives to, 230-232, 231t
Sapien XT valve, 720t
SAPPHIRE study, 563
Saquinavir, for HIV infection, 729t
Sarcoidosis, cardiac, 337-338
    treatment of, 338
Saturated fat, and coronary heart disease, 443-444
SAVE ONCO trial, 591-592
SAVE trial, 247t, 248
SBP (systolic blood pressure), and heart failure risk stratification, 285, 285t
SBP (systolic blood pressure) levels
    for boys, 530t-531t
SCA (senile cardiac amyloidosis), 336-337
Scandinavian Simvastatin Survival Study (4S) trial, 146, 541
SCANDSTENT trial, 216t
SCD. See Sudden cardiac death (SCD).
SCD-HeFT trial
    amiodarone in, 258
    implantable cardioverter-defibrillators in, 270-272, 397-398, 399t
    population subgroups in, 409f
    survival curves in, 400f
SCH530348, 115
SCIPIO trial, 326
Scleroderma, and pulmonary arterial hypertension, 596
SCORPIUS trial, 216t
Screening
    of at-risk family members for hypertrophic cardiomyopathy, 336
    for cardiovascular disease in HIV-positive patients, 731
    for hypertrophic cardiomyopathy, 336
SDHAF2 mutation, in pheochromocytoma, 491t
SDHB mutation, in pheochromocytoma, 491t, 494
SDHC mutation, in pheochromocytoma, 491t
SDHD mutation, in pheochromocytoma, 491t
SEARCH study, 63, 424
Seattle Heart Failure Model (SHFM), 316-317
Second messengers, 96
Secondary prevention
    of coronary events with ischemic heart disease, 139f, 144-149
        ACE inhibitors in, 147
        antiplatelet therapy in, 144-146, 146f
        β-blockers in, 147
        cardiac rehabilitation in, 144
        coronary artery bypass graft in, 147-149
        coronary revascularization in, 147-149
        lipid-lowering therapy in, 146-147, 148f
    of global cardiovascular disease, 75-77, 77f
    implantable cardioverter-defibrillators for, 396, 398t
Secondary prevention centers, 740
Secondary prevention programs, 741, 741b
Sectral. See Acebutolol (Sectral).
Seguin prosthesis, 695t
Self-expanding stents
    for aortoiliac disease, 546-547, 547f
    for carotid artery stenosis, 563

Self-expanding stents (Continued)
    for femoral-popliteal disease, 548, 548f-549f
Semuloparin, for thromboprophylaxis, 591-592
sEng (soluble endoglin), in preeclampsia, 521-522, 522f
Senile cardiac amyloidosis (SCA), 336-337
SENIORS study, 251t, 252
Senning operation, 633t
Sensing, by pacemaker, 752
Sensitivity
    and diagnostic cutoffs, 2-3, 2f
    of pacemaker, 752
    of test, 1-2, 2f
Sensitivity analysis, 26-27
    one-way, 26, 26f-27f
    probabilistic, 27, 29f
    two-way, 26-27, 28f
SEPIA-ACS1-TIMI 42 trial, 163
Sequential design, open or closed, 6
Sequential stopping boundaries, 9-10, 11f
Serotonin, in pulmonary arterial hypertension, 604
SESAMI trial, 216t
SFA (superficial femoral artery) disease, 545f, 547-549, 548f-549f
sFlt1 (soluble fms-related tyrosine kinase 1), in preeclampsia, 521, 522f, 525-526
SHARP trial, 430
SHEP (Systolic Hypertension in the Elderly Program), 555
SHFM (Seattle Heart Failure Model), 316-317
SHIFT trial, 264
Shock(s)
    cardiogenic, after STEMI, 195, 195f
    with implantable cardioverter-defibrillators, 759, 759f
        inappropriate, 759-760, 760t
    pulmonary artery catheters for, 748t
SICCO trial, 143
Sicilian gambit, 344, 345f
Signal-averaged ECG, for risk of sudden cardiac death, 398, 400t
Sildenafil citrate
    for heart failure, 264
    in pregnancy and lactation, 622t-623t, 629
    for pulmonary arterial hypertension, 601-602
Simulation studies, 16-17
Simvastatin
    for carotid artery disease, 556
    for chronic stable angina, 146
    clinical trials of, 423-424
    dosage of, 422
    drug interactions with, 422, 423t
    for peripheral artery disease, 541
    pharmacodynamics and pharmacokinetics of, 60t, 422t
    in pregnancy, 627
Single-blind trials, 6
Single-vessel small thoracotomy direct-vision bypass grafting (SVST), 227-228, 228f
Sinus bradycardia, after STEMI, 198
Sinus node reentrant tachycardia, 367, 371
Sinus rhythm, maintenance of, 375-379
    adjunctive therapy for, 377
    nonpharmacologic approaches to, 377
    pacing for, 378
    pharmacologic approaches to, 375-377, 375t
        choice of drug in, 376, 376f
        initiation and monitoring of, 376-377
Sinus tachycardia, inappropriate, 367
    catheter ablation for, 386
    pharmacologic treatment of, 371
    in pregnancy, 628
Sinus venosus defects, 637

SIRIUS trial, 143-144, 215, 216t
SIROCCO II trial, 548-549
Sirolimus
    with cardiac transplantation, 311t
    molecular structure and mechanism of action of, 220f
Sirolimus-eluting stent(s), 215, 216t
    with biodegradable polymers, 221
    for chronic stable angina, 143-144
    for femoral-popliteal disease, 548-549
SIRTAX trial, 215-217
Sitagliptin, labeling of, 35b
Sitaxsentan, for HIV-related pulmonary arterial hypertension, 735
Site management, for clinical trial, 38
Sitostanol, 430
Sitosterol, 430
SK (streptokinase), 123, 123t
    in pregnancy and lactation, 622t-623t, 626
    for STEMI, 186, 188t
Skin cancer, after cardiac transplantation, 314
SKS stenting, for bifurcation lesion, 223
SLCO1B1 gene
    and clinical efficacy of simvastatin, 424
Sliding valvuloplasty, for posterior leaflet prolapse, 705
Small-access coronary revascularization, 227-230, 227t
SMART (Second Manifestation of Arterial Disease) study, 565-566
SMART (Strategies for Management of Anti-Retroviral Therapy) study, 732
SMASH trial, 195
SMASH-VT multicenter trial, 391
SMILE study, 247t, 248
Smoking
    and chronic stable angina, 137-138
    and global cardiovascular disease, 80
    with HIV infection, 733
Smoking cessation
    cardiac rehabilitation and, 741b
    for carotid artery disease, 555
    after NSTE-ACS, 166t, 168
    for peripheral artery disease, 542-543, 543b, 543f
    after STEMI, 205t, 206
Sobrero, Ascanio, 83
Society of Thoracic Surgeons (STS) risk score, for transcatheter aortic valve implant, 716
Sodium
    dietary
        and hypertension in children, 534
        label language for, 471, 471t
        and resistant hypertension, 504
        tips for reducing, 471
    and heart failure risk stratification, 286t
Sodium channels, 344
"Sodium free," 471t
Sodium intake, for hypertension, 468-469, 469t
Sodium nitroprusside
    for acute decompensated heart failure, 293, 294f-295f
    for acute hypertensive crisis due to pheochromocytoma, 493, 493t
    for acute pulmonary edema, 300, 301f
    for aortic dissection, 613
    for hypertensive emergencies, 514t-515t
    in pregnancy and lactation, 622t-623t
Sodium restriction, for heart failure, 243, 243t
    acute decompensated, 297
    pathophysiologic mechanisms and, 242-243
Soluble endoglin (sEng), in preeclampsia, 521-522, 522f
Soluble fms-related tyrosine kinase 1 (sFlt1), in preeclampsia, 521, 522f, 525-526

SOLVD Prevention trial, 246, 247t, 248
SOLVD Treatment trial, 246, 247t, 248, 258
Sotalol (Betapace), 352-353
    adverse reactions to, 353, 375t
    clinical applications of, 352-353
    clinical pharmacology of, 353
    dosage and administration of, 375t
        modification in disease states of, 353
    drug interactions with, 353
    for heart failure, 259
    indications for, 101
    mechanism of action of, 353
    pharmacodynamic properties and cardiac
        effects of, 98t
    in pregnancy, 628-629
    properties of, 102t
    for sustained monomorphic ventricular
        tachycardia, 410t, 411
SPACE trial, 563-564
SPAF trial, 618
SPARCL trial, 556-557
Specificity, 1-2, 2f
    and diagnostic cutoffs, 2-3, 2f
SPIRIT FIRST study, 217t
SPIRIT trial, 558
SPIRIT-II study, 217t
SPIRIT-III study, 217t
SPIRIT-IV study, 217-218, 217t
Spironolactone (Aldactone)
    for heart failure, 243t
        acute decompensated, 291
        clinical efficacy of, 253
        pathophysiology and, 253
        practical considerations with, 254
        with preserved ejection fraction, 260
        randomized controlled trials of, 253t
    for hypertension, 482, 482t
        in children, 536t
        resistant, 505-507, 506f-507f
    in pregnancy and lactation, 622t-623t, 623
    for primary aldosteronism, 497
    for STEMI
        during convalescence, 193
        in long-term management, 206
St. Jude Medical mechanical valve, 695-697,
        695t, 696f
    complication rates with, 697, 697t, 698f
St. Jude Medical mitral valve device, 722t, 723f,
        724
St. Jude Medical Toronto-SPV stentless porcine
        bioprosthesis, 695t, 696f, 699
St. Thomas' Atherosclerosis Regression Study
        (STARS), 429, 429t
STABLE trial, 615
Stages of Change model, 448
Standardized normal statistic (Z_1), 9-10, 11f
Standards for Reporting of Diagnostic
        Accuracy (STARD), 1-2
Stanol(s), 430
Staphylococcus aureus, endocarditis due to
        methicillin-sensitive, 654
Staphylococcus viridans, endocarditis due to,
        654
STAR trial, 575-576, 576t
STARD (Standards for Reporting of Diagnostic
        Accuracy), 1-2
Starr, Albert, 691
Starr-Edwards valve, 695-697, 695t
STARS study, 429, 429t
Statewide system, for STEMI, 69
Statin(s), 60-63, 421-433
    for abdominal aortic aneurysms, 608
    available, 421-422
    with bile acid sequestrants, 428-430, 429t
        clinical efficacy of, 429, 429t
        effects on lipids and lipoproteins of, 429
        safety/compliance issues for, 429-430
    for cardiac syndrome X, 169

Statin(s) (Continued)
    for carotid artery disease, 556-557
    for chronic stable angina, 147-149
    dosage of, 422, 422t
    drug interactions with, 60-61, 422-423, 423t
    effects on lipids and lipoproteins of, 60-63,
        422t
    efficacy of, 423-424
        angiographic trials of, 423, 424f
        large-scale clinical trials of, 423-424, 425t
    with ezetimibe and cholesterol absorption
        inhibitors, 430
        effect on lipids and lipoproteins of, 430
        efficacy of, 430
        safety of, 430
    with HIV infection and HAART, 733, 733f
    indications for, 60, 421
    mechanism of action of, 60, 421
    mechanism of benefit of, 424-431, 426b
    for noncardiac vascular surgery, 544
    after NSTE-ACS, 167-168, 167f-168f
    for peripheral artery disease, 541
    pharmacodynamics and pharmacokinetics
        of, 60, 60t, 422-424, 422t
    pharmacogenetics of, 61-63
        future directions for, 63
        genetic polymorphism in, 54t, 62t
            and adverse effects, 63
        genome-wide association studies in, 62t,
            63
            APOC1 gene in, 62t, 63
            CLMN gene in, 62t, 63
        key genes in, 54t, 61t
            APOE as, 61, 62t
            CETP as, 61-62
            HMGCR as, 61
            KIF6 as, 62-63, 62t
            LDLR as, 62
            PCSK9 as, 61, 62t
        therapeutic implications of, 63
    with plant stanol esters, 430-431
        effects on lipids and lipoproteins of,
            430-431
        efficacy against coronary heart disease of,
            430-431
        safety of, 431
    in pregnancy, 627
    for primary vs. secondary prevention of
        cardiovascular disease, 421, 425t
    for renal artery stenosis, 574
    residual risk for, 434-435
    safety of, 424-431, 428b
        for liver, 424-426, 427f, 428b
        for muscle, 427-428, 428b
    after STEMI, 206
    for thoracic aortic atheroembolism, 618
    for thromboprophylaxis, 593
Statin-fibrin combination, for mixed
        dyslipidemia, 436
Statin-niacin combination, for mixed
        dyslipidemia, 436-437
Statin–omega-3 fatty acids combination, for
        mixed dyslipidemia, 437-438
Statistics, for clinical trial, 38
Stavudine (d4T), for HIV infection, 730t
Stem cell(s)
    cardiac
        age, cardiac disease and, 327-330
        endogenous, 326-327, 327f-330f
        hematopoietic stem cell
            transdifferentiation to, 323
        in myocardial repair, 322, 324f
    hematopoietic, 322
        in myocardial repair, 322, 324f
        transdifferentiation of, 323-324, 325f
Stem cell niches, 327, 328f-329f
STEMI. See ST-segment elevation myocardial
        infarction (STEMI).

Stent(s)
    for aortoiliac disease, 546-547, 547f
    carotid artery, 562-565
        indications for, 562, 562f
        in normal-risk symptomatic patients,
            563-565, 565f
        serial steps during, 559f
        in symptomatic and asymptomatic
            patients at high surgical risk, 563
    coronary. See Coronary stent(s).
    for femoral-popliteal disease, 547-548,
        548f-549f
    renal artery, 574-577
Stented bovine pericardial prosthesis, 695t,
        696f
Stented porcine valve bioprosthesis, 695t, 696f
Stented xenografts, 697
    characteristics of, 696t
    currently available, 695t, 696f
Stent-grafts
    for aortic aneurysms
        abdominal, 606-607, 607f
        thoracic, 612-613
    for aortic dissection, 615-616, 616f
Stentless porcine valve prosthesis, 695t, 696f
Stentless xenografts, 697-699
    characteristics of, 696t
    currently available, 695t, 696f
Step-down therapy, for antihypertensives, 486
Step-down unit, for STEMI, 190-192
STICH trial, 261
Stimulation threshold, 752, 754f
STRATEGY trial, 216t
Stratification levels, 6
STRENGTH study, 63
Streptococcus bovis, endocarditis due to, 655t
Streptococcus viridans, endocarditis due to,
        654, 655t
Streptokinase (SK), 123, 123t
    in pregnancy and lactation, 622t-623t, 626
    for STEMI, 186, 188t
Streptomycin, for infective endocarditis, 656t
Stress echocardiography, for chronic stable
        angina, 133-134, 137t
Stress electrocardiography, for chronic stable
        angina, 132, 133b, 134f-135f, 137t
Stress myocardial perfusion scintigraphy, for
        chronic stable angina, 134-135, 135b, 137t
STRESS study, 143, 214
Stress testing, for chronic stable angina, 136,
        137t
Stroke
    due to atrial fibrillation, 378, 378b, 378t
    epidemiology of, 553
    infective endocarditis with, 659t-660t,
        660-661
    risk of, 553
Structural heart disease, catheter ablation
        for ventricular tachycardia with, 391-392,
        391f
Structural valve degeneration (SVD), 696b
    aortic, 701, 701f
    mitral, 708
STS (Society of Thoracic Surgeons) risk score,
        for transcatheter aortic valve implant, 716
ST-segment elevation myocardial infarction
        (STEMI), 178-213
    Chain of Survival for, 178-179
    defined, 178
    emergency department management of,
        179-181
    early risk assessment in, 181-190
    medications used in, 181-184
        analgesia as, 181-182
        anticoagulant agents as, 182-183,
            183f-184f
        antiplatelet agents as, 182, 182f
        β-blockers as, 183-184

ST-segment elevation myocardial infarction (STEMI) *(Continued)*
nitroglycerin as, 181
oxygen as, 181
patient evaluation in, 180-181
patient triage in, 179-180
reperfusion therapy in, 184-190
fibrinolytic therapy as, 185-186, 187b, 188f, 188t
general concepts of, 184-185
in hospitals without on-site cardiac surgery, 190, 191b
percutaneous coronary intervention as, 186-190, 189f, 189t-190t
pharmacoinvasive management as, 190
predicted transfer and door-to-balloon time for, 185, 187f
risk of bleeding and, 185
risk stratification and, 185, 186f
stents in, 190
thrombus aspiration in, 190
time from symptom onset to, 185
epidemiology of, 178, 179t
exercise testing after, 740
hospital management of, 190-204
for arrhythmias, 198-199
brady-, 198-199, 198t
supraventricular, 199
ventricular, 199, 200f
for coronary artery bypass surgery, 202
for deep venous thrombosis and pulmonary embolism, 201
for hemodynamic disturbances, 193-196, 194f
due to cardiogenic shock, 195
hemodynamic assessment in, 193
due to hypotension, 193, 194f
due to low-output state, 193, 195f
due to pulmonary congestion, 193-194
due to right ventricular infarction, 196, 196f
for hemorrhagic complications, 201-202, 202b
for ischemic stroke, 200-201, 201f
location of, 190-192, 191b
for mechanical complications, 196-198
left ventricular aneurysm and left ventricular thrombus as, 197-198
left ventricular free wall rupture as, 197, 197t
mechanical support devices for, 198
mitral regurgitation as, 196-197, 197t
ventricular septal rupture as, 197, 197t
medications in, 192-193
antithrombotic agents as, 192
β-blockers as, 192
calcium channel blockers as, 193
for glycemic control, 193
nitroglycerin as, 192
renin-angiotensin-aldosterone system blockers as, 192-193
for recurrent chest pain, 199-200
due to pericarditis, 200
due to recurrent ischemia or infarction, 199-200
risk stratification in, 202-204, 203f
assessment of electrical substrate in, 204
echocardiography in, 202-203
exercise testing in, 202
invasive evaluation for, 204
left ventricular function in, 203-204
myocardial perfusion imaging in, 203
myocardial viability in, 204
routine measures in, 192
long-term management of, 204-207
for functional status, 207
follow-up visit in, 207

ST-segment elevation myocardial infarction (STEMI) *(Continued)*
physical activity in, 205t, 207
psychosocial impact in, 207
return to work and disability in, 207
medications in, 205t, 206-207
antiplatelet agents as, 205t, 206
β-blockers as, 205t, 206
and hormone replacement therapy, 207
renin-angiotensin-aldosterone system blockers as, 205t, 206
statins as, 206
risk factor control in, 204-206, 205t
blood pressure control in, 205t, 206
diabetes management in, 205t, 206
lipid management in, 205t, 206
smoking cessation in, 205t, 206
weight management in, 204, 205t
overview of, 178
prehospital management of, 178-179
destination protocols in, 179, 180f
emergency medical services and systems of care for, 179
fibrinolysis in, 179, 180f
out-of-hospital arrest in, 179
symptom recognition in, 178
primary and secondary prevention of, 178
quality improvement for, 71-72
systems of care for, 68-69, 68f
catheterization laboratory activation in, 68-69
Mission: Lifeline program in, 69
need for, 67-68
prehospital diagnosis in, 68-69
regional transfer protocols in, 69
selected programs developing, 68, 69t
statewide systems as, 69
transport to primary percutaneous coronary intervention centers in, 68-69
"Stunned" myocardium, 133-134
Subarachnoid hemorrhage (SAH), hypertensive emergencies with, 516
Subgroup analyses, 13
Sudden cardiac death (SCD), 396
defined, 396
epidemiology of, 396, 408, 409f
due to hypertrophic cardiomyopathy, 335, 335f
implantable cardioverter-defibrillators for prevention of, 396-407
cardiac resynchronization, 401, 403f
indications for, 401-404, 403b, 403f
primary, 397-398
clinical trials of, 397-398, 399t, 400f
with comorbidities, 400-401, 402f
risk stratification for, 398-400, 400t
secondary, 396, 398t
systems and technology for, 396-406, 397f
model of, 408, 409f
risk stratification for, 398-400, 400t
autonomic function (baroreflex slope) in, 398, 400t
ejection fraction in, 398, 400t
electrophysiologic studies in, 398, 400t
genetic testing in, 400
left ventricular scar burden in, 398-400, 400t
nonsustained ventricular arrhythmias in, 398, 400t
signal-averaged ECG in, 398, 400t
T-wave alternans in, 398, 400t
Suicide ventricle, 699
Sular (nisoldipine), for hypertension, 479t
Sulfhydryl depletion hypothesis, of nitrate tolerance, 87-88

Supera stent, for femoral-popliteal disease, 548
Superficial femoral artery (SFA) disease, 545f, 547-549, 548f-549f
Superficial venous thrombosis, 586-587
Superior treatment, 22-23
Superior Yield of the new Strategy of Enoxaparin, Revascularization and Glycoprotein IIb/IIIa Inhibitors (SYNERGY) trial, 160-161
Superiority trials, 8f, 9
Superoparaseptal space, 383-384
Supralimus stent, 221
Supraventricular arrhythmia, after STEMI, 199
Supraventricular tachyarrhythmias, catheter ablation for, 383-386
Supraventricular tachycardias (SVTs), 365-371
antidromic, 383
atrial flutter as, 369-371, 370f
long-term management of, 370
multifocal, 370
short-term management of, 370
calcium channel blockers for, 92
catheter ablation for accessory pathway–mediated, 383-385, 384f
circus movement, 383
evaluation of therapy for, 365
inappropriate sinus tachycardia as, 367, 371
junctional ectopic tachycardia as, 371
orthodromic, 383
paroxysmal, 366
long-term therapy of, 369, 369f
management of acute episodes of, 367-369, 368f, 369t
mechanism of, 366-369, 366f-367f
pharmacology of, 365, 366t
in pregnancy, 628
Surgical embolectomy, for pulmonary embolism, 590
Surgical myectomy, for LVOT obstruction, 332, 333f, 334t
Surgical Treatment for Ischemic Heart Failure (STICH) trial, 261
Surrogate endpoint, 9, 10f
for cardiovascular device trials, 45
Surveillance
after ERASR, 577
postmarket
for medical devices, 48-50, 48b
for new drugs, 35-36
of renovascular disease, 577-578
safety, 38
SVD (structural valve degeneration), 696b
aortic, 701, 701f
mitral, 708
SVGs (saphenous vein grafts), 222, 231t
alternatives to, 230-232, 231t
SVR (systemic vascular resistance), in acute decompensated heart failure, 290
SVST (single-vessel small thoracotomy direct-vision bypass grafting), 227-228, 228f
SVTs. *See* Supraventricular tachycardias (SVTs).
SWORD trial, 259, 352-353, 356
Sympathetic nervous system, in heart failure, 283
Sympathomimetic drugs, hypertensive emergencies due to, 518
Symplicity HTN-2 trial, 578
Symptom recognition, for STEMI, 178
Syndrome X
cardiac, 168-169, 169b, 170f
β-adrenergic blockers for, 100
metabolic, 168
SYNERGY stent, 221
SYNERGY trial, 160-161
System, defined, 67

Systemic perfusion, in acute decompensated heart failure, 287
Systemic vascular resistance (SVR), in acute decompensated heart failure, 290
Systems of health care
  defined, 67
  experience to date with, 68-70
    for heart failure, 69-70
    for out-of-hospital cardiac arrest, 70
    for STEMI, 68-69, 68f
      catheterization laboratory activation in, 68-69
      Mission: Lifeline program in, 69
      prehospital diagnosis in, 68-69
      regional transfer protocols in, 69
      selected programs developing, 68, 69t
      statewide systems as, 69
      transport to primary percutaneous coronary intervention centers in, 68-69
  vs. health care systems, 67
  lessons learned about, 72
  need for, 67-68
  and quality improvement
    experience to date with, 71-72
      for heart failure, 72
      for out-of-hospital cardiac arrest, 72
      for STEMI, 71-72
    theory of, 70-71
  for STEMI, 179
  and systems theory, 67
Systems theory, 67
Systems thinking, 67
System-specific barriers, to lifestyle modifications for hypertension, 469
Syst-Eur trial, 555
Systolic anterior motion (SAM), of mitral valve, 332-333
Systolic blood pressure (SBP), and heart failure risk stratification, 285, 285t
Systolic blood pressure (SBP) levels
  for boys, 530t-531t
  for girls, 531t-532t
Systolic Hypertension in the Elderly Program (SHEP), 555

T

TAAs. See Thoracic aortic aneurysms (TAAs).
Tachyarrhythmias, catheter ablation for, 383-395
  indications for, 383, 384b
  practical considerations with, 383, 384f
  results of, 383, 384t
  for supraventricular tachyarrhythmias, 383-386
    accessory pathway–mediated tachycardias as, 383-385, 384f
    atrial fibrillation as, 386-390, 387f-388f
    atrial flutter as, 386, 386f
    atrial tachycardia as, 385-386
    atrioventricular node reentry tachycardia as, 385, 385f
  for ventricular tachyarrhythmias, 390-392
    idiopathic ventricular tachycardia as, 390-391
    ventricular fibrillation and polymorphic ventricular tachycardia as, 392
    ventricular tachycardia in patients with structural heart disease as, 391-392, 391f
Tacrolimus, with cardiac transplantation, 311t
TACTICS-TIMI trial, 164, 164f, 170-171
Tadalafil
  in pregnancy, 629
  for pulmonary arterial hypertension, 602
Tailor prosthesis, 695t
Takeuchi procedure, 633t

TALISMAN trial, 549
TAMARIS trial, 549
TandemHeart device, 224
TAO trial, 163
Tarka (trandolapril/verapamil ER), for hypertension, 485t
TASC (Trans-Atlantic Inter-Society Consensus Document), 545, 545f
Task shifting, 78
TAVI. See Transcatheter aortic valve implant (TAVI).
Taxus Element stent, 219-220
Taxus paclitaxel-eluting stent, 215
TAXUS study, 215, 216t
Taxus-Express, 215
Taxus-Liberte, 215
Taztia. See Diltiazem.
3TC (lamivudine), for HIV infection, 730t
TCP (transcutaneous pacing), 758, 758f
TECAB (totally endoscopic coronary bypass), 229, 230f
TEE (transesophageal echocardiography), of infective endocarditis, 652, 653b, 653t, 654f
Tekamlo (aliskiren/amlodipine), for hypertension, 485t
Tekturna (aliskiren)
  for heart failure, 263-264
  for hypertension, 483-484, 483t
Tekturna HCT (aliskiren/hydrochlorothiazide), for hypertension, 485t
Telmisartan (Micardis), for hypertension, 479t
Telmisartan/amlodipine (Twynsta), for hypertension, 485t
Telmisartan/hydrochlorothiazide (Micardis HCT), for hypertension, 485t
Temporary pacemakers, 752-758
  complications and troubleshooting with, 758
  indications for, 752-758, 758f
  placement of, 758
Tenecteplase (TNK), 123t, 124
  for STEMI, 186, 188t
Tenofovir, for HIV infection, 730t
Tenoretic (atenolol/chlorthalidone), for hypertension, 485t
Tenormin. See Atenolol (Tenormin).
Terazosin (Hytrin), for hypertension, 483t
  due to pheochromocytoma, 491-493, 492t
Terutroban, 115
  for carotid artery disease, 558
Test treatments, 5-6, 5b
Tetracycline
  for abdominal aortic aneurysms, 608
  for neoplastic pericarditis, 673
Tetralogy of Fallot (TOF), 643-645
  epidemiology of, 643
  pathophysiology of, 643, 643f
  presentation in adults of, 643
  recommendations for, 645
  repair of
    atrial arrhythmias after, 644
    pulmonary artery stenosis after, 644-645, 644f-645f
    with pulmonary valve replacement, 644
    risk of death after, 643
    risk of worsening functional capacity after, 643
    RVOT obstruction after, 644-645, 644f-645f
    ventricular failure after, 643, 643t
  RVOT in, 643
    after repair, 644-645, 644f-645f
TEVAR (thoracic endovascular aortic repair), 612-613
Teveten (eprosartan mesylate), for hypertension, 479t
Teveten HCT (eprosartan mesylate/hydrochlorothiazide), for hypertension, 485t

TG(s). See Triglycerides (TGs).
TGF-β (transforming growth factor-β), in Marfan syndrome, 613
TH (therapeutic hypothermia), after cardiac arrest, 417
Thalitone. See Chlorthalidone (Hygroton, Thalitone).
Therapeutic hypothermia (TH), after cardiac arrest, 417
Therapeutic Lifestyle Changes diet, 192
Therapeutic strategies
  phases of evaluation of new, 3-4, 4t
  tools for assessment of, 1-32
    clinical trials as, 3-11
    comparative effectiveness research as, 19-23
    cost-effectiveness analysis as, 23-30
    meta-analysis as, 15-19
    trials that test equivalence of, 8-9, 8f
ThermoCool device, 722t
Thermodilution measurements, in acute decompensated heart failure, 290
Thiazide diuretics
  for carotid artery stenosis, 555
  for heart failure, 243-245, 243t
  for hypertension, 477t, 480-481, 480t
    in children, 536t
    in combination products, 485t
    monitoring and adverse effects of, 485t
    resistant, 505, 506f
  for peripheral edema in pregnancy, 623
  for primary aldosteronism, 497
Thiazide-like diuretics
  for heart failure, 243t
  for hypertension, 480-481
Thiazolidinediones (TZDs), with heart failure, 262
Thienopyridine derivatives, mechanisms of action of, 109
Thoracic aortic aneurysms (TAAs), 608-613
  etiology of, 608
  in Marfan syndrome, 608, 613
  medical management of, 613
  natural history of, 608
  surgical management of, 608-613
    of aortic arch, 609-611, 611f
    of aortic root, 609, 610f
    of ascending aorta, 609, 609f
    Bentall procedure for, 609
    cerebral protection with, 611
    complications of, 612
    composite aortic graft for, 609, 610f
    David-I technique for, 609
    David-V technique for, 609
    of descending aorta, 609, 612-613
    in Ehlers-Danlos syndrome, 608
    elephant trunk technique for, 612, 612f
    hemiarch repair for, 609, 611f
    hybrid procedure for, 611-612, 612f
    interposition prosthetic Dacron graft for, 609, 609f
    in Loeys-Dietz syndrome, 608
    in Marfan syndrome, 608
    Ross procedure for, 609
    timing of, 608
    total aortic arch repair for, 609-611, 611f
    transluminally placed endovascular stent-graft for, 612-613
    valve-sparing root repair for, 609, 610f
Thoracic aortic atheroembolism, 617-618
Thoracic endovascular aortic repair (TEVAR), 612-613
Thoracic endovascular stent-graft, for aortic dissection, 615-616, 616f
Thoracoscopic minimally invasive direct coronary bypass, 228
3F valve, 699

Thrombin generation, mechanism of, 115-117, 116f
Thrombin inhibitors, direct. See Direct thrombin inhibitors (DTIs).
Thrombocytopenia, heparin-induced, 117, 587, 588f
Thromboembolic disease, venous. See Venous thromboembolism (VTE).
Thromboembolic prophylaxis, for atrial fibrillation, 378, 378b, 378t
Thrombophilias, inherited, 580-581
Thromboprophylaxis, 591-593
  duration of and extension after discharge of, 593, 593t
  with hip replacement, knee replacement, and hip fracture, 592, 592b
  in-hospital, 592
  mechanical, 592-593
  in patients with cancer, 591-592
  in pregnancy, 624-626
  unconventional agents for, 592-593
    with statins, 593
    with vitamin E, 592-593
Thrombosis
  anticoagulant therapy for, 115-120
    direct thrombin inhibitors as, 118, 119f
      argatroban as, 120
      bivalirudin (hirulog) as, 120
      hirudin (lepirudin) as, 118-120
    low-molecular-weight heparin as, 117-118
      dosages of, 118
      indications for, 118
      mechanisms of action of, 117-118
      side effects and contraindications to, 118
    with oral anticoagulants, 121-123
      novel agents as, 122, 122f
      warfarin as, 121-122
    unfractionated heparin as, 115-117
      dosages of, 117
      indications for, 117
      mechanisms of action of, 115-117, 116f
      side effects and contraindications to, 117
  antiplatelet therapy for, 107-115
    aspirin as, 107-109
      dosages of, 109
      indication for, 108-109
      mechanism of action of, 107-108, 108f
      side effects and contraindications to, 109
    glycoprotein IIB/IIIA receptor antagonists as, 114-115
      dosages of, 114-115
      indications for, 114
      mechanisms of action of, 114
      side effects and contraindications to, 115
    novel agents in, 115, 116f
    P2Y$_{12}$ receptor antagonists as, 109-114
      dosages of, 112-113
      indication for, 111-112, 112t
      mechanism of action of, 109-111, 110f, 110t
      side effects and contraindications to, 113-114
  factor Xa inhibitors for, 121
  fibrinolytics for, 122-123
    dosages of, 123
    indications for, 123, 123t
    mechanisms of action of, 122
    side effects and contraindications to, 123, 124b
  and ischemic cardiovascular heart disease, 107-123
  platelet-mediated, 107, 107f
Thrombus, with prosthetic heart valve, 49f
Thrombus aspiration, for STEMI, 190

THUNDER trial, 548-549
THVs (transthoracic heart valves), 717-718
Thyroid dysfunction, 499
  presentation and diagnosis of, 499
  principles of treatment of, 499
Tiazac. See Diltiazem.
Ticagrelor, 110t
  vs. clopidogrel, 57
  dosage of, 113
  indication for, 112
  international regulation of, 37b
  mechanism of action of, 111
  for NSTE-ACS, 157
  side effects and contraindications to, 113-114
  for STEMI
    in acute phase, 182
    with PCI, 189f
Ticlopidine, 110t
  for chronic stable angina, 144
  dosage of, 112
  mechanism of action of, 109-111
  side effects and contraindications to, 113
Tilting disk mechanical valve, 695-697, 695t, 696f
Time horizon, of cost-effectiveness analysis, 28-29, 29f
TIME trial, 171
TIMI 3B trial, 164, 164f
TIMI 9 trial, 119
TIMI risk score, 153, 154t, 181, 186f
  with HIV infection, 732
Timolide (timolol maleate/ hydrochlorothiazide), for hypertension, 485t
Timolol (Blocadren)
  for hypertension, 481t
  indications for, 101
  pharmacodynamic properties and cardiac effects of, 98t
  pharmacology of, 250
  properties of, 102t
  for survivors of acute myocardial infarction, 99
Timolol maleate/hydrochlorothiazide (Timolide), for hypertension, 485t
Tipping-point approach, to implementing change, 70-71
Tipranavir, for HIV infection, 729t
TIPS study, 80
TIPS-K trial, 80
Tirofiban
  dosage of, 115
  indications for, 114
  mechanism of action of, 114
  for NSTE-ACS, 158
  with PCI for STEMI, 189t
Tissue plasminogen activator (tPA), 123, 123t
  in pregnancy, 626
Tissue-biomaterial interaction, 48
Titanium-nitride oxide stent, 220-221
TMEM127 gene, and pheochromocytomas, 490
TMLR (transmyocardial laser revascularization), for ischemic heart disease with heart failure, 261-262
TNK (tenecteplase), 123t, 124
  for STEMI, 186, 188t
TNT trial, 61, 63, 424, 425t
Tobacco use
  and chronic stable angina, 137-138
  and global cardiovascular disease, 80
  with HIV infection, 733
  quitting. See Smoking cessation.
TOF. See Tetralogy of Fallot (TOF).
Tolvaptan, for acute decompensated heart failure, 302
TOPCARE-AMI trial, 324
TOPCARE-DCM trial, 325
TOPCAT study, 254

TOPCAT trial, 260, 260t
Toprol. See Metoprolol (Lopressor, Toprol).
Torcetrapib
  for chronic stable angina, 149
  for low HDL cholesterol, 439
Tornado diagram, 26, 27f
Tornado plot, 26, 27f
Toronto-SPV stentless porcine bioprosthesis, 695t, 696f, 699
Torsades de pointes, 413-414
  catheter ablation for, 392
  causes of, 413, 414b
  ECG of, 413, 413f
  magnesium for, 413-414
Torsemide (Demadex)
  for heart failure, 243t
  for hypertension, 480t
  in pregnancy and lactation, 622t-623t
Total product life cycle approach, 47, 47f
Totally endoscopic coronary bypass (TECAB), 229, 230f
Toxin-induced pericardial disease, 674, 675t
Toxoplasma gondii, after cardiac transplantation, 312
TP receptor antagonists, 115
tPA (tissue plasminogen activator), 123, 123t
  in pregnancy, 626
TR. See Tricuspid regurgitation (TR).
TRACE trial, 247t
TRACER trial, 115
Training effect, 742
Training heart rate, 743, 743f
Trandate. See Labetalol (Trandate, Normodyne).
Trandolapril (Mavik)
  for heart failure, 246t
  for hypertension, 478t
Trandolapril/verapamil ER (Tarka), for hypertension, 485t
Transapical valves, 721, 721f
Transarterial transcatheter device, for patent ductus arteriosus, 645-646
Trans-Atlantic Inter-Society Consensus Document (TASC), 545, 545f
Transcatheter aortic valve implant (TAVI), 714
  access site evaluation for, 716
  for bicuspid aortic valve, 640
  currently available implants for, 714-715, 715f
  implantation procedure for, 717-721, 717f
  measurement of aortic valve annulus for, 716-717
  new access approaches for, 719
  new applications of, 719
  next generation of, 720-721, 720f, 720t
  patient evaluation and imaging prior to, 715-717, 715f
  patient outcomes with, 717-719, 718f-719f, 719t
  potential complications of, 719-720
  transapical valves in, 721
Transcatheter closure techniques, for ventricular septal defect, 646, 647f
Transcatheter pulmonary valve, for tetralogy of Fallot, 644
TRANSCEND trial, 479
Transcutaneous pacing (TCP), 758, 758f
Transdifferentiation, of hematopoietic stem cells, 323-324, 325f
Transesophageal echocardiography (TEE), of infective endocarditis, 652, 653b, 653t, 654f
Transfer protocols, for STEMI, 69
Transfer time, predicted, for STEMI, 185
Transforming growth factor-β (TGF-β), in Marfan syndrome, 613
Transition probabilities, 25
Transitional artery, 230-231
Translational blocks, 3-4, 3f

Translational science, spectrum of, 3-4, 3f
Transluminally placed endovascular stent-graft, for thoracic aortic aneurysms, 612-613
Transmyocardial laser revascularization (TMLR), for ischemic heart disease with heart failure, 261-262
Transradial access, for cardiac catheterization, 223-224
Transthoracic echocardiography (TTE)
    of infective endocarditis, 652, 653b, 653t, 654f
    of pulmonary embolism, 584, 585f
Transthoracic heart valves (THVs), 717-718
Transvenous pacing (TVP), 758, 758f
Traumatic pericardial disease, 674
Treatment effects
    detection of, 13-15, 15f-16f
    measures of, 12-13, 14t
Treatment IND, 35
Triage, for STEMI, 179-180
Trial-based cost-effectiveness analyses, 24-25
Triamcinolone
    for pericardial disease with renal failure, 674
    for postpericardial injury syndrome, 673
    for recurrent pericarditis, 668
Triamterene (Dyrenium)
    for acute decompensated heart failure, 291
    for heart failure, 243t
    for hypertension, 480t
Tribenzor (olmesartan medoxomil/amlodipine/ hydrochlorothiazide), for hypertension, 485t
Tricuspid insufficiency, 687
Tricuspid regurgitation (TR), 687
    functional, 708
    indications for surgical management of, 708
    with mitral valve disease, 709
    in pregnancy, 623-624
Tricuspid stenosis, 687
    indications for surgical management of, 708
Tricuspid valve disease, 687
Tricuspid valve repair, 708
Tricuspid valve replacement, 708
Tricuspid valve surgery, 708
    indications for, 708
    results of, 708
    surgical approach for, 708
    timing of, 687
    valve repair as, 708
    valve replacement as, 708
Triglycerides (TGs), elevated
    HIV infection and, 730, 733
    therapy to manage, 434-441
        non–HDL-c reduction in, 435, 435t
        rationale for, 434-435, 435f
        statin-fibrate, 436
        statin-niacin, 436-437
        statin–omega 3 fatty acids, 437-438
        therapy to modify HDL in, 435-436
Trimetazidine, for chronic angina, 106
Trimethaphan, for hypertensive emergencies, 514t-515t
Trimethoprim-sulfamethoxazole, after cardiac transplantation, 312
Triple therapy, for heart failure, 246-248
Triple-blind trials, 6
TRITON trial, 111-112
TRITON-TIMI 38 trial
    cost-effectiveness analysis in, 25
    indications in, 111-112
    NSTE-ACS in, 156-157
    pharmacogenetics in, 53, 56-57
    STEMI in, 182
TRIUMPH study, 601-602

Trizivir (abacavir/lamivudine/zidovudine), for HIV infection, 729-730, 730t
Troponins
    in heart failure, 284, 284f
    for STEMI, 181
Truvada (emtricitabine/tenofovir), for HIV infection, 729-730, 730t
T-stenting, for bifurcation lesion, 223, 223f
TTE (transthoracic echocardiography)
    of infective endocarditis, 652, 653b, 653t, 654f
    of pulmonary embolism, 584, 585f
T-type calcium channels, 90
Tuberculous pericarditis, 672-673
TVP (transvenous pacing), 758, 758f
T-wave alternans, and risk of sudden cardiac death, 398, 400t
2 x 2 table, 1-2, 2f
Two-stent approach, for bifurcation lesion, 223
Two-way sensitivity analysis, 26-27, 28f
Twynsta (telmisartan/amlodipine), for hypertension, 485t
Type I errors, 1-2, 2f, 9-11
Type II errors, 1-2, 2f, 9-11
TYPHOON trial, 216t
Tyramine, and MAO inhibitors, hypertensive emergencies due to, 518
TZDs (thiazolidinediones), with heart failure, 262

U

UA (unstable angina). See Non–ST-elevation acute coronary syndrome (NSTE-ACS).
UFH. See Unfractionated heparin (UFH).
U.K. Small Aneurysm Trial, 606
Ulcer, penetrating atherosclerotic, of aorta, 617
Ultrafiltration, for acute decompensated heart failure, 291-292
ULV (upper limit of vulnerability), 759, 759t
Unblinded trials, 6
Undersensing, 752, 754f
Unfractionated heparin (UFH), 115-117
    dosages of, 117
    indications for, 117
    mechanisms of action of, 115-117, 116f
    for NSTE-ACS, 159-161, 160t-161t, 161f, 163t
    in pregnancy and lactation, 622t-623t, 625
    side effects and contraindications to, 117
    for STEMI
        in acute phase, 182-183, 183f-184f
        during convalescence, 192
        with PCI, 190t
    for thromboprophylaxis, 591
    for venous thromboembolism, 587
Uniretic (moexipril/hydrochlorothiazide), for hypertension, 485t
United Network of Organ Sharing (UNOS), 309, 309t
Univasc (moexipril), for hypertension, 478t
UNLOAD trial, 291-292
"Unsalted", 471t
Unsaturated fat diets, for hyperlipidemia, 444-445, 444t
Unstable angina (UA). See Non–ST-elevation acute coronary syndrome (NSTE-ACS).
Upper limit of vulnerability (ULV), 759, 759t
U.S. Carvedilol Heart Failure Trials, 250, 251t
U.S. product approval, use of foreign data for, 46
Use dependence, of antiarrhythmic drugs, 344
Utilities, 23

V

V stenting, for bifurcation lesion, 223f
VA 309 trial, 560, 561t
VACS study, 144, 565
VAD. See Ventricular assist device (VAD).
VAHIT trial, 436
Valganciclovir, after cardiac transplantation, 312
Val-HeFT trial, 246-250, 247t, 255, 258
VALIANT trial, 5, 247t, 248, 272
Valid scientific evidence, for premarket approval, 43
"Valsalva grafts," for thoracic aortic aneurysms, 609
Valsartan (Diovan)
    for heart failure, 245-248, 246t, 250
    for hypertension, 479t
        in children, 536t
    for maintenance of sinus rhythm, 377
    for STEMI
        during convalescence, 192-193
        in long-term management, 206
Valsartan/amlodipine (Exforge), for hypertension, 485t
Valsartan/hydrochlorothiazide (Diovan HCT), for hypertension, 485t
Valturna (aliskiren/valsartan), for hypertension, 485t
VALUE trial, 94, 95f
Valve degeneration, structural, 696b
    aortic, 701, 701f
    mitral, 708
Valve dysfunction, nonstructural, 696b
Valve prostheses, 694-699
    annuloplasty devices as, 695t
    autografts as, 696t
    characteristics of, 694-695, 696t
    currently available, 694-695, 695t, 696f
    homografts as, 699
        characteristics of, 696t
        currently available, 695t, 696f
    mechanical, 695-697
        characteristics of, 696t
        currently available, 695t, 696f
        valve-related complications with, 697, 697t, 698f
    pregnancy with, 626
    valve-related complications of, 695, 696b
    xenografts as
        stented, 697
            characteristics of, 696t
            currently available, 695t, 696f
        stentless, 697-699
            characteristics of, 696t
            currently available, 695t, 696f
Valve surgery, 691-713
    aortic, 699-702
        for aortic insufficiency/regurgitation, 683, 700
            in asymptomatic patients, 683
            overall approach to, 683, 684f
            in symptomatic patients with LV dysfunction, 683
            in symptomatic patients with normal LV function, 683
        for aortic stenosis, 699-700
            in asymptomatic patients, 678
            in elderly patients, 678
            in low-grade stenosis, 677-678
            overall approach to, 678, 678b, 679f
            in symptomatic patients, 677
        aortic valve repair for, 702
        aortic valve replacement as, 700-701
            choice of prosthesis for, 701, 701f
            indications for, 678, 678b

Valve surgery (Continued)
    patient-prosthesis mismatch in, 701
    surgical technique for, 700, 700f
  indications for, 699-700
  for mixed aortic valve disease, 699-700
  overview of, 699-700
  results of, 702
    early, 702
    late, 702
  for atrial fibrillation, 711
  for endocarditis, 709-710
  historical background of, 691, 692t
  indications for, 691-692
  with ischemic heart disease, 710-711
    aortic stenosis in CABG patients as, 710
    incidental coronary disease in valve
      surgery patients as, 710
    incidental valve disease in coronary
      surgery patients as, 710
    mitral regurgitation in CABG patients as,
      710-711, 711f
  mitral, 702-708
    Carpentier's functional classification and,
      703-704, 703f, 703t
    indications for, 704
    for mitral insufficiency/regurgitation, 686,
      704
      in asymptomatic patients, 686
      in symptomatic patients, 686
    for mitral stenosis, 680-681, 704
      in asymptomatic patients, 680,
        680f
      with left atrial or left atrial appendage
        thrombosis, 680-681
      overall approach to, 680-681
      in patients with mild symptoms, 680,
        681f
      in patients with moderate to severe
        symptoms, 680, 681f
    mitral valve repair as, 704-706
      annuloplasty in, 704-705
      leaflet prolapse repair techniques in,
        705
      other techniques in, 706
      principles of, 703f, 704
      restricted leaflet techniques in,
        705-706
    mitral valve replacement as, 706
      choice of prosthesis for, 706, 706f
      chordal-sparing, 706
    overview of, 702-704, 702f
    preoperative evaluation for, 704
    results of, 706-708
      early, 706-707
      late, 707-708, 707f
    surgical anatomy for, 703, 703f
  for multiple valve dysfunctions, 709
    aortic and mitral, 709
    mitral and tricuspid, 709
  optimal timing of, 676-690
    for aortic insufficiency, 683
      in asymptomatic patients, 683
      overall approach to, 683, 684f
      in symptomatic patients with LV
        dysfunction, 683
      in symptomatic patients with normal LV
        function, 683
    for aortic stenosis, 676-678
      in asymptomatic patients, 678
      in elderly patients, 678
      in low-grade stenosis, 677-678
      overall approach to, 678, 678b, 679f
      in symptomatic patients, 677
    for mitral insufficiency, 686
      in asymptomatic patients, 686
      in symptomatic patients, 686
    for mitral stenosis, 680-681

Valve surgery (Continued)
    in asymptomatic patients, 680, 680f
    with left atrial or left atrial appendage
      thrombosis, 680-681
    overall approach to, 680-681
    in patients with mild symptoms, 680,
      681f
    in patients with moderate to severe
      symptoms, 680, 681f
    for pulmonary valve disease, 687-688
    for tricuspid valve disease, 687
  overview of, 691, 692t
  postoperative care after, 699
  preoperative evaluation and optimization of,
    692-694
    cardiac catheterization in, 692-693
    echocardiography in, 692
    history and physical in, 692
    medical therapy in, 693-694
    other testing in, 693
  prostheses for, 694-699
    annuloplasty devices as, 695t
    autografts as, 696t
    characteristics of, 694-695, 696t
    currently available, 694-695, 695t, 696f
    homografts as, 699
      characteristics of, 696t
      currently available, 695t, 696f
    mechanical, 695-697
      characteristics of, 696t
      currently available, 695t, 696f
      valve-related complications with, 697,
        697t, 698f
    stented xenografts as, 697
      characteristics of, 696t
      currently available, 695t, 696f
    stentless xenografts as, 697-699
      characteristics of, 696t
      currently available, 695t, 696f
    valve-related complications of, 695, 696b
  reoperation in, 709
  statistics on, 691, 693f
  surgical approaches for, 694
    via median sternotomy, 694
    minimally invasive, 694, 694f
  tricuspid, 708
    indications for, 708
    results of, 708
    surgical approach for, 708
    timing of, 687
    valve repair as, 708
    valve replacement as, 708
Valve thrombosis, 696b
Valve-related complications, 695, 696b
Valvular endocarditis, operated, 696b
Valvular heart disease
  aortic insufficiency as, 681-683
    aortic dissection with, 614
    assessment of severity of, 681-683, 682t
    and mechanical circulatory support, 318
    in pregnancy, 623-624
    timing of surgical intervention for, 683
      in asymptomatic patients, 683
      overall approach to, 683, 684f
      in symptomatic patients with LV
        dysfunction, 683
      in symptomatic patients with normal LV
        function, 683
  aortic stenosis as, 676-678
    assessment of severity of, 676-677,
      677t
    in CABG patients, 710
    in pregnancy, 624
    timing of surgical intervention for, 676-678
      in asymptomatic patients, 678
      in elderly patients, 678
      in low-grade stenosis, 677-678

Valvular heart disease (Continued)
    overall approach to, 678, 678b, 679f
    in symptomatic patients, 677
  future directions for, 688
  heart failure with, 262
  with ischemic heart disease, 710-711
    aortic stenosis in CABG patients as, 710
    incidental coronary disease in valve
      surgery patients as, 710
    incidental valve disease in coronary
      surgery patients as, 710
    mitral regurgitation in CABG patients as,
      710-711, 711f
  and mechanical circulatory support, 318
  mitral insufficiency/regurgitation as,
    683-687
    assessment of severity of, 683-685, 685t
    overall approach to, 686-687, 687f
    functional (ischemic), 686-687
    timing of intervention for, 686
      in asymptomatic patients, 686
      in symptomatic patients, 686
  mitral stenosis as, 678-681
    assessment of severity of, 678-680, 679b,
      680t
    indications for surgical intervention in,
      704
    in pregnancy, 624
    surgical approaches to, 681, 681t
    timing of intervention for, 680-681
      in asymptomatic patients, 680, 680f
      with left atrial or left atrial appendage
        thrombosis, 680-681
      overall approach to, 680-681
      in patients with mild symptoms, 680,
        681f
      in patients with moderate to severe
        symptoms, 680, 681f
  optimal timing of interventions for, 676-690
    for aortic insufficiency, 683
    for aortic stenosis, 676-678
    for mitral insufficiency, 686
    for mitral stenosis, 680-681
  overview of, 676
  percutaneous treatment for, 714-727
    aortic valve implantations in, 714
      access site evaluation for, 716
      currently available, 714-715, 715f
      measurement of aortic valve annulus
        for, 716-717
      new access approaches for, 719
      new applications of, 719
      next generation of, 720-721, 720f, 720t
      patient evaluation and imaging prior to,
        715-717, 715f
      patient outcomes with, 717-719, 718f-719f,
        719t
      potential complications of, 719-720
      transapical valves in, 721, 721f
      transcatheter implantation procedure
        for, 717-721, 717f
    for mitral valve therapy, 721-726, 722t
      chamber remodeling in, 722t, 724, 724f
      chordal implantation in, 722t, 725, 725f
      direct annuloplasty in, 722t, 724-725,
        725f
      leaflet repair in, 722-724, 722f-723f, 722t
      mitral valve replacement in, 725-726,
        726f
      ventricular remodeling in, 722t, 725
    overview of, 714
  in pregnancy, 623-624
  pulmonary artery catheters for, 748t
  right-sided, 687-688
    pulmonary, 687-688
    tricuspid, 687
  surgical treatment of. See Valve surgery.

Valvular pulmonary stenosis (VPS), 640-641, 641f
  in pregnancy, 624
  recommendations for, 641
Vancomycin, for infective endocarditis, 655t-657t
VANQWISH study, 164, 164f
Varenicline (Chantix), for smoking cessation in peripheral artery disease, 542-543, 543f
Variability
  between-trial, 16
  within-trial, 16
Vascular surgery
  hypertensive emergencies after, 518-519
  perioperative medical therapy for noncardiac, 544
    antiplatelet therapy as, 544
    β-blockers as, 544
    statin therapy as, 544
Vascular wall inflammation paradigm, of pulmonary arterial hypertension, 596, 598f, 599
Vaseretic (enalapril/hydrochlorothiazide), for hypertension, 485t
Vasoactive therapy, for acute decompensated heart failure, 292-296
  digoxin as, 296
  dobutamine as, 293-294, 294f, 295t
  dopamine as, 295-296, 295f
  epinephrine and norepinephrine as, 296
  milrinone as, 294-295, 294f
  nesiritide as, 292-293, 293f
  nitroglycerin as, 292, 292t
  nitroprusside as, 293, 294f-295f
Vasoconstriction monolayer model, of pulmonary arterial hypertension, 596, 598f, 599
Vasodilator(s)
  for hypertension, 483, 483t
    in children, 536t
  for hypertensive emergencies, 514t-515t
Vasopressin receptor antagonists, for heart failure, 263-264
Vasospastic angina, β-adrenergic blockers for, 97
Vasotec. See Enalapril (Renitec, Vasotec).
Vaughan Williams antiarrhythmic classification, 344, 345f
V-binding site, of calcium channel blockers, 90
Vegetation, in infective endocarditis, 652, 653f
Venous thromboembolism (VTE), 580-595
  chemotherapy-associated, 580, 581t
  defined, 580
  diagnosis of, 582-586
    for deep vein thrombosis, 582-583
      algorithm for, 583, 583f
      clinical likelihood assessment in, 582
      clinical presentation in, 582-583
      imaging in, 583, 583f
      laboratory testing in, 582-583
    for pulmonary embolism, 583-586
      algorithm for, 585-586, 586f
      chest CT in, 584, 584f-585f
      chest radiography in, 583
      clinical presentation in, 583-586, 584t
      ECG in, 583
      echocardiography in, 584, 585f
      laboratory testing in, 583
      lung scanning in, 584
      MRI in, 585
  epidemiology and risk factors for, 580-581, 581t-582t
  management of, 586-591
    advanced therapy in basic vs., 589-591

Venous thromboembolism (VTE) (Continued)
    for deep vein thrombosis, 589-590
    for pulmonary embolism, 590
  anticoagulation in, 587-589, 587b
    direct factor XA and factor IIA inhibitors for, 589
    duration of, 590, 590f
    with fondaparinux, 588
    and heparin-induced thrombocytopenia, 587, 588f
    with low-molecular-weight heparin, 588
    with unfractionated heparin, 587
    with warfarin, 588-589, 588b
  inferior vena cava filters for, 591
  spectrum of disease and, 586-587
  pathophysiology and natural history of, 582, 582f
  in pregnancy, 624-626
  prevention of, 591-593
    duration of prophylaxis and extension after discharge in, 593, 593t
    with hip replacement, knee replacement, and hip fracture, 592, 592b
    in-hospital prophylaxis in, 592
    mechanical prophylaxis for, 592-593
    in patients with cancer, 591-592
    unconventional prophylaxis for, 592-593
      with statins, 593
      with vitamin E, 592-593
  risk stratification for
    chest CT in, 584, 584f-585f
    echocardiography in, 584, 585f
    overall, 586, 586f, 586t-587t
Venous thrombosis
  deep. See Deep vein thrombosis (DVT).
  superficial, 586-587
Ventilation-perfusion lung scans, for pulmonary embolism, 584
Ventor transapical valve, 721, 721f
Ventricular arrhythmias
  with acute decompensated heart failure, 298
  implantable cardioverter-defibrillators for, 759, 759f, 759t
  nonsustained, and risk of sudden cardiac death, 398, 400t
  after STEMI, 199, 200f, 204
Ventricular assist device (VAD)
  for acute decompensated heart failure, 299
  bi-, 315
  left, 315
  after STEMI, 198
Ventricular asystole, after STEMI, 198-199
Ventricular dyssynchrony, in heart failure, 273
Ventricular fibrillation (VF)
  catheter ablation for, 392
  idiopathic, 408
  due to STEMI, 179, 204
  and sudden cardiac death, 408, 409f
Ventricular pacing, for LVOT obstruction, 334-335
Ventricular remodeling, in percutaneous mitral valve repair, 722t, 725
Ventricular repolarization, after STEMI, 204
Ventricular scar burden, and risk of sudden cardiac death, 398-400, 400t
Ventricular septal defects (VSDs), 646-647
  closure of
    indications for, 646
    for perimembranous defects, 647
    transcatheter techniques for, 646, 647f
  pathophysiology of, 646, 646f
  post-MI ventricular septal rupture with, 647, 648f
  recommendations for, 647
Ventricular septal rupture (VSR)
  after myocardial infarction, 647, 648f
  after STEMI, 197, 197t

Ventricular tachyarrhythmias, catheter ablation for, 390-392
Ventricular tachycardia (VT)
  acute management of, 408-414
  catheter ablation for
    exercise-induced, 390
    idiopathic, 390-391
    intrafascicular verapamil-sensitive reentrant, 390-391
    polymorphic, 392
    repetitive monomorphic, 390
    with structural heart disease, 391-392, 391f
  in heart failure, 284
  polymorphic, 413-414, 414b, 414f
    catheter ablation for, 392
    causes of, 413, 414b
    ECG of, 413, 413f
    magnesium for, 413-414
  in pregnancy, 629
  after STEMI, 199, 204
  and sudden cardiac death, 408, 409f
  sustained monomorphic with pulse, 408-413
    amiodarone for, 411-413
      algorithm for, 412f
      clinical trials of, 411-412, 411f
      recommended dose of, 410t
    cardioversion for, 413
    clinical presentations and symptoms of, 409
    etiology of, 408-409
    evaluation to exclude potentially reversible causes of, 413
    lidocaine for, 409-410, 410t
    magnesium for, 413
    overdrive ventricular pacing for, 413, 413f
    pharmacologic treatment of, 409, 410t
    procainamide for, 410-411, 410t
    sotalol for, 410t, 411
Verapamil (Covera, Verelan), 92-93
  for atrial fibrillation, 373t
  with β-adrenergic blockers, 99
  contraindications to, 93
  dose of, 93
  drug interactions with, 94
  for hypertension, 479t
  for maintenance of sinus rhythm, 377
  for paroxysmal supraventricular tachycardia, 368, 369t
  pharmacodynamic effects of, 91t
  pharmacokinetics of, 92
  for postinfarct protection, 92
  in pregnancy, 93, 622t-623t
    for mitral stenosis, 624
  side effects of, 93
  after STEMI, 193
  for supraventricular tachycardia, 92
"Very low sodium," 471t
VF. See Ventricular fibrillation (VF).
V-HeFT II trial, 246, 247t
Viabahn stent, for femoral-popliteal disease, 548
Viacor percutaneous transvenous mitral annuloplasty device, 722t, 723f, 724
Videoscopic approaches, for valve surgery, 694
Violative device, 50
Visken. See Pindolol (Visken).
Vitamin E, for thromboprophylaxis, 592-593
Vitamin K antagonists, for carotid artery disease, 58
VKORC1 gene
  in pharmacogenetics of warfarin therapy, 57-59, 58t
  testing for, 59

VKORC1 gene *(Continued)*
    therapeutic implications of, 59-60
    and therapeutic modifications, 59-60
    and warfarin dose-response, 589
VMAC study, 292
von Hippel–Lindau disease,
    pheochromocytomas in, 490, 491t
Vorapaxar, 115
VPS (valvular pulmonary stenosis), 640-641,
    641f
    in pregnancy, 624
    recommendations for, 641
VSDs. *See* Ventricular septal defects (VSDs).
VSR (ventricular septal rupture)
    after myocardial infarction, 647, 648f
    after STEMI, 197, 197t
VT. *See* Ventricular tachycardia (VT).
VTE. *See* Venous thromboembolism (VTE).

W

Waist circumference, 446-448
WARCEF study, 258
Warfarin, 57-60, 121-122
    for carotid artery disease, 557-558
    dosages of, 121
    drug interactions with, 57
    for heart failure, 258
    indications for, 57, 121
    mechanisms of action of, 57, 121
    monitoring of, 57
    after NSTE-ACS, 166
    for peripheral artery disease, 541
    pharmacogenetics of, 57-59, 58f
        future directions for, 60
        genetic polymorphism in, 54t, 58t
        key genes in, 54t
            CYP2C9 as, 58t, 59
            CYP4F2 as, 58t, 59
            VKORC1 as, 57-59, 58t
        testing for, 59
            cost effectiveness of, 59
        therapeutic implications of, 59-60
            therapeutic modifications as, 59-60
    pharmacology of, 57
    in pregnancy and lactation, 622t-623t, 625
    for pulmonary arterial hypertension, 599
    side effects and contraindications to,
        121-122
    after STEMI, 207
    for thoracic aortic atheroembolism, 618

Warfarin *(Continued)*
    for thromboembolism prophylaxis
        with atrial fibrillation, 378, 378b
        with hip or knee replacement, 592
    for venous thromboembolism, 588-589,
        588b
WARIS II study, 121, 207
Warnings, on new drug labels, 35
WARSS study, 558
WATCH trial, 258
Watchman device, 388, 389f
Waterston shunt, 633t
WAVE trial, 541
Weakness, in acute decompensated heart
    failure, 287
Weight control, after NSTE-ACS, 166t
Weight loss
    determination of calorie levels for,
        448
    goals for, 448
    for hypertension in children, 534
Weight management
    cardiac rehabilitation and, 741b
    after STEMI, 204, 205t
Weighted average, in meta-analysis, 15
Wells rule, for pulmonary embolism, 583,
    584t
Wells score, for deep vein thrombosis, 582
WHI (Women's Health Initiative), 443-444
WHO (World Health Organization), Essential
    Drug List of, 78
Whole blood–compatible systems, LDL
    apheresis using, 456-457, 457f, 457t
"Windows of opportunity," in medical device
    failures, 47-48
Wisconsin Sleep Cohort Study, 502
WISE trial, 169
Withdrawal studies, 7
Within-trial variability, 16
Wolff-Parkinson-White (WPW) syndrome,
    accessory pathways in, 383
Women, NSTE-ACS in, 171-172
Women's Health Initiative (WHI), 443-444
Women's Health Study, 592-593
Women's Ischemia Syndrome Evaluation
    (WISE) trial, 169
World Health Organization (WHO), Essential
    Drug List of, 78
World Trade Organization, 37
WOSCOPS study, 425t
WPW (Wolff-Parkinson-White) syndrome,
    accessory pathways in, 383

X

Xact stent, for carotid artery stenosis,
    563
Xarelto. *See* Rivaroxaban (Xarelto).
Xenografts
    stented, 697
        characteristics of, 696t
        currently available, 695t, 696f
    stentless, 697-699
        characteristics of, 696t
        currently available, 695t, 696f
Xience, 217-218
Ximelagatran, 122
Xuezhikang (XZK), 428

Y

Y stenting, for bifurcation lesion, 223f
Yacoub, Magdi, 609

Z

Z_1 (standardized normal statistic), 9-10, 11f
Zalcitabine (ddC), for HIV infection, 730t
Zaroxolyn (metolazone)
    for heart failure, 243t, 245
    for hypertension, 480t
Zebeta. *See* Bisoprolol (Zebeta).
Zenith Dissection Endovascular System,
    615
ZEST study, 217t
Zestoretic (lisinopril/hydrochlorothiazide), for
    hypertension, 485t
Zestril. *See* Lisinopril (Prinivil, Zestril).
Ziac (bisoprolol/hydrochlorothiazide), for
    hypertension, 485t
    in children, 536t
Zidovudine (azidothymidine, AZT), for HIV
    infection, 730t
    myocardial effects of, 734
Zidovudine/lamuvidine (Combivir), for HIV
    infection, 729-730, 730t
Zilver PTX stent, for femoral-popliteal disease,
    548-549
Zotarolimus, molecular structure and
    mechanism of action of, 220f
Zotarolimus-eluting stents, 217-218, 217t
Zyban (bupropion hydrochloride), for smoking
    cessation in peripheral artery disease,
    542-543, 543f

Feu d'ange